SCHAFFER AND AVERY'S

DISEASES OF THE NEWBORN

SCHAFFER AND AVERY'S

DISEASES OF THE NEWBORN

SIXTH EDITION

H. William Taeusch, M.D.

Professor, Department of Pediatrics
Charles R. Drew University
and University of California—Los Angeles
Los Angeles, CA

Roberta A. Ballard, M.D.

Professor of Pediatrics
University of California—San Francisco
San Francisco, CA

Mary Ellen Avery, M.D.

Thomas Morgan Rotch Professor of Pediatrics,
Harvard Medical School
Formerly, Physician-in-Chief,
Children's Hospital
Boston, MA

W. B. SAUNDERS COMPANY
Harcourt Brace Jovanovich, Inc.

Philadelphia   London   Toronto
Montreal   Sydney   Tokyo

W. B. Saunders Company
Harcourt Brace Jovanovich, Inc.

The Curtis Center
Independence Square West
Philadelphia, PA 19106

Library of Congress Cataloging-in-Publication Data

Schaffer and Avery's diseases of the newborn.—6th ed./[editors]
H. William Taeusch, Roberta A. Ballard, Mary Ellen Avery.
    p. cm

Rev. ed. of: Schaffer's diseases of the newborn. 5th ed. 1984.
    Includes bibliographical references and index.

ISBN 0-7216-2476-6

1. Infants (Newborn)—Diseases.   I. Taeusch, H. William.
    II. Ballard, Roberta A.   III. Avery, Mary Ellen.
    IV. Schaffer's diseases of the newborn.
    V. Title: Diseases of the newborn.
[DNLM: 1. Infant, Newborn, Diseases.   WS 420 S296]
RJ254.S3 1991   618.92′01—dc20   DNLM/DLC   90-9247

Editor: Lisette Bralow
Developmental Editor: Lawrence J. McGrew
Designers: Maureen Sweeney and Dorothy Chattin
Production Manager: Linda R. Garber
Manuscript Editors: Carol DiBerardino, David Prout and Jeanne M. Carper
Illustration Coordinator: Lisa Lambert
Indexer: Mark Coyle
Cover Designer: Maureen Sweeney

Schaffer and Avery's Diseases of the Newborn, 6th Edition   ISBN 0-7216-2476-6

Printed in the United States of America

Last digit is the print number: 9   8   7   6   5   4   3

DEDICATION

To contributors, past and present, whose collective wisdom endows this sixth edition with an unparalleled cumulative experience to be shared with our readers.

CONTRIBUTORS

Randal A. Aaberg, M.D.
Assistant Clinical Professor, Urology, University of Texas Health Sciences, San Antonio, Texas.
Prenatal Diagnosis and Management of Urinary Abnormalities; Developmental Abnormalities of the Kidneys; Tumors of the Kidney; Hydronephrosis, Megaureter, and Other Abnormalities of the Upper Urinary Tract; Developmental Abnormalities of the Lower Urinary Tract; Renal Vascular Thrombosis and Renal Cortical and Medullary Necrosis; Urinary Tract Infection and Vesicoureteral Reflux

Michael D. Amylon, M.D.
Associate Professor of Pediatrics, Stanford University School of Medicine, Stanford, California. Director, Bone Marrow Transplant Service, Children's Hospital at Stanford, Stanford, California.
Hemostatic Disorders in the Newborn

Sudhir K. Anand, M.D.
Professor of Pediatrics, Charles Drew School of Medical Sciences; Associate Professor of Pediatrics, UCLA School of Medicine, Los Angeles, California. King/Drew Medical Center, Los Angeles, California. Head of Pediatric Nephrology, Harbor—UCLA Medical Center, Torrance, California.
Disorders of the Kidney and Genitourinary System—Introduction, Embryology, and Morphology; Maturation of Renal Function; Clinical Evaluation of Renal Disease; Prenatal Diagnosis and Management of Urinary Abnormalities; Developmental Abnormalities of the Kidneys; Cystic Diseases of the Kidneys; Tumors of the Kidney; Hydronephrosis, Megaureter, and Other Abnormalities of the Upper Urinary Tract; Developmental Abnormalities of the Lower Urinary Tract; Abnormalities of the External Genitalia; Normal Foreskin and Circumcision; Acute Renal Failure; Renal Vascular Thrombosis and Renal Cortical and Medullary Necrosis; Hypertension; Urinary Tract Infection and Vesicoureteral Reflux; Nephrotic Syndrome and Glomerulonephropathies; Renal Tubular Disorders

Constantine S. Anast (Deceased)
Formerly Professor of Pediatrics, Harvard Medical School, and Head, Division of Endocrinology, Department of Pediatrics, Children's Hospital, Boston, Massachusetts
Disorders of Calcium and Phosphorus Metabolism

Mary Ellen Avery, M.D.
Thomas Morgan Rotch Professor of Pediatrics, Harvard Medical School, Boston, Massachusetts.
History and Epidemiology; Placental Function and Diseases; The Placenta, Fetal Membranes, and Umbilical Cord; Malformations of the Mediastinum and Lung Parenchyma

Philip L. Ballard, M.D., Ph.D.
Professor of Pediatrics, Senior Staff, Cardiovascular Research Institute, University of California—San Francisco, California.
Hormonal Influences on Fetal Development

Roberta A. Ballard, M.D.
Professor of Pediatrics, University of California—San Francisco, San Francisco, California. Chief, Department of Pediatrics, Director, Newborn Services, Mount Zion Hospital and Medical Center, San Francisco, California.
Diabetes Mellitus; Preeclampsia; Other Maternal Conditions Affecting the Fetus; Resuscitation in the Delivery Room; Hydrops Fetalis

Stephen Baumgart, M.D.
Associate Professor of Pediatrics, University of Pennsylvania, School of Medicine, Philadelphia, Pennsylvania. Senior Staff Physician, Division of Neonatology, Department of Pediatrics, Children's Hospital of Philadelphia, Philadelphia, Pennsylvania.
Temperature Regulation of the Premature Infant

Xylina Bean, M.D.
Associate Professor of Pediatrics, Charles R. Drew University and University of

California—Los Angeles, Los Angeles California.
Associate Director, Neonatology, King/Drew Medical Center, Los Angeles, California.
Maternal Substance Abuse

Richard L. Berkowitz, M.D.
Professor and Chairman, Mount Sinai Medical School, New York, New York. Chief of Obstetrics and Gynecology, Mount Sinai Medical Center, New York, New York.
Assessment of Fetal Well-Being

Stephanie A. Berman, L.C.S.W.
Supervisor, Perinatal Social Services, University of California—San Francisco Medical Center, San Francisco, California.
Caring for Parents of Infants in Intensive Care

Merton Bernfield, M.D.
Clement A. Smith Professor of Pediatrics, Professor of Anatomy and Cellular Biology, Harvard Medical School, Boston, Massachusetts. Director, Joint Program in Neonatology, Chief, Department of Newborn Medicine, Children's Hospital, Brigham and Women's Hospital, Beth Israel Hospital, Boston, Massachusetts.
General Strategies of Fetal Development

Diana W. Bianchi, M.D.
Assistant Professor of Pediatrics, Harvard Medical School, Boston, Massachusetts. Assistant in Medicine (Genetics, Newborn Medicine), The Children's Hospital, Boston, Massachusetts.
Prenatal Genetic Diagnosis

William J. Byrne, M.D.
Clinical Associate Professor of Pediatrics, University of California, San Francisco, California. Director, Division of Gastroenterology and Nutrition, Children's Hospital—Oakland, Oakland, California.
General Considerations (The Gastrointestinal System); Fetal, Transitional, and Neonatal Physiology

(The Gastrointestinal System); Disorders of the Teeth, Mouth, and Neck; Disorders of the Esophagus; Disorders of the Stomach; Disorders of the Intestines and Pancreas; Disorders of the Umbilical Cord, Abdominal Wall, Urachus, and Omphalomesenteric Duct; Ascites and Peritonitis; Disorders of the Liver; Nutrition in the Newborn

V. Charlton, M.D., M.S.
Professor of Pediatrics, University of California, San Francisco, California. Attending Neonatologist, Director, Extracorporeal Membrane Oxygenation Program, University of California Medical Center, San Francisco, California.
Fetal Growth; Nutritional Issues

Robin Dawn Clark, M.D.
Assistant Professor of Pediatrics, Division of Genetics, Loma Linda University School of Medicine. Head, Section of Clinical Genetics, Loma Linda University Medical Center, Loma Linda, California.
Congenital Anomalies

Ronald I. Clyman, M.D.
Professor of Pediatrics, Senior Staff, Cardiovascular Research Institute, University of California—San Francisco, San Francisco, California.
Patent Ductus Arteriosus in the Premature Infant

F. Sessions Cole, M.D.
Professor of Pediatrics and Associate Professor of Cell Biology and Physiology, Washington University School of Medicine, Seattle, Washington. Director, Division of Newborn Medicine, St. Louis Children's Hospital; Director of Newborn Services, Barnes and Jewish Hospitals; Medical Director, St. Louis Children's Hospital Transport Team; Pediatrician-in-Chief, Jewish Hospital.
Immunology; Fetal/Neonatal Human Immunodeficiency Virus Infection; Viral Infections of the Fetus and Newborn; Bacterial Infections of the Newborn; Other Specific Bacterial Infections; Fungus Infections; Protozoal Infections: Congenital Toxoplasmosis and Malaria; Infections with Spirochetal and Parasitic Organisms

Anthony Corbet, M.B.
Associate Professor, Department of Pediatrics, Baylor College of Medicine, Houston, Texas. Staff Neonatologist, Texas Children's Hospital; St. Luke's Episcopal Hospital; Texas Woman's Hospital; Ben Taub General Hospital; Methodist Hospital, Houston, Texas.

Lung Development and Function; Control of Breathing; Pulmonary Physiology of the Newborn; Principles of Respiratory Monitoring and Therapy; Disorders of the Transition; Airblock Syndromes; Chronic Lung Disease— Bronchopulmonary Dysplasia; Neonatal Pneumonias; Diseases of the Airways; Malformations of the Mediastinum and Lung Parenchyma; Accumulation of Fluid in the Pleural Space; Disorders of the Chest Wall and Diaphragm

Arthur E. D'Harlingue, M.D.
Associate Neonatologist, Children's Hospital—Oakland, Oakland, California.
General Considerations (The Gastrointestinal System); Nutrition in the Newborn; Vitamins and Trace Mineral Disorders

Nancy B. Esterly, M.D.
Professor of Pediatrics, Professor of Dermatology, Medical College of Wisconsin, Milwaukee, Wisconsin. Head, Division of Dermatology, Department of Pediatrics, Children's Hospital of Wisconsin, Milwaukee, Wisconsin.
Congenital and Hereditary Disorders of the Skin; Infections of the Skin; Common Benign Skin Disorders; Nevi and Cutaneous Tumors

Donna Jane Eteson, D.M.D.
Lecturer, Section of Orthodontics, UCLA School of Dentistry, Los Angeles, California. Clinical Assistant Professor, Department of Developmental Dentistry, University of Southern California School of Dentistry, Los Angeles, California.
Congenital Anomalies

Delbert A. Fisher, M.D.
Professor (Emeritus) of Pediatrics, University of California—Los Angeles, Los Angeles, California.
Disorders of the Thyroid Gland

George Franco, M.D.
Assistant Clinical Professor, UCLA Department of Pediatrics, Los Angeles, California. Staff Neonatologist, Santa Monica Hospital Medical Center, Santa Monica, California.
Acid Base, Fluid, and Electrolyte Management

Michael D. Freed, M.D.
Associate Professor of Pediatrics, Harvard Medical School, Boston, Massachusetts. Senior Associate in Cardiology, Chief of In-Patient

Cardiovascular Service, Children's Hospital, Boston, Massachusetts.
General Considerations (Cardiovascular System); Congenital Cardiac Malformations; Cardiomyopathies; Cardiac Dysrhythmias

Robert H. Friesen, M.D.
Associate Clinical Professor of Anesthesia and Pediatrics, University of Colorado School of Medicine, Denver, Colorado. Associate Director of Anesthesiology, Children's Hospital, Denver, Colorado.
Anesthesia and Analgesia; Issues for the Fetus and Newborn

Joan McIver Gibson, Ph.D.
Adjunct Professor of Bioethics, University of New Mexico Schools of Law and Medicine, Albuquerque, New Mexico. Medical Ethicist, St. Joseph Healthcare System, Albuquerque, New Mexico.
Ethical and Legal Issues in Newborn Care

Bertil E. Glader, Ph.D., M.D.
Professor of Pediatrics, Stanford University School of Medicine, Stanford, California. Professor of Pediatrics, Stanford University Medical Center, Director, Division of Hematology/Oncology, Children's Hospital at Stanford, Stanford, California.
Hemostatic Disorders in the Newborn; Leukocyte Disorders in the Newborn; Erythrocyte Disorders in Infancy

William Good, M.D.
Assistant Professor, Department of Ophthalmology, University of California, San Francisco, California. University of California; San Francisco General Hospital, San Francisco, California.
Disorders of the Eye

Peter A. Gorski, M.D.
Division Head, Behavioral and Developmental Pediatrics, Assistant Professor of Pediatrics and Psychiatry, Northwestern University Medical School, Chicago, Illinois. Division Chief, Behavioral and Developmental Pediatrics, Evanston Hospital, Evanston, Illinois; Attending Staff, Children's Memorial Hospital, Chicago, Illinois.
Behavioral Assessment of the Newborn

Amarylis C. Gutierrez-Pickett, Pharm.D.
Clinical Pharmacist Supervisor, King/ Drew Medical Center, Los Angeles, California. Assistant Professor of Medicine, Drew University School of Medicine, Los Angeles, California
Appendix 1: Drugs

Thomas N. Hansen, M.D.

Professor of Pediatrics, Head, Section of Neonatology, Baylor College of Medicine, Houston, Texas. Chief, Neonatology Service, Texas Children's Hospital; Deputy Chief, Pediatric Service, The Methodist Hospital; Director of Nurseries, St. Luke's Episcopal Hospital; Director of Nurseries, Ben Taub General Hospital; Director of Neonatology Service, Houston, Texas.

Lung Development and Function; Control of Breathing; Pulmonary Physiology of the Newborn; Principles of Respiratory Monitoring and Therapy; Disorders of the Transition; Airblock Syndromes; Chronic Lung Disease—Bronchopulmonary Dysplasia; Neonatal Pneumonias; Diseases of the Airways; Malformations of the Mediastinum and Lung Parenchyma; Accumulation of Fluid in the Pleural Space; Disorders of the Chest Wall and Diaphragm

Creig S. Hoyt, M.D.

Professor of Ophthalmology and Pediatrics, University of California—San Francisco, San Francisco, California. Vice-Chairman, Department of Ophthalmology, University of California—San Francisco, San Francisco, California.

Disorders of the Eye

Adrian D. Hurley, Pharm.D.

Pharmacy Supervisor, Inpatient Pharmacy, King/Drew Medical Center, Los Angeles, California.

Appendix 1: Drugs

Mark M. Jacobs, M.D.

Assistant Professor, Obstetrics, Gynecology, and Reproductive Sciences, University of California—San Francisco, San Francisco, California. Attending Physician, University of California Hospitals and Clinics, San Francisco, California.

Other Maternal Conditions Affecting the Fetus

Bruce R. Korf, M.D., Ph.D.

Assistant Professor of Neurology, Harvard Medical School, Boston, Massachusetts. Director, Clinical Genetics Program, Assistant in Neurology, Children's Hospital, Boston, Massachusetts.

Mechanisms of Genetic Disease; Chromosomal Abnormalities; Other Genetic Disorders; Genetic Counseling

Martin A. Koyle, M.D.

Associate Professor of Surgery/Pediatric Urology, University of Colorado School of Medicine, Denver, Colorado. Pediatric Urologist, The Children's Hospital; Rose Hospital; and University Hospital, Denver, Colorado.

Prenatal Diagnosis and Management of Urinary Abnormalities; Developmental Abnormalities of the Kidneys; Tumors of the Kidney; Hydronephrosis, Megaureter, and Other Abnormalities of the Upper Urinary Tract; Developmental Abnormalities of the Lower Urinary Tract; Abnormalities of the External Genitalia; Normal Foreskin and Circumcision; Renal Vascular Thrombosis and Renal Cortical and Medullary Necrosis; Urinary Tract Infection and Vesicoureteral Reflux

Rosemary Leake, M.D.

Professor of Pediatrics, UCLA, Los Angeles, California. Chief of Neonatology, Harbor—UCLA Medical Center, Los Angeles, California.

Growth Disorders

Harvey L. Levy, M.D.

Associate Professor of Neurology, Harvard Medical School, Boston, Massachusetts. Senior Associate in Medicine, Children's Hospital; Pediatrician, Massachusetts General Hospital; Assistant Neurologist, Massachusetts General Hospital, Boston, Massachusetts.

Screening of the Newborn; Inborn Errors of Metabolism

Helen Liley, M.B., Ch.B.

Instructor in Pediatrics, Harvard Medical School, Boston, Massachusetts. Assistant in Medicine (Newborn Medicine), Children's Hospital, Boston; Brigham and Women's Hospital; Beth Israel Hospital; Boston, Massachusetts.

General Strategies of Fetal Development

Denise M. Main, M.D.

Assistant Professor in Residence, Department of Obstetrics, Gynecology, and Reproductive Sciences, University of California—San Francisco, School of Medicine, San Francisco, California. Associate Chief, Perinatal Services, Children's Hospital of San Francisco, San Francisco, California

Prevention of Preterm Birth

Katherine K. Matthay, B.A., M.D.

Associate Professor of Pediatrics, University of California—San Francisco, School of Medicine, San Francisco, California. University of California Medical Center, San Francisco, California.

Congenital Malignant Disorders

Marie C. McCormick, M.D. Sc.D.

Associate Professor of Pediatrics, Joint Program in Neonatology, Harvard Medical School, Boston, Massachusetts. Senior Associate in Medicine, Children's Hospital; Associate Pediatrician, The Brigham and Women's Hospital; Associate in Pediatrics, The Beth Israel Hospital, Boston, Massachusetts.

Long-Term Costs of Perinatal Disabilities

John H. Menkes, M.D.

Professor Emeritus, Department of Neurology and Pediatrics, University of California School of Medicine, Los Angeles, California.

Neurologic Evaluation of the Newborn Infant; Perinatal Central Nervous System Trauma; Intracranial Hemorrhage: Pathogenesis and Pathology; Malformations of the Central Nervous System; Paroxysmal Disorders; Diseases of the Motor Unit; Miscellaneous Neurologic Disorders Presenting in the Newborn

J. Lawrence Naiman, M.D.

Clinical Professor of Pediatrics, Stanford University School of Medicine, Stanford, California. Director of Blood Services, Central California Region, American Red Cross, San Jose, California.

Erythrocyte Disorders in Infancy

Frank A. Oski, M.D.

Given Professor of Pediatrics, Chairman, Department of Pediatrics, Johns Hopkins University School of Medicine, Baltimore, Maryland. Physician-in-Chief, Johns Hopkins Hospital Children's Center, Baltimore, Maryland.

General Considerations (Disorders of Bilirubin Metabolism); Physiologic Jaundice; Unconjugated Hyperbilirubinemia; Kernicterus; Obstructive Jaundice Due to Biliary Atresia and Neonatal Hepatitis; Other Conjugated Hyperbilirubinemias; Differential Diagnosis of Jaundice

Robert Petersen, M.D.

Assistant Professor of Ophthalmology, Harvard Medical School, Boston, Massachusetts. Senior Staff Associate, Children's Hospital, Boston, Massachusetts.

Disorders of the Eye

Daniel H. Polk, M.D.

Assistant Professor in Pediatrics, UCLA School of Medicine, Los Angeles, California. Division of Neonatology, Harbor—UCLA Medical Center, UCLA

School of Medicine, Torrance, California.
Disorders of the Adrenal Gland; Abnormalities of Sexual Differentiation; Disorders of the Thyroid Gland; Disorders of Carbohydrate Metabolism

J. Usha Raj, M.D.
Associate Professor of Pediatrics, UCLA School of Medicine, Los Angeles, California. Associate Professor of Pediatrics, Director, Well Baby and Intermediate Care Nurseries, Harbor—UCLA Medical Center, UCLA School of Medicine, Torrance, California.
Acid Base, Fluid, and Electrolyte Management

Douglas K. Richardson, M.D., M.B.A.
Instructor in Pediatrics, Joint Program in Neonatology, Harvard Medical School, Boston, Massachusetts. Assistant Neonatologist, The Children's Hospital; Assistant Neonatologist, Brigham and Women's Hospital; Assistant Neonatologist, Beth Israel Hospital, Boston, Massachusetts.
Long-Term Costs of Perinatal Disabilities

James M. Roberts, M.D.
Professor, Obstetrics, Gynecology and Reproductive Sciences, and Senior Staff, Cardiovascular Research Institute, University of California—San Francisco, San Francisco, California.
Preeclampsia

Robert Schwartz, J.D.
Professor of Law, University of New Mexico, Albuquerque, New Mexico.
Ethical and Legal Issues in Newborn Care

Mandel R. Sher, M.D.
Clinical Assistant Professor, Pediatrics, Division of Allergy and Immunology, University of South Florida, St. Petersburg, Florida.
Rheumatic Disorders

John C. Sinclair, M.D.
Professor, Department of Pediatrics, McMaster University, Hamilton, Ontario, Canada. McMaster University Medical Centre, Hamilton, Ontario, Canada.
Evaluation of Therapeutic Recommendations

Lawrence M. Solomon, M.D.
Professor and Head, Department of Dermatology, University of Illinois, Chicago, Illinois.
Congenital and Hereditary Disorders of the Skin; Infections of the Skin; Common Benign Skin Disorders; Nevi and Cutaneous Tumors

H. William Taeusch, M.D.
Professor of Pediatrics, Charles R. Drew University and University of California—Los Angeles, Los Angeles, California. Director of Neonatology, King/Drew Medical Center, Los Angeles, California.
Initial Evaluation: History and Physical Examination of the Newborn; Disorders of the Kidney and Genitourinary System—Introduction, Embryology, and Morphology

Robert M. Ward, M.D.
Associate Professor of Pediatrics, University of Utah, Salt Lake City,

Utah. Medical Director, Newborn Critical Care Services, Primary Children's Medical Center, Salt Lake City, Utah.
Pharmacologic Principles and Practicalities; Appendix 1: Drugs

Linda J. Weaver, M.S.
Clinical Nurse Specialist/Practitioner, Intensive Care Nursery, Mt. Zion Hospital and Medical Center, San Francisco, California.
Issues in Nursing Care of the Newborn

Isabelle A. Wilkins, M.D.
Assistant Professor, Obstetrics, Gynecology, and Reproductive Science and Pediatrics, University of Texas Medical School at Houston, Houston, Texas. Attending Staff, Hermann Hospital, St. Joseph Hospital, Memorial Hospital System, Southwest Houston, Texas; LBJ Hospital, Johnson City, Texas.
Assessment of Fetal Well-Being

Victor Y. H. Yu, M.D., M.Sc. (Oxon)
Clinical Associate Professor of Paediatrics, Monash University, Melbourne, Victoria, Australia. Director of Neonatal Intensive Care, Coordinator of the Growth and Development Clinic, Monash Medical Centre, Melbourne, Victoria, Australia.
Aftercare of High-Risk Infants and Long-Term Outcome

Theodore Zwerdling, M.D.
Research Scholar, Children's Hospital Medical Center, Cincinnati, Ohio.
Leukocyte Disorders in the Newborn

PREFACE TO THE 6TH EDITION

THE GROWTH AND DEVELOPMENT OF DISEASES OF THE NEWBORN

In a foreword to the first edition of Alexander Schaffer's *Diseases of the Newborn* in 1960, Harry H. Gordon wrote that "Dr. Ethel C. Dunham, a pioneer in this field, posed the problem as follows: one must learn new facts about the newborn; one must spread more widely what is already known; one must make it possible to apply these facts. Dr. Schaffer's book is an important direct step toward these goals. Out of his extensive experience as a critical clinician and teacher he has written a book to help physicians judge the significance of symptoms in newborn infants. Appraisal of the neonate is most difficult, but careful history and careful physical examination are, as in all medicine, the basic modalities with which a physician must deal. The art is to know how to interpret findings, how to know when laboratory assistance is required. Direct experience with large numbers of newborn infants and understanding of their physiology are the bases for expert clinical judgment. Neither is a substitute for the other."

Schaffer and Avery wrote in the Preface to the Fourth Edition in 1977, "during the few decades of practice of pediatrics and observation of the problems of newborn infants that preceded the publication of the first edition, the senior author witnessed a decline in infant mortality from 47 per 1000 in 1940 to 26 per 1000 live births in 1960. By 1974, that number was further reduced to 16.5 per 1000 live births and the contributions of deaths under 28 days reached an all-time low of 12.1 per 1000 live births." It seems appropriate in 1991 to update that experience by commenting that deaths in the first year of life in the United States in 1989 reached an all-time low of 9.7 per 1000 live births (which represented a 79 per cent decline from 1940), and in 1989 the rate of deaths under 28 days was 5.4 per 1000 in the state of Massachusetts, less than half the number in 1974.

These striking changes have been seen in most of the developed countries of the world, with an all-time low infant mortality rate achieved in Japan of 4.4 deaths per 1000 live births. It is sobering indeed to realize that in the United States, major differences persist in the mortality rates by race as well as by region. Thus the comment of Ethel Dunham "to spread more widely what is already known" is as relevant today as it was in the 1950s.

When the first edition of *Diseases of the Newborn* appeared in 1960, the beautifully documented clinical observations introduced a generation of pediatricians to the normal and abnormal events that could be observed by an astute clinician.

In the Preface to the Third Edition (1971), edited by Schaffer and Avery, with contributions by Milton Markowitz and Laurence Finberg, Schaffer wrote "our prediction made 11 years ago that neonatology would become an accredited pediatric specialty has come true. Neonatologists abound and many more nurseries would utilize their services if there were enough of them available. In this past 6-year period, advances in large numbers and of great utility have been made."

The fourth edition (1977) marked the turning point from the era when several individuals could assemble most of what was known about diseases of the newborn to the recognition that the field has expanded to the extent that multiple authors were required to give voices of authority in the expanding field. Twenty-nine individuals contributed to the fourth edition. Schaffer and Avery asked, "What factors have been responsible for the increased interest in the fate of the newly born and for the remarkable advances in understanding of their problems? Evidence for the interest is abundant in the genesis of neonatal intensive care units, regional programs to make such care widely available, training programs for neonatologists, and we might add a number of excellent textbooks on the physiology of the newborn infant and disorders of infants. Monographs describing problems of one or another organ system may indeed be replacing more comprehensive textbooks devoted to a description of most disorders, but we hope our readers will continue to find a single text, now requiring a group of authors, however superficial its coverage of certain subjects, to be a welcome starting place for investigating and understanding the problem to be solved. . . ."

Quoting further from the Preface to the Fourth Edition (1977), "Understanding of problems in human development has received a major thrust from advances in other disciplines, and perhaps importantly from a new technology. We worried about hypoxia and hyperoxia in the 1940s, we measured oxygen concentration in incubators in the 1950s, but we could not measure the most important variable, the oxygen tension in the blood, until the 1960s. When it became possible by microchemical methods to measure not only blood gases, but also many other substances, we could practice modern scientific medicine to aid in the diagnosis and treatment of our small patients.

"We have also seen the application of some fundamental advances in molecular biology to the management of our fetal and newborn patients. For example, the ability to identify the abnormal globin changes in trace amounts of fetal hemoglobin now permits prenatal diagnosis of sickle cell disease and beta-thalassemia. Indeed, most prenatal diagnosis today depends on the application of biochemical detection of enzyme abnormalities or of chromosome identification, which were outgrowths of support of basic cellular biology."

After Schaffer's death at 79 years of age in 1981, the publishers asked Avery if she would continue the tradition of a clinically oriented textbook to be called *Schaffer's Diseases of the Newborn*, fifth edition. Recognizing the enormous task of bringing the textbook up to date, Avery recruited Dr. H. William Taeusch, then Director of the Joint Program in Neonatology at Harvard Medical School, to assist with the editing. Some of the original descriptions written by Schaffer and the original references he cited were included in that edition published in 1984.

In the planning of a sixth edition, Avery and Taeusch recruited Roberta A. Ballard, Professor of Pediatrics at the University of California at San Francisco, to become a co-editor and to help recruit a new group of contributors. We agreed to maintain a strong clinical emphasis but wanted to emphasize some of the basic biologic concepts that elucidate the pathophysiology of disease and direct present and future therapy. Much of the new science and technology of the 1970s and 1980s has been applied to the benefit of low-birth-weight infants, with an ever-greater reduction in their rates of mortality and morbidity. This trend also resulted from the explosion of information regarding prenatal diagnosis. In this edition, 30 years after the first edition, we have tried to integrate the relevant basic science within each chapter, and have maintained an organ system approach to overall organization, not unlike the organization used by Schaffer in the first edition in 1960. We have included some case histories and commentary in situations in which we believed they illustrate significant aspects of diagnosis or management. We have retained a few of the original illustrations, since some of the photographs of physical findings are timeless.

We have emphasized much more the development of *Diseases of the Newborn* than its growth, although its growth has been finite from 855 pages in the first edition to some 1200 in this edition. Obviously, much of the earlier work has been condensed or deleted; we do not pretend that a single text can ever completely describe all information relevant to the diagnosis and care of infants. We have used our judgment in selection and emphasis and hope that our readers will find the volume current and useful. We are grateful, of course, for the suggestions of many readers in the past and look forward to hearing from our next group of readers.

No textbook emerges without the efforts of many individuals, too numerous to acknowledge individually. They include the secretaries and administrative assistants in the three institutions of the editors, as well as the contributors, and the editors and production people at the W. B. Saunders Company.

We would like to acknowledge the support provided by our respective institutions, the Harvard Medical School and Children's Hospital, Boston; University of California, San Francisco, and Mount Zion Hospital and Medical Center; and University of California, Los Angeles, and King/Drew Medical Center.

Mary Ellen Avery, M.D.
Boston, Massachusetts

CONTENTS

VI INFECTIONS AND IMMUNOLOGIC DEFENSE MECHANISMS   305

F. Sessions Cole and H. William Taeusch

VII NEUROMUSCULAR DISORDERS   395

John H. Menkes and Mary Ellen Avery

VIII THE RESPIRATORY SYSTEM 461

Anthony Corbet, Thomas Hansen, and Roberta A. Ballard

IX PATENT DUCTUS ARTERIOSUS 563

Ronald I. Clyman and Roberta A. Ballard

XVII METABOLIC AND ENDOCRINE/EXOCRINE SYSTEMS   927

Daniel H. Polk and H. William Taeusch

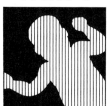

PART I

INTRODUCTION

HISTORY AND EPIDEMIOLOGY

1

Mary Ellen Avery

■ EARLY HISTORY OF CARE OF INFANTS*

In the late nineteenth century and the early part of the twentieth century, deaths from infectious diseases in the first years of life were so common that it is not surprising to find so few students of premature birth and so few articles concerning the special needs of low-birth-weight infants. These small babies were not expected to live. In fact, in the 1940s some authorities thought of birth weights under 3 pounds as incompatible with life, although rare exceptions have always been noted, as in the case of the Dionne quintuplets, each of whom weighed under 3 pounds. Dr. Allan Dafoe, who delivered them on May 28, 1934, wrote, "There were no scales small enough to measure accurately the separate weights of the babies, but on May 29 (second day) their combined weight was 13 pounds 6 ounces." They were born about 2 months early. Marie, the smallest, weighed 1½ pounds. Yvonne, the largest, weighed nearly 3 pounds. (Accurate scales arrived on the 6th day.)

As many infectious diseases came under control, physicians turned more attention to newborn babies. As far as we know, Pierre Budin in Paris published one of the first articles on premature infants in 1888. At about the same time, German physicians, one of whom was Heinrich Finkelstein in Berlin, became interested in the problems of premature infants and initiated special programs for their care. In Helsinki in 1912, Arvo Ylppo pioneered the research on prenatal and postnatal growth and the pathology of prematurity. Julius Hess, an American physician who studied in Europe, was the founder of the first center in the United States that specialized in the care of premature infants, at Michael Reese Hospital in Chicago in 1922. The criterion of 2500 g (5½ pounds) birth weight was used to distinguish a premature from a term infant, and not until much later was the concept of gestational age widely accepted as being a more accurate measure of the stage of development of an infant than weight

alone. Those physicians who were first concerned with premature infants noted very early that these children were unable to maintain their own body temperatures. Various devices, including double-walled metal tubs with the space between the walls filled with circulating hot water, were in use in Europe and Russia in the mid-nineteenth century. Other devices, such as hot-water bottles and electrically heated cribs, were the predecessors of our more modern incubators. Occasionally, the whole room in which many babies were cared for was kept at high temperatures, paving the way for the modern requirements that constant year-round temperature and humidity be maintained in the nurseries where premature infants are cared for.

It is not surprising that much attention was focused on ways to feed these immature infants, particularly since some of them were too weak to suckle. Etienne Tarnier is credited with introducing the practice of tube feeding for premature infants at the Maternity Hospital in Paris in 1884. Many other devices for oral and nasal feeding of premature infants have been advocated, but not until this past decade has research made total intravenous nutrition possible.

The first physicians to care for premature infants considered human milk indispensable for their welfare. In fact, in 1828 Friedrich Meissner in Leipzig, Germany, was so convinced of the benefits of human milk that he advised that the infant be fed mother's milk and be given enemas of milk and at least two milk baths daily.

A number of physicians, puzzled by the inability of many infants to tolerate cow's milk, proceeded to compare the chemical composition of human milk and cow's milk, with the expectation that they could modify cow's milk to make it a suitable substitute for mother's milk. In this regard, a number of extreme views were taken, including the idea that cow's milk contained an indigestible protein, casein, and that diluting it with three or four parts of water to keep the protein under 1 per cent would improve the infant's tolerance to this formula. Later it was believed that a higher percentage of protein was necessary to support adequate growth.

---

*Portions of this chapter appeared in: Avery ME, Litwack G: Born Early. Boston, Little, Brown, and Company, 1983.

Over the subsequent years, many pediatricians have continued the quest for optimal nutrition for babies of different gestational ages and birth weights, but no universal recommendations have emerged.

Some of the early students of care of premature infants recognized that any epidemic of respiratory tract infection and diarrheal disease could be lethal among such infants. In fact, special units for care of premature infants were established to avoid the dangers of acquired infection and epidemics within nurseries by providing separate facilities from other patients who might bring infection to the babies. In the early 1900s, the guidelines for care of premature infants specified that incubators that could be easily disinfected should be constructed, that rooms should not be crowded, that personnel should wear gowns and should wash their hands before handling an infant, and that infants with infections should be isolated from other infants.

It was not until after World War II that a new generation of pediatricians focused their attention on the medical needs of premature infants and, working with pathologists, began to study systematically the causes of death that occurs immediately after birth. Examination of the infants after death showed that not infrequently their lungs were airless, and when examined microscopically they revealed a material, hyaline membrane, in the terminal air spaces that should not have been there. From this discovery, the condition was named hyaline membrane disease; thereafter, the label respiratory distress syndrome was applied to describe the outstanding clinical feature of the disorder. The first obvious assumption was that the material in the lungs was aspirated from the amniotic fluid, but the absence of it in the lungs of infants who were stillborn made that an improbable explanation. Herbert Miller made this point in an article in 1949, suggesting that the affected infants acquired the membranes postnatally. Thereafter, many pathologists and pediatricians, through careful study of the infants during their first 2 or 3 days of life, and examination of the infants' lungs after death, clarified this condition as a functional immaturity of the lung with respect to synthesis of pulmonary surfactants. Because of improved understanding, deaths from hyaline membrane disease have decreased from about 10,000 per year in the United States in the 1950s to about half that number by the late 1980s.

Meanwhile, the 1940s were marked by the construction of many new nurseries and the introduction of more modern incubators that increased the amount of oxygen in the infants' environment. At that time it was evident that some of the infants had a newly recognized eye condition, called retrolental fibroplasia, which by the late 1940s became the leading cause of blindness in this country. The epidemic of this new condition led to enormous speculation about its origin and to a number of studies, which culminated in the work by Norman Ashton in England and Arnall Patz in Washington. When they exposed kittens to environments containing high levels of oxygen, the kittens acquired the condition. Although oxygen undoubtedly plays a role in retrolental fibroplasia, more recent experience with very immature infants indicates that other as yet undefined circumstances contribute to its severity.

Increased attention to the needs of small babies resulted in a gradual reduction in their mortality. As more very small babies lived, new problems came into focus. Some could be defined for the first time because of the availability of chemical techniques that allowed measurements on very small samples of blood. The application of these newer methods of measurement permitted study of the physiologic adaptations of the infant to extrauterine life. Parallel to increased attention to the babies themselves was the evolution of a field of perinatal physiology, stimulated largely through the work of Sir Joseph Barcroft and his colleagues in England in the 1930s and 1940s, and subsequently by many of their students and colleagues in the 1950s and thereafter. The book *The Physiology of the Newborn Infant* by Clement Smith brought many of these observations to the attention of pediatricians in 1945, and again in the three subsequent editions of his classic text.

The fetal lamb became the experimental model because the animal could be delivered from the uterus with umbilical cord intact and continue to receive oxygen and remove carbon dioxide across the placenta, since the uterus of the ewe does not contract under these circumstances. More recently, it has been possible to place catheters in vessels in the fetal lamb in the uterus for more physiologic studies of fetal life. The events surrounding delivery could then be witnessed in a carefully controlled manner with suitable measurements made to define qualitatively and quantitatively changes in the heart and lungs at birth. From these studies, many suggestions emerged for less direct measurements on the infants that were possible without jeopardizing their condition.

One of the major advances of recent years has been the evolution of perinatal-neonatal intensive care facilities in centers with adequate staff and enough babies who require care to maintain a high level of experience. A model system for the regionalization of perinatal health care was described by McCormick and associates (1985). The impact of antepartum risk identification and transfer of management of high risk pregnancies to tertiary care centers was to decrease even further neonatal mortality and morbidity.

■ RAPID ADVANCES IN NEONATAL CARE: PHASE 1 (1960–1975)

The first edition of *Diseases of the Newborn,* which was published in 1960, presented the observations of Alexander Schaffer and a few of his colleagues in diagnosis and management of newborn infants and, in so doing, provided a description of the state of neonatology in the late 1950s, and stimulated another generation to try to augment the scientific base of a new subspecialty that had long been relatively neglected in medical research and education. Consider for example that neonatal mortality was *20.5/1000* live births in 1950 compared with *7.5/1000* live births in the United States in 1985 (Fig. 1–1).

The major diagnostic tools in the 1960s were cultures, blood counts, urinalyses, radiographs, and biopsies. Little was known of the pathophysiology of many major disorders of infancy. The pulmonary hyaline membrane syndrome of the newborn was diagnosed by chest film and

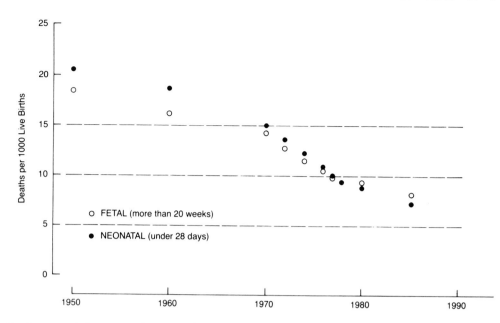

FIGURE 1–1. *Note that fetal death rates and neonatal death rates have been reduced by approximately one-half since 1970. Fetal death rates exceeded neonatal death rates for the first time in the period from 1978 to 1980. (Fetal death rate 9.4, neonatal death rate 8.9, 1978 to 1980; fetal death rate 81, neonatal death rate 7.1, 1983 to 1985.) (From Monthly Vital Statistics Report. National Center for Health Statistics 29, September 17, 1981, and Health United States, 1987. U.S. Department of Health and Human Services, DHHS Pub. No. (PHS) 88–1232, Hyattsville, MD, March 1988.)*

follow-up of clinical course. Surfactant deficiency, described the year before (1959), was not sufficiently recognized to warrant much discussion in the early 1960s. Blood gases were not available, respirators were not used, and half the infants, in whom the diagnosis was made, died.

Mother's milk was recommended for term infants, but if the mother did not wish to nurse her infant, she was assured the baby would thrive on evaporated milk diluted with water (2 parts to 3), with 5 to 10 per cent added carbohydrate. Premature infants had been observed to have fat intolerance, hence were given half-skimmed milk with added carbohydrate to achieve an average intake of 120 calories/kg/day. Very little discussion related to infants smaller than 3 pounds (1300 g), since only 28 per cent survived in 1954.

In the early 1960s, serial amino acid measurements in the blood of the infants receiving the accepted half-skimmed milk formula revealed transient elevations of phenylalanine and tyrosine that could be damaging to the developing brain. A baby's own mother's milk is now known to be most appropriate for even the smallest infants. Banking of breast milk, which was common in the 1950s, was markedly decreased when formulas of modified cow's milk became available. Breast-milk banks have little chance of reappearing now that we know viruses can be transmitted by breast milk, and infants without maternal antibody protection can become infected.

■ RAPID ADVANCES IN NEONATAL CARE: PHASE 2 (1975–   )

Surely the major changes in care of premature infants have come about as the result of miniaturization of equipment such as respirators; microchemical determinations that permit controlled intravenous alimentation; awareness of the appropriate thermal environment that can be servo-controlled by the infant; and devices to monitor blood gases, pulse, respirations, and blood pressure. Most importantly, we now have physicians who specialize in the care of sick infants and nurses who do likewise and not

only provide care for the infants but are interactive and supportive of the infants' families. This package of services called neonatal intensive care is available to most of the population in the United States through regionalization and maternal referrals for delivery in centers with perinatal programs.

Risks of transport are significant for the infant. They can be minimized by insistence on a well-equipped ambulance and an experienced physician-nurse team to accompany each infant during transport.

High-risk infants (or mothers expected to have such infants) are transferred to perinatal centers (level III units) that essentially combine a high-risk obstetric service with a neonatal intensive care unit. Around-the-clock sophisticated medical and ancillary services should be available. The level II unit is a large community hospital (i.e., one in which there are approximately 1000 deliveries/year) that provides intermediate care to infants who have returned from intensive care units for convalescence and growth or to problem newborns who do not require intensive care. Most babies in the United States are born in either a level II or a level I (primary care only) hospital. Intermediate care for infants and services relating to the needs of their parents should be more highly developed and better provided in the level II units. For every intensive care bed, there should be four to six intermediate care beds, with the exact number based on an estimate of length of stay (see Table 1–1).

The crescendo of interest in newborn infants in the 1980s followed the availability of appropriate equipment for their care, significant support for research into causes of abnormalities, and the presentation of evidence that even very-low-birth-weight infants could survive and be normal. If some could survive, why not most all of them? Prevention of adverse outcomes, with a possible 75-year survival rate, became very appealing to physicians, nurses, and most health-care workers. Neonatology became the largest subspecialty within pediatrics, and neonatologists developed their own subspecialties as their research interests required focus on a given organ system and the mobilization of tools of cellular and molecular biology.

Changes in practice evolved from the relative isolation of sick infants to involvement of family members, primary care nurses, and consultations with other concerned members of society, including general pediatricians and ethicists.

New questions came into focus, such as how small is too small? What is our responsibility with respect to mobilization or discontinuation of life support systems in the face of major or irreversible medical problems? As of the late 1980s, most neonatologists choose to individualize difficult decisions in consultation with the most concerned adults, chiefly parents, nurses, and primary care physicians. A consensus is almost always reached. Pressures to provide guidelines continue, from the two extremes of prolonging all life as long as possible, to setting specific limits when the outcome seems hopeless. It seems probable that in an increasingly cost-conscious society, a lower limit of gestational age (e.g., 23 to 24 weeks) can be defined as eligibility for neonatal intensive care, based not only on the odds of survival but on the likelihood of minimal later morbidity.

■ DEFINITIONS OF TERMS USED IN CARE OF THE NEWBORN

In a clarification of definitions by the World Health Organization (WHO) in 1974, Dr. Peter Dunn wrote, "The perinatal period occupies less than 0.5 per cent of the average life span, yet accounts in many countries for more deaths than the next 30 years. With the reduction in infant and childhood mortality, attention is increasingly being focused on the prevention of perinatal mortality."

The definitions agreed on by a WHO group in 1974 for reporting purposes remain appropriate in the 1980s. The perinatal period extends from the 28th completed week of pregnancy to the 7th day of life. Clearly, some infants survive after only 25 weeks' gestation, and, in the future, recording of these births and deaths will be appropriate in societies that are prepared to provide intensive care for newborns. Of course, infant deaths also occur after 7 days, and in this country neonatal deaths are often defined as deaths that occur within 28 days of birth, or, for local hospital purposes, deaths that occur before discharge from hospital after preterm birth.

A reason to maintain the WHO nomenclature for worldwide comparisons relates to the incomplete records available in some societies for very immature infants. Although infants born before 28 weeks' gestation account for fewer than 1 per cent of live births, careful recording of births and deaths and inclusion in national statistics penalize the countries that have the best reporting.

Preterm. Preterm is defined as less than 37 completed weeks', or 259 days', gestation. The definition is, of course, arbitrary, but it is based on the greater likelihood of conditions associated with immaturity, such as hyaline membrane disease, in the group of infants born before 259 days. For most developed countries, 37 completed weeks of gestation corresponds to a birth weight of 3000 g.

Stillbirth and Fetal Death. By definition, early fetal death occurs at less than 20 completed weeks of gestation, intermediate fetal death occurs at more than 20 and less than 28 completed weeks, and late fetal death occurs after 28 weeks. The term stillbirth is usually applied to late fetal deaths.

Live Birth. WHO defines live birth as "the complete expulsion or extraction from its mother of a product of conception, irrespective of the duration of pregnancy, which after such separation, breathes or shows any other evidence of life, such as beating of the heart, pulsation of the umbilical cord, or definite movement of voluntary muscles, whether or not the umbilical cord has been cut or the placenta is attached; each product of such a birth is considered liveborn."

Term. This defines births that occur from 37 to less than 42 completed weeks, measured from the day of onset of the last normal menstrual period (259 to 293 days, with an average of 280 days).

Post-Term. This refers to births that occur at 42 or more completed weeks (294 days).

Early Neonatal Death. This describes the death of a live-born infant during the first 7 completed days of life.

Late Neonatal Death. This refers to the death of a live-born infant after 7 but before 28 completed days of life.

In-Hospital Death. Although this term is not included in the WHO system, we have found that it is useful in recent years to record as in-hospital neonatal mortality any death that occurs within a hospital period that is continuous from birth. Therefore, infants who die at 3 to 6 months or later and who have been hospitalized continuously from birth because of complications and chronic disease following respiratory distress syndrome, congenital anomalies, and other conditions are included in this category.

■ EPIDEMIOLOGY

The outlook for a successful outcome of pregnancy has improved dramatically over the past five decades (see Fig. 1–1). A rough chronology of major advances is listed in Table 1–1. The impact of new knowledge and its application has resulted in an impressive reduction in deaths in the first year of life on the national scene, with a 50 per cent reduction in mortality rates from 1970 to 1985, and a 15 per cent reduction in the rate of low-birth-weight infants. Most of the reduction in infant mortality has been attributed to the decline in birth-weight–specific mortality, presumably related to improvements in perinatal care (Fig. 1–2). The number of deaths from respiratory distress syndrome and hyaline membrane disease (RDS/HMD) in the United States in three different 5-year periods is shown in Table 1–2.

RACE

Overall, the mortality rate of nonwhite infants in the first year of life is twice as high as that of white infants.

TABLE 1–1. Diagnostic and Therapeutic Advances in Perinatology

		PEDIATRICS	OBSTETRICS
1950–1960	Infections	Nursery infection control Widespread use of antibiotics	Control of endometritis Near elimination of maternal mortality in childbirth
	Rh disease	Exchange transfusions	Serum antibody testing Amniocentesis for bilirubin pigments
	Surgery	PDA, imperforate anus, TE fistula	Avoidance of midforceps delivery, improved maternal anesthesia
1961–1970	Toxicology	Chloramphenicol, sulfonamides, oxygen	Thalidomide, diethylstilbestrol
	Rh disease/jaundice	Phototherapy	Prevention of isoimmunization
	Regionalization	High-risk infants: neonatal intensive care units, intermediate care units	High-risk mothers: perinatal centers
	Monitoring	Intra-arterial blood gases, blood pressure Continuous heart and respiratory rate monitoring	Fetal heart rate monitoring, fetal scalp pH Maternal estrogen excretion
1971–1980	Amniotic fluid testing	Improved genetic counseling	Detection of fetal genetic disorders
	Infection	Cord blood serologies for detection of chronic fetal infections	Rubella immunization
	Respiratory disease	Ventilator support with continuous distending airway pressure Microtesting of blood samples Transcutaneous O_2 and CO_2 monitoring	Amniotic fluid testing for RDS risk Prenatal glucocorticoids to accelerate fetal lung maturation Improved suctioning techniques for removal of meconium in the upper airway
	Genetics	Neonatal screening: PKU, hypothyroidism, and other metabolic diseases	Heterozygote definition (Tay-Sachs) Fetal diagnosis of hemoglobinopathies
	Imaging	CAT scanning and ultrasonography	Fetal ultrasonography
	Prematurity	Intravenous hyperalimentation	Suppression of premature labor
1980–1989	Respiratory disease	Psychological support of parents of ICU infants Surfactant replacement Selective use of extracorporeal membrane oxygenator for severe cardiopulmonary failure	
	Cardiac disorders	Indomethacin for closure of ductus Total correction of heart malformations in infancy O_2 saturation monitoring	
	Genetics		Expanded molecular diagnosis Percutaneous fetal blood sampling Expanded use of fetal ultrasonography
	Prematurity	Cryotherapy for retinopathy of prematurity	Improved access to prenatal care

The higher rate of preterm births (12.8 per cent in nonwhite compared with 7.4 per cent for whites) was a large factor in the Massachusetts experience reported by Wise and co-workers (1985). The weight-specific mortality is actually lower in black infants under 2.5 kg (Table 1–3).

The reasons for the advantage of blacks when they are born prematurely may relate to biologic factors such as their accelerated lung maturation. The marked disadvantages in the first year of life of black infants born with weights over 2.0 kg are thought to be related to adverse socioeconomic factors (Miller and Jekel, 1987).

The causes of infant deaths, by race, are shown in Table 1–4. Note that the largest differences that confer disadvantage on blacks are short gestation and gastrointestinal diseases.

MATERNAL AGE

In general, the best outcome of pregnancy takes place when the mother is over age 20 and under age 35. Extension of maternal age in either direction has generally been thought to result in an increase in infant mortality. Berkowitz and co-workers (1990) have reported that, although pregnancy complications are increased, mortality need not be increased in pregnancies of healthy middle-class women. An association between the percentage of mothers under age 20 years and infant mortality in 4 countries is shown in Table 1–5. Since pregnancy among

adolescents occurs more commonly among mothers of lower socioeconomic status and more often among nonwhites than whites, assigning relative importance to these and other factors that coexist with young maternal age has been a challenge.

Several reasons are often cited for the rise in teenage pregnancies, principally the growing number of teenagers

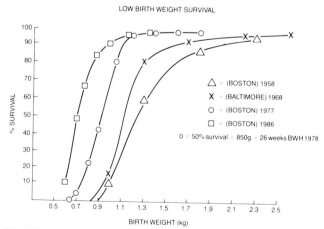

FIGURE 1–2. Birth data are shown from two centers in four time periods and illustrate the dependency of survival on birth weight. Note that a difference of 300 g (approximately 1½ weeks gestation) in 1977 could alter chances of survival from less than 5 per cent to more than 95 per cent. (BWH = Brigham and Women's Hospital [inborn infants].)

TABLE 1–2. Annual RDS/HMD Specific Mortality (United States Vital Statistics)

	1969–1973	1974–1978	1979–1983
White	7880	5945	3837
Black	1989	1897	1345
Total	9993	7962	5271
Rates/1000 live births	2.89	2.47	1.46
Per cent change in rates within 5-year period	+2.7	−9.4	−8.8

TABLE 1–3. Birth-Weight–Specific Infant Mortality Rates, Per Cent*

	1960		1980	
BIRTH-WEIGHT	W†	B†	W	B
<1000	92	88	75	72
1000–1499	58	48	25	17
1500–1999	24	18	7.9	5.7
2000–2499	6.2	5.9	2.7	2.1
2500–2999	1.7	2.5	.85	.98
3000–3499	.88	1.7	.43	.66
3500–3999	.69	1.7	.31	.56
4000–4499	.70	2.1	.31	.59
>4500	1.12	2.8	.51	1.22

*Rates are for singleton infants.
†W, white; B, black.

(From National Center for Health Statistics: Vital statistics of the United States, Vol. II, 1960. U.S. Government Printing Office, Washington, DC, 1963.)

and the increase in sexual activity. In the United States, over 900,000 teenage women between ages 15 and 19 become pregnant each year and almost 25,000 are 15 years old or younger. Adolescent mothers contribute 19 per cent of the births but have 26 per cent of the low-birth-weight infants. These mothers have increased risks for death in childbirth, toxemia, anemia, and neurologic disorders in their offspring. On the average, infants born to adolescent mothers may be less well nurtured, have a greater risk of child abuse, and receive less health supervision as children. Similarly, adolescent mothers who have infants are more prone to marital dissolution and emotional disturbances. Obviously, causes and effects are difficult to unravel, but there is little doubt that for a young woman between 15 and 19 years of age, pregnancy may contribute to what Smith described in 1980 as ''a dismal future of unemployment, poverty, dropping out of school, family breakdowns, emotional stress, dependency on public health agencies, and health problems for mother and child.''

Pregnancy after age 40 years is associated with another set of hazards for the baby. For pregnant women over 40 years, a sharp increase in deaths around the time of birth (perinatal mortality) occurs with each subsequent year of age. After 40 years of age, the hazards are greater if it is the woman's first pregnancy rather than a subsequent pregnancy. One of the risks of pregnancy after age 40 years is the approximately 2.6 per cent incidence of Down syndrome in the baby compared with an overall incidence of 0.15 per cent. Another problem relates to diminished elasticity of the pelvic structures, which results in difficulties with delivery. Diagnostic amniocentesis for detection of chromosomal abnormalities such as Down syndrome can alert the mother to that possibility and provide her with the option of abortion. Skillful obstetric management can reduce these hazards around the time of delivery.

PRENATAL CARE

Numerous studies have documented the higher incidence of prematurity and growth retardation in infants of mothers from a lower socioeconomic group and among the findings is a specific association of these developmental problems with lack of prenatal care (Miller and Jekel, 1987; Wise et al., 1985).

Many confounding factors complicate the interpretation of these and similar findings. Indeed, we do not know what aspects of prenatal care have a significant bearing on the outcome of a pregnancy. It seems reasonable to give much credit to health education. The mothers who want to do what is best for their babies are probably the ones who elect prenatal care. Early detection of risk factors, hypertension, and poor or excessive weight gain surely dictates appropriate interventions, which on the whole improve the outcome of pregnancy.

TABLE 1–4. Infant Mortality Rates and Black to White Ratios for Major Cause Groups*

	ICD CODES†	PROVISIONAL		FINAL 1985			
		1986	1985	Total	White	Black	B/W Ratio
All causes		1,039.2	1,057.0	1,064.5	931.5	1,819.0	1.95
Certain perinatal conditions	760–4, 766, 770–9	266.2	264.5	282.7	232.1	567.5	2.45
Congenital anomalies	740–759	218.9	236.7	227.7	230.6	233.3	1.01
Sudden infant death syndrome	798.0	130.4	129.6	141.3	125.6	223.1	1.78
Respiratory distress syndrome	769	94.4	100.7	98.2	90.5	149.8	1.66
Short gestation and low birth weight	765	87.9	83.3	86.6	62.3	217.9	3.50
Intrauterine hypoxia–birth asphyxia	768	24.2	28.4	30.8	26.1	58.2	2.23
Pneumonia and influenza	480–487	18.0	17.9	18.7	14.8	39.0	2.64
Birth trauma	767	8.6	7.5	8.7	7.4	16.3	2.20
Certain gastrointestinal diseases	008–9, 535, 555–8	5.9	4.8	5.4	3.5	14.9	4.26
All other causes	Residual	184.7	183.9	164.4	138.6	299.0	2.16

*Rates per 100,000 live births. Data from National Center for Health Statistics: Vital statistics of the United States Vol. II, 1980. U.S. Government Printing Office, Washington, DC, 1985.
†*International Classification of Diseases* (ICD), ninth revision.

(From Wegman, M. E.: Annual summary of vital statistics, 1986. Pediatrics 80:817, 1987.)

TABLE 1–5. Association of Infant Mortality in Four Countries with Per cent of Mothers Under Age 20 Years

COUNTRY	1985 INFANT MORTALITY PER 1000 LIVE BIRTHS	PER CENT MOTHERS UNDER AGE 20
Japan	5.5	1.1
Finland	6.3	5.0
United Kingdom	9.3	8.9
United States	10.4	14.8

(Mortality data from Wegman, M. E.: Annual summary of vital statistics, 1986. Pediatrics 80:817, 1987.)

■ THE FUTURE OF THE CARE OF THE NEWBORN

Much attention is now focused on the national embarrassment of the relatively high infant mortality rate in the United States compared with other developed nations, and the persistently high mortality among nonwhite infants. Goals set in 1979 for the year 1990 were not met and will require a concerted federal and state effort to reduce the social and economic barriers to access to prenatal care in the next decade (Table 1–6).

■ GLOBAL PERSPECTIVES

There is increasing worldwide attention to the disparities in infant mortality and the circumstances that are deemed

TABLE 1–6. 1990 Federal Priority Objectives for Pregnancy and Infant Health

Improved Health Status
1. National infant mortality rate (IMR) should be reduced to no more than 9 deaths per 1000 live births.
2. The neonatal death rate should be reduced to no more than 6.5 deaths per 1000.
3. The perinatal death rate should be reduced to no more than 5.5 deaths per 1000.
4. No county, racial, or ethnic group should have an IMR in excess of 12 deaths per 1000.
5. No county, racial, or ethnic group should have a maternal mortality rate of more than 5 deaths per 100,000 live births.

Reduced Risk Factors
6. Low-birth-weight (LBW) babies (less than 2500 g) should constitute not more than 5 per cent of live births.
7. No county, racial, or ethnic group should have an LBW rate that exceeds 9 per cent.
8. The majority of infants should leave hospitals in car safety seats.

Increased Public Awareness
9. Eighty-five per cent of women of child-bearing age should be able to choose foods wisely and should understand the hazards of smoking, alcohol, and drugs during pregnancy and lactation.

Improved Services and Protection
10. All women and infants should be served at a level appropriate to their need by a regionalized system of perinatal care.
11. The proportion of women in any county, racial, or ethnic group who obtain no prenatal care during the first trimester of pregnancy should not exceed 10 per cent.
12. All newborns should be screened for metabolic disorders for which effective tests and treatments are available.
13. All infants should be able to participate in comprehensive primary health care.

(From Public Health Service, Promoting health/preventing disease: objectives for the nation. Washington, DC: Department of Health and Human Services, Public Health Service, 1980. In Centers for Disease Control, National Center for Health Statistics: Progress toward achieving the 1990 objectives for pregnancy and infant health. MMWR 37:406, 1988.)

responsible. The lowest rates ever recorded were set in the mid-1980s when Japan achieved an infant mortality rate of 5.5 per 1000 live births, followed closely by Finland and Sweden, with the United States well behind at 10.6, and New Zealand, Italy, Austria, Israel, Greece, and Czechoslovakia even further behind. On the other hand, all of these so-called developed countries have vastly lower infant mortality rates than most of the countries in the world. According to data collected by the United Nations Children's Fund in 1986, at least 39 countries reported infant mortality rates of greater than 100 per 1000 live births. These included many of the countries of sub-Saharan Africa and Southeast Asia. The situation in Central and South America is also disturbing inasmuch as Brazil reports a mortality rate of 65 per 1000 live births; Honduras, 71 per 1000; Guatamala, 61 per 1000; and Ecuador, 64 per 1000.

MATERNAL PERSPECTIVES

In some societies, the maternal mortality rate is also shockingly high. In the developed countries, the maternal mortality rate is approximately 1 per 10,000 births, whereas among the poorest countries it is more than 100 times as high.

Priorities must differ in the context of the existing situations in each country. In a careful examination of the problem in the Zaria area of northern Nigeria, Harrison commented that preventing stillbirths of term infants who died in utero before their mothers arrived at the hospital is the highest priority.

Although there is recognition that the prevention of low birth weight by preterm delivery is clearly important, the high mortality of normal-birth-weight babies remains the central concern. Among the factors that contribute to the problem are the observation that in a traditional sub-Saharan society, African women are accorded a very inferior status. They take a limited part in the decision-making process, even when it involves childbearing. The decision to transfer a desperately ill pregnant woman to a hospital is nearly always made by the husband, and in his absence others may be unwilling to make the decision. There is a traditional dislike of operative deliveries, so that even when labor is obstructed, consent to relieve the obstruction by cesarean section may require prolonged discussion. Marriage soon after puberty is widely practiced among the illiterate traditional majority of individuals. Most of the girls of this age are underdeveloped and also nutritionally deprived so that pelvic contraction is common. A further problem is that young primigravidae are often shy about their pregnancies, strive to conceal the fact, and therefore have no prenatal care. Home delivery is nearly always preferred by that particular population.

Although the biosocial issues that have an impact on the outcome of pregnancy are complex, some of the solutions are straightforward. It is fair enough to say that major structural changes in the existing political, economic, and cultural milieu are necessary for major improvements to occur over the long term. It is also clear that providing facilities for antenatal care and an educational program that promotes its use can make an immediate difference. The development of facilities for performing cesarean section safely has to be a priority, as does availability of safe blood transfusions.

PEDIATRIC PERSPECTIVES

Experiences in developed and developing countries suggest that perinatal mortality may be reduced by 30 to 40 per cent within a few years by the application of some straightforward, common sense interventions. These include the recognition of risk factors and the identification of women who are likely to have difficulty during the perinatal period so that they may be delivered in safe settings. It also means applying current knowledge available, such as ensuring the availability of appropriate resuscitation and thermal environment for an infant, the encouragement of timely breast-feeding, and the minimizing of the risk of infection by making hand-washing a consistent practice. It is extraordinary to realize that in some hospital-based intensive care nurseries or even routine care nurseries, the caretakers move from baby to baby without washing hands between examinations. In many nurseries, no sinks are readily available except those at a considerable distance, and even then they may not be equipped with soap or disposable towels. The high prevalence of nosocomial infection in such environments is not surprising. In fact, the leading cause of death in many such settings is acquired infection in the period after delivery. Encouraging mothers to care for their own infants is of course an important intervention to provide where possible, and is widely practiced in some of the developing countries. If individuals other than the mother are to care for babies, they must be required to wash their hands, be encouraged not to insert their fingers into the babies' mouths, and be encouraged to make sure that sheets, blankets, and other objects with which the baby comes in contact have been washed and preferably sterilized. It is essential to realize that where the infant mortality rate is high, it can be reduced by at least one-third, if not one-half, through the application of the straightforward caretaking measures just cited.

Clearly, a major contribution to the reduction in the mortality of both term and low-birth-weight babies that has taken place in the developed countries has been the use of better incubators, temperature control devices, and respirators, and the ability to monitor blood gases, and to have microchemical determinations promptly available. Since the availability of such advanced equipment and the highly trained personnel to work with it cannot be reproduced in all settings where babies are born, it is inappropriate to assign its availability the highest priority.

TABLE 1–7. Fertility Rates and Birth Rates Between 1790 and 1985 (United States Vital Statistics)

YEAR	BIRTH RATE (PER 1000)	BIRTHS PER WOMAN (FERTILITY RATE)
1790	55	8
1900	30	—
1940	20	2.3
1950	22	3.2
1957	22	3.7
1970	19	2.5
1985	15.5	1.8

Each society must identify its own problems and ascertain the most appropriate, feasible interventions. In 1979, the United States Public Health Service defined a list of objectives for 1990, which were not achieved (see Table 1–6). Nothing will improve, however, without the advocacy of those who care about the health of mothers and infants in any social context. We should be encouraged by the remarkable success that has been achieved in the Scandinavian countries and Japan, and realize that maternal mortality is almost always preventable, and infant mortality should be less than 5/1000 live births. Fortunately, when infant mortality falls, fertility rates also fall since there is less need for a woman to have multiple pregnancies if there is reasonable assurance of the survival of each infant. This observation has been duplicated in every society in which there has been a reduction in infant mortality, including the United States (Table 1–7). The coupling of efforts to reduce maternal and infant mortality with advice on family planning and child spacing would seem to be the important goal for the next decades. Universal access to prenatal care is a high priority. Stimulated by the leadership shown by WHO, UNICEF, and the International Pediatric Association, as well as local pediatric societies and religious groups, the goals for the year 2000 could be attainable. At least, we should not rest until we see progress in reaching them being made in all parts of the world.

■ REFERENCES

AAP Special Report: Barriers to Care. Elk Grove Village, Ill., American Academy of Pediatrics, 1989.

Braverman, P., Oliva, G., Miller, M. G., et al.: Adverse outcomes and lack of health insurance among newborns in an eight-county area of California, 1982 to 1986. N. Engl. J. Med. *321*:508, 1989.

Behrman, R. E.: Premature births among black women. N. Engl. J. Med. *317*:763, 1987.

Berkowitz, G. S., Skouron, M. L., Lapinski, R. H., et al.: Delayed child bearing and the outcome of pregnancy. N. Engl. J. Med. *322*:659, 1990.

Cloherty, J. P., and Stark, A. R. (Eds.): Manual of Neonatal Care. Boston, Little, Brown and Company, 1980.

Editorial. Maternal health in sub-Saharan Africa. Lancet *1*:255, 1987.

Gould, J. B., Davey, B., and Stafford, R. S.: Socioeconomic differences in rates of cesarean section. N. Engl. J. Med. *321*:233, 1989.

Harrison, K. A.: Childbearing, health and social priorities: A survey of 2274 consecutive hospital births in Zaria, Northern Nigeria. Brit. J. Obstet. Gynaecol. *92* (Suppl 5):1, 1985.

Kiely, J. L., Paneth, N., and Susser, M.: An assessment of the effects of maternal age and parity in different components of perinatal mortality. Am. J. Epidemiol. *123*:444, 1986.

Kleinman, J. D., and Kessel, S. S.: Racial differences in low birth weight. N. Engl. J. Med. *317*:749, 1987.

Lee, K-S., and Corpuz, M.: Teenage pregnancy: Trend and impact on rates of low birth weight and fetal, maternal, and neonatal mortality in the United States. Clin. Perinatol. *15*:929, 1988.

Mahler, H.: The safe motherhood initiative: A call to action. Lancet *i*:668, 1987.

McCormick, M. C., Shapiro, S., and Starfield, B. H.: The regionalization of perinatal services. Summary of the evaluation of a national demonstration program. J.A.M.A. *253*:799, 1985.

Miller, H. C., and Jekel, J. F.: The effect of race on the incidence of low birth weight: Persistence of effect after controlling for socioeconomic, educational, marital, and risk status. Yale J. Biol. Med. *60*:221, 1987.

Modanlou, H., Dorchester, W., Freeman, R., and Rommal, C.: Perinatal transport to a regional perinatal center in a metropolitan area: Maternal vs. neonatal transport. Am. J. Obstet. Gynecol. *138*:1157, 1980.

Murray, J. L., and Bernfield, M.: The differential effect of prenatal care on the incidence of low birth weight among blacks and whites in a prepaid health care plan. N. Engl. J. Med. *319*:1385, 1988.

National Commission to Prevent Infant Mortality: *Death Before Life: The Tragedy of Infant Mortality*. August, 1988.

Perelman, R., and Farrell, P.: Analysis of causes of neonatal death in the U. S. with specific emphasis on fetal hyaline membrane disease. Pediatrics *70*:570, 1982.

Philip, A., Little, G., Polivy, D., and Lucey, J.: Neonatal mortality risk for the eighties: Importance of birthweight/gestational age groups. Pediatrics *68*:122, 1981.

Smith, P., and Mumford, P. (Eds.): Adolescent Pregnancy. Boston, C. K. Hall and Company, 1980, p. 18.

Wegman, M. E.: Annual summary of vital statistics—1986. Pediatrics *80*:817, 1987.

Wise, P. H., Kotelchuck, M., and Mills, M.: Racial and socioeconomic disparities in childhood mortality in Boston. N. Engl. J. Med. *313*:360, 1985.

ETHICAL AND LEGAL ISSUES IN NEWBORN CARE 2

Joan McIver Gibson and Robert Schwartz

■ BASIC PRINCIPLES OF ETHICS

In late 1983, after several years of occasionally acrimonious discussion among medical organizations and advocacy organizations for the developmentally disabled, the American Academy of Pediatrics, the Association for Retarded Citizens, the National Association of Children's Hospitals and Related Institutions, the American Association on Mental Deficiency and several other organizations issued the following joint policy statement that provides the basic principles of treatment of disabled infants:

> *Medical Care: When medical care is clearly beneficial, it should always be provided. When appropriate medical care is not available, arrangements should be made to transfer the infant to an appropriate medical facility. Consideration(s) such as anticipated or actual limited potential of an individual and present or future lack of available community resources are irrelevant and must not determine the decisions concerning medical care. The individual's medical condition should be the sole focus of the decision. . . .*
>
> *It is ethically and legally justified to withhold medical or surgical procedures which are clearly futile and will only prolong the act of dying. However, supportive care should be provided, including sustenance as medically indicated and relief of pain and suffering. The needs of the dying person should be respected. The family should also be supported in its grieving.*
>
> *In cases where it is uncertain whether medical treatment will be beneficial, a person's disability must not be the basis for a decision to withhold treatment. At all times during the process when decisions are being made about the benefit or futility of medical treatment, the person should be cared for in the medically most appropriate ways.*

These guidelines reflect what, in any discussion of ethical values issues, nearly always is the overarching principle: *respect for persons.* Serving this notion that all persons possess intrinsic dignity and worth are the somewhat more focused principles of *autonomy, beneficence,* and *justice.* In the health-care context, autonomy requires that persons be treated as self-determining and self-defining agents and that their wishes be respected wherever possible. Legal issues, such as informed consent, the right to privacy and confidentiality, and advance directive legislation (e.g., Living Will laws and Durable Powers of Attorney for Health-Care Decisions) rest on this principle. However, its direct applicability to infants is problematic,

because surrogate decision-making on their behalf cannot apply the now-preferred *substituted judgement standard,* which seeks to base all decisions on the expressed or, at least, inferred wishes of the patient. Rather, in cases involving infants, reference to the principle of autonomy usually is restricted to *ownership-of-decision* issues: the right of parents to bear primary responsibility for such decision-making as well as the physician's right to professional independence and authority.

The more traditional *best-interest standard* reflects the historical role of the health-care professional as one who has primary responsibility for assessing the patient's quality of life, whether the patient is an adult or an infant. As the substituted judgement standard rests on the principle of autonomy, so the best-interest standard rests on the ethical principle of *beneficence,* which exhorts physicians and others first to do no harm, to prevent and remove sources of harm, and to do good wherever possible. Issues of abuse and neglect, as well as calculations of relative benefits and burdens of treatment options, are fundamentally issues of beneficence. Of special concern for newborns is the medical uncertainty of some of these treatment options that give rise to moral uncertainty when clear-cut conclusions about benefits and burdens are impossible. Protecting infants from inappropriate experimentation, from wrongful treatment, and from treatment that is futile and unjustifiably prolongs life are all beneficence-driven duties on which there seems to be widespread agreement. What is difficult, of course, is the question: Does a proposed treatment fit such a category or not?

Finally, issues of *distributive justice,* i.e., of fair and equitable distribution of resources, of equal and appropriate access to basic health-care services, and of affordability of health-care services, have a special urgency when applied to certain age-specific health problems, such as those of seriously ill newborns and the rapidly increasing percentage of elderly persons living to an older age. Treatment in neonatal intensive care units is labor intensive, technologically sophisticated, and expensive. Shortages of beds in neonatal intensive care units can actually inflict harm on infants who must be transported over extremely long distances when the needed resources are not available locally. Macroeconomic policies that seek to redistribute existing resources in light of these broad demographic factors may have a significant effect on neonatal care as it is currently being delivered.

An anencephalic infant is diagnosed at 30 weeks' gestation during an otherwise normal pregnancy. The parents request that the infant's organs be used for transplants. At the same medical center, a seriously ill infant in need of a heart transplant awaits a suitable donor.

All of the ethical principles described above interact intensely in problems of organ procurement and transplantation in infant patients. Virtually everyone agrees that the intrinsic dignity and worth of all infants, both donors and recipients, must be respected. Often, however, it is difficult to know how to do this. For example, is it ethical to harvest organs from an anencephalic infant, even with the parents' consent, while the donor is alive?

Proponents of using anencephalic infants as organ donors argue that these infants comprise a unique exception and that they are not "persons" as usually defined, because of the virtual absence of major portions of the brain. Therefore, they argue, the traditional practices through which respect of person is observed do not apply. Nor, they continue, must we change the existing definition of brain death or related statutes and practices based on that definition in order to enable harvesting of organs from anencephalic infants.

Those who oppose this view counter that the frequently expressed discomfort associated with such procedures stems directly from our fundamental belief that these infants must be accorded at least the same level and kind of respect and dignity as other infants precisely *because* of their extremely vulnerable condition.

There is general agreement that the primary decision-makers in cases involving infants ought to be parents and guardians, especially with respect to organ donation. There is equal agreement that the best interests of all infants involved must be served. However, in any given case, who should make such best-interest decisions? This question arises frequently in discussions of ethical issues faced in neonatal intensive care units. Unless cardiopulmonary support measures are taken to maintain tissue oxygenation in an anencephalic infant, the organs sustain extensive hypoxic ischemic injury that makes the heart and liver unsuitable for transplant. Should such infants, then, receive "customary" care (no alteration of the ordinary course of treatment of a terminally ill infant), following the dictum of avoiding harm or producing needless suffering, and respecting the infant's right to die? Or, in seeking to apply the dictum to help wherever possible, should efforts be made to maintain the viability of the organs to improve the outlook of prospective recipients even though the anencephalic infant's terminal course may be slowed? How best to support the wishes of the parents also presents a dilemma. For many grieving parents of anencephalic infants, the potential benefit to another family offered by organ donation seems an avenue to achieving some good from their own tragedy.

In Europe, Holzgreve (1987) has reported success in transplanting kidneys of sustained anencephalic infants. However, in the United States, the question of harvesting organs from live-born anencephalic infants is moot, since these infants do not meet the legal requirements for brain death as defined by the United States Uniform Determi-

nations of Death Act, and since brain-stem function is initially demonstrable. Some efforts have been made to change the law in the United States, but at this time, organs derived from anencephalic infants are not suitable for transplantation (Peabody, 1989).

Issues of cost effectiveness and allocation of resources are perhaps nowhere more numerous than in high-technology areas where advances themselves create needs and shortages. The technology of transplantation frequently has proved to be cost effective when compared with other life-sustaining therapies, yet it has generated costs of its own. Whether to diminish the need by scaling down the frequency of certain procedures or to diminish the shortage by increasing the supply of available organs is not yet a settled issue—something that can be said of many of the health-care resource choices facing today's physicians, their patients, and policy-makers. Another related issue involves the question of when therapeutic experimental procedures become nontherapeutic and should be considered only experimental.

■ BASIC LEGAL PRINCIPLES

The basic legal principles are largely driven by the related ethical principles. Principles of malpractice and abuse and neglect law respond primarily to the duty to see that harm is avoided or prevented, while the doctrine of informed consent recognizes the right of the patient's surrogate to assume independent decision-making authority and responsibility to the greatest extent possible. Unfortunately, actual cases do not divide themselves neatly into clear-cut ethical and legal categories. As the following case and discussion illustrate, such concepts are most helpful when used as guides for understanding and analyzing specific cases rather than as recipes that are guaranteed to yield the "right" decision.

A preterm infant is born 12 hours after premature rupture of the membranes at 24 weeks' gestation. No cesarean section was done. The infant was septic at birth, and ultrasound study on the 2nd day of life showed massive intracranial hemorrhage. The baby, however, survived. During follow-up at 1 year of age, cerebral palsy was found. The parents sued the physicians involved for not having performed a cesarean section to prevent intracranial hemorrhage.

BASIC PRINCIPLES OF MALPRACTICE

With few exceptions, in the United States the law of doctor-patient relationships is state law. Although there are some consistencies, there are also substantial differences from state to state. As a general rule, the law of professional negligence (medical malpractice) is the same whether the patient is an adult or an infant. If a physician fails to exercise the duty of due care—i.e., fails to do what a reasonable physician would do under the circumstances—and that failure causes damage to the patient, the physician (and, indirectly, the physician's insurer) may be legally obligated to compensate the patient for the damages. In the above-mentioned case, if a reasonable physician would *not* be expected to perform a cesarean section at 24 weeks of gestation, or the failure to do so cannot be assigned as the cause of the intracranial hemorrhage, then the physician would not be liable for negligence in failing to perform the surgery.

No one is liable for malpractice in accidents in the absence of carelessness, and no one is liable because a course of treatment was unsuccessful or a procedure happened to do more harm than good in a particular case. An honest error in judgment is not grounds for malpractice, nor is a decision to employ some treatment that is not used by a majority of physicians, as long as a respectable minority of physicians might have taken the same action. A physician is liable only when he or she has been so careless as to perform an act that no reasonable physician would have done, and that act caused damage in fact.

Because errors in the treatment of newborns may yield tremendous financial damages—the patients have a longer life expectancy than elderly heart transplant patients, for example, and the cost of their continued medical care is extremely high—neonatologists are understandably fearful of high malpractice awards. Laws establishing limits on damages have been promulgated recently in many states, and procedural limitations have been imposed on some malpractice cases, which should assuage some of the fear among practitioners. It must be remembered that the major factor in the genesis of such suits, on the whole, is the lack of any other financial remedy for the families of these children in the society.

GENERAL PRINCIPLES OF INFORMED CONSENT

Someone ultimately must be responsible for determining the medical treatment provided to children, and the law has generally recognized the parent or guardian as possessing the formal authority over health-care decisions that directly affect the child. This practice is based on the presumption that parents are most likely to render an appropriate substituted judgment and are most likely to act in the best interest of their children. Except in an emergency, no treatment should be given to a newborn without appropriate consent. Consent should come from a parent, unless a different guardian has been legally appointed.

When a guardian has been appointed, the scope of the guardianship ought to be determined with care. Although parents naturally possess legal authority over their children, they may not appoint a guardian. A guardianship can be created only by action of a court. In creating a guardianship for a child, the court may authorize the guardian to give consent for the performance of a particular procedure or to exercise all of the authority of a parent of the child. To determine, in any given situation, whether or not a guardian has the authority to make a particular decision, it is necessary to have access to the "letters of guardianship" issued by the court.

The doctrine of informed consent provides that the authorized decision-maker must give informed, voluntary, and competent consent. Generally, a decision-maker is *informed* if that person has been provided with all of the information that a reasonable person would want to have in order to make a contemplated decision. That information should include the risks and benefits of the treatment, the alternative treatments and their risks and benefits, and the likely course if no treatment is provided. It is not necessary (and may be wrong) to provide information in such detail that the important factors are obscured. For example, it is *not* necessary to tell a patient (or a patient's decision-maker) of a very small chance of a trivial risk, but the chance of a serious adverse consequence ought to be revealed. Ultimately, the test is one of reasonableness. In any case, the information ought to be provided in such a way that the decision-maker will understand it, and that person's questions should be answered.

A decision-maker is acting *voluntarily* if the action is taken without any coercion or undue inducement. The choice must be truly a choice for the consent to be valid. For example, threatening to discharge a child or to cease providing other, unrelated treatment unless the parents consent to treatment may render the consent involuntary and, hence, invalid. Similarly, inducing a parent to consent by offering that parent substantial payment in return for permitting the treatment may vitiate an otherwise proper consent.

Finally, the law has had difficulty defining the *competency* of the decision-maker necessary to make a decision consistent with the principle of informed, voluntary, and competent consent. The mother in the above-mentioned case is clearly unwilling to voluntarily consent to withdrawal of care, and her wishes must be respected. Generally, when the decision-maker is (1) capable of understanding the risks, benefits, and alternatives of treatment and (2) acts consistently with values associated with that type of decision-maker, that person is competent to give (or withhold) consent—even if the decision made is perceived as unwise or harmful by health-care workers or others.

In the event of differences in opinion (as in case no. 3), we defer to the mother. Usually, in time, when the mother sees no improvement, she concurs with the staff.

Consent is a process that culminates in a decision; it is not a printed form. Except when the patient is a research subject or where local institutional rule requires it, consent need not be in writing. The written consent form does provide evidence of the consent, but it is not the consent itself. Adequate consent is often obtained orally, with no written record. Indeed, apparent consent that is supported by a written document may turn out to fail to have been informed, voluntary, or competent. In those cases, the written document has no more value than a check written against insufficient funds—it is either worthless or evidence of fraud.

The only time consent is not required is when there is an emergency and, thus, a need to act immediately to preserve the life or health of the patient. The emergency exception applies only when a decision-maker is not available to consent to treatment. The law has two alternative justifications for such an exception: Either consent is waived because it is impossible to obtain, or it is presumed because of the high level of certainty that consent would be given if it could be.

GENERAL APPLICATION OF ABUSE AND NEGLECT STATUTES

In the United States, child protection statutes vary substantially from state to state, but they generally permit state intervention—usually by a state social service agency—when intervention is necessary to protect the life or safety of a child. Most often, these statutes permit the state agency or local police agencies to take immediate custody of a threatened child and then to provide whatever services are necessary to overcome the threat to the child. A judicial hearing must be accorded the parents and the child soon after the state takes physical custody. Children removed from their parents (or others) and put in the custody of the state are thus cared for by the state, which has authority to act temporarily in the place of the parents. The process of state intervention under abuse or neglect generally can be commenced by any person who has knowledge of the abuse or neglect. Although, these statutes are most commonly invoked in cases of physical abuse or life-threatening neglect (e.g., parents' failure to provide food or clothing for their child), they can also be invoked whenever a parent or guardian fails to provide adequately the necessities of life, including appropriate medical care.

CASE NO. 3

A preterm infant is born at 30 weeks' gestation to a mother with abruptio placentae. The infant has severe hyaline membrane disease and is anemic and hypotensive. The parents are Jehovah's Witnesses and refuse consent for blood transfusion.

One common form of application of the neglect statutes to medical neglect is its application to parents who deny consent for treatment of their children because of the parents' religious beliefs. Although a competent adult may decide to forego any treatment for any reason, even if the decision will lead to death, parents cannot make martyrs of their children. Thus a Jehovah's Witness who declines to consent to a needed blood transfusion for a child is medically neglecting that child. In these cases, the state protective services agency may take custody of the child for the purpose of consenting to the treatment only; for all other purposes all parental rights may be left in the hands of the sincere and well-meaning parents. Although there have been some recent successful criminal actions against parents who deny their children treatment because of their own religious beliefs, such extensive state intrusion into child-rearing prerogatives is controversial in this country, especially when there are means other than criminal prosecution to protect the interests of children.

CASE NO. 4

A term infant is born with Down syndrome and duodenal atresia. Without surgery the infant will die. The parents refuse consent for surgery, and the baby dies.

Although the propriety of providing certain kinds of treatment to very severely ill newborns has been the subject of medical discussion for some time, it first became a matter of public discussion, public policy, and law during the 1980s, with the case of "Baby Doe." The discussion that followed led the federal Department of Health and Human Services (DHHS) to issue regulations governing the treatment of seriously ill newborns. The government reasoned that failure to treat seriously ill newborns because of their birth defects constituted discrimination against them because they possessed a handicap (the birth defect itself) and was thus a violation of a federal statute prohibiting any institution receiving federal funding from discriminating on the basis of the handicapped status of a program participant. Because the regulations initially provided for a highly intrusive federal presence in the newborn nursery, virtually all medical organizations opposed them. Physicians' groups responded in two primary ways. First, they argued that the decisions made in individual cases were made by parents (who gave or withheld consent), not by the physicians or the institutions. Second, they argued that DHHS allegations of discrimination greatly oversimplified the medical decision-making process, in which the illness itself (and, thus, the handicapping condition) was the subject of the treatment decision.

The first attempt by the DHHS to develop a scheme to deal with what became known as "Baby Doe cases" was found to be procedurally defective by a lower federal court. The DHHS corrected the defect and issued a second set of proposed regulations that never became final. Instead, after extensive comments on the second proposal, the DHHS issued yet a third set of regulations. This set was ultimately rejected by the Supreme Court, presumably because its issuance was beyond the power of the DHHS.

While the challenges to these intrusive regulations were wending their way through the courts, the medical societies and those who favored the proposed regulations agreed on a compromise that would provide some protection to seriously ill newborns but limit government intrusion into the sensitive family medical decision-making process. This compromise was enacted into law as a part of the Child Abuse Amendments of 1984, and it provided that states must have processes for investigating and resolving cases of suspected medical neglect (including instances of withholding of medically indicated treatment from disabled infants with life-threatening conditions). The statute (and the regulations issued to enforce it) define "withholding of medically indicated treatment" as

> . . . the failure to respond to the infant's life-threatening condition by providing treatment (including appropriate nutrition, hydration, and medication) which, in the treating physician's or physicians' reasonable medical judgment, will be most likely to be effective in ameliorating or correcting all such conditions, except that the term does not include the failure to provide treatment (other than appropriate nutrition, hydration, or medication) to an infant when, in the treating physician's or physicians' reasonable medical judgment,
>
> A. the infant is chronically and irreversibly comatose;
> B. the provision of such treatment would
>   (i) merely prolong dying,
>   (ii) not be effective in ameliorating or correcting all of the infant's life-threatening conditions, or
>   (iii) otherwise be futile in terms of the survival of the infant; or
> C. the provision of such treatment would be virtually futile in terms of the survival of the infant and the treatment itself under such circumstances would be inhumane.

Although the statute and the regulations have toothless enforcement mechanisms, this definition may articulate the current social, ethical, and medical consensus in the United States. There is a presumption in favor of treatment of seriously ill infants, but that presumption can be overcome if it is believed that the infant will never become conscious (e.g., a hydrancephalic infant, for example, even if the infant is not terminally ill), if the prospective treatment definitely will not save the life of the child (e.g., apparent need for heart surgery in an infant with trisomy 18 and a diaphragmatic hernia), or if it is extremely unlikely that the prospective treatment will save the life of the infant. In this last case, however, withholding treatment should occur only if the treatment would impose such a burden of pain or discomfort on the patient that providing the treatment would be inhumane (e.g., the case of a seriously neurologically handicapped child, in which a tiny hope of continued life could be realized only through highly invasive, painful surgery).

Although the Child Abuse Amendments may create as much ambiguity as they eliminate (and they do explicitly depend on "reasonable medical judgment"), they clearly contemplate the continued provision of appropriate nutrition and hydration. The Senate Committee that considered the statute, however, pointed out in its report that "there are many ways to provide nutrition in addition to oral feedings, and health care professionals must provide nourishment to the infant in the medically appropriate manner." The Child Abuse Amendments also clearly indicate that the infant's interest alone is to be considered in making decisions concerning treatment, not the parents' interest, the physicians' interest, the family's interest, or society's interest. Treatment cannot be withheld from a newborn solely because that newborn will become too much of a burden for the family (or society) to bear.

■ CONCLUSION

As is generally the case, good ethics and good medicine make good law. The "Principles of Treatment of Disabled Infants" endorsed by the American Academy of Pediatrics form the basis of the Child Abuse Amendments, and both refer, directly and indirectly, to appropriate medical conduct. A physician who acts consistently with the requirements of good medicine and good medical ethics—as physicians define good ethics—is acting consistently with the law. Such a physician is acting with respect for patients and their families and in their best interests. If the ethical and legal requirements appear ambiguous, that is merely a reflection of the ambiguity in the descriptions of medically appropriate care for newborns.

■ REFERENCES

Ashwal, S., and Schneider, S.: Brain death in the newborn. Clin. Perinatol. *16*:501, 1989.

Bowen v. American Hospital Association, 476 U.S. 610 (1986).

Brett, A. S., and McCullough, L. B.: When patients request specific interventions: Defining the limits of the physician's obligation. N. Engl. J. Med. *315*:1347–1351.

Cranford, R. E.: The persistent vegetative state: The medical reality (getting the facts straight). Hastings Cent. Rep. *18*(1):27, 1988.

Department of Health and Human Services. Child abuse and neglect prevention and treatment program. Fed. Regist. *50*:14878, 1985.

Department of Health and Human Services. Nondiscrimination on the basis of handicap relating to health care for handicapped infants. Fed. Regist. *49*:1622, 1985.

Guidelines for the determination of death: Report of the medical consultants on the diagnosis of death to the President's Commission for the Study of Ethical Problems in Medicine and Biomedical and Behavioral Research. J.A.M.A *246*:2184, 1981.

Holder, A. R.: Parents, courts and refusal of treatment. J. Pediatr. *103*:515, 1983.

Holtzgreve, W., Beller F. K., Buchholz, B., et al.: Kidney transplantation from anencephalic donors. N. Engl. J. Med. *316*:1069, 1987.

Kopelman, L. M., Irons, T. G., and Kopelman, A.E.: Neonatologists judge the "Baby Doe" regulations. N. Engl. J. Med. *318*:677, 1988.

Lantos, J. D., Miles, S. H., Silverstein, M. D., and Stocking, C. B.: Survival after cardiopulmonary resuscitation in babies of very low birth weight: Is CPR futile therapy? N. Engl. J. Med. *398*:91–95, 1988.

Leikin, S.: When parents demand treatment. Pediatr. Ann. *4*:266–268, 1989.

Medaris, D. N., Jr., and Holmes, L. B.: Editorial. On the use of anencephalic infants as organ donors. N. Engl. J. Med. *321*:391, 1989.

The Medical Task Force on Anencephaly: The infant with anencephaly. N. Engl. J. Med. *322*:669, 1990.

National Commission for the Protection of Human Subjects of Biomedical and Behavioral Research. Report and Recommendations. Research involving children. Washington, D. C., Government Printing Office, 1977. (DHEW publication no. (OS) 77-0004.)

Paris, J. J., Crone, R. K., and Reardon, F.: Physician's refusal of requested treatment. N. Engl. J. Med. *322*:1012, 1990.

Peabody, J. L., Emery, J. R., and Ashwal, S.: Experience with anencephalic infants as prospective organ donors. N. Engl. J. Med. *321*:34, 1989.

U. S. Child Abuse Prevention and Adoption Reform Act. Amendment no. 3385. Congressional Record: Senate S8951–S8956, 1984.

Uniform Determination of Death Act. 7180 of the Health and Safety Code. Uniform Law Annot. *12*:310, 1980.

Volpe, J. J.: Brain death determination in the newborn. Pediatrics *80*:293, 1987.

Walters, J. W., and Ashwal, S.: Organ prolongation in anencephalic infants: Ethical and medical issues. Hastings Cent. Rep. *18*(5):19, 1988.

Truog, R. D., and Fletcher, J. C.: Editorial. Anencephalic newborns. Can organs be transplanted before brain death? N. Engl. J. Med. *321*:387, 1989.

EVALUATION OF THERAPEUTIC RECOMMENDATIONS

3

John C. Sinclair

That pediatricians can differ in their beliefs about effective treatment is not a new phenomenon. What *is* new is the accelerating pace of therapeutic innovation resulting from the explosion of new knowledge concerning the causes, natural history, diagnosis, treatment, and prevention of diseases of the newborn and older child. Today's pediatrician needs up-to-date information concerning ever more powerful therapies, and more importantly, the ability to "separate the wheat from the chaff" when it comes to evaluating the validity and applicability of therapeutic recommendations.

What standards of evidence should be met before new tests or treatments are widely applied in clinical practice? The history of the development of perinatal and neonatal medicine has included both triumphs and disasters. The fact that therapeutic innovations can be effective, useless, or even harmful has been amply demonstrated in this field. One need only cite, as examples of the latter, the unsuspected and initially undetected occurrence of retrolental fibroplasia following the uncritical introduction of unrestricted oxygen therapy, kernicterus resulting from the use of sulfisoxazole, and the gray baby syndrome due to intoxication with chloramphenicol. These examples, taken from the 1940s and 1950s, serve to remind us that it may be not just unhelpful but actually disastrous to apply untested new treatments on a wide scale.

In the present era, the problem persists. For example, concerning the supportive care of premature newborn infants, we know on the basis of well-designed clinical research that keeping them warmer than we did previously reduces neonatal mortality; but a recent and alarming report (Lucas et al., 1988) of an association between low but asymptomatic neonatal glucose levels in low-birth-weight infants and impaired later neurodevelopment exposes the fact that there has never been an experimental test of the effect of contrasting policies of neonatal glycemic control on neurodevelopmental outcome in such patients. Concerning the treatment of diseases of the newborn and infant, recent well-designed clinical research has shown the effects of surfactant replacement for the treatment or prevention of respiratory distress syndrome (RDS), and cryotherapy for the treatment of stage 3⁺ retinopathy of prematurity; but can we point to research of comparable caliber to justify the use of tolazoline in persistent pulmonary hypertension, extracorporeal membrane oxygenation in severe pulmonary disorders, or (to choose a common, everyday problem in neonatal inten-

sive care) phenobarbital as the preferred first drug in the treatment of neonatal seizures?

For many, if not most, therapies in use at present, valid evidence of their effectiveness is lacking. Based on past experience, we can predict that many of the therapies that are presently incorporated into clinical practice will fall into disuse in the future. In fact, seven stages in the typical career of an innovative treatment or technology have been described (McKinlay, 1981):

1. Promising report
2. Professional and organizational adoption
3. Public acceptance and state (third-party) endorsement
4. Incorporation into standard practice, observational reports
5. Rigorous evaluation using randomized controlled trials
6. Professional denunciation
7. Abandonment and replacement by a newer technology

This sequence of events demonstrates a failure to properly evaluate new therapies or diagnostic technologies at an early stage of their diffusion. The case of intrapartum electronic fetal heart rate monitoring is a much studied example of widespread diffusion of a new technology before rigorous evaluation (Shy et al., 1987). In this chapter, a scheme for the evaluation of new therapies is described, and the application of this scheme in the field of perinatology is demonstrated.

■ THE MEASUREMENT ITERATIVE LOOP

A framework for such evaluation, called the "measurement iterative loop," is shown in Figure 3–1 (Tugwell et al., 1985). This scheme identifies distinct research and evaluation questions that constitute a logical progression: What is the burden of disease? What are the causes of health problems contributing to the burden? What is the effectiveness of treatment (a function of treatment efficacy, screening and diagnostic accuracy, physician and patient compliance, and coverage)? What are the costs in relation to the effects of the treatment? What interventions or programs should be selected for widespread use? What are the effects on quality of care and patient outcomes? How has the disease burden been affected? This chapter focuses particularly on the efficacy and effectiveness of treatment.

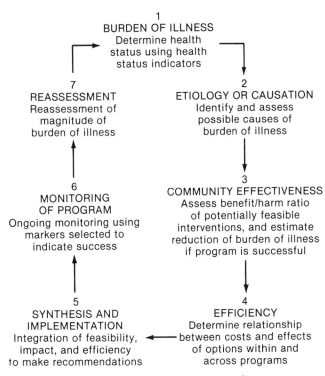

1
BURDEN OF ILLNESS
Determine health
status using health
status indicators

7
REASSESSMENT
Reassessment of
magnitude of
burden of illness

2
ETIOLOGY OR CAUSATION
Identify and assess
possible causes of
burden of illness

6
MONITORING
OF PROGRAM
Ongoing monitoring using
markers selected to
indicate success

3
COMMUNITY EFFECTIVENESS
Assess benefit/harm ratio
of potentially feasible
interventions, and estimate
reduction of burden of illness
if program is successful

5
SYNTHESIS AND
IMPLEMENTATION
Integration of feasibility,
impact, and efficiency
to make recommendations

4
EFFICIENCY
Determine relationship
between costs and effects
of options within and
across programs

FIGURE 3–1. The measurement iterative loop.

EVALUATING THE EFFICACY OF TREATMENT

The clinical questions to be asked about any treatment are

1. What is the magnitude of the baseline risk? (i.e., without treatment, what proportion of patients will experience an adverse outcome?)

2. Is there an effect of treatment? (i.e., is there an effect that is real and not due to chance?)

3. What are the direction and size of treatment effect?

4. What is the duration of treatment effect?

5. Are there unwanted side effects that are attributable to the treatment?

6. What are the economic costs?

7. Do the clinical benefits of treatment outweigh the unwanted side effects and/or economic costs?

8. To whom are these results applicable?

To obtain answers to these questions is not a simple matter. Research may sometimes result in a wrong answer because of systematic error (bias) or random error (imprecision). Even valid conclusions from research can be of limited generalizability to clinical practice. Thus, the physician needs to be concerned not just with the proclaimed results of clinical research concerning treatment but also with the methodologic issues of bias, precision, and applicability.

EXPRESSING THE EFFECT OF TREATMENT

Table 3–1 displays the structure of a typical study that seeks to evaluate treatment. There are two exposure groups (labeled as treated or control) and two possible outcome categories (labeled as event or no event). An event may be any outcome such as occurrence of disease, complication of disease, or death. Such a study design permits answers to clinically relevant questions about the effect of treatment cited above:

1. The magnitude of risk in the absence of treatment is given by the event rate in the control group, $c/c + d$.

2. The effect of treatment is given by comparing the event rate in the treated group with that in the control group. This comparison is expressed as either the *relative risk* (RR), $a/a + b \div c/c + d$, or the *risk difference* (RD), $a/a + b - c/c + d$. (Another measure of the association between treatment and outcome is given by the relative odds or odds ratio, $a/c \div b/d$. The odds ratio, an approximation of the relative risk at low prevalence, is used to estimate strength of association between outcome and exposure in case-control studies, in which relative risk cannot be calculated. However, in cohort studies including randomized clinical trials, strength of association is directly estimated as relative risk. Odds ratio is not considered further in this chapter.)

The relative risk and the risk difference convey different (and to some extent complementary) information. The relative risk indicates the *relative*, but not absolute, magnitude of reduction in the event rate. The complement of the relative risk $(1 - RR)$ gives the proportionate risks reduction. Thus, a relative risk of 0.75 represents a 25 per cent reduction in the rate of events in the treated group relative to the rate of events in the controls.

The risk difference, on the other hand, indicates the *absolute* magnitude of reduction of risk. For example, a risk difference of -0.10 represents an absolute 10 percentage point reduction of events in the treated group. The reciprocal of the risk difference (1/RD) indicates the number of patients who must be treated in order to prevent the event in one patient. This latter measure is particularly relevant when considering whether to use a treatment that is effective but whose effect is bought at considerable cost (in the form of either clinical side effects or economic cost). In the example here, 1/0.10, ten patients need to be treated to prevent one with an event.

When outcome data are reported on a continuous scale (e.g., blood pressure measured in mm Hg), a different measure of effect, the mean difference, is computed.

CONTROLLING BIAS

The fundamental goal of clinical research concerning the efficacy and safety of treatment is that it should obtain an unbiased answer to the question posed. By bias we mean a force that leads to an answer that is systematically different from the truth.

Most studies on treatment or prevention use designs that can be classified into one of four categories. These designs are listed below in order of ascending methodologic rigor:

1. Single case reports or case series without controls

TABLE 3–1. Structure of a Study to Evaluate the Effect of a Treatment

		OUTCOME	
		Event	No event
EXPOSURE	Treated	a	b
	Control	c	d

2. Nonrandomized studies using historical controls (e.g., comparing current patients who receive the innovative treatment with previous patients, from the same institution or from the literature, who did not)

3. Nonrandomized studies using concurrent controls (e.g., comparing contemporaneous patients who did or did not receive the experimental treatment)

4. Randomized controlled trials

The case report and case series (without controls) are the designs most prone to bias. The absence of a control group generally leads to an overestimate of the effect of treatment: Any improvement in the clinical course of patients in a case series is attributed to treatment, even when the improvement would have occurred in the absence of treatment.

Studies that utilize controls provide a much more valid basis for reaching conclusions about the effect of treatment. However, the performance of a controlled study is not, in itself, a sufficient guarantee of a valid result. Biases can seriously impair studies using either historical or nonrandomized concurrent controls (Sackett, 1979). Sacks and colleagues (1982) surveyed reports of controlled studies of six different therapies and found that for each therapy, studies utilizing historical controls were much more likely to find an apparent benefit than studies utilizing randomized controls. The difference was due to the fact that the control group in the historical control studies had worse outcomes than the controls in the randomized control studies; the treated patients in the two types of studies generally had similar outcomes. Historical control groups tend to fare poorly in part because they typically include all patients who meet the diagnostic criteria, even poor-risk or noncompliant patients or patients who have other adverse characteristics that might exclude them from enrollment in prospective randomized trials.

The randomized trial is based on principles originally developed for agricultural research by R.A. Fisher in the 1920s and subsequently applied to clinical research in the pioneering work of Bradford Hill, William Silverman, and others in the 1940s and 1950s. The randomized trial is the strongest design for evaluating the effect of treatment. It offers maximum protection against selection biases that can invalidate comparisons between groups of patients because of "confounding." A confounder is extraneous to the question being posed, is unequally distributed between the treatment groups being compared, and is itself a determinant of the outcome. In nonrandomized studies, the investigator tries to control confounding by strategies such as exclusion, stratification at the time of sampling, matching, stratification in the analysis, adjustment and standardization, and modeling. However, these techniques require that the source of confounding be known. In clinical medicine, the confounders are often unknown; a presently unknown confounder may be discovered tomorrow. It is the unique property and strength of randomization that it has the capacity to allocate not only known but also unknown confounders in an unbiased manner.

Methodologic standards for the design, conduct, and analysis of randomized trials continue to be refined (Chalmers et al., 1981; Department of Clinical Epidemiology and Biostatistics, McMaster University, 1981; Reisch et al.,

1989; Tyson et al., 1983). Several features of the design deserve emphasis:

1. There must be an a priori hypothesis, stated in quantitative terms, susceptible to disproof. This requires a predetermined sample size based on estimates of the hypothesized clinical effect of the new treatment, and the investigators' predetermined probabilities of missing a real treatment effect, and of incorrectly identifying the treatment as being effective. (The reader of a report of a randomized trial that did not find a statistically significant effect of treatment may well wonder whether the trial was large enough to have found a clinically significant difference [e.g., relative risk reduction of 25 or 50 per cent] if it had occurred. Such postfacto consideration of the results of completed trials is aided by tables prepared by Detsky and Sackett [1985].)

2. The allocation process should be truly random and impervious to code-breaking or tampering. (Quasi-random allocation procedures such as alternation and day of week are not preferred.)

3. When feasible, blinding of both physician and patient to the treatment allocation should be accomplished. (Among other advantages, this defends against co-intervention bias—the selective use of additional screening, diagnostic, or therapeutic procedures in one group more than in the other.)

4. Outcome measurements should be made by observers who are blinded to the treatment allocation.

5. All patients randomized must be accounted for in the primary analysis.

The methodologic criterion (item 5) that all patients randomized must be accounted for in the primary analysis has specific application in the case of *competing risks*. For example, the risk for neonatal death and that for chronic lung disease are competing risks; chronic lung disease cannot occur if the patient has died early. An intervention that is effective in reducing the incidence of neonatal death (e.g., mechanical ventilation) may also increase the incidence of chronic lung disease among survivors. An unbiased view of the effect of mechanical ventilation requires that outcomes be related to the number of patients exposed to the intervention—i.e., the number of patients with the event as a proportion of the number randomized in each arm of the trial. In the case of competing risks, outcomes expressed in this way can then be aggregated— e.g., *either* neonatal death *or* chronic lung disease—to obtain a global view of the effect of the intervention. Note that the incidence of chronic lung disease among survivors of mechanical ventilation, taken alone, would give a biased impression of the treatment effect if mechanical ventilation also caused an important difference in the neonatal death rate.

Of the above-mentioned criteria, the avoidance of bias in treatment allocation is arguably the most fundamental requirement. Chalmers and associates (1983) obtained empirical evidence of the importance of unbiased allocation by surveying 145 reports of controlled studies of the treatment of myocardial infarction. This group of papers included 57 in which the randomization process was blinded (i.e., neither the investigator nor the patient knew the treatment assignment until after the patient had been enrolled in the study and informed consent had been obtained), 45 in which the randomization process may

TABLE 3–2. Articles on Treatment or Prevention of Diseases of the Newborn, by Study Design

STUDY DESIGN	NUMBER OF ARTICLES	PER CENT
Randomized trials	57	(24)
Concurrent controls, nonrandomized	69	(29)
Historical controls, nonrandomized	24	(10)
No controls (case series or case reports)	84	(36)
Total	234	(100)

have been unblinded in that the patient could be selected or rejected for the study after the physician knew the treatment assignment, and 43 in which historical or nonrandomized concurrent controls were used. It was found that studies in which the assignment of controls was unblinded or nonrandom suffered from dissimilar distributions of prognostic variables (typically favoring the experimental group) and were also more likely to find a significant difference (again in favor of the experimental group). Treatment assignment in randomized trials should occur only after the patient has been accepted and formally enrolled in the study; then random assignment should be performed according to a prearranged scheme such as a telephone call to a statistical center, or consecutively arranged blinded medications or treatment instructions contained in opaque envelopes.

Table 3–2 indicates the relative frequency of use of different study designs in a recent survey of the literature on treatment or prevention of diseases of the newborn (Schmidt, et al., 1987). An increased use of randomized controlled trials is apparent in published reports of research. In neonatology, the use of randomized trials has increased to the point where they currently account for close to 25 per cent of published studies concerning treatment and prevention of diseases of the newborn (Kirpalani et al., 1989). A review of the 4434 abstracts submitted to the Society for Pediatric Research and American Pediatric Society annual meeting for the years 1988 and 1989 shows that 122 abstracts reported randomized trials of various aspects of management of the newborn, although the use of randomized trials was quite uneven across neonatal subspecialties. More than 5000 reports of randomized controlled trials in neonatology and perinatology have been registered to date in the Oxford Database of Perinatal Trials (Oxford Electronic Publishing).

EXAMPLE: EXPRESSING THE EFFECT OF TREATMENT, AND THE CONTROL OF BIAS

The outcome data of the Auckland trial (Liggins and Howie, 1972; Crowley, 1989) of antepartum glucocorticoid therapy to prevent RDS in premature infants are shown in Table 3–3. This was a randomized controlled trial of betamethasone therapy in mothers in whom premature delivery threatened or was planned before 37 weeks' gestation. The risk of RDS in the absence of betamethasone therapy is given by the RDS rate in the control group, $84/538 = 15.6$ per cent. The effect of treatment expressed as the relative risk is $49/532 \div 84/538 = 0.59$. This tells us that risk of RDS after glucocorticoid treatment is reduced to 59 per cent of the risk in the control group—i.e., a relative risk reduction of

41 per cent. Alternatively, the effect of treatment can be expressed as the risk difference, $49/532 - 84/538 = -0.064$. This tells us that the risk of RDS has been reduced, in absolute terms, by 6.4 per cent; the reciprocal $(1/0.064)$ indicates that approximately 16 patients need to be treated to prevent one case of RDS.

These estimates of treatment effect are likely to be unbiased, because

1. The investigators employed the strongest design for the control of selection bias, the randomized trial.

2. The allocation process was truly random and probably impervious to code-breaking or tampering (a pharmacist at arm's length from the trial controlled the randomization).

3. The active and control injections appeared to be identical so that neither the patient nor the health-care professionals knew the identity of the treatment.

4. The diagnosis of RDS was made using objective clinical and radiologic criteria; however, it is not certain whether assessors were blind to treatment allocation.

5. Virtually all randomized patients were included in the analysis.

The issue of competing risks would arise in this trial if glucocorticoid treatment also substantially affected the fetal death rates: RDS could not occur if the fetus were not born alive. This issue is resolved by computing both the fetal death rates and the RDS rates as a proportion of the number randomized in each arm of the trial. In this instance, there is no important difference in the incidence of stillbirth, and this competing risk, therefore, does not explain the reduction in incidence of RDS.

ESTIMATING PRECISION

Randomized trials are concerned with *estimation* (estimating the size of effect of treatment) as well as with *hypothesis-testing* (testing whether an effect is real or due to chance). Although a randomized trial offers the most powerful design for providing an unbiased estimate of the size of difference in outcomes of the treatment regimens being compared, the estimate can be imprecise.

The confidence interval (Bulpitt, 1987) displays the uncertainty in the study's estimate of the size of effect by presenting the upper and lower bounds for the anticipated true treatment difference. The 95 per cent confidence interval indicates that if the study were to be repeated 100 times, the true value would be included within the calculated confidence interval on 95 occasions.

The confidence interval tends to widen when the data are very variable, the sample size is small, or both. Thus,

TABLE 3–3. Effect of the Administration of Betamethasone Prior to Preterm Delivery on RDS and Stillbirth without Lethal Malformation

TREATMENT GROUP	n	RDS	STILLBIRTH
Betamethasone	532	49 (9.2 per cent)	31 (5.8 per cent)
Control	538	84 (15.6 per cent)	28 (5.2 per cent)
Relative risk		0.59	1.12
(95% CI)		(0.42, 0.82)	(0.68, 1.84)
Risk difference		−6.4	+0.6
(95 per cent CI)		(−10.3, −2.5)	(−2.1, +3.3)

CI = confidence interval.

imprecision in estimation is a particular problem in trials that enroll only small numbers of patients. As the number of patients increases, the confidence interval narrows.

The *clinical* significance of a true treatment effect depends on the size of treatment effect and on the complications and costs of treatment. Weighing these considerations is a matter of clinical judgement. The declaration of *statistical* significance, on the other hand, is a determination that a treatment effect is real—i.e., unlikely to be due to chance. A clinically significant difference may be suggested in a study whose sample size is too small to achieve statistical significance. Alternatively, a difference that is so small that it is of little or no clinical importance can be rendered statistically significant if the sample size is very large. In evaluating treatment recommendations, therefore, the clinician will be most impressed by the demonstration of treatment effects that are both clinically and statistically significant.

EXAMPLE: ESTIMATING PRECISION

Returning to the data shown in Table 3–3, we can ask "How precise is the estimate of treatment effect in this study?" Precision can be expressed by calculating the 95 per cent confidence interval around the "point estimate" for treatment effect. We calculated previously that the relative risk of RDS was reduced by betamethasone treatment to 0.59. The 95 per cent confidence interval attached to this estimate is 0.42 to 0.82. This interval would contain the true value for the effect of betamethasone treatment in 95 of 100 replications of this trial. Similarly, we calculated previously that the risk of RDS, in absolute terms, was reduced by 6.4 per cent; the confidence interval around this estimate is 2.5 to 10.3 per cent.

JUDGING APPLICABILITY

The applicability of the results of a trial depends on the appropriateness of generalizing the trial's conclusion to a particular clinical practice. This, in turn, depends on the physician's answers to the questions:

1. Were the study patients recognizably similar to his or her own?
2. Is the intervention feasible in practice?
3. Were all clinically relevant outcomes reported?

Underlying these specific questions is the more general issue of whether the trial is of the "management" or "explanatory" type (Sackett and Gent, 1987). The conceptual distinction is that a management trial determines the *effectiveness* of an intervention in actual clinical practice, whereas an explanatory trial determines the *efficacy* of an intervention under optimal or narrowly defined conditions. The primary analysis of a management trial, based on all patients randomized, takes into account such real-life problems as diagnostic errors that are appreciated only after treatment, patients with additional diseases or with outcomes not obviously caused by the treatment being studied, and patients who die early before treatment takes hold. The primary analysis of a management trial is sometimes described as an "intention-to-treat" analysis,

thus reflecting the clinical reality that a management decision to treat does not necessarily mean that the full course of treatment will be received as prescribed. Moreover, with some treatments, the patient may die before the treatment is given. For example, it may take several hours to prepare a granulocyte transfusion, leading to a significant delay in treatment. Such an important treatment effect can only be identified by counting all deaths in a study instead of only those occurring after treatment.

The limits of applicability of the results of a randomized trial are generally determined by the range of variation among entry characteristics and intervention policies as described in the index trial. The wider these limits, the wider the limits of applicability of the conclusions. It is not warranted, however, to extend the results beyond the limits tested in the trial. A famous example of inappropriate application in neonatal practice was the extrapolation of the restricted oxygen policy to all premature infants after the report in 1954 that oxygen restriction greatly reduced the incidence and severity of retrolental fibroplasia. The fact that all infants who entered the trial had to be at least 48 hours old was overlooked in making this recommendation. It was estimated subsequently (Cross, 1973) that 16 deaths (mainly from respiratory disorders in the first days of life) were caused for every case of retrolental fibroplasia prevented, even though the original trial demonstrated no mortality due to oxygen restriction. The extension of a study's results to a different patient population, therefore, should be done first under the auspices of a new randomized trial.

Even when a randomized trial exists that appears to be applicable to one's patient, there remains the issue that the conclusions from clinical research based on groups of patients do not necessarily apply to each individual patient. Indeed, in virtually all randomized trials that prove a therapy to be effective, there are some treated patients who do not benefit or are even harmed; conversely, in trials that generate a negative result, there are nevertheless some treated patients that appear to have benefited. These considerations have prompted the recent development of the strategy of randomized trials in individual patients— so-called N-of-1 trials—in which a single patient undergoes a series of pairs of treatments (one active and one placebo or alternative treatment per pair) with the order determined by random allocation (Guyatt et al., 1986). The results of such a trial apply without reservation to the patient who was the participant in the trial; however, the N-of-1 design does not provide information on how to treat other patients with the same disorder.

Applicability also depends on the range of outcomes that are evaluated in a trial of a new treatment. Although the investigator may assess only a single outcome, many interventions have the capacity to affect more than one outcome of clinical importance. Before a new therapy is adopted for widespread use, we need evidence concerning its effect on all the major outcomes it is likely to influence. This is an exceedingly difficult dictum to carry over into practice, since neither investigators nor clinicians are wise enough to know all the places they should look. Moreover, some effects are not expressed until considerable time has elapsed. Nevertheless, a few suggestions can be made:

1. Concerning choice of outcome, the reader should beware of what has been called the "substitution game,"

in which a risk factor (e.g., blood cholesterol level) is substituted for events of prime clinical importance (i.e., heart attack, stroke). This issue arises also when an intermediate outcome (e.g., alveolar-arterial oxygen ratio) is substituted for the more relevant clinical outcomes of death or major morbidity.

2. Although scientific rationale can provide a strong lead in determining "where to look" in assessing the effects of a new therapy, one should not easily dismiss apparent effects for which no scientific rationale presently exists. This is particularly true if the effect has been exposed in a well-designed and conducted randomized trial (e.g., the demonstration that sulfisoxazole causes an increase in the incidence of and death from kernicterus in premature infants) (Silverman et al., 1956).

3. Total mortality, as well as mortality from the specific disease under investigation, should be considered.

4. Long-term follow-up to determine late outcomes should be undertaken.

EXAMPLE: JUDGING APPLICABILITY

Do the data shown in Table 3–3 entirely justify the widespread use of antenatal glucocorticoid treatment of mothers who threaten to deliver prematurely? Liggins and Howie (1972) were careful, from the outset, to point to the need for further trials that would refine treatment indications and that would assess multiple outcomes including both early and late effects. Such trials have examined the effects of glucocorticoids by gestational age at treatment, by status of the membranes (whether intact or ruptured), and by presence or absence of maternal hypertension. The effect of glucocorticoids has been assessed in male and female fetuses. Trials have examined the effects on major neonatal problems such as infection, periventricular hemorrhage, and necrotizing enterocolitis. Effects on perinatal mortality (all causes) and on neurologic abnormality at follow-up have been assessed. Even length of stay in hospital and cost savings have been estimated. Thus, the clinician is now armed with a wide range of clinically important information concerning the indications for, and likely clinical effects of, antepartum glucocorticoid treatment.

WHY RESULTS OF RANDOMIZED CONTROLLED TRIALS MAY DIFFER

Does phenobarbital prevent intraventricular hemorrhage? Does vitamin E prevent bronchopulmonary dysplasia? The reader of the recent clinical literature may well be perplexed at the apparently conflicting answers that have been obtained in randomized trials.

In considering this issue, it is first necessary to be satisfied that the trials are addressing the same question— i.e., that they enroll comparable patients, test the same (or closely similar) intervention, and define and measure the same outcome. Having been satisfied that this is so, there are two commonly cited reasons why the results of randomized trials may differ (Horwitz, 1987):

1. There may be a failure to control bias in individual trials (systematic error).

2. There may be variation in the results of individual trials owing to chance, particularly in trials of small sample size (random error). If we consider a theoretical population of identical trials of an efficacious drug, having typically set power for avoiding the incorrect acceptance of the null hypothesis of no treatment effect at 80 per cent, then one in five trials incorrectly reports the drug as having no benefit. In fact, many trials have power closer to only 50 per cent (Freeman et al., 1978) and half of such trials miss a true treatment effect. Alternatively, in a population of trials of a drug that has no real efficacy, 1 in 20 (α = 0.05) incorrectly finds a significant treatment effect. Thus, to place the result of an apparently unbiased but small trial in context, the physician needs access to all the relevant (and unbiased) trials that have tested the same intervention.

META-ANALYSIS

A formal overview of a series of comparable trials of an intervention (sometimes termed a "meta-analysis" [Sacks et al., 1987]) seeks to obtain a summary estimate of the effect of that intervention on each outcome of interest. A valid overview requires that all clinically relevant trials be identified by predefined inclusion and exclusion criteria. There is some evidence of a publication bias favoring trials claiming so-called "positive" results (as compared with those claiming "no difference"); to ensure that a meta-analysis represents all trials to date, the method requires a search for unpublished as well as published trials. Next, the trials are examined for their methodologic quality; those whose methods fail to meet predefined criteria for methodologic quality are excluded. Then, and only then, the results of the included trials are tabulated, and a summary estimate of treatment effect is calculated. This summary effect (sometimes termed a "typical effect") is some form of weighted average across trials; the weights are inversely related to the variance in the estimate of treatment effect provided by each participating trial. The variance in any single trial is a function of the number of patients studied, the homogeneity of the patients on entry to the trial, the homogeneity of the response in untreated (control) patients, and the homogeneity of response in treated patients.

The results of a meta-analysis of randomized trials have several uses: (1) A meta-analysis provides increased statistical power, especially when individual trials are all relatively small; this increased power can resolve uncertainty arising from disagreement between individual trials as to whether a treatment effect is real or due to chance. (2) A meta-analysis provides increased precision in the estimate of effect size; this increased precision can be critical in weighing benefits of a treatment against clinical side effects, in choosing between alternative treatments when more than one has a true beneficial effect, and in quantitating the cost-effectiveness of the treatment. (3) A meta-analysis can also be useful in exploring the differences between studies in their results and in generating hypotheses (not posed at the start of individual trials) about the source of such differences. (4) A meta-analysis provides an existing structure for the incorporation of new evidence from comparable trials performed in the future.

TABLE 3–4. Effect of Glucocorticoid Prior to Preterm Delivery on RDS

STUDY	GLUCOCORTICOID		CONTROL		RELATIVE RISK	95% CI	RISK DIFFERENCE %	95% CI
	n	%	n	%				
(Liggins and Howie) 1972	49/532	(9.2)	84/538	(15.6)	0.59	(0.42, 0.82)	− 6.4	(−10.3, − 2.5)
(Block et al) 1977	5/69	(7.3)	12/61	(19.7)	0.37	(0.14, 0.99)	−12.4	(−24.1, − 0.7)
(Morrison et al) 1978	6/67	(9.0)	20/59	(33.9)	0.26	(0.11, 0.61)	−24.9	(−38.8, −11.1)
(Papageorgiou et al) 1979	7/71	(9.9)	23/75	(30.7)	0.32	(0.15, 0.70)	−20.8	(−33.3, − 8.3)
(Schutte et al) 1979	11/64	(17.2)	17/58	(29.3)	0.59	(0.30, 1.15)	−12.1	(−27.0, +2.8)
(Taeusch et al) 1979	7/56	(12.5)	14/71	(19.7)	0.63	(0.28, 1.46)	− 7.2	(−19.9, +5.5)
(Doran et al) 1980	4/81	(4.9)	10/63	(15.9)	0.31	(0.10, 0.95)	−10.9	(−21.1, − 0.8)
(Teramo et al) 1980	3/38	(7.9)	3/42	(7.1)	1.11	(0.24, 5.15)	+ 0.8	(−10.8, +12.3)
(Collaborative Group) 1981	42/371	(11.3)	59/372	(15.9)	0.71	(0.49, 1.03)	− 4.5	(− 9.5, +0.4)
(Schmidt et al) 1984	9/34	(26.5)	10/31	(32.3)	0.82	(0.39, 1.75)	− 5.8	(−27.9, +16.4)
(Morales et al) 1986	30/121	(24.8)	63/124	(50.8)	0.49	(0.34, 0.70)	−26.0	(−37.7, −14.3)
(Gamsu et al) 1989	7/131	(5.3)	16/137	(11.7)	0.46	(0.20, 1.08)	− 6.3	(−13.0, +0.3)
Typical effect					0.54	(0.46, 0.64)	− 8.1	(−10.4, −5.8)

*Typical effects calculated by Professor Bracken, Perinatal Epidemiology Unit, Yale University.

(Adapted from Crowley, P.: Promoting pulmonary maturity *In* Chalmers, I., Enkin, M., and Keirse, M. [Eds.]: Effective Care in Pregnancy and Childbirth. New York, Oxford University Press, 1989.)

EXAMPLE: META-ANALYSES OF ALL TRIALS OF GLUCOCORTICOID TREATMENT FOR PREVENTION OF RDS

Between 1972 and 1989, at least 12 randomized trials were reported, enrolling almost 3300 cases of threatened preterm delivery (Table 3–4). The summary or "typical" estimate of treatment effect based on all trials confirms the original finding of Liggins and Howie (1972) that glucocorticoid treatment reduces the incidence of RDS. Note that there is considerable variation between trials, both in the "point estimate" of treatment effect (due to the play of chance, and to variable success in control of bias) and in the width of the 95 per cent confidence intervals (due to differences in sample size). Note also, however, that despite such differences between the individual trials, the confidence interval around the "typical" estimate of treatment effect is narrower than for that of any single trial.

Similar meta-analyses have been conducted to assess the effect, across trials, of the typical effect of glucocorticoid treatment with respect to a range of maternal, fetal, and neonatal outcomes (Crowley, 1989). These overviews indicate that glucocorticoid treatment is effective in reducing the incidence of RDS in both male and female fetuses. Such treatment reduces the incidence of both periventricular hemorrhage and necrotizing enterocolitis. Overall, there is no effect on the incidence of fetal or neonatal infection, although there is a statistically nonsignificant trend of an increase in the rate of infection if a steroid is given after rupture of membranes. Most importantly, the overview shows that there is an important reduction in early neonatal deaths (all causes) and a trend (not quite significant) toward a decrease in the rate of neurologic abnormality at follow-up.

Overviews of randomized trials of perinatal interventions (such as that shown in Table 3–4) are included in The Oxford Database of Perinatal Trials and in two related publications: *Effective Care in Pregnancy and Childbirth*, edited by I. Chalmers, M., Enkin, 1989, and *Effective Care of the Newborn Infant*, Sinclair, J. C., and Bracken, M. B., eds., in preparation, Oxford University Press.

■ REFERENCES

Bulpitt, C. J.: Confidence intervals. Lancet 1:494–497, 1987.

Chalmers, T. C., Smith, H., Blackburn, B., et al.: A method for assessing the quality of a randomized controlled trial. Controlled Clin. Trials 2:31–49, 1981.

Chalmers, T. C., Celano, P., Sacks, H. S., and Smith, H.: Bias in treatment assignment in controlled clinical trials. N. Engl. J. Med. 309:1358–1361, 1983.

Cross, K. W.: Cost of preventing retrolental fibroplasia. Lancet 2:954–956, 1973.

Crowley, P.: Promoting pulmonary maturity. *In* Chalmers, I., Enkin, M., and Keirse, M. (Eds.): Effective Care in Pregnancy and Childbirth. New York, Oxford University Press, 1989, pp. 746–764.

Department of Clinical Epidemiology and Biostatistics, McMaster University Health Sciences Center: How to read clinical journals: V. To distinguish useful from useless or even harmful therapy. Can. Med. Assoc. J. 124:1156–1162, 1981.

Detsky, A. S., and Sackett, D. L.: When was a "negative" clinical trial big enough? How many patients you needed depends on what you found. Arch. Intern. Med. 145:709–712, 1985.

Freeman, J. A., Chalmers, T. C., Smith, H., and Kuebler, R. R.: The importance of beta, the type II error and sample size in the design and interpretation of the randomized control trial. N. Engl. J. Med. 299:690–694, 1978.

Guyatt, G., Sackett, D. L., Taylor, D. W., et al.: Determining optimal therapy—randomized trials in individual patients. N. Engl. J. Med. 314:889–892, 1986.

Horwitz, R. I.: Complexity and contradiction in clinical trial research. Am. J. Med. 82:498–510, 1987.

Kirpalani, H., Schmidt, B., McKibbon, K. A., et al.: Searching MEDLINE for randomized clinical trials involving care of the newborn. Pediatrics 83:543–546, 1989.

Liggins, G. L., and Howie, R. N.: A controlled trial of antepartum glucocorticoid treatment for prevention of the respiratory distress syndrome in premature infants. Pediatrics 50:515–525, 1972.

Lucas, A., Morley, R., and Cole, T. J.: Adverse neurodevelopmental outcome of moderate neonatal hypoglycemia. Br. Med. J. 297:1304–1308, 1988.

McKinlay, J. B.: From "promising report" to "standard procedure": Seven stages in the career of a medical innovation. Milbank Q. 59:374–411, 1981.

Reisch, J. S., Tyson, J. E., and Mize, S. G.: Aid to the evaluation of therapeutic studies. Pediatrics 84:815–827, 1989.

Sackett, D. L.: Bias in analytic research. J. Chron. Dis. 32:51–63, 1979.

Sackett, D. L., and Gent, M.: Controversy in counting and attributing events in clinical trials. N. Engl. J. Med. 316:450–455, 1987.

Sacks, H., Chalmers, T. C., and Smith, H.: Randomized versus historical controls for clinical trials. Am. J. Med. 72:233–240, 1982.

Sacks, H. S., Berrier, J., Reitman, D., et al.: Meta-analysis of randomized controlled trials. N. Engl. J. Med. 316:450–455, 1987.

Schmidt, B., Kirpalani, H., and Sinclair, J. C.: Unpublished observations, 1987.

Silverman, W. A., Andersen, D. H., Blanc, W. A., and Crozier, D. N.: A difference in mortality rate and incidence of kernicterus among premature infants allotted to two prophylactic antibacterial regimens. Pediatrics 18:614, 1956.

Shy, K. K., Larson, E. B., and Luthy, D. A.: Evaluating a new technology: The effectiveness of electronic fetal heart rate monitoring. Ann. Rev. Public Health 8:165–190, 1987.

Tugwell, P., Bennett, K. J., Sackett, D. L., and Haynes, R. B.: The measurement iterative loop: A framework for the critical appraisal of need, benefits and costs of health interventions. J. Chron. Dis. 38:339–351, 1985.

Tyson, J. E., Furzan, J. A., Reisch, J. S., and Mize, S. G.: An evaluation of the quality of therapeutic studies in perinatal medicine. J. Pediatr. 102:10–13, 1983.

PART II

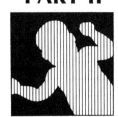

MAJOR INFLUENCES ON FETAL GROWTH AND DEVELOPMENT

GENERAL STRATEGIES OF FETAL DEVELOPMENT

4

Helen Liley and Merton Bernfield

The sequence of human development can be viewed as a progression of successive stages. These stages involve the generation of cells that organize and specialize, yielding tissues that show new functional properties and structural complexities. Development is a cellular process, in which various factors orchestrate the behavior of single cells so that they become the functional tissues that make up organs. The development from zygote to neonate is the change from independent cells to tissues and organs that are assemblies of cells that function in concert. As organs emerge, they become increasingly interdependent for normal function. This chapter attempts to show how developmental biology, which addresses the control of cells, merges with classical embryology, which considers the assembly of cells into organs.

■ THE FIVE MILESTONES OF HUMAN EMBRYOGENESIS

Human development begins with the formation of the gametes and consists of five stages (Fig. 4–1). These are (1) fertilization, the formation of the fertilized zygote by union of the egg and sperm; (2) cleavage, the rapid set of cell divisions initiated by the fusion of egg and sperm; (3) implantation, the invasion of the embryo into maternal tissue; (4) gastrulation, the movement of cells that creates the basic body plan; and (5) organogenesis, the relatively lengthy process of formation of individual organs. This progression occurs early in human development. Organogenesis, the final stage, begins in the 3rd week after

fertilization. Growth of the embryo ensues, achieved largely by increasing the number of cells and by deposition of extracellular materials.

Gametogenesis produces highly specialized male and female gametes that have undergone meiosis and thus contain a haploid number of chromosomes. The general schemes by which egg and sperm form are similar; the major differences are the duration of meiosis and the amount of cytoplasm. During meiosis, the genome of the gamete precursor cell undergoes extensive recombination as a result of crossing-over between homologous chromosomes in the first meiotic division. The genotype of each gamete is further varied because the chromosomal homologues sort independently of each other at the end of the first division. These processes cause the genetic complement of each human gamete to be unique. DNA present in the mitochondria of the egg, the source of mitochondria in the zygote, provides another source of genetic diversity because each zygote inherits mitochondrial DNA only from its mother.

The gametes are highly differentiated cells. The sperm head contains condensed DNA and is topped by the acrosome, a membrane-bound structure containing enzymes used to penetrate the ovum. The neck contains numerous mitochondria to provide energy for the motion generated by the flagellum tail. Unlike the sperm, the egg is large; in fact, it is the largest human cell. Eggs contain stores of RNA and ribosomes that enable protein synthesis to start rapidly following fertilization. Egg differentiation includes the production of a covering layer, the zona pellucida, that protects the egg, if fertilized, during its passage through the fallopian tube.

FERTILIZATION

Fertilization restores the diploid number of chromosomes, determines sex, and initiates the developmental sequence. Fertilization of the egg occurs in the fallopian tube near the ovary by fusion of a recently ovulated egg with a sperm that has undergone capacitation induced by uterine fluids. Capacitation involves changes in the membrane covering the acrosome, allowing release of hydrolytic enzymes that enable the sperm to penetrate the zona pellucida. The sperm head attaches to the surface of the egg and their plasma membranes fuse. The egg reacts to this contact with depolarization of its plasma membrane and polymerization of the zona pellucida, changes that prevent the entry of other sperm. The fertilized egg completes meiosis, a process which began during the fetal life of its mother. Once in the egg cytoplasm, the nucleus of the sperm enlarges. The male and female haploid nuclei fuse and their chromosomes intermingle, forming the zygote or fertilized egg.

CLEAVAGE

The zygote undergoes rapid cell divisions or cleavages to form a ball of cells, the morula, which then develops an internal cavity, the blastocyst. The first division of the zygote occurs about 30 hours after fertilization and repeated cleavages produce smaller cells, called blastomeres. The absence of cell growth between these divisions distinguishes them from most cell divisions at later stages. The divisions occur as the zygote, still surrounded by the zona pellucida, is transported along the fallopian tube toward the uterus. About 3 days after fertilization, the morula, now a solid ball of 16 to 32 cells, enters the uterine cavity. On the 4th day, a fluid-filled cavity develops within the morula, creating the blastocyst. Meanwhile, the internal cells divide at a greater rate than the outer cells so that the blastocyst consists of two distinct cell populations, an outer trophoblast and an inner cell mass. The trophoblast cells will form the extraembryonic structures, the amnion and the chorion. The cells of the inner cell mass will produce the embryo and the yolk sac, which later contributes chorionic mesoderm to the trophoblast. Because of this contribution, chorionic villous sampling

can allow the biopsy of cells derived both from the trophoblast shell and from the inner cell mass.

Development to this point can occur without maternal influence after in vitro fertilization, and results in the pre-embryo. The term pre-embryo was recently coined to refer to the multicellular organism before it implants.

IMPLANTATION

The blastocyst begins to implant into the endometrial lining of the uterus, thus initiating the formation of the placenta. On about the 5th day, the zona pellucida degenerates, exposing an adhesive region on the trophoblast cells overlying the inner cell mass. This region adheres to endometrial cells that have been prepared by steroid hormone stimulation of the ovarian cycle. At about the 7th day, implantation begins as the trophoblast cells invade between the uterine lining cells. Thus, by the end of the 1st week, the blastocyst is superficially implanted within the uterus, but it does not have functional connections with the mother. The trophoblast then differentiates into two layers—the syncytiotrophoblast, an outer layer lacking cell boundaries, and the cytotrophoblast, an inner, cellular layer. As the syncytiotrophoblast continues to invade, it produces chorionic gonadotropin that converts the corpus luteum in the ovary into the corpus luteum of pregnancy. Steroid hormones produced by the corpus luteum then maintain the lining of the uterus to support subsequent development of the embryo.

During the 2nd week of human development, the trophoblast cells further differentiate and begin to form the placenta and the extraembryonic membranes including the amniotic sac. The embryo will subsequently grow into the cavity formed by the amniotic sac. The amniotic sac enlarges and obliterates the chorionic cavity that is formed by the surrounding chorion, another derivative of the trophoblast. Implantation is normally completed by the end of the 2nd week.

GASTRULATION

Gastrulation begins at about the 15th day, coincident with the first missed menstrual period. During the formation of the extraembryonic membranes, the inner cell mass flattens to form two epithelial sheets, the embryonic endoderm and ectoderm, that lie between the primary yolk sac and the amniotic cavity. The events of gastrulation convert these two flat circular layers of the embryonic disc into a three-dimensional organism and create a basic body plan. This plan has three axes, anterior-posterior, dorsal-ventral, and left-right. During gastrulation, the embryo forms three distinct germ layers: the ectoderm, the mesoderm, and the endoderm.

Gastrulation begins at a midline groove, the primitive streak. This groove forms in the embryonic ectoderm near the posterior end of the embryonic disc. A population of embryonic ectoderm cells migrates into this groove and begins to fill the potential space between the cell sheets of embryonic ectoderm and endoderm. These cells, which migrate anteriorly and laterally, form the embryonic mesoderm or mesenchyme. A cord of these cells coalesces anterior to the primitive streak to form the midline notochord that lengthens, causing the embryonic disc to be-

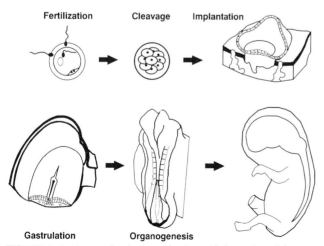

FIGURE 4–1. *Human development begins with formation of the gametes and consists of five stages (see text).*

come elongated. By the end of the 3rd week, when gastrulation is completed, the embryo has three layers and has each of the three body axes.

ORGANOGENESIS

Cells form specific tissues and organs by differentiation, the acquisition of specialized cell structure and function, and morphogenesis, change in shape and location. The ectoderm, the first layer to undergo organogenesis, begins to form the central nervous system on the 18th day of gestation. The ectoderm will form the brain, its accessory organs, the adrenal medulla, and the melanocytes. It also forms the epidermis and its derivatives, the sweat and mammary glands. Neurulation, the initial step in formation of the central nervous system, occurs by thickening and folding of the ectoderm in the dorsal midline to form the neural tube, a continuous canal running from the head to the tail end of the embryo. Because the neural tube grows at a greater rate than the rest of the embryo, the relatively flat embryonic disc takes on increasing convexity, so that the originally dorsal ectoderm ultimately almost surrounds the embryo.

The originally ventral endoderm becomes enveloped by the other two germ layers and folds to form a tube that later becomes the gut epithelium and its derivatives. These derivatives, which include the liver, pancreas, salivary glands, and lungs, form as outgrowths from the tube. By the 30th day, the embryo has become rounded and elongated, and the organ anlagen are nearly in their final positions relative to one another.

The mesoderm organizes into specialized regions, the major ones being in the center of the embryo between the base of the head and the tail. The mesoderm consists of loose connective tissue, the mesenchymal cells. In some places, these cells interact with epithelia of ectodermal and endodermal origin to form various organs. The somite (or paraxial) mesoderm is adjacent to the notochord. It condenses into segments or somites, each of which soon splits into three parts. These are the dermatome, which forms the dermis; the myotome, which forms the muscles of the limbs and trunk; and the sclerotome, which forms the skeleton of the vertebral column.

Lateral to the somites is the intermediate (or nephrogenic) mesoderm, which will form the urogenital system and its associated glands. Lateral to the intermediate mesoderm is the lateral plate mesoderm, which will form the serous linings, the lymphatic and blood vascular systems, and the bone marrow. In response to cues from surface ectoderm, this mesoderm will form the bones and cartilage of the limbs.

Although organogenesis begins during the 3rd week, it is a lengthy process and the different organs develop at different rates. The earliest organ system to become functional is the cardiovascular system, which begins early in the 4th week of development to bring nutrients and oxygen from the uterine lining to the developing embryo. The last organ system to begin to develop is the urogenital system. The development of particular organs is described in standard textbooks of human embryology, a few of which are listed in the references.

By term, most organs have achieved their adult shape but almost none have achieved their adult histoarchitec-ture. The growth and development of most organs is not complete until the end of adolescence. However, maturation of several organs is accelerated around the time of birth to enable the fetus to accommodate to extrauterine life. These developmental changes are induced at different times and rates and by a variety of stimuli. For example, before birth various stimuli, including increased levels of cortisol, increase surfactant production in the lung. At birth, changes in afterload caused by absence of the placenta, dilation of the pulmonary vasculature, and closure of the ductus arteriosus induce changes in the molecular and cellular structure of the heart. After birth, as the infant is exposed to new antigens, and as maternally derived immunoglobulins decline, B-cell production of immunoglobulins gradually increases.

■ DEVELOPMENTAL BIOLOGY AND THE PROCESSES INVOLVED IN EMBRYOGENESIS

To develop functioning tissues and organs, cells must control their own fate and direct the behavior of other cells. Developmental biology is the study of how cells accomplish these ends.

GENES CONTROL DEVELOPMENT

The blueprint for development is encoded in DNA, which is present in all nucleated cells in the body. With rare exceptions, such as in B cells where immunoglobulin genes undergo rearrangement, each diploid cell contains identical DNA sequences. However, each cell type expresses only about 1% of its genes. The programming of each cell type to acquire distinct patterns of gene expression is one of the processes needed for the formation of functioning tissues and organs.

CELLS COMMIT TO DISTINCT DEVELOPMENTAL FATES

The zygote and its early daughter cells are capable of giving rise to any type of cell in the body. These totipotent cells give rise to lineages of progressively more specialized cells (Fig. 4–2). The cells that begin the formation of organs have a less extensive repertoire but can still develop into multiple different cell types. For example, as the lung starts to develop, epithelial cells bud from the foregut endoderm. They eventually form the wide range of specialized epithelial cells found in the airways and acini. The cells of the splanchnic mesoderm, into which the bud grows, will become fibroblasts, smooth muscle cells, and chondrocytes. The processes by which cells become specialized are known as determination and differentiation.

Determination, or commitment, is the process of gradual reduction of developmental options that eventually renders the cells capable of becoming only a single cell type. The cells become committed to a particular type of differentiation. These changes in the developmental potential of cells are heritable by daughter cells and are irreversible. Although determination is induced by factors in the environment of cells, changes in the environment can induce new determination events but cannot reverse

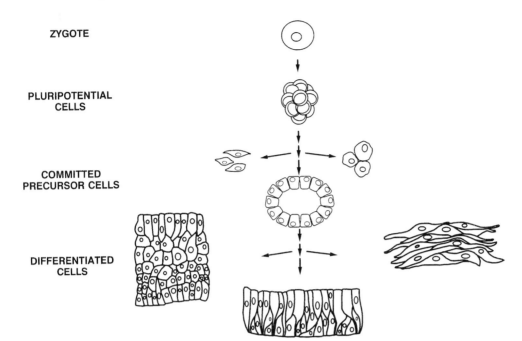

ZYGOTE

PLURIPOTENTIAL
CELLS

COMMITTED
PRECURSOR CELLS

DIFFERENTIATED
CELLS

FIGURE 4–2. The zygote and its early daughter cells can give rise to any type of cell in the body. The potential developmental fates of later generations of cells becomes restricted by the stepwise process of determination. Eventually, determination renders cells capable of becoming only a single cell type. Concurrently, through the process of differentiation, cells acquire individual phenotypes that enable them to fulfill specialized functions.

existing ones. Determination does not result from a loss of DNA but from stable changes in how and when genes are expressed. Importantly, a cell becomes determined before one can recognize changes in phenotype. Thus, one cannot establish when a cell has become committed until after the commitment has occurred.

CELLS BECOME SPECIALIZED IN FORM AND FUNCTION

In contrast to determination, which narrows developmental options, differentiation is the acquisition of characteristics that enable cells to fulfill specialized functions. For example, neural crest cells eventually differentiate into cells with a wide variety of specialized functions, including conduction and transmission of signals, mechanical support, nutrition of other cells, and hormone production.

The expression of differentiated characteristics is influenced by a cell's hormonal milieu and physical environment. For example, if cells are dissociated and grown in culture dishes, they rarely perform their full range of specialized functions exactly as they did in vivo. However, these changes in environment do not reverse a cell's commitment. A pancreatic islet cell cannot be made into a thyroid epithelial cell or vice versa.

Determination and differentiation occur in a series of overlapping steps. Indeed, cells frequently have some differentiated characteristics even though they have not yet undergone their final determination. For example, cells from embryonic bone have characteristics that distinguish them as osteogenic cells, yet they are able to develop into osteoblasts, osteoclasts, and osteocytes. They also give rise to a population of stem cells, the osteoprogenitor cells. Stem cells differ from embryonic cells in that they persist into adult life and have extensive capacity for self-renewal, but they give rise to at least one and often several types of differentiated progeny.

ACQUISITION OF SPECIALIZED FUNCTION AND THE GENERATION OF UNIQUE FORMS

The development of functioning organs requires not only that cells acquire specialized roles but that they

arrange themselves correctly. A type I pneumocyte cannot perform its most important function, gas exchange, unless it is organized properly with respect to its adjacent cells, including type II pneumocytes to provide surfactant, capillary endothelial cells to conduct blood, and fibroblasts to produce scaffolding. To form functioning organs, the behavior of populations of cells must be coordinated. Thus the genome of cells not only contains information needed for a variety of specialized functions but also for the plan that will orchestrate the formation of organs and the whole organism. The origins of this plan may reside in a number of genes that act as switches (Blau, 1988).

When activated, these genes permit or inhibit the expression of other genes that alter the expression of yet more genes. Thus, these genes may form a regulatory hierarchy in which activation of "master" genes turns on entire developmental sequences. Such genes may also repress developmental sequences, but evidence for this is not as clear. The number of master genes required to regulate development is not known. A small number of genes, probably fewer than the number of differentiated cell types, likely acts in various sequences and combinations to control the many steps of determination and differentiation.

Some of the genes regulating development in organisms with short life cycles, such as the fruit fly, *Drosophila melanogaster,* have been identified. Genes that may regulate some of the early processes of mammalian development have been identified because they share sequences with the *Drosophila melanogaster* genes (Dressler and Gruss, 1988; Gehring, 1987). The functions of most of these genes in mammals are still unknown, but their temporal and spatial patterns of expression suggest that, like their insect counterparts, they control formation of tissue patterns and organs. Examples of the genes that control development in *Drosophila melanogaster* include genes of the homeo box family that code for proteins controlling the identity of body segments, genes of the paired box family that code for proteins controlling segmentation, and genes for proteins with multiple "zinc-finger" DNA-binding motifs that may control cell determination. Putative genes involved in regulating development have also been identified and their roles explored in mammals by gene transfer (Gossler et al., 1989). For example, candidate genes from committed, though as yet undifferentiated, cells have been introduced into uncommitted recipient cells so that the effects of the genes on cell lineage could be explored.

CELL SPECIALIZATION AND SELECTIVE GENE ACTIVATION

Products of regulatory genes act at many levels to control the expression of many hundreds of other genes at precise times during development. Sites of regulation include the synthesis, processing, and degradation of numerous RNA and protein molecules. This large repertoire of mechanisms is used both to control where genes are transcribed and to diversify their products.

DNA Structure. RNA synthesis is regulated by factors that change the conformation (or shape) of DNA. These include nuclear proteins that control DNA-folding, specific chemical modifications of DNA, short DNA sequences in or near genes themselves (so-called *cis*-acting factors), and proteins that interact with DNA sequences to increase or decrease transcription (so-called *trans*-acting factors). The products of genes can also control protein synthesis by affecting RNA processing, messenger RNA stability and transport, and transfer RNA availability. In addition, various modifications of proteins can alter their location, activity, and rate of degradation. Each of these post-translational modifications can affect the cell's phenotype.

DNA Conformation. DNA is a linear polymer, but it exists in cells as a double helical strand that is highly and precisely contorted. Slight differences in its folding appear to profoundly affect gene expression. Some of the folding is controlled by histones, which are small, highly basic proteins that bind tightly to the negatively charged DNA. Histone-DNA complexes, in which DNA strands are looped at regular intervals around several histone molecules, form chromatin. Chromatin is contorted into higher order filamentous structures, also by interactions with histone proteins. A third level of DNA conformation is heterochromatin, a highly condensed form of DNA. One of the X chromosomes in each mammalian female cell is almost entirely heterochromatin. Other chromosomes, although not entirely condensed, can also develop lengthy regions of heterochromatin.

These methods of progressively increasing the order of DNA folding produce stable decreases in the likelihood of gene transcription. The folding must be undone to allow DNA replication, but the patterns of folding can be passed on to many generations of daughter cells. Little is known about how these patterns are maintained and inherited.

Chemical Modification of DNA. Physiologic methylation of certain DNA bases, the cytidines, also affects the local conformation of segments of DNA (Cedar, 1988). Methylation alters the binding of regulatory factors, histones, and other proteins. So-called housekeeping genes, which are expressed in nearly all cells, are predominantly unmethylated. In contrast, tissue-specific genes are typically almost fully methylated during early development in germ line and somatic cells, but they become unmethy-

lated in those cells that can express them. Moreover, daughter cells inherit specific methylation patterns. The factors responsible for site-specific changes in methylation are unknown. Furthermore, because methylation of DNA does not occur in some eukaryotic organisms, there must be other mechanisms for selecting genes for transcription.

Protein Interactions with DNA: **Cis-** and **Trans-Acting Factors.** So-called *trans*-acting factors are proteins that transiently interact with DNA to activate or suppress transcription. They appear to change the local conformation of DNA and thus alter the binding of RNA synthetic enzymes. *Trans*-acting proteins bind to specific DNA sequences, designated as *cis* elements. *Cis* elements are promoters, which by definition, include the site where transcription is initiated, and enhancers, which are more distant from the gene and can act on more than one gene. DNA-folding may bring *cis* elements together to allow protein-binding, enabling distant elements to interact (Dynan, 1989; Schüle et al., 1988).

Some genes have multiple promoters, each used in different tissues or at different times (Schibler and Sierra, 1989). The alternative promoters can be affected distinctly by *trans*-acting factors to vary the rate of transcription, and their transcripts can have differing rates of degradation or translation, leading to diverse expression of the same gene. Less commonly, use of an alternative promoter changes the translation initiation codon, and, therefore, the primary structure of the protein.

Other DNA sequences can also produce tissue- or development-specific variations of a protein. For example, short sequences determine where messenger RNA molecules can be spliced, thus determining which sections of the transcript are removed (Breitbart et al., 1987). Alternative splicing and alternative promoters are mechanisms whereby a wide variety of myosin and troponin isoforms are produced from a limited number of genes. These different isoforms are expressed in different sites and at different times in development to vary the functional properties of cardiac and skeletal muscles.

Certain other sequences in genes can render their transcripts susceptible, in certain circumstances, to degradation (Klausner and Harford, 1989). For example, a sequence in transferrin transcripts causes them to be less stable when the cells expressing them are exposed to iron.

Various proteins produced or activated in response to extracellular signals can serve as *trans*-acting factors. Examples of *trans*-acting factors include steroid hormone receptors. Hormone-binding causes these receptors to interact with regulatory elements common to many inducible genes.

There are probably only a limited number of *trans*-acting factors, and their effects are also regulated. For example, modifications of the DNA, *cis* elements, and cooperative binding of different *trans*-acting factors can permit, amplify, reduce, or negate the effects of transcriptional activation.

GENERATION OF TISSUE AND ORGAN FORMS

The generation of tissue and organ forms requires coordination of multiple gene products. Although genes control expression of specific proteins, and can act as switches to begin formation of tissue patterns, such as segments and limbs, how they dictate these patterns is not known. Establishment of patterns requires interaction between cells. Morphogenesis, the process whereby cells organize into correct arrangements to form functional organs, involves the basic mechanisms whereby cells control and are controlled by the behavior of their neighbors. Although there is enormous diversity in the structure and function of organs, cells regulate multiple gene products to produce a limited repertoire of behaviors that control all of morphogenesis.

The Cellular Behaviors of Morphogenesis. In order to form organs, cells must adhere, change in shape, and change in number. These behaviors are coordinated and propagated by the insoluble extracellular matrix and the diffusible peptide growth factors.

Cell Adhesion. Embryonic tissues can be dissociated into suspensions of single cells that, under certain circumstances, can reassemble and reform structures resembling the original tissue. This property depends on the ability of cells to adhere to and to recognize one another.

Cell adhesion and recognition behaviors are vital to the establishment of tissue boundaries, the migration of cells along specific pathways, and the relative placement of cells. Cell adhesion and cell recognition are accomplished by cell adhesion molecules. Subsequently, specialized cell junctions arise that maintain and stabilize the adhesions and allow intercellular communication.

Cell Adhesion Molecules. A variety of cell adhesion molecules have been identified, and have been characterized to varying degrees (Edelman, 1986; Ekblom, 1986; Takeichi, 1988). All have extracellular domains that interact with other cell adhesion molecules, and intracellular domains that interact with the cytoskeleton. The molecules can be grouped based on whether or not they require calcium ions to mediate adhesion and whether the molecule they bind to on adjacent cells is identical (homophilic) or nonidentical (heterophilic). Examples include E-cadherin (also known as uvomorulin or ECAM [epithelial cell adhesion molecule]), a calcium-dependent cell adhesion molecule that is found initially on blastomeric cells and cells of the inner cell mass. Its distribution changes during development and ultimately it is confined to epithelial cells, where it forms part of the junctional complex between cells. Another example is N-cadherin (NCAM) (originally neural cell adhesion molecule). Binding with NCAM is calcium independent. It is found on endoderm, mesoderm, and ectoderm of the early embryo, but it is later confined to neural cells, smooth muscle, and motor end-plates.

Each cell adhesion molecule has a specific tissue and developmental distribution. The expression of cell adhesion molecules is regulated in ways that are important in morphogenesis. For example, the density, distribution, and number relative to other cell adhesion molecules can all be regulated. In addition, in some cases the extracellular domains of cell adhesion molecules may be altered by post-translational modifications and their cytoplasmic domains can be varied by differential splicing of messenger RNAs. These changes can lead to altered binding with other cell adhesion molecules and altered interactions with the cytoskeleton (Cunningham et al., 1987).

Cell Junctions. Once simple epithelial cells form a sheet or tube, they become connected at their lateral borders by a junctional complex that encircles the apex of each cell. It has several components. The tight junction, or zonula occludens, the most apical part of the complex, appears earliest in development and acts to polarize the epithelium. Tight junctions act as a fence to limit the diffusion of membrane constituents between the apical and lateral membranes and to selectively regulate the passage of ions between cells. The extent of this gating function varies widely between epithelia.

The intermediate junction (zonula adherens) also encircles the cell within the junctional complex and connects to the actin network in the cell (see the section, Change in Cell Shape).

Spot desmosomes (macula adherens) appear to act as rivets between lateral cell membranes. These junctions also consist of a membrane domain and a cytoplasmic plaque that is anchored to the structural cytokeratin network within the cell.

Gap junctions provide passageways connecting adjacent cells. They are assembled from subunits of hydrophobic proteins to form channels within the plasma membrane that admit various ions and molecules with a molecular mass of less than 500 daltons. The intercellular transfer of these small molecules may regulate and coordinate the differentiation of certain cell types.

Change in Cell Shape. When a cell differentiates, it acquires a specific shape that is one of its differentiated characteristics. Cell shape results, in part, from a cytoplasmic framework, the cytoskeleton. This framework is composed of polymers of fibril-forming proteins and various accessory proteins organized together into microfilaments, intermediate filaments, and microtubules (Table 4–1). The accessory proteins affect filament assembly or link the filaments to one another or to other cell components. The cytoskeleton is not a permanent structure but changes rapidly in response to cellular events. In addition to its role in cell shape, the cytoskeleton (1) interacts extensively with cell membranes and regulates the mobility of integral proteins within the membrane; (2) organizes the cytoplasm by binding various organelles; (3) forms specialized regions of cells, such as microvilli; and (4) contributes to secretory mechanisms.

The other influences on cell shape are various external factors, which include cell–cell and cell–matrix adhesion. These adhesions are transduced by a variety of transmembrane signaling systems. Changes in shape are generally initiated by changes in linkages between membrane proteins and the microfilament network and are maintained by microfilaments and microtubules.

Cell culture evidence suggests that specific cell shape is needed to maintain differentiated cell function. The details of how cell shape exerts these effects are not known but may include traction of cytoskeletal components on the nucleus and organelles, and activation of various second messenger systems.

Cell shape has other important effects during morphogenesis. Cells can move when they change shape. If the cells are linked together, as in an epithelial sheet, then a change in cell shape results in a change in the form of the entire sheet. If the cells are not linked, then a change in their shape can begin a locomotory sequence, in which

TABLE 4–1. Major Classes of Cytoskeletal Components

	COMPOSITION	FUNCTIONS
Microfilaments	Actin and diverse group of actin-binding proteins	Contractile systems necessary to generate tension and for cell extension movement and division Mechanical support for cell structures and extensions by lamellipodia, microvilli Interactions with cell adhesion molecules, extracellular matrix receptors
Microtubules	Alpha and beta tubulins	Strength and motility of cilia and flagella Anchorage of nucleus Formation of mitototic spindle
Intermediate filaments	Vimentin, desmin, cytokeratins, and others (characteristic of cell type)	Tension bearing

coordinated adhesion of the leading edge to the substratum and change in cell shape together result in cell migration.

Change in Cell Number. Localized differences in rates of proliferation change the shape of developing organs. Higher rates of mitosis of some groups of cells relative to others initiate the formation of many organs and lead to the development of specialized forms, such as branches and lobes. Both the rate of mitosis and the plane of cleavage, which determines the position of the daughter cells relative to one another, are important. Also, mitosis can yield two identical progeny or be asymmetrical, yielding two different daughter cells (O'Farrell et al., 1989).

The local control of proliferation of cells is complex. It is mediated partly by peptide growth factors and growth inhibitory factors and partly by changes in the extracellular matrix. The molecular mechanisms whereby these local environmental influences affect cell proliferation are also not well understood. Two families of intracellular proteins, the H_1 kinases and the cyclins, appear to interact to control the transition of all eukaryotic cells into and out of mitosis. How the local regulatory factors that affect the proliferation of cells influence these and other proteins awaits discovery (Murray and Kirschner, 1989).

Cell death at specific localized sites is a normal event in morphogenesis, illustrated in the interdigital areas of the limb buds, where the death of cells allows separation of the digits. In the developing central and peripheral nervous system, cell death is a ubiquitous phenomenon. Survival or death of a neuron appears to be determined by events in its projection field. Another example of localized cell death is the death of the intimal cell layer of the ductus arteriosus when it closes after birth. Cell death in this case may be secondary to failure of nutrition due to cessation of blood flow through the vessel. Cell death had also been presumed to cause loss of epithelia at several sites during organogenesis. However, loss of some of these epithelia is now thought to result from the conversion of epithelium to mesenchymal cells, e.g., the medial palatine epithelium at the time of palatal fusion.

The Extracellular Coordinating Molecules. Morphogenesis is wholly dependent on the molecules that organize the behavior of individual cells into morphologically and functionally defined groups. Two classes of molecules can serve this function—the extracellular matrix components and the peptide growth factors. These molecules are the predominant influences on the differentiation, proliferation, shape, and migration of cells. The extracellular matrix components are large, multidomain molecules that are extensively cross-linked to each other, predominantly by noncovalent bonds, to form an insoluble matrix that spans multiple cells. The growth factors are small, soluble peptides that can diffuse locally to affect groups of cells.

Thus, extracellular matrix composites and peptide growth factors differ in fundamental ways, yet they share biologic effects. They both act (1) locally, influencing a particular population of cells; (2) via autocrine or paracrine mechanisms, influencing their tissue of origin or adjacent tissues; and (3) at the cell surface, by binding receptors. The insoluble matrix can modulate the effect of the otherwise diffusible growth factors. The matrix binds some growth factor peptides, and thus can partition their effects, protect them from degradation, or serve as a reservoir for growth factors.

Extracellular Matrix Components. All cells undergoing morphogenesis produce and deposit an insoluble mesh, the extracellular matrix, beyond their cell membranes. Each cell type produces a specific type of matrix. For example, parenchymal cells produce a basal lamina, and mesenchymal cells produce an interstitial matrix (Fig. 4–3). The major components of each matrix are the structural proteins, which include the collagens and elastin, the adhesive glycoproteins, and the proteoglycans. However, the exact composition and organization of matrices vary from tissue to tissue and change during development (McDonald, 1988).

The Collagens. The collagens provide resiliency to all matrices. There are at least 12 genetically distinct forms of collagen, each sharing a characteristic triple helix, and most are formed by assembly of nonidentical subunits transcribed from several genes. These heterotrimers are generally polymerized into macroscopic fibrils. Some collagen types (e.g., Type IV, the predominant collagen in basal laminae) do not form fibrils but produce a chicken wire–like mesh. Collagen fibrils have great tensile strength because of intermolecular cross-linking of the molecules.

Elastin. Elastin is a constituent of the matrix in organs like the lung, skin, and aorta in which considerable elasticity is required. Elastin is composed of a single type of hydrophobic polypeptide that forms random coils. These are highly cross-linked to produce multimers that can both stretch and recoil.

Adhesive Glycoproteins. These large proteins contain multiple distinct polypeptide domains that bind tightly to various other matrix molecules and to specific cell surface receptors. The most abundant types, laminin, found pre-

MAJOR EXTRACELLULAR MATRIX COMPONENTS

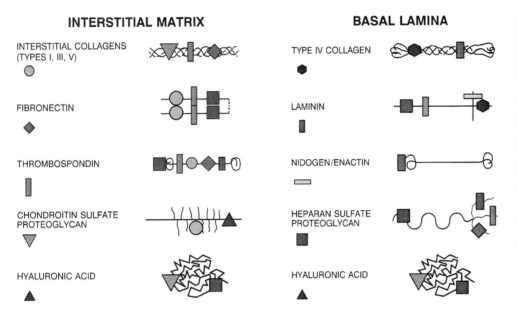

INTERSTITIAL MATRIX

INTERSTITIAL COLLAGENS
(TYPES I, III, V)

FIBRONECTIN

THROMBOSPONDIN

CHONDROITIN SULFATE
PROTEOGLYCAN

HYALURONIC ACID

BASAL LAMINA

TYPE IV COLLAGEN

LAMININ

NIDOGEN/ENACTIN

HEPARAN SULFATE
PROTEOGLYCAN

HYALURONIC ACID

FIGURE 4–3. *Mesenchymal cells produce an interstitial matrix, and parenchymal cells produce a basal lamina. Both of these extracellular matrix types contain collagens, adhesive glycoproteins (such as fibronectin, thrombospondin, laminin, and nidogen), and glycosaminoglycan-containing molecules (the proteoglycans and hyaluronic acid). The interstitial matrix and the basal lamina each contain characteristic molecular species of these large, extensively cross-linked, insoluble components. Major matrix components are shown. The symbols represent each component, and molecular interactions are indicated. For example, the interstitial collagens bind chondroitin sulfate proteoglycan, thrombospondin, and fibronectin.*

dominantly in the basal lamina, and fibronectin, located in the interstitial matrix, typify matrix adhesive glycoproteins. Each contains specific amino acid sequences that are recognized by cell surface receptors, notably arg-gly-asp in fibronectin and tyr-ile-gly-ser-arg in laminin, and the heparin-binding regions of both fibronectin and laminin.

Proteoglycans. Surrounding and bound to the protein components of the matrix are proteoglycans and hyaluronate. Proteoglycans consist of glycosaminoglycan chains covalently linked to a core protein. Hyaluronate is a large linear glycosaminoglycan. These polysaccharides are composed of alternating hexuronate and *N*-acetyl hexosamine residues. The glycosaminoglycans can bind many large and small molecules, including water, and can occupy a huge volume for their mass, thus allowing diffusion of nutrients, metabolites, and hormones across the extracellular matrix. Variations in the core proteins and in the glycosaminoglycan chains permit considerable diversity of the proteoglycans. For example, the proteoglycans organize components of the basal lamina, lubricate joints, provide turgor to the dermis, stabilize collagen fibrils, and resist compressive forces in cartilage (Ruoslahti, 1988).

Peptide Growth Factors. These factors were originally identified by their ability to stimulate proliferation of cultured cells and, thus, are usually referred to as growth factors. However, they can have a much wider range of actions, including altering responsiveness to other hormones or growth factors, inducing or repressing differentiation, and changing the composition of the extracellular matrix. Although usually autocrine or paracrine in action, some, such as the insulin-like growth factors, circulate in blood and may have endocrine functions. The actions of combinations of growth factor peptides are not necessarily predictable from an analysis of their actions when examined separately, and their effects can differ after changes in differentiation of the target cells (Mercola and Stiles, 1988; Slack, 1989).

There are several families of peptide growth factors. Examples are given in Table 4–2. Each family has several members that share at least one amino acid sequence and activity and may be recognized by the same receptor. Related forms are found in a wide variety of animal species. Some oncogenes also encode family members of growth factors or their receptors. Oncogenes are genes whose products confer on cells properties common to cells of many malignant tumors.

Any list of peptide growth factors is likely to be incomplete because this is a rapidly expanding field of research. Examples other than those in Table 4–2 include a group of neurotropic growth factors that promote growth and prevent programmed death of neurons in both the peripheral and central nervous systems. The cytokines, which include the interferons, the interleukins, and tumor necrosis factor, are structurally unrelated but together control the determination and differentiation of bone marrow–derived cells.

Localization of growth factors and their mRNAs has provided valuable insights into the functions of these factors in development but requires cautious interpretation because their actions are complex. For example, the presence of the mRNA as a factor in a developing tissue does not prove that the message is translated, that the active form of the factor is secreted, that it encounters functional receptors, or what other influences might modify its actions.

The Receptors for Peptide Growth Factors and Matrix Components. The actions of both growth factor peptides and matrix components in changing cell behavior are mediated through binding to receptors, which are proteins with extracellular, *trans*-membrane, and intracellular domains. In each case, binding can lead to altered production of various proteins. However, the steps between receptor-binding and the alteration of transcription, translation, and protein-processing are not yet well understood. The receptors for peptide growth factors and matrix components have different properties.

TABLE 4–2. Examples of Peptide Growth Factors

FAMILY	EXAMPLES	EXAMPLES OF FUNCTIONS
Epidermal growth factors	EGF TGF-alpha	Stimulate proliferation of many embryonic cells Promote expression of differentiation of many mature cells, especially epithelial cells
Platelet-derived growth factors	PDGF-A PDGF-B PDGF-AB	Mitogenic for mesenchymal cells Chemotactic for vascular endothelial cells
Transforming growth factor-beta	TGF-beta 1 TGF-beta 2	Induction of other growth factors Cause accumulation of matrix components
	Inhibins Activins Müllerian growth factor Inhibitory factor	Control development of the genital tract
Heparin-binding growth factors (fibroblast growth factors)	Acidic FGF Basic FGF KFGF FGF5	Promotion of angiogenesis Mitogens for mesodermal and neurectodermal cells
Insulin-like growth factors	IGF-1 IGF-2	Mitogenic for some cells Promote differentiation of others, e.g., muscle, cartilage
	Relaxin	Maturation of female reproductive tract

Binding of the soluble peptide growth factors to their receptors is specific and of high affinity. It leads to activation of intracellular signaling mechanisms and, often, to internalization and degradation or recycling of the receptor. Members of the epidermal growth factor, insulin-like growth factor, and platelet-derived growth factor families have receptors that activate intracellular pathways by phosphorylating tyrosines in various enzymes.

Because the matrix is insoluble, its receptors act differently (Buck and Horowitz, 1987). Matrix receptors often interact with more than one type of matrix component, and can have small intracellular domains that interact with components of the cytoskeleton. Binding does not lead to internalization or degradation of the receptor. Although different matrix receptors, such as the syndecans or the members of the integrin superfamily, can bind cells to virtually identical matrix components, each may have distinct effects on cell behaviors.

Developmental Strategies

Nature versus Nurture on a Cellular Level. The overall sequence of development involves the generation of precursor cells to produce progeny that become determined and differentiated and organize into functional tissues and organs. Multicellular organisms use two strategies to accomplish these processes—mosaic and regulative development.

In mosaic development, cells are instructed by events within themselves corresponding to their intrinsic nature. Information dictating cellular development is derived from cellular genes and is independent of the behavior or even the existence of neighboring cells. Cell diversity is achieved by genetically induced changes in lineages. Some invertebrates, such as nematodes, develop primarily in this manner.

In regulative development, cells in a developing organism influence or nurture the development of other cells or tissues. These cell-cell interactions have profound effects on the determination, differentiation, and morphogenetic behavior of cells. Regulative development allows for a great degree of developmental plasticity. However, as a cell matures, its responses to its neighbors are affected to an increasing degree by previous cell-cell interactions and, therefore, by its own intrinsic nature. Thus, the degree of plasticity diminishes with increasing maturity of the organism. This regulative strategy predominates in vertebrates.

Developmental Strategies Are Time Dependent and Sequential. Both cell lineage and cell interactions dictate development in mammals, but responses to these influences are not stereotyped; rather, they undergo changes during development. Changes in cell behavior induced by any interaction will modify the cell's response to all subsequent interactions. Thus, the response to a developmental influence is critically dependent on the history of the target cell, specifically how and when it was previously influenced. Thus, the sequential changes in phenotype of cells in developing tissues occur in parallel with changes in their potential patterns of response. This concept underlies the familiar differential effect of various teratogens. For example, the distinct phenotypes caused by thalidomide exposure resulted from effects on different tissues. The tissues that were affected depended on when during gestation exposure occurred, and thalidomide had essentially no teratogenic effect if exposure was sufficiently late.

■ NORMAL ORGAN FORM AND FUNCTION

The generation of organ form and function is affected by other developing organs, just as the behaviors of cells are governed partly by adjacent cells. Normal growth of the lung, for example, is dependent on growth of the chest wall and the fetal breathing movements of the diaphragm. How physical factors such as distention, compression, and stretch regulate behaviors of cells to form and deform organs is not well understood but is likely to be mediated in part through the extracellular matrix and intercellular junctions.

MALFORMATIONS

Earlier sections of this chapter have shown that the cell is the simplest functional unit of morphogenesis and that a limited number of cell behaviors form all organs. Conceptually, congenital anomalies have been divided into malformations, deformations, and disruptions. However, in all of these, the anomalies result partly because the spatial and temporal distributions of expression of the molecules that govern cell behavior, such as the growth factors, matrix molecules, and their receptors, are altered. In the case of the abnormal collagen gene in type I osteogenesis imperfecta, the mechanism is known and directly affects expression of a matrix component; but most of the defects are unknown, and it is likely that many are indirect.

Mutations of the genes that regulate segmentation and other aspects of pattern formation may also account for some congenital anomalies. As discussed earlier, these genes may be near the top of a hierarchy of genes that regulate the patterns of expression of other genes including those for growth factors, matrix molecules, and factors that control cell lineage. The pattern-forming genes of *Drosophila melanogaster* have been identified and characterized because mutant forms of them cause anomalies. To date, no human genes that determine body form have been identified or linked to congenital anomalies. However, mutation or abnormal expression of these pattern-forming genes early in gestation could account for malformations of single organs and for multiple malformation sequences.

PREMATURE BIRTH AND ABNORMAL DEVELOPMENT

When birth occurs prematurely, developmental influences occur out of sequence. There is sufficient flexibility in development of many organs for them to attain full size, form, and function despite their incomplete development when an infant is born in the late second or early third trimester. However, the delivery and postnatal support of premature infants frequently result in the superimposition of tissue damage on the events of development.

Tissue repair can modify developmental processes, and the results of repair may differ in mature and in developing tissue. For example a variety of agents, including hyperoxia, affect the lung differently early in development than in a mature individual. In preterm infants, these agents can induce coarse emphysema and scarring and reduced alveolar number, whereas in adults hyperoxia induces diffuse interstitial fibrosis. The responses differ but are both mediated through the controls that cells exert over one another.

Developmental processes can also modify tissue repair, presumably because the same types of cell behaviors and molecular controls are operating. Additionally, developing tissues may contain cells that are less committed than those in adult tissues. The developing tissues may therefore have a greater capacity to restore normal architecture at a site of injury. Although the mechanism is unclear, the rapid and remarkably complete repair of some developing tissues such as skin, cartilage, and bone of the fetus and infant is well known.

■ REFERENCES

Alberts, D., Bray, D., Lewis, J., Roberts, K., and Watson, J. D.: Molecular biology of the cell. New York and London, Garland, 1989.

Blau, H. M.: Hierarchies of regulatory genes may specify mammalian development. Cell 53:673–674, 1988.

Breitbart, R. E., Andreadis, A., and Nadal-Ginard, B.: Alternative splicing: A ubiquitous mechanism for the generation of multiple protein isoforms from single genes. Annu. Rev. Cell Biol. 56:467–495, 1987.

Buck, C. A., and Horowitz, A. F.: Cell surface receptors for extracellular matrix molecules. Annu. Rev. Cell Biol. 3:179–205, 1987.

Carraway, K. L., and Carraway, C. A. C.: Membrane–cytoskeleton interactions in animal cells. Biochim. Biophys. Acta 988:147–171, 1987.

Cedar, H.: DNA methylation and gene activity. Cell 53(1):3–4, 1988.

Chen, S., Teicher, L. C., Kazim, D., Pollack, R. E., and Wise, L. S.: Commitment of mouse fibroblasts to adipocyte differentiation by DNA transfection. Science 244:582–585, 1989.

Cunningham, B. A., Hemperly, J. J., Murray, B. A., et al.: Neural cell adhesion molecule: Structure, immunoglobulin-like domains, cell surface modulation and alternative RNA splicing. Science 236:799–806, 1987.

Dressler, G. R., and Gruss, P.: Do multigene families regulate vertebrate development? Trends Genet. 4:214–219, 1988.

Dynan, W. S.: Modularity in promoters and enhancers. Cell 58:1–4, 1989.

Edelman, G. M.: Cell adhesion molecules in the regulation of animal form and tissue pattern. Annu. Rev. Cell Biol. 2:81–116, 1986.

Ekblom, P., Vestweber, D., and Kemler R.: Cell–matrix interactions and cell adhesion during development. Annu. Rev. Cell Biol. 2:27–47, 1986.

Gaunt, S. J., Sharpe, P. T., and Duboule, D.: Spatially restricted domains of homeo-gene transcripts in mouse embryos: Relation to a segmented body plan. Development 104S:169–179, 1988.

Gehring, W. J.: Homeo boxes in the study of development. Science 236:1245–1252, 1987.

Gossler, A., Joyner, A. L., Rossant, J., et al.: Mouse embryonic stem cells and reporter constructs to detect developmentally regulated genes. Science 244:463–465, 1989.

Hall, P. A., and Watt, F. M.: Stem cells: The generation and maintenance of cellular diversity. Development 106:619–633, 1989.

Klausner, R. D., and Harford, J. B.: Cis-trans models for post-transcriptional gene regulation. Science 246:870–872, 1989.

Maniatis, T., Goodbourn, S., and Fischer, J. A.: Regulation of inducible and tissue-specific gene expression. Science 236:1237–1245, 1987.

McDonald, J. A.: Extracellular matrix assembly. Annu. Rev. Cell Biol. 4:183–207, 1988.

Mercola, M., and Stiles, C. D.: Growth factor superfamilies and mammalian embryogenesis. Development 102:451–460, 1988.

Metcalf, D.: The molecular control of cell division, differentiation, commitment and maturation in haemopoietic cells. Nature 339:27–30, 1989.

Murray, A. W., and Kirschner, M. W.: 1989 Dominoes and clocks: The union of two views of the cell cycle. Science 246:614–621, 1989.

O'Farrell, P. H., Edgar, B. A., Lakich, D., and Lehner, C. F.: Directing cell division during development. Science 246:635–640, 1989.

Pelton, R. W., Nomura, S., Moses, H. L., and Hogan, B. L.: Expression of transforming growth factor beta-2 RNA during murine embryogenesis. Development 106:759–767, 1989.

Rizzino, A.: Transforming growth factor-β: Multiple effects on cell differentiation and extracellular matrices. Devel. Biol. 130:411–422, 1988.

Ross, R.: Platelet-derived growth factor. Lancet i:1179–1182, 1989.

Ruoslahti, E.: Structure and biology of proteoglycans. Annu. Rev. Cell Biol. 4:229–255, 1988.

Sadler, T.: Langman's Medical Embryology. 6th edition. Baltimore, Williams and Wilkins, 1990.

Schibler, U., and Sierra, F.: Alternative promoters in developmental gene expression. Annu. Rev. Genet. 21:237–257, 1989.

Schüle, R., Muller, M., Kaltschmidt, C., and Renkawitz, R.: Many transcription factors interact synergistically with steroid receptors. Science 242:1418–1420, 1988.

Slack, J. M. W.: Peptide regulatory factors in embryonic development. Lancet i:1312–1315, 1989.

Takeichi, M.: The cadherins: Cell–cell adhesion molecules controlling animal morphogenesis. Development 102:639–655, 1988.

Yarden, Y., and Ullrich, A.: Growth factor receptor tyrosine kinases. Annu. Rev. Biochem. 57:443–478, 1988.

HORMONAL 5
INFLUENCES ON FETAL
DEVELOPMENT

Philip L. Ballard

The physiology of the fetal endocrine system differs from that of the adult with regard to the hormonal milieu, production sites, plasma levels, rates and pathways of degradation, and biologic function. The unique endocrine environment of the fetus and placenta is important for both normal growth and differentiation of the fetus and for timely parturition. Although there are major differences in endocrine physiology and regulated genes between the fetus and adult, the basic cellular mechanisms of hormone action do not change during development.

■ SITES OF PRODUCTION AND ACTION

Autocrine. Some hormones act primarily on the cells where they are synthesized. Hormones are synthesized within the cells, secreted at the cell surface into the extracellular domain, and then bind to specific cell surface receptors on the same cell. This interaction initiates a series of intracellular events, as described below, which modify growth, differentiation, or function of the cell.

Paracrine. In this system, hormones are secreted by one cell type and act on adjacent neighboring cells of another type. This mechanism provides for cell-cell communication within a tissue and is involved in regulating both growth and differentiation. In the fetal lung and other tissues, for example, insulin-like growth factors (IGF) are produced and secreted by mesenchymal cells and influence the growth of adjacent epithelial cells.

Endocrine. Most hormones are produced in a specific cell type of a tissue, secreted into the circulation, and exert their regulatory effects on distant tissues. Included in this category are polypeptide hormones synthesized in the hypothalamus, pituitary, placenta, and other tissues as well as the steroid hormones (androgens, estrogens, progestins, mineralocorticoids, vitamin D, and glucocorticoids). The steroid hormones and many of the protein hormones are bound to specific binding proteins in the serum, providing a hormone reservoir that is less susceptible to degradation. For most hormones, the plasma concentration of free (unbound) hormones represents the physiologically active hormones available to target cells. After secretion, the activity of hormones may be modified by metabolism in the circulation or tissues. For example, inactive cortisone may be converted to active cortisol by target tissues (e.g., lung and liver), and T_4 can undergo deiodination to either active T_3 or inactive reverse T_3 (rT_3) in the adult and fetus, respectively.

CELLULAR MECHANISMS

The signal inherent in a hormone is expressed through the binding of a hormone to its receptor, which initiates a series of biochemical events within the cell leading to altered replication or function. In general, the steps in this process of signal transduction are identical for adult and fetal cells, although different genes and/or proteins of a given cell type may be responsive during the developmental process. Furthermore, in the fetus, developmental immaturity or deficiency of specific components in the signal transduction system can alter hormone responsiveness.

MEMBRANE RECEPTORS

The protein, peptide, and biogenic amines exert their effects on cells by binding to specific receptor proteins located on the cell membrane. The receptors are membrane-spanning proteins with an extracellular domain containing the binding site for the hormone and a cytoplasmic domain that transmits the hormonal signal to intracellular molecules. For many hormonal systems, binding of hormone to receptor results in increased intracellular levels of a second messenger, such as cyclic adenosine monophosphate (cAMP). Membrane receptors are capable of moving within the cell membrane and may aggregate and be endocytosed after binding of the hormone. Receptors are also substrates for various protein kinases, and in some cases phosphorylation is dependent on the binding of hormones. These processes can produce a transient deficiency or inactivity of receptors (down regulation) and relative unresponsiveness of the cells to continued hormonal exposure. For example, down regulation and hormone refractoriness may be observed clinically with continued administration of a beta agonist.

One of the best described membrane receptor systems is that for beta-adrenergic agonists. The receptor has been isolated, purified, and sequenced, and complementary DNAs have been cloned for studying receptor structure, function, and regulation (Lefkowitz and Caron, 1988). The cytoplasmic domain of the receptor is associated with G proteins, which either activate or inhibit the catalytic component of adenyl cyclase. In the case of activation, binding of the hormone results within minutes in increased production of cAMP from adenosine triphosphate (ATP); the response is transient and levels rapidly return to near baseline values. cAMP, in turn, binds to the regulatory subunit of protein kinase A, releasing and activating the catalytic subunit. This enzyme phosphorylates specific cellular proteins resulting in either activation or inactivation with subsequent effects on either enzyme activity (e.g., glycogen phosphorylase), intracellular structure (e.g., in the cytoskeleton), or gene expression in the nucleus. This sequence of events is summarized in Figure 5–1.

INTRACELLULAR RECEPTORS

Thyroid hormones, steroid hormones, and certain polypeptide hormones enter target cells and bind to specific receptors in the cytoplasm, on the nuclear membrane, or within the nucleus. In the case of steroid hormones, interaction with a receptor protein modifies receptor structure and increases its affinity for specific binding sites (response elements) on regulated genes. This alters the rate of gene transcription and subsequently the levels of the encoded protein. Hormones can also alter mRNA levels by influencing stability or efficiency of translation of the transcript. When the hormone is removed, steroid dissociates from the receptor through the law of mass action, and the response is reversed. Whereas binding of hormones to membrane receptors often produces responses within minutes (e.g., adrenocorticotropic hormone [ACTH] stimulation of cortisol production), steroid and other hormones that regulate gene expression require several hours to increase the content of specific messenger RNAs and the encoded proteins. The mechanism of steroid hormone action is depicted in Figure 5–2.

Evans (1988) has established that the receptors for steroid hormones and thyroid hormones have striking structural similarities. In particular, the region of the receptor involved in DNA binding is quite homologous among the various proteins. This finding suggests an evolutionary relationship between these receptors as well as similarities in their mechanism of action at target genes.

POSTRECEPTOR EVENTS

Hormones have diverse effects on cells, but their mechanism of action is in general limited to one of three categories: (1) directly modifying an enzyme or a protein and altering function (e.g., phosphorylation), (2) activating specific genes that increase synthesis and content of the encoded protein, or (3) repressing the expression of a gene. All three processes occur during fetal life. One effect of beta agonists in the fetal lung is secretion of surfactant from type II cells, and this response occurs within minutes on hormone exposure, presumably reflecting phosphorylation of specific proteins involved in the exocytic process (Walters, 1985). Catecholamines also stimulate production of pulmonary surfactant lipids and proteins, and this response involves de novo RNA and protein synthesis over a longer time scale (Ballard, 1989). Glucocorticoid treatment of fetal lung induces a number of proteins but also inhibits the synthesis of others (Odom et al., 1989); the stimulatory and inhibitory effects of glucocorticoids appear to be mediated through distinct nucleotide sequences (response elements) in the promoter region of the regulated genes.

Hormonal responsiveness of a cell is determined by both the levels of circulating hormone and the concentration and activity of cellular receptors and other mediating proteins. In the undisturbed adult organism, for example, responsiveness is determined primarily by the level of circulating hormone that normally fluctuates over a relatively limited range (e.g., diurnal variation). As hormone levels increase, the percentage of receptors occupied by hormone also increases, often in a nearly linear fashion, resulting in a highly responsive and tightly regulated stimulus-response system. In the fetus, particularly early in gestation, hormonal responsiveness is limited by developmental deficiencies in hormone levels, number of receptors, necessary cofactors, or mediating proteins. In the adrenergic system, for example, low receptor number and altered ratio of G protein subunits result in relative insensitivity of fetal tissues to adrenergic stimulation. Furthermore, cells may be hormonally unresponsive at certain points in development owing to alterations in chromatin structure that prevent receptor-hormone binding.

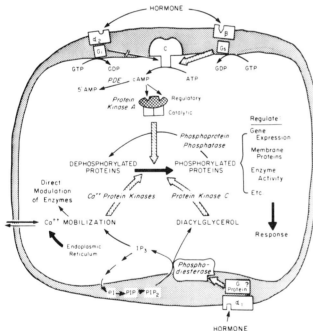

FIGURE 5–1. *Molecular mechanism of catecholamine action. This model applies for a variety of hormones that act through either cAMP or IP3 as secondary messengers. ATP = adenosine-5'-triphosphate; cAMP = adenosine-3',5'-cyclic monophosphate; 5'-AMP = adenosine-5'-monophosphate; C = catalytic subunit of adenylate cyclase; GTP = guanosine-5'-triphosphate; GDP = guanosine-5'-diphosphate; G = guanine nucleotide regulatory protein (stimulatory or inhibitory); PI = phosphatidylinositol; PIP = phosphatidylinositol-4-phosphate; PIP$_2$ = phosphatidylinositol-4,5-diphosphate; IP$_3$ = inositol triphosphate; PDE = phosphodiesterase. (From Ballard, P. L.: Mechanism of hormone action. In Rudolph, A. M., and Hoffman, J. I. E. [Eds.]: Pediatrics. Norwalk, Conn., Appleton & Lange, 1987.)*

■ UNIQUE FEATURES OF THE FETAL ENDOCRINE SYSTEM

The endocrine environment of the fetus is unique with regard to the endocrine organs, the presence of certain hormones, changing and often high circulating concentra-

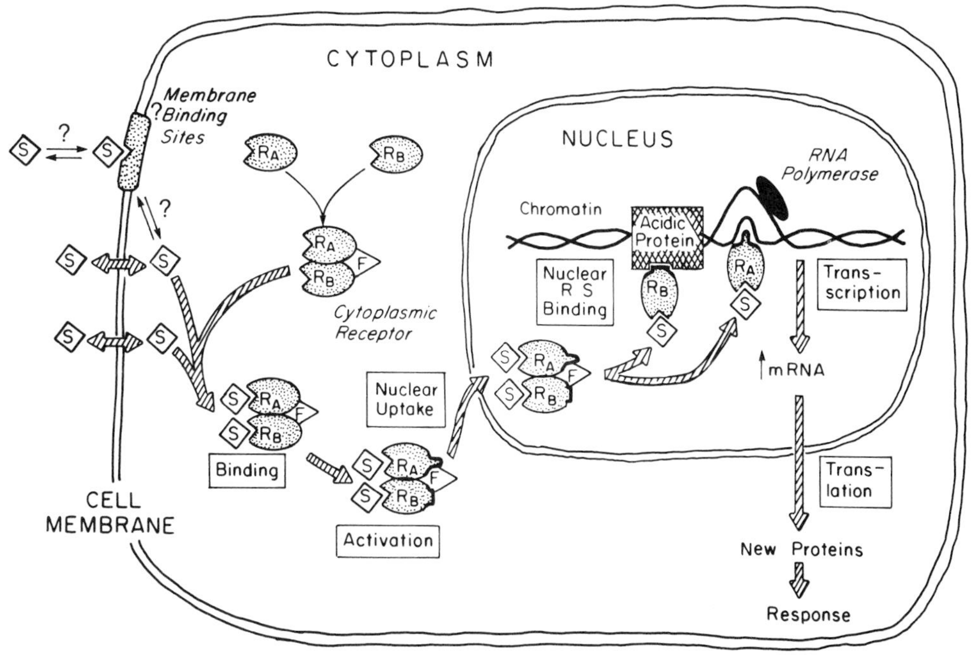

FIGURE 5–2. Molecular mechanism of action of steroid hormones in their target cells. This model applies in general to glucocorticoids, estrogens, androgens, progestins, mineralocorticoids, and vitamin D. S = steroid; R_A = subunit A of receptor; R_B = subunit B of receptor; RS = receptor-steroid complex. (From Ballard, P. L.: Mechanism of hormone action. In Rudolph, A. M., and Hoffman, J. I. E. [Eds.]: Pediatrics. Norwalk, Conn., Appleton & Lange, 1987.)

tions of hormones, hormone metabolism, and specialized responses related to in utero development. Although the pattern of fetal growth and development is not generally dependent on hormones, the timing of these events is highly regulated. This becomes particularly important in the premature infant who has received insufficient exposure to critical hormones and thus is not fully prepared for extrauterine life.

HORMONES AND SOURCES

During the first trimester of gestation, the fetal testes produce an inhibitor of müllerian duct differentiation. Müllerian inhibiting factor (MIF) is a glycoprotein with a MW of approximately 72,000, which acts locally through paracrine mechanisms to cause involution of the müllerian structures and may inhibit oocyte meiosis in the ovary (Ueno et al., 1988). The cellular mechanism of action of MIF is uncertain but may involve dephosphorylation of a membrane protein.

During pregnancy, steroid hormones are produced through complex interaction of mother, fetus, and placenta. Progesterone is initially synthesized by the maternal corpus luteum, whereas during the second and third trimester, the placenta is the major source. Progesterone is synthesized from maternal low-density lipoprotein (LDL) and occurs independent of the fetus. The high levels of progesterone appear to serve at least two functions: suppressing uterine activity and decreasing maternal immune responses against fetal antigens.

The adult zone of the fetal adrenal produces cortisol (in increasing amounts during gestation), and the inner fetal zone acts in concert with the placenta to produce estrogens and their precursors. The fetal zone is deficient in delta-5,3-beta-OH dehydrogenase and delta-4,5,3-ketosteroid isomerase and has considerable steroid sulfokinase activity, resulting in production of dehydroepiandrosterone sulfate (DHAS) from pregnenolone supplied by the placenta. DHAS undergoes 16-hydroxylation in

the fetal liver and then is transported to the placenta where it and DHAS (of both fetal and maternal origin) are the major substrates for estrogen synthesis. Much of the estrogen, predominantly estriol, enters the maternal circulation and subsequently is excreted in the urine. High levels of estrogen also accumulate in the fetus and amniotic fluid, but the function of estrogen in the fetus is uncertain. Estrogen biosynthesis is greatly reduced in infants with steroid sulfatase deficiency; development of the fetus under these circumstances, though, appears to be normal.

In addition to production of progesterone, the placenta synthesizes a number of polypeptide hormones throughout pregnancy. These include human chorionic somatomammotropin (hCS), human chorionic gonadotropin (hCG), human chorionic corticotropin (hCC), human chorionic thyrotropin (hCT), beta endorphin, α-melanocyte–stimulating hormone (α-MSH), and both beta and alpha lipotropin. The placenta also produces most, if not all, of the releasing hormones synthesized by the hypothalamus. Thus, the placenta contributes to the circulating pool of pituitary and hypothalamic hormones in the fetus. In addition to the placenta, other fetal tissues, particularly the gut and pancreas, synthesize a number of the releasing hormones characteristic of the hypothalamus. The presence of extrahypothalamic peptides is established, but their role in fetal development is not certain.

Another unique source of hormone production in the fetus is the para-aortic chromaffin system. These extramedullary paraganglia, the largest of which are referred to as the organs of Zuckerkandl, are located along the abdominal and pelvic sympathetic plexuses during fetal life and disappear completely in the first years after birth. By the second trimester of gestation, this tissue actively produces norepinephrine but relatively little epinephrine due to low levels of phenylethanolamine-N-methyl transferase. The chromaffin cells of the para-aortic system as well as the sympathetic nerve cells are derived from a neuroectodermal stem cell and are responsive to nerve growth factor.

The catecholamine responses at birth are due in part to the para-aortic chromaffin system as well as increased postganglionic sympathetic neuronal and adrenal medullary catecholamine secretion. Circulating catecholamines (norepinephrine, epinephrine, and dopamine) increase exponentially after delivery and cord cutting. In the newborn sheep, which lacks para-aortic chromaffin tissue, the increased circulating norepinephrine is derived predominantly from the spillover of postganglionic sympathetic neurons, while the increased epinephrine derives solely from adrenal medullary secretion. Lacking complete organ sympathetic innervation and maturation of adrenergic receptor mechanisms, the fetus and newborn exhibit profound dependence on circulating catecholamines for maintenance of cardiovascular and metabolic homeostasis in response to physiologic stress such as the transition to extrauterine life (Padbury and Martinez, 1988). Adrenalectomized animals, deficient in the normally increased levels of circulating epinephrine in the newborn period, are impaired in their ability to increase cardiac output and myocardial contractility, secrete surfactant, and mobilize energy substrates for successful postnatal adaptation. It is not known precisely how long this dependence on circulating catecholamines persists postnatally, but basal myocardial function and the high resting cardiac output characteristic of the first weeks of life remain dependent on an intact sympathoadrenal system. Survival during hypoxic stress in newborn rats has been shown to be dependent on similar mechanisms (Slotkin and Seidler, 1988).

In addition to the anterior and posterior lobes of the pituitary, the fetus has an intermediate lobe that regresses after birth and is not found in adults. In animals, however, the intermediate lobe is maintained through adult life. The intermediate lobe secretes primarily alpha-MSH and beta-endorphin, which are derived from proopiomelanocortin (POMC). In the anterior lobe of the pituitary, POMC is cleaved primarily to beta-lipotropin and ACTH. By the second trimester of gestation, the fetal neurohypophysis contains arginine vasopressin (AVP), oxytocin, and arginine vasotocin (AVT). The pituitary gland contains AVT throughout fetal life, but this hormone disappears after birth. AVT is also present in the pineal glands of both fetuses and adults.

ONTOGENY

The function of hormones in the fetus is determined primarily by the developmental pattern of the hormones and/or their receptor system. In general, most endocrine systems of the fetus are functional by the end of the first trimester, although circulating levels of many hormones increase substantially only during the third trimester. One exception to this pattern is illustrated by the hypothalamic-pituitary-gonad axis. Secretion of hypothalamic gonadotropin-releasing hormone (Gn-RH) becomes active in the first trimester, resulting in pulsatile release of LH and FSH, which stimulates production of testosterone or estradiol by the fetal gonads. Throughout the rest of fetal life and through childhood, until the onset of puberty, this hormonal axis remains quiescent. Control of this hormonal system is felt to reside in the central nervous system.

Hormones known to influence terminal differentiation (acquisition of specialized functions by cells) have developmental patterns consistent with this role. For example, cortisol is detected in fetal plasma at low levels during the second trimester and then increases exponentially during the third trimester (Murphy, 1982). Glucocorticoid receptors are detected relatively early in gestation in many fetal tissues and appear to be fully functional. The influence of endogenous cortisol on fetal development, therefore, is determined by the rate of adrenal production of cortisol and perhaps by postreceptor responsiveness in target tissues. Similarly, plasma levels of T_3 and T_4 increase only during the third trimester, whereas thyroid hormone receptors are present throughout the second trimester (Fisher and Klein, 1981; Gonzales and Ballard, 1981). Prolactin levels in plasma and amniotic fluid increase throughout the third trimester to levels much greater than those found in the adult or in the mother. By contrast, levels of growth hormone increase during the first two-thirds of pregnancy, and then decline toward term.

The adrenergic response system appears to be constrained throughout most of gestation. The catecholamine response to the stress of delivery is greater at term than in preterm deliveries, and in the fetal lung and heart, for example, the number of beta-adrenergic receptors and the ability to provoke cAMP are low in the midgestation fetus as compared with the adult (Davis et al., 1987).

METABOLISM

In the human fetus the levels of circulating cortisol (an active glucocorticoid) and cortisone (inactive) are similar. Whereas most adult tissues, particularly the liver, readily convert cortisone to cortisol, fetal tissues generally lack this ability because of deficiency of the enzyme 17-beta-hydroxysteroid dehydrogenase or cofactors NADP and NADPH. The low enzymatic activity in most tissues reduces the possible contribution of cortisone to tissue glucocorticoid activity. In the fetal lung of animals, the ability to convert cortisone to cortisol increases markedly during the third trimester, coincident with lung maturation (Nicholas et al., 1978). Lung tissue from the human fetus is similarly responsive to cortisone and cortisol during explant culture, reflecting rapid conversion of cortisone to cortisol (Gonzales et al., 1986; Liley et al., 1989). In this tissue, therefore, cortisone contributes to the pool of circulating glucocorticoids. Administered corticosteroids are rapidly cleared from the fetal circulation by metabolism in the maternal liver, whereas similar doses to the newborn infant are metabolized very slowly because of liver immaturity.

Thyroid hormone metabolism also varies markedly in the fetus when compared to that of the adult (see Chapter 109). In the fetus, T_4 is deiodinated preferentially to inactive reverse T_3 rather than the active metabolic T_3. This occurs in most fetal tissues but particularly the placenta. In fetal sheep, at least, the switch from production of rT_3 to T_3 is regulated by endogenous cortisol (levels increase markedly in late gestation) and is stimulated precociously by administered glucocorticoids (Thomas et al., 1978). The generalized inactivation of T_4 during most of fetal life would appear to have at least two beneficial effects in the fetus: first, to protect most fetal tissues from the catabolic effects of thyroid hormone and, second, to provide a mechanism whereby selected tissues could increase their exposure to active T_3 by increasing local T_3 production. Moreover, several fetal tissues in animals are relatively unresponsive to administered T_3 with regard to thermogenesis, a function that is not needed by the fetus before birth.

HORMONES AND TISSUE DEVELOPMENT

The developmental processes of organogenesis and subsequent maturation of tissue structure and function are, for the most part, programmed and occur in the absence of hormonal influences. Chapter 4 reviews current understanding of the genetic control of tissue development, which involves coordination and interaction of multiple gene products. Maintenance of the differentiated state appears to be an active process requiring continued synthesis of specific regulatory proteins. Hormones and growth factors have three general roles in the process of differentiation. First, they modulate the rate of tissue development by virtue of increased concentrations and/or tissue responsiveness during normal gestation. Hormonal effects involve both enzyme induction, resulting in differentiated tissue function (e.g., pulmonary surfactant production), and repression of specific genes (e.g., hepatic alpha-fetoprotein) with loss of a fetal-specific protein. Within a given tissue, the response to a particular hormone typically involves a specific subset of cellular proteins (e.g, sugar-metabolizing enzymes of the intestine), providing a coordinated maturational response. Second, hormones can accelerate the normal timetable of development resulting in precocious organ maturation. This accelerating effect is observed with exogenous hormone treatment and at times of increased hormone production, such as during chronic in utero stress, during both premature and term labor and delivery, in the immediate postnatal period, and, in animals, around the time of weaning. The third area of hormonal influence relates to tumorigenesis in which there is loss of growth control and dedifferentiation. A number of oncogenes have been recently described whose overexpression is associated with the genesis of cancer. The oncogenes of retroviruses represent slightly mutated cellular genes that have been obtained by the virus and that are constitutively expressed on viral infection. Many of the oncogenes encode growth factors, their receptors, other hormone receptors, or proteins involved in signal transduction (Drucker et al., 1989). For example, oncogenes encode for proteins related to epidermal growth factor receptor (erbB), platelet-derived growth factor (sis), fibroblast growth factor (int-2), the G proteins of adenyl cyclase (ras), and thyroid hormone receptor (erbA). Thus, appropriate expression of hormones, growth factors, and receptors is important in both initial differentiation and maintenance of the differentiated state. Table 5–1 gives a partial listing of hormones that probably have a role in fetal development.

INTRINSIC TIMETABLE

Experiments of nature, such as anencephaly with panhypopituitarism, indicate that fetal growth and development proceed in a near-normal fashion in the absence of hypothalamic and pituitary input. Although such fetuses are still exposed to hormones from the mother and placenta, circulating levels of many hormones are much lower than in normal fetuses. When fetal tissue is placed in explant culture in the absence of serum or added hormones, growth, structural development, and biochemical differentiation continue at a rate equal to or greater than that in in vivo. Fetal lung, for example, undergoes airway branching, formation of peripheral air spaces, and cytodifferentiation of epithelial cells into surfactant-producing type II cells (Fig. 5–3). These findings in vivo and in vitro suggest that tissue growth and differentiation are independent of circulating hormones and proceed as a result of gene expression apparently determined by cell lineage and cell interactions. It is likely that tissue interactions, which are essential for normal development, are mediated in part through the production of growth factors and possibly other regulators acting in an autocrine or a paracrine fashion. The primary role of circulating hormones in the fetus is to modulate the rate of differentiation, in part as a response to changes in the fetal environment.

SEXUAL DIFFERENTIATION

The patterns of hormonal secretion and response vital to sexual differentiation are described in Chapter 108. Figure 5–4 summarizes the major events in sexual differentiation.

Besides affecting sexual development, the patterns of sex steroid secretion may have important effects on other organ systems. In experimental animals, the surge of circulating androgens near midgestation appears to influence the subsequent pattern of lung maturation. Male fetuses have a transient developmental delay in the production of pulmonary surfactant, which can be abolished by treatment with antiandrogen agents (Nielsen et al., 1982). These experimental observations may relate to the situation in human infants where males have an increased risk for respiratory distress syndrome (RDS) and may be less responsive to prenatal betamethasone treatment.

TERMINAL DIFFERENTIATION

The major role of circulating hormones in development relates to the rate of tissue maturation in late gestation. Increasing levels of hormones modulate normal tissue maturation and accelerate the process in stressful conditions (e.g., placental insufficiency, prolonged rupture of membranes, premature labor), a process which has been described as preparation for birth. Several different hormones, as described below, are involved in the stress response, and in several tissues there is an interaction between hormones to stimulate maturation. Many of the problems encountered by the premature infant may be thought of as developmental deficiencies or immaturity of critical functions in select tissues. Table 5–2 lists diseases that result from immature hormonally regulated systems.

GLUCOCORTICOIDS

Endogenous cortisol, and in some tissues, cortisone, is the most important hormone regulating tissue maturation. Cortisol levels increase continually through the third trimester, and are elevated in both acutely and chronically

TABLE 5–1. Hormones of the Fetus That Influence Growth or Differentiation (in Vitro and/or in Vivo)

HORMONE OR GROWTH FACTOR	SOURCES	FETAL EFFECTS
Adrenocorticotropic hormone (ACTH)	Pituitary, placenta	Activates fetal adrenal gland.
Androgens (testosterone)	Testes, adrenals, liver	Produces male sexual differentiation. Delays lung maturation?
β-Endorphin	Pituitary, placenta	Maintains vasoregulation?
Calcitonin	Thyroid	Promotes bone mineralization and anabolism?
Catecholamines	Adrenal	Produces lung differentiation. Increases cardiac output, thermogenesis, and glycogen and fat mobilization.
Human chorionic corticotropin (hCC)	Placenta	Regulates fetal adrenal cortex.
Human chorionic gonadotropin (hCG)	Placenta	Luteotropic; stimulates steroid production by the fetal testes and adrenals.
Human chorionic somatomammotropin (hCS), human placental lactogen (hPL)	Placenta	Promotes secretion of insulin-like growth factors (IGFs)?
Cortisol	Adrenal adult zone	Needed for parturition and differentiation of numerous tissues.
Eicosanoids (prostaglandins, leukotrienes, and thromboxanes)	Most tissues	Initiates uterus contraction; regulates vessel tone and lung maturation; activates fetal adrenals.
Epidermal growth factor (EGF)	Multiple tissues	Regulates epithelial cell division.
Estrogens (estrone, estradiol, and estriol)	Placenta	Regulates lung differentitation? Increases uteroplacental blood flow.
Fibroblast growth factors (FGFs)	Fibroblasts	Regulate cell division.
Insulin-like growth factors (IGFs)	Multiple tissues	Regulate cell division (and differentiation?).
Interferon-gamma	White blood cells, other cell type	Differentiates lungs and other tissues?
α-Melanocyte-stimulating hormone (α-MSH)	Pituitary and placenta	Activates fetal adrenals.
Müllerian-inhibiting factor (MIF)	Testes (Sertoli cells)	Activates involution müllerian ducts.
Nerve growth factor (NGF)		Needed for development and maintenance of neurons and Sertoli cells?
Parathyroid hormone	Parathyroids	Produce 1,25-vitamin D.
Platelet-derived growth factor (PDGF)	Platelets, other tissues	Needed for cell replication.
Progesterone	Placenta	Precursor for fetal steroids, needed for pregnancy maintenance.
Prolactin	Pituitary	Needed for water balance and lung development?
Releasing hormones (TRH, SRIF, CRF, gonadotropin releasing hormone [GRH])	Hypothalamus, placenta, gut	Augment output of fetal pituitary hormones and placental hormones?
Thyroid hormones (T$_4$, T$_3$)	Thyroid, liver	Activate lung and heart differentiation.
Transforming growth factor (TGF)	Multiple tissues	Regulates cell division, deposition of extracellular matrix, and differentiation.
Vasopressin, vasotocin	Neurohypophysis, pineal	Maintain placental and lung water transport. Stimulate ACTH release from fetal pituitary?
Vitamin D	Maternal skin, liver, kidney	Placental calcium transport.

stressful situations. Glucocorticoids are known to have the following effects in fetal and newborn tissues of animals:

1. In the lung, glucocorticoids accelerate structural development and the appearance, accumulation, and secretion of surfactant (see Chapter 49).

2. In some species, they increase pulmonary receptors for insulin, EGF, and beta-adrenergic agonists.

3. They induce the adrenal medullary enzyme phenylethanolamine-N-methyl transferase, which catalyses epinephrine synthesis from norepinephrine.

4. In animals, but probably not in the human fetus, they induce the hepatic enzyme that catalyzes production of T$_3$ from T$_4$.

5. They decrease the sensitivity of the ductus arteriosus (in fetal sheep) to dilating prostaglandins, facilitating closure of the ductus in response to increased oxygen concentration.

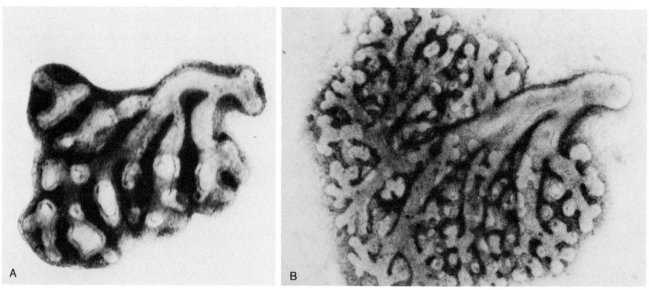

FIGURE 5–3. Development of the fetal lung in vitro. Intact lungs from 14-day rat fetuses were cultured as explants in medium without hormones for 1 day (A) and 4 days (B). (From Gross, I., and Wilson, C. M.: Fetal rat lung maturation: Initiation and modulation. J. Appl. Physiol. 55:1725 – 1731, 1983.)

6. They accelerate secretory activity of the fetal pancreas.

7. In the liver, they stimulate glycogen deposition, induce gluconeogenic and other enzymes important in postnatal function, and repress hematopoietic cells and production of alpha-fetoprotein.

8. In the placenta of sheep, they promote estrogen biosynthesis, which in turn stimulates prostaglandin $F_{2\alpha}$ production and subsequently the initiation of parturition.

9. They influence the rate of myelination in the brain, accelerating or retarding this process depending on species, timing, and dose.

10. They induce glutamine synthetase activity in the embryonic neural retina.

11. In suckling or weaning animals, they induce brush border enzymes, such as peptidases, sucrase, maltase, and

alkalane phosphatase, which are required for normal function of the adult intestine.

12. They inhibit cell division in some but not all tissues.

Experimentally, these findings with glucocorticoids arise from studies with administered hormone ablation procedures (e.g., hypophysectomy or adrenalectomy), which delay organ maturation, and temporal associations between circulating corticosteroids and inducible responses. A prepartum rise in circulating fetal corticosteroids occurs in all species that have been studied, and the experimental manipulations of steroid treatment or withdrawal provide consistent results in a variety of animal models.

In many tissues, the maturational effects of glucocorticoids require or are synergistic with effects of other hormones such as T_3 and catecholamines (cAMP). Although it is not possible to extrapolate all of the findings in animals to the human infant, a number of these regulatory events appear to occur in the human and have clinical implications (see Table 5–2).

The effects and physiologic role of glucocorticoids are well described with regard to maturation of the fetal lung. Studies with explant cultures of human tissue have established that glucocorticoids affect both lung structure and production of surfactant by type II cells (Gonzales et al., 1986). Treatment accelerates differentiation of the epithelial cells into type II cells (loss of glycogen and the appearance of apical microvilli and intracellular lamellar bodies), reduces mesenchymal volume, narrows the intra-alveolar septal distance, and increases maximal lung volume and compliance. Surfactant production and secretion are increased, and the response includes all of the known components of pulmonary surfactant (saturated phosphatidylcholine and the three surfactant-associated proteins). The response to glucocorticoids in fetal lung is mediated by glucocorticoid receptors and involves increased gene expression (i.e., increased content of messenger RNA) for the surfactant-associated proteins. Glucocorticoids increase the activity of choline phosphate cytidylyltransferase (via increased levels of lipid cofactor), the rate-limiting

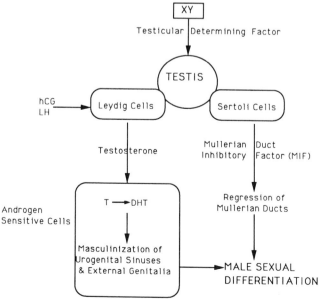

FIGURE 5–4. Outline of hormonal effects in fetal sexual differentiation.

TABLE 5–2. Abnormalities of the Newborn That May Be Related to Hormonal Conditions

ABNORMALITY	HORMONE	ETIOLOGY (KNOWN OR POSTULATED)
Male pseudohermaphrodism	Testosterone	Genetic defects in testosterone biosynthesis, metabolism (5α-reducase), or responsiveness (receptor deficiency or abnormality).
Testicular feminization	Dihydrotesterone	Decreased receptors in androgen target tissues yield female phenotype in genetic male.
Female pseudohermaphrodism (congenital hyperplasia)	Cortisol, insulin	Enzymatic defects in cortisol biosynthesis with excess androgen.
Infant diabetic mother	Insulin	Fetal hyperinsulinemia increases growth and fat deposition and delays lung development.
Infant leprechaunism	Insulin	Decreased insulin receptors with intrauterine growth retardation.
Congenital hypothyroidism	T_4, T_3	Hormone deficiency alters development of brain, heart, lung, and other tissues.
Respiratory distress syndrome	Cortisol, T_3, catecholamines, prolactin?	Developmental deficiency in one or more hormones may delay lung development.
Transient tachypnea of newborn	Cortisol, catecholamines, arginine vasopressin, and others?	Decreased hormone levels or responsiveness of lung epithelium for fluid clearance.
Lung hypoplasia	Unknown growth factor	Presumed decreased production of lung factors.
Persistent pulmonary hypertension of newborn	?	Stress-related hormones may delay pulmonary vascular development in utero.
Patent ductus arteriosus	Cortisol, prostaglandins?	Possible imbalance in levels and/or responsiveness for dilating and constricting prostaglandins.
Necrotizing enterocolitis	Cortisol, glucagon?	Developmental deficiency in hormones may delay gut development.

enzyme of the choline incorporation pathway, and stimulate production of fatty acid synthetase, the rate-limiting enzyme for fatty acid production from malonyl coenzyme A. Prenatal treatment of rats with dexamethasone causes a precocious increase in antioxidant enzyme activities in the fetal lung, but at present there are no data in the human. It is likely that glucocorticoids have other maturational effects in the lung, since a number of as yet unidentified proteins are induced by glucocorticoid treatment of cultured tissue. The clinical effects of prenatal corticosteroid therapy are discussed in Chapters 3 and 53. The improved survival rates in treated infants result from precocious maturation of the lung as well as other organs.

THYROID HORMONES

Levels of both T_3 and T_4 increase in the human fetus during the third trimester. Although thyroid hormones are important for normal postnatal growth, the athyroid human fetus also grows normally and does not display signs or symptoms of hypothyroidism seen in children and adults (see Chapter 109). However, thyroid hormones may play an important role in the maturation of the fetal lung and perhaps other tissues. Surfactant production and structural pulmonary development are retarded in hypothyroid sheep fetuses. Treatment with thyroid hormone accelerates phospholipid synthesis in cultured lung (Ballard, 1989), and thyroid hormones are necessary for maximal response to cortisol treatment in fetal sheep (Schellenberg et al., 1988). The in vitro effects of thyroid hormone on lipid synthesis are receptor-mediated, indicating that physiologic levels of hormones can be effective in vivo. At present, the enzymatic sites of thyroid hormone action are not known. Combined treatment with both glucocorticoid and thyroid hormone results in an additive or synergistic stimulation of phospholipid synthesis in cultured tissue (Fig. 5–5). In vivo, cortisol treatment of sheep fetuses also increases circulating T_3 concentrations via increased conversion from T_4. These and other observations on the interactions of glucocorticoids and thyroid hormones led to recent clinical trials of prenatal therapy with betamethasone plus thyrotropin-releasing hormone (TRH) for prevention of RDS. Initial results indicate little benefit in incidence of RDS, but an unexpected reduction in chronic lung disease for treated infants (Morales et al.,

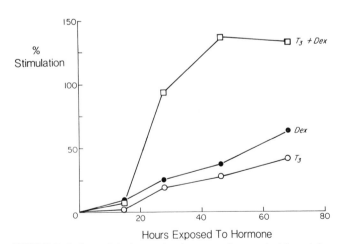

FIGURE 5–5. Synergistic interaction between glucocorticoids and thyroid hormones in phosphatidylcholine synthesis. Explant cultures of fetal rabbit lung were treated with dexamethasone and/or T_3 for the times shown; data are expressed as per cent stimulation over control. (From Ballard, P. L., Hovey, M. L., and Gonzales, L. K.: Thyroid hormone stimulation of phosphatidylcholine synthesis in cultured fetal rabbit lung. J. Clin. Invest. 74:898–905, 1984.)

1989; Ballard et al., 1990). The mechanism of this response is not understood, but may involve beneficial alterations in lung structure.

Thyroid hormones are also important for cardiac development. In the sheep fetus, thyroidectomy during late gestation blunts the increase in heart rate, cardiac output, and oxygen consumption normally seen after birth, and replacement T_3 therapy before birth is corrective. This T_3 effect appears to be mediated through beta-adrenergic receptor concentration and responsiveness to endogenous catecholamines (Birk et al., 1988). The normal hypertrophic growth of the myocardium is also dependent on thyroid hormones but apparently does not involve the beta-adrenergic system.

CATECHOLAMINES

Circulating catecholamine concentrations increase dramatically with labor and delivery, and amniotic fluid levels, which probably reflect production by the fetus, are generally elevated in complicated pregnancies. A well-described effect of catecholamines on terminal differentiation is in the fetal lung. Treatment with beta-adrenergic agonists causes a prompt increase in surfactant secretion both in vivo and in isolated type II cells, and endogenous catecholamines contribute to release of surfactant at the time of birth. For example, the amount of surfactant in airways of fetal animals is decreased by blockade of the beta-adrenergic receptors with an irreversible antagonist, by treatment with an inhibitor of catecholamine biosynthesis, and by adrenalectomy.

A second effect of catecholamines is to stimulate the rate of surfactant synthesis. In cultured lung tissue, treatment with analogs of cAMP, beta agonists, or other agents that induce cAMP increases synthesis of surfactant phospholipids and surfactant-associated proteins A and B. Alveolar structure in cultured lung explants is also modified by these treatments, probably resulting from altered ion and fluid transport.

A third effect of catecholamines is reduction of lung fluid. In fetal animals, beta agonists decrease fluid accumulation in the air spaces by inhibiting the chloride pump and promoting fluid reabsorption through a sodium pump in epithelial cells. The physiologic relevance of these responses has been demonstrated in the fetal lamb where there is a close correlation between fluid flux and endogenous levels of catecholamines during labor. Responsiveness to catecholamines normally increases during the third trimester; the response is markedly blunted in thyroidectomized fetuses but restored by combined treatment with T_3 and hydrocortisone but not by treatment with either hormone alone (Barker et al., 1988a and 1989). These findings suggest that increasing concentrations of cortisol and T_3 during development enhance the sensitivity of epithelial cells for responding to catecholamines. This system illustrates the interaction of hormones in regulating a developmental process important for successful adaptation to extrauterine life. Clinical aspects of lung fluid are discussed in Chapter 51.

All three catecholamine effects in fetal lung are mediated by beta-adrenergic receptors and increased intracellular levels of cAMP. Protein kinase A is activated by cAMP, resulting in phosphorylation of specific cell proteins that affect the secretory process (surfactant) and ion channels or pumps (fluid flux) or regulate gene expression (synthesis of surfactant components). Obviously, this chain of intracellular events can be modified at various levels to affect the response. For example, glucocorticoid treatment increases adrenergic receptor concentration and accordingly the sensitivity to catecholamines (in animals) and may also affect the G protein of adenyl cyclase (Cheng et al., 1980; Bottari et al., 1988). In fetal sheep, chronic infusion of glucose delayed the developmental increase in lung beta-adrenergic receptor concentration (Warburton et al., 1988). Clinically, it is conceivable that exposure of the fetus to xanthines or other inhibitors of cAMP phosphodiesterase would enhance cAMP responses and lung maturation.

Catecholamines are also involved in increasing myocardial contractility and systemic vascular resistance, and in triggering the onset of thermogenesis through mobilization of energy substrates. Infants born prematurely are thus at increased risk with regard to cardiac function and thermal stability due to both decreased metabolic reserves and suboptimal catecholamine levels.

INSULIN

The infant of a diabetic mother is at increased risk for a number of abnormalities including macrosomia with organomegaly, placental hypertrophy, polyhydramnios, congenital anomalies, and intrauterine death (see Chapter 9). Based on these observations and animal models of diabetes, it is generally felt that fetal hyperinsulinemia delays the appearance of pulmonary surfactant and may alter surfactant composition (and therefore its function) and/or alveolar structure. One possible explanation for this effect relates to the mitogenic activity of insulin and the general biologic principle that cell differentiation (e.g., production of surfactant) is associated with decreased cell division. Thus, under the stimulation of increased circulating insulin, lung type II cells may remain in an active cell cycle, not entering the G_0 stage when specialized cell products are synthesized. Another possible explanation is an inhibitory effect of insulin on synthesis of surfactant per se. Experiments with cultured lung tissue found that insulin can inhibit synthesis of surfactant protein A, which is required for normal surfactant structure and function (Snyder and Mendelson, 1987). A third possible explanation suggested by in vitro studies is that insulin blocks cortisol stimulation of lung structure and type II cell function. Infants of diabetic mothers also have an increased incidence of respiratory distress due to delayed fluid clearance. The mechanism of this abnormality is not known but could relate to either increased cell division or antagonism of glucocorticoid effects in the lung.

The inhibitory effects of insulin on lung development are presumably mediated by plasma membrane receptors. High-affinity binding sites have been described for whole fetal lung tissue and on isolated adult type II cells of the rat. Receptor levels may be influenced by other hormones in the fetus, although down regulation of receptors by insulin appears not to occur. This latter observation could indicate that the fetus of a diabetic pregnancy is subject to both hyperinsulinemia and increased receptor concentration.

EICOSANOIDS

These compounds, which include prostaglandins, thromboxanes, and leukotrienes, are produced from arachidonic acid (released from phospholipids) in the placenta and various fetal tissues. Although many effects of prostaglandins are paracrine, these hormones are present in the circulation, and levels of some (e.g., PGE_2) are much higher in the fetus than the adult, reflecting in part decreased metabolic clearance by the poorly perfused fetal lung. Synthesis of prostaglandins is increased by a variety of stimuli, many of which involve perturbation of cell membrane integrity, and production is inhibited by glucocorticoids (induction of lipocortin, which blocks phospholipase A_2) and drugs such as xanthine derivatives that block synthetic enzymes. Effects of prostaglandins are mediated through membrane receptors (primarily on the cell surface) and, at least in part, by the generation of cAMP.

In addition to their important role in initiation of parturition, prostaglandins have several known effects in maturational events of the cardiopulmonary system. Prostaglandins, in particular PGE_2, maintain the patency of the ductus arteriosus in fetal life; in fetal sheep, sensitivity to PGE_2 decreases during late gestation and in response to glucocorticoid treatment, allowing increased responsiveness to the contracting influence of oxygen (Clyman et al., 1981).

The increased incidence of patent ductus arteriosus in premature infants (and closure with prenatal glucocorticoid and postnatal indomethacin treatment) probably results from changing prostaglandin levels and sensitivity. Prostaglandins also influence the tone of the pulmonary vessels in utero and after birth. Maintenance of pulmonary vasoconstriction in the fetus is due in part to leukotrienes produced within the lung. The rapid fall in pulmonary vascular resistance at the time of birth results in part from the vasodilating effects of prostacyclin as well as other agents (e.g., PGD_2, bradykinin, and histamine) that are released by stretching the lung. Thus, altered prostaglandin production or responsiveness could conceivably contribute to the development of persistent pulmonary hypertension in some newborn infants.

Prostaglandins may also have physiologic roles in other aspects of lung development. Treatment of fetal sheep with inhibitors of prostaglandin synthesis increases fetal breathing movements, and in some studies decreases both the rate of lung fluid production and its surfactant content. In newborn lambs, treatment with PGE_2 produces hyperventilation and apnea (Guarra et al., 1988). In cultured lung tissue, PGE_2 and PGE_1, presumably acting through cAMP, stimulate syntheses of surfactant lipids and surfactant protein A and promote the release of surfactant from type II cells. Thus, endogenous prostaglandins may contribute to lung growth (via fluid production and breathing movements) and maturation of the surfactant system in utero. Conceivably, the administration of inhibitors of prostaglandin synthesis such as tocolytics might adversely affect lung maturation in the human fetus.

ARGININE VASOPRESSIN AND ARGININE VASOTOCIN

Although AVP and AVT are present in the pituitary gland of the human fetus, it is not known whether they have a unique physiologic role in the fetus. In addition to conserving water for the fetus, vasopressin is increased in response to hypoxic stress to levels greater than those occurring with osmolar stimuli. As a stress response hormone, AVP may contribute to maintenance of fetal blood pressure during hemorrhage or hypoxia. Administration of AVP to fetal animals decreases production of fetal lung fluid without affecting fluid osmolarity (Ross et al., 1984; Hooper et al., 1989). This response was greater in older fetuses, indicating developmental changes in responsiveness. Plasma AVP is elevated in infants delivered vaginally compared with cesarean section deliveries, and exposure to labor reduces the incidence of respiratory distress after birth. It is possible, therefore, that increased levels of endogenous AVP or AVT associated with labor and delivery contribute to the clearance of lung water.

ATRIAL NATRIURETIC PEPTIDE

Fluid production, and possibly other lung functions, may be influenced by atrial natriuretic peptide (ANP) which is synthesized and secreted from atrial myocytes under glucocorticoid regulation. Recent studies indicate ANP is also synthesized in pulmonary type II cells of newborn rats, and high-affinity binding sites occur within lung tissue (Matsubara et al., 1988). In fetal sheep, infusion of ANP or saline decreases lung fluid production. In the human, plasma concentrations of ANP are higher in term newborns than in adults and are further elevated in infants with RDS (Shaffer et al., 1986). Thus, ANP, whose levels are regulated by cortisol, may have a developmental influence in fluid production by both the kidney and lung. ANP also has vasorelaxant properties and thus could have an effect on pulmonary blood flow and the occurrence of patent ductus arteriosus in the newborn (Hargrave et al., 1990; Pesonen et al., 1990).

Recent studies indicate that ANP is also synthesized in a number of extra-atrial tissues such as adrenal, gut, pancreas, nerve, and endocrine cells of the adult animal. The presence of ANP receptors in many of these same tissues suggests possible autocrine or paracrine roles of ANP in addition to its regulation of water and salt homeostasis. Possible roles of ANP in developing tissues other than the lung have not yet been investigated.

NEUROPEPTIDES

A variety of regulatory peptides are synthesized and secreted by a diffuse endocrine system of small granule cells of the intestine, pancreas, thyroid, lung, and other organs. Products of these cells are the biogenic amines and neuropeptides such as bombesin (gastrin-releasing peptide), bombesin-related compounds, calcitonin, calcitonin gene–related peptides, leucine enkephalin, somatostatin, and cholecystokinin. The neuroendocrine cells and their products are present in the fetus from early gestation, increase during fetal life, and then generally decline during childhood. The developmental pattern and distribution of these endocrine and paracrine systems suggest that the neuropeptides may have a role in fetal growth and/or development. At present, specific biologic functions have not been defined.

Activin and inhibin are protein hormones, recently

isolated from the adult ovary, which regulate in opposite manner both secretion of follicle-stimulating hormone (FSH) and gonadotropin-mediated steroidogenesis. These hormones may also influence early embryogenesis and cell differentiation in the fetus. For example, activin (also termed "erythroid differentiation factor") and inhibin, acting antagonistically, modulate hemoglobin production in human bone marrow and an erythroid cell line, and expression of the inhibin gene occurs in several tissues other than the ovary (e.g., bone marrow, thymus, placenta, and adrenal cortex).

OTHER HORMONES

Other hormones have less well-defined roles in tissue differentiation. Levels of prolactin are very high in the fetus, increase throughout the third trimester, and correlate with lung maturity (and the occurrence of RDS). In fetal lambs, at least, treatment with prolactin increases the stimulatory effect of T_3 and cortisol on lung development, but prolactin alone has no effect (Schellenberg et al., 1988). Prolactin may also play a role in water regulation in the fetus and across the placenta. A role for α-MSH, derived from proopiomelanocortin (POMC) of the intermediate lobe of the fetal pituitary, in activation of the fetal adrenal has been proposed; this effect may occur before adrenal activation by ACTH. Beta-endorphin, another cleavage product of POMC, is present in fetal serum and levels increase during gestation. This hormone may contribute to the circulatory responses to stress but its role is not well defined.

FETAL GROWTH

Growth of the fetus is determined primarily by genetic factors, the capacity of the mother to provide nutrients, and the ability of the placenta to transfer nutrients. Relatively little is known regarding the role of hormones and growth factors in the complex process of fetal growth. Whereas growth hormone and thyroid hormones are important for postnatal growth, they appear to have no growth-promoting role in utero. In fact, growth retardation is not a feature of anencephaly, which often involves complete absence of hypothalamic and pituitary hormones.

In recent years a number of different and related growth-promoting factors have been identified and studied. The biologic responses to these proteins depend on the target cells and may involve differentiation, stimulation of replication, or growth inhibition. It is likely that tissue growth in the fetus is determined in large part by an interplay of locally produced growth factors. Studies in cell lines indicate that stimulation of cell division requires both competence factors (e.g., platelet-derived growth factor [PDGF] and fibroblast growth factor [FGF]), which render growth-arrested cells capable of entering the cell cycle (G_0 to G_1), and progression factors (e.g., insulin-like growth factors), which promote entry into the DNA synthesis phase of the cell cyle.

Insulin. One fetal hormone known to influence fetal growth is insulin. It is present in the human fetal pancreas and circulation by 10 weeks of gestation and its levels are influenced by the blood glucose concentration. The rare condition of congenital absence of the pancreas is associated with marked reduction in birth length and weight. The syndrome of leprechaunism, which involves a genetic deficiency of insulin receptors and therefore lack of responsiveness, is also characterized by severe growth retardation. In animals, experimental hypoinsulinism leads to fetal growth retardation, and infusion of insulin increases fetal weight and causes organomegaly. Infants of diabetic mothers with poorly controlled disease are often macrosomic, and this overgrowth is not observed when the diabetes is well controlled. In severe diabetes, with vascular disease and decreased uterine blood flood, fetuses are growth retarded due to nutrient deprivation. Infants with the Beckwith-Wiedemann syndrome are macrosomic with generalized organomegaly and appear to be hypersensitive to circulating insulin. The mechanism of insulin action in fetal growth is not fully defined but probably includes a direct stimulation of cell division through insulin receptors (insulin promotes cell division in culture), enhanced glucose and amino acid uptake into cells, and possible interactions with the insulin-like growth factors.

Insulin-Like Growth Factors. Insulin-like growth factors (IGFs, or somatomedins) are a family of proteins that are structurally related to insulin, have some insulin-like metabolic activities, and mediate the action of growth hormone on postnatal growth. They circulate bound to specific binding proteins and act via cell membrane receptors. IGFs and their receptors are present in most fetal tissues (except the brain) and undoubtedly have a role in both organ and somatic growth. There is a correlation between size at birth and levels of IGFs in cord blood consistent with a physiologic role. Production of IGFs by tissues is developmentally controlled and cell specific. For example, in the lung, mRNA for IGFII is high in the fetus, decreases markedly by term, and is not detected in adult lung; by contrast, IGFI mRNA is found in both fetal and adult tissue (Scott et al., 1985). IGFII mRNA is found only in lung mesenchymal cells, indicating the cellular site of synthesis, whereas immunostaining occurs in epithelial cells but not mesenchymal fibroblasts. These and other findings suggest that IGFs are produced by certain cell types (e.g., fibroblasts), secreted, and stimulate proliferation of neighboring cells after binding to cell surface receptors. Agents or hormones that influence either IGFs or their receptors could potentially influence the rate of fetal growth. For example, secretion of IGF by cultured lung tissue is inhibited by cortisol (Stiles and D'Encole, 1990). This finding may reflect one aspect of the general reciprocal relationship between cellular proliferation and differentiation that is modulated by glucocorticoids (i.e., promotion of maturation at the expense of growth).

Epidermal Growth Factor. Epidermal growth factor (EGF) was first identified as a protein from the mouse submaxillary gland, which accelerated eruption of the incisors and eyelid opening in the newborn animal. EGF has generalized effects on epithelial growth and keratinization in several species and in a variety of cell types (mammary epithelial cells, chondrocytes, corneal cells, vascular smooth muscle cells, prostatic cells, glial cells, fibroblasts, and epithelial cells of the female reproductive organs). In vitro, EGF stimulates DNA synthesis in cultured cells. In explant culture of fetal lung, EGF stimulates both cell division and phospholipid biosynthesis. Infusion of EGF into fetuses stimulates epithelial growth in many tissues, with major effects on the weight of the placenta, intestine, kidneys, and adrenals, but does not affect general somatic growth. These observations suggest that endogenous EGF may have a role in growth and maturation of the kidney, adrenal cortex, intestine, and lung.

Nerve Growth Factor. Nerve growth factor (NGF) was also first isolated from mouse salivary glands but has been detected in various tissues, including human placenta. Treatment of chick embryos with NGF increases the size of sensory and sympathetic ganglia due to survival of neurons that normally degenerate. Sympathetic ganglia of newborn animals contain more NGF than adult ganglia and are more responsive in terms of transformation of sympathetic neuroblasts into differentiated neurons. It has been postulated that locally produced NGF is important in the maturation of adrenergic neurons, the sympathetic nervous system, and fetal brain development in general. Administration of T_4 to rats increases NGF in brain and other tissues, suggesting a possible mechanism for postnatal T_4 effects on brain development. NGF and its receptor are also present in the testes of rats but the possible role of EGF in this tissue is not known (Persson et al., 1990).

Other Growth Factors. Basic fibroblast growth factor (B-FGF) and related proteins (A-FGF, K-FGF, int-2, and FGF-5) appear to play an important role in early embryonic induction, angiogenesis of myocardial and vascular disease, and wound healing. They are mitogenic for vascular endothelial cells through an autocrine mechanism and also promote endothelial cell migration and invasion and production of plasminogen activator—all necessary features of angiogenesis in vivo. Platelet-derived growth factor (PDGF), in combination with other growth factors, stimulates division of glial cells, muscle cells, ovarian granulosa cells, pancreatic beta cells, and certain cell types of the immune system.

The transforming growth factors, in particular TGF-beta, have multiple effects on a variety of tissues. For example, TGF-beta stimulates growth and extracellular matrix production by fibroblasts, promotes a switch from chondrocytic to osteoblastic phenotype, and inhibits the synthesis of surfactant components in cultured lung. TGF-beta mRNA appears to be localized to epithelial cells adjacent to the mesenchyme of cartilage, bone, teeth, and other tissues consistent with a paracrine mechanism of action on these connective tissue cells. These findings suggest that TGF-beta may act in the fetus as both a growth stimulator (e.g., of bone) and differentiation inhibitor (e.g., in the lung). It is also conceivable that TGF-beta (and other growth factors) play a role in the disordered growth and repair process that is a part of bronchopulmonary dysplasia in infants.

■ REFERENCES

Ballard, P. L.: Hormonal regulation of pulmonary surfactant. Endocr. Rev. *10*(2):165–181, 1989.

Ballard, R. A.: Antenatal glucocorticoid therapy: Clinical effects. *In* Hormones and Lung Maturation, vol. 28. Monographs on Endocrinology. Berlin, Springer-Verlag, 1986, pp. 137–172.

Ballard, R. A., Ballard, P. L., Creasy, R., et al.: Prenatal thyrotropin-releasing hormone plus corticosteroid decreases chronic lung disease. Clin Res. *38*:192A, 1990.

Ballard, P. L., Hovey, M. L., and Gonzales, L. K.: Thyroid hormone stimulation of phosphatidylcholine synthesis in cultured fetal rabbit lung. J. Clin. Invest. *74*:898–905, 1984.

Barker, P. M., Brown, M. J., Ramsden, C. A., et al.: The effect of thyroidectomy in the fetal sheep on lung liquid readsorption induced by adrenaline or cyclic AMP. J. Physiol. *407*:373–383, 1988.

Barker, P. M., Markiewicz, M., Parker, K. A., et al.: Induction of the adrenaline-dependent reabsorption of lung liquid in the fetal sheep by synergistic action of triiodothyronine and hydrocortisone. Proc. Physiol. Soc. *146P*:137, 1989.

Birk, E., Rudolph, A. M., and Roberts, J. M.: Fetal thyroidectomy reduces postnatal myocardial beta-adrenergic receptor responses in newborn lambs. Pediatr. Res. *23*:431A, 1988.

Bottari, S. P., King, I. N., Liley, H. G., et al.: Changes in G-proteins may determine development of adrenergic sensitivity in human lung. Clin. Res. *36*:239A, 1988.

Cheng, J. B., Goldfien, A., Ballard, P. L., et al.: Glucocorticoids increase pulmonary β-adrenergic receptors in fetal rabbit. Endocrinology *107*:1646–1648, 1980.

Clyman, R. I., Mauray, F., Roman, C., et al.: Glucocorticoids alter the sensitivity of the lamb ductus arteriosus to prostaglandin E₂. J. Pediatr. *98*:126–128, 1981.

Davis, D. J., Dattel, B. J., Ballard, P. L., et al.: β-Adrenergic receptors and cyclic adenosine monophosphate generation in human fetal lung. Pediatr. Res. *21*:142–147, 1987.

Drucker, B. J., Harvey, J., Mamon, B. S., et al.: Oncogenes, growth factors and signal transduction. N. Engl. J. Med. *321*:1383–1391, 1989.

Evans, R. M.: The steroid and thyroid hormone receptor superfamily. Science *240*:889–895, 1988.

Fisher, D. A., and Klein, A. H.: Thyroid development and disorders of thyroid function in the newborn. N. Engl. J. Med. *304*:702–707, 1981.

Gonzales, L. W., and Ballard, P. L.: Identification and characterization of nuclear 3,5,3′-triiodothyronine-binding sites in fetal human lung. J. Clin. Endocrinol. Metab. *53*:21–28, 1981.

Gonzales, L. W., Ballard, P. L., Ertsey, R., et al.: Glucocorticoids and thyroid hormones stimulate biochemical and morphological differentiation of human fetal lung in organ culture. J. Clin. Endocrinol. Metab. *62*:678–691, 1986.

Gross, I., and Wilson, C. M.: Fetal rat lung maturation: Initiation and modulation. J. Appl. Physiol. *55*:1725–1731, 1983.

Guarra, F. A., Savich, R. D., Wallen, K. D., et al.: Prostaglandin E₂ causes hyperventilation and apnea in newborn lambs. J. Appl. Physiol. *64*:2160–2166, 1988.

Hargrave, B., Roman, C., Morville, P., et al.: Pulmonary vascular effects of exogenous atrial natriuretic peptide in sheep fetuses. Pediatr. Res. *27*:140–143, 1990.

Hooper, S. B., Wallace, M. J., and Harding, R.: Development of the lung liquid secretory response to vasopressin in fetal sheep. Fetal and Neonatal Physiology *118A*:7, 1989.

Lefkowitz, R. J., and Caron, M. C.: Adrenergic receptors: Models for the study of receptors coupled to guanine nucleotide regulatory proteins. J. Biol. Chem. *263*:4993–4996, 1988.

Liley, H. G., White, R. T., Warr, R. G., et al.: Regulation of messenger RNAs for the hydrophobic surfactant proteins in human lung. J. Clin. Invest. *83*:1191–1197, 1989.

Matsubara, H., Mori, Y., Umeda, Y., et al.: Atrial natriuretic peptide gene expression and its secretion. Biochem. Biophys. Res. Commun. *156*(2):619–627, 1988.

Morales, W. J., O'Brien, W. F., Angel, J. F., et al.: Fetal lung maturation: The combined use of corticosteroids and thyrotropin-releasing hormone. Obstet. Gynecol. *73*:111–116, 1989.

Murphy, B. E. P.: Human fetal serum cortisol levels related to gestational age: Evidence of a midgestational fall and a steep late gestational rise independent of sex or mode of delivery. Am. J. Obstet. Gynecol. *144*:276–280, 1982.

Nicholas, T. E., Johnson R. G., Lugg, M. A., et al.: Pulmonary phospholipid biosynthesis and the ability of the fetal rabbit lung to reduce cortisone to cortisol during the final ten days of gestation. Life Sci. *22*:1517–1522, 1978.

Nielsen, H. C., Zinman, H. M., and Torday, J. S.: Dihydrotestosterone inhibits fetal rabbit pulmonary surfactant production. J. Clin. Invest. 69:611–919, 1982.

Odom, M. W., Ertsey, R., Ballard, P. L.: Hormonal effects on protein synthesis in human fetal lung. Pediatr. Res. 26:321A, 1989.

Padbury, J. F., and Martinez, A. M.: Sympathoadrenal system activity at birth and integration of postnatal adaptation. Semin. Perinatol. 12:163–172, 1988.

Persson, H., Lievre, C. A-L., Soder, O., et al.: Expression of β-nerve growth factor receptor mRNA in sertoli cells downregulated by testosterone. Science 247:704–707, 1990.

Pesonen, E., Merritt, A. T., Heldt, G., et al.: Correlation of patent ductus arteriosus shunting with plasma atrial natriuretic factor concentration in preterm infants with respiratory distress syndrome. Pediatr. Res. 27:137–139, 1990.

Ross, M. G., Ervin, G., Leake, R. D., et al.: Fetal lung liquid regulation by neuropeptides. Am. J. Obstet. Gynecol. 150:421–425, 1984.

Schellenberg, J. C., Liggins, G. C., Manzai, M. K., et al.: Synergistic hormonal effects on lung maturation in fetal sheep. J. Appl. Physiol. 65:94–100, 1988.

Scott, J., Cowell, J., Robertson, M. E., et al.: Insulin-like growth factor-II gene expression in Wilms' tumour and embryonic tissues. Nature 317:260–262, 1985.

Shaffer, S. G., Geer, P. G., and Goetz, K. L.: Elevated atrial natriuretic factor in neonates with respiratory distress syndrome. J. Pediatr. 109:1028–1033, 1986.

Slotkin, T. A., and Seidler, F. J.: Adrenomedullary catecholamine release in the fetus and newborn: Secretory mechanisms and their role in stress and survival. J. Devel. Physiol. 10:1–16, 1988.

Snyder, J. M., and Mendelson, C. R.: Insulin inhibits the accumulation of the major lung surfactant apoprotein in human fetal lung explants maintained in vitro. Endocrinology 120:1250–1257, 1987.

Stiles, A., and D'Ercole, J.: Insulin-like growth factors and the lung. Am. J. Respir. Cell Molec. Biol. 3:93–100, 1990.

Thomas, A. L., Krane, E. J., and Nathanielsz, P. W.: Changes in the fetal thyroid axis after induction of premature parturition by low-dose continuous intravascular cortisol infusion to the fetal sheep at 130 days of gestation. Endocrinology 103:17–23, 1978.

Ueno, S., Manganaro, T. F., and Donahoe, P. K.: Human recombinant müllerian-inhibiting substance inhibition of rat oocyte meiosis is reversed by epidermal growth factor in vitro. Endocrinology 123:1652–1659, 1988.

Walters, D. V.: The role of β-adrenergic agents in the control of surfactant secretion. Biochem. Soc. Trans. 13:1089–1090, 1985.

Warburton, D., Parton, L., Buckley, S., et al.: Combined effects of corticosteroid, thyroid hormones, and β-receptor binding in fetal lamb lung. Pediatr. Res. 24:166–170, 1988.

■ SUGGESTED READINGS

Albrecht, E. D., and Pepe, G. J.: Placental steroid hormone biosynthesis in primate pregnancy. Endocr. Rev. 11:124–150, 1990.

Ballard, P. L.: Hormones and Lung Maturation, vol. 28. In Monographs on Endocrinology. Berlin, Springer-Verlag, 1986.

Ballard, P. L.: Mechanism of hormone action. In Hoffman (Eds.): Pediatrics. Norwalk, Conn., Appleton & Lange, 1987, pp. 1447–1453.

Ballard, P. L.: Hormonal regulation of pulmonary surfactant. Endocr. Rev. 10:165–181, 1989.

Browne, C. A., and Thorburn, G. D.: Endocrine control of fetal growth. Biol. Neonate 55:331–346, 1989.

Challis, J. R. G., and Brooks, A. N.: Maturation and activation of hypothalamic-pituitary-adrenal function in fetal sheep. Endocr. Rev. 10:182–204, 1989.

Evans, R. M.: The steroid and thyroid hormone receptor superfamily. Science 240:889–895, 1988.

Fisher, D. A.: The unique endocrine milieu of the fetus. J. Clin. Invest. 78:603–611, 1986.

Jones, C. T. (Ed.): The Biochemical Development of the Fetus and Neonate. Oxford, Elsevier Biomedical Press, 1982, pp. 65–619.

Jones, C. T. (Ed.): Perinatal endocrinology. In Baillière's Clinical Endocrinology and Metabolism, vol. 3. London, Baillière Tindall, 1989, pp. 579–886.

Lefkowitz, R. J., and Caron, M. C.: Adrenergic receptors: Models for the study of receptors coupled to guanine nucleotide regulatory proteins. J. Biol. Chem. 263:4993–4996, 1988.

Pepe, G. J., and Albrecht, E. D.: Regulation of the primate fetal adrenal cortex. Endocr. Rev. 11:151–199, 1990.

PRENATAL GENETIC DIAGNOSIS

6

Diana W. Bianchi

As a result of the ever-expanding number of prenatal diagnostic tests that are performed on pregnant women, we know quite a lot about our patients long before we ever touch them. It is the aim of this chapter to discuss the common methods of prenatal genetic diagnosis, the information they convey, and the implications for the newborn.

■ MATERNAL SERUM ALPHA-FETOPROTEIN SCREENING

Maternal alpha-fetoprotein (AFP) screening is rapidly becoming part of routine obstetric care. It is used to identify a high-risk pregnancy in a low-risk population. AFP is one of the major proteins in fetal serum. Its precise physiologic role is currently unknown. It can be detected as early as 4 weeks' gestation, when it is synthesized by the yolk sac (Bergstrand, 1986). Subsequently, it is produced in the fetal liver and peaks in the fetal serum between 10 and 13 weeks' gestation. AFP is then excreted into the fetal urine or leaks into the amniotic fluid through the skin prior to keratinization at 20 weeks. It is also present in cerebrospinal fluid. AFP in maternal serum is exclusively fetal in origin (Crandall, 1981). Maternal serum AFP peaks at 32 weeks' gestation owing to increased placental permeability for the protein (Ferguson-Smith, 1983). Most clinical assays are performed at 16 weeks' gestation. Accurate gestational dating and maternal weight are critical to the interpretation of results.

In 1972, Brock and Sutcliffe observed that there were markedly increased levels of AFP in the amniotic fluid of fetuses with anencephaly and open neural tube defects. Subsequently, it was shown that elevated amniotic fluid AFP levels were associated with increased maternal serum AFP (Ferguson-Smith, 1983). The possibility of a screening test for open neural tube defects became apparent. In the initial collaborative efforts aimed at studying maternal serum AFP, results were expressed as multiples of the median (MoM) to allow comparison between laboratories. It is now a convention to describe results >2.5 MoM as abnormally high and <0.6 as abnormally low. Both require further investigation.

If the AFP is elevated, many physicians opt to repeat the test before advancing to more invasive procedures. In some medical centers, the patient is offered an ultrasonographic examination to verify gestational age, determine fetal viability, and diagnose many of the structural abnormalities that can be associated with an elevated AFP. Although the AFP test was developed to screen for neural tube defects, abnormally high results are not specific for

this condition (Table 6–1). If the ultrasonographic examination is unrevealing, the patient undergoes amniocentesis to assay the amniotic fluid for the presence of AFP and acetylcholinesterase, which are elevated in open spina bifida (Crandall et al., 1983). While an elevated AFP is compatible with a normal diagnosis, a study of 277 infants with elevated maternal serum AFP and normal amniotic fluid AFP revealed an increased incidence of intrauterine growth retardation and non–neural tube anomalies (Burton and Dillard, 1986).

More recently, maternal serum AFP screening has been utilized to detect chromosomally abnormal fetuses, following an observation that a low AFP value was more likely in a trisomy 18 or 21 fetus than in a normal fetus (Merkatz et al., 1984). Several prospective studies have demonstrated that, by expressing risk for Down syndrome as a combined function of maternal age and AFP value, and offering amniocentesis to all women with a risk of 1:270 or greater (the equivalent risk in a 35-year-old woman based on age alone), about a third of otherwise unexpected Down syndrome fetuses will be detected (Dimaio et al., 1987; Palomaki and Haddow, 1987). The etiology of low AFP values is probably due to decreased hepatic production in the affected fetus. Although it would make sense to ascribe this to a small liver, a recent study found no association between fetal weight and low AFP values in chromosomally abnormal fetuses (Librach et al., 1988). The differential diagnosis of a decreased AFP level is shown in Table 6–2. Since a low AFP value detects only a third of Down syndrome fetuses, a normal AFP value does not rule out trisomy 21. Abnormal levels of other placental products are associated with an increased risk for chromosome abnormalities. In particular, persistently elevated levels of human chorionic gonadotropin are found in the serum of women carrying fetuses with trisomy 21 (Bogart et al., 1987).

■ ULTRASONOGRAPHY

The routine use of ultrasound imaging in pregnancy has been controversial (Bakketeig et al., 1984; Eik-Neis et al., 1984). Nevertheless, it remains the best noninvasive method for gestational dating, definition of fetal anatomy, serial measurements of fetal growth, and evaluation of dynamic parameters such as cardiac contractility, fetal urine production, and fetal movement. Additionally, it has been suggested that antenatal visualization of the fetus promotes maternal-infant bonding (Fletcher and Evans, 1983). Despite controversies, it has been estimated that 40 per cent of obstetric patients undergo at least one ultrasonographic examination during pregnancy (Hill et

TABLE 6–1. Differential Diagnosis of an Abnormally High Maternal Serum Alpha-Fetoprotein

Incorrect gestational dating
Multiple pregnancy
Threatened abortion
Fetomaternal hemorrhage
Anencephaly
Open spina bifida
Anterior abdominal wall defects
Congenital nephrosis
Acardia
Lesions of the placenta and umbilical cord
Turner syndrome
Cystic hygroma
Renal agenesis
Polycystic kidney disease
Epidermolysis bullosa
Hereditary persistence (AD trait)

al., 1983). The advent of antenatal ultrasonography has had a large impact on the types of patients who present to the neonatal intensive care unit.

It is beyond the scope of this chapter to discuss the numerous indications for ultrasonography. Within the context of prenatal genetic diagnosis, ultrasonography may be utilized to detect congenital anomalies. In 2 to 3 per cent of live births, a malformation is present (Nelson and Holmes, 1989). In approximately 10 per cent of infants with anomalies, the central nervous system is involved (Hill et al., 1983). Ultrasonography is particularly useful in the diagnosis of anencephaly, microcephaly, encephalocele, and hydrocephalus. By 20 weeks' gestation, the fetal facial structures may be examined for cyclopia, cleft lip, or micrognathia. A nuchal fat pad is suggestive of Down syndrome (Benacerraf et al., 1987), whereas cystic hygroma may be seen in Turner syndrome, Noonan syndrome, familial pterygium colli, or chromosome abnormalities (Chervenak et al., 1983). The cardiovascular structures may be reliably examined after 20 weeks' gestation. The presence of four cardiac chambers, the dynamic relationships between the cardiac valves, and the location of the vessels allow such diagnoses as hypoplastic left heart, double outlet right ventricle, tricuspid atresia, tetralogy of Fallot, and Ebstein anomaly to be made. Pericardial effusion and arrhythmias may be similarly observed.

Gastrointestinal anomalies occur in about 0.6 per cent of live births, and one-third of them are associated with chromosome abnormalities (Barss et al., 1985). The decrease in fetal swallowing seen in some cases of bowel obstruction (from atresia, stenosis, annular pancreas, or diaphragmatic hernia) may lead to polyhydramnios that results in a uterine size greater than expected for gestational dates. Although gastroschisis and omphalocele are readily diagnosed, they may be confused with each other, and their differing prognoses may cause considerable parental anxiety (Griffiths and Gough, 1985). Gastroschisis usually occurs as an isolated anomaly; infants do

TABLE 6–2. Differential Diagnosis of Abnormally Low Maternal Serum Alpha-Fetoprotein

Incorrect gestational dating
Trisomy 21
Trisomy 18
Intrauterine growth retardation

well after surgical repair. The kidneys are identifiable by 14 weeks' gestation, but the presence of perirenal fat and large adrenals may obscure the diagnosis of renal agenesis (Hill et al., 1983). Renal cysts, hydronephrosis, and obstructive uropathy are easily visualized. Oligohydramnios is indicative of poor renal function. Multiple standard curves now exist for fetal anthropometric measurements (Elejalde and Elejalde, 1986; Saul et al., 1988). These are particularly helpful in the diagnosis of skeletal dysplasias and evaluation of growth retardation. Fetal genitalia may be reliably determined by 24 weeks' gestation (Birnholz, 1983). Additionally, ultrasonographic examination is of benefit in the diagnosis and management of multiple pregnancies (Fig. 6–1).

Although there have been no documented adverse outcomes related to ultrasound exposure during human pregnancy, the reported experimental biologic effects of altered immune response, cell death, change in cell membrane functions, free radical formation, and reduced cell reproductive potential prompted an NIH consensus panel to recommend against routine ultrasonographic screening (NIH Consensus Development Panel, 1984). This is an area where further study is necessary.

The accuracy of ultrasonographic diagnosis has been addressed in several papers. In one study of 1737 referrals, 244 malformations were correctly diagnosed. Six results were falsely called abnormal (0.3 per cent), and 16 were incorrectly called normal (0.9 per cent) (Campbell and Pearce, 1983). In 596 women referred for ultrasonography, 81 had fetal anomalies diagnosed, with a falsely abnormal rate of 0.6 per cent and a falsely normal rate of 0.5 per cent (Sabbagha et al., 1985). The limitations of ultrasonography were delineated in a study correlating anatomic pathology at autopsy with prenatal diagnosis (Rutledge et al., 1986). Fifty-two malformations in 45 fetuses were correctly diagnosed antenatally, but 90 additional malformations were missed.

Finally, continuous ultrasonographic fetal imaging is important in improvement of the safety and efficacy of the more invasive diagnostic procedures such as amniocentesis, chorionic villus sampling, and percutaneous umbilical blood sampling, which are discussed in the following sections.

■ AMNIOCENTESIS

Amniocentesis refers to the removal of up to 20 ml of amniotic fluid from the pregnant uterus between 11 and 17 weeks' gestation. Contained within this fluid are cellular components (desquamated fetal epithelial and macrophage-like cells), which serve as a source of chromosomes, DNA, or enzymes. The majority of these cellular elements are nonviable. Hence, amniocytes generally require tissue culture under specific conditions to provide enough material for diagnosis (Gosden, 1983). Herein lies one of the major disadvantages of the procedure—results are received late in the second trimester after fetal quickening has occurred. In contrast, the amniotic fluid itself may be assayed immediately after removal for the presence of alpha-fetoprotein, acetylcholinesterase, bilirubin, lecithin, sphingomyelin, or phosphatidylcholine.

The indications for genetic amniocentesis are: (1) maternal age ≥35 years at the time of conception because

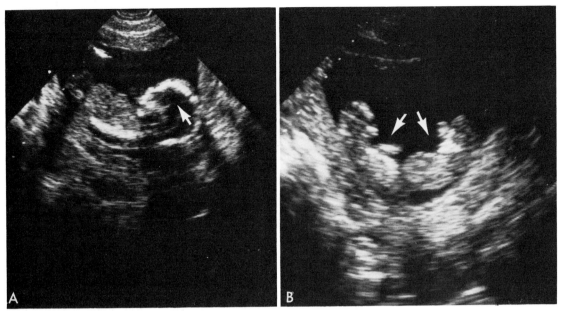

FIGURE 6–1. Appearance on ultrasonographic examination (B-mode scan, 5.0 MHz) of a singleton pregnancy (A) at approximately 4 months' gestation and a twin pregnancy (B) at approximately 12 weeks' gestation. The arrow in A points to the fetal cranium; the arrows in B indicate the fetuses. (Courtesy of Dr. Jason Birnholz.)

of the increased risk for fetal chromosome abnormalities, (2) a previous pregnancy that resulted in an infant with chromosome abnormalities, (3) either parent with a balanced chromosome translocation, (4) an abnormally high or low maternal serum alpha-fetoprotein level, (5) a family history of a child with a neural tube defect, (6) a family history of a metabolic disorder for which the enzyme defect is known, (7) a maternal history of X-linked disorder, or (8) a family history of a disorder for which DNA diagnosis is available.

Extensive clinical experience with amniocentesis has accrued since the results of the first large-scale randomized trials were published in the 1970s (National Institute of Child Health and Human Development [NICHHD] National Registry, 1976; Simpson et al., 1976). Most institutions in the United States currently quote a 1 to 2 per cent incidence of minor complications, such as amniotic fluid leakage, uterine cramping, or vaginal spotting, following the procedure; a 0.5 to 1.0 per cent incidence of more serious complications, such as chorioamnionitis and miscarriage, also exists. There is a significant inverse relationship between procedural experience and risk of miscarriage (Verjaal and Leschot, 1981).

In a series of 3000 amniocenteses performed at a single institution over 8 years, there was a diagnostic accuracy rate of over 99 per cent. Chromosome abnormalities were detected in 2.4 per cent of 2404 women with advanced maternal age, 1.2 per cent of 240 women who had previously had an infant with trisomy 21, and 9.1 per cent of 55 women with other cytogenetic indications (Golbus et al., 1979).

With amniocentesis, since results are received relatively late in the pregnancy, research efforts have focused on evaluation of the procedure if performed between 12 and 15 weeks' gestation. At the present time, there are no significantly increased risks associated with early amniocentesis (Nevin et al., 1990). Despite the fact that a smaller amount of amniotic fluid is withdrawn, there does not

appear to be any increased difficulty in obtaining enough cells to make a diagnosis (Hanson et al., 1987). In many medical centers, early amniocentesis is being offered as an alternative to chorionic villus sampling.

■ CHORIONIC VILLUS SAMPLING

Despite the wealth of experience with amniocentesis, its usefulness has been somewhat limited by the timing of the procedure, as previously discussed. Since the publication of the first English language report on sampling of the chorion (Kazy et al., 1982), there has been enormous medical and scientific interest in first-trimester prenatal diagnosis.

Chorionic villus sampling (CVS) involves the aspiration of the chorion frondosum between 9 and 11 weeks' gestation (Fig. 6–2). The fact that the procedure is performed so early is an advantage, as most women at this point do not have external manifestations of pregnancy and have not yet perceived fetal movement. The chorionic villi are composed of syncytiotrophoblast and mesenchymal core cells that are actively growing and dividing. In contrast to the dying epithelial cells shed into the amniotic fluid, chorionic villus cells do not require prolonged culture to provide enough mitoses for a cytogenetic diagnosis. Karyotype results are generally available within one week of the procedure. Initially, direct preparations derived from syncytiotrophoblasts were used for analysis, but the number of false-positive results proved unacceptable. Cultured preparations derived from the cells of the mesenchymal core are more closely related in embryonic origin to the actual fetus; however, they too carry a small risk of falsely abnormal results. It is currently recommended that both direct and cultured preparations be utilized for cytogenetic analysis. *Mosaicism*, defined as the presence of two or more cell lines carrying different chromosomal constitutions, is a true biologic (not technical) problem in CVS. In one large study, 1.7 per cent of 1000 cases had a chromosome abnormality that was present in the villus but not in the fetus (Hogge et al., 1986).

The indications for CVS are the same as those for amniocentesis with two exceptions: neural tube defects cannot be diagnosed by this procedure, and AFP screening is not routinely offered at this point in gestation. In fact, there is evidence showing that the fetomaternal hemorrhage associated with placental biopsy results in elevated maternal serum AFP immediately after the procedure (Brambati et al., 1988).

CVS is performed by one of two methods. International experience has accumulated with the transcervical technique, but the inherent risks of fetal and maternal infection appear to be greater due to the impossibility of sterilizing the cervix. Under ultrasonic guidance, a flexible catheter is passed through the endocervix and placed into the chorion frondosum. A small segment of placenta is then aspirated into sterile tissue culture medium and the catheter is withdrawn (Jackson, 1985). In contrast, the transabdominal technique uses a needle to obtain villus material; sterilization of the skin surface is straightforward (Brambati et al., 1988). With either method, about 10 to 50 mg of tissue are obtained. Subsequently, the villi are dissected from maternal decidua and processed for tissue culture or DNA extraction.

The safety and accuracy of these relatively new techniques are being closely monitored. A randomized NIH clinical trial compared amniocentesis with CVS (Rhoads et al., 1989). Also, an international newsletter published the results of ongoing experience with CVS. As of January

TABLE 6–3. Chorionic Villus Sampling—Advantages and Disadvantages as Compared with Amniocentesis

Advantages
Performed in first trimester—results available quickly
Cells obtained are mitotically active
Amount of tissue obtained is preferable for DNA analysis
Disadvantages
Miscarriage rate possibly higher
Increased fetomaternal hemorrhage following procedure
Risk of isoimmunization
One per cent incidence of chromosomal mosaicism
Risk of serious maternal infection

1990, 67,288 patients had undergone the procedure. About half of these have delivered infants without an increased number of congenital anomalies or percentage of premature births. The risks of miscarriage after CVS are 3.0 per cent overall, with 3.4 per cent transcervical and 2.5 per cent transabdominal (Jackson, 1990).

The advantages and disadvantages of CVS are summarized in Table 6–3. For patients at high risk for single gene disorders amenable to DNA diagnosis (e.g., cystic fibrosis, sickle cell anemia, or Duchenne muscular dystrophy), CVS is probably the preferred prenatal diagnostic method. On the other hand, for patients with relatively low risk (e.g., a 35-year-old woman being tested for chromosome abnormalities), an amniocentesis may be more appropriate. It is of concern that there have been several reports of serious maternal sepsis associated with transcervical CVS (Blakemore et al., 1985; Barela et al., 1986). The 1 per cent incidence of mosaicism in villus samples may necessitate further invasive techniques such as umbilical blood sampling to confirm or refute diagnoses. While the prospects of first-trimester diagnosis are genuinely exciting, more information is needed on the long-term implications for the fetus and neonate.

■ PERIPHERAL UMBILICAL BLOOD SAMPLING

Peripheral umbilical blood sampling (PUBS) was first described as a means of obtaining fetal immunoglobulin M (IgM) values in the diagnosis of congenital toxoplasmosis (Daffos et al., 1985). Under continuous ultrasonographic imaging, the insertion site of the umbilical cord into the placenta is identified. Using a 20-gauge needle, the umbilical vein is punctured, the sample is withdrawn, and the umbilical cord is observed for signs of hemorrhage. The technique has been used diagnostically in many clinical settings (Table 6–4) (Forestier et al., 1988). With regard to genetic diagnosis, the lymphocytes are a source of cells for a rapid karyotype. This is helpful in two situations: (1) when anomalies have been noted on ultra-

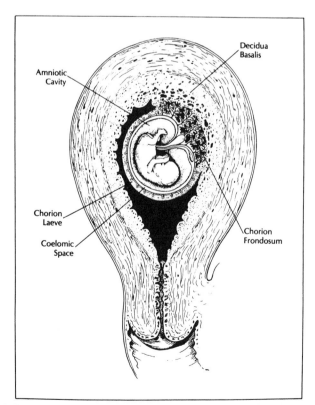

FIGURE 6–2. *A pregnant uterus containing a fetus at about 9 weeks' gestation. The chorion frondosum, if biopsied, can provide fetal cells for chromosome, enzyme, or DNA analysis. (From Jackson, L.G.: First trimester diagnosis of fetal genetic disorders. Hosp. Prac., March 15, 1985, p. 40.)*

TABLE 6–4. Indications for Fetal Blood Sampling

Diagnosis of:
   Hemoglobinopathies
   Bleeding disorders
   Immunodeficiency
   Congenital infection
   Acid-base abnormalities
   Fetal blood type incompatibility
   Metabolic disorders
   Chromosome abnormalities

sonographic examination but it is too late in gestation to perform an amniocentesis (antenatal diagnosis of trisomy 13 or 18 influences delivery room management), and (2) for confirmation of a fetal karyotype when amniocentesis or CVS has shown mosaicism (Gosden et al., 1988).

■ FUTURE DIRECTIONS

All nucleated fetal cells from the same individual contain identical genetic information. As a result of this fact, research efforts are focused on noninvasive methods for fetal cell isolation. An attractive potential population are the rare fetal cells that cross the placenta and circulate. Fetal gene sequences have been detected in circulating nucleated erythrocytes obtained from maternal venous blood samples at 16 weeks' gestation (Bianchi et al., 1990).

■ REFERENCES

Bakketeig, L. S., Eik-Neis, S. H., Jacobsen, G., et al.: Randomised controlled trial of ultrasonographic screening in pregnancy. Lancet 2:207, 1984.

Barela, A. I., Kleinman, G. E., Golditch, I. M., et al.: Septic shock with renal failure after chorionic villus sampling. Am. J. Obstet. Gynecol. 154:1100, 1986.

Barss, V. A., Benacerraf, B. R., and Frigoletto, F. D.: Antenatal sonographic diagnosis of fetal gastrointestinal malformations. Pediatrics 76:445, 1985.

Benacerraf, B. R., Gelman, R., and Frigoletto, F. D.: Sonographic identification of second trimester fetuses with Down's syndrome. N. Engl. J. Med. 317:1371, 1987.

Bergstrand, C. G.: Alphafetoprotein in paediatrics. Acta Paediatr. Scand. 75:1, 1986.

Bianchi, D. W., Flint, A. F., Pizzimenti, M. F., et al.: Isolation of fetal DNA from nucleated erythrocytes in maternal blood. Proc. Natl. Acad. Sci. USA 87:3279, 1990.

Birnholz, J. C.: Determination of fetal sex. N. Engl. J. Med. 309:942, 1983.

Blakemore, K. J., Mahoney, M. J., and Hobbins, J. C.: Infection and chorionic villus sampling. Lancet 2:338, 1985.

Bogart, M. H., Pandian, M. R., and Jones, O. W.: Abnormal maternal serum chorionic gonadotropin levels in pregnancies with fetal chromosome abnormalities. Prenat. Diagn. 7:623, 1987.

Brambati, B., Lanzani, A., and Oldrini, A.: Transabdominal chorionic villus sampling. Clinical experience of 1159 cases. Prenat. Diagn. 8:609, 1988.

Brock, D. J. H., and Sutcliffe, R. G.: Alpha feto protein in the antenatal diagnosis of anencephaly and spina bifida. Lancet 2:197, 1972.

Burton, B. K., and Dillard, R. G.: Outcome in infants born to mothers with unexplained elevations of maternal serum alphafetoprotein. Pediatrics 77:582, 1986.

Campbell, S., and Pearce, J. M.: Ultrasound visualization of congenital malformations. Br. Med. Bull. 39:322, 1983.

Chervenak, F. A., Isaacson, G., and Blakemore, K. J.: Fetal cystic hygroma. Cause and natural history. N. Engl. J. Med. 309:822, 1983.

Crandall, B. F.: Alpha-fetoprotein: The diagnosis of neural tube defects. Pediatr. Ann. 10:38, 1981.

Crandall, B. F., Robertson, R. D., and Lebherz, T. B.: Maternal serum alpha-fetoprotein screening for the detection of neural tube defects. West. J. Med. 138:524, 1983.

Daffos, F., Capella-Pavlovsky, M., and Forestier, F.: Fetal blood sampling during pregnancy with use of a needle guided by ultrasound: A study of 606 consecutive cases. Am. J. Obstet. Gynecol. 153:655, 1985.

Dimaio, M. S., Baumgarten, A., Greenstein, R. M., et al.: Screening for fetal Down's syndrome in pregnancy by measuring maternal serum alphafetoprotein levels. N. Engl. J. Med. 317:342, 1987.

Eik-Neis, S. H., Okland, O., Aure, J. C., et al.: Ultrasound screening in pregnancy: A randomised controlled trial. Lancet 1:1347, 1984.

Elejalde, B. R., and Elejalde, M. M.: The prenatal growth of the human body determined by the measurement of bones and organs by ultrasonography. Am. J. Med. Genet. 24:575, 1986.

Ferguson-Smith, M. A.: The reduction of anencephalic and spina bifida births by maternal serum alpha-fetoprotein screening. Br. Med. Bull. 39:365, 1983.

Fletcher, J. C., and Evans, M. I.: Maternal bonding in early fetal ultrasound examinations. N. Engl. J. Med. 308:392, 1983.

Forestier, F., Cox, W. L., Daffos, F., et al.: The assessment of fetal blood samples. Am. J. Obstet. Gynecol. 158:1184, 1988.

Golbus, M. S., Longman, W. D., Epstein, C. J., et al.: Prenatal genetic diagnosis in 3000 amniocenteses. N. Engl. J. Med. 300:157, 1979.

Gosden, C. M.: Amniotic fluid cell types and culture. Br. Med. Bull. 39:348, 1983.

Gosden, C., Nicolaides, K. H., and Rodeck, C. H.: Fetal blood sampling in investigation of chromosome mosaicism in amniotic fluid cell culture. Lancet 1:613, 1988.

Griffiths, D. M., and Gough, M. H.: Dilemmas after ultrasonographic diagnosis of fetal abnormality. Lancet 1:623, 1985.

Hanson, F. W., Zorn, E. M., and Tennant, F. R.: Amniocentesis before 15 weeks' gestation: Outcome, risks, and technical problems. Am. J. Obstet. Gynecol. 156:1524, 1987.

Hill, L. M., Breckle, R., and Gehrking, W. C.: The prenatal detection of congenital malformations by ultrasonography. Mayo. Clin. Proc. 58:805, 1983.

Hogge, W. A., Schonberg, S. A., and Golbus, M. S.: Chorionic villus sampling: Experience of the first 1000 cases. Am. J. Obstet. Gynecol. 154:1249, 1986.

Jackson, L. G.: First trimester diagnosis of fetal genetic disorders. Hosp. Prac., March 15, 1985, p. 39.

Jackson, L. G.: CVS Newsletter No. 29, January 1988.

Kazy, Z., Rozovsky, I. S., and Bakharev, V. A.: Chorion biopsy in early pregnancy: A method of early prenatal diagnosis for inherited disorders. Prenat. Diagn. 2:39, 1982.

Librach, C. L., Hogdall C. K., and Doran, T. A.: Weights of fetuses with autosomal trisomies at termination of pregnancy: An investigation of the etiologic factors of low serum alphafetoprotein values. Am. J. Obstet. Gynecol. 158:290, 1988.

Merkatz, I. R., Nitowsky H. M., Macri, J. N., et al.: An association between low maternal serum alphafetoprotein and fetal chromosome abnormalities. Am. J. Obstet. Gynecol. 148:886, 1984.

Nelson, K., and Holmes, L. B.: Malformations due to presumed spontaneous mutations in newborn infants. N. Engl. J. Med. 320:19, 1989.

Nevin, J., Nevin, N. C., Dornan, J. C., et al.: Early amniocentesis: Experience of 222 consecutive patients, 1987–1988. Prenat. Diagn. 10:79, 1990.

National Institute of Child Health and Human Development (NICHHD) National Registry: Midtrimester amniocentesis for prenatal diagnosis: Safety and accuracy. J.A.M.A. 236:1471, 1976.

NIH Consensus Development Panel: The use of diagnostic ultrasound imaging during pregnancy. J.A.M.A. 252:669, 1984.

Palomaki, G. E., and Haddow, J. E.: Maternal serum alphafetoprotein, age, and Down syndrome risk. Am. J. Obstet. Gynecol. 156:460, 1987.

Rhoads, G., Jackson, L., Schlesselman, S., et al.: The safety and efficacy of chorionic villus sampling for early prenatal diagnosis of cytogenetic abnormalities. N. Engl. J. Med. 320:609, 1989.

Rutledge, J. C., Weinberg, A. G., and Friedman, J. M.: Anatomic correlates of ultrasonographic prenatal diagnosis. Prenat. Diagn. 6:51, 1986.

Sabbagha, R. E., Sheikh, Z., Tamura, R., et al.: Predictive value, sensitivity, and specificity of ultrasonic targeted imaging for fetal anomalies in gravid women at high risk for birth defects. Am. J. Obstet. Gynecol. 152:822, 1985.

Saul, R. A., Stevenson, R. E., Rogers, R. C., et al.: Growth references from conception to adulthood. Proc. Greenwood Genetic Ctr. Supplement 1, 1988.

Simpson, N. E., Dallaire, L., Miller J. R., et al.: Prenatal diagnosis of genetic disease in Canada: Report of a collaborative study. Can. Med. Assoc. J. 115:739, 1976.

Verjaal, M., and Leschot, N. J.: Risk of amniocentesis and laboratory findings in a series of 1500 prenatal diagnoses. Prenat. Diagn. 1:173, 1981.

PLACENTAL FUNCTION AND DISEASES: THE PLACENTA, FETAL MEMBRANES, AND UMBILICAL CORD

Mary Ellen Avery*

The placenta, an essential and unique organ in the mammalian reproductive system, is the only fetal tissue whose sole function is to provide an optimal environment for fetal growth. It has a life span of approximately 266 days in the human, during which time it must grow, differentiate, serve as the organ of fetal gas exchange, provide nutrients for fetal growth, and regulate both fetal and maternal metabolism by means of its own hormone production. To support its own growth and metabolism, the placenta utilizes about one-third of the oxygen and glucose delivered to the uterus via the maternal circulation.

Throughout its life span the placenta differentiates in a manner that adapts to the changing requirements of the fetus. For example, the uptake rates of glucose and amino acids per gram of placental weight increase toward term. Trace minerals are also transported in increased amounts toward term even after placental growth has slowed or ceased. Additionally, maternal immunoglobulins are transported to the human fetus in the last trimester in preparation for the transition to extrauterine life and serve to protect the fetus and newborn against many infectious agents.

This complex organ, so central in fetal life, is now the object of intense study. The reader should refer to Diczfalusy (1985) and Redline and Driscoll (1989) for an overview on placental function.

■ ANATOMY OF THE PLACENTA

The human placenta at term is a disc-like, roughly circular organ that weighs approximately 500 g or about 17% of fetal weight (after the cord and membranes have been excised). It measures 15 to 20 cm in diameter, and is 2 to 3 cm thick. About half the weight of the placenta represents maternal blood and about 15 per cent represents fetal blood. The insertion of the cord varies and may be central, marginal, or incorporated into the fetal mem-

branes (velamentous). Figure 7–1 shows the development of the placenta in the uterus through gestation.

The placenta is of extraembryonic origin. Within 72 hours of fertilization, differentiation of the blastula occurs yielding five embryo-producing cells and 53 cells that are destined to form trophoblasts. After implantation the trophoblasts proliferate rapidly and invade the surrounding endometrium, which forms the decidua (later shed at parturition). As the invasion of the endometrium by the trophoblasts proceeds, the maternal blood vessels are eroded and form lacunar spaces filled with maternal blood. The vascular channels are lined with trophoblasts and solid cellular columns grow into the lacunar space to form primary villous stalks. The villi may be seen in the placenta as early as the 12th day after fertilization. Angiogenesis occurs within the mesenchymal cores of the villi, so that by the 17th day both the fetal and maternal blood vessels are functional and the placental circulation is established when the fetal heart can pump blood. Since the human maternal blood is in direct contact with the placental villous surface, the placenta is classified as hemochorial.

The villi that contact the decidua basalis proliferate to form the chorion frondosum, or fetal discoid placenta, whereas those that contact the decidua parietalis degenerate to form the chorion laeve. Some of the villi extend from the chorionic plate to the decidua and serve as anchoring villi. Others branch and end freely in the intervillous space. At the end of the third month the chorion laeve and its adjacent amnion form an avascular membrane that serves solute and fluid transport as well as prostaglandin formation near the time of onset of labor.

The principal cell type associated with placental function is the trophoblast. The villous trophoblast may be mononuclear (cytotrophoblast) or multinuclear (syncytiotrophoblast). Cytotrophoblasts are known to coalesce to form multinucleated syncytiotrophoblasts, which cover the surface of the villi. It is the latter that are the most active in the production of placental hormones and the initial sites of nutrient transport from the mother to the fetus.

As gestation progresses and the placenta ages, the syncytiotrophoblasts predominate as the cytotrophoblasts

*I am grateful to Professor Maureen Young and Drs. Dorothy Villee, Raymond Redline, Elliott Main, and Michael Fant for their suggestions and review of the manuscript.

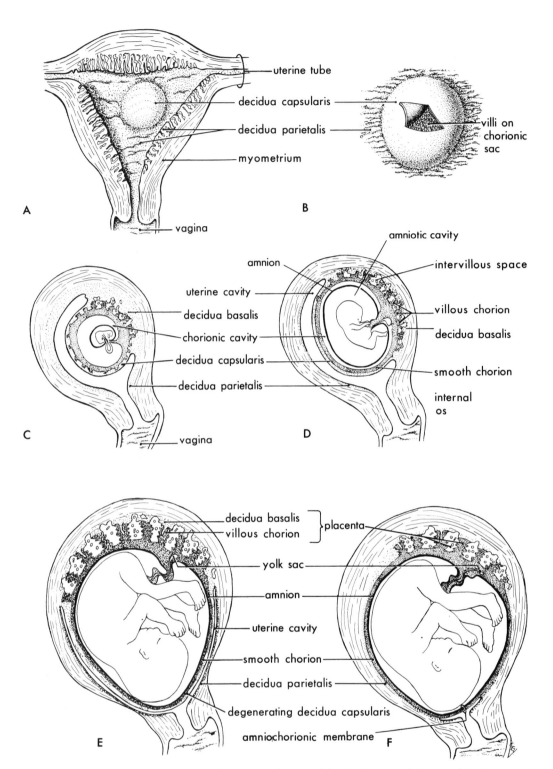

FIGURE 7–1. A, Drawing of a frontal section of the uterus showing the elevation of the decidua capsularis caused by the expanding chorionic sac of a 4-week embryo, implanted in the endometrium on the posterior wall. B, Enlarged drawing of the implantation site. The chorionic villi have been exposed by cutting an opening in the decidua capsularis. C to F, Drawings of sagittal sections of the gravid uterus from the 4th to 22nd weeks, showing the changing relations of the fetal membranes to the decidua. In F, the amnion and chorion are fused with each other and the decidua parietalis, thereby obliterating the uterine cavity. Note that the villi persist only where the chorion is associated with the decidua basalis; here they form the villous chorion (fetal portion of the placenta). (From Moore, K.L.: The Developing Human: Clinically Oriented Embryology, 4th ed. Philadelphia, W. B. Saunders Company, 1988.)

undergo terminal differentiation. Fetal capillaries are also oriented closer to the basement membrane underlying the syncytium.

■ PLACENTAL CIRCULATION

The placenta serves as the organ of gas exchange, nutrient transfer, and excretion of metabolic wastes for the fetus. Consequently, it receives more than 50 per cent of the cardiac output of the fetus. Maternal arterial blood reaches the placenta through funnel-shaped openings in the chorionic plate under slightly reduced arterial pressure. The blood enters the intervillous space in spurts and bathes the chorionic villi of the placenta. The fetal blood flows through the placenta through the two umbilical arteries that carry desaturated blood from the fetus to the capillary bed of the finger-like villi. The vessels form a dense capillary network in the terminal divisions of the villi, which are perfused by the better oxygenated blood from the maternal circulation. The oxygenated blood that leaves the villi exits the placenta via the umbilical vein and returns to the fetus through the ductus venosus (Figs. 7–2 and 7–3).

Optimal placental function, therefore, is dependent upon both the maternal and fetal components of its circulation. For example, clinical conditions associated with decreased uterine blood flow such as maternal hypertension lead to decreased nutrient delivery to the placenta and subsequent growth retardation of both the placenta and the fetus. The regulation of both the maternal and fetal components of the placental circulation are areas of active investigation.

■ PLACENTAL IMMUNOLOGY

The fetus can be regarded as a "natural transplant" that the mother tolerates throughout gestation. In general, the fetal circulation is separate from the maternal circulation, although it is evident that minute communications between the two circulations can occur. Numerous studies have shown that some maternal cells enter the fetal circulation and fetal cells enter the maternal circulation. In addition to red cells, maternal leukocytes and platelets have been found crossing the placenta from mother to fetus, and enough lymphocytes can pass into the fetus to cause a graft-versus-host reaction, although very rarely.

Several theories have been set forth to explain maternal tolerance of the fetal presence. The fetus is immunologically immature but still capable of producing antibodies very early in life. Likewise, the mother during pregnancy has in some respects moderately diminished immunologic capacity. She is, however, certainly capable of producing antifetal antibodies. An example occurs in erythroblastosis fetalis where maternal antibodies to fetal red cells cross the placenta and produce hemolysis in the fetus.

Active immunoregulation may prevent the mother from recognizing and responding to fetal antigens. For example, maternal and fetal lymphocytes have reduced responses

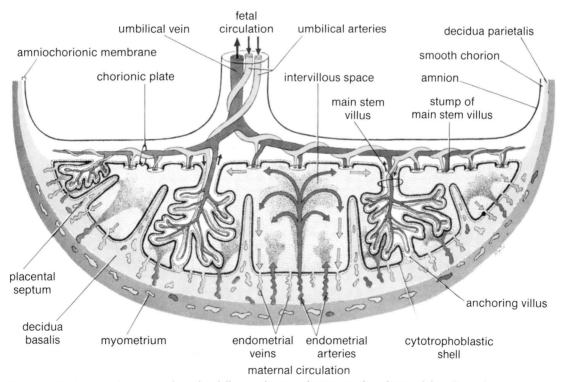

FIGURE 7–2. Schematic drawing of a section through a full-term placenta, showing (1) the relation of the villous chorion (fetal placenta) to the decidua basalis (maternal placenta), (2) the fetal placental circulation, and (3) the maternal placental circulation. Maternal blood flows into the intervillous spaces in funnel-shaped spurts, and exchanges occur with the fetal blood as the maternal blood flows around the villi. The in-flowing arterial blood pushes venous blood out into the endometrial veins, which are scattered over the entire surface of the decidua basalis. Note that the umbilical arteries carry deoxygenated fetal blood to the placenta and that the umbilical vein carries oxygenated blood to the fetus. Note that the cotyledons are separated from each other by decidual septa of the maternal portion of the placenta. Each cotyledon consists of two or more main stem villi and their many branches. In this drawing only one main stem villus is shown in each cotyledon, but the stumps of those that have been removed are indicated. (From Moore, K.L.: The Developing Human: Clinically Oriented Embryology, 4th ed. Philadelphia, W. B. Saunders Company, 1988.)

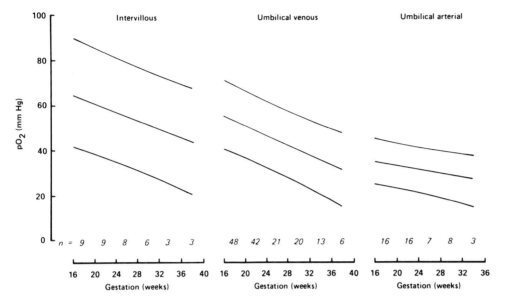

FIGURE 7–3. PO_2 (mean and 95 per cent confidence intervals) in intervillous, umbilical venous, and umbilical arterial blood. The results did not differ by method of blood sampling. There were significant negative correlations with gestation in each compartment (intervillous r = −0.44, N = 38, P <0.005; umbilical venous r = 0.61, N = 150, P <0.0001; umbilical arterial r = −0.36, N = 50, P <0.01). (From Soothill, P.W., Nicolaides, K. H., Rodeck, C. H., and Campbell, S.: Effect of gestational age on fetal and intervillous blood gas and acid-base values in human pregnancy. Fetal Therapy 1:168, 1986, reviewed in Obstet. Gynecol. Surv. 43:1–35, 1988.)

to each other in mixed lymphocyte reactions (Finn et al., 1977). Partial immunologic identity is not required between mother and fetus since totally allogeneic blastocyst transfers (oocyte donors) thrive in both humans and in experimental animals. At least three classes of immunoregulation have been proposed: (1) maternal bone-marrow–derived cells with suppressor function, (2) surface properties of trophoblasts that protect it from attack (syncytiotrophoblasts express no human lymphocyte antigens [HLAs] and invasive cytotrophoblasts express a nonpolymorphic unique HLA antigen), and (3) local production of suppressor factors or hormones. Clearly more research is indicated to ascertain which of these (or other) possibilities occurs.

■ PLACENTAL HORMONES

Human chorionic gonadotropin (hCG) was the first pregnancy hormone found by Ascheim and Zondek (1927) in the urine of pregnant women. The placental source of the hormone was established by demonstrating its production by trophoblasts in tissue culture (Gey et al., 1938). It is thought to be produced primarily by syncytiotrophoblasts and achieves its highest plasma concentration at 8 to 10 weeks' gestation. The major known role of chorionic gonadotropin is to maintain the function of the corpus luteum. It presumably also acts on fetal testes to promote testosterone synthesis and secretion, which are essential for the development of the male phenotype.

Human placental lactogen (hPL), first described in 1961 by Ito and Higashi (1961), is detectable in the syncytiotrophoblast by the 3rd week after ovulation. Maternal serum levels rise progressively throughout gestation. It has been thought that hPL influences fetal metabolism indirectly by altering glucose and lipid metabolism in the mother, thus making glucose available for fetal uptake. It also promotes the growth of the mammary glands in preparation for lactation. Most hPL is secreted into the maternal circulation. Plasma levels in the maternal circulation are about 5 to 10 μg/ml, whereas fetal levels are in the range of 400 to 500 ng/ml. This has encouraged the notion that its target tissues are located primarily in the mother, although recent studies have shown this not to be the case. Recep-

tors specific for hPL have been identified in human fetal tissues. hPL stimulates glycogen synthesis, amino acid transport, and production of insulin-like growth factor I in the fetus. Other direct effects of hPL on fetal growth will undoubtedly emerge from future studies.

The syncytiotrophoblast is also the site of increased steroid hormone production during pregnancy. The high levels of estriol and estradiol in blood and urine result from its synthesis in the placenta utilizing precursors from both the mother and the fetus. The ovary is not an important source of estrogens after the first few weeks of pregnancy. The dependence of estrogen synthesis on an intact fetoplacental unit has allowed estriol secretion to be used as a marker of fetal and placental well-being. The hyperestrogenic state ends with parturition.

Progesterone is synthesized by the placenta from maternal cholesterol. The progesterone produced by the placenta serves as a precursor for other steroid hormones produced by the fetal adrenal glands.

Other hormones produced by the placenta include human chorionic thyrotropin (hCT) and adrenocorticotropic hormone (ACTH). Hypothalamic-like releasing hormones, such as luteinizing hormone–releasing hormone (LHRH), corticotropin-releasing factor (CRF), and somatostatin, have been identified in both the cytotrophoblast and syncytiotrophoblast. Additionally, a number of peptide growth factors, such as insulin-like growth factors (IGFs) I and II and fibroblast growth factors (FGFs), are produced by the placenta and presumably play important roles in regulating placental growth, metabolism, and angiogenesis. An ever-increasing number of chorionic peptides with hormonal activity are being identified, but little is known about their function (Siler-Khodr, 1988).

Hormones that increase in maternal plasma during pregnancy are listed in Table 7–1.

■ CONCEPT OF THE FETAL-PLACENTAL-MATERNAL UNIT

The interactions between fetal, placental, and maternal tissues are complex. With respect to estrogen synthesis, for example, the placenta is the main source of the great increase in estrogens during pregnancy. It achieves this

TABLE 7–1. Hormones That Increase in Maternal Plasma During Pregnancy

β-Estradiol
Estriol
Progesterone
Aldosterone
Cortisol
Deoxycorticosterone
Renin
Angiotensinogen
Angiotensin II
Human placental lactogen
Human chorionic gonadotropin
Human chorionic thyrotropin
Chorionic adrenocorticotropic hormone
Catecholamines
Prolactin

production from prehormones that are supplied by both maternal and fetal plasma.

The fetal source of these prehormones is the fetal adrenal cortex, which is as large in a term fetus as in an adult, and is composed of a fetal zone (80 per cent) and an adult zone (20 per cent). The fetal zone secretes large amounts of dehydroepiandrosterone sulfate and 16α-hydroxydehydroepiandrosterone sulfate, which are precursors of placental estrogens.

Cortisone, produced in the placenta from maternal cortisol, is converted back to cortisol in the fetal lung where it regulates the time of differentiation of the alveolar type II cell as well as other lung structures. Cortisol is an important physiologic stimulus to differentiation of epithelial cells in the intestines and distal renal tubules as well as the lungs.

■ PLACENTAL TRANSPORT

In general, molecules with molecular weights under 500 move between the fetal and maternal circulations by specific transport mechanisms located in the placenta. The exceptions are substances that presumably pass through leaks in the placental vasculature and some microorganisms. They include rubella, poliomyelitis, human immunodeficiency virus (HIV), cytomegalovirus, *Toxoplasma*, and *Treponema pallidum*. Substances that go from maternal to fetal blood must traverse the trophoblast, stroma, and fetal capillaries.

Oxygen and carbon dioxide cross by diffusion. The average PO_2 of umbilical venous blood is 27 mm Hg, and arterial blood 15 mm Hg. The average PO_2 in the intervillous space is about 30 to 35 mm Hg, but with regional variations depending on the location of the sampling needle with respect to the jet of maternal arterial blood. During gestation, intervillous PO_2 falls and PCO_2 rises. As PO_2 falls, cord hemoglobin concentration increases so that the fetal blood oxygen content remains stable from 16 to 40 weeks (Soothill et al., 1986).

Glucose is the main source of energy for the fetus, providing about 50 per cent of the requirement. The remainder comes from amino acids and lactate. The primary source of glucose is from the mother, and it is transported by facilitated diffusion to the fetus. Glucose is stored in the lung as glycogen until late gestation (22 to 24 weeks) and in the liver as hepatic glycogen until parturition. Liver glycogen stores are the primary source of energy for the infant in the first hours after birth.

The nutrition of the fetus requires availability of all nutrients from the mother. The fetus depends on transport of free amino acids across the placenta for synthesis of enzymes, hormones, hemoglobin, and all proteins; the latter constitute about 12 per cent of body weight. The uptake of amino acids is mediated by facilitated diffusion and active transport.

The chorionic villus is capable of maintaining concentrating gradients of nutrients between the fetus and mother. Substances that are not synthesized by the fetus may be at higher concentrations in fetal than maternal blood. These include ascorbic acid, iron, and some amino acids (Van Dijk, 1988).

The placenta is also required to assure that the net exchange of water is toward the fetus. Although the average hydrostatic pressure in fetal capillaries is 35 mm Hg compared to only 10 mm Hg in the intervillous space, cellular sodium and hydrogen pumps can increase the local concentration of ions to produce sufficient osmotic pressure for water to enter the fetal circulation. Moreover, the placenta produces peptides that specifically regulate the release of decidual prolactin, which is thought to play a role in the regulation of fluid homeostasis in the fetus.

■ DRUGS AND PREGNANCY

Most drugs ingested during pregnancy or their metabolites cross the placenta. All sedatives and analgesics affect the fetus to some extent. Fetal drug addiction is well-known from maternal use of heroin, morphine, and cocaine (see Chapter 26). Fetal injury from maternal ethanol ingestion probably occurs from transport of acetaldehyde across the placenta. Studies with perfused human placental cotyledons further demonstrate the capacity of the placenta to oxidize ethanol to acetaldehyde and release it into the perfusate on the fetal side (Karl et al., 1988).

■ AMNIOTIC FLUID

Amniotic fluid increases in volume throughout gestation from 30 ml at 10 weeks to 1000 ml at 37 weeks. The major source of amniotic fluid after 16 weeks is fetal urine. In the absence of kidneys, oligohydramnios (low fluid volume) is present. The fetal lung is another source of amniotic fluid, and presumably some fluid is secreted by the amnion. Polyhydramnios (excess fluid volume) occurs in some central nervous system malformations, such as anencephaly, and in any circumstance in which fetal swallowing is impaired, such as esophageal atresia and neuromuscular disorders. Near term, the fetus normally swallows 400 to 500 ml per day of amniotic fluid. Congenital anomalies account for approximately half of the cases of polyhydramnios; other causes include maternal diabetes, fetal infection, and multiple gestation.

The osmolarity of amniotic fluid decreases from 24 weeks (about 275 mOsm/kg water) to term (about 250 mOsm/kg water). Presumably, the increasing volume of dilute fetal urine accounts for the decrease. Amniotic fluid has slightly less Na^+, K^+, and Cl^- than maternal or fetal serum. Sugar is much lower than in maternal serum, averaging 32 mg/dl compared to 79 mg/dl in serum. Total proteins are only 0.23 mg/dl compared with 6.1 g/dl in serum. Amniotic fluid is similar to interstitial fluid in its low concentrations of large molecules, such as lipoproteins, fibrinogen, and some immunoglobulins. The average pH is 7.07. Tracheal effluent contributes its more acid secretion (pH 6.43) with a carbon dioxide level of 4.4 mEq/l, compared with 18.4 mEq/l for amniotic fluid. The lung also contributes surface-active lipoproteins that are components of the pulmonary surfactant. Recognition of this fact has permitted assessment of lung maturity by measurement of the phospholipid profiles, lecithin-to-sphingomyelin ratio, saturated phosphatidyl- choline, or the surfactant-associated proteins. In isoimmunization, fetal bilirubin is also present in amniotic fluid, and the associated change in optical density is used as an index of fetal hemolysis. Measurement of alpha-fetoprotein has been used to detect various congenital anomalies (see Chapter 12).

Solid components of amniotic fluid include epithelial cells sloughed from fetal skin, kidneys, and the gastrointestinal tract with later gestational age. In the presence of fetal stress, meconium may contaminate the amniotic fluid. Infection with *Listeria* may produce greenish fluid that resembles meconium.

The fetal membranes, once thought to function as an inert mesothelial barrier, are now known to be metabolically active. They possess the capacity for metabolizing steroid hormone as well as synthesizing prostaglandin E_2 and $F_{2\alpha}$. Phospholipase A_2 is present, which can catalyze the release of arachidonic acid, the probable rate-limiting step in prostaglandin synthesis. The observation that stripping membranes or amniotomy stimulates labor makes it apparent that some mediators of labor are released by stretching the cells in the amnion and/or chorion. Many peptides have been isolated from these tissues as well as the decidua. They include prolactin, a somatostatin-like peptide (relaxin), and platelet-activating factor (Bryant-Greenwood and Greenwood, 1988). The role these hormones or others have in orchestrating labor is not yet fully understood (Mitchell, 1988).

■ UMBILICAL CORD AND PLACENTA

The umbilical cord extends from the fetal surface of the placenta to the fetal umbilicus. Its diameter is 1 to 2½ cm with an average length of 55 cm but with a very wide range of 30 to 100 cm. The vessels within the cord are longer than the cord and therefore are tortuous. They can produce bends that appear as false knots. The two arteries are smaller than the vein, and all vessels are surrounded in a matrix of Wharton jelly. The cord itself has no nerves, but there are cholinesterase-positive nerves in the periarterial plexus in the cord. Some of these nerves can be traced to the placenta, but they do not enter it.

EXAMINATION OF
THE CORD AND PLACENTA

The cord should be inspected for evidence of true knots, which can occur during delivery and compromise gas exchange to the fetus. The number of umbilical arteries should be observed since approximately 1 in 200 infants has only 1 umbilical artery and if so, there is a 20 to 40

per cent chance of associated malformations, particularly of the genitourinary system. The prevalence of a single umbilical artery in twins is about five times greater than in singletons. Screening for urinary tract abnormalities in infants with only one umbilical artery yielded positive results in 18 per cent of the cases (Leung and Robson, 1989).

Maternal conditions that can affect the appearance of the cord include diabetes mellitus, which is associated with cord edema and umbilical vein thrombi, and maternal cigarette smoking, associated with a cord of smaller diameter and less tense consistency. In intrauterine growth retardation there can be associated reduction in size of the cord and particularly in the amount of Wharton jelly. In addition, the placenta may have a reduction in cell number, protein content, and glycogen. Conditions associated with small placentas include preeclampsia or maternal hypertension of other etiology, such as vascular disease, and a single umbilical artery. Conversely, placentas of smoking mothers are of average size or even slightly heavier than those of nonsmokers even though the infants may be growth-retarded. Presumably, chronic hypoxia from increased levels of carboxyhemoglobin produces the physiologic equivalent of residence at high altitudes. Blood flow to the placenta is reduced during maternal smoking (Christianson, 1979).

In the presence of oligohydramnios, the fetal surface of the placenta may show thickening in several areas (amnion nodosum). The fetal surface may be discolored by meconium or show hematomas or vascular tears. Vascular communications may be present in twin pregnancies and lead to a twin-to-twin transfusion, with one infant plethoric and the other anemic.

Areas of infarction are commonly seen after 37 weeks. If present earlier, they are considered abnormal. Multiple areas of infarction probably account for about one-third of the cases of fetal growth retardation (Elliott and Knight, 1974).

Abnormalities in placental attachment and position can be disastrous, as in placenta previa and membranous insertion of the umbilical cord.

Placental abruption, or separation of the placenta (usually partial), is associated with maternal hemorrhage and disseminating intravascular coagulation and, often, markedly impaired placental perfusion that leads to fetal distress. This represents a major cause of fetal and neonatal morbidity caused by associated preterm birth and/or hypoxia.

Chorioamnionitis, frequently associated with premature rupture of membranes, and/or premature labor are a manifestation of intrauterine infection. In some instances, infection probably predisposes one to the rupture of membranes. Frequently, the amniotic fluid is cloudy, and the fetal membranes become opaque. Histologic examination permits estimates of duration of infection and its severity. The usual organisms are those of the vaginal and maternal rectal flora.

Amnionic bands may result from disruption of the amnion with formation of fibrous bands. When they constrict a limb of the fetus, intrauterine amputation may result. An incomplete constriction may lead to edema distal to the site of compression.

■ MULTIPLE BIRTHS

Twins occur in about 1 in 90 pregnancies, and triplets in 1 in 800 pregnancies in the United States. About one-third of the twins are from one zygote and thus are monozygotic, or identical. The two embryos usually each have their own amniotic sac, but develop with one chorionic sac and a common placenta. Twins that originate from two zygotes (dizygotic) may be of the same or different sexes. They each have their own amnion and chorion, although sometimes the chorions are fused and can make the distinction from monozygotic twins difficult by inspection of the placenta alone.

If the developing embryonic cell mass does not divide completely, the twins may be conjoined. This event occurs in about one in every 40 monozygotic twin pregnancies.

TWIN-TWIN TRANSFUSION

Transfusion from one homozygous twin to another can result in anemia in the donor twin and polycythemia in the recipient. Significant hemorrhage is seen only in monochorionic monozygous twins (approximately 70 per cent of all monozygous twins). In approximately 15 per cent of these pregnancies, there is a twin-twin transfusion. Bleeding occurs because of vascular anastomosis in monochorionic placentas. The anemic donor twin is usually smaller than the polycythemic recipient. Polyhydramnios is frequently seen in the recipient twin and oligohydramnios is seen in the donor. Twin-twin transfusions should be suspected when the hemoglobin concentration of identical twins differs by more than 5 g/dl.

■ NEONATAL BLOOD VOLUME

The infant at birth contains 70 to 95 ml of blood/kg of body weight, depending largely on the redistribution of blood between the fetus and placenta at the time of birth. If the umbilical cord is clamped before the first breath, and before the fetus can receive placental blood by gravity, the infant's blood volume may be 30 per cent less than it would have been with late cord clamping. Most of the placental transfusion occurs within 3 minutes of delivery. The optimal timing of cord clamping is not clear. Delayed clamping can induce a fluid shift to the extracellular space and delay clearance of lung liquid. It can also increase the red cell volume and exaggerate physiologic jaundice. On the other hand, very early cord clamping can result in a low blood volume and, later, anemia.

■ REFERENCES

Ascheim, S., and Zondek, B: (Anterior pituitary hormone and ovarian hormone in the urine of pregnant women.) Klin. Wochenschr. 6:248, 1927.

Boyd, P. A., and Scott, A.: Quantitative structural studies on human placentas associated with pre-eclampsia, essential hypertension and intrauterine growth retardation. Br. J. Obstet. Gynaecol. 92:714, 1985.

Bryant-Greenwood, G. D., and Greenwood, F. C.: The human fetal membranes and decidua as a model for paracrine interactions. In McNellis, D., et al. (Eds.): The Onset of Labor, Ithaca, N.Y., Perinatology Press, 1988.

Christianson, R. E.: Gross differences observed in the placentas of smokers and nonsmokers. Am. J. Epidemiol. 110:178, 1979.

Diczfalusy E: The early history of the feto-placental unit, or the rise and fall of the placental empire. In Jaffe, R. B., Dell'Aqua, S. (Eds): The Endocrine Physiology of Pregnancy and the Peripartal Period. New York, The Raven Press, 1985.

Elliott, K., and Knight, J. (Eds.): Size at Birth. Ciba Foundation Symposium 27. Amsterdam, Excerpta Medica, 1974.

Fant, M., Munro, H., and Moses, A. C.: An autocrine/paracrine role for insulin-like growth factors in the regulation of human placental growth. J. Clin. Endocrinol. Metabol. 63:499, 1986.

Finn, R., Davis, J. C., St. Hill, C. A., et al.: Fetomaternal bidirectional mixed lymphocyte reaction and survival of fetal allograft. Lancet 1:200, 1977.

Gey, G. O., Jones, G. E. S., Hellman, L. S.: The production of a gonadotrophic substance (prolan) by placental cells in tissue culture. Science 88:306, 1938.

Head, J. R., Drake, B. L., and Zuckermann, F. A.: Major histocompatibility antigens on trophoblast and their regulation: Implications in the maternal-fetal relationship. Am. J. Reprod. Immunol. 15:12, 1987.

Hill, D. J.: Insulin as a growth factor. In Somatomedins and other peptide growth factors. 89th Ross Conference on Pediatric Research 75. Columbus, Ohio, Ross Laboratories, 1985.

Hunziker, R. D., and Wegmann, T. G.: Placental immunoregulation. CRC Crit. Rev. Immunol. 6:245, 1986.

Ito, Y., and Higashi, K.: Studies on prolactin-like substance in human placenta. II. Endocrinol. Jpn. 8:279, 1961.

Karl, P. C., Gordon, H. J., Lieber, C. S., et al.: Acetaldehyde production and transfer by the perfused human placental cotyledon. Science 242:273, 1988.

Leung, A. K. C., and Robson, W. L. M.: Single umbilical artery. A report of 159 cases. Am. J. Dis. Child. 143:108, 1989.

McKay, D. G., Hertig, A. T., Adams, E. C., et al.: Histochemical observations on the human placenta. Obstet, Gynecol. 12:1, 1958.

Margolis, A. J., and Orcutt, E.: Pressures in human umbilical vessels in utero. Am. J. Obst. Gynec. 80:573, 1960.

Mitchell, B. F. (Ed.): The Physiology and Biochemistry of Human Fetal Membranes. Ithaca, N.Y., Perinatology Press, 1988.

Moore, K. L.: The Developing Human, 4th ed. Philadelphia, W. B. Saunders Company, 1988.

Munro, H. N.: Role of the placenta in ensuring fetal nutrition. Fed. Proc. 45:2500, 1986.

Page, A. W., Villee, C. A., and Villee, D. B.: Human Reproduction: Essentials of Reproductive and Perinatal Medicine, 3rd ed. Philadelphia, W. B. Saunders Company, 1981.

Ramsey, E. M., Corner, G. W., and Donner, M. W.: Serial and cineradioangiographic visualization of maternal circulation in the primate (hemichorial) placenta. Am. J. Obstet. Gynecol. 86:213, 1963.

Redline, R. W., and Driscoll, S. H.: The placenta and adnexa. In Reed, G. B., Claireaux, A. E., and Bain, A. D. (Eds.): Diseases of the Fetus and Newborn. London, Chapman and Hall, 1989.

Seeds, A. E.: Current concepts of amniotic fluid dynamics. Am. J. Obstet. Gynecol. 138:575, 1980.

Siler-Khodr, T. M.: Chorionic peptides. In McNellis, D., et al. (Eds.): The Onset of Labor: Cellular and Integrative Mechanisms. Ithaca, N.Y., Perinatology Press, 1988, p. 213.

Soothill, P. W., Nicolaides, K. N., Rodeck, C. H., et al.: Effect of gestational age on fetal and intervillous blood gas and acid values in human pregnancy. Fetal Therapy 1:168, 1986.

Strang, L. B.: Neonatal Respiration: Physiological and Clinical Studies. Oxford, Blackwell Scientific Publications, 1977.

Tullassay, T., Seri, I., and Rascher, W.: Atrial natriuretic peptide and extracellular volume contraction after birth. Acta Paediatr. Scand. 76:444, 1987.

Van Dijk, J. P.: Regulatory aspects of placental iron transfer—a comparative study. Placenta 9:215, 1988.

Young, M.: The handling of amino-acids by the feto-placental unit. In Lindblad, B. S. (Ed.): Perinatal Nutrition. New York, Academic Press, 1988.

Young, M., Boyd, R. D. H., Longo, L. D., and Telegdy, G.: Placental Transfer Methods and Interpretations. Philadelphia, W. B. Saunders Company, 1981.

FETAL GROWTH: 8
NUTRITIONAL ISSUES

V. Charlton

■ PATTERN OF NORMAL FETAL GROWTH

CHANGES IN WEIGHT AND LENGTH

Fetal growth does not occur at a uniform rate but rather changes over gestation (Moore, 1988). The rate of increase in crown-rump length occurs most rapidly early in gestation and then continues at a steady, somewhat slower pace. Fetal weight gain, viewed as a percentage increase in fetal weight, is also greatest in the earliest stages of gestation when the fetus is actively increasing its mass. However, this represents only a small increase in absolute weight. Absolute weight increases most steeply during the last half of gestation. These changing growth patterns can be appreciated in Table 8–1. Fetal weight and crown-rump length are presented, beginning with fetuses of 9 weeks conceptual age and extending up to near-term fetuses of 36 weeks. Early in gestation the change in crown-rump length is approximately 50 mm per month. This later declines to 40 mm per month. Fetal weight increases 460 per cent between 9 and 12 weeks, but this represents an absolute increase of only 37 g. In contrast, fetal weight increases 800 g between 32 and 36 weeks, yet this is an increase of only 38 per cent.

The rapid increase in absolute fetal weight and the increases in total length and head circumference that occur in later gestation are seen in Figure 8–1. These graphs were constructed by Usher and McLean (1969) from information on size at birth at various gestations for infants in Montreal. Mean values ± 2 standard deviations are given. Over the majority of the intervals shown, fetal size increases linearly. However, during the last few weeks of gestation, size begins to level off.

ORGAN GROWTH

The rate of increase in total fetal size is not necessarily matched by the growth rate of individual organs. Organ growth varies so that body proportions change over gestation. The relative size of the fetal head decreases from almost 50 per cent of fetal length at 9 conceptual weeks to 25 per cent near term, while the contribution of limb length to overall length increases (Moore, 1988). Organ weights as a percentage of body weight also change. For example, between midgestation (20 to 24 weeks) and term, there are: an increase in liver weight from 3.7 to 5.1 per cent of total fetal weight; an increase in small intestinal weight from 0.5 to 1.0 per cent; and a decrease in skeletal weight from 22 to 18 per cent (Shah and Rajalakshmi, 1988; Widdowson, 1974).

BODY COMPOSITION

Further, as the fetus develops from midgestation to term, there is a change in body composition (Apte and Iyengar, 1972; Ziegler et al., 1976). The percentage of fetal weight that is water decreases from 89 to 74 per cent, and the absolute accretion rate of major body constituents changes markedly, as can be seen in Table 8–2. Along with the higher rates of accretion, there are increases in the per cent both of body weight that is lipid (rising from <1 to 11 per cent) and of protein (increasing from 9 to 12 per cent). Tissue concentrations of calcium, magnesium, and phosphorus also increase by 17 to 40 per cent, while sodium and chloride concentrations decrease slightly (Ziegler et al., 1976). Fetal iron stores triple (Apte and Iyengar, 1972). At the end of gestation, some slowing in the rates of fetal tissue accretion again occurs, coincident with the plateauing in overall growth.

■ ROLE OF NUTRIENTS IN FETAL GROWTH AND DEVELOPMENT

Throughout gestation, the quantity and balance of nutrients available to the fetus affect the patterns of fetal development and growth. Early in gestation, when the absolute increase in fetal weight is small, abnormalities in nutrient supply are associated with abnormal embryogenesis and organ development. Later in gestation, abnormalities in nutrient supply have a more pronounced effect on the growth rate, influencing both the total size and growth of specific organs.

EARLY GESTATION
NUTRITIONAL DEFICIENCIES

Maternal deficiencies and excesses of trace vitamins and minerals during early pregnancy result in fetal dys-

TABLE 8–1. Average Fetal Weight and Length at Different Ages

CONCEPTUAL AGE (weeks)	WEIGHT (g)	CROWN-RUMP LENGTH (mm)
9	8	50
12	45	87
16	200	140
20	460	190
24	820	230
28	1300	270
32	2100	300
36	2900	340

Weights are from fixed fetuses and are approximately 5 per cent greater than fresh weights. (Adapted from Moore, K. L.: The fetal period. In Moore, K. L.: The Developing Human, 4th ed. Philadelphia, W. B. Saunders Company, 1988, pp. 87–103.)

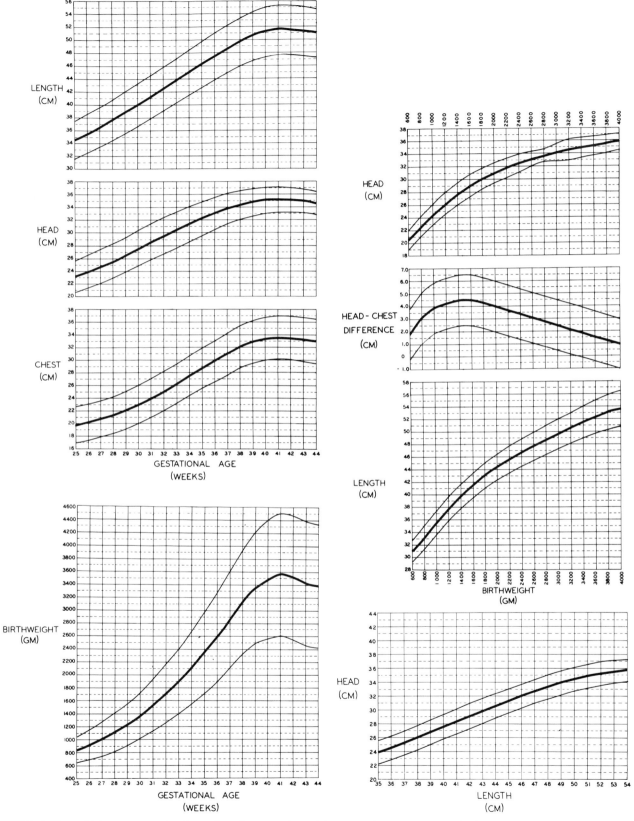

FIGURE 8–1. Size at birth versus gestational age. Smooth curve values of the mean plus or minus 2 standard deviations (3rd and 97th percentiles) for white infants at sea level (Montreal). (From Usher, R., and McLean, F.: Intrauterine growth of live born Caucasian infants at sea level. J. Pediatr. 74:901, 1969.)

TABLE 8–2. Daily Increments in Body Weight and Constituents of the Reference Fetus

GESTATION (weeks)	WEIGHT (g)	PROTEIN (g)	LIPID (g)	Ca (mg)	P (mg)	Mg (mg)	Na (meq)	K (meq)	Cl (meq)
24–25	11.4	1.25	0.5	61	39	1.8	0.9	0.5	0.8
29–30	23.1	2.76	2.6	138	89	3.7	1.7	1.0	1.3
34–35	31.4	4.23	4.4	258	162	6.0	2.2	1.3	1.4
39–40	17.1	2.50	5.0	302	179	5.0	1.0	0.6	0.3

(Adapted from Ziegler, E., O'Donnell, A., Nelson, S., et al.: Growth 40:329, 1976.)

genesis (Hurley, 1980). Examples of such abnormalities in experimental animals are listed in Table 8–3. Besides fetal abnormalities, reduced maternal fertility and increased numbers of preterm offspring and stillbirths are observed in animals with deficiencies of specific vitamins and minerals (e.g., riboflavin, folate, thiamine, pantothenic acid, vitamin C, vitamin E, and zinc).

In the human, microcephaly and eye anomalies have been reported in the offspring of vitamin A–deficient mothers. Vitamin D deficiency leads to fetal rickets. Zinc deficiency has been linked to low birth weight and, when severe, malformations of the central nervous system (Hurley, 1980; Worthington-Roberts, 1985).

Mothers giving birth to infants with neural tube defects (NTDs) have been found to have low blood cell levels of folate, riboflavin, and vitamin C (Smithells et al., 1976). Further, prospective studies in Britain have indicated that prophylactic ingestion of a multivitamin and iron supplement for several months, before and after conception, markedly reduces the rate of recurrence of NTD pregnancies (Smithells et al., 1981 and 1989). In contrast, a recent retrospective American study found no effect of periconceptual maternal vitamin intake on the incidence of NTDs (Mills et al., 1989). These differences may be due to the lower routine intake of vitamins in Britain, the higher incidence of NTDs there, and the normally health-conscious diet of Californian mothers who were the majority of the American subjects.

NUTRITIONAL EXCESSES

Increased maternal vitamin intake has also been associated with fetal abnormalities in the human, such as of vitamin A, which may cause fetal genitourinary malformations and neural tube defects when taken in excess (Bernhardt and Dorsey, 1974; Gal et al., 1972). Recently, vitamin A analogues used to treat severe acne (e.g., isotretinoin) have also been associated with a constellation of defects including CNS malformations, microtia, and cardiac defects (Lammer et al., 1985).

Excessive intake of vitamin D during pregnancy may cause hypercalcemia in the infant. The infant may also have supravalvular aortic stenosis and/or peripheral pulmonic arterial stenoses. Hypotonia, irritability, vomiting, and dehydration may be present when the serum calcium is elevated and may resolve with low calcium and low vitamin D intake and appropriate hydration.

The findings of hypercalcemia are indistinguishable from those of Williams syndrome, although the latter can occur in the absence of a history of excessive intake of vitamin D. It is thought to represent a hypersensitivity to the vitamin.

Derangements in macronutrient availability early in pregnancy can also lead to fetal dysgenesis. Hyperglycemia and related metabolic abnormalities in lipid and protein metabolism have been associated with an increased risk of multiple fetal anomalies in diabetics (Cousins, 1983). These include fetal cardiac disease, anal atresia, vertebral abnormalities, microcolon, caudal regression syndrome, and NTDs. Hyperphenylalaninemia in mothers with phenylketonuria has been associated with a high incidence of CNS abnormalities and poor growth in utero in their nonphenylketonuric offspring (Lipson et al., 1984).

LATE GESTATION

Later in gestation, during the period when absolute growth and tissue accretion rates are high, wide variation in fetal size becomes apparent. In Figure 8–1, the range in weight encompassed between 2 standard deviations above and below the mean is approximately 2000 g at term.

TABLE 8–3. Abnormalities of Fetal Development in Animals Associated with Maternal Deficiencies and Excesses of Trace Nutrients

NUTRIENT	SPECIES STUDIED	RESULTING FETAL ABNORMALITY
Deficiency		
Vitamin A	Rat, pig	Defects in eyes, cardiovascular system, urogenital system, and lungs.
Vitamin D	Rat, cow	Fetal rickets.
Riboflavin	Rat, pig	Bone and rib anomalies, fused or missing digits, hydrocephaly, and cleft palate.
Folate	Rat	Eye defects, hydrocephaly, cleft lip, and failure of closure of the thoracic and abdominal walls.
Vitamin B_{12}	Rat	Hydrocephaly.
Magnesium	Rat	Anemia, red cell abnormalities, and multiple malformations.
Iron	Rat	Anemia, reduced tissue iron, and hyperlipidemia.
Copper	Sheep	Spastic paralysis, blindness, CNS anomalies, anemia.
	Guinea pig	Ataxia.
Zinc	Rat	Stunted growth, short limbs, missing digits and tail, and hydrocephaly.
Manganese	Rat	Severe ataxia.
Excess		
Vitamin A	Rat, mouse, guinea pig, pig, rabbit, monkey	Severe anomalies of skull and brain, cleft lip, cleft palate, and eye defects.
Vitamin C	Guinea pig	Increased fetal mortality.
Vitamin D	Rat	Growth retardation, multiple fractures, and abnormal bone development.
	Rabbit	Cranial, facial, and aortic lesions.
Calcium	Rat	Low birth weight and neonatal hypocalcemia.

(Adapted from Hurley, L.: Developmental Nutrition. Englewood Cliffs, N.J., Prentice Hall, 1980.)

FACTORS INFLUENCING VARIABILITY IN FETAL SIZE

The differences in fetal size are influenced both by inherent fetal genetic variation and by extrinsic maternal and environmental factors. Studies comparing weights of monozygotic twins, who share a genotype and womb environment, and dizygotic twins, who are genetically different but share the intrauterine environment, have suggested that the fetal genotype normally accounts for only 10 to 18 per cent of the variation in birth weight (Yates, 1988). The remainder of variation is due to extrinsic environmental, maternal, and placental factors (Table 8–4). Most of these factors affect the delivery of nutrients and oxygen to the fetus (Charlton, 1986; Gross, 1989). Their association with fetal growth suggests that availability of adequate substrates is a major determinant of intrauterine growth. The estimated variation in fetal size attributable to some of these extrinsic factors include maternal height and prepregnancy weight, 8 per cent; total weight gain during pregnancy, 3 to 6 per cent; weight gain from midpregnancy to term, 3 per cent; and maternal age, education, and a prior low birth weight infant, 8 per cent (Metcoff et al., 1981). Reductions in fetal weight of 2 per cent are induced by maternal alcohol and coffee consumption and of 3 to 6 per cent by varying levels of cigarette smoking (Fisher et al., 1983; Metoff et al., 1981; Mochizuki et al., 1984; Socol et al., 1982; Worthington-Roberts, 1985).

It should be noted that the growth curves presented in Figure 8–1 were collected at sea level using white infants. Because of variations in populations and environment,

TABLE 8–4. Maternal, Placental, and Environmental Factors Affecting Fetal Growth

MATERNAL FACTORS
1. Maternal nutrient levels and nutrient stores: *Reduced by* inadequate or poorly balanced nutrient intake, low prepregnancy weight, small maternal size, poor gestational weight gain, poor late-pregnancy weight gain, recent pregnancy, young maternal age, hypoglycemia, chronic illness, and alcoholism. *Increased by* good dietary intake, normal prepregnancy weight, and good gestational weight gain.
2. Oxygen levels: *Reduced by* cyanotic heart disease, hemoglobinopathies, respiratory failure, and smoking.
3. Uteroplacental blood flow: *Reduced by* hypertension, renal disease, vascular disease, cocaine, smoking, and caffeine.
4. Multiple gestation: Decreases substrates available for each fetus.
5. Medications: Fetal growth reduced by antimetabolites, phenytoin, warfarin, and beta blockers.
6. Previous low-birth-weight infant: Increases risk for low birth weight.

PLACENTAL FACTORS
1. Placental size and surface area: Reduced substrate transfer with decreased size and surface area.
2. Structural abnormalities: Reduced transfer area with infarcts, villous changes, and abnormal cord insertion.
3. Transport: Alcohol reduces placental amino acid and zinc transport.

ENVIRONMENTAL FACTORS
1. Socioeconomic and educational status: Low socioeconomic and educational status is associated with reduced birth weight.
2. Altitude: High altitude reduces maternal oxygen levels.
3. Toxins: Can lead to abnormal fetal development, e.g., methyl mercury.

(Adapted from Charlton, 1986; Fisher et al., 1983; Gross, 1989; Metcoff et al., 1981; Mochizuki et al., 1984; Socol et al., 1982; Van den Berg 1981; Woods et al., 1987.)

data collected in other locations differ. Lower mean birth weights at 40 weeks' gestation have been reported in Denver (3230 g) and in Baltimore (3280 g), presumably reflecting differences in altitude and population composition (Naeye and Dixon, 1978). The growth curve appropriate for each population should be used when assessing infant size.

THE UNDERGROWN FETUS

Infants at the extremes of the range in growth, either too small or too large, are at increased risk of perinatal mortality versus infants of normal growth (see Chapter 25). Inadequate growth in utero has commonly been defined as a birth weight less than 2 standard deviations below the mean for gestation (approximately the third percentile) on fetal weight curves. Some authors use a less restrictive definition of a birth weight below the 10th percentile. Infants whose size falls below these levels are termed "intrauterine growth retarded," "small for gestational age," or "small for dates." Unfortunately, these definitions, based on birth weight alone, do not differentiate infants who are also reduced in length or head circumference and completely overlook long, wasted infants whose birth weight is slightly above the defined cut off. A plea has recently been made for a fresh approach to categorizing normal and abnormal intrauterine growth, including some indicator of weight for length (Miller and Jekel, 1989).

Infants who are small for gestational age are a heterogeneous group. Some appear symmetrically growth retarded, with proportionally reduced size in weight, length, and head circumference. These infants have a slow growth rate beginning early in gestation and are more likely to have marked genetic constraints on growth, a dysmorphic syndrome, a chromosomal disorder, or a congenital infection (Campbell, 1974). Most growth-retarded infants, however, are asymmetrically growth retarded. Their severest growth reductions are in weight and perhaps length, but there is relative sparing of head growth. Despite this relative sparing, absolute head size is usually decreased for gestation (Kramer et al., 1989). In fact, growth-retarded infants who have died in the newborn period have been found to have a 19 to 20 per cent decrease in cerebral size and cellularity and a 35 to 37 per cent reduction in size and cellularity of the cerebellum (Chase et al., 1972).

The asymmetric form of growth retardation is usually due to extrinsic influences on the fetus and becomes apparent later in gestation, when growth should be most rapid. These infants have a malnourished, wasted appearance, and the individual organs most reduced in size are those compromised by postnatal malnutrition—the liver, spleen, thymus, and adrenals. This growth pattern again suggests an etiologic role for malnutrition in poor fetal growth (Naeye, 1965). Animal studies indicate that key organs, such as the brain, maintain somewhat better growth because they are given a larger share of the available nutrients, through preferential blood distribution patterns and increased rates of blood flow (Charlton, 1986).

Growth-retarded infants also have undergrown placentas (Molteni et al., 1978), and they are at increased risk for perinatal complications, such as birth asphyxia, hypoglycemia, meconium aspiration, and polycythemia (see Chapter 25.) In addition, long-term sequelae of growth retardation occur. As a group, these infants tend to remain short during childhood (Fitzhardinge and Steven, 1972a), and they have an increased incidence of neurologic deficits. Learning difficulties and poor fine motor coordination have been reported in 25 per cent of the cases as well as speech deficits in 30 per cent (Fitzhardinge and Steven, 1972b). The severity of the sequelae appears to correlate with the duration and severity of the compromise in fetal growth. If the growth of the fetal head (as determined by ultrasonographic measurements of the biparietal diameter) slows before 34 weeks' gestation, the growth insult is such that the child tends to remain short. If head growth slows before 26 weeks' gestation, there are also persistent perceptual and motor deficits (Harvey et al., 1982).

It should be remembered that normal fetal growth plateaus near term. Even under normal conditions, fetal requirements eventually outstrip substrate supply so that high rates of growth cannot be maintained. After birth and adjustment to ex utero conditions, rapid growth resumes.

THE LARGE FETUS

Excessive growth in utero has been defined as a birth weight either greater than two standard deviations above the mean for gestation (the 97th percentile) or above the 90th percentile. Infants with weights above these levels are termed "large for gestational age" or "large for dates."

Infants who are large for gestational age can be either normal, large infants or infants whose growth has been stimulated by abnormal conditions in utero. These abnormal conditions usually involve exposure to increased levels of glucose and/or hyperinsulinism, suggesting that a surplus of substrate and increased glucose metabolism promote fetal growth. Examples are infants of diabetic mothers (Willman et al., 1986) and infants with Beckwith-Wiedemann syndrome. The latter includes pancreatic hyperplasia and hyperinsulinism (Jones, 1988). Placental size tends to be increased in these large infants (Molteni et al., 1978), but higher rates of substrate utilization raise the demand for oxygen (Milley et al., 1984; Phillips et al., 1985). These fetuses are at risk for birth asphyxia and birth trauma. Postnatal complications include hypoglycemia and polycythemia.

■ FETAL NUTRITIONAL NEEDS DURING THE PERIOD OF RAPID GROWTH

To avoid these extremes in growth, with their adverse sequelae, a balanced quantity of nutrients must reach the fetus during the latter part of gestation. Normal caloric entry into the human fetus near term has been estimated as approximately 90 to 100 kcal/kg/day. Of this, 40 kcal/kg/day are utilized for growth (Sparks et al., 1980). The major nutrients that provide these calories are glucose and amino acids.

GLUCOSE

Glucose is the major source of energy for the fetus and a large source of carbon. It is also the major substrate used by the fetal brain (Jones, 1979). Glucose crosses the placenta by facilitated diffusion, and fetal uptake of glucose is proportional, over a wide range, to maternal glucose levels and the concentration gradient between mother and fetus (Hauguel et al., 1986; Kennaugh and Hay, 1987). Glucose levels in the human fetus at birth are 70 to 80 per cent of maternal venous values, with fetal umbilical venous concentrations reported as 55 to 85 mg/dl (Morriss et al., 1975). Studies of cesarean sections indicate that if all the glucose entering the fetus were completely oxidized, glucose use could account for approximately 80 per cent of fetal oxygen consumption (Morriss et al., 1975).

Availability of glucose appears to play a major role in fetal growth. Growth-retarded newborns have low cord blood levels of glucose (Haymond et al., 1974), and both low fasting maternal glucose levels and rapid maternal utilization of glucose have been found in women giving birth to small infants (Langer et al., 1986; Raman, 1981). The association between increased levels of glucose and insulin and increased fetal size has been mentioned. In women with diabetes, the chance of fetal macrosomia is increased two-fold when mean maternal glucose levels exceed 130 mg/dl (Willman et al., 1986).

In third-trimester fetal sheep, the total quantity of glucose taken up across the umbilical circulation normally averages 27 g/day. In experimentally growth-retarded fetal lambs, total glucose uptake falls by up to 50 per cent. However, the quantity of glucose taken up per kilogram of fetal weight declines by only 10 to 30 per cent, suggesting that fetal growth adapts in response to the substrate supply (Charlton, 1986).

AMINO ACIDS

Amino acids serve as the source of nitrogen for the fetus and as a major source of carbon. They are utilized during anabolism and are rapidly catabolized, as indicated by a high fetal urea production rate. They are actively transported into the fetus against a concentration gradient, resulting in higher amino acid levels in the fetus than in the mother (Kennaugh and Hay, 1987; Rosso, 1983). Total fetal amino acid concentrations average 2.3 mmol/l in the midtrimester human, and with the decrease in maternal amino acids during pregnancy, fetal levels average 2.4 times maternal. While fetal amino acid levels are higher than maternal, there is a direct correlation between fetal and maternal values for most amino acids in the human (Soltesz et al., 1985). Amino acid abnormalities in maternal blood will, therefore, be magnified in the fetus. This undoubtably relates to the previously mentioned high incidence of malformations in nonphenylketonuric infants born to mothers with phenylketonuria (Lipson et al., 1984).

Poor fetal growth has been associated with decreased total plasma amino acid levels in the mother and decreased maternal levels of specific amino acids (Metcoff et al., 1981). Further, growth-retarded human fetuses have been found to have decreased cord blood levels of total and specific amino acids (Cetin et al., 1988).

In third-trimester fetal sheep, approximately 20 g of amino acids are taken up across the umbilical circulation each day. With maternal malnutrition, fetal umbilical uptake of amino acids decreases, and amino acids are diverted from fetal protein synthesis to use as oxidative fuels (Charlton, 1986; Kennaugh and Hay, 1987).

LACTATE

Under conditions of normal oxygenation, lactate has been identified as an additional major fetal nutrient in sheep (Charlton and Creasy, 1976a). It is produced by placental metabolism and excreted into the fetal and maternal circulations. Further, it is produced by fetal metabolism and utilized as a substrate by fetal organs such as the heart and gastrointestinal tract (Sparks et al., 1982). In sheep, fetal umbilical uptake of lactate averages 7 g/day (Charlton, 1986). Lactate is also produced by the human placenta, and cord blood measurements, made at elective repeat cesarean section, suggest that it is taken up across the umbilical circulation by the human fetus (Charlton and Creasy, 1976b).

FATS, KETONES, AND ACETATE

Fats are a major source of calories postnatally, but there is great species variation in the extent to which fatty acids are transferred across the placenta. In the human, there appears to be some placental lipid transport and also lipid synthesis within the fetus (Rosso, 1983). Essential fatty acids and acetate, which can be used to synthesize lipids and cholesterol, cross the human placenta (Plotz et al., 1968). In the fetal lamb, acetate uptake across the umbilical circulation has been documented in quantities that could explain up to 10 per cent of fetal oxygen consumption (Charlton and Creasy, 1976c). Ketone transfer in animals is usually low but increases slightly when maternal levels are elevated (Morriss et al., 1974). In the human, fetal cord blood levels of ketones have been found to correlate with maternal levels (Bencini and Symonds, 1972).

RELATION BETWEEN MACRONUTRIENT SUPPLY AND GROWTH-PROMOTING HORMONES

The effects of macronutrients on fetal growth may in part be mediated by their effects on growth-promoting hormones. The increased insulin levels in macrosomic infants have been mentioned, but the somatomedins, or insulin-like growth factors (IGFs), appear to play a larger role in fetal growth (Sara, 1988). Cord blood levels of IGFs show a correlation with birth weight in the human, and growth-retarded infants have low IGF levels (Engstrom and Heath, 1988). In animals, malnutrition during pregnancy leads to decreased fetal levels of IGFs as well as decreased fetal growth (D'Ercole, 1987).

In the human fetus, the predominant IGFs are a variant form of IGF1 and IGF2. The IGFs are produced in all fetal tissues, and their production is independent of growth hormone regulation. Placental lactogen may regulate IGF production in some species, but in the human it has been suggested that IGF biosynthesis is regulated by availability of substrate to the cell. This would provide a local mechanism for controlling cellular growth (Sara, 1988).

TRACE MINERALS AND VITAMINS

Besides macronutrients, micronutrients are needed for normal late fetal growth. The high accretion rates of some minerals in late gestation were already given in Table 8–2. Adequate fetal supply of key minerals, such as calcium, phosphorus, and iron, enter the fetus by active transport, and near term, fetal blood levels of these minerals exceed maternal. Nonetheless, fetal anemia and depleted iron stores can occur with maternal iron deficiency (Hurley, 1980).

Both fat- and water-soluble vitamins are needed by the fetus. Fat-soluble vitamins (A, D, E, and K) cross the placenta by diffusion, and fetal levels are less than or equal to maternal levels. Because water-soluble vitamins (B and C) cross the placenta by active transport, fetal levels are greater than maternal (Rosso, 1983). Specific vitamin abnormalities can present as derangements in the newborn period. Fetal thiamine deficiency can lead to congenital beriberi with cardiac failure, aphonia, and/or a pseudomeningitis. Excess fetal vitamin C can lead to high rates of ascorbate metabolism and neonatal scurvy (Hurley, 1980).

OXYGEN

To allow utilization of all the substrates discussed in this chapter, sufficient oxygen must also enter the fetus. In animal studies, it has been estimated that 20 per cent of normal fetal oxidative metabolism is consumed by growth (Clapp et al., 1981). Since oxygen enters the fetus rapidly by simple diffusion, oxygen levels are usually adequate. However, in fetuses with abnormal growth, both small and large, there may be evidence of decreased oxygenation, indicated by low cord blood oxygen tensions, increased hemoglobin levels, and increased erythropoietin levels (Charlton, 1986; Georgieff et al., 1989).

■ MATERNAL NUTRITION DURING PREGNANCY

NORMAL WEIGHT GAIN

To provide the fetus with the proper quantity and mix of substrates, the normal pregnant woman in a developed country is expected to gain approximately 25 pounds (10 to 12 kg). Of this, approximately 38 per cent is fetal and placental weight, 30 per cent is increase in maternal blood volume and extracellular fluid, 9 per cent is amniotic fluid, and the remainder is made up of new maternal tissue (e.g., uterus and breasts) plus fat stores for lactation (Pitkin, 1981). Maternal weight gain during the first and second trimesters goes mainly toward maternal components (blood, extracellular fluid, tissue, and fat stores) and the placenta, while weight gain during the third trimester goes mainly toward fetal tissue. This is why maternal weight gain during late pregnancy is a specific risk factor influencing fetal size (Van den Berg, 1981).

CALORIC AND DIETARY NEEDS

The extra nutritional intake required by the mother to achieve this increase in weight and optimum fetal growth has been estimated at 80,000 kcal in developed countries. The National Research Council of the American Academy of Sciences (1980) has, therefore, recommended an intake of 300 kcal/day. over nonpregnant needs, or an approximate total caloric intake of 2500 kcal/day. As Table 8–5 shows, the Academy of Sciences also recommends that protein intake be increased up to a total of about 75 g/day. Excessive protein intake, however, is undesirable and may lead to an increased incidence of preterm births (Susser, 1981). During pregnancy it is recommended that the intake of most vitamins should be increased by 15 to 30 per cent, folate should be increased by 100 per cent, and calcium and iron increased by 50 to 100 per cent.

In some nations, apparently normal fetal growth is achieved with lower maternal caloric intakes than those recommended by the American National Research Council. Caloric needs during pregnancy have, therefore, been recently investigated in a large seven-country study, which included developed and developing nations (Durnin, 1987). The results of the study suggest that in some populations actual maternal caloric needs are lessened by maternal physiologic adaptations, including decreased basal metabolic rate, activity levels, body temperature, and fat stores. Below maternal caloric intakes of around 1800 kcal/day, however, fetal growth can no longer be protected (Whitehead, 1988).

ATTEMPTS TO IMPROVE FETAL GROWTH

MATERNAL DIETARY SUPPLEMENTATION

To try to improve fetal size and outcome, trials of dietary supplementation have been carried out in different parts of the world. Supplementation rates of up to 1000 kcal and 40 g of protein per day have been given. The benefits of supplementation have been variable, and

where an effect has been seen, it has been only in the range of a 100 to 300 g increase in birth weight (Whitehead, 1988). However, even these small increases can have a marked effect in reducing the incidence of low birth weight in some populations (e.g., from 28 to 5 per cent in Gambia) (Nutrition Reviews, 1984). A number of questions have also been raised about these studies with respect to the mother's ingestion of the supplement instead of her regular diet, rather than consuming it as additional intake, and the prior level of maternal physiologic adaptation to malnutrition (Whitehead, 1988).

NONDIETARY APPROACHES

In developed nations, in settings in which maternal oral nutrition is considered sufficient, fetal growth retardation continues to occur. Therefore, other approaches have been taken to help augment delivery of substrates to the fetus and even bypass a possibly poorly functioning placenta (Harding and Charlton, 1989). Variable success has been achieved with nutritional therapies such as intravenous infusion of glucose and amino acids into the mother, infusion of amino acids into the amniotic fluid, and infusion of amino acids directly into the fetal peritoneal cavity. Non-nutritional therapies aimed at improving uterine blood flow (such as bed rest and maternal aspirin therapy) have been used, as well as maternal oxygen therapy to improve fetal-placental oxygenation. To date, the advantages and risks of each of these therapies are still undefined.

■ SUMMARY

In summary, the substrates available to the developing fetus play an important role in fetal development and growth. To provide the best nutritional environment for the fetus, the mother should be optimally treated for any underlying medical conditions, should be in good nutritional status prior to pregnancy, and should consume an adequate, balanced diet during pregnancy that results in a normal gestational weight gain.

■ REFERENCES

Apte, S., Iyengar, L.: Composition of the human fetus. Br. J. Nutr. 27:305–312, 1972.

Bercini, F., and Symonds, E.: Ketone bodies in fetal and maternal blood during parturition. Aust. N.Z. Obstet. Gynecol. 12:176–178, 1972.

Bernhardt, I., and Dorsey, D.: Hypervitaminosis A and congenital renal anomalies in a human infant. Obstet. Gynecol. 43:750–755, 1974.

Campbell, S.: The assessment of fetal development by diagnostic ultrasound. Clin. Perinatol. 2:507–525, 1974.

Cetin, I., Marconi, A., Bozzetti, P., et al.: Umbilical amino acid concentrations in appropriate and small for gestational age infants: A biochemical difference present in utero. Am. J. Obstet. Gynecol. 158:120–126, 1988.

Charlton, V.: Nutritional supplementation of the growth retarded fetus: Rationale, theoretical considerations, and in vivo studies. In Milunsky, A., Friedman, E., Gluck, L. (Eds.): Advances in Perinatal Medicine, vol. 5. New York, Plenum Press, 1986, pp. 1–42.

Charlton, V., and Creasy, R.: Lactate and pyruvate as fetal metabolic substrates. Pediatr. Res. 10:231–234, 1976a.

Charlton, V., and Creasy, R.: Unpublished observations, 1976b.

Charlton, V., and Creasy, R.: Acetate as metabolic substrate in the fetal lamb. Am. J. Physiol. 230:357–361, 1976c.

Chase, P., Welch, N., Dabiere, C., et al.: Alterations in human brain biochemistry following IUGR. Pediatrics 50:403–411, 1972.

TABLE 8–5. Recommended Average Daily Dietary Intake*

	NONPREGNANT	ADDITION DURING PREGNANCY
Energy, kcal	2000–2100	+300
Protein, g	46	+20
Fat-Soluble Vitamins		
Vitamin A, μg	800	+500
Vitamin D, μg	5–10	+5
Vitamin E, mg	10	+2
Water-Soluble Vitamins		
Vitamin C, mg	60	+10
Thiamin, mg	1.0–1.1	+0.4
Riboflavin, mg	1.2–1.3	+0.3
Niacin, mg	15	+2
Vitamin B_6, mg	1.6	
Folate, μg	180	+220
Vitamin B_{12}, μg	2.0	+0.2
Minerals		
Calcium, mg	1200	+400
Phosphorus, mg	1200	+400
Magnesium, mg	280	+40
Iron, mg	15	+30–60
Zinc, mg	12	+3
Iodine, μg	150	+25

* Values are for females of childbearing years, greater than 19 years of age, and of average weight (120 lbs or 55 kg) and height (64 inches or 163 cm)

(From National Research Council, Food and Nutrition Board: Recommended Dietary Allowances, 10th rev. ed. Washington, D.C., National Academy of Sciences, 1989.)

Clapp, J., Szeto, H., Larrow, R., et al.: Fetal metabolic response to experimental placental vascular damage. Am. J. Obstet. Gynecol. *140*:446–451, 1981.

Cousins, L.: Congenital anomalies among infants of diabetic mothers. Am. J. Obstet. Gynecol. *147*:333–338, 1983.

D'Ercole, A.: Somatomedins/insulin-like growth factors and fetal growth. J. Develop. Physiol. *9*:481–495, 1987.

Durnin, J.: Energy requirements of pregnancy. Lancet *2*:895–896, 1987.

Engstrom, W., and Heath, J.: Growth factors in early embryonic development. *In* Cockburn, F. (Ed.): Fetal and Neonatal Growth: Perinatal Practice, vol. 5. New York, John Wiley and Sons, 1988, pp. 11–32.

Fisher, S., Atkinson, M., Jacobsen, S., et al.: Selective fetal malnutrition: The effect of in vivo ethanol exposure upon in vitro placental uptake of amino acids in the non-human primate. Pediatr. Res. *17*:704–707, 1983.

Fitzhardinge, P., and Steven, E.: The small for date infant I. Later growth patterns. Pediatrics *49*:671–681, 1972a.

Fitzhardinge, P., and Steven, E.: The small for date infant II. Neurological and intellectual sequelae. Pediatrics *50*:50–57, 1972b.

Gal, I., Sharman, I., and Pryse-Davies, J.: Vitamin A in relation to human congenital malformations. Adv. Teratol. *5*:143–159, 1972.

Georgieff, M., Widness, J., Mills, M., et al.: The effect of prolonged intrauterine hyperinsulinemia on iron utilization in fetal sheep. Pediatr. Res. *26*:467–469, 1989.

Gross, T.: Maternal and placental causes of intrauterine growth retardation. *In* Gross, T., and Sokol, R. (Eds.): Intrauterine Growth Retardation. A Practical Approach. Chicago, Year Book, 1989, pp. 57–67.

Harding, J., and Charlton, V.: Treatment of the growth retarded fetus by augmentation of substrate supply. Semin. Perinatol. *14*:211–223, 1989.

Harvey, D., Prince, J., Bunton, J., et al.: The abilities of children who were small for gestational age. Pediatrics *69*:296–300, 1982.

Hauguel, S., Desmaizieres, V., and Challier, J.: Glucose uptake, utilization and transfer by the human placenta as a function of maternal glucose concentration. Pediatr. Res. *20*:269–273, 1986.

Haymond, M., Karl, I., and Pagliara, A.: Increased gluconeogenic substrates in the small for gestational age infant. N. Engl. J. Med. *291*:322–328, 1974.

Hurley, L.: Nutritional influences on embryonic and fetal development: Fat-soluble vitamins, water-soluble vitamins, major mineral elements, trace elements. *In* Hurley L.: Developmental Nutrition. Englewood Cliffs, N.J., Prentice Hall, 1980, pp. 125–227.

Jones, D.: Energy metabolism in developing brain. Semin. Perinatol. *3*:121–129, 1979.

Jones, K.: Beckwith-Wiedemann syndrome. *In* Graham, J. M., Jr. (Ed.): Smith's Recognizable Patterns of Human Malformation. Philadelphia, W. B. Saunders Company. 1988, pp. 136–139.

Kennaugh, J., and Hay, W.: Nutrition of the fetus and newborn. West. J. Med. *147*:435–448, 1987.

Kramer, M., McLean, F., Olivier, M., et al.: Body proportionality and head and length "sparing" in growth retarded neonates: A critical reappraisal. Pediatrics *84*:717–723, 1989.

Lammer, E., Chen, D., Holar, R., et al.: Retinoic acid embryopathy. N. Engl. J. Med. *313*:837–841, 1985.

Langer, O., Damus, K., Maiman, M., et al.: A link between relative hypoglycemia-hypoinsulinemia during oral glucose tolerance tests and intrauterine growth retardation. Am. J. Obstet. Gynecol. *155*:711–716, 1986.

Lipson, A., Beuhler, B., Bartley, J., et al.: Maternal hyperphenylalaninemia fetal effects. J. Pediatr. *104*:216–220, 1984.

Metcoff, J., Costiloe, J. P., Crosby, W., et al.: Maternal nutrition and fetal outcome. Am. J. Clin. Nutr. *34* (Suppl. 4):708–721, 1981.

Miller, H., and Jekel, J.: Malnutrition and growth retardation in newborn infants. Pediatrics *83*:443–444, 1989.

Milley, R., Rosenberg, A., Phillips, A., et al.: The effect of insulin on ovine fetal oxygen extraction. Am. J. Obstet. Gynecol. *149*:673–677, 1984.

Mills, J., Rhoads, G., Simpson, J., et al.: The absence of a relation between the periconceptual use of vitamins and neural-tube defects. N. Engl. Med. *321*:430–435, 1989.

Mochizuki, M., Maruo, T., Masuko, K., et al.: Effect of smoking on fetoplacental-maternal system during pregnancy. Am. J. Obstet. Gynecol. *149*:413–420, 1984.

Molteni, R., Stys, S., and Battaglia, F.: Relationships of fetal and placental weight in human beings: Fetal/placental weight ratios at various gestational ages and birth weight distributions. J. Reprod. Med. *21*:327–334, 1978.

Moore, K.: The fetal period. *In* Moore, K. L. (Ed.): The Developing Human, 4th ed. Philadelphia, W. B. Saunders Company, 1988, pp. 87–103.

Morriss, F., Boyd, R., Makowski, E., et al.: Umbilical V-A differences of acetoacetate and β-hydroxybutyrate in fed and starved ewes. Proc. Soc. Exp. Biol. Med. *145*:879–883, 1974.

Morriss, F., Makowski, E., Meschia, G., et al.: The glucose/oxygen quotient of the term human fetus. Biol. Neonate *25*:44–52, 1975.

Naeye, R.: Malnutrition-probable cause of fetal growth retardation. Arch. Pathol. *79*:284–291, 1965.

Naeye, R., and Dixon, J.: Distortions in fetal growth standards. Pediatr. Res. *12*:987–991, 1978.

National Research Council, Food and Nutrition Board: Recommended Dietary Allowances, 9th rev. ed. Washington, D.C., National Academy of Science, 1980, pp. 16–30.

Nutrition Reviews Editorial: Nutrition intervention in pregnancy. Nutr. Rev. *42*:42–44, 1984.

Phillips, A., Rosenkrantz, T., Porte, P., et al.: The effects of chronic fetal hyperglycemia on substrate uptake by the ovine fetus and conceptus. Pediatr. Res. *19*:659–666, 1985.

Pitkin, R.: Assessment of nutritional status of mother, fetus and newborn. Am. J. Clin. Nutr. *34*(Suppl 4):658–668, 1981.

Plotz, E., Kabara, J., Davis, M., et al.: Studies on the synthesis of choleterol in the brain of the human fetus. Am. J. Obstet. Gynecol. *4*:534–538, 1968.

Raman, L.: Influence of maternal nutritional factors affecting birth weight. Am. J. Clin. Nutr. *34* (Suppl. 4) :775–783, 1981.

Rosso, P.: Nutritional needs of the human fetus. Clin. Nutr. *2*:4–8, 1983.

Sara, V.: The role of somatomedins in fetal growth. *In* Lindbland, B. (Ed.): Perinatal Nutrition. New York, Academic Press, 1988, pp. 63–74.

Shah, R., and Rajalakshmi, R.: Studies on human fetal tissues. I. Fetal weight and tissue weights in relation to gestational age, fetal size, and maternal status. Indian J. Pediatr. *55*:261–271, 1988.

Smithells, R., Sheppard, S., and Schorah, C. J.: Vitamin deficiencies and neural tube defects. Arch. Dis. Child. *51*:944–950, 1976.

Smithells, R., Sheppard, S., Schorah, C. J., et al.: Apparent prevention of neural tube defects by periconceptual vitamin supplementation. Arch. Dis. Child. *56*:911–918, 1981.

Smithells, R., Sheppard, R., Wild, J., et al.: Prevention of neural tube defect recurrences in Yorkshire: Final report. Lancet *2*:498–499, 1989.

Socol, M., Manning, F., Murata, Y., et al.: Maternal smoking causes fetal hypoxia: Experimental evidence. Am. J. Obstet. Gynecol. *142*:214–218, 1982.

Soltesz, G., Harris, D., MacKenzie, I., et al.: The metabolic and endocrine milieu of the human fetus and mother at 18–21 weeks of gestation I. Plasma amino acid concentration. Pediatr. Res. *19*:91–93, 1985.

Sparks, J., Girard, J., and Battaglia, F.: An estimate of the caloric requirements of the human fetus. Biol. Neonate *38*:113–119, 1980.

Sparks, J., Hay, W., Bonds, D., et al.: Simultaneous measurements of lactate turnover rate and umbilical lactate uptake in the fetal lamb. J. Clin. Invest. *70*:179–192, 1982.

Susser, M.: Prenatal nutrition, birth weight and psychological development. Am. J. Clin. Nutr. *34* (Suppl. 4):784–803, 1981.

Usher, R., and McLean, F.: Intrauterine growth of live born Caucasian infants at sea level. J. Pediatr. *74*:901–910, 1969.

Van den Berg, B.: Maternal variables affecting fetal growth. Am. J. Clin. Nutr. *34* (Suppl. 4):722–726, 1981.

White, R. A., Preus, M., Watters, G. V., et al.: Familial occurrence of the Williams syndrome. J. Pediatr. *91*:614, 1977.

Whitehead, R.: Birth from the nutritional point of view. *In* Lindblad, B. (Ed.): Perinatal Nutrition. New York, Academic Press, 1988, pp. 197–206.

Widdowson, E.: Change in body proportion and composition during growth. *In* Davis, J., and Dobbing, J. (Eds.): Scientific Foundation in Pediatrics. Philadelphia, W. B. Saunders Company, 1974, pp. 153–163.

Willman, S., Leveno, K., Guzick, D., et al.: Glucose threshold for macrosomia in pregnancy complicated by diabetes. Am. J. Obstet. Gynecol. *154*:470–475, 1986.

Woods, R., Plessinger, M., and Clark, K.: Effect of cocaine on uterine blood flow and fetal oxygenation. J.A.M.A. *257*:957–961, 1977.

Worthington-Roberts, B.: Nutrition deficiencies and excesses. Impact on pregnancy, part 2. J. Perinatol. *5*:12–21, 1985.

Yates, J.: The genetics of fetal and postnatal growth. *In*: Cockburn, F. (Ed.): Fetal and Neonatal Growth. New York, John Wiley and Sons, 1988, pp. 1–10.

Ziegler, E., O'Donnell, A., Nelson, S., et al.: Body composition of the reference fetus. Growth *40*:329–341, 1976.

DIABETES MELLITUS 9

Roberta A. Ballard

The deleterious effects of maternal diabetes mellitus on development and outcome of the fetus and newborn have long been recognized, and the opportunity to improve this outcome has been one of the first challenges to be met by a coordinated perinatal-neonatal approach to management. The prevalence of insulin-dependent (Type I) diabetes mellitus is estimated at 0.1 to 0.5 per cent of all pregnancies in the United States, with an additional 3 to 12 per cent of women experiencing transient biochemical abnormalities that produce gestational diabetes. Diabetes mellitus is not only a disturbance of glucose metabolism, since insulin has multiple effects on metabolism of proteins and fatty acids. However, it is in the area of carbohydrate metabolism where most of the investigation has occurred and where the clinical effects are most apparent.

■ DIAGNOSIS

Many perinatologists have recommended that, if possible, women should be routinely screened for diabetes during pregnancy, but all agree that women who have any of the risk factors of being overweight, previous delivery of a macrosomic or stillborn infant, or family history of diabetes as well as all women over 25 years of age should be screened. Evaluation of the risk for the fetus can be done best by considering that there are two conditions in which pregnancies may be complicated by diabetes mellitus: (1) diabetes existing before pregnancy and (2) gestational diabetes. The risk assessment of White (1949), as modified by the American College of Obstetrics and Gynecology (1986), is presented in Table 9–1. Through joint perinatal-neonatal management and increased understanding of the mechanisms of diabetes and its metabolic effects, the perinatal mortality from diabetes has been decreased ten-fold over the past four decades, (Table 9–2) compared with a four- to five-fold decrease in overall perinatal mortality during this period of time (Fig. 9–1). It is felt that perinatal mortality associated with carefully managed diabetes is now approaching the expected mortality in the general population. At present, congenital anomalies comprise the leading cause of perinatal mortality in infants of diabetic mothers.

■ METABOLIC DISTURBANCES IN THE MOTHER

NORMAL PREGNANCY

The maternal glucose-insulin balance that occurs during normal pregnancy favors hyperglycemia because, despite some degree of hyperinsulinism secondary to islet cell hyperplasia, pregnancy is apparently associated with insulin resistance. This resistance is thought to be related to

TABLE 9–1. Classification of Diabetes in Pregnancy

PREGESTATIONAL DIABETES

Class	Age at Onset (year)		Duration (year)	Vascular Disease	Therapy
A	Any		Any	–	A-1, diet only A-2, insulin
B	>20		<10	–	Insulin
C	10–19	or	10–19	–	Insulin
D	<10		>20	Benign retinopathy	Insulin
F	Any		Any	Nephropathy	Insulin
R	Any		Any	Proliferative retinopathy	Insulin
H	Any		Any	Heart disease	Insulin

GESTATIONAL DIABETES

Class	Fasting Glucose Level		Postprandial Glucose Level
A-1	<105 mg/dl	and	<120 mg/dl
A-2	>105 mg/dl	and/or	>120 mg/dl

From American College of Obstetrics and Gynecology: Management of diabetes mellitus in pregnancy. Technical Bulletin No. 92, May 1986.

changes in other maternal hormones, such as human placental lactogen, progesterone, cortisol, and possibly prolactin. In addition, disposal of glucose after carbohydrate intake appears to be impaired, causing somewhat higher maternal glucose levels. Glucagon is suppressed by glucose during pregnancy, and secretory responses of glucagon to amino acids are not increased above nonpregnancy levels. Lipid metabolism is also altered, with more glucose being converted to triglyceride in pregnant, compared with nonpregnant, women. The effect of this process is to conserve calories and enhance fat deposition.

GESTATIONAL DIABETES

Depending upon the diagnostic criteria used, approximately 3 to 12 per cent of previously nondiabetic pregnant women develop some glucose intolerance during the

TABLE 9–2. Perinatal Mortality and White's Classification for Diabetes

WHITE'S CLASS	NO. OF CASES	PERINATAL MORTALITY	
		Deaths	Per 1000
B	465	13	27.9
C	257	7	27.2
D, R, & F	321	10	31.2
R/F*	96	6	62.5
TOTAL	1,139	36	31.6

*Obtained from reports that separately identify class R/F.
From Hunter, D. J. F.: Diabetes in pregnancy. In Chalmers, I., Enkin, N., and Keirse, M. J. N. C.: Effective Care in Pregnancy and Childbirth, vol. 1. Oxford, Oxford Medical Publishers, 1989, p. 579.

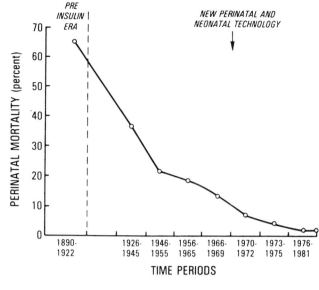

FIGURE 9–1. Perinatal mortality rate among newborn infants of diabetic mothers from 1890 to 1981. Data plotted from numerical reports of Craigin and Ryder (1916), DeLee (1920), Williams (1925), Pedersen (1977), Gabbe (1978), and Jorge et al. (1981). (From Creasy, R.K., and Resnick, R.: Maternal Fetal Medicine: Principles and Practice, 2nd ed. Philadelphia, W. B. Saunders Company, 1989.)

second half of gestation. The mechanism of this is not fully understood; however, follow-up studies indicate that about 40 to 60 per cent of overweight women with glucose intolerance during pregnancy develop overt diabetes within the subsequent 10 to 20 years.

DIABETES MELLITUS

The general insulin resistance of pregnancy makes hyperglycemia in women with true diabetes mellitus very difficult to control, particularly after the first trimester. It is not unusual for a diabetic woman's insulin requirement to increase up to three-fold during pregnancy. In addition, hepatic ketone production increases during pregnancy; therefore, the development of ketoacidosis may both be more rapid and occur at relatively low blood glucose levels. It is most important that diabetic women be well educated about this problem during pregnancy, especially if they experience any signs of dehydration or infection. Ketoacidosis is, by far, the most serious metabolic disturbance that can affect the fetus, with a mortality rate of 50 per cent in fetuses of women who have had a serious episode of ketoacidosis.

Women with diabetes mellitus are also more likely to develop hypoglycemia during pregnancy. This is attributed to two factors: (1) increased placental-fetal utilization of glucose and (2) limitation of hepatic gluconeogenesis due to a relative lack of alanine, a major substrate. In hypoglycemia, the risk is primarily to the mother, since the fetus appears to be protected at the mother's expense. Both hyperglycemia and hypoglycemia are even more difficult to control in pregnant adolescents (even without the complicating social factors) than in adult women. It is highly desirable that a nutritionist be closely involved in the management of pregnant diabetics.

The incidence of preeclampsia is also greatly increased in pregnant diabetics (see Chapter 10), presumably because of the problems with diabetic control.

■ METABOLIC EFFECTS ON THE FETUS AND NEWBORN

The Pedersen hypothesis (1977) is now generally accepted. Pedersen suggested that maternal and, hence,

fetal hyperglycemia results in fetal hyperinsulinism secondary to hypertrophy of the fetal pancreatic islet cells. Menon and associates (1990) have demonstrated that some animal insulin bound by anti-insulin antibody actually crosses the placenta to the fetus and thus contributes to fetal hyperinsulinemia. The expanded hypothesis considers, in addition, that the beta cells may be more sensitive to the insulinogenic effect of amino acids and that the combination of hyperinsulinism with increases in amino acids, lipids, and ketones is the cause of the macrosomia and organomegaly that occur in infants of diabetic mothers. Insulin is considered to be a growth hormone of the fetus, responsible for acceleration of protein synthesis and deposition of glycogen and fat.

NEONATAL HYPOGLYCEMIA

One of the metabolic problems common to these infants is hypoglycemia, which is related to the degree of maternal control (or lack of it). Hypoglycemia is most likely to occur between 1 and 5 hours after birth, as the supply of maternal glucose is withdrawn and the infant's levels of circulating insulin remain elevated. These infants therefore require close monitoring for blood glucose concentration during the first hours after birth (see Chapter 110). Infants of diabetic mothers also appear to have disorders of both catecholamine and glucagon metabolism and seem unable to mount normal compensatory responses to hypoglycemia. In the past, these infants were treated with glucagon; however, this treatment frequently results in very high blood glucose levels that trigger insulin secretion and repeated cycles of hypoglycemia-hyperglycemia. Current recommendations, therefore, include early feeding when possible, along with infusion of intravenous glucose.

Ordinarily, blood glucose levels can be controlled satisfactorily with an infusion of 10 per cent glucose. If greater amounts of glucose are required, bolus administration of 5 ml/kg of 10 per cent glucose is recommended, with gradually increasing concentrations of glucose administered every 30 to 60 min, if necessary. Close monitoring to correct the hypoglycemia while avoiding hyperglycemia and consequent stimulation of insulin secretion is important. Since it is difficult to measure insulin levels accurately in the newborn (because of the placental crossover of insulin antibodies), measurements of C-peptide have been useful as an indicator of "level of control." C-peptide is a byproduct of the conversion of proinsulin to insulin and is secreted by the beta cells in the pancreas in equimolar amounts to insulin. Increased levels of C-peptide can be found in the umbilical cords of infants whose mothers' diabetes has not been tightly controlled. Figure 9–2 shows the relationship of cord serum C-peptide levels to gestational age in infants of nondiabetic and diabetic mothers.

MACROSOMIA

Although macrosomia clearly is most marked in infants of women with poor diabetic control, it is also becoming apparent that about 30 per cent of infants whose mothers' diabetes had been fairly well controlled fall above the 90th percentile in weight for gestational age. Some of these infants have exposure to excess insulin due to the transplacental passage of animal insulin–anti-insulin antibody complex, which has been associated with macrosomia (Menon et al., 1990; Schwartz, 1990). In addition, it is probable that macrosomia reflects other aspects of maternal energy intake and expenditure associated with increased maternal levels of amino acids and free fatty acids. The most reliable predictors of macrosomia are maternal obesity and weight gain during pregnancy, followed by the mother's own birth weight. These factors must therefore be considered in assessment of whether macrosomia in an infant of a diabetic mother is secondary to poor control of the maternal diabetes. Obviously, very large infants are more prone to birth trauma and more likely to be delivered by emergency cesarean section and thus are subject to the increased morbidity and mortality associated with these situations.

Macrosomic infants have organomegaly, particularly involving the liver, adrenal glands, and heart. Brain growth is not excessive, and therefore the head of the infant may appear relatively small compared with the rest of the

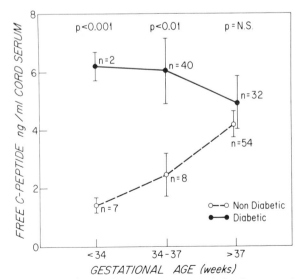

FIGURE 9–2. *Relation of cord serum C-peptide levels to gestational age in infants of nondiabetic and diabetic mothers (mean ± S.E.M.). (From Sosenko, I., et al., N. Engl. J. Med. 301:859, 1979. Reprinted by permission of the New England Journal of Medicine.)*

infant's body. Infants with marked *cardiomegaly* may have hypertrophic cardiomyopathy, which may cause congestive heart failure. On echocardiogram, hypertrophic cardiomyopathy may be indistinguishable from hypertrophic subaortic stenosis, showing thickening of the anterior wall of the right ventricle and intraventricular septum as well as some left ventricular hypertrophy. Ordinarily, cardiomegaly related to macrosomia of the diabetic infant resolves by about one month of age.

■ OTHER PROBLEMS

Infants of diabetic mothers (IDMs) are known to have hypocalcemia and hypomagnesemia. However, there is no evidence that either these findings or hypoglycemia contribute to the generalized jitteriness seen in these infants. In addition, polycythemia is common and frequently associated with dehydration. These infants also have increased total body water and fat content. Therefore, careful attention to hydration is necessary to prevent the development of intravascular thrombosis. In particular, renal vein thrombosis has been associated with birth to a diabetic mother (Avery et al., 1957). Hyperbilirubinemia is also common, with more than 20 per cent of IDMs having prolonged hyperbilirubinemia. In addition, the transition from fetal to adult hemoglobin in these infants is delayed until after birth, instead of occurring normally between 28 and 34 weeks' gestation (Perrine et al., 1985).

■ OTHER PERINATAL RISKS

Studies of the adverse outcomes for diabetic pregnancies have noted an increased incidence of spontaneous abortion only in women with poor glycemic control (Sutherland and Pritchard, 1986). This is probably related to the increased number of anomalies also seen in these infants. Women in good control do *not* have an increased rate of spontaneous abortion over normal controls. The greater number of preterm deliveries reported is generally related to elective early delivery, since delivery prior to 36 weeks' gestation was previously recommended to prevent later in utero demise. Stillbirth, previously a major problem for diabetic pregnancies, appears to be much better prevented now by virtue of improved control of maternal glucose levels and careful monitoring of fetal well-being, especially after 32 weeks' gestation (see Chapter 12). Intrauterine growth retardation occasionally may occur when microvascular disease is present in the fetus, particularly in association with nephropathy in the mother.

■ RESPIRATORY DISTRESS SYNDROME

Robert and colleagues (1976) reported a five-fold increase in the risk of respiratory distress syndrome (RDS) in infants of diabetic mothers, compared with infants of nondiabetic mothers matched for gestational age, route of delivery, and other maternal complications. It seems clear that hyperglycemia and fetal reactional hyperinsulinism both contribute to delaying fetal lung maturation (Bourbon and Farrell, 1985). Current obstetric management approaches, including tight control of maternal glucose levels and careful fetal surveillance with use of stress and nonstress tests, have been successful in bringing pregnancies closer to term and thus reducing the incidence of RDS. With better understanding of amniotic fluid indicators of pulmonary maturation, the incidence of RDS in infants of diabetic mothers is now approaching that of the general population. It is known, however, that these infants may have RDS even with a lecithin-to-sphingomyelin ratio (L/S) of 2 or greater. However, infants appear to be free of RDS if phosphatidyl glycerol is present in the amniotic fluid or if the L/S ratio is greater than 3. The mechanism responsible for this is not well understood (see Chapter 49). The course of infants of diabetic mothers is also complicated by respiratory distress secondary to wet lung, i.e., delayed clearance of pulmonary fluid, since many of them are delivered without labor by cesarean section. Wet lung now contributes more to morbidity in these infants than does RDS (Fig. 9–3).

■ CONGENITAL ANOMALIES

Congenital anomalies have emerged as the principal cause of perinatal mortality among infants of diabetic mothers. Molsted-Peterson and co-workers (1964) reported an incidence of congenital anomalies of 6.4 per cent in a group of 853 infants cared for over a period of 37 years. This was much higher than a rate of 2.1 per cent in a control group collected over a 6-month period. Apparently, the risk of congenital anomalies in infants of diabetic mothers is increased approximately three- to five-fold (Table 9–3). The greatest number of affected infants are those with cardiac anomalies, but vertebral anomalies with caudal regression syndrome occur in a significant percentage (Fig. 9–4) as well as central nervous system defects, particularly holoprosencephaly. Anencephaly and meningomyelocele also occur. In addition, some infants have a small left colon (microcolon), which later resolves.

The Atlanta Birth Defects Case-Control Study found the relative risk for major malformations among infants of

TABLE 9–3. Malformations Associated with Maternal Diabetes and Their Estimated Risk Ratio (Frequency Relative to Non-diabetic Women)

MALFORMATION	RISK RATIO
Sacral dysgenesis	200–600
Situs inversus	84
Ureter duplex	23
Renal agenesis	6
Cardiac anomalies*	4
Anencephalus	3
Holoprosencephaly	40–400

*Cardiac anomalies, for example, constitute the greatest problem in IDMs because of their higher frequency in the general population. Therefore, despite the fact that their relative risk (expressed as risk ratio) is only moderately increased, their occurrence, in terms of actual number, is greater.

From Mills, J. L.: Congenital malformation in diabetes. *In* Gabbe, S. G., and Oh, W. (Eds.): Report of the 93rd Ross Conference on Pediatric Research. Columbus, Ohio, Ross Laboratories, 1987, p. 13.

insulin-dependent diabetic mothers to be 7.9 per cent, with a relative risk for major central nervous system and cardiovascular system defects of 15.5 and 18.0 per cent, respectively. The study reported, however, that the highest relative risk (20.6 per cent) for major cardiovascular defects occurred among infants of women with gestational diabetes who developed insulin dependence in the third trimester. The absolute risk for this group of infants was 9.7 per cent (Becerra et al., 1990). Since there was no consistent routine for screening for diabetes mellitus during the study (1968 to 1980), it is likely that some of these women who were thought to develop gestational diabetes

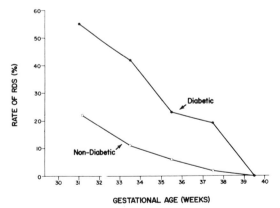

FIGURE 9–3. Rate of respiratory distress syndrome (RDS) versus gestational age. Each rate represents the rate for all infants born in the week before and the week after the gestational age designated. The high rate of respiratory distress in infants of diabetic mothers in the 1960s was related to the degree of prematurity. Elective cesarean section was carried out at 36 to 37 weeks' gestation to avoid late fetal deaths. A change in the management of mothers that maintains close control of blood sugar levels and tries to prolong pregnancy to term has resulted in a major reduction in RDS and in fetal and neonatal deaths. Obstetric management includes nonstress tests and ultrasonograms at intervals from 32 weeks. Amniocentesis to measure L/S ratio or saturated phosphatidylcholine at 36 to 37 weeks allows prediction of the risk of respiratory distress in a given infant. About 25 per cent of diabetic mothers are delivered by cesarean section because of fetal distress.

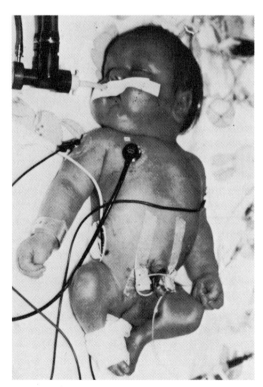

FIGURE 9–4. Newborn with caudal regression syndrome, flexion contractures, and hypoplasia of the lower extremities. The mother had Type I diabetes and and Hb A$_{1c}$ concentration of 13.5 per cent when first seen for prenatal care at 12 weeks' gestation. (From Creasy, R.K., and Resnick, R.: Maternal-Fetal Medicine: Principles and Practice, 2nd ed. Philadelphia, W. B. Saunders Company, 1989.)

were, in fact, women with previously unrecognized, true diabetes mellitus in an early stage.

There is evidence in animals (Baker et al., 1980; Sadler et al., 1980) that the malformations that occur in infants of diabetic mothers are caused by excessive glucose and other metabolic derangements. Whole-embryo cultures of mice exposed to diabetic levels of glucose demonstrate a high incidence of neural tube defects, and uncontrolled diabetes in the rat produces lumbosacral malformations analogous to those that occur in the infants of diabetic women. Control of diabetes during the period of organogenesis reduces the incidence of these defects (Baker et al., 1980).

CONTROL OF GLUCOSE IN THE HUMAN

There are also indications that the incidence of congenital anomalies in human pregnancies is related to diabetic control. A significant correlation has been found between elevated hemoglobin A_{1c} levels in the first trimester with the incidence of congenital anomalies (Miller et al., 1981). In infants of women with normal hemoglobin A_{1c} levels, the incidence of anomalies was similar to that in the general population. There is increasing evidence that the incidence of anomalies is reduced when maternal diabetes is well controlled prior to conception (Kitzmiller et al., 1988). In a randomized trial comparing three groups of women according to degree of control of blood glucose levels: "very tight" (blood sugars maintained below 5.6 mMol/l), "tight" (levels between 5.6 and 6.7 mMol/l), and "moderate" (levels between 6.7 and 8.9 mMol/l), Farrag (1987) found that very tight control was associated with a high incidence of episodes of hypoglycemia in early pregnancy and does not appear to confer any benefits in pregnancy outcomes. On the other hand, in comparing moderate versus tight control, he found tight control to be associated with a lower incidence of cesarean section and fewer infants with birth weights above the 90th percentile. In addition, he noted a trend in those with moderate control toward decreased urinary tract infection, hypertension, preterm labor, RDS, and overall perinatal mortality. Since it has been established that good control during pregnancy is associated with a decrease in the other metabolic problems of the newborn, there is adequate evidence that expert surveillance and interdisciplinary collaboration in the management of diabetic mothers can achieve excellent results. It is important, however, for the responsible caregivers to define a program of care that minimizes disruption to the woman's daily life and that is individualized for each woman's specific circumstances if an optimal opportunity for successful reproduction is to be achieved.

■ OUTCOME

Adverse neurodevelopmental outcome of infants of diabetic mothers appears to be limited to some suggestion of decreased I.Q. among infants whose mothers demonstrated acetonuria during their pregnancy (Churchill et al., 1969; Stehbens et al., 1977). There does not appear to be any disadvantage in developmental outcome compared to the normal population in term infants who have no anomalies, although more large for gestational age infants

are found to be obese at 7 years of age. The risk of juvenile-onset diabetes is less than 2 per cent (Zamora, 1976) and in fact is higher among infants with diabetic fathers (6 per cent).

■ ACKNOWLEDGMENT

The Editorial Review of John L. Kitzmiller is gratefully acknowledged.

■ REFERENCES

American College of Obstetrics and Gynecology: Management of diabetes mellitus in pregnancy. Technical Bulletin No. 92, May 1986.

Avery, M. E., Oppenheimer, E. M., and Gordon, H. H.: Renal vein thrombosis in newborn infants of diabetic mothers. N. Engl. J. Med. 256:1134, 1957.

Baker, S., Eglar, J. M., Klein, S. H., et al.: Meticulous control of diabetes during organogenesis prevents congenital lumbosacral defects in rats. Diabetes 30:955, 1980.

Becerra, J. E., Khoury, M. J., Cordero, J. F., et al.: Diabetes mellitus during pregnancy and the risks for specific birth defects: A population-based case-control study. Pediatrics 85:1, 1990.

Bourbon, J. R., and Farrell, P. M.: Fetal lung development in the diabetic pregnancy. Pediatr. Res. 19:253, 1985.

Chalmers, I., Enkin, N., and Keirse, M. J. N. C. (Eds.): Effective Care in Pregnancy and Childbirth. Oxford, Oxford Medical Publications, 1989.

Churchill, J. A., Berendes, H. W., and Nemore, J.: Neuropsychological deficits in children of diabetic mothers. Am. J. Obstet. Gynecol. 105:257, 1969.

Cornblath, M., and Schwartz, R.: Infant of the diabetic mother. In Cornblath, M. (Ed.): Disorders of Carbohydrate Metabolism in Infancy, 3rd ed. Philadelphia, W. B. Saunders Company, 1976, pp. 115–154.

Craigin, E. B., Ryder, G. H.: Obstetrics. A Practical Textbook for Students and Practitioners. Philadelphia, Lea and Febiger, 1916.

Dehee, J. B.: The Principles and Practice of Obstetrics. 3rd ed. Philadelphia, W. B. Saunders Company, 1920.

Farquhar, J. W.: Control of the blood sugar level in the neonatal period. Arch. Dis. Child. 29:519, 1954.

Farquhar, J. W.: The child of the diabetic woman. Arch. Dis. Child. 34:76, 1959.

Farrag, O. A. M.: Prospective study of 3 metabolic regimens in pregnant diabetics. Aust. N.Z. J. Obstet. Gynaecol. 27:6, 1987.

Fuhrmann, K., Reiher, H., Semmler, K., et al.: The effect of intensified conventional insulin therapy before and during pregnancy on malformation rate in offspring of diabetic mothers. Exp. Clin. Endocrinol. 83:173, 1984.

Gabbe, S. G.: Management of diabetes mellitus in pregnancy. Am. J. Obstet. Gynecol. 153:824, 1985.

Gabbe, S. G., Lowensohn, R. I., Mestman, J. H., et al.: Lecithin/sphingomyelin ratio in diabetic pregnancy. Obstet. Gynecol. 66:521, 1977.

Gabbe, S. G., Lowensohn, R. I., Wu, P. Y. K., and Guerra, G.: Current patterns of neonatal morbidity and mortality in infants of diabetic mothers. Diabetes Care 1:334, 1978.

Hunter, D. J. F.: Diabetes in pregnancy. In Chalmers, I., Enkin, N., and Keirse, M. J. N. C. (Eds.): Effective Care in Pregnancy and Childbirth. Oxford, Oxford Medical Publications, 1989.

Jorge, C. S., Artal, R., Paul, R. H., et al.: Antepartum fetal surveillance in diabetic pregnant patients. Am. J. Obstet. Gynecol. 141:641, 1981.

Kitzmiller, J. L., Brown, E. R., Phillipe, M., et al.: Diabetic nephropathy and perinatal outcome. Am. J. Obstet. Gynecol. 141:741, 1981.

Kitzmiller, J. L., Gavin, L. A., Gin, D. G., et al.: Managing diabetes and pregnancy. Curr. Probl. Obstet. Gynecol. Fertil. 12:107, 1988.

Kitzmiller, J. L., Younger, M. D., Hare, J. W., et al.: Continuous subcutaneous insulin therapy during early pregnancy. Obstet. Gynecol. 66:606, 1985.

Kucera, J.: Rate and type of congenital anomalies amongst offspring of diabetic women. J. Reprod. Med. 7:61, 1971.

Menon, R. K., Cohen, R. M., Sperling, M. A., et al.: Transplacental passage of insulin in pregnant women with insulin-dependent diabetes mellitus. N. Engl. J. Med. 323:309, 1990.

Miller, E., Hare, J. W., Clotherty, J. P., et al.: Elevated maternal hemoglobin A_{1c} in early pregnancy and major congenital anomalies in infants of diabetic mothers. N. Engl. J. Med. *304*:1331, 1981.

Milunsky, A., Alpert, E., Kitzmiller, J. L., et al.: Prenatal diagnosis of neural tube defects. VIII. The importance of serum alpha-fetoprotein screening in diabetic pregnant women. Am. J. Obstet. Gynecol. *142*:1030, 1982.

Molsted-Pedersen, L., Tygstrug, I., and Pedersen, J.: Congenital malformations in newborn infants of diabetic women. Lancet *1*:1124, 1964.

Oppenheimer, E. H., and Esterly, J. R.: Thrombosis in the newborn: Comparison of infants of diabetic and non-diabetic mothers. J. Pediat. *67*:549, 1965.

Pederson, J.: The Pregnant Diabetic and Her Newborn, 2nd ed. Baltimore, Williams & Wilkins, 1977, p. 9.

Perrine, S. P., Greene, M. F., and Faller, D. V.: Delay in the fetal globin switch in infant of diabetic mothers. N. Engl. J. Med. *312*:338, 1985.

Robert, M. F., Neff, R. K., Hubbell, J. P., et al.: Association between maternal diabetes and the respiratory distress syndrome in the newborn. N. Engl. J. Med. *294*:357, 1976.

Sadler, T. W.: Effects of maternal diabetes on early embryogenesis. The teratogenic potential of diabetic serum. Teratology *21*:339, 1980.

Schwartz, R.: Hyperinsulinemia and macrosomia. N. Engl. J. Med. *323*:340, 1990.

Stehbens, J. A., Baker, G. L., and Kitchell, M.: Outcome at ages 1, 3, and 5 years of children born to diabetic women. Am. J. Obstet. Gynecol. *56*:144, 1977.

Stronge, J. M., Foley, M. E., and Drury, M. I.: Diabetes mellitus and pregnancy. N. Engl. J. Med. *314*:58, 1986.

Sutherland, H. W., and Pritchard, C. W.: Increased incidence of spontaneous abortion in pregnancies complicated by maternal diabetes mellitus. Am. J. Obstet. Gynecol., *155*:135, 1986.

White, P.: Pregnancy complicating diabetes. Am. J. Med. *7*:609, 1949.

Williams, J. W.: Obstetrics: A Textbook for the Use of Students and Practitioners. New York, D. Appleton, 1925.

Yatscoff, R. H., Mehta, A., and Dean, H.: Cord blood glycosylated hemoglobin: Correlation with maternal glycosylated hemoglobin and birthweight. Am. J. Obstet. Gynecol. *152*:861, 1985.

Zamora, J.: Considerations on genetic counselling. *In* New, M. I., and Fiser, R. H. (Eds.): Diabetes and Other Endocrine Disorders during Pregnancy and in the Newborn. New York, Alan R. Liss, 1976, pp. 1–12.

PREECLAMPSIA 10

Roberta A. Ballard and James M. Roberts

Hypertension in pregnancy remains a significant cause of morbidity and mortality for both mother and infant. There are two etiologically distinct entities that account for most hypertensive disorders of pregnancy: preeclampsia and chronic hypertension. Chronic hypertension may be present and observable prior to pregnancy or is diagnosed before the 20th week of gestation and serves as an additional predisposing factor to superimposed pregnancy-induced hypertension.

■ ECLAMPSIA

Eclampsia was recognized by Hippocrates as a convulsive disorder that occurs in pregnant women. In the early nineteenth century, it was first distinguished from epilepsy, and the associated proteinuria was recognized in the 1840s. With the introduction of methods for measuring blood pressure around the turn of the century, it was recognized that women with eclampsia also had hypertension. This entity remains the leading cause of maternal death in the United States, England, and Wales (Kaunitz et al., 1985). In a review of eclampsia by Doll and Hanington (1961), the international incidence of eclampsia with seizures at was cited as 1.2 to 2.2 per 1000 deliveries. Eclampsia in the United States currently occurs in less than 1.0 per 1000 deliveries.

■ PREECLAMPSIA

Preeclampsia is diagnosed on the basis of a blood pressure increase accompanied by proteinuria or edema or both, but *without* seizures, and it is an important cause of fetal and neonatal morbidity and mortality (Chamberlain et al., 1978; MacGillivray, 1983). It is estimated that 5 to 7 per cent of pregnancies in the United States are affected by preeclampsia. In addition, women with underlying microvascular disease, such as diabetes, collagen vascular disease, or idiopathic hypertension, are also affected. The incidence of preeclampsia is increased in twin pregnancies, hydatidiform mole, and fetal hydrops. It is cured by delivery of the infant and appears to be completely reversible. Recurrence is infrequent (only 10 per cent), and therefore, collagen vascular disease, diabetes, or other causes of hypertension should be suspected and investigated in any woman who appears to have a second episode of preeclampsia.

DIAGNOSIS

Preeclampsia is a perplexing syndrome that affects many, and perhaps most, organ systems. It occurs primarily in first pregnancies after the 20th week of gestation, and the affected woman usually presents first with signs rather than symptoms. Symptoms are variable and may mimic many other kinds of problems, including abdominal pain, backache, and headache (Table 10–1). The diagnosis of preeclampsia or eclampsia is made on the basis of blood pressure elevation of >15 mm Hg (diastolic) or >30 mm Hg (systolic), compared with values early in the pregnancy. If the early blood pressure is not known, a blood pressure of >140/90 in late pregnancy is considered indicative. In addition, the diagnosis requires proteinuria of >0.3 g/24 hours and/or edema. Other signs and symptoms that are of concern and require close management include blood pressure >160 mm Hg (systolic) or >110 mm Hg (diastolic), proteinuria >3.5 g/24 hours, oliguria with increased serum creatinine, evidence of retinal hemorrhage, cerebral or visual disturbances, pulmonary edema or cyanosis, and most serious, central nervous system involvement resulting in seizures.

HELLP SYNDROME

Redman and colleagues (1978) first described a reduction in platelet count as an early manifestation of preeclampsia. It has been postulated that circulating platelets are activated when collagen is exposed to damaged vascular endothelium. Weinstein (1986) identified a group of patients with the findings of hemolysis (*H*), elevated liver enzymes (*EL*), and low platelet count (*LP*). These findings are considered indicative of a fairly severe form of preeclampsia that occurs early in the third trimester, even though patients in whom they appear do not necessarily exhibit hypertension on presentation. Associated findings in women with the HELLP syndrome may include jaundice, elevated BUN and creatinine levels, and severe right-upper-quadrant pain. Clotting factors other than platelets are usually normal. The patients have a firm, tense liver with some evidence of subcapsular hematoma. They may also be affected by hypoglycemia. It is therefore important to obtain serial platelet counts and liver enzymes during pregnancy in patients with mild to moderate preeclampsia.

PATHOPHYSIOLOGY

The 40 per cent increase in plasma blood volume that occurs normally in pregnancy does not occur in women with preeclampsia. The common pathologic changes are

TABLE 10–1. Signs and Symptoms of Preeclampsia-Eclampsia

Cerebral	Headaches, dizziness, tinnitus, change in respiratory rate, tachycardia, and fever
Visual	Diplopia, scotomata, blurred vision, and amaurosis
Gastrointestinal	Nausea, vomiting, epigastric pain, and hematemesis
Renal	Oligura, anuria, hematuria, and hemoglobinuria

necrosis and hemorrhage, compatible with reduced organ perfusion. Among the organs particularly affected is the kidney, in which a lesion called glomeruloendotheliosis occurs. This lesion is not found in any other form of hypertension. The process involves primarily the renal glomerulocapillary endothelium, which is edematous and may virtually occlude the capillary lumen, with inclusions in the basement membrane. Decidual vessels are also affected, with characteristic changes occurring in the spiral arteries that supply the placental site. Some vessels may be occluded by a lesion called atherosis (Fig. 10–1), which may be noted as early as the first trimester but which always occurs by 20 weeks' gestation. In addition, cardiovascular changes occur, including increased total peripheral resistance and decreased plasma volume.

Changes in renal function include decreased glomerular filtration rate, renal blood flow, and urate clearance. Proteinuria results from a nonselective increase in glomerular permeability. Glomerular filtration is reduced, but tubular handling of sodium remains relatively normal and thus reduces the filtered load of sodium and net sodium retention. Hyperuricemia is the earliest and most consistent change in renal function. It is secondary to altered tubular function, similar to that seen with hypovolemia. The renin-angiotensin-aldosterone system, although considered a potential candidate, does not appear to have a simple relationship with the hypertension of preeclampsia. Coagulation changes secondary to activation of intravascular coagulation with formation of microthrombi further compromise tissue perfusion. Disseminated intravascular coagulation (DIC) occurs in preeclampsia in approximately 10 per cent of patients with severe disease (Roberts and May, 1976).

Since the levels of procoagulants are normal in most patients with preeclampsia, the coagulation changes that occur may be secondary rather than primary pathogenic factors. The etiologic basis for these changes is a matter of controversy, but it is possible that either the vascular changes of preeclampsia or vasospasm may initiate the phenomenon.

Preeclamptic women also have increased sensitivity to pressor agents. Although attempts have been made to identify an endogenous pressor agent that causes increased vasoconstriction and hypertension, it is now very clear that these women are extremely sensitive to any pressor substances. It is known that reduced plasma volume, activation of coagulation mechanisms, and increased sensitivity to pressors all precede the diagnostic clinical changes.

PATHOGENESIS

The underlying pathogenesis of preeclampsia is not understood at this time, and various etiologic explanations—from parasites to prostaglandins and other circulating factors—have been suggested. Since preeclampsia can occur in abdominal pregnancy (thus ruling out the uterus) and occurs in association with hydatidiform mole (thus ruling out a role for the fetus), it has been considered a trophoblast-related disease. In addition, since it occurs almost exclusively in first pregnancies (unless there is other underlying disease), it has been suggested that exposure to paternal antigen may be protective. It appears that multiparous women who have a first pregnancy with a new partner share the same risk of preeclampsia as those having first pregnancies. Proposed unifying hypotheses include the following: (1) preeclampsia may be a "hyperdynamic" condition (Easterling and Benedetti, 1989) and (2) endothelial-cell injury is a central pathophysiologic change in preeclampsia and that the blood of preeclamptic women contains a factor produced by the poorly perfused trophoblast that injures endothelial cells (Roberts, 1989).

■ EFFECTS ON THE FETUS

Estimates of increased fetal-neonatal mortality due to maternal eclampsia range from two- to five-fold, a significant portion of which is associated with the frequent necessity for preterm delivery. In mild to moderate disease, there appears to be little risk to the fetus, and therefore, management is aimed at minimizing the severity of the progression of the maternal disease. Since preeclampsia is associated with increased incidence of placental abruption, this emergency contributes to the number of preterm deliveries with attendant hypovolemia and asphyxia and, hence, to morbidity and mortality in the infants. Clearly, the most severe outcome relates to infants who have been exposed in utero to maternal seizures. The long-term effects range from fetal death, due to interruption of placental perfusion at the time of seizure, to other signs of hypoxic ischemic damage, such as long-term neurologic deficits, acute tubular necrosis resulting from poor renal perfusion, and necrotizing enterocolitis as a result of poor gastrointestinal perfusion.

Intrauterine Growth Retardation. Significant morbidity is associated with intrauterine growth retardation, which

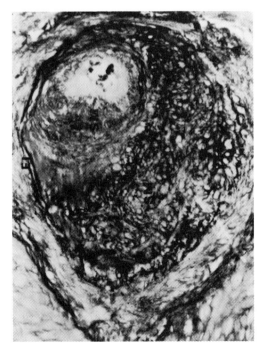

FIGURE 10–1. Atherosis: Numerous lipid-laden cells (L) and fibrin deposition (F) are present in the media of this occluded decidual vessel. (From Sheppard, B.D., and Bonnar, J.: Uteroplacental arteries and hypertensive pregnancy. In Bonnar, J., MacGillivray, I., Symonds, G. (Eds.): Pregnancy Hypertension. Baltimore, University Park Press, 1980.)

occurs in moderate to severe cases of preeclampsia after about 28 weeks' gestation (see Chapter 25). These infants show some changes related to chronic hypoxia and, in addition, tolerate labor very poorly and are often born through meconium that contributes further to the degree of perinatal asphyxia. They may also have polycythemia and blood hyperviscosity, and associated hypoglycemia due to decreased glycogen stores and inability to mobilize glucose. They may be subject to prolonged hypoglycemia until adequate nutrition is established.

Respiratory Distress Syndrome. Gluck and Kulovich (1973) were the first to call attention to the protective effect of maternal stress on fetal lung maturation. Yoon and co-workers (1980) reported that the incidence of respiratory distress syndrome (RDS) was less among infants of mothers with hypertensive disease, controlled for gestation. In infants of less than 32 weeks' gestation, the incidence of RDS was reduced from 40.8 to 26.1 per cent. Nevertheless, the incidence of RDS was still significant. There was no difference in morbidity and mortality among infants with RDS, and mortality was actually increased in the group *without* RDS. Hypovolemia, asphyxia, and meconium aspiration are probably contributing factors.

Effect of Maternal Drugs. Since preeclamptic mothers often require treatment with high doses of magnesium or other drugs to control blood pressure, their infants may have hypermagnesemia with apnea and slow responsiveness as well as hypotension.

Thrombocytopenia. These infants may share in the coagulation problems of their mothers. About 25 to 50 per cent of infants born to mothers with thrombocytopenia also have platelet counts <150,000/mm^3 at birth, but their platelet counts rise rapidly to normal levels thereafter.

Neutropenia. Infants born to mothers with preeclampsia and particularly the HELLP syndrome may have neutropenia. The cause of this finding is not clear, but it is thought to be related to agents that cause endothelial damage in the mother and cross the placenta (Weinstein, 1986).

MANAGEMENT

In the management of pregnancies complicated by preeclampsia, delay in delivery is always for the sake of the fetus. The appropriate timing of delivery is an area in which close cooperation between the obstetrical and neonatal providers is very important for guaranteeing the best outcome for both mother and infant. Attempting to control maternal blood pressure and to avoid seizures is a primary concern, since there presently is no cure for preeclampsia, and its course is progressive. Cornerstones for successful management of the fetus include close fetal assessment in conjunction with maternal surveillance and intervention by delivery if the fetus shows signs of losing reactivity.

Cesarean section is necessary in many cases, since the fetus often is unable to tolerate labor.

The administration of prenatal glucocorticoid in the presence of immature fetal lungs can be beneficial as long as the fetus is monitored closely for signs of distress.

Resuscitation. Finally, it is essential that staff who are skilled in resuscitation be present at the delivery of these infants, particularly for preterm deliveries, so an infant with meconium aspiration, asphyxia, and/or hypovolemia can be dealt with rapidly.

■ REFERENCES

Brazie, J. E., Grumm, J. K., and Little, V. A.: Neonatal manifestations of severe maternal hypertension occurring before the thirty-sixth week of pregnancy. J. Pediatr. *100*:265, 1982.

Chamberlain, F., Philipp, E., Howlett, B., et al.: British Births 1970, vol. 2. London, Heinemann. pp. 80–107.

Chesley, L. C.: Hypertension in pregnancy. Definitions, familial factor, and remote prognosis. Kidney Intl. *18*:234, 1980.

Collins, R., and Wallenburg, H. C. S.: Pharmacological prevention and treatment of hypertensive disorders in pregnancy. In Chalmers, I., Enkin, M., and Keirse, M. J. N. C. (Eds.): Effective Care in Pregnancy, vol. 1. Oxford, Oxford University Press, 1989, pp. 512–531.

Cunningham, F. G., and Gant, N. F.: Prevention of preeclampsia—a reality? N. Engl. J. Med. *321*:606–607, 1989.

Doll, R., and Hanington, E.: International survey of eclampsia and preeclampsia 1958–1959. Epidemiologic aspects. Pathol. Microbiol. (Basel) *24*:531, 1961.

Easterling, T. R., and Benedetti, T. H.: Preeclampsia: A hyperdynamic disease model. Am. J. Obstet. Gynecol. *160*:1447, 1989.

Gant, N. F., and Worley, R. J.: Hypertension in Pregnancy: Concepts and Management. New York, Appleton-Century-Crofts, 1980.

Gluck, L., and Kulovich, M. V.: Lecithin/sphingomyelin ratio in amniotic fluid in normal and abnormal pregnancy. Am. J. Obstet. *115*:539, 1973.

Hubel, C. A., Roberts, J. M., Taylor, R. N., et al.: Lipid peroxidation in pregnancy: New perspectives on preeclampsia. Am. J. Obstet. Gynecol. *161*:1025–1034, 1989.

Kaunitz, A. M., Hughes, J. B., Grimes, D. A., et al.: Causes of maternal mortality in the United States. Obstet. Gynecol. *65*:605–612, 1985.

Knutzen, V. K., and Davey, D. A.: Hypertension in pregnancy: Perinatal mortality and causes of fetal death. S. Afr. Med. J. *51*:675–678, 1977.

Kleikner, H. B., Giles, H. R., and Corrigan, J. J.: The association of maternal and neonatal thrombocytopenia in high-risk pregnancies. Am. J. Obstet. Gynecol. *128*:235, 1977.

MacGillivray, I.: Preeclampsia. In Beller, F., and MacGillivray, I (Eds.): The Hypertensive Disorders of Pregnancy. London, W. B. Saunders Company, 1983.

Redman, C. W. G., Bonnar, J., and Berlin, L.: Early platelet consumption in preeclampsia. Br. Med. J. *1*:467, 1978.

Roberts, J. M., May, W. J.: Consumptive coagulopathy in severe preeclampsia. Obstet. Gynecol. *48*:163, 1976.

Roberts, J. M., Taylor, R. N., Musci, T. J.: Preeclampsia: An endothelial cell disorder. Am. J. Obstet. Gynecol. *161*:1200–1204, 1989.

Roberts, J. M.: Pregnancy-related hypertension. In Creasy, R. K., and Resnick, R. (Eds.): Maternal-Fetal Medicine: Principles and Practice, 2nd ed. Philadelphia, W. B. Saunders Company, 1989, p. 718.

Wallenburg, H. C. S.: Detecting hypertensive disorders of pregnancy. In: Chalmers, I., Enkin, M., and Keirse, M. J. N. C. (Eds.): Effective Care in Pregnancy, vol. 1. Oxford University Press, 1989, pp. 382–402.

Weinstein, L.: Preeclampsia/eclampsia with hemolysis, elevated liver enzymes, and thrombocytopenia. Obstet. Gynecol. *66*:657, 1985.

Weinstein, L.: The HELLP syndrome, a severe consequence of hypertension in pregnancy. J. Perinatol. *6*:316, 1986.

Yoon, J. J., Kohl, S., and Harpers, R. G.: The relationship between maternal hypertensive disease of pregnancy and the incidence of idiopathic RDS. Pediatrics *65*:735, 1980.

OTHER MATERNAL CONDITIONS AFFECTING THE FETUS

11

Mark M. Jacobs and Roberta A. Ballard

Predicting the adverse effects on fetal health and well-being of maternal medical problems may seem a daunting task. If several common features of maternal-fetal physiology are understood, however, the practitioner can in most cases identify the major risk factors. The important components of maternal-fetal exchange are adequate function of the maternal lungs, blood, blood vessels, and heart. The placenta must have adequate surface area, and there should be sufficient relaxation of the uterus to allow exchange of gases, substrates, and wastes between the fetus and mother.

The degree of fetal risk associated with a maternal medical problem is directly related to the degree of organ function impairment. For example, a 40-year-old woman with well-controlled asthma, normal lung function, and arterial oxygen saturation would have little fetal risk unless an acute exacerbation of her asthma occurred. On the other hand, an 18-year-old with cystic fibrosis, a vital capacity of 2 l and room-air arterial oxygen saturation of 89 per cent is at high risk for fetal problems.

After the fetus at risk is identified, a plan for management of the primary maternal medical problem and a program of fetal surveillance can be designed. There is now a confusing array of high-tech methods for evaluating fetal health in utero, all with their passionate advocates and almost all of unproven efficacy. However, there are some points of agreement regarding assessing the fetus when maternal medical problems complicate pregnancy. First is that assessment of fetal growth is the best way to estimate the function of the fetal-placental unit over weeks to months. Less-than-expected fetal growth should prompt an intensive program of close fetal surveillance, which usually includes kick counts and electronic fetal monitoring. When a fetus falls four or more weeks behind in growth or amniotic fluid volume begins to fall, the risk of distress and death is high (see Chapter 12).

High-risk pregnancies are best managed by the obstetrician or perinatal specialist with support from internists, pediatricians, and anesthesiologists. Pediatric consultation should be obtained as soon as an unhealthy fetus is identified, if the maternal condition worsens, or when delivery is contemplated. Many pediatricians are reluctant to become involved with obstetric decision-making, and many obstetricians may feel "crowded" by an assertive pediatrician. This situation is unfortunate because unambiguous estimates of neonatal morbidity and mortality, which should be derived from local experience, can greatly simplify decision-making by the patient and her obstetrician.

■ CIRCULATORY ADAPTATION TO PREGNANCY

Normal function of the maternal heart and lung is critical to fetal well-being, and even short periods of dysfunction may kill or seriously injure a healthy fetus. Chronic problems may result in reduced fetal growth and increased risk of fetal distress during labor. To understand the risks of heart disease during pregnancy, it is first necessary to review the hemodynamic alterations that occur normally.

During pregnancy there is increased demand for cardiac work in response to increased metabolic demands. Even in women without heart disease, these changes may result in signs and symptoms that are difficult to distinguish from those associated with early heart failure. The mechanisms of these alterations are still undefined; however, increased estrogen and progesterone are felt to be important contributing factors. The major changes that occur include the following:

1. *Increased blood volume,* total body water, and sodium. Excess sodium retention reaches 500 to 900 mEq by delivery and is associated with another 8 to 10 l of fluid accretion. Maternal blood volume increases during the first and second trimesters and plateaus in the third trimester. Total blood volume expansion is 40 to 45 per cent in singleton pregnancies and 50 to 60 per cent in multiple gestations. Total red cell volume also increases, beginning in the second trimester (Fig. 11–1). The total increase in red cells is 20 to 33 per cent, which represents a total hemoglobin increase of approximately 85 g. Since plasma volume expansion is greater than red cell volume expansion, hemoglobin is actually decreased; this phenomenon has been called the "physiologic anemia of pregnancy."

2. *Increased cardiac output.* Cardiac output is increased 40 per cent above the nonpregnant resting value. Heart rate increases 15 beats/minute early in gestation and remains elevated. Stroke volume is also increased but to a smaller degree. The pregnant woman's cardiac output and blood pressure fluctuate widely with positional changes. When supine, the uterus obstructs caval flow, and cardiac output is significantly less than in a sitting or lateral recumbent position, producing the so-called supine

hypotension syndrome. Supine hypotension can be exacerbated by anesthesia, labor, dehydration, and multifetal pregnancy. If systolic pressure is reduced to less than 90 mm Hg, fetal compromise can occur.

During labor, cardiac output increases progressively, though modestly, and the patient with compensated cardiac disease usually does well. Uterine contractions can cause an additional increase in cardiac output, which can be eliminated if labor is in the lateral position and adequate analgesia is provided. Cardiac output peaks immediately after delivery, and this is the period of maximum danger for women who have impaired cardiac function.

3. *Distribution of cardiac output.* There are alterations in the distribution of blood flow to various maternal organs, with increased flow to the uterus, kidney, and skin.

4. *Intravascular pressure.* Both systolic and diastolic blood pressures decrease slightly in the second trimester and then rise slowly toward term. Patients who do not experience this midtrimester reduction in blood pressure are at increased risk of developing hypertension later in gestation.

■ HEART DISEASE IN PREGNANCY

Diagnosis. Based on these hemodynamic alterations it is not surprising that cardiovascular findings are normally altered during pregnancy. As many as 80 per cent of normal pregnant women have some peripheral edema. A third heart sound and systolic murmurs also commonly occur. A systolic murmur of Grade III or more, however, deserves further evaluation, as does any diastolic murmur. Pulsations of the neck veins are prominent in pregnancy, but neck-vein distention that lasts throughout the cardiac cycle is *not* normal.

Because cardiac work is increased during pregnancy, even compensated heart disease tends to worsen. However, since cardiac output increases gradually, sudden decompensation is unusual. Also, since more than half of the increased output is present by 12 weeks, patients doing well by that time should be reassured. Although labor and delivery result in a moderate increase in cardiac work, there appears to be no advantage to cesarean birth

if adequate pain relief is provided and pushing (Valsalva's maneuver) in the second stage is minimized. The most dangerous time for patients with impaired cardiac function is the immediate postpartum period, when rapid alterations take place in blood volume, vascular capacity, peripheral resistance, and systemic and pulmonary pressures.

Specific Cardiac Lesions. Lesions that produce right-to-left shunts are the most dangerous for fetus and mother. Because systemic pressure drops during pregnancy and fluctuates widely during labor and delivery, the risk of increased shunting is high. Myocardial infarction, although rare, is also extremely dangerous. Maintaining desired concentrations of cardiac and other drugs may be difficult because of increased intravascular volume and drug metabolism and decreased gastrointestinal function.

Congenital Heart Disease in Pregnancy. Increasing numbers of women born with congenital heart disease are reaching child-bearing age. Although all abnormalities carry an increased risk of maternal morbidity and mortality during pregnancy, some constitute a greater risk than others (Table 11–1). In addition, the presence of congenital cardiac anomalies in either a parent or sibling increases the risk of cardiac or other congenital anomalies in the fetus (Table 11–2). When an anomaly is transmitted as an autosomal dominant trait, such as in idiopathic hypertrophic subaortic stenosis, the child has a 50 per cent chance of developing the same abnormality.

Management During Pregnancy. A team approach to the pregnant woman with cardiovascular disease optimizes outcome for mother and fetus. Moderate activity and dietary restriction is usually necessary. Because pregnant women with heart disease tolerate infections poorly, they should be immunized prior to pregnancy and antibiotic prophylaxis against endocarditis liberally used during dental or surgical procedures and delivery.

■ MATERNAL SEIZURE DISORDERS

It is estimated that between 0.3 and 0.6 per cent of pregnant women have epilepsy. The effect of pregnancy on seizures is unpredictable. In one series, seizure frequency increased in 45 per cent of patients, was reduced in 5 per cent, and remained unchanged in 50 per cent

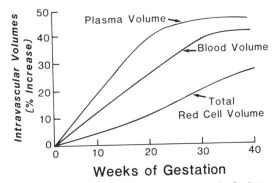

FIGURE 11–1. *Schematic of the per cent increases in the intravascular volumes that occur during pregnancy. Plasma volume increases by approximately 50 per cent and total red cell volume by approximately 25 per cent, causing a 40 per cent increase in total blood volume. (From McAnulty, et al.: Cardiovascular disease. In Burrow, G.N., and Ferris, T.F.: Medical Complications During Pregnancy, 3rd ed. Philadelphia, W. B. Saunders Company, 1988.)*

TABLE 11–1. High-Risk Maternal Cardiovascular Disorders

DISORDER	MATERNAL MORTALITY RATE* (%)
Aortic valve disease	10–20
Coarctation of the aorta	5
Eisenmenger syndrome	30–70
Marfan syndrome	25–50 (estimated)
Mitral stenosis with atrial fibrillation	14–17
Peripartal cardiomyopathy	15–60
Primary pulmonary hypertension	50
Tetralogy of Fallot	12

*These figures, compiled from 18 references, represent different study periods and disorders of varying severity; therefore, they must be regarded as approximations.

From Creasy, R. K., and Resnick, R. (Eds.): Maternal-Fetal Medicine: Principles and Practice, 2nd ed. Philadelphia, W. B. Saunders Company, 1989.

TABLE 11–2. Congenital Heart Disease in the Offspring of a Parent with Congenital Heart Disease

CONGENITAL HEART DEFECT IN A PARENT	RISK OF CONGENITAL HEART DISEASE IN OFFSPRING IF ONE PARENT IS AFFECTED*†
Intracardiac Shunts	
ASD	3–11%
VSD	4–22%
PDA	4–11%
Obstruction to Flow	
Left-sided obstruction‡	3–26%
Right-sided obstruction	3–22%
Complex Abnormalities	
Tetralogy of Fallot	4–15%
Ebstein's anomaly	Uncertain
Transposition of the great arteries	Uncertain

*The higher number in each range comes from one large series. The incidence of congenital heart disease in the offspring tends to be closer to the lower numbers for most other reported series.

†The risk in obstructive lesions is decreased by corrective surgery prior to pregnancy.

‡Includes coarctation, aortic stenosis, discrete subaortic stenosis, supravalvular stenosis. It does not include IHSS; with this the child has a 50 per cent chance of having IHSS.

From Burrow, G. N., and Ferris, T. F. (Eds.): Medical Complications During Pregnancy, 3rd ed. Philadelphia, W. B. Saunders Company, 1988.

(Knight and Rhind, 1975). When seizure frequency increased, this occurred in the first trimester, with reversion to the prepregnancy pattern at the end of gestation.

Management. The objective is to keep the pregnant epileptic woman seizure-free while minimizing the known adverse effects of maternal medications both on other aspects of the pregnancy and particularly on the fetus. The interaction between maternal epilepsy, metabolism of anticonvulsant agents, teratogenesis, and the fetal effects on maternal metabolism of anticonvulsants is complex, and management of many of these issues is still controversial. Hormones directly affect the seizure threshold: estrogens appear to activate seizure foci, and progestins may dampen activity.

Changing Drug Requirements. It is often difficult to maintain adequate anticonvulsant therapy during pregnancy. Phenytoin and phenobarbital requirements increase during pregnancy and then decline again after delivery. Similar findings have been noted for other anticonvulsants. Possible reasons include the changes in plasma and extracellular fluid volume normally experienced during pregnancy, poor compliance with anticonvulsant regimen (sometimes related to nausea and vomiting), and changes in plasma protein binding as well as in absorption and excretion of drugs. In addition, if women receive folic-acid therapy, plasma phenytoin may be reduced below the therapeutic range. The increased metabolic capacity of the maternal liver, as well as fetal and/or placental metabolism, may also affect the drug dose necessary.

Other Effects. There is a significant increase in maternal bleeding during pregnancy in the presence of epilepsy, but no increase in other significant medical conditions. There does not appear to be any difference in the frequency of preeclampsia. The spontaneous abortion rate does not appear to be increased, but stillbirth is more likely. The offspring of epileptic women have a higher incidence of epilepsy, mental retardation, and microcephaly.

Teratogenesis. Information in the literature about the teratogenesis of anticonvulsant drugs is contradictory. However, it does appear that the risk of congenital malformations is increased among infants of epileptic mothers who are receiving anticonvulsants. Trimethadione is considered a teratogen for humans, as is valproic acid (which is associated with a 1 per cent incidence of neural tube defects in the fetus). There does not appear to be any increase in malformations among infants whose mothers have been taking phenobarbital. Maternal use of phenytoin during pregnancy has been associated with a specific syndrome, the fetal hydantoin syndrome, characterized by prenatal and postnatal growth deficiency, microcephaly, dysmorphic facies, and mental deficiency. It is believed to occur in up to 10 per cent of infants exposed to phenytoin in utero. This syndrome, however, resembles the fetal alcohol syndrome and is not unlike that attributed to other anticonvulsants. Therefore, it is not clear that this complex is related specifically to hydantoin alone. A clinical or subclinical coagulopathy may also occur in infants whose mothers received anticonvulsants during pregnancy. There is no evidence of coagulopathy in the mother, but factors II, VII, IX, and X are decreased in the newborn and are thought to represent a deficiency of vitamin K–dependent clotting factors. Bleeding may occur in utero, resulting in stillbirth, and vitamin K_1 should be administered to the newborn immediately after birth. It has also been proposed that infants born to mothers receiving high doses of phenytoin should have prothrombin time measured in cord blood, so that fresh frozen plasma can be administered, if necessary. After delivery, infants should be inspected for possible congenital malformations and receive vitamin K. Breast-feeding should be encouraged.

■ DISORDERS OF THE THYROID

INCIDENCE

Thyroid disorders, in general, are more frequent in women than men and represent a common endocrine abnormality during pregnancy. Both hyperthyroidism and hypothyroidism in the mother put the infant at risk and require careful management by the perinatal-neonatal team. Table 11–3 presents an overview of the approach to infants who are thought to be at risk for abnormal thyroid function because of maternal thyroid abnormalities. The most frequently described problem is the syndrome of postpartum thyroiditis, which has been reported to complicate as many as 5 per cent of all pregnancies. The diagnosis of thyroid disease in pregnancy is complicated by the natural changes that occur in immunologic status of the mother and fetus and that complicate assessment of any of the autoimmune thyroid disorders.

HYPERTHYROIDISM

Hyperthyroidism occurs in approximately 0.2 per cent of pregnancies and results in a significant increase in the

TABLE 11–3. Approach for Infants Judged To Be at Risk for Abnormal Thyroid Function

POSSIBLE THYROID ABNORMALITY	CORD BLOOD ANALYSIS	ASSESSMENT AT BIRTH	ASSESSMENT AT 2–7 DAYS OF LIFE
Congenital hyperthyroidism because mother has: Graves disease with hyperthyroidism; and may have been treated with PTU, methimazole, ^{131}I, or iodides, or surgery History of maternal Graves disease or Hashimoto disease	T$_4$, RSH, TSAb	Physical examination for IUGR,* goiter, exophthalmos, tachycardia, bradycardia, size of anterior fontanel, synostosis, congenital anomalies Gestational age by dates, ultrasonography during pregnancy, or Dubovitz examination Plot intrauterine growth by gestational age Neurologic examination Bone age (knee) For selected cases: EKG, auditory and visual evoked potentials, motor conduction velocity tests, skull x-rays	T$_4$, TSH, TSAb (if available) determinations: If normal, given no Rx; observe and repeat T$_4$, T$_3$, TSH at 7–10 days† If hypothyroid, repeat T$_4$, TSH; if abnormal, Rx at 7–10 days‡ If hyperthyroid, begin Rx with PTU (8 mg/kg) and propranolol
Congenital or early childhood hypothyroidism because mother has: Graves disease with excessive PTU therapy Hashimoto disease ?Acute (subacute) thyroiditis Familial genetic defect in thyroxine synthesis Rx with iodides or lithium for nonthyroidal illness Exposure to ^{131}I while pregnant	T$_4$, RSH, ThyAb	Same as for suspected hyperthyroidism	T$_4$, TSH, ThyAb determinations: If hypothyroid, perform thyroid ultrasound scan to define presence, size, location of thyroid tissue If hypothyroidism confirmed, begin Rx with Synthroid (0.05 mg/d)

*IUGR = intrauterine growth retardation.
†The children of mothers who receive PTU may not develop neonatal Graves disease at age 7–10 days.
‡Children who receive PTU in utero may have transient or longer-lasting hypothyroidism.
From Creasy, R. K., and Resnick, R. (Eds.): Maternal-Fetal Medicine: Principles and Practice, 2nd ed. Philadelphia, W. B. Saunders Company, 1989.

prevalence of both low-birth-weight delivery and a trend toward increased neonatal mortality. The most common cause of thyrotoxicosis (85 per cent of cases) in women of child-bearing age is Graves disease, but other causes include acute (or subacute) thyroiditis (transient), Hashimoto disease, hydatidiform mole, choriocarcinoma, toxic nodular goiter, and toxic adenoma. Graves disease has a peak incidence during the reproductive years, but patients with Graves disease may actually have remissions during pregnancy, and then postpartum exacerbations. The unique feature of these pregnancies, however, is that the fetus may also be affected, regardless of the mother's concurrent medical condition. Thyroid function is difficult to evaluate in the fetus, and the status of the fetus may not correlate with that of the mother.

DIAGNOSIS

The differential diagnosis of thyrotoxicosis becomes more difficult during pregnancy, since normal pregnant women may have a variety of hyperdynamic signs and symptoms. These may include intolerance to heat, nervousness, irritability, emotional lability, and increased perspiration, along with tachycardia and anxiety. Laboratory data are also difficult to evaluate, because total serum thyroxin values are normally elevated during pregnancy as a result of estrogen-induced increases in thyroxine-binding globulin (TBG). Thus, if TBG is increased, resin triiodothyronine uptake may be in the euthyroid to slightly increased range in a patient who has true hyperthyroidism.

Hollingsworth (1989) has reviewed the assessment of thyroid function tests in nonpregnant and pregnant women, along with the differential diagnosis of hyperthyroidism during pregnancy.

PATHOGENESIS OF GRAVES DISEASE

The pathogenesis of Graves disease is not completely understood, but it probably represents an overlapping spectrum of disorders that are characterized by production of polyclonal antibodies. It has been appreciated since the 1960s (Sunshine et al., 1965) that abnormal thyroid-stimulating immunoglobulins, which appear to be immunoglobulin G (IgG), are present in pregnant women with Graves disease and cross the placenta easily to cause neonatal hyperthyroidism in some infants (McKenzie and Zakarija, 1978). The clinical spectrum of Graves disease in utero is quite broad and may result in stillbirth or preterm delivery. Some affected infants have widespread evidence of autoimmune disease, including thrombocytopenic purpura and generalized hypertrophy of the lymphatic tissues. Thyroid storm can occur shortly after birth, or infants may have disease that is transient in nature, lasting from 1 to 5 months. Infants born to mothers who have been treated with thioamides may appear normal at birth but subsequently develop signs of thyrotoxicosis at 7 to 10 days of age, when the effect of thioamide suppression of thyroxine synthesis is no longer present. The measurement of thyroid-stimulating antibodies (TSAbs) is useful in predicting whether the fetus will be affected.

MANAGEMENT OF THE MOTHER

Since radioactive iodine therapy is contraindicated during pregnancy, treatment of the pregnant woman with thyrotoxicosis involves a choice between antithyroid drugs and surgery. The therapeutic goal is to achieve a euthyroid or, perhaps slightly hyperthyroid, state in the mother while preventing fetal hypothyroidism or hyperthyroidism. Either propylthiouracil (PTU) or methimazole may be used to treat thyrotoxicosis during pregnancy. However, because methimazole therapy may be associated with aplasia cutis in the offspring of treated women and because propylthiouracil crosses the placenta more slowly than methimazole, PTU has become the drug of choice during pregnancy. Ordinarily, the disease can be controlled with doses of 300 mg per day. Once the disorder is under control, however, it is important to keep the dose as low as possible, preferably less than 100 mg daily, since these drugs do cross the placenta and block fetal thyroid function and may produce hypothyroidism in the fetus. In women with cardiovascular effects, the use of beta blockers may be appropriate to achieve rapid control of thyrotoxicosis. Since administration of propranolol to pregnant women has been associated with intrauterine growth retardation and impaired responses of the fetus to anoxic stress as well as postnatal bradycardia and hypoglycemia, the dosages must be closely controlled. Iodides have also been used, particularly in combination with beta-blocking agents, to control thyrotoxicosis. However, long-term iodide therapy presents a risk to the fetus. Because of the inhibition of the incorporation of iodide into thyroglobulin, the fetus can develop a large, obstructive goiter. Surgery during pregnancy is best reserved for cases in which a woman is hypersensitive to antithyroid drugs or there is poor compliance with medication or, in rare cases, when drugs are ineffective in controlling the disease.

EFFECTS ON THE NEWBORN

Approximately 1 per cent of infants born to mothers with some degree of thyrotoxicosis will themselves have thyrotoxicosis (Fig. 11–2). Assessment of fetal risk in utero, includes measurement of thyroid-stimulating immunoglobulins, with expectation that if the titers are high, there is increased risk of thyrotoxicosis. Additional assessment of the fetus should pay particular attention to elevated resting heart rate and poor fetal growth. Daneman and Howard (1980) reported on the outcome of nine infants with neonatal thyrotoxicosis and noted normal growth but a high incidence of craniosynostosis and intellectual impairment. It may, therefore, be necessary to treat the asymptomatic mother with thioamides and propranolol (and thyroid replacement) during pregnancy in order to treat the infant and prevent serious neonatal morbidity and long-term problems.

Mothers with thyrotoxicosis who are taking normal doses of thioamides may safely breast-feed their infants, although thioamides do appear in breast milk in very low amounts. Currently, there does not appear to be any long-term adverse outcome for infants whose mothers have received propylthiouracil during pregnancy.

HYPOTHYROIDISM

Maternal hypothyroidism ordinarily can be classified as primary in nature, since secondary hypothyroidism due to pituitary disease is rare in young women, accounting for less than 5 per cent of the cases. The principal causes of hypothyroidism in pregnant women are chronic lymphocytic thyroiditis and previous treatment for Graves disease. Other causes include previous therapy with ^{131}I, subtotal thyroidectomy, or exposure to excessive doses of PTU. Ordinarily, maternal hypothyroidism occurring during pregnancy is relatively mild, since severe hypothyroidism results in failure of ovulation. This makes diagnosis particularly difficult during pregnancy. Many women will have an increased requirement for thyroxine replacement during pregnancy (Mandel et al., 1990). Pregnancies complicated by untreated hypothyroidism may be associated with increased fetal loss or prolongation of gestation.

Treatment with replacement doses of thyroid hormone is usually well tolerated and easily titrated. The clinician must be aware of the fact that the increased thyroid-binding globulin levels in maternal plasma may result in movement of thyroid hormone from the fetus to the mother with a decrease in severity of her disease during the pregnancy. Hypothyroidism has occurred in the fetus when the mother has received ^{131}I inadvertently during pregnancy. There is currently no reliable method for diagnosing hypothyroidism in utero (see Chapter 109).

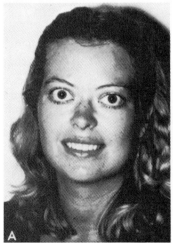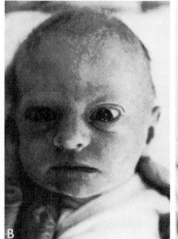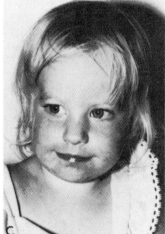

FIGURE 11–2. A, Hypothyroid 21-year-old mother who developed Graves disease at age 7 and was treated by subtotal thyroidectomy. She was given maintenance therapy with daily levothyroxine sodium (Synthroid), 0.15 mg, through pregnancy. B, Her infant baby girl was born at term with severe Graves disease, goiter, and exophthalmos that persisted for 6 months. C, Child was normal at age 20 months. (From Creasy, R.K., and Resnick, R.: Maternal-Fetal Medicine: Principles and Practice, 2nd ed. Philadelphia, W. B. Saunders Company, 1989.)

■ REFERENCES

Amino, N., Mori, H., Iwatani, I., et al.: High prevalence of transient postpartum thyrotoxicosis and hypothyroidism. N. Engl. J. Med. *306*:849, 1982.

Aminoff, N. J.: Neurologic disorders. *In* Creasy, R. K., and Resnick, R. (Eds.): Maternal-Fetal Medicine: Principles and Practice, 2nd ed. Philadelphia, W. B. Saunders Company, 1989.

Burrow, G. N.: The management of thyrotoxicosis in pregnancy. N. Engl. J. Med. *313*:562, 1986.

Burrow, G. N.: Thyroid diseases. *In* Burrow, G. N., and Ferris, T. F. (Eds.): Medical Complications During Pregnancy, 3rd ed. Philadelphia, W. B. Saunders Company, 1988.

Daneman, D., and Howard, N. J.: Neonatal thyrotoxicosis: Intellectual impairment and craniosynostosis in later years. J. Pediatr. *97*:257, 1980.

Donaldson, J. O.: Neurologic complications. *In* Burrow, G. N., and Ferris, T. F. (Eds.): Medical Complications During Pregnancy, 3rd ed. Philadelphia, W. B. Saunders Company, 1988.

Hollingsworth, D. R.: Endocrine disorders in pregnancy. *In* Creasy, R. K., and Resnick, R. (Eds.): Maternal-Fetal Medicine: Principles and Practice, 2nd ed. Philadelphia, W. B. Saunders Company, 1989.

Knight, A. H., and Rhind, E. G.: Epilepsy and pregnancy. A study of 153 pregnancies and 59 patients. Epilepsia *16*:99, 1975.

Mandel, S. J., Larsen, P. R., Seely, E. W., et al.: Increased need for thyroxine during pregnancy in women with primary hypothyroidism. N. Engl. J. Med. *323*:91, 1990.

McAnulty, J. H., Metcalf, J., and Ueland, K.: Cardiovascular disease. *In* Burrow, G. N., and Ferris, T. F. (Eds.): Medical Complications During Pregnancy, 3rd ed. Philadelphia, W. B. Saunders Company, 1988.

McKenzie, J. M., and Zakarija, M.: Pathogenesis of neonatal Graves' disease. J. Endocrinol. Invest. *2*:183, 1978.

Mestman, J. H.: Thyroid disease in pregnancy. Clin. Perinatol. *12*:1651, 1985.

Nelson, K. B., and Ellenberg, J. H.: Maternal seizure disorders. Outcome of pregnancy and the neurologic abnormalities in the children. Neurology *32*:1247, 1982.

Sunshine, P., Kusomoto, H., and Kriss, J. P.: Survival time of long-acting thyroid stimulator in neonatal thyrotoxicosis. Implications of diagnosis and therapy of the disorder. Pediatrics *36*:869, 1965.

Ueland, K.: Cardiac diseases. *In* Creasy, R. K., and Resnick, R. (Eds.): Maternal-Fetal Medicine: Principles and Practice, 2nd ed. Philadelphia, W. B. Saunders Company, 1989.

Zakarija, M., McKenzie, J. M., Munro, D. S., et al.: Delayed onset of neonatal Graves' disease due to interactions of thyroid-stimulating antibody (TSAb) and a thyroid-directed inhibitor. Clin. Res. *30*:494A, 1982.

ASSESSMENT OF FETAL WELL-BEING 12

Isabelle A. Wilkins and Richard L. Berkowitz

■ ULTRASONOGRAPHY DURING PREGNANCY

The availability of ultrasound and its frequent use in pregnant women has probably been the most significant advance in obstetrics over the past 10 to 15 years. This modality has literally changed the practice of obstetrics in both the high-risk and low-risk patient.

Ultrasound provides a great deal of information about the intrauterine contents, including the volume of amniotic fluid, placental texture and location, and the size and number of fetuses (Fig. 12–1). Fetal anatomy and biophysical parameters can also be studied, particularly in the second and third trimesters. Common indications for an ultrasound examination include dating a pregnancy of uncertain gestational age, the diagnosis and follow-up of

multiple gestation, and the detection of possible intrauterine growth retardation (IUGR) and a variety of fetal morphologic anomalies (Table 12–1). Although gestational age assessment and the diagnosis of multiple gestation is extremely accurate in the first and second trimester, the detection of fetal anomalies and IUGR are usually accomplished in the second and third trimesters.

The ultrasonic detection of congenital anomalies has allowed obstetricians to counsel patients, initiate therapy, and time delivery (Vintzileos et al., 1987). For example, the parents of a fetus with lethal disorders, such as Potter syndrome or anencephaly, should be offered elective termination if these conditions are detected in the second trimester. If lesions such as an omphalocele are discovered, chromosomal studies should be obtained, because aneuploidies are known to be frequently associated with

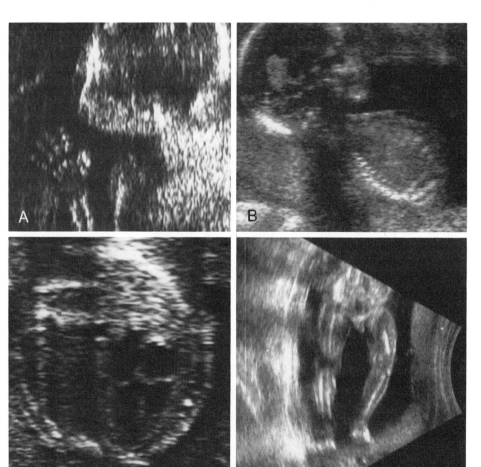

FIGURE 12–1. *Typical ultrasound images: A, 20-week fetus with hand, forearm, and skull visible. B, Fetus at 20 weeks in profile. C, Four-chamber view of a fetal heart at 20 weeks. D, Male fetus with bladder and legs visible.*

TABLE 12–1. Indications for Ultrasound Examination

- Gestational age assessment.
- Placental localization.
- Evaluation of fetal growth.
- Suspected or known multiple gestation.
- Suspected or known polyhydramnios or oligohydramnios.
- Suspected or known fetal anomaly.
- Biophysical examination for fetal well-being.
- Fetal lie.
- Late registration for prenatal care.
- Discrepancies between uterine size and clinical dates.
- Adjunct to procedures such as amniocentesis, external version, chorionic villus sampling, and intrauterine transfusion.

this defect, and their presence affects prognosis (Carpenter et al., 1984). If specific types of arrhythmias are detected, they may be treated with drugs given to the mother and the fetus followed ultrasonographically for signs of a return to normal sinus rhythm (Kleinman et al., 1980). Finally, fetuses with conditions such as isolated hydrocephalus may benefit from early delivery if the size of the head begins to increase rapidly (Chervenak et al., 1985).

The ultrasonic assessment of placental location has drastically changed the management of women with vaginal bleeding late in pregnancy. The diagnosis of placenta previa can be definitively made without resorting to potentially dangerous pelvic examinations. On the other hand, abruptio placentae (premature separation of the placenta) is inconsistently seen sonographically.

Characteristics of placental texture are possible to detect with ultrasound, but their clinical value is uncertain in most situations. The quantity and pattern of calcifications in the placenta has been classified into a grading system. More advanced degrees of calcification and separation of cotyledons are seen as pregnancy progresses. Some chronic maternal disorders may be associated with an acceleration of this process. However, attempts to correlate advanced placental maturation with lung maturity or placental insufficiency have not been consistently successful.

A controversy currently confronting obstetricians is whether all pregnant women should be screened with ultrasound. Most congenital anomalies occur in women with no known risk factors. Multiple gestation and IUGR may be suspected clinically rather late in gestation. These conditions could all potentially profit from early diagnosis. At this point, however, the benefits of a universal screening program have not been conclusively demonstrated in a population of low-risk women.

Another important role of ultrasound is an adjunct to invasive fetal procedures. Chorionic villus sampling, amniocentesis, and in utero transfusions for Rh disease have been refined or made possible by using ultrasound guidance.

Other modalities are also available for imaging the fetus, though their usefulness is less established. Traditional radiographic techniques are currently almost never used to study fetal anatomy or number. Magnetic resonance imaging is a developing technology, but at present, its use in evaluating the fetus is limited by the lack of a real-time mode. On the other hand, fetal echocardiography, a specialized form of ultrasound, is widely used to evaluate the structure and rhythm of the fetal heart. A

detailed examination by a specialist is indicated when congenital heart disease is suspected either by history or by an abnormal screening ultrasound study (Kleinman and Santalli, 1983).

■ DOPPLER FLOW STUDIES

One of the newest techniques for assessing fetal health is through the use of Doppler flow studies. Flow has been measured and related to clinical outcome in uterine and umbilical arteries (Trudinger et al., 1985). Currently, flow through fetal carotid, renal, and cerebral arteries has also been studied. Echocardiographers have used flow in the aorta, across the heart valves, and through the ductus arteriosus to correlate with their anatomic findings. Work in this area has centered on conditions in which alterations in fetal blood flow can be expected to correlate with the severity of stress in utero. Thus, conditions such as intrauterine growth retardation, placental insufficiency, and maternal hypertension as well as fetal heart disease have received a large share of attention.

The primary use of Doppler flow studies is to detect increased resistance in the umbilical and uterine circulations by demonstrating decreased flow during diastole (Fig. 12–2). Thus far, the most productive use of this diagnostic tool has been in assessing the degree of compromise in fetuses that are growth-retarded because of uteroplacental compromise rather than constitutional factors.

■ BIOCHEMICAL MARKERS

Biochemical markers of placental function used in the past, such as maternal estriol and human placental lactogen levels, have now been supplanted by fetal heart rate testing and biophysical parameters.

Fetal acid-base studies obtained from scalp sampling are used in some hospitals in laboring patients as adjuncts to fetal heart rate monitoring. However, in the antepartum patient, the fetal blood necessary for this test is obtainable only through percutaneous umbilical blood sampling (PUBS). This technique uses ultrasound to direct a needle introduced through the maternal abdomen into the um-

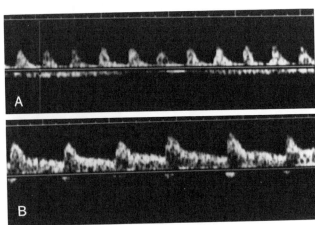

FIGURE 12–2. Doppler waveforms in the umbilical artery of 2 fetuses. A, Abnormal pattern with decreased diastolic flow in a severely growth-retarded fetus. B, Normal pattern with normal diastolic flow indicating low resistance.

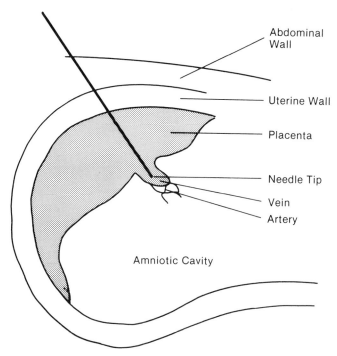

FIGURE 12–3. *In a percutaneous umbilical blood sampling (PUBS) procedure, a needle is advanced into the umbilical vein at its insertion into the placenta under ultrasound guidance in order to obtain a sample of fetal blood. (From Daffos, F., et al.: Am J Obstet Gynecol 153:655, 1985. Reprinted with permission from the American College of Obstetricians and Gynecologists.)*

bilical vein at a fixed point, such as its insertion into the placenta (Fig. 12–3).

PUBS has proved to be invaluable for a number of prenatal diagnostic indications (Daffos et al., 1985). Hematocrit or rapid fetal karyotype determinations are two common indications for this test. Some fetal infections, such as toxoplasmosis, can also be diagnosed with this modality (Daffos et al., 1988). To a lesser degree, PUBS has also been used to assess fetal well-being via acid-base studies. In the latter case, the results may be reassuring in certain situations, but this approach is of limited overall usefulness in ongoing pregnancies because of its invasiveness and the possibility of rapid changes in fetal status. Investigations of other biochemical and hematologic markers of progressive conditions such as IUGR using fetal blood obtained by PUBS are still in the preliminary stages (Cox et al., 1988).

■ LUNG MATURITY STUDIES

One important neonatal complication that is predictable by antenatal testing is respiratory distress syndrome (RDS) related to prematurity. Chemical analysis of amniotic fluid can reliably predict whether an infant delivered soon after the analysis is at significant risk for this disorder (Hamilton et al., 1984). Such testing may therefore be indicated prior to elective delivery to avoid what would be in those cases an iatrogenic complication.

The most common setting in which this issue arises is an elective repeat cesarean section. Recently, opinion has shifted away from doing an amniocentesis for fetal lung studies in all such cases. The American College of Obstetricians and Gynecologists has issued guidelines for deciding which patients may be safely delivered without performing lung maturity studies (ACOG Committee of Obstetrics, 1986). Briefly, the recommendations exclude from amniocentesis a group of patients at term by strict dating criteria who are not diabetic—a condition known to delay lung maturity.

Another group of patients who may benefit from amniocentesis for fetal lung maturity studies are those who *require* delivery prior to term. Knowing the status of fetal pulmonary maturity may influence the timing of obstetric decisions in these cases. However, if early delivery is being contemplated, it is often because of a situation such as maternal medical illness that necessitates delivery irrespective of fetal status. Similarly, if the mother is in active preterm labor, her fetus may deliver despite all attempts at delay.

Nonetheless, the analysis of fluid can be very helpful. Fluid collected vaginally from a patient with ruptured membranes may also be tested, but these assays are probably less reliable. Once fluid is obtained several tests may be performed, the two most common being the lecithin-sphingomyelin (L/S) ratio and quantification of the amount of phosphatidylglycerol (PG) (Table 12–2). Each test has a false-positive rate of less than 2 per cent and a false-negative rate that is quite a bit higher.

When the fetal lungs are known to be immature by amniotic fluid testing or are presumed to be immature because of extremely early gestational age, corticosteroids administered to the mother may enhance pulmonary maturity. Several studies (Liggins and Howie, 1972; Collaborative Group on Antenatal Steroid Therapy, 1981; Avery et al., 1986) have demonstrated a decreased incidence of RDS in these newborns. These drugs are not effective unless delivery is delayed at least 24 hours after its administration, and the effects may only last 7 days. However, in carefully selected cases, corticosteroids have a significant impact. In addition, the incidence of intraventricular hemorrhage, necrotizing enterocolitis, and patent ductus arteriosus may also be reduced in treated infants. Whether these are independent effects or a consequence of decreased respiratory problems is not established.

Many questions remain concerning the role of corticosteroids in special circumstances. For example, are multiple courses of these drugs indicated in women whose delivery is delayed 7 days or more? Are they effective in multiple gestation? Finally, their effectiveness has not been prospectively studied in newborns born prior to 28 weeks' gestation.

An area of particular controversy is the role of corticosteroids in the management of the patient with premature rupture of the membranes (PROM). PROM is felt by most investigators to reduce the incidence of RDS, and this effect may not be further enhanced by the addition of corticosteroids. Studies of this issue have been divided in

TABLE 12–2. Lung Maturity Tests

- Lecithin-sphingomyelin (L/S) ratio.
- Phosphatidylglycerol (PG) measurement.
- Foam stability tests.
- Delta OD$_{450}$.
- Shake test.
- Fluorescence polarimetry.
- Slide agglutination PG test.
- Measures of surfactant proteins

their conclusions. Unfortunately, there is a small but demonstrable increase in infectious complications in the treatment group for both mother and newborn in many of these series.

Future investigations in this area will no doubt include studies of other hormones that play a role in pulmonary maturation, particularly prolactin and thyroxine. The combination of thyrotropin-releasing hormone and corticosteroids was found to be superior to corticosteroids alone in preventing RDS in one recent study (Morales et al., 1989).

■ ANTEPARTUM FETAL HEART RATE TESTING

Antepartum fetal heart rate testing is the cornerstone of the assessment of fetal well-being. These tests—the nonstress test and the oxytocin challenge test—are much like fetal heart rate monitoring in labor in that, if either one is negative, it is an excellent predictor of fetal well-being in utero (Freeman et al., 1982; Phelan, 1981). Their main drawback is that a positive or abnormal test is not specific for fetal distress.

The oxytocin challenge test (OCT) was the first such test developed and is the standard against which other tests are judged. To perform this test, a dilute oxytocin solution is given intravenously causing mild uterine contractions. A 10-minute window that includes three contractions is then evaluated for fetal heart rate abnormalities similar to those that may be seen in labor. The presence of good baseline variability and the absence of decelerations is reassuring, and the risk of death in utero over the subsequent 7 days for fetuses with these findings is extremely low. A positive or ominous test, on the other hand, is one in which late decelerations follow each contraction. Although a positive test is considered an indication for delivery by most obstetricians, between 10 and 50 per cent of these fetuses tolerate labor well and thus may represent false positives.

A variation of the OCT is the nipple stimulation test. Rather than administering intravenous oxytocin, the patient gently manipulates the nipple of one of her breasts which releases endogenous oxytocin and causes uterine contractions. The advantage of this test over the traditional OCT is ease of administration. However, the release of endogenous oxytocin is less controlled, and it has been associated with hyperstimulation of the uterus.

The nonstress test (NST) measures accelerations in fetal heart rate associated with fetal movement (Fig. 12–4). Two or three accelerations in 20 minutes defines a reactive or reassuring test and, again, fetal mortality over the next 7 days is extremely low for fetuses with this finding. However, if the fetus fails to move or have the necessary accelerations in 20 minutes, the likelihood of a false-positive result is high. Approximately 80 per cent of such fetuses are normal and not asphyxiated.

There is some controversy as to the best initial screening test to use in high-risk pregnancies. Although the OCT is considered to be more definitive, the convenience of the NST has made it the initial test used in most centers. When the NST is nonreactive, the OCT is typically used as the backup test.

Both of these tests have limitations. Although the NST

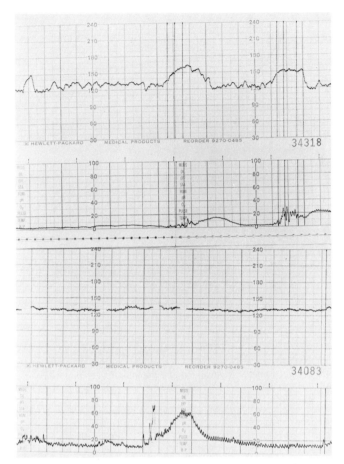

FIGURE 12–4. Nonstress tests: Top two traces, Reactive, accelerations in the fetal heart rate accompanied by fetal movement. Bottom two traces, Nonreactive, no accelerations in fetal heart rate over baseline.

can be reactive in extremely immature fetuses, a nonreactive test may simply reflect neurologic immaturity rather than asphyxia (Druzin et al., 1985). The OCT has specific contraindications, such as PROM, preterm labor, and placenta previa, because of the possibility of initiating labor. Finally, the interpretation of both of these tests is somewhat subjective and may, on occasion, be difficult.

■ FETAL BIOPHYSICAL PROFILE

This widely used test was developed as an alternative to the oxytocin challenge test and a refinement of the nonstress test. Its design was modeled on the Apgar score and consists of five measures for which a score from 0 to 2 is assigned (Table 12–3). A total score of 8 or greater is reassuring and a score of 4 or less is indicative of asphyxia (Manning et al., 1981). Four of the measures are obtained by ultrasound—fetal breathing, tone, movements, and amniotic fluid volume. The fifth is a nonstress test.

With widespread utilization of this test, it has become apparent that the five measures are not of equal value. For example, diminished amniotic fluid volume correlates well with chronic hypoxic states, whereas fetal tone is present until the fetus is moribund and thus is a late predictor of distress. The probable advantage of the biophysical profile (BPP) over traditional antepartum fetal heart rate testing is the decrease in the number of false-

TABLE 12–3. Biophysical Profile Scoring

BIOPHYSICAL VARIABLE	NORMAL (score = 2)	ABNORMAL (score = 0)
Fetal breathing movements	At least one episode of FBM of at least 30-second duration in 30-min observation.	Absent FBM or no episode of ≥30 seconds in 30 minutes
Gross body movements	At least three discrete body/limb movements in 30 minutes (episodes of active continuous movement considered as a single movement).	Two or fewer episodes of body/limb movements in 30 minutes.
Fetal tone	At least one episode of active extension with return to flexion of fetal limb(s) or trunk. Opening and closing of hand considered normal tone.	Either slow extension with return to partial flexion or movement of limb in full extension of absent fetal movement.
Reactive FHR	At least two episodes of FHR acceleration of ≥15 bpm and of at least 15-second duration associated with fetal movement in 20 minutes.	Less than two episodes of acceleration of FHR or acceleration of <15 bpm in 40 minutes.
Qualitative AFV	At least one pocket of AF that measures at least 1 cm in two perpendicular planes.	Either no AF pockets or a pocket <1 cm in two perpendicular planes.

FBM = fetal breathing movements; FHR = fetal heart rate; AFV = amniotic fluid volume; bpm = beats per minute; AF = amniotic fluid.
From Manning, F. A., Lange, M. B., Morrison, I., et al.: Fetal biophysical profile score and the nonstress test: A comparative trial. Obstet. Gynecol. 64:326, 1984.

positive tests associated with the latter (Manning et al., 1984). Furthermore, if a nonstress test is nonreactive and all other parameters of the BPP are normal, an OCT, which may be undesirable in certain clinical settings, can be avoided. Finally, at early gestational ages, when an NST may be nonreactive because of neurologic immaturity, the other four measures are still reliable.

Perhaps the single most important contribution of the biophysical profile is to underscore the value of the assessment of amniotic fluid volume (Vintzileos et al., 1987). In the absence of ruptured membranes, an abnormally decreased fluid volume is worrisome, and further evaluation is indicated. In retrospect, oligohydramnios may well have been present in many of the patients with falsely reassuring NSTs in the early clinical trials.

■ FETAL HEART RATE IN LABOR

Fetal heart rate monitoring in labor is part of good modern obstetrical care. However, routine electronic fetal heart rate monitoring (EFM) has been associated with significant controversy. Although this modality has been invaluable in the care of high-risk patients, it has not been conclusively shown to improve fetal or neonatal morbidity or mortality in low-risk patients who are carefully monitored by auscultation (Thacker, 1987). In clinical trials of universal EFM, low-risk patients who did not have EFM had one-on-one nursing with frequent auscultatory fetal heart rate checks and careful assessment of other clinical parameters. Although this type of monitoring may be

equally as effective as EFM, in hospitals where nursing personnel is at a premium, providing this type of labor-intensive alternative may be impractical.

In certain high-risk situations, electronic fetal monitoring is clearly indicated. Mothers with conditions such as diabetes, sickle cell anemia, or preeclampsia all have an increased incidence of fetal distress in labor and should be monitored continuously. Those who develop problems in labor, such as detection of meconium-stained amniotic fluid, chorioamnionitis, fixed heart rate, or decelerations noted by auscultation, should also receive EFM.

Interpretation of an electronic tracing depends on evaluating several factors (Freeman and Garite, 1981). The first is beat-to-beat variability in the fetal heart rate. Decreased variability may be an early sign of fetal distress. Accelerations of the fetal heart rate are always reassuring, but some types of decelerations may be ominous.

Decelerations are classified by their temporal relationship with uterine contractions, and the various classes of deceleration have very different prognoses (Fig. 12–5). Type I, or early decelerations, have a simultaneous onset with the contractions. These represent a vagal response to compression of the fetal head and are of virtually no significance. Type II, or late decelerations, are more worrisome. In these the peak of the deceleration occurs after the preceding uterine contraction. Late return to the baseline heart rate represents myocardial depression after an episode of fetal hypoxia. Type III, or variable decelerations, are of variable onset and shape and generally represent umbilical cord compression. The severity of variable decelerations is classified by their duration and degree of bradycardia, and by associated findings, such as beat-to-beat variability. Their severity reflects their seriousness. Mild variable decelerations are usually of little significance, whereas severe variable decelerations may be as serious as late decelerations.

Since the interpretation of electronic fetal heart rate

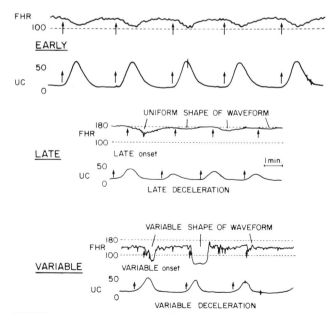

FIGURE 12–5. Early, late, and variable average fetal heart rate responses are recorded on the ordinate, with time on the abscissa. Uterine contractions (mm Hg) are shown in relation to the heart rate changes. (FHR = fetal heart rate. UC = uterine contractions.)

tracings is somewhat subjective and because tracings tend to overpredict fetal distress, some centers use fetal capillary pH as a second-line test. The fetal scalp is visualized through a specially designed speculum, an area is cleaned and knicked with a scalpel, a bead of blood is then collected into a capillary tube and the pH determined. If the latter is less than 7.20 expeditious delivery is indicated, whereas a value of greater than 7.25 is normal. The intermediate zone warrants close observation and possibly a repeat sample analysis in approximately 20 minutes.

Acute fetal distress in utero is initially treated by altering possible precipitating factors. If relative hypotension results from the administration of epidural anesthesia, intravenous fluids are given to the mother. Uterine hyperstimulation from oxytoxin administration can be corrected. General measures may also be helpful such as administering oxygen to the mother in order to increase the oxygen content of the blood flowing to the placenta. Finally, the patient can be repositioned on her left side to maximize uterine blood flow. If these measures fail, delivery is generally indicated. Recently, other measures to resuscitate the fetus in utero have been described (Patriarco et al., 1987). Tocolytic agents, such as terbutaline or magnesium sulfate, have been given rapidly to the mother in an attempt to abate uterine contractions and maximize uterine blood flow. In many cases, this treatment results in a return to a normal fetal heart rate tracing, thus eliminating the necessity for an emergency cesarean section or difficult forceps delivery.

The fetal heart rate tracing obtained by electronic fetal monitoring can be influenced by many factors other than fetal asphyxia. Narcotics given to the mother for pain relief in labor may decrease beat-to-beat variability. Baseline fetal tachycardia occurs when sympathomimetic drugs are administered to the mother to prevent preterm delivery. Tachycardia may also be an effect of maternal fever or intra-amniotic infection, and these fetuses often have a decrease in beat-to-beat variability. Thus, caution must be maintained not to overread abnormalities of fetal heart rate in these circumstances.

■ REFERENCES

ACOG Committee of Obstetrics: Assessment of fetal maturity prior to repeat cesarean delivery or elective induction of labor. Maternal-Fetal Medicine, No. 22, March 1986.

Avery, M. E., Aylward, G., Creasy, R., et al.: Update on prenatal steroid for prevention of respiratory distress. Report of a conference—September 26–28, 1985. Am. J. Obstet. Gynecol. *155*:2, 1986.

Carpenter, M. W., Curci, M. R., Dibbins, A. W., et al.: Perinatal management of ventral wall defects. Obstet. Gynecol. *64*:646, 1984.

Chervenak, F. A., Berkowitz, R. L., Tortora, M., et al.: The management of fetal hydrocephalus. Am. J. Obstet. Gynecol. *151*:933, 1985.

Collaborative Group on Antenatal Steroid Therapy. Effect of antenatal dexamethasone administration on the prevention of respiratory distress syndrome. Am. J. Obstet. Gynecol. *141*:276, 1981.

Cox, W. L., Daffos, F., Forestier, F., et al.: Physiology and management of intrauterine growth retardation: A biologic approach with fetal blood sampling. Am. J. Obstet. Gynecol. *159*:36, 1988.

Daffos, F., Capella-Pavlovsky, M., and Forestier, F.: Fetal blood sampling during pregnancy with use of a needle guided by ultrasound: A study of 606 consecutive cases. Am. J. Obstet. Gynecol. *153*:655, 1985.

Daffos, F., Forestier, F., Capella-Pavlovsky, M., et al.: Prenatal management of 746 pregnancies at risk for congenital toxoplasmosis. N. Engl. J. Med. *318*:271, 1988.

Druzin, M. L., Fox, A., Kogut, E., and Carlson, C.: The relationship of the nonstress test to gestational age. Am. J. Obstet. Gynecol. *153*:386, 1985.

Freeman, R. K., Anderson, G., and Dorchester, W.: A prospective multi-institutional study of antepartum fetal heart rate monitoring. II. Contraction stress test versus nonstress test for primary surveillance. Am. J. Obstet. Gynecol. *143*:778, 1982.

Freeman, R. K., and Garite, T. J.: Fetal Heart Rate Monitoring. Baltimore, Williams and Wilkins, 1981.

Hamilton, P. R., Hauschild, D., Broekhaizen, F. F., et al.: Comparison of lecithin: Sphingomyelin ratio, fluorescence polarization, and phosphatidylglycerol in the amniotic fluid in the prediction of respiratory distress syndrome. Obstet. Gynecol. *63*:52, 1984.

Kleinman, C. S., Hobbins, J. C., Jaffe, C. C., et al.: Echocardiographic studies of the human fetus: Prenatal diagnosis of congenital heart disease and cardiac dysrrhythmias. Pediatrics *65*:1059, 1980.

Kleinman, C. S., and Santalli, T. V.: Ultrasonic evaluation of the fetal human heart. Semin. Perinatol. *7*:90, 1983.

Liggins, G. C., and Howie, R. N.: A controlled trial of antepartum glucocorticoid treatment for prevention of the respiratory distress syndrome in premature infants. Pediatrics *50*:515, 1972.

Manning, F. A., Baskett, T. F., Morrison, I., et al.: Fetal biophysical profile scoring: A prospective study in 1,184 high-risk patients. Am. J. Obstet. Gynecol. *140*:289, 1981.

Manning, F. A., Lange, M. B., Morrison, I., et al.: Fetal biophysical profile score and the nonstress test: A comparative trial. Obstet. Gynecol. *64*:326, 1984.

Morales, W. J., O'Brian, W. F., Angel, J. L., et al.: Fetal lung maturation: The combined use of corticosteroids and thyrotropin-releasing hormone. Obstet. Gynecol. *73*:111, 1989.

Patriarco, M. S., Viechnicki, B. M., Hutchinson, T. A., et al.: A study on intrauterine fetal resuscitation with terbutaline. Am. J. Obstet. Gynecol. *157*:384, 1987.

Phelan, J. P.: The nonstress test: A review of 3,000 tests. Am. J. Obstet. Gynecol. *139*:7, 1981.

Romero, R., Pilu, G., Jeonty, P., et al.: Prenatal Diagnosis of Congenital Anomalies. East Norwalk, Conn., Appleton and Lange, 1987.

Thacker, S. B.: The efficacy of intrapartum electronic fetal monitoring. Am. J. Obstet. Gynecol. *156*:24, 1987.

Trudinger, B. J., Giles, W. B., and Cook, C. M.: Flow velocity waveforms in the maternal uteroplacental and fetal umbilical placental circulations. Am. J. Obstet. Gynecol. *152*:155, 1985.

The Use of Diagnostic Ultrasound Imaging in Pregnancy. National Institutes of Health. Consensus Development Conference, February 6–8, 1984.

Vintzileos, A. M., Campbell, W. A., Nochimson, D. J., et al.: The use and misuse of the fetal biophysical profile. Am. J. Obstet. Gynecol. *156*:527, 1987.

Vintzileos, A. M., Campbell, W. A., Nochimson, D. J., et al.: Antenatal evaluation and management of ultrasonically detected fetal anomalies. Obstet. Gynecol. *69*:640, 1987.

PREVENTION OF PRETERM BIRTH

13

Denise M. Main

The preterm delivery rate in the United States has remained almost stable over the past 30 years, despite advances in obstetric diagnosis and treatment of the major causes of premature birth. Although it was hoped that the introduction of tocolytic therapy, improved detection of multiple gestation and placenta previa with new ultrasound techniques, and the marked decrease in untreated syphilis would reduce preterm births dramatically, over 9 per cent of live births in the United States still occur before 37 weeks' gestation and 6 per cent before 36 weeks' gestation (US Department of Health and Human Services, 1990). Similarly, government-funded medical assistance and nutritional supplementation programs have had no discernible impact on the national preterm delivery rate.

■ RISK FACTORS ASSOCIATED WITH PRETERM BIRTH

Many of the risk factors associated with preterm birth have been known for at least 20 years (Committee to Study the Prevention of Low Birth Weight, 1985; Main, 1988). Among these, reproducible factors include demographic and behavioral risks, inadequate health care, medical conditions predating pregnancy, and current pregnancy complications (Table 13–1). Some of the more frequent and important factors are reviewed in the following sections.

TABLE 13–1. Risk Factors Associated with Preterm Birth

DEMOGRAPHIC
  Age
  Race
  Socioeconomic status
  Marital status

BEHAVIORAL
  Smoking
  Other substance abuse
  Poor nutrition
  Excessive physical activity

HEALTH CARE
  Absent or inadequate prenatal care

MEDICAL RISKS PREDATING PREGNANCY
  Poor obstetric history
  Uterine or cervical malformations, myomas, DES exposure
  Selected medical conditions

CURRENT PREGNANCY COMPLICATIONS
  Multiple gestations
  Abnormalities in amniotic fluid volume
  Vaginal bleeding
  Fetal abnormalities
  Serious infection
  Abdominal surgery

SOCIOECONOMIC FACTORS

A variety of socioeconomic characteristics are related to the incidence of low birth weight (LBW), and, although often less well documented, to preterm birth. Maternal age of 19 years and younger or 40 years and older, unmarried status, limited educational achievement, and race other than white are all factors associated with increased risk. The most striking, perplexing, and distressing factor is maternal race. A black woman is at least two times more likely to deliver a live-born baby who weighs less than 2500 g than a white, Mexican, Cuban, Chinese, Japanese, or Native American woman (US Department of Health and Human Services, 1989). The low birth weight rate of 12.4 per cent among black women also compares unfavorably with the 8.7 per cent rate for Puerto Rican women, the ethnic group with the second highest LBW rate. Furthermore, the percentage of infants born in the very-low-birth-weight (VLBW) category, i.e., less than 1500 g, those at highest risk for neonatal mortality, is disproportionately high among blacks. In 1987, 2.73 per cent of black and 0.94 per cent of white infants were in this very-high-risk group. Not surprisingly, the preterm delivery rate (<37 weeks' gestation) is also approximately twice that for whites (17.9 per cent versus 8.5 per cent in 1987). It is distressing how little is known about the factors that may explain these marked racial and ethnic discrepancies in the LBW and preterm birth rates. They do not appear to be accounted for by differences in age, parity, educational attainment, marital status, prenatal care, nutrition, smoking, and substance abuse (Kleinman and Kessel, 1987; Shiono, 1986a). However, adequate prenatal care appears to be of greater relative benefit for black women as compared with white women (Murray and Bernfield, 1988).

TOBACCO AND COCAINE

Cigarette smoking lowers birth weight in a dose-related fashion. Although much of this results from relative intrauterine growth retardation, cigarette smoking also is associated with decreased gestational age (Meyer et al., 1976; Shiono et al., 1986b). This risk persists even after adjusting for potentially confounding variables such as mother's weight, height, hospital status, age, parity, birth place, previous pregnancy history, weight gain, time of onset of prenatal care, sex of child, and caffeine and alcohol use. In the United States, where 30 per cent of all women smoke, it has been estimated that 13 to 20 per cent of all preterm births can be attributed to maternal smoking (Committee to Study the Prevention of Low

Birth Weight, 1985). Smoking also increases the frequency of preterm premature rupture of the membranes (PPROM), placental abruption and previa, and fetal death—specific adverse outcomes that can lead to preterm delivery. With the recent increase in use of cocaine during pregnancy, it is becoming clear that cocaine also may affect both birth weight and gestational age (see Chapter 26). (Chouteau et al., 1988).

PRIOR OBSTETRIC OUTCOME

The incidence of preterm birth correlates strongly with prior obstetric outcome. A history of one previous preterm birth is associated with a recurrence risk of 17 to 40 per cent, with the risk increasing with the number of preterm births and decreasing with the number of term deliveries (Bakketeig and Hoffman, 1981; Keirse et al., 1978). There is also a definite increase in subsequent preterm deliveries in women who have experienced one or more second-trimester abortions. One spontaneous or legally induced first-trimester abortion does not increase the risk for prematurity. There is still debate over whether or not multiple first-trimester induced abortions are associated with a higher preterm delivery rate.

CERVICAL INCOMPETENCE

Whether secondary to trauma from a prior obstetric or gynecologic procedure, a result of diethylstilbestrol (DES) exposure in utero, or of unknown cause, cervical incompetence classically leads to painless second-trimester cervical dilatation and abortion. Once dilatation has occurred, preterm labor or rupture of membranes or both can follow, making it difficult to establish the cause of the preterm birth. Because of differences in definitions and populations, the absolute contribution of this factor to preterm delivery is unclear; estimates of its incidence range from 1 in 125 to 1 in 2000 deliveries. Most obstetricians consider cervical cerclage the therapy of choice for this condition.

CURRENT PREGNANCY COMPLICATIONS

Multiple gestation pregnancy represents perhaps the clearest risk factor for preterm birth. In 1987, 43.9 per cent of all white plural pregnancies and 52.2 per cent of all black plural pregnancies ended before 37 weeks' gestation (US Department of Health and Human Services, 1990). Additional current pregnancy complications that predispose the mother to delivery of preterm or LBW infants include placenta previa and abruption, abnormalities in amniotic fluid volume, abdominal surgery, and fetal abnormalities.

Numerous associations have been made between vaginal colonizations and preterm delivery. Organisms implicated in at least some studies include group B streptococcus, *Chlamydia trachomatis, mycoplasma,* other anaerobes, and gonococcus (Roveno and Mazor, 1988). In addition, a significant proportion of women who present with preterm labor (mean 16 per cent, range 3 per cent to 48 per cent) or PPROM (mean 28 per cent, range 15 per cent to 43 per cent) demonstrate occult intra-amniotic infections diagnosed by amniotic fluid culture.

UNDERLYING MEDICAL CONDITIONS

Women with certain underlying medical conditions are also at great risk for preterm birth. Examples of such high-risk conditions include diabetic nephropathy, collagen vascular diseases, and lupus erythematosus. These pregnancies often result in preterm birth because of maternal hypertension, deteriorating kidney function, or fetal growth retardation or distress.

■ SCREENING TO IDENTIFY WOMEN AT RISK FOR PRETERM DELIVERY

Given the wide variety of known risk factors associated with low birth weight and preterm delivery, it is not surprising that a number of investigators have developed screening systems to identify women likely to deliver preterm infants (Kaminski et al., 1973, Creasy et al., 1980b). It is disappointing, however, that these systems, when tested in the United States, have identified at best only half of the women who deliver preterm infants (sensitivities 0.26 to 0.56) (Main, 1987). Furthermore, women identified as high risk by these systems have only a 9 to 18 per cent likelihood of delivering prior to term. Intermittent monitoring for uterine activity while women are waiting for routine prenatal visits may improve our ability to identify women at risk for preterm labor (Main et al., 1988).

EARLY DETECTION OF PRETERM LABOR

Although it is unlikely that any system will be sufficiently sensitive and predictive to identify women who require prophylactic treatment for preterm labor, many recommend that women identified as being at high risk on the basis of risk-screening receive increased education and more intensive antepartum surveillance (Herron et al., 1982). Uterine monitoring at home to detect contractions may be of benefit for select, very-high-risk patients (Katz et al., 1986; Morrison et al., 1987). These approaches are designed to facilitate the early diagnosis of preterm labor and thus, possibly, increase the likelihood of effective tocolytic treatment. However, some researchers using similar approaches in different settings have failed to document their efficacy (Goldenberg et al., 1990; Iams et al., 1988; Main et al., 1989).

■ PROXIMATE CAUSES OF PRETERM BIRTH

Broadly categorized, there are four acute obstetric conditions that result in preterm delivery. These are preterm labor; PPROM; maternal medical or obstetric complications; and fetal distress or demise. Meis and colleagues (1987) recently studied the relative contributions of preterm labor and PPROM in different populations. Using two samples of approximately 1500 women each, one group receiving public assistance and the other having private insurance, this study showed significant differences in the obstetric factors leading to preterm birth. In the group receiving public assistance, 34 per cent of preterm births were due to preterm labor, 46 per cent to PPROM, and 20 per cent to medical complications. In contrast, in the group having private insurance, 55 per cent of the preterm births resulted from preterm labor, 27 per cent from PPROM, and 18 per cent from medical complications.

■ DIAGNOSIS AND TREATMENT OF PRETERM LABOR

Preterm labor is defined as regular uterine contractions associated with cervical change, occurring prior to 37 weeks' gestation. The most widely used definition of labor requires a minimum of eight contractions per hour or four in 20 minutes (Gonik and Creasy, 1986). The amount of cervical change and whether it represents change from a previous examination or only while under observation for contractions is less standardized. The less the cervical change, the higher the success rate of tocolytic (and placebo) therapy. Most placebo-controlled studies of tocolytics have required cervical dilatation of at least 2 cm and/or effacement of at least 80 per cent, and/or progressive cervical change under observation. Many physicians also limited treatment to women with maximal cervical dilatation or ≤ 5 cm, because a much lower success rate is achieved in the presence of more advanced cervical dilatation.

Evaluation of the efficacy of tocolytic agents as compared with that of placebo treatment (often bed rest, hydration, and/or sedation) has been mostly limited to small studies of beta-mimetic agents. Interpretation of this research has been hampered by the difficulty in defining basic terms: What is considered a successful outcome in the use of tocolytic agents? Is a successful outcome considered to be achievement of 37 weeks' gestation? Or is it at 34 to 35 weeks' gestation, after which almost all babies do well? Or should delivery be delayed 48 hours to allow for corticosteroid administration? Or should success be considered only as a reflection of improved perinatal morbidity and mortality data?

When one looks at the aggregate of data from 16 randomized trials with beta-mimetic agents involving a total of 484 treated patients, it is apparent that delivery can be delayed for at least 48 hours in approximately 75 per cent of the cases, with approximately 50 per cent reaching at least 37 weeks' gestation (King et al., 1988). These results are significantly better than those achieved with placebo (approximately 60 per cent of cases of preterm labor stop for 48 hours, and 36 per cent of cases of preterm labor stop until term). These success rates with placebo treatment demonstrate the relative inaccuracy of the diagnosis of preterm labor, even when cervical change is required as an indicator for diagnosis. There is no evidence that tocolytic therapy improves perinatal morbidity or mortality, factors that would require much larger sample sizes for accurate assessment because of their reduced prevalence.

Prerequisites for use of tocolytic agents include (1) the presence of preterm labor, (2) a gestational age at which treatment will benefit the fetus, and (3) absence of maternal or fetal contraindications to treatment. Prior to 34 weeks' gestation, there is obstetric consensus that a fetus is likely to benefit from inhibition of labor. It is more difficult to demonstrate benefit from tocolytic therapy after 34 weeks' gestation (Korenbrot et al., 1984). Nonetheless, tocolytic agents are often prescribed until 36 or 37 weeks'

gestation. In this later preterm gestational age range, the decision to inhibit labor is more often made on a case-by-case basis, depending on fetal lung maturation and other factors. Maternal and fetal contraindications to tocolytic therapy include eclampsia or severe preeclampsia, major maternal hemorrhage, chorioamnionitis, a dead or seriously compromised fetus, or a fetus with anomalies incompatible with life.

CLASSES OF TOCOLYTIC AGENTS

There are four classes of tocolytic agents currently in use: beta-mimetic agents, magnesium sulfate, prostaglandin inhibitors, and calcium channel blockers. To understand their respective mechanisms of action, it is necessary first to review briefly the regulatory mechanisms of smooth muscle contractility. The key process in actin-myosin interaction, and thus contraction, is myosin light-chain phosphorylation. This reaction is controlled by myosin light-chain kinase. The activity of tocolytic agents can be explained on the basis of their effects on the factors regulating the activity of this enzyme, notably calcium and cAMP. Calcium is essential for the activation of myosin light-chain kinase and binds to the kinase as calmodulin-calcium complex. Intracellular calcium levels are regulated by two general mechanisms: (1) influx across the cell membrane, and (2) release from intracellular storage sites. The proposed mechanisms of action for tocolytic agents are summarized in Table 13–2 (Caritis et al., 1988).

USE OF TOCOLYTIC AGENTS IN THE UNITED STATES

The two classes of tocolytics most widely used in the United States are beta-mimetics, specifically terbutaline and ritodrine, and magnesium sulfate. Several prospective, randomized studies have suggested a comparable efficacy for these two types of agents when used for initial intravenous tocolysis (Beall et al., 1985; Hollander et al., 1987). Irrespective of the first agent chosen, the alternative agent is successful in 80 to 90 per cent of cases that fail to respond to the first choice. The optimal duration for initial intravenous treatment with either beta-mimetics or magnesium sulfate has not been established. Therapy commonly is administered for 12 to 48 hours. Following successful inhibition of labor with the intravenous agent, either oral terbutaline or ritodrine is prescribed. These oral agents have been shown to prolong the interval from primary to recurrent preterm labor, if it recurs (Brown and Tejani, 1981; Creasy, 1980a). Indomethacin has been used for short courses of therapy, especially prior to 32 weeks' gestation. Long-term use and primary use are limited because of concerns about fetal toxicity. Although nifedipine is a potent inhibitor of uterine contractions, experience with its use is still limited. Use of nifedipine is presently restricted in many centers.

SIDE EFFECTS OF TOCOLYTIC AGENTS

Ritodrine and Terbutaline. Ritodrine and terbutaline affect multiple maternal and fetal organs, because beta-adrenergic receptors are ubiquitous. Although relatively

TABLE 13–2. Proposed Mechanisms of Action for Tocolytic Agents

AGENT CLASS	SPECIFIC AGENTS	MECHANISMS
Beta-mimetics	Ritodrine Terbutaline	Interact with membrane receptors, causing activation of adenylate cyclase to produce cAMP
		Promote placental progesterone production which, in turn, reduces gap junction formation
Magnesium sulfate	Same	Mechanisms only partially understood, but include the following:
		Extracellular and membrane magnesium modulates calcium intake by competing for calcium binding sites and by stimulating cAMP production
		Intracellular magnesium stimulates ATPase, which promotes calcium uptake by the sarcoplasmic reticulum
Prostaglandin inhibitors	Indomethacin	Inactivate cyclo-oxygenase, the enzyme needed to produce PGG_2, the first prostaglandin intermediate
Calcium channel blockers	Nifedipine	Inhibit calcium cell entry by blocking voltage-dependent calcium channels

beta$_2$ specific, these agents produce significant cardiovascular effects, including increases in heart rate, cardiac output, and pulse pressure and decreases in diastolic blood pressure and peripheral vascular resistance. These changes can predispose the patient to pulmonary edema, a potentially life-threatening complication. In addition, beta-mimetics produce multiple metabolic effects, including increases in blood glucose, insulin, lactate, and free fatty acids and a decrease in plasma potassium. With continuing therapy over 24 hours, most of these changes return toward pretreatment levels. Side effects such as chest pain, shortness of breath, and nausea occur more frequently when infusion rates are increased rapidly (Caritis et al., 1983).

Ritodrine and terbutaline freely cross the placenta, increasing fetal heart rate and affecting fetal metabolism. Umbilical blood flow and fetal acid-base status are unchanged. Uterine blood flow is not substantially affected. Metabolic effects present at birth, however, include neonatal hyperinsulinemia, hypoglycemia, and hypokalemia. One group of investigators has noted increased neonatal ventricular septal thickness following in utero exposure to ritodrine (Nuchpuckdee et al., 1986). In the 41 newborns, studied, this effect appeared dependent on the duration of in utero exposure and returned to normal by 3 months of age in all subjects. Fetal echocardiographic evaluation of nine fetuses exposed to long-term terbutaline therapy failed to demonstrate any difference with regard to intraventricular septal thickness or other cardiac measurements as compared with controls matched for gestational age (Srensen and Brlum, 1988). Long-term follow-up of fetuses exposed to ritodrine or terbutaline in utero is limited. The few studies addressing long-term morbidity, however, have found no differences in neurologic, developmental, behavioral, or growth parameters (Polowczyk et al., 1984; Hadders-Algra et al., 1986).

Magnesium Sulfate. As a potent peripheral vasodilator, intravenously administered magnesium sulfate can cause flushing, sweating, and the sensation of warmth. Additional potential maternal side effects include nausea, vomiting, palpitations, dizziness, and dryness of mouth. Pulmonary edema can also occur with magnesium sulfate. Significant magnesium toxicity includes loss of tendon reflexes, and, with higher levels, respiratory and/or cardiac arrest. Magnesium freely crosses to the fetus with equilibration of maternal and fetal blood levels. It is very uncommon for the drug to result in neonatal depression when doses are maintained within therapeutic levels, although isolated cases have been reported (Lipsitz, 1971).

Indomethacin. Use of indomethacin as a tocolytic agent has been limited in the United States because of potential fetal side effects, including prenatal closure of the ductus arteriosus, persistent fetal circulation, oliguria, and lung hypoplasia. Concern about closure of the ductus in utero is based on experimental animal studies and isolated case reports in humans. Most of the case reports are retrospective; and confounding factors, such as asphyxia, were either present or could not be excluded. All cases occurred when indomethacin therapy was given after 34 weeks' gestation, often after prolonged therapy with the drug. However, a recent echocardiographic study of fetuses exposed in utero to short-term maternal use of indomethacin demonstrated evidence of ductal constriction in 7 of 14 fetuses (Moise et al., 1988). At re-evaluation of the fetuses within 24 hours of discontinuing indomethacin therapy, the constriction had resolved. Indomethacin has also been shown to cause oligohydramnios, meconium-staining, and an increased rate of fetal death in monkeys whose mothers received the drug in the last days of pregnancy (Novy, 1978). A decrease in mean urine production, as measured by bladder size, has been reported in fetuses exposed to short-course indomethacin therapy (Kirshon et al., 1988). Despite case reports and experimental evidence, three recent series containing information on a total of 510 patients have demonstrated no adverse neonatal effects (Dudley and Hardie, 1985; Neibyl and Withe, 1986; Zuckerman et al., 1984). Nonetheless, most recommend that indomethacin be used only as a second-line tocolytic agent and that its use be limited to courses of 48 hours to 72 hours prior to 32 weeks' gestation.

Nifedipine. Two small randomized studies suggest that nifedipine is at least as effective a tocolytic agent as intravenous ritodrine (Read and Wellby, 1986; Ferguson, et al., 1990). Maternal cardiovascular and metabolic side effects appear less severe than with intravenous beta-mimetic tocolysis (Ferguson, et al., 1989). Although there have been no reported adverse fetal effects, the relatively limited number of published reports of experiences with this agent relegates it to a second line or experimental agent at many centers.

■ PRETERM PREMATURE RUPTURE OF MEMBRANES (PPROM)

PPROM refers to the leakage of amniotic fluid through the cervix at least 1 hour prior to the start of labor and prior to 37 weeks' gestation. The diagnosis is usually determined by (1) history of leakage of fluid through the vagina, (2) visual observation of a collection, or pool, of fluid in the vagina upon speculum examination, (3) an increase in vaginal pH (this test is approximately 90 to 98 per cent accurate.) and (4) a positive "fern" test. (When amniotic fluid is placed on a clean slide and allowed to air dry, a pattern of microscopic arborization is produced. This finding is present in 85 to 98 per cent of cases.)

The cause of PPROM is often unexplained. It appears that membranes that rupture prior to term have local defects. These defects may be due to infection, nutritional deficiencies, genetic factors, or other unknown causes. The management of PPROM remains one of the most controversial areas in obstetrics. In general, the management options include a conservative approach of "letting nature take its course," a recourse to immediate delivery, or aggressive schemes to attempt to delay delivery and/or accelerate fetal lung maturation. The choice of which therapeutic modality is most appropriate is based on balancing the relative risks from PPROM, specifically infection and asphyxia from cord compression or prolapse, against the risks of prematurity. Although research efforts regarding management of this difficult obstetric complication are limited, recent studies suggest that tocolytic therapy may not be beneficial (Garite et al., 1987; Weiner et al., 1988).

In contrast, antibiotic therapy appears to prolong time to delivery and reduce neonatal infection rates. Five randomized controlled trials have been reported, at least at scientific meetings. All demonstrated significant benefit: pregnancy prolongation in four; reduced neonatal infection in three; and reduced maternal infection in one. Antibiotics used were either mezlocillin or ampicillin, with or without erythromycin or gentamicin. Further research is needed regarding specific agents, dosage, and combination therapy with corticosteroids.

■ REFERENCES

Bakketeig, L. S., and Hoffman, H. J.: Epidemiology of preterm birth: Results from a longitudinal study of births in Norway. *In* Elder, M. G., and Hendricks, C. H., (eds.): Preterm Labor. London, Butterworths, 1981.

Beall, M. H., Edgar, B. W., Paul, R. H., et al.: A comparison of ritodrine, terbutaline, and magnesium sulfate for the suppression of preterm labor. Am. J. Obstet. Gynecol. 153:854, 1985.

Brown, S., and Tejani, N.: Terbutaline sulfate in the prevention of the recurrence of preterm labor. Obstet. Gynecol. 57:22, 1981.

Caritis, S. N., Danby, M. J., and Chan, L.: Pharmacological treatment of preterm labor. Clin. Obstet. Gynecol. 31:635–651, 1988.

Caritis, S. N., Lin, L. S., Toig, G., et al.: Pharmacodynamics of ritodrine in pregnant women during preterm labor. Am. J. Obstet. Gynecol. 147:752, 1983.

Chouteau, M., Brickner, N., and Leppert, P.: The effect of cocaine abuse on birthweight and gestational age. Obstet. Gynecol. 72:351–354, 1988.

Committee to Study the Prevention of Low Birth Weight. Preventing Low Birthweight. Washington, DC, National Academy Press, 1985.

Creasy, R., Golbus, M., Laros, R., Jr., et al.: Oral ritodrine maintenance in the treatment of preterm labor. Am. J. Obstet. Gynecol. 137:212, 1980a.

Creasy, R. K., Gummer, B. A., and Liggins, G. C.: System for predicting spontaneous preterm birth. Obstet. Gynecol. 55:692–695, 1980b.

Dudley, D. K. L., and Hardie, M. J.: Fetal and neonatal effects of indomethacin used as a tocolytic agent. Am. J. Obstet. Gynecol. 151:181–184, 1985.

Ferguson, J. E., Dyson, D. G., Holbrook, K. H., et al.: Cardiovascular and metabolic effects associated with nifedipine and ritodrine tocolysis. Am. J. Obstet. Gynecol. 161:788, 1989.

Ferguson, J. E., Dyson, D. C., Schutz, B. A., and Stevenson, D. K.: A comparison of tocolysis with nifedipine or ritodrine: Analysis of efficacy & maternal, fetal and neonatal outcome. Am. J. Obstet. Gynecol. 163:105, 1990.

Garite, T. J., Keegan, K. A., Freeman, R. K., et al.: A randomized trial of ritodrine tocolysis versus expectant management in patients with premature rupture of the membranes at 25 to 30 weeks of gestation. Am. J. Obstet. Gynecol. 157:388, 1987.

Goldenberg, R. L., Davis, K. O., Copper, K. L., et al.: The Alabama preterm birth prevention project. Obstet. Gynecol. 75:933, 1990.

Gonik, B., and Creasy, R. K.: Preterm labor: Its diagnosis and management. Am. J. Obstet. Gynecol. 154:3, 1986.

Hadders-Algra, M., Touwen, B. C. L., and Huisjes, H. J.: Long-term follow-up of children prenatally exposed to ritodrine. Br. J. Obstet. Gynaecol. 93:156, 1986.

Herron, M. A., Katz, M., and Creasy, R. K.: Evaluation of a preterm birth prevention program: Preliminary report. Obstet. Gynecol. 59:452–456, 1982.

Hollander, D. E., Nagey, D. A., and Pupkin, M. J.: Magnesium sulfate and ritodrine hydrochloride: A randomized comparison. Am. J. Obstet. Gynecol. 156:433, 1987.

Iams, J. C., Johnson, F. F., and O'Shaughnessy, R. W.: A prospective random trial of home uterine activity monitoring in pregnancies at increased risk of preterm labor, Part II. Am. J. Obstet. Gynecol. 159:595–603, 1988.

Kaminski, M., Goujard, J., and Rumeau-Rouquette, C.: Prediction of low birthweight and prematurity by a multiple regression analysis with maternal characteristics known since the beginning of pregnancy. Int. J. Epidemiol. 2:195–204, 1973.

Katz, M., Newman K.B., Gill V.J.: Assessment of uterine activity in ambulatory patients at high risk for preterm labor and delivery. Am. J. Obstet. Gynecol. 154:44–47, 1986.

Keirse, M., Rush, R., Anderson, A., et al.: Risk of pre-term delivery in patients with previous pre-term delivery and/or abortion. Br. J. Obstet. Gynaecol. 85:81–85, 1978.

King, J. F., Grand, A., Keirse, M. J. N., et al.: Beta-mimetics in preterm labour: An overview of the randomized controlled trials. Br. J. Obstet. Gynaecol. 95:211–222, 1988.

Kirshon, B., Moise, K. J., Jr., Wasserstrum, N., et al.: Influence of short-term indomethacin therapy on fetal urine output. Obstet. Gynecol. 72:51–53, 1988.

Kleinman, J. C., and Kessel, S. S.: Racial differences in low birth weight: Trends and risk factors. N. Engl. J. Med. 3:749–754, 1987.

Korenbrot, C. C., Aalto, L. H., and Laros, R. K., Jr.: The cost effectiveness of stopping preterm labor with beta-adrenergic treatment. N. Engl. J. Med. 310:691–696, 1984.

Lipsitz, P. H.: The clinical and biochemical effects of excess magnesium in the newborn. Pediatrics 47:501–505, 1971.

Main, D. M.: Epidemiology of preterm birth. Clin. Obstet. Gynecol. 31:521–532, 1988.

Main, D. M., and Gabbe, S. G.: Risk scoring for preterm labor: Where do we go from here? Am. J. Obstet. Gynecol. 157:789, 1987.

Main, D. M., Richardson, D. K., Hadley, C. B., et al.: Controlled trial of a preterm labor detection program: Efficacy and costs. Obstet. Gynecol. 74:873, 1989.

Main, D. M., Katz, M., Chiu, G., et al.: Intermittent weekly contraction monitoring to predict preterm labor in low-risk women: A blinded study. Obstet. Gynecol. 72:757–761, 1988.

McGregor, J. A., French, J. I., Reller, B., et al.: Adjunctive erythromycin treatment for idiopathic preterm labor: Results of a randomized double-blinded placebo-controlled trial. Am. J. Obstet. Gynecol. 154:198, 1986.

Meis, P. J., MacErnest, J., and Moore, M. L.: Causes of low birthweight births in public and private patients. Am. J. Obstet. Gynecol. 156:1165–1168, 1987.

Meyer, M. B., Jonas, B. S., and Toascia, J. A.: Perinatal events associated with maternal smoking during pregnancy. Am. J. Epidemiol. 103:464–476, 1976.

Moise, K. J., Jr., Huhta, J. C., Sharif, D. S., et al.: Indomethacin in the treatment of premature labor. N. Engl. J. Med. 319:327–331, 1988.

Morales, W. J., Angel, J. F., O'Brien, W. F., et al.: A randomized study of antibiotic therapy in idiopathic preterm labor. Obstet. Gynecol. 72:829, 1988.

Morales, W. J., Angel, J. F., O'Brien, W. F., et al.: Use of ampicillin and corticosteroids in premature rupture of the membranes: A randomized study. Obstet. Gynecol. 73:721, 1989.

Morrison, J. C., Martin, J. N., Martin, K. W., et al.: Prevention of preterm birth by ambulatory assessment of uterine activity: A randomized study. Am. J. Obstet. Gynecol. 156:536–543, 1987.

Murray, J. L., and Bernfield, M.: The differential effect of prenatal care on the incidence of low birth weight among blacks and whites in a prepaid health care plan. N. Engl. J. Med. 319:1385–1391, 1988.

Neibyl, J. R., and Withe, F. R.: Neonatal outcome after indomethacin treatment for premature labor. Am. J. Obstet. Gynecol. 155:747–749, 1986.

Newton, E. R., Dinsmoor, M. J., and Gibbs, R. S.: A randomized, blinded, placebo-controlled trial of antibiotics in idiopathic preterm labor. Obstet. Gynecol. 72:829, 1989.

Novy, M. T.: Effects of indomethacin on labor, fetal oxygenation, and fetal development in Rhesus monkeys. Adv. Prostaglandin Thromboxane Leukotriene Res. 4:285–289, 1978.

Nuchpuckdee, P., Brodsky, N., Porat, R., et al.: Ventricular septal thickness in neonates after in utero ritodrine exposure. J. Pediatr. 109:687–691, 1986.

Papiernik, E., Bouyer, J., Dreyfus, J., et al.: Prevention of preterm births: A perinatal study in Haguenau, France. Pediatrics 76:154, 1985.

Polowczyk, D., Tejani, N., Lauersen, N., et al.: Evaluation of seven- to nine-year-old children exposed to ritodrine in utero. Obstet. Gynecol. 64:485, 1984.

Read, M. W., and Wellby, D. E.: The use of a calcium channel blocker (nifedipine) to suppress preterm labour. Brit. J. Obstet. Gynaecol. 93:933, 1986.

Roveno, R., and Mazor, M.: Infection and preterm labor. Clin. Obstet. Gynecol. 31:443, 1988.

Shiono, P. H., and Klebanoff, M. A.: Ethnic differences in very preterm delivery. Am. J. Public Health 76:1317–1321, 1986a.

Shiono, P. H., Klebanoff, M. A., and Rhoads, G. G.: Smoking and drinking during pregnancy. J. Am. Med. Assoc. 255:82, 1986b.

Srensen, K. E., Brlum, K. G.: Fetal cardiac function in response to long-term maternal terbutaline treatment. Acta Obstet. Gynecol. Scand. 67(2):105–107, 1988.

US Department of Health and Human Services, Public Health Service: Vital Statistics of the United States, 1983, Vol. I (Natality). Hyattsville, Md., National Center for Health Statistics, 1988.

US Department of Health and Human Services. Report of the Secretary's Task Force on Black and Minority Health, Publication 0-487-637 (QL3). Vol 6 (Infant mortality and low birthweight). Hyattsville, Md.: National Center for Health Statistics, 1985.

Weiner, C. P., Renk, K., and Klugman, M.: The therapeutic efficacy and cost-effectiveness of aggressive tocolysis for premature labor associated with premature rupture of the membranes. Am. J. Obstet. Gynecol. 159:16–22, 1988.

Zuckerman, H., Shalev, E., Gilad, G., et al.: Further study of the inhibition of premature labor by indomethacin. J. Perinat. Med. 12:19, 1984.

ANESTHESIA AND ANALGESIA: ISSUES FOR THE FETUS AND NEWBORN

14

Robert H. Friesen

■ OBSTETRIC ANESTHESIA AND ANALGESIA

Obstetric anesthesia and analgesia is a unique and challenging field in which the goals of maternal safety and comfort during childbirth are shared with that of preserving the well-being of the fetus and newborn. Drugs and techniques administered to the mother may have direct or indirect effects on the baby. Current aspects of these issues are discussed in this chapter.

INTRAVENOUS ANALGESIA AND SEDATION

Most sedative and narcotic drugs cross the placenta readily, primarily by passive diffusion, and can cause dose-related neonatal depression. Barbiturates are rarely used for maternal sedation for this reason. Diazepam has minimal effects on the newborn when small doses are given to the mother. Among the narcotics, meperidine is associated with less neonatal depression than is morphine (Way et al., 1965) and remains the most commonly used parenteral narcotic in obstetrics. The timing of meperidine administration in relation to delivery of the newborn is important, with the greatest neonatal depression observed 2 to 3 hours after maternal intravenous injection (Kuhnert et al., 1979). Preterm newborns are more easily depressed by maternal sedatives and narcotics than are term newborns.

REGIONAL ANALGESIA AND ANESTHESIA

Regional analgesia and anesthesia with local anesthetics are widely used during labor and delivery. Such techniques provide the mother with excellent pain relief without sedation and exert minimal effects on the fetus and newborn. Several regional blocks can be employed, including lumbar epidural, subarachnoid (spinal), caudal epidural, pudendal, and paracervical. Recently, epidural narcotic analgesia has been introduced for labor and delivery. When these techniques are used, important issues that affect the status of the fetus and newborn must be considered.

Maternal Hypotension. Sympathetic blockade with accompanying maternal hypotension and decreased uteroplacental blood flow is the most common undesired side effect of lumbar epidural and subarachnoid anesthesia. Maternal hypotension can usually be prevented by prior intravenous administration of 15 to 20 ml/kg of dextrose-free balanced salt solution and, for epidural block, incremental injection of local anesthetic solutions at a rate not exceeding 5 ml/30 seconds (Shnider and Levinson, 1986). Aortocaval compression by the gravid uterus causes supine maternal hypotension and reduces uterine arterial and venous blood flow (Kerr et al., 1964; Bieniarz et al., 1968), so the mother should be kept in the lateral position, or left uterine displacement (usually by means of a wedge under the right hip) should be employed. If hypotension develops, the mother should receive oxygen and be placed in a slight Trendelenburg position. Ephedrine, 5 to 15 mg administered intravenously, is the drug of choice for treatment of persistent maternal hypotension. Drugs that are direct alpha-adrenergic agonists, such as phenylephrine and epinephrine, should not be used to treat maternal hypotension because they cause uterine vasoconstriction and reduction in uteroplacental blood flow. Treatment of maternal hypotension is summarized in Table 14–1.

Effects of Local Anesthetics on the Newborn. When used for uncomplicated epidural anesthesia for labor and delivery, lidocaine, bupivacaine, and chloroprocaine do not exert adverse effects on neonatal Apgar scores or acid-base status (Abboud et al., 1982; Abboud et al., 1983). Lidocaine has been associated with neurobehavioral impairment of the newborn (Kuhnert et al., 1984; Scanlon et al., 1974), but those effects were subtle and have not been consistently observed (Abboud et al., 1982; Abboud et al., 1983). Although baseline fetal heart rate and beat-to-beat variability of fetal heart rate are not affected, late deceleration patterns of fetal heart rate

TABLE 14–1. Treatment of Maternal Hypotension

1. Administer 15 to 20 ml/kg balanced salt solution IV
2. Left uterine displacement for aortocaval decompression
3. Administer oxygen by face mask
4. Place patient in slight Trendelenburg position
5. Administer ephedrine 5–15 mg IV

appear to be more common during epidural anesthesia with bupivacaine (Abboud et al., 1982).

In the event of accidental maternal vascular injection, all local anesthetics can cause central nervous system depression and seizures. Amide local anesthetics cause myocardial depression, with bupivacaine being more cardiotoxic than lidocaine (Clarkson and Hondeghem, 1985). Fetal plasma levels of local anesthetics are directly related to maternal plasma levels.

Paracervical Block. This block, which provides analgesia during the first stage of labor, is associated with fetal anesthetic toxicity, manifested by a high incidence of bradycardia and acidosis. When fetal bradycardia occurs a few minutes after administration of the block, fetal blood levels of local anesthetic are high and are significantly greater than maternal levels (Asling et al., 1970). This implies rapid uptake of the local anesthetic by the uterine artery, located near the injection site. Duration of bradycardia is up to 15 minutes (Asling et al., 1970) and is probably limited by transfer of the local anesthetic across the placenta to the mother (Morishima, 1967). Neonatal depression can occur if the neonatal blood level is still elevated. If feasible, delay of delivery for 30 to 60 minutes following local anesthetic–related fetal bradycardia may reduce this risk (Morishima and Adamsons, 1967).

Similar fetal and neonatal depression can occur following accidental injection of local anesthetic into the fetal head, which can occur during attempted paracervical, pudendal, and caudal blocks.

Epidural Narcotics. Narcotics, usually 100 μg fentanyl, can be added to lumbar epidural local anesthetic blocks for enhanced analgesia during labor and cesarean section. Studies have not shown statistically significant fetal or neonatal effects attributable to this technique, but some suggest that subtle ventilatory depression of the newborn may occur (Cohen et al., 1987; Benlabed et al., 1988; Schlesinger and Miletich, 1988).

GENERAL ANESTHESIA

General anesthesia is often preferred for emergency cesarean section for fetal distress because the risk of maternal hypotension is less than during regional anesthesia. To minimize the effects of anesthetic drugs on the fetus, anesthesia is not induced until the patient is prepped and draped and the surgeon is ready to make the incision.

Thiopental is the usual choice for induction of anesthesia. It crosses the placenta readily but has minimal effect on the newborn if the mother's dose is less than 4 mg/kg (Kosaka et al., 1969). Muscle relaxants, employed to facilitate tracheal intubation and to relax abdominal muscles, do not cross the placenta and, thus, do not affect the baby. Narcotics are generally not administered until the umbilical cord is clamped.

Anesthetic concentrations of inhalation anesthetics can cause neonatal depression and uterine relaxation. However, subanesthetic concentrations of nitrous oxide and the potent inhalation anesthetics are not associated with such problems and can be safely administered to the mother during the few minutes after thiopental induction

prior to delivery of the baby (Shnider and Levinson, 1986).

Controlled ventilation is necessary to maintain adequate maternal oxygenation during general anesthesia for cesarean section. However, it is imperative to avoid hyperventilation of the mother before delivery of the baby. Hypocapnia decreases uterine and umbilical blood flow, increases the affinity of maternal hemoglobin for oxygen, and may be associated with fetal hypoxemia and acidosis (Levinson et al., 1974).

■ NEONATAL ANESTHESIA AND ANALGESIA

Neonatal anesthesia has progressed remarkably during the past 20 years. Great strides have been made in the development of monitoring devices, the understanding of neonatal physiology, and the medical and surgical treatment of diseases of the newborn. The number of pediatric anesthesiologists has increased 10-fold, and anesthesia for the newborn is notably safer now. The issues discussed in this chapter are of current interest to the specialty.

RESPONSE TO PAIN

Provision of adequate anesthesia and analgesia to the newborn has been hampered by long-held misconceptions regarding the newborn's neurophysiologic maturity and by a paucity of studies documenting the newborn's response to pain. Although the newborn does display functional immaturity of several organ systems, including the neurologic system, there is no question that he perceives and reacts appropriately to pain, even at 26 weeks of conceptual age (Dargassies, 1977). Acceptance of this fact and confidence in our ability to safely prevent pain have been slow to develop. However, the newborn's response to pain and the consequences of that response are better documented now than they were during the early years of neonatal anesthesia (Anand and Hickey, 1987a; Porter, 1989).

Major Surgery. It has become increasingly evident that the paralyzed, but inadequately anesthetized, newborn displays a marked stress response to major surgical procedures, measurable by cardiovascular, hormonal, and metabolic parameters. Yaster (1987) studied newborns undergoing major surgical operations. Those patients who were inadequately anesthetized (<10 μg/kg fentanyl) responded to surgical stimuli with significant increases in heart rate and systolic blood pressure.

Anand and colleagues (1987b) followed the intraoperative and postoperative hormonal and metabolic responses of two groups of preterm newborns undergoing ligation of patent ductus arteriosus. One group was lightly anesthetized with 50 per cent nitrous oxide and immobilized with a muscle relaxant. This group displayed a major stress response to surgery (Fig. 14–1), characterized by significant elevations of plasma levels of catecholamines, corticosteroids, and glucagon. Metabolically, this group exhibited a marked and sustained hyperglycemia and an intraoperative rise and postoperative fall in blood levels of gluconeogenic substrates. A catabolic response, as indicated by a rise in the urinary 3-methylhistidine/creatinine

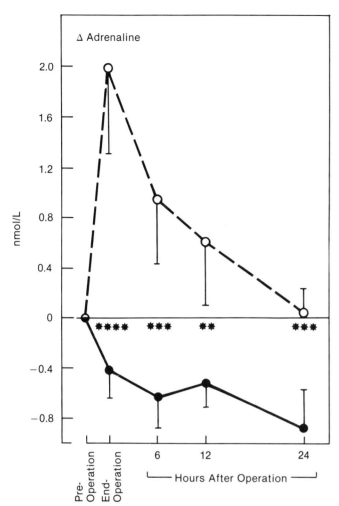

FIGURE 14–1. *The stress response of the inadequately anesthetized preterm newborn during major surgery can be prevented by general anesthesia with fentanyl. (○, 50% N_2O; ●, 50% N_2O + 10 μg/kg fentanyl; all asterisks, statistically significant differences.) (Reprinted with permission from Anand, K.J.S., Sippell, W.G., and Aynsley-Green, A.: Randomised trial of fentanyl anaesthesia in preterm babies undergoing surgery: Effects on the stress response. Lancet 1:243–248, 1987.)*

ratio, was evident on the 2nd and 3rd postoperative days. Administration of intravenous fentanyl, 10 μg/kg, to a second group of similar patients prevented these changes and reduced the number of postoperative clinical complications.

Circumcision and Minor Procedures. The stress response of newborns undergoing minor surgical procedures during inadequate anesthesia can also be deleterious. Williamson and Williamson (1983) and Maxwell and associates (1987) studied two groups of awake newborns undergoing circumcision. The patients who were not provided analgesia displayed prolonged crying, increased heart rate and blood pressure, and decreased transcutaneous Po_2 or oxygen saturation. These changes were significantly less in similar groups of newborns who underwent dorsal penile nerve block with lidocaine prior to circumcision. Use of dorsal penile nerve block also attenuated the behavioral disruptions observed following circumcision without local anesthesia (Dixon et al., 1984).

Chest tube insertion and cutdown for vascular access, procedures performed in the neonatal intensive care unit

(NICU), must be assumed to trigger responses similar to those of circumcision. Accordingly, adequate intravenous or local analgesia should be used for such procedures. On the other hand, the unchecked use of analgesia or sedation for every noxious stimulus in the NICU is probably not warranted either; overdosage and oversedation are genuine hazards. In this regard, the topical application of local anesthetic cream (Soliman et al., 1988; Halperin et al., 1989) to the skin prior to arterial, venous, or lumbar puncture may prove to be a safe and effective means of providing analgesia without sedation.

Pulmonary Hypertension and Stress. Although the newborn's pulmonary vascular resistance falls at birth, it does not decrease to normal childhood levels during the neonatal period. Pulmonary hypertension and fluctuations in pulmonary vascular resistance occur in several diseases of the newborn. In patients with these diseases, a variety of noxious stimuli can cause abrupt increases in pulmonary vascular resistance and clinical deterioration. Chest physiotherapy and tracheal suctioning of preterm newborns with respiratory distress syndrome was associated with increased plasma catecholamines, a hormonal stress response that was diminished by sedation with phenobarbital (Greisen et al., 1985). Fentanyl, 25 μg/kg, was shown to significantly attenuate the increases in pulmonary artery pressure and pulmonary vascular resistance as well as other circulatory stress responses that accompanied tracheal suctioning in infants after repair of congenital heart defects (Hickey et al., 1985). A similar stabilizing effect on the pulmonary vasculature was achieved by continuing fentanyl anesthesia during the postoperative period in critically ill newborns with congenital diaphragmatic hernia (Vacanti et al., 1984). Thus, anesthetic doses of fentanyl significantly blunt the pulmonary hemodynamic response to stressful stimuli and may be beneficial in diseases in which pulmonary hypertension is a problem.

Tracheal Intubation and Intracranial Pressure. Although the perianesthetic period does not appear to be one of greater risk for the development of intracranial hemorrhage in preterm newborns (Strange et al., 1985; Friesen et al., 1987a), specific procedures associated with fluctuations of cerebral blood flow and intracranial pressure may occur during that time. One such procedure is tracheal intubation. In a study of preterm newborns requiring anesthesia for surgical operations, anterior fontanel pressure was observed to increase markedly during laryngoscopy and intubation in awake patients (Friesen et al., 1987b). Those patients exhibited a vigorous motor response, in the form of coughing and sustained forced expiratory effort, to intubation. In contrast, newborns who were paralyzed with pancuronium and anesthetized prior to laryngoscopy and intubation did not have significant changes in anterior fontanel pressure (Fig. 14–2). This situation is analogous to that of a study by Perlman and colleagues (1985) of preterm newborns with respiratory distress syndrome who required mechanical ventilation. Wide fluctuations in the velocity of cerebral blood flow, presumably due to fluctuations in intrathoracic pressure, were observed in newborns breathing out of synchrony with their ventilators. Muscle relaxation with pancuronium eliminated the fluctuations in the cerebral blood flow and

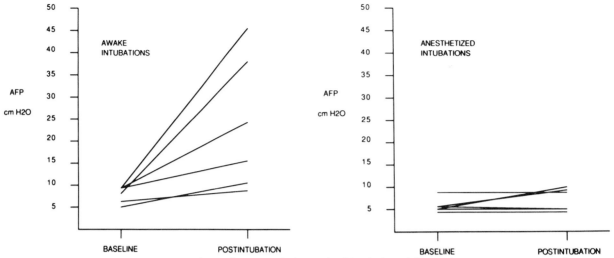

FIGURE 14-2. The marked increase in anterior fontanel pressure during tracheal intubation of the awake preterm neonate can be prevented by general anesthesia and muscle relaxation. (Reprinted with permission from the International Anesthesia Research Society from Friesen, R. H., Honda, A. T., and Thieme, R. E.: Changes in anterior fontanel pressure in preterm neonates during tracheal intubation. Anesth. Analg. 66:874–878, 1987.)

reduced the incidence and severity of intracranial hemorrhage.

These observations have led the author to recommend that, during anesthetic management of preterm newborns, tracheal intubation should be performed only after paralysis and anesthesia have been induced, unless a specific indication for intubation with the patient awake (such as in the case of a moribund or unstable patient, a gastric or small bowel obstruction, or a difficult airway) exists. A similar recommendation regarding intubation in the NICU or delivery room is probably not warranted at this time because patients in those settings usually require intubation during periods of clinical deterioration or resuscitation. However, neonatologists should be aware of the effects of tracheal intubation in the awake patient and should consider the use of pancuronium and mask ventilation prior to intubation in selected patients at greatest risk for intracranial hemorrhage.

ANESTHETICS AND ANALGESICS IN CURRENT USE

General Anesthetics. Early in the development of pediatric anesthesia, anesthetizing a preterm newborn was considered to be an uncommon emergency procedure entailing high risk. Hypovolemia, sepsis, respiratory failure, and cardiovascular immaturity frequently resulted in hypotension during anesthesia. Such problems, combined with the misconception that newborns did not sense pain well, created a setting in which anesthesiologists provided cardiovascular stability and immobility by using muscle relaxants and minimal or no anesthetic. Clinical research has since established that adequate anesthesia can be provided to preterm and term newborns without causing significant cardiovascular depression.

Nitrous oxide was, because of its cardiovascular stability, the most commonly used anesthetic in newborns for many years. However, it is a weak inhalation anesthetic that fails to prevent the stress response to surgery (Anand et al., 1987b). Furthermore, its use is contraindicated in many commonly encountered disease states of the newborn, including conditions requiring high amounts of oxygen, pneumothorax, pulmonary interstitial emphysema, necrotizing enterocolitis, and bowel obstruction or perforation. When this agent is not contraindicated, the role of nitrous oxide now is limited to supplementing other anesthetics.

Fentanyl, an intravenously administered synthetic narcotic, has been extensively studied as a neonatal anesthetic. A dose of 10 μg/kg in preterm newborns prevents the hemodynamic response to surgical stimuli for 75 minutes (Yaster, 1987) and, when added to 50 per cent nitrous oxide, blocks the hormonal and metabolic stress response to surgery (Anand et al., 1987b). Even at high doses of 30 to 50 μg/kg, fentanyl's cardiovascular effects are minimal (Robinson and Gregory, 1981). At anesthetic doses, fentanyl is a profound ventilatory depressant, and postoperative mechanical ventilation is required. Because it is slowly eliminated by the newborn (Collins et al., 1985; Koehntop et al., 1986), its effects are prolonged.

The concentration of an inhalation anesthetic required to prevent a motor response to painful stimulation in 50 per cent of subjects is known as its minimum alveolar concentration. The minimum alveolar concentration of halothane is reported to be 0.87 per cent in term newborns (Lerman et al., 1983) and 0.55 per cent in preterm newborns (Berry and Gregory, 1987), and that of isoflurane to be 1.6 per cent in term newborns (Cameron et al., 1984) and about 1.3 per cent in preterm newborns (LeDez and Lerman, 1987a). Cardiovascular depression can be a problem in newborns receiving these anesthetics. Even at concentrations at or below the minimum alveolar concentration, systolic blood pressure decreases by 25 to 30 per cent (Friesen and Henry, 1986; LeDez and Lerman, 1987a; Lerman et al., 1983). This sensitivity to the cardiovascular depressant effects of inhalation anesthetics is age related (Fig. 14–3) (Cook et al., 1981; Rao et al., 1986; Krane and Su, 1987) and is probably due to the immaturity of the neonatal myocardium, which has fewer contractile elements, immature sympathetic innervation, lower norepinephrine stores, and poorer compliance than the myocardium of the adult (Friedman, 1972). This cardiovascular depression can be minimized by the administration of atropine (Friesen and Lichtor, 1982) and

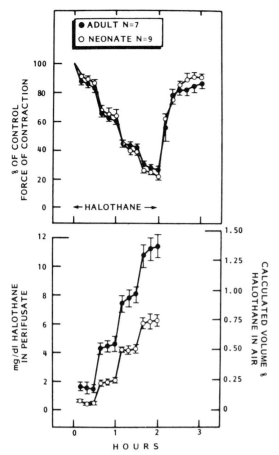

FIGURE 14–3. *The newborn mammal is far more sensitive to the myocardial depressant effects of inhalation anesthetics than is the mature mammal. In this study, the concentration of halothane (lower graph) required to depress atrial contractility (upper graph) in the newborn rat was only half that required in the adult. (Reprinted with permission from Rao, C. C., Boyer, M. S., Krishna, G., and Paradise, R. R.: Increased sensitivity of the isometric contraction of the neonatal isolated rat atria to halothane, isoflurane, and enflurane. Anesthesiology 64:13–18, 1986.)*

intravenous fluids or by using lower doses of halothane or isoflurane combined with a low dose of fentanyl. Inhalation anesthetics are eliminated rapidly and their effects are short lived after administration ceases.

The newborn's requirement for the intravenous anesthetic ketamine has not been extensively studied. An induction dose of 2 mg/kg is associated with cardiovascular stability (Friesen and Henry, 1986) and does not appear to raise intracranial pressure in preterm newborns (Friesen et al., 1987c) as it does in adults. Transient ventilatory depression follows ketamine administration.

Local Anesthetics. Traditional dose limitations for local infiltration and nerve blocks in children and adults are 4 mg/kg of lidocaine solution or, because of delayed absorption and slower rise in plasma concentration, 7 mg/kg of lidocaine mixed with epinephrine. Although specific dose recommendations for newborns are not available, greater caution is indicated during administration of local anesthetics. Newborns have low serum concentrations of alpha$_1$ acid glycoprotein, the plasma protein that binds local anesthetics (LeDez et al., 1986). The resulting increased free fraction of local anesthetics and their prolonged elimination by the newborn (LeDez et al., 1987b)

may place newborn patients at greater risk of local anesthetic toxicity. Nevertheless, dorsal penile nerve block for neonatal circumcision results in safe lidocaine plasma levels (Maxwell et al., 1987), and even conservative dosage guidelines allow satisfactory local anesthesia for vascular cutdown and chest tube insertion. Such uses should be encouraged. Topical cutaneous application of a eutectic mixture of prilocaine and lidocaine provides effective analgesia for venous cannulation and similar procedures in children (Soliman et al., 1988; Halperin et al., 1989), but it has not been evaluated in newborns.

Parenteral Analgesics. Intravenous fentanyl, 1 to 2 μg/kg, or morphine, 0.05 to 0.1 mg/kg, is a useful analgesic for pain that does not require general or local anesthesia. These medications can enjoy wide application in the neonatal intensive care unit. Narcotics have minimal direct cardiovascular effects, but they are potent ventilatory depressants and, like most drugs, have prolonged elimination phases in the newborn (Collins et al., 1985; Koehntop et al., 1986; Lynn and Slattery, 1987). Appropriate monitoring and vigilance for cumulative effects on ventilation and consciousness should be practiced. Usually, doses should not be repeated for several hours.

■ REFERENCES

Abboud, T. K., Khoo, S. S., Miller, F., et al.: Maternal, fetal, and neonatal responses after epidural anesthesia with bupivacaine, 2-chloroprocaine, or lidocaine. Anesth. Analg. 61:638–644, 1982.

Abboud, T. K., Kim, K. C., Noueihed, R., et al.: Epidural bupivacaine, chloroprocaine, or lidocaine for cesarean section—maternal and neonatal effects. Anesth. Analg. 62:914–919, 1983.

Anand, K. J. S., and Hickey, P. R.: Pain and its effects in the human neonate and fetus. N. Engl. J. Med. 317:1321–1329, 1987a.

Anand, K. J. S., Sippell, W. G., and Aynsley-Green, A.: Randomised trial of fentanyl anaesthesia in preterm babies undergoing surgery: Effects on the stress response. Lancet 1:243–248, 1987b.

Asling, J. H., Shnider, S. M., Margolis, A. J., et al.: Paracervical block anesthesia in obstetrics. II. Etiology of fetal bradycardia following paracervical block anesthesia. Am. J. Obstet. Gynecol. 107:626–634, 1970.

Benlabed, M., Midgal, M., Dreizzen, E., et al.: Neonatal pattern of breathing after cesarean section with or without epidural fentanyl. Anesthesiology 69:A651, 1988.

Berry, F. A., and Gregory, G. A.: Do premature infants require anesthesia for surgery? Anesthesiology 67:291–293, 1987.

Bieniarz, J., Crottogini, J. J., and Curuchet, E.: Aortocaval compression by the uterus in the late human pregnancy. II. An arteriographic study. Am. J. Obstet. Gynecol. 100:203–217, 1968.

Cameron, C. B., Robinson, S., and Gregory, G. A.: The minimum anesthetic concentration of isoflurane in children. Anesth Analg. 63:418–420, 1984.

Clarkson, C. W., and Hondeghem, L. M.: Mechanism for bupivacaine depression of cardiac conduction: Fast block of sodium channels during the action potential with slow recovery from block during diastole. Anesthesiology 62:396–405, 1985.

Cohen, S. E., Tan, S., Albright, G. A., and Halpern, J.: Epidural fentanyl/bupivacaine mixtures for obstetric analgesia. Anesthesiology 67:403–407, 1987.

Collins, C., Koren, G., Crean, P., et al.: Fentanyl pharmacokinetics and hemodynamic effects in preterm infants during ligation of patent ductus arteriosus. Anesth. Analg. 64:1078–1080, 1985.

Cook, D. R., Brandom, B. W., Shiu, G., and Wolfson, B.: The inspired median effective dose, brain concentration at anesthesia, and cardiovascular index for halothane in young rats. Anesth. Analg. 60:182–185, 1981.

Dargassies, S. S.: Neurological development in the full-term and premature neonate. Amsterdam, Excerpta Medica, 1977, pp. 248–256.

Dixon, S., Synder, J., Holve, R., and Bromberger, P.: Behavioral effects of circumcision with and without anesthesia. J. Dev. Behav. Pediatr. 5:246–250, 1984.

Friedman, W. F.: The intrinsic physiologic properties of the developing heart. Prog. Cardiovasc. Dis. 15:87–111, 1972.

Friesen, R. H., and Henry, D. B.: Cardiovascular changes in preterm neonates receiving isoflurane, halothane, fentanyl, and ketamine. Anesthesiology 64:238–242, 1986.

Friesen, R. H., Honda, A. T., and Thieme, R. E.: Perianesthetic intracranial hemorrhage in preterm neonates. Anesthesiology 67:814–816, 1987a.

Friesen, R. H., Honda, A. T., and Thieme, R. E.: Changes in anterior fontanel pressure in preterm neonates during tracheal intubation. Anesth. Analg. 66:874–878, 1987b.

Friesen, R. H., and Lichtor, J. L.: Cardiovascular depression during halothane anesthesia in infants: A study of three induction techniques. Anesth. Analg. 61:42–45, 1982.

Friesen, R. H., Thieme, R. E., Honda, A. T., and Morrison, J. E., Jr: Changes in anterior fontanel pressure in preterm neonates receiving isoflurane, halothane, fentanyl, or ketamine. Anesth. Analg. 66:431–434, 1987c.

Greisen, G., Frederiksen, P. S., Hertel, J., and Christensen, N. J.: Catecholamine response to chest physiotherapy and endotracheal suctioning in preterm infants. Acta Pediatr. Scand. 74:525–529, 1985.

Halperin D. L., Koren, G., Attias, D., et al.: Topical skin anesthesia for venous, subcutaneous drug reservoir and lumbar punctures in children. Pediatrics 84:281–284, 1989.

Hickey, P. R., Hansen, D. D., Wessel, D. L., et al.: Blunting of stress responses in the pulmonary circulation of infants by fentanyl. Anesth. Analg. 64:1137–1142, 1985.

Kerr, M. G., Scott, D. B., and Samuel, E.: Studies of the inferior vena cava in late pregnancy. Br. Med. J. 1:532–533, 1964.

Koehntop, D. E., Rodman, J. H., Brundage, D. M., et al.: Pharmacokinetics of fentanyl in neonates. Anesth. Analg. 65:227–232, 1986.

Kosaka, Y., Takahashi, T., and Mark, L. C.: Intravenous thiobarbiturate anesthesia for cesarean section. Anesthesiology 31:489–506, 1969.

Krane, E. J., and Su, J. Y.: Comparison of the effects of halothane on newborn and adult rabbit myocardium. Anesth. Analg. 66:1240–1244, 1987.

Kuhnert, B. R., Harrison, M. J., Linn, P. L., and Kuhnert, P. M.: Effects of maternal epidural anesthesia on neonatal behavior. Anesth. Analg. 63:301–308, 1984.

Kuhnert, B. R., Kuhnert, P. M., Tu, A. L., and Lin, D. C. K.: Meperidine and normeperidine levels following meperidine administration during labor. II. Fetus and neonate. Am. J. Obstet. Gynecol. 133:909–914, 1979.

LeDez, K. M., and Lerman, J.: The minimum alveolar concentration (MAC) of isoflurane in preterm neonates. Anesthesiology 67:301–307, 1987a.

LeDez, K. M., Strong, A., Reider, M., Burrows, F. A., and Lerman J.: Effect of age on the pharmacokinetics of intravenous lidocaine in pediatrics. Anesthesiology 67:A500, 1987b.

LeDez, K. M., Swartz, J., Strong, A., Burrows, F. A., and Lerman, J.: The effect of age on the serum concentration of alpha-1 acid glycoprotein in newborns, infants, and children. Anesthesiology 65:A421, 1986.

Lerman, J., Robinson, S., Willis, M. M., and Gregory, G. A.: Anesthetic requirements for halothane in young children 0–1 month and 1–6 months of age. Anesthesiology 59:421–424, 1983.

Levinson, G., Shnider, S. M., deLorimier, A. A., and Steffenson, J. L.: Effects of maternal hyperventilation on uterine blood flow and fetal oxygenation and acid-base status. Anesthesiology 40:340–347, 1974.

Lynn, A. M., and Slattery, J. T.: Morphine pharmacokinetics in early infancy. Anesthesiology 66:136–139, 1987.

Maxwell, L. G., Yaster, M., Wetzel, R. C., and Niebyl, J. R.: Penile nerve block for newborn circumcision. Obstet. Gynecol. 70:415–418, 1987.

Morishima, H. O., Adamsons, K.: Placental clearance of mepivacaine following administration to the guinea pig fetus. Anesthesiology 28:343–348, 1967.

Perlman, J. M., Goodman, S., Kreusser, K. L., and Volpe, J. J.: Reduction in intraventricular hemorrhage by elimination of fluctuating cerebral blood-flow velocity in preterm infants with respiratory distress syndrome. N. Engl. J. Med. 312:1353–1357, 1985.

Porter, F.: Pain in the newborn. Clin. Perinatol. 16:549–564, 1989.

Rao, C. C., Boyer, M. S., Krishna, G., and Paradise, R. R.: Increased sensitivity of the isometric contraction of the neonatal isolated rat atria to halothane, isoflurane, and enflurane. Anesthesiology 64:13–18, 1986.

Robinson, S., and Gregory, G. A.: Fentanyl-air-oxygen anesthesia for ligation of patent ductus arteriosus in preterm infants. Anesth. Analg. 60:331–334, 1981.

Scanlon, J. W., Brown, W. U., Weiss, J. B., and Alper, M. H.: Neurobehavioral responses of newborn infants after maternal epidural anesthesia. Anesthesiology 40:121–128, 1974.

Schlesinger, T. S., and Miletich, D. J.: Epidural fentanyl and lidocaine during cesarean section: Maternal efficacy and neonatal safety using impedance monitoring. Anesthesiology 69:A649, 1988.

Shnider, S. M., and Levinson, G.: Obstetric anesthesia. In Miller, R. D. (Ed): Anesthesia. 2nd ed. New York, Churchill Livingstone, 1986, pp. 1681–1728.

Soliman, I. E., Broadman, L. M., Hannallah, R. S., and McGill, W. A.: Comparison of the analgesic effects of EMLA (eutectic mixture of local anesthetics) to intradermal lidocaine infiltration prior to venous cannulation in unpremedicated children. Anesthesiology 68:804–806, 1988.

Strange, M. J., Myers, G., Kirklin, J. K., et al.: Surgical closure of patent ductus arteriosus does not increase the risk of intraventricular hemorrhage in the preterm infant. J. Pediatr. 107:602–604, 1985.

Vacanti, J. P., Crone, R. K., Murphy, J. D., et al.: The pulmonary hemodynamic response to perioperative anesthesia in the treatment of high-risk infants with congenital diaphragmatic hernia. J. Pediatr. Surg. 19:672–679, 1984.

Way, W. L., Costley, E. C., and Way, E. L.: Respiratory sensitivity of the newborn infant to meperidine and morphine. Clin. Pharmacol. Ther. 6:454–461, 1965.

Williamson, P. S., and Williamson, M. L.: Physiologic stress reduction by a local anesthetic during newborn circumcision. Pediatrics 71:36–40, 1983.

Yaster, M.: The dose response of fentanyl in neonatal anesthesia. Anesthesiology 66:433–435, 1987.

PART III

Mary Ellen Avery

GENETIC DISEASES

MECHANISMS OF 15
GENETIC DISEASE

Bruce R. Korf

The human genome encodes the information needed to build a complex organism from a single cell. This information, stored in the sequence of four bases in a total of 3×10^9 base pairs of DNA, provides instructions for the synthesis of approximately 100,000 different proteins in a precise temporal order. Moreover, the DNA sequence is faithfully reproduced each time a cell divides. The fidelity of human development is especially remarkable when viewed in these terms. Small variations in coding sequence or genome organization are usually tolerated, but when variations are larger or occur in critical regions, the program is disrupted and a genetic disorder may result.

■ ORGANIZATION OF THE HUMAN GENOME

Although the exact number of genes in the human genome is not known, it is estimated to be in the range of 50,000 to 100,000. These genes are arranged in linear order on molecules of DNA that, in turn, are packaged into 23 pairs of chromosomes. Each chromosome consists of a single DNA molecule encompassing tens of millions of base pairs and many thousands of genes. The arrangement of specific genes on a particular chromosome is identical in all people. Considerable progress has been made in the past 15 years in mapping the human genome (Fig. 15–1). At recent count, approximately 4000 to 5000 human genes have been identified, and over 1000 have been localized to a particular chromosome or chromosome segment (McKusick, 1988). What is known, however, is only a small segment of the total. A national commitment to mapping the human genome was launched in 1988.

Not all of the chromosomal DNA encodes genetic information. A proportion of the noncoding DNA consists of short sequences repeated thousands of times. These tend to be clustered near the centromeres of chromosomes and are believed to play a structural role. Other repeated sequences are interspersed among expressed genes; their role is unknown. Noncoding sequences also flank genes and serve to regulate their expression. Finally, the coding

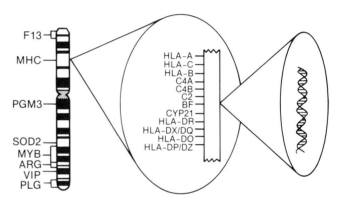

FIGURE 15–1. Map of human chromosome number 6. The entire chromosome is shown at the left, with the location of a number of genetic loci indicated. A close-up map of the major histocompatibility complex (MHC), which consists of many separate genes, is shown at the center. Each gene is represented by a sequence along a single DNA molecule that runs the entire length of the chromosome (right).

regions of most genes are interrupted by noncoding regions of unknown function (these are called introns, see later).

In addition, not all cellular DNA resides in the nucleus. Each mitochondrion contains multiple copies of a circular double-stranded DNA molecule. This DNA encodes a set of ribosomal and transfer RNAs, as well as 13 mitochondrial polypeptides important for oxidative phophorylation, although most are encoded by nuclear DNA. Several human genetic disorders are now known to be the result of mutations in mitochondrial DNA (Wallace, 1986). These tend to be transmitted by maternal inheritance (Egger and Wilson, 1983).

GENE STRUCTURE AND REGULATION

The usual flow of genetic information is from DNA to RNA to protein (Fig. 15–2). The process whereby this occurs was elucidated in the 1950s and 1960s and is the centerpiece of our understanding of genetics and cell biology (see Alberts et al., 1983 and Darnell et al., 1986

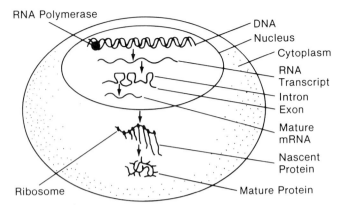

FIGURE 15–2. *Flow of genetic information from DNA through protein. DNA is transcribed into RNA in the nucleus, catalyzed by RNA polymerase. Introns are spliced out of the RNA and the mature mRNA is transported to the cytoplasm. Ribosomes bind to the mRNA, and the message is translated into protein. The mature protein is complexed with molecules such as sugars and is then transported to its destination within the cell or exported out.*

for complete description). It has subsequently been learned that genetic information can also flow from RNA to DNA, mainly as part of the life cycle of certain RNA-containing viruses, but no major role for such a process has yet been identified in normal cell physiology.

The amino-acid sequence of a protein is encoded in the base sequence of one of the two strands of the DNA double helix. Each amino acid is represented by a triplet of bases, so that the amino acid sequence of a protein is "read" from one end of a gene to the other. The specific amino acid represented by a given base triplet is the same in most forms of life. The process of copying the base sequence of DNA into RNA is called transcription, and it is catalyzed by enzymes called RNA polymerases. The ultimate product is a strand of messenger RNA (mRNA) whose sequence is the same as the coding strand of DNA. After processing in the nucleus, mRNA is transported to the cytoplasm where it is translated into protein on the ribosome. The protein molecules are then processed by enzymes that add molecules such as sugars, and the molecules are finally transported to their ultimate destinations within the cell or exported out.

The DNA comprising most genes includes more bases than are required to encode the amino acids of the corresponding protein products. These extra bases are accounted for by segments of DNA that do not encode protein, interspersed between blocks of coding DNA within a gene. The noncoding regions are referred to as introns, and the coding sequences as exons. During transcription, the entire gene, including both introns and exons, is transcribed into RNA. The large RNA molecule is then processed within the nucleus so that the introns are clipped out and the exons spliced together to form a mature mRNA. Most eukaryotic genes have introns. The number of introns in a gene, their location within the gene, and their base sequence tend to be the same in all individuals. Some genes have dozens of introns, in which case a primary transcript many thousands of base pairs long may be processed to an mRNA of a thousand or fewer nucleotides. The function of introns that justifies this apparent waste is unknown.

The regulation of gene expression is not fully under-

stood, but some details are beginning to fall into place. RNA polymerase binds at a site referred to as a promoter, which is a specific base sequence located just prior to the region where transcription begins. Other base sequences located upstream from this site are involved in allowing the polymerase to bind and initiating transcription. These sequences bind specific protein molecules that activate the transcription of specific genes. The regulation of gene expression thus involves an interplay of proteins, themselves the products of genes, with specific base sequences situated adjacent to genes.

■ GENETIC DISORDERS

The intricate structure and complex function of the genome render it susceptible to disruption. Such disruptions can range from the loss or gain of entire chromosomes to the change of a single base pair within a gene. The consequences vary likewise. Some alterations of the genome are incompatible with survival in utero, and they lead to miscarriage. Others produce specific and distinct clinical syndromes, and still others have no detectable clinical impact. Recent advances in molecular genetics have produced an explosive increase in our knowledge about the molecular basis of human genetic disorders, and have provided sensitive means of diagnosis (Orkin, 1986; White and Caskey, 1988).

ALTERATIONS OF CHROMOSOME STRUCTURE

The loss or gain of entire chromosomes or large chromosome segments typically has profound effects. Specific clinical syndromes are described in the chapter on chromosomal abnormalities. Most gross chromosomal abnormalities are lethal, either early in development or early in the postnatal period. Exactly why this is so is not known. Proteins encoded by genes in duplicated or deleted segments have in some cases been shown to be produced in proportion to the number of gene copies present. The presence of aberrant quantities of specific proteins in a cell apparently disrupts a finely balanced process of regulation and development.

SINGLE GENE MUTATIONS

Long before DNA was recognized as the genetic material, it was known that some human disorders are transmitted from generation to generation in accordance with the laws of Mendel. Three major modes of genetic transmission are observed. In autosomal dominant transmission, a trait is passed from generation to generation and can be given to both sons and daughters by either parent. Only a single copy of the gene needs to be altered to produce the full phenotype of the disorder. Autosomal recessive traits tend to occur within sibships, the parents being unaffected carriers. Both gene copies must be altered in offspring for the disorder to become manifest. Sex-linked traits are transmitted with a sex chromosome (generally the X). The hallmark of X-linkage is lack of transmission from a father to his sons, since the sons do not receive an X from their father.

Even before the era of molecular genetics, some insights

had been gained into the biochemical basis of mendelian inheritance. Recessively transmitted disorders, first recognized by Sir Archibald Garrod in the first decade of this century, are usually due to deficiencies of specific enzymes. Phenylketonuria, for example, involves the accumulation of phenylalanine due to deficiency of the enzyme that is required for its metabolism, phenylalanine hydroxylase. Since even small amounts of functional enzyme are sufficient to carry out most reactions, individuals with a single copy of an impaired gene are generally asymptomatic. If two such individuals have children together, and a child receives the abnormal gene copy from each parent, no functional enzyme may be made and a clinical problem may result.

The first human genetic disorder to be understood at the molecular level was sickle cell anemia. Linus Pauling (1949) suggested that this disorder might be due to a change in the structure of hemoglobin, and it was subsequently demonstrated that sickle cells differ from normal cells by a single amino-acid substitution in the beta-globin chain. Subsequently, this exchange of valine for glutamic acid was traced to a single base-pair change in the beta-globin gene, resulting in a change of coding sequence.

As knowledge of the structure of specific genes has accumulated, a variety of genetic changes, or mutations, has been discovered (Fig. 15–3). The simplest are single base-pair changes that occur within exons and change the amino acid inserted into a particular site of a protein. The consequences of amino-acid substitution depend on the chemical properties of the substituted amino acid and the region of the protein involved in the substitution. Changes involving amino acids with different properties, such as charged versus uncharged, occurring at sites with critical functions, tend to have the greatest impact. On the other hand, substitutions involving similar types of amino acids, or involving regions of the protein with a less critical role, may result in no detectable change of protein function.

Single base-pair changes can result in changes of the level of expression of a protein rather than of its functional properties. This may occur by a number of mechanisms (Orkin, 1987). For example, three sets of base triplets encode instructions to end translation of an mRNA rather than to insert an amino acid into a protein. A mutation that changes a normal amino acid code to such a stop code causes translation to terminate prematurely, resulting in a truncated, unstable protein. Base-pair changes at intron-exon boundaries can upset normal RNA processing, resulting in deficient production of mRNA. Finally, base-pair changes involving transcriptional regulatory sequences can lead to decreased levels of transcription.

Not all base-pair changes result in changes of a protein product. Since not all DNA encodes protein, mutations involving noncoding sequences may have no impact. It has been found that any two individuals differ at one base pair in every hundred, on average. Some of these differences involve gene products and account for phenotypic differences among people. Most involve noncoding DNA, however, and are of no apparent consequence.

In addition to base-pair changes, some mutations consist of deletions of DNA. Such deletions may range from a single base pair to an entire chromosome region. Loss of a single base pair can have profound effects on protein structure. Since the genetic code involves triplets of bases,

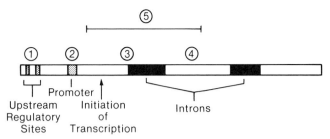

FIGURE 15–3. *Block diagram of a gene, indicating sites that may be disrupted by mutation. (1) Deletion or point mutation at upstream regulatory sites results in decreased transcription. (2) Mutation at promoter site results in decreased transcription. (3) Mutation at intron-exon boundary results in defective processing and decreased or abnormal protein product. (4) Point mutation within exon results in protein with abnormal structure or truncated size. (5) Deletion results in severely abnormal, truncated protein.*

the loss of a single base pair alters the "reading frame" of triplets and, therefore, completely changes the amino acids encoded after that point. Losses of blocks of DNA within genes may result in deletions of blocks of amino acids from proteins and, consequently, abnormal protein function (Koenig et al., 1987). Deletions involving regulatory sequences may lead to deficient transcription.

Large deletions may affect sets of closely linked genes. Deletions visible with the microscope must include over a million base pairs, comprising as many as 10 to 20 genes. Submicroscopic deletions may include smaller numbers of genes. The larger deletions typically result in multiple congenital anomaly syndromes, which are usually lethal. Smaller deletions may be exhibited as distinctive syndromes or as the simultaneous occurrence of two or more mendelian disorders in an individual (Schmickel, 1986).

MOLECULAR DIAGNOSIS OF HUMAN GENETIC DISORDERS

The use of recombinant DNA technology has led to great advances in the understanding of the structure of genes and the regulation of their expression. This technology allows fragments of human DNA to be inserted into bacterial cells. The bacterial colonies grown from these cells each contain a single piece of inserted human DNA, which can then be studied in detail. Until the advent of recombinant DNA technology, diagnosis of genetic disorders was based on clinical observation and testing of blood, urine, or tissues. As "cloned" DNA sequences corresponding to specific genes become available, diagnosis of genetic disorders can be based on direct analysis of the structure of a gene. This allows diagnosis to be done at any time in life, using readily available tissues such as white blood cells. It also enables prenatal diagnosis using fetal cells obtained from chorionic villus biopsy or amniocentesis as a source of DNA (see Chapter 6). A list of disorders that may be exhibited in the newborn period for which DNA diagnosis is now feasible is provided in Tables 15–1 and 15–2.

DNA may be analyzed for the presence of a mutation by a variety of means, the details of which are beyond the scope of this text (Caskey, 1987). In general, two approaches are used. First is direct study of the sequence of a gene in an individual. This is possible when the gene responsible for a disorder has been cloned and the types

TABLE 15–1. Diagnosis of Genetic Disorders by Direct Analysis of a Cloned Gene

DISORDER	TYPES OF MUTATIONS	REFERENCE
Duchenne and Becker muscular dystrophy	Deletions in dystrophin gene in over 65 per cent cases	Koenig et al., 1987
Sickle cell anemia	Point mutation in beta-globin gene	Orkin, 1987
Thalassemia	Deletion or point mutation in alpha- or beta-globin genes	Orkin, 1987
Hemophilia A	Deletion or point mutation in factor VIII gene	Pecorara et al., 1987
Hemophilia B	Deletion or point mutation in factor IX gene	Poon et al., 1987
Alpha$_1$-antitrypsin deficiency	Point mutation in alpha$_1$-antitrypsin gene	Hejtmancik et al., 1986
Ornithine transcarbamylase deficiency	Deletion or point mutation of OTC gene	Rozen et al., 1985
Lesch-Nyhan syndrome	Deletion or point mutation in hypoxanthine guanine phosphoribosyl transferase gene	Wilson et al., 1983
21-hydroxylase deficiency	Deletion or point mutation of 21-hydroxylase gene	White et al., 1987

of mutations commonly responsible for disorders involving that gene are known. Testing for a particular mutation affords accurate and rapid diagnosis.

The list of cloned genes associated with genetic disorders is growing rapidly (see Table 15–1), but genes responsible for most genetic disorders remain unknown. DNA studies can be helpful in the diagnosis of some of these disorders, however, using the principle of genetic linkage. This method relies on the use of cloned DNA segments that have been found to reside near a gene responsible for a disorder. Such marker genes can be used to track a chromosome carrying a disease gene through a family and to predict whether specific individuals in the family are likely to have inherited the disease gene or its normal counterpart. Such testing requires the study of many members of a family. The accuracy depends on the proximity of the marker genes to the disease gene locus. In spite of these limitations, however, diagnosis by linkage analysis is widely used in a variety of genetic disorders for which knowledge of the underlying molecular defect is not yet available (see Table 15–2).

Marker genes have also been used as starting points for "chromosome walking" toward a mutant gene. This affords a means of cloning a gene without prior knowledge of the gene product, a process referred to as "reverse

TABLE 15–2. Diagnosis of Disorders Using Genetic Linkage Analysis

DISORDER	CHROMOSOME LOCUS	REFERENCE
Neurofibromatosis 1	Long arm of 17	Collins et al., 1988
Myotonic dystrophy	Long arm of 19	Bartlett et al., 1987
Cystic fibrosis	Long arm of 7	Spence et al., 1987
Adult polycystic kidney disease	Short arm of 16	Breuning et al., 1987

genetics" (Orkin, 1986). So far, genes for Duchenne muscular dystrophy, chronic granulomatous disease, retinoblastoma, cystic fibrosis, and neurofibromatosis have been cloned by this means (Friend et al., 1986; Monaco et al., 1986; Rommens et al., 1989; Royer-Pakora et al., 1986; Viskochil et al., 1990; Wallace et al., 1990).

THERAPY OF GENETIC DISORDERS

Treatment of genetic disorders is usually based on the correction of symptoms through medication or surgery. For some metabolic disorders, symptoms can be ameliorated or avoided by dietary changes to reduce intake of substances that cannot be metabolized or to supply those that cannot be synthesized. The classic example is restriction of phenylalanine intake for children with phenylketonuria. Children that are so treated virtually escape the otherwise inevitable mental retardation that accompanies this disorder. Organ transplantation has also been undertaken to provide tissue able to carry out a deficient metabolic process. This has been attempted using bone marrow for children with mucopolysaccharidosis (Krivit and Whitley, 1987) and liver for urea cycle defects, tyrosinemia, and a number of other inborn errors of metabolism. Promising results have been achieved in several instances, particularly when the transplantation has been done early in life. Laboratory experiments are under way in an effort to insert functional genes into cells using recombinant DNA methods. The major challenges to be overcome are attaining physiologic levels of expression and targeting gene therapy to proper cells. This approach has not yet been used in clinical applications, but provides long-range hope for treatment of a wide range of inherited disorders (Ledley, 1987; Valle, 1987).

■ REFERENCES

Alberts, B., Bray, D., Lewis, J., et al.: The Molecular Biology of the Cell. New York, Garland Publishing, Inc., 1983.

Bartlett, R. J., Pericak-Vance, M. A., Yamaoka, L., et al.: A new probe for the diagnosis of myotonic dystrophy. Science 235:1648–1650, 1987.

Breuning, M. H., Reeders, S. T., Brunner, H., et al.: Improved early diagnosis of adult polycystic kidney disease with flanking DNA markers. Lancet 2:1359–1361, 1987.

Caskey, C. T.: Disease diagnosis by recombinant DNA methods. Science 326:1223–1229, 1987.

Collins, F. S., Ponder, B. A., Seizinager, B. R., and Epstein, C. J.: Invited editorial: The von Recklinghausen neurofibromatosis region on chromosome 17—Genetic and physical maps come into focus. Am. J. Hum. Genet. 44:1–5, 1988.

Darnell, J., Lodish, H., and Baltimore, D.: Molecular Cell Biology. New York, Scientific American Books, 1986.

Egger, J., and Wilson, J.: Mitochondrial inheritance in a mitochondrially mediated disease. N. Engl. J. Med. 309:142, 1983.

Friend, S. H., Bernards, R., Rogelj, S., et al.: A human DNA segment with properties of the gene that predisposes to retinoblastoma and osteosarcoma. Nature 323:643–646, 1986.

Hejtmancik, J. F., Sifers, R. N., Ward, P. A., et al.: Prenatal diagnosis of alpha-1-antitrypsin deficiency by restriction fragment length polymorphisms, and comparison with oligonucleotide probe analysis. Lancet 2:767–769, 1986.

Hoffman, E. P., Fischbeck, K. H., Brown, R. H., et al.: Characterization of dystrophin in muscle-biopsy specimens from patients with Duchenne's or Becker's muscular dystrophy. N. Engl. J. Med. 318:1363, 1988.

Koenig, M., Hoffman, E. P., Bertelson, C. J., et al.: Complete cloning of the Duchenne muscular dystrophy (DMD) cDNA and preliminary genomic organization of the DMD gene in normal and affected individuals. Cell 50:509–517, 1987.

Krivit, W., and Whitley, C. B.: Bone marrow transplantation for genetic diseases. N. Engl. J. Med. 316:1050, 1987.

Ledley, F. D.: Somatic gene therapy for human disease: Background and prospects. J. Pediatr. 110:1–8, 1987.

McKusick, V. A.: The morbid anatomy of the human genome. I. General considerations. Medicine 65:1–33, 1986.

McKusick, V. A.: The morbid anatomy of the human genome. II. Chromosome 1 to 12. Medicine 66:1–63, 1987.

McKusick, V. A.: The morbid anatomy of the human genome. III. Chromosome 13 to X, inclusive. Medicine 66:237–296, 1987.

McKusick, V. A.: The morbid anatomy of the human genome. IV. Applications and the future. Medicine 67:1–19, 1988.

McKusick, V. A.: Mendelian Inheritance in Man. Baltimore, The Johns Hopkins University Press, 1988.

Monaco, A. P., Neve, R. L., Colletti-Feener, C., et al.: Isolation of candidate cDNAs for portions of the Duchenne muscular dystrophy gene. Nature 323:646–650, 1986.

Orkin, S. H.: Reverse genetics and human disease. Cell 47:845–850, 1986.

Orkin, S. H.: Disorders of hemoglobin synthesis: The thalassemias. In Stamatoyannopoulos, G., Nienhuis, A. W., Leder, P., and Majerus, P. W. (Eds.): The Molecular Basis of Blood Diseases. Philadelphia, W. B. Saunders Company, 1987, pp. 106–126.

Pauling, L., Itano, H. A., Singer, S. J., and Wells, I. C.: Sickle cell anemia: A molecular disease. Science 110:543, 1949.

Pecorara, M., Casarino, L., Mori, P. G., et al.: Hemophilia A: Carrier detection and prenatal diagnosis by DNA analysis. Blood 70:531–535, 1987.

Poon, M.-C., Chui, D. H. K., Patterson, M., et al.: Hemophilia B (Christmas disease) variants and carrier detection analyzed by DNA probes. J. Clin. Invest. 79:1204–1209, 1987.

Rommens, J. M., Iannuzzi, M. C., Kerem, B. S., et al.: Identification of the cystic fibrosis gene: chromosome walking and jumping. Science 245:1059–1065, 1989.

Royer-Pakora, B., Kunkel, L. M., Monaco, A. P., et al.: Cloning the gene for an inherited disorder—chronic granulomatous disease—on the basis of its chromosomal location. Nature 322:32–38, 1986.

Rozen, R., Fox, J., Fenton, W. A., et al.: Gene deletion and restriction fragment length polymorphisms at the human ornithine transcarbamylase locus. Nature 313:815–817, 1985.

Schmickel, R. D.: Contiguous gene syndromes: A component of recognizable syndromes. J. Pediatr. 109:231–241, 1986.

Spence, J. E., Buffone, G. J., Rosenbloom, C. L., et al.: Prenatal diagnosis of cystic fibrosis using linked DNA markers and microvillar intestinal enzyme analysis. Hum. Genet. 76:5–10, 1987.

Valle, D.: Genetic disease: An overview of current therapy. Hosp. Pract. 22:167–182, 1987.

Viskochil, D., Buchberg, A. M., Xu, G., et al.: Deletions and a translocation interrupt a cloned gene at the neurofibromatosis type 1 locus. Cell 62:187–192, 1990.

Wallace, D. C.: Mitochondrial genes and disease. Hosp. Pract. 21:77–92, 1986.

Wallace, M. R., Marchuk, D. A., Andersen, L. B., et al.: Type 1 neurofibromatosis gene: Identification of a large transcript disrupted in three NF1 patients. Science 249:181–186, 1990.

White, R., and Caskey, C. T.: The human as an experimental system in molecular genetics. Science 240:1483–1488, 1988.

White, P. C., New, M. I., and Dupont, B.: Congenital adrenal hyperplasia. N. Engl. J. Med. 316:1580–1596, 1987.

Wilson, J. M., Young, A. B., and Kelley, W. N.: Hypoxanthine-guanine phosphoribosyltransferase deficiency: Molecular basis of the clinical syndromes. N. Engl. J. Med. 309:900–910, 1983.

CHROMOSOMAL ABNORMALITIES 16

Bruce R. Korf

The advent in 1956 of simple and reliable means of visualizing human chromosomes opened an era of rapid discovery of clinical disorders due to chromosomal abnormalities. The first of these was Down syndrome (trisomy 21), although it is sobering to note that in 1932 Waardenburg suggested that the disorder then known as mongolism might be due to a chromosomal aberration. Waardenburg's prophecy was based on the stereotyped complex of features that constitute this syndrome; the tendency for chromosomal abnormalities to result in consistent patterns of multiple malformations remains the hallmark of this class of disorders.

■ THE HUMAN KARYOTYPE

The normal human karyotype consists of 46 chromosomes, including 22 pairs of autosomes and two sex chromosomes, either two X's or an X and a Y. During the formation of germ cells the homologous chromosomes pair and then separate so that each spermatocyte or oocyte receives one member of each pair. In this process of meiosis the homologues exchange segments, allowing for genetic recombination. The diploid number of 46 is restored by fertilization.

A standard display of the human chromosome complement is shown in Figure 16–1. Each chromosome pair has a distinctive size, centromere position, and staining pattern. The designation of groups A, B, C, D, E, F, G, and sex chromosomes is a reference to the early days of cytogenetics prior to the development of chromosome banding methods. It is now routine to individually identify each chromosome by number, utilizing a standardized nomenclature to describe particular chromosome regions (ISCN, 1985).

METHODS OF STUDYING CHROMOSOMES

Each chromosome consists of a single DNA molecule comprising tens of millions of base pairs. The DNA is relatively extended in the nucleus in nondividing cells and becomes highly compacted during mitosis. This compaction is responsible for the characteristic size and shape of individual chromosomes. It is therefore necessary to study dividing cells in order to visualize individual chromosomes. Some tissues, for example, placenta or bone marrow, contain sufficient dividing cells for direct analysis, but in most cases it is necessary to culture cells to obtain an adequate number for analysis (Table 16–1).

CHROMOSOME BANDING AND SPECIAL STUDIES

The development of banding techniques in the late 1960s led to a second wave of discovery of new chromosomal syndromes (Yunis, 1977). These staining methods exploit characteristic regional differences in degree of compaction or chemical structure along the chromosome. Identification of each chromosome by banding is now standard practice in all cytogenetics laboratories. An array of special staining methods exists to help elucidate chromosomal abnormalities involving particular regions (Table 16–2). A standard chromosome preparation includes about 400 bands distributed on the 23 pairs of chromosomes. If cells are grown under specific conditions, chromosomes that are not fully compacted can be obtained, resulting in the appearance of many more, finer, bands. Such extended, or high-resolution, analysis permits the detection of more subtle chromosome rearrangements that might be missed on a 400-band analysis. A number of clinical syndromes have been identified with such rearrangements (see Table 16–3), and high-resolution studies are indicated when such syndromes are suspected.

■ CHROMOSOME ABNORMALITY SYNDROMES

EPIDEMIOLOGY

The vast majority of chromosomally abnormal conceptuses die before reaching term (Boue et al., 1973). Those that do survive represent the few whose genetic imbalance is minor enough to be compatible with life in utero. Many of these die immediately post term, or in early life. It is estimated that at least 15 per cent of recognized pregnancies end in miscarriage, and an unknown number of very early pregnancies end prior to implantation. Of the 15 per cent, at least half have a chromosomal anomaly. Thus, upwards of 10 per cent, and probably a higher proportion, of human conceptuses have a chromosomal abnormality. In contrast, the frequency of live-born infants with chromosomal anomalies is about 1 in 200 (Hook and Porter, 1977).

BASIC SCIENCE

The most easily recognized syndromes are those due to loss or gain of a single chromosome, referred to as aneuploidy. These include trisomies 8, 9, 13, 18, 21, XXX, XXY and XYY and monosomy X. They are believed

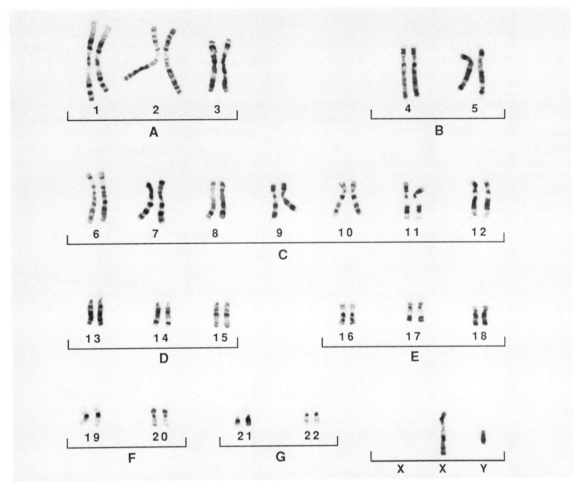

FIGURE 16–1. G-banded human male karyotype. The 46 chromosomes are arranged into 23 pairs, each with a specific banding pattern.

to arise from an error in chromosome separation during meiosis or mitosis, referred to as nondisjunction (Therman, 1986). Meiotic nondisjunction results in a germ cell with an extra or a missing chromosome, which on fertilization produces a monosomic or trisomic zygote. Mitotic nondisjunction results in two cell lines, one trisomic and one monosomic. The latter often dies off, leaving trisomic cells descended from the one in which nondisjunction occurred. If the event takes place after first cleavage, some normal cells will also exist, and the embryo is said to be mosaic.

In addition to the classic aneuploidy syndromes, there are innumerable examples of infants born with gains or losses of small chromosome regions. These may arise sporadically, owing to unknown mechanisms, or may occur as a result of a balanced translocation in a parent. Such a translocation involves the exchange of segments between two nonhomologous chromosomes. Little or no genetic material is gained or lost, so the carriers of a balanced rearrangement are usually phenotypically normal. Various combinations of the rearranged chromosomes may be transmitted to offspring, however, resulting in a high frequency of miscarriage and possibly the birth of a child with an unbalanced rearrangement (Ford and Clegg, 1969).

DOWN SYNDROME

Definition. Down syndrome is an association of congenital anomalies that includes a characteristic facies. Affected individuals usually have reduced intellectual capacity, although this is variable.

TABLE 16–1. Sources of Dividing Cells for Chromosomal Analysis

Chorionic villus	Direct analysis or culture for prenatal testing
Amniotic fluid	Cell culture for prenatal testing
Peripheral blood	Culture of phytohemagglutinin-stimulated lymphocytes; standard tissue for chromosomal analysis
Skin biopsy	Cell culture of fibroblasts; used to examine for mosaicism
Bone marrow	Direct analysis of dividing cells; rapid cytogenetic diagnosis but quality inferior to analysis of cultured lymphocytes

TABLE 16–2. Major Types of Chromosome Banding and Staining Methods

G-banding	Standard choice for banded chromosomal analysis
Q-banding	Fluorescent banding, pattern similar to G-banding
R-banding	Reverse banding, pattern opposite to G- and Q-banding
C-banding	Dark staining at the centromeres of chromosomes
NOR staining	Staining at nucleolus-organizer region of chromosomes 13, 14, 15, 21, 22
Distamycin/DAPI	Bright staining at centromeres of 1, 9, 15, 16, Y; often used to identify marker derived from 15

Epidemiology. Down syndrome is the most common trisomy compatible with live birth, with an incidence of approximately 1 in 700 to 1 in 1000. Infant mortality is high, so that the prevalence in the general population is 1 in 3000. The cause of this disorder is the presence of an extra copy of chromosome 21 material. The abnormality is sporadic (not familial) in most instances. In about 93 per cent of cases there is a complete extra copy of 21 in all cells, resulting from meiotic nondisjunction. In about 5 per cent the extra 21 results from translocation, in which one parent has a balanced translocation between 21 and some other chromosome, most commonly 14. Segregation of the translocation chromosome to the same cell with the normal 21 leads to trisomy if that germ cell fertilizes a normal cell. The remaining 3 per cent are mosaics, having various proportions of trisomy 21 and normal cells resulting from mitotic nondisjunction. This group may be of normal intelligence, depending on the number of trisomic cells present.

The risk of trisomy 21 due to meiotic nondisjunction increases sharply with maternal age, beginning in the mid-30s (Hook, 1981; Hassold and Chiu, 1985) (Fig. 16–2). Since most pregnancies occur in younger woman, however, the majority of children with Down syndrome are born to younger mothers. A weaker paternal age effect may exist, but data are not as clear.

Natural History. Most pediatricians are familiar with the phenotype of Down syndrome in the neonatal period (Fig. 16–3) (Warkany et al., 1966; Jackson et al., 1976; Preus, 1977; Bersu, 1980). There is an increased frequency of prematurity, and birth weight is usually somewhat decreased. Head circumference is likewise smaller than average. The head tends to be brachycephalic, the neck short, and the nuchal skin excessive. The face is usually rounded with a flat profile. The palpebral fissures slant upward and outward, and epicanthal folds are often present. The epicanthal folds and flat nasal bridge may give the appearance of hypertelorism, but interorbital distance is usually not increased. Small white spots, referred to as Brushfield spots, may be visible on the iris. Ears tend to be small and ear canals atretic. In older

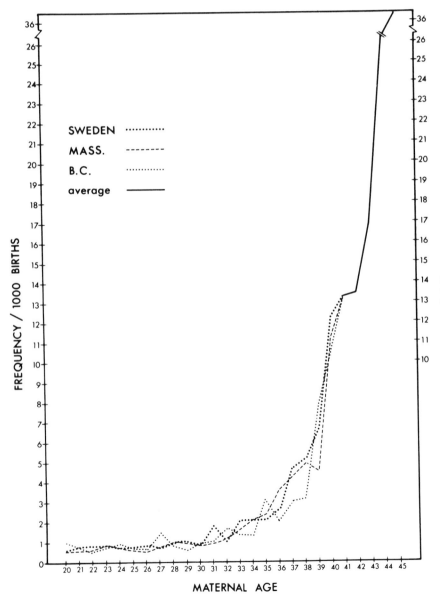

FIGURE 16–2. *Graph of frequency of Down syndrome as a function of maternal age. (Fraser, F. C., and Nora, J. J.: Genetics of Man, Philadelphia, Lea & Febiger, 1986, p. 35.)*

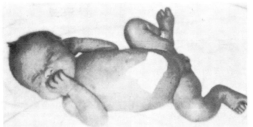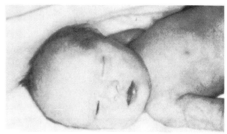

FIGURE 16–3. Newborn with Down syndrome (trisomy 21), illustrating some of the characteristic facial features, including up-slanting palpebral fissures and flat profile.

children the tongue is often protuberant, but this is less regularly the case in newborns. Hands are short, and there is often a single transverse palmar crease and incurved fifth finger (clinodactyly). Ulnar loop patterns predominate on the fingertips. Virtually all these babies are profoundly hypotonic. This may impair feeding and is sometimes the first indication that the baby has a problem. Polycythemia in the first days of life has been noted, as has transient congenital leukemoid reaction that resolves by age 5 months (Miller and Cosgriff, 1983; Lin et al., 1980).

Diagnosis. Although the clinical diagnosis of Down syndrome is often straightforward, cytogenetic studies should *always* be obtained. Even experienced geneticists have encountered infants in whom definitive diagnosis is difficult, and incorrect clinical diagnoses of Down syndrome have been made. Cytogenetic studies not only provide confirmation of the diagnosis but also distinguish simple trisomy, which has a low recurrence risk, from translocation, which may be familial.

Trisomy 21 is easily detected by cytogenetic analysis of amniotic fluid or chorionic villus cells, affording accurate prenatal diagnosis. This is typically offered to women aged 35 or older, in whom the risk of trisomy 21 exceeds the risk of complications of amniocentesis. Screening tests based on finding low maternal serum alpha-fetoprotein (DiMaio et al., 1987) or excessive nuchal skin in the fetus visualized by ultrasound (Benacerraf et al., 1987) are so far not sufficiently sensitive or specific to provide accurate population screening of all pregnancies.

Prognosis. The prognosis in the neonatal period is related to the occurrence of visceral malformations. The most common of these are congenital heart disease and gastrointestinal malformations. At least 40 per cent have congenital heart defects, of which the most characteristic are endocardial cushion defects, followed by ventricular or atrial septal defects (Park et al., 1977). These defects may cause congestive heart failure in the neonatal period. Gastrointestinal malformations include duodenal stenosis or atresia, esophageal atresia, anal atresia, and megacolon. Both the cardiac and the gastrointestinal problems are often amenable to surgical correction. Early recognition of these problems can greatly enhance survival of children with Down syndrome in the neonatal period. Similarly, children who present with cardiac or gastrointestinal malformations should be examined for the presence of other signs of Down syndrome.

Infants with Down syndrome who survive the neonatal period have an excellent prognosis for longer-term survival. Their height is usually two standard deviations below

that expected (Cronk et al., 1988). Most affected children walk between 2 and 4 years, while average age for speech is 4 to 6 years. Common childhood problems include frequent respiratory infections, especially serous otitis media. Secondary sexual development is normal, although males are infertile owing to interstitial fibrosis of the testes and hypoplasia of seminiferous tubules (Zellweger et al., 1987). There is a 10- to 30-fold increased risk of leukemia compared with the general population. Down syndrome adults may develop premature senility in middle age. Changes in the brain are very similar to those in Alzheimer disease. Some affected individuals live into their 50s (Robison et al., 1984).

Children with Down syndrome are almost always pleasant and lovable. They may be educable to higher levels than had been described at a time before early educational opportunities were made available to them.

Management. Congenital heart disease can usually be corrected surgically in the first weeks of life. Bowel obstruction likewise requires surgical relief. Primary hypothyroidism may coexist and requires thyroid replacement. Since the atlantoaxial joint is unstable in about 10 to 15 per cent of Down syndrome individuals, a screening lateral cervical radiograph has been recommended at about age 6 years before sports that could impose stress on the head are permitted (Peuschel et al., 1987). Davidson (1988) points out, however, that radiographs are not necessarily predictive, and in most cases, neurologic signs precede dislocations for weeks or even months.

Early-intervention programs for groups of children with Down syndrome have been helpful. Speech therapy and physical therapy may be indicated.

TRISOMY 18 (EDWARDS SYNDROME)

Definition. This syndrome is characterized by micrognathia, low-set ears, flexion deformity of fingers, and congenital heart disease. Trisomy 18 is second to trisomy 21 in frequency, occurring in about 1 in 3000 to 1 in 4000 live births. Most cases are associated with complete trisomy for chromosome 18. A minority of individuals are mosaics or have partial trisomy due to translocations.

Natural History. Most of these infants are small for gestational age, and many are born post term. Characteristic craniofacial features (Fig. 16–4) include a prominent occiput, small mouth and narrow palate, and low-set malformed ears (Warkany et al., 1966; Butler et al., 1965; Taylor, 1968; Hodes et al., 1978). There is usually a typical clenching of the hands, with the second finger overlapping the third and the fifth overlapping the fourth.

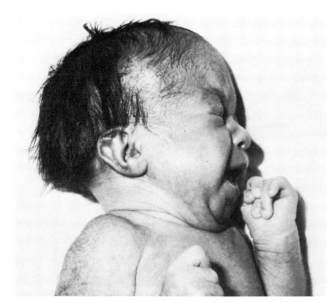

FIGURE 16—4. *Newborn with trisomy 18, with typical facial appearance and clenched hands.*

Fingernails are hypoplastic, and dermal ridges on the fingertips are mostly arches. Rocker-bottom feet are often present. Infants with many of these features, but normal chromosomes, have been described (Simpson and German, 1969). Some have the Pena-Shokeir I syndrome, which is inherited as an autosomal recessive trait (Muller and de Jong, 1986).

Virtually all infants with trisomy 18 have congenital heart disease, most typically ventricular septal defects and valve anomalies. Neurologic function in these infants is markedly abnormal. They suck poorly, are either hypotonic or hypertonic, and may have seizures.

Diagnosis. The clinical syndrome is strongly suggestive of the diagnosis, which should be confirmed by chromosomal analysis.

Prognosis. A large proportion of infants with trisomy 18 die in the immediate neonatal period, mostly as a result of cardiac disease. Some examples of prolonged survival have been reported, generally associated with mosaicism. Significant cognitive impairment occurs in most of these individuals.

Prevention. Prenatal diagnosis should be undertaken in subsequent pregnancies, since the risk of recurrence is 1 to 2 per cent.

TRISOMY 13 (PATAU SYNDROME)

Definition. Trisomy 13 results in a constellation of severe malformations. It is the least frequent of the live-born autosomal trisomies, occurring in about 1 in 10,000 live births. Most affected have simple trisomy, but some are mosaics or translocation trisomics.

Natural History. These babies tend to be of low birth weight, although not as dramatically so as for trisomy 18. Craniofacial features can be very abnormal (Fig. 16–5). These include microphthalmia, hypotelorism, cleft lip and

palate, low-set ears, and scalp skin defects near the vertex (Warkany et al., 1966; Taylor, 1968; Addor et al., 1975; Hodes et al., 1978). The cleft lip is usually bilateral and often lacks the premaxillary tissue below the nose. In some instances the eyes may be fused in a single orbit, or cyclopia may be present. These facial features suggest the occurrence of holoprosencephaly, which is commonly found in association with trisomy 13. Hands tend to be clenched, and there may be postaxial polydactyly. Rocker-bottom feet occur in this syndrome as well. Cardiac, renal, and gastrointestinal malformations are very commonly associated with trisomy 13.

A major point in the differential diagnosis of trisomy 13 is Meckel-Gruber syndrome. Infants affected with this autosomal recessive disorder also may have holoprosencephaly, postaxial polydactyly, and renal anomalies (Salonen, 1984). They often, but not always, have encephalocele. In the absence of a family history of Meckel-Gruber syndrome, chromosome studies are required to distinguish this disorder from trisomy 13.

Prognosis: As with trisomy 18, most infants with trisomy 13 die in the neonatal period. Surgical emergencies may necessitate operation to permit survival long enough

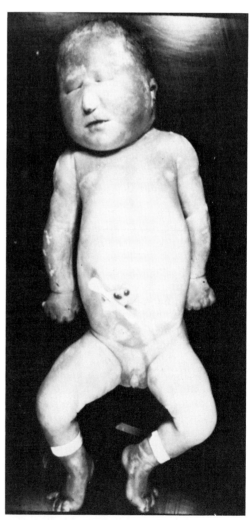

FIGURE 16—5. *Stillborn with trisomy 13. The facial appearance is that of cebocephaly, which is associated with holoprosencephaly. There is an extra digit on the ulnar border of the right hand.*

for the diagnosis to be confirmed. Those who survive, often chromosomal mosaics (Mankinen et al., 1976), generally have severe mental and physical developmental impairment.

Prevention. Prenatal examination of the karyotype of fetal cells should be done in subsequent pregnancies. The risk of recurrence is about 1 per cent.

SEX CHROMOSOME ANOMALIES

The sex chromosome abnormality most likely to come to attention in the newborn is Turner syndrome, associated with a 45, X karyotype (Coco and Bergada, 1977). These infants are often small for gestational age and have excessive nuchal skin. Many have lymphedema, especially in the dorsa of the hands and feet. Turner syndrome should be included in the differential diagnosis of nonimmune hydrops. Cardiac malformations, including coarctation of the aorta, are common, as are renal anomalies. Long-term problems include complications of congenital heart disease, short stature, and primary amenorrhea. Psychomotor development is quite variable, although some form of cognitive impairment, particularly visual-perceptual difficulty, is common (Bender et al., 1984). Cytogenetic investigations should include careful search for mosaic cell lines, including an abnormal Y chromosome, since individuals with a Y may have testicular tissue at risk for later development of gonadoblastoma.

TRIPLOIDY

Triploidy results from fertilization by two sperm, fusion of a polar body with a zygote, or fertilization involving a diploid sperm or egg. Most triploid fetuses result in hydatidiform moles without embryos and are aborted. Some live births of triploid infants do occur (Wertelecki et al., 1976). These newborns are usually small for gestational age, with large placentas having hydatidiform degeneration. There are often facial clefts and ocular anomalies. Males may have hypospadias and cryptorchidism, in some cases to the extent of ambiguous genitalia. Syndactyly of the third and fourth digits is characteristic. Most triploid infants die in the neonatal period, but longer survival with milder manifestations may occur, particularly for mosaics.

OTHER CHROMOSOMAL SYNDROMES

The loss or gain of an entire chromosome is usually lethal in utero. Only trisomies 8, 9, 13, 18, 21, X, and Y and monosomy X are occasionally found in live-born infants. Duplication or deficiency states for smaller chromosome regions are much more likely to be compatible with survival, at least to birth. Some are common enough to be associated with specific syndromes, such as cri-du-chat syndrome, which is due to deletion of the tip of the short arm of chromosome 5. For the most part, though, the clinical manifestations of these chromosomal anomalies are sufficiently rare and variable as to elude even experienced geneticists trying to make a clinical diagnosis. Moreover, the effects vary with the size of the deleted or duplicated region, and unbalanced translocation may result in the simultaneous deletion of one segment and duplication of another. Therefore, many children have unique syndromes reflecting their particular chromosomal abnormality.

Some of the better defined duplication and deficiency syndromes are described in Table 16–3. There are, in addition, a number of well-illustrated compendia of clinical syndromes associated with chromosomal anomalies (de Grouchy and Turleau, 1984; Schinzel, 1984). In spite of the difficulty, it is worth some effort to clinically identify a specific chromosomal syndrome. As the resolution of cytogenetic analysis increases, it becomes possible to identify small but significant losses or gains of chromosomal material. The probability of finding such an abnormality increases if a specific chromosomal region can be targeted for high-resolution analysis using clinical information.

Many of these chromosomal abnormalities are the result of familial balanced translocations segregating at meiosis to produce unbalanced gametes. Others appear to be sporadic events of deletion or duplication of chromosomal material. Cytogenetic studies should always be performed, if possible, on the parents of a child with a partial trisomy or deletion. The identification of a balanced translocation in a parent obviously has profound implications for recurrence risk. It also may reveal the origin of a small piece of translocated material in the child, which might otherwise elude identification.

■ INDICATIONS FOR CHROMOSOMAL ANALYSIS

The indications for chromosomal analysis in the newborn may therefore be summarized as follows: (1) infant

TABLE 16–3. Major Syndromes Resulting from Deletion or Trisomy of Chromosomes or Parts of Chromosomes*

3q trisomy	Hirsutism and synophrys resembling Cornelia de Lange syndrome
4p deletion	Wolf-Hirschhorn syndrome; microcephaly, broad nasal bridge, hypertelorism
5p deletion	Cri-du-chat syndrome; microcephaly, catlike cry, hypertelorism
8 trisomy	Osteoarticular anomalies, developmental delay; most often mosaic
8q deletion	Langer-Gideon syndrome (band q22–24); exostoses, bulbous nose, abnormal hair
9 trisomy	Microdolichocephaly, upslanting palpebral fissures
9p trisomy	Microbrachycephaly, bulbous nose
9p deletion	Trigoncephaly, upslanting palpebral fissures, short nose
11p deletion	Aniridia, Wilms' tumor, genitourinary anomalies (band p13)
12p trisomy	Hypotonia, flat facies; also tetrasomy 12p seen in some cases, with mosaicism confined to skin
13q deletion	Retinoblastoma (band q14); limb anomalies, genital anomalies, CNS malformations
15q deletion	Prader-Willi or Angelman syndrome (band q11)
17p deletion	Miller-Dieker syndrome (band p13); lissencephaly, characteristic facies
18p deletion	Characteristic facies, large ears
18q deletion	Midface hypoplasia, digital anomalies
21q deletion	Characteristic facial features
22q deletion	Cat-eye syndrome; coloboma, anal atresia, preauricular skin tags
Fragile-X	X-linked mental retardation, macro-orchidism; fragile site on X chromosome when cells grown in low-folate medium

*p = short arm; q = long arm.

with a recognizable chromosomal anomaly syndrome, and (2) presence of at least two "significant" congenital anomalies not diagnostic of a known nonchromosomal syndrome. "Significant" anomalies include major visceral or structural malformations, not including minor variants such as single transverse palmar crease. It is important to stress that cytogenetic studies should be performed on *all* infants suspected of having a chromosomal anomaly, even if the clinical diagnosis seems clear. As noted earlier, some mendelian disorders can be confused with trisomy syndromes. In such cases, a family may be falsely reassured in a subsequent pregnancy by a normal prenatal karyotype only to discover that a nonchromosomal disorder with a 25 per cent recurrence risk has affected another child. It is also important to perform cytogenetic studies on stillborn fetuses and abortuses, if possible. This can reveal anomalies that identify couples at risk for recurrence, which next time might be compatible with live birth.

Infants with multiple congenital anomalies are often medically unstable, and there may be considerable pressure to identify a specific chromosomal syndrome for prognostic purposes. It must be remembered, however, that there is a range of phenotypic consequences of chromosomal syndromes. Chromosomal studies are but a part of the evaluation of a critically ill malformed infant, and should be done as carefully as possible to detect both major trisomies and more subtle rearrangements. Decisions on appropriate medical interventions should be based on a thorough assessment of the type and number of malformations as well as the potential for survival and developmental outcome given these anomalies.

▪ REFERENCES

Addor, C., Cox, J. N., Cabrol, C., and Crippa, L.: Patau's syndrome: A pathological and cytogenetic study of two cases. I. Anatomicopathological aspects. J. Genet. Hum. 23:83, 1975.

Benacerraf, B. R., Gelman, R., and Frigoletto, F. D., Jr.: Sonographic identification of second-trimester fetuses with Down's syndrome. N. Engl. J. Med. 317:1371, 1987.

Bender, B., Puck, M., Salbenblatt, J., and Robinson, A.: Cognitive development of unselected girls with complete and partial X monosomy. Pediatrics 73:175, 1984.

Bersu, E. T.: Anatomical analysis of the developmental effects of aneuploidy in man: The Down syndrome. Am. J. Med. Genet. 5:399, 1980.

Boue, J., Boue, A., and Lazar, P.: The epidemiology of human spontaneous abortions with chromosomal anomalies. In Blandau, R. J. (ed.) Aging Gametes. Basel; A. Karger, 1973, pp. 330–348.

Butler, L. J., Snodgrass, G. J. A. I., France, N. E., et al.: E(16–18) trisomy syndrome: Analysis of 13 cases. Arch. Dis. Child. 40:600, 1965.

Buyse, M. L. (Ed.): Birth Defects Encyclopedia. Cambridge, Mass., Blackwell Scientific Publications, Inc., 1990.

Coco, R., and Bergada, C.: Cytogenetic findings in 125 patients with Turner's syndrome and abnormal karyotypes. J. Genet. Hum. 25:95, 1977.

Cronk, C., Crocker, A. C., Pueschel, S. M., et al.: Growth chart for children with Down syndrome: 1 month to 18 years of age. Pediatrics 81:102, 1988.

Davidson, R. G.: Atlantoaxial instability in individuals with Down syndrome: A fresh look at the evidence. Pediatrics 81:857, 1988.

de Grouchy, J., and Turleau, C.: Clinical Atlas of Human Chromosomes. 2nd ed. New York, John Wiley & Sons, 1984.

DiMaio, M. S., Baumgarten, A., Greenstein, R. M., et al.: Screening for Down's syndrome by measuring maternal serum alpha-fetoprotein levels. N. Engl. J. Med. 317:342, 1987.

Ford, C. E., and Clegg, H. M.: Reciprocal translocations. Br. Med. Bull. 25:110, 1969.

Hassold, T., and Chiu, D.: Maternal age-specific rates of numerical chromosome abnormalities with special reference to trisomy. Hum. Genet. 70:11, 1985.

Hodes, M. E., Cole, J., Palmer, C. G., and Reed, T.: Clinical experience with trisomies 18 and 13. J. Med. Genet. 15:48, 1978.

Hook, E. B.: Rates of chromosome abnormalities at different maternal ages. Obstet. Gynecol. 58:282, 1981.

Hook, E. B., and Porter, I. H.: Population Cytogenetics. New York, Academic Press, 1977.

International System for Human Cytogenetic Nomenclature (ISCN) (1985). Basel, S. Karger, 1985.

Jackson, J. F., North, E. R. III, and Thomas, J. G.: Clinical diagnosis of Down's syndrome. Clin. Genet. 9:483, 1976.

Lin, H.-P., Menaka, H., Lim, K.-H., and Yong, H.-S.: Congenital leukemoid reaction followed by fatal leukemia. Am. J. Dis. Child. 134:939, 1980.

Mankinen, C. B., and Sears, J. W.: Trisomy 13 in a female over 5 years of age. J Med. Genet. 13:157, 1976.

Miller, M., and Cosgriff, J. M.: Hematological abnormalities in newborn infants with Down syndrome. Am. J. Med. Genet. 16:173, 1983.

Muller, L. M., and de Jong, G.: Prenatal ultrasonographic features of the Pena-Shokeir I syndrome and the trisomy 18 syndrome. Am. J. Med. Genet. 25:119, 1986.

Park, S. C., Mathews, R. A., Zuberbuhler, J. R., et al.: Down syndrome with congenital heart malformation. Am. J. Dis. Child. 131:29, 1977.

Preus, M.: A diagnostic index for Down's syndrome. J. Med. Genet. 12:47, 1977.

Pueschel, S. M., Findley, T. W., Furia, J., et al.: Atlantoaxial instability in Down syndrome: Roentgenographic, neurologic, and somatosensory evoked potential studies. J. Pediatr. 110:515, 1987.

Robison, L. I., Nesbit, M. E., Jr., and Sather, H. N.: Down syndrome and acute leukemia in children: A 10-year retrospective survey from Children's Cancer Study Group. J. Pediatr. 105:235, 1984.

Salonen, R.: The Meckel syndrome: Clinicopathological findings in 67 patients. Am. J. Med. Genet. 18:671, 1984.

Schinzel, A.: Catalogue of Unbalanced Chromosome Aberrations in Man. Berlin, Walter de Gruyter, 1984.

Simpson, J. L., and German, J.: Developmental anomaly resembling the trisomy 18 syndrome. Ann. Genet. 12:107, 1969.

Taylor, A. I.: Autosomal trisomy syndromes: A detailed study of 27 cases of Edwards' syndrome and 27 cases of Patau's syndrome. J. Med. Genet. 5:227, 1968.

Therman, E.: Human Chromosomes. New York, Springer:Verlag, 1986.

Warkany, J., Passarge, E., and Smith, L. B.: Congenital malformations in autosomal trisomy syndromes. Am. J. Dis. Child. 112:502, 1966.

Wertelecki, W., Graham, J. M., Jr., and Sergovich, F. R.: The clinical syndrome of triploidy. Obstet. Gynecol. 47:69, 1976.

Yunis, J. J. (ed.): New Chromosomal Syndromes. New York, Academic Press, 1977.

Zellweger, H., and Patil, S. R.: Down Syndrome. In Vinken, P. J., Bruyn, G. W., and Klawans, H. L. (eds.): Handbook of Clinical Neurology. Vol. 50. Malformations. Amsterdam, Elsevier Science Publishers, 1987.

SCREENING OF THE NEWBORN 17

Harvey L. Levy

In most of the metabolic disorders, the clinical consequences develop postnatally. They result from biochemical abnormalities that appear when the infant is no longer protected by intrauterine maternal-fetal exchange. The infant with phenylketonuria (PKU), for instance, has essentially a normal blood phenylalanine level at birth but within a few hours develops hyperphenylalaninemia. If this and other biochemical abnormalities of PKU are not corrected or at least controlled by dietary treatment, the infant shows signs of developmental delay by 3 or 4 months of age and subsequently becomes mentally retarded. When dietary therapy is begun and the blood phenylalanine level controlled from the first weeks of life, mental retardation is prevented.

PKU was the first of the metabolic disorders known to benefit from early dietary therapy. This fact was established by the late 1950s. The challenge then became to detect PKU in all affected infants before irreversible brain damage occurred. This meant conducting neonatal screening for a biochemical marker of the disease.

In 1962, Guthrie met this challenge by developing a simple bacterial inhibition assay for phenylalanine that required only a very small amount of whole blood in filter paper. Thus, infants in newborn nurseries could be routinely tested for PKU from blood specimens obtained by lancing the heel and blotting a few drops of blood onto a filter paper card. This blood–filter paper specimen could be mailed to a central laboratory for PKU testing. An increased phenylalanine concentration in the specimen suggested PKU in the infant.

By the mid 1960s, many states began routine newborn PKU screening programs. Infants with PKU were identified in larger numbers than anticipated and were showing normal development while on treatment. The success of PKU screening led to the addition of tests for other metabolic disorders, including galactosemia, maple syrup urine disease, and homocystinuria—all of which are similar in principle to PKU. These additional tests could be applied to the same blood–filter paper specimen obtained for PKU screening. More recently, a test for congenital hypothyroidism has been added. Currently, still other tests, such as those for congenital adrenal hyperplasia, biotinidase deficiency, sickle cell disease, hyperlipidemia, congenital toxoplasmosis, and congenital AIDS, are being added or being considered as additions to the process of routine newborn screening. Furthermore, screening of urine soaked into filter paper has been a valuable adjunct to blood screening in identifying many metabolic disorders not otherwise identifiable and, most recently, neuroblastoma. Thus newborn screening is not only expanding within the field of metabolic disorders but is beginning to include screening for nonmetabolic genetic disorders, infectious diseases, and even cancer. Table 17–1 lists the frequencies of the disorders for which newborn screening is currently performed or strongly considered.

▪ SCREENING PROGRAMS

Specimen. The blood specimen is obtained from the heel of the infant, as depicted in Figure 17–1. This simple specimen, conceived and introduced by Guthrie, has had an enormous impact on newborn screening. The specimen is not only easily obtained but also easily and inexpensively sent by mail to a central testing facility. There are no complications in obtaining this specimen from the newborn, contrary to early fears that this would produce problems such as infection or excessive bleeding. The major considerations are that the specimen is obtained from *every newborn prior to nursery discharge* or by the 4th day of life (whichever is first) and that all circles on the filter paper card are fully saturated with blood.

With the growing practice of early nursery discharge, often during the 1st or 2nd day of life, there is concern that some infants with a metabolic disorder will not have ingested sufficient protein for amino acid elevation to occur and, therefore, may not be identified. Recent information, however, indicates that most, if not all, newborns with PKU have an elevated blood phenylalanine concentration during the first day of life and should not be overlooked by newborn screening. The markers for maple syrup urine disease, as well as for congenital hypothyroidism and galactosemia, are also usually present in very early blood specimens. It is important to obtain a blood specimen for routine screening from *all newborns* prior to hospital discharge, regardless of how soon after birth

TABLE 17–1. Approximate Frequencies of Disorders Included in or Considered for Newborn Screening

DISORDER	FREQUENCY
Congenital hypothyroidism	1:4000
Phenylketonuria	1:12,000
Galactosemia	1:60,000
Maple syrup urine disease	1:200,000
Homocystinuria	1:300,000
Biotinidase deficiency	1:70,000
Congenital adrenal hyperplasia	1:12,000
Sickle cell disease	1:4000
Cystic fibrosis	1:3000
Duchenne muscular dystrophy	1:8000
Congenital toxoplasmosis	1:10,000
Hyperlipidemia	1:500
Alpha$_1$-antitrypsin deficiency	1:8000
Neuroblastoma	1:4000

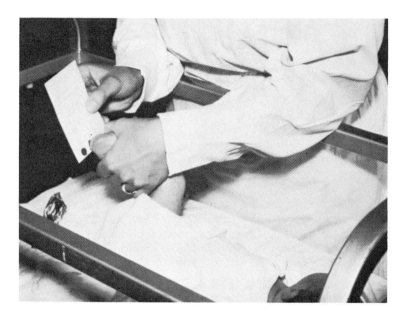

FIGURE 17–1. Filter paper specimen of blood collected from the heel of a neonate for routine newborn screening. (From Avery, M. E., and Taeusch, H. W. [eds.]; Diseases of the Newborn. 5th ed. Philadelphia, W. B. Saunders Company, 1984, p.61.)

discharge occurs. In addition, to be certain that an infant with a disorder is not missed, a repeat blood–filter paper specimen should be obtained no later than 2 weeks of age from infants whose initial specimen was obtained within the first 24 hours of life.

Screening Laboratory. Newborn screening tests are usually performed in a centralized state, provincial, or regional laboratory. In the United States, for example, the blood specimen is most often mailed to the state public health laboratory. It may be tested in that laboratory or sent to a neighboring state laboratory that serves as the regional testing facility for several states. A few states contract with one or more large private or medical center laboratories within the state to conduct the testing. The screening laboratory performs the basic screening tests and notifies the attending physician (or collaborating state program) of abnormal results. Confirmatory testing is also conducted in some screening laboratories.

Screening Tests. The testing procedure begins with the punching of small discs (each ⅛ inch in diameter) from the filter paper specimen. This process may be performed manually with a paper punch or with a semi-automated punch indexer machine. In the bacterial assays for PKU and other inborn errors of metabolism (galactosemia, homocystinuria, and maple syrup urine disease), the discs are placed on agar gels that contain bacteria, growth media, and other necessary factors. Each bacterial plate is constituted for response to a particular metabolite; the amount of bacterial growth around the disc is proportional to the concentration of the metabolite in the blood. For instance, in the Guthrie test for PKU, the disc from the blood specimen of an affected newborn is surrounded by a large zone of bacterial growth (Fig. 17–2). Guthrie and others have developed a number of these bacterial assays, at least five of which are currently used in newborn screening (Table 17–2).

A radioimmunoassay for thyroxine (T_4) or thyroid-stimulating hormone (TSH) is the screening test for congenital hypothyroidism (Table 17–2). A disc from the filter paper–blood specimen is placed in a test tube. For the T_4

assay, the tube contains radioactive (^{125}I) T_4, anti-T_4 antibodies, and a chemical to prevent binding of T_4 to thyroxine-binding globulin. T_4 in the blood competes with the (^{125}I) T_4 for binding to anti-T_4 antibody. When the T_4 concentration in the blood is low (e.g., in congenital hypothyroidism), more antibody binding sites are occupied by (^{125}I) T_4, resulting in less free (^{125}I) T_4. Free and bound T_4 are separated, and the gamma radioactivity in one of the fractions is counted. Following computerized integration, a T_4 level is assigned to each blood specimen. Any specimen with a low T_4 value is tested for the TSH level, also by radioimmunoassay. An elevated TSH concentration combined with a low T_4 level indicates primary hypothyroidism. In many programs, the radioimmunoassay for TSH is used as the primary screening test for hypothyroidism.

Several other screening tests are also used in some

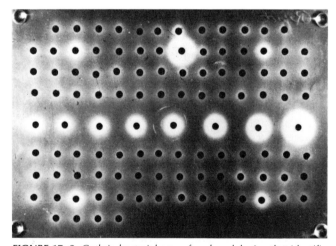

FIGURE 17–2. Guthrie bacterial assay for phenylalanine that identifies PKU in the neonate. Small discs from the filter paper blood specimen are placed on an agar gel. Note the large growth around the disc in the center of the second row from the top, which indicated PKU in this infant. The center row of discs are control specimens containing increasing amounts of phenylalanine from 2 mg/dl (a normal value) on the left to 20 mg/dl on the right. The remaining discs are from normal neonates and are surrounded by growth zones smaller than or no larger than that surrounding the 2 mg/dl control disc.

TABLE 17–2. Tests Used in Newborn Screening

TYPE OF TEST	TEST MARKER	DISORDER
Bacterial assay	↑ Phenylalanine	Phenylketonuria
	↑ Galactose (-1-P)	Galactosemia
	↑ Methionine	Homocystinuria
	↑ Leucine	Maple syrup urine disease
	↑ Tyrosine	Tyrosinemia
	↑ Histidine	Histidinemia
Radioimmunoassay	↓ T_4, ↑ TSH	Congenital hypothyroidism
	↑ 17-hydroxyprogesterone	Congenital adrenal hyperplasia
Protein electrophoresis	S hemoglobin	Sickle cell disease
	↓ Alpha$_1$-antitrypsin	Alpha$_1$-antitrypsin deficiency
Enzyme assay	↓ Galactose-1-phosphate uridyl transferase (GALT)	Galactosemia
	↓ Biotinidase	Biotinidase deficiency
Enzyme-linked immunosorbent assay (ELISA)	↑ Creatine phosphokinase	Duchenne muscular dystrophy
	Toxoplasma antibody (IgM)	Congenital toxoplasmosis
	HIV antibody (IgG)	AIDS
	↑ Trypsinogen	Cystic fibrosis
	↑ Apolipoportein B	Hyperlipidemia
	↑ Vanillylmandelic acid, homovanillic acid	Neuroblastoma
Fluorometric assay	↓ Phenylalanine	Phenylketonuria

↑, Increase; ↓, decrease.

programs (Table 17–2). Hemoglobin electrophoresis of blood eluted from the filter paper disc is employed for sickle cell disease screening. The Beutler enzyme spot assay for galactose-1-phosphate uridyl transferase is often used to screen for galactosemia. An enzyme assay for biotinidase is used to screen for biotinidase deficiency. Enzyme immunoassays, including the enzyme-linked immunosorbent assay (ELISA) method, are becoming available and are in more frequent use to screen for congenital toxoplasmosis, cystic fibrosis, hyperlipoproteinemia, and neuroblastoma; for epidemiologic studies of AIDS; and even for specific sickle cell disease. Several programs in North America screen for PKU with a fluorometric assay for phenylalanine.

Confirmatory Tests. An abnormal finding in a newborn screening test is *not diagnostic* of a disorder. It only indicates that the infant might have a disorder. Abnormalities in the newborn specimen can also be transient or produced by artifacts. Accordingly, when an abnormality is identified, *additional tests* must be performed so that a disorder can be either confirmed or ruled out.

In screening for congenital hypothyroidism, the original newborn blood specimen with a low T_4 level can be used for the TSH assay, as noted previously. Confirmation of PKU, galactosemia, or other inborn errors of metabolism requires additional specimens. Consequently, a repeat blood specimen (filter paper or plasma) and often a urine specimen are necessary for specific testing when the newborn blood specimen suggests an abnormality of this type.

DNA analysis with allele-specific oligonucleotide probes may be used for the confirmation of many disorders identified by newborn screening. Analysis of DNA in fetal nucleated red cells found in the maternal circulation is a promising approach (Bianchi et al., 1990). The combination of gene amplification by the polymerase chain reaction (PCR) and hybridization with specific gene probes allows for the application of DNA analysis to the blood–filter paper specimen and could result in confirmatory testing for PKU and other genetic disorders in the newborn screening specimen (Fig. 17–3).

Physician Contact. The pediatrician or other physician of record should be contacted immediately when the newborn blood specimen illustrates such a striking abnormality that a metabolic disorder is strongly suspected. Thus, as noted in Table 17–1, a very low level of T_4 combined with an elevated TSH concentration indicates congenital hypothyroidism; and a markedly elevated level of phenylalanine, galactose, methionine, or leucine indicates PKU, galactosemia, homocystinuria, or maple syrup urine disease, respectively. If the infant is well, confirmatory testing should be performed; and if a disorder is confirmed, the infant should be evaluated at a center that specializes in the disorder. If the infant is ill, he or she should be admitted to a special care nursery, preferably in a center that has a pediatric metabolic unit experienced in the diagnosis and treatment of inborn errors of metabolism. Specimens for confirmatory testing should be collected, and therapy for the illness should be initiated without delay.

Less striking abnormalities illustrated in the newborn blood specimen can be followed up by a letter to the

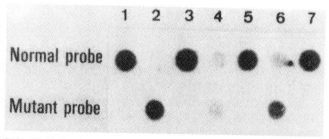

FIGURE 17–3. Genotype analysis of PCR-amplified genomic DNA from newborn filter paper blood specimens. DNA was extracted from each specimen, and a section of the phenylalanine hydroxylase gene was amplified by the polymerase chain reaction (PCR). The amplified DNA was hybridized to allele-specific P-labelled oligonucleotides. Numbers 1, 3, 5, and 7 are from infants with PKU who do not have the specific mutation represented by the mutant oligonucleotide. Their DNA hybridized to the normal probe but not to the mutant probe. Number 2 is from an infant with the mutation represented by the mutant probe. This DNA hybridized to it but not to the normal probe. Numbers 4 and 6 are from infants who carry two mutant alleles (compound heterozygotes), one of which is the mutation represented by the mutant probe.

physician requesting a repeat specimen. The physician should be notified of these results as soon as possible.

Most infants with a positive screening result, particularly when this result is only mildly or moderately abnormal, do not have a disorder. Transient or nonspecific abnormalities are quite frequent. Though all infants with an abnormal screening result must have repeat testing, the families should be informed that an initial positive result may have no medical implications. This can alleviate excessive anxiety and prevent unnecessary diagnostic procedures and treatment.

It is important to emphasize that the physician should contact the screening laboratory whenever the results of repeat testing have not been received or when an infant has symptoms that suggest a metabolic disorder or other disorder for which screening can be conducted. The screening laboratory can check the results of the newborn or repeat testing, or may be able to perform additional tests on the blood–filter paper specimen.

■ DISORDERS

Phenylketonuria (PKU). This metabolic disorder should *always* be identified by newborn blood screening (see Chapter 18). Most newborns with an elevated blood phenylalanine level have either PKU, a variant such as non-PKU hyperphenylalaninemia, a pterin defect with secondary hyperphenylalaninemia, or a transient elevation of phenylalanine. Infants with galactosemia who are acutely ill may also have an increased concentration of phenylalanine.

Urine screening, either by ferric chloride testing for phenylketone identification or by Guthrie bacterial assay, is *unreliable* for the detection of PKU in newborns and should *never* be used for this purpose. The newborn infant with PKU rarely has detectable phenylketones and often does not have increased phenylalanine in the urine, unlike the older infant or child.

Treatment for PKU should *never* be given on the basis of a positive screening test alone. The dietary therapy is complicated and can be hazardous to an infant who does not have PKU. Only after repeat testing and confirmation of PKU should treatment be given and then only in collaboration with or directly by a metabolic center.

Congenital Hypothyroidism. This is the most frequent of the disorders identified by routine newborn screening. It occurs in about 1:4000 to 1:5000 screened infants, as compared with the approximately 1:12000 frequency of PKU.

The screening procedure for congenital hypothyroidism is reliable for identifying the affected infants, whether the primary screen is for a low T_4 level or for a high TSH concentration. Nevertheless, affected infants are missed in the screening process. This may be due to lack of the "marker" (either low T_4 or high TSH) in the specimen or to laboratory error by misreading or overlooking the abnormal result.

False-positive results are frequent. As many as 3 per cent of screened infants have a low T_4 not due to congenital hypothyroidism. Most of these are premature infants with a normal TSH concentration in whom the low T_4 is transient. Nevertheless, to avoid missing an infant with congenital hypothyroidism, screening programs usually require a repeat blood specimen from each of these infants.

Infants with a positive screening test should neither be "labeled" as having congenital hypothyroidism nor treated for this disorder until confirmation testing is at least in progress. If the newborn blood specimen contains a high TSH concentration as well as a low T_4 level, treatment can be initiated before the results of the confirmatory tests are known. If the TSH concentration in the blood specimen of the newborn is normal, however, treatment should be withheld until confirmatory test results are available.

Galactosemia. Newborn screening for this disorder is advisable. Without routine newborn screening, up to 30 per cent of affected infants either are not diagnosed until they become terminally ill with sepsis (see Chapter 18) or die without being diagnosed. In addition, other disorders of galactose metabolism, particularly galactokinase deficiency, may not be identified until the development of irreversible cataracts.

An assay for galactose (and galactose-1-phosphate), such as Paigen *Escherichia coli*–phage assay, is preferable to a specific enzyme assay such as the Beutler spot test for galactose-1-phosphate uridyltransferase. The former is more reliable for the detection of galactosemia and also identifies other galactose metabolic disorders.

The most rapid confirmatory test for a positive newborn screening result is urine testing for nonglucose-reducing substance. In almost all cases, this element is strongly positive in galactosemia and at least moderately positive in galactokinase or epimerase deficiency. If the urine contains reducing substance and the infant has clinical signs of galactosemia, milk feedings (breast or formula) should be discontinued; and blood specimens for confirmatory testing should be obtained. These confirmatory tests should include the measurement of blood galactose and galactose-1-phosphate and erythrocyte galactose-1-phosphate uridyltransferase activity. If the urine is negative for reducing substance, the newborn screening result is likely to be false positive or to indicate an enzyme variant, probably one that is benign. Nevertheless, repeat blood testing should be performed.

Homocystinuria. The newborn blood screening marker for detection of this disorder is an increased level of methionine, as identified by the Guthrie assay (Table 17–2). This screening test is included in some programs, and affected newborns have been detected. Infants with homocystinuria have also been missed in newborn screening, usually because their blood methionine concentration was not increased. Most of these infants later become hypermethioninemic and can be identified in a blood specimen obtained at 2 weeks of age or later.

Newborn infants may have slight transient increases in the blood methionine concentration. At 3 to 6 weeks of age, these transient increases can be quite marked. To confirm homocystinuria, a repeat blood specimen is required. If the methionine concentration is again increased, quantitative amino acid analysis of plasma and urine should be performed. In the homocystinuric infant, there usually is detectable homocystine in plasma and urine, increased methionine in plasma, and reduced cystine.

Newborn screening for methionine elevations also identifies a rare inborn error known as hypermethioninemia (see Chapter 18). On confirmatory testing, these infants have markedly increased methionine in plasma with no homocystine in plasma or urine and a normal plasma cystine concentration.

Maple Syrup Urine Disease. The marker for this disorder is increased leucine in the newborn blood specimen (Table 17–2). Newborns with classic maple syrup urine disease virtually always have a four-fold or greater elevation of leucine. Transient increases in the blood leucine concentration are infrequent and usually no more than twice the normal concentration.

Maple syrup urine disease can be a fulminant disease associated with severe ketoacidosis and profound neurologic effects (see Chapter 19). Consequently, the finding of a substantially increased leucine level in the newborn blood specimen indicates the need for an immediate call to the attending physician. If the infant is ill, confirmatory plasma and urine specimens should be obtained and emergency therapy initiated. If the infant has maple syrup urine disease, the plasma contains markedly increased concentrations of leucine, isoleucine, allo-isoleucine, and valine (the branched-chain amino acids); and the urine will be strongly positive for ketones and contain large quantities of the branched-chain ketoacids and amino acids. The characteristic odor reminiscent of maple syrup may not yet be present on the body or in the urine of a newborn with maple syrup urine disease.

Milder variants of maple syrup urine disease can be missed in newborn screening. The newborn with the intermediate variant may have not yet developed an elevated blood leucine level or may have such a slight increase that it is overlooked. In the intermittent variant, the blood leucine concentration is elevated only during acute metabolic episodes.

Sickle Cell Disease. In a number of state newborn screening programs, the newborn blood specimen is tested for hemoglobin abnormalities. The major goal is to identify the infant with sickle cell disease before the onset of life-threatening pneumococcal septicemia. Oral penicillin prophylaxis has been proved effective and is recommended (Gaston, et al., 1986).

When sickle hemoglobin is found, it is important to perform confirmatory testing so that the infant with the disease is differentiated from the far greater number of infants who only carry the mutant gene (sickle cell trait). Infants with sickle cell trait do not develop the complications of this disease and should not be stigmatized as having sickle cell disease.

■ OTHER SCREENING

Cord Blood. Umbilical cord blood can be screened for maternal metabolic disorders that may affect the fetus and result in neonatal abnormalities. Paramount among these abnormalities is maternal PKU (see Chapter 18). Cord blood contains the increased phenylalanine transferred from the maternal circulation. Disorders intrinsic to the infant can also be screened in cord blood when the abnormality is present in erythrocytes. Among these disorders is galactosemia, in which cord blood has increased galactose-1-phosphate and no activity of galactose-1-phosphate uridyltransferase.

Routine cord blood screening was conducted in Massachusetts for over 10 years. A filter paper card was soaked with umbilical cord blood at delivery of the infant and sent to the state screening laboratory. Initially, this specimen was screened for galactosemia and maternal PKU. Subsequently, galactosemia screening was discontinued, since this disease could be effectively screened in the newborn blood specimen. Screening for maternal PKU continued, and screening for other maternal metabolic disorders, such as maternal histidinemia, was added. This led to valuable information about these disorders and their relation to the fetus. The information was of limited value to the families, however, and cord blood screening has been discontinued.

Urine. Routine newborn urine screening is conducted in Massachusetts, Rhode Island and Quebec, and was formerly conducted in Australia. This screening identifies infants who have disorders that are not identifiable by blood screening. Among these are organic acid disorders such as methylmalonic acidemia (see Chapter 18), certain aminoacidopathies such as several of the urea cycle disorders that are not identified by blood screening (see Chapter 18), and renal transport disorders such as cystinuria and Hartnup disorder.

The specimen is obtained by the parent when the infant is about 3 weeks old. The usual method of collection consists of pressing a wet portion of the diaper onto a filter paper card that the parent receives when leaving the hospital with the newborn infant. The filter paper specimen is mailed to the screening laboratory, where it is tested by either paper or thin-layer chromatography. Figure 17–4 depicts several abnormalities identified by newborn urine screening. This type of urine specimen, collected from 6-month-old infants, is used in routine screening for neuroblastoma in Japan.

■ SPECIFIC ISSUES OF NEWBORN SCREENING

SPECIMEN COLLECTION

Early Discharge. The identification of PKU and other amino acid disorders in newborn screening depends on the presence of an amino acid elevation in the newborn blood specimen. This elevation occurs after birth and results from protein ingestion as well as amino acid release by catabolic processes. With early discharge from the nursery, on the 1st or 2nd day of life, there is concern that the newborn with a metabolic disorder will have a normal result in screening because insufficient protein has been ingested.

This concern appears to be largely unfounded with regard to the identification of PKU. Recent studies indicate that virtually all infants with PKU have an elevated blood phenylalanine level during the 1st day of life. Early development of hyperphenylalaninemia is probably a consequence of proteolysis or the high content of protein in colostrum (early breast milk), or both. On the other hand, some newborns with non-PKU hyperphenylalaninemia

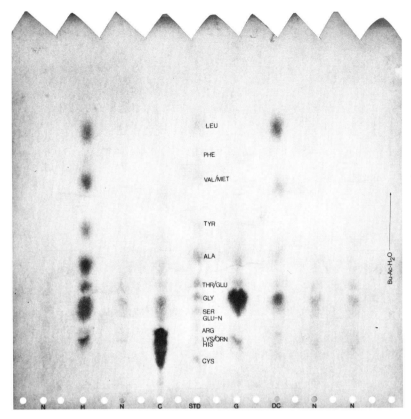

FIGURE 17–4. A triketohydrindene hydrate (Ninhydrin)–stained paper chromatogram from newborn urine screening that depicts the amino acid pattern of normal urine (N) and several abnormalities, including Hartnup's disease (H), cystinuria (C), and hyperglycinemia (G). DC is a specimen contaminated by diaper rash cream. The center lane (STD) contains reference amino acids.

take longer to develop an increased blood phenylalanine level. Although most of these infants have a benign condition, a few have a serious disorder such as a pterin defect.

An occasional infant with congenital hypothyroidism might be missed if newborn screening relies only on a blood specimen obtained during the 1st day of life, since the T$_4$ level in the hypothyroid infants tends to decrease postnatally. Infants with homocystinuria and variant forms of other metabolic disorders might also be missed in the testing of an early specimen.

The American Academy of Pediatrics recommends a repeat blood specimen at 2 to 4 weeks of age from every infant initially tested before 24 hours of age. Most important, a newborn blood specimen should be obtained from every infant prior to nursery discharge, regardless of how early discharge occurs. A metabolic disorder is far more likely to be missed because a newborn blood specimen was never obtained than because it was obtained too early.

Routine Follow-Up (Repeat) Screening. Obtaining a second or follow-up blood specimen from all infants at 4 to 6 weeks of age was recommended when newborn screening began and was common practice in most screening programs during the 1960s. After several years, however, it became apparent that very few infants with PKU were identified through the use of this specimen and many screening programs abandoned routine follow-up specimen collection. A survey disclosed that only four infants with PKU were identified among over 2.3 million follow-up specimens tested in the United States; and at least three of these four infants should have been detected by initial newborn blood screening. By comparison, 290

infants with PKU were identified among 3.4 million initial newborn blood specimens tested in these surveyed states. Routine follow-up screening is not justifiable for PKU detection and is probably unjustified in screening for other metabolic disorders.

Informed Consent. During the 1970s there was lively discussion about the need for informed consent for newborn screening. Advocates argued that parents should decide whether newborn screening is to be performed and that public health laws mandating newborn screening are intrusive. This advocacy has waned, primarily because of the virtually insurmountable difficulty in obtaining truly informed consent from the parents of all newborn infants.

The issue of informed consent has implications that go beyond practicality. A major question is whether specific informed consent should be required for routine newborn screening when it is not required for other newborn tests (e.g., serum bilirubin) that are often necessary. Most would agree that mandatory screening without specific informed consent is justifiable for disorders such as congenital hypothyroidism and PKU that cause mental retardation and for which there is proven preventive treatment. However, as it becomes possible to use the newborn specimen to screen for many other abnormalities, particularly genetic disorders in which the phenotype may be variable and for which there may be little or no treatment, the issue of informed consent may again become prominent.

■ SCREENING PROGRAMS

Central Laboratories. Newborn screening should be conducted by large laboratories rather than by many small laboratories. This usually means that a single state laboratory or a regional laboratory serving several states should perform the screening. The mass analysis that results from consolidated screening decreases costs and also enhances accuracy, since there is much greater exposure to and thus familiarity with specimen abnormalities. Perhaps most important, a large central laboratory can include both a professional and administrative unit that can continually monitor the process of specimen collection and repeat testing.

Missed Cases. Infants with PKU, congenital hypothyroidism, and other screened metabolic disorders have been missed in newborn screening. Laboratory or program error is the usual cause of these missed cases. In some instances, a specimen was never collected, particularly when the infant was transferred to a neonatal intensive care unit at another hospital. In other instances, mistakes occurred because the laboratory was not properly supervised or resulted from logistical difficulties of mass screening in which very large numbers of specimens and results were processed daily. Thus, physicians must exercise clinical judgement and not fall into the trap of excluding a diagnosis because an infant has presumably been screened. Specific testing for metabolic disorders should be performed in any infant or child with symptoms that suggest the presence of such a disorder, regardless of the assumed or even actual newborn screening result.

Metabolic Disorders Not Screened. A frequent error is the assumption that routine newborn screening covers metabolic disorders in general and that a normal screening result excludes most, if not all, of these disorders. Actually, most screening programs in North America test only for PKU and congenital hypothyroidism. Other programs in the United States and many in Europe and Japan include screening for galactosemia, homocystinuria, and maple syrup urine disease; but most metabolic disorders are not covered by newborn screening. As previously noted, all infants and children with symptoms that suggest a metabolic diagnosis should undergo specific testing.

■ OTHER DISORDERS CONSIDERED FOR SCREENING

Biotinidase Deficiency. Biotinidase deficiency is a recently discovered disorder of recycling of biotin, a vitamin cofactor for carboxylases. Lack of biotinidase activity produces a deficiency of intracellular free biotin, which results in an organic acid disorder known as multiple carboxylase deficiency. The clinical features of the disorder include developmental delay, seizures, hearing loss, alopecia, and dermatitis. Death during infancy has also been reported. Treatment with biotin alone has been effective in controlling the symptoms, although the developmental delay is not reversible. The initiation of biotin therapy in early infancy, however, prevents all of the features of the disorder. For this reason, a screening test for biotinidase deficiency that is applicable to the newborn blood specimen has been developed and added to a number of newborn screening programs in the United States, Japan, and Europe. The frequency of identified newborns in these programs has a wide range, from 1:30,000 to 1:235,000. Almost all infants were asymptomatic when

identified and have remained normal on biotin treatment. The test for this disorder seems to be a very worthwhile addition to newborn screening.

Duchenne Muscular Dystrophy. Duchenne muscular dystrophy disorder can be detected by newborn blood screening. The test is an assay that identifies increased creatine phosphokinase (CPK) activity. Several areas in France and Germany and large screening programs in Pittsburgh and Manitoba include this test. The gene and gene product (protein) defects in this disorder have been identified, but the absence of therapy that will prevent the clinical manifestations seems to militate against routine newborn screening for this disorder at the present time.

Congenital Adrenal Hyperplasia. Infants with the salt-losing form of this disorder can die precipitously, often without a specific diagnosis. Male infants with congenital adrenal hyperplasia are usually not diagnosed in infancy, and even some females, virtually all of whom have ambiguous genitalia, are unrecognized early in infancy. Accurate gender assignment and initiation of hormonal therapy as soon after birth as possible are critical to a favorable prognosis in congenital adrenal hyperplasia. Thus, newborn screening is a valuable aid in early diagnosis and prompt therapy. A radioimmunoassay for 17α-hydroxyprogesterone, which is increased in congenital adrenal hyperplasia, can be performed on the newborn blood specimen and has been added to routine newborn screening in several state programs and in a number of other countries. An ELISA for 17α-hydroxyprogesterone is also available. It is becoming clear that the frequency of congenital adrenal hyperplasia and the value of newborn screening detection justify adding this test to routine screening programs.

Cystic Fibrosis. The frequency and severity of this disorder have made it prominently considered for routine newborn detection.

Early identification of the disorder can alert parents and physicians to monitor for growth, institute pancreatic enzyme replacement, and treat vigorously any pulmonary infection. Siblings of affected infants should have a sweat test, usually at 1 or 2 months of age, when the collection of sweat is more reliable than in newborns. Alternately, DNA analysis of siblings reliably identifies those with the disorder.

Much debate concerns the use of DNA analysis for prenatal diagnosis, since the major genotype occurs in only approximately 70 per cent of patients (Kerem et al., 1989). The remainder may result from 20 or more different genotypes. This polymorphism is of interest in predicting disease severity but lessens the value of first trimester amniocentesis for prenatal diagnosis (Pool, 1990).

Hyperlipidemia. Recognition that hyperlipidemia, particularly increased low-density lipoprotein, is a major cause of early cardiovascular disease among adults has led to an interest in newborn screening for identification of at-risk infants. Evidence that hyperlipidemia may be controlled by diet and medication has spurred this interest. Until recently, however, there was no reliable marker for newborn screening. For instance, the cholesterol level varies widely in early infancy and was found not to correlate with later serum cholesterol levels. Investigators are now studying increased apolipoprotein B in the newborn as a marker for genetically determined hyperlipidemia. Apolipoprotein B, a major apolipoprotein of low-density lipoproteins, can be measured in the newborn blood specimen by an ELISA method. This could become a very important addition to routine newborn screening.

Neuroblastoma. Neuroblastoma is the most frequent solid tumor of childhood. It is characterized by the excretion of increased vanillylmandelic acid and homovanillic acid. In Japan, screening for neuroblastoma has been conducted with filter paper–urine specimens collected when the infant is six months of age. The marker is increased vanillylmandelic acid and homovanillic acid as determined by high-performance liquid chromatography of urine eluted from the paper or increased vanillylmandelic acid identified by directly spot testing the filter paper specimen. This type of screening has resulted in the early detection of neuroblastoma in many clinically normal infants. In most, the tumor was localized and could be completely removed at surgery. These infants have remained well. Only a very few infants already had advanced and inoperable cancer. In general, it seems that urine screening has been valuable in the early identification and treatment of neuroblastoma.

Screening for neuroblastoma represents an opportunity to add the new dimension of early identification of cancer to screening of infants. Nevertheless, there are a number of questions. Arranging for the routine collection of a specimen when infants are 6 months old presents logistical difficulties, particularly in the United States. The most effective screening test, high-performance liquid chromatography, is labor intensive and expensive. The simpler spot test has relatively high rates of false-positive and false-negative results. Perhaps the recently developed ELISA test for vanillylmandelic acid and homovanillic acid will address these problems. Thin-layer chromatography, used for this purpose in Quebec, may be a more practical alternative. Finally, neuroblastoma screening may lead to diagnosis and surgery in some infants in whom the neuroblastoma is of the regressive type and may never become symptomatic. Consequently, most programs are likely to await further study and experience before adopting routine screening for neuroblastoma.

Congenital Toxoplasmosis. Screening for congenital toxoplasmosis has been added to the tests applied to the newborn blood specimen in two states, Massachusetts and New Hampshire. The test is an ELISA that captures toxoplasma-specific IgM antibodies. The objective is to identify newborns with prenatally acquired toxoplasmosis who are clinically recognizable either because they are asymptomatic or have occult damage. There is evidence that a number of these infants will develop neurologic sequelae or suffer recurrent chorioretinitis with progressive visual impairment and blindness. Treatment with sulfadiazine and pyrimethamine is effective against actively multiplying parasites and may prevent the development of these clinical sequelae. Among the 300,000 newborns who have been screened for congenital toxoplasmosis, 30

have been positive, a frequency of 1:10,000. Most of these infants were asymptomatic and, on treatment, have remained asymptomatic.

Acquired Immunodeficiency Syndrome (AIDS). Although there is as yet no truly effective treatment for AIDS, there is need for continuing epidemiologic surveillance of the frequency and distribution of infected individuals. Virtually all such surveys, however, are probably biased against identifying AIDS, since individuals who believe they might have AIDS may not agree to be tested. Screening newborn blood specimens routinely for antibodies to human immunodeficiency virus (HIV) avoids this bias and serves as a proxy for the frequency and distribution of AIDS in the childbearing segment of the population, since HIV-specific IgG antibodies in the newborn blood specimen reflect maternal infection. This screening is currently conducted as a national collaborative effort among newborn screening programs in the United States. Anonymity is maintained so that the identity of positive infants is unknown. Universal voluntary screening of pregnant women in high-risk areas, with informed consent, is now recommended.

Alpha₁-Antitrypsin Deficiency. In the 1970s, there was much interst in newborn screening for alpha₁-antitrypsin deficiency. The association of this deficiency with cirrhosis in infants and obstructive lung disease in young adults had been discovered in the 1960s. It was believed that presymptomatic identification such as in newborns could lead to measures that might reduce the risk of lung disease, even if there was no preventive therapy for the liver disease. The prophylactic measures that were suggested included the avoidance of areas in which the air is polluted or smoke filled. In Sweden, 200,000 infants were screened by electroimmunoassay applied to the newborn blood specimen, and approximately 1:2000 were found to have PiZZ, the type of alpha₁-antitrypsin deficiency associated with disease. Only three of these infants subsequently developed cirrhosis; it is still too early to determine the frequency of lung disease in this affected population. Consequently, uncertainty over the risk of disease even in PiZZ alpha₁-antitrypsin deficient individuals and the lack of clearly preventive therapy for either the hepatic or the pulmonary sequelae caused the interest in newborn screening for alpha₁-antitrypsin deficiency to wane. Recent evidence that injections of recombinant alpha₁-antitrypsin produce normal blood levels in deficient individuals and may protect them from lung disease could renew interest in newborn screening for this disorder (Wewers et al., 1987).

Histidinemia. Among the Guthrie bacterial assays that can be applied to the newborn blood–filter paper specimen is one for histidine (Table 17–2). This assay identifies an increased histidine concentration, the marker for histidinemia. It had been included in the New York State screening program and in programs in Austria and Japan, and led to the identification of many histidinemic infants. However, there seems to be little need for this screening, since histidinemia is probably benign in most, if not all, affected individuals (see Chapter 18).

■ REFERENCES

Bianchi, D. W., Flint, A. F., Pizzimenti, M. F., et al.: Isolation of fetal DNA from nucleated erythrocytes in maternal blood. Proc. Natl. Acad. Sci. *87*:3279, 1990.

Bickel, H., Guthrie, R., and Hammersen, G. (Eds.): Neonatal Screening for Inborn Errors of Metabolism. Berlin, Springer-Verlag, 1980.

Committee for the Study of Inborn Errors of Metabolism: Genetic Screening. Programs, Principles, and Research. Washington, National Academy of Sciences, 1975.

Committee on Genetics, American Academy of Pediatrics: New issues in newborn screening for phenylketonuria and congenital hypothyroidism. Pediatrics *69*:104, 1982.

Committee on Genetics, American Academy of Pediatrics: Newborn screening fact sheets. Pediatrics *83*:449, 1989.

Committee on Genetics, American Academy of Pediatrics; and Committee on Neonatal Screening, American Thyroid Association: Newborn screening for congenital hypothyroidism: recommended guidelines. Pediatrics *80*:745, 1987.

Consensus conference: Newborn screening for sickle cell disease and other hemoglobinopathies. J. A. M. A. *258*:1205, 1987.

Dankert-Roelse, J. E., te Meerman, G. J., Martijn, A., et al.: Survival and clinical outcome in patients with cystic fibrosis, with or without neonatal screening. J. Pediatr. *114*:362–367, 1989.

Gaston, M. H., Verter, J. I., Woods, G., et al.: Prophylaxis with oral penicillin in children with sickle cell anemia: A randomized trial. N. Engl. J. Med. *314*:1593, 1986.

Hoff, R., Berardi, V. P., Weiblen, B. J., et al.: Seroprevalence of human immunodeficiency virus among childbearing women. Estimation by testing samples of blood from newborns. N. Engl. J. Med. *318*:525, 1988.

Kerem, B., Rommens, J. M., Buchanan, J. A., et al.: Identification of the cystic fibrosis gene: Genetic analysis. Science *245*:1073, 1989.

Kolata, G.: Panel urges newborn sickle cell screening. Science *236*:259, 1987.

Levy, H. L.: Phenylketonuria—1986. Pediatr. Rev. *7*:269, 1986.

Levy, H. L.: Genetic Screening. Adv. Hum. Genet. *4*:1, 1973.

Levy, H. L., and Hammersen, G.: Newborn screening for galactosemia and other galactose metabolic defects. J. Pediatr. *92*:871, 1978.

McCabe, E. R. B., Huang, S.-Z., Seltzer, W. K., et al.: DNA microextraction from dried blood spots on filter paper blotters: Potential applications to newborn screening. Hum. Genet. *75*:213, 1987.

Meryash, D. L., Levy, H. L., et al.: Prospective study of early neonatal screening for phenylketonuria. N. Engl. J. Med. *304*:294, 1981.

Nishi, M., Miyake, H., Takeda, T., et al.: Effects of the mass screenings for neuroblastoma in Japan. A study of 68 cases. Eur. J. Pediatr. *147*:308, 1988.

Ohta, T., Migita, M., Yasutake, T., et al.: Enzyme-linked immunosorbent assay for apolipoprotein B on dried blood spot derived from newborn infant: Its application to neonatal mass screening for hypercholesterolemia. J. Pediatr. Gastroenterol. Nutr. *7*:524, 1988.

Pang, S., Wallace, M. A., Hofman, L., et al.: Worldwide experience in newborn screening for classical congenital adrenal hyperplasia due to 21-hydroxylase deficiency. Pediatrics *81*:866, 1988.

Pool, R.: CF screening delayed for a while, perhaps forever. Science *247*:1296, 1990.

Sepe, S. J., Levy, H. L., and Mount, F. W.: An evaluation of routine follow-up blood screening of infants for phenylketonuria. N. Engl. J. Med. *300*:606, 1979.

Sveger, T.: Liver disease in alpha-1-antitrypsin deficiency detected by screening of 200,000 infants. N. Engl. J. Med. *294*:1316, 1976.

Sveger, T.: The natural history of liver disease in α_1-antitrypsin deficient children. Acta Paediatr. Scand. *77*:847, 1988.

Wewers, M. D., Casolaro, M. A., Sellers, S. E., et al.: Replacement therapy for alpha-1-antitrypsin deficiency associated with emphysema. N. Engl. J. Med. *316*:1055, 1987.

Wilcken, B., and Chalmers, G.: Reduced morbidity in patients with cystic fibrosis detected by neonatal screening. Lancet *2*:1319, 1985.

Wolf, B., and Heard, G. S.: Worldwide experience in newborn screening for biotinidase screening. Pediatrics *85*:512, 1990.

INBORN ERRORS OF METABOLISM

18

Harvey L. Levy

GENERAL CONSIDERATIONS

The inborn errors of metabolism are among the most exciting and challenging disorders for the specialist to deal with in medicine. This is particularly true for those that cause clinical disease in the newborn infant or that are identified by routine newborn screening. As newly recognized inborn errors are added to an already long list, it becomes increasingly obvious that they represent not only a substantial percentage of known genetic disorders but also a growing percentage of newborn disease.

Three factors account for the increased recognition that inborn errors of metabolism are an important part of neonatal medicine: (1) the greater appreciation of clinical signs of these disorders in the newborn, (2) the increased availability of reliable methods for detecting and measuring biochemical substances in physiologic fluids, and (3) the emergence of newborn screening for metabolic disorders as a routine procedure that identifies biochemical disorders in infants who may be *clinically normal* and in whom timely treatment will *prevent* clinical manifestations (see Neonatal Screening).

The inborn error of metabolism is genetic in origin. As in other genetic disorders, the basic abnormality is a mutant gene. The gene, acting as a template, directs the synthesis of a complementary mRNA (messenger RNA) that passes from the nucleus, where it was synthesized, to the cytoplasm, there attaching itself to ribosomes and directing the arrangement of amino acids into a polypeptide chain.* An abnormality (mutation) in the gene results in an abnormality in the polypeptide chain or perhaps even failure of polypeptide synthesis.

In an inborn error, this results in absence of the enzyme protein or a protein that is functionally and structurally abnormal. The functional deficiency may be inadequate binding of substrate or, less commonly, insufficient binding of coenzyme. Regardless of the cause, enzyme deficiency results in accumulation of substrate and reduced synthesis of product (see Fig. 58–3). Metabolic byproducts of the substrate (secondary metabolites) may also accumulate as a result of the increased substrate concentration.

An example of this is phenylketonuria (PKU), as illustrated in Figure 18–3 (see p. 128). Deficient activity of phenylalanine hydroxylase results in increased concentrations of phenylalanine and related metabolites in body fluids and tissues and a decrease in the concentration of tyrosine, the product of phenylalanine hydroxylation. In PKU, the phenylalanine hydroxylase enzyme (apoen-

zyme) is abnormal. Phenylalanine hydroxylation may also be impaired if the cofactor required for this reaction, tetrahydrobiopterin (BH_4), is deficient. This may result from a defect in dihydropteridine reductase, which catalyzes the regeneration of BH_4 from quininoid dihydropteridine (qBH_2), or a defect in the synthesis of biopterin, a precursor of BH_4.

The basis of the clinical abnormalities in the inborn errors of metabolism is presumed to be the accumulation of substrate and/or related metabolites, which may be toxic to certain organs when given in increased concentrations. The mechanism(s) by which toxicity occurs is not known.

The excitement surrounding the inborn errors of metabolism has been generated by the recognition that a number of them can be treated and the irreversible clinical complications prevented. Thus, early diagnosis and treatment can prevent such damage as mental retardation, liver disease, and eye disease. Furthermore, the potential for preventing certain types of heart and kidney disease that can be due to metabolic disorders renders the field that much more exciting.

At present, there are two forms of specific therapy. The most frequent is a dietary change that results in lowered concentrations of the putative toxic metabolites and normalization of the levels of the deficient product. The second type of therapy is the administration of a large amount of a specific vitamin that is used as a cofactor by the deficient enzyme system. This therapy, which activates the enzyme, is possible only when the defect is in binding of the coenzyme or in production of the cofactor. Optimal effectiveness from either of these therapeutic modes, however, is often possible only when the metabolic disorder is identified in the newborn by routine screening or prompt recognition of the clinical signs followed by appropriate biochemical testing.

Prenatal diagnosis of an inborn error of metabolism (see Prenatal Genetic Diagnosis) has potential therapeutic value. For this diagnosis, the fetus must be known to be at risk for a specific metabolic disorder, usually because the disorder has occurred previously in the family. The diagnosis is made by amniocentesis and examination of the cultured amniotic cells or the fluid, or measurement of enzyme activity in biopsied chorionic villi. The only therapy for an affected pregnancy in most instances is termination, which, while not actually treatment, may be extremely important to the family. A significant alternative to abortion is intrauterine therapy for the fetus, which is administered to the mother. Vitamin B_{12} treatment has been successful for a fetus with B_{12}-responsive methyl-

---

*For the few mitochondrial genes these events occur within the mitochondrion.

120

malonic acidemia, and (prenatal) biotin has protected a fetus with multiple carboxylase deficiency (Roth et al., 1982). Prenatal therapy may be applicable to other metabolic disorders.

Other forms of therapy, such as liver transplantation, have also been successful for certain metabolic disorders. This is one of the most important areas presently being investigated, and substantial advances can be anticipated in the years ahead. The technique of recombinant DNA is particularly promising for the production of enzymes that could be effectively administered. Perhaps even more promising is the possibility that molecular genetic technology will lead to somatic gene therapy (Ledley, 1987).

▪ SPECIFIC DIAGNOSIS

Whenever the possibility of an inborn error of metabolism is suspected in a newborn because of clinical signs in the infant or the discovery of a family history of a disorder, it is important to conduct laboratory tests that can detect metabolic disorders in the newborn. It is especially important to be certain that the proper blood and/or urine specimens are submitted. Since some of these tests are complicated, they may not be available in certain states or regions. This is particularly true for organic acid analyses. In this case, the physician should check with a medical center laboratory or a screening facility to determine where they can be performed. Certain large laboratories perform comprehensive screening for inborn errors and will accept specimens from throughout the United States as well as from other countries. The American Academy of Pediatrics has published a list of these facilities with the names and addresses of individuals who can be contacted (American Academy of Pediatrics, Committee on Nutrition, 1976).

The type of specimen that is appropriate for testing depends on the inborn error of metabolism suspected. For instance, phenylketonuria (PKU) is far more likely to be detected by examining a blood specimen than a urine specimen. Conversely, argininosuccinic acidemia is far more readily identified by testing urine than by examining blood. For other diseases, such as galactosemia, both blood and urine tests are desirable for a definitive diagnosis. In general, however, whenever there is any reason to suspect an inborn error of metabolism, both blood and urine should be submitted for examination. The filter-paper blood specimen collected for routine neonatal screening may be sufficient for a specific diagnosis in some instances, although plasma, serum, or liquid whole blood is usually preferable. Similarly, a urine specimen blotted into filter paper may be sufficient for the detection of certain disorders, but a liquid urine specimen is often desirable. The laboratory at which the testing will be performed should be consulted for information about the type of specimen(s) that should be obtained.

Certain clinical signs in the newborn should alert one to the possibility that an inborn error of metabolism is present. These signs, listed in Table 18–1, include pro-

TABLE 18–1. Major Clinical Signs in the Neonatal Period That Suggest the Presence of an Inborn Error of Metabolism

SIGNS	POSSIBLE DISORDER(S)
Jaundice Hepatomegaly Lethargy Weight loss Poor feeding	Galactosemia Tyrosinemia
Lethargy Hypotonicity or spasticity Vomiting Poor feeding Metabolic acidosis	Maple syrup urine disease Methylmalonic acidemia Isovaleric acidemia Propionic acidemia (Other) organic acidemias
Lethargy Poor feeding Hypotonicity Hyperammonemia	Urea cycle disorder
Lethargy Poor feeding Hypotonicity Poor respirations	Nonketotic hyperglycinemia
Obstipation (meconium ileus) Abdominal distention Vomiting	Cystic fibrosis

longed and unexplained jaundice, lethargy, weight loss or lack of weight gain, vomiting, poor feeding, and neurologic features such as convulsions or hypotonia. On occasion, a distinctive odor can be appreciated. Two general laboratory findings, hyperammonemia and metabolic acidosis, may be associated with one or more of these clinical signs and may be present in several different inborn errors of metabolism. Thus, among the first tests that should be obtained when one or more of these clinical signs appear are the determination of blood ammonia and of the state of acid-base balance. If the blood ammonia level is increased, there would be reason to suspect one of the urea cycle disorders. In the event of metabolic acidosis, maple syrup urine disease or one of the inborn errors of organic acid metabolism may be present. These disorders are discussed in more detail later.

A newborn with an organic acid metabolic disorder may have hyperammonemia and metabolic acidosis, although the hyperammonemia in this instance is usually less severe than that with the urea cycle disorders. Conversely, metabolic acidosis is usually not present with a urea cycle disorder.

It is important to remember that routine newborn screening for metabolic disorders, even when multiple testing is performed, does not cover most inborn errors of metabolism (see Neonatal Screening). Thus, any newborn with signs of a metabolic disorder (Table 18–1) should be tested for an inborn error by the comprehensive examination of blood *and* urine. Delays in the diagnosis and treatment of these disorders are often due to the mistaken notion that an infant who has received newborn screening with presumed negative results cannot have a metabolic disorder. This misconception can result in tragedy to the families of these patients—tragedy that is preventable.

CARBOHYDRATE DISORDERS

■ GALACTOSEMIA

Galactosemia is an inborn error of metabolism that usually produces clinically recognizable illness within the first few days of life. Observations from routine newborn screening for galactosemia indicate, however, that this disorder is frequently overlooked in the assessment of the sick newborn, despite the fact that a simple urine test for reducing substances can quickly lead to the diagnosis. Early diagnosis and the prompt institution of relatively simple dietary therapy prevents neonatal death from galactosemia and leads to a normal, or near-normal, life in an infant who otherwise faces the possibilities of cataracts, cirrhosis, and mental retardation.

The salient clinical features of galactosemia in the newborn include jaundice, hepatomegaly, lethargy, poor feeding, excessive and continuing weight loss, and vomiting. By the age of 10 to 14 days, many galactosemic infants become septic, usually with *Escherichia coli,* unless dietary treatment has been given. Sepsis in a galactosemic infant is usually accompanied by meningitis and is almost always fatal despite antibiotic therapy. If sepsis does not intervene, the untreated newborn may recover from the clinical illness but will later develop the chronic complications of cataracts, cirrhosis, and mental retardation.

The urine of the untreated galactosemic newborn yields strongly positive results for reducing substance (galactose) but yields negative results on specific testing for glucose. Albuminuria and hyperaminoaciduria may also be present. The diagnosis is confirmed by specific testing of blood, which will reveal markedly increased concentrations of galactose and galactose-1-phosphate and the absence of erythrocyte galactose-1-phosphate uridyltransferase (GALT) activity. Treatment consists of eliminating all foods containing lactose from the diet. The prognosis for normal physical and mental development is good when treatment is begun early in the neonatal period and is continued throughout life.

The presence of increased galactose in blood and urine may be due to a defect in either of two other galactose metabolic enzymes. These two entities, galactokinase deficiency and uridine diphosphate galactose 4-epimerase deficiency, are discussed in the following section, and the term galactosemia refers only to the deficiency in GALT activity. Even within galactosemia, however, there are a number of variants, each representing a different genetic disorder. These variants, listed in Table 18–2, may or may not result in clinical disease, depending on the amount of residual enzyme activity and perhaps other factors that are as yet undetermined. Since galactose-1-phosphate accumulates in blood and galactose may be present in urine in the variants as in classic galactosemia, the initial diagnostic processes are identical, as is the therapy.

Incidence. The average frequency of galactosemia throughout the world is about one case per 50,000 infants, as based on data from routine newborn screening. This frequency varies from one case per 30,000 in some countries (e.g., Switzerland) to less than one case per 100,000 in other countries. These differences in the observed frequency, to some extent, may be a result of differences in screening effectiveness. It has become clear that infants with galactosemia may be missed, often due to poor selection of screening methods but on occasion even in well-organized and well-conducted programs that use optimal screening methods.

Etiology. Galactosemia is a genetic disorder transmitted as an autosomal recessive trait. The mutant gene encodes an altered protein that has little or no GALT activity. This defective enzyme may also have a different electrophoretic mobility from the normal enzyme (Table 18–2), indicating that the structure of the enzyme protein is abnormal, possibly in the substitution of a single amino acid residue, as in the case of sickle hemoglobin. The gene for GALT has now been cloned (Reichardt and Berg, 1988) and in all likelihood the mutations responsible for galactosemia will soon be identified.

Heterozygotes (carriers) usually have about 50 per cent of normal erythrocyte GALT activity, as expected, and often have abnormalities in the galactose tolerance curve. Nevertheless, they are clinically normal and do not have detectable galactose and/or galactose-1-phosphate in their blood or galactose in their urine when they are on a normal diet.

Pathology. In the newborn or young infant, the liver is enlarged and there is a striking fatty change without excess glycogen deposition. This fatty change should lead to the suspicion of galactosemia in an undiagnosed newborn who dies with hepatomegaly, lethargy, and perhaps, sepsis. Blood obtained from the heart postmortem and spotted on filter paper (PKU-type specimen) can be sent to a newborn screening laboratory for galactosemia testing. In addition, the original newborn blood specimen that was submitted for routine metabolic screening (see Chapter 17) can be recovered from the screening laboratory and tested (or re-tested) for galactosemia.

Later in infancy or childhood, the alterations of portal cirrhosis are seen, including periportal fibrosis and bile duct regeneration. This may progress to full-blown nodular cirrhosis of the Laennec type. The ocular lenses may show the characteristic opacification of cataract formation.

The neuropathology of galactosemia has only been reported in two older children. The findings included scattered areas of hypomyelination in the cerebral white matter and loss of Purkinje cells in the cerebellum (Haberland et al., 1971).

Pathogenesis. Galactose enters the body as a result of the ingestion of milk or milk products. Lactose, the disaccharide of milk, is hydrolyzed by intestinal lactase to its monosaccharide constituents, glucose and galactose. These monosaccharides are transported through the intestinal wall into the portal system and carried to the liver. There the galactose is phosphorylated and, as galactose-1-phosphate, is exchanged for the glucose moiety of uridine diphosphate glucose to form uridine diphosphate galactose (Fig. 18–1). The glucose-1-phosphate released

TABLE 18–2. Characteristics Regarding Variants of Galactose-1-Phosphate Uridyl Transferase (GALT)

VARIANT	ERYTHROCYTE TRANSFERASE ACTIVITY (% of Normal)	STARCH-GEL ELECTROPHORETIC MOBILITY (Related to Normal)	OTHER BIOCHEMICAL CHARACTERISTICS	CLINICAL CHARACTERISTICS
"Classic"	0*	—	—	Disease†
Durate	50*	Faster	—	Benign
"Negro"	0*	—	10% activity in liver and intestine	Disease
Indiana	0–45	Slower	Unstable in heparinized blood and isotonic phosphate buffer	Disease
Rennes	7	Slower	—	Disease
Los Angeles	140	Faster	—	Benign

*This represents the activity in individuals homozygous for the variant.
†Jaundice, other neonatal signs with complications of cataracts, liver disease, and mental retardation.

is eventually converted to carbon dioxide through the glucose monophosphate shunt. The uridine diphosphate galactose may serve as galactose donor for the synthesis of galactolipids and galactoproteins of cell membranes and brain or may be epimerized to uridine diphosphate glucose for re-entry into the cycle.

This metabolic pathway involves several enzymes (Fig. 18–1) that are normally expressed in virtually all tissues including erythrocytes. In galactosemia, activity of the GALT enzyme is markedly deficient or undetectable. As a result, galactose-1-phosphate accumulates in body cells. The accumulated galactose-1-phosphate inhibits the activity of galactokinase (product or feedback inhibition), and galactose also accumulates. Galactose-1-phosphate remains within the cell, and it is detectable only in erythrocytes or in other cells. Galactose, however, freely exchanges between intracellular and extracellular spaces and, as a result, is detectable within cells and in extracellular compartments such as plasma or serum and urine.

Galactose in the ocular lens is converted to galactitol, establishing an osmotic gradient that draws fluid into the lens. This causes swelling of the lens, denaturation and precipitation of lenticular protein, and eventually, cataract formation. It is believed that the damage to other organs, primarily brain, liver, and kidney, results from intracellular toxicity of galactose-1-phosphate. According to this concept of pathogenesis, galactose-1-phosphate accumulates in neurons, hepatocytes, and renal tubular cells, causing damage that eventually results, respectively, in mental retardation, cirrhosis, and renal tubular dysfunction characterized by the renal Fanconi syndrome.

There are a number of secondary abnormalities for which there is as yet no clear explanation. Most prominent among these is the marked hypoglycemia that is often present when there is acute neonatal illness from galactosemia. This may be due to reduced gluconeogenesis as a direct result of the enzyme deficiency, but it is perhaps more likely that the hepatocellular disease results in impaired gluconeogenesis and hypoglycemia, as occurs in liver disease from other causes. The hepatocellular disease does account for the marked aberrations in liver function and, probably, for the hyperaminoacidemia in which tyrosine and methionine are notably elevated but that also includes almost all the measurable free amino acids in blood.

Diagnosis. The phenotype associated with galactosemia in the newborn varies widely from clinical normality to very severe and often precipitous disease characterized by marked jaundice, hepatosplenomegaly, vomiting, lethargy, and weight loss that, if untreated, results in sepsis and death. This clinical spectrum is usually associated with a range of GALT activity that varies from undetectable in the very ill infant to 10 per cent of normal activity in the newborn who is clinically normal. However, occasionally an infant with no detectable activity remains free of neonatal illness. Furthermore, the black infant may have the "Negro variant," in which GALT is virtually undetectable in erythrocytes but present in low activity in liver and in which there also may be no symptoms in the neonatal period. Thus, routine newborn screening for galactosemia is very valuable in the early identification of infants who

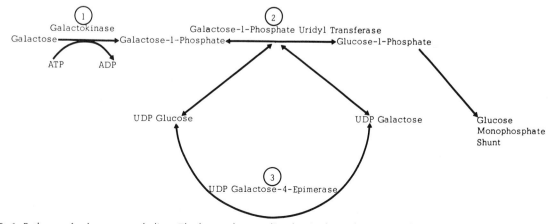

FIGURE 18–1. Pathway of galactose metabolism. The known human disorders in this pathway are indicated by the numbered enzyme deficient in each disorder.

would otherwise not be diagnosed until clinical illness occurs or who may be overlooked despite illness.

In the infant who is ill, the greatest immediate danger appears to be sepsis, most often due to *E. coli*. As a result of routine newborn screening, it is now known that a number of newborns with galactosemia have died because of sepsis and were not recognized as having galactosemia until abnormalities in the screening test directed attention to the disorder.

The clinically ill newborn usually develops jaundice on the 2nd or 3rd day of life. The jaundice increases, and by the 5th or 6th day of life the infant has hepatomegaly, perhaps splenomegaly, vomiting, excessive weight loss, lethargy, and occasionally, diarrhea. Cataracts are not obvious at this time, although careful ophthalmologic examination reveals a "water drop" clouding of the optic lenses. If milk is not withdrawn, these clinical signs worsen and sepsis may intervene, at which point death may be unavoidable. In the absence of sepsis, the signs of disease may spontaneously disappear, despite the continuation of the feeding of milk. These infants will develop the chronic abnormalities of galactosemia later in infancy or in childhood.

Laboratory Investigations

Galactosuria and Melituria. Within less than 1 hour after the ingestion of milk, galactose-1-phosphate can be demonstrated in whole blood and galactose appears in blood and urine. The diagnosis can be readily made by testing a blood–filter paper blood specimen (PKU specimen) for galactose and galactose-1-phosphate, using either a bacterial or a chemical assay. These procedures may be most efficiently performed in a central state or regional laboratory that conducts routine newborn screening for metabolic disorders. The large amount of urinary galactose can be detected as reducing substance by a strongly positive reaction to Benedict solution. This is most readily shown by testing the urine with a test tablet for reducing substance.*

When testing the urine, one should be aware that the commonly used dipstick method does not identify galactose because it utilizes glucose oxidase for the test result and thus is specific for glucose. When this is the only method used in the nursery or in the laboratory that tests urine specimens from the nursery, galactosemia is missed. Accordingly, whenever a urinalysis is performed in the newborn, the test for urinary sugar should always be one that detects reducing substances rather than the dipstick type. If there is reducing substance in the urine, a dipstick test for glucose should then be performed. In galactosemia, this latter test will be negative or at most only slightly positive, consistent with the fact that most or all of the reducing substance is galactose. The identity of galactose in urine can be verified by a chromatographic method for sugars or by a specific chemical or bacterial assay.

Two facts should be kept in mind when examining urine from an infant suspected of having galactosemia. The first is that normal newborns may excrete detectable amounts of reducing substance, mostly lactose or glucose. Occasionally, the quantity is sufficient to produce a strong reaction with Benedict solution. These infants have a

normal result on blood testing for galactosemia. The other fact is that the urine remains free of galactose in galactosemic infants unless milk is fed. This obvious fact may be overlooked when evaluating a sick newborn who is receiving only intravenous fluids. This infant, however, has increased erythrocyte galactose-1-phosphate levels, so an appropriate blood test (e.g., an assay that responds to galactose-1-phosphate as well as to galactose) will be positive and will verify suspected galactosemia.

Proteinuria. Albumin is usually present during acute illness due to galactosemia and disappears within 2 to 4 days after milk is withdrawn. The albuminuria varies from a trace to a moderately large amount.

Formed Elements in the Urine. Red blood cells, white blood cells, and casts of various kinds may be present in the urine.

Hyperaminoaciduria. A marked increase in the excretion of virtually all free amino acids in the urine occurs during acute illness. Although this hyperaminoaciduria is accompanied by an increased concentration of blood amino acids, it is far in excess of what is expected in "overflow" from blood and is caused by the renal tubular damage and resulting impaired renal transport of amino acids. The hyperaminoaciduria is not a specific type but is similar to that seen in small premature infants or in those with renal tubular malabsorption due to other causes of the renal Fanconi syndrome. When milk is withdrawn, the hyperaminoaciduria disappears in 2 to 4 days.

Galactose Tolerance. After the oral administration of a loading dose of galactose (1.25 to 1.50 g/kg), the blood galactose and galactose-1-phosphate concentrations increase to an inordinately high level (100 to 200 mg/dl) and remain markedly elevated for 5 hours or more.

Galactose tolerance tests probably should not be performed in infants with proven galactosemia or in those even suspected of having galactosemia. The marked accumulations of galactose and galactose-1-phosphate, as well as the hypoglycemia, that occur after a loading dose of galactose in galactosemic infants and children could result in irreversible organ damage. For clinical diagnosis and therapy, galactosemia can be very adequately studied on the basis of response to a milk feeding, which produces elevations in blood galactose and galactose-1-phosphate that are less dramatic and more rapidly resolved than those that occur after a galactose load. A milk feeding will differentiate infants with GALT variants from those with classic galactosemia (Fig. 18–2). Furthermore, enzyme assays using erythrocytes or cultured skin fibroblasts almost always determine the specific type and degree of galactosemia.

Liver Function. One of the first signs of galactosemia is neonatal jaundice. By the 3rd to 5th day of life, jaundice is often quite substantial, with total serum bilirubin concentrations of approximately 14 to 18 mg/dl. If the galactosemia remains untreated, the serum bilirubin level will usually continue to increase, and by 7 to 9 days of life it may be as high as 20 mg/dl or higher. The hyperbilirubinemia frequently leads to exchange transfusion in the undiagnosed newborn. It is often stated that the bilirubin is predominantly of the direct-reacting (conjugated) type, suggesting that the hyperbilirubinemia is due to liver damage, perhaps obstructive in nature. Recent observations, however, indicate that the early hyperbilirubinemia

---

*Clinitest (Miles Inc., Diagnostic Division, Elkhart, IN 46515).

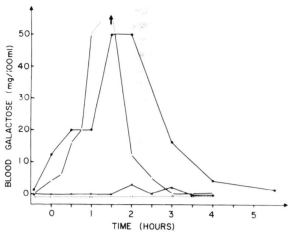

FIGURE 18–2. Galactose tolerance curves following the ingestion of milk that contains 0.78 g of galactose (in the form of lactose) per kilogram of body weight for normal control subjects (△····△); a Duarte/ "classic" galactosemia mixed heterozygous patient (▲—▲); a "classic" galactosemic patient on dietary treatment (●—●); and a patient with Rennes variant on dietary treatment (○—○). (From Hammersen, G., Houghton, S., and Levy, H. L.: Rennes-like variant of galactosemia; Clinical and biochemical studies. J. Pediatr. 87:50–57, 1975. Reproduced by permission of the Journal of Pediatrics.)

of the galactosemic newborn may be predominantly of the indirect-reacting (unconjugated) type. This can still be explained by inhibition of the bilirubin conjugating mechanism by galactose-1-phosphate or other toxic metabolites that accumulate in galactosemia. Coagulopathy with increased prothrombin time and partial thromboplastin time is also usually present within the 1st week of life in untreated galactosemia and can be quite severe, even life threatening. Other indicators of liver damage, such as elevated levels of serum glutamic-oxaloacetic transaminase and of serum alkaline phosphatase, may be present, but often these findings do not appear until the 2nd week of life. Within 2 to 3 days after the withdrawal of milk, the serum bilirubin concentration begins to recede, and other markers of liver dysfunction begin to return to normal.

Renal Function. Basic kidney function seems to remain intact, despite impaired tubular transport of amino acids. The blood urea nitrogen concentration, the specific gravity of the urine, and the excretion of electrolytes remain within normal limits.

Blood Elements. There is usually little or no alteration in the indices of hematologic function. In particular, evidence of hemolysis is almost always absent. Hemoglobin usually remains normal, as does the reticulocyte count. If neonatal sepsis intervenes, however, any of the hematologic signs of this dire complication may be present. These signs include anemia, evidence of hemolysis, alterations in the white blood cell count, and thrombocytopenia.

Treatment. Treatment consists of the elimination of milk and milk products from the diet at the moment the diagnosis is established. This means that breast-feeding or feeding of any milk-containing formula or of whole milk must cease, and a nonmilk formula must be substituted. Two types of formulas are used. One is soybean based, and several of these products are readily available. The carbohydrate source in soybean-based formulas is su-

crose, a disaccharide consisting of glucose and fructose. The other type of acceptable formula is casein hydrolysate based, in which the carbohydrate source is usually glucose. If there is substantial hypoglycemia and if the infant is feeding poorly or is dehydrated, it is wise to institute nonspecific intravenous fluid therapy for replacement and maintenance. If the infant is ill, cultures (blood, urine, and cerebrospinal fluid) should be obtained, and antibiotic therapy effective against E. coli and other gram-negative organisms should be given *before* the results of the cultures are available. This is particularly important, since galactosemia is so often associated with sepsis.

The galactosemic individual will probably have to remain on a diet that excludes milk and milk products for the remainder of his or her life. In contrast to infants with many other inborn errors of metabolism, galactosemic patients may readily ingest protein-rich foods such as meats and fish. Thus, the diet in galactosemia can be relatively easily administered and tolerated. It should be monitored at regular intervals in a specific pediatric metabolic unit.

Prognosis. Unless the diagnosis is made during the 1st week or two of life, the infant may die with sepsis. Should the infant survive and not receive treatment until late in infancy or childhood, the cirrhosis and cataracts that develop may remain or they may regress on treatment after having been present for surprisingly long periods of time.

Early diagnosis and treatment prevents cataracts and chronic liver disease. The prognosis with respect to mental development is not yet known with certainty; however, there appears to be little doubt that the frank mental deficiency observed in untreated or late-treated galactosemia is to a great extent, if not entirely, a result of the disease. This mental deficiency is largely or completely preventable by early and correct treatment.

Despite the benefits of early treatment, it is now known that even these infants may later develop certain chronic complications of galactosemia (Buist et al., 1988). These complications include speech defects (Waisbren et al., 1983), learning disabilities (Buist et al., 1988), ovarian failure (Kaufman et al., 1981) and, occasionally, a progressive neurologic disability with tremors and ataxia (Lo et al., 1984). The cause of these complications is unknown. One theory is that they are due to a deficiency of uridine diphosphate galactose, which has been documented in erythrocytes and cultured fibroblasts from treated patients (Ng et al., 1987). The uridine diphosphate galactose levels are restored to normal when cultured fibroblasts from these patients are exposed to uridine. Treating patients with oral uridine has also resulted in an increase of the erythrocyte uridine diphosphate galactose levels to normal values. Uridine therapy as an adjunct to milk avoidance in galactosemia is currently under investigation to determine whether or not this method might prevent these complications.

CASE STUDY

A male infant was born to a primigravida mother after a normal pregnancy and full-term gestation. Delivery was by breech extraction under spinal anesthesia. Apgar scores were 6 at 1 minute and 9 at 5 minutes. Birth measurements were as follows: weight, 3180 g (7 pounds); length, 50 cm; and head circumference, 35.5 cm. Breast-feeding was attempted but was abandoned on the 3rd day, and the infant was formula-fed thereafter.

Jaundice was noted on the 4th day, with total serum bilirubin level at 15.8 mg/dl (1.2 mg/dl direct reactive). Phototherapy was instituted. On the 6th day, the total serum bilirubin level was 14.0 mg/dl, but the patient was lethargic and had excessive weight loss. Sepsis was suspected, and cultures of blood, cerebrospinal fluid, and urine were initiated. Antibiotic therapy was begun. The cerebrospinal fluid contained a total sugar concentration of 235 mg/dl, and the blood total sugar concentration was 300 mg/dl. The sugar was not further characterized, and a form of neonatal diabetes mellitus was initially suspected. On the 7th day, the state newborn screening laboratory reported by telephone that the results of screening tests on the routine blood specimen (obtained on the 3rd day) indicated the diagnosis of galactosemia. Specifically, this specimen contained a very large amount of galactose and galactose-1-phosphate (greater than 50 mg/dl) and the enzyme spot screening test for GALT revealed no evidence of activity. Blood amino acid analysis at this time revealed a generalized increase with particularly prominent increases in methionine and tyrosine. The infant was immediately switched from regular formula to a casein hydrolysate–based formula.

By the 9th day, the infant began to improve with a reduction in the degree of jaundice and an initiation of weight gain. The cultures that were obtained on the 6th day were reported as negative, so the antibiotic therapy was discontinued. Ophthalmologic examination with a slit-lamp disclosed a small amount of opacity in both lenses consistent with the early cataract formation found in galactosemia but thought to be reversible.

On the 10th day (3 days after milk was withdrawn), the blood galactose and galactose-1-phosphate level was only 4 mg/dl, and by the 13th day, neither galactose nor galactose-1-phosphate was detectable in blood or urine. Blood and urine amino acid levels were also normal. At this time, the patient was no longer jaundiced, was gaining weight, and was active. He was discharged on the 21st day.

At home, the casein hydrolysate–based formula was continued. The infant was allowed to have all baby foods and, later, other solid foods that did not contain milk or milk products. When he was weaned from the bottle, he was given fruit juices as a substitute and a daily calcium supplement to supply calcium needs that are ordinarily fulfilled by normal milk intake.

His growth and development have been normal. He has no signs of liver disease, and his ocular lenses are clear with no evidence of cataracts. He did have delayed speech with some minor speech and language difficulties, but these were overcome with speech therapy. He is now 14 years old, is physically normal, and has normal intelligence.

Confirmatory enzyme studies of erythrocytes revealed no detectable GALT activity in this boy and approximately 50 per cent of normal activity in each parent. These findings are consistent with the autosomal recessive mode of inheritance known to be present in galactosemia.

Comment. This patient developed many of the characteristic findings of galactosemia in the newborn nursery, including unexplained jaundice, lethargy, and excessive weight loss. Galactosemia was not initially recognized because the elevated sugar in his blood and cerebrospinal fluid was mistakenly assumed to be glucose. Simple urine tests for reducing substance and for glucose (the latter would have been negative) would have established the diagnosis of galactosemia, but unfortunately, these were

not performed. However, routine newborn screening in the state does include testing for galactosemia, so a potential tragedy was avoided.

■ GALACTOKINASE AND URIDINE DIPHOSPHATE GALACTOSE-4-EPIMERASE DEFICIENCIES

Galactose may appear in blood and urine as a result of deficient activity of galactokinase or uridine diphosphate galactose-4-epimerase (see Fig. 18–1). Galactokinase deficiency has been identified in the newborn as well as in older children. In contrast to galactosemia, this condition is not associated with an accumulation of galactose-1-phosphate. In the untreated state, cataracts develop during infancy or early childhood; but, unlike galactosemia, galactokinase deficiency produces no neonatal symptoms, and other complications such as liver disease and mental retardation do not occur. The diagnosis is suspected when a large amount of galactose alone is discovered in the blood and urine and is confirmed by the demonstration of markedly reduced or absent galactokinase activity in erythrocytes. The treatment is identical with that for galactosemia in that milk and milk products are excluded from the diet. Neonatal screening in which an assay for galactose is performed should detect galactokinase deficiency as well as galactosemia. It is important to identify and treat this disorder in the neonatal period in order to prevent the formation of cataracts.

Uridine diphosphate galactose-4-epimerase (epimerase) deficiency has been described in only a few families. The affected infants or older individuals accumulate a small amount of galactose in blood and a much larger amount of galactose-1-phosphate in erythrocytes. In most affected infants, no signs of disease have been noted. It is likely that they have a localized enzymatic defect. Two reported infants, however, have had jaundice, hepatomegaly and failure to thrive identical to infants with galactosemia (Henderson et al., 1983; Sardharwalla et al., 1988). They are considered to have a generalized defect in epimerase. They were treated with milk withdrawal, but both became mentally retarded, suggesting that in clinically expressing (generalized) epimerase deficiency, additional therapy may be necessary. The diagnosis is confirmed by the demonstration of reduced epimerase activity in erythrocytes.

■ GLYCOGEN STORAGE DISEASES

At least eight different inherited abnormalities of glycogen metabolism can lead to the same effect—an excessive accumulation of glycogen in tissues. Some of these may produce clinical abnormalities in the neonatal period, whereas others do not become symptomatic until later in life. The three types that can produce neonatal findings are discussed in the subsequent paragraphs.

TYPE I (VON GIERKE DISEASE)

In this rare disorder, there is a striking accumulation of glycogen in liver and kidneys. It is due to either a deficiency in glucose-6-phosphatase activity or a defect in the microsomal uptake of glucose-6-phosphate. Both forms are inherited as autosomal recessive traits.

Clinical Findings. The affected newborn has hepatomegaly and may be hypoglycemic. Otherwise, the newborn period is usually normal but by several months of age abdominal enlargement appears because of massive hepatomegaly, loss of appetite, and vomiting. In some instances, "sinking spells" (sudden onset of lethargy) and even convulsions due to hypoglycemia are noted.

Diagnosis. Type I glycogen storage disease is suspected because of hepatomegaly. Withdrawal of food for a few hours leads to hypoglycemia, lactic acidemia, and pyruvic acidemia. The hypoglycemia is unresponsive to the administration of epinephrine and glucagon. Other laboratory findings include elevated serum triglycerides, phospholipids, cholesterol, and uric acid. Liver biopsy reveals liver cells that contain vacuoles filled with glycogen. In type 1a disease, reduced or absent glucose-6-phosphatase activity is demonstrated by enzyme assay of liver tissue. In type 1b disease, liver glucose-6-phosphatase activity is normal but is inactive in vivo because of a defect in the microsomal uptake of glucose-6-phosphate, the substrate for the enzyme (Nordlie and Sukalski, 1986).

Prognosis. Without continuous therapy to control the hypoglycemia, affected infants fail to grow adequately and some die within the first years of life. Those who are less severely affected survive but have stunted growth, persistent hypoglycemia, and a bleeding diathesis. If the affected individuals live beyond age 4 years, the abdomen becomes less prominent, and the prognosis progressively improves. In type 1b disease, neutropenia, neutrophil dysfunction, and recurrent infections are a distinctive feature (Narisawa et al., 1987).

Treatment. Affected infants are given frequent feedings during the day and continuous nasogastric feedings through the night to counteract the hypoglycemia (Folk and Greene, 1984). The feedings may need to be given every 3 or 4 hours. Older children are treated with uncooked corn starch made up in a slurry every 4–6 hours (Chen et al., 1984). Hypoglycemic crises must be treated vigorously with glucose infusions.

TYPE II (GENERALIZED GLYCOGENOSIS; POMPE DISEASE)

Type II glycogen storage disease usually comes to attention because of its effects on the heart. There is massive cardiomegaly accompanied by an extremely abnormal electrocardiogram. There is also marked hypotonia, although the muscles are firm and of normal mass. The tongue may be enlarged, and there is a failure to thrive. Diagnosis is confirmed by muscle biopsy demonstrating increased concentration of glycogen with normal structure. Enzyme confirmation is obtained by demonstration of virtual absence of alpha-glucosidase in leukocytes. There is no known effective treatment.

TYPE III ("DEBRANCHER" DISEASE)

Patients with Type III glycogen storage disease may have a clinical appearance that is similar to that of babies with Type I glycogen storage disease. Hepatomegaly develops early in infancy, and growth retardation may be striking. There is also hypoglycemia and hyperlipidemia. Unlike those with Type I disease, however, these patients may have splenomegaly but no renal involvement.

The enzyme deficiency is in amylo-1,6-glucosidase (debrancher) activity. The diagnosis is confirmed by complicated enzyme studies of muscle and liver. The disorder is inherited as an autosomal recessive trait. Treatment includes frequent feedings to offset the hypoglycemic tendency (Slonim et al., 1984). The prognosis may be good, since Type III disease is milder than Type I disease and the hepatomegaly may disappear at puberty.

■ ESSENTIAL BENIGN FRUCTOSURIA

Fructosuria appears in infants who have an inherited deficiency of fructokinase, an enzyme that phosphorylates fructose to fructose-1-phosphate. The disorder is transmitted as an autosomal recessive trait. The diagnosis is made through discovery of urinary reducing substance that is identified as fructose and through demonstration of prolonged and high curves of blood fructose concentration after the oral or intravenous administration of fructose. The disorder is benign, and no treatment is required.

■ HEREDITARY FRUCTOSE INTOLERANCE

This inborn error of fructose metabolism is inherited as an autosomal recessive trait and produces clinical abnormalities when fruit or sucrose, a disaccharide that consists of fructose and glucose, is ingested. Following fructose ingestion, fructose and fructose-1-phosphate accumulate in the body, a result of deficient aldolase B activity. Soon after even the first ingestion of fructose, infants with this condition develop poor feeding, vomiting, failure to thrive, and hepatomegaly. Symptoms such as lethargy and clinical findings such as pallor, hemorrhage, and jaundice may also be present.

The diagnosis is suspected when an infant with these findings has a history of fructose (or sucrose) ingestion. Formerly, this did not occur until about the 2nd month of life or later, when fruit is first added to the infant's diet. Fructose ingestion may now occur much earlier in life, however, since a number of formulas (particularly those that are soybean based) contain sucrose as the source of carbohydrate. Thus, clinical illness from hereditary fructose intolerance can occur early in the neonatal period.

Laboratory. The laboratory findings include the presence of reducing substance in the urine (which consists of both fructose and glucose); hyperaminoaciduria; abnormal liver function test results such as elevations in serum glutamic-oxaloactic transaminase, serum alkaline phosphatase, and prothrombin time; hypokalemia; and hypophosphatemia. Blood amino acid analysis may reveal increased tyrosine and methionine, and the diagnosis may be confused with hereditary tyrosinemia (see Hereditary Tyrosinemia, in this chapter).

Diagnosis. The differential diagnosis in an infant with this clinical picture who has ingested fructose includes galactosemia, hereditary tyrosinemia, sepsis, neonatal hepatitis, and liver dysfunction of unknown origin. Galactosemia and sepsis are respectively excluded on the basis of negative tests for galactose and galactose-1-phosphate in blood (see Galactosemia) and negative cultures. The other possibilities are more difficult to exclude, and the diagnosis of hereditary fructose intolerance may be confirmed by an intravenous fructose tolerance test. For this test, a fructose dose of 0.2 to 0.3 gm/kg is given in a single injection. Within 20 to 40 minutes, blood glucose and serum phosphate decrease markedly. A fructose tolerance test should be performed *only* in a hospital under carefully controlled conditions with intravenous fluid administered, since marked hypoglycemia and, perhaps, hypokalemia can occur precipitously in an affected infant. The finding of decreased liver aldolase activity by direct enzyme assay provides definitive evidence for the diagnosis. Cloning and characterization of the aldolase B gene (Rottman et al., 1984; Tolan and Penhoet, 1986) have resulted in the identification of mutations that produce hereditary fructose intolerance (Cross et al., 1988). Consequently, the diagnosis can now be confirmed and the mutation identified by molecular genetic techniques.

Treatment. When the diagnosis is established, treatment must begin immediately by withdrawal of sources of fructose from the diet. This includes the elimination of all fruits, sugar, and formulas that contain sucrose.

Prognosis. Following treatment, the symptoms and signs, except hepatomegaly, usually resolve almost immediately. Fatty changes in the liver may persist for many months, but this also eventually resolves.

AMINO ACID DISORDERS

In evaluating clinical illness, metabolic tests usually include blood and/or urine amino acid analysis. Newborn screening also includes the measurement of specific amino acids. Consequently, amino acid disorders are among the most frequently identified inborn errors of metabolism. It is neither necessary nor desirable to discuss all of the 40 or more inborn errors in this category. Many are very rare and not likely to be encountered. Others are quite likely to be seen either because of clinical presentation in the newborn period or as a result of routine newborn screening (see Chapter 17). Early recognition is important since irreversible damage can often be prevented by therapy that begins during the first days or weeks of life. Identification of the specific disorder may be difficult, however, and confirmation requires an experienced laboratory with on-site direction by a physician or other professional who specializes in pediatric metabolic disorders. This type of laboratory should be contacted before specific therapy is given and whenever a question concerning the diagnosis of one of these disorders arises.

■ PHENYLKETONURIA

Phenylketonuria (PKU) is an inborn error of amino acid metabolism involving phenylalanine. It should always come to attention as a result of routine newborn screening (see Chapter 17). Treatment must begin in the neonatal period or no later than early infancy if mental retardation is to be prevented.

Incidence. The general frequency is about one in 12,000 individuals. Among different countries, the frequency varies between one per 6,000 to less than one per 200,000. The frequency also varies among different ethnic groups (Scriver and Clow, 1980). The highest frequencies are reported in Ireland, among Americans of Irish descent, and in Yemenite Jews in Israel. Relatively high frequencies are also reported in Eastern Europe. On the other hand, the frequency in Japan is less than one per 200,000, and PKU is rarely found among blacks and Ashkenazi Jews. Approximately 1 to 2 per cent of individuals institutionalized for mental retardation have PKU.

Etiology and Pathogenesis. PKU is inherited as an autosomal recessive trait. Approximately 2 per cent of most populations carry the gene. In affected PKU individuals (those who inherit two mutant genes), the genetic abnormality results in an almost total lack of phenylalanine hydroxylase activity, which in turn results in an inability to convert phenylalanine to tyrosine (Fig. 18–3). This produces a marked accumulation of phenylalanine in the

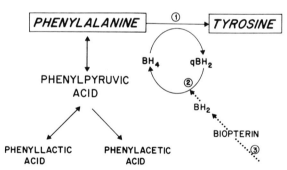

FIGURE 18–3. *Pathway of phenylalanine hydroxylation. The hydroxylating enzyme, phenylalanine hydroxylase (1), requires tetrahydrobiopterin (BH₄) for activity. The reduced pterin is oxidized to quininoid dihydrobiopterin (qBH₂) in this reaction. The qBH₂ is reduced back to BH₄ via activity of dihydropteridine reductase (2). Dihydrobiopterin (BH₂) also enters this cycle as a reduced product of biopterin. The pathway of biopterin synthesis is controlled by several enzymes, among which two, 6-pyruvoyl-tetrahydropterin synthase (3) and GTP cyclohydrolase are involved in inborn errors of pterin metabolism.*

The most frequent cause of increased phenylalanine concentration and the accumulation of phenylpyruvic acid and other metabolites is a defect in the apoenzyme phenylalanine hydroxylase. This produces phenylketonuria (PKU), atypical PKU, and mild hyperphenylalaninemia. In rare cases, phenylalanine and metabolite accumulations are caused by a defect in dihydropteridine reductase or a defect in the synthesis of biopterin, both of which result in BH₄ deficiency. This produces a marked reduction in phenylalanine hydroxylase activation and must be differentiated from PKU.

blood, urine, and tissues when the diet is normal. In children and adults with untreated PKU, phenylalanine metabolites, including phenylpyruvic acid, phenylactic acid, phenylacetic acid, phenylacetylglutamine, and *o*-hydroxyphenylacetic acid are also increased in blood and urine. In the newborn, however, there may be little or no urinary excretion of these metabolites, since their formation depends on activity of phenylalanine transaminase, an enzyme that may not become active until the infant is several months of age.

The brain damage in untreated PKU is probably a direct result of the accumulation of phenylalanine or its metabolites or both. When these concentrations are controlled by a special diet, mental retardation and other neurologic signs do not appear. However, the precise cause of the brain toxicity is unknown (Kaufman, 1976). Theories regarding pathogenesis include:

1. Direct toxic effect of phenylalanine or one of its metabolites
2. Deficiency of other brain amino acids due to inhibition of amino acid transport at the blood-brain barrier produced by increased phenylalanine
3. Reduction in synthesis of neurotransmitters due to increased phenylalanine in the brain
4. Reduced protein synthesis in brain caused by phenylalanine-induced disaggregation of polyribosomes
5. Inhibition by phenylalanine or phenylpyruvate of key glucose metabolic enzymes in brain.

Regardless of the immediate pathogenic mechanism, reduction in the accumulation of phenylalanine and its metabolites by a low-phenylalanine diet is the most effective therapy available.

Diagnosis. PKU should always be identified in the newborn by routine newborn screening. PKU cannot otherwise be suspected since the clinical signs of developmental delay and mental retardation do not appear until later in infancy or childhood (Levy, 1986). By then, much of the brain damage is irreversible. The frequency of prenatal, perinatal, and neonatal complications is no greater among phenylketonuric infants than in the general newborn population. Affected newborns usually appear to be normal.

Identification in the newborn is based on an increased concentration of phenylalanine in the blood. If PKU is known to be present in the family, usually in a sibling, the suspicion of PKU should be high, since the disorder is inherited. For example, if a sibling has PKU, each parent is presumed to carry the gene, and the probability that the newborn will have PKU is one in four. Regardless of family history, however, a PKU test should be performed on every newborn infant. In most infants with PKU, the blood phenylalanine concentration, normally 2 mg/dl (120 μM) or less, will be at least 6 mg/dl (360 μM) or greater by the 3rd day of life. An occasional infant with PKU, however, will have only a slightly increased phenylalanine level in the screened blood specimen. In order not to overlook this infant, one must obtain another blood specimen for PKU screening from any newborn infant whose blood phenylalanine concentration is greater than 2 mg/dl.

It is important to remember that urine from a newborn

with PKU rarely has a detectable increase in phenylalanine metabolites. Thus, the urine ferric chloride test for phenylpyruvic acid is almost always negative and ineffective in detecting PKU in the newborn period, although it may identify PKU in older infants and children. Consequently, a urine test is *not* reliable in the detection of PKU in the newborn infant.

Upon identification by newborn screening, the infant with an increased blood phenylalanine level should be referred to a pediatric metabolic center that is experienced in the diagnosis and treatment of PKU. If a referral such as this is impossible, at least direct contact with this type of center should be established so that the proper confirmatory and treatment procedures are initiated as soon as possible. For confirmation, all amino acids should be measured in blood by an accurate quantitative technique (e.g., amino acid analyzer). A specific elevation of the phenylalanine concentration to 20 mg/dl (1200 μM) or greater when the infant is on a normal diet indicates that classic PKU is present. When the confirmatory blood phenylalanine concentration is increased but less than 20 mg/dl, another degree of phenylalanine hydroxylase deficiency or type of biochemical defect may be present (Table 18–3). Since the defect in PKU results in failure of phenylalanine to convert to tyrosine (Fig. 18–3), the blood tyrosine concentration in the phenylketonuric infant is usually at the lower end of the normal range.

The phenylalanine hydroxylase gene has been cloned, and its cDNA with restriction enzymes has been used to examine the haplotypes determined by restriction fragment length polymorphism (RFLP) at the gene locus in normal and PKU populations. With this technique, chromosomes bearing either normal or mutant PKU alleles can be followed in many families with PKU. Consequently, prenatal diagnosis for PKU is now possible by examining cultured amniocytes obtained by amniocentesis. This can be done, however, only if the family is "informative," i.e., if there is already an affected individual in the family (usually a child) and each parent is heterozygous for RFLP haplotypes at the phenylalanine hydroxylase locus so that the two chromosomes from each parent can be separated. Despite the availability of prenatal diagnosis for PKU, most families have elected not to have it. The decision with regard to an affected fetus would be either to continue the pregnancy with knowledge that the baby will have PKU or terminate the pregnancy, and most families consider PKU a treatable disorder for which they would not terminate a pregnancy.

The mutations in the phenylalanine hydroxylase gene that cause PKU are now being identified (Levy, 1989). At least seven different PKU-linked mutations are known. Still other mutations will undoubtedly be found. The existence of many different mutations makes it quite certain that PKU has arisen in different areas of the world rather than having spread from one area.

In the near future it will be possible to determine the precise gene mutations(s) responsible for PKU in virtually every affected newborn. This will be accomplished using the allele-specific oligonucleotide (ASO) method, in which oligonucleotide probes with sequences that represent each of the known PKU-linked mutations as well as the normal probe will be applied to DNA from the identified infant. Hybridization occurring with a mutant probe will indicate

TABLE 18–3. Metabolic Disorders Associated with an Increased Blood Phenylalanine (Phe) Concentration

DISORDER	BLOOD PHE (mg/dl)	ENZYME DEFECT	TREATMENT
PKU	>20	Phe hydroxylase (<1%)	Diet
Atypical PKU	12≥20	Phe hydroxylase (2–3%)	Diet
Mild hyphe*	>2–<12	Phe hydroxylase (2–5%)	None
Transient hyphe*	>2–20	?	None
Tetrahydrobiopterin deficiencies	12–20	DHPR (<1%) PTS (<20%) GTP cyclohydrolase (<4%)	Neurotransmitter precursors

*Hyphe = Hyperphenylalaninemia.

the mutation that produced PKU in the infant. With the polymerase chain reaction (PCR) technique for amplification of the phenylalanine hydroxylase gene, the ASO method can even be applied to the newborn blood-filter paper specimen used in neonatal screening.

Treatment. When the diagnosis of PKU is confirmed, the infant should be given a low-phenylalanine diet. For optimal benefit, the diet should begin within the first 3 weeks of life. This treatment regimen must be planned and carefully monitored by physicians, nutritionists, and others experienced and knowledgeable in the treatment of PKU (Koch and Wenz, 1987). A special low-phenylalanine or phenylalanine-free formula is substituted for regular infant formula or breast-feeding. A small amount of milk or regular formula is added to the special formula in order to supply the infant with the amount of phenylalanine required for protein synthesis and cellular homeostasis. If these requirements are not satisfied, phenylalanine depletion accompanied by a very low blood phenylalanine concentration and severe complications occur. These complications include growth retardation, brain damage, and even death. The amount of milk necessary as a dietary supplement varies from one infant to another and is adjusted on the basis of the blood phenylalanine concentration. For optimal therapeutic effects, this concentration should be maintained within the range of 4 to 10 mg/dl (240 to 600 μM). Foods added to the diet later in infancy should be low in protein, generally fruits and vegetables.

Breast-feeding can be continued while the infant is provided with a safe low-phenylalanine diet (McCabe and McCabe, 1986). In fact, the best metabolic control is often achieved with a breast-feeding regimen. About two or three breast-feedings per day are allowed, and the other feedings must consist of a special phenylalanine-free formula. The precise number of breast-feedings per day and the amount of special formula are determined by the blood phenylalanine levels in the treated infant.

The current policy in most centers is to recommend continuation of a low-phenylalanine diet. This is in contrast to the former policy of recommending discontinuation of the diet when the child reached 5 or 6 years of age and is in response to recent information that I.Q. scores decrease in some children who discontinue the diet (Schmidt et al., 1987). Whether the diet should continue into adult years or can be safely discontinued after childhood has not yet been determined.

■ HYPERPHENYLALANINEMIAS

Inborn errors of metabolism other than phenylketonuria are also associated with reduced activity of phenylalanine hydroxylase. These defects result in mild to moderate degrees of increase in the blood phenylalanine level, rather than the more severe increase associated with PKU (see Table 18–3). These entities are sometimes included under the rubric of phenylketonuria, but they are distinct entities.

ATYPICAL PHENYLKETONURIA

An infant whose blood phenylalanine concentrations in the untreated state are consistently greater than 12 mg/dl (720 μM) but less than 20 mg/dl (1200 μM) is considered to have atypical PKU. The frequency of atypical PKU is less than that of phenylketonuria, approximating 1:40,000. The extent to which clinical complications may occur in this disorder is not known, although it is believed that if it is left untreated, either lowered intellectual performance or a mild degree of mental retardation may result. Most centers administer a low-phenylalanine diet to these infants just as in PKU. Because these infants have a greater tolerance for phenylalanine than those with PKU, their diet must be monitored with particular care.

MILD PERSISTENT HYPERPHENYLALANINEMIA

Mild hyperphenylalaninemia, like atypical PKU, is usually genotypically distinct from PKU. The untreated infant with mild persistent hyperphenylalaninemia has a blood phenylalanine concentration consistently higher than the normal 2 mg/dl (120 μM), but no greater than 12 mg/dl (720 μM). The frequency of this entity seems to be about 1:25,000 but it has wide ethnic variation. It seems to be clinically benign and, consequently, probably does not require treatment (see Table 18–3). For this reason, it is important to differentiate mild persistent hyperphenylalaninemia from atypical and classic PKU.

TETRAHYDROBIOPTERIN DEFICIENCY

From 0.25 to 1 per cent of infants with hyperphenylalaninemia have a defect in synthesis of tetrahydrobiopterin (BH_4), the cofactor required by phenylalanine hydroxylase. When BH_4 is not available in sufficient amounts, hydroxylations of tyrosine and tryptophan as well as of phenylalanine are reduced. Thus, neurotransmitters such as dopamine and norepinephrine (products derived from tyrosine hydroxylation) and serotonin (derived from tryptophan hydroxylation) are deficient.

Infants with tetrahydrobiopterin deficiency are often incorrectly diagnosed as having PKU or atypical PKU. The correct diagnosis is often suspected only when, unlike infants with PKU, they show signs of severe brain damage despite treatment with a low-phenylalanine diet. These signs include lethargy, delayed development, and seizures. The brain damage probably results from the deficiencies in neurotransmitters, although other factors may also be important.

At least three genetically distinct metabolic defects are known to cause BH_4 deficiency. Each is inherited as an autosomal recessive trait. The first described, *dihydropteridine reductase (DHPR) deficiency* (Kaufman et al., 1975), results in lack of BH_4 regeneration from qBH_2 (see Fig. 18–3). The other two *6-pyruvoyl-tetrahydropterin synthase (PTS)* (Shintaku et al., 1988) and *GTP cyclohydrolase deficiencies* (Naylor et al., 1987) result in reduced biopterin synthesis. The diagnosis of each is established by enzyme assay in cultured skin fibroblasts, erythrocytes, or biopsied liver.

All newborn infants with any degree of hyperphenylalaninemia should be tested for a defect in tetrahydrobiopterin synthesis. The most convenient test is the measurement of neopterin and biopterin in urine. In cyclohydrolase deficiency both neopterin and biopterin are markedly reduced. In PTS deficiency, urinary biopterin is very low, so the neopterin-to-biopterin ratio is high. In DHPR deficiency, urinary biopterin is increased, so the neopterin-to-biopterin ratio is low. In PKU, this ratio is essentially unchanged from that seen in normal infants. This analysis can be performed with urine dried on filter paper as well as a random liquid urine specimen. To be certain that DHPR deficiency is not overlooked, a corner of the newborn blood-filter paper specimen is also sent for measurement of DHPR activity.

The current treatment for tetrahydrobiopterin deficiency consists of supplying the immediate precursors of the deficient neurotransmitters. Thus, L-dopa (and carbidopa) are given so that the infant can synthesize dopamine and norepinephrine, and hydroxytryptophan is given to stimulate serotonin synthesis. This therapy has not reversed the severe neurologic signs in affected children, although it has increased the activity and muscle tone in some patients. In several instances, this therapy has been beneficial in preventing the neurologic sequelae when begun in the newborn period. In addition, folinic acid (citrovorum factor; 5-formyltetrahydrofolate) has produced clinical improvement in patients with DHPR deficiency and probably should be included in the treatment of these infants (Irons et al., 1987). Other modes of therapy, such as treatment with BH_4 or BH_4 analogues, are currently under investigation.

■ MATERNAL PHENYLKETONURIA

Women with PKU who do not receive the low-phenylalanine diet during pregnancy bear children with microcephaly, mental retardation, low birth weight, and often congenital heart disease (Lenke and Levy, 1980). The microcephaly may be quite striking in the newborn and has often led to an extensive evaluation prior to nursery discharge when the mother has not been known to have PKU. An evaluation for neonatal microcephaly should always include a maternal blood phenylalanine measurement (PKU test of the mother). This should be performed even if the mother is not mentally retarded, since an occasional phenylketonuric individual will be mentally normal despite not receiving treatment for PKU.

These abnormalities in the offspring occur whether or not the offspring has PKU (most such offspring do not have PKU) and are presumed to be a consequence of fetal damage from one or more of the PKU-related maternal metabolites that cross the placenta (Levy, 1987). The fetal damage in maternal PKU, therefore, is due to the aberrant intrauterine environment and not to a genetic defect in the offspring.

Maternal PKU is becoming an important problem since, as a result of newborn screening programs and early treatment of PKU, there are now many young women with PKU who are mentally normal and who are capable of reproducing. Will all offspring of these women be mentally retarded?

Women with classic PKU whose blood phenylalanine concentrations are 20 mg/dl (1200 μM) or greater and perhaps some women with atypical PKU seem to be at greatest risk of bearing damaged offspring. Women with mild hyperphenylalaninemia may be at less risk or may be at no greater than normal risk of having retarded children (Levy and Waisbren, 1983).

Treatment during pregnancy with a low-phenylalanine diet that controls the maternal biochemical abnormalities may prevent fetal damage in maternal PKU. Several such cases with normal offspring have been reported. Treatment during pregnancy has not always resulted in normal offspring, however, and one determinant may be how soon in relation to pregnancy treatment begins (Rohr et al., 1987). For optimal results, treatment may have to begin before conception so that it is in effect throughout pregnancy (Drogari et al., 1987).

■ MAPLE SYRUP URINE DISEASE

Maple syrup urine disease, or branched-chain ketoaciduria, is an inborn error of metabolism involving the branched-chain amino acids (leucine, isoleucine, and valine) and their ketoacid analogues. It is inherited as an autosomal recessive trait and is rare, occurring in approximately one per 200,000 infants. The metabolic defect is due to reduced activity of an enzyme complex known as branched-chain α-ketoacid dehydrogenase (see Figure 18–3). This defect results in increased concentrations of the branched-chain amino acids, particularly leucine, and their corresponding ketoacids.

Clinical Characteristics. There are three degrees of severity of maple syrup urine disease (MSUD). The first described and the most severe is the *classic* form in which the enzymatic defect is complete or almost complete. The infant with this form of the disorder becomes lethargic on the 2nd or 3rd day of life after normal prenatal, perinatal, and early neonatal courses. By the 4th or 5th day of life, he or she develops lethargy, poor feeding, vomiting, and weight loss. Neurologic signs such as hypotonia or hypertonia, seizures, and loss of basic reflexes then appear. Metabolic acidosis with ketonuria due to the accumulation of ketoacids is evident by this time. If vigorous treatment is not begun, the clinical course rapidly declines, and death ensues within the first weeks of life.

The *intermediate variant* of maple syrup urine disease is associated with 2 to 5 per cent of normal enzyme activity. Affected infants are usually asymptomatic during the neonatal period and remain clinically normal until they are several months old, when developmental delay is evident. Subsequently, the affected child has episodes of metabolic acidosis, usually precipitated by acute febrile illnesses, and becomes mentally retarded.

The *intermittent variant* is characterized by 5 to 15 per cent residual enzyme activity. These infants are also clinically normal during the neonatal period and usually remain asymptomatic through infancy and childhood, except when there is an acute febrile episode or trauma, such as surgery or an accident. At these times the branched-chain amino acids and ketoacids accumulate and severe ketoacidosis with all the acute signs of severe maple syrup urine disease may appear. Several affected children have died during these acute episodes.

Diagnosis. The most effective means of diagnosing maple syrup urine disease is routine newborn screening. In an infant with the classic or intermediate form, this may represent the only chance for instituting therapy before death or irreversible brain damage.

Most newborn screening programs in North America do not test for MSUD. Consequently, the diagnosis often depends upon clinical suspicion. If MSUD is suspected because of clinical signs or family history, blood should be analyzed for amino acids and urine for both amino acids and organic acids. During acute episodes the branched-chain amino acid concentrations in blood are many times greater than normal. Leucine, the most markedly increased amino acid, may have a level as high as 4,000 μM (53 mg/dl) as compared to the normal upper limit of 120 μM (1.6 mg/dl). The urine may have an odor reminiscent of maple syrup. The branched-chain ketoacid concentrations in the urine are very high and may be detected by a screening test using the dinitrophenylhydrazine reagent. When this reagent is acidified and added to urine containing a large concentration of ketoacids, dinitrophenylhydrazones form, causing the clear solution to become cloudy and form a precipitate; there is no change in a normal urine. Amino acid analysis of urine reveals increased branched-chain amino acid concentrations.

In the intermediate variant of maple syrup urine disease, the only findings may be mildly increased branched-chain amino acid concentrations in blood except during acute episodes, when the ketoacidosis appears. In the intermittent variant, blood and urine amino acid levels, including leucine, are normal and ketoacids are absent—except, again, during an acute episode. The intermittent variant, therefore, may be particularly difficult to diagnose and usually is suspected only when an acute episode has occurred.

Confirmation of the diagnosis depends upon demonstration of the enzyme defect in leukocytes or cultured fibroblasts. The branched-chain ketoacid dehydrogenase complex has several components, and it is clear that MSUD can result from a defect in any one of the major components (Indo et al., 1988). Recently, there has been substantial progress in identifying these components and in cloning the genes that encode them (Hu et al., 1988). It is likely that in the near future the specific component defect will be identifiable in each infant with MSUD.

Prenatal diagnosis is possible for all forms of MSUD.

Treatment. During acute illness, treatment must be immediate. This is especially urgent in the newborn. The affected infant requires intensive care and neurologic monitoring. Peritoneal dialysis or hemodialysis is effective in clearing the accumulated metabolites and should be performed as soon as possible. Intravenous glucose and bicarbonate must be given, the former to provide adequate calories so that catabolism is reduced, and the latter to control acidosis. Anticonvulsant medication may be required for seizures. All protein intake is discontinued until the branched-chain amino acid levels return to normal or near normal, and the urine is free of ketoacids.

The chronic treatment of MSUD is dietary. The diet is reduced in branched-chain amino acid content, especially leucine, and is difficult to prepare and administer. Dietary therapy should be provided at a pediatric metabolic unit staffed by physicians, nutritionists, and others who have the knowledge and experience required to treat this disorder. The diet consists of a special medical formula, free of branched-chain amino acids, composed of other essential amino acids and some nonessential minerals, carbohydrate, and fat. It is supplemented with a small amount of milk or formula so that the infant has sufficient quantities of the branched-chain amino acids to support protein synthesis. Allowable foods include those low in protein, such as fruits and vegetables.

Thiamine (vitamin B_1) might be helpful in the treatment of certain infants and children with MSUD (Fernhoff et al., 1985). A coenzymatically active derivative of thiamine is necessary for branched-chain dehydrogenase activity. Large amounts of thiamine might stimulate this activity in some individuals with classic MSUD or the variants, although thiamine therapy is usually adjunctive and cannot replace dietary restriction.

■ SULFUR AMINO ACID ABNORMALITIES

There are several disorders within this group, each due to a specific metabolic block in the methionine pathway. Some are associated with severe clinical disease and others appear to be benign. Each is inherited as an autosomal recessive trait. Newborn screening only partially addresses these disorders.

HYPERMETHIONINEMIA

Several infants with methionine adenosyltransferase (MAT) deficiency have been described (Fig. 18–4). All have had markedly elevated concentrations of methionine in blood without other amino acid abnormalities. The enzyme defect is expressed only in the liver; cultured skin fibroblasts have normal activity. Affected individuals have remained clinically normal, suggesting that this disorder may be benign (Gahl et al., 1987). A subgroup of hypermethioninemia has been described in which liver MAT activity is normal. These children have a normal neonatal course but subsequently develop clinical features ranging from mental retardation and proximal muscle weakness to fatty liver. An enzyme defect has not yet been identified in these patients (Gaull et al., 1981).

Normal newborns receiving a *high protein diet* may

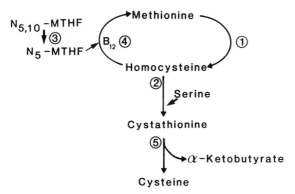

FIGURE 18–4. *Transsulfuration in methionine metabolic pathway. The inborn errors in this diagram include (1) hypermethioninemia due to methionine adenosyltransferase deficiency; (2) homocystinuria due to cystathionine β-synthase deficiency; (3) methionine remethylation defect due to N5,10-methylenetetrahydrofolate reductase deficiency and to (4) B₁₂ metabolic defect; and (5) cystathioninemia due to cystathionase deficiency.*

have increased concentrations of methionine. This is a transient state that usually disappears 2 or 3 days after the protein intake is lowered. Even if increased protein intake continues, the hypermethioninemia spontaneously disappears by the age of 3 months. No clinical abnormality is known to result from transient hypermethioninemia. With the trend back to breast-feeding and, consequently, a lower protein intake, transient hypermethioninemia is much less frequent than it formerly was.

Increased blood methionine concentrations may also occur in association with neonatal *liver disease.* This is most frequently noted in neonatal hepatitis but is also seen with liver disease due to hereditary tyrosinemia, galactosemia, and hereditary fructose intolerance. The hypermethioninemia (and tyrosinemia) of liver disease is presumably secondary to hepatocellular damage. The amino acid abnormalities are important in that they may serve as indicators of liver disease and perhaps also as measures of the severity of damage.

HOMOCYSTINURIA

This disorder results from a deficiency of cystathionine β-synthase enzyme activity. This enzyme is responsible for the conversion of homocysteine to cystathionine (see Fig. 18–4). The most striking biochemical abnormality in affected newborns is an increased blood methionine level, since homocysteine tends to be remethylated back to methionine. There is also a small accumulation of homocystine in blood and urine while cystine is reduced or absent in blood. Later in infancy and in childhood, the homocystine accumulation becomes more prominent, and the hypermethioninemia is less striking. The frequency of this disorder is approximately one per 200,000 infants.

Clinical Characteristics. The newborn with homocystinuria is usually normal. Detection of the disease at this early age, therefore, depends on routine newborn screening or suspicion due to family history. Unfortunately, routine newborn screening has proved to be unreliable for identification of homocystinuria, and a number of affected infants have been missed. When untreated, homocystinuria leads to mental retardation, dislocation of the

ocular lenses (ectopia lentis), skeletal abnormalities including osteoporosis and elongated limbs, and thromboembolism. Most of these clinical complications are highly variable, however. Some individuals have normal intelligence, others have little or no skeletal involvement, and still others avoid thrombotic complications. On the other hand, ectopia lentis seems to be almost invariable.

The propensity for thromboembolic complications in this disease may result in cerebrovascular incidents, even in infancy. Thus, infants with a stroke should always be tested for homocystinuria.

Diagnosis. The diagnosis of homocystinuria is based on increased methionine and the presence of homocystine in blood and urine. The demonstration of homocystine may require careful, quantitative analysis of amino acids, preferably with an amino acid analyzer. Less sensitive methods such as thin-layer or paper chromatography or screening methods such as the urine cyanide-nitroprusside test may be insufficient to detect the small amount of homocystine present in the affected newborn or young infant. The diagnosis is confirmed by demonstrating reduced cystathionine β-synthase activity in cultured cells. The gene for this enzyme has been cloned (Kraus et al., 1986). This should lead to more specific molecular diagnosis in the near future. Prenatal diagnosis is also available (Fowler et al., 1982).

Treatment. Treatment consists of pyridoxine (vitamin B₆) supplementation or a special low-methionine diet supplemented with cystine. Approximately 50 per cent of homocystinuric individuals respond to pharmacologic doses of pyridoxine. In these individuals, pyridoxine hydrochloride (25 to 200 mg/day), perhaps in association with a low-protein or modified low-methionine diet, may be all that is necessary to control the biochemical manifestations. Infants unresponsive to pyridoxine require a special methionine-restricted diet. This diet is complicated and difficult to prepare and administer. It should be given only at a pediatric metabolic center. Treatment begun early in infancy may prevent most if not all the clinical complications. Even when begun after the clinical complications have appeared, treatment has sometimes been beneficial.

METHIONINE REMETHYLATION DEFECTS

Methionine homeostasis requires that methionine be remethylated from homocysteine (see Fig. 18–4). The major pathway for methionine remethylation is via the enzyme N5-methyltetrahydrofolate-homocysteine methyltransferase (methionine synthase), which transfers methyl from methyltetrahydrofolate to homocysteine. This enzyme requires methyl-B₁₂, one of two coenzymatically active vitamin B₁₂ products, as a cofactor.

Either of two metabolic blocks can result in a reduction of methionine remethylation. One is a primary defect in N5,10-methylenetetrahydrofolate reductase (MTHFR), an enzyme that is responsible for the synthesis of N5-methyltetrahydrofolate. Thus, MTHFR deficiency limits the availability of methyltetrahydrofolate. The metabolic consequences of reduced methionine remethylation follow: homocystine accumulates in blood and urine, and the blood methionine level is reduced. Failure to thrive and mental retardation have been described in this disease. Treatment consists of folinic acid and, possibly, methionine supplementation.

The other block is due to reduced activity of methionine synthase secondary to lack of sufficient methyl-B_{12}. Vitamin B_{12} deficiency as a result of breast-feeding from a vegetarian mother may cause this (Higginbottom et al., 1978). Such infants fail to thrive and present with megaloblastic anemia at 3 to 5 months of age. Vitamin B_{12} treatment is curative. More often reported as a cause of this block is an inborn error in B_{12} metabolism. These infants have normal serum total B_{12} levels, but their cells cannot synthesize sufficient amounts of methyl-B_{12} from precursor B_{12}. The clinical phenotype varies widely. The most severely affected have intrauterine growth retardation with low birth weight and microcephaly. They grow poorly after birth and usually come to attention at 2 to 4 months of age with failure to thrive, microcephaly, developmental delay, and megaloblastic anemia. Infants that are less affected have a normal neonatal course and do not present until later in infancy or childhood. Their presentation includes developmental delay and megaloblastic anemia. All of these infants have accumulations of homocystine in blood and urine, and usually a low blood methionine level. In one category of these disorders (cbl C, D, F), methylmalonic acid also accumulates; whereas in the other category (cbl E, G), methylmalonic aciduria is absent. The biochemical abnormalities and the megaloblastosis may respond partially or completely to pharmacologic doses of B_{12} (hydroxocobalamin). This treatment may also produce clinical benefit.

CYSTATHIONINEMIA

This inborn error is caused by deficient activity of the enzyme cystathionase, resulting in increased cystathionine in blood and urine (see Fig. 18–4). As in homocystinuria, there are two forms of this disorder, one that is biochemically responsive to pyridoxine (vitamin B_6) and another that shows no such response, even to massive amounts of pyridoxine. The former is much more frequent than the latter. The diagnosis of either form depends on the demonstration of persistently increased cystathionine levels in urine and the presence of cystathionine in blood. Present evidence indicates that cystathioninemia is probably benign, although the author has seen hyperactivity and learning disabilities develop in several children. Therapy consists of pyridoxine hydrochloride supplementation in oral doses of 25 to 200 mg/day for the B_6-responsive form. Treatment has not been given in the B_6-nonresponsive form.

▪ TYROSINEMIA

An increase in the concentration of tyrosine may occur either transiently or as a persistent condition in the newborn.

TRANSIENT NEONATAL TYROSINEMIA

This formerly occurred in as many as 5 to 10 per cent of all newborns. As with transient hypermethioninemia,

the recent reduction in protein intake through wider use of breast-feeding has substantially decreased the frequency of transient tyrosinemia. It is initiated by delayed maturation of parahydroxyphenylpyruvic acid oxidase, an enzyme that metabolizes parahydroxyphenylpyruvic acid, a product of tyrosine oxidation (Fig. 18–5). Reduced activity of this enzyme results in the accumulation of tyrosine and parahydroxyphenylpyruvate as well as secondary metabolites such as parahydroxyphenyllactate and parahydroxyphenylacetate. The blood tyrosine level is often markedly increased, sometimes in excess of 1100 μM or 20 mg/dl (the normal blood tyrosine concentration is less than 120 μM or 2.2 mg/dl). Tyrosine and the aforementioned metabolites are present in excessive quantities in the urine (Avery et al., 1967).

There are several interesting characteristics of this common entity. First, transient tyrosinemia is much more frequent among premature than full-term infants. This is presumably related to the tendency toward immaturity of many enzyme systems in premature infants. Second, a high-protein intake stimulates the metabolite accumulations. Hence, the tyrosinemia usually appears after the 1st week of life and reaches its peak during the 2nd or 3rd month. Third, ascorbic acid (vitamin C) therapy activates the enzyme in most infants and thus eliminates the biochemical abnormalities.

There is a debate about whether this finding causes clinical problems. Some centers have reported slightly reduced intellectual performance among children who had transient neonatal tyrosinemia (Rice et al., 1989), whereas

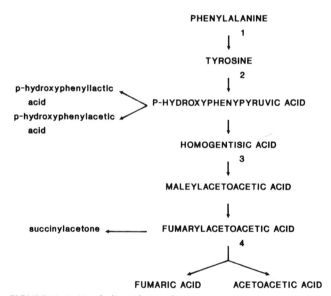

FIGURE 18–5. Metabolic pathway of tyrosine. Tyrosine is a nonessential amino acid, synthesized from phenylalanine via phenylalanine hydroxylase. The inborn errors represented in this pathway include: (1) phenylketonuria (PKU) due to phenylalanine hydroxylase deficiency (see Figure 18–4); (2) tyrosinemia II due to cytosolic tyrosine transaminase deficiency; (3) alcaptonuria due to homogentisic acid oxidase deficiency; and (4) tyrosinemia I due to fumarylacetoacetate hydrolase deficiency. In tyrosinemia I the unstable fumarylacetoacetic acid is converted to succinylacetone, which accumulates in that disease and serves as a marker for the diagnosis. Tyrosine and the tyrosine metabolites such as p-hydroxyphenyllactic and p-hyroxyphenylacetic acid also accumulate, the latter is excreted in large quantities. This is probably a secondary biochemical effect in tyrosinemia I, perhaps due to inhibition of both tyrosine transaminase and p-hydroxyphenylpyruvic acid oxidase by succinylacetone.

other centers have found no such reduction (Martin et al., 1974). No physical problems have been reported. It is probably advisable to limit the protein intake of infants to less than 3 g/kg/day and to maintain a daily vitamin C intake of at least 25 mg/day in order to lessen the chances that significant tyrosinemia will occur.

Tyrosinemia can occasionally confuse the results of newborn screening for phenylketonuria. A markedly elevated blood tyrosine level may be associated with an increased concentration of phenylalanine, presumably because tyrosine can compete with phenylalanine for phenylalanine hydroxylase (see Fig. 18–3). When this occurs, an increased phenylalanine concentration in the newborn blood specimen may be incorrectly interpreted as an indication of phenylketonuria. If a complete blood amino acid analysis is performed, however, the differentiation between phenylketonuria and tyrosinemia is unmistakable, since phenylketonuria is associated with a normal or reduced tyrosine concentration and tyrosinemia causes a markedly increased tyrosine concentration. This type of analysis should be performed on all infants whose newborn screening results suggest phenylketonuria.

TYROSINEMIA I

Type I, or hereditary, tyrosinemia is inherited in an autosomal recessive manner. It is rare except among those of French-Canadian ancestry, in whom a relatively high frequency has been found. The metabolic defect is in deficient activity of fumarylacetoacetate hydrolase, the final enzyme in the tyrosine degradative pathway (see Fig. 18–5). Deficient activities of parahydroxyphenylpyruvic acid oxidase and tyrosine transaminase have been reported in the liver of patients, but these are almost certainly secondary defects. On the other hand, these defects probably account for the most prominent amino acid findings, increased tyrosine in blood and increased tyrosine and tyrosine metabolites in urine. Methionine is also markedly increased in blood as is the serum alpha-fetoprotein concentration. The presence in urine of succinylacetone, a breakdown product of fumarylacetoacetate, is a primary finding and characteristic of the disorder (Sassa and Kappas, 1983).

Clinical Characteristics. Tyrosinemia I has two presentations. The most dramatic is the acute phenotype, characterized by severe liver disease apparent within the 1st or 2nd week of life or, at the latest, within the first 2 or 3 months. Hepatomegaly and jaundice appear. Liver function test results are abnormal, with a coagulopathy demonstrated by increased prothrombin and partial thromboplastin times particularly prominent. Ascites often develops. This presentation is usually associated with a rapidly progressive course characterized by deteriorating liver function, bleeding, and death within the 1st or 2nd year of life.

Often the presentation is later in infancy, referred to as the chronic phenotype. These infants are usually clinically normal until the end of the 1st year of life or into the 2nd year when jaundice and hepatomegaly are noted. Liver function is abnormal, and the renal Fanconi syndrome, with glycosuria, generalized hyperaminoaciduria, and proteinuria, is present. The hepatic disease progresses to cirrhosis and hypophosphatemic rickets develops. If untreated, death from liver failure or bleeding complications very often occurs, usually during the first few years of life.

Mental retardation does not occur, and the nervous system seems to be spared in most cases of tyrosinemia I. However, in a recent report from Quebec, nearly half the patients had neurologic crises characterized by hypertonic posturing, paralysis, or pain. The oldest patient among those with neurologic crises was 19 years of age (Mitchell et al., 1990).

Diagnosis. The diagnosis of tyrosinemia I can be difficult. Liver disease from several causes, including hepatitis, galactosemia, and hereditary fructose intolerance, may be associated with increased tyrosine and tyrosine metabolites as well as increased methionine. Consequently, these biochemical abnormalities are not specific for tyrosinemia I. Urinary succinylacetone is specific, however, and serves as a marker for the disorder. The diagnosis is confirmed by finding markedly reduced activity of fumarylacetoacetate hydrolase in erythrocytes or cultured skin fibroblasts (Kvittingen et al., 1983).

Prenatal diagnosis is possible on the basis of succinylacetone in amniotic fluid (Gagne et al., 1982) or reduced activity of fumarylacetoacetate hydrolase in cultured amniocytes (Kvittingen et al., 1985) or chorionic villi (Kvittingen et al., 1986).

Treatment. Treatment includes therapy for the complications of liver disease as well as control of the amino acid abnormalities through the use of a special diet. This diet, low in both tyrosine and phenylalanine as well as methionine, reverses the renal abnormalities and the rickets but, except in a few isolated instances, has not been effective in arresting the progression of the liver disease.

Even when liver disease stabilizes, many children with this disorder have developed hepatocellular carcinoma (Weinberg et al., 1976). To avoid this complication as well as that of progressive liver disease and liver failure, liver transplantation is increasingly performed. Most liver transplants for this disorder have been successful (Esquivel et al., 1989).

TYROSINEMIA II

Only a few cases of this disorder have been described. It seems to be transmitted as an autosomal recessive trait. The metabolic defect is a deficiency of cytosolic tyrosine transaminase (Fig. 18–5) with normal mitochondrial tyrosine transaminase. This results in increased tyrosine in the cytoplasm, some of which enters the mitochondria and is converted to parahydroxyphenylpyruvic acid. Because of different expressions of parahydroxyphenylpyruvate oxidase among body tissues, the mitochondrial parahydroxyphenylpyruvic acid may or may not be further metabolized. Thus, in addition to increased tyrosine, these patients also have accumulations of tyrosine metabolites in urine (tyrosyluria). Despite these accumulations, which are even more striking than those in tyrosinemia I, there are no abnormalities of liver, kidney, or bone. This may be explained by the absence of succinylacetone, which accumulates in tyrosinemia I and may be the toxic factor in that disease.

Most reported patients with tyrosinemia II, however, have been mentally retarded. The mental retardation appears to be similar to that seen in phenylketonuria, with developmental delay during the 1st year of life and obvious intellectual retardation noted by the 2nd or 3rd year. In addition, affected individuals have two other striking features, painful hyperkeratotic lesions on the hands and feet and keratitis with corneal ulcerations resulting in photophobia and increased lacrimation. The skin and eye lesions can be controlled by a diet restricted in tyrosine and phenylalanine that reduces the levels of tyrosine and tyrosine metabolites. If tyrosinemia II is analogous to phenylketonuria, the diet would have to be initiated during the first weeks of life in order to prevent the mental retardation.

■ UREA CYCLE DISORDERS

Five of the six disorders in the urea cycle may produce dramatic clinical symptoms and signs during the neonatal period. These seem to be associated with the large accumulation of ammonium that results from a block in the urea cycle, which is responsible for converting ammonium to urea (Fig. 18–6). The blood ammonium concentration exceeds 100 μM (180 μg/dl) and is usually much greater than 200 μM (360 μg/dl) in the newborn with the severe or neonatal form of any of these disorders. These infants are normal at birth but by the 2nd or 3rd day of life develop marked lethargy and hypotonia. Their clinical condition then rapidly progresses to seizures and coma. Hepatomegaly with little or no liver dysfunction is often present. Patients with the later onset form of these disorders are normal in the neonatal and early infancy period but present in later infancy or childhood with episodes of Reye syndrome or chronic signs such as lethargy, failure to thrive, hepatomegaly, and developmental delay.

The sick newborn requires immediate lifesaving measures. These include hemodialysis to reduce the blood ammonium as quickly as possible and supportive parenteral therapy. Chronic treatment for the recovered newborn and the infant who presents with the later onset

phenotype consists of a low-protein diet along with a special formula and specific organic acid medications, discussed below.

N-ACETYLGLUTAMATE SYNTHETASE DEFICIENCY

This disorder is due to a defect in the enzyme required for the production of N-acetylglutamate, an effector for carbamyl phosphate synthetase, the first enzyme in the urea cycle. One patient has been described (Bachmann et al., 1981). He had marked hyperammonemia with the neonatal phenotype as described above. Two siblings had died during the neonatal period.

CARBAMYL PHOSPHATE SYNTHETASE DEFICIENCY

Carbamyl phosphate synthetase (CPS) deficiency is an autosomal recessive disorder of the first step in the urea cycle. Most affected infants present with severe hyperammonemic neonatal illness typical of urea cycle disorders; others have the later onset phenotype. In the neonatal form, the blood ammonium level is usually increased 10- to 20-fold, but the later onset form is associated with more modest elevation. Blood amino acid analysis reveals markedly reduced levels or the absence of citrulline; arginine may also be reduced. The diagnosis is confirmed by enzyme analysis in the liver obtained by biopsy. Treatment consists of a low-protein diet accompanied by an essential amino acid mixture and citrulline supplementation with the addition of two organic acids, sodium phenylacetate and sodium benzoate. Despite therapy, most of the patients have died during an acute hyperammonemic episode or have suffered severe brain damage from recurrent episodes. Consequently, liver transplantation should be considered once the patient has been stabilized (Tuchman, 1989).

ORNITHINE TRANSCARBAMYLASE DEFICIENCY

Ornithine transcarbamylase (OTC) deficiency is caused by deficient activity of OTC, the second enzyme in the urea cycle. It is probably the second most frequent of the urea cycle disorders. Since the gene for OTC is located on the X chromosome, the disorder is inherited as an X-linked trait, unlike most inborn errors which are autosomal recessive. Accordingly, male infants with OTC deficiency, who are hemizygotes (since they have only one X chromosome), have virtually no OTC activity and usually become profoundly hyperammonemic and develop the neonatal phenotype during the first days of life. As in CPS deficiency, the blood ammonium level at this time is usually elevated at least 10-fold, and amino acid analysis of blood reveals little or no citrulline. Glutamine and alanine are increased secondary to the increased body ammonium. A key finding is increased orotic acid in urine. Orotic acid is derived from carbamyl phosphate, a cosubstrate of OTC (see Fig. 18–6), which presumably is increased in OTC deficiency. Increased orotic acid distinguishes OTC deficiency from CPS deficiency, which is associated with a normal or reduced level of urinary orotic

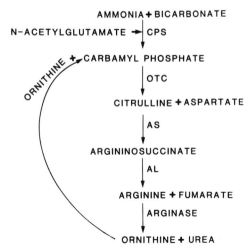

FIGURE 18–6. Urea cycle: Ammonia is metabolized to urea through a series of five major enzymatic reactions. There is an inborn error of metabolism for each of the enzymes. CPS = carbamylphosphate synthetase, OTC = ornithine transcarbamylase, AS = argininosuccinate synthetase, and AL = argininosuccinate lyase.

acid. The diagnosis of OTC deficiency is confirmed by enzyme assay in biopsied or postmortem liver.

OTC deficiency once was an almost universally fatal disease in males, but recently developed treatment consisting of hemodialysis combined with intravenous therapy that includes phenylacetate, benzoate, and arginine allows infants to survive the neonatal period (Msall et al., 1984). Anticipatory treatment from birth of at-risk male newborns that includes protein restriction and medications prevents illness in the affected infants. Chronic therapy with low-protein diet, essential amino acid supplements, and organic acid medications has permitted these children to survive, but recurrent hyperammonemic episodes despite treatment have resulted in brain damage with mental retardation in most of them (Brusilow et al., 1984). To prevent this damage and to circumvent the enormous difficulty of continuous therapy and frequent emergency medical attention, liver transplantation is increasingly recommended. This cures the metabolic disease and has been tolerated without unusual problems (Largillière et al., 1989).

The female with OTC deficiency is a heterozygote (since she has a second X chromosome with a normal gene for OTC). Due to random inactivation of the X chromosome in females (Lyon hypothesis), the affected female may have any degree of OTC deficiency varying from very mild to very severe. Thus, she may be asymptomatic or develop hyperammonemia with clinical illness in infancy or childhood. The signs, which usually mimic the Reye syndrome, include vomiting, lethargy, ataxia, and hepatomegaly. Illness usually coincides with an increase in protein in an acute febrile illness. Treatment for symptomatic females is the same as for males.

Cloning of the gene for OTC has allowed prenatal diagnosis on the basis of haplotype identification (Spence et al., 1989). This is particularly important when the fetus is male.

CITRULLINEMIA

Citrullinemia is an autosomal recessive disorder caused by a deficiency in argininosuccinate synthetase (AS), the third enzyme in the urea cycle (see Fig. 18–6). It may present as acute neonatal disease identical to other urea cycle disorders or as chronic disease with developmental delay later in infancy or childhood. There may also be a benign variant of citrullinemia. There is marked hyperammonemia in the sick newborn but a less severe degree of hyperammonemia in the older infant. The major amino acid abnormality is a markedly increased level of citrulline in blood and urine. The urine also contains increased orotic acid. The diagnosis is confirmed by enzyme assay in cultured skin fibroblasts or biopsied liver. Treatment consists of a low-protein diet with organic acid medication. Supplementation with arginine may also be helpful in the treatment of this disorder. Cloning of the gene for this enzyme has led to extensive investigation of the gene defect in this disease (Beaudet et al., 1986). Prenatal diagnosis is available.

ARGININOSUCCINIC ACIDEMIA

Argininosuccinic acidemia (ASA) is probably the most frequent urea cycle disorder. It is transmitted as an auto-somal recessive trait characterized by deficient activity of argininosuccinate lyase (AL), the fourth enzyme in the urea cycle (see Fig. 18–6). There are at least three forms of this disorder. The most severe presents in the newborn with marked hyperammonemia and accumulations of argininosuccinate in blood and urine. Arginine is usually reduced in blood, and orotic acid is increased in urine. These newborns have the clinical features of the neonatal phenotype. Few have survived, although therapy with massive amounts of arginine has produced dramatic recovery and, if given early in the course of the disease, might sustain almost all neonatally-affected infants (Brusilow and Batshaw, 1979). A later onset form presents during the 3rd or 4th month of life with developmental lag and hepatomegaly. The neurologic disease in this form may progress, and convulsions usually appear. These infants have moderate hyperammonemia and argininosuccinate in blood, urine, and CSF. Treatment consists of a low-protein diet and supplementation with arginine. The third form appears to be clinically benign but may produce learning disability and seizures later in childhood. These infants have been discovered by routine newborn screening on the basis of increased urinary argininosuccinate. They have normal or only slightly increased concentrations of blood ammonium. Treatment consists of reducing the protein intake.

The diagnosis of ASA can be readily confirmed by enzyme studies of erythrocytes. Similar studies can also be performed in cultured skin fibroblasts as well as tissues such as liver, kidney, and brain obtained postmortem. The precise enzymatic differences among infants with these different clinical pictures have not been clearly defined. The gene for AL has been cloned (O'Brien et al., 1986). Prenatal diagnosis is available (Vimal et al., 1984).

HYPERARGININEMIA

Hyperargininemia is an autosomal recessive disorder caused by deficient activity of arginase, the fifth and final enzyme in the urea cycle (see Fig. 18–6). Only a few cases have been reported. Unlike the other urea cycle disorders, it does not produce neonatal disease. The clinical picture is that of progressive neurologic involvement with developmental delay appearing in late infancy, and mental retardation, ataxia, and spasticity in childhood. Spastic diplegia is almost always present. Laboratory findings include mild hyperammonemia, increased arginine in blood and urine on amino acid analysis, and increased orotic acid in urine. The diagnosis is confirmed by enzyme assay in erythrocytes. Treatment consists of a low-protein diet and organic acid medications.

TRANSIENT HYPERAMMONEMIA OF THE NEWBORN

Transient hyperammonemia was first recognized in premature or small-for-gestational-age infants, but it also occurs in term infants. The cause is unknown. Other than the markedly increased blood ammonium level, laboratory findings are normal. Notably, amino acid levels are normal with no amino acid evidence of a urea cycle defect, and urine orotic acid is not increased. Affected newborns develop hyperammonemia within the first 24 hours of life instead of the 2nd or 3rd day of life, as in a urea cycle disorder, but otherwise have the clinical picture of the neonatal phenotype of a urea cycle disorder including lethargy, hypotonia, and coma (Hudak et al., 1985).

The diagnosis is based on finding a very high level of blood ammonium, often in excess of 600 μM (1,000 μg/dl), without other laboratory evidence of a urea cycle defect. Treatment must be aggressive and consists of hemodialysis or peritoneal dialysis as well as parenteral fluids with phenylacetate and benzoate. Without aggressive therapy, many of these infants die in the neonatal period. With successful therapy, however, the infant should completely recover without residual brain damage.

■ HYPERGLYCINEMIA

The term "hyperglycinemia" should not imply a specific disorder but a biochemical abnormality common to a number of disorders that may produce neonatal disease. When increased glycine is associated with ketosis and metabolic acidosis, the general term "ketotic hyperglycinemia" has been applied. This includes several inborn errors of organic acid metabolism in which the hyperglycinemia is a secondary feature. Hyperglycinemia may also be present as a specific finding in the absence of ketosis or acidosis. When so, it usually indicates a disorder known as nonketotic hyperglycinemia.

KETOTIC HYPERGLYCINEMIA

Many of the organic acidemias (e.g., propionic acidemia and methylmalonic acidemia) are associated with hyperglycinemia. Signs of metabolic acidosis may appear during the first 2 or 3 days of life. These include lethargy, tachypnea, vomiting, and poor feeding. Amino acid analysis reveals a glycine concentration two to four times normal in blood and markedly increased in urine. Lysine and other amino acids such as glutamine and alanine may also be increased. CSF glycine is increased to the same degree as the blood glycine (i.e., the CSF-to-plasma ratio for glycine is unaltered). Tests for urinary ketones are usually positive. The basic disorder in these infants involves a defect in the metabolism of an organic acid, and the disease should be considered in that category. Thus, "ketotic hyperglycinemia" is an obsolete term.

NONKETOTIC HYPERGLYCINEMIA

Hyperglycinemia as a specific finding in the absence of ketoacidosis denotes a disorder called nonketotic hyperglycinemia (NKH). There are several distinct clinical phenotypes in this disorder, and different molecular defects seem to account for the spectrum of disease observed.

ACUTE NEONATAL TYPE

The clinical presentation in the acute neonatal type of NKH, an autosomal recessive disorder, is one of the most striking in neonatal medicine. The infant, born after a normal pregnancy and delivery, appears to be normal for the first 24 to 36 hours of life. At this time, he or she becomes noticeably lethargic and, by the end of the 2nd

day of life, is hypotonic and poorly responsive or perhaps unresponsive. Supportive measures become necessary. Seizures, usually generalized, develop by the 3rd or 4th day. There are no other clinical findings. Notably, there is no hepatomegaly or other organomegaly. Routine laboratory data are surprisingly normal for such a serious clinical state. In particular, there is no evidence of acidosis, urine is negative for ketones, and blood glucose and ammonium are normal. Amino acid studies, however, reveal increased glycine concentrations in blood and urine. The CSF glycine increase is even more striking than the blood increase, often 20 to 40 times normal. This inordinate increase in CSF glycine produces an increased CSF-to-plasma glycine ratio. Organic acids, including short-chain fatty acids, are normal. Glycine cleavage enzyme activity is absent or barely detectable in the liver and less than 20 per cent of normal in the brain.

The defect in this disorder seems to be in the glycine cleavage enzyme. Japanese studies have identified different components of this enzyme complex and have begun to elucidate the abnormalities in NKH (Hayasaka et al., 1987). The complex consists of at least four proteins. In the neonatal form of the disorder, the P, or pyridoxal phosphate-containing, protein is most often defective. Cloning of the genes for these proteins should soon be accomplished and should allow for more definitive molecular identification of the defect.

There is no effective therapy. Exchange transfusion and peritoneal dialysis have not produced clinical improvement. Strychnine therapy in the form of strychnine sulfate 100 μg/kg/day may improve muscle tone and responsiveness but does not prevent the profound and progressive brain damage. Supplementation of the diet with L-serine has been reported to result in dramatic benefit to one infant (Wijburg et al., 1988). Sodium benzoate reduces the peripheral accumulation of free glycine by conjugating with glycine to form hippurate (benzoylglycine). When given in huge amounts (250 mg to 1 g/kg/day), sodium benzoate reduces CSF glycine and may reduce seizure frequency (Wolff et al., 1986). Infants with this disorder either die within the first few weeks of life or survive to develop progressive neurologic deterioration, severe myoclonic seizures with a hypsarrhythmic electroencephalographic pattern, and only a minimally functioning state.

INFANTILE TYPE

The infants of this type of NKH are clinically normal until 1 to 2 months of age, when poor head control and other signs of developmental lag become evident. There are no abnormal physical findings. Myoclonic seizures develop by 3 to 4 months of age. As in the acute neonatal disease, amino acid analysis reveals specifically increased concentrations of glycine in blood, urine, and CSF with an increased CSF-to-plasma glycine ratio. The glycine concentrations, however, are usually less markedly increased than in the acute neonatal disease. Several of these children have had a peculiar transient comatose reaction to the administration of valine; the pathogenesis of this response is unknown. The defect in the glycine cleavage complex seems to be in the T or H protein component rather than the P component (Hayasaka et al., 1987). There is no known treatment for this form of NKH. The disease is not progressive, and the children develop a stable mental retardation.

OTHER FORMS

Several children with NKH have had only mild to moderate mental retardation without seizures. An unusual type of spinal motor neuron disease involving the legs and beginning in childhood or adolescence has been described in association with NKH. There might also be a benign form, although this has not been clearly documented.

ORGANIC ACID DISORDERS

The term "organic acid" applies to acidic molecules that do not contain nitrogen. Often they are intermediary metabolites within amino acid metabolic pathways that appear after the amino group has been removed. The disorders of organic acid metabolism are considered separately from the disorders of amino acid metabolism, however, because of two important distinctions. First, *metabolic acidosis* is a prominent feature of the organic acid disorders, whereas acidosis is rarely seen in a primary aminoacidopathy. Second, in an organic acid disorder, the organic acid(s) rather than an amino acid is the primary abnormality expressed. Thus, if metabolic testing is performed only for amino acids, as is often the case, an organic acid disorder will be overlooked.

The most frequently identified organic acid disorders in the newborn are due to defects in the metabolic pathways of the branched-chain amino acids (leucine, isoleucine, and valine). The most prominent of these disorders, maple syrup urine disease, was described previously in this chapter because unlike other organic acid disorders, specific amino acid abnormalities are also present. Other disorders in these pathways include isovaleric acidemia, 3-hydroxy-3-methylglutaryl-CoA lyase deficiency, propionic acidemia, and methylmalonic acidemia, which will be discussed now. Pyruvic acidemia, a defect in glucose metabolism, the multiple carboxylase deficiencies, glutaric acidemia, and the mitochondrial myopathies, in which lactic acidosis is prominent, will also be described. Other very rare organic acid disorders are not be considered, but any of them may cause disease in the newborn or in early infancy. Thus, any sick newborn, especially one with metabolic acidosis, should receive an organic acid analysis of urine. This analysis should only be performed in laboratories that utilize gas chromatography with access to mass spectrometry. Otherwise, many organic acid disorders will be missed.

■ ISOVALERIC ACIDEMIA

Isovaleric acidemia, an autosomal recessive disorder, has been termed the "sweaty foot syndrome" because of the offensive odor noted on the body and in the blood and urine of affected individuals. It is caused by a defect

■ HISTIDINEMIA

Histidinemia, an autosomal recessive disorder, results from a defect in the enzyme histidase which catalyzes the conversion of histidine to urocanic acid. It does not produce neonatal disease and is probably benign, but it is included here because it is identified in some newborn screening programs. The major biochemical finding is a three-to-seven-fold increase in the blood histidine level and an even greater increase in urinary histidine. Metabolites of histidine such as imidazolepyruvic, imidazolelactic and imidazoleacetic acids are also present in urine. A low-histidine diet is available for treatment, but there is no clear evidence that treatment is necessary.

in the leucine metabolic pathway at the point at which isovaleryl-CoA is converted to beta-methylcrotonyl-CoA (Fig. 18–7). Isovaleric acid, a short-chain fatty acid, accumulates and is detectable in blood, urine, and CSF. The free isovaleric acid is presumably responsible for the unique odor reminiscent of dried sweat or rancid cheese.

Clinical Characteristics. Metabolic acidosis and the odor are the characteristic features of this disease. In the early onset form of the disorder, acidosis usually appears in the neonatal or early infancy periods accompanied by

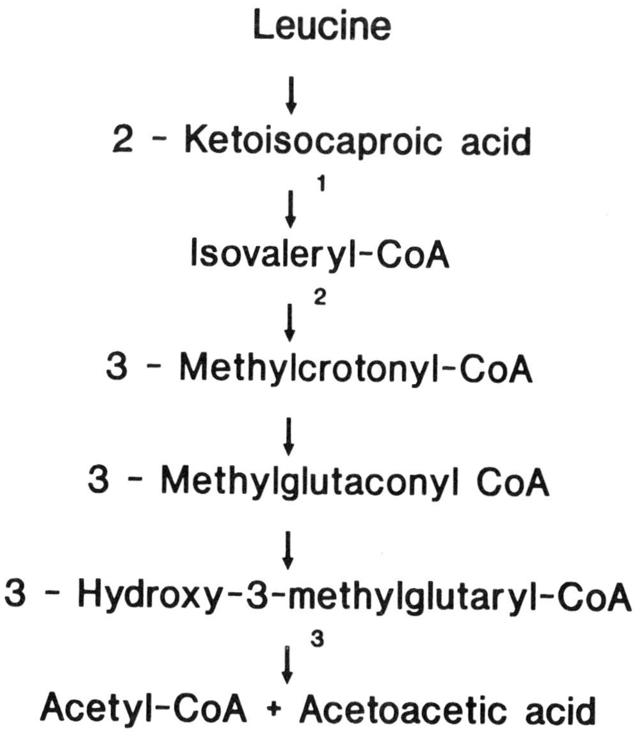

Leucine
↓
2 - Ketoisocaproic acid
↓ 1
Isovaleryl-CoA
↓ 2
3 - Methylcrotonyl-CoA
↓
3 - Methylglutaconyl CoA
↓
3 - Hydroxy-3-methylglutaryl-CoA
↓ 3
Acetyl-CoA + Acetoacetic acid

FIGURE 18–7. Metabolic pathway of leucine degradation: Several organic acid metabolic disorders involve this pathway. The enzyme blocks of three of the major disorders in this pathway include (1) branched-chain alpha-ketoacid dehydrogenase (maple syrup urine disease), (2) isovaleryl-CoA dehydrogenase (isovaleric acidemia), and (3) 3-hydroxy-3-methylglutaryl-CoA lyase (3-hydroxy-3-methylglutaryl-CoA lyase deficiency).

vomiting, lethargy, and weight loss. There are no specific abnormalities on physical examination. With general supportive therapy, these acute symptoms disappear, and the infant remains clinically normal until infection, a high-protein intake, or other intercurrent event precipitates another episode of metabolic acidosis. Thus, as with other organic acid disorders, recurrent metabolic acidosis is the usual history. Death can occur during one of these episodes. Mental retardation often develops unless specific therapy is initiated in infancy (Berry et al., 1988).

Diagnosis. The diagnosis is made on the basis of increased isovaleric acid in blood and the presence of isovalerylglycine in urine. Other laboratory findings during acute episodes include ketonuria and leukopenia or pancytopenia. Amino acids may be normal, or there may be a mild increase in glycine. The diagnosis is confirmed by demonstrating markedly reduced activity of the enzyme isovaleryl-CoA dehydrogenase in leukocytes or cultured skin fibroblasts. Prenatal diagnosis is available.

Treatment. Aside from supportive therapy during acute episodes, isovaleric acidemia may be controlled with a low-leucine diet and the supplementation of glycine, which conjugates with isovaleryl-CoA to form isovalerylglycine and thereby reduces the level of the presumably toxic free acid (Naglak et al., 1988). The mental retardation can be prevented by prompt institution of this diet.

■ 3-HYDROXY-3-METHYLGLUTARYL-CoA LYASE DEFICIENCY

3-Hydroxy-3-methylglutaryl-CoA lyase deficiency is a recessive disorder caused by a block in the final enzyme of the leucine catabolic pathway (see Fig. 18–7). Since acetoacetic acid, a major ketone in the body, is a product of the reaction catalyzed by this enzyme, acute episodes of metabolic acidosis in this organic acid disorder are not accompanied by ketonuria.

Clinical Characteristics. The disorder often presents in the early neonatal period with vomiting, lethargy, hypotonia, metabolic acidosis and severe nonketotic hypoglycemia (Gibson, et al., 1988). There may be rapid progression to coma.

Diagnosis. Metabolic acidosis and hypoglycemia without urinary ketones should raise suspicion of this disorder. Urine organic acid analysis reveals a characteristic pattern of abnormal organic acids that include 3-hydroxy-3-methylglutaric, 3-methylglutaconic, 3-hydroxyisovaleric, and 3-methylglutaric acids. The diagnosis is confirmed on the basis of deficient enzyme activity in leukocytes or cultured skin fibroblasts. Prenatal diagnosis is available.

Treatment. During acute episodes, therapy must be aimed at correcting the hypoglycemia and acidosis with intravenous glucose and bicarbonate. Chronic treatment involves frequent caloric feedings to avoid hypoglycemia and leucine restriction so that the organic acid accumulations are minimized.

■ PROPIONIC ACIDEMIA

The prominent feature of propionic acidemia, an autosomal recessive disorder, is recurrent metabolic acidosis, usually beginning in the neonatal period. The metabolic defect is at the distal segment of the isoleucine and valine degradative pathways. As shown in Figure 18–8, these branched-chain amino acids are degraded to propionyl-CoA which, in propionic acidemia, cannot be converted to methylmalonyl-CoA because of deficient propionyl-CoA carboxylase activity. The amino acids threonine and methionine as well as cholesterol and odd-chain fatty acid are also metabolized to propionic acid. The defect results in an increased level of propionic acid in blood, but even more striking is the presence of metabolites such as hydroxypropionate, hydroxyisovalerate, methylcitrate, and propionylglycine in urine.

Clinical and Laboratory Characteristics. The usual history is that of severe metabolic acidosis presenting in the newborn or young infant. The infant is tachypneic, lethargic, feeds poorly, may vomit, and fails to gain weight. Unless intravenous therapy is begun, the clinical condition worsens and the infant may lapse into a coma. Blood pH is low, sometimes even less than 7.0. Blood bicarbonate is usually less than 15 mmol/L. Ketonuria is present, often to a high degree. The blood ammonia level is increased. Blood amino acid analysis usually reveals an increased glycine concentration ("ketotic hyperglycinemia"), but other amino acid concentrations are normal. Analysis of serum for short-chain fatty acids discloses an increased concentration of propionic acid. The diagnosis is usually made on the basis of urine organic acid analysis, which reveals the aforementioned characteristic metabolites (Wolf et al., 1981).

The diagnosis is confirmed on the basis of markedly reduced or absent propionyl-CoA carboxylase activity in cultured skin fibroblasts or leukocytes. The genes for the two subunits (alpha and beta) of this multimeric enzyme have been cloned (Lamhonwah et al., 1986), and mutations that produce propionic acidemia are being defined (Ohura et al., 1989). Prenatal diagnosis for propionic acidemia is available.

Treatment. Without prompt treatment of the acute episodes, death often occurs in the neonatal period. If the infant survives but does not receive specific treatment, the usual sequelae are recurrent acidosis, failure to thrive, frequent infections, and mental retardation. These chronically ill children often die within the first few years of life.

Treatment of the acute acidotic episodes consists of supportive intravenous fluids that should include amino acids in carefully calculated amounts as well as supplemental L-carnitine (Kahler et al., 1989). The infant often recovers rapidly. If the acidosis is particularly severe or prolonged, bicarbonate is added. Chronic therapy includes a low-protein diet and a special formula free of the offending amino acids. Adequate calories and other nutrients must also be provided. Supplemental biotin (5 to 10 mg/day) is recommended by some, since propionyl-CoA carboxylase is a biotin-dependent enzyme, but this is not of proven therapeutic benefit. Carnitine, an amine that forms readily excreted esters with certain organic

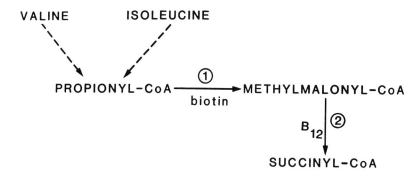

FIGURE 18–8. *Metabolism of propionic acid and methylmalonic acid: This organic acid pathway begins with propionyl-CoA, which derives from the amino acids valine and isoleucine. Normally, propionyl-CoA is carboxylated to methylmalonyl-CoA. In propionic acidemia, propionyl-CoA carboxylase activity is reduced, and propionic acid and its metabolites accumulate. Under normal conditions, methylmalonyl-CoA is converted to succinyl-CoA. In methylmalonic acidemia, however, methylmalonyl-CoA mutase activity is deficient, and methylmalonic acid and its metabolites accumulate.*

① **PROPIONYL-CoA CARBOXYLASE**
② **METHYLMALONYL-CoA MUTASE**

compounds (notably propionyl-CoA) and thereby removes them from the body, has been a valuable addition in the treatment of this disease (Roe and Bohan, 1982).

CASE 18–1

A male infant, one of dizygotic twins, was born to a gravida 3, para 2 mother after an uneventful full-term pregnancy. Labor and delivery were normal. Birth weight was 2820 gm. Apgar scores were 9 at 1 and 5 minutes. On the evening of the 2nd day of life, his very observant mother noted that he was irritable, that he fed poorly from the breast, and that his breathing was rapid. By the third day of life, he had marked tachypnea and was increasingly lethargic. Blood gases at this time revealed pH 7.25 and TCO_2 10. Cultures of blood and CSF were negative. His twin brother remained normal. Family history at this time revealed that a sibling born 6 years before died at 13 days of age after a neonatal course that was characterized by lethargy, tachypnea, poor feeding, and dehydration. There was no specific diagnosis in this sibling, and no metabolic studies were performed.

Physical examination on the 3rd day revealed a tachypneic newborn with poor skin turgor and mild hepatomegaly. Urine was strongly positive for ketones. Complete blood count revealed leukopenia with a white blood count of only 5500. Blood ammonia was 394 μg/dl (normal 40 to 75 μg/dl). All other laboratory data were normal, including serum electrolytes, serum creatinine, liver function indicators, and blood urea nitrogen.

Supportive therapy with intravenous fluids was begun. Within 12 hours, the patient's blood gases became normal, and he was markedly improved with increasing activity and subsiding tachypnea. Specific metabolic studies were initiated at this time. Blood amino acid analysis disclosed slight hyperglycinemia but otherwise normal findings. Thus, maple syrup urine disease was eliminated. Urine organic acid analysis revealed no methylmalonic acid (ruling out methylmalonic acidemia) and no elevation of lactic acid (ruling out pyruvic acidemia). A more elaborate urine organic acid analysis (by gas chromatography) was pending. There was no body odor, so isovaleric acidemia was unlikely. The working diagnosis was propionic acidemia.

Intravenous therapy was maintained, and the infant continued to improve. On the 6th day of life, he began to accept clear fluids orally. Blood ammonia became normal by the 9th day, and 1.0 g/kg/day protein feedings were begun. He tolerated these well, and by discharge at 18 days of age he was tolerating 2.0 g of protein/kg/day without difficulty. The diagnosis of propionic acidemia was substantiated by the characteristic urinary findings of increased hydroxypropionate, hydroxyisovalerate, methylcitrate, and propionylglycine as determined by gas chromatographic analysis.

Chronic treatment consists of a low-protein diet and oral biotin supplementation of 10 mg daily. For the first six months of life, the infant's daily protein intake was 1.5 to 2.0 g/kg. His growth was at the third percentile, and his development was about 1 month delayed. He had numerous episodes of metabolic acidosis, however, usually associated with an acute febrile respiratory illness. Consequently, his daily protein intake was reduced to 1.0 g/kg.

During the 2nd year of life, he began to refuse food. By his 3rd year, he had signs of severe protein malnutrition. He then received a feeding gastrostomy and dramatically improved in growth, development, and general appearance. He is now 9 years old and clinically stable, although he is mildly retarded and hyperactive.

■ METHYLMALONIC ACIDEMIA

Methylmalonic acidemia is an autosomal recessive organic acid disorder that presents either as severe metabolic acidosis in the newborn or as acute metabolic acidosis in the previously well young infant. The enzymatic defect is in methylmalonyl-CoA mutase, a vitamin B_{12}–dependent enzyme responsible for the conversion of methylmalonyl-CoA to succinyl-CoA (see Fig. 18–8). The block in this metabolic step results in a marked accumulation of methylmalonic acid in blood, urine, and CSF.

Clinical and Laboratory Characteristics. The most striking presentation is in the newborn (Matsui et al., 1983). This is usually fulminant and rapidly lethal. The newborn is noted to be lethargic and to feed poorly, generally on the 2nd or 3rd day of life. There may be hepatomegaly but no other physical findings. Studies reveal severe metabolic acidosis. The blood ammonia level may be markedly increased. Many of the amino acids in blood are elevated. Analysis of urine organic acids discloses a huge concentration of methylmalonic acid, also demonstrable in serum. Urinary organic acid metabolites similar to those seen in propionic acidemia may also be present.

In the delayed presentation, the previously well, 2- or 3-month-old infant becomes lethargic, vomits, and refuses to feed. This usually coincides with an increase in the amount of dietary protein. Metabolic acidosis, hyperammonemia, and often hyperglycinemia are present. Urine analysis for organic acids reveals increased methylmalonic acid as the predominant finding.

The diagnosis is confirmed by finding reduced or absent methylmalonyl-CoA mutase activity in cultured skin fibroblasts. The gene for this enzyme has been cloned (Ledley et al., 1988), and mutations in methylmalonic acidemic patients are being defined. Prenatal diagnosis is available.

Treatment. The fulminant neonatal presentation or the acute phase of the delayed presentation requires aggressive therapeutic measures. Hemodialysis or peritoneal dialysis may be lifesaving. Protein intake should cease, and intravenous fluids containing very large amounts of calories as well as bicarbonate to counteract the acidosis should be given. Vitamin B_{12} (cyanocobalamin or hydroxocobalamin) 1 mg intramuscularly should be administered to cover the possibility that the type of methylmalonic acidemia presenting is B_{12}-responsive.

Chronic therapy consists of a special diet that includes low-protein foods and a formula free of offending amino acids. About 50 per cent of affected infants who have the delayed presentation respond to the administration of vitamin B_{12} with marked reduction in the levels of blood and urine methylmalonic acid. These B_{12}-responsive patients have a defect in the synthesis of adenosylcobalamin (adenosyl-B_{12}), the specific B_{12} cofactor for methylmalonyl-CoA mutase. They should receive weekly or biweekly injections of vitamin B_{12} and a modified low-protein diet.

Other Causes. Methylmalonic acid may be present in urine (and blood) of infants who have a more extensive B_{12} metabolic defect (see the previous section on "Sulfur Amino Acid Abnormalities"). These infants also have amino acid abnormalities such as homocystinuria(-emia), cystathioninuria(-emia), and hypomethioninemia. Methylmalonic acid may also appear in the urine of vitamin B_{12}–deficient infants breast-fed by strictly vegetarian mothers or as a transient finding in normal breast-fed infants (Shih et al., 1976). Finally, there appears to be a benign form of mutase deficiency in which the infant has persistent but mild methylmalonic acidemia. These healthy infants have generally been identified by routine newborn urine screening. No treatment is indicated for this condition (Ledley et al., 1984).

■ PYRUVIC ACIDEMIA

Pyruvate is an intermediary metabolite in the degradation of glucose. Complete or aerobic glycolysis produces acetyl-CoA and oxaloacetate from pyruvate, both of which enter the tricarboxylic acid (Krebs) cycle and support maximal energy production. Two inherited enzyme deficiencies in pyruvate oxidation have been described. The most frequent is pyruvate dehydrogenase complex deficiency which limits acetyl-CoA formation. This may be an X-linked disorder (Brown et al., 1989). The other is pyruvate carboxylase deficiency, which limits the formation of oxaloacetate.

Clinical and Laboratory Characteristics. Infants with pyruvic acidemia from either defect who present in the neonatal period develop tachypnea, lethargy, and hypotonia during the first few days of life. Laboratory data reveal profound metabolic acidosis and increased blood

lactate and pyruvate. Urine is positive for ketones. On organic acid analysis, the urine is found to contain huge amounts of lactate and beta-hydroxybutrate. Blood amino acid analysis reveals an increased concentration of alanine but is otherwise normal. The diagnosis is confirmed by enzyme studies of leukocytes or cultured skin fibroblasts or of postmortem tissue.

Treatment. Therapy consists of intravenous infusion with fluids and large amounts of bicarbonate. Glucose should be given but only in maintenance amounts since more than that increases the accumulation of pyruvate and lactate. Caloric support should primarily consist of even-chain fatty acids. These infants have usually died in early infancy or have suffered chronic neurologic damage.

■ MULTIPLE CARBOXYLASE DEFICIENCY

Multiple carboxylase deficiency is a biochemical syndrome produced by an extraordinary requirement for the vitamin biotin. It is expressed as deficient activities of the four biotin-requiring carboxylase enzymes in the body, which are pyruvate carboxylase, propionyl-CoA carboxylase, beta-methylcrotonyl-CoA carboxylase, and acetyl-CoA carboxylase. The metabolites that accumulate as a result of these deficient activities include lactic and pyruvic acids, hydroxypropionate, and other metabolites associated with propionic acidemia, and beta-methylcrotonylglycine. This pattern of organic acid abnormalities is unique to multiple carboxylase deficiencies and should be recognized by urine organic acid analysis.

Clinical and Laboratory Characteristics. There are two clinically distinct expressions of multiple carboxylase deficiency, each due to a different enzyme defect. The first expression is early onset or neonatal and is due to a defect in the enzyme holocarboxylase synthetase, which binds biotin to the carboxylases. Affected infants present in the neonatal period with vomiting, lethargy, and other signs of severe metabolic acidosis. Laboratory findings include hypoglycemia, acidosis, ketonuria, and hyperammonemia.

The second expression, known as *biotinidase deficiency*, has a later onset and is due to a defect in biotinidase, the enzyme responsible for intracellular recycling of biotin (Wolf et al., 1985). These patients often present in infancy with developmental delay, hypotonia, seizures, alopecia, eczema, and hearing loss. Biotinidase deficiency may come to attention in the newborn period before symptoms appear, however, since some newborn screening programs include this among the disorders for which the newborn blood specimen is screened (see Chapter 17). Laboratory findings in the symptomatic infant include lactic acidosis and ketonuria. These are usually absent in the presymptomatic state.

Diagnosis. The characteristic organic aciduria of multiple carboxylase deficiency as determined by organic acid analysis calls attention to either holocarboxylase synthetase deficiency in the sick newborn or to biotinidase deficiency in the chronically ill infant. The diagnosis of either is confirmed by demonstrating the enzyme defect.

Holocarboxylase synthetase is measured in cultured skin fibroblasts. Biotinidase can be measured in serum, whole blood, red blood cells, or cultured skin fibroblasts.

Treatment. The acutely ill newborn requires intravenous fluids including glucose for caloric support and bicarbonate to correct the metabolic acidosis. These infants should be given biotin in doses of 10 to 80 mg/day (Packman et al., 1981).

Infants and children found to have biotinidase deficiency should be treated with biotin 10 mg/day. This reverses some of the manifestations in the symptomatic infant and prevents clinical disease in the presymptomatic newborn (Wolf et al., 1985).

■ GLUTARIC ACIDEMIA

Glutaric acid is an intermediate in the metabolism of the amino acids lysine, hydroxylysine, and tryptophan. Two inherited disorders involving glutaric acid degradation have been described. The first of these, *glutaric acidemia type I*, is a primary defect in glutaric acid metabolism and results from a deficiency in glutaryl-CoA dehydrogenase.

Glutaric aciduria type II is a much more dramatic condition causing metabolic acidosis with lethargy and hypotonia in the newborn and is described in the next section on the mitochondrial myopathies.

A striking clinical feature of glutaric aciduria type I is macrocephaly at birth (Goodman et al., 1987). The enlarged head usually suggests hydrocephalus (Iafolla and Kahler, 1989) and leads to studies such as a CAT scan which reveals changes similar to those seen in subdural effusions but, in glutaric acidemia, are due to bilateral atrophy of the temporal lobes (Amir et al., 1987). This is often unrecognized, and many of these infants have been subjected to dry subdural taps before the metabolic disorder has been identified. Other than macrocephaly, the newborn with glutaric acidemia I seems to be normal. Later in infancy or early childhood, however, progressive neurologic deterioration begins with choreoathetosis and dystonia due to basal ganglia involvement. Many of the affected children are mentally retarded.

Laboratory Characteristics and Treatment. The laboratory features include chronic metabolic acidosis and a characteristic organic aciduria that features increased glutaric acid, hydroxyglutaric acid, and glutaconic acid. The diagnosis is confirmed by demonstrating decreased activity of glutaryl-CoA dehydrogenase in cultured skin fibroblasts (Amir et al., 1989). Treatment consists of a special diet reduced in lysine and tryptophan. Prenatal diagnosis is available.

A large number of riboflavin-responsive children with glutaric acidemia I have been discovered among the Pennsylvania Amish (Morton et al., 1989).

■ MITOCHONDRIAL MYOPATHIES

This is a category of disorders that are due to defects in the electron transport system (respiratory chain) of the mitochondrion. Skeletal and cardiac muscles are strikingly involved because of their dependence on mitochondrially generated energy, but other organs of the body are also dysfunctional. Two of these disorders present in the newborn and are considered here.

GLUTARIC ACIDURIA II

Glutaric aciduria type II is the second of the autosomal recessive disorders in which there is increased urinary glutaric acid. Unlike glutaric acidemia type I (see above), glutaric aciduria II has a striking neonatal presentation with profound metabolic acidosis and nonketotic hypoglycemia, often present on the 1st day of life (Goodman et al., 1983). The newborn is lethargic and markedly hypotonic. Cardiomyopathy is often present. Some of these infants also have congenital anomalies, notably polycystic kidneys. Omphalocele and anomalies of the external genitalia have also been reported. Many die in the neonatal period. Those who survive develop poorly and usually die during infancy.

The basic defect is in the electron-transfer flavoprotein (ETF), which accepts electrons from the various dehydrogenases, or in ETF ubiquinone oxidoreductase, which transfers electrons from ETF to the ubiquinone pool of the cellular respiratory chain. With either defect, electron transfer from the dehydrogenases is impaired, and their functions are compromised. Consequently, organic acids, such as glutaric acid and the dicarboxylic acids, which accumulate when fatty acid oxidation is blocked, are excreted in the urine. Other laboratory findings include hypoglycemia and lactic acidosis.

There is no effective treatment for this disorder. Supportive therapy with intravenous fluids and the inclusion of carnitine might offer temporary help. Prenatal diagnosis is available.

SENGER SYNDROME

Senger syndrome is characterized by bilateral congenital cataracts, mitochondrial myopathy with severe hypotonia, cardiomyopathy, and intermittent lactic acidosis (Cruysberg et al., 1986). The cataracts and hypotonia are neonatal features, whereas the cardiomyopathy may not appear until later in infancy. Conduction defects have accompanied the cardiomyopathy and have caused sudden death in some of these children. The specific metabolic defect has not yet been identified, although the striking mitochondrial abnormalities noted on electron microscopy of skeletal muscle indicate that the primary defect is in the mitochondrion.

Laboratory findings have included lactic acidosis, which may be present only during acute illness, and sometimes dicarboxylic aciduria noted on organic acid analysis. However, there is no characteristic laboratory feature nor confirmatory test. The diagnosis is based on clinical findings and muscle histopathology.

Treatment is supportive and symptomatic. Some of these infants die in the neonatal or infancy periods with cardiac decompensation or sudden death. Others have growth and developmental delay but live into childhood. Still others have normal growth and development and have survived into adult years.

■ REFERENCES

General Considerations

American Academy of Pediatrics, Committee on Nutrition: Special diets for infants with inborn errors of amino acid metabolism. Pediatrics 57:783, 1976.

Cederbaum, S. D.: Introduction to recombinant DNA. Pediatrics 74:408, 1984.

Ledley, F. D.: Somatic gene therapy for human disease: background and prospects. J. Pediatr. 110:1, 167, 1987.

Roth, K. S., Yang, W., Allan, L., et al.: Prenatal administration of biotin in biotin responsive multiple carboxylase deficiency. Pediatr. Res. 16:126, 1982.

Carbohydrate Disorders

Galactosemia

Buist, N., Waggoner, D., Donnell, G., et al.: The effect of newborn screening on prognosis in galactosemia. Results of an international survey. Am. J. Hum. Genet. 43:A3, 1988.

Haberland, C., Perou, M., Brunngraber, E. G., et al.: The neuropathology of galactosemia. A histopathological and biochemical study. J. Neuropathol. Exp. Neurol. 30:431, 1971.

Kaufman, F. R., Kogut, M. D., Donnell, G. N., et al.: Hypergonadotrophic hypogonadism in female patients with galactosemia. N. Engl. J. Med. 304:994, 1981.

Lo, W., Packman, S., Nash, S., et al.: Curious neurologic sequelae in galactosemia. Pediatrics 73:309, 1984.

Ng, W. G., Xu, Y. K., Kaufman, F. R., et al.: Deficit of uridine diphosphate galactose in galactosaemia. J. Inherited Metab. Dis. 12:257, 1989.

Reichardt, J. K. V., and Berg, P.: Cloning and characterization of a cDNA encoding human galactose-1-phosphate uridyltransferase. Mol. Biol. Med. 5:107, 1988.

Waisbren, S. E., Norman, T. R., Schnell, R. R., and Levy, H. L.: Speech and language deficits in early-treated children with galactosemia. J. Pediatr. 102:75, 1983.

Galactokinase and Uridine Diphosphate Galactose-4-Epimerase Deficiencies

Henderson, M. J., Holton, J. B., and MacFaul, R.: Further observations in a case or uridine diphosphate galactose-4-epimerase deficiency with severe clinical presentation. J. Inherited Metab. Dis. 6:17, 1983.

Sardharwalla, I. B., Wraith, S. E., Bridge, C., et al.: A patient with severe type of epimerase deficiency galactosemia. J. Inherited Metab. Dis. 11(Suppl. 2):249, 1988.

Glycogen Storage Diseases

Chen, Y. T., Connblath, M., and Sidbury, J. B.: Cornstarch therapy in type 1 glycogen storage disease. N. Engl. J. Med. 310:171, 1984.

Folk, C. C., and Greene, H. L.: Dietary management of type 1 glycogen storage disease. J. Am. Diet. Assoc. 84:293, 1984.

Narisawa, K., Igarishl, Y., and Tada, K.: Glycogen storage disease type 1b: Genetic disorder involving the transport system of intracellular membrane. Enzyme 38:177, 1987.

Nordlie, R. C., and Sukalski, K. A.: Multiple forms of type 1 glycogen storage disease: Underlying mechanisms. Trends Biochem. Sci. 11:85, 1986.

Slonim, A. E., Coleman, R. A., and Moses, W. S.: Myopathy and growth failure in debrancher enzyme deficiency: Improvement with high-protein nocturnal enteral therapy. J. Pediatr. 105:906, 1984.

Hereditary Fructose Intolerance

Cross, N. C. P., Tolan, D. R., and Cox, T. M.: Catalytic deficiency of human aldolase B in hereditary fructose intolerance caused by a common missense mutation. Cell 53:881, 1988.

Rottmann, W. H., Tolan, D. R., and Penhoet, E. E.: Complete amino acid sequence for human aldolase B derived from cDNA and genomic clones. Proc. Natl. Acad. Sci. USA. 81:2738, 1984.

Tolan, D. R., and Penhoet, E. E.: Characterization of the human aldolase B gene. Mol. Biol. Med. 3:245, 1986.

Suggested Readings

Allen, J. T., Holton, J. B., Lennox, A. C., et al.: Early morning urine galactitol levels in relation to galactose intake: A possible method of monitoring the diet in galactokinase deficiency. J. Inherited Metab. Dis. 11(Suppl. 2):243, 1988.

Baerlocher, K., Gitzelmann, R., Steinmann, B., et al.: Hereditary fructose intolerance in early childhood: A major diagnostic challenge. Helv. Paediatr. Acta 33:465, 1978.

Donnell, G. N., Koch, R., Fishler, K., et al.: Clinical aspects of galactosaemia. In Burman, D., Holton, J. B., and Pennock, C. A. (Eds.): Inherited disorders of carbohydrate metabolism. Lancaster, MTP Press, 1980, pp. 103–115.

Kerr, M. M., Logan, R. W., Cant, J. S., et al.: Galactokinase deficiency in a newborn infant. Arch. Dis. Child. 46:864, 1971.

Levy, H. L., Sepe, S. J., Walton, D. S., et al.: Galactose-1-phosphate uridyl transferase deficiency due to Duarte/galactosemia combined variation: Clinical and biochemical studies. J. Pediatr. 92:390, 1978.

Levy, H. L., Sepe, S. J., Walton, D. S., et al.: Sepsis due to Escherichia coli in neonates with galactosemia. N. Engl. J. Med. 297:825, 1977.

Thalhammer, O., Gitzelmann, R., and Pantlitschko, M.: Hypergalactosemia and galactosuria due to galactokinase deficiency in a newborn. Pediatrics 42:441, 1968.

Phenylketonuria

Guttler, F.: Hyperphenylalaninemia. Diagnosis and classification of the various types of phenylalanine hydroxylase deficiency in childhood. Acta Pediatr. Scand. 280(Suppl.):7, 1980.

Holtzman, N. A.: Ethical issues in prenatal diagnosis of phenylketonuria. Pediatrics 74:424, 1984.

Kaufman, S.: Phenylketonuria: Biochemical mechanisms. In Agranoff, B. W., and Aprison, M. H. (Eds.): Advances in Neurochemistry, vol. 2. New York, Plenum Press, 1976, pp. 1–132.

Koch, R., and Wenz, E.: Phenylketonuria. Ann. Rev. Nutr. 7:117, 1987.

Kwok, S. C. M., Ledley, F. D., DiLella, A. G., et al.: Nucleotide sequence of a full-length complementary DNA clone and amino acid sequence of human phenylalanine hydroxylase. Biochemistry 24:556, 1985.

Ledley, F. D., Koch, R., Jew, K., et al.: Phenylalanine hydroxylase expression in liver of a fetus with phenylketonuria. J. Pediatr. 113:463, 1988.

Levy, H. L.: Phenylketonuria—1986. Pediatr. Rev. 7:269, 1986.

Levy, H. L.: Molecular genetics of phenylketonuria and its implications. Am. J. Hum. Genet. 45:667, 1989.

McCabe, E. R. B., and McCabe, L.: Issues in the dietary management of phenylketonuria: Breast-feeding and trace-metal nutriture. Ann. N.Y. Acad. Sci. 477:215, 1986.

Schmidt, H., Mahle, M., Michel, U., et al.: Continuation vs. discontinuation of low-phenylalanine diet in PKU adolescents. Eur. J. Pediatr. 146(Suppl. 1):A17, 1987.

Scriver, C. R., and Clow, C. L.: Phenylketonuria: Epitome of human biochemical genetics. N. Engl. J. Med. 303:1336 and 1394, 1980.

Scriver, C. R., and Clow, C. L.: Avoiding phenylketonuria: Why parents seek prenatal diagnosis. J. Pediatr. 113:495, 1988.

Scriver, C. R., Kaufman, S., and Woo, S. L. C.: Mendelian hyperphenylalaninemia. Ann. Rev. Genet. 22:301, 1988.

Hyperphenylalaninemias

Irons, M., Levy, H. L., O'Flynn, M. E., et al.: Folinic acid therapy in the treatment of dihydropteridine reductase deficiency. J. Pediatr. 110:61, 1987.

Kaufman, S., Berlow, S., Summer, G. K., et al.: Hyperphenylalaninemia due to a deficiency of biopterin. A variant form of phenylketonuria. N. Engl. J. Med. 299:673, 1978.

Kaufman, S., Holtzman, N. A., Milstien, S., et al.: Phenylketonuria due to a deficiency of dihydropteridine reductase. N. Engl. J. Med. 293:785, 1975.

Naylor, E. W., Ennis, D., Davidson, G. F., et al.: Guanosine triphosphate cyclohydrolase I deficiency: Early diagnosis by routine urine pteridine screening. Pediatrics 79:374, 1987.

Shintaku, H., Niederwieser, A., Leimbacher, W., et al.: Tetrahydrobiopterin deficiency: Assay for 6-pyruvoyl-tetrahydropterin synthase activity in erythrocytes, and detection of patients and heterozygous carriers. Eur. J. Pediatr. 147:15, 1988.

Maternal Phenylketonuria

Drogari, E., Smith, I., Beasley, M., et al.: Timing of strict diet in relation to fetal damage in maternal phenylketonuria. Lancet 2:927, 1987.

Lenke, R. R., and Levy, H. L.: Maternal phenylketonuria and hyperphenylalaninemia. An international survey of the outcome of untreated and treated pregnancies. N. Engl. J. Med. 303:1202, 1980.

Levy, H. L.: Maternal phenylketonuria. Review with emphasis on pathogenesis. Enzyme 38:312, 1987.

Levy, H. L., and Waisbren, S. E.: Effects of maternal phenylketonuria and hyperphenylalaninemia on the fetus. N. Engl. J. Med. 309:1269, 1983.

Rohr, F. J., Doherty, L. B., Waisbren, S. E., et al.: The New England Maternal PKU Project: Prospective study of untreated and treated pregnancies and their outcomes. J. Pediatr. 110:391, 1987.

Waisbren, S. E., and Levy, H. L.: Effects of untreated maternal hyperphenylalaninemia on the fetus: Further study of families identified by routine cord blood screening. J. Pediatr. 116:926, 1990.

Maple Syrup Urine Disease

Clow, C. L., Reade, T. M., and Scriver, C. R.: Outcome of early and long-term management of classical maple syrup urine disease. Pediatrics 68:856, 1981.

Fernhoff, P. M., Lubitz, D., Danner, D. J., et al.: Thiamine response in maple syrup urine disease. Pediatr. Res. 19:1011, 1985.

Hammersen, G., Wille, L., Schmidt H., et al.: Maple syrup urine diseases: Treatment of the acutely ill newborn. Eur. J. Pediatr. 129:157, 1978.

Hu, C. W. C., Lau, K. S., Griffin, T. A., et al.: Isolation and sequencing of a cDNA encoding the decarboxylase (E1) α precursor of bovine branched-chain α-keto acid dehydrogenase complex. J. Biol. Chem. 263:9007, 1988.

Indo, Y., Akaboshi, I., Nobukuni, Y., et al.: Maple syrup urine disease: A possible biochemical basis for the clinical heterogeneity. Hum. Genet. 80:6, 1988.

Naylor, E. W., and Guthrie, R.: Newborn screening for maple syrup urine disease. Pediatrics 61:262, 1978.

Sulfur Amino Acid Abnormalities

Fowler, B., Borresen, A. L., and Boman, N.: Prenatal diagnosis of homocystinuria. Lancet 2:875, 1982.

Gahl, W. A., Finkelstein, J. D., Mullen, K. D., et al.: Hepatic methionine adenosyltransferase deficiency in a 31-year-old man. Am. J. Hum. Genet. 40:39, 1987.

Gaull, G. E., Benden, A. N., Vulovic, D., et al.: Methioninemia and myopathy: A new disorder. Ann. Neurol. 9:423, 1981.

Higginbottom, M. C., Sweetman, L., and Nyhan, W. L.: A syndrome of methylmalonic aciduria, homocystinuria, megaloblastic anemia and neurologic abnormalities in a vitamin B₁₂–deficient breast-fed infant of a strict vegetarian. N. Engl. J. Med. 299:317, 1978.

Kraus, J. P., Williamson, C. L., Firgaira, F. A., et al.: Cloning and screening with nanogram amounts of immunopurified mRNAs: cDNA cloning and chromosomal mapping of cystathionine β-synthase and β subunit of propionyl-CoA carboxylase. Proc. Natl. Acad. Sci. U.S.A. 83:2047, 1986.

Levy, H. L., Mudd, S. H., Schulman, J. D., et al.: A derangement in B₁₂ metabolism associated with homocystinemia, cystathioninemia, hypomethioninemia and methylmalonic aciduria. Am. J. Med. 48:390, 1970.

Mudd, S. H., Levy, H. L., and Skovby, F.: Disorders of trans-sulfuration. In Scriver, C. R., Beaudet, A. L., Sly, W. S., et al. (Eds.): The Metabolic Basis of Inherited Disease. New York, McGraw-Hill, 1989, pp 693–734.

Schuh, S., Rosenblatt, D. S., Cooper, B. A., et al.: Homocystinuria and megaloblastic anemia responsive to vitamin B₁₂ therapy—an inborn error of metabolism due to a defect in cobalamin metabolism. N. Engl. J. Med. 310:686, 1984.

Shih, V. E., Axel, S. M., Tewksbury, J. C., et al.: Defective lysosomal release of vitamin B₁₂ (cbl F): A hereditary cobalamin metabolic disorder associated with sudden death. Am. J. Med. Genet. 33:555, 1989.

Whitehead, P. D., Clayton, B. E., Ersser, R. S., et al.: Changing incidence of neonatal hypermethioninemia: Implications for the detection of homocystinuria. Arch. Dis. Child. 54:593, 1979.

Wilcken, B., and Turner, G.: Homocystinuria in New South Wales. Arch. Dis. Child. 53:242, 1978.

Tyrosinemia

Avery, W. E., Clow, C. L., Menkes, J. M., et al.: Transient tyrosinemia of the newborn. Dietary and clinical aspects. Pediatrics 39:160, 1967.

Esquivel, C. O., Mieles, L., Marino, I. R., et al.: Liver transplantation for hereditary tyrosinemia in the presence of hepatocellular carcinoma. Transplant. Proc. 21:2445, 1989.

Gagne, R., Lescault, A., Grenier, A., et al.: Prenatal diagnosis of tyrosinaemia: Measurement of succinylacetone in amniotic fluid. Prenat. Diagn. 2:185, 1982.

King, G. S., MacKenzie, F., and Pettit, B. R.: Neonatal and prenatal diagnosis of hereditary tyrosinaemia. Lancet 2:1279, 1983.

Kvittingen, E. A., Guibaud, P. P., Divry, P., et al.: Prenatal diagnosis of hereditary tyrosinaemia type I by determination of fumarylacetoacetase in chorionic villus material. Eur. J. Pediatr. 144:597, 1986.

Kvittingen, E. A., Halvorsen, S., and Jellum, E.: Deficient fumarylacetoacetate fumarylhydrolase activity in lymphocytes and fibroblasts from patients with hereditary tyrosinaemia. Pediatr. Res. 14:541, 1983.

Kvittingen, E. A., Steinmann, B., Gitzelmann, R., et al.: Prenatal diagnosis of hereditary tyrosinaemia by determination of fumarylacetoacetase in cultured amniotic fluid cells. Pediatr. Res. 19:334, 1985.

Martin, H. P., Fischer, H. L., Martin, D. S., et al.: The development of children with transient neonatal tyrosinemia. J. Pediatr. 84:212, 1974.

Mitchell, G., Larochelle, J., Lambert, M., et al.: Neurologic crisis in hereditary tyrosinaemia. N. Eng J. Med. 322:432, 1990.

Rice, D. N., Houston, I. B., Lyon, I. C. T., et al.: Transient neonatal tyrosinaemia. J. Inher. Metab. Dis. 12:13, 1989.

Sassa, S., and Kappas, A.: Hereditary tyrosinaemia and the heme biosynthetic pathway—profound inhibition of δ-aminolevulinic acid dehydratase activity by succinylacetone. J. Clin. Invest. 71:625, 1983.

Weinberg, A. G., Mize, C. E., and Worthen, H. G.: The occurrence of hepatoma in the chronic form of hereditary tyrosinemia. J. Pediatr. 88:434, 1976.

Urea Cycle Disorders

Bachmann, C., Krähenbühl, S., and Colombo, J. P.: N-acetylglutamate synthetase deficiency: A disorder of ammonia detoxication. N. Engl. J. Med. 304:543, 1981.

Beaudet, A. L., O'Brien, W. E., Bock, H. G. O., et al.: The human argininosuccinate synthetase locus and citrullinemia. In Harris, H., and Hirschhorn, K. (Eds.): Advances in Human Genetics, vol. 15. New York, Plenum, 1986, pp. 161–196.

Brusilow, S. W., and Batshaw, M. L.: Arginine therapy of argininosuccinase deficiency. Lancet 1:124, 1979.

Brusilow, S. W., Danney, M., Waber, L. J., et al.: Treatment of episodic hyperammonemia in children with inborn errors of urea synthesis. N. Engl. J. Med. 310:1630, 1984.

Hudak, M. L., Jones, M. D., Jr., and Brusilow, S. W.: Differentiation of transient hyperammonemia of the newborn and urea cycle enzyme defects by clinical presentation. J. Pediatr. 107:712, 1985.

Largillière, C., Houssin, D., Gottrand, F., et al.: Liver transplantation for ornithine transcarbamylase deficiency in a girl. J. Pediatr. 115:415, 1989.

Msall, M., Batshaw, M. L., Suss, R., et al.: Neurologic outcome in children with inborn errors of urea synthesis—outcome of urea-cycle enzymopathies. N. Engl. J. Med. 310:1500, 1984.

O'Brien, W. E., McInnes, R., Kalumuck, K., et al.: Cloning and sequence analysis of cDNA for human argininosuccinate lyase. Proc. Natl. Acad. Sci. U.S.A. 83:7211, 1986.

Spence, J. E., Maddalena, A., O'Brien, W. E., et al.: Prenatal diagnosis and heterozygote detection by DNA analysis in ornithine transcarbamylase deficiency. J. Pediatr. 114:582, 1989.

Tuchman, M.: Persistent acitrullinemia after liver transplantation for carbamylphosphate synthetase deficiency. N. Engl. J. Med. 320:1498, 1989.

Vimal, C. M., Fensom, A. H., Heaton, D., et al.: Prenatal diagnosis of argininosuccinicaciduria by analysis of cultured chorionic villi. Lancet 2:521, 1984.

Hyperglycinemia

Hayasaka, K., Tada, K., Fueki, N., et al.: Nonketotic hyperglycinemia: Analyses of glycine cleavage system in typical and atypical cases. J. Pediatr. 110:873, 1987.

Tada, K.: Nonketotic hyperglycinemia: Clinical and metabolic aspects. Enzyme 38:27, 1987.

Wijburg, F. A., deGroot, C. J., Schutgens, R. B. H., et al.: Clinical effects of serine medication in nonketotic hyperglycinaemia due to deficiency of P-protein of the glycine cleavage complex. J. Inherited Metab. Dis. 11(Suppl.2):218, 1988.

Wolff, J. A., Kulovich, S., Yu, A. L., et al.: The effectiveness of benzoate in the management of seizures in nonketotic hyperglycinemia. Am. J. Dis. Child. 140:596, 1986.

Histidinemia

Coulombe, J. T., Kammerer, B. L., Levy, H. L., et al.: Histidinaemia. Part III. Impact; a prospective study. J. Inherited Metab. Dis. 6:58, 1983.

Scriver, C. R., and Levy, H. L.: Histidinaemia. Part I. Reconciling retrospective and prospective findings. J. Inherited Metab. Dis. 6:51, 1983.

Isovaleric Acidemia

Berry, G. T., Yudkoff, M., Segal, S.: Isovaleric acidemia: Medical and neurodevelopmental effects of long-term therapy. J. Pediatr. 113:58, 1988.

Naglak, M., Salvo, R., and Segal, S.: The treatment of isovaleric acidemia with glycine supplement. Pediatr. Res. 24:9, 1988.

3-Hydroxy-3-Methylglutaryl-CoA Lyase Deficiency

Gibson, K. M., Brever, J., et al.: 3-Hydroxy-3-methylglutaryl-coenzyme. A lyase deficiency: Review of 18 reported patients. Eur. J. Pediatr. 148:180, 1988.

Propionic Acidemia

Kahler, S. Q., Millington, D. S., Cederbaum, S. D., et al.: Parenteral nutrition in propionic and methylmalonic acidemia. J. Pediatr. 115:235, 1989.

Lamhonwah, A. M., Barankiewicz, T. J., Willard, H. F., et al.: Isolation of cDNA clones coding for the alpha and beta chains of human propionyl-CoA carboxylase: Chromosomal assignment and DNA polymorphisms associated with PCCA and PCCB genes. Proc. Natl. Acad. Sci. U.S.A. 83:4864, 1986.

Ohura, T., Kraus, J. P., and Rosenberg, L. E.: Unequal synthesis and differential degradation of propionyl CoA carboxylase subunits in cells from normal and propionic acidemia patients. Am. J. Hum. Genet. 45:33, 1989.

Roe, C. R., and Bohan, T. P.: L-Carnitine therapy in propionic acidaemia. Lancet 1:1411, 1982.

Wolf, B., Hsia, Y. E., Sweetman, L., et al.: Propionic acidemia: A clinical update. J. Pediatr. 99:835, 1981.

Methylmalonic Acidemia

Ledley, F. D., Levy, H. L., Shih, V. E., et al.: Benign methylmalonic aciduria. N. Engl. J. Med. 311:1015, 1984.

Ledley, F. D., Lumetta, M. R., Zoghbi, H. Y., et al.: Mapping the human methylmalonyl CoA mutase (MUT) locus on chromosome 6. Am. J. Hum. Genet. 42:839, 1988.

Matsui, S. M., Mahoney, M. J., and Rosenberg, L. E.: The natural history of the inherited methylmalonic acidemias. N. Engl. J. Med. 308:857, 1983.

Shih, V. E., Coulombe, J. T., Maties, M., et al.: Methylmalonic aciduria in the newborn. N. Engl. J. Med. 295:1320, 1976.

Pyruvic Acidemia

Aleck, K. A., Kaplan, A. M., Sherwood, W. G., et al.: In utero central nervous system damage in pyruvate dehydrogenase deficiency. Arch. Neurol. 45:987, 1988.

Brown, R. M., Dahl, H. H. M., and Brown, G. K.: X-chromosome localization of the functional gene for the E1 alpha subunit of the human pyruvate dehydrogenase complex. Genomics 4:174, 1989.

Byrd, D. J., Krohn, H.-P., Winkler, L., et al.: Neonatal pyruvate dehydrogenase deficiency with lipoate responsive lactic acidaemia and hyperammonaemia. Eur. J. Pediatr. 148:543, 1989.

Oizumi, J., Ng, W. G., and Donnell, G. N.: Pyruvate carboxylase defect: Metabolic studies on cultured skin fibroblasts. J. Inher Metab. Dis. 9:120, 1986.

Robinson, B. H., MacMillan, H., Petrova-Benedict, R., et al.: Variable clinical presentation in patients with defective E1 component of pyruvate dehydrogenase complex. J. Pediatr. 111:525, 1987.

Multiple Carboxylase Deficiency

Packman, S., Sweetman, L., Baker, H., et al.: The neonatal form of biotin-responsive multiple carboxylase deficiency. J. Pediatr. 99:418, 1981.

Wolf, B., Grier, R. E., Secor McVoy, J. R., et al.: Biotinidase deficiency: A novel vitamin recycling defect. J. Inherited Metab. Dis. 8(Suppl. 1):53, 1985.

Wolf, B., Heard, G. S., Jefferson, L. G., et al.: Clinical findings in four children with biotinidase deficiency detected through a statewide neonatal screening program. N. Engl. J. Med. 313:16, 1985.

Glutaric Acidemia

Amir, N., Elpeleg, O. N., Shalev, R. S., et al.: Glutaric aciduria type I: Enzymatic and neuroradiologic investigations of two kindreds. J. Pediatr. 114:983, 1989.

Amir, N., El-Peleg, O., Shalev, R. S., et al.: Glutaric aciduria type I: Clinical heterogeneity and neuroradiologic features. Neurology 37:1654, 1987.

Goodman, S. I., Frerman, F. E., and Loehr, J. P.: Recent progress in understanding glutaric acidemias. Enzyme 38:76, 1987.

Iafolla, A. K., and Kahler, S. G.: Megalencephaly in the neonatal period as the initial manifestation of glutaric aciduria type I. J. Pediatr. 114:1004, 1989.

Morton, H., Bennett, M., Nichter, C., et al.: Glutaric aciduria type I of the Amish. Am. J. Hum. Genet. 45:A9, 1989.

Mitochondrial Myopathies

Cruysberg, J. R. M., Sengers, R. C. A., Pinckers, A., et al.: Features of a syndrome with congenital cataract and hypertrophic cardiomyopathy. Am. J. Ophthalmol. 102:740, 1986.

Goodman, S. I., Reale, M., and Berlow, S.: Glutaric acidemia type II: A form with deleterious intrauterine effects. J. Pediatr. 102:411, 1983.

OTHER GENETIC DISORDERS 19

Bruce R. Korf

■ DEFECTS INVOLVING CONNECTIVE TISSUE

MARFAN SYNDROME

Marfan syndrome (arachnodactyly) is a hereditary disorder of connective tissue with many somatic manifestations. Inheritance is autosomal dominant, but those who carry the gene show great differences in the severity and variety of features expressed and occasionally fail to show any manifestations of the mutant gene (nonpenetrance), making counseling difficult. About 15 to 25 per cent of patients do not have an affected relative and presumably represent new mutations. Since many of the features are not present at birth, the condition is often difficult to diagnose at this stage unless there is an affected near relative. The prevalence is 1 per 12,000 population in the United States, or about 20,000 affected individuals.

Basic Science. Many of the pathologic alterations in Marfan syndrome can be attributed to an abiotrophy of connective tissue (i.e., to its imperfect structure leading to precocious weakening under stress). The specific defect leading to this connective tissue weakness is for the most part unknown (Pope and Nicholls, 1987). A single patient with Marfan syndrome having a defect in the alpha-2 chain of type I collagen has been described (Byers et al., 1981), but linkage to this and some other collagen genes has been excluded for other families (Francomano et al., 1988). Recent evidence suggests that abnormalities in the microfibrillar fiber system may be related to the pathogenesis of Marfan syndrome (Hollister et al., 1990).

Natural History and Diagnosis. The diagnosis is made on the basis of clinical findings. The fingers tend to be long compared with the size of the hands (arachnodactyly). The upper-to-lower segment ratio is usually more than two standard deviations below the mean, and the arm span is greater than length. The head is long and narrow (dolichocephaly), the palate high and arched, and there is a tendency for kyphoscoliosis and pectus carinatum or excavatum. Joints are hyperextensible. Over the course of months or years, abnormalities of other organs and systems may appear. These include eye defects (of which myopia and subluxation of the lens are most frequent), and cardiac disorders. The latter include mitral valve prolapse, dilation of the aortic root, and eventually, aortic aneurysm, which is a hazard in active adolescents.

The disorder will be looked for carefully in infants in a family in which the diagnosis of Marfan syndrome has been made in a parent or other near relative. It may be suspected if the newborn has inordinately long, thin, tapering fingers and toes, especially if these are accompanied by dolichocephaly, joint laxity, myopia, and the aforementioned skeletal disproportions (Gross et al., 1989). Echocardiography usually reveals a characteristic picture of increased aortic compliance (Child et al., 1981). One does not expect to find the cardiac and severe ocular abnormalities to be fully developed within the first months of life, but they have been seen this early.

The differential diagnosis includes homocystinuria (autosomal recessive), which can be ruled out by the absence of excess homocystine in the urine, and congenital contractural arachnodactyly, also dominantly inherited, in which the arachnodactyly is accompanied by multiple joint contractures and large, floppy ears. The distinction is important, as these patients do not develop the severe ocular and cardiac complications of Marfan syndrome, and the contractures improve with age.

Treatment. The use of beta blockers such as propranolol in treating those with aortic root dilation or aneurysm has been recommended (Pyeritz, 1983). The child with Marfan syndrome requires close medical follow-up for early detection and management of orthopedic, cardiac, and ophthalmologic complications. If the aorta is damaged, grafts may be helpful (Gott et al., 1986).

Prognosis. Prognosis is variable, depending on whether or not cardiac and vascular complications supervene; there is no way of predicting which children will ultimately show these manifestations. Murdoch and colleagues (1972) have calculated the life expectancy of persons with Marfan syndrome. The average age at death was 32 years. This rather dismal outlook may improve with increased awareness of the condition and continuing progress in management of the cardiovascular complications.

Prenatal Diagnosis. Prenatal ultrasonography can detect an increase in femur length relative to cranial biparietal diameter. Cardiac valvular abnormalities can also be identified prenatally.

CASE 19–1

(This is case J. G. of Bolande and Tucker [1964].)
This 1-month-old white male infant was admitted with a diagnosis of congenital Marfan syndrome. During breech extraction of the 3.5 kg baby, the left femur was fractured. Both mother and father are unusually tall and slender. On examination, the infant measured 58 cm and weighed 3.5 kg. The head was narrow and long, the ears were soft and floppy, and there

147

was an entropion of the right eye. A grade I systolic murmur was heard in the third left intercostal space. The extremities were long and thin, with extremely long hands, fingers, feet, and toes, and a flail wrist on the left (Fig. 19–1). Bilateral inguinal hernias were visible. Deep tendon reflexes were absent. Fluoroscopy revealed cardiac enlargement and pulmonary vascular congestion. The murmur became louder and harsher, cardiac failure ensued, dislocation of the right lens became obvious, the lungs became emphysematous, and the infant died after about 5 weeks in hospital.

OSTEOGENESIS IMPERFECTA

Osteogenesis imperfecta (OI) is a heterogeneous group of disorders involving bone fragility. Four major types are recognized on clinical and genetic grounds (Sillence et al., 1979). Biochemical and molecular genetic studies of collagen molecules and collagen genes are rapidly clarifying this classification scheme and providing powerful diagnostic tools (Byers, 1989).

Dominant OI with Blue Sclerae (Type 1). In this type, often referred to as OI tarda, brittle bones and blue sclerae usually appear after birth, although fractures occasionally occur prenatally. About 40 per cent of these

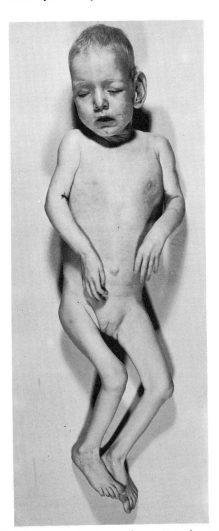

FIGURE 19–1. Infant with Marfan syndrome. Note the extremely long arms and hands, legs, and feet; the long, narrow skull; the very large ears; and the dropped left wrist.

patients have severe hearing impairment as adults. OI Type 1 has a frequency of about one per 28,000 births. About 15 per cent have a negative family history and probably represent new mutations.

Lethal Perinatal OI (Type 2). This is the classic OI congenita. Shortening and bowing of the upper and lower limbs are present at birth, and radiographs show characteristic crumpling of the femora, marked angulation of the tibiae and sometimes the femora, fractures of the long bones, beaded ribs, and poor ossification of the vault and base of the skull that resembles a membranous bag. The sclerae are usually blue. Affected infants expire in the newborn period, perhaps from damage to the poorly protected brain. The condition has been detected in utero in the second trimester, so prenatal diagnosis is possible. Infants with hypophosphatasia may present with similar appearing skeletal manifestations. This disorder can be ruled out by finding normal or increased levels of serum alkaline phosphatase activity.

The frequency is about 1 in 62,000 births. Most cases are sporadic, and molecular studies have indicated the occurrence of de novo mutations in type I collagen genes in several patients (Byers et al., 1988; Willing et al., 1988).

Progressively Deforming OI with Normal Sclerae (Type 3). Fractures are often present at birth, but the bones do not show the crumpled appearance evident in type 2. The sclerae are usually not blue. There is a progressive deformity of the limbs during childhood and of the spine during late childhood and adolescence. There is marked ligamentous laxity, and about one in four children show easy bruising. About half the patients have dentinogenesis imperfecta. The frequency is about 1 in 200,000 births. Both autosomal dominant and autosomal recessive inheritance have been described.

Dominant OI Without Blue Sclerae (Type 4). This autosomal dominant type resembles type 1 except for the lack of blue sclerae. Occasionally, fractures occur before birth. Dentinogenesis imperfecta is common, but deafness is not.

■ STORAGE DISEASES

This is a group of disorders characterized by an inability to break down specific compounds caused by the deficiency of appropriate enzymes. The hallmark of these disorders is the progressive accumulation of substrate, leading to loss of neurologic function, organomegaly, and skeletal dysplasia in various combinations. It is rare to recognize these disorders in the newborn; most do not become clinically apparent before the first few months of life, or even later. Some which occasionally present in newborns are described in Table 19–1. Other storage diseases, including GM_2 gangliosidosis (Tay-Sachs and Sandhoff diseases), metachromatic leukodystrophy, and mucopolysaccharidoses are not listed since presentation in the newborn period would be unusual. The diagnosis of these disorders is based on assay of the appropriate lysosomal enzymes.

TABLE 19–1. Lysosomal Storage Disease That May Present in Newborns as an Autosomal Recessive Trait

DISORDER	CHARACTERISTICS
GM₁ gangliosidosis	Hypotonia, poor suck reflex, coarse facial features, hepatomegaly, cherry red spot, deficiency of beta galactosidase.
Gaucher disease	Hepatosplenomegaly, spasticity, oculomotor palsy, Gaucher cells in bone marrow, deficiency of beta glucosidase.
Niemann-Pick Disease	Hepatosplenomegaly, failure to thrive, hypotonia, foam cells in bone marrow, deficiency of sphingomyelinase.
Krabbe Disease	Irritability, stiffening of body, seizures, tonic spasms, deficiency of galactocerebroside beta galactosidase.
I-Cell Disease (mucolipidosis II)	Coarse facial features, skeletal anomalies, stiff joints, cardiomegaly, hepatosplenomegaly.

FAMILIAL HYPERLIPIDEMIAS

At least six distinct disorders are recognized within this group. These are classified as types I through VI. Each type is characterized by a particular pattern of lipoprotein abnormality. Inheritance is either autosomal dominant or autosomal recessive. All except type II present in childhood or adult years. Although type II rarely presents in the neonatal period, an awareness of this disorder is important, since in some instances it may be desirable to begin dietary therapy in early infancy so that later clinical complications might be prevented. Only type II will be described in this discussion.

Type II hyperlipidemia, known as familial hypercholesterolemia, is the best-known and most frequent hyperlipidemia. The inheritance is autosomal dominant. In the homozygous state it is characterized by extremely high concentrations of cholesterol and low-density lipoprotein (LDL) in plasma and a moderately increased plasma triglyceride concentration. Xanthomas (yellowish fatty nodules) are present on the eyelids or over the elbows, extensor tendons of the hands, and the Achilles tendon. These xanthomas may be present at birth. Ischemic heart disease and other complications of severe atherosclerosis develop in childhood or during adolescence.

Type II hyperlipidemia is rare in the homozygous state, but in the heterozygous (carrier) state it may have a frequency as high as 1 per cent of the population. These individuals will have increased plasma cholesterol, triglyceride, and LDL. The degree of increase, however, will be far less than that in the homozygous state. These individuals tend to develop premature atherosclerosis with ischemic heart disease and other complications. These clinical problems usually appear in the middle adult years.

The biochemical defect in type II hyperlipidemia appears to be a deficiency of cellular LDL receptor activity. Thus, LDL cannot enter peripheral cells in the normal manner and is thereby increased in the circulation. This increased LDL with its cholesterol is picked up by reticuloendothelial cells, and in this manner forms the basis for atheromas. The usual therapy is a low-cholesterol diet so that the amount of body cholesterol can be reduced. Other therapeutic measures are sometimes used, but their effectiveness has not been proved.

LYSOSOMAL STORAGE DISEASES

In these inherited disorders, the defective enzymes are located in the lysosomes of the cell, in contrast to other inborn errors of metabolism in which the enzyme in question is in the mitochondria or cytosol of the cell.

There are several categories of these disorders. These categories include (1) the lipidoses, in which lipid material accumulates in cells, often neurons, (2) the mucopolysaccharidoses, in which the cellular accumulation is a mucopolysaccharide, (3) generalized glycogen storage disease (Pompe disease), and (4) other diseases of complex carbohydrate metabolism (fucosidosis, mannosidosis, aspartylglucosaminuria, and Wolman disease).

Most of the lysosomal storage diseases present later than the neonatal period. However, several may produce neonatal findings, which will be discussed. In addition, Tay-Sachs disease (GM₂ gangliosidosis) will be described, since it is a prominent lipidosis.

TAY-SACHS DISEASE

This is the best known of the lipidoses. It is transmitted as an autosomal recessive trait and is most frequent among Ashkenazi Jews, although it may also occur in other ethnic groups. GM₂ ganglioside accumulates in neurons because of a deficiency in hexosaminidase-A activity. This results in severe and progressive mental and motor deterioration, which begins between 3 and 6 months of age. Death is inevitable, usually occurring by 3 years of age, following a tragic clinical course that includes deafness, blindness, convulsions, and spasticity. There is no treatment for this disease. Antenatal diagnosis is available. A number of different mutations that are responsible for Tay-Sachs disease have recently been identified and now can be used to improve the precision of carrier detection and diagnosis (Triggs-Raine et al., 1990).

GM₁ GANGLIOSIDOSIS (TYPE 1)

This is one of the few lipidoses that presents in the neonate. In this autosomal recessive disease, GM₁ ganglioside accumulates in neurons. There are foam cells throughout the reticuloendothelial system and in other visceral organs such as the kidney. The enzyme defect is in β-galactosidase activity. Shortly after birth, the infant becomes lethargic, sucks poorly, and loses weight. He is noted to have dysmorphic facial features and hepatosplenomegaly. Growth and development are severely limited, and severe neurologic impairment develops during the first year of life. The symptoms are progressive, and death occurs by 2 years of age.

GAUCHER DISEASE (TYPE 2)

Gaucher disease of the infantile, or type 2, form usually presents at 3 to 4 months of age with hepatosplenomegaly and failure to thrive. Occasionally, the affected infant is abnormal at birth, with lethargy and poor feeding as well as hepatosplenomegaly. Glucocerebroside accumulates in the brain and other organs owing to a deficiency of glucocerebrosidase activity. The infants show progressive deterioration and usually die by 1 or 2 years of age. There is no treatment. Enzyme replacement has been attempted but so far this has not proved clinically beneficial. Bone marrow transplantation has been attempted in a few cases, with some evidence of clinical response (Hobbs et al., 1987).

NIEMANN-PICK (TYPE A)

In the infantile, or Type A, form of Niemann-Pick disease, the infant may have hepatomegaly within the first days of life. Feeding difficulties ensue, and severe progressive neurologic involvement with hepatosplenomegaly develops during the next few months with death by 3 years of age. The accumulating lipid is sphingomyelin, which is found in increased quantities in the brain and viscera of patients. Sphingomyelinase appears to be the defective enzyme. The disease is inherited as an autosomal recessive trait and is most frequent among Ashkenazi Jews. There is no specific treatment.

WOLMAN DISEASE

This disease is characterized by vomiting, failure to thrive, and hepatosplenomegaly during the first week or two of life. An additional and striking finding is calcification of the adrenal glands. Triglycerides and cholesterol ester are the predominant lipids that accumulate in this disease. These accumulations are noted in the liver and spleen; plasma cholesterol and triglyceride levels are normal. The enzyme defect in this autosomal recessive disease is in acid lipase. The disease is progressive, with death usually occurring by 3 to 6 months of age. There is no specific therapy.

I-CELL DISEASE

This autosomal recessive disease, often referred to as mucolipidosis II, is one of the few lipidoses that is expressed at birth. These infants have somewhat low birth weight, coarse facies, and orthopedic abnormalities such as clubfeet, congenital hip dislocation, thoracic deformities, and kyphosis. Affected males have congenital inguinal hernias. Cultured skin fibroblasts from these patients contain very large lysosomes that are filled with mucopolysaccharide material. Levels of lysosomal hydrolases are increased in body fluids and decreased in cultured fibroblasts, suggesting that in this disease the hydrolases are structurally deficient and therefore unable to remain in or re-enter cells. The diagnosis of I-cell disease is made on the basis of the characteristic clinical phenotype and the measurement of increased hydrolase activities in serum and urine. There is no specific treatment, and most of the children die by the age of 6 years.

■ MISCELLANEOUS INBORN ERRORS OF METABOLISM

MENKES STEELY-HAIR DISEASE

Clinical Characteristics. This disease, also referred to as kinky-hair syndrome, is inherited as an X-linked recessive trait. Affected males often express the disease at birth. Delivery may be premature at 34 to 36 weeks' gestation with appropriate birth weight.

The newborn infant may be lethargic and feed poorly. Temperature instability as manifested by hypothermia may also be present in the newborn. These problems continue, and by the age of 2 months, the infant has poor weight gain and is flaccid. By the age of 4 to 5 months, the infant has developmental delay, marked temperature instability, and often, convulsions. At this time or even before, his hair becomes depigmented and sparse. The hair strands break easily, leaving short stubbles that feel like "steely" hair. Microscopic examination of the hair strand reveals changes of pili torti. The clinical course is one of progressive neurologic deterioration, with death usually occurring during the first year of life.

Etiology. Menkes disease appears to be a disorder of copper metabolism or transport. Levels of copper may be low in the liver and brain and very high in the kidney and intestinal mucosa. Copper is also increased in cultured skin fibroblasts. Orally administered copper is poorly absorbed, but intravenously or intramuscularly administered copper is handled normally. The mechanism for this disease may be the trapping of copper in certain tissues, particularly intestinal mucosa and kidney, perhaps by metallothionein, a copper-binding protein.

Diagnosis and Treatment. The diagnosis of Menkes disease is based on the characteristic clinical phenotype and the presence of reduced levels of copper and ceruloplasmin in serum. Liver biopsy with the demonstration of reduced copper concentration provides further evidence of this disease as does the demonstration of increased copper in cultured skin fibroblasts. Treatment with parenterally administered copper raises the serum copper and ceruloplasmin concentrations to normal levels but has neither improved the clinical manifestations nor stemmed the progression of the disease.

HYPOPHOSPHATASIA

Hypophosphatasia is characterized by deficient mineralization of bones and low activity of serum and other tissue alkaline phosphatase. The infantile form of hypophosphatasia is a recessively inherited disorder that appears in three distinct patterns. Type 1 has its onset in utero with severe skeletal abnormalities, craniostenosis, hypercalcemia, and hypophosphatasia. These most severely affected infants usually die in their first year. Type 2 is a later more gradual onset of rickets and premature loss of teeth. Type 3 may be asymptomatic, although adults with this rare type have low values for serum phosphatase. In some adults, a milder form of this disorder is inherited as a dominant trait.

Other forms of hypophosphatasia have included an infant with the clinical features of the disorder but normal levels of plasma alkaline phosphatase. However, that patient hydrolyzed phosphoethanolamine more slowly than normal (Scriver and Cameron, 1969). She suffered from repeated midshaft femoral fractures that healed slowly in later life.

Levels of alkaline phosphatase may be normal in the intestines and placenta, but low in the liver, bone, and kidneys.

Management. No way has been found to correct this metabolic defect. Warshaw and co-workers (1971) showed that long-chain triglycerides cause an elevation in serum alkaline phosphatase. Therapy with steroids or vitamin K has been ineffective.

Prevention. Prenatal diagnosis can be definitive in the most severely affected individuals. Low alkaline phosphatase activity in chorionic villus samples has been reported.

NEPHROGENIC DIABETES INSIPIDUS

This is an inherited defect in which there is lack of response to antidiuretic hormone (ADH) by the renal tubule. There is excessive loss of water from the kidneys because the renal tubules cannot reabsorb water. Chemical abnormalities in the blood are secondary to this water loss.

Etiology. This is an X-linked genetic disease. Males are hemizygotes and are more frequently and usually much more severely affected than females. The few females who have had clinical evidence of nephrogenic diabetes insipidus are presumably heterozygotes who by Lyon randomization have inherited an unusually large number of cells with the defect.

Diagnosis. Affected infants usually come to attention within the first few months of life. Failure to thrive with unexplained fever are the most frequent clinical signs at presentation. Diarrhea or constipation may also be present. Further history reveals that there is polyuria and that the infant may also be almost continuously thirsty (polydipsia). Recurrent urinary tract infection has been noted in some infants. On examination, the infant is dehydrated and might show signs of developmental delay. In older children, mild mental retardation is frequent, and hydronephrosis as well as hydroureters may be present.

The urine output is voluminous, and the urine specific gravity is usually below 1.010. Except when infection is present, the urine is otherwise normal. There is no glycosuria or proteinuria, and urine amino acids are normal. Serum sodium, chloride, and creatinine and blood urea nitrogen levels are elevated. Plasma ADH levels are normal or elevated. Injections of vasopressin fail to increase the urine specific gravity or decrease urine output.

Treatment. There is no specific therapy. Adequate hydration must be maintained. In acute episodes of dehydration, this may require parenteral therapy that consists of a minimum of glucose (so as not to promote solute diuresis) and a low sodium-chloride content.

Diuretics such as the chlorothiazides may reduce urine flow and increase urine concentration when given chronically to patients with nephrogenic diabetes insipidus. This effect is enhanced when the patient is maintained on a low-sodium diet.

NEONATAL MYASTHENIA GRAVIS

Approximately 12 per cent of the offspring of women with myasthenia gravis will have transient neonatal myasthenia gravis.

Etiology. Neonatal myasthenia gravis is caused by the passive transfer of antiacetylcholine receptor antibody across the placenta. The antibody blocks the nicotinic acetylcholine receptor at the neuromuscular junction, resulting in a lack of response by the muscle to the nerve impulse. For reasons unknown, the fetus generally appears to be protected from the effects of this blocking action, since fetal movements and other characteristics of pregnancy are normal in most cases. At birth or shortly after birth, however, clinical effects become apparent.

Diagnosis. The infant is usually normal at delivery with good Apgar scores. Within hours of birth, however, weakness is noted. This is most commonly manifested by difficulty in feeding. The infant is hungry and begins to suck vigorously, but sucking weakens so rapidly that adequate nourishment is impossible. Generalized weakness and hypotonia are present, sometimes producing respiratory difficulty. Many infants have a weak cry and flat facial expression. Features of permanent myasthenia gravis, such as oculomotor paresis and ptosis, are usually absent.

The most important feature of family history is maternal myasthenia gravis. An intravenous injection of 0.5 mg or an intramuscular injection of 1 to 2 mg of edrophonium chloride will confirm the diagnosis. There is a clear improvement in suck and muscle strength within 10 to 15 minutes of this injection. Neostigmine methylsulfate, 0.1 mg/kg intramuscularly, may also be used as a therapeutic test. The duration of the maximum effect with neostigmine is often approximately 30 minutes.

Treatment and Prognosis. In 20 per cent of the cases, the symptoms are mild and drug therapy is unnecessary. Adequate nutrition can be maintained with frequent small feedings. In severely affected infants, respirations and feeding should be carefully supported. Neostigmine methylsulfate, 0.1 mg intramuscularly, should be initially administered 20 minutes prior to feeding. More exact dosages should be determined by the response in terms of respirations and feeding. If oral doses are used when adequate swallowing has been established, they should be 10 times the intramuscular doses. The need for medication may persist for several weeks. Periodic attempts to withdraw the drug should be made.

The outlook for the newborn with myasthenia gravis is good, provided one makes the diagnosis promptly and treats properly. The symptoms may persist for as short a time as a few hours or for as long as 7 weeks. Once muscle strength has returned, it never again is lost.

CONGENITAL MYASTHENIA

Congenital myasthenia can present in an infant in the absence of a maternal history of myasthenia. Five subtypes have been noted, distinguished by structural or ultrastructural anomalies of the neuromuscular junction:

1. A sporadic form caused by a deficiency of acetylcholine esterase
2. An autosomal recessive defect in acetylcholine resynthesis
3. An autosomal recessive defect in acetylcholine mobilization

4. An autosomal dominant prolongation of the open-time of acetylcholine ion channels

5. A familial form of decreased numbers of receptors and abnormal end-plate morphology.

The majority of these infants present before 2 years of age, and some have had decreased fetal movements. The usual presentation is with bulbar symptoms and poor response to inhibitors of acetylcholine esterase. Spontaneous remissions have been seen, but the usual course is lifelong.

CYSTIC FIBROSIS

Cystic fibrosis is an inherited disorder that affects many different organs of the body, most notably the lungs and pancreas. It is characterized by excessive sodium and chloride secretion in sweat glands, airways, and other epithelium.

Incidence. The disease is inherited in an autosomal recessive manner. In the United States, it is far more common among whites than among blacks, having an incidence of approximately 1 per 1600 in whites to 1 per 30,000 in blacks. In general, it has a similar frequency among most white Europeans. It is very rare in Orientals. The risk of producing a child with cystic fibrosis in the Caucasian population varies with the family history (Table 19–2).

Pathophysiology. The most prominent biochemical abnormality found is increased concentrations of sodium and chloride in sweat. The viscosity of mucus secreted by many exocrine glands is markedly increased. This leads to inspissated mucus in many organs, including the trachea and bronchial tree, the pancreas, the intestinal tract, the bile ductules and ducts of the liver, and the testes. The viscid mucus in the tracheobronchial system leads to chronic pulmonary infection. In other organs, the outflow tracts become chronically obstructed, and the secretions collect within the organ, causing tissue damage. In the pancreas, this results in a reduction in the flow of digestive

TABLE 19–2. Risks of Producing a Child with Cystic Fibrosis (CF)*

ONE PARENT	OTHER PARENT	RISK OF CYSTIC FIBROSIS IN EACH PREGNANCY
With no CF history	With no CF history	1:1600
With no CF history	With 1st cousin having CF	1:320
With no CF history	With aunt or uncle having CF	1:240
With no CF history	With sib having CF	1:120
With no CF history	With CF child by previous marriage	1:80
With no CF history	With parent having CF	1:80
With no CF history	Has CF	1:40
With sib having CF	With sib having CF	1:9
With CF child	With CF child	1:4

*Based on prevalence of cystic fibrosis of 1:1600 in the Caucasian population, its mode of inheritance being autosomal recessive with complete penetrance. (From Bowman, B. H., and Mangos, J. A.: N. Engl. J. Med. 294:937, 1976. Reprinted by permission of the New England Journal of Medicine.)

enzymes to the intestine. In the liver, biliary cirrhosis may eventually occur.

The basic defect in cystic fibrosis (CF) is an abnormality in chloride channels on the apical surface of epithelia. A defect in secretion of chloride in response to beta-adrenergic agonists characterizes cells from CF patients. As of 1989, the chloride channels have not been isolated or characterized (Boat et al., 1989).

In 1985, the gene for most CF patients was identified on chromosome 7. After a worldwide effort, groups from Toronto and Michigan in 1989 identified and characterized the gene and its product, cystic fibrosis transport regulator (CFTR). The gene consists of 250,000 base pairs, and has a single missing codon for phenylalanine, located at a binding site for ATP. This deletion in the gene has been found in about 70 per cent in CF patients. Other mutations are being sought (Rommens et al., 1989; Kerem et al., 1989).

The advances in molecular biology have opened the way to prenatal diagnosis and to better understanding of the protean manifestations of the disease. As of 1989, they do not point to any new therapeutic approaches.

Clinical Manifestations. Most infants with cystic fibrosis appear to be normal during the neonatal period. However, an occasional affected infant will have meconium ileus. When this is present, the diagnosis of cystic fibrosis is almost certain. The meconium plug syndrome has also been described in neonates with cystic fibrosis. Occasionally, excessive sweating is evident in the neonate. The sweat will contain increased electrolyte quantities. This sweat may be noted to have a "salty taste" by the mother when she kisses the infant. Respiratory infections may also present during the first days of life, with the most consistent feature being hyperinflation of the chest. Failure to gain weight and hypoproteinemia may become evident in the weeks after birth. Bulky and fatty stools, usually the first signs of the deficiency of pancreatic enzymes, may be noted during the early months of life. Prolonged obstructive jaundice may also be an early manifestation of the disease.

Diagnosis. The collection of sweat by iontophoresis for analysis of sodium and chloride, or measurement of electrical conductivity, which depends on the concentrations of these ions, is the definitive diagnostic test. It may be difficult to collect a sufficient amount of sweat from infants in the first weeks of life for these chemical assays, although in expert hands this is usually possible. If an infant has an affected sibling or any signs or symptoms suggesting cystic fibrosis, sweat analysis is essential before making or excluding the diagnosis.

Treatment. No consensus exists on how vigorous one should be in treating the asymptomatic infant with cystic fibrosis. Most would agree on a normal diet and the addition of water-soluble vitamins. The prompt identification and treatment of pulmonary infections is imperative and probably preferable to chemoprophylaxis. Some hold that the initial staphylococcal pneumonia is so harmful that antibiotics should be given daily in an attempt to prevent it. Pancreatic supplements are recommended as tolerated.

Prognosis. Each year the prognosis for this disease improves, in part because of wider recognition and detection of milder cases and in part, no doubt, in relation to therapy. Many afflicted individuals are now adults, and some of the females are parents. Sterility in the males is very common. The severity of the disease varies greatly among siblings; hence, prognostication about the life span of an affected infant is unwise.

■ REFERENCES

Adams, R. D., and Lyon, G.: Neurology of Hereditary Metabolic Diseases of Children. New York, McGraw-Hill, 1982.

Antonowicz, I., Ishida, S., and Shwachman, H.: Studies in meconium: Disaccharidase activities in meconium from cystic fibrosis patients and controls. Pediatrics 56:782, 1975.

Barlow, C. F.: Neonatal myasthenia gravis. Am. J. Dis. Child. 135:209, 1981.

Blumenthal, I., and Fielding, D. W.: Hypoproteinaemia, oedema, and anaemia: An unusual presentation of cystic fibrosis in dizygotic twins. Arch. Dis. Child. 55:812, 1980.

Boat, T. J., Welsh, A., and Beuadet, A. L.: Cystic fibrosis. In Scriver, C. R., Beaudet, A. L., Sly, W. S., et al. (Eds.): The Metabolic Basis of Inherited Disease. New York, McGraw-Hill, 1989, pp 2649–2682.

Bolande, R. P., and Tucker, A. S. Pulmonary emphysema and other cardiorespiratory lesions as part of the Marfan abiotrophy. Pediatr 33:356, 1964.

Breslow, J. L.: Pediatric aspects of hyperlipidemia. Pediatrics 62:510, 1978.

Brody, J. S.: The interface of basic science and clinical medicine. Cell. Mol. Biol. 1:347–348, 1989.

Byers, P. H., Siegel, R. C., Peterson, K. E., et al.: Marfan syndrome: Abnormal alpha-2 chain in type I collagen. Proc. Nat. Acad. Sci. 78:7745–7749, 1981.

Byers, P. H., Tsipouras, P., Bonadio, J. F., et al.: Perinatal lethal osteogenesis imperfecta (OI type II): A biochemically heterogeneous disorder usually due to new mutations in the genes for type I collagen. Am. J. Hum. Genet. 42:237–248, 1988.

Byers, P. H.: Osteogenesis imperfecta: An Update. Growth, Genetics and Hormones 4:1–5, 1988.

Child, A. H., et al.: Aortic compliance in connective tissue disorders affecting the eye. Ophthal. Paediatr. Genet. 1:59, 1981.

Cipolloni, C., Boldnni, A., et al.: Neonatal mucolipidosis II (I-cell disease): Clinical, radiological and biochemical studies in a case. Helv. Paediatr. Acta 35:85, 1980.

Crocker, A. C.: Inborn errors of lipid metabolism: Early identification. Clin. Perinatol. 3:99, 1976.

Danks, D. M., Campbell, P. E., et al.: Menkes's kinky hair syndrome. An inherited defect in copper absorption with widespread effects. Pediatrics 50:188, 1972.

Donaldson, J. O., Penn, A. S., et al.: Antiacetylcholine receptor antibody in neonatal myasthenia gravis. Am. J. Dis. Child. 135:222, 1981.

Drachman, D. B.: Myasthenia gravis. N. Engl. J. Med. 298:136, 186, 1978.

Elias, S. B., Butler, I., et al.: Neonatal myasthenia gravis in the infant of a myasthenic mother in remission. Ann. Neurol. 6:72, 1979.

Fenichel, G. M.: Clinical syndromes of myasthenia in infancy and childhood. Arch. Neurol. 35:97, 1978.

Francomano, C. A., Streeten, E. A., Meyers, D. A., et al.: The Marfan Syndrome: Exclusion of genetic linkage to three major collagen genes. Am. J. Med. Genet. 29:457–462, 1988.

Goldstein, J. L., and Brown, M. S.: The LDL receptor locus and the genetics of familial hypercholesterolemia. Ann. Rev. Genet. 13:259, 1979.

Gott, V. T., Pyeritz, R. E., Magovern, G. J., et al.: Surgical treatment of aneurysms of the ascending aorta in Marfan Syndrome. N. Eng. J. Med. 314:1070, 1986.

Gross, D. M., Robinson, L. K., Smith, L. T., et al.: Severe perinatal Marfan syndrome. Pediatrics 84:83–89, 1989.

Hen, J., Jr., Dolan, T. F., Jr., and Touloukian, R. J.: Meconium plug syndrome associated with cystic fibrosis and Hirschsprung's disease. Pediatrics 66:466, 1980.

Hobbs, J. R., Jones, K. H., Shaw, P. J., et al.: Beneficial effect of pretransplant splenectomy on displacement bone marrow transplantation for Gaucher's syndrome. Lancet 1:1111–1115, 1987.

Hollister, D. W., Godfrey, M., Sakai, L. Y., Pyeritz, R. E.: Immunohistologic abnormalities of the microfibrillar fiber system in the Marfan syndrome. N. Engl. J. Med. 323:152–159, 1990.

Holmes, L. B., Driscoll, S. G., et al.: Contractures in a newborn infant of a mother with myasthenia gravis. J. Pediatr. 96:1067, 1980.

Iavarone, A., Dolfin, G., Bracco, G., et al.: First trimester prenatal diagnosis of Wolman disease. J. Inherit. Metab. Dis. 12(Suppl):299, 1989.

Ida, H., Eto, Y., Maesawa, K. Fetal GMI-gangliosidosis: morphological and biochemical studies. Brain Dev 11:394, 1989

Kerem, B., Rommens, J. M., Buchanan, J. A., et al.: Identification of the cystic fibrosis gene: Genetic analysis. Science 245:1073–1080, 1989.

Knox, G. E., Palmer, M. D., and Huddleston, J. F.: Fetal cystic fibrosis presenting as dystocia due to midgut volvulus with lethal perforation. Am. J. Obstet. Gynecol. 131:698, 1978.

Kolodny, E. H.: Current concepts in genetics. Lysosomal storage diseases. N. Engl. J. Med. 294:1217, 1976.

Labadie, G. U., Hirschhorn, K., et al.: Increased copper metal-lothionein in Menkes cultured skin fibroblasts. Pediatr. Res. 15:257, 1981.

Lott, I. T., DiPaolo, R., et al.: Abnormal copper metabolism in Menke's steely-hair syndrome. Pediatr. Res. 13:845, 1979.

Maesaka, H., Niitsu, N., et al.: Neonatal hypophosphatasia with elevated serum parathyroid hormone. Eur. J. Pediatr. 125:71, 1977.

Menkes, J. H.: Textbook of Child Neurology, 3rd ed. Philadelphia, Lea & Febiger, 1985, p. 94.

Muenzer, J.: Mucopolysaccharidoses. A review. Adv. Pediatr. 33:269, 1986.

Murdoch, J. L., Walker, B. A. Halpern, B. L., et al.: Life expectancy and causes of death associated in the Marfan syndrome. N. Engl. J. Med. 286:804, 1972.

Nooijen, J. L., De Groot, C. J., et al.: Trace element studies in three patients and a fetus with Menkes' disease. Effect of copper therapy. Pediatr. Res. 15:284, 1981.

Pazzaglia, U., Beluffi, G., Campbell, J., et al.: Mucolipidosis II: Correlation between radiological features and histopathology of the bones. Pediat Radiol 19:406, 1989.

Percy, A. K.: The inherited neurodegenerative disorders of childhood: Clinical assessment. J. Child. Neurol. 2:82–97, 1987.

Poenaru, L., Castelnau, L., Tome, F., et al.: A variant of mucolipodosis. II. Clinical biochemical, and pathological investigations. Eur. J. Pediat. 147:321, 1988.

Pope, F. M., and Nicholls, A. C.: Molecular abnormalities of collagen in human disease. Arch. Dis. Child. 62:523, 1987.

Pyeritz, R. E.: Propranolol retards aortic root dilatation in Marfan syndrome. Circulation 68(Suppl. 3):111, 1983.

Pyeritz, R. E., and McKusick, V. A.: The Marfan syndrome. Diagnosis and management. N. Eng. J. Med. 300:772–777, 1979.

Riordan, J. R., Rommens, J. M., Kerem, B., et al.: Identification of the cystic fibrosis gene: Cloning and characterization of complementary DNA. Science 245:1066–1073, 1989.

Rommens, J. M., Iannuzzi, M. C., Kerem, B., et al.: Identification of the cystic fibrosis gene: Chromosome walking and jumping. Science 245:1059–1065, 1989.

Schreiner, R. L., Skafish, P. R., et al.: Congenital nephrogenic diabetes insipidus in a baby girl. Arch. Dis. Child. 53:906, 1978.

Schmidt, H., Ulrich, J. H., von Lengerke, J., et al.: Radiological findings in patients with mucopolysaccharidase I (H/S) Hurler-Scheie syndrome. Pediatr. Radiol. 17:409, 1987.

Scriver, C. R., and Cameron, D.: Pseudohypophosphatasia. N. Engl. J. Med. 281:604, 1969.

Silence, D. O., Senn, A. S., and Danks, D. M.: Genetic heterogeneity in osteogenesis imperfecta. J. Med. Genet. 16:101–106, 1979.

Spatz, R. A., Doughty, R. A., et al.: Neonatal presentation of I-cell disease. J. Pediatr. 93:954, 1978.

Stanbury, J. B., Wyngaarden, J. B., Fredrickson, D. S., et al.: The Metabolic Basis of Inherited Disease, 5th ed. New York, McGraw-Hill, 1983.

Takahashi, Y., Orii, T.: Severity of GMI gangliosidosis and urinary oligosaccharide excretion. Clin. Chem. Acta 179:153, 1989.

Ten Bensel, R. W., and Peters, E. R.: Progressive hydronephrosis, hydroureter, and dilatation of the bladder in siblings with congenital diabetes insipidus. J. Pediatr. 77:439, 1970.

Triggs-Raine, B. L., Feigenbaum, A. S. J., Natowicz, M., et al.: Screening for carriers of Tay-Sachs disease among Ashkenazi Jews. N. Engl. J. Med. 323:6–12, 1990.

Van Regemorter, N., Dodion, J., Druart, C., et al.: Congenital malformations in 10,000 consecutive births in a university hospital: Need for genetic counseling and prenatal diagnosis. J. Pediatr. *104*:386. 1984.

Warren, R. C., McKenzie, C. F., Rodeck, C. H., et al.: First trimester diagnosis of hypophosphatasia with monoclonal antibody to the liver/bone/kidney isoenzyme of alkaline phosphatase. Lancet *2*:856, 1985.

Warshaw, J. B., Littlefield, J. W., Fishman, W. H., et al.: Serum alkaline phosphatase in hypophosphatasia. J. Clin. Invest. *50*:2137, 1971.

Willing, M. C., Dohn, D. H., Starman, B., et al.: Heterozygosity for a large deletion in the alpha-2 (I) collagen gene has a dramatic effect on type I collagen secretion and produces perinatal lethal osteogenesis imperfecta. J. Biol. Chem. *263*: 8398–8404, 1988.

Wolfish, N. M., and Heick, H.: Hyperparathyroidism and infantile hypophosphatasia: effect of prednisone and vitamin K therapy. J. Pediatr. *95*:1079, 1979.

Wolman, M.: Proposed treatment for infants with Wolman disease. Pediatrics *10*:1074, 1989.

GENETIC COUNSELING **20**

Bruce R. Korf

The occurrence of a genetic disorder or congenital malformation in a newborn represents for most families an enactment of their worst nightmare. Providing medical support for the child and moral support for the family is the job of the entire medical team. The role of genetic counseling was articulated by the American Society of Human Genetics (Fraser, 1974) as helping the family to: "(1) Comprehend the medical facts, including the diagnosis, the probable course of the disorder, and the available management; (2) appreciate the way heredity contributes to the disorder . . . ; (3) understand the options for dealing with the risk of recurrence; (4) make the best possible adjustment to the disorder . . . and/or the risk of recurrence of this disorder."

■ DIAGNOSIS OF GENETIC DISORDERS

The time and mode of diagnosis of infants with inherited disorders or congenital malformations can vary widely. In some instances, a specific disorder may be known to run in a family, and transmission to a child may be no surprise. At other times, the problem may be detected by prenatal ultrasound examination or chromosomal analysis. In such cases, the genetic counseling process begins well before birth, in the former case, perhaps before conception. Finally and probably most commonly, a baby may be recognized as having problems shortly after birth, which come as a surprise to both the family and the medical team. This situation poses the greatest challenge, both in terms of arriving at a diagnosis and in helping the family adjust.

Immediately after birth, the focus of attention is the newborn. There is a need to assess the extent of the infant's medical problems and determine the feasibility of treatment. Some biochemical disorders are amenable to medical therapy, such as dietary restriction of specific amino acids or sugars. Likewise, many infants with congenital malformations can be treated surgically. There remain many problems, however, for which treatment is unavailable. In any case, the family will be interested in prognosis. Are the baby's apparent problems his or her only difficulties, or are there other components of the disorder yet to be detected? Does the disorder progress? Is the disorder compatible with normal cognitive development? How long can the child be expected to survive?

To a large extent, answers to questions about natural history require knowledge of etiology, permitting prognostic information to be based on past experience. It may also be possible to anticipate specific medical problems before they become clinically apparent. Prognostic information based on diagnosis must be used with care, however. There is often wide variation in the degree of expression of a genetic disorder from individual to individual. Case reports published in the medical literature are often biased toward more severe or dramatic problems; more mildly affected individuals generally receive less attention. Also, data on long-term outcome are necessarily derived from individuals diagnosed many years ago, when standards of medical care were different from today. Prognosis must therefore be individualized to a particular child. This is necessarily the case when the etiology is not known, but should be remembered even when the etiology is known.

GENETIC DIAGNOSIS OF PERINATAL DEATH

Many inherited disorders are so severe as to be incompatible with survival, and may result in miscarriage, stillbirth, or perinatal death. There is an urgent need to examine such infants or fetuses and, when appropriate, obtain tissue samples for chromosomal, biochemical, or DNA studies (Wigglesworth, 1987; Winter et al., 1988). Information obtained in this manner can be instrumental in making a diagnosis that can be the basis for genetic counseling and future prenatal diagnosis.

■ RECURRENCE RISK ASSESSMENT

As time passes after the birth of a child with an inherited disorder, most families become increasingly concerned with the likelihood of recurrence in future pregnancies. It is the job of the genetic counselor to provide this information, gleaned from a review of the family history and knowledge of recurrence risks associated with particular disorders. The counselor must also educate the family regarding options for dealing with this recurrence risk.

REVIEW OF THE FAMILY HISTORY

The major goal in taking a family history is to determine if a disorder "runs in the family." The first and most important question is whether similar problems have occurred to others in the family. Rarely, the answer to this provides sufficient information to establish a diagnosis and determine the mode of inheritance. More often, it is necessary to probe deeply into the medical background of both parents, siblings, aunts and uncles, cousins, and grandparents. Couples usually do not have all the information at their disposal during the initial interview. It may be necessary for them to inquire of relatives and, in some cases, arrange for medical records to be obtained for review. Even clearcut Mendelian disorders may go unmentioned in a first attempt to gather family history.

In some instances, a Mendelian pattern of genetic transmission may be identified. Autosomal dominant traits are passed from generation to generation, from either mothers or fathers to either sons or daughters

(Fig. 20–1A). On average, about half the offspring of an individual with an autosomal dominant trait inherits the mutant gene, although the degree of expression may vary from person to person, even within a sibship. Autosomal recessive traits tend to occur among sibs, and to be absent in parents or other relatives (Fig. 20–1B). Rare autosomal recessive disorders occur more frequently in the offspring of consanguineous matings, reflecting inheritance of a rare mutant allele through both parents from a common ancestor. Yet consanguinity is infrequent even in families with autosomal recessive disorders, and the occurrence of parental consanguinity does not prove that a disorder is recessively inherited.

X-linked inheritance involves transmission of genes on the X chromosome. The hallmark is lack of male-to-male transmission, since fathers do not transmit an X chromosome to their sons (Fig. 20–1C). X-linked recessive disorders tend to be transmitted from asymptomatic carrier females to, on average, half their sons. X-linked dominant disorders can be expressed in both males and females. Because the male has only a single X chromosome, such disorders may be expressed in more severe form in males, indeed sometimes so severe as to lead to death in utero.

Some chromosomal disorders tend to recur among members of a kindred. These usually take the form of balanced translocations, chromosome rearrangements that involve no loss or gain of genetic material but that predispose to abnormal chromosome segregation at meiosis. The usual clue in the family history is the occurrence of multiple early pregnancy miscarriages in translocation carriers as well as the occasional birth of a child with multiple congenital anomalies (Fig. 20–2). Chromosome analysis of any such children and both parents are indicated when such a family history is obtained.

Aside from Mendelian traits and chromosomal rearrangements, there are many disorders that tend to cluster in families. These include common medical problems, such as diabetes mellitus and hypertension, but also rare disorders presenting in infancy, such as myelodysplasia and congenital heart disease. These disorders are subject to multifactorial inheritance, in which some combination of multiple genes and environmental factors contribute to the occurrence of the disorder (Carter,

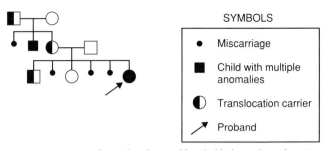

SYMBOLS

●	Miscarriage
■	Child with multiple anomalies
◑	Translocation carrier
↗	Proband

FIGURE 20–2. *Hypothetical pedigree of familial balanced translocation.*

1969). In most cases, the specific genes involved have not been identified.

RECURRENCE RISK COUNSELING

Determination of the recurrence risk is most straightforward in the case of Mendelian disorders. If a parent has an autosomal dominant trait, there is a 50 per cent risk of the disorder in any subsequent pregnancy. A couple having had a child with an autosomal recessive disorder have a 25 per cent risk for future pregnancies. For an X-linked recessive disorder, the risk in future pregnancies to a carrier mother is 50 per cent for sons; daughters are not affected but have a 50 per cent risk of being carriers themselves.

Recurrence risks associated with chromosome disorders depend on the nature of the chromosomal anomaly. Major trisomies, such as trisomy 13, 18, and 21, rarely recur. From empiric data, the risk of trisomy in a future offspring to a couple having had a child with trisomy is about 1 per cent (Lister and Frota-Pessoa, 1980) when the child is born to a mother less than 30 years old. This is the risk of trisomy for any chromosome, regardless of the specific chromosome involved in the abnormality in the proband. Thus, for example, parents of a child with trisomy 21 have a 1 per cent risk of having a subsequent child with trisomy, which could involve 13, 18, or 21. For mothers over 30 years old at the time of birth of the trisomic child, the recurrence risk is derived from empiric figures based on maternal age.

If a child has a translocation, inversion, or deletion, both parents should be studied to determine if this abnormality is familial. If it is, recurrence is possible, although the precise risk depends on the nature of the chromosome rearrangement. Recurrence risk data exist for some of the more common rearrangements, such as translocations between chromosomes 14 and 21 (Lister and Frota-Pessoa, 1980). For more unusual abnormalities it may be impossible to find published data about the frequency of liveborn chromosomally abnormal offspring. Some information may be inferred from reproductive outcomes of other members of the family known to carry the abnormality (Stene and Stengel-Rutkowski, 1982).

Recurrence risks of disorders associated with multifactorial inheritance are determined from empiric data. The risk tends to be increased in families with a prior history of the disorder and may be higher in couples of a specific racial or ethnic background in which the trait is particularly common. Tables of empiric risk data should be consulted for counseling (Emery and Rimoin, 1983) (Table 20–1).

The greatest challenge in recurrence risk determination is posed when a couple have had a child with a disorder

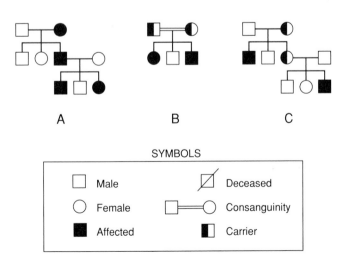

A   B   C

SYMBOLS

□	Male	⊘	Deceased
○	Female	□—○	Consanguinity
■	Affected	◧	Carrier

FIGURE 20–1. *Pedigrees illustrating patterns of Mendelian transmission: A, Autosomal dominant, B, autosomal recessive, and C, sex-linked recessive.*

TABLE 20–1. Rates (%) of Recurrence of the Same Defect in a Child of Given Relationship to an Affected Person*

DEFECT	f/1000	SEX RATIO	♂	Parent	♀	Brother	Sister	Sib	2 Sibs	Parent + Sib	2nd Degree	3rd Degree
Heart malformation												
VSD	2.5			4.0				3.0				
PDA	1.2			4.0				2.5				
Tetralogy	1.1			4.0				2.4				
ASD	1.1			2.5				2.5				
PS	0.8			3.5				2.0				
AS	0.4			4.0				2.0				
Coarctation	0.6			2.0				2.0				
Transposition	0.5							2.0				
Legg-Perthes†	0.7	5.2				3.6	4.3	3.8				
Anencephaly‡	3.0	0.6				3.2	6.5	5.4	10			0.3–1.3
Spina bifida‡	3.0	0.8		3.0		3.8	3.1	3.4				
			♂ 5.5		18.9	3.8	9.2					
Pyloric stenosis	3.0	5.0						6.0				
			♀ 2.4		7.0	2.7	3.8					
Scoliosis, idiopathic (adolescent onset)	1.8	0.15					5.0				3.7	1.5
Talipes equinovarus	1.2	2.0				2.0	6.0	2.9			0.5	0.2
			♂	6.0				♂ 1.8				
Dislocated hip§	5.0	0.3								36	1.5	0.3
			♀	17.0				♀ 11.4				
Cleft lip ± palate	1.0	1.6		4.0		3.9	5.0	4.3	9	15?	0.7	0.4
Cleft palate	0.45	0.7		5.8		6.3	2.3	2.9		15?	0.4	0.3
Hirschsprung disease	0.2	3.7				7.0	12.0	7.0				
Schizophrenia	8.0	1.0		15.0				10–15			2.0	1.5
Manic depressive (bipolar)	6.0	0.8		14.0				14.0				

*To find the probability of occurrence for a child whose mother has pyloric stenosis, look up pyloric stenosis, parent, ♀. The probability is 18.9% for a male and 7% for a female child.
†Attack rate to age 15.
‡Rates given are for anencephaly and/or spina bifida.
§Neonatal diagnosis.
(From Fraser, F. C., and Nora, J. J.: Genetics of Man, 2nd ed. Philadelphia, Lea & Febiger, 1986, p. 188.)

not known to be familial. If the disorder is usually transmitted as an autosomal recessive trait, the couple must be counseled that the recurrence risk is 25 per cent. If it is an autosomal dominant trait, both parents should be evaluated to determine if one is affected. For some disorders, such as myotonic dystrophy, a parent may have the trait in a form so mild that they were previously unaware of being affected. If, after thorough examination, neither parent is found to be affected, it may be concluded that the trait is either due to new mutation in the child, or nonpenetrance in the parent. The implication of concluding that a child represents a new mutation is that the recurrence risk for the parents is very low, perhaps no greater than the general population risk. Recent studies have indicated that some inherited disorders may recur in children of unaffected parents due to germ-line mosaicism (Bakker et al., 1987).

If the etiology of a child's problem is not known and there is no prior family history of a similar disorder, it may be impossible to determine the exact recurrence risk. Even in the absence of proof that the disorder is genetically transmissible, the child may have a previously undescribed autosomal or sex-linked recessive disorder. It is extremely important to counsel that the disorder could *possibly* recur in future pregnancies, although the exact risk is not known. It should also be noted that all pregnancies face a 3 per cent risk of the child having a congenital anomaly of some kind.

RISK PERCEPTION

The principles associated with Mendelian, chromosomal, and multifactorial inheritance are complex. Given the diverse backgrounds of individuals being counseled, and the emotional stresses they usually bring to the counseling session, it should not be surprising that recurrence risk information is not always understood or remembered (Griffin et al., 1976; Lippman-Hand and Fraser, 1979; Abramovsky et al. 1980). Moreover, the reaction of an individual to a specific risk depends on factors such as past experience with the disorder, perception of risk prior to counseling, and general attitude toward the concept of "risk" (Wertz et al., 1986). Genetic counseling is best done with both members of a couple present and without distractions such as supervising young children during the session. A written summary of the session should be provided to the family, and it is helpful to offer a follow-up session to repeat information and answer questions.

OPTIONS

In addition to informing a family about recurrence risks, the genetic counselor must explain the options available to modify that risk. These include such possibilities as artificial insemination (in the case of autosomal recessive disorders or dominant disorders if the father is affected). The possibility of prenatal diagnosis should also be raised. Although prenatal diagnosis is often viewed as a prelude to pregnancy termination if a fetus is found to be affected, there are many other reasons that a couple may want to avail themselves of prenatal testing. These include reassurance or the need to plan for the medical needs of a child with a disorder. The reaction of a couple to the possibility of a genetic disorder cannot be predicted because it depends on innumerable individual factors including attitude, background, and knowledge. It is a canon of genetic counseling to be *nondirective,* that is, to provide information in as neutral a manner as possible, leaving the decision as to course of action to the individuals being counseled.

■ ADJUSTMENT

The reaction of a couple who have had a child with a genetic disorder commonly includes a mixture of fear, guilt, anger, confusion, and disappointment. As they evaluate and treat the child, the members of the medical team must also contribute to an emotional healing process in the parents and other family members. This begins with keeping the family informed of efforts to arrive at a diagnosis, explaining therapeutic options, and providing updates on the child's progress and prognosis.

The process of gathering medical information provides a number of opportunities to educate the family and help assuage some of their negative emotions. For example, in taking a pregnancy history, the main goal is to identify an event or exposure that might have contributed to the child's problems. There are a number of well-documented teratogenic agents and congenital infections that produce more or less well-defined neonatal syndromes. In most cases, however, pregnancy-related events cannot be clearly related to the infant's problems. Everybody can identify something that happened during pregnancy, such as some medication taken or some alcohol consumed, which consciously or subconsciously they may blame for the disorder in their child. It should be assumed that this is the case for *every* family, and it is the job of the genetic counselor to be thorough in obtaining a pregnancy history and, where possible, provide facts to allay feelings of guilt. Similarly, individuals often have erroneous theories about genetic causes of a child's problems. The counselor must be alert to such attempts at explanation, which may result in feelings of guilt on the part of one parent, and help to correct such misconceptions.

The process of genetic counseling must occur over a period of time, beginning with the recognition of a genetic disorder in a family and continuing through future pregnancies. Contributions are made both by genetic counselors and by other professionals such as nurses, social workers, members of the clergy, and psychiatrists who interact with the family (Wood, 1974). The effort is most likely to be helpful if there is a physician who establishes a long-term relationship with the family and if other consultants communicate frequently with one another.

Parent support groups are often of great help. Attention to the day-to-day needs of handicapped children is improved by parent-to-parent education. In addition, national organizations prepare information for parents that can be a useful supplement to the advice provided directly by physicians.

For example the following agency could be consulted:

March of Dimes
1275 Mamaroneck Ave.
White Plains, NY 10605
(914) 428–7100

or

Center for Birth Defects Information Services
Dover Medical Building
30 Springdale Ave., Box 1776
Dover, MA 02030
(508) 785–2525

■ REFERENCES

Abramovsky, I., Godmilow, L., Hirschhorn, K., et al.: Analysis of a follow-up study of genetic counseling. Clin. Genet. *17*:1–12, 1980.

Bakker, E., Van Broeckhoven, C., Bonten, E. J., et al.: Germline mosaicism and Duchenne muscular dystrophy mutations. Nature *329*:554–556, 1987.

Carter, C. O.: Genetics of common disorders. Br. Med. Bull. *25*:52–57, 1969.

Emery, A. E. H., and Rimoin, D. L.: Principles and Practice of Medical Genetics. Edinburgh, Churchill Livingstone, 1983.

Fraser, F. C.: Genetic counseling. Am. J. Hum. Genet. *26*:636–659, 1974.

Griffin, M. L., Kavanagh, C. M., and Sorenson, J. R.: Genetic knowledge, client perspectives, and genetic counseling. Soc. Work Health Care *2*:171–180, 1976.

Kelly, T. E.: Clinical Genetics and Genetic Counseling, 2nd ed. Chicago, Year Book Medical Publishers, 1986.

Lippman-Hand, A., and Fraser, F. C.: Genetic counseling—The postcounseling period: I. Parent's perceptions of uncertainty. Am. J. Med. Genet. *4*:51–71, 1979.

Lister, T. J., and Frota-Pessoa, O.: Recurrence risks for Down syndrome. Hum. Genet. *55*:203–208, 1980.

Murphy, E. A., and Chase, G. A. Principles of Genetic Counseling. Chicago, Year Book Medical Publishers, 1975.

Nelson, K., and Holmes, L. B.: Malformations due to presumed spontaneous mutations in newborn infants. N. Engl. J. Med. *320*:19, 1989.

Schuett, V. E.: National Survey of Treatment Programs for PKU and Selected Other Inherited Programs for Metabolic Diseases. Washington, D.C., U.S. Department of Health and Human Services, DHHS Publication No. HRS-M-CH-89-5, 1989.

Stene, J., and Stengel-Rutkowski, S.: Genetic risks for familial reciprocal translocations with special emphasis on those leading to 9p, 10p, and 12p trisomies. Ann. Hum. Genet. *46*:41–74, 1982.

Wertz, D. C., Sorenson, J. R., and Heeren, T. C.: Clients' interpretation of risks provided in genetic counseling. Am. J. Hum. Genet. *39*:253–264, 1986.

Wigglesworth, J. S.: Investigation of perinatal death. Arch. Dis. Child. *62*:1207–1208, 1987.

Winter, R. M., Knowles, S. A. S., Bieber, F. R., et al.: The Malformed Fetus and Stillbirth. A Diagnostic Approach. New York, John Wiley and Sons, 1988.

Wood, J. W.: The pediatrician as genetic counselor. Ped. Clin. N. Am. *21*:401–405, 1974.

CONGENITAL 21 ANOMALIES

Robin Dawn Clark and Donna Jane Eteson

When considered individually, congenital anomalies are rare; when considered collectively, their impact is great. Between 2 and 4 per cent of all newborns have a significant birth defect (Marden et al., 1964). However, 25 per cent of all perinatal deaths are now caused by lethal malformations compared to 8 per cent in 1940. In full-term infants, congenital malformations account for nearly half of the mortality rate (Goldenberg et al., 1983). As prematurity and intrauterine growth retardation are defeated by advances in perinatology, congenital anomalies will become the major source of morbidity and mortality in the intensive care nursery. For this reason, pediatricians must learn to recognize the various patterns of congenital anomalies along with their causes and consequences. The study of clinical genetics is, of necessity, an integral part of the training of a pediatrician.

■ CLASSIFICATION OF CONGENITAL ANOMALIES

When birth defects are grouped in terms of their causes, four major categories emerge (Kalter and Warkany, 1983). **Environmental** or nongenetic agents, such as maternal medication or disease and congenital infection, account for approximately 6 per cent of all major defects. **Multifactorial** conditions, such as pyloric stenosis, due to both genetic and environmental factors, make up 20 per cent of significant anomalies. **Single gene** disorders, so-called mendelian traits, contribute 7.5 per cent of all defects. **Chromosome** anomalies cause an additional 6 per cent. By far, the majority of birth defects have an unknown cause.

Unfortunately, this classification system is more useful to the epidemiologist than to the clinician at the bedside. A child with a cleft palate, for instance, may have been exposed to a teratogen (environmental agent), may have an isolated malformation (multifactorial), may have a monogenic trait such as **Van der Woude syndrome** of lip pits and clefting, or may have a chromosome deletion syndrome. This classification system does not help the clinician to distinguish among the various possible causes.

For the purpose of establishing a diagnosis, which is most important for clinical management, prognosis, and counseling, a morphogenetic classification system has proved more useful (Jones, 1988). The first question to be answered is, are intrinsic or extrinsic forces responsible for a given defect? If normal morphogenesis is altered or interrupted by an extrinsic agent—such as a virus—the recurrence risk (i.e., chance of having another affected child) would usually be low. Two major types of defects, deformations and disruptions, usually fall into this extrinsic category.

Deformations are caused by mechanical forces that alter the course of (but do not stop) otherwise normal development. The term mechanical forces usually refers to various types of intrauterine constraint; however, the lack of normal mechanical forces can also lead to a deformed structure. For instance, the absence of normal fetal movement in amyoplasia (Hall, 1985) can lead to deformations of the limbs through disuse. It is important to use the term deformation specifically in this way and not, as it is so commonly applied, as a synonym for any type of congenital anomaly.

Disruptions are caused by destructive forces that interfere with or interrupt normal morphogenesis. Disruptions can be caused by all types of teratogenic agents, such as infection, drugs, chemicals, maternal disease, and thermal injury. They also include amputations caused by amniotic bands. Vascular events, such as emboli from an infarcted placenta, can lead to disruptions in poorly perfused tissues (e.g., a porencephalic cyst).

Malformations, on the other hand, are caused by intrinsically abnormal morphogenesis. Malformations can be isolated, such as a neural tube defect or cleft lip, or they may appear in conjunction with other defects. A **malformation sequence** results when a single malformation initiates a chain of subsequent defects. Holoprosencephaly is a good example (Fig. 21–1). Because midline facial structures are induced by the developing brain, holoprosencephaly often leads to absence of the nasal septum, columella, and premaxilla with a cleft palate. In males, the penis can be very small, probably owing to absent hypophyseal hormone production. A **syndrome** is a recognizable pattern of malformations without such a causal link between the defects, such as **Cornelia de Lange syndrome** (see Fig. 21–21) of mental retardation, typical facies, and limb reduction defects.

Finally, a **dysplasia** results from abnormal morphogenesis affecting only tissues of a certain type. As an example, ectodermal dysplasias involve hair, teeth, sweating, tears, and skin.

Infants may have various combinations of deformations, disruptions, malformations, or dysplasias. A successful evaluation determines which mechanism was primary and which was secondary. The stillborn boy in Figure 21–2 had a single primary **malformation,** posterior urethral valves, which led to decreased amniotic fluid and in utero compression causing **deformations:** Potter facies and pulmonary hypoplasia. In addition, the massively

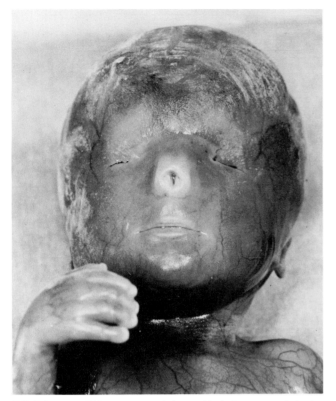

FIGURE 21–1. *This premature infant with holoprosencephaly has cebocephaly, which is characterized by the absence of midline facial structures and a single nostril.*

dilated urinary tract caused a "prune belly" and significant vascular compromise leading to a **disruption** of the lower extremities (Carey et al., 1982). This case provides an example of the clinical utility of this classification scheme. By examining the layers of deformations, disruptions, and malformations, a clear picture emerges of the events leading to the multiple congenital anomalies in this child.

■ EVALUATING THE NEWBORN WITH CONGENITAL ANOMALIES

The process of evaluating a newborn with multiple congenital anomalies involves a detailed search for other defects in the infant and other family members. It is helpful to list all anomalies systematically, taking note of the time in embryogenesis when the defect would have most likely occurred. Minor anomalies, such as epicanthal folds or a single transverse palmar crease, are commonly encountered and usually have no cosmetic or functional consequences. On the other hand, they may be an indication of a significant defect. When two minor anomalies are present, there is a 10 per cent chance of encountering at least one major anomaly. When three minor anomalies are detected, 85 per cent of infants have multiple major anomalies (Marden et al., 1964). Some syndromes may be recognized only in the form of a combination of minor anomalies. **Down syndrome** may fit this pattern.

Clinical photographs are a very effective way of documenting the unusual appearance of a particular child. Every nursery should have a simple camera for this purpose. Permission from the parents to photograph the infant should be sought. In our experience, parents usually

agree that a photograph, rather than a written account, provides a clearer description of their baby's problems, and therefore, they give consent. These photographs can prove to be an invaluable resource, especially if the appearance of the infant changes with age or the child dies. Many diagnoses have been made retrospectively in this way.

In addition to photographs, a thorough examination of the infant can include a detailed cardiac examination, an ophthalmologic examination through dilated pupils, a brain stem auditory evoked response, a computed tomography (CT) or ultrasound study of the brain, a renal ultrasound study, and a chromosome analysis. When the limbs or the spine is involved, a complete set of radiographs should include a lateral view of the spine, which can reveal defects (e.g., coronal clefting or beaked vertebrae) that are not visible on an anteroposterior (AP) view. In the event of a lethal malformation, the importance of performing an autopsy on the infant should be stressed to the parents.

The patient's history often holds the essential clues to the cause of an obscure syndrome. A maternal history must include information about drug or alcohol exposure, the presence or absence of fetal movement, and vaginal

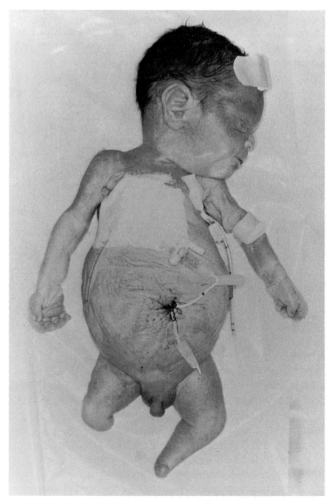

FIGURE 21–2. *In this infant, a primary malformation causing urethral stenosis led to oligohydramnios, Potter sequence, and subsequent deformations. The dilated kidneys, ureters, and bladder, which resulted in a "prune belly," disrupted the vascular supply to the lower extremities, leading to bilateral transverse terminal defects.*

bleeding or amniotic fluid loss as well as previous miscarriages, stillbirths, or infertility. A detailed family history can be very valuable. Consanguinity is frequently occult and often this information is revealed only after many attempts are made to extract it. Consanguinity may be of key significance because it increases the chance of the transmission of an autosomal recessive trait. Information about other similarly affected children, unexplained infant deaths, mental retardation, other birth defects, or hereditary conditions should be sought from parents and, if possible, grandparents who frequently have more reliable and extensive knowledge of family history. Parents should be examined for milder versions of their infant's problems such as a bifid uvula when the baby has a cleft palate. It must be stressed that a careful physical examination and detailed maternal and family histories are often more important than any laboratory test in establishing a diagnosis. Nevertheless, the lack of a positive family history does not rule out a genetic cause (Nelson and Holmes, 1989).

■ GENETIC COUNSELING

The goal of genetic counseling is to educate the patient about a genetic disorder, its pattern of inheritance, and prognosis in order to make appropriate choices in family planning. Parental guilt and cultural superstitions are among the many impediments to this process. Many Latin Americans believe that viewing a lunar eclipse during pregnancy or the mixing of "bad blood" between the parents (such as Rh factor discrepancies) causes birth defects. College-educated professionals are also susceptible to "magical thinking." Frequently there is the unspoken belief that a baby with a congenital anomaly is in some way a retribution for a previous transgression such as an elective abortion.

Reliable counseling is possible only when a definitive diagnosis has been established. The natural impulse to reassure a worried parent can cause more harm than good if it creates a false impression of hope. In one unfortunate case of premature counseling, a mother had been reassured, by an eager but inexperienced physician, that each of her baby's anomalies (cleft lip, omphalocele, polydactyly, and scalp defect) could be repaired and that the infant would then be normal. A few minutes later, bilateral anophthalmia was noted by the clinical geneticist, who then had to explain to the mother the high probability of trisomy 13 and the associated poor outcome.

The timing of the counseling session is also important. Information received immediately after birth is often forgotten and should be repeated later. The information is best retained when it is presented several times in both verbal and written forms. A follow-up appointment to discuss chromosome or other test results, including autopsy reports, is often an appropriate time to review genetic implications.

Because genetic counseling is fraught with such difficulties, it is best done by qualified counselors or medical geneticists.

■ DEFORMATIONS

Deformations, which result from the application of abnormal mechanical forces on an otherwise normal developmental process, are relatively common (Graham, 1988). Two per cent of all newborns have some type of deformation, ranging from a dislocated hip to an abnormally molded breech head. They can occur from 20 weeks' gestation until after birth and are caused by a variety of maternal (extrinsic) and fetal (intrinsic) factors. When the deformation is due to extrinsic causes, the recurrence risk is frequently low. Deformations usually respond well to therapy, and some even resolve spontaneously.

The deformed organ can be identified because all structural elements are present, although they are distorted in shape. The complete absence of any body part, such as a missing thumb, rules out deformation as the cause.

A primigravida or small woman has a higher chance of having an infant with a fetal deformation. A structurally abnormal uterus, present in 1 to 2 per cent of all women, can limit fetal mobility. For example, the fetus can become entrapped in one horn of a bicornate uterus. This type of constraint has led to craniosynostosis. Often, the mother recalls that the baby's kicks were always located in the same area. Uterine sacculations and fibromas can also cause in utero constraint. Multiple gestation leads to deformation through fetal crowding and abnormal lie.

MALPRESENTATION

The breech position, present in about 3 per cent of term singleton deliveries, accounts for 30 per cent of all deformations. In the vertex position, the fetal head is molded more or less evenly by the pelvis. In the breech position, the downward tug of the uterine fundus deforms the head anteriorly and posteriorly causing a long narrow shape, a prominent occiput, and an overhanging, even wrinkled, forehead. The shoulders may be forced up against the ears, making the latter protrude. The legs, especially when extended in the frank breech position, may deform the rib cage or the mandible, causing micrognathia or facial asymmetry (Fig. 21–3). The knees when hyperextended can dislocate causing genu recurvatum. Other significant problems often related to the breech position include torticollis, scoliosis, hip dislocation, and equinovarus.

Confounding factors must be considered when evaluating a breech baby. First, the breech position occurs more commonly in the presence of fetal malformations, hypotonia, and central nervous system (CNS) or muscle disease. Therefore, the physician should not be too quick to attribute all defects to the breech position. Only after noting a patulous anus and a poor urinary stream on a second examination was it clear to one author (R. D. C.) that a breech baby with scaphocephaly and dislocated hips actually had sacral agenesis as the primary problem. Without normal muscle power, the lower extremities could not propel the fetus into the vertex position.

Secondly, any decrease in amniotic fluid volume, whether because of chronic leakage or decreased fetal urinary output, will make it difficult for the fetus to attain the vertex position. When evaluating the breech baby, it is important to note the amount of amniotic fluid and the baby's ability to urinate.

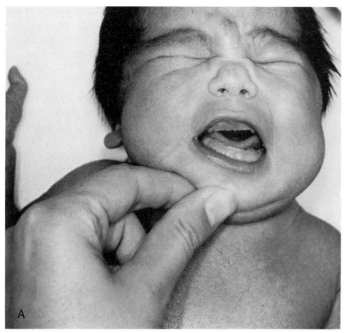

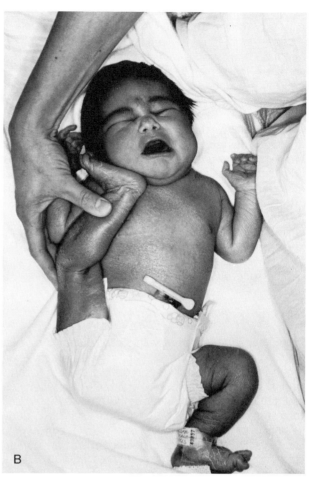

FIGURE 21–3. A, The upward displacement of the right alveolar ridge is a deformation caused by pressure from the right foot due to the infant's breech position in utero (B).

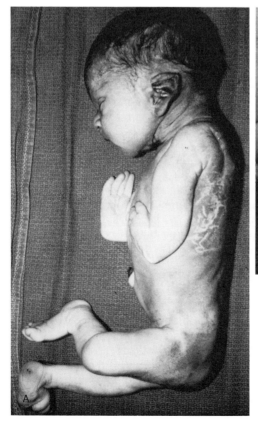

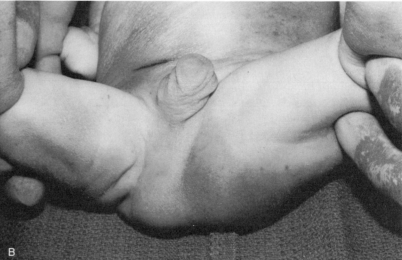

FIGURE 21–4. A, This infant with Potter sequence also has other multiple congenital anomalies—note the absent forearms—in addition to the expected flat facies and large ears. B, There is no anus or urethral meatus. The penis is absent (karyotype 46,XY), but an empty scrotum is present. A persistent atretic cloaca caused these perineal anomalies and the resulting oligohydramnios.

OLIGOHYDRAMNIOS

Potter sequence of oligohydramnios, fetal constraint, flat facies, and pulmonary hypoplasia is frequently associated with the breech position. This condition has many causes—chronic amniotic fluid leakage, renal agenesis or dysplasia, and posterior urethral valves. It can be associated with other defects and chromosome anomalies (Curry et al., 1984). Rarely, a malformation, such as a persistent atretic cloaca, interferes with formation of the genitalia, urethra, and anus (Koffler et al., 1978). The infant with Potter sequence shown in Figure 21–4 had no perineal orifices.

CLUBFOOT

The term clubfoot is used to describe a number of abnormalities, the most common of which is talipes equinovarus wherein the foot is plantar flexed and the forefoot curves inward. Clubfoot, which occurs in about 1 in 1000 births, is probably due to in utero constraint in one-third to one-half of cases. Severe cases are thought to be malformations rather than deformations. The sex ratio is 2 males:1 female. Clubfoot is also present in association with a variety of neuromuscular disorders including spina bifida and arthrogryposis. From 10 to 20 per cent of cases of clubfoot are complicated by other anomalies. There are over 150 syndromes in which clubfoot has been described. In isolated clubfoot, the risk to future siblings is 3 per cent, which supports a multifactorial pattern of inheritance.

Serial casting by a pediatric orthopedist is often an effective treatment. Serial casting is begun in the first days of life, when the infant's ligaments remain lax because of presence of maternal hormones. About 50 per cent of the cases of clubfoot will be normal after some months of casting; 50 per cent will require some surgery, usually to release contractures and restore a more normal alignment. Following surgery, casts are required for 8 to 12 weeks, with continued splinting for several more months. Treatment is very effective, although some calf atrophy and mild (1 to 2 cm) limb shortening can occur with or without surgery.

CONGENITAL DISLOCATED HIP

The dislocated or subluxed hip occurs in approximately 5 of 1000 births. Females are most usually affected. The dislocated hip is commonly associated with intrauterine constraint. About 50 per cent are associated with breech presentation (Graham, 1988). However, there is also a genetic factor. When a parent is affected, the offspring has a 12 per cent risk. This risk is somewhat higher for daughters and lower for sons. When a previous child is affected, the overall risk for subsequent siblings is 6 per cent (Wynne-Davies, 1973).

The diagnosis is based primarily on the physical examination. In the Barlow maneuver, an unstable hip can be dislocated from the acetabulum. In the Ortolani maneuver, a dislocated hip is repositioned into the acetabulum. Both maneuvers produce a palpable "clunk" as the hip is either dislocated or relocated. Minor clicks are frequently noted and are not of diagnostic significance. The gluteal creases may also be asymmetric with short-ening of one leg. Treatment is most successful when it is begun early and the hip is splinted in a position of flexion and moderate abduction. Surgery is usually reserved for late diagnoses.

IATROGENIC CAUSES

Neonatologists should recognize and try to prevent common iatrogenically induced deformations associated with prematurity. A towel rolled into the shape of a doughnut or a half-empty bag of intravenous fluid can be used as a pillow to prevent a dolichocephalic head shape and long face. Prolonged intubation may lead to a long narrow palatal groove, or a deviated nasal septum.

▪ DISRUPTIONS

Disruptions cause the destruction of otherwise normal tissue by interrupting normal morphogenic processes. All teratogenic agents, including drugs, chemicals, radiation, thermal injury, infection, and maternal disease, are disruptive. In addition, any cause of fetal injury, such as early amniotic rupture and vascular accidents, acts by disrupting normal morphogenesis.

MEDICATIONS AND DRUGS

The use of medications and drugs in pregnancy is common. Forty per cent of women take medications in the first trimester and only 20 per cent of pregnant women use no drugs at any time during gestation (Golbus, 1980). In spite of this, drugs and chemicals are believed to cause only 2 to 3 per cent of congenital anomalies. Several general principles of teratology help explain this discrepancy (Wilson, 1977).

First, exposure must occur at the critical time, usually within the period of embryogenesis, which takes place during the first 12 weeks. Second, teratogens usually produce a specific embryopathy, which may vary, however, with dosage and other factors. Diethylstilbestrol (DES) causes abnormalities of the cervix and uterus. Isotretinoin (Accutane), a retinoic acid derivative, causes central nervous system malformations, microtia or anotia, and aortic arch anomalies (Fig. 21–5) (Lammer et al., 1985). The case against Bendectin, Agent Orange, and other purported teratogens was weakened considerably by the wide variety of defects for which they were held responsible.

Third, teratogens are species specific. What is teratogenic in the mouse may not be so in humans. As the human experience with thalidomide demonstrated, the converse may also be true. Thalidomide, a drug used to suppress vomiting in early pregnancy in the 1960s, was never approved for use in the United States. Although no malformations are seen with prenatal exposure in the mouse, in humans thalidomide is one of the most potent teratogens known. The most striking malformation is phocomelia, but malformations of the eyes, ears, teeth, and intestines can also be present.

In spite of many more known teratogens in animals, there are very few proven teratogens in humans. However, because of the background risk for all birth defects and the difficulty of performing unbiased, prospective,

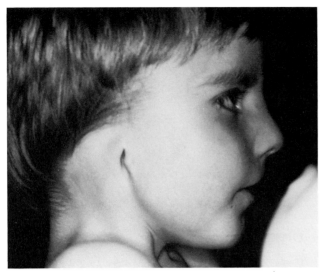

FIGURE 21–5. Isotretinoin (Accutane) embryopathy caused the severe ear anomaly and micrognathia seen in this boy. (Courtesy of Dr. Edward Lammer.)

controlled human studies, it may be impossible to prove that a drug is safe for use in pregnancy. Similarly, if the teratogenic potential of a commonly used drug, like diazepam (Laegreid et al., 1989), is weak, its association with specific birth defects may be difficult to ascertain.

Finally, a genetically determined predisposition may contribute to the teratogenic potential of an agent. This may account, at least in part, for the fact that not all fetuses exposed at the critical time in embryogenesis are adversely affected. This genetic variability has been demonstrated in dizygotic and heteropaternal (different fathers) twins exposed to the same teratogen in utero who have been discordant for its effects (Phelan et al., 1982).

The drugs and chemicals known to be teratogenic in humans are summarized in Table 21–1. The effects of intrauterine infections are summarized in Table 21–2.

RADIATION

Animal studies have consistently shown that fetal radiation damage is related to dose and gestational age. The risk for malformation, growth retardation, or mental retardation does not appear to be increased in infants born to mothers receiving diagnostic radiation delivering 5 rads or less to the fetus (Brent, 1986). In humans, disturbances of growth have been observed in infants receiving 25 rads during early gestation. At 50 rads, growth retardation, decreased head circumference, and mental retardation have been observed. Small size for gestational age, microcephaly, microphthalmia, cataracts, retinal pigmentary changes, genital anomalies, and skeletal malformations were observed in infants exposed to 250 rads between weeks 3 and 20 of gestation (Dekaban, 1968). Anomalies have been observed only in infants with growth retardation or a CNS abnormality (Brent, 1986). Risks for genetic damage (mutagenesis) and carcinogenesis to the radiation-exposed fetus have not been determined.

THERMAL INJURY

The risk for fetal injury by maternal hyperthermia is unknown; however, case reports and experimental data

point to its significance as a teratogenic agent in humans. In animals, severe maternal hyperthermia (an increase of at least 1.5 to 3° C) during early gestation has produced neural tube defects, microphthalmia, microcephaly, spinal cord dysmorphogenesis, and minor distal limb anomalies (Edwards, 1967). Retrospective studies in human pregnancies have discovered CNS, craniofacial, and minor limb defects in infants whose mothers had febrile illness (40° C [104° F] or greater) of one or more days duration or who had hyperthermia owing to a prolonged sauna or very hot tub bath at 4 to 14 weeks after conception (Jones, 1988). Maternal hyperthermia occurring at about 3 to 4 weeks of gestational age was associated with nearly 10 per cent of neural tube defects (Fisher, 1981). In addition, hyperthermia due to influenza has been associated with spontaneous abortion, stillbirth, and prematurity.

MATERNAL DISEASE

Infants of insulin-dependent diabetic mothers are at an increased risk for malformations, including neural tube defects, situs inversus, and cardiovascular, genitourinary, and musculoskeletal defects. The incidence of major malformations has been estimated to be between 6 and 18 per cent (Molsted-Pedersen et al., 1964; Chung and Myrianthopoulos, 1975). The mechanism of action is unknown. However, animal studies have revealed that neither insulin nor hyperglycemia is teratogenic. A vascular pathogenesis has been proposed, as those women in White classes D and F (those with vascular disease) have the highest rates of malformation (Mills, 1982). When the maternal hemoglobin A_{1c} is 8.5 or less before the 14th week of pregnancy, the incidence of defects is about 3.4 per cent, whereas at levels greater than 8.5, the incidence is 22.4 per cent (Miller et al., 1981). The infants of gestational or non-insulin-dependent diabetics do not appear to have an increased number of malformations.

Infants of diabetic mothers account for 16 per cent of the newborns with **sacral agenesis** or caudal dysplasia sequence (caudal regression syndrome). This disorder, however, occurs in only about 1 in 350 children of diabetic mothers (Pederson, 1977) as compared with cardiac anomalies, which are much more frequent at 1 in 40. Caudal dysplasia sequence consists of varying degrees of sacral dysplasia and the resulting neurologic impairment, leading to urinary incontinence, patulous anus, and sensory and motor deficiencies of the lower limbs.

Untreated maternal phenylketonuria (PKU) or hyperphenylalaninemia, which acts as a potent human teratogen, has a frequency of approximately 1 in 20,000 pregnant women (Levy and Waisbren, 1983). It causes spontaneous abortion, mental retardation, microcephaly, congenital heart defects, and low birth weight (Lipson et al., 1984). Maternal PKU should be considered in families in which all children have unexplained mental retardation or microcephaly regardless of the mother's intelligence. Women with untreated PKU are not invariably severely mentally retarded, and because newborn screening for the disease was not available until the early 1960s, they may be unaware of their condition. Furthermore, as restriction of protein intake was often discontinued in childhood, even those who had been diagnosed at birth could later be unaware of their diagnosis.

TABLE 21–1. The Effects of Teratogenic Agents in Humans

TERATOGEN	MANIFESTATIONS	RISK	REFERENCES
Alcohol	Growth retardation Microcephaly Mental retardation Short palpebral fissures Long philtrum Thin, smooth upper lip Nail hypoplasia Cerebral palsy	30 to 50 per cent in chronically alcoholic women Binge drinkers may also be at risk	Jones et al., 1973
Anticoagulants Warfarin	Nasal hypoplasia Stippled epiphyses Low birth weight Developmental delay Blindness, optic atrophy microphthalmia Deafness CNS anomalies	17 to 30 per cent	Hall et al., 1980b Iturbe-Alessio et al., 1986
Anticonvulsants Phenytoin (Dilantin)	Prenatal/postnatal growth retardation Mental retardation Mild craniofacial dysmorphism Nail hypoplasia, distal phalanx hypoplasia Cleft lip and palate Possible relationship with neural crest tumors	10 per cent have full-blown syndrome of growth retardation, mental retardation, and mild craniofacial dysmorphism. An additional 30 per cent have some features of the condition	Hanson, 1986
Paramethadione (Trimethadione)	V-shaped eyebrows Cleft lip and/or palate Cardiac defects Tracheoesophageal fistula Mental retardation	83 per cent of infants born alive have at least 1 major malformation 28 per cent are mentally retarded	Zackai et al., 1975
Valproic acid (Depakene)	Spina bifida (with exposure in first 30 days) Developmental delay (71 per cent) Micrognathia (83 per cent) Prominent metopic ridge (71 per cent) Minor ear anomalies (57 per cent)	1 to 2 per cent have spina bifida	Lammer et al., 1987 Ardinger et al., 1988
Antithyroid medications Propylthiouracil Iodine Methimazole	Fetal goiter hyperthyroidism hypothyroidism Scalp defects Imperforate anus	12 per cent risk for goiter	Briggs et al., 1986
Cytotoxic agents Aminopterin Methotrexate (folic acid antagonists)	Prenatal growth retardation Microcephaly Frontal upsweep of hair Prominent eyes Micrognathia Cleft palate	Risk unknown	Shepard, 1989

Table continued on following page

TABLE 21–1. The Effects of Teratogenic Agents in Humans *Continued*

TERATOGEN	MANIFESTATIONS	RISK	REFERENCES
Diethylstilbestrol	Cervical and uterine anomalies Vaginal adenosis Vaginal adenocarcinoma Infertility in both sexes Hypotrophic testes, epididymal cysts	>50 per cent of females 0.14 to 1.4 in 1000 25 per cent of males	Herbst, 1981
Lead	Increased rate of stillbirth and abortion Possible effect on fetal CNS development	Risk unknown	Shepard, 1989
Lithium	Cardiac anomaly, especially Ebstein anomaly	8.2 per cent (15 in 183) 2.7 per cent	Warkany, 1988
Methyl mercury	Microcephaly Mental retardation Blindness Deafness Spasticity Seizures Eye anomalies	60 per cent	Harada, 1986
Retinoic acid (Accutane)	Cerebellar defects, cranial nerve deficiencies, hydrocephalus, microcephaly Microtia, anotia Aortic arch anomalies Retina and optic nerve involvement Cleft palate	25 per cent risk of anomalies 40 per cent risk of miscarriage with 1st trimester exposure	Lammer et al., 1985 Lammer et al., 1988
Steroid hormones	Clitoral enlargement, labioscrotal fusion in females Sexual precocity in males		Wilson and Brent, 1981
Streptomycin	Hearing loss due to cochlear or vestibular injury or VIII nerve damage		
Tetracycline	Discolorations of deciduous teeth with 2nd or 3rd trimester exposure		Toaff and Ravid, 1966 Cohlan, 1977
Thalidomide	Microtia Phocomelia Duplication of toes Preaxial digital deficiencies in hands Intestinal atresias Congenital heart defects Renal, anal, genital anomalies	20 per cent of exposed infants have anomalies	Lenz, 1988 Mellin and Katzenstein, 1962

TABLE 21–2. Teratogenic Congenital Infections

INFECTIOUS AGENT (RATE OF SIGNIFICANT CONGENITALLY ACQUIRED DISEASE IN THE NEWBORN)	MANIFESTATIONS	RISK TO THE FETUS WHEN INFECTION OCCURS DURING PREGNANCY	COMMENTS	REFERENCES
Herpes viruses Cytomegalovirus (1 in 500)	Prenatal growth retardation Microcephaly, mental retardation Hydrocephaly Intracranial calcification of ependymal area Chorioretinitis, blindness, optic atrophy Seizures Jaundice, direct hyperbilirubinemia Hepatosplenomegaly Thrombocytopenia	0.5–2 per cent of live births have congenital infection 10 per cent of infected infants are symptomatic at birth Another 10 per cent may have late-appearing sequelae, especially deafness	25% of children with microcephaly had congenital cytomegalovirus	Emanuel and Kenny, 1988 Reynolds et al., 1986 Stagno and Whitley, 1985a
Herpes simplex (HSV) (1 in 300,000)	Stillbirth, abortion Hydranencephaly, microcephaly, mental retardation Chorioretinitis Deafness With 3rd trimester infection: Fetal growth retardation Scarring, vesicles, aplasia cutis	25 per cent risk of spontaneous abortion when primary genital infection occurs in 1st 20 weeks of gestation	Of newborns with herpes simplex infection (1 in 2500 to 1 in 5000 deliveries), 95 per cent acquire the virus during delivery, not earlier in gestation	Stagno and Whitley, 1985b Baldwin and Whitley, 1989
Varicella (1 to 5 in 25,000)	Hypoplasia of the extremities Cortical atrophy Skin lesions Ocular abnormalities	Risk for malformations is low with maternal varicella Exposure during the first 20 weeks most often associated with fetal abnormalities		Fuccillo, 1986 Stagno and Whitley, 1985b
Rubella (<1 in 100,000)	Hearing loss (most frequent) Mental retardation Congenital heart defects Cataracts, microphthalmia, glaucoma Growth retardation Thrombocytopenia Hepatosplenomegaly Osteolytic metaphyseal lesions	80 per cent chance of fetal malformation with 1st trimester exposure 40 per cent chance of fetal malformation with exposure at 13 to 14 weeks		South and Sever, 1985
Syphilis	Abortion, stillbirth Fetal growth retardation Hydrops Anterior or posterior uveitis Hepatosplenomegaly Periostitis of long bones	Untreated maternal syphilis results in congenital infection in 75 to 95 per cent of cases	Late manifestations: Hemolytic anemia Hutchinson teeth Mulberry molar Saddle nose, nasal discharge ("snuffles") Saber shins Maculopapular rash Osteochondritis Interstitial keratitis of the eye	Grossman, 1986
Toxoplasmosis (1 in 4000)	Fetal growth retardation Hydrocephalus, hydranencephaly Microcephaly, seizures, deafness Periventricular calcifications Microphthalmia, anophthalmia Chorioretinitis, cataracts Hepatosplenomegaly, jaundice	40 per cent risk for congenital infection, but only 15 per cent of infected infants have overt or severe disease and 20 per cent have mild disease	Late manifestations: Deafness Microcephaly Low IQ	Sever et al., 1988 Larsen, 1986

Although the risk to the fetus increases with the mother's phenylalanine level, even women in whom the condition is fairly well controlled may have children who are affected (Lenke and Levy, 1980). The best outcome occurs when preconceptional dietary restriction is continued throughout gestation. Ninety-five per cent of women on unrestricted diets with phenylalanine levels of 20 mg per deciliter or greater had at least one mentally retarded child and 81 per cent had only mentally retarded children. When the phenylalanine level was within the treatment range of 3 to 10 mg/dl, which corresponds to a protein-restricted diet, 32 per cent had at least one mentally retarded child and 13 per cent had only mentally retarded children.

EARLY AMNION RUPTURE SEQUENCE

Rupture of the amnion in early embryogenesis can cause hemorrhage and necrosis of previously normal limb, trunk, and craniofacial structures. Entrapment of fetal parts, especially digits and extremities, in residual bands of amnion leads to congenital amputations and deep circumferential constriction rings (Fig. 21–6). The early amnion rupture sequence occurs in from 1 in 1300 (Ossipoff and Hall, 1977) to 1 in 10,000 (Baker and Rudolph, 1971) live births. The defects are usually asymmetric. Distal structures can be swollen because of obstruction of venous and lymphatic return. Structures proximal to the band, however, are normal. The hypoplastic thumb shown in Figure 21–7 was at first thought to be due to an amniotic constriction until the missing metacarpal was discovered. This infant also had ipsilateral agenesis of the lung that could not be explained by amniotic bands but probably had a vascular cause.

The **limb-body wall complex** (Van Allen et al., 1987), part of the spectrum of the early amnion rupture sequence, occurs when the extraembryonic coelom persists beyond the normal 60 days. The amnion, normally adherent to the umbilical cord and contiguous with the periumbilical skin, attaches to the body abnormally at the head, chest, or abdomen. Amniotic or placental adhesions to the head have been seen with anencephaly, oblique facial clefts, and encephaloceles (Fig. 21–8). Large ventral wall defects or thoracoschisis leads to evisceration (Fig. 21–9). Associated limb and internal anomalies usually have a vascular cause, although constriction rings can be seen.

VASCULAR INSUFFICIENCY

Fetal vascular deficiency, due to thrombus, embolus, hemorrhage, hypoplasia, or aplasia of the blood vessels, causes ischemia and hypoxia in dependent tissues. The severity and variety of the resulting anomalies depend on the time and location of the disruption.

Placental thrombi have been associated with absence of distal limb structures (Hoyme et al., 1982). Emboli are

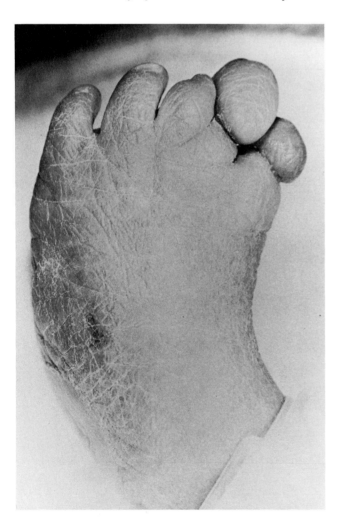

FIGURE 21–6. The deep circumferential constriction rings, the terminal amputation of the third toe, and the distal swelling of the first two digits are typical of the disruption caused by an amniotic band.

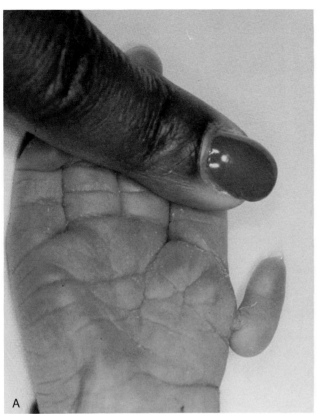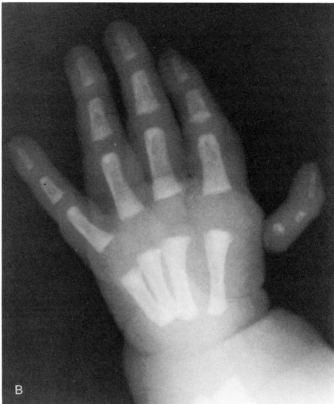

FIGURE 21–7. A, This hypoplastic thumb was initially interpreted as an amniotic band defect. However, the radiograph (B) demonstrates the absence of the first metacarpal—a defect proximal to the presumed constriction—which rules out the amniotic band disruption sequence.

believed to be responsible for these limb defects. Radial aplasia has been associated with anomalies of the radial artery (Van Allen et al., 1982).

Gastroschisis, a defect in the abdominal wall to the right of the umbilical cord, may be due to interruption of blood flow in the omphalomesenteric artery at the base of the cord. Infarction and necrosis of this area allow ventral herniation of the intestines. A more proximal defect in the omphalomesenteric artery causes additional defects, especially multiple intestinal atresias (Hoyme et al., 1983).

The **Poland sequence** of unilateral absence of the sternal head of the pectoralis major muscle and ipsilateral syndactyly and brachydactyly of the hand is thought to be caused by a vascular defect in the proximal subclavian artery prior to 6 weeks' gestation (Bouwes Bavinck and Weaver, 1986). **Möbius syndrome** of unilateral or bilateral palsies of the 6th and 7th cranial nerves may be similarly caused by an interruption of the basilar artery. The infant in Figure 21–10 had a severe vascular disruption that caused many left-sided defects, such as cleft lip, dysplastic ear, facial palsy, severe hypoplasia of the arm, vertebral anomalies, absent lung, and a complex cardiac defect with left-sided hypoplastic heart.

Other defects believed to have a vascular cause include porencephalic cyst, hydranencephaly, hemifacial microsomia (hypoplasia of the mandibular ramus and ear), sirenomelia, **DiGeorge syndrome,** and **Klippel-Feil anomaly** (segmentation defects of the cervical spine). The increase in the number of congenital anomalies in monozygotic twins has been attributed in part to their shared placenta and co-mingled blood supply.

■ MALFORMATIONS

The existence of thousands of multiple malformation syndromes can make finding the correct diagnosis extremely difficult. It is best to search through the differential diagnosis of the rarest malformations first. If the baby has an unusual anomaly, e.g., duplicated thumbs, and a more common one, e.g., postaxial polydactyly of the hand, the differential diagnosis is substantially smaller for the unusual anomaly than for the common one. The rarer the malformation, the more useful or discriminating it is in leading the physician to the diagnosis. Some anomalies such as single transverse palmar crease, low-set ears, clinodactyly, and epicanthal folds are encountered so frequently that they are of limited use in establishing a diagnosis.

The computer has made it possible to search quickly for similar cases reported in the medical literature by using different combinations of the various anomalies to aid in the search. The London Dysmorphology Database (Oxford University Press) is a software package that includes information and references on hundreds of rare dysmorphic syndromes (Winter et al., 1984). In addition, such databases maintain registries of "unknowns"—those unreported cases without a known diagnosis.

The multiple malformation syndromes discussed in this section are grouped by their rarest or most prominent malformation. It should be kept in mind when considering a potential diagnosis that individual cases of a given syndrome will vary, and a typical or expected anomaly need not be present in every instance.

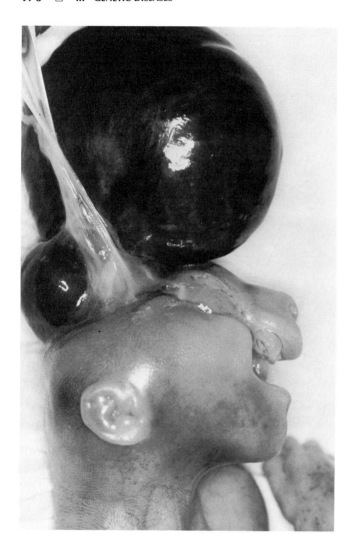

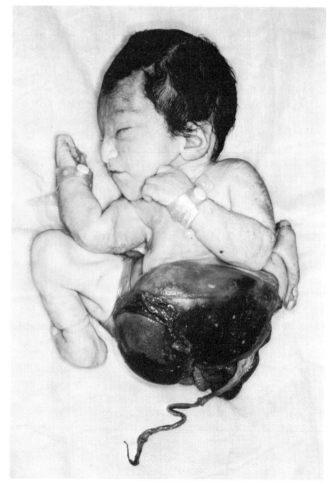

FIGURE 21–8. This stillborn infant with early amnion disruption sequence has an abnormal attachment of amnion to the head. There are bilateral oblique facial clefts (note that the nares are intact unlike the typical bilateral cleft lip) and a large neural tube defect.

FIGURE 21–9. The limb-body wall defect, one form of the early amnion disruption sequence, is illustrated in this infant with flat facies, a ventral wall defect, a hypoplastic leg, and an amniotic membrane surrounding the right leg. Constriction rings are evident above the right ankle.

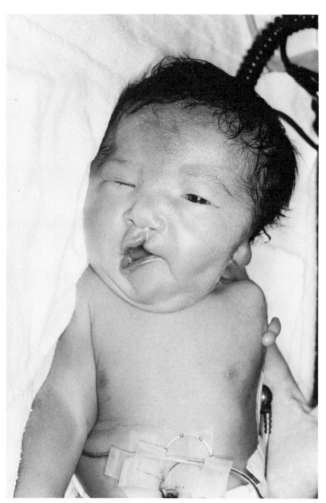

FIGURE 21–10. *There are many left-sided defects, such as cleft lip, dysplastic ear, facial nerve paralysis, missing arm, absent lung and hypoplastic left heart, that are consistent with a vascular disruption sequence.*

CENTRAL NERVOUS SYSTEM MALFORMATIONS

Hydrocephalus is frequently associated with spina bifida, but when isolated, it occurs in about 1 in 1700 live births. It is usually a sporadic event with a low recurrence risk of 1 to 2 per cent. One-third of cases are due to aqueductal stenosis. Autosomal recessive inheritance is rare, but an X-linked recessive form makes up about 2 per cent of all cases and 7 to 27 per cent of cases in males. This X-linked condition is associated with aqueductal stenosis; hypoplasia or absence of the pyramids; hypoplastic, flexed, adducted thumbs; spasticity; and mental retardation (Halliday et al., 1986). Without a positive family history, it is very difficult to make the diagnosis of X-linked hydrocephalus in a male with aqueductal stenosis. In this circumstance, the recurrence risk is about 6 per cent for all sibs but 12 per cent for male sibs (Burton, 1979).

Hydrocephalus also occurs in the autosomal recessive **hydrolethalus syndrome** named for the association of hydrocephalus, polyhydramnios, and lethality. A variety of CNS defects include aqueductal stenosis, cerebellar hypoplasia, agenesis of the corpus callosum, holoprosencephaly, and Dandy-Walker malformation. The eyes are

small, and there may be clefts of the lip or palate and polydactyly of the hands and feet (Aughton and Cassidy, 1987).

A posterior encephalocele is an important finding in several syndromes. **Meckel syndrome** is a lethal autosomal recessive condition with occipital encephalocele, cystic dysplasia of the kidneys, fibrosis of the liver, and postaxial polydactyly. Cleft lip and palate, microphthalmia, and other brain malformations such as hydrocephalus, holoprosencephaly, and anencephaly may occur (Salonen, 1984). There have been several reports in which the only cranial abnormality was hydrocephalus. Meckel syndrome can be misdiagnosed as a simple neural tube defect, or it can be confused with trisomy 13; therefore, a renal ultrasound and chromosome analysis are recommended.

Walker-Warburg syndrome is a lethal autosomal recessive disorder that is known by several names: **HARD ± E** (*h*ydrocephalus-*a*gyria-*r*etinal *d*ysplasia-*e*ncephalocele) and **COMS** (*c*erebro-*o*cular-*m*uscular dystrophy-*s*yndrome). The syndrome includes hydrocephalus, agyria, macrogyria, polygyria, absent midline CNS structures, cerebellar malformation with hypoplastic vermis, and posterior encephaloceles. The eye anomalies include microphthalmia, colobomas, persistent hyperplastic primary vitreous, and retinal detachment and dysplasia. There is hypotonia with elevation of serum creatine kinase and myopathic changes on electromyography (Dobyns et al., 1989).

CRANIAL MALFORMATIONS

Craniosynostosis, the premature fusion of one or more cranial sutures, occurs as a single anomaly or infrequently as a part of a multiple malformation syndrome. Cohen (1986) has extensively reviewed this subject in a monograph. The frequency is estimated to be 1 in 2500 live births (Hunter and Rudd, 1976). The infant's head shape depends on which sutures are closed (Table 21–3).

Kleeblattschädel is a severe form of craniosynostosis in which multiple fused sutures produce a cloverleaf configuration (Fig. 21–11). Many syndromes (chromosomal, monogenic, and sporadic) and disruptions are associated with kleeblattschädel (Cohen, 1988). **Thanatophoric dysplasia** accounts for 40 per cent of all cases of Kleeblattschädel, and **Pfeiffer syndrome** accounts for another 20 per cent.

TABLE 21–3. Head Shapes Resulting From Cranial Suture Synostosis

SUTURE	SHAPE	DESCRIPTION
Sagittal	Scaphocephaly	Long, narrow cranium with prominent forehead and occiput
Coronal (bilateral)	Brachycephaly	Short, wide cranium; may be tall
Coronal (unilateral)	Plagiocephaly	Asymmetric skull with flattening of half of the forehead and contralateral flattening of the occiput. Asymmetry of orbits and ears
Metopic	Trigonocephaly	Pointed, prominent forehead

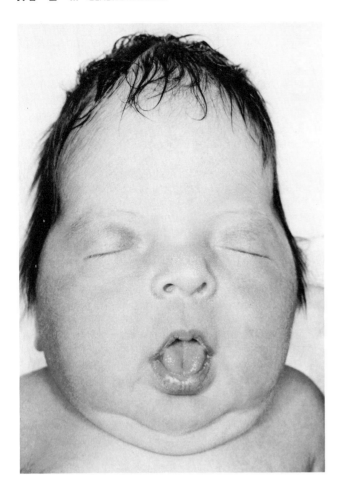

FIGURE 21–11. *This newborn girl with craniosynostosis has kleeblatt-schädel, or cloverleaf skull. In more severe cases, the orbits can be very shallow, causing protrusion of the eyes.*

Simple sagittal suture synostosis (involving one suture only) is the most common type of craniosynostosis and comprises over 50 per cent of simple synostosis. Coronal synostosis is the next most common type of craniosynostosis, occurring in about 25 per cent of cases. Males are more commonly affected in sagittal suture synostosis, whereas females are more frequently affected in coronal suture synostosis. About 2 per cent of cases of simple sagittal craniosynostosis and 8 per cent of cases of simple coronal craniosynostosis are familial.

Over 50 syndromes have been described in which craniosynostosis is a feature (Cohen, 1986). Table 21–4 lists some of the more common syndromes. These should not be strictly classified by which sutures are involved because synostosis is not specific to any suture in any syndrome.

Mental retardation has been reported in all of the craniosynostoses; however, the true frequency is not known. The risk for mental retardation may increase as more sutures are involved and the occurrence of increased intracranial pressure increases. In synostosis of a single suture, the rate of mental retardation is low (2 to 5 per cent) (Shillito and Matson, 1968). Early surgical intervention may reduce the risk of mental retardaton.

Evaluation of the newborn with an abnormal cranial shape includes palpation for sutural ridging and skull x-ray studies. A prenatal history of uterine constraint suggests deformation rather than synostosis; however, synostosis may result from prolonged constraint. Family members must be examined for similar anomalies. The craniofacial region should be examined for other abnormalities such as midface hypoplasia, prominent eyes, and palatal defects. Extracranial skeletal defects, especially of the hands and feet, should be sought. A complete neurologic and neurosurgical evaluation is indicated. Early surgical intervention is recommended to improve cranial contours and to allow more normal growth of the brain and cranium.

CLEIDOCRANIAL DYSPLASIA

Cleidocranial dysplasia is an autosomal dominant disorder noted for defects of the skull, clavicles, and teeth (Forland, 1962). Multiple other skeletal defects that are not limited to membranous bones can occur in the syndrome. Defects of the clavicles may be asymmetric and range from complete absence to lateral hypoplasia. With the more severe defects, the shoulders may be approximated at the midline. At birth, extremely large fontanels are present. Closure is delayed, and occasionally, a protective helmet has been required. Wormian bones are present on radiographs. Dental anomalies may present the most significant problem for these patients in childhood. Two-thirds of cases are familial, and family members should be examined when the condition is suspected. Cesarean section is required in about 35 per cent of affected women owing to the small diameter of the pelvic outlet.

TABLE 21–4. Syndromes Containing Craniosynostosis

SYNDROME	CRANIOFACIAL DEFECTS	OTHER DEFECTS	INHERITANCE
Crouzon	Brachycephaly, midface hypoplasia with relative prognathism, high narrow palate, shallow orbits, proptosis, conductive hearing loss	Cervical vertebral fusion Stiffness of elbows	Autosomal dominant
Apert	Tall, brachycephalic skull, large anterior fontanel, midface hypoplasia, beaked nose, high, narrow palate with thick alveolar ridges, cleft palate, conductive hearing loss, hydrocephalus	Cutaneous and bony syndactyly of digits 2, 3, and 4 of hands and feet; cardiovascular defects 9% Infrequent: T E fistula, esophageal atresia, pyloric stenosis	Autosomal dominant, typically occurs as a new mutation
Pfeiffer	Tall, brachycephalic skull, kleeblattschädel, hypoplasia, ocular hypertelorism, down-slanting palpebral fissures, beaked nose, high-arched palate, hydrocephalus, choanal atresia	Broad thumbs and great toes Infrequent: Pyloric stenosis, malpositioned anus Patients with cloverleaf skull have poor prognosis, even with craniofacial surgery	Autosomal dominant
Saethre-Chotzen	Brachycephaly, plagiocephaly, low frontal hairline, ptosis, prominent ear crus, mild hearing loss	Partial cutaneous syndactyly Infrequent: Congenital heart defects, renal anomalies, cryptorchidism	Autosomal dominant
Carpenter	Sagittal and lambdoid synostosis, dystopia canthorum, mental deficiency but normal intelligence has also been reported	Brachydactyly, cutaneous syndactyly, postaxial polydactyly (hands), preaxial polydactyly (feet), congenital heart defects in 33 per cent Infrequent: cryptorchidism, hydronephrosis, accessory spleens	Autosomal recessive
Greig cephalopolysyndactyly	Scaphocephaly, craniosynostosis in 5 per cent, frontal bossing, hypertelorism	Broad thumbs and great toes, cutaneous syndactyly, pre- and postaxial polydactyly	Autosomal dominant
Antley-Bixler	Brachycephalic, trapezoidal head shape, dysplastic ears, choanal atresia, depressed nasal bridge	Arachnodactyly, radiohumeral synostosis, joint contractures Infrequent: Congenital heart defect, renal anomalies, genital anomalies, imperforate anus, vertebral anomalies	Autosomal recessive
Craniofrontonasal dysplasia	Coronal synostosis, frontonasal dysplasia (bifid nasal tip, hypertelorism, widow's peak)	Mild cutaneous syndactyly, grooved nails, broad thumbs, scoliosis, sloping shoulders	X-linked versus autosomal dominant
Thanatophoric dysplasia	Kleeblattschädel, depressed nasal bridge, midface retrusion	Disproportionate short stature with very short limbs and narrow thorax. Lethal in neonatal period	Sporadic, probably a dominant trait seen only as a new mutation

NATAL TEETH

Natal teeth are teeth that are erupted at birth or that erupt in the first month of life. Bodenhoff and Gorlin (1963) have extensively (and charmingly) reviewed the folklore and facts on this subject. The incidence of natal teeth is about 1 in 2000; however, the estimates of incidence vary widely. Natal teeth may be part of the normal complement of primary (deciduous) teeth or they may be supernumerary, which must be determined radiographically. The most common natal teeth are the mandibular central incisors. Natal teeth may be mobile because the roots are not completely formed. However, about 70 per cent of natal teeth are firmly fixed. When the teeth are mobile, extraction may be necessary because of the risk of aspiration. Supernumerary teeth should be extracted.

The cause of natal teeth is unknown. About 15 per cent of cases are familial. Infrequently, natal teeth are associated with several syndromes, including chondroectodermal dysplasia or **Ellis–van Creveld syndrome, Hallermann-Streiff syndrome,** and pachyonychia congenita.

CLEFT LIP WITH OR WITHOUT CLEFT PALATE

Cleft lip with or without cleft palate occurs in approximately 1 in 700 to 1000 live births. Cleft lip may be only a small notch on one side of the lip or a complete opening into the floor of the nasal cavity. Clefts are most frequent on the left side but may be bilateral and involve the alveolar ridge. The great majority occur as isolated malformations with a multifactorial cause that includes both genetic and environmental factors and a 3 to 5 per cent recurrence risk. Cardiac defects are common, occurring in about 7 per cent of those with oral clefts (Geis et al., 1981). Growth hormone deficiency is encountered in 4 per cent of children with oral clefts (Rudman et al., 1978). On the whole, 7 to 13 per cent of those with isolated cleft lip and 2 to 11 per cent of those with cleft lip and palate have other congenital anomalies (Gorlin et al., 1990). Only 1 per cent of cleft lip and cleft palate cases are associated with multiple malformation syndromes (Bixler, 1981), although there are over 150 such syndromes (Cohen, 1978).

The surgical repair of cleft lip usually should be performed when the infant weighs 10 lbs, is 10 weeks old, and has a hemoglobin of 10 grams (the rule of 10s). Feeding can be a problem if the baby cannot create a seal on the nipple to generate negative pressure (see the section entitled Cleft Palate). Optimum therapy for cleft lip or cleft palate requires a multidisciplinary approach involving pediatrics, genetics, plastic surgery, otolaryngology, audiology, pediatric dentistry, orthodontics, prosthodontics, speech therapy, and social services.

Van der Woude syndrome of lower lip pits and oral clefts is an autosomal dominant trait with a frequency of 1 in 100,000 in the white population (Cervenka et al., 1967). The lip pits, which can be expressed as discrete protrusions, mounds, depressions, or dimples (Fig. 21–12), communicate with salivary glands and can ooze saliva. The syndrome can be expressed as any combination of lip pits, cleft lip, or cleft palate. Lip pits are also encountered in the **popliteal pterygium syndrome.** This autosomal dominant syndrome includes pterygia or webbing in the popliteal area, synechiae between upper and lower eyelids or the alveolar processes, an unusual pinched appearance at the base of the nail of the hallux, and cleft lip and cleft palate.

The **EEC syndrome** (Fig. 21–13) of ectrodactyly (split or cleft hands or feet), ectodermal dysplasia, and clefting, is an autosomal dominant trait. Renal anomalies are also frequently noted in this condition (Rollnick and Hoo, 1988).

Hypertelorism–hypospadias syndrome, also called the **Opitz, Opitz G, or BBB syndrome,** is an autosomal dominant condition that is more commonly recognized in males, although females can be mildly affected (Cappa et al., 1987). In addition to cleft lip with or without cleft palate, swallowing dysfunction can lead to severe feeding difficulties and aspiration in infancy. Anal anomalies have also been noted (Tolmie et al., 1987).

HMC syndrome, for *h*ypertelorism, *m*icrotia, and *c*lefting, also called Bixler syndrome, is a rare autosomal recessive trait (Bixler et al., 1969). Hearing loss, stenotic external auditory canals, and cardiac defects are also observed in this condition.

CLEFT PALATE

Cleft palate alone, which occurs less frequently than cleft lip and cleft palate at 1 in 2500 live births, is associated with multiple malformation syndromes in 8 per cent of cases. Isolated cleft palate is usually a multifactorial condition, although an X-linked form of cleft palate with ankyloglossia exists (Lowry, 1970; Moore et al., 1987).

Feeding the infant with cleft palate is made easier by using soft pliable premie (red) or orthodontic (Nuk) nipples with an enlarged cross-hatched opening. The long black lamb's nipple is too stiff, and by delivering the milk directly to the posterior pharynx, does not promote a normal suck. Soft bottles (evenflow bags [Playtex], and cleft lip and cleft palate nurser [Mead Johnson]) can be squeezed gently to help deliver milk. Infant feeding obturators can be made by pedodontists or orthodontists to prevent collapse of the palatal segments when the alveolar ridge

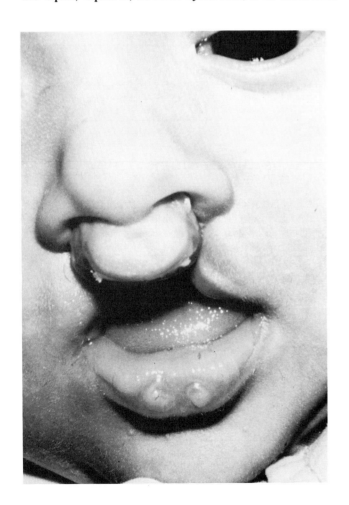

FIGURE 21–12. *This infant with van der Woude syndrome has a bilateral cleft lip and two fistulas, also called pits, in the lower lip. Note that all midline structures are present.*

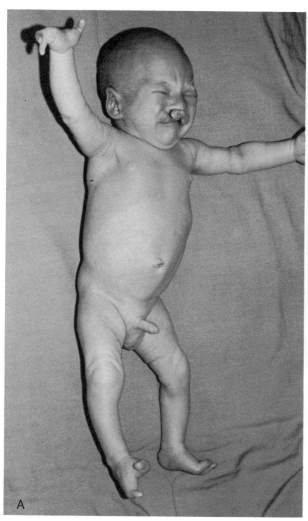

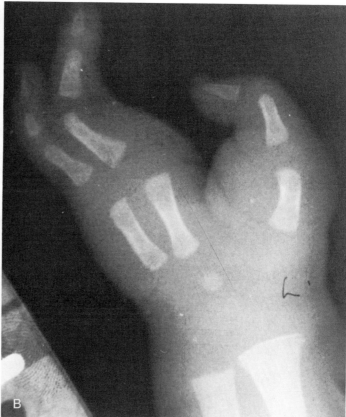

FIGURE 21–13. A, This infant with ectrodactyly (split or cleft hands and feet), bilateral cleft lip and palate, and scant hair has the EEC or ectrodactyly-ectodermal dysplasia-clefting syndrome. B, The radiograph shows the absent middle rays.

is also cleft. Breast-feeding is sometimes possible with lactation aids (Lactaid) and a motivated mother. Feeding in a vertical position helps minimize nasal regurgitation. Surgical repair usually is performed between 12 and 24 months. Because of frequent ear infections, hearing loss, speech problems, dental malocclusion, and psychosocial factors, a multidisciplinary craniofacial team approach is recommended from birth.

Cleft palate is frequently associated with micrognathia or mandibular hypoplasia in what is known as the **Pierre Robin sequence.** This is not a diagnostic entity, and can be seen in several syndromes, especially **Stickler syndrome.** Also known as autosomal dominant arthro-ophthalmopathy, **Stickler syndrome** can be difficult to diagnose at birth. In addition to cleft palate and micrognathia, there are prominent eyes, myopia, deafness, flat face, hypotonia, and prominent joints. Changes resulting from spondyloepiphyseal dysplasia are more apparent later in childhood (Stickler et al., 1965).

Intubation or tracheostomy may be required in **Pierre Robin sequence** if airway obstruction is sufficient to raise carbon dioxide tension with its associated hypoxia and pulmonary hypertension. Feeding can also be a major problem. Aspiration is a serious concern. The tongue can easily fall back and obstruct the airway, making a vertical feeding position helpful. Gavage feeding is sometimes

necessary, but it should be accompanied by the use of a pacifier for oral stimulation. In time, growth of the mandible occurs and breathing and feeding become easier.

Velo-cardio-facial syndrome, an autosomal dominant trait, should be considered when cleft palate and heart defects, especially ventricular septal defect, occur together. Neonatal hypocalcemia occurs in 13 per cent of patients. The fingers are slender and tapering. The nose is prominent and tubular. Microcephaly and eye abnormalities may also occur (Williams et al., 1985).

Smith-Lemli-Opitz syndrome, a rare and frequently lethal autosomal recessive condition, should be considered when cleft palate occurs with the ambiguous genitalia seen in affected males (Fig. 21–14). Intrauterine growth retardation, microcephaly, hypoplastic thumbs, soft tissue syndactyly of the second and third toes, postaxial polydactyly, pyloric stenosis, and cardiac defects are common. The face has an unusual appearance with epicanthal folds, prominent nasal bridge, thick alae nasi, and small chin.

Cleft palate occurs in the **cervico-oculo-acoustic,** or **Wildervanck, syndrome,** a triad of Klippel-Feil anomaly (fused cervical vertebrae), congenital sensorineural deafness, and Duane anomaly (abducens palsy with retractio bulbi). Renal anomalies may also be present. The condition is found almost exclusively in females, but the pattern of inheritance remains unresolved.

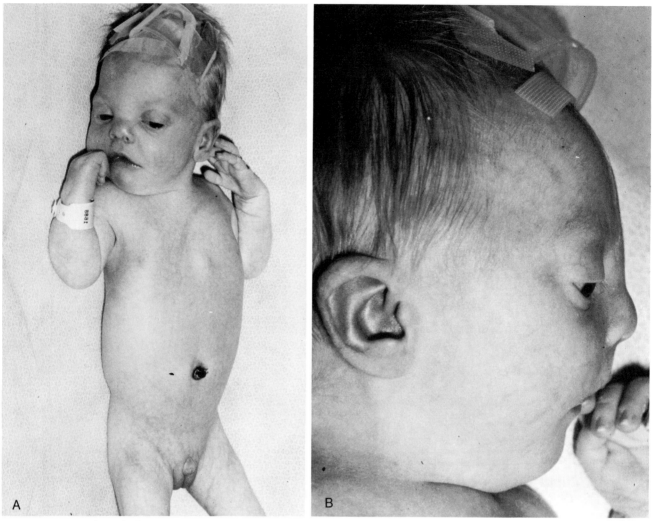

FIGURE 21–14. A, This male (karyotype 46,XY) with Smith-Lemli-Opitz syndrome has ambiguous genitalia, cleft palate, and unusual facies. B, The profile is noteworthy for the small chin and the continuous line from the forehead to the nose without the normal angle at the nasal bridge.

Otopalatodigital syndrome type I, an X-linked condition, includes mental retardation, cleft palate, conductive deafness, and a short nose with a broad nasal bridge and hypertelorism, giving the infant a pugilistic appearance. The feet are striking, with a short bulbous hallux and widely spaced toes. The toes have been compared with those of a tree frog. All patients are below the 10th percentile for height (Dudding, et al., 1967).

ATYPICAL CRANIOFACIAL CLEFTS

Typical oral clefts of the lip and palate must be distinguished from the more unusual midline, oblique, or horizontal facial clefts that are associated with unique patterns of malformations (Kawamoto, 1976).

Midline cleft lip is generally of two types: those with complete absence of the premaxilla (Fig 21–15) and those with a midline notch in the upper lip (Fig. 21–16). In premaxillary agenesis, the nasal septum, columella, philtrum, and premaxillary process may be missing or hypoplastic. Because this condition is part of the **holoprosencephaly sequence,** a CT or magnetic resonance imaging (MRI) scan of the head and chromosome analysis should be performed in every case. Premaxillary agenesis is often

incorrectly described as a bilateral cleft lip, which can be misleading because the differential diagnosis, recurrence risk, and prognosis for the two conditions are completely different.

The second type of midline cleft lip is due to failure of fusion of the medial nasal processes that make up the philtrum. The upper lip can be notched, or a true cleft can extend beyond the vermillion border. These clefts are typical of the **oral-facial-digital syndrome** (see Fig. 21–16), which also includes lobulated or bifid tongue, thick oral frenulas, cleft palate, brachydactyly, syndactyly, and polydactyly, especially of the hallux. There are two main types: oral-facial-digital syndrome type I seems to be an X-linked dominant trait and is only seen in females; Mohr syndrome, or oral-facial-digital syndrome type II, is an autosomal recessive trait (Rimoin and Edgerton, 1967).

Oblique facial clefts usually have no relationship to the embryology of the face and typically represent disruptions, often from amniotic bands. The clefts can extend into the orbit, causing anophthalmia, and beyond, disrupting the supraorbital ridge and eyebrow (see Fig. 21–8).

Horizontal clefts through the mouth, causing macrostomia, may be bilateral or unilateral. They are frequently associated with the facial and preauricular tags, mandib-

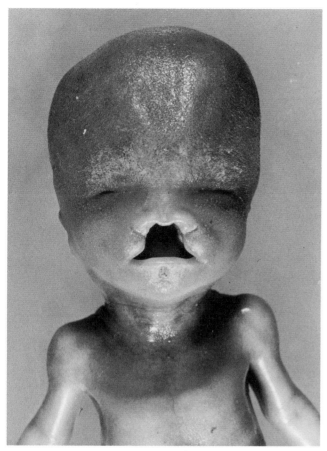

FIGURE 21–15. This infant with the hydrolethalus syndrome has microphthalmia and premaxillary agenesis. The complete absence of the columella, philtrum, and primary palate makes holoprosencephaly more likely. Premaxillary agenesis should not be described as a bilateral cleft lip (see Fig. 21–12).

ular hypoplasia, and ear anomalies of **Goldenhar syndrome.**

EAR ANOMALIES

Anomalies of the external ear are relatively common. In the study by Melnick and Marianthopoulos (1979), external ear malformations, and branchial sinuses and tags together had an incidence of about 1 in 90 births. Malformations of the pinna occurred in about 1 in 670 births, and about 80 per cent of these malformations were

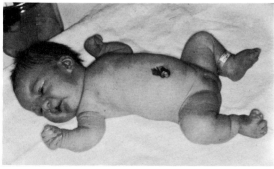

FIGURE 21–16. The oral-facial-digital syndrome type II (Mohr syndrome) is present in this girl with a midline cleft lip and preaxial polydactyly of the feet.

isolated defects. About 1 in 200 infants with a preauricular pit will have severe hearing loss (Fraser et al., 1980). It is recommended that all patients with minor ear anomalies be evaluated for hearing loss (Aase, 1980).

Numerous syndromes have ear anomalies as a feature. **Hemifacial microsomia (first and second branchial arch syndrome, Goldenhar syndrome, oculo-auriculo-vertebral dysplasia)** consists of microtia with preauricular tags, and hypoplasia and aplasia of the mandibular ramus and condyle. In addition, other facial anomalies include microphthalmia, epibulbar dermoids, and macrostomia (Fig. 21–17). Defects are not limited to the facial region, and vertebral and other skeletal anomalies, cardiac defects, and renal malformations also are seen. The facial defects may be bilateral but are asymmetric. The incidence is estimated at 1 in 3500 to 5600 live births (Grabb, 1965; Poswillo, 1974). There is a slight predilection for males, and the anomalies usually occur on the left side. In the classic type of hemifacial microsomia defined by Tenconi and Hall (1983) as unilateral involvement without eye anomalies, the risk for vertebral, cardiac, and renal defects was 3 to 6 per cent. However, in the **Goldenhar syndrome** (defined by the presence of epibulbar dermoids), vertebral defects occurred in 40 per cent of patients, cardiac defects occurred in 10 per cent, and none of the 10 patients studied had renal defects. The cause is unknown; however, vascular disruptions have been proposed as one cause (Poswillo, 1974). Hemifacial microsomia has a low recurrence risk and may represent more than one disorder.

Treacher Collins syndrome (mandibulofacial dysostosis) is a well-described autosomal dominant syndrome with a wide variability of expression. As opposed to hemifacial microsomia, it is a bilaterally symmetric disorder. Down-slanting palpebral fissures, lower lid colobomas with absence of lower lashes, malar hypoplasia and aplasia, anomalous external ears, and mandibular hypoplasia with a large antegonial notch produce a characteristic facial appearance (Fig. 21–18). Conductive deafness occurs in about 40 per cent of patients (Jones, 1988). In infancy, respiratory difficulty may occur as a result of the retrusive mandible, which requires a tracheostomy. Cleft palate is present in about 30 per cent of patients (Gorlin et al., 1990). Congenital heart defects are an occasional finding. Two disorders with similar facial anomalies have, in addition, limb anomalies. In **Miller syndrome,** there are postaxial (ulnar ray) limb reduction defects (Miller et al., 1979), whereas in **Nager acrofacial dysostosis** (Halal et al., 1983), the limb deficiencies are preaxial (radial ray). Autosomal recessive inheritance has been proposed for Miller syndrome, and both autosomal dominant and recessive inheritance have been proposed for Nager acrofacial dysostosis.

Microtia in association with hypertelorism and facial clefting **(HMC syndrome)** is an autosomal recessive syndrome (Bixler et al., 1969). Cardiac and renal anomalies were reported in the original cases. **Branchio-oto-renal syndrome** is an autosomal dominant syndrome with ear anomalies, preauricular pits, branchial cleft sinuses, deafness (conductive, sensorineural, or mixed), and renal anomalies (Melnick, et al., 1978). Branchio-oto-dysplasia is now thought to represent a variation of the same disorder (Heimler and Leiber, 1986). About 2.5 per cent

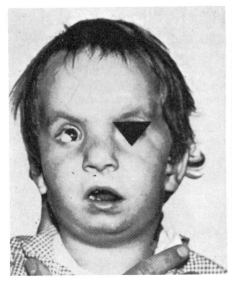
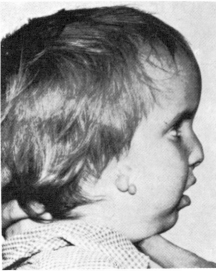

FIGURE 21–17. A, *Hemifacial microsomia (Goldenhar syndrome) with bilateral involvement in a young boy. An epibulbar dermoid is present in the temporal area of the right eye. There is slight macrostomia on the left. B, The patient's right ear is severely malformed and only rudimentary tags are present. (From Gorlin, R.J., et al.: J. Pediatr. 63:991, 1963.)*

of children with profound hearing loss have branchio-oto-renal syndrome (Fraser et al., 1980). It is recommended that audiologic and renal studies be done in all patients with familial branchial arch malformations.

CHARGE syndrome includes *c*oloboma, *h*eart defect, *a*tresia choanae, *r*etarded growth and/or development, *g*enital anomalies, and *e*ar anomalies. Other malformations include CNS anomalies, tracheoesophageal fistula, renal anomalies, cleft lip and cleft palate, micrognathia, and omphalocele (Pagon et al., 1981). The external ear anomalies are distinct. The ears are short, wide, and cupped with more intact superior structures and hypoplastic or missing antihelix, antitragus, and lobule (Davenport et al., 1986).

ANOMALIES OF THE NECK

Anomalous developments of the branchial arches may become manifest in a great variety of forms. The most obvious of these are (1) skin tags, (2) pits, (3) fistulas, and (4) cysts. They are located for the most part in two sites, the preauricular region and anywhere along the anterior border of the sternocleidomastoid muscle, from mastoid to manubrium.

Skin tags should be removed for cosmetic reasons. Pits may be ignored. Fistulas may discharge mucoid or purulent material; they may penetrate deep in the neck to terminate near the pharynx and rarely may open into the pharynx. Cysts usually lie at the angle of the mandible but may be found low, just above the clavicle. Fistulas should be removed by careful, thorough dissection. Cysts should be extirpated early because they are prone to infection.

Branchial cysts (also called branchiogenic, lateral cervical, or cervical thymic cysts) arise in the embryo from either the branchial groove, the thymic stalk, or the pharyngeal pouch. They may be present at birth or may appear suddenly at any age. They lie beneath the sternomastoid muscle, but their anterior edge may bulge out from the muscle's anterior margin. They demonstrate a strong tendency to become infected and pus-filled.

KLIPPEL-FEIL ANOMALY

Klippel-Feil anomaly consists of cervical vertebral segmentation defects, often described as "fusion," which may result in a short, webbed neck, limitation of head movement, and a low posterior hairline. Although recognized for centuries, the anomaly derived its eponym from the report by Klippel and Feil in 1912. Four subtypes have

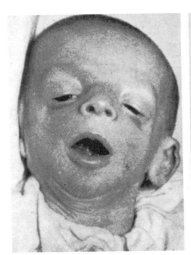
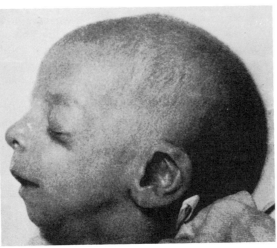

FIGURE 21–18. A, *Treacher Collins syndrome is evident from the down-slanting palpebral fissures and malar hypoplasia. Note the notch in the right lower lid. B, Mandibular hypoplasia and mild external ear dysmorphism are evident. (From McKenzie and Craig: Arch. Dis. Child. 30:391, 1955.)*

been described, which vary in severity and location of defects (Raas-Rothschild et al., 1988). The etiology is heterogeneous. Most cases are sporadic; however, familial occurrences, both autosomal dominant and recessive, have been reported. Mild manifestations are evident in 7 of 1000 newborns, whereas the severe expression of this condition is seen in 3 of 100,000 births.

Klippel-Feil anomaly may occur in isolation or with other defects including strabismus, sensorineural and/or conductive hearing loss, cleft palate, congenital heart defects, and various neurologic abnormalities with occasional mental retardation (Gorlin et al., 1990). Two syndromes should be considered in the differential diagnosis. **Rokitansky-Küster-Hauser syndrome,** also known as **MURCS** association, includes *müllerian duct aplasia, renal aplasia,* and *cervicothoracic somite dysplasia.* **Wildervanck syndrome** of cervical anomalies, deafness, and Duane anomaly is typically seen only in females.

LIMB ANOMALIES

The extremities, especially the hands, display a wide variety of malformations, such as oligodactyly, polydactyly, brachydactyly, and syndactyly, that may occur in isolation or as part of syndromes (Temtamy and McKusick, 1978). Deformations of the limbs, of course, may also occur (see the section entitled Clubfoot).

Oligodactyly (missing digits) and transverse terminal defects are seen in the early amnion disruption sequence, the previously mentioned **EEC syndrome,** and several other syndromes. The **hypoglossia-hypodactyly,** or **aglossia-adactyly, syndrome** consists of a small or absent tongue and a variety of limb defects. Glossopalatine ankylosis is a rare finding (Fig. 21–19). Hypoglossia-hypodactyly can also be seen with the cranial nerve deficiencies (VI and VII) of **Möbius syndrome.** These two sporadic conditions may have a similar cause.

Scalp defect–ectrodactyly syndrome, or **Adams-Oliver syndrome,** is also associated with often asymmetric transverse terminal defects of the hands and feet (Sybert, 1985). The aplasia cutis of the scalp may overlie a bony defect (Fig. 21–20). This autosomal dominant trait is highly variable and may be nonpenetrant. The scalp and extremities of the parents should be examined carefully for small scarred areas at the vertex or minimal digital hypoplasia. Oligodactyly is also seen frequently in the sporadic **Cornelia de Lange,** or **Brachmann–de Lange,** syndrome (Fig. 21–21), with prenatal growth deficiency, hirsutism, mental retardation and characteristic facies, including synophrys, short anteverted nose, thin downturned upper lip, and prominent philtrum (Hawley et al., 1985).

Hypoplasia of the thumbs can be associated with defects of the radius as in the autosomal recessive **thrombocytopenia–absent radius syndrome.** In this condition, the ulna may be absent and other skeletal anomalies are common. The thrombocytopenia is transient and only present in infancy. Cardiac anomalies are seen in one-third of cases. The thumbs are always present in contrast to **Fanconi pancytopenia syndrome** in which they may

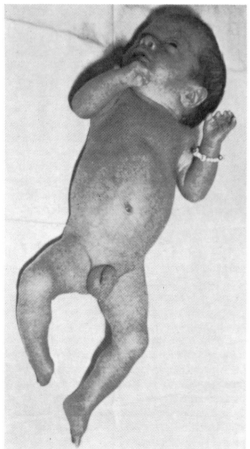

A

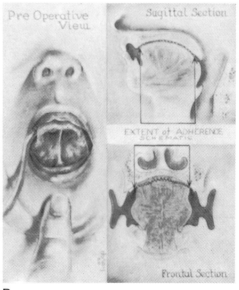

B

FIGURE 21–19. *A, This infant has the transverse terminal limb defects of the hypoglossia-hypodactylia syndrome. B, Instead of the more common hypoglossia, there is glossopalatine ankylosis. (From Wilson, R.A., et al.: Pediatrics 31:1051, 1963. Reproduced by permission of Pediatrics.)*

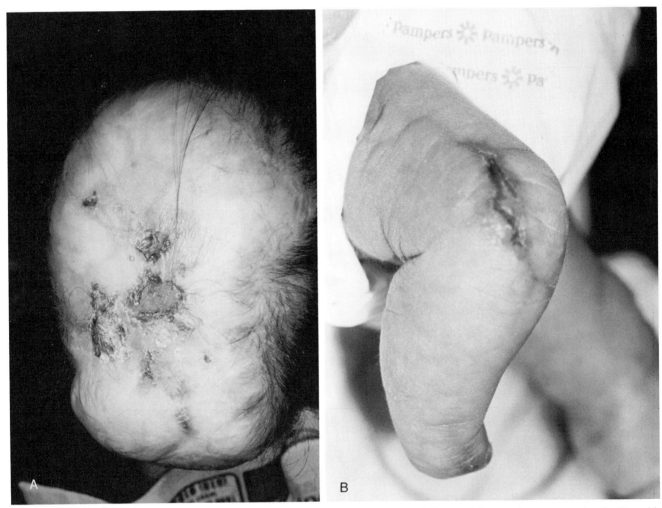

FIGURE 21–20. A, This child with scalp defect–ectrodactyly syndrome has a large area of alopecia following the near-complete healing of her scalp defect. The underlying bony defect is also almost totally resolved. B, There is a transverse terminal defect at the ankle and aplasia cutis at the knee.

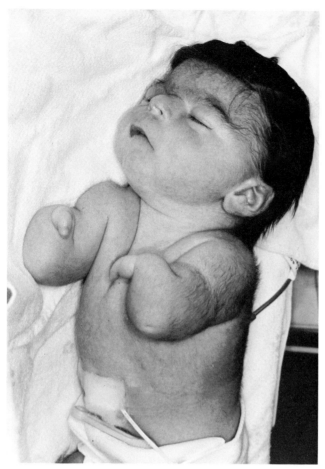

FIGURE 21–21. This infant with Cornelia de Lange syndrome has a thin, down-turned upper lip with a long, prominent philtrum. The infant is hirsute, with short forearms and monodactyly.

be absent. This autosomal recessive disorder consists of short stature of prenatal onset, hyperpigmentation, and multiple malformations, including mainly renal, genital, and radial defects. There is an increased risk for leukemia and other cancers. Pancytopenia is not present in infancy but occurs at about 8 years of age. Cytogenetic abnormalities consist of an increased number of chromatid breaks and gaps and hypersensitivity to mitomycin C.

Holt-Oram syndrome is an autosomal dominant disorder of the thumb and includes radial defects and various cardiac anomalies, usually an atrial septal defect. The typical hand malformation is a triphalangeal thumb, but any degree of absent or rudimentary thumb can be seen. The upper limbs can be variably affected, with phocomelia in the severe cases. Some patients also exhibit a defect in ocular adduction (Duane anomaly).

Robert syndrome is a frequently lethal, autosomal recessive cause of limb reduction, varying from radial hypoplasia to phocomelia of all four extremities. Commonly, there is cleft lip and palate, severe prenatal growth deficiency, and mental retardation. In about one-half of cases, cytogenetic findings are unusual: there is premature centromeric separation of sister chromatids.

Goltz syndrome, or **focal dermal hypoplasia** (Fig. 21–22), is primarily a disorder of the skin, eyes, and digits. Focal areas of fatty herniation or indentations occur because of skin atrophy. Streaks of hypopigmentation or

hyperpigmentation, microphthalmia, iris coloboma, and syndactyly of the middle and ring fingers are common. Many other digital anomalies may be present, such as polydactyly, ectrodactyly, and hypoplasia. This condition is present almost exclusively in females and may represent an X-linked dominant trait with lethality in males.

Postaxial (ulnar ray) polydactyly is frequently encountered as an isolated malformation in blacks (3.6 in 1000 infants) that is inherited as an autosomal dominant trait. This type of polydactyly is also seen in some bone dysplasias, such as **Ellis–van Creveld syndrome, short rib polydactyly,** and **asphyxiating thoracic dystrophy.** Postaxial polydactyly is seen in the previously discussed **Meckel syndrome** and in **Mohr syndrome (oral-facial-digital syndrome** type II, see Fig. 21–16). It is common in the **Laurence-Moon-Bardet-Biedl syndrome** along with obesity, hypogenitalism, retinitis pigmentosa, and mental retardation. This autosomal recessive trait produces a high rate of cardiovascular and renal anomalies and dysfunction.

Preaxial polydactyly or bifid thumb is much rarer (8 in 100,000 infants) than postaxial polydactyly. In its mildest form, it becomes manifest as a broad distal phalanx. Very broad and deviated thumbs are seen in the **Pfeiffer acrocephalo-syndactyly syndrome** of craniosynostosis and soft-tissue syndactyly. The previously discussed **oto-palatodigital syndrome** also includes broad thumbs. **Rubinstein-Taybi syndrome,** which is exhibited by broad thumbs, beaked nose, down-slanting palpebral fissures and mental subnormality, is a sporadic condition.

HEMIHYPERTROPHY

In hemihypertrophy, which is more appropriately described as hemihyperplasia, typically some or all structures on one side of the body are larger in circumference and/or length. The cause of hemihypertrophy is heterogeneous. The majority of cases are sporadic and not part of a syndrome, but **Beckwith-Wiedemann syndrome** should be considered in the differential diagnosis. Various chromosome anomalies have also been noted infrequently. Other abnormalities reported in association with hemihypertrophy have been well summarized by Gorlin and associates (1990). Whether or not other associated findings are present, hemihypertrophy carries a significant risk for embryonal tumors, especially Wilms tumor, adrenal cortical carcinoma, hepatoblastoma, and others. Hoyme and associates (1987) determined that in isolated congenital hemihypertrophy, the chance of developing a tumor is 3.8 per cent. Tumors have occurred on the side contralateral to the hypertrophy, and they have been seen in cases in which hemihypertrophy was limited to the face. Gorlin and colleagues (1990) recommend that abdominal ultrasound examinations and alpha-fetoprotein tests should be performed every 6 months until age 4 and then less frequently until age 7.

Beckwith-Wiedemann syndrome of somatic gigantism, macroglossia, omphalocele, and posterior ear pits and creases is associated with hemihypertrophy in 13 per cent of cases. Hypoglycemia and polycythemia can be seen in the neonatal period. A chromosome anomaly, duplication of 11p15, has been described in several patients. The risk of embryonal tumors is 7.5 per cent in this

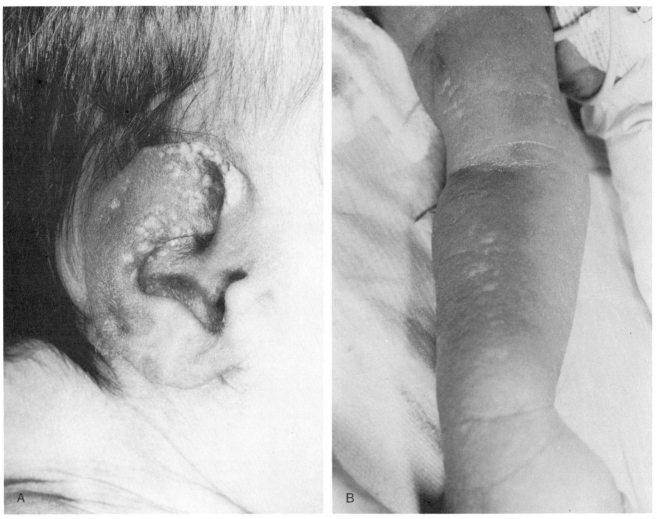

FIGURE 21–22. A, The speckled hypopigmentation in Goltz syndrome or focal dermal hypoplasia is evident in this ear with a "moth-eaten" appearance. B, The focal depressions and indentations are due to areas of skin hypoplasia, especially of the dermis.

syndrome. Tumors are not limited to those patients with Beckwith-Wiedemann syndrome who have hemihypertrophy, although the risk is probably greater in that group.

ARTHROGRYPOSIS

Multiple congenital contractures, or **arthrogryposis multiplex congenita,** which occur in 1 in 5000 to 10,000 births, has many causes. It should not be considered a diagnosis in itself but rather a clinical sign. Decreased movement in utero (fetal akinesia), whatever the cause, can lead to arthrogryposis. Over 70 nonchromosomal syndromes exhibit some degree of congenital contractures (Hall, 1983).

The evaluation of the infant with arthrogryposis should be directed at the four main causes of this condition: muscle, nerve (including CNS), or connective tissue abnormalities and mechanical forces that limit movement in utero (deformations). Laboratory data from electromyography, muscle biopsy, skeletal radiographs, imaging studies of the CNS, and chromosome analysis can be very helpful.

Therapy is directed at increasing mobilization and function of the joints. Soon after birth, passive range of motion exercises, splinting, and casting are usually recommended

by pediatric orthopedists and occupational therapists. Surgery is sometimes required to stabilize joints and release contractures. The worst prognosis occurs in those with concomittant CNS abnormalities. The best prognosis is associated with **autosomal dominant distal arthrogryposis** and in utero deformations.

In approximately one-third of infants with multiple congenital contractures, the muscles are replaced with fat and fibrous tissue in what is known as **amyoplasia.** This sporadic condition is characterized by rigidity of the joints, bilateral symmetric limb involvement, flat midline facial hemangiomas, and dimples at the elbows and knees. The distinctive posture of the arms—internally rotated at the shoulder, extended at the elbow, and flexed at the wrist (the so-called "policeman's tip" appearance)—is helpful in making the diagnosis. For unknown reasons, gastroschisis, amniotic band constrictions, and monozygotic twinning (with discordance for the contractures) are commonly associated with amyoplasia.

The **multiple pterygium syndrome** (Fig. 21–23), another cause of multiple congenital contractures, is usually an autosomal recessive condition, although autosomal dominant inheritance has been documented. This diagnosis may be difficult to make at birth because the characteristic webs, finger contractures, and facies become

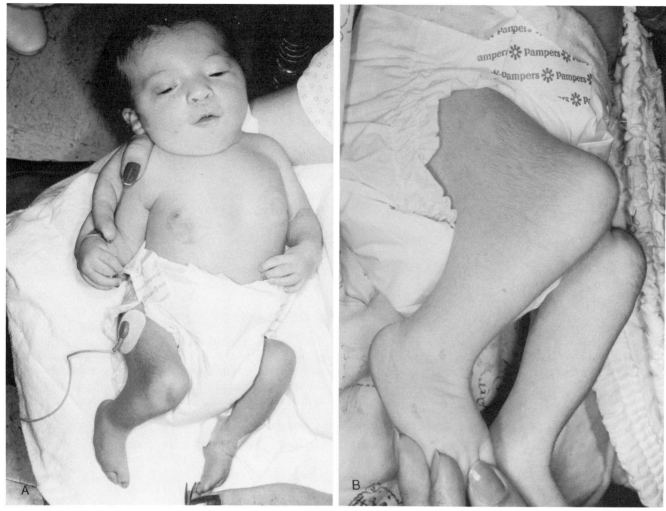

FIGURE 21–23. A, *This child with congenital contractures or arthrogryposis has the multiple pterygium syndrome. The neck is short, the chest is broad, the fingers are deviated radially, and the knees are webbed, as seen in detail in B.*

more pronounced with time (Thompson et al., 1987). At birth, the fingers are tightly fisted and later develop camptodactyly. The facial appearance that is typical of this syndrome exhibits micrognathia, posteriorly rotated, low-set ears, and down-slanting palpebral fissures with ptosis. Cleft palate occurs in approximately one-third of cases. Pterygia, or webs, which need not be present at birth, involve many areas, especially the lateral neck, elbows, and knees. The feet may have an equinovarus or rocker-bottom appearance. Scoliosis and kyphosis are common. Radiographs show frequent vertebral anomalies with failure to fuse posteriorly.

The **cerebro-oculo-facio-skeletal syndrome** is an autosomal recessive cause of congenital contractures and carries a poor prognosis. The infants with this condition are of normal birth weight but subsequently fail to grow or gain weight, with death usually occurring before age 5. Microcephaly and intracranial calcifications are useful signs. The palpebral fissures are short, with frequent cataracts or microphthalmia.

The **Pena-Shokeir syndrome,** which consists of multiple ankyloses, camptodactyly, short umbilical cord, pulmonary hypoplasia, oligohydramnios, and intrauterine growth retardation, probably includes many conditions that follow the common final pathway of fetal akinesia

(Hall, 1986). A specific recurrence risk is difficult to ascertain given the genetic heterogeneity of this condition; however, autosomal recessive inheritance was implicated in the original report of two affected sisters and many subsequent publications. The empiric risk is about 10 to 15 per cent.

DIAPHRAGMATIC HERNIA

A diaphragmatic hernia, when it occurs as an isolated malformation, is associated with a 1 to 2 per cent recurrence risk. However, other anomalies, especially neural tube defects, oral clefts, and omphaloceles, are frequently present. David and Illingworth's study (1976) of 143 patients with diaphragmatic hernia in Southwest England showed that 50 per cent had other malformations. Heart defects are so often seen that a thorough cardiac evaluation prior to surgery is prudent even in the absence of a murmur. The authors are aware of an infant, without a cardiac murmur, who had a successful surgical repair of a diaphragmatic hernia only to die later of an unrecognized left-sided hypoplastic heart. In spite of the high association with other anomalies, the number of recognized syndromes that include diaphragmatic hernia is relatively small. Rare familial cases of autosomal recessive isolated diaphragmatic hernia have been reported (Norio et al., 1984). Diaphragmatic hernia is an uncommon feature of **Poland anomaly** and the **VATER association** (see the discussion in the next section) (Frias and Felman, 1974, McCredie and Reid, 1978). Toriello and associates (1985) presented a study of a male infant with unilateral agenesis of the lung and diaphragm whose sister had bilateral pulmonary and diaphragmatic agenesis.

Finally, it is important for the neonatologist to be aware of **Fryns syndrome** (Moerman et al., 1988), an autosomal recessive condition that is almost always lethal. In this disorder, diaphragmatic hernia is associated with cleft palate, hypoplastic nails and terminal phalanges, cystic kidneys, genital and CNS anomalies, and facial dysmorphism.

IMPERFORATE ANUS

Imperforate anus is a feature of many multiple malformation syndromes (Pinsky, 1978; Tolmie et al., 1987; Boocock and Donnai, 1987) (Table 21–5), although in approximately 50 per cent of infants it occurs as an isolated event. Associated abnormalities are more common when the malformation is high. In one study of 169 cases of imperforate anus, a family history of a similar malformation was found in 9 per cent of infants (Boocock and Donnai, 1987).

The acronym **VATER** is used to describe the frequent association of *v*ertebral, *a*nal, *t*racheoesophageal, *r*enal and *r*adial anomalies (Weaver et al., 1986). Cardiac and other limb anomalies also occur, in which case the acronym becomes **VACTERL** association. Usually, three or more of the major abnormalities must be present to make this diagnosis. The disorder is typically sporadic and the prognosis for normal development is good. The cause is unknown.

Exstrophy of the common cloaca, into which ureters, ilium, and rudimentary hindgut open, leads to the **OEIS** association—*o*mphalocele, *e*xstrophy of the bladder, *i*mperforate anus, and *s*pinal defects (Evans et al., 1985; Carey et al., 1978). The pubic rami fail to unite. Males may have absent penis or cryptorchidism, whereas females may have atretic vagina or bifid uterus. This condition seems to be more common in identical twins (Redman et al., 1981). There is some similarity in appearance with the **limb-body wall complex.**

Another acronym, the **FG syndrome,** uses the initials of the two families in which this X-linked condition was first described (Opitz and Kaveggia, 1974). Affected male infants are hypotonic, macrocephalic, and have anal anomalies varying from an imperforate, stenosed, or anteriorly placed anus to severe constipation. Cardiac lesions and agenesis of the corpus callosum have been noted. Infants suffer from failure to thrive, and some die in infancy. At a later age, mental retardation, upswept hair at the forehead, and prominent fingerpads can be appreciated (Thompson et al., 1985). The diagnosis can be difficult when imperforate anus is not present.

The **Pallister-Hall syndrome,** which is almost always lethal, consists of imperforate anus, postaxial polydactyly, hypopituitarism, hypothalamic hamartoblastoma, multiple buccal frenula, and laryngeal and epiglottal defects (Hall, 1980a). The hamartoblastoma is not always evident early. If it is suspected that this condition is present, MRI or CT scans should be repeated. All cases have been sporadic (Graham et al., 1986).

■ DYSPLASIAS

The term dysplasia is used to describe congenital anomalies that are confined to organs deriving from one tissue type. **Marfan syndrome,** a connective tissue dysplasia, becomes manifest by aortic enlargement, ectopia lentis, joint laxity, tall stature, and arachnodactyly. Ectodermal dysplasias involve abnormalities of the hair, teeth, nails, and skin. Skeletal dysplasias affect the bones, typically resulting in disproportionate short stature. Myopathies such as Duchenne muscular dystrophy are dysplasias of muscle. The implication in each of these examples is that the defect is unique to one tissue type.

A more liberal definition of a dysplasia would include those syndromes in which a unique morphogenetic error affects a progenitor tissue and the many different tissues that derive from it. For instance, **Waardenburg syndrome,** which consists of white forelock, deafness, heterochromia of the irides, and partial albinism, is probably due to a defect in the migration of neural crest cells. The increased incidence of both **Hirschsprung aganglionic megacolon** and cleft lip in this condition can be explained by the absence of critical tissues derived from neural crest. In this way, neurofibromatosis and tuberous sclerosis would be considered, quite appropriately, dysplasias.

TABLE 21–5. Syndromes That May Include an Anal Malformation

SYNDROME	OTHER DEFECTS
Hypertelorism-hypospadias syndrome	Hypertelorism, hypospadias, and swallowing defects
Townes-Brocks syndrome	Hand, foot, and ear anomalies
Cryptophthalmos syndrome	Palate, ear, renal, laryngeal, genital, digital, and eye malformations
Kaufman-McKusick syndrome	Congenital heart disease, polydactyly, and hydrometrocolpos
Johanson-Blizzard syndrome	Hypoplastic nasal alae, exocrine pancreatic insufficiency, deafness, and hypothyroidism
FG syndrome	Macrocephaly, hypotonia, mental retardation, and characteristic facies
VATER association	Vertebral, anal, tracheoesophageal, renal, and radial limb defects
PIV syndrome	Polydactyly, imperforate anus, and vertebral anomalies
Jarcho-Levin syndrome	Rib and vertebral defects; respiratory failure in infancy
Ivic syndrome	Radial defects, strabismus, thrombocytopenia, and deafness
Pallister-Hall syndrome	Hypothalamic hamartoblastoma, hypopituitarism, and postaxial polydactyly
Meckel syndrome	Encephalocele, polydactyly, and cystic kidneys
Cat eye syndrome	Ocular coloboma, ear and renal anomalies, and occasional mental retardation

(Modified from Tolmie J. L., Coutts, N., and Drainer, I.K.: Congenital anal anomalies in two families with Opitz 6 syndrome. J. Med. Genet. 24:688–691, 1987.)

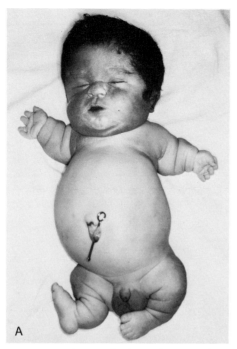
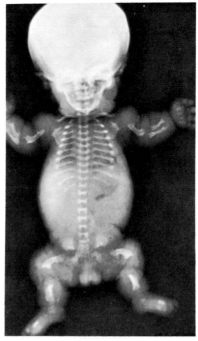

FIGURE 21–24. A, This postmortem photograph of a newborn with thanatophoric dysplasia shows the severe shortening of the extremities and the narrow thorax. The deep creases and folds on the extremities are characteristic of the condition, as is the gap between the middle and ring fingers. B, The key radiographic features of thanatophoric dysplasia are curved "telephone receiver" femurs and inverted U-shaped lumbar vertebrae. (From Aegerter, E., and Kirkpatrick, J. A.: Orthopedic Diseases. 3rd ed. Philadelphia, W.B. Saunders Company, 1968.)

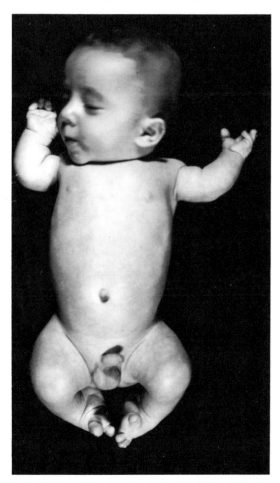

FIGURE 21–25. In addition to short-limbed dwarfism, this infant with diastrophic dysplasia has medially deviated great toes (hallux varus), talipes equinovarus, and proximally displaced "hitchhiker" thumbs. (Courtesy of Dr. Robert Wilkinson, Children's Hospital, Boston.)

SKELETAL DYSPLASIAS

The skeletal dysplasias comprise a large group of generalized disorders of cartilage and/or bone growth that frequently produce disproportionate short stature (dwarfism). Over 100 distinct disorders have now been described from a group which, in the 1960s, would probably have been misdiagnosed as **achondroplasia** (short-limb dwarfism) or **Morquio syndrome** (short-trunk dwarfism). It is beyond the scope of this chapter to discuss all the skeletal dysplasias, and the reader is directed to several comprehensive texts (Maroteaux, 1979; Spranger et al., 1974; Taybi et al., 1990; and Wynne-Davies and Hall, 1985). Selected dysplasias are listed in Table 21–6.

Many, but not all, of the skeletal dysplasias are recognizable at birth. Some are uniformly fatal in the newborn period (e.g., **thanatophoric dysplasia;** Fig. 21–24) and must be distinguished from those that may have early neonatal problems but have a good prognosis for survival with aggressive therapy (e.g., **Ellis–van Creveld syndrome**).

Many of these disorders may be diagnosed using clinical and radiographic criteria alone. Classically, the approach to the differential diagnosis begins with a clinical assessment of body proportion; that is, are the limbs most affected (short-limb dwarfism) or is the trunk primarily affected (short-trunk dwarfism)? Are the segments of the limbs proportionately short or is there more shortening of the proximal (rhizomelia), middle (mesomelia), or distal (acromelia) segment? Many of the skeletal dysplasias have other anomalies such as cleft palate and clubfeet (**diastrophic dysplasia,** Fig. 21–25), congenital heart defects and polydactyly (**Ellis–van Creveld syndrome**), cataracts (**rhizomelic chondrodysplasia punctata,** Fig. 21–26), and fractures (**osteogenesis imperfecta,** Fig. 21–27) that may provide clues to the differential diagnosis.

TABLE 21–6. Skeletal Dysplasias Recognized at Birth

NAME	SKELETAL ANOMALIES	EXTRASKELETAL ANOMALIES	RADIOGRAPHIC FEATURES	INHERITANCE	COMMENTS
Lethal Disorders					
Thanatophoric dysplasia	Large cranium, with or without Kleeblatt-schädel Depressed nasal bridge Midface hypoplasia Small chest Very short limbs	Hydrocephalus CNS anomalies Congenital heart defect	Short-cupped ribs Platyspondyly U-shaped vertebral bodies on anteroposterior view Short, curved long bones, "telephone receiver" femurs Metaphyseal widening	AD	Most common lethal bone dysplasia: 1 in 40,000 births
Achrondrogenesis type I	Very short limbs Short trunk Barrel-shaped chest	Hydropic appearance Prominent abdomen Congenital heart defect	Poorly ossified skull Absence of ossification of vertebral bodies Short, thin horizontal ribs, fractures Absence of pubic ossification Very short long bones with concave ends, spurs	AR	
Achondrogenesis type II (includes hypochondrogenesis)	Very short limbs Short trunk Barrel-shaped chest	Hydropic appearance Prominent abdomen	Short ribs Absence of ossification of vertebral bodies Very short long bones with cupped, flared metaphyses	AR	
Short rib polydactyly type I (Saldino-Noonan)	Short limbs Narrow chest Postaxial polydactyly	Hydropic appearance Heart defect Anal atresia Kidney defect Genital anomaly	Very short ribs Short long bones with metaphyseal spurs Small iliac bones	AR	
Short rib polydactyly type II (Majewski)	Narrow chest Short extremities pre- and/or postaxial polydactyly	Hydropic appearance Cleft lip/cleft palate Heart defect Renal cysts Genital anomalies	Very short ribs Very small tibia	AR	
Osteogenesis imperfecta, type II	Soft calvarium Small chest Short, bowed limbs	Fragile skin Blue sclerae	Osteoporosis Multiple fractures "crumpled" long bones Beaded ribs	AD	1 in 60,000 births Various defects in type I collagen 6 per cent recurrence risk due to parental gonadal mosaicism (Byers and Bonadio, 1985; Byers, 1988)
Nonlethal Disorders					
Achondroplasia	Large calvarium Depressed nasal bridge Midface hypoplasia Rhizomelia "Trident hands"	Occasional hydrocephalus Spinal cord impingement at foramen magnum has been associated with apnea, sudden death in infancy (Pauli et al., 1984)	Small foramen magnum Short cupped ribs Decreased interpedicular distance in lumbosacral region on anteroposterior view, short pedicles Squared-off ilia, small sacrosciatic notches Wide metaphyses	AD	Most common nonlethal bone dysplasia: 1 in 10,000 births Peripheral hypotonia with delayed motor milestones first 2 yrs Revised developmental chart available (Todorov et al., 1981) Frequent otitis media, hearing loss CT evaluation of cervical spine recommended (Reid et al., 1987)
Diastrophic dysplasia	Short limbs "Hitchhiker thumbs" Clubfeet Joint contractures	Acute swelling of pinnae in early infancy leading to cauliflower ear Cleft palate (50 per cent of cases)	Scoliosis Short broad long bones with metaphyseal flaring Ovoid first metacarpal Odontoid hypoplasia	AR	Contractures recalcitrant to traditional orthopedic treatment

TABLE 21–6. Skeletal Dysplasias Recognized at Birth *Continued*

NAME	SKELETAL ANOMALIES	EXTRASKELETAL ANOMALIES	RADIOGRAPHIC FEATURES	INHERITANCE	COMMENTS
Nonlethal Disorders *(Continued)*					
Kniest dysplasia	Flat face Short trunk Symphalangism Short extremities with prominent joints	Congenital myopia Retinal detachment Deafness Cleft palate	Platyspondyly Coronal clefts of lumbar vertebral bodies in infancy Short long bones with rounded, broad metaphyses	AD	Abnormality of type II collagen C-propeptide (Poole et al., 1988)
Metatrophic dysplasia	Narrow chest Long trunk in infancy (becomes short with severe scoliosis) Tail-like appendage at sacrum Prominent joints, contractures		Platyspondyly with wide intervertebral spaces in infancy Diamond-shaped vertebrae on lateral view Short tubular bones with metaphyseal flare and epiphyseal dysplasia	AR	
Chondroectodermal dysplasia (Ellis–van Creveld)	Narrow chest Postaxial polydactyly Short limbs, acromelia is most marked	Dental anomalies Natal teeth Multiple frenuli Heart defect Nail hypoplasia	Short tubular bones Cone epiphyses Low iliac wings with hooklike projections at acetabulum	AR	Death may occur in infancy because of congenital heart defect and pulmonary insufficiency
Spondyloepiphyseal dysplasia congenita	Flat face Short neck Barrel chest Rhizomelia Clubfeet	Myopia, retinal detachment Cleft palate	C_1 to C_2 instability Retarded epiphyseal ossification Platyspondyly Retarded ossification of pubic bones	AD	Type II collagen defect
Chondrodysplasia punctata, rhizomelic type	Rhizomelia Joint contractures Flat face Depressed nasal bridge with short nose	Cataracts Severe mental retardation Ichthyosiform erythroderma	Epiphyseal and extraepiphyseal calcification in infancy Wide coronal clefts of vertebral bodies	AR	Failure to thrive Poor prognosis, with most dying in 1st year Elevated plasma phytanic acid Deficient activity of peroxisomal enzymes Acyl-CoA: dihydroxy-acetone-phosphate acyltransferase (Heymans et al., 1985)
Chondrodysplasia punctata, Conradi-Hünermann type	Asymmetric shortening of limbs Flat face Depressed nasal bridge with short nose Joint contractures	Hydramnios, hydrops Cataracts (20 per cent of patients) Atrophic skin changes/alopecia	Asymmetric shortening of long bones Calcific stippling of ends of long bones, carpal and tarsal regions, spine scoliosis	AD	
Asphyxiating thoracic dysplasia	Long, narrow chest, with or without postaxial polydactyly Short extremities (childhood)	Respiratory insufficiency Nephropathy Intestinal malabsorption Retinal degeneration Cysts of liver, pancreas, kidney	Cephalocaudal shortening of iliac bones Metaphyseal irregularity	AR	Increased mortality in infancy due to respiratory distress

AD, autosomal dominant; AR, autosomal recessive.

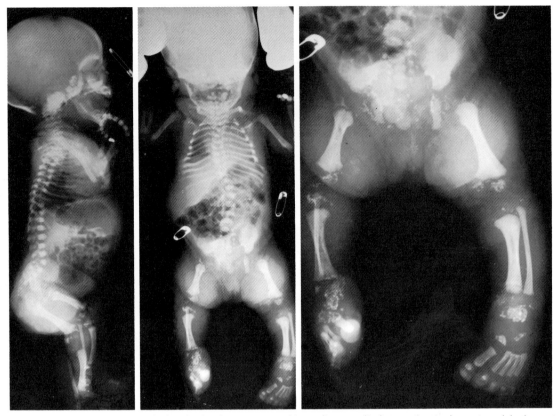

FIGURE 21–26. Radiographs of an infant with chondrodysplasia punctata, rhizomelic type, display symmetric shortening of the humeri and femora and calcific stippling of the epiphyses. (Courtesy of Dr. E.M. Savignac.)

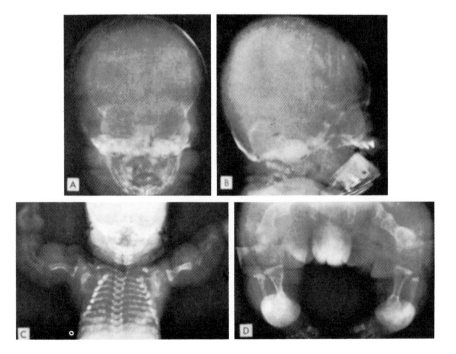

FIGURE 21–27. Radiographs of a newborn infant with osteogenesis imperfecta, type II, show poor ossification of the skull (A and B). The beaded ribs (C) and crumpled femora (D) are a result of multiple fractures in utero. (From Aegerter, E., and Kirkpatrick, J. A., Jr.: Orthopedic Diseases, 3rd ed. Philadelphia, W.B. Saunders Company, 1968.)

When a definitive diagnosis cannot be ascertained by clinical and radiographic examinations, microscopic examination of bone and cartilage should be undertaken, especially in the case of neonatal death. Growth plate (cartilage-bone interface) of rib, vertebrae, and long bone should be preserved.

For an exhaustive list of syndromes, the reader is referred to the *Birth Defects Encyclopedia,* edited by M. L. Buyse (Blackwell Scientific Publications, 3 Cambridge Center, Cambridge, Massachusetts 02142), or the Center for Birth Defects Information Services, Inc., Dover Medical Building, 30 Springdale Avenue, Dover, Massachusetts 02030.

■ REFERENCES

Aase, J. M.: Microtia—Clinical observations. Birth Defects 16(4):289–297, 1980.

Ardinger, H. H., Atkin, J. F., Blackston, R. D., et al.: Verification of the fetal valproate syndrome phenotype. Am. J. Med. Genet. 29:171–185, 1988.

Aughton, D. J., and Cassidy, S. B.: Hydrolethalus syndrome: Report of an apparent mild case, literature review and differential diagnosis. Am. J. Med. Genet. 27:935–942, 1987.

Baird, P. A., Robinson, G. C., and Buckler, W. St. J.: Klippel-Feil syndrome: A study of mirror movement detected by electromyography. Am. J. Dis. Child. 113:546, 1967.

Baker, C. J., and Rudolph, A. J.: Congenital ring constrictions and intrauterine amputations. Am. J. Dis. Child. 121:393–400, 1971.

Baldwin, S., and Whitley, R. J: Teratogen update: Intrauterine herpes simplex virus infection. Teratology 39:1–10, 1989.

Bergsma, D. (Ed.): Birth Defects Compendium. 2nd ed. New York, A. R. Liss, Inc., 1979.

Bixler, D.: Genetics and clefting. Cleft Palate J. 18:10–18, 1981.

Bixler, D., Christian, J. C., and Gorlin, R. J.: Hypertelorism, microtia and facial clefting: A newly described inherited syndrome. Am. J. Dis. Child. 118:495–500, 1969.

Bodenhoff, J., and Gorlin, R. J.: Natal and neonatal teeth: Folklore and fact. Pediatrics 32:1087–1093, 1963.

Boocock, G. R., and Donnai, D.: Anorectal malformation: familial aspects and associated anomalies. Arch. Dis. Child. 62:576–579, 1987.

Borgoankas, D.: Chromosomal Variation in Man: A Catalog of Chromosomal Variates and Anomalies. 5th ed. New York, A. R. Liss, Inc., 1989.

Bouwes Bavinck, J. N., and Weaver, D. D.: Subclavian artery supply disruption sequence: Hypothesis of a vascular etiology for Poland, Klippel-Feil and Möebius anomalies. Am. J. Med. Genet. 23:903–918, 1986.

Brent, R. L.: Radiation teratogenesis. In Sever, J. L., and Brent, R. L. (Eds.): Teratogen Update: Environmentally Induced Birth Defect Risks. New York, A. R. Liss, Inc. 1986, pp. 145–163.

Briggs, G. G., Freeman, R. K., and Yaffe, S. J.: Drugs in Pregnancy and Lactation. 2nd ed. Baltimore: Williams & Wilkins, 1986, pp. 281–283, 382–385.

Burton, B. K.: Empiric recurrence risks for congenital hydrocephalus. Birth Defects 15(5C):107–115, 1979.

Byers, P. H.: Osteogenesis imperfecta: An update. Growth: Genetics and Hormones 4(2):1–5, 1988.

Byers, P. H., and Bonadio, J. F.: The molecular basis of clinical heterogeneity in osteogenesis imperfecta: Mutations in type I collagen genes have different effects on collagen processing. In Lloyd, J. and Scriver, C. R. (Eds.): Metabolic and Genetic Disease in Pediatrics. London, Butterworths, 1985, pp. 56–90.

Cappa, M., Borrelli, P., Marini, R. and Neri, G.: The Opitz syndrome: A new designation for the clinically indistinguishable BBB and G syndromes. Am. J. Med. Genet. 28:303–309, 1987.

Carey, J. C., Eggert, L., and Curry, C. R.: Lower limb deficiency and the urethral obstruction sequence. Birth Defects 18[3B]:19–28, 1982.

Carey, J. C., Greenbaum, B., and Hall, B. D.: The OEIS complex (omphalocele, exstrophy, imperforate anus, spinal defects). Birth Defects 14[6B]:253–263, 1978.

Cervenka, J., Gorlin, R. J., and Anderson, V. E.: The syndrome of pits of the lower lip and cleft lip or cleft palate: Genetic considerations. Am. J. Hum. Genet. 19:416–432, 1967.

Chung, C. S., and Myrianthopoulos, N. C.: Factors affecting risks of congenital malformations II: Effect of maternal diabetes. Birth Defects 11(10):23–38, 1975.

Cohen, M. M., Jr.: Syndromes with cleft lip and cleft palate. Cleft Palate J. 15:306–328, 1978.

Cohen, M. M., Jr.: Craniosynostosis: Diagnosis, Evaluation, and Management. New York, Raven Press, 1986.

Cohen, M. M., Jr.: Craniosynostosis update 1987. Am. J. Med. Genet. 4:99–148, 1988.

Cohlan, S. Q.: Tetracycline staining of teeth. Teratology 15:127–130, 1977.

Curry, C. J. R., Jensen, K., Holland, J., et al.: The Potter sequence: A clinical analysis of 80 cases. Am. J. Med. Genet. 19:679–702, 1984.

Davenport, S. L. H., Hefner, M. A., and Thelin, J. W.: CHARGE syndrome. Part I. External ear anomalies. Int. J. Pediatr. Otorhinolaryngol. 12:137–143, 1986.

David, T. J., and Illingworth, C. A.: Diaphragmatic hernia in the southwest of England. J. Med. Genet. 13:253–262, 1976.

Dekaban, A. S.: Abnormalities in children exposed to X-irradiation during various stages of gestation: Tentative timetable of radiation injury to the human fetus. J. Nucl. Med. 9:471–477, 1968.

Dobyns, W. B., Pagon, R. A., Armstrong, D., et al.: Diagnostic criteria for Walker-Warburg syndrome. Am. J. Med. Genet. 32:195–210, 1989.

Dudding, B. A., Gorlin, R. J., and Langer, L. O.: The oto-palato-digital symptom: A new symptom-complex consisting of deafness, dwarfism, cleft palate, characteristic facies, and a generalized bone dysplasia. Am. J. Dis. Child. 113:214–221, 1967.

Edwards, M. J.: Congenital defects in guinea pigs following induced hyperthermia during gestation. Arch. Pathol. 84:42–48, 1967.

Emanuel, I., and Kenny, G. E.: Cytomegalic inclusion disease of infancy. Pediatrics 38(6, part I):957–965, 1988.

Evans, J. A., Darvill, K. D., Trevenen, C., et al.: Cloacal exstrophy and related abdominal wall defects in Manitoba: Incidence and demographic factors. Clin. Genet. 27:241–251, 1985.

Fisher, N. L.: Occipital encephalocele and early gestational hyperthermia. Pediatrics 68:480–483, 1981.

Forland, M.: Cleidocranial dystosis: A review of the syndrome and a report of a sporadic case with hereditary transmission. Am. J. Med. 33:792–799, 1962.

Fraser, F. C., Sproule, J. R., and Halal, F.: Frequency of the branchio-oto-renal (BOR) syndrome in children with profound hearing loss. Am. J. Med. Genet. 7:341–349, 1980.

Frias, J. L., and Felman, A. H.: Absence of the pectoralis major, with ipsilateral aplasia of the radius, thumb, hemidiaphragm and lung: An extreme expression of Poland anomaly? Birth Defects 10[5]:55–59, 1974.

Fuccillo, D. A.: Congenital varicella. In Sever, J. L., and Brent, R. L. (Eds.): Teratogen Update: Environmentally Induced Birth Defect Risks. New York, Alan R. Liss, Inc., 1986, pp. 101–105.

Geis, N., Seto, B., Bartoshesky, L., et al.: The prevalence of congenital heart disease among the population of a metropolitan cleft lip and palate clinic. Cleft Palate J. 18:19–23, 1981.

Golbus, M. S.: Teratology for the obstetrician: Current status. Obstet. Gynecol. 55:269–277, 1980.

Goldenberg, R. L., Humphrey, J. L., Hale, C. B., et al.: Lethal congenital anomalies as a cause of birth-weight–specific neonatal mortality. J.A.M.A. 250:513–518, 1983.

Gorlin, R. J., Cohen, M. M., Jr., and Levin, L. S.: Syndromes of the Head and Neck. 3rd ed. New York, Oxford University Press, 1990.

Grabb, W. C.: The first and second arch syndrome. Plast. Reconstr. Surg. 36:485–508, 1965.

Graham, J. M., Jr.: Smith's Recognizable Patterns of Human Deformation. 2nd ed. Philadelphia, W. B. Saunders, Company, 1988.

Graham, J. M., Jr., Saunders, R., Fratkin, J., et al.: A cluster of Pallister-Hall syndrome cases (congenital hypothalamic hamartoblastoma syndrome). Am. J. Med. Genet. 2(Suppl.):53–63, 1986.

Grossman, J. J., III: Congenital syphilis. In Sever, J. L., and Brent, R. L. (Eds.): Teratogen Update: Environmentally Induced Birth Defect Risks. New York, A. R. Liss, Inc., 1986, pp. 113–117.

Halal, F., Herrmann, J., Pallister, P. D., et al.: Differential diagnosis of Nager acrofacial dysostosis syndrome: Report of four patients with Nager syndrome and discussion of other related syndromes. Am. J. Med. Genet. 14:209–224, 1983.

Hall, J. G.: Arthrogryposes (congenital contractures). In Emery, A. E. H., and Rimoin, D. L. (Eds.): Principles and Practice of Medical Genetics. New York, Churchill Livingstone, 1983, pp. 781–811.

Hall, J. G.: In utero movement and use of limbs are necessary for normal growth: A study of individuals with arthrogryposis. *In* Papadatos, C. J., and Bartsocas, C. S. (Eds.): Endocrine Genetics and Genetics of Growth. New York, A. R. Liss, Inc., 1985, pp. 155–162.

Hall, J. G.: Invited editorial comment: Analysis of Pena Shokeir phenotype. Am. J. Med. Genet. *25*:99–117, 1986.

Hall, J. G., Pallister, P. D., Clarren, S. K., et al.: Congenital hypothalamic hamartoblastoma, hypopituitarism, imperforate anus and postaxial polydactyly—a new syndrome. Parts I and II. Am. J. Med. Genet. *7*:47–83, 1980a.

Hall, J. G., Pauli, R. M., and Wilson, K. M.: Maternal and fetal sequelae of anticoagulation during pregnancy. Am. J. Med. *68*:122–140, 1980b.

Halliday, G., Chow, C. W., Wallace, D., and Danks, D. M.: X-linked hydrocephalus: A survey of a 20-year period in Victoria, Australia. J. Med. Genet. *23*:23–31, 1986.

Hanson, J. W.: Teratogen update: Fetal hydantoin effects. Teratology *33*:349–353, 1986.

Harada, M.: Congenital Minamata disease: Intrauterine methylmercury poisoning. *In* Sever, J. L., and Brent, R. L. (Eds.): Teratogen Update: Environmentally Induced Birth Defect Risks. New York, A. R. Liss, Inc., 1986, pp. 127–130.

Hawley, P. P., Jackson, L. G., and Kurnit, D. M.: Sixty-four patients with Brachmann–de Lange syndrome: A survey. Am. J. Med. Genet. *20*:453–459, 1985.

Heimler, A., and Leiber, E.: Branchio-oto-renal syndrome: Reduced penetrance and variable expressivity in four generations of a large kindred. Am. J. Med. Genet. *25*:15–27, 1986.

Herbst, A. L.: Diethylstilbestrol and other sex hormones during pregnancy. Obstet. Gynecol. *58*(5, Suppl):35S–40S, 1981.

Heymans, H. S. A., Oorthys, J. W. E., Nelck, G., et al.: Rhizomelic chondroplasia punctata: Another peroxisomal disorder. Letter to the Editor. N. Engl. J. Med. *313*:187–188, 1985.

Hoyme, H. E., Jones, K. L., Van Allen, M. I., et al.: Vascular pathogenesis of transverse limb reduction defects. J. Pediatr. *101*:839–843, 1982.

Hoyme, H. E., Jones, M. C., and Jones, K. L.: Gastroschisis: Abdominal wall disruption secondary to early gestational interruption of the omphalomesenteric artery. Sem. Perinatol. *7*:294–298, 1983.

Hoyme, H. E., Procopio, F., Crooks, W., et al.: The incidence of neoplasia in children with isolated congenital hemihypertrophy (abstract). Proceedings of the Greenwood Genetic Center *6*:126, 1981.

Hunter, A. G. W., and Rudd, N. L.: Craniosynostosis. I. Sagittal synostosis: Its genetics and associated clinical findings in 214 patients who lacked involvement of the coronal suture(s). Teratology *14*:185–193, 1976.

Iturbe-Alessio, I., Fonseca, M. C., Mutchinik, O., et al.: Risks of anticoagulant therapy in pregnant women with artificial heart valves. N. Engl. J. Med. *315*:1390–1393, 1986.

Jones, K. L.: Smith's Recognizable Patterns of Human Malformation. 4th ed. Philadelphia, W. B. Saunders Company, 1988.

Jones, K. L., Smith, D. W., Ulleland, C. N., et al.: Pattern of malformation in offspring of chronic alcoholic mothers. Lancet *1*:1267–1271, 1973.

Kalter, H., and Warkany, J.: Congenital malformations: Etiologic factors and their role in prevention. N. Engl. J. Med. *308*:424–431, 491–497, 1983.

Kawamoto, H. K.: The kaleidoscopic world of craniofacial clefts: Order out of chaos (Tessier Classification). Clin. Plast. Surg. *3*:529–572, 1976.

Koffler, H., Aase, J. M., Papile, L.-A., et al.: Persistent cloaca with absent penis and anal atresia in one of identical twins. J. Pediatr. *93*:821–822, 1978.

Laegreid, L., Olegard, R., Walstrome, J., and Conradi, N.: Teratogenic effects of benzodiazepine use during pregnancy. J. Pediatr. *114*:126–131, 1989.

Lammer, E. J., Chen, D. T., Hoar, R. M., et al.: Retinoic acid embryopathy. N. Engl. J. Med. *313*:837–841, 1985.

Lammer, E. J., Hayes, A. M., and Schuniot, A.: Unusually high risk for adverse outcomes of pregnancy following fetal isotretinoin exposure. Am. J. Hum. Genet. *43*(3 suppl.):A58, 1988.

Lammer, E. J., Sever, L. E., and Oakley, G. P., Jr.: Teratogen update: Valproic acid. Teratology *35*:465–473, 1987.

Larsen, John W.: Congenital toxoplasmosis. *In* Sever, J. L., and Brent, R. L. (Eds.): Teratogen Update: Environmentally Induced Birth Defect Risks. New York, A. R. Liss, Inc., 1986, pp. 97–100.

Lee, C. M., Jr., and Mattheis, H.: Congenital lumbar hernia. Arch. Dis. Child. *32*:42, 1957.

Lenke, R. R., and Levy, H. L.: Maternal phenylketonuria and hyperphenylalanimenia. N. Engl. J. Med. *303*:1202–1208, 1980.

Lenz, W.: A short history of thalidomide embryopathology. Teratology *38*:203–215, 1988.

Levy, H. L., and Waisbren, S. E.: Effects of untreated maternal phenylketonuria and hyperphenylalaninemia on the fetus. N. Engl. J. Med. *309*:1269–1274, 1983.

Lipson, A., Buehler, B., Bartley, J., et al.: Maternal hyperphenylalaninemia fetal effects. J. Pediatr. *104*:216–220, 1984.

Lowry, R. B.: Sex-linked cleft palate in a British Columbia Indian family. Pediatrics *46*:123–128, 1970.

Marden, P. M., Smith, D. W., and McDonald, M. J.: Congenital anomalies in the newborn infant, including minor variations. J. Pediatr. *64*:357–371, 1964.

Maroteaux, P.: Bone Diseases of Children. Philadelphia, J. B. Lippincott Co., 1979.

McCredie, J., and Reid, I. S.: Congenital diaphragmatic hernia associated with homolateral upper limb malformation. J. Pediatr. *92*:762–765, 1978.

Mellin, G. W., and Katzenstein, M.: The saga of thalidomide. N. Engl. J. Med. *267*:1184–1193, 1238–1244, 1962.

Melnick, M., Hodes, M. E., Nance, W. E., et al.: Branchio-oto-renal dysplasia and branchio-oto dysplasia: Two distinct autosomal dominant disorders. Clin. Genet. *13*:425–442, 1978.

Melnick, M., and Myrianthopoulos, N. C.: External ear malformations: Epidemiology, genetics and natural history. Birth Defects *15*(9):1–137, 1979.

Miller, E. M., Hare, J. W., Cloherty, J. R., et al.: Major congenital anomalies and elevated hemoblobin A$_{1c}$ in early weeks of diabetic pregnancy. N. Engl. J. Med. *304*:1331–1334, 1981.

Miller, M., Fineman, R., and Smith, D. W.: Postaxial acrofacial dysostosis syndrome. J. Pediatr. *95*:970–975, 1979.

Mills, J. I.: Malformations in infants of diabetic mothers. Teratology *25*:385–394, 1982.

Moerman, P., Fryns, J.-P., Vandenberghe, K., et al.: The syndrome of diaphragmatic hernia, abnormal face and distal limb anomalies (Fryns syndrome): Report of two sibs with further delineation of this multiple congenital anomaly (MCA) syndrome. Am. J. Med. Genet. *31*:805–814, 1988.

Molsted-Pedersen, L., Tygstrup, I., and Pedersen, J.: Congenital malformations in newborn infants of diabetic women. Lancet *1*:1124–1126, 1964.

Moore, G., Ivens, A., Chambers, J., et al.: Linkage of an X-chromosome cleft palate gene. Nature *326*(6108):91, 1987.

Nelson, K., Holmes, L. B.: Malformations due to presumed spontaneous mutations in newborn infants. N. Engl. J. Med. *320*:19, 1989.

Norio, R., Kääriäinen, H., Rapola, J., et al.: Familial congenital diaphragmatic defects: Aspects of etiology, prenatal diagnosis, and treatment. Am. J. Med. Genet. *17*:471–483, 1984.

Opitz, J. M., and Kaveggia, E. G.: The FG syndrome: An X-linked recessive syndrome of multiple congenital abnormalities and mental retardation. Z. Kinderheilkd. *117*:1–18, 1974.

Ossipoff, V., and Hall, B. D.: Etiologic factors in the amniotic band syndrome: A study of 24 patients. Birth Defects *13*(3D):117–132, 1977.

Pagon, R. A., Graham, J. M., Jr., Zonana, J., and Yong, S. L.: Coloboma, congenital heart disease, and choanal atresia with multiple anomalies: CHARGE association. J. Pediatr. *99*:223–227, 1981.

Palant, D. J., and Carter, B. L.: Klippel-Feil syndrome and deafness. Am. J. Dis. Child. *123*:218, 1972.

Pauli, R. M., Scott, C. I., Wassman, E. R., Jr., et al.: Apnea and sudden unexplained death in infants with achondroplasia. J. Pediatr. *104*:342–348, 1984.

Pederson, J.: The Pregnant Diabetic and Her Newborn. 2nd ed. Baltimore, Williams & Wilkins Company, 1977.

Phelan, M. C., Pellock, J. M., Nance, W. E.: Discordant expression of fetal hydantoin syndrome in heteropaternal dizygotic twins. N. Engl. J. Med. *307*:99–102, 1982.

Pinsky, L.: The syndromology of anorectal malformation (atresia, stenosis, ectopia). Am. J. Med. Genet. *1*:461–474, 1978.

Poole, A. R., Pidoux, I., Reiner, A., et al.: Kneist dysplasia is characterized by an apparent abnormal processing of the c-propeptide of type II cartilage collagen resulting in imperfect fibril assembly. J. Clin. Invest. *81*:579–589, 1988.

Poswillo, D.: Otomandibular deformity: Pathogenesis as a guide to reconstruction. J. Maxillofac. Surg. *2*:64–72, 1974.

Rass-Rothschild, A., et al.: Klippel-Feil anomaly with sacral agenesis: An additional subtype, type IV. J. Craniofac. Genet. Dev. Biol. 8:297–301, 1988.

Redman, J. F., Seibert, J. J., and Page, B. C.: Cloacal exstrophy in identical twins. Urology 17:73–74, 1981.

Reid, C. S., Pyeritz, R. E., Kopits, S. E., et al.: Cervicomedullary compression in young patients with achondroplasia: Value of comprehensive neurologic and respiratory evaluation. J. Pediatr. 110:522–530, 1987.

Reynolds, D. W., Stagno, S., and Alford, C. A.: Congenital cytomegalovirus infection. In Sever, J. L., and Brent, R. L. (Eds.): Teratogen Update: Environmentally Induced Birth Defect Risks. New York, A. R. Liss, Inc., 1986, pp. 93–95.

Rimoin, D. L., and Edgerton, M. T.: Genetic and clinical heterogeneity in the oral-facial-digital syndromes. J. Pediatr. 71:94–102, 1967.

Rimoin, D. L., and Sillence, D. O.: The skeletal dysplasias: Nomenclature, classification and clinical evaluation. In Akesson, W. H., Bornstein, P., and Glimcher, M. (Eds.): Heritable Disorders of Connective Tissue. St. Louis, C. V. Mosby, 1982, p. 324.

Rollnick, B. R., and Hoo, J. J.: Genitourinary anomalies are a component manifestation in the ectodermal dysplasia, ectrodactyly, cleft lip/palate (EEC) syndrome. Am. J. Med. Genet. 29:131–136, 1988.

Rudman, D., Davis, T., Priest, J. H., et al.: Prevalence of growth hormone deficiency in children with cleft lip or palate. J. Pediatr. 93:378–382, 1978.

Salonen, R.: The Meckel syndrome: Clinicopathological findings in 67 patients. Am. J. Med. Genet. 18:671–689, 1984.

Sever, J. L., Ellenberg, J. H., Ley, A. C., et al.: Toxoplasmosis: Maternal and pediatric findings in 23,000 pregnancies. Pediatrics 82:181–192, 1988.

Shepard, T. H.: Catalog of Teratogenic Agents. 6th ed. Baltimore, Johns Hopkins University Press, 1989.

Shillito, J., and Matson, D. D.: Craniosynostosis: A review of 519 surgical patients. Pediatrics 41:829–853, 1968.

Shulman, B. H., and Terhune, C. B.: Epiphyseal injuries in breech delivery. Pediatrics 8:693, 1951.

Smith, D. W.: Recognizable Patterns of Human Malformation. 3rd ed. Philadelphia, W. B. Saunders Company, 1982.

South, M. A., and Sever, J. L.: Teratogen update: The congenital rubella syndrome. Teratology 31:297–397, 1985.

Spranger, J. W., Langer, L. O., Jr., and Wiedemann, H.-R.: Bone Dysplasias: An Atlas of Constitutional Disorders of Skeletal Development. Philadelphia, W. B. Saunders Company, 1974.

Stagno, S., and Whitley, R. J.: Herpes virus infections of pregnancy. Part I: Cytomegalovirus and Epstein-Barr virus infection. N. Engl. J. Med. 313:1270–1274, 1985a.

Stagno, S., and Whitley, R. J.: Herpes virus infections of pregnancy. Part II: Herpes simplex virus and varicella-zoster virus infections. N. Engl. J. Med. 313:1327–1330, 1985b.

Stern, R.: When a uniquely effective drug is teratogenic: The case of isotretinoin. N. Engl. J. Med. 320:1007–1009, 1989.

Stickler, G. B., Belau, P. G., Farrell, F. J., et al.: Hereditary progressive arthro-ophthalmopathy. Mayo Clin. Proc. 40(6):433–455, 1965.

Sybert, V. P.: Aplasia cutis congenita: A report of 12 new families and review of the literature. Pediatr. Dermatol. 3:1–14, 1985.

Taybi, H., Lachman, R., et al.: Radiology of Syndromes and Metabolic Disorders. 3rd ed. Cambridge, Mass., Blackwell, 1990.

Temtamy, S., and McKusick, V.: The genetics of hand malformations. Birth Defects 14(3):i–xviii, 1–619, 1978.

Tenconi, R., and Hall, B. D.: Hemifacial microsomia: Phenotype classification, clinical implications and genetic aspects. In Harvold, E. P., Vargervick, K., and Chierici, G.: Treatment of Hemifacial Microsomia. New York, A. R. Liss, Inc., 1983, pp. 39–49.

Thompson, E. M., Baraitser, M., and Lindenbaum, R. H.: The FG syndrome: 7 new cases. Clin. Genet. 27:582–589, 1985.

Thompson, E. M., Donnai, D., Baraitser, M., et al.: Multiple pterygium syndrome: Evolution of the phenotype. J. Med. Genet. 24:733–749, 1987.

Toaff, R., and Ravid, R.: Tetracyclines and the teeth. Lancet 2:281–282, 1966.

Todorov, A. B., Scott, C. I., Jr., Warren, A. E., and Leeper, J. D.: Developmental screening tests in achondroplastic children. Am. J. Med. Genet. 9:19–23, 1981.

Tolmie, J. L., Coutts, N., and Drainer, I. K.: Congenital anal anomalies in two families with the Opitz G syndrome. J. Med. Genet. 24:688–691, 1987.

Toriello, H. V., Higgins, J. V., Jones, A. S., et al.: Pulmonary and diaphragmatic agenesis: Report of affected sibs. Am. J. Med. Genet. 21:87–92, 1985.

Van Allen, M. I., Curry, C., and Gallagher, L.: Limb body wall complex: I. Pathogenesis. Am. J. Med. Genet. 28:529–548, 1987.

Van Allen, M. I., Hoyme, H. E., and Jones, K. L.: Vascular pathogenesis of limb defects: I. Radial artery anatomy in radial aplasia. J. Pediatr. 101:832–838, 1982.

Warkany, J.: Teratogen update: Lithium. Teratology 38:593–596, 1988.

Weaver, D. D., Mapstone, C. L., and Yu, P.-L.: The VATER association: Analysis of 46 patients. Am. J. Dis. Child. 140:225–229, 1986.

Williams, M. A., Goldberg, R. B., and Shprintzen, R. J.: Male to male transmission of the velo-cardio-facial syndrome: A case report and review of 60 cases. J. Craniofac. Dev. Biol. 5:175–180, 1985.

Wilson, J. G.: Current status of teratology. In Wilson, J. G., and Fraser, F. C. (Eds.): Handbook of Teratology. Vol. 1. New York, Plenum Press, 1977, pp. 47–96.

Wilson, J. G., and Brent, R. L.: Are female sex hormones teratogenic? Am. J. Obstet. Gynecol. 141:567–580, 1981.

Winter, R. M., Baraitser, M., and Douglas, J. M.: A computerized database for the diagnosis of rare dysmorphic syndromes. J. Med. Genet. 21:121–124, 1984.

Wynne-Davies, R.: Heritable Disorders in Orthopaedic Practice. Oxford, Blackwell, 1973.

Wynne-Davies, R., and Hall, C. M.: Atlas of Skeletal Dysplasias. New York, Churchill Livingstone, 1985.

Zackai, E. H., Mellman, W. J., and Neiderer, B.: The fetal trimethadione syndrome. J. Pediatr. 87:280–284, 1975.

PART IV

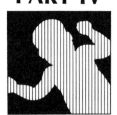

THE NEWBORN— STABILIZATION AND INITIAL EVALUATION

RESUSCITATION IN THE DELIVERY ROOM 22

Roberta A. Ballard

■ PHYSIOLOGY OF BIRTH

During normal gestation, labor, and delivery, powerful biochemical and mechanical forces act upon the fetus to prepare it to adapt to extrauterine life. However, a myriad of adverse circumstances—genetic, maternal, and fetal—that vary in duration, degree, and implication for outcome can occur during the antepartum and intrapartum periods and impair the infant's ability to make this adaptation successfully. Hence, there is a need for resuscitative efforts to assist in this process. The approach to the resuscitation of any infant depends on a keen appreciation of the historical factors behind the need, an understanding of the physiologic mechanisms of adaptation, and sensitivity to the individual infant's responses, as well as skill in resuscitative techniques. Thus, successful resuscitation depends on much more than the "mechanical" application of practiced routines; it requires a clear understanding of basic physiologic principles and excellent assessment skills as well as the essential equipment and practiced teamwork.

"STRESS" OF BIRTH

As pointed out by Lagercrantz and Slotkin (1986), "At first thought, being born would seem to be a terrible and dangerous ordeal. The human fetus is squeezed through the birth canal for several hours, during which the head sustains considerable pressure, and the infant is intermittently deprived of oxygen. . . . then delivered from a warm, dark, sheltered environment into a cold, bright hospital room . . . (in response) the fetus produces unusually high levels of the "stress" hormones, adrenalin and noradrenalin, . . . typically used to prepare the body to fight or flee from a perceived threat to survival." Surely, the process of labor and delivery is the time of greatest jeopardy that occurs during life, but would avoidance of this stress and the consequent elevation of catecholamine

levels lead to better outcomes? Catecholamines clearly contribute to the regulation of many processes important to the infant's adaptation at birth, including resorption of lung liquid, release of surfactant into the alveoli, mobilization of readily usable fuel for nutrition, defense against cold stress, and modulation of cardiac output to ensure the preferential flow of blood to vital organs, such as the heart and brain. Perhaps, as some have suggested, elevated levels of catecholamines even promote attachment between mother and child by increasing the appearance of alertness of the infant (Fig. 22–1).

The normal preterm infant has lower catecholamine levels at birth than the normal term infant, which contributes to the disadvantages of preterm infants in establishing ventilation and maintaining temperature. In both term and preterm infants, catecholamine levels are higher with delivery after labor and also higher in girls than in boys. Levels are proportionately very much higher in each of these groups when there is asphyxia (Greenough et al., 1987; Newnham et al., 1984). In addition to catecholamines, the endogenous opiate peptides (enkephalins and endorphins) also probably modulate the cardiovascular response to stress and play a role in the infant's adaptation at birth (Martinez et al., 1988). It is hoped that increased understanding of the interaction of these and other agents will eventually allow optimal preparation of the fetus for labor. This understanding may also provide insight on which interventions to use during labor and at birth to ensure an optimal outcome.

TRANSITION FROM FETAL TO NEONATAL CIRCULATION

Prior to birth, the placenta serves as the gas-exchange organ for the fetus and also provides a low-resistance "shunt" compared with the high resistance of the fetus' peripheral circulation. As a result, the fetus normally has two large right-to-left shunts: one from the right atrium to

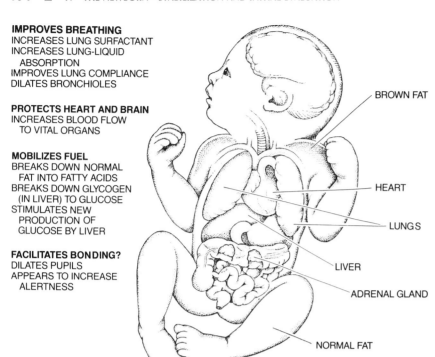

IMPROVES BREATHING
INCREASES LUNG SURFACTANT
INCREASES LUNG-LIQUID
  ABSORPTION
IMPROVES LUNG COMPLIANCE
DILATES BRONCHIOLES

PROTECTS HEART AND BRAIN
INCREASES BLOOD FLOW
  TO VITAL ORGANS

MOBILIZES FUEL
BREAKS DOWN NORMAL
  FAT INTO FATTY ACIDS
BREAKS DOWN GLYCOGEN
  (IN LIVER) TO GLUCOSE
STIMULATES NEW
  PRODUCTION OF
  GLUCOSE BY LIVER

FACILITATES BONDING?
DILATES PUPILS
APPEARS TO INCREASE
  ALERTNESS

BROWN FAT

HEART

LUNGS

LIVER

ADRENAL GLAND

NORMAL FAT

FIGURE 22–1. Adaptational effects of a catecholamine surge during delivery include promotion of normal breathing, alteration of blood flow to protect the heart and brain against potential asphyxia, immediate mobilization of fuel for energy and, possibly, enhancement of maternal-infant attachment. (From Lagercrantz, H., and Slotkin, T. A.: The "stress" of being born. Sci. Am. 254:100, 1986.)

the left atrium through the foramen ovale, and the second from the pulmonary artery to the aorta across the ductus arteriosus (Fig. 22–2). In utero, as a result of constricted pulmonary arterioles that produce high pulmonary vascular resistance, only a small percentage of the fetal cardiac output flows through the lungs. The fetus accommodates well to a normal PO_2 of 20 to 25 mm Hg in its best-oxygenated blood, which comes through the umbilical vein from the placenta. As a result of the right-to-left shunts through the foramen ovale and the ductus arteriosus, the best-oxygenated blood streams from the umbilical vein to the inferior vena cava, through the foramen ovale into the left atrium and ventricle, and then out the aorta, thus supplying best-oxygenated blood to the brain and myocardium of the fetus (Fig. 22–2).

At delivery, two major changes occur in this system: First, the umbilical cord is clamped, eliminating the placenta as a gas-exchange organ as well as a low-resistance "shunt." The second major change is the initiation of respiration by the fetus. Expansion of the lungs results in a marked drop in pulmonary vascular resistance that is furthered by the increased level of oxygenation that occurs as the infant begins to breathe (Fig. 22–3). With these changes, the flow of blood to the left atrium via the pulmonary veins increases, so that left atrial pressure exceeds right atrial pressure and functionally closes the foramen ovale. When pulmonary vascular resistance drops to a level lower than the systemic vascular pressure, the ductus arteriosus is functionally closed.

At birth, the lungs normally are partially filled with fluid. Therefore, the initial breaths taken by the infant must inflate the lungs and effect a change in vascular pressures so that lung water is absorbed into the pulmonary arterial system and cleared from the lung. At the same time, inflation is a powerful mechanism for the release of pulmonary surface-active material, which increases compliance of the lung and enables stabilization of functional residual capacity (Taeusch et al., 1974; Massaro and Massaro, 1983).

FETAL RESERVE

Since the fetus is normally relatively hypoxemic (PO_2 of 20 to 24 mm Hg) and during labor is subjected to stresses associated with both increased oxygen consumption and interrupted gas exchange, the fetus is at particular risk for asphyxia at the time of birth. However, the fetus has several compensatory mechanisms that help protect it: fetal hemoglobin has greater oxygen affinity than adult hemoglobin, fetal tissues have an increased ability to extract oxygen, and the fetus has greater tissue resistance to acidosis than does the adult. In addition, as mentioned in the discussion of "stress," the fetus has mechanisms that compensate for asphyxia. These include bradycardia and the "diving reflex" (similar to that found in diving mammals), which allows a preferential distribution of blood flow to the brain, adrenal glands, and heart and away from the lungs, gut, liver, spleen, kidney, and carcass. The fetus is also capable of decreasing oxygen consumption and switching to anaerobic glycolysis, as long as liver glycogen stores are adequate.

■ ASPHYXIA

PHYSIOLOGY

Asphyxia is defined as a combination of *hypoxemia, hypercapnia,* and *metabolic acidemia.* If lung expansion does not occur in the minutes following birth and the infant is unable to establish ventilation and pulmonary perfusion, a progressive cycle of worsening hypoxemia, hypercapnia, and metabolic acidemia evolves. Pulmonary vascular resistance remains high, the ductus arteriosus remains widely patent (Fig. 22–4), and right-to-left shunting through the foramen ovale also persists. Once this process begins, it tends to be self-perpetuating and may result in serious tissue acidosis, which ultimately may lead to irreversible organ damage. Asphyxia may be caused by maternal, placental, or fetal factors that reduce the fetal affected the infant's level of asphyxia at the moment of birth.

DELIVERY ROOM ASSESSMENT

When called to the delivery room to care for an infant who has failed to establish normal ventilation, the physician must rapidly determine whether the infant's problem (1) is due to asphyxia that began because of maternal and fetal conditions before or during labor and delivery or (2) represents a condition that was initiated in the newborn infant following birth. In the first case, the asphyxia represents a process that must be interrupted rapidly and that should respond to standard resuscitation. In the latter case, the infant was probably vigorous at birth and then, in attempting to establish respiration, developed apnea, cyanosis, or bradycardia. Differential diagnosis in the second infant with asphyxia after delivery requires rapid assessment of conditions that might be causing obstruction of the airway.

Obstruction of the airway may be due to (1) meconium aspiration or severe pneumonia that will respond to suctioning; (2) intrathoracic malformations that interfere with ventilation, e.g., cystic adenomatoid malformation and

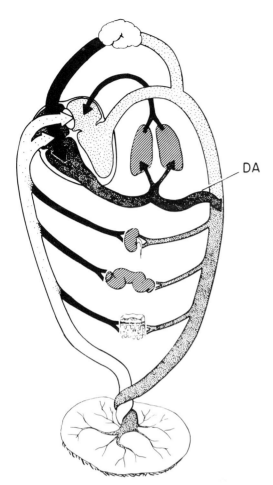

FIGURE 22–2. The fetal circulation. *Oxygenated blood leaves the placenta by way of the umbilical vein (vessel without stippling). It flows into the portal sinus in the liver (not shown), and a variable portion of it perfuses the liver. The remainder passes from the protal sinus through the ductus venosus into the inferior vena cava, where it joins blood from the viscera (represented by kidney, gut, and skin). About half of the inferior vena cava flow passes through the foramen ovale to the left atrium, where it mixes with a small amount of pulmonary venous blood. This relatively well-oxygenated blood* (light stippling) *supplies the heart and brain by way of the ascending aorta. The other half of the inferior vena cava stream mixes with superior vena cava blood and enters the right ventricle (blood in the right atrium and ventricle has little oxygen, which is denoted by heavy stippling). Because the pulmonary arterioles are constructed, most of the blood in the main pulmonary artery flows through the ductus venosus (DV) so that the descending aorta's blood has less oxygen* (heavy stippling) *than blood in the ascending aorta* (light stippling). *(From Avery, G. N.: Neonatology. Philadelphia, J. B. Lippincott, 1987.)*

reserve (Table 22–1). Since the duration of asphyxia is critical to the outcome of the infant, it is important to evaluate rapidly all of the factors contributing to the asphyxia and to interrupt the process as early as possible.

Figure 22–5 demonstrates the classic cardiopulmonary changes in an infant suffering from asphyxia, as described by Dawes (1968). The initial phase of asphyxia is marked by increased respiratory effort *(primary hyperpnea)*. This is followed by *primary apnea*, which lasts approximately 1 minute. Rhythmic gasping then begins and is maintained at a rate of 8 to 10 gasps per minute for several minutes, after which the gasps become weaker and slower until they cease, which is called *secondary apnea*. Obviously, some variation occurs in the period of gasping, as a result of prior maternal and fetal conditions that may have

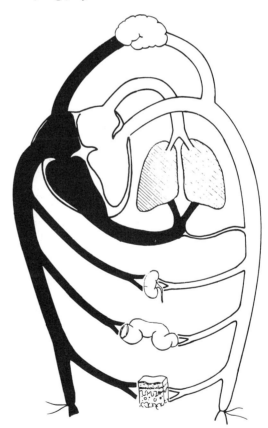

FIGURE 22–3. The circulation in the normal newborn. *After expansion of the lungs and ligation of the umbilical cord, pulmonary blood flow increases and left atrial and systemic arterial pressures rise while pulmonary arterial and right heart pressures fall. When the left atrial pressure exceeds right atrial pressure, the foramen ovale closes so that all of the inferior and superior vena cava blood leaves the right atrium, enters the right ventricle, and is pumped through the pulmonary artery toward the lung. With the rise in systemic arterial pressure and fall in pulmonary arterial pressure, flow through the ductus arteriosus becomes left to right, and the ductus constricts and closes. The course of the circulation is the same as in the adult. (From Avery, G. N.: Neonatology. Philadelphia, J. B. Lippincott, 1987.)*

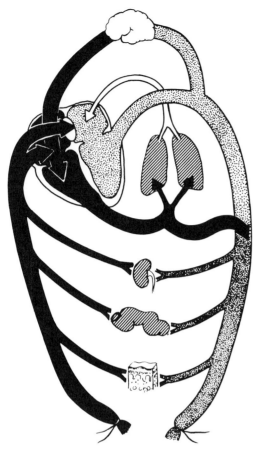

FIGURE 22–4. The circulation in an asphyxiated newborn with incomplete expansion of the lungs. *Pulmonary vascular resistance is high, pulmonary blood flow is low (normal number of pulmonary vein), and flow through the ductus arteriosus is high. With little pulmonary arterial flow, left atrial pressure drops below right atrial pressure, the foramen ovale opens, and vena caval blood flows through the foramen into the left atrium. Partially venous blood goes to the brain via the ascending aorta. The blood of the descending aorta that goes to the viscera has less oxygen than that of the ascending aorta (heavy stippling) because of the reverse flow through the ductus arteriosus. Thus, the circulation is the same as in the fetus except that there is less well-oxygenated blood in the inferior vena cava and umbilical vein. (From Avery, G. N.: Neonatology. Philadelphia, J. B. Lippincott, 1987.)*

diaphragmatic hernia; or (3) congenital malformations of the airway, e.g., laryngeal web. In addition, pneumothorax should always be considered in an infant who is initially vigorous at birth. Obviously, if asphyxia is due to malformations, standard resuscitation and establishment of ventilation must be accompanied by interventions to correct the underlying cause.

UNIVERSAL PREREQUISITES FOR RESUSCITATION

Skilled Personnel. In the United States, 4 million babies per year are born in 5000 hospitals with delivery services. Ninety per cent of these hospitals are small, Level 1 services; 5 per cent are Level 2; and another 5 per cent are Level 3 (Bloom and Cropley, 1987). Thus, the majority of infants are born in hospitals that do not have sophisticated perinatal programs. In their combined program for neonatal resuscitation, the American Heart Association (AHA) and the American Academy of Pediatrics (AAP) emphasize the basic principle that effective resus-

citation must begin with the awareness that *well-trained personnel must be immediately available in any setting where an infant is likely to be delivered.** Identification and training of staff is, therefore, the first step in preparation for neonatal resuscitation. The second step is close communication between obstetricians and pediatricians to identify high-risk women before labor if possible, to prevent abnormal labors, and to focus planning for the resuscitation of infants thus identified. Understanding the special needs of different kinds of infants enables caregivers to anticipate and prepare for various types of resuscitation appropriately.

Resuscitation of the newborn infant is best done in the delivery room or immediately adjacent to it, so that the time lapse between delivery and initiation of resuscitation is minimized.

Equipment. The equipment that should be available for neonatal resuscitation is listed in Table 22–2, and is divided into (1) items needed in every institution for resuscitation of low-risk term infants with unexpected problems and (2) additional equipment required for resuscitation of high-risk or known preterm infants.

■ MANAGEMENT AT DELIVERY

ASSESSMENT OF DEGREE OF ASPHYXIA

The Apgar score (Table 22–3) was originally introduced to help quantitate the initial evaluation of newborn infants. Apgar scores should be assigned at 1, 5, and 10 minutes, and if the infant still requires resuscitation, at 15 and 20 minutes as well. The scoring process requires the discipline to evaluate several aspects of the infant at once within the 1st minute of life and also serves as a framework around which to gear resuscitative efforts, since the score is an

---

*The American College of Obstetrics and Gynecology, the American Society of Anesthesiology, the American Academy of Family Physicians, and the Canadian Pediatric Society have also stated their support for this principle.

TABLE 22–1. Conditions Affecting Fetal Reserve

DETERMINANTS	COMMON DISORDERS
Maternal	
Infection	Amnionitis
Lungs	Pneumonia, asthma, ARDS*
Heart	Arrhythmia, structural defect, failure
Blood	Anemia, hemoglobinopathy
Blood vessels	Systemic lupus erythematosus, diabetes, hypertension, hypotension
Uterus	Hypertonus, malformation, rupture
Other	Genetic, drugs, deformities, preterm labor, multiple gestation, abnormal fetal presentation
Placental	
Age	Postmaturity
Size, morphology	Abruptio placentae, placenta previa
Fetal	
Umbilical cord	Knot, entanglement, prolapse, compression, thrombosis
Blood	Anemia
Metabolic	Inborn error, aneuploidy
Other	Infection, hydrops, malformations

*Adult Respiratory Distress Syndrome
(Adapted from Jacobs, M., and Phibbs, R.: Clin. Perinatol. *16*(4):785, 1989.)

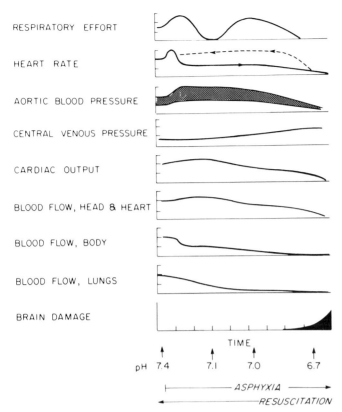

RESPIRATORY EFFORT

HEART RATE

AORTIC BLOOD PRESSURE

CENTRAL VENOUS PRESSURE

CARDIAC OUTPUT

BLOOD FLOW, HEAD & HEART

BLOOD FLOW, BODY

BLOOD FLOW, LUNGS

BRAIN DAMAGE

TIME

pH   7.4   7.1   7.0   6.7

⊢————— ASPHYXIA ————→

←————————— RESUSCITATION

FIGURE 22–5. The sequence of cardiopulmonary changes with asphyxia and resuscitation. *Time is on the horizontal axis: Asphyxia progresses from left to right; resuscitation proceeds from right to left. Units of time are not given. If there is complete interruption of respiratory gas exchange, the entire process of asphyxia from extreme left to right could occur in about 10 minutes. It could take much longer with an asphyxiating process that only partly interrupts gas exchange or does so completely, but only for repeated brief periods. With resuscitation, the process reverses, beginning at the point to which asphyxia has proceeded. (Adapted from Dawes, G.: Foetal and Neonatal Physiology. Chicago, Year Book Publishers, 1968 and Avery, G. N.: Neonatology. Philadelphia, J. B. Lippincott, 1987.)*

indicator of responsiveness to therapy as well as a way of defining infants who are at high risk for further difficulty. It is not surprising that the score at 5 minutes and later is more predictive of survival and neurologic status than the 1-minute score, since the ability to interrupt and reverse the process indicates not only successful intervention but also that the process was not established for a long period in utero.

OVERVIEW OF RESUSCITATION

Initial resuscitation of the depressed newborn always includes maintenance of body temperature and rapidly drying and placing the infant under a radiant heater. Clearing the airway is essential; this may be done using a bulb syringe, or, in the case of the infant born through thick, particulate material, by endotracheal suction. A nasogastric tube may be passed into the stomach. The infant is placed on an open bed near a table with all of the equipment (see Table 22–2) available and then assessed for further intervention. A double-clamped segment of umbilical cord should be obtained for cord blood gas analysis.

AMERICAN HEART ASSOCIATION– AMERICAN ACADEMY OF PEDIATRICS (AHA-AAP) APPROACH TO RESUSCITATION

The AHA-AAP approach to resuscitation of the newborn infant takes the same type of clinical information that is gathered from the Apgar score and uses it to develop a schema for approaching resuscitation of the term infant (Fig. 22–6).

Infants with a Score of 7 or Above. These vigorous infants generally do not require resuscitation other than some brief period of oxygen blown over the face. In approaching these infants who are not at risk for retrolental fibroplasia, it is important to remember (1) that administration of oxygen is accompanied by decreased pulmonary vascular resistance and increased pulmonary blood flow, and (2) that at birth, the newborn infant's lungs are normally full of fluid, which is cleared by resorption into the pulmonary arterial system. Excessive suctioning of clear fluid from the nasopharynx is not helpful and may, in fact, contribute to atelectasis.

Infants with a Score of 4 to 6. These infants require stimulation and administration of 100 per cent oxygen by face mask; in addition, they may require some use of bag and mask ventilation to expand the lungs. Most infants respond to these measures and begin spontaneous respi-

TABLE 22–2. Equipment for Neonatal Resuscitation

LOW-RISK AND TERM INFANTS
Radiant warmer to maintain temperature control
Stethoscope
Source of warm, humidified oxygen
Suction source
Suction catheters and DeLee trap
Nasogastric tube and syringe
Oral airway
Apparatus for bag and mask ventilation of infant, either anesthesia bag or Ambu bag with masks for different size infants
Laryngoscope with pencil handle
Endotracheal tubes (Portex)—sizes 2.5, 3.0, and 3.5
Fluids (D_5W, $D_{10}W$, normal saline)
Medications (naloxone hydrochloride [Narcan], sodium bicarbonate, atropine, calcium gluconate, epinephrine)
Clock or stopwatch
Tubes for obtaining blood gases or other samples
Equipment for placing umbilical catheter
Equipment for micro-technique for measuring blood gases
Portable x-ray equipment
HIGH-RISK AND PRETERM INFANTS
All of the equipment listed earlier, plus
Spotlight
Manometer for gauging pressure being used in ventilation
Blender for delivering oxygen in concentrations ranging from room air to 100 per cent, with heated nebulizer
Oxygen analyzer
EKG electrodes
Heart rate monitoring equipment
Blood pressure monitoring equipment
Transcutaneous oxygen and carbon dioxide monitoring equipment
Hemoglobin saturation monitor
Blood gas syringes, heparinized and ready to use
Blood gas laboratory immediately available (10-minute processing time)
Volume expander (5 per cent human albumin) and/or blood available on emergency basis
Umbilical artery catheter must be set up and ready to insert, with vascular pressure monitor
Emergency medications with estimated dosages calculated

TABLE 22–3. Apgar Scoring System

FEATURES EVALUATED	0 POINTS	1 POINT	2 POINTS
Heart rate	0	<100	>100
Respiratory effort	Apnea	Irregular, shallow, or gasping respirations	Vigorous and crying
Color	Pale, blue	Pale or blue extremities	Pink
Muscle tone	Absent	Weak, passive tone	Active movement
Reflex irritability	Absent	Grimace	Active avoidance

ration. It is important to empty the stomach of any infant who is receiving bag and mask ventilation.

Infants with a Score of 1 to 3. These infants usually require intubation and expansion of the lung. However, if staff skilled in intubation and the appropriate equipment are not immediately available, initial bag and mask ventilation usually is adequate to sustain the infant. Further resuscitative steps depend on the heart-rate response to ventilation.

Infants with an Apgar Score of 0. Virtually no live born infant should be assigned this score; and resuscitation of an infant who truly has an Apgar score of zero, indicative of cardiac arrest prior to delivery, is probably a subject for ethical discussion. However, it is frequently impossible in the excitement that surrounds the delivery of an asphyxiated infant to make absolutely certain that there is no heartbeat, and in such circumstances, resuscitation should proceed immediately as for an infant in the previous group with an Apgar score of 1 to 3, with the addition of cardiac compression.

The primer for resuscitation techniques is the manual prepared by the American Heart Association in conjunction with the American Academy of Pediatrics (Bloom and Cropley, 1987). It provides very complete and well-illustrated instructions on how to proceed with mask ventilation, cardiac compression, and intubation. Figure 22–7 shows the landmarks of the larynx that should be visualized for successful intubation of the newborn. If an infant does not respond to adequate ventilation and cardiac compression with an increase in heart rate to >80 after 30 seconds of positive-pressure insufflation, then the administration of medications should be considered. Figure 22–8 contains the chart developed by the AHA-AAP for administration of drugs, including epinephrine, volume expanders, sodium bicarbonate, dopamine, and naloxone. Table 22–4 provides the recommended drug dosages for neonatal resuscitation.

Expansion of the Lungs. Frequently, the only requirement for initiation of resuscitation of the newborn is adequate expansion of the lung. It is obvious that the airway must be cleared prior to attempts to expand the lung. Initial inflation of the gasless, fluid-filled lung is best accomplished by application of a relatively high inflation pressure (sufficient to move the chest, usually 25 to 40 cm H_2O) over a relatively long time (0.5 to 1 second). The object is to inflate the lung as well as to trap some gas during exhalation and thereby create a functional

residual capacity. This process occurs over a series of breaths. The term infant with a strong chest wall and larger terminal airways is better able to generate the necessary forces to achieve lung inflation than is the premature infant who may need to be assisted. Lung inflation also stimulates surfactant secretion in mature lungs, and this response is enhanced by large-volume inflation. When intubation is necessary, it should be remembered that no attempt should last longer than 30 to 45 seconds before returning to bag and mask ventilation to support the child.

Administration of Epinephrine. If the infant does not respond to intubation and ventilation with an increase in heart rate, epinephrine should be administered endotracheally.

Umbilical Vessel Catheterization. In the high-risk or significantly asphyxiated infant, it is important to place an umbilical catheter, preferably in the umbilical artery, to obtain arterial blood gases and other samples as well as to monitor arterial pressure. Changes in arterial pulse pressure and mean pressure can thus be followed during the resuscitation and provide important indicators of cardiovascular responsiveness. In addition, appropriate medications can be administered easily through the catheter.

Correcting Metabolic Acidosis. Whenever possible, samples for cord blood gas determination should be obtained. In addition, the infant's blood gases should be measured immediately and the results known prior to the infusion of sodium bicarbonate; and, certainly, no bicarbonate should be given unless ventilation has been established and $PaCO_2$ is normal or low. The most severely asphyxiated infants are those with an arterial pH of 7.0 or less and a calculated base deficit of 25 mEq/l or greater in the presence of a marked elevation of $PaCO_2$. By means of artificial ventilation alone, this calculated deficit can be reduced by approximately 10 mEq/l if the infant's circulation is normal and oxygenation is achieved. This effect results from a significant bicarbonate shift that occurs when $PaCO_2$ exceeds 70 mm Hg and therefore must be taken into consideration in calculations for correcting base deficit. Some additional correction occurs with ventilation at pH levels above 7.0, and therefore, the dose of bicarbonate administered should always be no more than one-quarter of the initially calculated value. Blood gas studies should be repeated prior to giving additional increments of bicarbonate. The equation for calculation of base replacement is:

$$mEq\ Base = \frac{0.3 \times weight\ in\ kilograms \times base\ deficit\ in\ mEq/l}{4}$$

Bicarbonate should always be diluted 1:1 with sterile water and administered very slowly. Arterial blood pressure should be measured both before and after bicarbonate is given, since the administration of sodium bicarbonate may unmask hypovolemia that has not been apparent because of peripheral vasoconstriction.

Support of the Cardiovascular System. Many conditions that produce asphyxia or preterm birth may be associated with loss of a large volume of blood, and the

Overview of
Resuscitation in the Delivery Room

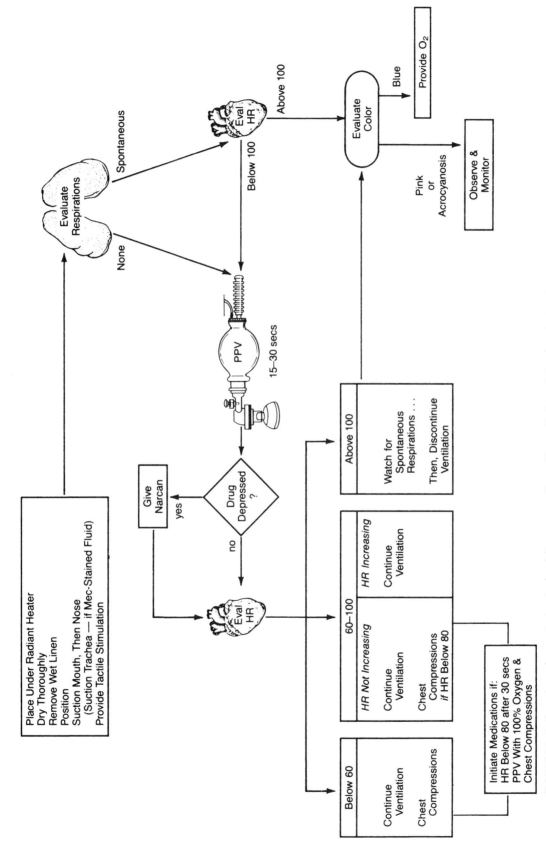

FIGURE 22–6. *Overview of resuscitation in the delivery room. (From Bloom, R. S., and Cropley, C: American Heart Association–American Academy of Pediatrics Textbook of Neonatal Resuscitation. Dallas, American Heart Association National Center, 1987. Reproduced with permission. © Textbook of Neonatal Resuscitation, 1987. Copyright American Heart Association.)*

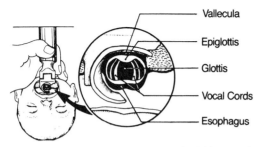

FIGURE 22–7. Landmarks of the larynx that should be visualized for intubation of the newborn. (From Bloom, R. S., and Cropley, C: American Heart Association–American Academy of Pediatrics Textbook of Neonatal Resuscitation. Dallas, American Heart Association National Center, 1987. Reproduced with permission. © Textbook of Neonatal Resuscitation, 1987. Copyright American Heart Association.)

asphyxiated infant is even less able to compensate for large losses of blood volume than the normal infant. However, the majority of asphyxiated infants are *not* hypovolemic, and it is often a challenge to assess the infant's circulatory status to determine whether hypovolemia is the cause of hypotension or whether the infant is suffering cardiovascular depression because of some other problem. Physiologic variables to be remembered are

1. The association of falsely high arterial blood pressure readings with acidosis (which may respond to sodium bicarbonate administration, as mentioned above).

2. The association of hypocapnia with hypotension, so that infants who are being overventilated may have falsely low arterial blood pressure readings.

3. That an infant with normal blood pressure who has poor perfusion may be maximally vasoconstricted, and therefore, significant hypotension may be masked.

4. That an infant who is distressed and in pain may have a falsely elevated blood pressure level.

5. That the normal range of blood pressure for very small prematures may be low (see Appendix). The physician should assume that the blood pressure is normal in infants with good oxygenation and good peripheral perfusion and no signs of circulatory collapse.

6. That monitoring an infant's hematocrit levels over time can be enormously helpful. A drop in hematocrit during the first 2 hours after birth may be an indication of hypovolemia, since infants have the ability to mobilize fluid rapidly.

7. That preterm newborn infants ordinarily do not exhibit tachycardia as a sign of shock, and therefore, a rapid heart rate generally is not useful as an indicator of volume status.

Support of the circulatory system and treatment of hypovolemic shock are best accomplished by the administration of small (10 ml/kg) transfusions of whole blood. However, it is often appropriate to give an initial infusion of 10 ml/kg of normal saline and note the infant's response

TABLE 22–4. Medications for Neonatal Resuscitation

MEDICATION	CONCENTRATION TO ADMINISTER	PREPARATION	DOSAGE/ROUTE*	TOTAL DOSE/INFANT			RATE/PRECAUTIONS
Epinephrine	1:10,000	1 ml	0.1–0.3 ml/kg IV or IT	Weight 1 kg 2 kg 3 kg 4 kg		Total ml's 0.1–0.3 ml 0.2–0.6 ml 0.3–0.9 ml 0.4–1.2 ml	Give rapidly
Volume expanders	Whole blood 5% albumin Normal saline Ringer lactate	40 ml	10 ml/kg IV	Weight 1 kg 2 kg 3 kg 4 kg		Total ml's 10 ml 20 ml 30 ml 40 ml	Give over 5 to 10 minutes
Sodium bicarbonate	0.5 mEq/ml (4.2 per cent solution)	20 ml or two 10-ml prefilled syringes	2 mEq/kg IV	Weight 1 kg 2 kg 3 kg 4 kg	Total dose 2 mEq 4 mEq 6 mEq 8 mEq	Total ml's 4 ml 8 ml 12 ml 16 ml	Give *slowly*, over at least 2 minutes Give only if infant is being effectively ventilated
Naloxone	0.4 mg/ml	1 ml	0.25 ml/kg IV, IM, SQ, IT	Weight 1 kg 2 kg 3 kg 4 kg		Total ml's 0.25 ml 0.50 ml 0.75 ml 1.00 ml	Give rapidly
	1.0 mg/ml	1 ml	0.1 ml/kg IV, IM, SQ, IT	1 kg 2 kg 3 kg 4 kg		0.1 ml 0.2 ml 0.3 ml 0.4 ml	
Dopamine	$6 \times \dfrac{\text{weight} \quad \text{desired dose}}{(\text{kg}) \times (\mu g/kg/min)}{\text{desired fluid (ml/hr)}} = \begin{array}{l}\text{mg of dopamine}\\\text{per 100 ml of}\\\text{solution}\end{array}$		Begin at 5 μg/kg/min (may increase to 20 μg/kg/min if necessary) IV	Weight 1 kg 2 kg 3 kg 4 kg		Total μg/min 5–20 μg/min 10–40 μg/min 15–60 μg/min 20–80 μg/min	Give as a continuous infusion using an infusion pump Monitor heart rate and blood pressure closely Seek consultation

*IM—Intramuscular; IT—intratracheal; IV—intravenous; SQ—subcutaneous.

(From Bloom, R. S., and Cropley, C. S.: American Heart Association—American Academy of Pediatrics Textbook of Neonatal Resuscitation. Dallas, American Heart Association National Center, 1987. Reproduced with permission. © Textbook of Neonatal Resuscitation, 1987. Copyright American Heart Association.)

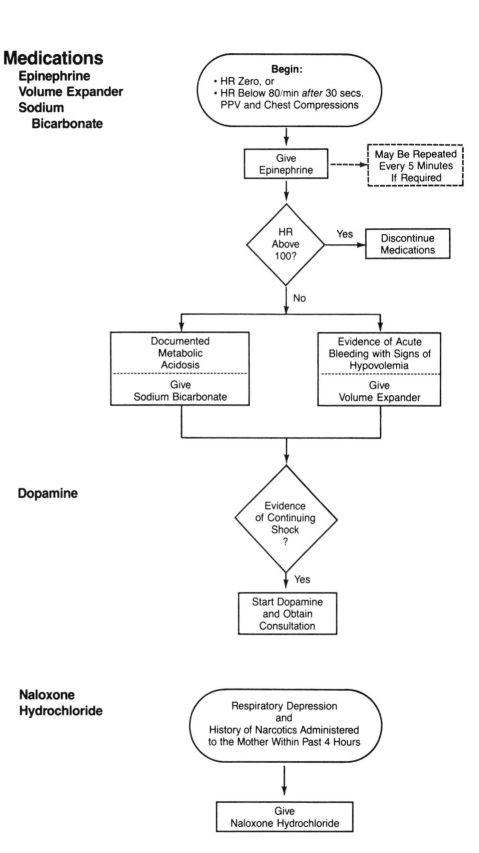

Medications
 Epinephrine
 Volume Expander
 Sodium
  Bicarbonate

Dopamine

Naloxone
Hydrochloride

FIGURE 22–8. Schedule for administration of drugs for resuscitation of the newborn. (From Bloom, R. S., and Cropley, C: American Heart Association–American Academy of Pediatrics Textbook of Neonatal Resuscitation. Dallas, American Heart Association National Center, 1987. Reproduced with permission. © Textbook of Neonatal Resuscitation, 1987. Copyright American Heart Association.)

in blood pressure, peripheral perfusion, and oxygenation. Five per cent albumin in saline may also be used while awaiting the availability of either packed red cells or whole blood. In administering volume replacement, it is of the utmost importance that it be given slowly, since some vascular beds (particularly those of the brain) may already be maximally dilated in response to systemic hypotension, and excessive pressure may be transmitted to the fragile capillaries and lead to intracranial hemorrhage.

Myocardial Failure. In infants who have had prolonged or severe asphyxia, myocardial failure due to poor contractility may occur, evidenced by hypotension that persists after initial resuscitation. Such infants may respond to an inotropic agent such as dopamine at a starting dose of 2.5 to 5 μg/kg/min and increased as needed up to 15 to 20 μg/kg/min to produce an adequate response. It may be useful in these infants to pass a second umbilical catheter through the umbilical vein, via the ductus venosus, into the right atrium to monitor central venous pressure in addition to arterial pressure.

Continuation of Support After Resuscitation. One of the factors essential to successful resuscitation is the ability to identify the infant who has continuing difficulties after resuscitation and, thus, to facilitate prevention of a relapse. This applies particularly to the premature infant with respiratory distress syndrome who initially responds favorably to treatment with ventilation and sodium bicarbonate but then requires continued cardiorespiratory support to prevent his or her respiratory distress from becoming severe and causing another cycle of hypoxia and acidosis. Another example is the infant born after undergoing an episode of fetal distress, who may have reactive pulmonary vasculature. If such an infant is allowed to become hypoxic, pulmonary vasoconstriction may occur (or worsen) and progress to persistent pulmonary hypertension of the newborn.

■ THINGS TO AVOID IN RESUSCITATION

Successful resuscitation of a newborn infant involves not only interrupting the cycle of hypoxia and acidemia and bringing the infant back toward the physiologic norm but also avoiding iatrogenic damage. There are, therefore, some important "rules" of resuscitation:

1. *Don't panic if an endotracheal tube cannot be placed immediately.* Concentrate on bag and mask ventilation and call for help. Don't assume that medication is a substitute for ventilation.

2. *Don't do excessive suctioning of clear fluid from the infant's nasopharynx.* Fluid is normally absorbed into the lungs.

3. *Don't use excessive oxygen concentrations to resuscitate the premature infant unless the infant clearly requires it.*

4. *Don't use too much ventilatory pressure to expand the infant's lungs.* Initially this may be significantly higher than it is within 30 to 45 minutes after birth. Use good clinical judgment. Watch the infant's chest and listen to breath sounds. Try reducing ventilation with hand ventilation to ensure that the lowest pressure necessary is being used. Excessive pressure on lungs that are normalizing may decrease venous return to the heart and decrease cardiac output and cause injury to lung tissue.

5. *Don't give volume or sodium bicarbonate automatically.* Each of these agents has been associated with production of intracranial hemorrhage in animal models.

6. *Don't focus or rely too heavily on cardiac resuscitation,* since the usual problem in neonatal resuscitation is the need for ventilatory support.

7. *Don't spend more than 5 minutes on umbilical artery catheter placement* if an infant is dying. Place an umbilical venous line temporarily. Administer epinephrine through the endotracheal tube.

8. *Don't withhold oxygen from the term or post-term infant with meconium aspiration or asphyxia,* since these infants may have reactive pulmonary blood vessels and develop pulmonary vasoconstriction if oxygen administration is not generous.

■ SPECIAL CONDITIONS REQUIRING ATTENTION DURING RESUSCITATION

EXTREMELY PREMATURE INFANT (<1000 g)

Resuscitation of the very premature infant begins in utero, and therefore, whenever possible, such infants should be born in a perinatal center with skilled staff from the obstetric, anesthetic, and neonatal teams in attendance. The fragility of these infants requires gentleness in handling and a high level of skill in the staff performing the resuscitation. Because of their relatively large surface area, attention to immediate drying and temperature control is of even greater importance for these infants than for the normal newborn. When possible, they should be moved to a small warm room adjacent to the delivery room and carefully dried and placed under a radiant warmer for resuscitation. It is essential that the gas used for very small infants, even for resuscitation, be warmed and humidified. Many of these infants require immediate intubation as part of their resuscitation, and in many centers, such infants are intubated routinely to enhance the clearance of lung water and the release of surfactant. If infants are intubated routinely, it is of great importance to avoid overventilation, which may cause interstitial emphysema and/or pneumothoraces as well as interfere with cardiac output. Other centers observe tiny infants briefly and provide respiratory support, particularly in the form of oxygen and continuous distending pressure via nasal prongs, if there is any evidence of respiratory deterioration. Particularly if the infants are known to be surfactant deficient, it would appear appropriate to initially intubate these tiny infants, treat them with surfactant, and then carefully evaluate their status to determine whether or not further respiratory support is needed. In resuscitating very small infants, it is also important to avoid hyperoxia; therefore, it is recommended that the oxygen blender be set at 40 per cent when resuscitation is begun, then turned down as rapidly as possible, and thereafter increased only if the infant has clinical signs of cyanosis.

Most of these tiny infants also benefit from having an umbilical artery catheter placed so that the initial monitoring of their blood gases does not require painful procedures for obtaining blood or for the administration of fluid, drugs, or volume. Arterial blood pressure monitoring is important in this group of infants as an adjunct to assessing adequacy of circulating blood volume. It should be realized, however, that the range of mean blood pressure for the tiny infant is wide and initially may be as low as 24 to 25 mm Hg. In an infant who is well oxygenated at low inspired oxygen concentrations and who has good peripheral perfusion, low blood pressure alone should never be used as the basis for volume administration. Careful administration and monitoring of blood glucose concentrations are also critical.

Finally, it is important to move these infants from the resuscitation area to the nursery with as little disruption of their support systems as possible. Therefore, a resuscitation bed that is fully equipped to be moved from the delivery area to the nursery is essential to maintain stabilization. It also enables continuous observation of these fragile infants whose course may change rapidly during the first few hours after birth.

MECONIUM ASPIRATION

It is estimated that approximately 11 per cent of all pregnancies are complicated by passage of meconium and that 2 per cent of infants have some degree of aspiration syndrome, ranging from some minor initial tachypnea to very severe meconium-aspiration pneumonia with pulmonary hypertension. There are two reasons why it is essential that skilled personnel are present at the delivery of an infant born through meconium:

1. It is critical that any *particulate* matter be removed from the infant's airway as rapidly as possible. A combined approach of suctioning of the nasopharynx on the perineum, followed by intubation and gentle tracheal suction, appears to be the most effective procedure for preventing obstruction of the airway and pneumonitis. It should be noted that it is *not* necessary to intubate an infant who is simply born through fluid that is stained with meconium but does not contain particulate material. Unnecessary intubation can cause iatrogenic damage. The most severe meconium-aspiration pneumonias occur when an infant has passed a large amount of meconium in utero and is asphyxiated and gasping, thus moving large amounts of meconium into the thoracic airways prior to birth.

2. The passage of meconium indicates that an infant has been in trouble at some period in time. This group of infants is more susceptible to having reactive pulmonary vessels, which may reconstrict with hypoxia. They require careful initial evaluation and close observation to ensure that oxygenation is adequate and to prevent the gradual development of hypoxia and consequent pulmonary vasoconstriction, setting off the cycle that ultimately may result in persistent pulmonary hypertension of the newborn.

HYDROPS

The evaluation and resuscitation of the infant with hydrops, as for very small premature infants, begins with interdisciplinary management by the perinatal team to assess the fetus and to arrive at decisions as to optimal time of delivery (see also Chapter 88, Hydrops). Ultrasound evaluation is recommended to determine whether or not the infant would benefit from removal of excessive fluid from either the abdominal or thoracic cavity prior to delivery. In preparing for resuscitation of a hydropic infant, it is critical that equipment be set up and a member of the team assigned to perform either paracentesis or thoracentesis, or both, immediately after the birth, if the amount of fluid should interfere with the ability to ventilate the infant. In addition, it is essential to have either whole blood or packed red cells available at the resuscitation site if the cause of the hydrops is related to anemia. It is critical to realize that these infants have extremely stiff lungs and may require high ventilatory pressures, including high end-expiratory pressure, for initial stabilization. It is usually necessary to continue administering oxygen at high pressures until the infant begins to mobilize and clear fluid. In severe cases, it may also be appropriate to have a dose of diuretic already drawn up and ready to administer in the delivery room. It is always appropriate to catheterize both the umbilical vein and umbilical artery so that central venous pressure, as well as systemic pressures, can be measured for evaluation of volume status. In addition, for severely anemic infants the hematocrit can be augmented by immediate, isovolemic exchange transfusion through the two catheters. Staff should be aware that skin electrodes and saturation monitors frequently do not function accurately when used for infants with hydrops.

INFANTS WITH SEVERE MALFORMATIONS

Sometimes the resuscitation team is faced with an infant who has apparent, severe malformations. Resuscitation should proceed in a normal fashion unless (1) the staff present at the delivery have enough experience and skill to recognize that the malformations are associated with conditions incompatible with life; and (2) there has been some foreknowledge of the possibility of malformations and the family has requested that there be no resuscitation of a severely malformed infant. Otherwise, it is appropriate to proceed with the resuscitation and stabilize the infant so that an accurate diagnosis can be made and the family can see the baby and participate in further decision-making about their child.

■ CONTROVERSIES IN RESUSCITATION

Administration of Sodium Bicarbonate. The routine use of sodium bicarbonate to treat asphyxiated infants is clearly fraught with danger ranging from problems associated with hypernatremia and high osmotic load to those related to rapid shifts in volume and circulatory status of the infant. Complete avoidance of sodium bicarbonate, however, may delay an infant's recovery from severe asphyxia. Therefore, it is probably most reasonable to give bicarbonate with extreme caution.

Intubation of the Extremely-Low-Birth-Weight Infant (<1000 g). Although many centers have adopted a policy to intubate and ventilate at birth all infants weighing less than 1000 g, there remains some controversy. Other centers prefer to stabilize and watch vigorous, extremely low-birth-weight infants (James, 1987) and only give respiratory support if signs of respiratory distress syndrome develop. The last-mentioned centers recommend that an

TABLE 22–5. Prevalence Rate of Cerebral Palsy by Apgar Score and Birth Weight

Apgar Score	INFANTS < 2500 g			INFANTS > 2500 g		
	Mortality in 1st Year (Per Cent)	Per Cent of Survivors with Cerebral Palsy	Number of Cerebral Palsy Cases	Mortality in 1st Yr (Per Cent)	Per Cent of Survivors with Cerebral Palsy	Number of Cerebral Palsy Cases
7–10 @ 1 minute	3.8	0.6	13	<1	0.2	53
0–3 @ 1 minute	50	2.9	9	6	1.5	22
0–3 @ 5 minutes	75	6.7	5	15	4.7	13
0–3 @ 10 minutes	85	3.7	1	34	16.7	11
0–3 @ 15 minutes	92	0	0	52	36.0	9
0–3 @ 20 minutes	96	0	0	59	57.1	8

(Modified from Nelson, K. B., and Ellenberg, J. H.: Apgar scores as predictors of chronic neurologic disability. Pediatrics 68:36, 1981. Reproduced by permission of Pediatrics)

infant who is having retractions and other signs of distress have nasal prongs inserted for continuous positive airway pressure and oxygen administration to facilitate stabilization of the chest wall. As mentioned earlier, however, it may become standard procedure to treat extremely low-birth-weight infants prophylactically with surfactant; if so, intubation undoubtedly will be necessary.

Duration of Resuscitation. Resuscitation should rarely be continued beyond 15 to 20 minutes in an infant whose initial Apgar score is truly 0 and who does not respond rapidly to adequate ventilation, appropriate cardiac compression, and drugs. In infants who respond after this period of time, the incidence of death or very severe, irreversible, neurologic damage is unacceptably high.

■ LONG-TERM OUTCOME

The two central questions to be considered in thinking about the outcome of an infant after perinatal asphyxia are (1) what is the contribution of perinatal asphyxia to mental retardation and cerebral palsy in the population, and (2) how often does documented perinatal asphyxia result in cerebral palsy and mental retardation? Severe mental retardation without cerebral palsy does not appear to be related to perinatal asphyxia (Paneth and Stark, 1983), and only 10 to 15 per cent of children with mental retardation were subject to perinatal asphyxia. In addition, it is known that at least 50 per cent of infants with cerebral palsy had no documented respiratory depression at the time of birth.

The attempt to delineate which cases of perinatal asphyxia lead to cerebral palsy began in 1862 when Little noted the association of suboptimal perinatal events with subsequent poor neurologic outcome. A number of studies since that time have attempted to relate outcome to Apgar score, to the interval between birth and spontaneous respiration, and to various biochemical and biophysical markers of oxygen deprivation. The Collaborative Perinatal Project, conducted from 1959 to 1966 (Niswander et al., 1975), reported on the outcome of 49,000 infants as correlated with Apgar scores (Table 22–5). The conclusions of this study were that low Apgar scores are risk factors for cerebral palsy; however, (1) 55 per cent of children with cerebral palsy had Apgar scores of 7 to 10 at 1 minute; (2) 73 per cent of children with cerebral palsy had Apgar scores of 7 to 10 at 5 minutes; (3) of 99 children who had Apgar scores of 0 to 3 at 10, 15, or 20 minutes, only 12 (12 per cent) had cerebral palsy. However, the mortality rate in the last group was more than 50 per cent in infants weighing >2500 g and more than 90 per cent in infants of <2500 g; (4) eleven of the 12 infants with cerebral palsy were mentally retarded.

Hypoxic Ischemic Encephalopathy. Sarnat and Sarnat (1975) developed a clinical staging system for evaluating hypoxic-ischemic encephalopathy (HIE) (Table 22–6), and Robertson and Finer (1985) reported on the follow-up of infants after HIE (Table 22–7). Robertson

TABLE 22–6. Clinical Staging of Posthypoxic Encephalopathy

FACTOR	STAGE I	STAGE II	STAGE III
Level of consciousness	Alert	Lethargic	Comatose
Muscle tone	Normal	Hypotonic	Flaccid
Tendon reflexes	Increased	Present	Depressed or absent
Myoclonus	Present	Present	Absent
Complex reflexes			
Sucking	Active	Weak	Absent
Moro response	Exaggerated	Incomplete	Absent
Grasping	Normal to exaggerated	Exaggerated	Absent
Oculocephalic response (doll's eyes)	Normal	Overreactive	Reduced or absent
Autonomic function			
Pupils	Dilated	Constricted	Variable or fixed
Respiration	Regular	Variations in rate and depth, periodic	Ataxic, apneic
Heart rate	Normal or tachycardia	Bradycardia	Bradycardia
Seizures	None	Common	Uncommon
EEG	Normal	Low voltage, periodic and/or paroxysmal	Periodic or isoelectric

(Modified from Sarnat, H. B., and Sarnat, M. S.: Neonatal encephalopathy following fetal distress. Arch. Neurol. 33:696, 1975. Copyright 1975, American Medical Association.)

TABLE 22–7. Outcome 3 to 5 Years After Hypoxic-Ischemic Encephalopathy (HIE)

SEVERITY OF HIE	NUMBER OF INFANTS	INFORMATION AVAILABLE AT 3 TO 5 YEARS	NUMBER OF DEATHS	OUTCOME AT 3 TO 5 YEARS (SURVIVORS)	
				Normal	Handicapped
Mild	79	69	0	69	0
Moderate	119	103	6*	75	22
Severe†	28	28	21	0	7
Total	226	200	27	144	29
				% of Survivors	
Per cent	100	88.5	13.5	83.2	16/8

*One death was due to an unrelated accident.
†All infants died or became handicapped.

(Using classification from Sarnat, H. B., and Sarnat, M. S.: Neonatal encepalopathy following fetal distress. Arch. Neurol. 33:696, 1975. Adapted from Robertson, C., and Finer, N.: Term infants with hypoxic-ischemic encephalopathy: outcome at 3–5 years. Dev. Med. Child Neurol. 27:473, 1985.)

and Finer found that 100 per cent of infants with severe HIE either died or had significant handicap. Among those with moderate HIE, 26 per cent died or were handicapped; and among those with mild HIE, none died subsequently or were handicapped. Robertson and associates (1989) also noted no difference in school performance (at 8 years of age) between neurologically unimpaired children who suffered mild or moderate HIE and a matched peer group.

Holden and colleagues (1982) noted that the incidence of seizures increased 17 times in infants with cerebral palsy compared with that found in the normal population. Evaluation using a modified Amiel-Tison examination (1973) at the time of discharge (around 2 weeks of age) can be predictive of abnormal outcome (Piecuch et al., 1987). Others (Perlman and Tack, 1988) have attempted to use injury to other organs as an indicator to help predict eventual outcome. They found that oliguria in the perinatal period was significantly associated with signs of HIE, including seizures, death, and long-term neurologic deficit. In general, it can be assumed that an infant who has experienced an asphyxial event severe enough to produce permanent brain damage will have evidence of significant damage to other organs within hours to days after birth.

Sunshine (1989) concludes, in addition, that infants with perinatal asphyxia should be evaluated for structural abnormalities with current imaging techniques and that, if identified, an attempt should be made to determine whether the abnormalities can be explained on the basis of intrapartum asphyxia or are developmental aberrations or abnormalities that occurred prior to labor. In addition, he points out that infants who are small for gestational age comprise a significant percentage of the total patients who experience neonatal asphyxia, HIE, and seizures as well as cerebral palsy. Therefore, attempts to improve outcome should focus on recognition of infants who are small for gestational age and on possible types of intervention in pregnancies complicated by intrauterine growth retardation. Others have attempted to predict the degree of perinatal brain damage by measurement of substances presumed to be released in response to hypoxia and acidemia, including vasopressin, erythropoietin, and hypoxanthine. Whether cerebral palsy and mental retardation can result from perinatal asphyxia in the absence of neonatal encephalopathy is unknown, but most experts would doubt it. By the same token, it is known that many infants with moderate degrees of perinatal asphyxia do not exhibit encephalopathy, whereas others with similar degrees of fetal distress have severe encephalopathy.

The most accurate prediction comes from a full knowledge of perinatal and neonatal events, combined with biochemical and imaging studies and careful repeated clinical evaluations in the first years of life.

■ REFERENCES

American Academy of Pediatrics Committee on Drugs: Emergency drug doses for infants and children. Pediatrics 81:462, 1988.

Amiel-Tison, C.: Neurologic disorders in neonates associated with abnormalities of pregnancy and birth. Curr. Probl. Pediatr. 3:1, 1973.

Apgar, V.: A proposal for new method for evaluation of the newborn infant. Anesth. Analg. 32:260, 1953.

Blair, E., and Stanley, J.: Intrapartum asphyxia: A rare cause of cerebral palsy. J. Pediatr. 112:515, 1988.

Bloom, R. S., and Cropley, C. S.: American Heart Association—American Academy of Pediatrics Textbook of Neonatal Resuscitation. Dallas, American Heart Association National Center, 1987.

Cabal, L. A., Devaskar, U., Siassi, B., et al.: Cardiogenic shock associated with perinatal asphyxia in preterm infants. J. Pediatr. 96:705, 1980.

Carson, B. S., Lasey, B. W., Bowes, W. A., et al.: Combined obstetric and pediatric approach to prevent meconium aspiration syndrome. Am. J. Obstet. Gyencol. 126:712, 1976.

Corbet, A., Cregan, J., and Frink, J.: Distention-produced phospholipid secretion in postmortem in situ lungs of newborn rabbits. Am. Rev. Respir. Dis. 128:695, 1983.

Cunningham, A. S., Lawson, E. E., Martin, R. J., and Pildes, R. S.: Tracheal suction and meconium: A proposed standard of care. (Discussion) J. Pediatr. 116:153, 1990.

Dale, H. H., and Evans, C. L.: Effects on the circulation of changes in carbon dioxide content of the blood. J. Physiol. 56:125, 1972.

Dawes, G.: Foetal and Neonatal Physiology. Chicago, Year Book Publishers, 1968.

Drew, J. H.: Immediate intubation at birth of the very low birth weight infant: Effect on survival. Am. J. Dis. Child. 136:207, 1982.

Ellis, W. G., Goetzman, B. W., and Lindenberg, J. A.: Neuropathologic documentation of prenatal brain damage. Am. J. Dis. Child. 12:858, 1988.

Falcilia, H. S.: Failure to prevent meconium aspiration syndrome. Obstet. Gynecol. 71:349, 1988.

Greenough, H., Lagercrantz, H., Pool, J., et al.: Plasma catecholamine levels in preterm infants: Effect of birth asphyxia and Apgar score. Acta Paediatr. Scand. 76:54, 1987.

Gregory, G. A., Gooding, C. A., Phibbs, R. H., et al.: Meconium aspiration in infants: A prospective study. J. Pediatr. 85:807, 1974.

Hack, M. N., and Fanaroff, A. A.: Changes in the delivery room care of the extremely small infant (less than 750 g). Effects on morbidity and outcome. N. Engl. J. Med. 314:660, 1986.

James, L. S.: Emergencies in the delivery room. In Fanaroff, A. A., and Martin, R. J. (Eds.): Neonatal-Perinatal Medicine. 4th ed. St. Louis, CV Mosby, 1987, pp. 360–378.

Karlberg, P.: The adaptive changes in the immediate postnatal period, with particular reference to respiration. J. Pediatr. 56:585, 1960.

Kitterman, J. A., Phibbs, R. H., and Tooley, W. H.: Catheterization of umbilical vessels in newborn infants. Pediatr. Clin. North Am. 17:895, 1970.

Lagercrantz, H., and Slotkin, T. A.: The "stress" of being born. Sci. Am. 254:100, 1986.

Lindemann, R.: Resuscitation of the newborn with endotracheal administration of epinephrine. Acta Paediatr. Scand. 73:210, 1984.

Linder, N., Aranda, J. V., Tsur, M., et al.: Need for endotracheal intubation and suction in meconium-stained neonates. J. Pediatr. 112:613–615, 1988.

Little, W. J.: On the influence of abnormal parturition, difficult labours, premature birth, and asphyxia neonatorum on the mental and physical condition of the child, especially in relation to deformities. Trans. Obstet. Soc. (London) 3:293, 1861–1862.

Martinez, A., Padbury, J., Shames, L., et al.: Naloxone potentiates epinephrine release during hypoxia in fetal sheep: Dose response and cardiovascular effects. Pediatr. Res. 23:343, 1988.

Massaro, G. D., and Massaro, D.: Morphologic evidence that large inflations of the lung stimulate secretion of surfactant. Ann. Rev. Resp. Dis. 127:235, 1983.

Nelson, K. B.: What proportion of cerebral palsy is related to birth asphyxia? J. Pediatr. 112:572, 1988.

Newnham, J. P., Marshall, C. L., Padbury, J. F., et al.: Fetal catecholamine release with preterm delivery. Am. J. Obstet. Gynecol. 149:888, 1984.

Niswander, K. R., Gordon, M., and Drage, J. S.: The effect of intrauterine hypoxia on the child surviving to 4 years. Am. J. Obstet. Gynecol. 121:892, 1975.

Paneth, N., and Fox, H. E.: The relationship of Apgar score to neurologic handicap: A survey of clinicians. Obstet. Gynecol. 61:547, 1983.

Paneth, N., and Stark, R. I.: Cerebral palsy and mental retardation in relation to indicators in perinatal asphyxia. Am. J. Obstet. Gynecol. 147:960, 1983.

Perlman, J. M., and Tack, E. D.: Renal injury in the asphyxiated newborn infant: Relationship to neurologic outcome. J. Pediatr. 113:875, 1988.

Phibbs, R. H.: Delivery room management of the newborn. In Avery, G. B. (Ed.): Neonatology. 3rd ed. Philadelphia, J. B. Lippincott, 1985, pp. 215–234.

Piecuch, R., Leonard, C., et al.: Predicting neurodevelopmental outcome in infants with severe perinatal asphyxia. Pediatr. Res. 21:401A, 1987.

Robertson, C., and Finer, N.: Term infants with hypoxic-ischemic encephalopathy: Outcome at 3–5 years. Dev. Med. Child Neurol. 27:473, 1985.

Robertson, C. M. T., Finer, N. N., and Grace, M. G. A.: School performance of survivors of neonatal encephalopathy associated with birth asphyxia at term. J. Pediatr. 114:753, 1989.

Rosen, M. G.: Factors during labor and delivery that influence brain disorders. In Freeman, J. M. (Ed.): Prenatal and Perinatal Factors Associated with Brain Disorders. Bethesda, MD, NIH Publication No. 85–1149, April, 1985, pp. 237–262.

Rossi, E. M., Philipson, E. H., Williams, T. G., et al.: Meconium aspiration syndrome: Intrapartum and neonatal attributes. Am. J. Obstet. Gynecol. 161:1106–1110, 1989.

Ruth, V., Sutti-Ramo, I., Granstrom, M.-L., et al.: Prediction of perinatal brain damage by cord plasma vasopressin, erythropoietin and hypoxanthine levels. J. Pediatr. 113:880, 1988.

Sarnat, H. B., and Sarnat, M. S.: Neonatal encephalopathy following fetal distress. Arch. Neurol. 33:696, 1975.

Sola, A., Spitzer, A. R., Morin, F. C., et al.: Effects of arterial carbon dioxide tension on the newborn lamb's cardiovascular responses to rapid hemorrhage. Pediatr. Res. 17:70, 1983.

Strang, L. B.: Neonatal Respiration: Physiological and Clinical Studies. Oxford, U. K., Blackwell Scientific Publications, 1977.

Sunshine, P.: Epidemiology of perinatal asphyxia. In Stevenson, D. K., and Sunshine, P. (Eds.): Fetal and Neonatal Brain Injury. Toronto, Philadelphia, B. C. Decker, Inc., 1989.

Taeusch, H. W., Wyszogrodski, I., Wang, N. S., et al.: Pulmonary pressure-volume relationships in premature fetal and newborn rabbits. J. Appl. Physiol. 37:809, 1974.

Thiebault, D. W., Hall, T. K., Sheehan, M. B., et al.: Postasphyxial lung disease in newborn infants with severe perinatal acidosis. Am. J. Obstet. Gynecol. 150:393, 1984.

Vyas, H., Millner, A. D., Hopkin, I. E., et al.: Physiologic responses to prolonged and slow-rise inflation in the resuscitation of the asphyxiated newborn infant. J. Pediatr. 99:635, 1981.

Walters, D. V., and Olver, R. E.: The role of catecholamines in lung liquid absorption at birth. Pediatr. Res. 12:239, 1978.

Weil, M. H., Rackrow, E. C., Trevino, R., et al.: Difference in acid base state between venous and arterial blood during cardiopulmonary resuscitation. N. Engl. J. Med. 315:153, 1986.

Wiswell, T. E., Tuggle, J. M., and Turner, B. S.: Meconium aspiration syndrome: Have we made a difference? Pediatrics 85:715–721, 1990.

INITIAL EVALUATION: 23 HISTORY AND PHYSICAL EXAMINATION OF THE NEWBORN

H. William Taeusch

The goals of the history and physical examination are simple—to gain rapport with the parents and to evaluate the current and future well-being of the infant. With the birth of a sick or an anomalous infant, the history and physical exam may have to be done concurrently, along with informing the parents of the infant's initial and subsequent course. Specifics of the examination of various systems are given throughout this book. Therefore, the points relevant to newborns, particularly sick and anomalous infants, are emphasized in this chapter.

■ EMERGENCY ASSESSMENT

Assessment of the newborn includes routine evaluation of a healthy full-term infant nearing the time of discharge or emergency assessment of a gray, evidently lifeless, 500-g newborn in the delivery room. The impressions gained in the first seconds and minutes often dictate the speed with which further assessment and treatment must occur. A rapid assessment including both a brief history and physical examination is warranted whenever an infant has an acute change in status. Obviously, the evaluation should not impede attention to the infant's immediate needs. It is a novice's mistake to suspect overwhelming sepsis, then to take several hours to do the history and physical examination and a leisurely lumbar puncture before assuring that antibiotics have been received by the infant. Another mistake is to wait for a chest radiograph when an infant has hypotension with a clinically evident tension pneumothorax. A third mistake is to allow an infant to suffer thermal and oxygen insufficiency while hidden under sterile drapes during a protracted insertion of an umbilical artery catheter. A list of perinatal and postnatal conditions necessitating emergency assessment is given in Table 23–1. Delivery room assessment and resuscitation are discussed in Chapter 22.

■ HISTORY

The first interview with the parents should occur before birth. With rapidly expanding genetic diagnostic capabili-

ties and identification of high-risk fetuses with prenatal ultrasonography, the need and the frequency of pediatricians meeting with the parents before birth are increasing.

The first evaluation of the newborn infant is often said to be the most important routine exam that the infant receives in his or her lifetime. If the infant is sick or has anomalies, this truism is particularly pertinent. However, for well infants, remarkably few studies have examined which elements of the initial history and physical exam are most important and which professional personnel should conduct these exams. If the infant is born at term with no complications, under optimal circumstances, the parents are delighted with the good news. If the infant requires intensive care (about 3 per cent of livebirths), the tendency to focus on ventilators, monitors, lab tests, radiographs, and ultrasounds downgrades the importance of the history and thereby the opportunity for meaningful

TABLE 23–1. Neonatal Conditions Requiring Emergency Assessment

Potentially lethal conditions	Anencephaly or hydranencephaly, severe hydrops with hypoplastic lungs, extremely low birth weight (pre-viability), known 13 to 18 trisomies, and nonresponsiveness to resuscitation.
Respiratory conditions	
Airway obstruction	Mucus, meconium, blocked endotracheal tube, webs, cysts, tongue, stenosis, tumors, and vascular rings.
Space-occupying lesions	Pneumothorax, pleural effusions, hypoplastic lungs, tracheoesophageal fistula, diaphragmatic hernia, adenomatoid malformation, and tumors.
Insufficient respiratory drive	Immaturity, asphyxia, maternal drugs, and CNS damage or infection.
Parenchymal disease	Respiratory distress syndrome, meconium aspiration pneumonia, and infectious pneumonitis.
Cardiovascular conditions	Hypovolemia or hypotension, bradycardia or other arrhythmia, hydrops and congestive heart failure, decreased pulmonary blood flow, and anemia or hyperviscosity.

interaction with the parents. Frequently, infants enter the neonatal intensive care unit (NICU) without the parents' having been able to anticipate this occurrence. When the parents first visit the NICU, they confront a strange environment in which the life of their infant is entrusted to nurses and doctors not known to them. Both parents may be exhausted and anxious in the hours after the delivery, at the time they become aware the infant is seriously ill. Some parents are fatalistic and accept opinions about diagnosis and prognosis less out of trust than a belief that they can little affect events. Others attempt to exert control over the caregivers in the belief that their infant's plight can be fixed if they (the parents) can only force the correct decisions and treatments to be made.

Therefore, the style with which the initial interview is conducted must be adapted to the parents' needs as well as to those of the infant, and the interview serves several purposes. First, it allows the collection of information that affects the management of the infant. Second, a therapeutic bond may be formed with the parents, the first stage in enlisting them as allies rather than adversaries in the days, weeks, and possibly months ahead while the infant is in the NICU. Third, an initial assessment of the adequacy of the home and the parents with regard to the care of the infant can be made. Fourth, the interview provides the opportunity for the parents to receive an initial report on the status of the infant.

If the infant is being transferred to another hospital, giving the mother a belonging of the infant (e.g., a bracelet or Polaroid picture) can help her to contend with the birth and immediate loss (to the NICU) of her infant. Realistically allaying parental anxiety about their infant's condition on the first interview is often not possible, but the manner and conduct of the history-taking can help the parents feel that their infant will receive competent care. Frightening though the illness or anomaly may be, the parents' conception of their infant's problem may be even more frightening, and thus, some reassurance can be offered in most cases, especially after the parents have seen their infant. Novice caregivers, as a symptom of their own insecurity, may emphasize data in these discussions. This tactic, particularly at the first meeting, usually does more harm than good. The error of the opposite approach is to patronize the parents in an abbreviated interview. The worst mistake is to minimize contact with the parents altogether.

Usually, parents are justly intolerant of the professional who waits until after all history-taking, examinations, and lab data are in hand before giving them any notion of the problems. It may be wise to start an interview with an overview and follow with the history-taking. At the conclusion of the interview, one should outline the next steps (diagnostic and therapeutic), real and potential problems, seek questions from the parents, and close with plans for the next contact.

The initial history and physical examination are screening tools. All systems and areas of the body are evaluated in a feed-forward mode: that is to say, if the initial screen is positive, e.g., with the heart or lungs, then that system immediately receives a more thorough evaluation, not only through the physical examination, but also through expansion of the history and lab examinations. The equally weighted and relentlessly thorough history and physical exam of the compulsive novice are rightfully replaced by a balanced exam suitable for the individual circumstances of the infant.

The examiner throughout the history and physical examination is seeking answers to a series of questions, the first and most important of which is whether the infant is acutely ill. Next one asks whether there is a problem with regard to:

- Any specific organ system
- Infection
- Inadequate oxygen or nutrients (acute or chronic)
- Abnormal in utero environment
- Growth
- Anomalies or genetic disease
- Trauma
- Maturity
- Transition from in utero existence
- Home environment

Physical examination and laboratory evaluations are never complete with sick infants in an intensive care setting. Information is constantly appearing from diagnostic studies from secretaries, physicians, nurses, respiratory therapists, family members, and so forth. Integration of these data with clear and appropriate communication is one of the hardest tasks to learn. One of the best techniques is the use of careful, succinct, system- or problem-oriented, dated and timed notes in the infant's hospital chart, including information about what has been told to the parents and their particular concerns.

MATERNAL HISTORY

The history of the newborn is principally the history of the mother's pregnancy, general health, and prior pregnancies. Table 23–2 outlines the array of maternal conditions that can affect the newborn, and these are discussed in more detail throughout the book. Maternal influences on the fetus are thoroughly reviewed by Creasy and Resnick (1989).

Some of these maternal factors deserve emphasis. The major problem of newborns throughout the world is that of low birth weight and prematurity. The complex and interrelated factors are summarized in Table 23–3, and each of these factors is important to note. If present in the maternal history, their relative weight has to be individualized since none of the items listed is necessarily associated with preterm delivery.

Prenatal Care. The reasons why only some women receive prenatal care are of vital interest. While it is clear that birth weight–specific mortality in the United States is among the world's lowest, our high neonatal mortality is directly dependent on a high low-birth-weight delivery rate. Deficient or absent prenatal care is associated with an increased risk of prematurity. All who care for mothers and infants share a responsibility for disseminating these facts and uncovering and correcting the reasons why prenatal care is so often missed in this country.

Duration of Pregnancy. Estimates of gestational length should be obtained from the date of the mother's last menstrual period, date of quickening (16 to 18 weeks),

TABLE 23–2. Maternal History

SOCIAL, EDUCATIONAL, AND ECONOMIC FACTORS
Age, race, primary language, work, stress, education, religion, reasons for becoming pregnant, preparation for infant care, home support, health care access, and history of child abuse.

BEHAVIORAL FACTORS AND HABITS
Smoking, drugs, alcohol, and exercise (duration and amount).

EXPOSURE TO TOXINS OR TERATOGENS
Radiation, radiochemicals, hormones (including diethylstilbestrol), thyroid suppressants, aminopterin, anticancer agents, mercury, chlorobiphenyls and other organic substances, hydantoins, coumarin, and accutane.

NUTRITION
Diet, vitamin and mineral supplements, and weight gain.

GENETIC/FAMILIAL DISORDERS
(See Table 23–4).

CHRONIC MEDICAL PROBLEMS PREDATING PREGNANCY

OUTCOME OF PRIOR PREGNANCIES
Fetal death, twins, prematurity, blood group incompatibilities, and birth weight or gestational age of prior children.

PRENATAL CARE
Number of visits, trimester of first visit, ultrasound examinations, and location.

PROBLEMS OF CURRENT PREGNANCY*
CNS or psychiatric, endocrine (diabetes, thyroid status, or thyroid medication), metabolic (cholestasis), cardiopulmonary (mitral insufficiency or asthma), hypertensive disorders, preeclampsia, hematologic (anemia, Rh incompatibility, and idiopathic or alloimmune thrombocytopenia), third-trimester bleeding (placenta previa, abruptio placentae, or ruptured uterus), immunologic (lupus), surgery or trauma, infections, medications (tocolytics, glucocorticoids, antibiotics, or antihypertensives), renal, neoplastic, and reproductive (incompetent cervix and hydramnios or oligohydramnios).

SPECIAL TESTS DURING PREGNANCY
Ultrasound exams, karyotyping, alpha-fetoprotein, chorionic villus biopsy, percutaneous umbilical blood sampling of the fetus, stress and nonstress testing, amniotic fluid testing for bilirubin, fetal lung maturity, and biophysical profile.

INFECTION SCREENING
Rubella, syphilis, AIDS, toxoplasmosis, herpes, hepatitis B, cytomegalovirus, tuberculosis, and gonorrhea (for close contacts as well as mother).

ONSET AND EVENTS OF LABOR
Fetal heart rate monitoring, fetal scalp pH, meconium, rupture of membranes, amnioinfusion, fever, maternal oxygen, vena cava decompression, blood pressure, ventilation, analgesia or anesthesia, other medications, and duration of stages of labor (1 = onset to full cervical dilatation, 2 = dilatation to delivery, and 3 = delivery to delivery of placenta), and mode of delivery.

*Pregnancy-associated diseases and fetal exposure to tobacco, marijuana, alcohol, or illicit drugs are now included on the U.S. standard certificates of livebirth and fetal death (Freedman, 1988).

and the first appearance of fetal heart sounds (18 to 20 weeks with a fetoscope) and ultrasound size standards. Nägele's rule allows one to estimate the time of term delivery by subtracting 3 calendar months from the first day of the last menstrual period and adding 7 days. The fundus is usually at the umbilicus by the 5th month after the last menstrual period.

Genetic and Familial Factors. A history of genetic and familial disorders is becoming increasingly important as diagnosis of genetic disease of the fetus during pregnancy becomes more widely available (see Part III). Table 23–4 illustrates a screening history adapted from the one recommended by the American College of Obstetricians and Gynecologists.

Onset and Events of Labor. The timing and events that occur around the onset of labor are important.

Examples include a car accident, premature rupture of membranes, progression of labor pains, or sharp near-continuous low back pain with vaginal bleeding. Indications for risk of acute or chronic infections to the fetus should be sought. Has the mother had a recent infection? Did she have a fever around the time of delivery? Has she received antibiotics? How long did labor last and how long were the membranes ruptured?

The fetal heart rate in conjunction with uterine contractions is the best signal during labor of the condition of the fetus (see Chapter 12). Adjuncts include use of fetal scalp pH.

The presentation of the fetus in the birth canal and the route of delivery are of obvious importance. Breech position occurs in about 8 per cent of women in labor. In about 25 per cent of breech deliveries, conditions such as

TABLE 23–3. Principal Risk Factors for Low Birth Weight*

I. Demographic risks
  A. Age (<18 or >35)
  B. Race
  C. Low socioeconomic status
  D. Unmarried
  E. Low level of education
II. Medical risks predating pregnancy
  A. Parity (0 or >4)
  B. Low weight for height
  C. Genitourinary problems, renal insufficiency, or surgery
  D. Selected diseases, e.g., diabetes and hypertension
  E. Nonimmune status, e.g., rubella
  F. Poor obstetric history, including previous low-birth-weight baby or multiple abortions
  G. Maternal genetic factors, e.g., the mother herself was a low-birth-weight infant
III. Medical risks in current pregnancy
  A. Multiple pregnancy
  B. Poor weight gain
  C. Short interpregnancy interval
  D. Hypotension
  E. Hypertension, preeclampsia, or toxemia
  F. Infections, e.g., rubella, symptomatic bacteriuria, or cytomegalovirus
  G. First- or second-trimester bleeding
  H. Placental problems, such as placenta previa or abruptio placentae
  I. Hyperemesis
  J. Oligo- or polyhydramnios
  K. Anemia or abnormal hemoglobin
  L. Isoimmunization
  M. Fetal anomalies
  N. Incompetent cervix
  O. Spontaneous premature rupture of membranes
IV. Behavioral and environmental risks
  A. Smoking
  B. Poor nutritional status
  C. Alcohol and other substance abuse, particularly cocaine
  D. Diethylstilbestrol exposure and other toxins
  E. High altitude
V. Health care risks
  A. Insufficient prenatal care
  B. Iatrogenic prematurity
VI. Other possible correlates of premature labor
  A. Physical and psychosocial stress or abuse
  B. Uterine irritability
  C. Cervical changes before labor
  D. Infections, e.g., *Mycoplasma* and *Chlamydia*
  E. Plasma volume
  F. Progesterone
  G. Immune interactions between the mother and fetus

*Adapted from Institute of Medicine Committee to Study the Prevention of Low Birthweight: Preventing Low Birthweight. Washington, D.C., National Academy Press, 1985.

TABLE 23–4. Maternal Prenatal Genetic Screen*

1. Are you over 34 years of age?
2. Has anyone in your family or the father's family had: Down syndrome ("mongolism"), chromosome problems or abnormalities, back (midline) defects at birth or later in life (spina bifida), prolonged or excessive bleeding (hemophilia), muscle weakness problems (muscular dystrophy), or childhood lung problems (cystic fibrosis)?
3. Do you or does the baby's father have a birth defect? Do family members of you or the father have birth defects of any kind?
4. Have any members of your family, the father's family, or any of your prior infants had other problems that were inherited or "passed down" through family members to their children?
5. Do you or the baby's father have any close relatives with mental retardation or trouble learning in school?
6. Have you or the father ever been tested for these genetic problems [relevant to specific ethnic group]: Tay-Sachs disease, sickle cell trait or disease, or β-thalassemia?
7. Have you lost any early pregnancies (miscarriages)?

*Adapted from American College of Obstetricians and Gynecologists: Antenatal Diagnosis of Genetic Disorders. (ACOG Technical Bulletin No. 108) Washington, D.C., ACOG, 1987, p. 3.

placenta previa, malformations of the fetus or uterus, twinning, or premature labor may coexist. Risks of vaginal delivery for the fetus in the breech position include prolapse of the cord, trapping of the head at the level of the cervix, asphyxia, and trauma.

Amniotic Fluid. The infant at term is immersed in about 1 liter of amniotic fluid. Its sources are fetal urine, lung secretions, and transudate from surrounding membranes. Before birth, ultrasound assessment of amniotic fluid volume is part of the biophysical profile. While standards vary, normal volumes are associated with one or more pockets of fluid with a total vertical diameter of >4 cm. Oligohydramnios is indicated by less than 500 ml of fluid. Polyhydramnios indicates more than 2 liters of fluid at birth. Near term, the fetus drinks about 125 ml/kg body weight of amniotic fluid per day (equivalent to volume of postnatal milk intake). The fluid has a pH of 7.2 and is alkaline with respect to vaginal fluid. Therefore leakage of amniotic fluid from the vagina can be tested by checking the pH.

Oligohydramnios or polyhydramnios is most common when fetal swallowing or micturition is increased or decreased. Either condition can be a matter of degree and is best assessed with fetal ultrasound. Phelan and colleagues (1987) describe the simplest method in which the largest pocket of fluid visualized by ultrasound in each of four uterine quadrants is summed. If the sum is <6 cm, oligohydramnios is diagnosed. Conditions associated with oligohydramnios are renal abnormalities, lung hypoplasia, Potter facies, contractures and limb deformities, possibly maternal indomethacin use, and cord compression. Conditions listed in Table 23–5 are associated with polyhydramnios. High intestinal obstruction and anencephaly (presumably due to decreased clearance of amniotic fluid by swallowing) are the most common.

Timing of Umbilical Cord Clamping. Many events affect the relative volume of blood left in the newborn versus the placenta after birth. Prenatal asphyxia shifts blood from the placenta to the fetus, and in these cases, because of the need to suction meconium and resuscitate the infant, no delay in cord clamping appears to be useful.

TABLE 23–5. Conditions Associated with Polyhydramnios

- Agnathia
- Anencephaly and other CNS defects
- Beckwith-Wiedemann syndrome
- Chylothorax
- Conjoined twins
- Cystic adenomatoid malformation of the lung
- Diaphragmatic hernia
- Fetal akinesia
- Fetal death
- Hydrops
- Gastroschisis
- Hemangioma
- Maternal diabetes
- Obstructive teratoma
- Trisomies
- Tumors of the lungs, placenta, or ovaries
- Umbilical cord compression
- Upper gastrointestinal obstruction (e.g., duodenal atresia)
- Werdnig-Hoffman disease

In normal infants, if the cord is clamped within 5 seconds of delivery before a contraction compresses the placenta, and if the infant is held well above the mother's introitus before cord clamping, then the infant may well be hypovolemic. In contrast, if the obstetrician zealously "strips" the cord toward the infant and delays clamping it, the resulting shift of blood volume to the newborn may result in polycythemia, delayed absorption of lung fluid, and hyperbilirubinemia. Despite years of research, there is little consensus on the optimal timing of cord clamping. In the absence of asphyxia or isoimmunization, 30 to 45 seconds is a reasonable period while the infant is held at the level of the introitus. This interval usually allows for an inspiratory gasp on the part of the newborn and a uterine contraction on the part of the mother—both occurrences favoring transfer of blood from the placenta to the newborn (Table 23–6). The obstetrician can be gainfully employed in suctioning the nares and oropharnyx during this period. Few pediatricians and obstetricians note the timing and nature of the separation of the newborn infant from the placenta, although it would be helpful in infants with anemia or polycythemia.

Blood volumes are between 85 and 100 ml/kg of body weight in term infants and up to 110 ml/kg in preterm infants. Values can be 35 per cent higher with large shifts of blood volume from the placenta. At term, 75 to 100 ml (20 to 35 ml/kg) of blood is available to the newborn from the placenta.

TABLE 23–6. Factors Determining Neonatal and Placental Blood Volume

- Prenatal drugs (e.g., ergot derivatives)
- Maternal vascular disease (preeclampsia or diabetes)
- Placental and fetal size
- Maternal hypotension
- Fetal asphyxia or placental insufficiency
- Rate of umbilical artery constriction
- Gravity
- Uterine contractions (frequency, amplitude, duration, and baseline)
- Time of cord clamping
- Neonatal cardiac output
- Fetal blood volume (hydrops)
- Time of placental separation
- Route of delivery
- Cord compression
- Timing of first breaths relative to cord clamping

■ PLACENTA AND UMBILICAL CORD

The problems of the placenta are discussed in Chapter 7. The placenta at term (cord and membranes excised 2 cm from the insertion) weighs between 400 to 500 g, with about half the weight representing maternal blood and about 15 per cent composed of fetal blood. When the fetal-placental weight ratio at birth is >10, it implies that nutrient delivery and gas exchange may have been suboptimal. The cord may demonstrate one umbilical artery (0.7 per cent of live births), true knots, evidence of vascular rupture, cord compression, hematoma, or edema. In some infants with intrauterine growth retardation, the cord and chorionic plate may be stained greenish-brown, and diminished Wharton jelly may be present. The insertion of the cord may be central or marginal or incorporated into the membranes (velamentous), sometimes with vasa praevia (splitting of the vessels in the membranes before insertion into the placenta). The umbilical cord is usually >40 cm in length at term, and shorter cords may indicate relative fetal akinesia from a variety of causes, the inference being that fetal activity contributes to lengthening of the cord. Amniotic membranes may show evidence of banding or thickening, often in association with amniotic fluid infection. In twins, there may be no membrane between cord insertions (monochorionic, monoamniotic), a thin transparent membrane (diamniotic), or a thick but separable opaque membrane (dichorionic, diamniotic).

■ PHYSICAL EXAMINATION

The examiner always faces the dilemma of needing to be thorough versus needing to be gentle and quick in order not to destabilize the smallest and sickest infants. The physical examination of newborn infants is tailored to fit both the gestation and the postnatal age of an infant. The evaluation in the delivery room of a gasping 25-week premature infant is different from the routine exam at 12 hours of age of a full-term infant in the well baby nursery. (Compare Figures 23–1, 23–2, and 23–3 with the full-term infants in subsequent figures, then look at Figure 23–4). One needs patience to return frequently to do parts of the exam in order to stay within the limits of an infant's tolerance. It is fruitless to examine the abdomen of a crying infant and risky to do the same exam after a full feeding. At the same time, it is appropriately embarrassing to miss an imperforate anus or extra digits in an infant whose respiratory problems have captivated initial interest. An outline of a complete history and physical examination is given in Table 23–7.

NOSOCOMIAL INFECTION

Before touching an infant for any purpose, handwashing should be carried out after removal of rings and watches. The handwashing should occur immediately before and immediately after the examination. A "low level of mysophobia" is prevalent among nursery personnel, and this no doubt contributes to the nosocomial infection rate that approaches 100 per cent for small sick infants who have spent more than a month in an NICU. If the prevalence of handwashing is suboptimal in most nurseries, the use of insufficiently cleaned stethoscopes and other equipment is ever present. With concern provoked by the prevalence of AIDS, many nurseries now utilize universal precautions, meaning that a fresh gown and gloves are used for each direct contact of each patient, whether or not direct handling of bodily fluids occurs. Reason dictates that patients should receive at least the same protection against common nosocomial bacteria as caregivers afford themselves against the much smaller risk of AIDS.

VITAL SIGNS

Vital signs are usually assigned the first place in write-ups of the physical exam. For small sick newborns, single measurements are less important than trends, and these can be recorded as such. For example, "Axillary temperature was 34° C at 20:05 on arrival in the NICU and was

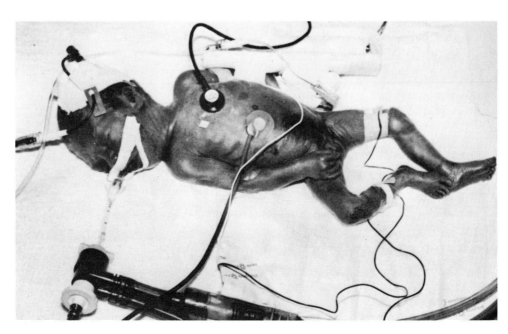

FIGURE 23–1. *The problems of physical examination are illustrated by comparing this 25-week, 710-g infant (A.W.) with respiratory distress syndrome with the full-term newborn in Figure 23–5. The story of this premature infant is the subject of a book entitled* Born Early. *(From* Born Early: The Story of a Premature Baby, *by Mary Ellen Avery, M.D., and Georgia Litwack. Copyright © 1983 by Mary Ellen Avery, M.D., and Georgia Litwack. By permission of Little, Brown and Company.)*

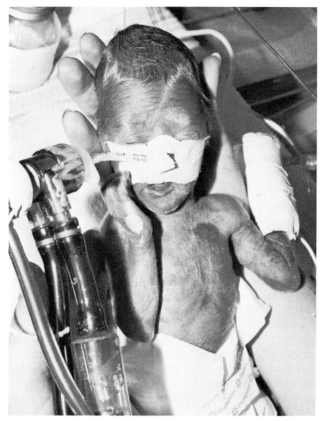

FIGURE 23–2. The infant (A.W.) is shown after the first week of life. Note the size of the skull relative to the adult hand supporting the head. Abundant lanugo hair is evident. (Courtesy of G. Litwack.)

flow. Intra-arterial catheters permit continuous blood pressure monitoring as a matter of routine. Infants being evaluated for a heart problem should have blood pressure measured in all four extremities to check primarily for problems of preductal coarctation and left ventricular and outflow tract hypoplasia. Blood pressure correlates directly with gestational age and birth weight. In general, hypotension must be considered for blood pressures below 35/25 with means <30 in infants <1000 g. In the first 12 hours, mean blood pressures as low as 23 may not be abnormal in the smallest liveborn infants (although the definition of "normal" in this group is a conundrum). In the smallest, sickest newborns, blood pressures are usually measured intra-arterially with transducers that often receive suboptimal calibration. The transducer must be at the level of the ventricles, and with lower blood pressures, errors with leveling may cause large errors in blood pressure readings. Trends in blood pressure, skin perfusion, recent clinical events, urine output, and arterial pH trends are essential inputs for the diagnosis of clinically significant hypotension. Hypertension is a consideration with mean pressures above 50 to 70 in preterm or term infants (see Appendix).

WEIGHT, LENGTH, AND HEAD CIRCUMFERENCE

Weight should be measured in grams for greatest accuracy. For infants from 500 to 800 g birth weight, differences of only 100 g are associated with differences in mortality of 50 per cent. Length is more easily measured with an inflexible meter rule beside the baby rather than

36.8° C after two hours in the servo-controlled overhead warmer supplemented with heat lamps." Without a good indication of the times of the measurements, vital signs for newborns have little meaning. Temperature for the most part is measured by axilla using electronic thermometers with disposable tips (see Chapter 27). Rectal temperatures, because of the greater risk of trauma or perforation, are useful only when core temperature may be in question.

For all spontaneously breathing infants, term and premature, respiratory rates normally fall within a range of 40 to 60 breaths per minute by 1 hour of age. Rarely, a term infant has a persisting respiratory rate of 100 on the 2nd day of life with no evident clinical, radiographic, or laboratory abnormality. In these cases, the respiratory rate becomes normal by the end of the 1st week. Persistent bradypnea is rare—seen only in extremely premature infants who are ill, or in those with persisting central hypoventilation (Ondine curse). Apneic episodes and periodic breathing should be described. In recording observations, description rather than opinion is preferable, e.g., "The infant had about six respiratory pauses of 4 to 7 seconds each without bradycardia or evident desaturation during a 5-minute period while lying undisturbed in apparent REM sleep."

Blood pressure is not usually routinely measured in well infants, and the cost-benefit analysis of this procedure for normal infants is unknown. For sick infants, blood pressure is assessed, for example, by direct intra-arterial measurement, oscillometry, auscultation, and Doppler

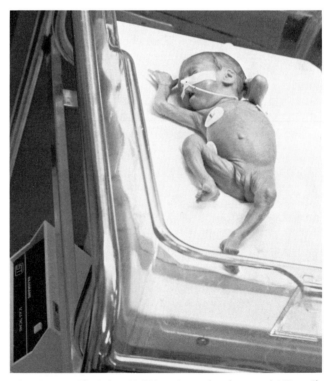

FIGURE 23–3. The infant (A.W.) at six weeks of age and 850 g. She required 33 days of ventilator support and had surgical ligation of a patent ductus arteriosus. With the head to the right, the infant manifests a strong spontaneous tonic neck reflex posture. The infant required an incubator for temperature control, but is shown here during a weight measurement. (Courtesy of G. Litwack.)

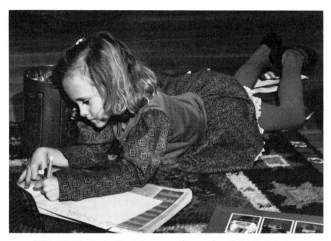

FIGURE 23–4. *A.W. at 5 years of age; the child is thriving.*

with a flexible measuring tape. Measurements of length carried out by one person using a measuring tape on a squirming infant are commonly inaccurate by several centimeters. The tonic neck reflex can occasionally help in straightening the leg during the measurement. The "ponderal index" (length in circles divided by the cube root of the weight in pounds) may be useful in identifying the occasional baby who is underweight for length and therefore small for gestational age, who nonetheless is not so identified by standard weight, gestation, and length norms. Head circumference is determined by placing a soft tape measure just above the eyebrows and finding the largest circumference over the occiput (Fig. 23–5).

GESTATIONAL AGE ASSESSMENT

The evaluation is best done by recording several estimates, that is, gestation duration based on last menstrual period, prenatal ultrasound estimates, and after birth, the gestation that matches the 50th percentile for head circumference, length, and weight and the estimate of gestation based on physical characteristics. These indicators can be combined to give an "obstetric" estimate of gestation and a "pediatric" estimate of gestation that can be combined into a "clinical" estimate. We believe that the physical assessments of gestation have been overemphasized because it is clear that the skin and the central nervous system, which contribute the most to the score, can be affected by factors other than the duration of gestation. None of the physical assessment examinations have been standardized to gauge gestation. The scoring examination by Ballard (1977) is one of the simplest and should be consulted for detailed assessments (see Chapter 25). As a rule of thumb, 24-week infants are about 600 g (usual limits of viability), 28-week infants are 1200 g (600 × 2), and 33-week infants are 1800 g (600 × 3).

OVERALL APPEARANCE

Observing the infant is the most important aspect of the physical examination. It is best performed with the infant quiet and nude. Occasionally, the two states are incompatible, in which case the infant can usually be quieted by rocking to-and-fro while the examiner makes faces and babbles. This time-honored method usually catches the surprised attention of the infant (and other

personnel who happen by). The state of alertness, the muscle tone, the activity, obvious anomalies or injuries, respiration, and the skin are assessed during inspection. The infant may appear sick or well, responsive or nonresponsive. The muscle tone should be sufficient for the hips, knees, and elbows to be flexed while the infant is lying supine or prone. Some spontaneous movements should be evident, and the well infant should appear alert at some point during the exam, unless the examiner is an extraordinarily boring person. The color should be pink, rather than sallow and pale or blue. Cyanosis may be generalized or limited to the distal extremities or to the lower part of the body, as is rarely seen with right-to-left shunting through a ductus arteriosus. When only the hands and feet are blue, the infant may be cold with resulting peripheral vasoconstriction. This appearance is called acrocyanosis.

The appearance of the small premature infant after stabilization is of course different from this description. The 900-g infant with respiratory distress syndrome may be intubated or ventilated and have an arterial line or peripheral intravenous lines in place. He or she usually has a thermistor attached for temperature regulation and

---

TABLE 23–7. History and Physical Examination Outline

TIME AND DATE OF HISTORY
ADDRESS AND PHONE NUMBERS FOR DAY AND NIGHT CONTACT
MATERNAL HISTORY
(See Table 23–2.)
NEONATAL COURSE
Delivery room events, resuscitation, Apgar scores, cord blood gases, evident anomalies, maternal condition after birth, gross appearance of placenta, results of initial lab tests, and other events before the physical examination below
NEWBORN PHYSICAL EXAMINATION
- Date and time of exam
- Weight and gross appearance of placenta
- Vital signs
- Overall appearance, symmetry, and general proportions
- Assessment of gestational length
- Height, weight, head circumference, and growth percentile
- Skin: bands, rash, birthmarks, tumors, and angiomas
- Head: size, shape, sutures, fontanels, and pressure
- Ears: tags, anatomy of folds, and placement on skull
- Eyes: size, spacing, coloboma, and cataracts
- Mouth: filtrum, size, and clefts
- Neck: fistula and swellings
- Lungs/chest: malformations or air entry
- Heart/vascular: pulses, rhythm, murmurs, and point of maximal intensity
- Abdomen: cord, vessels, masses, distention, scaphoid, bowel sounds, and musculature
- Extremities: extra digits, bands, duplications, or fusions
- Spine: scoliosis, sinus, or masses
- Genitourinary and anus
- Musculoskeletal: range of motion, movement, or pain
- Neurologic: movement, responses, tone, sensorium, cranial nerves, and reflexes
IMPRESSIONS/PROBLEMS
COMMON LAB RESULTS
- Initial neonatal blood gases and oxygen saturation, and FiO$_2$
- Complete blood count and hematocrit
- Blood sugar (Dextrostix)
- Cultures taken: blood or cerebrospinal fluid
- Screenings: syphilis, rubella, HIV, hepatitis, tuberculosis, genetic and metabolic diseases, and illicit drugs
INITIAL RADIOGRAPHY AND IMAGING RESULTS
PLAN
SIGNATURE AND TITLE

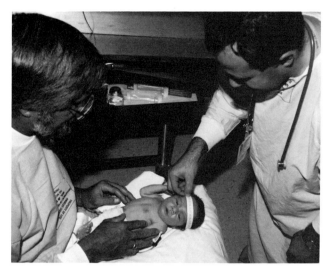

FIGURE 23–5. *Positioning of tape for head circumference measurement.*

leads attached for cardiac and respiratory monitoring. This infant may also be sedated or paralyzed by muscle relaxants. Regardless, the infant is usually flaccid and minimally responsive. The infant may be covered in various ways to minimize heat loss and restrained to maintain the vascular lines. Stimulation during the exam may cause arterial desaturation, silent crying attempts around the endotracheal tube, decreased blood pressure, tachycardia or bradycardia, and decreased skin perfusion. In these cases, continual information on gas exchange, blood pressure, temperature, ventilation, and heart rate is gained at the price of access to the infant, which in any case can be harmful, especially if the exam is lengthy and/or inept. Nonetheless, a careful head-to-foot examination can be gently and quickly carried out by one or two (not four or five) examiners. The cardiac and pulmonary exams are often difficult because of ventilator noise (water accumulation in the inspiratory tube) and because of difficulties obtaining a good seal on the chest of premature babies with stethoscope bells designed for larger babies. The examination of the abdomen using a single index finger is often easier than the exam of full-term infants because of the thinness and diminished tone of the anterior abdominal wall.

Anomalies and birth injuries are often apparent on inspection. Malformations and deformations are discussed in Chapter 21 and chromosomal problems are discussed in Chapter 16. The most common anomalies are listed in Table 23–8. Birth injuries occur with greater frequency in breech deliveries and with other abnormal presentations. The most common birth injuries are listed in Table 23–9.

The chest should be inspected for symmetry. A prominent left chest may indicate cardiac hypertrophy from an obstructive lesion. A visible cardiac impulse may indicate a patent ductus arteriosus with left-to-right shunt. A small chest with the infant manifesting respiratory distress or failure may indicate pulmonary hypoplasia or, in a more severe form, asphyxiating thoracic dystrophy.

Much information is obtained by watching the infant breathe. Regular respiratory movements of <60/min without suprasternal, intercostal, or subcostal retractions and absence of jaundice make pulmonary disease unlikely. Apneic spells versus periodic breathing can be observed.

TABLE 23–8. Most Common Anomalies Noted on the Initial Exam

ANOMALY	FREQUENCY (LIVE BIRTHS)
Skin tags	10–15/1000
Polydactyly	10–15/1000
Cleft lip or palate	1–4/1000
Congenital heart defects	1–4/1000
Congenital hip dislocation	1–4/1000
Down syndrome	1–4/1000*
Talipes equinovarus	1–4/1000
Spina bifidas, anencephaly, or encephalocele	1–4/10,000

*Increases with maternal age >33.

INSPECTION BY SYSTEM

After one gains a general impression of the infant's status and is convinced that emergency intervention (intubation, relief of pneumothorax, or transfusion) is unnecessary, one may continue observation of the infant by system, usually starting at the head and working caudad. Then the exam is repeated with palpation, auscultation, reflex testing, the shining of lights into various orifices, and finally, range of motion. Auscultation and abdominal exam require a quiet if not cooperative infant. The hip exam and the Moro reflex testing should be the finale as these assessments frequently leave the infant displeased with the whole concept of being examined.

SKIN

Vernix usually covers the skin especially in the skinfolds of the axillae, neck, and groin at birth. Post-term infants characteristically have little vernix, and the skin is dry, cracked, and wrinkled. The texture of the skin is evaluated with regard to scaliness, elasticity, thickness, and local or generalized edema (see also Part XVIII). One looks for hemangiomas, nevi, and urticarial, pustular, vesicular, nodular, or ischemic rashes. Particularly in those with vascular catheters, evidence of partial or complete arterial or venous obstruction should be sought at regular intervals. Dermal sinuses occur in the midline of the back from occiput to coccyx and near the ears and in the neck. Dimples, sinuses, hirsute areas, or cystic swellings suggest the presence of cranial or vertebral sinuses or underlying defects.

Ecchymoses or petechiae may relate to birth trauma and may herald a more-than-normal degree of hyperbili-

TABLE 23–9. Most Frequent Birth Injuries

- Decreased gas exchange: placental insufficiency, prolapsed cord, or premature placental separation*
- Broken clavicle
- Facial palsy
- Brachial plexus injuries (especially Erb palsy)
- Fractures of the humerus or skull
- Ruptured internal organs
- Testicular trauma
- Fat necrosis
- Lacerations or scalpel injury and cephalohematoma
- Scalp lesions from fetal scalp electrode, or forceps
- Bleeding of the cord or placenta: hypotension or shock

*Acute prepartum asphyxia of sufficient duration and severity to be associated with hypoxic-ischemic encephalopathy. The incidence for each of these conditions is roughly 1–3/1000 livebirths.

rubinemia as the blood products break down and are absorbed over 24 to 36 hours. Generalized and recurring petechiae especially those not on the head and necklace region may signify serious infectious or hematologic problems.

Common findings include milia, white papules less than 1 mm, that are scattered across the forehead. These and white vesicles with a red base (erythema toxicum) are transient and benign. In black infants, a similar but more dramatic benign condition is transient neonatal pustular melanosis. These conditions at times are impossible to differentiate from infectious pustules by inspection. Jaundice in the 3rd day of life or later is common, but jaundice that is evident on the 1st day of life is unusual and needs laboratory investigation.

HEAD

The commonest abnormalities are caput succedaneum and cephalohematoma. The first is edema of the scalp skin and crosses suture lines. Cephalohematomas are subperiosteal and therefore do not cross suture lines. Frequently, one gains the impression of a depressed skull fracture as one palpates the rim of a cephalohematoma. This (false) perception is so common that we do not routinely take skull radiographs of an infant with a cephalohematoma unless other worrisome signs are present as well. In the 1st day of life, molding of the head from descent through the birth canal may be present, and the skull plates are overriding. After a few days, one can better estimate the size of the fontanels and their flatness, fullness, or tenseness and the width of suture lines (Popich and Smith, 1972; Faix, 1982). One can note the fusion of the sagittal, metopic, or coronal sutures—totally, partially, or unilaterally. Large fontanels and split sutures are most often a normal variant, but they can be associated with increased intracranial pressure or conditions that impair bone growth. Likewise, small fontanels and overriding sutures are generally of little significance but may be associated with conditions in which brain growth has been retarded (Table 23–10). Unusual whorls or other hair patterns or asymmetries of the skull may indicate problems in global or regional brain development.

Craniotabes is a demineralized area or softening of the skull. In newborn infants when this is appreciated to a mild degree near the suture lines, it is commonly a normal variant. When it is present over most of the skull, it may be associated with conditions in which calcification has been deficient, e.g., syphilis or osteogenesis imperfecta.

Transillumination is useful for detecting severe hydrocephaly and hydranencephaly. The heads of premature infants normally have a greater degree of transillumination than the heads of term infants.

EYES

Eyes are difficult to examine in the newborn especially when instillation of silver nitrate has occurred. Its use, now not preferred over other antibacterials, is associated with swelling and conjunctivitis during the first 36 hours of life. Often a soothed infant with to-and-fro rocking during which the head is elevated, spontaneously opens his or her eyes, allowing inspection and the ability to assess visual tracking of the examiner's face or a bright object as it moves from side to side (Fig. 23–6). Gross vision can also be assessed by noting whether the infant turns to a diffuse light. Pupils should be equal, reactive to light, and symmetric. The corneae should be clear. The pupil can be inspected with a light and the pink retina (red reflex) discerned to rule out lenticular, anterior, or posterior chamber opacities. Fixed strabismus should be absent, and the eye movements for the most part should be coordinated. Eye movements can be assessed by checking for oculovestibular nystagmus by holding the infant under the axillae facing the examiner while the examiner turns in a circle. The infant's eyes have a slow deviation in the direction of spin with quick movements in the opposite direction. If other disease is present or a more complete exam is indicated, then the eyes should be dilated and the infant restrained for a complete retinal exam.

EARS

The ears are examined for placement and deformation. Low-set and/or posteriorly rotated ears may be associated with other more major anomalies. Usually, the tips of the ears are cephalad to a circumferential line around the skull through the inner and outer canthus of both eyes. Gross hearing is assessed by seeing whether the infant blinks to a loud noise (handclap) and whether the infant attends to an unusual sound (ringing a bell or tuning fork). In the

TABLE 23–10. Disorders Sometimes Associated with Abnormal Fontanel Size

TOO LARGE
- Skeletal disorders (e.g., hypophosphatasia or osteogenesis imperfecta)
- Chromosomal abnormalities
- Hypothyroidism
- Increased intracranial pressure or hydrocephalus

TOO SMALL
- Hyperthyroidism
- Craniosynostosis
- Microcephaly

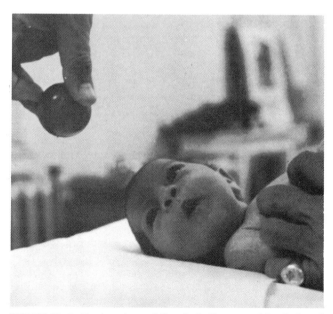

FIGURE 23–6. Head turning to follow ball. (Courtesy of Dr. B. Brazelton.)

immediate newborn period, the ear canals are usually occluded by vernix and are not routinely examined.

MOUTH AND LOWER FACE

The lips may be good indicators of whether or not the infant is cyanotic. Retention cysts on the alveolar ridge may appear like teeth, and in fact, natal teeth occur rarely and are usually shed in a few days. Retention cysts are called Epstein pearls, and these disappear in a few weeks. The frenulum, which in years past was occasionally cut to prevent "tongue-tie" can usually be ignored. The palate is examined for cleft, the tongue for size, and the sublingual area for masses. Both corners of the mouth should move symmetrically when the infant cries or grimaces, and asymmetry is most usually caused by a seventh cranial nerve palsy. A long philtrum, thin upper lip, cleft lip, cleft palate, and small jaw are other significant findings associated with abnormal fetal development sometimes caused by chromosomal abnormalities.

NOSE

Patency of each naris can be checked by listening at the orifice while the other naris is occluded with the mouth closed. Newborn infants breathe preferentially through the nose so that bilateral choanal atresia may cause severe respiratory distress. Flaring of the nostrils occurs whenever respiratory effort is increased regardless of cause.

Almost half of all infants have nonfunctional nasolacrimal ducts for 1 to 5 days. Swelling is common at the inner canthal region, but infection (dacryocystitis) is rare. More than 80 per cent open spontaneously by age 3 months.

NECK

The neck of the newborn always seems short. Very short and webbed necks may be associated with Klippel-Feil or Turner syndrome. The neck is palpated for cysts or masses. A thyroglossal duct cyst is usually palpable in the midline and retracts with tongue protrusion. The infant may have congenital muscular torticollis with or without a fibrous mass in the sternocleidomastoid muscle, associated with head tilt (see Chapter 21). A cystic hygroma is a spongy mass that may increase with increased intrathoracic pressure and may transilluminate. Hemangiomas are similar to hygromas upon palpation but frequently are associated with skin discoloration. Branchial cleft cysts may have associated fistulae. They are palpable anterior to the sternocleidomastoid and may retract with swallowing. Thyroid masses are usually visible and easily palpable with the head extended.

CHEST AND LUNGS

The circumference of the chest of the newborn is roughly equivalent to that of the head. Continued inspection of the chest may reveal a protruding xiphisternum (pectus carinatum), which is usually a normal variant. In contrast, a pigeon breast deformity (pectus excavatum) may be present at birth or associated with prolonged low-compliance respiration. While breathing, nasal flaring may be present along with retractions and "grunting," which is partial glottic closure at the first part of expiration. Suprasternal retractions and gasping, as opposed to substernal retractions, may indicate upper airway obstruction, and laryngoscopy should be performed rapidly. Almost any cardiopulmonary disease in the newborn period reduces lung compliance and is associated with subcostal retractions. The appearance of flaring, grunting, tachypnea, and retractions is called respiratory distress. Respiratory distress may be associated with pneumonia, delayed resorption of lung fluid, respiratory distress syndrome, or any number of cardiorespiratory problems.

Asymmetry of the chest may indicate fetal obstructive cardiac anomalies, a tension pneumothorax, or other forms of air trapping or mass lesions.

The nipples and underlying breast tissue are usually 1 cm in diameter in term infants, both boys and girls, and these may be asymmetric. Under maternal hormonal influence the breast bud may become as large as 3 to 4 cm and may excrete a watery whitish fluid for a few days or weeks ("witch's" milk). The enlargement occurs in both sexes, and is usually symmetric. Redness or asymmetry indicates probable infection, which requires the administration of antibiotics. Widely spaced nipples and accessory nipples should be noted.

Single-finger percussion can be useful for detection of consolidated pneumonias or pleural effusions. Suspicion of clinically significant pneumothorax should lead to instant confirmatory checks of blood pressure, auscultation, transillumination, emergency pleural taps, and chest radiographs. Transillumination is carried out with high-energy cuffed flashlights or fiberoptic transillumination devices in a darkened room. Some practice is necessary before one can clearly distinguish the normal from excessive coronas of pink transillumination around the closely applied light source.

Auscultation of the lungs is best carried out with a cleaned and warmed stethoscope bell. Rhonchi can be inspiratory or expiratory. Inspiratory stridor implies large airway obstruction, and expiratory prolongation indicates small airway obstruction. Rales are moist crackling sounds emulated by licking a thumb and forefinger and separating them close to one's ear. The burst of fine crackles on separation of the thumb and forefinger is of the same quality and intensity as rales in the newborn. Gurgling and bubbling sounds come from secretions in large airways and often indicate the need for tracheal suctioning. Harsher bubbling sounds may be from water accumulating in the tubing of a ventilator. Listening alternately in the right and left axillae may indicate diminished breath sounds on either the right or the left. These asymmetries may indicate unilateral pneumothorax or that an endotracheal tube has inadvertently advanced into the right mainstem bronchus. Rarely, bowel sounds may be heard high in the chest in the absence of breath sounds. If so, diaphragmatic hernia is suspected, and emergency radiologic examination and surgical consultation are mandatory. Meanwhile, a nasogastric tube should be inserted to prevent distention of stomach and bowel within the chest cavity.

HEART AND VASCULAR SYSTEM

The most common cardiac conditions in the newborn period include perinatal adaptations involving the ductus arteriosus (see Chapter 61), with right-to-left shunting through the ductus of term infants and persistent pulmonary hypertension and left-to-right shunting through the ductus of premature infants. Significant structural heart anomalies occur in the first week of life in about 1 per cent of livebirths. The commonest anomalies recognized in the first week of life are transpositions, hypoplastic left heart syndromes, tetralogy of Fallot, and coarctations. The commonest findings for an infant with heart disease in the newborn period are tachypnea and/or cyanosis—"an increased O_2 requirement." These findings are associated with the commonest pathophysiologic conditions associated with congenital heart disease: low output, congestive heart failure from shunts, obstruction to outflow, and insufficient pulmonary blood flow. The general appearance can often signal a cardiac problem, for example, the shocky underperfused infant on the 3rd day of life with a hypoplastic left ventricle versus the contented cyanotic infant in no distress with transposition of the great vessels. Other aspects of heart disease detectable from general inspection are the severity of signs, hypertrophy of the left chest, and rarely, venous engorgement (for example, in an infant with thrombosis of a central venous line leading to a vena cava syndrome).

Murmurs. These should first be checked in "noncardiac" areas such as the axilla (peripheral pulmonic stenosis), the neck (aortic obstruction), and the head and liver (atrioventricular malformations). Timing of the onset of murmurs is important. Frequently, murmurs that depend on pulmonary vascular tone (left-to-right shunt through a patent ductus arteriosus, for example) may not be heard until pulmonary vascular resistance has dropped in the 2nd to 3rd day of life in an infant with RDS or within 12 hours of birth in a normal full-term infant. The murmur of tricuspid insufficiency associated with a dilated heart after severe perinatal asphyxia may be present only in the first hours of life. Obstructive murmurs characteristically are heard from birth unless low cardiac output is present. Other characteristics that are important to note are the site where they are heard best, the timing of the murmur with regard to systole and diastole, the quality, and the loudness. The murmurs that are of low intensity, that occur near the sternum or only in noncardiac areas, and that occur early in systole, are often innocent.

A detailed history and physical exam including four-extremity blood pressures, a chest radiograph, blood gases, electrocardiogram, and ultrasound examination are usually sufficient to clarify whether congenital heart disease is present or not. Neonatologists and pediatricians who frequently care for newborns should be able to screen the heart with ultrasound as well as with chest radiographs, electrocardiograms, and auscultation.

CASE 23–1

Baby B was transferred to the NICU at 6 hours of age because of tachypnea. The history of pregnancy and delivery was unremarkable. On examination the infant was a well-formed full-term infant breathing at a rate of 78/minute. Lungs had occasional rales. The heart rate was 180/minute. A gallop rhythm was heard but no murmurs. The liver was palpable 4 cm below the costal margin and was thought to be enlarged. The physical

findings suggested heart failure, which was confirmed by a chest radiograph that showed an enlarged heart and pulmonary congestion. Arterial blood gases in 30 per cent oxygen revealed a Pa_{O_2} of 68, a P_{CO_2} of 48, and a pH of 7.2 with a base deficit. An electrocardiogram indicated a modest reduction of voltage in all leads. Ultrasound exam of the heart revealed a large heart with poor contractility. A number of diagnoses were entertained including various cardiomyopathies, pericardial effusion, and anomalous pulmonary venous drainage with obstruction. The infant was taken for cardiac catheterization where a large and inoperable AV malformation of the brain was diagnosed after injection of dye for cardiac angiography. After the infant returned to the unit a large bruit was easily heard with the stethoscope applied to the anterior fontanel or to the skull lateral to the eyes.

This case serves as a reminder that heart failure may occur from arteriovenous fistulas anywhere in the body.

ABDOMEN

The abdomen is assessed by inspection and palpation for organomegaly, masses, inflammation, and distention. Unusual flatness or a scaphoid shape to the abdomen may be associated with congenital diaphragmatic hernia. Examination by inspection, palpation, auscultation, transillumination, and ultrasound examination can usually discriminate air within or outside the gastrointestinal tract, and enlarged viscus or viscera, or a cystic or solid tumor. Normally, one palpates a 1- to 2-cm liver edge below the right costal margin, a spleen tip overlying the stomach, and the lower pole of the left kidney in the pelvic gutter (Fig. 23–7). One also looks for dilated veins on the abdominal wall indicating venous distention. Visible gastric or bowel patterns may be considered a certain sign of

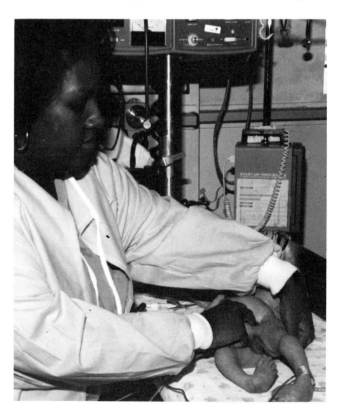

FIGURE 23–7. *Abdominal palpation is carried out using counterpressure in the flank with one hand. The lower pole of each kidney is usually palpable with this technique in the first days of life before abdominal muscle tone increases. Note the bilateral club feet.*

ileus or other obstruction. The umbilical stump should be examined for bleeding, abnormal vessels, increased or decreased Wharton jelly, meconium staining, polyps, granuloma, exudative discharge, or other evidence of inflammation (redness, tenderness, edema of abdominal wall, induration) or abnormal communication with intra-abdominal viscera. Omphaloceles and gastroschisis are readily apparent, but small umbilical hernias and diastasis recti abdominis may be less so.

Abdominal masses occur in about one of 1000 livebirths (Table 23–11). Most masses are benign, and a tentative diagnosis is made after history, physical examination, ultrasound, and radiography. Some masses are transitory and of little significance, e.g., intraluminal stool, gaseous dilatation of the stomach or colon, distended bladder, or large but normal kidneys (Table 23–12).

GENITAL SYSTEM

Maturation of the genitalia is apparent over the last 3 months of gestation, and these changes serve as one index on scoring of physical attributes for gestational age assignment. There is a surprising range of differences that nonetheless fall within the normal range. For a discussion of ambiguous genitalia, see Chapter 98. Penile length and clitoral size are assessed. A clear white mucus is often present in the vagina of term infants for the first few days as a result of estrogens from the mother. The location of the urethral meatus and presence or absence of palpable gonads are noted, and inguinal hernias are looked for. Most "congenital" hernias have an onset in appearance only after a month or two, and these are most common in premature infants. The anus should be checked for patency and distance from the genitalia. The perineum should be checked for palpable masses.

MUSCULOSKELETAL SYSTEM

The musculoskeletal system is assessed by observation and palpation for obvious trauma, inflammation, or malformation. The most common alterations in the musculo-

TABLE 23–11. Commonest Congenital Abdominal Masses

> **Renal** (55% of total abdominal masses)
> - Hydronephrosis
> - Multicystic or polycystic kidneys
> - Renal malformations
> - Renal vein thrombosis
> - Renal neoplasms
>
> **Genital** (15%)
> - Hydrometrocolpos
> - Ovarian cyst
>
> **Gastrointestinal** (15%)
> - Obstructions
> - Cysts or tumors
> - Duplications
>
> **Liver and Biliary** (5%)
> - Cysts
> - Tumors
>
> **Retroperitoneal** (5%)
> - Solid tumors
> - Anterior meningomyelocele
>
> **Adrenal** (5%)
> - Hemorrhage
> - Neuroblastoma

Data from Griscom, N. T.: The roentgenology of neonatal abdominal masses. Am. J. Roentgenol., *93*:447, 1965 and Kirks, D.: Radiol. Clin. North Am., *19*:527, 1981.

TABLE 23–12. Common Findings of Little Clinical Significance*

- *Head:* caput succedaneum, cephalohematoma, asymmetries, bony protrusions, or molding
- *Ears:* skin tags
- *Eyes:* position (close-set) or conjunctival hemorrhage
- *Nose:* asymmetric nares
- *Mouth:* ranula, sucking calluses, epulis, frenulum, natal teeth, or Epstein pearls
- *Face:* unusual features not consistent with known syndromes
- *Skin:* sparse petechiae on the head, erythema toxicum, mongolian spot, nevus flammeus, telangiectasia, nevi, inclusion cysts, bruises, prominent lanugo or vernix, milia, miliaria, dark pigmentation over genital skin, mild jaundice after 2nd day, peeling of skin, skin tags, or sacrococcygeal dimple
- *Neck:* relative absence
- *Chest:* nipple spacing, extra nipples, breast hypertrophy, witch's milk
- *Umbilicus:* erythema or umbilicus cutis
- *Abdomen:* evanescent masses
- *Heart:* evanescent murmurs and adventitious sounds
- *Genitalia:* mild hypospadias, prominent labia, mucous secretion, transient vaginal blood, or phimosis
- *Extremities:* extra digits, syndactyly, hips tight to abduction, or neck in extension after breech delivery
- *Neurologic system:* transient tone asymmetries or abnormality, jitters, or sudden jerky movements

*Some of the items on this list may in fact be associated with significant disease, e.g., jitteriness may be associated with metabolic problems or drug withdrawal. However, when findings on this list are mild and transient, they are most frequently not associated with significant disease. When in doubt, it is prudent to ask for another opinion and follow up.

skeletal system are deformations caused by adverse mechanical forces in utero. Oligohydramnios that limits fetal movement and neuromuscular problems of the fetus can both be associated with multiple contractures known as arthrogryposis. Most positional deformities are mild and resolve with time. The hips deserve special attention since the physical exam is the only method of detecting problems before permanent damage has occurred by 1 year of age or so. Examination of the hips should be undertaken repeatedly in the 1st year of life because a dislocation may not be demonstrable for several months after birth (see Chapter 21) (Place et al., 1978).

Congenital dislocation of the hips occurs in about one of 800 livebirths, more commonly in whites and females. Maternal hormones during pregnancy may contribute to joint capsule laxity particularly in the female fetus. The condition represents a spectrum of conditions from the dislocatable hip found in approximately 5 out of 100 livebirths, to the fixed dislocation that may occur in the second trimester associated with some forms of arthrogryposis. In utero conditions that limit hip movement as well as specific syndromes and chromosomal disorders may be associated with hip dislocation. It is often unilateral, occurring more commonly in the left hip, for reasons that are unclear.

There are two major tests (with a number of variations) for determining whether the femoral head is fixed in the acetabulum (Fig. 23–8). The Barlow test determines whether the femoral head can be dislocated posteriorly. As the knees are brought together (adducted) or held in midabduction, the examiner pushes laterally on the upper inner thigh (lesser trochanter). A click or clunk indicates that the femoral head slips over the lateral ridge of the

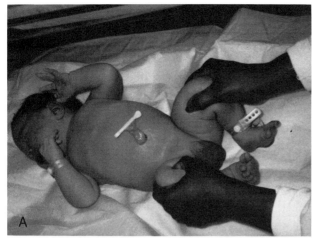

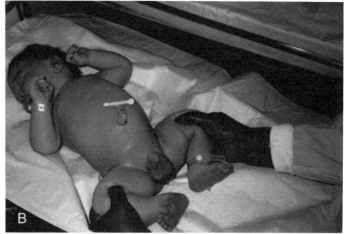

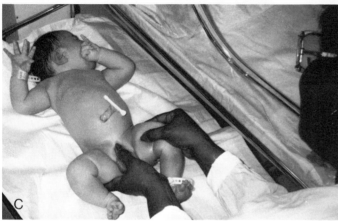

FIGURE 23–8. A, *The hips are checked with the Ortolani maneuver. The examiner's second and third fingers press up against the heads of the femurs and the hands press the shafts of the femurs toward the mattress while simultaneously abducting the hips. A palpable "clunk" during this maneuver indicates that the femoral head has slipped over the lip of the acetabulum and is dislocatable.* B *shows full abduction.* C, *For the Barlow maneuver, the examiner stabilizes the pelvis with her left hand and attempts to move the shaft of the femur upward and downward without flexing the hip. This maneuver checks whether the femoral head can be displaced posteriorly out of the acetabulum; instability of the femoral head is palpable during this maneuver with congenitally dislocated hips.*

acetabulum during this maneuver. With the examiner's fingers on the greater trochanter, the hip can be alternately pushed into and out of the acetabulum by alternating pressure with the thumb or the fingers. The Ortolani test is carried out by abducting the flexed hips while the examiner pushes upward on the posterior proximal femur. The knees are flexed to 90 degrees; downward pressure is exerted on the knee while the hips are simultaneously abducted. A positive test occurs with a click or clunk as the laterally dislocated femoral head is pushed over the acetabular ridge into the acetabulum. A modification of the Barlow maneuver is to move the thigh anteriorly and posteriorly while holding the midthigh firmly with one hand and stabilizing the pelvis with the other. With this maneuver, the femoral head can alternately be dislocated and relocated, and in my experience, this test has been successful where the other two have not.

Fixed dislocations that occurred early in fetal life can often not be detected by the tests outlined above because the femoral head is locked outside of the acetabulum because of joint capsule contractures. The diagnosis is made by palpation of the femoral head posteriorly and by detecting limitation of hip mobility, in association with other problems such as spina bifida or arthrogryposis.

The four extremities should be checked for fractures and the joints for hyper- or hypomobility. A hypotonic arm or wrist drop implies brachial palsy on the affected side. The digits should be examined for polydactylism, syndactylism, edema, unusual skin ridge whorls and creases, nail growth, and unusual digit placement or

contractures. Amputations or other evidence of amniotic bands may be present. A variety of malformations of the lower extremities are common. *Genu recurvatum* is characterized by abnormal hyperextensibility of the knee joint. The number of females who are affected is significantly greater than the number of males. Many more babies with genu recurvatum present by the breech position than is to be expected. The disorder may also occur as a feature in a number of disorders, such as the **Ehlers-Danlos, Marfan, Klinefelter, and Turner syndromes**, but usually it occurs as an in utero deformation not associated with other conditions. The extended leg or both legs describe a concave arc when hyperextended at the knee. Hyperextensibility is mild or severe; that is, the arc is shallow or deep. In severe cases, there may be actual posterior dislocation of the knee. Nothing need be done for cases of mild or moderate severity. Posterior splinting or, rarely, casting for 2 to 4 weeks is indicated for the most severe forms.

Pes calcaneovalgus is the absolutely flat and sometimes slightly convex foot that often lies at rest dorsiflexed at an acute angle to the foreleg. When gentle pressure is applied to the sole of the foot, dorsiflexion increases easily until its dorsal surface lies in contact with the shin.

These feet should be casted in the equinovarus position for 4 to 6 weeks, and this therapy should be repeated several times if necesary. Continued treatment with tarsosupinator shoes and, perhaps, with the Denis Browne bar may probably be needed for several years.

In *pes metatarsovarus*, the heel and posterior half of

the foot appear normal, but the forefoot angulates sharply inward. Thus, the outer border of the foot is convex, whereas its inner border is concave. If the foot can be straightened by gentle traction, with the thumb held firmly over the apex of the convexity, no immediate treatment is needed. If, however, the angulation is difficult or impossible to overcome, casting is probably indicated. Later use of corrective shoes may or may not be necessary.

Pes equinovarus is the classic clubfoot with sharp and tight hyperextension and incurving of the entire foot. It is often a solitary defect but not infrequently it is associated with congenital dislocation of the hip, myelomeningocele, arthrogryposis, or other defects. It requires immediate and long-term orthopedic care. Most cases can be corrected by casting and subsequent shoe corrections. A few cases will require open operation.

NEUROLOGIC SYSTEM

The neurologic examination is discussed in detail in Chapter 42. For most infants, the aim is to find whether or not a neurologic problem exists (Table 23–13). If present, the examination can be expanded to fully describe the findings. For a paralyzed 800-g infant on a ventilator, a complete neurologic exam is impossible. Nonetheless, it should not be deferred completely. For example, attention to head size, shape, or abnormality, fontanel size and pressure, pupil size and equality, lability of blood gases and blood pressure, variability of heart rate, and limb muscle mass are all available information about an infant's CNS status.

The quality and quantity of spontaneous movements are the best indicators of neuromuscular function and are assessed by inspection. Decreased tone may be one of the first detectable abnormalities in a full-term infant with sepsis. Tone is gestation- and illness-dependent, with smaller and sick infants having decreased tone. Tone may also differ in different muscle groups. The range of passive rotation of the neck is checked by turning the head to the left and right. Flexor tone in the neck and arms is assessed by pulling the infant toward a sitting position (Fig. 23–9). Extensor tone in the neck is evaluated by holding the infant prone. Shoulder tone is assessed by holding the infant in a vertical sling, i.e., under the axillae, and by the scarf maneuver (Fig. 23–10). Tone in the lower extremities is checked by the hip exam and by the heel-to-ear maneuver.

An array of primitive reflexes are present in the term

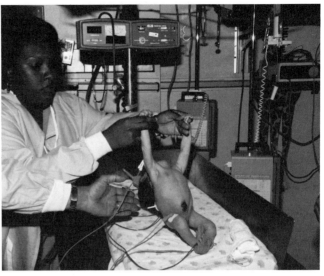

FIGURE 23–9. *Tone of the neck flexors is assessed by pulling the infant off the mattress by both hands. In this infant marked head lag is present.*

newborn infant, but their expression is highly dependent on state—the most optimal being a sleepy awake state. Premature infants have diminished responses with decreasing gestational age, although this belief may be confounded by the increasing frequency of illness with decreasing gestation and the fact that sick infants respond poorly to elicitation of these reflexes. The Moro and the tonic neck reflex disappear by 6 months of age, but others make their appearance as these wane—e.g., the parachute and the Landau reflexes.

The most obvious primitive reflex of the newborn is the Moro. The infant can be supported behind the upper back by the examiner's hand, then dropped back 1 cm or so to the mattress. The arms are flung open followed by a flexion and an adduction, i.e., an "embrace." The eyes open, as if in surprise, and the baby commonly emits a lusty cry making this reflex a good stopping point for the exam. The grasp reflex can be elicited in both hands and feet by placing a thumb on the infant's palm. With palmar pressure, the infant may open his or her mouth and yawn (palmar-mental reflex). By stimulating the dorsum of the feet the infant lifts the stimulated foot and places it on a surface (placing). By allowing the plantar surface of the other foot to contact a table top, the infant makes crude sequential walking movements (stepping). The tonic neck reflex is obtained by rotating the infant's head to the right or left while maintaining the supine infant's shoulders flat. The arm and leg to the side of the occiput flex, and the contralateral arm and leg extend (fencer's stance). When the infant is supported prone by the examiner's hand, tickling the area of the lateral spine causes the buttocks to swing to the side of stimulation (trunk incurvation reflex). Holding the infant in the same position and running a finger from the base of the spine toward the neck elicits spinal extension and, with a full bladder, micturition. Light pressure applied with the examiner's fingers to the soles of the feet causes the legs to extend (magnet reflex). Extending one of the infant's legs while the infant is supine and stimulating the plantar surface of the same foot causes the contralateral leg to flex, adduct, and extend (crossed extension reflex).

TABLE 23–13. Outline of Neurologic Screening Examination

- Appearance
- Behavior, state, or abnormal movements
- Visual responses
- Hearing responses
- Head size and shape
- Active and passive tone of major muscle groups:
  —suck and cry
  —neck
  —shoulders and upper extremities
  —trunk
  —lower extremities
- Cranial nerves
- Primitive neonatal reflexes
- Deep tendon reflexes

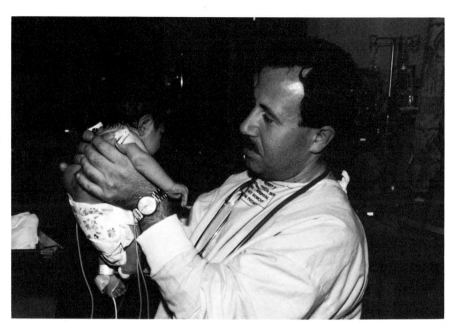

FIGURE 23–10. *The infant is held in a vertical sling. Muscle tone of the shoulder girdle is assessed with this maneuver. Extensor tone of the neck is checked. The infant may follow the face of the examiner. In older infants, "scissoring" of the lower extremities is suggestive of increased tone. With the infant held in this position while the examiner turns in a circle, oculovestibular nystagmus can be assessed.*

The deep tendon reflexes are best assessed using the tap of the examiner's index finger.

Other physical findings of clinical significance are listed in Table 23–14. Table 23–15 lists the various evaluations for a "typical" high-risk premature infant during hospitalization.

■ ULTRASOUND EXAMINATION

Whenever a problem is defined with anomalies or with the head, heart, abdomen, or kidneys, the physician should conduct a screening ultrasound examination. While the physician of newborns may not be an expert in imaging technique, he or she should be capable of doing a screening exam in the same way one carries out auscultation of the heart even when one is not a cardiologist. In this, obstetricians subspecializing in perinatology have surpassed neonatologists in their proficiency with ultrasound screening. Using a 5 MHz sector scanner, the examiner can gain useful information using only gain and depth controls.

Head. The head is examined in the coronal and parasagittal planes through the anterior fontanel. Ventricular size and the presence or absence of paraventricular and intraventricular blood are noted. A large degree of ventricular enlargement can be appreciated even by the relatively untrained examiner.

Heart. The examiner should be able to identify all four chambers by aiming the probe, held in a transverse plane, cephalad from the substernal area. Atria are smaller than the ventricles and are symmetric. At birth, the ventricles appear equally sized. Good contractility can be appreciated. Pericardial fluid may be noted by the presence of an echo-free area around the heart that is surrounded by the echo-dense pericardium.

Renal. The paravertebral areas and the locale of the bladder are examined. Presence, size, shape, and whether large cysts or dilated collection systems are noted. The bladder can be visualized if filled with urine.

■ LABORATORY SCREENING

At the time of the initial history and physical exam, the infant should be screened for a number of conditions that depend on the characteristics of the population being served. For example, in an inner-city population, we tend to screen particularly for the following conditions.

Syphilis. Standard immunologic tests for syphilis are a routine part of prenatal care in the United States. Because it is possible for exposure to occur between the first trimester and delivery, mothers or infants of high-risk populations should be screened at delivery as well.

Human Immunodeficiency Virus. We offer testing for the human immunodeficiency virus (HIV) antibody to the newborn of any mother who is positive for syphilis or hepatitis, from high-risk areas (Haiti, Dominican Republic, endemic parts of Africa, or inner cities of the United States), involved with prostitution, an intravenous drug abuser, or a mother with no prenatal care. Risk varies widely in different geographic areas.

TABLE 23–14. Common Physical Findings of Clinical Significance

- Apnea
- Tachypnea
- Grunting
- Bradycardia
- Cyanosis
- Hypotonia
- Decreased breath sounds
- Heart murmurs
- Organomegaly
- Evident anomalies other than ears and digits
- Jaundice
- Plethora or pallor
- Diffuse petechiae

TABLE 23–15. Changing Issues During Hospitalization of a "Typical" High-Risk Premature Infant

INITIAL EVALUATION
- Major malformations
- Severe cardiopulmonary conditions
- Viability
- Postasphyxial complex
- Hypotension
- Intrauterine growth and length of gestation
- Meeting with parents

MIDWEEK EVALUATION
- Patent ductus arteriosus
- Intraventricular hemorrhage
- Pneumothoraces and airleaks
- Jaundice
- Culture reports
- Meeting with parents

FIRST-WEEK EVALUATION
- Metabolic
- Renal
- Gastrointestinal issues, necrotizing enterocolitis
- Intraventricular hemorrhage
- Meeting with parents

FIRST-MONTH EVALUATION
- Chronic lung disease
- Cystic periventricular lesions or ventricular enlargement
- Retinopathy
- Nutritional status
- Nosocomial infection
- Meeting with parents

INTERMEDIATE CARE EVALUATIONS
- Parental issues
- Anemia
- Feeding
- Hydrocephalus
- Growth
- Chronic CNS disability
- Apnea

BEFORE-DISCHARGE EVALUATIONS
- Meeting with parents
- Special needs, e.g., home oxygen
- Primary care versus specialty medical follow-up planning
- Other support services
- Review of hospital course and global follow-up plans

Hepatitis B. We screen newborns whose mothers are involved in prostitution or come from high-risk areas (Asia, Africa, Pacific islands, or inner cities of the United States) and those with occupational exposure to blood products, those who have been rejected for blood donation, those who have received multiple frequent blood transfusions or any transfusion before 1985, IV drug users, those who have had no prenatal care, or those with a positive history of liver disease or who live with family members with liver disease or on dialysis. Current risk estimates for infants born in Los Angeles are approximately 3 per 1000 live-births (HIV and hepatitis data courtesy of Dr. L. Mascola, Los Angeles Department of Health Services).

Drug Abuse. Toxicology screens are carried out on urine for newborns whose mothers have an illicit drug history, who received little prenatal care, and (for our inner-city population) on all NICU admissions. The screen used in our hospital identifies metabolites of amphetamines, phencyclidine (angel dust), opiates, and cocaine. It does not identify alcohol or cannabis. Approximately 20 per cent of inner-city infants admitted to NICUs test positive for illicit drugs.

Tuberculosis. Mothers in the previously listed high-risk groups should be skin-tested near delivery, and positive results should be followed with a chest radiograph and a careful history for tuberculosis exposure and treatment.

Metabolic Diseases. The United States and most developed countries now have centralized screening programs for all newborn infants. These were initiated after judging them cost-effective primarily for phenylketonuria. These assays vary according to state and county, but most generally screen for thyroid disorders, galactosemia, and other metabolic diseases as well as phenylketonuria (Table 23–16).

■ WELL BABY CARE

The principles of routine care for normal infants are those of screening for disease, prophylaxis for common problems (eye care and vitamin K_1 oxide), education when needed about infant care, and anticipatory guidance. The initial and discharge history and exams are truncated versions of the above. A welcome current trend "demedicalizes" routine delivery and postpartum care. This concept means delivery in a "homey," rather than an operating room setting. More choices are offered to the parents concerning issues of childbirth, such as anesthesia and route and timing of delivery. The infant and mother are kept together as much as possible after birth. The mother and infant are now discharged from 1 to 3 days after a routine delivery. Fathers are often present during delivery, and liberal visiting policies that allow children to see their mother and new sibling are encouraged. Both before and after birth, nonmedically oriented classes are offered for discussing problems of both the mother and the infant. Forces in favor of these trends come from parents and (with regard to shorter hospital stays) financial considerations. Forces against these trends stem from administrative difficulties in handling the desires of parents and concerns about cross-infection.

The pediatrician usually sees the infant and the mother daily while in the hospital, often in conjunction with a nurse practitioner; a full examination is done within 24 hours of birth and again prior to discharge.

In most United States hospitals, in the delivery room, the newborn's eyes are instilled with erythromycin or 1 per cent silver nitrate drops from single-use containers for prophylaxis of gonococcal eye infection. Vitamin K_1 oxide, 0.5 to 1.0 mg, is given intramuscularly, to prevent hemorrhagic disease of the newborn. The infant is then bathed with a nonmedicated mild soap. No antiseptic is routinely applied to the umbilical cord stump.

TABLE 23–16. Available Newborn Screening Tests

DISEASE	APPROXIMATE FREQUENCY
Biotinidase deficiency	1/70,000
Congenital adrenal hyperplasia	1/12,000
Cystic fibrosis	1/2000 (white)
Duchenne muscular dystrophy	1/11,000
Galactosemia	1/70,000
Hemoglobinopathy	1/400 (black)
Homocystinuria	1/100,000
Hypothyroidism	1/4000
Maple syrup urine disease	1/275,000
Phenylketonuria	1/15,000

N.I.C.U. Patient Data Base
KING/DREW MEDICAL CENTER
County of Los Angeles • Department of Health Services

Imprint Patient's ID
MLK No.
Name
D.O.B

Census/Transport

Inborn ☐	Hospital ☐		Date of
Transport ☐	of Origin		Adm.
Referring Physician		Phone	Admission Weight (gms)

Discharge Data

Status: ☐ Alive ☐ Dead
Discharge Date:
Transferred to:

Maternal Data

MLK No. _____ Phone (__)_____

Address _____
    Street   City   State   ZIP

Age	Married ☐ Single ☐	Education	0-9	10-12	Grad	> HS	Habits	Yes	No
							Smokes > 10 cigs/day		
Race	White	Black	Hispanic	Asian	Other	Home Language	Alcoholic drinks > 3/day		
							Illicit drugs (hx or tox)		
							Drug(s) used:		

Pregnancy Data

Trimester	1	2	3		Yes	No
Number of Prenatal Care Visits				Previous Births < 4lb		
				Prenatal Tocolytics		
Parity (now): G____P____Ab____				Prenatal Steroids		
				C-Section		

Birth Data

Apgar Score	1 min		5 min	
Gestational Age (wks)				
Birth Weight (kg)				

Diagnoses

	Yes	No	?*
IVH (Grade III or IV)			
PDA requiring Indocin or Ligation			
NEC (pneumatosis or perforation)			
Post Asphyxial Encephalopathy			
Pneumothorax/PIE			
Retinopathy of Prematurity			

* Not determined

Procedures

	Yes	No	?*
UA Catheter			
Central Line			
Cut Down			
Chest tube			
Exchange Transfusion			

* Not known

Use Reverse Side for Additional Comments

Ventilator

RDS	None	CPAP +02	IMV <7 days	IMV >7 days
Days on Ventilator	None	≤7	8-14	15-21	≤22
BPD	None	Other Criteria	02 at 1 mo.	IMV > 1 mo.	IMV > 3 mo.

Sepsis

	Yes	No	Prob. Organism		
Congenital (<48°)					
Nosocomial (>48°)					
Number of episodes	1	2	3	≤4	

Major Anomalies/CHD	
Surgery (type)	
Other Major Dx.	

FIGURE 23–11. This one-page data collection form for discharge information of infants who have been in the neonatal intensive care unit can accompany the mother and be sent to multiple personnel involved in follow-up care. It helps when more detailed records are missing. (From Ekelem, I., and Taeusch, W.: Defining quality care indicators for the neonatal intensive care unit. J. Natl. Med. Assoc. 82:345–350, 1990.)

■ DISCHARGE PLANNING

Discharge from the intermediate care unit for premature infants can take place when the parents have made adequate preparations (actual and psychological) for the care of the infant. Meeting this need may take weeks of preparation on the part of the staff, and may include arranging in-home support and equipment, teaching feeding and medication techniques, and providing anticipatory guidance. Other criteria for discharge include adequate feeding and weight gain, and physiologic stability (e.g., absence of apnea and steady body temperature).

Detailed recording of the major events of the infant's stay—diagnoses, results of meetings with parents and case conferences, most recent evaluations, medications, and future needs—all should be summarized, and the information disseminated appropriately.

Most importantly, the primary physician should know the parents and the infant well by the time of discharge, so trust and confidence exist on both sides.

DISCHARGE SUMMARY

Our summary discharge data sheet for all infants leaving the neonatal intensive care unit is shown in Figure 23–11. This one-page data collection sheet contains approximately 70 fields that are easily entered (<5 minutes/page) on a microcomputer. We use an easily accessible database management program for sorting and analysis. Data are used for tracking, follow-up, morbidity and mortality analyses, quality control, census tracking, staff and equipment needs assessments, infection control, comparison with neighboring hospitals, teaching purposes, and obtaining demographic data for grant preparation.

■ FOLLOW-UP CARE

A variety of support groups are available for parents of infants with special problems. Pediatric follow-up care for normal infants is detailed in the *Guidelines for Health Supervision* published by the American Academy of Pediatrics and in standard pediatric texts (Avery and First, 1989). Follow-up care of high-risk infants is described in detail by Ballard (1988) and by Taeusch and Yogman (1987).

■ REFERENCES

American Academy of Pediatrics, Committee on Genetics: Newborn screening fact sheets. Pediatrics 83:449, 1989.

Avery, G.: Neonatology: Pathophysiology and Management of the Newborn. 3rd ed. Philadelphia, J. B. Lippincott, 1987.

Avery, M., and First, L.: Pediatric Medicine. Baltimore, Williams & Wilkins, 1989.

Avery, M., and Litwack, G.: Born Early. Boston, Little, Brown and Co., 1983.

Ballard, J. L., et al.: A simplified assessment of gestational age. Pediatr. Res. 11:374, 1977.

Ballard, R.: Pediatric Care of the ICN Graduate. Philadelphia, W. B. Saunders Company, 1988.

Barness, L.: Manual of Pediatric Physical Diagnosis. 4th ed. Chicago, Year Book, 1976.

Bates, B.: A Guide to Physical Diagnosis and History Taking. 4th ed. Philadelphia, J. B. Lippincott, 1987.

Boylan, P., and Parisi, V.: An overview of hydramnios. Sem. Perinatol. 10:136, 1986.

Cloherty, J., and Stark, A.: Manual of Neonatal Care. 2nd ed. Boston, Little, Brown and Co., 1985.

Coen, R., and Koffler, H.: Primary Care of the Newborn. Boston, Little, Brown and Co., 1987.

Creasy, R., and Resnick, R.: Maternal-Fetal Medicine: Principles and Practice. 2nd ed. Philadelphia, W. B. Saunders Company, 1989.

Crelin, E.: Anatomy of the Newborn—an Atlas. Philadelphia, Lea & Febiger, 1969.

Dunn, P., Evans, T., Thearle, M., et al.: Congenital dislocation of the hip: Early and late diagnosis and management compared. Arch. Dis. Child. 60:407, 1985.

Eden, R., and Boehm, F.: Assessment and Care of the Fetus. Norwalk, Conn., Appleton & Lange, 1990.

Ekelem, I., and Taeusch, H. W.: Defining quality of care indicators for the neonatal intensive care unit. J. Natl. Med. Assoc. 82:345, 1990.

Faix, R.: Fontanel size in black and white infants. J. Pediatr. 100:304, 1982.

Fanaroff, A., and Martin, R.: Neonatal-Perinatal Medicine. St. Louis, C. V. Mosby, 1987.

Freedman, M. A., Gay, G. A., Brookert, J. E., et al.: The 1989 revisions of the U.S. Standard Certificates of Live Birth and Death and the U.S. Standard Report of Fetal Death. Am. J. Public Health 78:168–171, 1988.

Gottfried, A., and Garter, J.: Infant Stress under Intensive Care: Environmental Neonatology. Baltimore, University Park Press, 1985.

Graham, J.: Smith's Recognizable Patterns of Human Deformation. Philadelphia, W. B. Saunders Company, 1988.

Gruebel-Lee, D.: Disorders of the Hip. Philadelphia, J. B. Lippincott, 1983.

Hoeckelman, R.: The Physical Examination of Infants and Children. In Bates, B. (Ed.): A Guide to Physical Exam and History Taking. 4th ed. Philadelphia, J. B. Lippincott, 1987, pp. 525–598.

Illingworth, R.: The Development of the Infant and Young Child. 2nd ed. Baltimore, Williams & Wilkins, 1963.

Larson, E.: A causal link between hand washing and risk of infection? Examination of the evidence. Infect. Control 9:28, 1988.

Levene, M., Bennett, M., and Punt, J.: Fetal and Neonatal Neurology and Neurosurgery. Edinburgh, Churchill Livingstone, 1989.

Lovery, J. P.: Human Placenta, Clinical Perspectives. Rockville, Md., Aspen, 1987.

Oski, F., DeAngelis, C., Feigin, R., et al.: Principles and Practice of Pediatrics. Philadelphia, J. B. Lippincott, 1990.

Phelan, J., Smith, C., Broussard, P., et al.: Amniotic fluid volume assessment using the four quadrant technique in the pregnancy between 36 and 42 weeks gestation. J. Reprod. Med. 32:540, 1987.

Place, M., Parkin, P. M., and Fitton, M.: Effectiveness of neonatal screening for congenital dislocation of the hip. Lancet 2:249, 1978.

Popich, G., and Smith, D.: Fontanels, range of normal size. J. Pediatr. 80:749, 1972.

Roberton, N.: Textbook of Neonatology, Edinburgh, Churchill Livingston, 1987.

Scanlon J.: A System of Newborn Physical Exam. Baltimore, University Park Press, 1979.

Schwartz, M., and Shaul, D.: Abdominal masses in the newborn. Pediatr. Rev. 11:172, 1989.

Staheli, L.: Management of congenital hip dysplasia. Pediatr. Ann. 18:24, 1989.

Taeusch, H. W., and Yogman, Y.: Follow-up Management of the High-Risk Infant. Boston, Little, Brown and Co., 1987.

Versmold, H. T., Kitterman, J. A., Phibbs, R. H., et al.: Aortic blood pressure during the first 12 hours of life in infants with birth weight 610 to 4220 grams. Pediatrics 67:607–613, 1981.

Volpe, J. (Ed.): Neonatal neurology (Preface). Clin. Perinatol. 16:xi, 1989.

Vulliamy, D., and Johnston, P.: The Newborn Child. 6th ed. Edinburgh, Churchill Livingstone, 1987.

Yu, V., and Wood, C.: Prematurity. Edinburgh, Churchill Livingstone, 1987.

Ziai, M., Clarke, T., and Merritt, A.: Assessment of the Newborn—A Guide for the Practitioner. Boston, Little, Brown and Co., 1984.

BEHAVIORAL ASSESSMENT OF THE NEWBORN 24

Peter A. Gorski

Thanks to the advanced state of contemporary neonatal medicine, scientific and clinical attention is increasingly directed toward functional understanding and support of the developing brain and central nervous system (CNS) of newborn infants. Today, neonatal intensive care units commonly treat infants who survive deliveries after only 24 to 26 weeks' gestation. Such infants face months of hospitalization, even in the absence of life-threatening physiologic instability. While providing necessary pulmonary, cardiac, nutritional, and metabolic support, the nursery should also offer a balance of sensory stimulation and protection for the immature brain and nervous system of these smallest newborns.

The science of brain-behavior relationships has exploded with insights into the nature of neonatal neurologic functioning—infant behavior. Normal or disturbed behavior may point to healthy or affected areas and mechanisms in the CNS (Pearson and Dietrich, 1985). As a result, research is beginning to inform clinical practice about the effects on infant neurobehavioral outcome from sensory patterns and caregiving protocols in the hospital environment.

This chapter is organized into three sections: (1) biological foundations of neonatal behavior, (2) environmental influences upon the organization of neonatal behavior, and (3) social importance of neonatal behavior to long-term survival, growth, and development.

■ BIOLOGICAL FOUNDATIONS OF NEONATAL BEHAVIOR

INTRINSIC ACTIVITY CYCLES

Much research has concentrated on the search for a basic cycle of human movement, rest, and alerting that might describe a fundamental characteristic of behavioral organization and underlying brain activity that exists from early fetal life. Robertson (1987) has documented the existence of spontaneous motility cycles in human newborns across all behavioral states of sleep and wakefulness. This cyclic variation in spontaneous movement every 1 to 10 minutes is observed in utero in human fetuses during the second half of gestation and perhaps earlier (deVries et al., 1982 and 1985; Robertson, 1985). These patterns of human cyclic motility are weaker and less regular during less organized behavioral states of active sleep and may be influenced by alterations in the metabolic environment

of the fetus and newborn (Robertson and Dierker, 1986). Most importantly, the finding of remarkable stability of these cycles of spontaneous movement from midgestation through the first 10 weeks of post-term life adds evidence for a dramatic shift in brain organization and behavioral self-regulation, not at the time of birth at 40 weeks, but after 50 postconceptual weeks. Previous studies of electrophysiologic organization of the CNS, structural maturation of the cerebral cortex, and behavioral development of infant crying and sleep patterns indicate relative CNS immaturity during the first 2 to 4 months post-term with respect to fundamental organization of cortical activity as well as of higher perceptual and cognitive processes (Brazelton, 1962; Conel, 1947; Parmelee, 1977; Parmelee et al., 1964). Therefore, despite the substantial environmental and physiologic changes that accompany birth, the human fetus and newborn share basic continuities of behavior and responsiveness.

In general, healthy full-term infants display a regular series of distinct states over a period of time. These were first described and systematized by Wolff (1959 and 1966). A number of other classification schemes have been published (Brazelton, 1984; Prechtl, 1974; Thoman, 1985). As an example, Brazelton has proposed a system with the following six states: (1) quiet sleep, (2) active sleep, (3) drowsiness, (4) alert inactivity, (5) active awake, and (6) crying. Each state can be distinguished on the basis of a number of distinct clusters of behavior (Table 24–1).

The study of behavioral states in infants has attracted wide interest as an indicator of the functional integrity of the CNS during the fetal, neonatal, and infant periods of development. Maturational changes in sleep-wake cycles have been studied, and neonatal state periodicities have been correlated with later neurodevelopmental, especially mental, outcome. These investigations have found that earlier maturation of electrophysiologic and behavioral patterns of quiet sleep in the neonatal period predict higher performance on cognitive tests at preschool and school age (Anders and Keener, 1985; Becker and Thoman, 1981; Nijhuis et al., 1982; Thoman et al., 1981).

While sleeping and waking states in infancy reflect the competency of the central nervous system, they also modulate the infant's interactions with the external environment (Thoman et al., 1979). A number of studies have documented the influence that an infant's state has on his or her response to stimulation; the response may be different, depending upon whether the infant is in a sleep,

TABLE 24–1. Neonatal State Classification Scale

STATE	CHARACTERISTICS
Quiet sleep	Regular breathing, eyes closed; spontaneous activity confined to startles and jerky movements at regular intervals. Responses to external stimuli are partially inhibited, and any response is likely to be delayed. No eye movements, and state changes are less likely after stimuli or startles than in other states.
Active sleep	Irregular breathing patterns, sucking movements, eyes closed but rapid eye movements can be detected underneath the closed lids. Infants also have some low-level and irregular motor activity. Startles occur in response to external stimuli and can produce a change of state.
Drowsiness	While the newborn is semidozing, eyes may be open or closed; eyelids often flutter; activity level variable and interspersed with mild startles. Drowsy newborns are responsive to sensory stimuli but with some delay, and state change frequently follows stimulation.
Alert inactivity	A bright alert look, with attention focused on sources of auditory or visual stimuli; motor activity is inhibited while attending to stimuli.
Active awake	Eyes open, considerable motor activity, thrusting movements of extremities, and occasional startles set off by activity; reactive to external stimulation with an increase in startles or motor activity. Discrete responses are difficult to distinguish due to general high activity level.
Crying	Intense irritability in the form of sustained crying, and jerky limb movement. This state is difficult to break through with stimulation.

(Data from Brazelton, T. B.: Neonatal Behavioral Assessment Scale, 2nd ed. London, Heinemann, 1984.)

drowsy, or alert state (Berg and Berg, 1979; Korner, 1972; Pomerleau-Malcuit and Clifton, 1973). For example, a visual stimulus that captures the attention of a quietly awake infant does not elicit a response from a more aroused, crying infant. Indeed, this arousal distinction applies not only between states but also within a particular state. A newborn infant displays a different pattern of responsiveness at the beginning of an alert period compared with the end of the period. This difference is analogous to the daytime pattern of adults who commonly go through periods of higher and lower arousal while awake. This pattern, called the basic rest-activity cycle (BRAC) by Aserinsky and Kleitman (1955), is distinct from the sleep-wake cycle and is theoretically related to the cyclic activity of the autonomic nervous system (ANS). The ANS mediates the infant's responsivity to the external environment and is responsible for regulating a number of homeostatic functions.

Among the ANS effects on homeostatic processes are its effects on cardiac and respiratory functions. The effect of the ANS on cardiac activity develops prenatally and through the 1st year of life. When cardiac activity first appears in the embryo, it shows no beat-to-beat variability, even during periods of increased movement (Berg and Berg, 1979). As the fetus develops, heart rate (HR) becomes more responsive to increased movement. The average HR of a full-term infant is between 120 and 160 beats per minute (Ashton and Connolly, 1971). Both the average and the variability of HR are affected by the

behavioral state of the infant, with higher, more variable rates seen in the more active states and lower, more regular rates found in the quiet states. During the first 2 to 3 months after birth, both the mean HR and the HR variability increase, followed by a decrease in both rate and variability between 3 and 6 months (Harper et al., 1976). In addition, the rise in HR variability is increasingly regulated by input from the ANS.

Respiratory activity, although not under direct ANS control, shows a pattern of development that is similar to that seen in cardiac activity. Before 30 weeks' gestational age, preterm infants show a constant semiregular pattern of respiration that is not affected by increased motor activity (Dreyfus-Brisac, 1968). By 40 weeks, respiration becomes more related to body activity, with quiet periods becoming more strongly associated with periods of regular respiration (Parmelee et al., 1967). In addition, the proportion of irregular to regular respirations decreases across the first 8 months of life (Parmelee et al., 1972).

Apnea and bradycardia are phenomena that also demonstrate the relative lack of organization of nervous system control over respiratory and cardiac functions, respectively. Both are rare in healthy full-term infants, but they occur much more frequently in preterm infants (Gabriel et al., 1976). The decrease in frequency of apnea and bradycardia parallels maturational changes in the structure and function of the infant's nervous system (Bronson, 1982). Parmelee and colleagues (1972) demonstrated that such changes in respiratory patterns were concurrent with changes in eye movement and body movement patterns which appear to reflect the maturation of inhibitory cortical mechanisms in infants.

Neonatal behavioral and psychophysiologic measures of state organization and cardiac variability are now among the most frequently applied methods in neonatal behavioral research. These techniques highlight maturational differences between preterm and term infants that could affect their responses to treatment practices. Consistent differences in the sleep characteristics of preterm infants distinguish them from full-term infants when tested at the same conceptual ages. Preterms have been found to have relatively longer bouts of quiet sleep, more movement in sleep states, more frequent REM episodes, and less consistent combinations of behavioral and physiologic criteria used to define infant sleep states (Anders and Keener, 1985; Davis and Thoman, 1987; Parmelee et al., 1967).

Less consensus exists across studies of waking behavior in preterm and full-term infants. Some report less alert time in preterm infants when compared with full-term infants at the same postconception ages (DiVitto and Goldberg, 1979; Lester et al., 1976). Others find them to be equally alert (Paludetto et al., 1982; Telzrow et al., 1982). Still other investigators find preterm infants to be more alert (Davis and Thoman, 1987; Palmer et al., 1982). Similar discrepancies are reported with respect to irritability and arousal levels (Aylward, 1982; Howard et al., 1976; McGehee and Eckerman, 1983; Michaelis et al., 1973).

Taken together, the findings suggest that the underlying difference in CNS organization between premature and full-term infants lies in an unevenness in the development of premature infants. Aspects of greater CNS maturity (more alertness and less sleep) coexist with characteristics of less CNS maturity (more nonalert waking activity and more frequent sleep-wake transitions). As Davis and Thoman (1987) conclude, premature infants exhibit irregular state development as compared with full-term infants, rather than either increased maturity or immaturity. These early neurobehavioral differences between infants of different gestational ages could reflect significant changes in brain organization that may continue throughout childhood development. Such functional differences may affect specific perceptual, cognitive, or emotional processes rather than intelligence. Current long-term follow-up studies of preterm infants tend to find that the mental development and neurologic status of preterm infants at school age does not differ from that of full-terms (Bakeman and Brown, 1980; Saint-Anne Dargassies, 1979), yet these same children are more likely to show visual-motor and spatial difficulties, with associated school underachievement (Hunt et al., 1982; Klein et al., 1985).

The infant cry state is itself attracting interest in the effort to develop predictive measures of CNS functioning (Lester, 1987). The association of unusual cry features with conditions related to nervous system damage has been recognized for years. Early research demonstrated the association of cry features, such as unusually high pitch and short duration, with brain damage as well as with illnesses that affect the nervous system and prenatal drug exposure. The cry characteristics were generally not key diagnostic criteria in these cases but served to substantiate a previous diagnosis (Blinick et al., 1971; Fisichelli and Karelitz, 1963; Karelitz and Fisichelli, 1962; Michelsson et al., 1977; Vourenkoski et al., 1966).

Analysis of cries may serve a useful diagnostic function. The cry characteristics of full-term infants with pre- and perinatal complications and infants who show signs of inadequate prenatal nutrition, for example, have been found to be much like those found among infants with more obvious signs of nervous system problems (Zeskind and Lester, 1978 and 1981). Successful prediction of developmental outcome from neonatal cry analyses corroborates a relation between the characteristics of the infant's cry and the functional integrity of the infant's nervous system (Lester, 1987).

Physiologic measures of autonomic regulation are linked to maturational and developmental characteristics of CNS organization in full-term and high-risk infants. Furthermore, new research identifies correlations between behavioral and physiologic indices of neurodevelopment. Neural control of heart rate patterns through parasympathetic pathways may be a marker of CNS integrity and reactivity (Porges et al, 1982). In particular, vagal activity, or respiratory arrhythmia, has been linked to CNS maturation, cognitive outcome following high-risk birth, intrinsic temperamental characteristics of individual children and emotional adaptation to stress in the parent-infant relationship (Coll et al., 1984; Field et al., 1988; Fox and Porges, 1985; Porges, 1983).

SENSORY-PERCEPTUAL FUNCTIONS

Sensory systems undergo rather rapid changes during the last trimester of pregnancy and the first several months after birth. Prenatally, the various senses begin to differentiate at separate times and then continue to develop at different rates through postnatal life. Estimation of the functional onset of a given sensory system is complicated by a number of factors. First, since peripheral structures mature before central ones, responsiveness in peripheral structures does not necessarily indicate that the full system is functional. Second, since a variety of methods (i.e., histologic, electrophysiologic, and behavioral) have been used to determine the onset of function, discrepancies in the estimation of actual time of functional onset may result. Despite these problems, there appears to be an orderly sequence in the functional development of the sensory systems of human infants. This sequence is cutaneous (tactile), vestibular, auditory, and visual across a variety of species, including the human (Gottlieb, 1971).

The path from first onset to functional maturity is marked by changes in the system's ability to respond to stimulation and by shifts in the system's organization (Turkewitz et al., 1983). Since the tactile, visual, and auditory senses are the avenues of communication between the infant and the world, a brief outline of some key aspects of development in these systems follows.

CUTANEOUS (TACTILE) SYSTEM

The earliest signs of human behavior appear as the reaction of a fetus to touch. Hooker's (1952) classic studies demonstrate that before 7½ weeks' gestational age, the human embryo shows no evidence of reflex activity, and no area of the skin is sensitive to tactile stimulation. During the next 7 weeks, however, almost the entire body surface becomes sensitive to touch, beginning with the lips and ending with the feet and legs. (The top and back of the head remain insensitive until birth. Thus, responses to somesthetic stimulation are the first human behaviors to develop, followed approximately 2 weeks later by responses to vestibular and proprioceptive stimulation. Being the first, it may prepare the organism for subsequent organization around environmental input and thus have fundamental importance for later development (Carmichael, 1954; Montagu, 1971).

Early tactile contact during infancy may influence growth rates, adaptability, learning, activity level, exploratory behavior, attachment, sociability, ability to withstand stress, and immunologic development (Brown, 1984; Field et al., 1986). Whether the human newborn is sensitive to pain stimuli induced by medical procedures, such as common heel sticks for blood or invasive surgical operations, has been debated (Anand and Hickey, 1987; Owens and Todt, 1984) (see Chapter 14). Neuroanatomic and physiologic studies declare the early fetal development of sensory nerve tract fibers responsive to pain (Anand and Hickey, 1987; Swafford and Allan, 1968). Neonatal circumcision has been the prototypic subject for demonstrating infant behavioral, physiological, and humoral responses to pain stimulation (Dixon et al., 1984; Gunnar et al., 1981; Williamson and Williamson, 1983). Nonnutritive sucking on pacifiers and parenteral use of sedatives and analgesics diminish irritable behavior and blunt heart rate and mean arterial pressure changes during and immediately following painful medical procedures (Anand et al., 1987; Anderson et al., 1983; Field and Goldson, 1984; Gunnar et al., 1984). Such interventions may help maintain physiologic homeostasis during stressful procedures. Preterm infants, in particular, may benefit from the resultant stability of cerebral and possibly pulmonary blood flow (Brazy, 1988; Perlman and Volpe, 1985). The potential for preventing some of the occurrence and consequences of intracranial hemorrhage or acute pulmonary vasoconstriction could have enormous impact on the developmental outcome of high-risk infants, and prevention may, in part, depend on increased recognition and control of pain in newborn infants.

AUDITORY SYSTEM

The auditory system becomes functional somewhere between the 25th and 27th week of gestation (Grimwade et al., 1971; Rubel, 1985; Starr et al., 1977). Moreover, sound is capable of penetrating the abdominal wall as well as the amniotic sac (Armitage et al., 1980; Bench, 1968; Bench et al., 1979). Low-frequency sounds (below 1000 Hz) pass most easily through the abdominal wall; as the frequency of the sounds increases, their intensity becomes progressively attenuated. Once the sound passes through the abdominal wall, its spectral composition is further altered by the fact that the sound-conducting medium is aquatic. From a functional standpoint, the auditory system is initially responsive to low and middle frequencies, and as development progresses, sensitivity to higher frequencies increases. These changes have been shown to be related to the growth of the basilar membrane, although more central changes may be responsible for them as well (Hecox and Deegan, 1985; Rubel, 1985). During development, the overall intensity of sound necessary for a response decreases. Roughly speaking, the infant's sensitivity to sounds is approximately 15 to 20 decibels lower than that of adults, although these thresholds change during the first months of life.

The prevailing view has been that the primary sounds available to the mammalian fetus are cardiovascular sounds. However, both internal sounds generated by the mother and externally generated sounds are clearly audible (Armitage et al., 1980). Thus, the fetus is exposed to internal and external sounds whose characteristics change during gestation both due to changes in the properties of the auditory environment of the mother and due to intrinsic changes in the auditory structures. Such exposure to sound during gestation may permit the infant to recognize his or her mother's voice right after birth. In fact, infants under 30 hours of age preferentially suck on a nonnutritive pacifier that triggers a recording of their mother's voice rather than a stranger's voice (DeCasper and Fifer, 1980).

From a behavioral standpoint, the full-term newborn is able to orient toward nonaversive sources of auditory stimulation by turning the head and eyes toward the sound and to turn away from an intense, aversive stimulus (Muir and Field, 1979; Turkewitz et al., 1966). This orienting behavior, characterized by a fairly long latency (7 to 8 seconds), gradually declines over the first 4 months of life and then reemerges by the 5th month as a short latency response (Muir and Clifton, 1985).

In addition to these basic auditory capacities, the young infant possesses the ability to make discriminations of basic sounds of spoken language. Such an ability is crucial for the acquisition of language since a linguistic system consists of a set of distinct classes of sounds, known as phonemes (e.g., "ba" and "pa"), that signal to the listener differences in meaning. The general findings from numerous studies are that similar to adults, infants are able to distinguish between phonemes that belong to different categories (Aslin et al., 1983). Moreover, the set of phonemes that infants are able to discriminate either diminishes or changes once they are exposed to their native linguistic environment.

VISUAL SYSTEM

The visual system offers an interesting paradox. On the one hand, it is the last system to start functioning during gestation and the least well-developed at birth. On the other hand, it is the system that is usually dominant in our everyday interactions with our environment and, as a result, has been the most investigated.

The retina differentiates during the first trimester of gestation. The retina consists of the fovea, located in the central region as well as rods and other peripheral structures. The fovea is composed of cones whose primary function is to mediate detail and color vision. The rods are responsible for the detection of changes in brightness and movement. Although differentiation of the foveal region occurs first, at birth the foveal region is quite immature and different from the adult fovea while the periphery is fairly similar to the adult periphery (Abramov et al., 1982).

The other major structures in the visual pathway also change considerably during postnatal development. The lateral geniculate nucleus (LGN) of the thalamus, a relay station between the eye and the visual cortex, undergoes important physiologic and anatomic changes. In primates, the LGN becomes more responsive with development. The most significant changes, however, occur in the visual cortex where the neurons undergo marked morphologic changes. These changes, which peak at 6 months postterm, consist of the growth and arborization of a large number of dendrites, presumably accompanied by synaptogenesis. In addition, the visual pathway is gradually myelinated. Myelination of the optic nerve is completed by 3 months of age while that of the visual cortex is completed somewhat later (Yakovlev and LeCours, 1967).

Nearly all basic functions of the visual system exhibit marked changes in the first 3 to 6 months of life. Accommodation (i.e., ability to focus objects) is poor between birth and 1 month of age and then improves through the 3rd month (Banks, 1980). In the 1st month infants tend to overaccommodate distant objects and underaccommodate near objects. Smooth-pursuit eye movements display similar changes. Prior to 6 weeks of age, infants do not display smooth pursuit of a moving target but track it with jerky (saccadic) eye movements. By the 8th week smooth pursuit appears and improves thereafter until the 3rd month when no saccades are present (Aslin, 1981).

One of the most important functions of the visual system is to detect patterned information. A traditional measure of the system's ability to do so has been visual acuity. Acuity is poor at birth and improves rapidly over the first 6 months of life. Acuity in a newborn infant is roughly equivalent to a Snellen value of 20/600, which is

30 times lower than normal adult acuity. There is also a steady increase in the range of detectable spatial frequencies and contrasts over the first 6 months of life. Thus, young infants are sensitive to only a fraction of the patterned information that adults are sensitive to and are able to perceive best only those objects that are close to them and that have high contrast (Banks and Salapatek, 1983).

Despite these limitations, young infants can fixate visually with a variety of stimuli with attributes such as intensity, number and size of elements, pattern, and flicker. Response to color is a somewhat controversial topic, but the most conservative estimate is that by 2 months of age infants probably possess red and green cones but lack blue cones and are therefore, at least dichromats; by 3 months it is less likely that they have a blue insensitivity (Banks and Salapatek, 1983; Fantz and Fagan, 1975; Fantz and Nevis, 1967; Lewkowicz, 1985).

TEMPERAMENT

The preceding discussion highlighted aspects of behavioral and neurobiological development that are common to all human infants. Differences in development were noted to be caused by idiosyncrasies of gestational age at birth or other medical risk factors. How then, can we account for the range and stability of differences in the behavior of infants born at the same gestation, and with similar medical courses? The pattern of behavioral and psychophysiologic responses to animate and inanimate stimuli that characterize each newborn is often referred to as temperament. Temperament describes the style without supplying the explanation of individual patterns of behavior.

Researchers tend to agree that temperamental dimensions reflect behavioral styles rather than discrete behavioral acts, have biological underpinnings, and enjoy continuity of expression relative to other aspects of behavior (Goldsmith et al., 1987). Infancy is commonly regarded as the time of clearest expression of temperamental characteristics, before the link between temperament and behavior becomes more complex as the child matures.

Disagreements exist about the extent to which an infant's behavior can be attributed to temperament, whether temperament is stable within individuals regardless of social contexts, and the nature of its inheritance (Goldsmith et al, 1987). Formal neonatal behavioral examination, standardized psychological assessment, and parents' reports all identify behavioral traits that together compose an image of the nature each infant brings into interaction with the caregiving world (Brazelton, 1984; Carey and McDevitt, 1978; Rothbart, 1981; Thomas et al., 1963). According to Chess and Thomas (1986), caregivers learn to relate to infants through nine behavioral categories of individual differences that comprise temperament (Table 24–2).

Chess and Thomas (1986) describe three functionally significant temperamental constellations that emerged from their sample during the New York Longitudinal Study. Perinatal medical risks were distributed equally across the three groups of children, and, thus, did not appear to determine temperament. About 40 per cent of all children were characterized by early and sustained

TABLE 24–2. Temperament Categories

CATEGORY	DESCRIPTION
Activity level	The motor level of a child's functioning. The ratio of active to inactive periods each day (e.g., infant may move often even during sleep).
Intensity of reaction	The general magnitude of response, regardless of affective direction (e.g., cries loudly for all needs, also vocalizes with audible vigor).
Quality of mood	The predominance of contented, positive behavior versus irritable, negative disposition, regardless of intensity (e.g., generally calm, smiling, easily engaged versus fussy).
Rhythmicity or regularity	The predictability or unpredictability of biological or behavioral patterns (e.g., sleep-wake cycle, hunger, feeding pattern, elimination schedule, crying, and alerting).
Threshold of responsiveness	The amount of stimulation required to elicit a response (e.g., rapidity of build-up to full cry when handled).
Approach or withdrawal	The initial response to a new stimulus (e.g., new food, toy, person, or room). Responses are observed through mood (e.g., smiling, grimacing, or crying) or activity (e.g., in infancy, by calming, squirming, or spitting).
Adaptability	The eventual response to a new or changed environment or condition (e.g., acceptance of bottle or baby-sitter).
Attention span and persistence	Two related categories describing the duration of effort at a task or activity and the continuation at task, despite attention to distractions (e.g., prolonged visual fixation and orienting).
Distractibility	The infant's susceptibility to changing attention or activity when presented with interfering stimuli (e.g., diverted from visual attention by extraneous sound stimulus).

(Adapted from Chess, S., and Thomas, A.: Temperament in Clinical Practice. New York, Guilford Press, 1986, pp. 273–278.)

rhythmicity, predominantly positive mood, mild intensity of reactions, positive approach to new stimuli, and positive adaptability over repeated exposures to change. About 10 per cent of the sample were infants and children with irregular behavior, intense and predominantly negative expressions, negative withdrawal from new stimuli and difficulty adapting to change even over time. Another 15 per cent were somewhere in between the two. These infants were distinguished by mildly negative initial withdrawal from new stimuli with slow, yet eventual adaptability after repeated contact. Thirty-five per cent of their sample could not readily be classified into those "easy," "difficult," or "slow-to-warm up" personalities.

Caregivers and children bring their individual temperaments into the relationship they create with each other. Similarities or differences can produce understanding and comfort or confusion and conflict. Whether stable or changed over time, temperament influences the ease, harmony, and pleasure between the child and his environment at each stage of development. In return, the child continuously learns to find those environments and relationships that best support his or her needs and style. These lessons begin immediately through the new relationship between newborn infant and parent. The neonatal period serves to launch parents' perceptions and infants' expectations in the direction of contented anticipation of the future or toward frustration and learned helplessness (Goldberg, 1979; Seligman, 1975).

■ ENVIRONMENTAL INFLUENCES

The preceding sections testified to the genetically influenced biologic foundations of behavior in human infants. This structural and functional development unfolds throughout the prenatal and neonatal period. Concurrently, the developing brain and nervous system are constantly exposed and responsive to various conditions, substances, and stimuli from the external environment. The course of behavioral development may be altered accordingly. This section illustrates some of the better-known sources of environmental influence upon the emerging behavioral organization of infants.

IN UTERO DRUG EXPOSURE

There has been long-standing concern as to the behavioral effects of narcotic drugs on the developing fetus. Heroin-addicted newborns are at high risk for sleep disturbances (as measured by electroencephalograms), growth retardation, CNS irritability associated with narcotic withdrawal, sudden infant death syndrome, and behavioral disorganization of state and alerting and motor processes (Chavez et al., 1979; Desmond and Wilson, 1975; Strauss et al., 1975). Similar findings have been reported for infants prenatally exposed to numerous other narcotic as well as nonnarcotic drugs (Chasnoff et al., 1982 and 1983; Doberczak et al., 1987; Ward et al., 1986). Quality of prenatal care, maternal nutrition, and home environment compound, or even exceed, the developmental risks associated with maternal drug addiction (Lifschitz et al., 1985).

The neurodevelopmental and behavioral effects of cocaine on the human infant are of serious concern, ranging from perinatal cerebral infarction to intrauterine growth retardation, abnormal sleep and feeding patterns, irritability, and tremulousness (Chasnoff et al., 1986; Chasnoff 1988; Dixon et al., 1990; Oro and Dixon, 1987). (See Chapter 26.)

Other substances that cross the placental circulation may contribute to neonatal behavioral disturbances and later developmental dysfunction. These include, among others, alcohol, caffeine, and compounds in cigarette smoke (Clarren and Smith, 1978; Emory et al., 1988; MacArthur and Knox, 1988; Shaywitz et al., 1981). We often cannot discriminate the extent to which the drugs directly cause long-term CNS damage; whether they act primarily to contribute to hypoxic ischemic conditions; or whether they serve as a proxy for a suboptimal home environment.

MATERNAL STRESS

Studies of the psychobiology of stress during pregnancy warn of possible noradrenergic and cholinergic perturbations resultant from severe psychological stress (Moyer et al., 1977). Such biochemical alterations during fetal development may in turn modify neuroanatomic and physiologic organization, resulting in neonatal behavioral disorders and developmental risk (Herrenkohl, 1986).

PERINATAL ENVIRONMENTAL INFLUENCES

Compounds that create regional depression of sensory pathways during labor may cross the placental circulation

and could cause CNS depression in the delivered newborn. However, studies that carefully control for the effects of parity and length of labor indicate that when applied in tightly controlled dosage, using the minimum quantities needed to achieve anesthesia, behavioral signs of neurologic depression are minimal and short-lived (Kraemer et al., 1972; Tronick et al., 1976). This finding has been replicated across studies that tested the effects of a variety of drugs and routes of administration (Horowitz et al., 1977; Lester et al., 1982; Murray et al., 1981). Current clinical concern, however, centers on the possibly disorganizing effect of obstetric medication on newborn sucking and feeding (Kuhnert et al., 1985; Sanders-Phillips et al., 1988).

After birth, infants are placed in any number of physical environments. Each caregiving locale presents a unique combination and pattern of sensory stimuli. The newborn's response and adaptation depend on the nature of the interaction between the infant's biobehavioral capacities and the sensory characteristics of the caregiving environment. Public attention has long been directed at alternative birthing environments in and out of hospital for full-term low-risk infants (Ballard et al., 1985). Meanwhile, professionals who treat high-risk and prematurely born infants have begun to investigate the sources and neurobehavioral impact of sensory stimulation intrinsic to the physical and human environment of neonatal intensive care units (NICU).

ENVIRONMENT OF THE NEONATAL INTENSIVE CARE UNIT (NICU)

Consequent to recent technological breakthroughs in neonatal medicine, neonatal mortality has dramatically decreased in the past half decade. The exogenous administration of natural or synthetic surfactant offers hope for even more accelerated progress toward reducing neonatal mortality and morbidity (Fujiwara et al., 1990; Merritt and Hallman, 1988). NICUs are increasingly populated by tiny newborns (<1000 g) who breathe spontaneously, oxygenate effectively, and are likely to survive well beyond the neonatal period. However, the physiologic immaturity of all their organ systems aside from their pulmonary alveoli demands prolonged hospitalization in high-risk neonatal medical centers. These infants are often medically stable, yet fragile, and their central nervous systems are appropriately immature given their gestational age at birth. Hospitalized for weeks or months during the critical period of preterm neurologic organization previously discussed in this chapter, these infants are chronically exposed to potentially positive or negative conditions in their environment. Evidence links acute fluctuations of systemic hemodynamics with environmental events and caregiver interventions (Gorski et al., 1984; Gorski and Huntington, 1988; Linn et al., 1985b; Long et al., 1980). Moreover, modern methods of monitoring cerebral blood flow, intracranial pressure changes, and brain oxygenation identify a direct relationship between central hypoxemia, apnea, bradycardia, and cerebral circulation and autoregulation (Brazy, 1988; Perlman and Volpe, 1985).

Over the past decade, investigators have systematically examined characteristics of NICUs, caregiving protocols including patterns of medical and social intervention, and infant behavioral and physiologic responses in interaction with this level of care (Gaiter, 1985; Gorski et al., 1979, 1983; Gottfried et al., 1981; High and Gorski, 1985; Lawson et al, 1977; Linn et al., 1985a). Since these studies did not impose changes in caregiver behavior, they provide representative views of the sensory conditions normally experienced by premature infants in a NICU. For example, results have depicted the NICU environment as one which provides both sensory overload and deprivation (High and Gorski, 1985). These studies found that infants experience a bombardment of stimuli from sheer numbers of different caregivers and procedures each day. At the same time, however, little social contact and long intervals of social isolation also characterize the nature of caregiver-infant interaction in NICUs. They also discovered an absence of temporal contingency between the sleep or awake state of infants in a NICU and the onset of either medical or, surprisingly, social interventions by NICU caregivers. These dissociated sensory experiences in the neonatal period might theoretically relate to subsequent developmental deficits of cross-sensory and sensory-motor integration in premature infants (Rose et al., 1978).

How and to what extent can caregivers influence developmental outcome by manipulating the NICU environment? Some investigators started from the theoretical premise that the NICU environment deprives infants of necessary stimulation and therefore tested the effects of supplemental sensory input (Bernbaum et al., 1983; Field et al., 1982 and 1986; Katz, 1971; Korner et al., 1975 and 1978; Korner and Schneider, 1983; Leib et al., 1980; Resnick et al., 1987; White and Labarba, 1976). Positive results from these studies include increased formula intake and weight gain; better motor, visual, and auditory functioning; altered sleep patterns; decreased apnea; and improved scores on developmental testing after hospital discharge. Other researchers who professed a belief that the NICU bombards infants with constant overstimulation designed methods of protecting infants from potentially damaging responses to sensory inputs from the environment while at the same time offering stimuli contingent with the infant's activity or physiologic status (Als et al., 1986; Barnard and Bee, 1983; Thoman and Graham, 1986). Their positive results include earlier weaning from ventilatory support, improved developmental scores on follow-up, enhanced motor organization, and increased time in quiet sleep.

Neonatal behavioral intervention programs represent a proactive effort to consider and support infant and family development at the beginning of extrauterine life. Methodologic weaknesses pervade the literature and weaken the generalizability and efficacy of current research in this field (Gilkerson et al., 1990). Common limitations include small sample sizes, insufficient demographic data to insure subject comparability prior to intervention, limited descriptions of routine and experimental protocols, simultaneous use of multiple interventions, limited involvement of parents, and short-term follow-up periods.

Much useful and positive experience also has resulted from these investigations. The work has advanced concern for the effects of the NICU environment on brain growth and behavior, while providing further explanation for the nearly universal discrepancy in function between prema-

ture and full-term infants when tested at the same postconceptual age during infancy (Als et al., 1988; Aylward, 1982; Ferrari et al., 1983).

NON-NUTRITIVE SUCKING

Stimulating non-nutritive sucking during gavage feedings has been utilized as a method of influencing neuromaturation through learned experience. Contemporary research on preterm human infants documents the benefits of this practice on a wide range of physiologic processes and health outcomes. For example, compared with control group infants, infants who were gavage-fed while simultaneously using a pacifier had fewer tube feedings, earlier onset of successful bottle and breast-feeding, a higher average daily weight gain, earlier discharge from hospital, and lower hospital care costs (Burroughs et al., 1981; Field et al., 1982).

Bernbaum and her co-workers (1983) found that non-nutritive sucking during gavage feeding accelerated the maturation of the sucking reflex, decreased intestinal transit time, and led to more efficient use of calories absorbed. Woodson and Hamilton (1988) linked improved growth in preterm infants to the finding that non-nutritive sucking sustains reduced heart rates. The behavioral calming effect produced during non-nutritive sucking may rechannel calorie consumption from aroused states, crying, and motor activity to sleep and growth.

■ THE SOCIAL SIGNIFICANCE OF NEONATAL BEHAVIOR

This chapter has reviewed evidence for the newborn infant's competence to perceive, respond to, and communicate with its environment. Newborn infants help adults succeed as caregivers by being readable, predictable, and responsive. No longer can professionals allow parents to feel totally responsible for all their infant's actions. The newborn, once thought to be a "blank slate to be written upon by his environment, his world a blooming, buzzing confusion" (James, 1890), now is respected as a social partner who can effectively engage and, to some extent, guide caregivers to support his or her growth and development.

Not all infants are lucky enough to be born after a full intrauterine gestation, without CNS pathology or behavioral dysfunction. Premature infants are generally less alert, less active, and less responsive than full-term infants during the neonatal period and the first few months of infancy (Brown and Bakeman, 1979; DiVitto and Goldberg, 1979). These infants challenge their caregivers to be more active in initiating social interaction or, paradoxically, less intrusive and more sensitive of their lower sensory thresholds (Beckwith and Cohen, 1978; Field, 1977). Whereas healthy full-terms quickly and consistently reward their parents for providing a satisfying or organizing response, premature infants and their parents risk repeated frustration and interactive failures. For example, when a caregiver holds and talks to an alert full-term newborn, the infant may calmly inhibit body movements and smoothly follow the adult's face while maintaining healthy skin color and breathing patterns. In contrast, the same social stimulation might exceed the premature infant's sensory threshold, causing the infant to startle, avert his or her gaze, and become cyanotic or tachypneic (Gorski, 1983).

Premature delivery and the NICU experience can themselves foster unique psychological stress on preterm parents. If the family of a high-risk infant is burdened further by social isolation, serious marital problems, a history of child abuse or neglect, or emotional depression, the parents may not be able to cope with the added stress of a behaviorally disorganized infant. Without professional intervention, such infants may be at increased risk for maltreatment (Hunter et al., 1978; Klein and Stern, 1971). Although few families are incapacitated to the point of actively harming their infants, many parents of medically vulnerable newborns continue to anxiously overprotect their infants long after such restriction is warranted and healthy (Gorski, 1988; Green and Solnit, 1964). Neonatal health-care professionals have an opportunity to note the psychological condition of the parents in addition to the medical status and behavior of the newborn. By offering attention and support to the family as well as to the newborn, caregivers can contribute most effectively to the quality of infant health and development following high-risk birth.

■ REFERENCES

Abramov, I., Gordon, J., Hendrickson, A., et al.: The retina of the newborn human infant. Science 217:265–267, 1982.

Als, H., Duffy, F. H., and McAnulty, G. B.: Behavioral differences between preterm and full-term newborns as measured with the APIB system scores: I. Inf. Behav. Dev. 11:305–318, 1988.

Als, H., Lawhon, G., and Brown, E.: Individualized behavioral and environmental care for the very low birthweight preterm infant at high risk for bronchopulmonary dysplasia: Neonatal intensive care unit and developmental outcome. Pediatrics 78:1123–1132, 1986.

Anand, K. J. S., and Hickey, P. R.: Pain and its effects in the human neonate and fetus. N. Engl. J. Med. 317:1321–1329, 1987.

Anand, K. J. S., Sippell, W. G., and Aynsley-Green, A.: Randomized trial of fentanyl anaesthesia in preterm babies undergoing surgery: Effects on the stress response. Lancet 1:243–248, 1987.

Anders, T. F., and Keener, M. A.: Developmental course of nighttime sleep-wake patterns in full-term and premature infants during the first year of life. I. Sleep 8:173–192, 1985.

Anderson, G. C., Burroughs, A. K., and Measel, C. P.: Nonnutritive sucking opportunities: A safe and effective treatment for preterm neonates. In Field, T., and Sostek, A. (Eds.): Infants Born at Risk. New York, Grune & Stratton, 1983, pp. 129–146.

Armitage, S. E., Baldwin, B. A., and Vince, M. A.: The fetal environment of sheep. Science 208:1173–1174, 1980.

Aserinsky, E., and Kleitman, N.: A motility cycle in infants as manifested by ocular and gross bodily activity. J. Appl. Physiol. 8:11–18, 1955.

Ashton, R., and Connolly, K.: The relation of respiration and heart rate to sleep states in the human newborn. Dev. Med. Child Neurol. 13:180–187, 1971.

Aslin, R. N.: Development of smooth pursuit in human infants. In Fisher, D. F., Monty, R. A., and Sanders, J. W. (Eds.): Eye Movements: Cognition and Visual Perception. Hillsdale, N.J., Erlbaum, 1981.

Aslin, R. N., Pisoni, D. B., and Jusczyk, P. W.: Auditory development and speech perception in infancy. In Haith, M. M., and Campos, J. J. (Eds.): Handbook of Child Psychology: Infancy and Developmental Psychobiology, vol. 2. New York, John Wiley, 1983, pp. 573–687.

Aylward, G. P.: Forty-week full-term and preterm neurologic differences. In Lipsitt, L. P., and Field, T. M. (Eds.): Infant Behavior and Development: Perinatal Risk and Newborn Behavior. Norwood, N.J., Ablex, 1982, pp. 67–83.

Bakeman, R., and Brown, J. V.: Early Interaction: Consequences for social and mental development at three years. Child Dev. 51:437–447, 1980.

Ballard, R. A., Ferris, C. B., Clyman, R. I., et al.: The hospital Alternative Birth Center: Is it safe? Experience in 1000 cases from 1976–1980. J. Perinatol. 5(3):61–64, 1985.

Banks, M. S.: The development of visual accommodation during early infancy. Child Dev. 51:646–666, 1980.

Banks, M. S., and Salapatek, P.: Infant visual perception. In Haith, M. M., and Campos, J. J. (Eds.): Handbook of Child Psychology: Infancy and Developmental Psychobiology, vol. 2. New York, John Wiley, 1983, pp. 435–571.

Barnard, K., and Bee, H.: The impact of temporally patterned stimulation on the development of preterm infants. Child Dev. 54:1156–1167, 1983.

Becker, P. T., and Thoman, E. B.: Rapid eye movement storms in infants: Rate of occurrence at 6 months predicts mental development at one year. Science 212:1415–1416, 1981.

Beckwith, L., and Cohen, S. E.: Preterm birth: Hazardous obstetrical and postnatal events as related to caregiver-infant behavior. Inf. Behav. Dev. 1:403–411, 1978.

Beckwith, L., and Parmelee, A. H.: EEG patterns of preterm infants, home environment, and later I.Q. Child Dev. 57:777–789, 1986.

Bench, J.: Sound transmission to the human fetus through the maternal abdominal wall. J. Genet. Psychol. 113:85–87, 1968.

Bench, J., Anderson, J., and Hoare, M.: Measurement system for fetal audiometry. J. Acoust. Soc. Am. 47:1602–1606, 1979.

Berg, W. K., and Berg, K. M.: Psychophysiologic development in infancy: State, sensory function, and attention. In Osofsky, J. D. (Ed.): Handbook of Infant Development. New York, John Wiley, 1979, pp. 283–343.

Bernbaum, J., Pereira, G., and Watkins, J.: Nonnutritive sucking during gavage feeding enhances growth and maturation in premature infants. Pediatrics 71:41–45, 1983.

Blinick, G., Tavolga, W. N., and Antopol, W.: Variations in birth cries of newborn infants from narcotic addicted and normal mothers. Am. J. Obstet. Gynecol. 110:948–958, 1971.

Brazelton, T. B.: Crying in infancy. Pediatrics 4:579–588, 1962.

Brazelton, T. B.: Neonatal Behavioral Assessment Scale. 2nd ed. London, Heinemann, 1984.

Brazy, J. E.: Effects of crying on cerebral blood volume and cytochrome aa_3. J. Pediatr. 112:457–461, 1988.

Bronson, G. W.: Structure, status and characteristics of the nervous system at birth. In Stratton, P. (Ed.): Psychobiology of the Human Newborn. Chichester, John Wiley, 1982, pp. 99–118.

Brown, C. C. (Ed.): The Many Facets of Touch. Skillman, N.J., Johnson & Johnson, 1984.

Brown, J. V., and Bakeman, R.: Relationships of human mothers with their infants during the first year of life: Effects of prematurity. In Bell, R. W., and Smotherman, W. P. (Eds.): Maternal Influences and Early Behavior. Holliswood, N.Y., Spectrum, 1979.

Burroughs, A. K., Anderson, G. C., Patel, M. K., et al.: Relation of nonnutritive sucking pressures to t_cPO_2 and gestational age in preterm infants. Perinat.-Neonatol. 5:54–62, 1981.

Carey, W. B., and McDevitt, S. C.: Revision of the infant temperament questionnaire. Pediatrics 61:735–739, 1978.

Carmichael, L.: The onset and early development of behavior. In Carmichael, L. (Ed.): Manual of Child Psychology. New York, John Wiley, 1954.

Chasnoff, I. J.: Newborn infants with drug withdrawal symptoms. Pediatr. Rev. 9:273–277, 1988.

Chasnoff, I. J., Bussey, M. E., Savich, R., et al.: Perinatal cerebral infarction and maternal cocaine use. J. Pediatr. 108:456–459, 1986.

Chasnoff, I. J., Hatcher, R., and Burns, W. J.: Polydrug- and methadone-addicted newborns: A continuum of impairment? Pediatrics 70:210–213, 1982.

Chasnoff, I. J., Hatcher, R., Burns, W. J., et al.: Pentazocine and tripelennamine ("t's and blue's"): Effects on the fetus and newborn. Dev. Pharm. Ther. 6:162–169, 1983.

Chavez, C. J., Ostrea, E. M., Stryker, J. C., et al.: Sudden infant death syndrome among infants of drug-dependent mothers. J. Pediatr. 95:407–409, 1979.

Chess, S., and Thomas, A: Temperament in Clinical Practice. New York, Guilford Press, 1986, pp. 273–281.

Clarren, S. K., and Smith, D. W.: The fetal alcohol syndrome. N. Engl. J. Med. 298:1063–1067, 1978.

Coll, C. G., Kagan, J., and Resnick, S. J.: Behavioral inhibition in young children. Child Dev. 55:1005–1019, 1984.

Conel, J. L.: The Postnatal Development of the Human Cerebral Cortex. Cambridge, Mass., Harvard University Press, 1947.

Davis, D. H., and Thoman, E. B.: Behavioral states of premature infants: Implications for neural and behavioral development. Dev. Psychobiol. 20(1):25–38, 1987.

De Casper, A. J., and Fifer, W. P.: Of human bonding: Newborns prefer their mother's voices. Science 208:1174–1176, 1980.

Desmond, M. M., and Wilson, G. S.: Neonatal abstinence syndrome: Recognition and diagnosis. Addict. Dis. 2:113–121, 1975.

deVries, J. I. P., Vissar, G. H. A., and Prechtl, H. F. R.: The emergence of fetal behaviour. I. Qualitative aspects. Early Hum. Dev. 7:301–322, 1982.

deVries, J. I. P., Vissar, G. H. A., and Prechtl, H. F. R.: The emergence of fetal behaviour. II. Quantitative aspects. Early Hum. Dev. 12:99–120, 1985.

DiVitto, B., and Goldberg, S.: The effects of newborn medical status on early parent-infant interaction. In Field, T. M., Sostek, A. S., Goldberg, S., and Shuman, H. H. (Eds.): Infants Born At Risk. New York, Spectrum, 1979.

Dixon, S. D., Bresnahan, K., and Zuckerman, B.: Cocaine babies: meeting the challenge of management. Contemp. Pediatr. 7(6):70–92, 1990.

Dixon, S., Snyder, J., Holve, R., et al.: Behavioral effects of circumcision with and without anesthesia. J. Dev. Behav. Pediatr. 5:246–250, 1984.

Doberczak, T. M., Thornton, J. C., Berstein, J., et al.: Impact of maternal drug dependency on birth weight and head circumference of offspring. Am. J. Dis. Child 141:1163–1167, 1987.

Dreyfus-Brisac, C.: Sleep ontogenesis in early human prematures from 24 to 27 weeks conceptional age. Dev. Psychobiol. 1:162–169, 1968.

Emory, E. K., Konopka, S., Hronsky, S., Tuggey, R., and Dave, R.: Salivary caffeine and neonatal behavior: Assay modification and functional significance. Psychopharm. Bull. 94:64–68, 1988.

Enhorning, G., Shennan, A., Pessinager, F., et al.: Prevention of neonatal respiratory distress syndrome by tracheal instillation of surfactant: A randomized clinical trial. Pediatrics 76:145–153, 1985.

Fantz, R. L., and Fagan, J. F.: Visual attention to size and number of pattern details by term and preterm infants during the first six months. Child Dev. 46:3–18, 1975.

Fantz, R. L., and Nevis, S.: Pattern preferences and perceptual-cognitive development in early infancy. Merrill-Palmer Q. 13:77–108, 1967.

Ferrari, F., Grosoli, M. V., Pontana, G., et al.: Neurobehavioral comparison of low-risk preterm and full-term infants at term conceptual age. Dev. Med. Child Neurol. 25:450–458, 1983.

Field, T. M.: Effects of early separation, interactive deficits, and experimental manipulations on mother-infant interaction. Child Dev. 48:763–771, 1977.

Field, T. M., and Goldson, E.: Pacifying effects of nonnutritive sucking on term and preterm neonates during heelstick procedures. Pediatrics 74:1012–1015, 1984.

Field, T. M., Healy, B., Goldstein, R., et al.: Infants of depressed mothers show "depressed" behavior even with nondepressed adults. Child Dev. 59:1569–1579, 1988.

Field, T. M., Ignatoff, E., Stringer, S., et al.: Nonnutritive sucking during tube feedings: Effects on preterm neonates in an intensive care unit. Pediatrics 70:381–384, 1982.

Field, T. M., Schanberg, S. M., Scafidi, F., et al.: Tactile/Kinesthetic stimulation effects in preterm neonates. Pediatrics 47:654–658, 1986.

Fisichelli, V., and Karelitz, S.: The cry latencies of normal infants and those with brain damage. J. Pediatr. 62:724–734, 1963.

Fox, N. A., and Porges, S. W.: The relation between neonatal heart period patterns and developmental outcome. Child Dev. 56:28–37, 1985.

Fujiwara, T., Konishi, M., Chida, S., et al.: Surfactant replacement therapy with a single post-ventilatory dose of a reconstituted bovine surfactant in preterm infants with respiratory distress syndrome: Final analysis of a multicenter, double-blind randomized trial and comparison with similar trials. Pediatrics 86:753–764, 1990.

Gabriel, M., Albani, M., and Schulte, F. J.: Apneic spells and sleep states in pre-term infants. Pediatrics 57:142–147, 1976.

Gaiter, J. L.: Nursery environments: The behavior and caregiving experiences of full-term and preterm newborns. In Gottfried, A. W., and Gaiter, J. L. (Eds.): Infant Stress Under Intensive Care. Baltimore, University Park Press, 1985, pp. 55–81.

Gilkerson, L., Gorski, P. A., and Panitz, P.: Hospital-based intervention for preterm infants and their families. In Meisels, S. J., and Shonkoff, J. P. (Eds.): Handbook of Early Intervention: Theory, Practice, and Analysis. Cambridge, Cambridge University Press, 1990.

Goldberg, S.: Premature birth: Consequences for the parent-infant relationship. Am. Sci. 67:214–220, 1979.

Goldsmith, H. H., Buss, A. H., Plomin, R., et al.: Roundtable: What is temperament? Four approaches. Child Dev. 58:505–529, 1987.

Gorski, P. A.: Premature infant behavioral and physiological responses to caregiving interventions in the intensive care nursery. In Call, J. D., Galenson, E., and Tyson, R. L. (Eds.): Frontiers of Infant Psychiatry. New York, Basic Books, 1983, pp. 256–263.

Gorski, P. A.: Fostering family development following preterm hospitalization. In Ballard, R. A. (Ed.): Pediatric Care of the ICN Graduate. Philadelphia, W.B. Saunders Company, 1988, pp. 27–32.

Gorski, P. A., Davison, M. F., and Brazelton, T. B.: Stages of behavioral organization in the high-risk neonate: Theoretical and clinical considerations. Sem. Perinat. 3:61–72, 1979.

Gorski, P. A., Hole, W. T., Leonard, C. H., et al.: Direct computer recording of premature infants and nursery care. Pediatrics 72:198–202, 1983.

Gorski, P. A., and Huntington, L.: Physiological measures relative to tactile stimulation in hospitalized preterm infants. Pediatr. Res. 23:210A, 1988.

Gorski, P. A., Leonard, C., Sweet, D., et al.: Caring for immature infants—a touchy subject. In Brown, C. C. (Ed.): The Many Facets of Touch. Skillman, N.J., Johnson & Johnson, 1984, pp. 84–91.

Gottfried, A. W.: Environment of newborn infants in special care units. In Gottfried, A. W., and Gaiter, J. L. (Eds.): Infant Stress Under Intensive Care. Baltimore, University Park Press, 1985, pp. 23–54.

Gottfried, A. W., Wallace-Lande, P., Sherman-Brown, S., et al.: Physical and social environment of newborn infants in special care units. Science 214:673–675, 1981.

Gottlieb, G.: Ontogenesis of sensory function in birds and mammals. In Tobach, E., Aronson, L. R., and Shaw, E. (Eds.): The Biopsychology of Development. New York, Academic Press, 1971, pp. 67–126.

Green, M., and Solnit, A.: Reactions to the threatened loss of a child: A vulnerable child syndrome. Pediatrics 34:58–66, 1964.

Grimwade, J. C., Walker, D. W., Bartlett, M., et al.: Human fetal heart rate changes and movement in response to sound and vibration. Am. J. Obstet. Gynecol. 109:86–90, 1971.

Gunnar, M. R., Fisch, R. O., Kovsvilc, S., et al.: The effects of circumcision on serum cortisol and behavior. Psychoneuroendocrinology 6:269–275, 1981.

Gunnar, M. R., Fisch, R. O., and Malone, S.: The effects of a pacifying stimulus on behavioral and adrenocortical responses to circumcision in the newborn. J. Am. Acad. Child Psych. 23:34–38, 1984.

Harper, R. M., Hoppenbrowers, T., Sterman, M. B., et al.: Polygraphic studies of normal infants during the first six months of life. 1. Heart rate as a function of state. Pediatr. Res. 10:945–951, 1976.

Hecox, K. E., and Deegan, D. M.: Methodological issues in the study of auditory development. In Gottlieb, G., and Krasnegor, N. A. (Eds.): Measurement of Audition and Vision in the First Year of Postnatal Life: A Methodological Overview. Norwood, N.J., Ablex, 1985, pp. 391–418.

Herrenkohl, L. R.: Prenatal stress disrupts reproductive behavior and physiology in offspring. Ann. N.Y. Acad. Sci., 474:120–128, 1986.

High, P. C., and Gorski, P. A.: Recording environmental influences on infant development in the intensive care nursery. In Gottfried, A. W., and Gaiter, J. L. (Eds.): Infant Stress Under Intensive Care. Baltimore, University Park Press, 1985, pp. 131–155.

Hooker, D.: The Prenatal Origins of Behavior. Lawrence, Kan., University of Kansas Press, 1952.

Horowitz, F. D., Ashton, J., Culp, R., et al.: The effects of obstetric medication on the behavior of Israeli newborn infants and some comparisons with Uruguayan and American infants. Child Dev. 48:1607–1623, 1977.

Howard, J., Parmelee, A. H., Kopp, C. B., et al.: A neurologic comparison of pre-term and full-term infants at term conceptional age. J. Pediatr. 88:995–1002, 1976.

Hunt, J. V., Tooley, W. H., and Harvin, D.: Learning disabilities in children with birth weights ≤1500 grams. Semin. Perinatatol. 6:280–287, 1982.

Hunter, R. S., Kilstrom, W., Kraybill, E. N., et al.: Antecedents of child abuse and neglect in premature infants: A prospective study in a newborn intensive care unit. Pediatrics 61:629–635, 1978.

James, W.: Principles of Psychology. Vol. I. F. Burkhardt (Ed.). Cambridge, Harvard University Press, 1981 [1890].

Karelitz, S., and Fisichelli, V.: The cry thresholds of normal infants and those with brain damage. J. Pediatr. 61:679–685, 1962.

Katz, V.: Auditory stimulation and developmental behavior of one premature infant. Nurs. Res. 20:196–201, 1971.

Klein, M., and Stern, L.: Low birth weight and the battered child syndrome. Am. J. Dis. Child 122:15–18, 1971.

Klein, N., Hack, M., Gallagher, J., et al.: Preschool performance of children with normal intelligence who were very low birth weight infants. Pediatrics 75:531–537, 1985.

Korner, A. F.: State as variable, as obstacle, and as mediator of stimulation in infant research. Merrill-Palmer Q. 18:77–94, 1972.

Korner, A. F., Guilleminault, C., and Van den Hoed, J.: Reduction of sleep apnea and bradycardia in preterm infants on oscillating water beds: A controlled polygraphic study. Pediatrics 61:528–533, 1978.

Korner, A. F., Kraemer, H., and Haffner, E.: Effects of waterbed flotation in premature infants: A pilot study. Pediatrics 5:361–365, 1975.

Korner, A. F., and Schneider, P.: Effects of vestibular-proprioceptive stimulation on the neurobehavioral development of preterm infants: A pilot study. Neuropediatrics 14:170–175, 1983.

Kraemer, H., Korner, A. F., and Thoman, E. B.: Methodological considerations in evaluating the influence of drugs used during labor and delivery on the behavior of the newborn. Dev. Psychol. 6:128–134, 1972.

Kuhnert, B. R., Linn, P. L., and Kuhnert, P. M.: Obstetric medication and neonatal behavior: Current controversies. Clin. Perinatol. 12:423–440, 1985.

Lawson, K., Daum, C., and Turkewitz, G.: Environmental characteristics of a neonatal intensive care unit. Child Dev. 48:1633–1639, 1977.

Leib, S., Benfield, G., and Guidubaldi, J.: Effects of early intervention and stimulation on the preterm infant. Pediatrics 66:83–89, 1980.

Lester, B. M.: Developmental outcome prediction from acoustic cry analysis in term and preterm infants. Pediatrics 80:529–534, 1987.

Lester, B. M., Als, H., and Brazelton, T. B.: Regional obstetric anesthesia and newborn behavior: A reanalysis toward synergistic effects. Child Dev. 53:687–692, 1982.

Lester, B. M., Emory, E. K., Hoffman, S. L., et al.: A multivariate study of the effects of high-risk factors on performance on the Brazelton Neonatal Assessment Scale. Child Dev. 47:515–517, 1976.

Lewkowicz, D. J.: Developmental changes in infants' response to temporal frequency. Dev. Psychol. 21:858–865, 1985.

Lifschitz, M. H., Wilson, G. S., Smith, E. O., et al.: Factors affecting head growth and intellectual function in children of drug addicts. Pediatrics 75:269–274, 1985.

Linn, P. L., Horowitz, F. D., Buddin, B. J., et al.: An ecological description of a neonatal intensive care unit. In Gottfried, A. W., and Gaiter, J. L. (Eds.): Infant Stress Under Intensive Care. Baltimore, University Park Press, 1985a, pp. 83–111.

Linn, P. L., Horowitz, F. D., and Fox, H. A.: Stimulation in the NICU: Is more necessarily better? Clin. Perinat. 12:407–422, 1985b.

Long, J., Lucey, J., and Philip, A.: Noise and hypoxemia in the intensive care nursery. Pediatrics 65:143–145, 1980.

MacArthur, C., and Knox, E. G.: Smoking in pregnancy: effects of stopping at different stages. Br. J. Obstet. Gynecol. 95:551–555, 1988.

McGehee, L. J., and Eckerman, C. O.: The preterm infant as a social partner: Responsive but unreadable. Infant Behav. Dev. 6:467–470, 1983.

Merritt, T. A., and Hallman, M.: Surfactant replacement: A new era with many challenges for neonatal medicine. Am. J. Dis. Child. 142:1333–1339, 1988.

Michaelis, R., Parmelee, A. H., Stern, E., et al.: Activity states in premature and term infants. Dev. Psychobiol. 6:209–215, 1973.

Michelsson, K., Sirvio, P., and Wasz-Hockert, O.: Sound spectrographic cry analysis of infants with bacterial meningitis. Dev. Med. Child Neurol. 19:309–315, 1977.

Montagu, A. Touching: The Human Significance of the Skin. New York, Columbia University Press, 1971.

Moyer, J. A., Herrenkohl, L. R., and Jacobowitz, D. M.: Effects of stress during pregnancy on catecholamines in discrete brain regions. Brain Res. 121:385–393, 1977.

Muir, D., and Clifton, R. K.: Infants' orientation to the location of sound sources. In Gottlieb, G., and Krasnegor, N. A. (Eds.): Measurement of Audition and Vision in the First Year of Postnatal Life: A Methodological Overview. Norwood, N.J., Ablex, 1985, pp. 167–194.

Muir, D., and Field, J.: Newborn infants orient to sounds. Child Dev. 50:431–436, 1979.

Murray, A. D., Dolby, R. M., Nation, R. L., et al.: Effects of epidural anesthesia on newborns and their mothers. Child Dev. 52:71–82, 1981.

Nijhuis, J., Prechtl, H., Martin, C., et al.: Are there behavioral states in the human fetus. Early Hum. Dev. 6:177–195, 1982.

Oro, A. S., and Dixon, S. D.: Perinatal cocaine and methamphetamine exposure: Maternal and neonatal correlates. J. Pediatr. 111:571–578, 1987.

Owens, M. E., and Todt, E. H.: Pain in infancy: Neonatal reaction to a heel lance. Pain 20:77–86, 1984.

Palmer, P. G., Dubowitz, L. M. S., Verghote, M., et al.: Neurological and neurobehavioural differences between preterm infants at term and full-term newborn infants. Neuropediatrics 13:183–189, 1982.

Paludetto, R., Mansi, G., Rinaldi, P., et al.: Behavior of preterm newborns reaching term without any serious disorder. Early Human Dev. 6:357–363, 1982.

Parmelee, A. H.: Remarks on receiving the C. Anderson Aldrich Award. Pediatrics 59:389–395, 1977.

Parmelee, A. H., Stern, E., and Harris, M. A.: Maturation of states in premature and young infants. Neuropediatrie 3:294–304, 1972.

Parmelee, A. H., Wenner, W. H., Akiyama, Y., et al.: Sleep states in premature infants. Dev. Med. Child Neurol. 9:70–77, 1967.

Parmelee, A. H., Wenner, W. H., and Schulz, H. R.: Infant sleep patterns from birth to 16 weeks of age. J. Pediatr. 65:576–582, 1964.

Pearson, D. T., and Dietrich, K. N.: The behavioral toxicology and teratology of childhood: models, methods, and implications for intervention. Neurotoxicology 6:165–182, 1985.

Perlman, J. M., McMenamin, J. B., and Volpe, J. J.: Fluctuating cerebral blood-flow velocity in respiratory-distress syndrome. N. Engl. J. Med. 310:204–209, 1984.

Perlman, J. M., and Volpe, J. J.: Episodes of apnea and bradycardia in the preterm newborn: Impact on cerebral circulation. Pediatrics 76:333–338, 1985.

Pomerleau-Malcuit, A., and Clifton, R. K.: Neonatal heart rate response to tactile, auditory, and vestibular stimulation in different states. Child Dev. 44:485–496, 1973.

Porges, S. W.: Heart rate patterns in neonates: A potential diagnostic window to the brain. In Field, T. M. and Sostek, A. S. (Eds.): Infants Born At Risk. New York, Grune & Stratton, 1983, pp. 3–22.

Porges, S. W., McCabe, P. M., and Yongue, B. G.: Respiratory-heart rate interactions: Psychophysiological implications for pathophysiology and behavior. In Cacippo, J. T. and Petty, R. E. (Eds.): Perspectives in Cardiovascular Psychophysiology. New York, Guilford Press, 1982, pp. 233–260.

Prechtl, H. F. R.: The behavioral states of the newborn infant: a review. Brain Research 76:1304–1311, 1974.

Resnick, M., Eyler, F., and Nelson, R.: Developmental intervention for low birth weight infants: Improved early developmental outcome. Pediatrics 80:68–74, 1987.

Robertson, S. S.: Cyclic motor activity in the human fetus after midgestation. Dev. Psychobiol. 18:411–419, 1985.

Robertson, S. S.: Human cyclic motility: Fetal-newborn continuities and newborn state differences. Dev. Psychobiol. 20:425–442, 1987.

Robertson, S. S., and Dierker, L. J.: The development of cyclic motility in fetuses of diabetic mothers. Dev. Psychobiol. 19:223–234, 1986.

Rose, S. A., Gottfried, A. W., and Bridger, W. H.: Cross-modal transfer in infants: Relationship to prematurity and socioeconomic background. Dev. Psychol. 14:643–652, 1978.

Rothbart, M. K.: Measurement of temperament in infancy. Child Dev. 52:569–578, 1981.

Rubel, E. W.: Auditory system development. In Gottlieb, G. and Krasnegor, N. A. (Eds.): Measurement of Audition and Vision in the First Year of Postnatal Life: A Methodological Overview. Norwood, N.J., Ablex, 1985, pp. 53–89.

Saint-Anne Dargassies, S.: Normality and normalization as seen in a long-term neurological follow-up of 286 truly premature infants. Neuropediatr. 10:226–244, 1979.

Sanders-Phillips, K., Strauss, M. E., and Gutberlet, R. L.: The effect of obstetric medication on newborn infant feeding behavior. Infant Behav. Dev. 11:251–263, 1988.

Seligman, M. R.: Helplessness: On Development, Depression, and Death. San Francisco, W. H. Freeman, 1975.

Shaywitz, S. E., Capanilo, B. K., and Hodgson, E. S.: Developmental language disability as a consequence of prenatal exposure to ethanol. Pediatrics 68:850–855, 1981.

Starr, A., Amlie, R. N., Martin, W. H., et al.: Development of auditory function in newborn infants revealed by auditory brainstem potentials. Pediatrics 60:831–839, 1977.

Strauss, M. E., Lessen-Firestine, J. K., Starr, R. H., et al.: Behavior of narcotic-addicted newborns. Child Dev. 46:887–893, 1975.

Swafford, L. I., and Allan, D.: Pain relief in the pediatric patient. Med. Clin. North Am. 52:131–136, 1968.

Telzrow, R. W., Kang, R. R., Mitchell, S. K., et al.: An assessment of the behavior of the preterm infant at 40 weeks conceptional age. In Lipsitt, L. P. and Field, T. M. (Eds.): Infant Behavior and Development:

Perinatal Risk and Newborn Behavior. Norwood, N.J., Ablex, 1982, pp. 85–96.

Thoman, E. B.: Sleep and waking states of the neonate (revised edition), 1985. (Available from E.B. Thoman, Box U-154, Dept. of Psychology/Behavioral Neuroscience, 3107 Horsebarn Hill Rd., University of Connecticut, Storrs, CT 06268).

Thoman, E. B., Acebo, C., Dreyer, C. A., et al.: Individuality in the interactive process. In Thoman, E. B. (Ed.): Origins of the Infant's Social Responsiveness. Hillsdale, N.J., Lawrence Erlbaum, 1979, pp. 305–338.

Thoman, E. B., Denenberg, V. H., Sieval, J., et al.: State organization in neonates: Developmental inconsistency indicates risk for developmental dysfunction. Neuropediatr. 12:45–54, 1981.

Thoman, E. B., and Graham, S.: Self-regulation of stimulation by premature infants. Pediatrics 78:855–860, 1986.

Thomas, A., Chess, S., Birch, H. G., et al.: Behavioral Individuality in Early Childhood. New York, New York University Press, 1963.

Tronick, E., Wise, S., Als, H., et al.: Regional obstetric anesthesia and newborn behavior: Effect over the first ten days of life. Pediatrics 58:94–100, 1976.

Turkewitz, G., Birch, H. G., Moreau, T., et al.: Effect of intensity of auditory stimulation on directional eye movements in the human neonate. Anim. Behav. 14:93–101, 1966.

Turkewitz, G., Lewkowicz, D. J., and Gardner, J. M.: Determinants of infant perception. In Rosenblatt, J., Beer, C., Hinde, R., et al. (Eds.): Advances in the Study of Behavior. New York, Academic Press, 1983, pp. 39–62.

Vourenkoski, V., Lind, J., Partanen, T., et al.: Spectrographic analysis of cries from children with maladie du cri du chat. Ann. Paediatrias Fenniae 12:174–180, 1966.

Ward, S. L. D., Schuetz, S., Krishna, V., et al.: Abnormal sleeping ventilatory pattern in infants of substance-abusing mothers. Am. J. Dis. Child 140:1915–1920, 1986.

White, J., and Labarba, R.: The effects of tactile and kinesthetic stimulation on neonatal development in the premature infant. Dev. Psychobiol. 9:569–577, 1976.

Williamson, P. S., and Williamson, M. L.: Physiologic stress reduction by a local anesthetic during newborn circumcision. Pediatrics 71:36–40, 1983.

Wolff, P. H.: Observations on newborn infants. Psychosom. Med. 221:110–118, 1959.

Wolff, P. H.: The causes, controls, and organization of behavior in the neonate. Psychol. Issues 5:1–105, 1966.

Woodson, R., and Hamilton, C.: The effect of nonnutritive sucking on heart rate in preterm infants. Dev. Psychobiol. 21:207–213, 1988.

Yakovlev, P. I., and LeCours, A.: The myelogenetic cycles of regional maturation of the brain. In Minkowski, A. (Ed.): Regional Development of the Brain in Early Life. Philadelphia, F. A. Davis, 1967, pp. 3–65.

Zeskind, P. S., and Lester, B. M.: Acoustic features and auditory perceptions of the cries of newborns with prenatal and perinatal complications. Child Dev. 49:580–589, 1978.

Zeskind, P. S., and Lester, B. M.: Cry features of newborns with differential patterns of fetal growth. Child Dev. 51:207–212, 1981.

GROWTH DISORDERS 25

Rosemary Leake

■ SIGNIFICANCE

The mortality rate of very growth-retarded term infants is five to six times that of normally grown infants of a similar gestational age. Preterm growth-retarded infants also appear to be at increased risk although studies with gestational-age–matched mortality figures are limited (Heinonen et al., 1985; Koops et al., 1982; Usher, 1970). Mortality among undergrown infants is commonly associated with congenital anomalies, intrauterine infection, perinatal asphyxia or asphyxia-related complications, such as hypothermia, hypoglycemia, pulmonary hemorrhage, and meconium aspiration (Ounsted et al., 1981). Premature infants who are growth retarded but free of infection, anomalies, and asphyxia in some respects may have an advantage over weight-matched premature infants who have appropriate weight for gestation. For example, decreased risk of respiratory distress, intraventricular hemorrhage, and apnea may occur in some growth-retarded premature infants (Teberg et al., 1988). In fact, the smallest infants who survive are inevitably both premature and small for gestational age (Ginsberg et al., 1990). Recognition of the undergrown fetus and newborn infant continues to be important as an indicator for the risk of asphyxia and neonatal death.

■ DEFINITION OF SIGNIFICANT GROWTH RETARDATION

Clifford (1954) was one of the first to describe a group of infants with striking physical similarities suggesting a growth disturbance (babies who are long and thin with alert expressions; decreased subcutaneous, subareolar, and thigh fat; prominent ribs; and long nails). Review of birth histories frequently revealed the presence of significant oligohydramnios, fetal distress, and perinatal asphyxia. These "dysmature" infants were growth-deprived near the end of pregnancy so that weight but not length was reduced. Battaglia and Lubchenco (1967) and Lubchenco and associates (1963, 1966) published standards for weight, length, and head circumference of infants born in Denver that allowed classification of infants into those appropriate for gestational age, small for gestational age, or large for gestational age, based on values for intrauterine weight and length at various gestational ages. Based on this work, significant growth retardation was defined as weight less than the 10th percentile for gestational age, as determined on a standard intrauterine growth curve. The definition is now sometimes additionally divided into severe (<3rd percentile) and moderate (<10th percentile) growth retardation.

■ HISTORY

Based on the initial observations of Clifford, Battaglia and Lubchenco, and Lubchenco and colleagues, a number of others (especially Amiel-Tison, 1968; Dubowitz, 1970; Farr, 1966; Gruenwald, 1963; Usher, 1966) have contributed to our understanding of growth retardation by improving the techniques used for estimating gestational age and by focusing on the importance of symmetric versus asymmetric retardation. Symmetric growth retardation produces a small infant with a proportionately small head and length. Asymmetric growth retardation results in a small infant whose head and length are relatively normal size for gestational age but whose weight-length ratio is reduced. Symmetric growth retardation is believed to begin early in gestation and, therefore, affects cell number. The asymmetric type generally occurs late in gestation and produces cell hypertrophy. Also, there are babies who demonstrate a combined type of intrauterine growth retardation affecting both cell number and producing cell hypertrophy (Miller, 1985). Clearly, some infants achieving heights and weights less than the 10th percentile are healthy and their smallness is genetically determined; additionally some term infants weigh more than the weights represented in the 10th percentile but are clearly malnourished as determined by their subcutaneous tissue; these infants may exhibit long-term sequelae of malnutrition (Hill et al., 1984). The concept of the ponderal index, defined as weight in grams $\times$ 100, divided by length in centimeters, helped to provide a definition for these infants as well as quantify "thinness" as weight in relation to length (Miller and Hassanein, 1971). Symmetric growth retardation produces a normal ratio of weight and length, whereas asymmetric growth retardation produces an infant that has a low ponderal index as determined by his or her low birth weight and normal or near-normal length.

Many terms were initially used to describe the condition of the undergrown infant, including smallness for gestational age, fetal malnourishment (Scott and Usher, 1966), chronic fetal distress (Gruenwald, 1963), intrauterine growth retardation (Wigglesworth, 1966) and pseudoprematurity (Soderling, 1953). The term pseudoprematurity was based on the recognition that in developed countries one-third of all infants classified as preterm infants by weight (<2500 g) were actually small for gestational age and, in fact, might be full term, i.e., 37 weeks' or more gestational age. Generally growth retardation is now termed intrauterine growth retardation (IUGR) when the condition is determined in the fetus (Wigglesworth, 1966), and the resultant newborn is said to be small for gestational age (SGA).

■ EPIDEMIOLOGY

The prevalence of IUGR varies with the population studied but is generally defined as 3 to 10 per cent for national populations in developed countries (Hobbins and

Berkowitz, 1977; Hobbins et al., 1978). Definitions of standards for normal growth should ideally include features such as maternal height, weight, age, ethnicity, geographic factors, birth number and socioeconomic background. It is important to differentiate infants on the basis of sex, since male infants weigh on average 200 g more than female infants by term. Few standards exist incorporating all of these factors; however, Figure 25–1 demonstrates the University of California growth chart for determining gestational age and expected growth measures; this chart also predicts normal growth as determined locally in Ohio and North Carolina. Using locally generated data for normal growth markedly increased the prevalence of SGA infants in several studies (Miller and Jekel, 1985, 1989; Raju et al., 1987). The Denver chart (Fig. 25–2) is not an accurate measure of growth retardation for babies at sea level (Miller and Jekel, 1985; Raju et al., 1987); the University of California growth curve, based on birth certificate data from 2,000,000 births, is in agreement with the Denver curves until about 32 weeks' gestational age; at that point, there is a gradual increase in the California 10th percentile weight until, by 36 weeks, California's 10th percentile weight exceeds that of the Denver chart by 200 g (Brar and Rutherford, 1988).

Growth standards for infants less than 30 weeks' gestational age are particularly inadequate. Assignment of gestational age based on the infant's skin and neurologic features overestimates the number of SGA infants among very immature infants.

Significant maternal risk factors for IUGR include low socioeconomic level, primiparity and/or a history of having borne a previous IUGR infant (Tejani and Mann, 1977). High altitude; low maternal height and weight (Naeye, 1979); poor pregnancy weight gain; smoking (Quigley et al., 1979); heroin, methadone, phencyclidine piperidine (PCP), cocaine, or alcohol use (Taeusch et al., 1973; Tze and Lee, 1975); and maternal diseases (found in 7 to 35 per cent of IUGR pregnancies) such as hemoglobinopathies, hypertensive cardiovascular diseases, toxemia, or advanced diabetes place the fetus at increased risk. The nature of the mother's work and the stress she undergoes during pregnancy may be risk factors as well.

Multiple births represent a special risk category; for example, approximately 20 per cent of twin gestations are significantly growth retarded. Growth generally progresses normally until the combined fetal weights exceed a total of 3000 g; therefore, growth retardation generally begins by 30 weeks' gestation for twins and 26 weeks' gestation for quadruplets (Naeye, 1964). Growth retardation can be severe at term, since the median weight for all twins at term is only at the 10th percentile.

Not surprisingly, maternal nutrition appears to influence fetal growth. Experience in third world countries suggests that it is the mother's total caloric intake rather than protein or fat intake that affects birth weight (Warshaw, 1986). Interestingly, birth weights following the Dutch famine during World War II did not deviate widely from normal; however, several studies show that both low

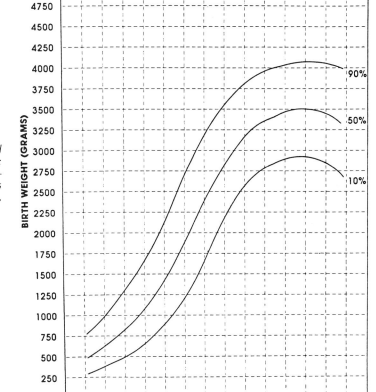

FIGURE 25–1. University of California growth chart. (Adapted from Williams, R. L., Creasy, R. K., Cunningham, G. C., et al.: Fetal growth and perinatal viability. Obstet. Gynecol. 59:624–632, 1982. Printed courtesy of the North Coast Perinatal Access System, HSE 1462, University of California, San Francisco, California 94143.)

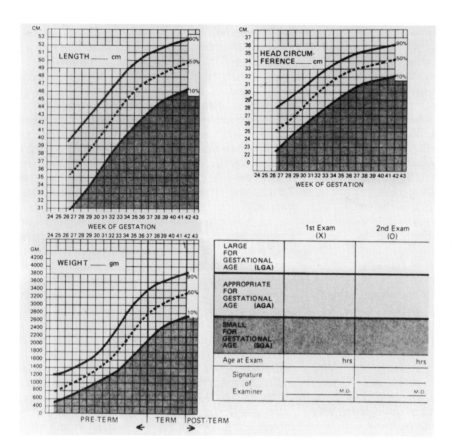

FIGURE 25–2. Colorado growth chart. (Adapted from Lubchenco, L. C., Hansman, C., and Boyd, E.: A practical classification of newborn infants by weight and gestational age. Pediatrics 37:403, 1966; Battaglia, F. C., and Lubchenco, L. C.: A practical classification of newborn infants by weight and gestational age. J. Pediatr. 71:159, 1967.)

prepregnancy weight (Bakketeig et al., 1979) and food supplementation programs (Lechtig, 1975) affect fetal weight.

■ ETIOLOGY AND NATURAL HISTORY

The etiology of growth retardation is discussed in detail in Chapters 7 and 8 of this volume. Briefly summarized, although 60 per cent of cases of IUGR are idiopathic, the remaining causes include chromosomal abnormalities and congenital anomalies (present in 5–10 per cent of all IUGR infants); viral infections (approximately 3 per cent of IUGR infants); high-dose radiation; alcohol; use of illicit drugs such as heroin, methadone, PCP, and cocaine; chronic maternal corticosteroid administration; phenytoin; smoking; and multiple births. Maternal diseases, such as congenital heart disease if associated with cyanosis or pulmonary hypertension, renal disease, hypertension (especially that associated with glomerulonephritis, multiparous preeclampsia without preceding hypertension and chronic hypertension) (Lin et al., 1982), may produce IUGR. Severe anemia, collagen vascular disease, and severe diabetes (especially Class D, F or R diabetes) are additional risk factors. Maternal smoking is a major contributor to IUGR, probably because of associated maternal norepinephrine and epinephrine release, with the resultant decrease in uteroplacental flow and increased maternal carboxyhemoglobin, which produces decreased fetal oxygenation (Quigley et al., 1979).

The natural history of IUGR has changed over the past several years, based on increasing knowledge of its various causes and on improved detection and growth monitoring capabilities provided by ultrasound. The birth of a SGA infant is no longer a surprise. Significant growth retardation is now often detected in the second trimester, chromosome analysis is conducted, and a diagnosis of symmetric or asymmetric growth retardation is made. A careful examination for fetal anomalies by ultrasound is often made, and serial evaluation of fetal movements may be carried out. An estimation of the placental size may be useful. A normal-sized placenta associated with growth retardation usually is linked to congenital anomalies, whereas a small placenta is generally associated with causes other than congenital anomalies (Winick et al., 1973). Maternal counseling and individualized approaches to the timing of labor and site and route of delivery are often possible based on conclusions drawn from data gathered from the intrauterine evaluation.

■ INITIAL MANAGEMENT AND TREATMENT

Despite improved detection and monitoring, the pediatrician first may be aware that an infant is small for gestational age when he or she receives an emergency call from the delivery room. Significant fetal heart rate decelerations are present in one-third of SGA infants with IUGR, and one-fifth of these infants exhibit fetal acidosis and low Apgar scores. These effects are generally believed to be secondary to decreased maternal-to-fetal-oxygen transfer from inadequate placentation (Low et al., 1982). Cordocentesis studies suggest that a significant number of growth retarded fetuses are chronically hypoxic, hypercapneic, acidotic, and hyperlacticemic (Soothill et al., 1987). These findings explain why some SGA infants appear to be asphyxiated following an atraumatic delivery; in these cases, fetal reserves appear to be chronically compromised. The resultant neonatal depression may be associated with the additional complications of hypothermia, pulmonary hemorrhage, postasphyxial seizures, disseminated intravascular coagulation, and hypocalcemia. A significant number (10 to 20 per cent) of SGA infants exhibit major congenital anomalies as well. Additionally, hypoglycemia, hyperviscosity (Gross et al., 1973), increased oxygen consumption, and abnormalities of glucose utilization are sometimes present. Classic respiratory distress syndrome is found infrequently in SGA infants who are compared with infants matched either for weight or for gestation, presumably because of increased fetal exposure to endogenous hormones that mature the lung, but meconium aspiration is common.

Treatment begins with optimal resuscitation. Despite the use of this approach, acidosis may be present and lactate levels are generally elevated. Maintenance of body temperature may be difficult to accomplish since the infant's markedly reduced subcutaneous tissue reduces the efficiency of thermoregulation. Interestingly, the infant's relatively mature skin makes estimates of neutral thermal environmental temperatures invalid if taken from tables with recommendations for environmental temperature based on birth weight (Hammerlund and Sedin, 1980). However, careful temperature maintenance may prove an important element in the prevention of pulmonary hemorrhage. Meconium aspiration is also preventible at times with aggressive, deep suctioning of the nasopharynx (Carson et al., 1976; Gregory, 1975). Pulmonary vasoconstriction may occur in response to chronic intrauterine hypoxia, and a delayed decrease in pulmonary vascular resistance is present in some SGA infants (Gierman et al., 1983). Additionally, ischemic myocardial damage may occur (Bucciarelli et al., 1977; Riemenschneider et al., 1976). Neurologic abnormalities are common in these infants; these abnormalities include hyperexcitability, tone aberrations, poor responsiveness on interaction, and exaggerated arm movements on the Moro reflex (Fredrickson and Brown, 1980; Michaelis et al., 1970). Additionally, hypoxic ischemic encephalopathy may be associated with seizures.

The SGA infant is at high risk for several metabolic problems. The greater the IUGR, the greater the hypermetabolic state (Hill and Robinson, 1968), probably because of the relationship of cell mass to cell number, and the percentage of body weight represented by the visceral organs as opposed to less metabolically active organs. Caloric needs may be increased for the IUGR as compared with normal infants when calculated on a per-kilogram basis because of the relatively high oxygen consumption associated with their aberrant tissue-weight distribution. Decreased body fat and, most particularly, the lack of brown fat leads to a risk for hypothermia. Hypoglycemia is a risk (Lubchenco and Bard, 1971) because of poor glycogen stores, decreased glucose production, increased metabolic demands, and a relatively large brain (Cornblath et al., 1964), which is the organ that uses 75 per cent of the body's glucose. There is abnormal handling of glucose precursors as well in that basal alanine levels are elevated in the SGA infant and the provision of alanine orally does not produce a gluconeogenic response (increased glucose or increased insulin) during the first day of life as it does for appropriately nourished infants (Williams et al., 1975).

Moreover, cordocentesis studies of human fetuses suggest that (mean) umbilical arterial and venous glucose levels are significantly lower in IUGR infants, and fetal hypoglycemia is proportional to the degree of fetal hypoxia. Since umbilical arterial and venous glucose samples are nearly identical, the intrauterine hypoglycemia appears to be due to a reduced glucose supply (Economides and Nicolaides, 1989). Hypocalcemia occurs because of perinatal asphyxia and aggressive use of sodium bicarbonate (Tsang et al., 1975). Hyperviscosity is present in nearly 20 per cent of all SGA infants (Humbert et al., 1969; Wirth et al., 1975), probably because of active erythropoietin production in response to fetal hypoxia (Finne, 1966). This theory is supported by cord blood erythropoietin levels, nucleated red blood cell counts, and a rapid decrease in the reticulocyte count following delivery in SGA infants (Philip and Tito, 1989).

There appears to be impaired cellular and humoral responses in SGA infants (Ferguson et al., 1974; Yang et al., 1984). These include decreased numbers of circulating T lymphocytes; deficiency in complement C'3 and nonspecific deficiency in white cell, phagocyte, and opsonic activity; and low levels of IgG, IgA, and (without intrauterine infection) IgM (Yeung and Hobbs, 1968).

Despite the fact that all infants have a risk of initial asphyxia and postasphyxial complications, all SGA infants are not alike. There is increasing recognition that growth retardation is generally symmetric (so-called Type I) or asymmetric (Type II) and that this division suggests the likely cause and affects the direction of the evaluation. Symmetric growth retardation generally begins early in pregnancy, affects most organs equally (including the brain), and usually represents teratogenic, infectious, or drug effects or long-standing nutritional inadequacy. Type II growth retardation, which is more common (representing roughly 80% of SGA infants), generally affects liver, kidney size, and subcutaneous tissue but spares the brain. This relative sparing may represent redistribution of the cerebral circulation to the brain in the face of stress.

Besides a careful examination of the placenta (Rolschan, 1978a, 1978b), a review of the maternal history, physical examination and estimation of gestational age, the work-up of the symmetric SGA infant may include chromosomal analysis; a sepsis work-up, including toxoplasmosis, syphilis, rubella, cytomegalovirus; herpes titers; and an IgM measurement (Alford et al., 1967; Alford, 1971; Jones, 1972; Matthews and O'Herlihy, 1978). Since asymmetric growth retardation is generally a result of maternal disease or placental pathology, the work-up may require no more than a careful history to determine whether or not the mother practices smoking or alcohol abuse, and an examination of the history and placenta, plus a careful plan for postnatal nutrition and developmental and neurologic follow-up examination.

▪ PROGNOSIS

Many SGA infants, especially of the Type II subgroup resulting from uterine constraint or placental insufficiency, exhibit rapid growth during the first months of extrauterine life (Cruise, 1973; Holmes et al., 1977). Growth in Type I SGA infants is less predictable, especially for those infants with decreased cell numbers secondary to the effects of

TABLE 25–1. Follow-Up of Premature Small-for-Gestational-Age Infants

AUTHORS	YEAR OF BIRTH	NUMBER		MEAN (g)		MEAN GA (wk)		FOLLOW-UP (yr)	MAJOR NEUROLOGIC PROBLEMS (%)		DQ	
		SGA	AGA	SGA	AGA	SGA	AGA		SGA	AGA	SGA	AGA
Commey and Fitzhardinge (1979)	1974 to 1975	71	0	1113		31.8		2	21		86 MDI 78 PDI	
Kumar et al. (1980)	1974 to 1977	13	37	1056		29.5		1	30	8	—	
Hack (1989)	1977 to 1982	102	379	1126	1204	32	29	2	6	11	89.9	92.8
Kitchen (1984)	1979 to 1980	10	83	871		27.1		2	30	9	83.0	94.4
Vohr (1983)	1973 to 1975	21	20	1190	1221	33	29	5	15	12	*	*
Calame (1983)	1971 to 1975	71	110	1640	1520	35	30	5	8	16	107	101
		35	35	1132	1179	32	29	1	23	26	96	100
Pena (1988)	1982 to 1983	20	20	1006	1294	30.8	30.6	1	30	5	95	100

*Information not available.
SGA, small for gestational age; AGA, average for gestational age.
(Modified from Teberg, A. J., Walther, F. J., and Pena, I. C.: Mortality, morbidity and outcome for the small-for-gestational-age infant. Semin. Perinatol. 12:84, 1988.)

intrauterine infection and for those with chromosomal abnormalities or congenital anomalies. Somatic growth appears fairly consistently compromised in preterm SGA infants (Babson, 1970; Fitzhardinge, 1972). In one series nearly half of the preterm SGA infants were < 3rd percentile for weight at 1 year of age (Kumar, 1980). Some of the problems with somatic growth may reflect the increased incidence of long-term feeding problems in growth retarded infants (Mullen, 1987).

Intrauterine growth retardation results from a variety of conditions, not all of which carry the same risk for long-term effects, and it is difficult to predict neurologic and intellectual outcome for a particular infant. Brain development involves neuronal mitosis in the first half of pregnancy and glial cell multiplication, dendritic and synaptic development and myelination during the period from 20 weeks' gestation to 2 years of age. Thus, the condition producing the intrauterine growth retardation and both intrauterine and extrauterine malnutrition may affect cell number and axonal and dendritic growth, depending on the timing of onset, duration, and extent of the malnutrition (Brandt, 1981; Lien et al., 1977). Studies of twins support the view that, in general, intellectual development and postnatal growth are influenced by the malnutrition that causes intrauterine growth retardation, the smaller twin being at higher risk (Churchill, 1965).

Tables 25–1 and 25–2 summarize the results of neurologic and developmental outcome studies for preterm and term SGA infants. In general, the incidence of significant neurologic deficits and learning and behavioral problems is significant in growth-retarded preterm infants,

averaging about 20 per cent. This number represents a higher prevalence of neurologic and developmental problems than in appropriately grown preterm infants. Growth retardation with an associated small head circumference is linked to an especially high risk of neurologic deficits and poor school achievement (Gross et al., 1978; Parkinson et al., 1981); this is not surprising, since head circumference reflects brain size in the absence of hydrocephalus. The combination of a history of neonatal illness and subnormal head growth at 8 months of age are particularly accurate predictors of a poor outcome for the SGA infant (Hack et al., 1989). Growth-retarded infants appear to have more complications in the nursery than controls with the appropriate size for gestational age (similar birth weight); this factor may add to the prevalence of long-term neurologic problems (Pena et al., 1988).

Several studies of term and preterm SGA infants suggest that male sex and/or the presence of asphyxia, intracranial hemorrhage and neonatal seizures predicted a poor outcome. Low socioeconomic level appears to be the most powerful determinant of cognitive outcome, however (Fitzhardinghe and Steven, 1972a, b; Low et al., 1978, 1982; Ounsted et al., 1981, 1983, 1984; Vohr et al., 1983; Westwood et al., 1983).

■ PREVENTION AND NEW APPROACHES

Prevention of intrauterine growth retardation requires a more complete understanding of fetal growth and of the nutritional and hormonal milieu of the fetus. Significant progress has been made in the area of early identification

TABLE 25–2. Follow-Up of Term Small-for-Gestational-Age Infants

STUDIES	YEAR OF BIRTH	NUMBER OF INFANTS		MEAN BIRTH WEIGHT (g OR %)		MEAN GESTATIONAL AGE (wk)		FOLLOW-UP (yr)	MINOR NEUROLOGIC PROBLEMS (%)		IQ/DQ	
		SGA	AGA	SGA	AGA	SGA	AGA		SGA	AGA	SGA	AGA
Neligan et al. (1976)	1960 to 1962	141	187	2537	3508	40.1	40.1	7	—	—	92.7	99.1
Hill et al. (1984)	1964 to 1965	33	13	—*	—	>37	>37	12 to 14	9.0	0	104	121
Rubin et al. (1973)	1960 to 1964	46	85	≤2500	>2500	>37	>37	7	—	—	97.5	103.3
Fitzhardinge et al. (1972a, b)	1960 to 1964	96	60	2144	>3%	40.0	≥38	5.6	16.7	1.7	99	104
Westwood et al. (1983)	1960 to 1964	33	33	2188	25 to 75%	40.0	38 to 42	13 to 19	—	—	103.6	108.7
Low et al. (1978)	early 1970s	76	88	2302	3485	39.1	40.3	6	23	17	105.2	104.4
Ounsted et al. (1984)	1970 to 1974	138	138	2180	3380	≤33	≤33	7	6.5	7.2	37.9	39.7
Walther (1988)	1976 to 1977	24	24	2372	3433	39.5	39.7	7	50	4.2	—	—

*Information not available.
SGA, small for gestational age; AGA, average for gestational age.
(Modified from Teberg, A. J., Walther, F. J., and Pena, I. C.: Mortality, morbidity and outcome for the small-for-gestational-age infant. Semin. Perinatol. 12:84, 1988.)

of the growth-retarded fetus. This diagnosis is warranted when the fetus is 3 or more weeks behind the normal standard for size for its gestational age and/or has a growth rate of < 2 cm/month. Once growth retardation is suspected, the fetal growth rate may improve with appropriate management of the mother, such as bed rest and increased nutrition. Moreover, tests of fetal well-being and combined neonatal and perinatal consultation regarding optimal timing and routes of delivery can be initiated.

There is accumulating evidence that a variety of cytokines may be important in fetal growth regulation; moreover, the administration of insulin clearly has a major role in the regulation of fetal growth in that it contributes to overgrowth in the infant of a diabetic mother. When insulin is not administered, undergrowth occurs, such as that seen in leprechaunism that is associated with the absence of insulin receptors. Experimental attempts to increase the nutrient supply directly to the fetus do not appear to have clinical usefulness at this time. However, there are preliminary studies that report short-term improvement in fetal oxygenation during periods of maternal hyperoxygenation in SGA infants (Nicolaides et al., 1987). This treatment also improves the aortic blood velocity, which is known to be reduced in SGA infants with fetal hypoxia (Soothill et al., 1987).

■ REFERENCES

Alford, C. A., Schaefer, J., Blankenship, W. J., et al.: A correlative immunologic, microbiologic and clinical approach to the diagnosis of acute and chronic infections in newborn infants. N. Engl. J. Med. 277:437, 1967.

Alford, C. A.: Immunoglobulin determinations in the diagnosis of fetal infection. Pediatr. Clin. North Am. 18:99, 1971.

Amiel-Tison, C.: Neurologic evaluation of the maturity of newborn infants. Arch. Dis. Child. 43:89, 1968.

Babson, S. G.: Growth of low birth weight infants. J. Pediatr. 77:11, 1970.

Bakketeig, L. S., Hoffman, H. J., and Horley, E. E.: The tendency to repeat gestational age and birth weight in successive births. Am. J. Obstet. Gynecol. 135:1086, 1979.

Battaglia, F. C., and Lubchenco, L. O.: A practical classification of newborn infants by weight and gestational age. J. Pediatr. 71:159, 1967.

Brandt, I.: Brain growth, fetal malnutrition and clinical consequence. J. Perinat. Med. 9:3, 1981.

Brar, H. S., and Rutherford, S. E.: Classification of intrauterine growth retardation. Semin. Perinatol. 12:2, 1988.

Bucciarelli, R. L., Nelson, R. M., Egan, E. A., et al.: Transient myocardial insufficiency of the newborn: A form of myocardial dysfunction in stressed neonates. Pediatrics 59:330, 1977.

Calame, A., Ducret, S., Juanin, L., et al.: High risk appropriate for gestational age (AGA) and small for gestational age (SGA) preterm infants. Helv. Paediatr. Acta 38:39, 1983.

Carson, B. S., Losey, R. W., Bowes, W. A., et al.: Combined obstetrics and pediatric approach to prevent meconium aspiration syndrome. Am. J. Obstet. Gynecol. 126:712, 1976.

Chandra, R. K.: Immunocompetence in low-birth-weight infants after intrauterine malnutrition. Lancet 2:1393, 1974.

Churchill, J. A.: The relationship between intelligence and birth weight in twins. Neurology 15:341, 1965.

Clifford, S. G.: Postmaturity—with placental dysfunction; clinical syndrome and pathologic findings. J. Pediatr. 44:1, 1954.

Commey, J. O. O., and Fitzhardinge, P. M.: Handicap in the preterm small-for-gestational age infant. J. Pediatr. 94:779, 1979.

Cornblath, M., Wybregt, S. H., Baens, G. S., et al.: Symptomatic neonatal hypoglycemia. VIII: Studies of carbohydrate metabolism in the newborn infant. Pediatrics 33:388, 1964.

Cruise, M. O.: A longitudinal study of low-birth-weight infants. J. Pediatr. 51:620, 1973.

Dubowitz, L. M. S., Dubowitz, V., and Goldberg, C.: Clinical assessment of gestational age in the newborn infant. J. Pediatr. 77:1, 1970.

Economides, D. C., and Nicolaides, K. H.: Blood glucose and oxygen tension levels in small-for-gestational-age fetuses. Am. J. Obstet. Gynecol. 160:385, 1989.

Farr, V., Mitchell, R. G., Neligan, G. A., et al.: The definition of some external characteristics used in the assessment of gestational age in the newborn infant. Dev. Med. Child. Neurol. 8:507, 1966.

Ferguson, A. C., Lawlor, G. J., Neumann, C. G., et al.: Decreased rosette-forming lymphocytes in malnutrition and intrauterine growth retardation. J. Pediatr. 85:717, 1974.

Finne, P. H.: Erythropoietin levels in cord blood as an indicator of intrauterine hypoxia. Acta Pediatr. Scand. 55:478, 1966.

Fitzhardinge, P. M., and Steven, E. M.: The small-for-date infant. I. Later growth patterns. Pediatrics 49:671, 1972a.

Fitzhardinge, P. M., and Steven, E. M.: The small for date infant. II. Neurologic and intellectual sequelae. Pediatrics 50:50, 1972b.

Fredrickson, W. T., and Brown, J. V.: Gripping and Moro responses: Differences between small-for-gestational age and normal weight term newborns. Early Hum. Dev. 4:69, 1980.

Gierman, C. A., Wu, P. Y. K., and Young, G.: Echocardiographic changes in neonatal polycythemia. J. Calif. Perinat. Assoc. 3:50, 1983.

Ginsberg, H., Goldsmith, J., and Stedman, C.: Intact survival of a 380-gram infant. J. Perinat. 10:330, 1990.

Gregory, G. A.: Resuscitation of the newborn. Anesthesiology 43:225, 1975.

Gross, G. P., Hathaway, W. E., and McGaughey, H. R.: Hyperviscosity in the neonate. J. Pediatr. 82:1004, 1973.

Gross, S. J., Kosmetatos, N., Grines, C. T., et al.: Newborn head size and neurologic status. Am. J. Dis. Child. 132:753, 1978.

Gruenwald, P.: Chronic fetal distress and placental insufficiency. Biol. Newborn 5:215, 1963.

Hack, M., and Fanaroff, A. A.: The outcome of growth failure associated with preterm birth. Clin. Obstet. Gynecol. 27:647, 1984.

Hack, M., Breslau, N., and Fanaroff, A. A.: Differential effects of intrauterine and postnatal brain growth failure in infants of very low birth weight. Am. J. Dis. Child. 143:63, 1989.

Hammerlund, K., and Sedin, G.: Transepidermal water loss in newborn infants. IV: Small for gestational age infants. Acta Paediatr. Scand. 69:377, 1980.

Haymond, M. W., Karl, I. E., and Pagliara, A. S.: Increased gluconeogenic substrates in the small-for-gestational age infant. N. Engl. J. Med. 291:322, 1974.

Heinonen, K., Matilainen, R., Koske, H., et al.: Intrauterine growth retardation (IUGR) in pre-term infants. J. Perinat. Med. 13:171, 1985.

Hill, J. R., and Robinson, D. C.: Oxygen consumption in normally grown, small-for-dates and large-for-dates new-born infants. J. Physiol. 199:685, 1968.

Hill, R. M., Verniaud, W. M., Deter, R. L., et al.: The effect of intrauterine malnutrition on the term infant. A 14-year progressive study. Acta Pediatr. Scand. 73:482, 1984.

Hobbins, J. C., and Berkowitz, R. L.: Ultrasonography in the diagnosis of intrauterine growth retardation. Clin. Obstet. Gynecol. 20:957, 1977.

Hobbins, J. C., Berkowitz, R. L., and Grannum, P. T.: Diagnosis and antepartum management of intrauterine growth retardation. J. Reprod. Med. 21:319, 1978.

Holmes, G. E., Miller, H. C., Hassanein, K., et al.: Postnatal somatic growth in infants with atypical fetal growth patterns. Am. J. Dis. Child. 131:1078, 1977.

Humbert, J. R., Abelson, H., Hathaway, W. E., et al.: Polycythemia in small for gestational age infants. J. Pediatr. 75:812, 1969.

Jones, W. R.: Cord serum immunoglobulin levels in "small for dates" babies. Aust. Pediatr. J. 8:30, 1972.

Kitchen, W., Ford, G., Orgill, A., et al.: Outcome in infants with birth weight 500 to 999 gm: A regional study of 1979 and 1980 births. J. Pediatr. 104:921, 1984.

Koops, B. L., Morgan, L. J., and Battaglia, F. C.: Neonatal mortality risk in relation to birth weight and gestational age. Update. J. Pediatr. 101:969, 1982.

Kumar, S. P., Anday, E. K., Sacks, L. M., et al.: Follow-up studies of very low birth weight infants (1,250 grams or less) born and treated within a perinatal center. Pediatrics 66:438, 1980.

Lechtig, A., Yarborough, C., Delgado, H., et al.: Effect of moderate maternal malnutrition on the placenta. Am. J. Obstet. Gynecol. 123:191, 1975.

Lien, N. M., Meyer, K. K., and Winick, M.: Early malnutrition and late adoption: a study of their effect on the development of Korean orphans adopted into American families. Am. J. Clin. Nutr. *30*:1734, 1977.

Lin, C. C., Lindheimer, M. D., River, P., et al.: Fetal outcome in hypertensive disorders of pregnancy. Am. J. Obstet. Gynecol. *142*:255, 1982.

Low, J. A., Boston, R. W., and Pancham, S. R.: Fetal asphyxia during the intrapartum period in intrauterine growth-retarded infants. Am. J. Obstet. Gynecol. *113*:351, 1972.

Low, J. A., Galbraith, R. S., Muir, D., et al.: Intrauterine growth retardation: A preliminary report of long term morbidity. Am. J. Obstet. Gynecol. *142*:670, 1978.

Low, J. A., Galbraith, R. S., Muri, D., et al.: Intrauterine growth retardation: A study of long-term morbidity. Am. J. Obstet. Gynecol. *142*:670–677, 1982.

Lubchenco, L. O., Hansman, C., Dressler, M., et al.: Intrauterine growth as estimated from liveborn birth-weight data at 24 to 42 weeks of gestation. Pediatrics *32*:793, 1963.

Lubchenco, L. O., Hansman, C., and Boyd, E.: Intrauterine growth in length and head circumference as estimated from live births at gestational ages from 26 to 42 weeks. Pediatrics *37*:403, 1966.

Lubchenco, L. O., and Bard, H.: Incidence of hypoglycemia in newborn infants classified by birth weight and gestational age. Pediatrics *47*:831, 1971.

Lubchenco, L. O., Searls, D. T., and Brazie, J. V.: Neonatal mortality rate: Relationship to birth weight and gestational age. J. Pediatr. *81*:814, 1972.

Matthews, T. G., and O'Herlihy, C.: Significance of raised immunoglobulin M levels in cord blood of small-for-gestational-age infants. Arch. Dis. Child. *53*:895, 1978.

Michaelis, R., Schulte, F. J., and Nolte, R.: Motor behavior of small for gestational age newborn infants. J. Pediatr. *76*:208, 1970.

Miller, H. C., and Hassanein, K.: Diagnosis of impaired fetal growth in newborn infants. Pediatrics *48*:511, 1971.

Miller, H. C., and Jekel, J. F.: Diagnosing intrauterine growth retardation in newborn infants. Perinatol. Neonatol. *9*:35, 1985.

Miller, H. C., and Jekel, J. F.: Malnutrition and growth retardation in newborn infants. Pediatrics *83*:443, 1989.

Mullen, M. K., Coll, C. G., Vohr, B. R., et al.: Mother-infant feeding interaction in full term small-for-gestational age infants. Pediatr. Res. *21*:183, 1987.

Naeye, R. L.: The fetal and neonatal development of twins. Pediatrics *33*:546, 1964.

Naeye, R. L.: Weight gain and the outcome of pregnancy. Am. J. Obstet. Gynecol. *135*:3, 1979.

Nicolaides, K. H., Campbell, S., Bradley, R. J., et al.: Maternal oxygen therapy for intrauterine growth retardation. Lancet *1*:942, 1987.

Ounsted, M., Moar, V., and Scott, W. A.: Perinatal morbidity and mortality in small-for-dates babies: The relative importance of some maternal factors. Early Hum. Dev. *5*:367, 1981.

Ounsted, M., Moar, V., and Scott, W. A.: Small for dates babies at the age of four years: Health, handicap and developmental status. Early Hum. Dev. *8*:243, 1983.

Ounsted, M. K., Moar, V., and Scott, A.: Children of deviant birthweight at the age of seven years: Health, handicap, size and developmental status. Early Hum. Dev. *9*:323, 1984.

Parkinson, C. E., Wallis, S., and Harvey, D.: School achievement and behaviour of children who were small-for-dates at birth. Dev. Med. Child. Neurol. *23*:41, 1981.

Parkinson, C. E., Scrivener, R., Graves, L., et al.: Behavioural differences of school-age children who were small-for-dates babies. Dev. Med. Child. Neurol. *28*:498, 1986.

Parmelee, A. H., Jr., and Schulte, F. J.: Development testing of preterm and small-for-date infants. Pediatrics *45*:21, 1970.

Pena, I. C., Teberg, A. J., and Finello, K. M.: The premature small for gestational age infant during the first year of life: Comparison by birth weight and gestational age. J. Pediatr. *113*:1066, 1988.

Philip, A. G., and Tito, A. M.: Increased nucleated RBC counts in SGA infants with very low birth weight. Am. J. Dis. Child. *143*:164, 1989.

Quigley, M. E., Sheehan, K. L., Wilkes, M. M., et al.: Effects of maternal smoking on circulating catecholamine levels and fetal heart rates. Am. J. Obstet. Gynecol. *133*:685, 1979.

Raju, T. N. K., Winegar, A., Seifert, L., et al.: Birth weight and gestational age standards based on regional perinatal network data: An analysis of risk factors. Am. J. Perinatol. *4*:253, 1987.

Riemenschneider, T. A., Nielsen, H. C., Ruttenberg, H. D., et al.: Disturbances of the transitional circulation: Spectrum of pulmonary hypertension and myocardial dysfunction. J. Pediatr. *89*:622, 1976.

Rolschan, J.: Circumvillate placenta and intrauterine growth retardation. Acta Obstet. Gynaecol. Scand. *72*(Suppl):11, 1978a.

Rolschan, J.: The relationship between some disorders of the umbilical cord and intrauterine growth retardation. Acta Obstet. Gynaecol. Scand. *72*(Suppl):15, 1978b.

Rubin, R. A., Rosenblatt, C., and Balow, B.: Psychological and educational sequelae of prematurity. Pediatrics *52*:353, 1973.

Scott, K. E., and Usher, R.: Fetal malnutrition: Its incidence, causes and effects. Am. J. Obstet. Gynecol. *94*:951, 1966.

Soderling, B.: Pseudoprematurity. Acta Paediatr. *42*:520, 1953.

Soothill, P. W., Nicolaides, K. H., and Campbell, S.: Prenatal asphyxia, hyperlacticaemia, hypoglycaemia and erythroblastosis in growth retarded fetuses. Br. Med. J. *294*:1051, 1987.

Taeusch, H. W., Jr., Carson, S. H., Wang, W. S., et al.: Heroin induction of lung maturation and growth retardation in fetal rabbits. J. Pediatr. *82*:869, 1973.

Teberg, A. J., Walther, F. J., and Pena, I. C.: Mortality, morbidity and outcome for the small-for-gestational age infant. Semin. Perinatol. *12*:84, 1988.

Tejani, N., and Mann, L. I.: Diagnosis and management of the small-for-gestational-age fetus. Clin. Obstet. Gynecol. *20*:943, 1977.

Tsang, R. C., Gigger, M., Oh, W., et al.: Studies in calcium metabolism in infants with intrauterine growth retardation. J. Pediatr. *86*:939, 1975.

Tze, W. J., and Lee, M.: Adverse effects of maternal alcohol consumption on pregnancy and fetal growth in rats. Nature *257*:479, 1975.

Usher, R., McLean, R., and Scott, K. E.: Judgment of fetal age. II: Clinical significance of gestational age and an objective method for its assessment. Pediatr. Clin. North Am. *13*:835, 1966.

Usher, R. H.: Clinical and therapeutic aspects of fetal malnutrition. Pediatr. Clin. North Am. *17*:169, 1970.

Villar, J., and Belizan, J. M.: Relative contributions of prematurity and fetal growth retardation to low birth weight in developing and developed societies. Am. J. Obstet. Gynecol. *143*:793, 1982.

Vohr, B. R., Oh, W., Rosenfeld, A. G., et al.: The preterm SGA infant: A two year followup study. Am. J. Obstet. Gynecol. *133*:425, 1979.

Vohr, B. R., and Oh, W.: Growth and development in preterm infants and small for gestational age. J. Pediatr. *103*:941, 1983.

Walther, F. J.: Growth and development of term SGA disproportionate infants at the age of 7 years. Early Human Dev. *18*:1–11, 1988.

Warshaw, J. B.: Intrauterine growth retardation. Pediatr. Rev. *8*:107, 1986.

Westwood, M., Kramer, M. S., Munz, D., et al.: Growth and development of full term nonasphyxiated small for gestational age newborns: followup through adolescence. Pediatrics *71*:376, 1983.

Wigglesworth, J. S.: Fetal growth retardation. Br. Med. Bull. *22*:13, 1966.

Winick, M., Brasel, J. A., and Velasco, E. G.: Effects of prenatal nutrition upon pregnancy risk. Clin. Obstet. Gynecol. *16*:184, 1973.

Wirth, F. H., Goldberg, K. E., and Lubchenco, L. O.: Neonatal hyperviscosity: Incidence and effect of partial plasma exchange transfusion. Pediatr. Res. *9*:372, 1975.

Yang, S.-L.: Altered immunologic development. *In* Lin, C. C., and Evans, M. I.: Intrauterine Growth Retardation. New York, McGraw-Hill Book Company, 1984.

MATERNAL SUBSTANCE ABUSE **26**

Xylina Bean

A dramatic increase has occurred during the past decade in the United States in the number of women of childbearing age who use legal and illegal substances that have adverse effects on pregnancy. Obstetric and neonatal problems associated with drug use during pregnancy were first described in significant numbers in the mid-1950s in the context of opiate abuse (Cobrinik et al., 1959). Since then, a variety of non-narcotic psychotropic substances have been shown to cause similar adverse perinatal effects (Jones et al., 1989). Psychotropic substances both legal (such as alcohol, cigarettes, and prescription drugs) and illegal (including heroin, amphetamine, cocaine, and phencyclidine) can cause obstetric complications and fetal injury and can have short- and long-term consequences for the newborn infant.

■ INCIDENCE

The number of women who abuse alcohol and drugs is unknown. In New York City the proportion of women in the known addicted population rose from 14 per cent in 1968 to 25 per cent in 1973, and it is now estimated that women represent 30 to 40 per cent of the total (Kaestner et al., 1986). Data from the Drug Abuse Program Office of Los Angeles County indicate that 43 per cent of the clients in drug treatment and 30 per cent of the clients in alcohol treatment are women. Nationally, women make up approximately 30 per cent of the drug treatment admissions and 25 per cent of alcohol treatment admissions. Women, however, are underrepresented in treatment because many treatment programs will not admit pregnant women.

National Institute of Drug Abuse Surveys conducted in 1982 estimated that 90,000 women from 19 to 25 years of age used heroin, and 970,000 women in this same age group used cocaine or other stimulants, an increase of 250 per cent from 1979 (NIDA, 1979, 1982). The present epidemic of drug abuse is attributable primarily to the marked increase in the use of cocaine (NIDA, 1986; Kozel and Adams, 1986). In 1982, 4.2 million women over age 12 years had used cocaine during the past year, and 1.4 million had used cocaine in the month prior to the survey. A recent survey conducted by the National Association for Perinatal Addiction Research and Education of 36 urban, suburban and rural hospitals found a consistent 11 per cent incidence of documented illicit drug use during pregnancy (Chasnoff, 1989). With the emergence of cocaine as a primary drug, perinatal substance abuse, previously thought to be a problem in a small number of women from urban ghettos, is recognized as a national problem involving women from all racial and socioeconomic groups.

■ DRUGS USED DURING PREGNANCY

COCAINE AND AMPHETAMINES

Cocaine and amphetamines are psychomotor stimulants with a long history of abuse. The neuropharmacology of these drugs is similar, and their clinical effects are indistinguishable. Cocaine, a member of the trophane family of alkaloids, is obtained from the *Erythroxylon* coca plant, which is indigenous to the mountain slopes of Central and South America. The coca leaf has been chewed for centuries by the natives of these areas to decrease fatigue and hunger and was introduced to Europe in the sixteenth century. The active ingredient, cocaine, was isolated by Albert Newman in 1860. Cocaine's ability to produce euphoria was exploited extensively in the United States in the late nineteenth and early twentieth centuries, when cocaine became an active ingredient in a number of elixirs and tonics. These over-the-counter preparations were widely utilized, and cocaine abuse became a major medical problem. The Harrison Act of 1914 regulated the distribution of narcotics and cocaine, which at that time was erroneously classified as a narcotic. In 1970, the older federal drug laws were replaced by the Comprehensive Drug Abuse Prevention and Control Act, and cocaine was classified with the opiates, barbiturates, and amphetamines as a Schedule II drug, i.e., one of "high abuse potential with restricted medical use." Cocaine use markedly decreased and, until recently, held the status of an exotic drug used primarily by those in sports and entertainment to enhance performance. The limitation on its importation made cocaine a relatively expensive drug, available primarily to the affluent. Its reputation as a "glamor" drug, the widely held misconception that cocaine is nonaddictive, and the development and marketing of "crack," a cheap version of cocaine, are the major factors in the resurgence of drug use (Adams and Durell, 1984; Adams and Kozel, 1985; Abelson and Miller, 1985).

Cocaine and other stimulants are now the drugs of choice for women (Washton, 1986), with an estimated 13 per cent of women in the United States between the ages of 18 and 25 years using cocaine regularly (Clayton, 1985; Tarr and Macklen, 1987). Women's use of cocaine cannot be disassociated from their sexuality and their relationship with men. The primary suppliers of cocaine to most women are their sexual partners, and sex is generally part of the price. This combination of women, sex, and drugs has resulted in a marked increase nationwide in the birth of infants exposed to cocaine in utero. A survey of 18 metropolitan hospitals conducted by the United States House Select Committee on Children, Youth and Families found three- to fourfold increases in deliveries of cocaine-exposed infants between 1985 and 1989 (Miller, 1989).

The pharmacologic action of cocaine relates to its ability to block reuptake of neurotransmitters by sympathetic nerve terminals, thereby allowing higher concentrations of neurotransmitters to interact with receptors (Ritchie and Green, 1985; Cregler and Mark, 1986). Cocaine interacts with three sets of neurotransmitters: norepinephrine, dopamine, and serotonin (Dackis and Gold, 1985; Jones, 1985). Cocaine, as the hydrochloride, is prepared by dissolving the alkaloid in hydrochloric acid to form a water-soluble salt. This results in a white powder that is used orally, intranasally (snorting), or intravenously (running). Intranasal use is favored typically by the white, affluent user. Intravenous users are more likely to have a past history of heroin abuse and often use the drug in combination with heroin (speedballing). Cocaine hydrochloride decomposes on heating and must be converted to the "freebase" for inhalation. "Freebasing" involves extraction of cocaine from aqueous solution into an organic solvent such as ether. "Crack," the most widely available form of freebase, is made by direct precipitation of the freebase with ammonia and baking soda to alkalinize the solution (Perez-Reyes et al., 1982; Siegel, 1985). Crack is almost pure cocaine, and when it is smoked, it readily enters the bloodstream to produce an effect similar to that occurring with intravenous use. Crack is popular in urban minority communities, where it may be smoked in combination with phencyclidine ("spacebasing"). Crack smoking appears to be particularly reinforcing and is associated with compulsive use, binges, and acceleration of the addictive process (Gawin and Ellinwood, 1988).

Amphetamines potentiate the action of norepinephrine, dopamine, and serotonin and are sympathomimetics similar to cocaine. Amphetamine (methylphenethylamine) was synthesized in 1887 and introduced into the United States in 1931 and the d,l-isomer marketed as Benzedrine. A number of other isomers soon followed, including dextroamphetamine (Dexedrine) and the n-methylated form, methamphetamine. Clinically the amphetamine isomers have the same effect and can be distinguished only in the laboratory (Jaffee, 1985). Amphetamines were initially marketed for the treatment of obesity and narcolepsy and continue to be used for treatment of attention-deficit disorders in children. Amphetamines are classified as Schedule II drugs, similar to cocaine and the narcotics. Amphetamines may have some ability to block reuptake of released neurotransmitters. However, in contrast to cocaine, they appear to exert their central nervous system effects primarily by enhancing the release of neurotransmitters from presynaptic neurons. They may also exert a direct stimulatory action on postsynaptic catecholamine receptors. Amphetamines are taken orally, inhaled, or injected. The clinical effects and toxicity of amphetamines are indistinguishable from those of cocaine. The primary difference is in the duration of action. The psychotropic effects of cocaine are of short duration, 5 to 45 minutes. The effects of amphetamines may last from 2 to 12 hours

(Gunne and Anggard, 1973; Robbins, 1979). Methamphetamine ("crystal") has been the primary form abused (Kramer et al., 1967; Smith, 1969). Amphetamines have always been popular among adolescents, especially adolescent females (MacDonald, 1987). The drug's popularity has been increasing owing to the appearance of a new smokable form of methamphetamine, "ice." Ice is currently the major drug abused in some parts of the United States, especially Hawaii and San Diego (Largent, 1989). "Crystal" and "ice" both can be produced locally and fairly cheaply. With increased restrictions on the importation of cocaine, a resurgence in amphetamine use can be expected. The popularity of amphetamines among women of child-bearing age places this group at very high risk for perinatal abuse (Dixon, 1989).

CLINICAL EFFECTS

Amphetamine and cocaine use results in a sense of well-being, increased energy, increased sexual achievement, and an intense euphoria or "high." The sympathomimetic action also has potentially devastating physiologic effects on the cardiovascular system. Cocaine has been associated with cerebral hemorrhage, cardiac arrest, cardiac arrhythmias, myocardial infarction, intestinal ischemia, and seizures (Gold et al., 1985a; Cregler and Mark, 1986; Mofenson and Caraccio, 1987; Gawin and Ellinwood, 1988; Farrar and Kearns, 1989). Chronic use is associated with anorexia, nutritional problems, and paranoid psychosis. Chronic use ultimately results in neurotransmitter depletion and a "crash" characterized by lethargy, depression, anxiety, severe insomnia, hyperphagia, and cocaine craving (Smith, 1986; Grabowski, 1984; Kleber and Gawin, 1987; Washton, 1989).

Women who use cocaine during pregnancy are at high risk for stillbirths (Critchley et al., 1988), spontaneous abortions (Chasnoff et al., 1985; Zuckerman et al., 1989; Burkett et al., 1990), abruptio placentae (Acker et al., 1983; Chasnoff et al., 1985; Chasnoff, Burns, and Burns, 1987), intrauterine growth deficiency (Oro and Dixon, 1987; MacGregor et al., 1987; Chouteau et al., 1988), anemia and malnutrition (Frank et al., 1988), and maternal death from intracerebral hemorrhage (Mercado et al., 1989). Other problems include evidence of fetal distress associated with abnormal fetal heart rate tracing and meconium staining. Increased risk of meconium aspiration syndrome, however, has not been described. These women are at high risk for premature labor, premature rupture of the membranes, and infections. The sex-for-drug connection has resulted in a high incidence of sexually transmitted diseases, especially syphilis (Burkett et al., 1990).

Infants born to these women may have problems of prematurity, low birth weight, and congenital infections, especially bacterial sepsis and congenital syphilis. These infants undergo drug withdrawal (Madden et al., 1986; Chasnoff et al., 1985; Ryan et al., 1987; Fulroth et al., 1989; Hadeed and Seigel, 1989), have abnormal EEGs and visual dysfunction (Doberczak et al., 1989; Oro and Dixon, 1987), and are at risk for seizures. Isolated cases of cerebral infarcts associated with high-dose use (Chasnoff et al., 1986) and of necrotizing enterocolitis (Telsy et al., 1988) have been reported. The incidence of sudden infant death syndrome (SIDS) appears to be greater in these infants (Chasnoff, 1987a; Chasnoff et al., 1985), and abnormal respiratory patterns are present (Ward, 1987). We do not find that the risk of respiratory distress syndrome (RDS) is affected specifically by cocaine use. Because the major risk of cocaine use during the third trimester is premature delivery, the frequency of RDS is greater in infants whose mothers use cocaine. There may be an increased risk for genitourinary anomalies (Chasnoff, 1988; Chavez, 1989). Long-term behavioral and learning problems are also being reported in these children (Howard et al., 1988; Chasnoff, 1989). The developmental problems in these children may be a combination of the direct teratogenic effect of cocaine on the developing brain and the equally "teratogenic" effect of drugs in the environment of the developing infant.

Many of the adverse perinatal outcomes with cocaine abuse are thought to be related to the effects of cocaine on uterine blood supply. An increase in maternal mean arterial blood pressure, a decrease in uterine blood flow, and a transient rise in fetal systemic blood pressure after an intravenous cocaine infusion have been found in fetal sheep (Moore et al., 1986). Additional animal studies demonstrated a significant fetal hypoxemia associated with changes in uterine blood flow with cocaine infusion (Woods et al., 1987). Maternal hypertension and intermittent fetal hypoxia contribute to the increased risk for abruptio placentae, intrauterine growth retardation, and congenital anomalies seen in cocaine-exposed infants.

Of all the problems attributed to cocaine use in the pregnant woman, the most common problem is that of premature delivery. Cocaine directly stimulates uterine contractions, with resulting increased risk for fetal distress and premature deliveries. Prematurity and intrauterine growth retardation (IUGR) also appear to be closely related to maternal life-style. In those populations studied in which the mother receives good prenatal care associated with drug treatment, the incidence of prematurity and IUGR is low (Chasnoff et al., 1985; Frank et al., 1988). However, in the presence of poor prenatal care and no documented drug treatment, the rates of premature birth and IUGR are high (Oro and Dixon, 1987; Chouteau et al., 1988, Cherukuri et al., 1988; Burkett et al., 1990). These findings have obvious implications for the development of effective treatment strategies to minimize adverse perinatal outcome in substance-abusing women.

The medical and obstetric complications of amphetamines are similar to those described for cocaine. Amphetamine toxicity has been described as more intense and prolonged than that seen with cocaine. Visual, auditory, and tactile hallucinations are common (Robbins, 1979; Schmidt, 1987), and microvascular damage has been seen in the brains of chronic users (Rothrock et al., 1988). Amphetamine withdrawal is characterized by prolonged periods of hypersomnia, depression, and intense, often violent, paranoid psychosis (Kramer et al., 1967; Smith et al., 1979). The pregnancies of amphetamine users are characterized by poor prenatal care, sexually transmitted diseases, and cardiovascular problems including abruptio placentae and postpartum hemorrhage (Eriksson et al., 1978, Larsson and Zetterstrom, 1979; Little et al., 1988). Neonatal problems include prematurity, IUGR, and both short- and long-term neurologic abnormalities (Oro and

Dixon, 1987; Dixon, 1989). Cardiovascular malformations have been described (Nora et al., 1970; Fein et al., 1987), but other studies have failed to show an increased risk (Briggs et al., 1975; Martin, 1977). Children of amphetamine abusers appear to be at high risk for social problems, including abandonment, abuse, and neglect (Eriksson et al., 1985; Eriksson et al., 1986). These children are described as exhibiting disturbed behavior, including hyperactivity, aggressiveness, and sleep disturbances. The children with the most severe problems were born to mothers who abused amphetamines throughout pregnancy and those being reared in homes with an addicted parent (Sussman, 1983; Billings et al., 1985).

NARCOTICS

Opium is obtained from the poppy *Papaver somniferum* indigenous to the Middle East and Southeast Asia. Opium derivatives have been used as analgesics for centuries and remain the most effective analgesics available. Morphine, first isolated from opium in 1803, is the major alkaloid of opium. Other derivatives include meperidine (Demerol), heroin, methadone, and codeine. The exact mechanism by which opiates produce their effects is unknown, but in the past decade specific opiate receptors have been identified in the brain. These receptors are associated with the naturally occurring opiate-like substances, the endorphins and enkephalins (Platt, 1986; Snyder, 1984). Morphine's potential for abuse and addiction was documented in the mid-1800s, shortly after it began to be used extensively. Opium along with cocaine was a common additive to popular patent medicines, and perinatal problems associated with opium were reported in the late 1800s; these involved women who became addicted as a result of abuse of these preparations. In 1914, the Harrison Act resulted in a marked decrease in the availability of opiate-containing medications (Deneau and Mule, 1981). Morphine addiction today is limited primarily to health care workers. However, since the 1950s, heroin, which had been synthesized in 1938, has become endemic in most major American cities.

Of the drugs known to be abused during pregnancy, heroin has been the most extensively studied. Heroin has been documented to have potentially devastating effects on the outcome of pregnancy. The majority of heroin-addicted pregnant women have poor general health with multiple medical problems associated with their drug abuse and addicted life-styles. Heroin can be ingested by smoking or by the intranasal or intravenous routes. Intranasal use is common among women, especially in the western United States, whereas the intravenous route is more popular among users on the eastern seaboard. Intravenous use places the addict at risk for multiple infectious complications including cellulitis, thrombophlebitis, hepatitis, AIDS, and endocarditis. Heroin addicts neglect general health and enter pregnancy with numerous major pre-existing problems including pyorrhea and untreated infections, especially sexually transmitted diseases such as gonorrhea, syphilis, herpes, and AIDS. The adverse effects of heroin abuse on pregnancy, the fetus, and newborn have been repeatedly described in the literature over the last 30 years (Cobrinik et al., 1959; Strauss et al., 1974; Connaughton et al., 1977; Ostrea and Chavez,

1979; Wapner et al., 1982). Obstetric complications include frequent abortions, abruptio placentae, chorioamnionitis, increased risk for cesarean section associated with breech presentatation, and fetal distress. Fetal distress with meconium passage, perinatal asphyxia, and low Apgar scores is common (Pinkert, 1985). More than 50 per cent of heroin-dependent women have no prenatal care. These mothers are more likely to deliver premature and intrauterine growth–retarded infants. The increased risk for prematurity and low birth weight is thought to be multifactorial. Heroin-addicted mothers are often malnourished. Heroin is an appetite suppressant and appears to interfere directly with the absorption of nutrients (Raye et al., 1980). Iron and folic acid deficiency anemia is common. The increased incidence of infection further contributes to IUGR and prematurity. Finally, because the drug supply for these mothers is often uncertain, the addict is subject to episodes of withdrawal and overdose, thereby subjecting the fetus to intermittent episodes of hypoxia in utero, hindering growth and increasing the risk for spontaneous abortion, stillbirth, and prematurity. Infants born to these mothers are, therefore, more likely to be of low birth weight, premature, and suffer from infection and perinatal asphyxia. The incidence of RDS is reportedly decreased in heroin, but not methadone, chronically exposed infants. This decrease may represent a direct effect of heroin on lung maturation but is more likely related to stress-induced accelerated lung maturation (Taeusch et al., 1973). The classic neonatal withdrawal or abstinence syndrome was first described in these infants, and long-term developmental and learning problems are common. The mortality rate in these infants is 3 to 4 per cent (Wapner and Finnegan, 1982). Mortality is rarely associated with withdrawal alone but occurs as a consequence of prematurity, infection, and severe perinatal asphyxia. Death in the postneonatal period is primarily related to SIDS, which has been documented to be several times greater in this population, child abuse, and neglect.

Because of the association between fetal withdrawal, perinatal asphyxia, and spontaneous abortions, detoxification of pregnant heroin abusers is rarely attempted, and most women are treated via methadone maintenance until termination of pregnancy (Newman et al., 1975). Women who receive methadone as part of a maintenance program that includes comprehensive prenatal care deliver infants of higher birth weight and gestational age. This favorable outcome is probably related to a stable intrauterine environment uncomplicated by periods of intoxication and withdrawal. Perhaps more important, provision of comprehensive prenatal care results in improvement in the general health and nutritional status of the mother (Rosner et al., 1982; Cooper et al., 1983; Suffet and Brotman, 1984). Methadone-dependent mothers who have inadequate prenatal care have many of the same problems seen in heroin-addicted mothers (Lee et al., 1985). Women in methadone maintenance programs usually do not continue after delivery, and the success of detoxification in this population is very low. Infants born to methadone-dependent women are generally larger at birth than those born to heroin-dependent women, but all growth measures, including head circumference, tend to be below those seen in infants born to socioeconomically comparable drug-free women. Infants who are chronically exposed to methadone have a greater incidence of neonatal drug withdrawal and exhibit more severe symptoms, often requiring pharmacologic treatment (Finnegan, 1982). Long-term follow-up studies of narcotic-exposed infants show significant developmental and learning deficits in both methadone- and heroin-exposed children (Wilson et al., 1973, 1979). The effects of methadone on the fetus appear to be related to the dose of the drug and the incidence of associated non-narcotic drug abuse (Reddy et al., 1971; Statzer and Wardell, 1972). Most drug abusers use multiple drugs including cigarettes, alcohol, Valium, cocaine, phencyclidine, and amphetamines (Blinick et al., 1976; Chasnoff et al., 1982; Lifschitz et al., 1985). Detoxification is safest between 14 and 28 weeks and should be done over several weeks with close toxicologic monitoring of other drug usage, "chipping," and obstetrical monitoring of fetal well-being (Mondanero, 1987).

Although the number of women addicted to stimulants now far exceeds the number of narcotic addicts, narcotic addiction continues to be an endemic problem in most major cities. The adverse effects on the fetus underscore the importance of appropriate identification and intervention. The advent of AIDS adds to the health risks faced by this population.

PHENCYCLIDINE (PCP)

Phencyclidine hydrochloride is an arylcyclohexamine developed in 1958 and marketed for the first time in 1963 as an anesthetic under the name Sernyl. The drug was withdrawn in 1968 after reports of delirium and hallucinations. It was remarketed in the early 1970s for veterinary use under the name Sernylan but again withdrawn after its abuse potential became evident. Phencyclidine is no longer manufactured legally and is included in the Comprehensive Drug Abuse Prevention and Control Act of 1970. The first reports of the illicit use of phencyclidine occurred in 1967 from the Haight-Ashbury district of San Francisco; however, epidemic use of PCP did not begin until the mid-1970s. By the early 1980s, PCP was described as the most frequently used hallucinogen by young adults in the United States (Jain et al., 1977; Cohen, 1977; Peterson and Stillman, 1978; Husson, 1984; Silber et al., 1988).

Phencyclidine, also known as angel dust, is a white crystalline powder soluble in water and alcohol. It can be snorted, taken orally, or injected intravenously. However, its popularity among young adults, especially women, is related to its ability to be smoked. PCP is usually smoked sprinkled (dusted) on cigarettes (lovely) or marijuana (sherm). The pharmacology of PCP is complex, and its exact mechanism of action is unknown. Phencyclidine receptors have been identified in the brain, but how they interact with PCP is unclear (Contreras et al., 1985). The effect of the drug is dose-related; low doses primarily cause euphoria associated with disturbances in body image. Moderate doses result in confusion, disorientation, and impaired sensory perception. High doses are followed by hypertension, seizures, hyperpyrexia, paranoid psychosis, coma, and death. Chronic use results in recurrent schizophrenia-like reactions, depressive anxiety, and an organic brain syndrome (Strasman, 1984).

There are limited data on the effects of phencyclidine on pregnancy and the newborn. Phencyclidine readily crosses the placenta and has been documented in both the fetus and the newborn as well as in breast milk (Kaufman et al., 1983; Golden et al., 1984). From 1981 to 1984 phencyclidine was the primary drug of abuse among women delivering at King/Drew Medical Center, located in the major area of PCP trafficking in Los Angeles during the early 1980s (Husson, 1984). Between 1981 and 1984, 165 infants were identified with a positive history and/or toxicology for PCP. Ninety-seven of these infants were born in 1984. The peak incidence of PCP deliveries correlated with the appearance in the community of cocaine, which by 1985 had completely replaced PCP as the drug of choice for substance-abusing women.

The effects of phencyclidine on the outcome of pregnancy are related to the amount that the mother uses. Most women smoked the drug in low doses, which has few side effects. The drug was cheap, and maintaining the habit required less money, so that the general health of the mother was better and she sought prenatal care at least in the initial phase of her addiction. Because of the anesthetic nature of the drug, precipitous deliveries at home, in ambulances, and in emergency rooms were more common. There was no increased incidence of other obstetric complications. Prematurity was not increased with PCP use but 40 per cent of the infants were small for gestational age. A severe neonatal abstinence syndrome was observed, with onset shortly after birth (Strauss, 1981). The neurologic findings in these infants were striking for the severity of the hypertonicity and hyperreflexia, often associated with spontaneous clonus and persisting for several weeks. The severity of the symptoms, often present at birth, raises the question of whether the neurologic findings represent drug withdrawal or drug effect, since PCP has been documented to persist in the body, and especially in fetal brains, for prolonged periods (Ahmad et al., 1987). Gastrointestinal symptoms, including abdominal distention, vomiting, and diarrhea, were also present in about 20 per cent of the infants. Phencyclidine continues to be identified in drug abusers in our institution but is now present in only 12 per cent of positive toxicology screens and is most often seen in combination with cocaine. The withdrawal syndrome seen in this new population of phencyclidine-exposed infants appears to be less intense, most likely related to a lower dose exposure, and the PCP now available on the streets of Los Angeles is less concentrated. Many of the positive toxicology serums are in women who consider cocaine their primary drug of abuse and use phencyclidine only inadvertently, since most drugs available on the street are adulterated or "cut." Phencyclidine withdrawal can be associated with significant neonatal morbidity due to the high incidence of associated gastrointestinal symptoms and the prolonged duration of symptoms. The mean duration of hospitalization in our population was 14 days (range, 10 to 21 days). We found no increased risk of congenital anomalies, in contrast to the report of Golden and co-workers (1987). Long-term outcome studies of chronically PCP exposed infants have shown them to be at high risk for severe developmental and behavioral problems (Howard et al., 1988; Chasnoff et al., 1983a).

ALCOHOL

First described in Europe by Lemoine in 1968 and subsequently recorded in a number of studies in the United States, the fetal alcohol syndrome (FAS) is an extensively documented teratogenic syndrome (Ulleland, 1972; Jones et al., 1973; Jones and Smith, 1978). FAS occurs in 1 to 2 in 1000 live births, making it the third major cause of mental retardation and the only cause that is known to be potentially preventable. The high incidence of FAS has led the government to add a warning label on beer, wine, hard liquor, and wine cooler containers effective as of November 1989:

GOVERNMENT WARNING: According to the Surgeon General, women should not drink alcoholic beverages during pregnancy because of the risk of birth defects. . . .

FAS consists of pre- and postnatal growth deficiency, microcephaly, and mental retardation associated with characteristic facies. The microcephaly is a reflection of the damage to brain tissues that results from alcohol exposure. The typical facial features consist of short palpebral fissures, flat nasal bridge, micrognathia, hypoplastic maxilla, and thin upper lip (Abel et al., 1983). Abnormal hand creases and cardiac anomalies have also been described. The subsequent degree of mental retardation correlates with the degree of physical stigmata (Smith, 1979; Streissguth et al., 1984). The postnatal growth deficiency is prominent in infancy, and persists into early childhood, and often is associated with unexplained vomiting. Speech and language problems are common in older children. Behavioral problems, including severe hyperactivity and attention-deficit disorders, contribute to the learning disabilities characteristically seen in these children (Iosub et al., 1981). FAS is estimated to occur in 30 to 40 percent of pregnant women who consume 3 ounces of absolute alcohol per day. These women also have a greater risk for abruptio placentae, spontaneous abortions, and stillbirths. Lesser degrees of alcohol consumption have been associated with IUGR, behavioral and neurologic abnormalities, and increased risk of congenital anomalies of the extremities and genitourinary tract (Streissguth et al., 1980; Mills and Graibard, 1987; Davis et al., 1982). A neonatal withdrawal syndrome with jitteriness and poor feeding has been reported in infants born to mothers who were intoxicated at the time of delivery (Pierog et al., 1970).

The adverse effects of alcohol on the fetus are related to the gestational stage at which exposure occurs, the amount of liquor the mother consumes, the presence of binge drinking, and the individual susceptibility of the fetus. There is no documented "safe" level of alcohol ingestion, and women should be advised to abstain from alcohol during pregnancy. The term "alcohol-related birth defects" (ARBD) is now used to reflect the range of anomalies associated with alcohol consumption in pregnancy.

CIGARETTES AND MARIJUANA

Cigarettes are the drug most often used during pregnancy; an estimated 25 percent of pregnant women smoke cigarettes. Cigarette smoking has been associated with an increased risk of spontaneous abortion, stillbirth, prematurity, and SIDS (Abel, 1984). The effect of cigarettes on fetal growth has been studied extensively. The degree of IUGR is related to the number of cigarettes smoked. One pack (20 cigarettes) per day correlates with a 280-g weight loss in a term newborn (Naeye, 1981; Stern and Susser, 1984). The exact mechanism of the adverse effect on pregnancy is unknown. Cigarettes contain a number of potentially toxic compounds. Most theories involve the induction of fetal hypoxia either from carbon monoxide production or from nicotine-induced vasospasm; however, a direct cytotoxic effect has not been ruled out.

Marijuana is the illegal drug that is probably most frequently used during pregnancy. Marijuana is derived from the hemp plant *Cannabis sativa,* with the most active ingredient being delta-9-tetrahydrocannabinol (delta-9-THC). Marijuana causes IUGR (Fried, 1982; Abel, 1980). Neurologic abnormalities similar to a mild withdrawal syndrome with hypertonicity, irritability, and jitteriness have been seen in the newborn (Fried et al., 1987) but without documented evidence of long-term sequelae (Fried and Watkinson, 1988). Marijuana is often used in combination with other drugs and potentiates the risk for prematurity and low birth weight (Abel, 1985; Tennes et al., 1985). FAS may be more common among women who abuse alcohol and marijuana (Hingston et al., 1982).

Polydrug abuse is the norm among substance-abusing women. These women routinely use cigarettes, alcohol, and their "primary" drug simultaneously, further increasing the risk of adverse pregnancy outcomes and fetal injury.

■ SPECIAL NEONATAL CONCERNS

NEONATAL ABSTINENCE SYNDROME

The neonatal abstinence or withdrawal syndrome is a combination of physiologic signs and symptoms seen in newborns who are withdrawn from an addictive drug at birth after repeated exposure in utero. The neonatal withdrawal syndrome has been studied most intensively in the context of opiate dependence. Withdrawal syndromes have been described for heroin, methadone, codeine, and meperidine (Desmond and Wilson, 1975; Newman et al., 1975; Kron et al., 1975; Mangurten and Benwara, 1980). As an increasing number of psychotropic drugs become available, withdrawal syndromes have been described for a variety of non-narcotic drugs, including alcohol, barbiturates, chlordiazepoxide (Librium), diazepam (Valium), ethchlorvynol (Placidyl), glutethimide (Doriden), and pentazocine (Talwin) (Kein et al., 1975; Webster, 1973; Goetz and Bain, 1974; Rumack and Walravens, 1973; Rementeria, 1977; Athinarazanan et al., 1976; Chasnoff et al., 1983b) as well as for amphetamines, cocaine, and phencyclidine (Tables 26–1 and 26–2).

The neonatal withdrawal syndrome is a multisystem disease. However, the most consistent symptoms described are neurologic: jitteriness, restlessness, tremulousness, and, on occasion, even seizures. Irritability, hypertonicity, and other manifestations of brain hyperactivity are also present. Gastrointestinal symptoms such as vomiting and diarrhea may lead to dehydration and failure to gain weight normally. In the immediate newborn period,

TABLE 26–1. Neonatal Abstinence Syndrome

DRUG	ONSET	PEAK	DURATION	SEVERITY
Alcohol	0–1 days	3–5 days	5–7 days	Mild
Heroin	0–3 days	3–7 days	2–4 weeks	Mild-moderate
Methadone	0–5 days	7–10 days	2–4 months	Mild-severe
Phencyclidine	0–2 days	5–7 days	2–6 months	Moderate-severe
Cocaine	0–3 days	3–5 days	2–8 weeks	Mild-moderate
Amphetamine	0–3 days	3–5 days	2–8 weeks	Mild-moderate

poor feeding is associated with poorly coordinated sucking and swallowing. After the acute stages, cocaine- and amphetamine-exposed infants are often described as having excessive appetites. Both cocaine and amphetamine have central appetite–suppressive effects, and this may reflect a "rebound" phenomenon. Because of the persistent increased hyperactivity in these infants the overeating is rarely associated with obesity. Other findings during the acute withdrawal phase may include high-pitched cry, sleep disturbances, fist sucking, excessive sweating, flushing, intermittent fever, tachypnea, and even respiratory distress. Clinically, neonatal withdrawal syndromes appear similar despite the diversity of the causative agents.

Heroin, cocaine, and amphetamine withdrawal usually occurs within the first 48 hours of birth in most infants, depending on the timing and amount of the mother's last dose. Gastrointestinal symptoms of vomiting and diarrhea are rarely seen in cocaine- and amphetamine-exposed infants. Cocaine-exposed infants may have staring episodes. Drowsiness may be very severe in amphetamine-exposed infants (Dixon, 1989). The acute phase lasts for about 2 weeks in most of these infants, though some mild symptoms persist for up to 4 weeks. Methadone withdrawal is often more severe and persistent than heroin withdrawal, although there does appear to be a dose relationship (Cooper et al., 1983). Mothers maintained on low-dose methadone (less than 40 mg daily) have infants with milder symptoms. Late presentation between 2 and 4 weeks of methadone withdrawal was described in the early reports (Kandall and Garner, 1972) but has not been reported subsequently. This phenomenon may have been related to the high doses of methadone commonly used at that time. Seizures are a rare complication in all withdrawal syndromes and are more often reported in association with methadone and barbiturates. Phencycli-

TABLE 26–2. Neonatal Abstinence Syndrome: Common Signs and Symptoms

NEUROLOGIC	RESPIRATORY
Restlessness	Depressed respirations
Tremors	Respiratory distress
Sleep disturbances	Rapid respirations
Convulsions	
Irritability	**AUTONOMIC**
Hypertonicity	High-pitched cry
Hyperactivity	Sneezing
Clonus	Fist-sucking
Staring episodes (cocaine)	Excessive yawning
Nystagmus (PCP)	Sweating
	Flushing of skin
GASTROINTESTINAL	Fever
Poor feeding	Nasal discharge
Vomiting	Skin abrasions
Diarrhea	
Abdominal distention	
Increased sucking	

dine withdrawal is often present at birth and is characterized by severe jitteriness and hypertonicity. The duration of withdrawal with PCP is similar to that for methadone and often persists for several weeks. Infants are rarely symptom-free at discharge; once discharged from the structured and stable nursery environment, they generally become more symptomatic. The most common prolonged symptoms are jitteriness, hypertonicity, hyperphagia, and sleep disturbances.

TREATMENT

Infants exposed to drugs prenatally may be born either under the influence of the drug or in withdrawal, depending on the timing of the mother's last dose. Respiratory depression is the primary symptom seen in infants born under the influence. If narcotics are suspected as the cause of respiratory depression, naloxone (Narcan) should be administered (AAP, 1989a). This agent is useful only in suspected opiate overdose and is not indicated for non-narcotic exposure. Narcan administration will immediately precipitate drug withdrawal. Early recognition of severely affected infants prevents progression of the withdrawal syndrome. Treatment of neonatal drug withdrawal is symptom oriented but usually does require hospitalization for a minimum of 5 to 14 days. Treatment in the nursery consists of providing a supportive environment, gentle handling, frequent feedings, and swaddling to control jitteriness. The majority of infants can be managed with supportive care only.

Severe symptoms, persistent diarrhea, vomiting, and failure to gain weight are indications for pharmacologic intervention. A number of medications, including paregoric, chlorpromazine (Thorazine), diazepam (Valium), and phenobarbital, have been used. In 1983, the American Academy of Pediatrics Committee on Drugs recommended phenobarbital as the drug of choice. Phenobarbital is administered in a dose of 5 to 10 mg/kg/day in two divided dosages, initially IM and then orally after good control has been achieved. Symptoms are usually under control within 24 to 48 hours. The therapeutic goal is to minimize the adverse effects of withdrawal, and clinical assessment of effectiveness is the best tool for monitoring. Serum levels done at 48 hours may be useful in avoiding toxicity. Once symptomatic control is achieved the drug should be continued until good weight gain is established, then slowly weaned. Weaning usually requires at least 1 week. An infant should remain in the hospital for at least 48 hours after discontinuation of therapy to assess the degree of residual withdrawal. Pharmacologic agents should be limited to those infants who do not respond to supportive care, and degree of symptomatology should be monitored with an abstinence scoring system (Finnegan, 1978). This system was developed for monitoring narcotic-exposed infants and may not capture all the symptoms seen in infants withdrawing from non-narcotics.

Once the infant is discharged from the nursery, symptoms can be expected to increase. Education and support of the caretakers are essential to avoid rehospitalization. Home use of sedatives should be avoided because of the potential for misuse by the caretaker. Extensive follow-up and home support services should be in place for these high-risk families.

BREAST FEEDING

Psychotropic drugs are low molecular weight and lipophilic, which means that they are readily excreted in breast milk (AAP, 1989b). Seizures and overdose symptoms have been reported in one infant whose mother used cocaine (Chasnoff et al., 1987). Amphetamines appear in large quantities in breast milk (Eriksson et al., 1978). Phencyclidine has also been found to readily cross into breast milk (Nicholas et al., 1982; Kaufman et al., 1983b). Because of the risk of toxicity, breast-feeding should be discouraged for known abusers of the above-named drugs with the exception of those mothers in drug treatment programs in which their drug use is monitored closely. Methadone is excreted in small quantities in breast milk and is considered safe if the mother is well controlled. Breast feeding longer than 3 to 6 months should be avoided because of the potential for increased exposure to methadone as the amount of milk consumption increases (Finnegan, 1978).

HUMAN IMMUNOVIRUS INFECTION (HIV)

Nationwide, intravenous drug abusers are the second largest risk group for HIV infection. Drug abusers also may be the primary source of infection for non–drug using heterosexuals as well as for children (Chamberland and Dondero, 1987; Rogers et al., 1987; Faloon et al., 1989). Pediatric AIDS is a perinatally acquired infection in 75 per cent of cases nationwide. The seropositivity rate among female intravenous drug users in New York City and northern New Jersey is estimated at 50 to 70 per cent compared to 5 to 20 per cent in California. Heroin and cocaine addicts often resort to prostitution to support their habit. Amphetamine and methamphetamine users often inject their drug several times daily. Alcohol decreases sexual inhibition, impairs judgment, and increases the chance of unsafe sexual activity. Every infant born to a substance abuser should be evaluated for HIV infection, and universal precautions must be strictly observed.

■ IDENTIFICATION AND INTERVENTION

The abuse of a variety of drugs during pregnancy has been documented to have adverse consequences for the mother, fetus, and newborn. The most effective tool for identification of high-risk behavior such as substance abuse is the prenatal history. Therefore, a drug and alcohol history should be routinely included as part of the initial contact with every pregnant patient. To be effective, such histories must be nonjudgmental and taken in the context of other life-style questions. When a positive history is obtained, intervention should begin immediately. The person taking the history should be prepared to offer preliminary counseling on risk reduction and concrete referrals for treatment programs.

A more controversial method of identification is routine drug screening of mothers and babies in cases in which drug abuse is suspected. Rapid reliable drug testing using urine or blood is readily available in most clinical laboratories. Drug screening should be combined with a history and should be a part of a well-delineated protocol that clearly defines which infants and mothers should be screened. Screening protocols should be based on well-defined high-risk behavior documented to be associated with perinatal drug abuse. High-risk behavior during the prenatal period includes a history of drug abuse, physical evidence of drug use (track marks or altered mental status), noncompliance with medical treatment and appointments, history of child abuse or children removed from the home, and history of a partner using drugs or excessive alcohol. A large percentage of drug abusers have no prenatal care or inadequate prenatal care (onset in last trimester or only a few visits), and this group has the highest rate of complicated deliveries. In addition, screening should include patients entering labor and delivery with complications associated with drug abuse such as hemorrhage, untreated sexually transmitted diseases and prematurity. Infants born to mothers who received no prenatal care and those born precipitously or prematurely should also be included. Screening should always be done in a manner to ensure as much as possible the right of privacy of the mother while allowing physicians to provide optimal medical care to both mother and infant (Chavkin and Kendall, 1990).

In the absence of intervention, infants discharged to mothers who abuse alcohol or illegal drugs are at high risk for subsequent physical abuse and neglect. Most states require some form of reporting to a child protective service agency. States differ in the aggressiveness with which they deal with this issue. In some states the child's drug exposure is prima facie evidence of abuse. However, in general the parent's addiction is evaluated in the context of its impact on her ability to care for the child.

As physicians caring for the mother and infant, our primary focus should be to ensure that all interventions are therapeutic and designed to foster the health of both patients.

■ REFERENCES

Abel, E.: Smoking and pregnancy. J. Psychoactive Drugs 16(4):327, 1984.

Abel, E.A., Jacobson, S., and Sherman, B.T.: In utero alcohol exposure: Functional and structural damage. Neurobehav. Toxicol. Teratol. 5:363, 1983.

Abel, E.L.: Effects of prenatal exposure to cannabinoids. In Pinker, M.G. (ed.): Current Research on the Consequences of Maternal Drug Abuse. Natl. Inst. Drug Abuse Res. Monogr. Ser. 59, 1985.

Abel, E.L.: Prenatal exposure to cannabis: A critical review of effects on growth development and behavior. Behav. Neural Biol. 29:137, 1980.

Abelson, H.J., and Miller, J.D.: A decade of trends in cocaine use in the household population. Natl. Inst. Drug Abuse Res. Monogr. Ser. 61:35, 1985.

Acker, D., Sachs, B.P., Tracy, K.J., and William, E.S.: Abruptio placentae associated with cocaine use. Am. J. Obstet. Gynecol. 146:220, 1983.

Adams, A.E.: Findings from the 1985 National Household Survey on Drug Abuse. N.Y. Acad. Sci. 3:10, 1988.

Adams, E.H., and Durell, J.: Cocaine: a growing public health problem. In Grabowski, J. (ed.): Cocaine: Pharmacology, Effects and Treatment of Abuse. Natl. Inst. Drug Abuse Res. Monogr. Ser. 50:9, 1984.

Adams, E.H., and Kozel, N.J.: Cocaine use in America: Introduction and Overview. Natl. Inst. Drug Abuse Res. Monogr. Ser. 61:1, 1985.

Adams, E.H., Gfroerres, J.C., Rouse, B.A., and Kozel, N.J.: Trends in prevalence and consequences of cocaine use. Adv. Alcohol Subst. Abuse. 6:49, 1986.

Ahmad, G., Halsall, L.C., and Bondy, S.C.: Persistence of phencyclidine in fetal brain. Brain Res. 415:194, 1987.

American Academy of Pediatrics (AAP) Committee on Drugs: Emergency drug doses for infants and children and naloxone use in newborns: clarification. Pediatrics 83(5):803, 1989a.

American Academy of Pediatrics Committee on Drugs: Neonatal drug withdrawal. Pediatrics 81:895, 1984.

American Academy of Pediatrics Committee on Drugs: Transfer of drugs and other chemicals into human milk. Pediatrics 84(5):924, 1989b.

Athinarazanan, P., Pierog, S., Nigan, S., and Glass, L.: Chlordiazepoxide withdrawal in the neonate. Am. J. Obstet. Gynecol. 124(2):212, 1976.

Beschner, G., and Thompson, P.: Women and drug abuse treatment: Needs and services. Natl. Inst. Drug Abuse Res. Monogr. Ser. 81:1057, 1981.

Besharov, D.: The children of crack—will we protect them? Public Welfare, Fall 1989.

Billings, L., Eriksson, M., Steneroth, G., and Zetterstrom, R.: Pre-school children of amphetamine-addicted mothers I: Somatic and psychomotor development. Acta Paediatr. Scand. 74:179, 1985.

Bingol, N., Fuchs, M., Diaz, V., et al.: Teratogenicity of cocaine in humans. J. Pediatr. 110:93, 1987.

Blinick, G., Wallach, R., Jerez, E., and Ackerman, B.D.: Drug addiction in pregnancy and the neonate. Am. J. Obstet. Gynecol. 125:135, 1976.

Briggs, G.G., Pharm, B.P., Samson, J.H., and Crawford, D.J.: Lack of abnormalities in a newborn exposed to amphetamine during gestation. Am. J. Dis. Child. 129:249, 1975.

Burkett, G., Yasin, S., and Palow, D.: Perinatal implications of cocaine exposure. J. Reprod. Med. 35(1): 35, 1990.

Chamberland, M.E., and Dondero, T.J.: Heterosexually acquired infection with human immunodeficiency virus (HIV): a view from the III International Conference on AIDS. Ann. Intern. Med. 107:763, 1987.

Chasnoff, I.J.: Drug use and women: Establishing a standard of care. Ann. N.Y. Acad. Sci. 562:208, 1989.

Chasnoff, I.J.: Drug use in pregnancy: Parameters of risk. Pediatr. Clin. North Am. 35(6):1403, 1988.

Chasnoff, I.J.: In utero cocaine exposure: Increased risk of SIDS. Pediatr. News 21:22, 1987a.

Chasnoff, I.J., Burns, K.A., and Burns, W.J.: Cocaine use in pregnancy: Perinatal morbidity and mortality. Neurobehav. Toxicol. Teratol. 9:291, 1987.

Chasnoff, I.J., Burns, W.J., Hatcher, R.P., and Burns, K.A.: Phencyclidine effects on the fetus and neonate. Devel. Pharmacol. Ther. 6:404, 1983a.

Chasnoff, I.J., Burns, W.J., Schnoll, S.H., and Burns, K.A.: Cocaine use in pregnancy. N. Engl. J. Med. 313(11):666, 1985.

Chasnoff, I.J., Bussey, M.E., Savich, R., and Stack, C.M.: Perinatal cerebral infarction and maternal cocaine use. J. Pediatr. 108(3):456, 1986.

Chasnoff, I.J., Chisum, G.M., and Kaplan, W.E.: Maternal cocaine use and genitourinary tract malformations. Teratology 87:201, 1988.

Chasnoff, I.J., Griffith, D.R., MacGregor, S., et al.: Temporal patterns of cocaine use in pregnancy: Perinatal outcome. JAMA 261(12):1741, 1989.

Chasnoff, I.J., Hatcher, R., and Burns, W.J.: Polydrug- and Methadone-addicted newborns: a continuum of impairment? Pediatrics 70(2):210, 1982.

Chasnoff, I.J., Hatcher, R., Burns, W., and Schnoll, S.: Pentazocine and tripelennamine ("T's and Blue's"): Effects on the fetus and neonate. Dev. Pharmacol. Ther. 6:162, 1983b.

Chasnoff, I.J., Lewis, D.E., and Squires, L.: Cocaine intoxication in a breast-fed infant. Pediatrics 80:836, 1987.

Chavez, G.F., Mulinare, J.F., Cordero, J.F.: Cocaine use during early pregnancy as a risk factor for congenital urogenital anomalies. J.A.M.A. 262(6):795, 1989.

Chavkin, W., and Kendall, S.R.: Between a "rock" and a "hard place": Perinatal drug abuse. Pediatrics 85(2):223, 1990.

Cherukuri, R., Minkoff, H., Feldman, J., et al.: A cohort study of alkaloidal cocaine ('crack') in pregnancy. Obstet. Gynecol. 72:147, 1988.

Chouteau, M., Namerow, P.B., and Leppert, P.: The effects of cocaine abuse on birth weight and gestational age. Obstet. Gynecol. 72(3):351, 1988.

Clarren, S.K., and Smith, D.W.: The fetal alcohol syndrome. N. Engl. J. Med. 298:1063, 1978.

Clarren, S.K., Alvord, E.C., Sumi, S.M., et al.: Brain malformations related to perinatal exposure to ethanol. J. Pediatr. 92(1):64, 1978.

Clayton, R.R.: Cocaine use in the U.S.: In a blizzard or just being snowed? In Kozel, N.J. and Adams, E.J. (eds.): Cocaine use in America: Epidemiologic and clinical perspectives. Natl. Inst. Drug Abuse Res. Monogr. Ser. 61:8, 1985.

Cobrinik, R.W., Hood, R.J., and Chusid, E.: The effect of maternal narcotic addiction on the newborn infant. Pediatrics 24:288, 1959.

Cohen, S.: Angel dust, JAMA *238*(6):515, 1977.

Committee on Substance Abuse, Academy of Pediatrics: Substance abuse. Pediatrics *86*:639–642, 1990.

Connaughton, J.F., Reeser, D., Schut, J., and Finnegan, L.P.: Perinatal addiction: outcome and management. Am. J. Obstet. Gynecol. *129*:679, 1977.

Contreras, P.C., Rafferty, M.F., Lessor, R.A., et al.: A specific alkylating ligand for phencyclidine (PCP) receptors antagonizes PCP behavioral effects. Eur. J. Pharmacol. *111*:405, 1985.

Cooper, J.R., Altman, F., Brown, B.S., and Czechowicz, D.: Effects of methadone on offspring and users. Research on the Treatment of Narcotic Addiction: State of the art. Nat. Inst. Drug Abuse. Treatment Ser. Dept. of HHS, 1983.

Cregler, L.L., and Mark, H.: Medical complications of cocaine abuse. N. Engl. J. Med. *315*:1495, 1986.

Critchley, H.O.D., Woods, S.M., Barson, A.J., et al.: Fetal death in utero and cocaine abuse: Case report. Br. J. Obstet. Gynaecol. *95*:195, 1988.

Dackis, C.A., and Gold, M.S.: New concepts in cocaine addiction: The dopamine depletion hypothesis. Neurosci. Biobehav. Rev. *9*:469, 1985.

Davis, P.J., Partridge, J.W., and Storrs, C.N.: Alcohol consumption in pregnancy. How much is safe? Arch. Dis. Child. *57*:940, 1982.

Deneau, G.A., and Mule, S.J.: Pharmacology of the opiates. *In* Lowinson, J.H., and Ruiz, P.: Substance Abuse: Clinical Problems and Perspectives. Baltimore, Williams & Wilkins, 1981, p. 129.

Desmond, M.D., and Wilson, G.: Neonatal abstinence syndrome: Recognition and diagnosis. Addict. Dis. *2*:113, 1975.

Dixon, S.D.: Effects of transplantation exposure to cocaine and methamphetamine on the neonate. West. J. Med. *150*:436, 1989.

Doberczak, T.M., Shanzer, S., Senie, R.T., and Kandall, S.R.: Neonatal neurologic and electroencephalographic effects of intrauterine cocaine exposure. J. Pediatr. *113*(2):354, 1989.

Eriksson, M., Larsson, G., Winbladh, B., and Zetterstrom, R.: The influence of amphetamine addiction on pregnancy and the newborn infant. Acta Paediatr. Scand. *67*:95, 1978.

Eriksson, M., Larsson, G., and Zetterstrom, R.: Amphetamine addiction and pregnancy II: Pregnancy, delivery, and the neonatal period. Sociomedical aspects. Acta Obstet. Gynaecol. Scand. *60*:253, 1981.

Eriksson, M., Stenoroth, G., and Zetterstrom, R.: Influence of pregnancy and child-rearing on amphetamine-addicted women: Five-year followup after delivery. Acta Psychiatr. Scand. *73*:634, 1986.

Falloon, J., Eddy, J.A., and Pizzo, P.: Human immunodeficiency virus infection in children. J. Pediatr. *114*(1):1, 1989.

Fantel, A.G., and Macphail, B.J.: The teratogenicity of cocaine. Teratology, *26*:17, 1982.

Farrar, H.C., and Kearns, G.L.: Cocaine: Clinical pharmacology and toxicology. J. Pediatr. *115*(5):665, 1989.

Fein, A.F., Shviro, Y., Manoach, M., and Nebel, L.: Teratogenic effect of D-amphetamine sulfate: Histodifferentiation and electrocardiogram pattern of mouse embryonic heart. Teratology *35*:27, 1987.

Finnegan, L.P. (ed.): Drug dependence in pregnancy: Clinical management of mother and child. A Manual for Medical Professionals and Paraprofessionals, prepared for the National Institute on Drug Abuse, Services Research Branch, Washington, D.C., U.S. Government Printing Office, 1978.

Finnegan, L.P.: In utero opiate dependence and sudden infant death syndrome. Clin. Perinatol. *6*:1, 163, 1979.

Finnegan, L.P.: Maternal and neonatal effects of drug dependence in pregnancy. *In* Lowinson, J.H., and Ruiz, P. (eds.): Substance Abuse: Clinical Problems and Perspectives. Baltimore, Williams & Wilkins, 1981, p. 545.

Fishburne, P.M.: National Survey on Drug Abuse: Main Findings:1979. Washington, D.C., National Institute on Drug Abuse (DHHS publication no. ADM 80-976), 1980.

Frank, D.A., Zuckerman, B.S., Amaro, H., et al.: Cocaine use during pregnancy: Prevalence and correlates. Pediatrics *82*(6):888, 1988.

Fried, P.A.: Marijuana use by pregnant women and effects on offspring: an update. Neurobehav. Toxicol. Teratol. *4*:451, 1982.

Fried, P.A., and Watkinson, B.: 12- and 24-month neurobehavioral follow-up of children prenatally exposed to marijuana, cigarettes and alcohol. Neurotoxicol. Teratol. *10*:305, 1988.

Fried, P.A., Watkinson, B., Dillon, R.F., and Dulberg, C.S.: Neonatal neurological status in a low-risk population after prenatal exposure to cigarettes, marijuana, and alcohol. J. Dev. Behav. Pediatr. *8*(6):318, 1987.

Fulroth, R., Phillips, B., and Durand, D.J.: Perinatal outcome of infants exposed to cocaine and/or heroin in utero. Am. J. Dis. Child. *143*:905, 1989.

Gawin, F.H., and Ellinwood, E.H.: Cocaine and other stimulants: actions, abuse, and treatment. N. Engl. J. Med. *318*(18):1173, 1988.

Gawin, F.H., and Kleber, H.D.: Abstinence symptomatology and psychiatric diagnosis in cocaine abusers. Arch. Gen. Psychiatry *43*:107, 1986.

Goetz, R., and Bain, R.: Neonatal withdrawal symptoms associated with maternal use of pentazocine. J. Pediatr. *84*(6):887, 1974.

Gold, M.S., Washton, A.M., and Dackis, C.A.: Cocaine abuse: neurochemistry, pharmacology and treatment. Natl. Inst. Drug Abuse Res. Monogr. Ser. *61*:130, 1985a.

Gold, M.S., Washton, A.M., and Dackis, C.A.: Patterns and consequences of cocaine use. Natl. Inst. Drug Abuse Res. Monogr. Ser. 61:85, 1985b.

Golden, N.L., Kuhnert, B.R., Sokol, R.J., et al.: Neonatal manifestations of maternal phencyclidine exposure. J. Perinat. Med. *15*:185, 1987.

Grabowski, J. (ed.): Cocaine: Pharmacology, effects and treatment of abuse. Natl. Inst. Drug Abuse Res. Monogr. Ser. *50*:9, 1984.

Gunne, L.M., and Anggard, E.: Pharmacokinetics studies with amphetamines: relationship to neuropsychiatric disorders. J. Pharmacokinet. Biopharm. *1*:481, 1973.

Hadeed, A.J., and Seigel, S.R.: Maternal cocaine use during pregnancy: Effects on the newborn infant. Pediatrics *84*(2):205, 1989.

Hanson, J.W., Streissguth, A.P., and Smith, D.W.: The effects of moderate alcohol consumption during pregnancy on fetal growth and morphogenesis. J. Pediatr. *92*:457, 1978.

Hingston, R., Alpert, J.J., and Day, N.: Effects of maternal drinking and marijuana use on fetal growth and development. Pediatrics *70*:539, 1982.

Howard, J., Kropenske, V., and Tyler, R.: The long-term effects on neurodevelopment in infants exposed prenatally to PCP. *In* Clout, D.H. (ed.): Phencyclidine: An update. Natl. Inst. Drug Abuse Res. Monogr. Ser. 6, 1988.

Husson, B.S.: Trends and epidemiology of drug abuse in Los Angeles County, California 1980–1983. Natl. Inst. Drug Abuse Res. Monogr. Ser. *1*:84, 1984.

Iosub, S., Fuchs, M., Bingol, N., and Gromisch, D.: Fetal alcohol syndrome revisited. Pediatrics *68*(4):475, 1981.

Jaffee, J.H.: Drug addiction and drug abuse. *In* Goodman, A., Goodman, L.S., and Gilman, A.G. (eds.): The Pharmacologic Basis of Therapeutics, 7th ed. New York, Macmillan, 1985, p. 550.

Jain, N.C., Budd, R.D., and Budd, B.S.: Growing abuse of phencyclidine: California "angel dust" N. Engl. J. Med. *297*:673, 1977.

Jones, C.L., and Lopez, R.E.: Direct and indirect effects on the infant of maternal drug abuse. *In* Hill G. (ed.): Public Health Service Report on the Content of Prenatal Care, Vol. II, Washington, D.C., US DHHS, 1989.

Jones, K.L., and Smith, D.W.: The fetal alcohol syndrome. N. Engl. J. Med. *298*:1063, 1978.

Jones, K.L., Smith, D.W., and Hanson, J.W.: The fetal alcohol syndrome: Clinical delineation. Ann. N.Y. Acad. Sci. *273*:130, 1976.

Jones, K.L., Smith, D.W., Streissguth, A.P., and Myianthopoulous, N.C.: Outcome in offspring of chronic alcoholic women. Lancet *1*:1076, 1974.

Jones, K.L., Smith, D.W., Ulleland, C.N., and Streissguth, P.: Pattern of malformations in offspring of chronic alcoholic mothers. Lancet *1*:1267, 1973.

Jones, R.T.: The pharmacology of cocaine. Natl. Inst. Drug Abuse Res. Monogr. Ser. *50*:34, 1985.

Kaestner, E., Frank, B., Marel, R., and Schneideler, J.: Substance use among females in New York State catching up with males. Adv. Alcohol Subst. Abuse 5:29, 1986.

Kamenski, M., Rumeau, C., and Schwartz, D.: Alcohol consumption in pregnant women and the outcome of pregnancy. Clin. Exp. Res. *2*(2):255, 1978.

Kandall, S.R., and Garner, I.M.: Late presentation of drug withdrawal symptoms in newborns. Am. J. Dis. Child. *127*:58, 1972.

Kaufman, K.R., Petrucha, R.A., Pitts, T.N., and Weekes, M.E.: PCP in amniotic fluid and breast milk: Case report. J. Clin. Psychiatry *44*(7):269, 1983.

Kleber, H.D., and Gawin, F.H.: Cocaine withdrawal. Arch. Gen. Psychiatry *44*:298, 1987.

Kozel, N.J., and Adams, E.H.: Epidemiology of drug abuse: An overview. Science *234*:970, 1986.

Kramer, J.C., Fischman, V.S., and Littlefield, D.C.: Amphetamine abuse: patterns and effects of high doses taken intravenously. JAMA *201*:305, 1967.

Kron, R.E., Litt, M., and Finnegan, L.P.: Narcotic addiction in the newborn: Differences in behavior generated by methadone and heroin. Int. J. Clin. Pharmacol. *12*:63, 1975.

Largent, D.R.: "Ice" Crystal Methamphetamine. California Dept. of Justice, Bureau of Narcotic Enforcement. September 1989.

Larsson, G., and Zetterstrom, R.: Amphetamine addiction and pregnancy: Psycho-social and medical aspects. Acta Psychiatr. Scand. *60*:334, 1979.

Lee, M.I., Stryker, J.C., and Sokol, R.J.: Perinatal care for narcotic-dependent gravidas. Perinatology/Neonatology Nov/Dec:35, 1985.

Lemoine, P., Harrousseau, H., Bortequ, J.P., and Menuet, J.C.: Les enfants de parents alcooliques: anomalies observes a propos de 127 cas. Quest. Med. *21*:476, 1968.

Lifschitz, M.H., Wilson, G.S., Smith, E.O., and Desmond, M.M.: Factors affecting head growth and intellectual function in children of drug addicts. Pediatrics *75*:269, 1985.

Little, B.B., Snell, L.M., and Gelstrap, L.C.: Methamphetamine abuse during pregnancy: Outcome and fetal effects. Obstet. Gynecol. *72*(2):541, 1988.

MacDonald, D.J.: Patterns of alcohol and drug use among adolescents. Pediatr. Clin. North Am. *34*(2):273, 1987.

MacGregor, S.N., Keith, L.G., Chasnoff, I.J., et al.: Cocaine use during pregnancy: Adverse perinatal outcome. Am. J. Obstet. Gynecol. *157*(3):686, 1987.

Madden, J.D., Payne, T.F., and Miller, S.: Maternal cocaine abuse and effect on the newborn. Pediatrics *77*:209, 1986.

Mahalik, M.P., Gautiere, R.T., and Mann, D.E.: Mechanism of cocaine-induced teratogenesis. Res. Commun. Subst. Abuse *5*:279, 1984.

Mangurten, H.H., and Benwara, R.: Neonatal codeine withdrawal in infants of non-addicted mothers. Pediatrics *65*:159, 1980.

Martin, J.C.: Effects on offspring of chronic maternal methamphetamine exposure. Dev. Psychol. *8*:397, 1977.

Mercado, A., Johnson, G., Calver, D., and Sokol, R.J.: Cocaine, pregnancy and postpartum hemorrhage. Obstet. Gynecol. *73*(3):467, 1989.

Miller, G.: Addicted infants and their mothers. A survey conducted for the House Select Committee on Children, Youth and Families, National Center for Clinical Infant Programs, Zero to Three. IX(5):20, 1989.

Mills, J.L., and Graibard, B.J.: Is moderate drinking during pregnancy associated with an increased risk for malformation? Pediatrics *80*(3):309, 1987.

Mofenson, H.C., and Caraccio, T.R.: Cocaine. Pediatr Annu. *16*:864, 1987.

Mondanero, J.: Chemical dependency, pregnancy and parenting: Assessments and treatment planning. In Current Issue in the Treatment of Chemically Dependent Women. National Institute of Drug Abuse Monograph. Washington, D.C., U.S. Government Printing Office, 1987.

Moore, T.R., Sorg, J., Thomas, C.K., et al.: Hemodynamic effects of intravenous cocaine on the pregnant ewe and fetus. Am. J. Obstet. Gynecol. *155*:883, 1986.

Naeye, R.L.: Maternal use of dextroamphetamine and growth of the fetus. Pharmacology *26*:117, 1983.

Naeye, R.L., Blanc, W., Leblanc, W., and Khatamee, M.A.: Fetal compilations of maternal heroin addiction: abnormal growth, infections and episodes of stress. J. Pediatr. *83*:1055, 1973.

Naeye, R.L., Ladis, B., and Drage, J.S.: Sudden infant death syndrome. Am. J. Dis. Child. *130*:1207, 1976.

National Institute of Drug Abuse (NIDA): Drug use among American high school students, college students and other young adults: National Trends through 1985. DHHS Pub. (ADM) 86-145. Washington, D.C., U.S. Government Printing Office, 1986.

National Institute of Drug Abuse (NIDA): Statistical Series, Trend Report Jan 1977–September 1980. Data from CODAP, US DHHS, Series E, No. 20, 1981.

National Institute of Drug Abuse (NIDA): Statistical Series Annual Data 1981, Data from CODAP, US DHHS, Series E. No. 25, 1982.

National Institute of Drug Abuse (NIDA): Services Research Branch Notes (1979). Estimate of Opiate-Addicted Births, U.S. DHEW, 1979.

National Institute of Drug Abuse (NIDA): National Household Survey on Drug Abuse: Population Estimates 1988, U.S. DHHS Pub. No. (ADM), 1989.

Neuman, L.L., and Cohen, S.N.: The neonatal narcotic withdrawal syndrome: A therapeutic challenge. Clin. Perinatol. *2*(1):99, 1975.

Nicholas, J.M., Lipshitz, J., and Schrieber, E.C.: Phencyclidine: Its transfer across the placenta as well as into breast milk. Am. J. Obstet. Gynecol. *143*:143, 1982.

Nora, J.J., Vargo, T.A., Nora, A.H., et al.: Dexamphetamine: A possible environment trigger in cardiovascular malformations. Lancet *1*:1290, 1970.

Oro, A.S., and Dixon, S.D.: Perinatal cocaine and methamphetamine exposure: Maternal and neonatal correlates. J. Pediatr. *111*:571, 1987.

Ostrea, E.M., and Chavez, C.J.: Perinatal problems (excluding neonatal withdrawal) in maternal drug addiction: A study of 830 cases. J. Pediatr. *94*(2):293, 1979.

Ouellette, E.M., Rosett, H.L., Rosman, N.P., et al.: Adverse effects on offspring of maternal alcohol abuse during pregnancy. N. Engl. J. Med. *297*:528, 1977.

Perez-Reyes, M., DiGuiseppi, S., Ondrusek, G., et al.: Free-base cocaine smoking. Clin. Pharmacol. Ther. *32*:459, 1982.

Pierog, S., Chandavasu, O., and Werler, J.: Withdrawal symptoms in infants with the fetal alcohol syndrome. J. Pediatr. *90*:630, 1970.

Pierson, P.S., Howard, P., and Kleger, D.: Sudden deaths in infants born to methadone-maintained addicts. JAMA *220*:1733, 1972.

Pinkert, T.M. (ed.): Current research on the consequences of maternal drug abuse. Natl. Inst. Drug Abuse Res. Monogr. Ser. 59, 1985.

Platt, J.J.: Heroin Addiction: Theory, Research, and Treatment. Malabar, Fla., Robert E. Kriegier Publishing Co., 1986.

Raye, J.R., Dubin, J.W., and Blechner, J.N.: Alterations in fetal metabolism subsequent to maternal morphine administration. Am. J. Obstet. Gynecol. *137*:505, 1980.

Reddy, A.M., Harper, R.G., and Stern, G.: Observations on heroin and methadone withdrawal in the newborn. Pediatrics *48*:353, 1971.

Resnick, R.B., and Kistenbaum, R.S.: Acute systemic effects of cocaine in man: a controlled study by intranasal and intravenous routes, Science *195*:696, 1977.

Ritchie, J.M., and Green, N.M.: Local anesthetics. In Goodman, A., Goodman, L.S., and Gilman, A.G. (eds.): The Pharmacological Basis of Therapeutics, 7th ed. New York, Macmillan, 1985, p. 309.

Rogers, M.F., Thomas, P.A., Starcher, E.T., et al: Acquired immunodeficiency syndrome in children: report of the Centers of Disease Control National Surveillance, 1982 to 1985. Pediatrics *79*:1008, 1987.

Rosett, H.L., Ouellette, E.M., and Weiner, L.: A pilot prospective study of the fetal alcohol syndrome at the Boston City Hospital, Part I: Maternal drinking. Ann. N.Y. Acad. Sci. *273*:118, 1976.

Rosner, M.A., Keith, L., and Chasnoff, I.: The Northwestern University Drug Dependence Program: The impact of intensive prenatal care on labor and delivery outcomes. Am. J. Obstet. Gynecol. *1*:23, 1982.

Rothrock, J.F., Rubenstein, B., and Lyden, P.D.: Ischemic stroke associated with methamphetamine inhalation. Neurology *38*:589, 1988.

Rumack, B., and Walravens, P.: Neonatal withdrawal following maternal ingestion of ethchlorvynol (Placidyl). Pediatrics *52*:716, 1973.

Ryan, L., Ehrlich, S., and Finnegan, L.: Cocaine abuse in pregnancy: effects on the fetus and newborn. Neurotoxicol. Teratol. *9*:295, 1987.

Schmidt, C.J.: Neurotoxicity of the psychedelic amphetamine, methyenedioxymethamphetamine. J. Pharmacol. Exp. Ther. *240*(1):1, 1987.

Schnoll, S.H., Daghestani, A.N., and Hansen, T.R.: Cocaine dependence. Resident Staff Physician *30*(11):24, 1984.

Siegel, R.K.: New patterns of cocaine use: Changing dose and routes. Natl. Inst. Drug Abuse Res. Monogr. Ser. *61*:204, 1985.

Siegel, R.K.: Cocaine smoking. J. Psychoactive Drugs *14*:277, 1982.

Silber, T.J., Losefsohn, M., Hick, J.M., et al.: Prevalence of PCP use among adolescent marijuana users. J. Pediatr. *112*(5):827, 1988.

Smith, D.E.: Cocaine-alcohol abuse: epidemiological, diagnostic and treatment considerations. J. Psychoactive Drugs *18*:117, 1986.

Smith, D.E.: The characteristics of dependence in high dose methamphetamine abuse. Int. J. Addict. *4*:453, 1969.

Smith, D.E., Wesson, D.R., and Busxon, M.E. (eds.): Amphetamine Use, Misuse, and Abuse. Boston, GK Hall, 1979.

Snyder, S.H.: Drug and neurotransmitter receptors in the brain. Science *224*:22, 1984.

Sokol, R.J., Miller, S.J., and Reed, G.: Alcohol abuse during pregnancy: an epidemiologic study. Clin. Exp. Res. *4*(2):135, 1979.

Statzer, D.E., and Wardell, J.N.: Heroin addiction during pregnancy. Am. J. Obstet. Gynecol. *113*:273, 1972.

Steiner, E., Villen, F., Hallberg, M., and Rane, A.: Amphetamine secretion in breast milk. Eur. J. Pharmacol. *27*:123, 1984.

Stern, Z.A., and Susser, M.: Intrauterine growth retardation: Epidemiological issues and public health significance. Semin. Perinatol. *8*:5, 1984.

Strasman, R.J.: Adverse reactions to psychedelic drugs: A review of the literature. J. Nerv. Ment. Dis. *172*:571, 1984.

Strauss, A.A., Mondanou, H.D., and Bosu, S.K.: Neonatal manifestations of maternal phencyclidine (PCP) abuse. Pediatrics *68*(4):550, 1981.

Strauss, M., Andresko, M., Stryker, J., et al.: Methadone maintenance during pregnancy: Pregnancy, birth, and neonate characteristics. Am. J. Obstet. Gynecol. *120*:895, 1974.

Streissguth, A.P.: Fetal alcohol syndrome: An epidemiological perspective. Am. J. Epidemiol. *107*(6):467, 1978.

Streissguth, A.P., Clarren, S.K., and Jones, K.L.: A 10-year follow-up of the first children described as having fetal alcohol syndrome. Clin. Exp. Res. *8*:21, 1984.

Streissguth, A.P., Landesman-Dwyer, S., Marlin, J.C., and Smith, D.W.: Teratogenic effects of alcohol in humans and laboratory animals. Science *209*:353, 1980.

Suffet, F., and Brotman, R.: A comprehensive care program for pregnant addicts: Obstetrical, neonatal, and child development outcomes. Int. J. Addict. *19*(2):199, 1984.

Sweet, A.Y.: Narcotic withdrawal syndrome in the newborn. Pediatr. Rev. *3*(9):285, 1982.

Taeusch, H.W., Carson, S.H., Wang, N.S., and Avery, M.E.: Heroin induction of lung maturation and growth retardation in fetal rabbits. J. Pediatr. *82*:869, 1973.

Tarr, J.E., and Macklen, M.: Cocaine. Pediatr. Clin. North Am. *34*(2):319, 1987.

Telsey, A.M., Merrit, T.A., and Dixon, S.D.: Cocaine exposure in a term neonate. Clin. Pediatr. *27*:547, 1988.

Tennes, K., and Blackard, C.: Maternal alcohol consumption, birth weight and minor physical anomalies. Am. J. Obstet. Gynecol. *138*:774, 1980.

Tennes, K.N., Avitable, N., Blackard, C., et al.: Marijuana: Prenatal and postnatal exposure in the human. *In* Pinker, M.H. (ed.): Current Research on the Consequences of Maternal Drug Abuse, NIDA Research Monograph 59, 1985.

Ulleland, C.N.: The offspring of alcoholic mothers. Ann. N.Y. Acad. Sci. *197*:167, 1972.

Van Dyke, C., and Byck, R.: Cocaine. Sci. Am. *246*:128, 1982.

Wapner, R.J., and Finnegan, L.P.: Perinatal aspects of psychotropic drug abuse. *In* Bolognese, R.J., Schwarz, R., and Schneicher, J. (eds.): Perinatal Medicine, 2nd ed. Baltimore, Williams & Wilkins, 1982, p. 394.

Washton, A.M.: Cocaine Addiction, Treatment, Recovery, and Relapse Prevention. New York, W.W. Norton & Co., 1989.

Washton, A.M.: Women and cocaine. Med. Aspects Hum. Sexuality *20*(3):57, 1986.

Webster, P.: Withdrawal symptoms in neonates associated with maternal antidepressant therapy. Lancet *2*:318, 1973.

Wilson, G.S., Desmond, M.M., and Verniaud, W.M.: Early development of infants of heroin-addicted mothers. J. Dis. Child. *126*:456, 1973.

Wilson, G.S., McCreary, R., Kean, J., and Baster, J.C.: The development of preschool children of heroin-addicted mothers: A controlled study. Pediatrics *63*:135, 1979.

Woods, J. R., Plessinger, M.A., and Clark, K.E.: Effects of cocaine on uterine blood flow and fetal oxygenation. JAMA *257*:957, 1987.

Zuckerman, B., Frank, D.A., Hingson, R., et al.: Effects of maternal marijuana and cocaine use on fetal growth. N. Engl. J. Med. *320*(12):762, 1989.

PART V

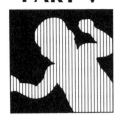

THE NEWBORN— GENERAL PRINCIPLES OF CARE

TEMPERATURE 27 REGULATION OF THE PREMATURE INFANT

Stephen Baumgart

The human newborn is considered homeothermic. Morbidity (i.e., poor brain and somatic growth) and mortality rates increase when core body temperature is permitted to fall much below 36° C (96.8° F). Moreover, even premature newborns respond adaptively to changes in their environment. Response to cold stress, however, may be insufficient to maintain core body temperature in premature infants and render them functionally poikilothermic, even in moderately temperate environments.

■ COLD STRESS: THE PROBLEM

The newborn frequently encounters the problem of severe heat loss for several reasons. First, the baby's exposed surface is much larger than the adult's relative to metabolically active body mass (Table 27–1). Especially for the very-low-birth-weight infant, the heat-dissipating area is five to six times greater proportionate to the adult. Second, the tiny baby's small size presents a much smaller heat sink to store thermal reserve. Finally, the radius of curvature of the body is less than in the adult, resulting in a thinner protective boundary layer of warm, humidified air.

Aside from these geometric considerations, characteristics of the premature infant's skin contribute to the problem of excessive heat loss. Especially in premature babies, the skin and subcutaneous fascia provide little

TABLE 27–1. Body Surface Area to Body Mass Ratio

	BODY WEIGHT (kg)	SURFACE AREA (m$_2$)	RATIO (cm$_2$/kg)
Adult	70	1.73	250
Premature infant	1.5	0.13	870
Very premature infant	0.5	0.07	1400

insulation against the flow of heat from the core to the surface. Moreover, the lack of a keratinized epidermal barrier exposes infants to vastly increased evaporative heat loss. In very-low-birth-weight infants (<1.0 kg), water lost to evaporation may be eight to ten times more than adult quantities. For these reasons, a major problem confronting small premature infants from birth is cold stress.

■ PHYSICAL ROUTES OF HEAT LOSS

Convection. Convective heat loss in newborn infants occurs when ambient air temperature is less than the infant's skin temperature. Convective heat loss includes (1) natural convection (passage of heat from the skin to the ambient still air), and (2) forced convection, where mass movement of air over the infant conveys heat away from the skin. The quantity of heat lost is proportional to the difference between air and skin temperatures, and to air speed. The effect of forced convection in disrupting the microenvironment of warm, humid air layered near an infant's skin usually is not appreciated in the nursery, where drafts, air turbulence, and consequently heat loss may occur even within the relatively protective environment of an incubator.

Evaporation. Passive transcutaneous evaporation of water from a newborn's skin (termed insensible water loss) results in the dissipation of 0.58 kcal/ml latent heat. As shown in Figure 27–1, transcutaneous water loss increases exponentially with decreasing size and gestation. The tiniest premature baby, least able to tolerate cold stress, may incur evaporative loss in excess of 4 kcal/hour. Evaporation is enhanced by low vapor pressure (high

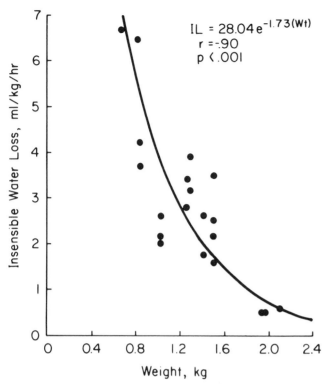

$$IL = 28.04 e^{-1.73(Wt)}$$
$$r = -.90$$
$$p < .001$$

FIGURE 27–1. Exponential rise in evaporative water loss from skin of very low birth weight infants. (Adapted with permission from Baumgart, S., et al.: Clin. Pediatr. 21(4):199–205, 1982).

temperature and low relative humidity) and air turbulence. The highest evaporative losses occur on the 1st days of life, and during the 1st week of life in infants of 25 to 27 weeks' gestation, evaporative heat losses are higher than radiant losses (Hammarlund et al., 1986).

Radiation. Radiant heat loss constitutes the transfer of heat from an infant's warm skin via infrared electromagnetic waves to the cooler surrounding walls. Radiant heat loss is proportional to the difference between skin and surrounding wall temperatures. An infant's posture may also affect radiant heat loss by increasing or reducing the effective radiating surface area of the baby exposed outward. In a humid environment, babies experience an ambient temperature determined 60 per cent by wall temperature and 40 per cent by air temperature.

Conduction. Conductive heat loss to cooler surfaces in contact with an infant's skin depends on the material of the surface and its temperature. Usually, babies are nursed on insulating mattresses that minimize conductive heat loss.

■ PHYSIOLOGY OF COLD RESPONSE

Afferents. Homeothermic response to a cold environment begins with sensation of temperature. Traditional physiology identifies two temperature sensitive sites: the hypothalamus and the skin. Sensation of cold by neonatal skin triggers a cold-adaptive response long before core sensors in the hypothalamus become chilled. Some investigators conjecture that neonatal cold reception resides primarily in the skin, whereas warm reception resides in the hypothalamus. Both sensors are probably integrated, however, since cold sensory response is inhibited by core sensor hyperthermia and vice versa. Peripheral skin cold sensation is teleologically important, since early detection aids in maintaining core temperature.

Central Regulation. Integration of multiple skin and hypothalamic temperature inputs probably occurs in the hypothalamus. No single control temperature seems to exist, however. Under different environmental conditions, temperature of the skin may fluctuate 8 to 10° C and temperature of the hypothalamus may vary ± 0.5° C. There exist also diurnal temperature fluctuations, variations with general sympathetic tone, and down-regulation with asphyxia, hypoxemia and other central nervous system defects. Premature infants may regulate core temperature near 37.5° C (99.4° F), whereas term infants may respond to maintain 36.5° C (97.7° F). Since important thermoregulatory processes are triggered by as little as ± 0.5° C, deviation at any temperature sensitive site is important.

Efferents. The effector limb of the neonatal thermal response is mediated primarily by the sympathetic nervous system, although infant motor behavior may also be involved. The earliest maturing response is vasoconstriction in deep dermal arterioles, resulting in reduced flow of warm blood from the infant's core to the exposed periphery. Additionally, reduction of blood flow effectively places a layer of insulating fat between the core and the exposed skin in the term infant. Reduced fat content in low-birth-weight babies, however, decreases the effective insulating properties of this strategy. Vasoconstriction nevertheless remains the newborn's first line of defense, and the response is present even in the most premature infant.

Brown fat constitutes a second sympathetic effector organ that provides a metabolic source of nonshivering thermogenesis (babies do not shiver). Brown fat located in axillary, mediastinal, perinephric, and other regions of the newborn is especially enervated and equipped with an abundance of mitochondria to hydrolyze and re-esterify triglycerides and to oxidize free fatty acids. In the term infant, these reactions are exothermic and increase metabolic rate by two-fold or more. Preterm babies, however, have little brown fat and may not be capable of more than a 25 per cent increase in metabolic rate despite the most severe cold stress (Hull, 1966).

Finally, evidence suggests that control of voluntary muscle tone, posture and increased motor activity with agitation may serve to augment heat production in skeletal muscle via glycogenolysis and glucose oxidation. Clinical observations of infant posture, behavior, skin perfusion and measurements of skin and core temperatures may ultimately provide the most useful guidelines for assessing infant comfort during incubation.

■ MODERN INCUBATION

The life-saving requirement of an appropriate thermal environment was demonstrated conclusively by Day and colleagues in 1966 and further defined by Silverman and associates (1966). Minor changes in heat balance exact an oxygen cost that can only be met by increased ventilation or increased inspired oxygen.

Thermal Neutral Zone. The thermal neutral zone is a narrow range of environmental temperatures within which newborn babies do not alter their metabolic rate in response to either peripheral cold stimulation or core hyperthermia. Rather, infants regulate temperature through vasomotor tone alone. A range of "critical" environmental temperatures relevant to modern incubators was identified by Hey and Katz (1970), (Figure 27–2 and Table 27–2). Below this range, an increase in the infant's minimal metabolic rate was observed. This range, therefore, was defined as the optimal incubator temperature. Several important considerations in regulating incubator temperature were included in these studies: (1) incubator wall temperature was maintained identical to air temperature, (2) relative humidity was controlled near 50 per cent, and (3) the environment was maintained in a steady state, uninterrupted by turbulence.

Many modern incubators, however, incorporate a single-walled design that results in higher radiant heat loss because the incubator's outside wall is exposed to cooler room air. Moreover, many nurseries do not humidify incubators artificially, fearing the occurrence of bacterial colonization. Finally, the incubator's steady state is frequently interrupted for nursing and medical procedures that require that doors be open to care for the infant. Although a useful concept, the thermal neutral zone must be rigorously defined in practical terms. Silverman, Sinclair, and Agate (1966) used a modified concept of the thermal neutral zone to simplify clinical application. Reasoning that infants sense environmental temperature first on the skin, electronic negative-feedback (servo-con-

trolled) regulation of the incubator's heater in response to skin temperature was employed. These authors demonstrated minimal metabolic expenditure near 36.5° C (97.7°F) abdominal skin temperature measured by a shielded thermistor in a less rigidly defined incubator environment. The importance of frequently checking core temperatures (axillary or rectal) must be emphasized, however, before delegating the infant's environment to such thermostatic control. In addition, Chessex and associates (1988) have demonstrated that incubator temperature may vary by more than 2° C when skin temperature servocontrol rather than air temperature control is used.

Finally, with the modern use of open radiant warmer beds (improving the means of access to the infant without interrupting heat delivery), skin temperature servocontrol has become the only practical method for approximating the thermal neutral zone (Malin and Baumgart, 1987). These variations in incubator design and technique, and the extension of infant warming to include very-low-birth-weight, critically ill premature babies have generated new problems for determining a universally accepted optimal environment.

Partitioning Infant Heat Losses and Heat Gains. Wheldon and Rutter (1983) demonstrated the special problems encountered in incubating very-low-birth-weight infants in a convection-warmed, closed-hood incubator environment (Fig. 27–3). The top graph demonstrates the thermal balance achieved by a series of 12 infants (mean weight 1.58 kg). Heat losses to radiation (R), convection (C) and evaporation (E) are modest, and their sum (Σ) is balanced by the infant's metabolic heat production (M). Used in this fashion, the incubator reduces physical heat losses such that the infant's minimal metabolism delicately balances the thermal environment.

In contrast, a very-low-birth-weight subject (1.08 kg) is evaluated in the bottom portion of Figure 27–3. As the incubator's servocontrol increases warming power (to accommodate massive evaporative heat loss), convective "loss" becomes a net "gain" (negative histogram bar). Radiant loss is diminished by warm walls inside the incubator. These conditions differ strikingly from those mentioned earlier: (1) the incubator is now truly warming the infant rather than modestly attenuating convective heat loss and (2) evaporative heat loss vastly exceeds the infant's metabolism. The very small infant's body temperature is balanced, therefore, between opposing physical parameters of evaporative and convective heat transfer: metabolism plays a secondary role.

The modern use of radiant warmers that are servocontrolled to maintain infant abdominal skin temperature between 36.5 and 37°C (97.7 to 98.6° F) also demonstrates the opposition of physical forces described earlier. Figure 27–4 (Baumgart, 1985) demonstrates the heat balance partition for 10 critically ill premature infants (mean weight 1.39 kg) nursed on open radiant warmer beds. Since ambient room air temperature is almost 10° C cooler than air inside an incubator, convective heat loss is nearly double the infant's metabolic heat production. Evaporation adds to the net physical heat loss. The infant's metabolism provides only one-third of the energy required to maintain body temperature, whereas the remainder is supplied by the servo-controlled radiant heat source. In

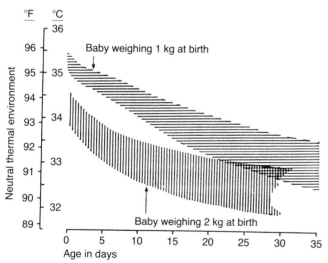

FIGURE 27–2. *The range of temperature needed to provide neutral environmental conditions for a baby lying naked on a warm mattress in draft-free surroundings of moderate humidity (50 per cent saturation) when mean radiant temperature is the same as air temperature. The hatched areas show the average neutral temperature range for a healthy baby weighing 1 kg. (≡) or 2 kg(|||) at birth. Optimum temperature probably approximates to the lower limit of neutral range as defined here. Approximately 1° C should be added to these operative temperatures to derive the appropriate neutral air temperature for a single-walled incubator when room temperature is less than 27° C (80° F), and more should be added if room temperature is very much less than this. (From Hey, E.N., and Katz, G.: Arch. Dis. Child. 45:328,1970.)*

TABLE 27–2. The Mean Temperature Needed to Provide Thermal Neutrality for a Healthy Baby Nursed Naked in Draft-Free Surroundings of Uniform Temperature and Moderate Humidity After Birth

BIRTH WEIGHT (kg)	OPERATIVE ENVIRONMENTAL TEMPERATURE*						
	35° C		34° C		33° C		32° C
1.0	For 10 days	→	After 10 days	→	After 3 weeks	→	After 5 weeks
1.5	—		For 10 days	→	After 10 days	→	After 4 weeks
2.0	—		For 2 days	→	After 2 days	→	After 3 weeks
>2.5	—				For 2 days	→	After 2 days

*To estimate operative temperature in a single-walled incubator, subtract 1° C from incubator air temperature for every 7° C by which this temperature exceeds room temperature.
(Data from Hey, E.: Thermal neutrality. Br. Med. Bull. *31*:72, 1975.)

this instance, radiant warming (not convection as in the incubator discussed earlier) delicately balances the infant's physical temperature environment. Wheldon and Rutter have demonstrated similar results in their studies.

Altering the Partition of Heat Balance. During this decade, several investigators have proposed the use of a variety of heat shields to reduce the opposition of large physical heat losses and gains in incubators and under radiant warmers. Double-walled incubators are available that reduce infant radiant heat loss by warming the interior wall via convection. Thin transparent plastic films have been proposed as blankets or tents over infants within incubators or under radiant warmers to reduce evaporation and convective turbulence by preserving the warm, humid microenvironment layered near the infant's skin. The possibility of a semipermeable membrane adherent to an infant's torso as an artificial barrier has also recently been investigated in this regard. These techniques, although occasionally useful, bear the risk of disrupting the heat partition unpredictably. Cases of hyperthermia have been reported. Their use should be restricted to carefully monitored settings where rigorous attention is given to all aspects of achieving safe thermal balance.

■ CONCLUSIONS

The very-low-birth-weight premature newborn is extremely vulnerable to harsh fluctuations in physical environment. These infants require frequent assessments of skin, core, and air temperatures and relative humidity to design an optimal strategy for thermal regulation. In caring for smaller babies, heat replacment is often required and refinement of techniques to accomplish replacement without inducing hyperthermia is needed.

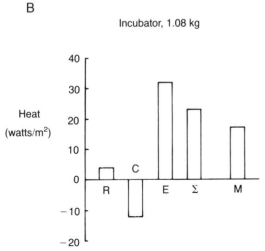

FIGURE 27–3. *A, Partition of heat losses and gains in 12 premature infants nursed within incubators. B, Partition in a 1.08-kg low-birth-weight newborn. (From Wheldon, A. E., and Rutter, N.: Early Hum. Dev. 6:131–143, 1982.)*

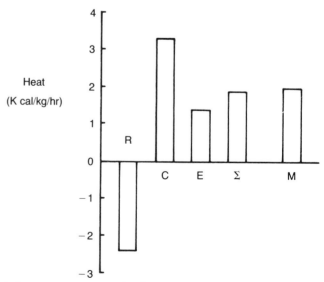

FIGURE 27–4. *Partitional calorimetry in 10 critically ill low-birth-weight premature newborns nursed under open radiant warmers. (From Baumgart, S.: Pediatrics 75:89–99, 1985. Reproduced by permission of Pediatrics.)*

■ REFERENCES

Baumgart, S.: Reduction of oxygen consumption, insensible water loss and radiant heat demand with use of a plastic blanket for low-birth-weight infants under radiant warmers. Pediatrics 74:1022–1028, 1984.

Baumgart, S.: Partitioning of heat losses and gains in premature newborn infants under radiant warmers. Pediatrics 75:89–99, 1985.

Baumgart, S., Fox, W. W., and Polin, R. A.: Physiologic implications of two different heat shields for infants under radiant warmers. J. Pediatr. 100:787–790, 1982.

Bell, E. F., and Rios, G. R.: A double-walled incubator alters the partition of body heat loss of premature infants. Pediatr. Res. 17:135–140, 1983.

Bell, E. F., and Rios, G. R.: Air versus skin temperature servocontrol of infant incubators. J. Pediatr. 103:954–959, 1983.

Bell, E. F., Weinstein, M. R., and Oh, W.: Heat balance in premature infants: comparative effects of convectively heated incubator and radiant warmer, with and without plastic heat shield. J. Pediatr. 96:460–465, 1980.

Bruck, K.: Heat production and temperature regulation. In Stave, U. (Ed.): Perinatal Physiology. New York, Plenum Publishing, 1978, pp. 455–498.

Chessex, P., Blouet, S., and Vaucher, J.: Environmental temperature control in very low birth weight infants (<1000 gms) cared for in double-walled incubators. J. Pediatr. 113:373, 1988.

Hammarlund, K., Strömberg, B., and Sedin, G.: Heat loss from the skin of preterm and full-term newborn infants during the first weeks after birth. Biol. Neonate 50:1–10, 1986.

Hey, E. N. and, Katz, G.: The optimum thermal environment for naked babies. Arch. Dis. Child. 45:328–334, 1970.

Knauth, A., Gordin, P., McNelis, W. and Baumgart, S.: A semipermeable polyurethane membrane as an artificial skin for the premature neonate. Pediatrics 83:945, 1988.

Malin, S., and Baumgart, S.: Optimal thermal management for low birth weight infants nursed under high-power radiant warmers. Pediatrics 79:47–54, 1987.

Marks, K. H., Lee, C. A., Bolan, C. D., and Maisels, M. J.: Oxygen consumption and temperature control of premature infants in a double-wall incubator. Pediatrics 68:93–98, 1981.

Mayfield, S. R., Bhatia, J., Nakamura, K. T., et al.: Temperature measurement in term and preterm neonates. J. Pediatr. 104:271–275, 1984.

Okken, A., Blijham, C., Franz, W., and Bohn, E.: Effects of forced convection of heated air on insensible water loss and heat loss in preterm infants in incubators. J. Pediatr. 101:108–112,1982.

Scopes, J. W.: Thermoregulation in the Newborn. In Avery, C. B. (Ed.): Neonatology, Pathophysiology and Management of the Newborn. 2nd ed. Philadelphia, J. B. Lippincott Company, 1981, pp. 171–181.

Silverman, W. A., Sinclair, J. C., and Agate, F. J.: The oxygen cost of minor changes in heat balance of small newborn infants. Acta Paediatr. Scand. 55:294, 1966.

Wheldon, A. E., and Rutter, N.: The heat balance of small babies nursed in incubators and under radiant warmers. Early Hum. Dev. 6:131–143, 1982.

■ SUGGESTED READINGS

Dawkins, M. J. R., and Hull, D.: The production of heat by fat. Sci. Am. 213:62, 1965.

Day, R. L., Caliguiri, L, Kaminski, C., et al.: Body temperature and survival of premature infants. Pediatrics 34:171, 1964.

Hull, D.: Brown adipose tissue. Br. Med. Bull. 22:92, 1966.

ACID BASE, FLUID AND ELECTROLYTE MANAGEMENT

28

J. Usha Raj and George Franco

At the moment of birth we are confronted with a sudden and dramatic change, thrust instantly from an aquatic into an arid environment. Neonatal physiology is uniquely and specifically adapted for this profound transition. Fluid and electrolyte management for newborn infants therefore requires of the physician an understanding of the adaptive processes utilized during this transitional period. Whereas for other patients the goal of fluid therapy is to achieve homeostasis, for the newborn the goal is rather to allow for a successful transition. In the case of the premature infant, this transition is made more difficult by the immaturity of important organ systems, and so a basic familiarity with certain aspects of fetal developmental physiology is necessary for clinical decision making.

■ BODY FLUID COMPARTMENTS IN THE FETAL AND NEONATAL PERIOD

CHANGES IN BODY WATER COMPOSITION DURING GROWTH

Total body water is distributed between an extracellular and an intracellular space. The extracellular space is further divided into the intravascular compartment (which is the plasma volume) and the interstitial compartment. The intracellular compartment includes the space in all cells, including red blood cells. Together, plasma and red cell volume add up to blood volume.

In the first few weeks of fetal life, 95 per cent of body weight is water (Friis-Hansen, 1961). As the cell mass and blood volume are small, most of this water is extracellular. As the fetus grows in utero, significant changes occur in the amount and distribution of water in the body. As cells proliferate and organs mature, the dry weight of cell mass and intracellular fluid (ICF) volume increase. This results in a concomitant decrease in the percentage of body weight that is water and a decrease in extracellular fluid (ECF) volume (Fig. 28–1). Therefore, a fetus born at 25 weeks' gestation may have 85 per cent of its body weight as water and 60 per cent of its body weight as extracellular water. However, by term, his or her total body water is only 78 per cent of body weight and the extracellular water is 45 per cent of body weight (Strauss, 1966).

As the fetus grows and there is a change in the fractional contribution of the various fluid compartments to total body weight, the total amount and distribution of the

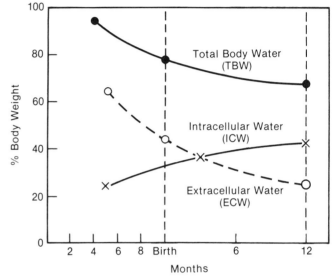

FIGURE 28–1. Changes in body fluid composition during fetal and neonatal life. (Adapted from Friis-Hansen, B.: Pediatrics 47 [Suppl.]: 264, 1971. Reproduced by permission of Pediatrics.)

solutes in the body also change (Fig. 28–2). The electrolyte composition of plasma and interstitial fluid is the same. The major difference between these two compartments of extracellular fluid is the protein content; the protein content of interstitial fluid is approximately two-thirds that of

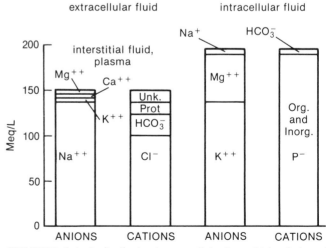

FIGURE 28–2. Ionic distribution in extracellular (interstitial and plasma) and intracellular fluid compartments.

plasma. The main cation in extracellular fluid is sodium, with potassium, calcium, and magnesium making up the balance. Chloride is the main anion, with protein, bicarbonate, and some undetermined anions constituting the balance. In the intracellular fluid compartment, potassium is the main cation, with magnesium and calcium contributing smaller fractions to the total cation pool. Organic and inorganic phosphates constitute the major fraction of anions, with bicarbonate contributing a very small fraction. As the fetus grows and the extracellular fluid compartment decreases, the amount of electrolytes in this compartment also decreases proportionately. This natural progression implies that a fetus born prematurely will have a greater amount of extracellular water and sodium in comparison with the term infant. Fluid and electrolyte composition of the fetus is significantly influenced by maternal fluid and electrolyte state and placental exchange. Maternal dehydration and overhydration during the immediate period before birth will affect body hydration in the newly born infant. Prematurely born newborns whose mothers have received large volumes of intravenous fluids as part of the treatment of preterm labor may have an excess of extracellular water and are likely to be hyponatremic (Rojas et al., 1984).

CHANGES IN BODY WATER AND ELECTROLYTE COMPOSITION AFTER BIRTH

Changes in body water composition continue after birth. However, if the fetus is born prematurely, total body cell mass and organ size do not increase at the same rate immediately after birth as in utero. Consequently, although the contraction of the extracellular water compartment continues, the intracellular water compartment does not increase in size immediately and the newborn infant loses weight in the first few days of life. The presence of lung disease such as respiratory distress syndrome, the immaturity of the gastrointestinal system, and the need to frequently change the composition and volume of intravenous fluids in the extremely premature infant usually result in a delay in achievement of adequate caloric intake. The smaller the gestational age and weight of the newborn, the greater is the fraction of birth weight that is lost in the immediate postnatal period. This fact is demonstrated in the growth curves constructed by Dancis and colleagues (1948) for low-birth-weight infants. It is interesting that even today, with our improved knowledge of enteral and parenteral nutrition for low-birth-weight infants, the Dancis growth curves, which were constructed in the 1940s, closely approximate the growth curves seen in newborn infants. Once nutritional intake is adequate, the newborn starts gaining weight, with contraction of the extracellular fluid compartment and expansion of the intracellular compartment (see Appendix 3).

Postnatal contraction of the extracellular fluid compartment is important for improvement of renal function and increase in urine output (Oh et al., 1966). If fluid and electrolyte overloading occurs in the first week of life, there may be a delay in the usual increase in urine output, and the expanded extracellular fluid compartment may predispose to the development of patent ductus arteriosus (PDA) and necrotizing enterocolitis (Bell et al., 1979, 1980). Lack of contraction of the extracellular fluid com-

partment may also lead to pulmonary edema with worsening gas exchange, necessitating an increase in and prolongation of oxygen and mechanical ventilation therapy (Spitzer et al., 1981).

▪ CHANGING RENAL FUNCTION IN THE NEONATAL PERIOD

DEVELOPMENT OF GLOMERULAR FILTRATION AND RENAL PERFUSION

The glomerular filtration rate (GFR) depends on the rate of plasma flow through the glomerular capillaries, the total capillary surface area, and the permeability of the capillaries to water. GFR is also affected by the gradient of hydrostatic and oncotic pressures across the glomerular membrane. In utero, the fetus does not have a full complement of nephrons until 35 weeks' gestation (McDonald and Emery, 1959), after which the number of nephrons does not change although the capillary surface area continues to increase following birth. Glomerular filtration rate is very low in utero, mainly owing to a very high renal vascular resistance and low renal plasma flow (Aperia and Herin, 1975; Ichikawa and Brenner, 1978). After birth, there is an immediate decrease in renal vascular resistance, resulting in increased renal plasma flow and glomerular filtration (Aperia et al., 1981). Thereafter, over the first few weeks of life, there is a continued increase in GFR as a result of several factors: a progressive rise in systemic blood pressures (Versmold et al., 1981), a further decrease in renal vascular resistance (Aperia and Herin, 1975; Ichikawa and Brenner, 1978), and a gradual decrease in hematocrit (Aperia et al., 1974).

At birth, GFR is lower in preterm infants than in term infants (Guignard, 1977). Although the rate at which GFR increases in the first weeks of life is similar in preterm and term infants, the actual values remain lower in the preterm infants throughout the first month of life (Leake et al., 1976). GFR is more dependent on extracellular fluid volume during infancy than later in life. An acute expansion of extracellular fluid volume results in an increase in GFR, largely due to an increase in renal plasma flow (Elinder et al., 1980). However, if an excess of intravenous fluid administration should result in an expanded extracellular fluid space together with hyponatremia, output might fall even though GFR would increase because of the increase in renal tubular sodium reabsorption.

SODIUM BALANCE

At term, the kidney is capable of efficient reabsorption of filtered sodium, which the newborn utilizes for growth. Although the full complement of cortical nephrons are present (which are salt-losing in function), filtered sodium is reabsorbed in the proximal tubule (Dean and McCance, 1949). In addition, a blunted renin feedback system results in relatively high aldosterone levels, which results in increased distal tubular reabsorption of sodium (Spitzer, 1982). The preterm infant is handicapped in two directions: (1) The kidney is not capable of efficient reabsorption of sodium, with resultant high urinary losses of sodium; and (2) in the event of a high sodium load being delivered to the kidney, it is not capable of increasing sodium excretion. The high fractional excretion of sodium, between 5 and 15 per cent, is due to deficient proximal tubular reabsorption and relative insensitivity of the distal tubule to high circulating levels of aldosterone. The inability of the preterm kidney to increase (Sulyok et al., 1979) sodium excretion above the relatively fixed high excretion rate is due to an inability of the preterm infant to increase GFR and an inability to redirect renal blood flow toward more mature, salt-losing cortical nephrons (Spitzer, 1982). Consequently, the preterm infant requires significant amounts of sodium to replace high baseline losses, but any excess sodium given will result in sodium and water retention.

WATER BALANCE

Sodium and water balance are linked in the kidney, as tubular water reabsorption is determined by the diffusional gradient created by active sodium transport. Independent of active sodium transport, the neonatal kidney is capable of regulating water balance to some extent and can dilute or concentrate the urine.

The diluting segment of the kidney, i.e., the ascending loop of Henle and the distal tubule, is well developed even in the premature infant (Robillard et al., 1979). A greater reabsorption of solute than of water by this portion of the kidney results in a dilute urine with urine osmolality as low as 30 to 50 mOsm/l. Despite this well-developed diluting ability, if a water load is given to a preterm infant, the delivery of filtrate to the diluting segment is insufficient and the infant tends to become water-loaded because GFR cannot be increased sufficiently.

The concentrating ability of the neonatal kidney is relatively limited. The final concentration of urine occurs in the collecting ducts. Antidiuretic hormone (ADH) makes the cells of the collecting ducts more permeable to water. However, for selective reabsorption of water but not of solutes to occur, the interstitium of the inner medulla has to be hypertonic. Hypertonicity of the medullary interstitium is maintained by the countercurrent mechanism of the loop of Henle. A relatively short loop of Henle and a distal tubule that is relatively insensitive to ADH (Edelman et al., 1959) results in a medullary interstitial osmolality no higher than 600 to 700 mOsm/l. Hence the neonatal kidney usually cannot concentrate urine beyond 700 mOsm/l.

These two major limitations, a low GFR leading to impaired excretion of water and a limited concentrating ability, result in a narrow margin of error in the administration of free water to the newborn.

ELECTROLYTE AND SOLUTE BALANCE

POTASSIUM

Potassium excretion remains low throughout gestation. Potassium is first filtered passively into the glomerulus and is then almost completely reabsorbed by the proximal tubule. Renal regulation of potassium in the body is done through excretion of potassium by the distal tubule, especially in response to aldosterone. In the distal tubule, sodium is reabsorbed in exchange for potassium, which is then excreted in the urine. In the extremely premature

infant, the mechanism of potassium excretion is impaired. First, because GFR is low, the amount of potassium that is filtered is low. Second, the distal tubule is relatively insensitive to aldosterone in the preterm kidney. This results in both sodium loss in the urine and a reduction in potassium excretion. This is manifested as a high urine sodium/potassium ratio (> 6) in the very premature infant (Sulyok et al., 1979). These two factors are sufficient to produce significant hyperkalemia in the preterm infant, when potassium administration is in excess of excretion. On occasion, when insensible water losses are high and the preterm infant becomes dehydrated, severe hyperkalemia can develop even in the absence of parenteral administration of potassium. The ability of the kidney to excrete potassium improves with increasing postnatal age.

Increased potassium losses in the urine can result when proximal tubular reabsorption of potassium is impaired, as in stressed newborns (Engle and Arant, 1984), or when diuretics are used.

GLUCOSE

Glomerulotubular balance for glucose is present very early in gestation (Brodehl et al., 1972). However, in the very premature infant a low renal threshold for glucose may exist (Stonestreet et al., 1980). Significant glucosuria will result in an excessive loss of water, sodium, and other solutes in the urine.

■ INSENSIBLE WATER LOSSES IN THE NEONATAL PERIOD

Free water loss occurs through passive evaporation from the skin and other epithelial surfaces exposed to air and is known as insensible water loss. Most of the evaporative water loss occurs through the skin, although losses from the respiratory system can be quite significant in infants who are tachypneic and in those who are breathing dry air. The major determinants of the magnitude of insensible water loss from the skin are the infant's environment, gestational age at birth, postnatal age, the relationship of body surface to size, and the metabolic rate.

After birth the infant is surrounded by an environment that is cooler and drier than the intrauterine milieu. Unless the surrounding air has 100 per cent humidity, an evaporative gradient is set up from the infant's skin to the ambient air. The lower the water vapor pressure in the ambient air, the greater is this evaporative gradient, resulting in greater evaporative water losses. Another factor that affects evaporative water losses is the presence of convective air currents. If the ambient air is still, the infant develops a microenvironment in which the air is humidified completely through his or her own evaporative water losses. However, if the infant is surrounded by convective air currents, the turbulence continuously disturbs this warm and humid layer of air, resulting in high evaporative water losses. Finally, when the infant is placed directly under a radiant warmer, the radiant heat may have a direct drying effect on skin water content, resulting in greater evaporative water losses. Insensible water losses also depend on gestational age. The mature infant has a well-cornified epithelial layer of skin. The keratin in the superficial epithelial cells and a lipid layer on the skin act as waterproofing agents, retarding evaporative water losses. The premature infant lacks this cornified layer, so that living epidermal epithelial cells are directly in contact with air, resulting in large evaporative water losses. Also, the premature infant lacks subcutaneous fat, and the capillaries in the interstitium underlying the skin are in close proximity to the ambient air. The large body surface area in relation to body weight and much larger total body water content predispose the premature infant to very large evaporative water losses (Hammarlund and Sedin, 1979).

Hyperthermia and an increased metabolic rate will increase insensible water loss by increasing skin blood flow. Postnatal age significantly affects the rate of skin evaporative water loss in premature infants. With age, the skin matures very rapidly, so that the evaporative water loss may decrease three- to fourfold by the end of the first week of life (Hammarlund and Sedin, 1983). Evaporative water loss and total body heat loss are linked. With increased evaporative water losses the infant loses considerable body heat, as 58 calories are lost for each 1 ml of water evaporated at 37°C. If the body is overheated by exposure to high ambient temperatures, the excess heat dissipation is achieved mainly via evaporative water and heat losses. However, if the ambient air temperature is lower than the neutral thermal range and the infant has to generate extra heat to maintain a normal core temperature, heat loss from the body to the cooler environment is mainly by radiation. Insensible water loss has been expressed in a variety of ways. Since evaporative water loss leads to heat loss and increased caloric expenditure, it has been expressed as ml/100 kcal/day. However, evaporative water loss is also dependent on body surface area and size, so it has been expressed as ml/m²/hr or ml/kg/hr. In general, insensible water loss is expressed as volume of water lost/kg body weight/hr.

The values for full-term mature infants with a resting metabolic rate have ranged from 0.7 to 1.6 ml/kg/hr (Hey and Katz, 1969; Oh and Karecki, 1972). With decreasing gestational age, the evaporative water loss increases exponentially, so that preterm infants between 25 and 26 weeks' gestation may have water losses that are 15 times higher than those in a full-term infant (Fig. 28–3).

This basal rate of insensible water loss may be increased or decreased by the various factors discussed. Temperature and humidity of the infant's environment are key factors modulating insensible water loss. Most preterm infants require additional heat in order to maintain body temperature in a physiologic range. The more immature the infant, the greater the need to heat the environment. The neutral thermal environment is that range of thermal environment in which an infant can maintain body temperature in the normal range without increasing heat production or evaporative water loss by more than 25 per cent. The range of neutral thermal environment for different-sized babies is shown in Figure 28–4 (Hey, 1971). The dark line indicates the optimum temperature and the shaded area the range of environmental temperature for naked (upper panel) and clothed (lower panel) infants. These values are obtained in a draft-free environment with 50 per cent humidity and no radiant heat losses, i.e., the infant is in a double-walled incubator, so that there is no radiant heat loss from the baby to the incubator wall.

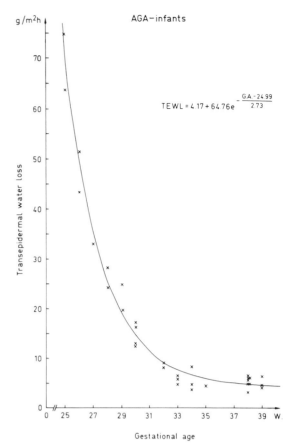

FIGURE 28–3. *Transepidermal water loss (TEWL) in newborn infants in relation to gestational age (G.A.). (AGA, appropriate for gestational age: W, completed weeks of gestation.) (From Hammarlund, K., and Sedin, G.: Acta Pediatr. Scand. 68:795–801, 1979.)*

It is interesting to note that elevation of the ambient temperature above the neutral thermal environment results in a significant increase in insensible water loss through an increase in evaporative heat loss. However, if the ambient temperature is below the neutral thermal range, the infant increases endogenous heat production to maintain body temperature but reduces the evaporative heat losses and therefore insensible water loss (Bell et al., 1980). (See also Chapter 27.)

The most efficient way to reduce insensible water loss is to place the infant in an environment with high relative humidity and ambient air in the neutral thermal range. Use of heat shields and double-walled incubators will also reduce evaporative water losses. Finally, keeping the environment undisturbed by reducing air drafts will preserve the humid warm-air blanket around the infant's body and thus reduce evaporative water losses. Although all these strategies will reduce evaporative water losses, in a very immature infant, on the first day of life, insensible water losses can be considerable. Unless counteracted, insensible water losses may result in severe hyperosmolar dehydration in a very short time. Osmolality of serum is normally 285 to 295 mOsm/l. The osmolality is determined by the number of osmotically active molecules (osmoles) dissolved in water. In the laboratory, osmolality is determined in a volume of plasma; as 1 L of plasma consists of 940 ml of water and 60 g of protein, the plasma value is lower than the true osmolality of blood. This difference is quite small, however, and an approxi-

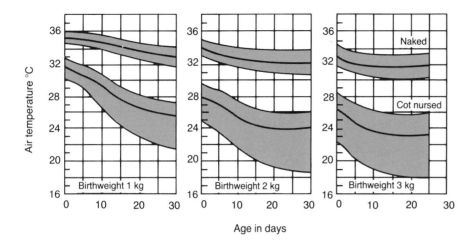

FIGURE 28–4. The range of temperature needed to provide neutral environmental conditions for a body lying either naked or dressed in a cot, in an environment that is draft free and with a relatively high humidity (50 per cent saturation) when mean radiant temperature is the same as air temperature. The dark line is the neutral temperature, and hatched area is the neutral thermal range. (From Hey, E.: The care of babies in incubation. In Hull, D., and Gairdner, D. [Eds.]: Recent Advances in Pediatrics. London, Churchill, 1971.)

mate estimate can be obtained by doubling the serum sodium concentration, as sodium and an equal number of anions are the main determinants of serum osmolality. In certain situations, such an estimation may be erroneous. For example, during a period of hyperlipidemia the volume of water in plasma is decreased further. If sodium is measured in a plasma sample, a marked hyponatremia will be present, which disappears when the lipid is extracted and sodium measured in plasma water. Increased concentrations of glucose and urea can also lead to erroneous estimation of plasma osmolality, if calculated from serum sodium concentrations alone. If plasma glucose concentration were 90 mg/100 ml, glucose would contribute 5 mOsm/L, and higher glucose levels in plasma would increase serum osmolality. The baby needs to maintain plasma osmolality in a normal range, and as the cellular metabolism of glucose cannot be increased, the osmotically active glucose draws water from the intracellular to the extracellular compartment to achieve osmotic equilibrium. This results in an expanded extracellular compartment and dilutional hyponatremia. Such shifts in fluid between the two compartments, with contraction of the intracellular compartment, can lead to intracranial hemorrhages. Additionally, hyperglycemia with increased plasma osmolality can lead to an osmotic diuresis and excessive losses of water and electrolytes.

■ FLUID AND ELECTROLYTE MANAGEMENT

The physiologic principles outlined in the previous sections must be used as the basis for gathering and interpreting actual patient data in order to properly diagnose and treat neonatal fluid and electrolyte problems. In applying them, one begins with an assessment of the patient.

PATIENT EVALUATION

PATIENT HISTORY

At birth, unless a specific congenital condition such as hydrops exists, the infant's fluid and electrolyte status is most importantly affected by maternal conditions. For example, the use of diuretics by the mother, attempts at induction of labor with oxytocin or hypotonic intravenous (IV) hydration can result in neonatal hyponatremia. The

presence of any particular disorders of birth is important: Was there asphyxia, potentially limiting renal function? Is there pulmonary disease or infection? Was there a trapped cord or abruption? Finally, in the days following birth, we need a history of the care the baby has received: Has there been feeding? Have radiant warmers been used? Are there any drainage tubes? What has the urine output been?

PHYSICAL EXAMINATION

Body weight is an important "laboratory value" to obtain when assessing fluid balance in a newborn. Accurate serial measurements of body weight plotted on a weight curve are essential. Fluid status can change rapidly and dramatically, especially in the smaller, very-low-birthweight infants. The difficulty of obtaining such measurements can be greatest in these cases, and the potential stresses imposed by the process may present a danger to the infant. This information must always be used in conjunction with information on serum electrolyte and urine output. Acute changes in body weight reflect changes in total body water.

Dry skin and mucous membranes are seen when 5 per cent dehydration occurs. Although difficult to assess for subtle changes in newborns, skin turgor and texture can be useful signs as time goes on, and changes are usually obvious at 10 per cent dehydration, as is a sunken fontanel, a sign unique to the neonate and one that should be looked for. Circulatory changes with tachycardia and low blood pressure occur very late, at about 15 per cent dehydration.

Signs of edema should be sought in dependent areas and in the pretibial and facial areas.

LABORATORY EVALUATION

Serum electrolyte determinations, mainly for sodium and potassium, are extremely important. Blood glucose determinations should be done routinely on all newborns until adequate nutrition is established and on an ongoing basis in sick infants.

Renal function is sometimes difficult to assess in the newborn because of the many factors influencing kidney performance (Arant, 1981). Urine specific gravity is important as well as the quantity of urine, although interpretation of this value requires factoring in many considerations. The creatinine at birth mainly reflects maternal values; it normally decreases postnatally, depending on gestational age, but should never increase.

GENERAL PRINCIPLES

As with any other age group, planning for fluid therapy in the newborn has three stages:
- Estimate the present fluid and electrolyte deficits or excesses, and calculate the proper replacements.
- Calculate the ongoing maintenance requirements (and any unusual continuing losses).
- Plan for continuing evaluation of the effectiveness of therapy and need for corrections.

ESTIMATE DEFICITS OR EXCESSES

Whenever possible, sequential data on body weight should be obtained. Accurate estimation of fluid status in the newborn period is quite difficult otherwise. Since a 5 to 10 per cent loss in body weight due to reduction of total body water is anticipated during the first week to 10 days of life, during this time weight should be plotted on the standard newborn growth curves to determine whether the change is appropriate or excessive. Once it has been established that the patient is normal, dehydrated, or overhydrated, the serum sodium can be used to classify the state as normonatremic, hypernatremic ($[Na^+] > 150$), or hyponatremic ($[Na^+] < 130$) and to calculate the deficit or surfeit of the electrolyte. Maintenance needs of the newborn after the 1st 48 hours are generally 2 to 3 mEq/kg/day.

Volume should be replaced with an urgency reflecting the degree of deficit and the pace of its development. Losses that occur acutely usually require a fairly brisk response, with IV therapy preferred in sick infants.

In hyponatremic states, sodium replacement can be estimated by assuming 70 per cent of total body weight (TBW) as the distribution space for sodium (obviously a rough estimate, since TBW is a changing value). Then one needs to calculate the amount of sodium required to raise the concentration of that space by the desired amount:

$$Na^+ \text{ deficit (mEq)} \approx 0.7 \times Kg \times ([Na^+]_{desired} - [Na^+]_{actual})$$

The sodium should be replaced on a schedule whereby about two thirds is replaced on the first day of treatment and the remainder on the second day. Repeated measurements are needed to assure that the estimated correction is working. Since the loss is assumed to be from the TBW, potassium, as the main intracellular electrolyte, will also need to be replaced but only after adequate renal function is established. High concentrations or rapid infusions of K^+ should be avoided. Generally, 2 to 4 mEq/kg/day is prescribed.

In hypernatremic dehydration, a more gradual correction should be planned. Rapid lowering of serum osmolality can lead to convulsions, brain swelling, and death. Both hypernatremia and too rapid correction of it have been associated with IVH in premature infants. Generally, $[Na^+]$ should be lowered by no more than about 10 mEq/day. The reverse of the calculation shown above can be used to estimate the amount of free water needed to bring $[Na^+]$ to normal:

$$H_2O \text{ deficit (liters)} \approx (0.7 \times Kg) \times \left(\frac{[Na^+]_{desired}}{[Na^+]_{actual}} - 1\right)$$

MAINTENANCE REQUIREMENTS

In calculating the maintenance requirements for a neonate, three factors must be considered.

First, consideration must be given to the infant's gestational age as well as the postnatal age. In all children, the days immediately following birth require an adjustment of total body water and sodium, as discussed previously. Therefore, it is perhaps more appropriate to speak of adaptive requirements rather than of maintenance requirements. Term infants are born well prepared with a surfeit of fluid volume and well-established glycogen stores, and they tolerate quite safely, if not quietly, the initial fast they must endure while awaiting the onset of lactation. Even some premature and low-birth-weight infants who are otherwise well have been found to survive thirst and fast in the initial days of life without becoming dangerously dehydrated (Hansen and Smith, 1953).

The goal of fluid therapy in term babies and in larger premature well babies in the first days of life should be simply prevention of dehydration and maintenance of adequate glucose homeostasis. Once fluid contraction has occurred, as evidenced by a weight loss of no more than 10 per cent over the first 3 days and some falling off of urine volume and an increase in concentration, fluid allowance can be increased to match losses—for a net zero balance and homeostasis.

The driving factor for intake on the first day is usually the serum glucose. If no nutritive intake is needed to combat hypoglycemia, the intake can be essentially zero. Otherwise, only the lowest intake consistent with the demands of intermediary metabolism needs to be offered. Small premature infants require stringent management, as is discussed later, whereas more mature infants are generally able to tolerate a wider latitude in fluid therapy. Even so, weight gain in the first 3 days of life indicates overhydration.

In an infant who is being maintained on intravenous therapy, a solution of 10 per cent glucose will usually provide adequate sugar given at a rate of 50 to 60 ml/kg/day. There is no requirement for salt on the first day of life.

Next, consideration must be given to the normal losses that constitute an infant's ongoing maintenance requirement. These are most importantly the insensible water losses and urine output. Fecal losses are negligible at this stage, and sweat losses are essentially nonexistent in most infants.

As discussed earlier, renal function may be limited but is not inadequate in newborns. The output will be dependent upon the solute load presented, when maximally concentrated at 700 to 800 mOsm/L; if a 25 mOsm/kg solute load were presented (typical for an infant on IV feeding solutions only), about 35 ml/kg/day of urine would be required at a minimum. A less concentrated urine would require 65 to 70 ml/kg/day.

An insensible loss of about 35 ml/kg/day is typical, so

a balance might be achieved at around 90 to 95 ml/kg/day. Over the first 2 or 3 days, fluid rates should be increased up to this range.

After the first day or so of life, electrolytes can be provided. The usual electrolyte intake of a feeding infant would be about 2 to 3 mEq/kg/ day of sodium, and so that seems a reasonable starting allowance for parenteral therapy. Potassium, 1 to 2 mEq/kg/day, is also given on the same basis. Both are normally given as the chloride salts. When on intravenous therapy, infants should have serum electrolytes determined daily and adjustments made accordingly.

Finally, certain factors may operate to modify the estimated requirements. Any alterations in renal function need to be accounted for, especially decreased functioning due to disease or hypoxia. Harmful overhydration will result rapidly, especially as the newborn already has increased body water. Insensible water losses are also variable. The use of radiant warmers can increase water requirements by 45 to 60 ml/kg/day because of insensible skin evaporative losses. Phototherapy increases insensible loss, probably by increasing skin blood flow, and also increases stool loss slightly because photodegradation products decrease stool transit time. An additional 20 ml/kg/day may be required under phototherapy.

Humidified air from ventilators and hoods can reduce evaporation from the lungs to near zero, and so decreases insensible losses by about 10 to 20 ml/kg/day.

The effects on fluid balance of particular disease states and clinical conditions will be discussed below, but consideration of ongoing requirements needs to address such special circumstances. Continuous losses, such as from gastrostomy drainage or chest tubes, need to be factored in. These usually have a significant electrolyte content, as can be determined by laboratory measurement, if necessary.

■ SPECIFIC CLINICAL CONDITIONS

THE VERY PREMATURE INFANT (25 TO 27 WEEKS' GESTATION)

The major problems of these infants relate to fluid and electrolyte management, respiratory distress syndrome that frequently evolves into chronic lung disease, infection, and intraventricular hemorrhage. As the infant's need for respiratory support is immediate and dramatic, the care giver frequently focuses on the management of respiratory insufficiency for the first few hours. Often, ventilator support is initiated in the delivery room, which is usually cool and dry, so that the infant arrives in the intensive care unit having experienced significant cold stress. Once in the intensive care unit, he or she is usually placed under an open radiant warmer, as rewarming efforts are made and also because easy access to the infant is needed to place various intravenous and intra-arterial lines and to make ventilator adjustments for optimal gas exchange. The infant may spend several hours under the radiant warmer before it is recognized that enormous insensible water losses have occurred. This cycle of events, namely immediate cold stress followed by excessive insensible water losses and dehydration, should be avoided.

Since thermoregulation and water homeostasis are linked, the regulation of the infant's temperature and fluid and electrolyte management should be considered together. In the delivery room, if the birth of an extremely premature infant is anticipated, the ambient air temperature must be raised to uncomfortable (for adults) levels of 30 to 32°C. As soon as the infant is delivered, care must be taken to reduce insensible water losses. As long as the infant is kept under a radiant warmer, insensible water losses may be as much as 15 ml/kg/hr in a 25 weeks' gestation infant, decreasing to 5 to 7.5 ml/kg/hr in the 27 weeks' gestation infant. With the use of heat shields and plastic wraps, these values can be decreased. The best approach is to place the infant in a double-walled Plexiglas incubator so heated that the temperature inside is within the neutral thermal range for the extremely small infant. The infant can be transferred into the incubator as soon as intubation and line placement have been accomplished. The environment should be well humidified to further decrease insensible water losses. This can be done by blowing warm mist generated via a nebulizer into the incubator. If the ambient air is in the neutral thermal range and the humidity is close to 100 per cent, insensible water losses will be decreased by 30 to 50 per cent.

If one adds to the insensible water losses the amount of water required for basal metabolism and urinary water losses, for infants between 25 and 27 weeks of gestation who are nursed under open radiant warmers or in humidified incubators, the volume of water required in the first few hours of life can range from 400 to 180 ml/kg/day. Basal glucose requirements are between 5 and 8 mg/kg/min; hence this large volume of fluid must be given as dilute glucose solutions—2 to 5 g/100 ml dextrose solutions. Also, as insensible water losses usually exceed urinary losses in the first few hours of life, the infant will require little or no sodium and potassium supplementation.

Immediately after birth, unless the infant is extremely stressed and asphyxiated, urine output is usually up to 2 ml/kg/hr. Over the first 2 to 3 days, urine output usually increases, reaching 5 to 7 ml/kg/hr. The fractional excretion of sodium is very high (10 to 15 percent), and hence urinary sodium losses are very high. Urinary potassium losses are usually not excessive, unless the kidneys have been damaged. In the presence of renal tubular necrosis, urine output can be as high as 10 to 15 ml/kg/hr with high urine sodium and potassium losses. After 2 to 3 days of life, the premature infant's skin is more mature and insensible water losses decrease. However, urinary water losses continue to increase. Therefore total water requirements will increase and electrolyte requirements will change. The infant now requires replenishment of urinary sodium losses, which can be very high, necessitating the use of 35 to 70 mEq/L saline solutions for intravenous fluid therapy. Oliguria is rare in very premature babies. Urine output continues in the face of severe dehydration, as the infant has an almost fixed high obligatory sodium loss in the urine. Also, as the infant loses weight, the extracellular fluid compartment contracts with preservation of the intravascular fluid compartment, so that renal perfusion is preserved. It is not uncommon, therefore, to find that an infant has lost as much as 20 to 25 per cent of body weight in 24 to 48 hours without any evidence of circulatory collapse. The most frequent complication resulting from suboptimal fluid and electrolyte therapy in the first 2 days of life is hyperosmolar dehydration associated with severe hypernatremia, without evidence of circulatory collapse, acidosis, or oliguria (Baumgart et al., 1982; Gruskay et al., 1988). Frequently this is associated with intraventricular hemorrhage. Hypernatremia, with serum sodium > 160 mEq/L, can result from an excessive loss of free water via the skin with relatively little sodium loss in urine. Hyperkalemia can develop even in the absence of potassium supplementation to the infant, as the immature kidney is not able to excrete potassium adequately. Hyperglycemia may result from excessive infusion of glucose and a relative insulin insufficiency and insulin resistance (Fisher, 1976). As the glucose utilization rate is low, infusion of glucose exceeding 5 to 8 mg/kg/min will invariably result in hyperglycemia in these infants. This may lead to glucosuria and an osmotic diuresis that will aggravate urinary losses of water and sodium.

After the first 24 to 48 hours of life, when urinary losses of water and sodium are very high, a common complication is dehydration associated with hyponatremia. If sodium replacement is being given at the "standard" 2 to 3 mEq/kg/day, serum sodium may fall below 120 mEq/L, rarely requiring treatment with sodium of up to 12 mEq/kg body weight/day. Always be sure that hyponatremia is not the result of excessive free water administration.

Finally, overzealous replacement of water and sodium may result in an absence of weight loss and a lack of contraction of the extracellular water compartment. This state invariably results in worsening of respiratory problems and may be associated with a significant left-to-right shunt across a patent ductus arteriosus. It is important, therefore, that the infant lose weight and contract the extracellular fluid compartment. This should occur gradually over several days, and total weight loss should not exceed 10 to 15 per cent of birth weight.

The following suggestions help avoid these complications.

First 24 hours: Calculate insensible water losses based on infant's gestational age, body weight, and environment. Replace this loss as free water. Urine losses are to be replaced as free water in the first day of life. Total water requirements will usually range from 100 to 180 ml/kg/day. Glucose infusion should run at the rate of 5 mg/kg/min. No sodium or potassium supplementation is needed. In the first 24 hours, follow urine output and, if a bed scale is available, weigh the infant every 8 hours and monitor serum electrolytes q 6–8 h. The infant should lose about 2 to 5 per cent of birth weight. Fluid and electrolyte requirements are to be calculated and written every 6 to 8 hours. Calcium supplementation should be aimed at keeping serum calcium between 8 to 9 mg/dl.

Day 2–4: Start replacing sodium losses. The aim should be to keep serum sodium between 130 and 145 mEq/L. Glucose infusion rate should remain relatively constant. Total water requirement may be as high as 180 ml/kg/day, and sodium requirement is usually 2 to 3 mEq/kg/L but rarely can be as high as 10 to 12 mEq/kg/day. Potassium can be added at 2 to 4 mEq/kg/day.

Day 4–7: During this period, nutritional intake should be gradually increased either enterally or parenterally. Furthermore, attempts must be made to determine whether renal tubular function is improving. Once the

water and electrolyte requirement for an 8- to 12-hour period has been calculated, the actual amount given to the infant should be reduced by 10 to 20 per cent. If the infant does not lose an excessive amount of weight or maintains body weight unchanged, the kidney is capable of increasing salt and water reabsorption. Such challenges must be continued each day so that water and sodium administration can be reduced.

■ ACID-BASE BALANCE IN THE FETUS AND NEWBORN

Although the principles of physical chemistry are no different in newborns, certain physiologic and anatomic limitations do exist, especially in premature infants, which restrict their ability to compensate for alterations in acid-base chemistry and to respond to therapeutic maneuvers, particularly in regard to brain blood flow.

PHYSIOLOGIC ACID-BASE CHEMISTRY

Acidity refers to the level of hydrogen ion concentration in body fluids. We measure $[H^+]$ using electrochemical meters that record pH, its inverse log;*

$$pH = \log_{10} \left\{ \frac{1}{[H^+]} \right\}$$

At the physiologic pH of 7.4, therefore, $[H^+] \approx 4 \times 10^{-8}$ Eq/l, making it a "trace substance," at a concentration four to seven orders of magnitude lower than most other physiologically important ions. The pH of a solution cannot be changed by simply adding or subtracting individual protons (or hydronium ions) even if there were a way to do this, since they do not really have an independent existence (Stewart, 1981). In solution, $[H^+]$ is dissociated from water and is in an equilibrium with $[OH^-]$. At any given temperature and solute concentration the product $[H^+] \times [OH^-]$ is a constant, K'_w, the ion product for water. $[H^+]$ is also in equilibrium with various weak organic acids, defined by their dissociation constants, and in electrical neutrality with various strong ions. It is thus a dependent variable (Stewart, 1981) that changes in response to changes in other variables, notably strong ion concentrations, especially $[Na^+]$ and $[Cl^-]$ and, very importantly, the dissociation of H^+ and HCO_3^- from H_2CO_3, carbonic acid. This relationship is expressed in the Henderson-Hasselbalch equation:

$$pH = 6.1 + \log_{10} \left\{ \frac{[HCO_3^-]}{[H_2CO_3]} \right\}$$

In turn, $[H_2CO_3]$ is derived from dissolved CO_2, the concentration of which is fixed by the pCO_2 as regulated by the lungs. A clinically useful form of the equation above can then be derived by applying the solubility coefficient of CO_2, $[HCO_3^-] = 0.0301 \times pCO_2$, and so:

---

*This awkward notation can distort some numerical relationships. A change of 0.1 "pH units" from 7.4 to 7.3 represents a change in $[H^+]$ of 1.03×10^{-8}, which is a significantly greater change than the 0.82×10^{-8} going from 7.4 to 7.5. Moreover, the change from 7.3 to 7.2 is 25 per cent greater than the change from 7.4 to 7.3!

$$pH = 6.1 + \log_{10}\left\{\frac{[HCO_3^-]}{0.0301 \times pCO_2}\right\}$$

This equation points out that hydrogen ion concentration in the patient is dependent upon the functioning of two regulatory systems. The pCO_2 is regulated by the lungs—the production of CO_2 being essentially constant, or in any case not able to be regulated—and so any change in pH caused by a change in pCO_2 is termed *respiratory*. The pCO_2 determines the amount of CO_2 dissolved in the body fluid. Dissolved CO_2 combines with water like a classic anhydride, in a reaction catalyzed by carbonic anhydrase, to form carbonic acid, with which it exists in an equilibrium defined by a constant. Carbonic acid dissociates into hydrogen and carbonate ions. Since the final concentration of the carbonic acid reflects an equilibrium value with $[H^+]$, it is the result of the multiple physiologic equilibria involving $[H^+]$ and other strong and weak acids in solution,* which are themselves the result of multiple physiologic processes involving their production during intermediary metabolism and their removal, chiefly through the kidneys. The changes in pH that reflect changes in $[HCO_3^-]$ are therefore termed *metabolic*.

Acidosis is a shift downward in pH, below 7.40; *alkalosis* is a shift above. Respiratory acidosis is a condition in which the pH is decreased owing to hypoventilation and resultant hypercarbia as seen in pulmonary insufficiency; the reverse, respiratory alkalosis, is an increase in pH due to hyperventilation and hypocarbia. Under conditions of hypoxemia, such as can occur in severe respiratory distress syndrome or in shock states, anaerobic metabolism leads to production of significant levels of lactic acidemia. This results in an equilibrium shift toward greater carbonic acid, reflecting a metabolic acidosis. The reverse, metabolic alkalosis, is most often caused by pharmacologic alterations in the kidneys' regulatory mechanisms, commonly through chronic diuretic therapy.

Whenever any stress disrupts the body's acid-base equilibrium, compensatory mechanisms are brought into play. Respiratory acidosis elicits a metabolic compensation in the kidneys, with net removal of negatively charged ionic species and a resultant increase in $[HCO_3^-]$. A spontaneously breathing patient may hyperventilate to raise a low pH during metabolic acidosis. In any case, the compensation is in the direction of normalcy, and the process does not lead to overcompensation. Such a situation would indicate a *mixed* acid-base disorder. An apparent lack of compensation may actually represent a mixed metabolic and respiratory disorder.

The body regulates acid-base homeostasis to very narrow limits within each body fluid compartment. The protein enzyme systems are adapted to these limits, and departures from normal can therefore cause deterioration of enzyme and hence cellular function, potentially causing tissue injury and organ dysfunction.†

---

*As Stewart (1981) points out, it is therefore misleading to speak of bicarbonate "stores," since bicarbonate is itself a dependent variable produced in essentially limitless supply by dissolved CO_2. Rather, its concentration reflects the body's overall metabolic disposition of many other strong and weak acids and bases.

†Not only enzymes are affected. The Gibbs-Donnan membrane equilibrium, the physical chemical basis for oncotic pressure, depends upon the charge density of plasma proteins, especially albumin, which can change significantly with variations in pH, resulting in important fluid shifts between compartments and changes in effective circulating volume.

CLINICAL EVALUATION OF ACID-BASE DISORDERS

The blood gas is the beginning of the evaluation. The pH and $PaCO_2$ are directly determined, and from these the $[HCO_3^-]$ is calculated.‡ From this information it can be determined whether the existing condition is acidosis or alkalosis, whether it is primarily respiratory or metabolic in origin, and whether it is an acute, uncompensated change or one of long enough duration for compensatory changes to have occurred.

The analysis of the blood gas values must then be considered in light of the patient's history and physical examination in order for a correct therapeutic response to be devised. Further laboratory evaluation may or may not be helpful, but history and physical data are essential. The treatment of acid-base problems generally demands correction of the underlying disorder, not just of the consequent pH change. For example, the correct response to the acidosis due to shock from hypovolemia involves the restoration of circulating volume; this requires a recognition of the shock state, a clinical rather than a laboratory diagnosis. The laboratory work-up then proceeds from the clinical evaluation. In a patient with respiratory distress, for example, arterial PaO_2 may be needed to reveal hypoxia when cyanosis is not apparent.

Measurement of an "anion gap" in the serum electrolytes may prove useful in the work-up of metabolic acidosis. Normally the difference between the concentration of Na^+, the major extracellular cation, and that of the anions Cl^- and HCO_3^- in the serum is about 8 to 16. In an acidotic patient, if the difference exceeds the upper limit of normal by about twice the $[HCO_3^-]$, this may be assumed to represent unmeasured anions, implicating acids, such as lactate, in the causation of acidosis. The etiology of an anion gap acidosis is often readily discerned from the clinical history and examination; if not, specific laboratory analyses of serum acids must be undertaken, depending upon the diagnoses clinically suspected.

RESPIRATORY ACIDOSIS

The etiology of respiratory acidosis is respiratory failure. The therapy is adequate ventilation.

It is important to note that the pH must be acid to support this diagnosis. A $PaCO_2$ of 60 mm Hg with a pH of 7.43 does not necessarily represent respiratory failure. Infants with bronchopulmonary dysplasia on chronic diuretic therapy, for example, may have a marked metabolic alkalosis. The elevated $PaCO_2$, therefore, may be the result of pulmonary insufficiency (a mixed metabolic alkalosis and respiratory acidosis), but it may also be in some degree a respiratory compensation for the metabolic disorder. In such circumstances, respiratory drive may be blunted.

METABOLIC ACIDOSIS

Metabolic acidosis results from the net accumulation of acid species in excess of bases. The disorder can arise rapidly, or it may develop from a more chronic imbalance.

---

‡ The calculation assumes that the pK' for the carbonic acid dissociation is constant, which is not true in sick infants (Karlowicz et al., 1984; Rosan et al., 1983), and very careful technique is required for reliable direct measurement of $[HCO_3^-]$; these errors can sometimes distort the interpretation of a patient's clinical status.

With any acute change in pH, as with lactic acidemia, there is a prompt compensatory increase in ventilation, which is sustained as required. Newborns are fully capable of such responses unless pulmonary function is impaired in some way. Renal adjustments occur over a longer period.

Acids accumulate in newborns through the normal metabolism of proteins and other substrates and during the incorporation of calcium into bone formation. These acids must be eliminated through the kidneys. A variety of renal disorders can result in the abnormal accumulation of normally produced acids. Less commonly, abnormal acids are produced by various inborn errors of metabolism.

Premature infants are able to compensate for acidemias through the usual renal ionic exchange and excretory mechanisms, although to some degree, particularly in the very-low-birth-weight infant, renal responses to acid-loading appear somewhat limited (Sulyok, 1971). There is a fairly rapid, gestational age–dependent maturation of this capacity postnatally (Svenningsen and Lindquist, 1974), with capacity more limited before 34 weeks. Excretion of titratable acid is relatively decreased in these patients, and although renal bicarbonate levels may not accurately reflect renal responses in acidosis (Stewart, 1981), it was noted early on that apparent bicarbonaturia is seen in spite of low basal serum bicarbonate levels (Tudvad et al., 1954). This limitation may, for example, result in mild acidemias with high dietary intake of nonmetabolizable acids (Shaw, 1989).

A syndrome of late metabolic acidosis of prematurity has been described (Kildeberg, 1964), which results from the high rates of intermediary metabolism accompanying the rapid growth of some patients. Newer formulas with lower casein:whey ratios require less from the limited kidneys, and the syndrome is now rarely seen.

ALKALI THERAPY

Out of concern for the deleterious effects of acidosis upon tissues and organs noted previously, direct correction of acidosis using alkali has been advocated in a variety of medical situations, particularly to correct the lactic acidosis due to hypoxia and hypoperfusion during CPR. The approach has been controversial, with recent studies questioning the effectiveness of such therapy and even suggesting that it may actually compound the problem (Graf et al., 1985; Stackpoole, 1986; Weil, 1985).

Sodium bicarbonate has been the most widely accepted alkali therapy (sodium carbonate and THAM have also been used), particularly in response to acidosis due to asphyxia. Because of the chemical equilibria outlined earlier, this therapy can be successful only in an open system in which ventilation is adequate to keep $PaCO_2$ low, allowing equilibrium to shift toward alkali generation. When ventilation is limited, as is often the case clinically, sodium bicarbonate infusion can produce increased CO_2. The resulting hypercapnia can actually decrease pulmonary perfusion, worsening oxygenation and acidosis (Steichen and Kleinman, 1977). $NaHCO_3$ infusions have also been shown to decrease myocardial performance (Dumont et al., 1984).

Clinically, pH is usually determined in arterial blood.

Within the tissues, however, poor perfusion also may produce a closed system, in which the $PaCO_2$ will be elevated by the addition of sodium bicarbonate. CO_2 diffuses rapidly across membranes, whereas HCO_3^- does not, exacerbating the intracellular pH balance. Such a process has been implicated in worsening cerebral acidosis and hypoxia in laboratory animals (Bureau et al., 1980).

BICARBONATE AND INTRAVENTRICULAR HEMORRHAGE

In premature newborns, sodium bicarbonate use has been linked with intraventricular hemorrhage (IVH). This association was first noted in 1967 (Usher, 1967). Earlier reports had shown improved outcome in RDS patients using therapy that included sodium bicarbonate infusions (Usher, 1963). Subsequent studies have failed to establish any therapeutic benefit from sodium bicarbonate in this setting (Corbet et al., 1977; Sinclair et al., 1968); several investigators have documented harmful effects attributable to its use, including deleterious reductions in cerebral blood flow (Lou et al., 1979) and an increased incidence of IVH in premature infants (Papile et al., 1978; Simmons et al., 1974).

This last issue has caused the greatest concern. Because stressed premature infants may be unable to autoregulate cerebral vascular pressure, rapid changes in perfusion pressure can cause the fragile vessels of the germinal matrix to rupture. $NaHCO_3$ therapy could potentially cause such injuries, since pressure fluctuations are known to occur when hyperosmolar solutions are infused (Huseby and Gumprecht, 1981). Since the greatest association of sodium bicarbonate with IVH has been seen with rapid administration of hyperosmolar solutions (Papile et al., 1978), more dilute solutions are considered safe if given slowly, although experimental verification for this is lacking. Furthermore, there is concern that because $NaHCO_3$ can cause increased $PaCO_2$ and possible hypoxemia (Baum and Robertson, 1975; Steichen and Kleinman, 1977), this could result in cerebral vascular dilatation, further potentiating IVH (Rahilly, 1980).

Since the administration of sodium bicarbonate entails recognizable risks, and since its beneficial effects are questionable, the accepted indications for its use have been considerably narrowed over time. The American Heart Association Guidelines for Neonatal Resuscitation (American Heart Association, 1986) now provide that $NaHCO_3$ *may* be used during CPR only in cases of *documented* metabolic acidosis. Its use in the acidosis associated with respiratory distress syndrome can no longer be recommended as a routine measure. Because hyperosmolality and sodium content appear to increase the risk of its use, sodium bicarbonate, if given at all, should be given slowly, and the standard 0.9 or 1 M solution should be diluted 1:2 to 1:4 with water. It is emphasized that such recommendations are largely arbitrary, with little experimental verification (Howell, 1987).

When acidosis is the result of abnormal electrolyte losses from renal or gastrointestinal disorders, replacement with sodium bicarbonate is therapeutic. Complications can nevertheless result from overly rapid correction. Since gastrointestinal losses can result in a net loss of sodium relative to chloride and other anions (Bower et al., 1988;

Stewart, 1981), maintenance sodium given as bicarbonate or acetate can be corrective and will not represent a hyperosmolar load.

RESPIRATORY ALKALOSIS

This disorder consists of an elevated pH due to an abnormally low $PaCO_2$. In the neonatal intensive care unit (NICU) it is almost always iatrogenic, from excessive mechanical ventilation. The treatment consists of appropriate ventilator management. From time to time infants are seen with mild spontaneous hyperpnea. Central nervous system drive is abnormal in these patients, and this occasionally may be a sequela of perinatal distress persisting beyond the resolution of any metabolic acidosis. It is usually self-limiting, requiring no specific therapy.

METABOLIC ALKALOSIS

Metabolic alkalosis is encountered much more frequently. It can develop relatively rapidly, for example, from continuous gastric suctioning or from the hyperemesis of pyloric stenosis—situations in which chloride ion is removed in excess of sodium, resulting in an equilibrium shift toward increased $[OH^+]$. Most often, however, alkalosis in the NICU is the result of chronic diuretic therapy.

With prolonged use of thiazide, mercurial, or loop diuretics, patients, among them newborn infants (Laudignon et al., 1989; Singh et al., 1984), may develop a variety of disorders, including an occasionally pronounced hypochloremic metabolic alkalosis (DeRubertis et al., 1970). This occurs frequently during the treatment of infants with bronchopulmonary dysplasia. Several mechanisms have been proposed, including increased $[HCO_3^-]$ due to contracted ECF, the so-called contraction alkalosis. However, chloride deficiency has been convincingly implicated as the principal basis for the syndrome (Kassirer et al., 1965), and it can be shown that chloride replacement alone can correct the disorder independent of volume replacement. (Rosen et al., 1988).

Therapy with potassium chloride is preferred, although NaCl also will correct the disorder, since there is almost always hypokalemia as well, brought on by the drug-induced kaliuresis. While serum $[K^+]$ is usually decreased, it may not accurately reflect the degree of total body potassium depletion, because K^+ is principally an intracellular ion. This condition is often accompanied by hyponatremia. The low $[Na^+]$ results from a shift of Na^+ into the ICF space to compensate for the depleted intracellular potassium (Fichman et al., 1971), possibly compounded by a magnesium deficit (Dykner and Wester, 1981). There may even be hyponatremia, with increased total body sodium and water retention. If total body sodium is known to be decreased, replacement is indicated. Most often, however, KCl will reverse the hyponatremia, correct the hypokalemia, and resolve the metabolic alkalosis without increasing total body sodium. Since chloride deficiency is the basis for the increased pH, ammonium chloride will also correct the alkalosis, but it will not relieve the other electrolyte imbalances. Adequate supplementation with KCl or treatment with potassium-sparing diuretics will prevent recurrence.

RESPIRATORY DISTRESS SYNDROME

THEORETICAL CONCERNS

In infants with respiratory distress syndrome (RDS), hypoventilation and hypoxia result in combined respiratory and metabolic acidosis that can lead ultimately to cardiovascular collapse and death. During the course of this disease, renal function may be compromised in a number of ways, just when transitional physiology demands a reduction in both total body water and sodium (Arant, 1982). If this results in excessive lung water, there will be further aggravation of already poor pulmonary function (Bland, 1982). All these considerations argue in favor of a restricted fluid intake during RDS.

In addition, excess fluid administration has been shown to influence the development of symptomatic patent ductus arteriosus in premature infants with RDS (Bell et al., 1980), whereas fluid restriction can be used to effect closure of an open ductus. Aggressive fluid therapy has also been linked to necrotizing enterocolitis (Bell et al., 1980), congestive heart failure, and intraventricular hemorrhage (Papile et al., 1978) and to the subsequent development of bronchopulmonary dysplasia (Brown et al., 1978; Spitzer et al., 1981). For these reasons, recent recommendations have emphasized the need for relatively restricted fluid input in RDS (Arant, 1982; Costarino and Baumgart, 1986, 1988; Oh, 1988). Past recommendations for aggressive fluid therapy (Usher, 1963) have been superseded as other improvements in the treatment of RDS obviate the benefits seen at that time.

A number of specific problems affect fluid balance during treatment of RDS. First, concomitant with respiratory distress syndrome, there is an alteration in renal function, often resulting in diminished urine output. It has been observed repeatedly that during the most severe stages of the disease, urine output is low and that a period of spontaneous diuresis is seen to either accompany (Cort, 1962; Torrado et al., 1974) or precede (Langman et al., 1981; Heaf et al., 1982) improvement in lung function. The basis for this phenomenon is unclear. Redistribution of an endogenous fluid load (Costarino, 1986) or compromise of renal function from hypoxia followed by recovery has been suggested. The effect of the pulmonary circulation on the regulation of ADH has also been implicated. By the same token, hypoxia, stress, and positive-pressure ventilation stimulate vasopressin release. However, ADH effect alone cannot fully explain the restricted output seen early in RDS, and its role may, in fact, be minimal (Engle et al., 1983). Loop diuretics can force a diuresis during the oliguric stage of respiratory distress syndrome and can improve lung function (Belik et al., 1987 Green et al., 1981, 1983a). Interestingly, when fluids are managed conservatively throughout the illness, this pattern of diuresis following oliguria is not seen (Lorenz et al., 1982). The effect may be, at least in part, iatrogenic, an artifact of fluid management.

Also to be considered are the effects of other interventions taken in the management of the disease such as the use humidified air in ventilators, evaporative losses from radiant warmers, and fluids used in the administration of other medications and the maintenance of indwelling lines.

PRACTICAL MANAGEMENT

GENERAL PRINCIPLES

A fluid plan must include methods for assessing the adequacy of therapy at each stage. *Recommendations for fixed schedules of fluid administration should no longer be considered appropriate for the management of infants with respiratory distress syndrome.*

The plan should be conservative—babies are born with more than enough fluid in their tissues. The goal is to provide the minimum of additional fluid and electrolytes needed to prevent dehydration and hyperosmolarity while allowing for the appropriate contraction of the patient's extracellular fluid volume and the maintenance of adequate serum glucose. Patients are maintained NPO while respiratory distress persists, so an umbilical artery catheter or a secure intravenous line will be required. The following recommendations apply to medium and large-sized premature infants (≥ 1250 g).

First Day. Initially, 10 per cent dextrose is given at a rate of 50 to 60 ml/kg/day. This provides 4 mg/kg/min of glucose, which will usually be adequate for a medium-sized premature infant with uncomplicated RDS. Higher glucose concentrations may be used, if needed, in preference to increasing the rate. No electrolytes are needed at this stage. Since in these patients all sodium losses are renal, replacement will not be required until diuresis has begun. Hyponatremia in the first day of life virtually always indicates fluid overload.

Subsequent Days. Body weight and serum electrolytes should be determined *at least* daily. Urine output and specific gravity should be recorded. Therapy is designed to allow a loss in body weight of from 10 per cent to no more than 15 per cent over the first three to seven days while maintaining normal serum electrolytes (Lorenz et al., 1982). The plans for water and for salts will be considered separately.

Water. Increase fluids if the weight loss exceeds 5 per cent in any one day, or 15 per cent overall. Decrease fluids if weight loss is less than 2 per cent daily for the first 3 days, or less than 7 to 10 per cent overall. Any weight gain during this time indicates fluid overload. Increase fluids if urine output drops below 0.5 ml/kg/hr in any 8-hour period after diuresis is established (early oliguria is common).

Salts. NaCl can be started when fluid volumes need to be increased if serum [Na$^+$] is normal, or sooner if serum [Na$^+$] is less than 135 mEq/L. Concentrations of 10 to 20 mEq/L will provide from 0.5 to 3 mEq/kg/day of sodium, depending on the fluid rate. (Remember that during the fluid contraction stage, the patient has an obligate net *negative* sodium balance.) Increase the amount of sodium being given if the weight loss exceeds the desired limits and [Na$^+$] is normal or low. Increase the amount of sodium being given if there is hyponatremia ([Na$^+$] < 135 mEq/L) and if there is no weight gain to indicate water overload. Decrease the amount of sodium being given if the desired weight loss does not occur or if there is any weight gain unless there is also hyponatremia.

Potassium chloride to provide 1 to 2 mEq/kg/day should be given when urine output is established.

Once fluid contraction to appropriate postnatal volumes has occurred, fluid therapy can be liberalized, and increasing nutrition will become the goal as the acute phase of RDS resolves. Over the next few days fluids usually will be increased to around 100 to 120 ml/kg/day, and as the respiratory disease resolves and parenteral or oral feedings are begun, volumes can be slowly increased as required to establish adequate calories for good growth and nutrition.

SPECIFIC ISSUES

Dehydration. Dehydration can occur if management is overly restrictive. This can happen very rapidly, especially in smaller infants. Clinically, dehydration may be suggested by skin texture and turgor, but until far advanced these can be difficult to assess in premature infants. Renal output is also an unreliable guide, since immature and compromised kidneys may maintain a diuresis even after ECF volume becomes depleted (conversely, in the prediuretic phase of RDS, there may be oliguria even though fluid volume is increased). Other signs of hypovolemia such as tachycardia, hypotension, or acidosis will be seen only after dehydration has become pronounced. Timely body weight and serum electrolyte measurements are therefore essential.

Diuretics. Increased lung water, whether from CHF or from other causes such as low oncotic pressure, contributes to the pathophysiology of RDS (Bland, 1982), and increased body water can contribute to the development of PDA.

Furosemide is the most commonly used diuretic in acute situations in the neonate. A dose of 1 mg/kg IV or IM or 2 mg/kg PO usually results in a brisk diuresis, usually within 2 hours. The drug is given at 8- or 12-hour intervals, and its half-life is significantly prolonged in infants compared with adults (Aranda et al., 1982).

Side effects of furosemide in infants include metabolic alkalosis, hyponatremia, and hypochloremia, generally from chronic administration. The chronic calciuria accompanying prolonged use of the drug can result in nephrolithiasis (Myracle et al., 1986) and bone demineralization (Venkataraman et al., 1983). It can also be ototoxic, exacerbating the risk associated with simultaneously administered aminoglycosides (Brummett, 1980).

Furosemide is a known stimulant of the renal release of prostaglandin E$_2$ (Friedman et al., 1978), a potent dilator of the ductus arteriosus, and has been shown to promote the appearance of PDA in RDS patients (Green et al., 1983b). However, the benefits of diuresis may outweigh the risk of PDA, since in the same study overall survival was actually increased in patients given furosemide.

There is some clinical evidence that the pulmonary effects of furosemide may not be a direct result of increased urine output (Najak et al., 1983; Belik et al., 1983; Yeh et al., 1984). *In vivo* data from anephric animals implicate a nondiuretic direct vascular effect on lung lymph flow (Bland et al., 1978), so that there is some theoretical benefit even in cases in which body water is not excessive.

The risks of furosemide seem to be associated primarily with long-term use, and although data showing significant reductions in morbidity from RDS with its use are lacking, there is good reason to think that it might be helpful in some cases. Nevertheless, it cannot be recommended as a routine treatment for RDS. In most cases, routine conservative fluid management should be sufficient, and diuretics should be used only when further reduction of fluid volume is judged necessary or when specific problems exist.

Hypovolemia. Hypovolemia is not a normal consequence of either prematurity or RDS. Blood pressure in otherwise stable premature infants, especially very small infants, may transiently dip to fairly low levels immediately after birth (to a mean < 30 mm Hg in very-low-birthweight infants) and spontaneously increase thereafter (Moscoso et al., 1983). Attempts to increase blood pressure in such cases with, for example, albumin infusions, are probably not helpful and have been shown to interfere with oxygen exchange in the lungs of these children (Barr et al., 1977).

Therefore, the finding of hypovolemia in a newborn infant with RDS should prompt a search for an etiology. There may be reduced blood volume secondary to cord compression or hemorrhage during the birth process, which would best be remedied by blood transfusion. Concurrent sepsis may require volume expansion to combat shock due to capillary leakage. Hypovolemia can also result from dehydration with overly conservative fluid management, particularly in very small babies. Low blood pressure due to poor cardiac output secondary to hypoxia and lactic acidosis does not imply hypovolemia and will respond best to correction of the hypoxia.

Whenever volume replacement is required in a premature infant, care should be exercised; rapid infusions of large volumes can lead to rapid fluctuations in blood pressure and have been implicated in causing intraventricular hemorrhage (Goldberg et al., 1980).

CHRONIC LUNG DISEASE

The presence of excess lung water and hyperreactive airways is the rationale for restricted fluid intake and diuretic therapy and the use of bronchodilators in the management of chronic lung disease. The following discussion pertains to premature infants more than 2 to 3 weeks of age with chronic lung disease.

Excessive fluid administration can increase lung water content by a variety of mechanisms. Intravascular volume overload can produce increased cardiac output and lung blood flow, with an increase in microvascular surface area and filtration pressures for fluid and solute filtration. An increased fluid intake can aggravate left-to-right shunting via a PDA and thus increase pulmonary blood flow. Also, small increases in left atrial pressure from excessive fluid administration can result in marked increases in lung fluid filtration. The impaired ability of the distorted lymphatic system to drain the filtered fluid is a contributing factor to increased pulmonary interstitial water content.

The goal of fluid and electrolyte therapy is to provide sufficient fluid and nutritional calories for growth and development, renal excretion of solutes, and insensible water losses, without any excess water intake. Depending on the infant, this may range from 100 to 150 ml/kg/day. Sodium and chloride intake is adjusted so that serum sodium concentration is in the low normal range: sodium 130 to 135 mEq/L and chloride 95 to 100 mEq/L. As most of the infants are also receiving diuretic therapy, the excessive losses of sodium, potassium, and calcium in the urine must be taken into consideration.

DIURETIC THERAPY

Diuretics are used in the management of hyperreactive airways and not as a means of reducing lung water content. Fluid and salt restriction is the best way to prevent pulmonary edema formation. Diuretics can reduce total airway resistance in patients with established chronic lung disease after a single intravenous injection or after 1 week of oral administration. After a single intravenous injection of furosemide, the improvement in airways resistance seems to be immediate and therefore unlikely to be due to diuresis. The mechanism of action of diuretics is therefore not clear. The ability of furosemide to improve dynamic compliance may be nondiuretic in nature and may relate to its vasoactive properties. Furosemide induces systemic venodilation and hence may also induce pulmonary venodilation, which would decrease venous engorgement and decrease microvascular pressures for fluid filtration. Decreased vascular congestion in the airways would also markedly improve airways conductance, resulting in decreased hyperinflation and CO_2 retention. For the management of infants with chronic lung disease, the most severe complications to anticipate and avoid are those resulting from chronic diuretic therapy. The most commonly used diuretics, furosemide and hydrochlorothiazide, lead to increased urinary loss of sodium, potassium, and chloride. Excess sodium loss can lead to hyponatremia. Prior to initiation of corrective measures, hyponatremia resulting from true total body sodium deficiency must be differentiated from dilutional hyponatremia resulting from excess water retention. A first step is to adjust the diuretics, either decreasing the dose of furosemide or replacing it with less potent salt-losing diuretics. However, if respiratory symptoms worsen when the diuretics are decreased and the beneficial nondiuretic effects of furosemide are lost, one may have to supplement the infant's diet with additional sodium. This must be done with extreme caution, with just enough supplementation to maintain serum sodium concentration in the low normal range (130 to 135 mEq/L) but not enough to cause excessive salt and water retention.

Increased potassium loss will result in total body potassium deficit. Since potassium is essentially an intracellular ion, this deficiency is not always manifest as a decreased level of potassium in plasma. In fact, plasma concentration of potassium is maintained in the normal range at the expense of intracellular potassium concentration. Excess chloride loss will lead to hypochloremia with bicarbonate retention. Both total body potassium deficit and hypochloremia will lead to a progressive metabolic alkalosis. Under normal circumstances, in the distal tubule of the kidney, potassium is excreted from the renal tubular cells in exchange for a sodium ion that is reabsorbed. If the renal tubular cells are deficient in potassium, sodium is exchanged for H^+ ions, resulting in a progressive metabolic alkalosis. This situation is frequently unrecognized, as most of the infants with chronic lung disease have chronic CO_2 retention with an associated compensatory metabolic alkalosis. If the potassium and chloride deficits are not corrected, they will lead to worsening metabolic alkalosis, which results in a vicious circle leading to more CO_2 retention.

Therefore, if an infant exhibits hypochloremia with metabolic alkalosis, even though serum potassium is within normal limits, both potassium and chloride must be supplemented. With adequate correction of these deficits, often both serum bicarbonate levels and CO_2 retention will decrease.

Excessive losses of calcium and phosphate in the urine will lead to poor bone mineralization. Chronic calcium excretion in the urine may lead to nephrocalcinosis and renal tubular damage. Renal stones may be visualized on renal ultrasound studies. Finally, use of furosemide may result in ototoxicity and hearing impairment.

■ FLUID AND ELECTROLYTE MANAGEMENT IN NEONATAL SURGICAL PATIENTS

The newborn requiring surgery may or may not have existing disturbances in body fluid and electrolyte composition. For example, a newborn infant with congenital pyloric stenosis and vomiting or a premature infant with necrotizing enterocolitis and bacteremia may have severe abnormalities in fluid and electrolyte status. Therefore, the first objective in an infant requiring surgery is determination of body fluid and electrolyte status and correction of any severe derangement prior to surgery. If necessary, surgery may have to be postponed for a few hours to a day or two, so that the infant's intraoperative and postoperative course is not further complicated by fluid and electrolyte disturbances.

The objective of intraoperative fluid and electrolyte management is to maintain homeostasis. During surgery is not the time to initiate long-term goals in fluid and electrolyte management or to correct any major imbalance.

Transport To and From the Nursery. The time spent in being transported to and from the operating room can be hazardous to a newborn. The major hazards are excessive cooling, increased insensible water losses, and accidental disconnection of intravenous, intratracheal, oxygen, and intra-arterial lines.

To minimize heat and water losses, the infant should be wrapped with plastic wrap, if necessary, and covered with a thermal blanket. If possible, he or she should be transported in a battery-operated transport unit, so that the heat source is not turned off. If this is not possible, warmed blankets and hot water bottles may be used. The infant's head should be covered with a cap to reduce heat losses from this surface. Plastic wrap and thermal blankets also reduce the air currents around the infant and thus lessen heat and water losses.

Maintenance and Support During Surgery. In the

operating room, it is essential to keep the temperature at about 89 to 92°F, a range that is usually uncomfortable for the surgeons but desirable for the infant. Warming all intravenous solutions will also help reduce heat losses.

During surgery, it is desirable that someone versed in neonatal respiratory and fluid and electrolyte problems be in attendance. This person could be a pediatric anesthesiologist or a neonatologist. Knowledge of the infant's ongoing problems will greatly aid in the intraoperative care.

Careful weighing of the infant immediately before and after surgery will pinpoint any major deficits or gains in total body water content. Monitoring the heart rate, blood pressure, urine output, skin and rectal temperature, transcutaneous PaO_2, blood pH, $PaCO_2$, and PaO_2 during surgery is essential. It is important to remember that systemic blood pressure may be maintained in the face of severe fluid losses due to intense peripheral vasoconstriction. Such a situation can be recognized by the presence of tachycardia and a low skin temperature and skin pO_2 with a relatively normal rectal temperature and blood pO_2. Therefore, fluid losses during surgery must be anticipated and replaced. However, fluid overloading must be avoided, as this may lead to worsening respiratory function or intraventricular hemorrhages in the premature infant.

Bowel surgery for correction of gastroschisis, omphalocele, or intestinal atresias necessitates exposure of the bowel and peritoneal cavity. Insensible water losses can be considerable from the exposed bowel, and this ongoing free water loss must be replaced appropriately. This can be done, in part, by increasing the administration of free water during the period when the bowel is exposed. A careful weighing of the infant after surgery will reveal the deficit or excess in water replacement. In situations in which the bowel is inflamed or traumatized, as in necrotizing enterocolitis and gastroschisis, there may be exudative losses of protein-rich fluid into the bowel wall and peritoneal cavity. In this circumstance, appropriate volumes of colloid-containing solutions must be given.

Postoperative Care. Immediately postoperatively, in some infants, urine output may decrease markedly owing to an increased secretion of ADH (Bennet et al., 1970). In infants undergoing cardiac surgery with hypothermia and the use of cardiopulmonary bypass, in the immediate postoperative period there may be excessive loss of fluids from the intravascular compartment into the interstitial compartment. This is usually due to a transient increase in capillary endothelial permeability. Consequently, the infant will require large volumes of fluids, either crystalloid or colloid solutions, to maintain an adequate intravascular volume and intracardiac filling pressures. This "leaky capillary" state usually lasts 24 hours, after which the fluid requirements slowly return to normal. During this phase, careful monitoring of central venous pressure, heart rate, systemic blood pressure, capillary filling time, acid-base status, heart size (by x-ray), and liver size (by palpation) will enable one to maintain the intravascular volume in a normal range. The infant's total body water and interstitial volume will increase excessively, but an inappropriate weight gain may be a necessary consequence of maintaining an adequate intravascular volume.

Neonatal Sepsis, Bowel Perforation, and Necrotizing

Enterocolitis. Neonatal sepsis with endotoxemia or bacteremia is associated with noncardiogenic shock. The presence of an increased capillary permeability to protein results in loss of fluid and protein from the intravascular space to the interstitial space. Hence, frequently the infant will be severely hypotensive and tachycardiac and will respond only to infusions of fluids (crystalloid or colloid solutions). This situation is analogous to the one described earlier. An adequate intravascular volume must be maintained to ensure adequate perfusion and oxygenation of tissues.

■ REFERENCES

American Heart Association–American Academy of Pediatrics: Guidelines for neonatal resuscitation. JAMA 255:2969, 1986.

Aperia A., and Herin P.: Development of glomerular perfusion rate and nephron filtration rate in rats 17–60 days old. Am. J. Physiol. 288:1319, 1975.

Aperia, A., Berggrvist, G., Broberger O., et al.: Renal function in newborn infants with high hematocrit values before and after isovolemic hemodilution. Acta Paediatr. Scand. 63:878, 1974.

Aperia, A., Broberger, O., Elinder, G., et al.: Postnatal development of renal function in preterm and full term infants. Acta Paediatr. Scand. 70:183, 1981.

Aranda, J.V., Lambert, C., Perez, J., et al.: Metabolism and renal elimination of furosemide in the newborn infant. J. Pediatr. 101:777, 1982.

Arant, B.S., Jr.: Fluid therapy in the neonate: Concepts in transition. J. Pediatr. 101:387, 1982.

Arant, B.S., Jr.: Nonrenal factors influencing renal function during the perinatal period. Clin. Perinatol. 8:225, 1981.

Barr, P.A., Bailey, P.E., Sumners, J., and Cassady, G.: Relation between arterial blood pressure and blood volume and effect of infused albumin in sick preterm infants. Pediatrics 60:282, 1977.

Baum, J.D., and Robertson, N.R.C.: Immediate effects of alkaline infusion in infants with respiratory distress syndrome. J Pediatr. 87:255, 1975.

Baumgart, S., Langman, C.B., and Sosulki, R.: Fluid, electrolyte and glucose maintenance in the very low birthweight infant. Clin. Pediatr. 21:199, 1982.

Belik, J., Spitzer, A.R., and Clark, B.J.: Effects of early furosemide administration in neonates with respiratory distress syndrome. Pediatr. Pulmonol. 3:219, 1987.

Belik, J., Spitzer, A.R., and Clark, B.J.: Furosemide therapy prior to spontaneous diuresis: Acute improvement in respiratory distress syndrome. Pediatr. Res. 17:304A, 1983.

Bell, E.F., Warburton, D., Stonestreet, B.S., and Oh, W.: Effect of fluid administration on the development of symptomatic patent ductus arteriosus and congestive heart failure in premature infants. N. Engl. J. Med. 302:598, 1980.

Bell, E.F., Warburton, D., Stonestreet, B.S., and Oh, W.: High volume fluid intake predisposes premature infants to necrotizing enterocolitis. Lancet 2:90, 1979.

Bell, E.F., Weinstein, M.R., and Oh, W.: Heat balance in premature infants. Comparative effects of convectively heated incubator and radiant warmer, with and without plastic heat shield. J. Pediatr. 96:460, 1980.

Bennet, E.J., Daughety, M.J., and Jenkins, M.T.: Fluid requirements for neonatal anaesthesia and operation. Anesthesiology 32:343, 1970.

Bland, R.D.: Edema formation in the newborn lung. Clin. Perinatol. 9:593, 1982.

Bland, R.D., McMillan, D.D., and Bressack, M.A.: Decreased pulmonary transvascular fluid filtration in awake newborn lambs after intravenous furosemide. J. Clin. Invest. 62:601, 1978.

Bower, T.R., Pringle, K.C., and Soper, R.T.: Sodium deficit causing decreased weight gain and metabolic acidosis in infants with ileostomy. J. Pediatr. Surg. 23:567, 1988.

Brodehl, J., Franken, A., and Gellissen, K.: Maximal tubular reabsorption of glucose in infants and children. Acta Paediatr. Scand. 61:413, 1972.

Brown, E.R., Stark, A., Sosenko, I., et al.: Bronchopulmonary dysplasia: Possible relationships to pulmonary edema. J. Pediatr. 92:982, 1978.

Brummett, R.E.: Drug-induced ototoxicity. Drugs 19:412, 1980.

Bureau, M.A., Begin, R., and Berthiaume, Y.: Cerebral hypoxia from bicarbonate infusion in diabetic acidosis. J. Pediatr. 96:968, 1980.

Corbet, A.J., Adams, J.M., and Kenny, J.D.: Controlled trial of bicarbonate therapy in high-risk premature newborn infants. J. Pediatr. 91:771, 1977.

Cort, R.L.: Renal function in the respiratory distress syndrome. Acta Pediatr. 57:313, 1962.

Costarino, A., and Baumgart, S.: Modern fluid and electrolyte management of the critically ill premature infant. Pediatr. Clin. North Am. 33(1):153, 1986.

Costarino, A.T., and Baumgart, S.: Controversies in fluid and electrolyte therapy for the premature infant. Clin. Perinatol. 15(4):863, 1988.

Dancis, J., O'Connell, J.R., and Holt, L.E., Jr.: A grid for recording the weight of premature infants. J. Pediatr. 33:570, 1948.

Dean, R.F.A., and McCance, R.A.: The renal response of infants to the administration of hypertonic solutions of sodium chloride and urea. J. Physiol. 109:81, 1949.

DeRubertis, F.R., Michelis, M.F., Beck, N., and Davis, B.B.: Complications of diuretic therapy: severe alkalosis and syndrome resembling inappropriate secretion of diuretic hormone. Metabolism 19:709, 1970.

Dumont, L., Stanley, P., and Chartrand, C.: The cardiovascular effects of hypertonic sodium bicarbonate in conscious dogs: Underlying mechanism for the action. Can. J. Physiol. Pharmacol. 62:314, 1984.

Dykner, T., and Wester, P.O.: Effects of magnesium infusions in diuretic induced hyponatremia. Lancet 1:585, 1981.

Edelmann, C.M. Jr., Troupkou, V., and Barnett, H.L.: Renal concentrating ability in newborn infants. Fed. Proc. 18:49, 1959.

Elinder, G., Aperia, A., Herin, P., et al.: Effect of isotonic volume expansion on glomerular filtration rate and renal hemodynamics in the developing kidney. Acta Physiol. Scand. 108:411, 1980.

Engle, W.D., and Arant, B.S., Jr.: Urinary potassium excretion in the critically ill neonate. Pediatrics 74:259, 1984.

Engle, W.D., Arant, B.S., Jr, Wiriyathian, S, and Rosenfeld, C.R.: Diuresis and respiratory distress syndrome: physiologic mechanisms and therapeutic implications. J. Pediatr. 102:(6):912, 1983.

Fichman, M.P., Vorherr, H., Kleeman, C.R., and Tefler, N.: Diuretic induced hyponatremia. Ann. Intern. Med. 75:853, 1971.

Fisher, D.A., Pyle, H.R., Porter, J.C., et al.: Studies of control of water balance in the newborn. Am. J. Dis. Child. 106:137, 1963.

Friedman, Z., Demers, L.M., Marks, K. H., et al.: Urinary excretion of prostaglandin E_2 following the administration of furosemide and indomethacin to sick low birthweight infants. J. Pediatr. 93:512, 1978.

Friis-Hansen, B.: Body water compartments in children: Changes during growth and related changes in body composition. Pediatrics 28:169, 1961.

Goldberg, R.N., Chung, D., Goldman, S.L., and Bancalari, E.: The association of rapid volume expansion and intraventricular hemorrhage in the preterm infant. J. Pediatr. 96:1060, 1980.

Graf, H., Leach, W., and Arieff, A.I.: Evidence for the detrimental effect of bicarbonate therapy in hypoxic lactic acidosis. Science 227:754, 1985.

Green, T.P., Thompson, T.R., Johnson, D.E., and Lock, J.E.: Diuresis and pulmonary function in premature infants with respiratory distress syndrome. J. Pediatr. 103:618, 1983a.

Green, T.P., Thompson, T.R., Johnson, D.E., and Lock, J.E.: Furosemide promotes patent ductus arteriosus in premature infants with the respiratory-distress syndrome. N. Engl. J. Med. 308(13):743, 1983b.

Green, T.P., Thompson, T.R., Johnson, D., and Lock, J.E.: Furosemide use in premature infants and appearance of patent ductus arteriosus. Am. J. Dis. Child. 135:239, 1981.

Gruskay, J.A., Costarino, A.T., Polin, R.A., and Baumgart, S.: Nonoliguric hyperkalemia in the premature infant less than 1000 grams. J. Pediatr. 113:381, 1988.

Guignard, J.P.: Assessment of renal function without urine collection. Arch. Dis. Child. 52:424, 1977.

Hammarlund, K., and Sedin, G.: Transepidermal water loss in newborn infants VIII. Relation to gestational age and postnatal age in appropriate and small for gestational age infants. Acta Paediatr. Scand. 72:721, 1983.

Hammarlund, K., and Sedin, G.: Transepidermal water loss in newborn infants III. Relation to gestational age. Acta Paediatr. Scand. 68:795, 1979.

Hansen, J.D.L., and Smith, C.A.: Effects of withholding fluid in the immediate postnatal period. Pediatrics 12:99, 1953.

Heaf, D.P., Belik, J., Spitzer, A.R., et al.: Changes in pulmonary function during the diuretic phase of respiratory distress syndrome. J. Pediatr. *101*(1):103, 1982.

Hey, E.N.: *In* Hull, D., and Gairdner, D. (eds.): The care of babies in incubation. Recent Advances in Pediatrics. London, Churchill, 1971.

Hey, E.N., and Katz, G.: Evaporative water loss in the newborn baby. J. Physiol. (Lond.) *200*:605, 1969.

Howell, J.H.: Sodium bicarbonate in the perinatal setting—revisited. Clin. Perinatal. *14*:807, 1987.

Huseby, J.S., and Gumprecht, D.G.: Hemodynamic effects of rapid bolus hypertonic sodium bicarbonate. Chest *79*:552, 1981.

Ichikawa, I., and Brenner, B.M.: Factors limiting glomerular filtration rate in the immature rat. Pediatr. Res. *12*:592, 1978.

Karlowicz, M.G., Simmons, M.A., Brusilow, S.W., and Jones, M.D.: Carbonic acid dissociation constant (pK') in critically ill newborns. Pediatr. Res. *18*:1287, 1984.

Kassirer, J.P., Berkman, P.M., Lawrenz, D.R., and Schwartz, W.B.: The critical role of chloride in the correction of hypokalemic alkalosis in man. Am. J. Med. *38*:172, 1965.

Kildeberg, P.: Disturbances of hydrogen ion balance occurring in premature infants. II. Late metabolic acidosis. Acta Paediatr. Scand. *53*:517, 1964.

Langman, C.B., Engle, W.D., Baumgart, S., et al.: The diuretic phase of respiratory distress syndrome and its relationship to oxygenation. J. Pediatr. *98*:462, 1981.

Laudignon, N., Ciampi, A., Coupal, L., et al.: Furosemide and ethacrynic acid: risk factors for the occurrence of serum abnormalities and electrolyte and metabolic alkalosis in newborns and infants. Acta Paediatr. Scand. *78*:133, 1989.

Leake, R.D.: Perinatal nephrobiology: A developmental perspective. Clin. Perinatol. *4*:321, 1977.

Leake, R.D., Trygstad, C., and Oh, W.: Inulin clearance in postnatal age. Pediatr. Res. *10*:759, 1976.

Lorenz, J.M., et al.: Water balance in very low birth weight infants: Relationship to water and sodium intake and effect on outcome. J. Pediatr. *101*:423, 1982.

Lou, H.C., Skov, H., and Pederson, H.: Low cerebral blood flow: A risk factor in the neonate. J. Pediatr. *95*:606, 1979.

McDonald, M.S., and Emery, J.L.: The later intrauterine and postnatal development of human glomeruli. J. Anat. *93*:331, 1959.

Moscoso, P., Goldberg, R.N., Jamieson, J., and Bancalari, E.: Spontaneous elevation in arterial blood pressure during the first hours of life in the very-low-birth-weight infant. J. Pediatr. *103*:114, 1983.

Myracle, M.R., McGahan, J.P., Goetzman, B.W., et al.: Ultrasound diagnosis of renal calcifications in infants on chronic furosemide therapy. J. Clin. Ultrasound *14*:281, 1986.

Najak, Z.D., Harris, E.M., Lazzara, A., and Pruitt, A.W.: Pulmonary effects of furosemide in preterm infants with lung disease. J. Pediatr. *102*:758, 1983.

Oh, W.: Renal function and fluid therapy in high risk infants. Biol. Neonate *53*(4):230, 1988.

Oh, W., and Karecki, H.: Phototherapy and insensible water loss in the newborn infant. Am. J. Dis. Child. *124*:230, 1972.

Oh, W., Oh, M.A., and Lind, J.: Renal function and blood volume in newborn infant related to placental transfusion. Acta Paediatr. Scand. *56*:197, 1966.

Papile, L., Burstein, J., Burstein, R., et al.: Relationship of intravenous sodium bicarbonate infusions and cerebral intraventricular hemorrhage. J. Pediatr. *93*:834, 1978.

Rahilly, P. M.: Effects of 2 percent carbon dioxide, and 100 percent oxygen on cranial blood flow of the human neonate. Pediatrics *66*:685, 1980.

Robillard, J.E., Matson, J.R., and Session, C.: Maturational changes in renal tubular reabsorption of water in the lamb fetus. Pediatr. Res. *13*:1172, 1979.

Rojas, J., Mohan, P., and Davidson, K.K.: Increased extracellular water volume associated with hyponatremia at birth in premature infants. J. Pediatr. *105*:158, 1984.

Rosen, R.A., Julian, B.A., Dubovsky, E.V., et al.: On the mechanism by which chloride corrects metabolic alkalosis in man. Am. J. Med. *84*:449, 1988.

Rosan, R.C., Enlander, D., and Ellis J.: Unpredictable error in calculated bicarbonate homeostasis during pediatric intensive care: the delusion of fixed pK'. Clin. Chem. *29*:69, 1983.

Shaw, J.C.: Nonmetabolizable base balance: effect of diet composition on plasma pH. J. Nutr. *119*:1789, 1989.

Simmons, M.A., Adcock, E.W., Bard, H., et al.: Hypernatremia and intracranial hemorrhage in neonates. N. Engl. J. Med. *291*:6, 1974.

Sinclair, J.C., Engel, K., and Silverman, W.A.: Early correction of hypoxemia and acidemia in infants of low birth weight: A controlled trial of oxygen breathing, rapid alkali and assisted ventilation. Pediatrics *42*:565, 1968.

Singh, S.R., Murphy, J.F., and Gray, O.P.: Metabolic alkalosis in a neonate after furosemide. Arch. Dis. Child. *59*:907, 1984.

Spitzer, A.: The role of the kidney in sodium homeostasis during maturation. Kidney Int. *21*:539, 1982.

Spitzer, A.R., Fox, W.W., and Delivoria-Papadopoulos, M.: Maximum diuresis—a factor in predicting recovery from respiratory distress syndrome and the development of bronchopulmonary dysplasia. J. Pediatr. *98*:476, 1981.

Stackpoole, P.W.: Lactic acidosis: The case against bicarbonate therapy. Ann. Intern. Med. *105*:276, 1986.

Steichen, J.J., and Kleinman, L.I.: Studies in acid-base balance: Effect of alkali therapy in newborn dogs with mechanically fixed ventilation. J. Pediatr. *91*:287, 1977.

Stewart, P.A.: How to Understand Acid-Base. New York, Elsevier North Holland, 1981.

Stonestreet, B.S., Rubin, L., Pollak, A., et al.: Renal functions of low birth weight infants with hyperglycaemia and glucosuria produced by glucose infusion. Pediatrics *66*:561, 1980.

Strauss, J.: Fluid and electrolyte composition of the fetus and newborn. Pediatr. Clin. North Am. *13*:1077, 1966.

Sulyok, E.: The relationship between electrolyte and acid-base balance in the premature infants during early postnatal life. Biol. Neonate *17*:227, 1971.

Sulyok, E., Nemeth, M., Tenyi, I., et al.: Postnatal development of renin-angiotensin-aldosterone system, RAAS, in relation to electrolytic balance in premature infants. Pediatr Res. *13*:817, 1979.

Svenningsen, N.W., and Lindquist, B.: Postnatal development of renal hydrogen excretion capacity in relation to age and protein intake. Acta Paediatr. Scand. *63*:721, 1974.

Torrado, A., Guignard, J.P., Prod'hom, L.S., and Gautier, E.: Hypoxaemia and renal function in newborns with respiratory distress syndrome(RDS). Helv. Paediat. Acta *29*:399, 1974.

Tudvad, F.H., McNamara, H., and Barnett, H.L.: Renal response of premature infants to administration of bicarbonate and potassium. Pediatrics *13*:4, 1954.

Usher, R.: Comparison of rapid versus gradual correction of acidosis in RDS of prematurity. Pediatr. Res. *3*:221, 1967.

Usher, R.: Reduction in mortality from respiratory distress syndrome of prematurity with early administration of intravenous glucose and sodium bicarbonate. Pediatrics *32*:966, 1963.

Venkataraman, P.S., Han, B.K., and Tsang, R.C.: Secondary hyperparathyroidism and bone disease in infants receiving long-term furosemide therapy. Am. J. Dis. Child. *137*:1157, 1983.

Versmold, H.T., Kitterman, J.A., and Phibbs, R.H.: Aortic blood pressure during the first 12 hours of life in infants with birth weight 610 to 4220 grams. Pediatrics *67*:607, 1981.

Weil, M.H.: Sodium bicarbonate during CPR: Does it help or hinder? Chest *88*:487, 1985.

Yeh, T.F., Shibii, A., Leu, S.T., et al.: Early furosemide therapy in premature infants (less than 2000 gm) with respiratory distress syndrome: A randomized controlled trial. J. Pediatr. *106*:603, 1984.

Zweymiller, E., and Preining, O.: The insensible water loss in the newborn infant. Acta Paediatr. Scand. (Suppl.) *205*, 1, 1970.

ISSUES IN NURSING CARE OF THE NEWBORN

29

Linda J. Weaver

With careful attention to details and intelligent cooperation on the part of a good nurse very many of these (premature infants) may be saved that otherwise would be absolutely hopeless.

—L. E. HOLT, 1897

Neonatal nursing is as old as birth itself. Very early pictorial representations of the lying-in chamber invariably depict attendants other than the midwife who are busy bathing the infant or warming swaddling clothes by the fire, while the exhausted mother rests after the ordeal of delivery (Dick, 1987). By 1900, the first nurseries for premature babies had been established in Europe, and besides swaddling and feeding the infants, nursing personnel had the never-ending task of filling the hot water bottles that provided heat for the incubator, or *couveuse* (Nelson, 1979). Today, the neonatal intensive care nurse presides over an array of computerized machinery, but the escalating technology is only an adjunct to the nurse's primary responsibility—care of a sick or premature infant.

■ CARE OF THE EXTREMELY-LOW-BIRTH-WEIGHT INFANT

Although at birth and immediately thereafter a great deal of attention is centered on the respiratory status of these fragile patients, we must remember that the infant as a whole is an "unfinished" being, who is not in any way ready for the environment into which he or she is placed. These tiny infants (<1000 g, <28 weeks' gestation) present unique nursing care problems.

MINIMAL HANDLING

The premature baby should be handled only when necessary, and then in the gentlest manner.

—C. G. KERLEY, 1920

Doctor Kerley's recommendation, in 1920, that premature infants receive minimal handling has come full circle after 2½ decades of aggressive management (1960s to mid-1980s) to almost constant hands-on care approaches (Hodgman, 1985). During the 1980s the sensitivity of the premature to the environment again received attention, and efforts were undertaken to try to "achieve a balance between 'hands-off' and 'hands-on' policies" (Silverman, 1987). To support the physiologic needs of

the very-low-birth-weight (VLBW) infant, nurses must give around-the-clock care, but interventions should be adjusted whenever possible to reduce stress on the infant.

Continuous monitoring of an infant's oxygenation shows decreases with any manipulation during the taking of vital signs, diaper changes, physical examinations, blood drawing, chest physiotherapy, suctioning, radiographic procedures, and other procedures (Danford et al., 1983; Dangman et al., 1976; Dingle et al., 1980) and even with close social interaction (Gorski et al., 1983). All of these observers found that 75 per cent of hypoxic time ($T_cPO_2<40$) observed in control infants was associated with handling. They concluded that handling the premature infant for any reason may cause significant stress and that multiple disturbances may result in an accumulative effect of more profound compromise. However, the amount of time during which oxygenation is compromised can be reduced by using monitoring information to identify care approaches and techniques that need to be altered to reduce stress or that are effective in minimizing it (Long et al., 1980b).

GENERAL GUIDELINES FOR MINIMIZING HANDLING

A number of nursing care approaches that minimize handling have emerged in response to the above observations.

Weighing. A VLBW infant should be weighed on admission to the neonatal intensive care nursery (NICU) to provide a baseline. Thereafter, unless the infant is on a bed scale, weekly weighing is usually adequate for very sick infants <1000 g, and is particularly desirable for those weighing <750 g. Fluid status can be managed with careful observations of intake and output and laboratory monitoring of serum electrolytes, urine specific gravity, and hematocrit until the infant's condition is stable enough to enable more frequent weighing without undue stress.

Controlling the Environment. When an infant is nursed under radiant heat, use of a nonpermeable transparent plastic wrap reduces insensible water loss and facilitates temperature control (Fitch et al., 1980). It may also help decrease auditory and tactile stimuli, although this has not been measured. The infant should be moved to a double-walled incubator as soon as possible to further decrease insensible water loss and sensory stimuli (Marks et al., 1981). Although sound levels in some incubators are high, the walls do muffle sudden, disturbing noises from the outside.

Vital Signs. VLBW infants should be examined and their vital signs determined once per shift, unless there are serious problems that require intervention. At the initial assessment, the reliability of the cardiac, respiratory, and blood pressure monitors can be determined. Subsequently, at intervals of 1 to 2 hours, vital signs can be read from the monitors without disturbing the infant. If axillary temperatures are being monitored, however, more frequent checking is necessary.

Physical Examinations. Before handling any sick infant, nursing or physician staff members should ask themselves whether the information to be gained justifies risking a drop in the baby's P_aO_2 and, if so, how to minimize the degree and duration of reduced oxygenation. The care plan should be coordinated among the caregivers (nurses and physicians), so that only one examination per day is necessary unless problems arise.

Positioning. Whenever possible, the infant should be cared for in the prone position with the head of the bed elevated slightly above the horizontal. Hutchinson and colleagues (1979) compared the lung mechanics of mechanically ventilated infants in the right lateral, supine, and prone positions and found that tidal volume, minute volume, and total work of breathing were significantly reduced in the prone position. (If the infant has an umbilical catheter in place, the prone position is contraindicated unless the catheter is on a pressure disconnect monitor. The auditory alarm of this monitor should *never* be silenced.) The basic nursing principle of frequently changing a patient's position to counteract the effects of immobility does apply to the ill very-low-birth-weight infant, but when an infant's position requires change, the manipulations should be correlated with the infant's sleep-wake cycle rather than with a set time schedule.

Suctioning. It is unfortunate that maintaining a patent airway, one of the most important aspects of ventilator care, requires one of the most potentially dangerous procedures. Suctioning has been associated with atelectasis (Brandstater and Muallem, 1968), bradycardia (Cabal et al., 1974), increased cerebral blood flow velocity and intracranial pressure (Perlman and Volpe, 1983), transient bacteremia (Storm, 1980), pneumothorax (Alpan et al., 1984), and hyperinflation, hyperoxia, and tracheal tissue damage (Cunningham et al., 1984). The components of the suctioning procedure, i.e., positioning, pre- and post-oxygenation, continuous or intermittent suction, and irrigation, have been studied in various combinations, but no agreement has been reached on a universally accepted "best" suctioning method. Practices vary from institution to institution.

Some principles, however, are especially applicable to the very-low-birth-weight infant (<1000 g):

1. *Suctioning should always be on an as-needed basis.* There is little need for suctioning during the first day or two in infants with respiratory distress syndrome (RDS), and during this period, if no secretions are obtained after suctioning in various positions, only routine suctioning every 8 hours is necessary.

2. *A two-person team* (nurse-nurse or nurse-respiratory therapist) *should perform the procedure.* This enables better stabilization of the infant.

3. *The infant's lungs should be reexpanded after suctioning.* In many infants, thoracic gas volume is reduced by suctioning, especially if the ventilator is disconnected for the procedure. Careful hand ventilation for a short time after suctioning may be necessary to achieve adequate reexpansion. Hand ventilation carries the risk of overventilating (barotrauma), and vigilant concern should be exercised to avoid this.

4. *Side-port endotracheal tube adaptors should be used in very labile infants.* Use of side-port adaptors eliminates the need to disconnect the ventilator during suctioning (Cabal et al., 1979; Zmora and Merrit, 1980).

5. *The catheter should not extend more than 1 cm beyond the tip of the endotracheal tube.* A sample tube can be used to premeasure the appropriate length for each infant's suctioning catheter. This procedure eliminates the trauma that accompanies the practice of advancing the catheter "until resistance is met," a frequently used guideline.

Minimal handling does not imply minimal care. The successful application of the minimal handling approach requires special diligence on the part of nursing staff in making observations and becoming attuned to the behaviors and responses of individual infants. Greater success can be achieved if nursing assignments can be consistent and enable the nurse and baby to familiarize themselves with each other. The approach requires heavy reliance on visual signs, and a nurse who spends 8 to 12 hours daily at an infant's bedside develops a sixth sense about that infant and an uncanny ability to detect subtle changes in the baby's condition before physiologic effects are detected by the monitoring devices. Speck and co-workers (1979) noted, "It is often the nurse who alerts us to the diagnosis (of sepsis) by observing subtle changes in color, tone, activity, or feeding difficulties in the infant." Efforts on the part of the nursing staff to achieve consistency among the staff, similar to training members of a research team to achieve inter-rater reliability, can further strengthen the effectiveness of minimal handling efforts.

SKIN CARE

The skin of premature infants is highly permeable and fragile (Kuller, 1984), and requires delicate care. Tobin (1984) advocates a conscientious effort to limit the amount of tape applied to the skin and recommends the use of an *artificial protective barrier* (such as Hollihesive) underneath adhesives when possible. This method works well under umbilical catheter "goalposts," around temperature probes, and under tape securing endotracheal tubes and allows the tape to be changed without disturbing the protective barrier. *Special monitor leads with little or no adhesive* are available for use in VLBW infants. Care should be taken not to place the leads on the chest or abdominal fields needed for radiographic studies, so that they do not need to be removed and replaced unnecessarily.

Alcohol preparations should not be used because alcohol further increases the permeability of the skin. Instead, an iodine preparation should be used for disinfection and then washed off carefully with sterile water. Similarly, alcohol should not be used to remove adhesive. With a little extra patience, adhesives can be removed gently with water-soaked cotton balls (Tobin, 1984). The ingredients of commercially available adhesive removers should be checked carefully before these products are used in the intensive care nursery. Some of these solvents can be rapidly absorbed through a premature infant's highly permeable skin and may prove toxic to the infant.

The foregoing discussion presents some highlights of minimal handling approaches to illustrate the application of this concept. Guidelines for minimal handling that meet specific population needs are best developed by the staff of individual units. These approaches should be practiced judiciously and the guidelines modified according to each infant's degree of prematurity and type of illness and applied flexibly rather than as fixed protocols.

CARE OF INFANTS WITH CHRONIC PROBLEMS

Chronic lung disease has emerged as an all-too-frequent sequela of "fetal-infant" survival, and many VLBW infants experience chronic respiratory distress that requires prolonged hospitalization. The nursing care of these infants presents special challenges and demands exceptional patience and persistence. They often have feeding difficulties, require management with bronchodilators and diuretics, and have increased susceptibility to infection (Platzker, 1988). They are also "irritable, difficult to console, and hard to cuddle" (Boynton and Jones, 1988). Nurses who can rise to the challenge of feeding a baby who refuses to eat, calm a dyspneic hypoxic infant, and work with their anxious families to provide appropriate support and teaching should be treasured.

■ EXPANSION OF THE NEONATAL NURSING ROLE

The need to provide intensive care for increasing numbers of sick infants has severely stretched the health care delivery system. In addition, changes in technology, physician roles, and residency training program requirements and the development of regionalized perinatal care have led to expanded nursing roles and advanced education that equip skilled nurses to assume responsibilities that formerly were the province of physicians. For example, nurses are increasingly relied upon for newborn resuscitation, infant transport, and primary patient management—including procedures such as spinal taps and chest tube placement (Johnson et al., 1979). By the early 1980s, nurses (called neonatal nurse practitioners) were practicing in some form of expanded role in 57 per cent of all tertiary neonatal units in the United States (Harper et al., 1982), and the demand for neonatal nurse practitioners has significantly increased.

During the early 1980s, individual ICNs developed expanded roles for skilled staff nurses that responded to their particular needs, i.e., unit-specific roles. However, these nurses have no specific credential, and their skills may not be readily applicable or appropriate for other units. Thus, the need to fill the demand for neonatal nurse practitioners and to provide a reliable standard of competence led to the establishment of training programs at several nursing schools throughout the country. These have included certificate programs of 9 to 12 months and 2-year graduate degree programs. Graduates of hospital-based or certificate programs may attain excellent clinical expertise but eventually find themselves unable to advance their careers within the professional nursing hierarchy. Academic programs that lead to the increasingly important master's degree usually include exposure to research methodology, teaching competency, and administrative strategies in addition to clinical experience. Graduates of these programs, although investing much more time, may have less clinical training during their 2-year course than those from nonacademic programs. There is a need for development of neonatal nurse clinician or practitioner programs that combine broad-based graduate nursing study with extensive clinical training.

National standards are still lacking for both educational curriculum and licensing. A few states have specific licensing procedures for neonatal nurse practitioners, but reciprocity is limited because the eligibility criteria vary greatly from state to state. The only national examination and credential is offered by the Nurses' Association of the American College of Obstetrics and Gynecology (NAACOG), which provides a voluntary certification examination to test the special knowledge of neonatal nurses functioning in expanded clinical roles. NAACOG certification candidates must meet clinical and didactic eligibility criteria and score favorably on a written examination. In addition, certification status must be renewed every 3 years through either approved continuing education or reexamination. It is hoped that NAACOG's efforts may provide a foundation for the development of uniform, mandatory education standards and licensing procedures for neonatal nurse practitioners, similar to those for registered nurses in general. The experience in addressing these issues in the United States over the next few years may provide useful approaches and curricula that can be applied elsewhere as other nations encounter similar problems in meeting increased demands for neonatal intensive care providers.

■ REFERENCES

Alpan, G., Glick, B., Peleg, O., et al.: Pneumothorax due to endotracheal tube suction. Am. J. Perinat. 1:345, 1984.

American Academy of Pediatrics, Committee on Fetus and Newborn: Neonatal nurse clinicians. Pediatrics 70:1004, 1982.

Boynton, C. A., and Jones, B.: Nursing care of the infant with bronchopulmonary dysplasia. In Merritt, T. A., Northway, W. H., Jr., and Boynton, B. R. (Eds.): Bronchopulmonary Dysplasia. Boston, Blackwell Scientific Publications, 1988.

Brandstater, B., and Muallem, M.: Atelectasis following tracheal suction in infants. Anesthesiology 31:468, 1968.

Cabal, L., Devaskar, S., Siassi, B., et al.: New endotracheal tube adaptor reducing cardiopulmonary effects of suctioning. Crit. Care Med. 7:552, 1979.

Cabal, L., Siassi, B., Blanco, C., et al.: Cardiovascular effect of airway suctioning in infants with H.M.D. on assisted ventilation. Pediatr. Res. 8:444A, 1974.

Cassady, G.: Through the looking glass—or, look before you leap. Pediatrics 70:1001, 1982.

Cunningham, M. L., Baun, M. M., and Nelson, R. M.: Endotracheal suctioning of premature neonates. J. Calif. Perinatal Assoc. *4:*49, 1984.

Danford, D., Miske, S., Headley, J., et al.: Effects of routine care procedures on transcutaneous oxygen in neonates: A quantitative approach. Arch. Dis. Child. *58:*20, 1983.

Dangman, B. C., Indyk, L., Hegyi, T., et al.: The variability of P_{O_2} in newborn infants in response to routine care. *In* Rooth, G., and Bratterly, L. (Eds.): Fifth European Congress of Perinatal Medicine. Uppsala, Sweden, Almquist and Wicksell International, 1976.

Dick, D.: Yesterday's Babies: A History of Babycare. Avon, The Bath Press, 1987.

Dingle, R. E., Grady, M. D., Lee, J. A., et al.: Continuous transcutaneous O_2 monitoring in the neonate. Am. J. Nurs. *80:*890, 1980.

Fitch, C. W., Korones, S. B., and Wade, J. E.: Diminished insensible water loss and radiant energy requirement with use of special heat shield. Pediatr. Res. *14:*597A, 1980.

Gorski, P. A., Hole, W. T., Leonard, C. H., et al.: Direct computer recording of premature infants and nursery care: Distress following two interventions. Pediatrics *72:*198, 1983.

Harper, R. G., Little, G. A., and Sia, C. G.: Scope of nursing practice in level III NICU's. Pediatrics *70:*875, 1982.

Hodgman, J. E.: Introduction. *In* Gottfried, A. W., and Gaiter, J. L.: Infant Stress Under Intensive Care. Baltimore, University Park Press, 1985.

Holt, L. E.: The Diseases of Infancy and Childhood. New York, D. Appleton and Co., 1897.

Hutchison, A. A., Ross, K. R., and Russell, G.: The effect of posture on ventilation and lung mechanics in preterm and light-for-date infants. Pediatrics *64:*429, 1979.

Johnson, P. J., Jung, A. L., and Baros, S. J.: Neonatal nurse practitioners. Part I-A, new expanded nursing role. Perinatology-Neonatology *3:*(1)34, 1979.

Kerley, C. G.: The Practice of Pediatrics, 2nd ed. Philadelphia, W. B. Saunders Company, 1920.

Kuller, J.: Skin care in the intensive care nursery: Part I, skin development and function. Neonatal Network *3:*(3)18, 1984.

Long, J. G., Lucey, J. F., and Philip, A. G. S.: Noise and hypoxemia in the intensive care nursery. Pediatrics *65:*143, 1980a.

Long, J. G., Philip, A. G. S., and Lucey, J. F.: Excessive handling as a cause of hypoxemia. Pediatrics *65:*203, 1980b.

Marks, K. H., Lee, C. A., Bolan, C. D., et al.: Oxygen consumption and temperature control of premature infants in a double-wall incubator. Pediatrics *68:*93, 1981.

Nelson, R. A.: Premature-infant care. Perinatology-Neonatology *3:*58, 1979.

Norris, S., Campbell, L., and Brenkert, S.: Nursing procedures and alterations in transcutaneous oxygen tension in premature infants. Nurs. Res. *31:*330, 1981.

Nurses' Association of the American College of Obstetricians and Gynecologists: Certification Program. Chicago, NAACOG Certification Corp., 1988.

Perlman, J. M., and Volpe, J. J.: Suctioning in the preterm infant: Effects on cerebral blood flow velocity, intracranial pressure, and arterial blood pressure. Pediatrics *72:*329, 1983.

Platzker, A. C. G.: Chronic lung disease of infancy. *In* Ballard, R. A. (Ed.): Pediatric Care of the ICN Graduate. Philadelphia, W. B. Saunders Company, 1988.

Silverman, W. A.: The "Hands-On or Hands-Off?" dilemma revisited. J. Perinat. *7(4):*277, 1987.

Speck, W. T., Fanaroff, A. A., and Klaus, M. H.: Neonatal infections. *In* Klaus, M. H., and Fanaroff, A. A. (Eds.): Care of the High-Risk Neonate, 2nd ed. Philadelphia, W. B. Saunders Company, 1979.

Storm, W.: Transient bacteremia following endotracheal suctioning in ventilated newborns. Pediatrics *65:*487, 1980.

Tobin, C. R.: Skin care in the intensive care nursery: Part II, dispelling common myths. Neonatal Network *3(3):*24, 1984.

Zmora, E., and Merritt, A.: Use of the side-hole endotracheal tube adaptor for tracheal aspiration. Am. J. Dis. Child. *134:*250, 1980. Volume 3, #3 Dec. 1984.

CARING FOR PARENTS OF INFANTS IN INTENSIVE CARE

30

Stephanie A. Berman

The extraordinary advances in neonatal care have made it possible for increasing numbers of sick and preterm infants to be treated successfully. Most of these children eventually go on to normal and productive lives. Many, however, require additional help and services after discharge home, and some will die in the days and months after birth. For each infant who dies or is disabled as well as for those whose lives become a testimony to the success of neonatology, there is a family whose life is forever altered. For each neonate who is rescued by a sophisticated neonatal transport team and whisked away to a high-risk tertiary unit, there is a bereft mother left behind at the referring hospital. She and other concerned family members watch as the care of their fragile newborn is assumed by health-care providers introduced to them just moments before. The intimacy of their childbirth has become a medical emergency shared with strangers.

In the days that follow, parents need to adjust to an environment totally foreign to them and with a specialized language few have heard before. Many are in unfamiliar cities and hospitals. Most worry about their other children, work, home, and insurance. The demands on a family whose baby is in intensive care are incalculable. Parents find themselves dependent on people they don't know for problems they don't understand. The response is, predictably, a loss of parenting control and a suspension of normalcy.

How families adapt to these abrupt changes depends to an important extent on the particular combination of coping skills and mechanisms they bring to this situation and its confounding problems. How the neonatal team can work together to help families identify and enhance these coping strengths is the subject of this chapter.

One of the difficulties confronting a family is the sheer number of people with whom they must interact in the course of their baby's hospitalization. This is especially problematic at regional tertiary centers, which are often teaching hospitals. For parents of an infant transferred to a tertiary care center, just the first 48 hours entails interaction with the physicians and nurses at the delivery; the nurse, doctor, and paramedics on the transport team; the neonatologist; resident and fellow at the center; and some six shifts of nurses and respiratory therapists along with social workers, billing staff, and others.

In contrast to a private pediatric practice, in which the family has a close and trusting relationship with their personal doctor, who orchestrates care and relates personally to them, neonatal intensive care requires a team approach to meet all of the family's needs. Ideally, the team members from different disciplines and perspectives work together to address the special needs intrinsic to the family's current crisis (Miles, 1979). Guidelines for supporting the families of high-risk infants are summarized in Table 30–1.

■ TEAM GOALS

Team goals for families remain relatively constant regardless of a baby's medical course and the length of stay.

TABLE 30–1. Guidelines for Supporting Families of High-Risk Infants

GOALS

1. To enable the family to cope with transient dependence on the medical care team.
2. To enable parents to assume responsibility for the care of their newborn at discharge.

STRATEGIES

Antepartum Approaches

1. Coordinate information among team members.
2. Provide concrete information to family.
3. Introduce neonatal team.
4. Orient family to the intensive care nursery.

Intensive Care Nursery

1. Coordinate information and assign responsibility for communication.
2. Meet with the family outside the unit (e.g., neonatologist, social worker, primary nurse, and resident).
3. Encourage family to participate in the infant's care.
4. Recognize stresses and coping strengths, and offer opportunities for counseling and support.

PREPARING FOR OUTCOME

Discharge Home

1. Coordinate follow-up plan and family meeting with team members.
2. Identify resources (e.g., medical needs, follow-up care, family support, and public health).
3. Arrange rooming-in prior to discharge.
4. Follow up with a telephone call after discharge to assess adjustment.

Death

1. Prepare family for the possibility of a fatal outcome.
2. Provide parenting opportunities (holding, extended visits, and privacy).
3. Mobilize family support (e.g., extended family and clergy).
4. Support the family's pace in decision-making (e.g., postmortem examination and funeral plans).
5. Offer resources (e.g., reading lists, support groups, and a staff resource person).
6. Follow up with a telephone call to assess adjustment.
7. Arrange a death conference.

They are, in essence, to help families cope with their transient dependence on the medical care providers and to work toward the parents' independence and assumption of responsibility for their infant's care. Restoring parental control depends in part on the team's willingness to empower families. Communicating information, sharing decision-making, and providing ongoing supportive care are the seminal elements for achieving this end. When the parents can master the crisis of having a sick or preterm baby, parents' feelings of self-worth are enhanced, and they can later resume their independence and their role as parents with increased confidence (Minde, 1984).

Teaching hospitals bring together medical providers with different levels of training, who are disparate in their abilities to work with families. The team approach of providing for the emotional and educational needs of families affords abundant opportunities for teaching through role modeling. Because parents are often isolated from friends and families, they rely on members of the health-care team for support. Whether it is the primary nurse, the neonatologist, or social worker on whom the parents come to depend most, is largely a function of "chemistry" and timing.

In a teaching center, where residents and neonatologists rotate on and off services, primary nurses are often the care providers with whom parents spend the most time and develop the strongest bond (Etzler, 1984). In units where a social worker is consistently available, the nurse and social worker can identify daily signs of family dysfunction and strength. Problems can be shared with team members, and approaches to solving them planned.

▪ INTERVENTION STRATEGIES

ANTEPARTUM PERIOD

Normal pregnancy is accompanied by physical and psychological changes that require adaptation by the parents, particularly with regard to their expectations about the infant. When there is a prospect of fetal abnormality, illness, or death, parents must readjust to these new circumstances. Their sucessful readjustment depends upon having a clear understanding of the risks to the mother, fetus, and newborn as well as the support systems and problem-solving skills available.

Providing Information. The most available strategy for adaptation to a threatening event is understanding. Concrete information about the status of a high-risk fetus should be shared with a family. Parents usually want to hear the news together; commonly they want a friend or relative with them as well. When presented with information about potential problems that are technical and complicated, parents are often scared, medicated, and distracted. They experience a flagging sense of control; everyone seems to know more about the mother's pregnancy and their baby than they do. Coordination of communications is important; team members need to share what has been discussed with the family, identify needs for follow-up, and assign responsibility for carrying out these tasks.

Introducing the Neonatal Team. Obstetric staff should introduce the family to appropriate members of the neonatal team who can prepare families for their baby's admission to the neonatal intensive care unit (NICU).

Orientation. When there is time available before delivery, orienting the family to the NICU can ready them for the events to come. Parents often appreciate talking with different team members, each reinforcing information from a different vantage point and adding perspective to the anticipated birth. When a prospective mother can be moved, a wheelchair visit to the nursery provides a critical desensitizing step. The sight of a preterm infant on a respirator or with multiple intravenous lines, while unsettling at first, helps prepare a family for what they may likely see later. Similarly, the sounds of monitors prove far less distracting if they have been experienced and explained. Once the baby has been delivered, parents who have been introduced to the nursery have some conceptual and factual framework to help them assess and cope with their baby's presence there.

NEONATAL PERIOD

Physicians in a neonatal intensive care unit are often pressed for time. Interruptions are the norm. A sick preterm infant frequently has a variable course. When parents hear a working diagnosis from a physician who stops by the bedside and the next day they hear from a nurse about information conveyed "at report," they sometimes feel they are receiving piecemeal and even conflicting information. When they receive information from residents unfamiliar to them and sometimes even to the problems they are attempting to explain, confusion and even alarm ensue.

Primary Caregivers. For infants who will probably remain in the NICU for more than a few weeks, it is important for the parents to know that some of the staff will care for their infant throughout the hospital stay. Usually, a nurse, senior physician, and/or social worker can fulfill this primary caregiver role. Primary caregivers need to maintain contact with the family and to join in some, if not all, of the family meetings, even if they are not providing direct care for the infant throughout the stay. They maintain continuity for the parents and remind those responsible for the day-to-day care of the infant of the long-term goals for the family.

The Family Meeting. Meeting with families outside the nursery environment and together with other members of the care team can be a most efficient mode of transmitting information. Family meetings are an opportunity to meet at a fixed point in time, to clarify what has happened and to discuss anticipated events. They provide a chance to assess a family's level of understanding and to identify issues that require review or elucidation. Once the parents grasp and integrate the medical information they receive, they can actively participate in decision-making and regain a sense of control over their circumstances.

Family meetings are cumbersome in that they require scheduling and organizing. At their best, however, they provide a common perspective for families and caregivers. They provide an overview of an infant's condition and also an opportunity for trainees to learn (by observing) styles of conveying technical information to parents.

When team members meet with a family, they have a clear understanding of the facts as presented and are better able to reinforce the information. When a family hears consistent information from their baby's nurse and more than one of the doctors, they are less anxious as well as less inclined to feel dependent upon one provider—some of whom invariably rotate off service.

Family meetings are also times to prepare for potential long-term disability or to brace parents for their infant's death. Miles and Carter (1982) defined voids in communication as "not stating what was wrong with the child, not communicating how sick the child was, not telling parents about tests and treatments, not talking with them, not giving emotional support, not encouraging repeated questioning, staff not telling their names or who they were, and suddenly sending parents out of the room without explanation." Family meetings can eliminate these problems. Issues that families are reluctant to raise can be broached by one of the team members, and parents' concerns can be revealed in a nonjudgmental and supportive atmosphere. Family meetings with NICU parents should be planned at least weekly. Soon after each meeting, a summarizing note should be placed in the chart. Parents vary widely in their ability to cope with the crisis of having a sick or preterm infant. Many experience persistent feelings of guilt and anxiety. Sometimes they become withdrawn and unavailable and thwart staff efforts to maintain open communication (Leander and Pettett, 1986). Supportive intervention by the NICU social worker can meet the needs of families burdened with such feelings. Parents appreciate interaction with a team member whose primary focus and skills are to meet their needs apart from the needs of the infant.

Sometimes normal feelings of guilt are exacerbated by the reality of a pregnancy and birth complicated by maternal drug and alcohol abuse, heavy smoking, or other potentially adverse activities. Mothers of infants born under such circumstances face disapproval from friends and family and often from hospital staff as well. Social service intervention is imperative here, and referral to child protective services is mandatory in most cases of documented drug abuse.

How families express their stress also varies widely. Medical care providers, by refraining from judgment, give a family opportunities to express their distress within the context of their personal coping styles. If, when interacting with families, staff appear to be overly judgmental, communication and trust can be jeopardized. Compassion, empathy, and understanding can enhance a family's ability to adjust. Facilitating adjustment, that is, helping the family resume its customary level of mental health is the focus of support for families (Baird, 1979).

Sometimes perinatal crises trigger underlying problems that result in depression and inability to function, and a parent with fragile mental health may decompensate. For such families, perinatal social workers may make referrals outside mental health professionals. In general, depression and disequilibrium are a part of the grieving process that accompanies the loss of a normal pregnancy and the idealized baby. With support and open communication, most parents adjust. Information about peer support groups, social services available from hospital staff, and outside mental health resources should be communicated to families. Parents can best decide when and if they need outside help. Reinforcing the family's own coping systems helps them marshal confidence in their ability to assume control of their lives after the immediate medical crisis (Baird, 1979).

■ DISCHARGE HOME

Discharge home, especially from a tertiary care nursery, creates anxiety and fear for parents. While discharge signals resumption of parental control, it also marks a disengagement from the experts and monitors and the hospital structure. When an NICU has unlimited visiting policies, many parents involve themselves quite early in routine infant care. Coupled with frequent visits and ongoing staff interaction, these parents are preparing themselves to care for their baby at home. Parents who have been unable to visit frequently are unprepared for the infant's discharge.

Ideally, a family discharge meeting can be held 7 to 10 days prior to the baby's proposed departure. Concerns can be reviewed, a discharge plan can be formulated, and parents can have time to organize their lives to accommodate the arrival of their infant. Parents should be offered a chance to room-in overnight with their baby prior to discharge (Minde, 1984).

Resources for follow-up at home need to be discussed. A public health nurse, together with the baby's pediatrician, can assess needs over time and introduce additional programs and resources gradually, should it become apparent that they are needed. At this time, parents find local community resources helpful. The name of a contact family of a recent premature or sick baby already at home may be quite helpful.

Choices for follow-up resources need to be presented. Families vary in their desire for independence and privacy as they leave the nursery experience. The most succesful discharge plan is one formulated in conjunction with the parents. Sometimes, in their eagerness to coordinate a thorough and comprehensive discharge plan, caregivers overwhelm families. Parents may surmise that staff think them unready to assume full charge of their recovering infant. Some families are reassured by numerous, closely spaced follow-up appointments. Others need time to adjust at home and to know their infants before they begin to relate to a new cast of medical providers. Interviewing and choosing a private pediatrician, while their infant is still in the NICU, is an important first step for parents in resuming control. A predischarge and an early postdischarge visit with the baby's pediatrician are essential and usually arranged as part of the discharge plan. Choices should be presented about follow-up resources and the timing of referrals.

The transition of an infant's care from hospital to family and community can be smoothed by the care team's ability to give control back to the parents. When a family has been kept well-informed and involved in decision-making during the hospital course, they feel trusted by staff and confident in their ability to carry out their parenting responsibilities. Comprehensive follow-up of high-risk infants and their families is essential (Ballard, 1988; Taeusch and Yogman, 1987).

■ NEONATAL DEATH

Parents need to know as soon as the staff expect that their baby may die. Admittedly, most infants who come to a high-risk center are gravely ill for a time. While experienced staff are accustomed to working with fragile newborns, parents often have no way to gauge the severity of their child's condition. The medical care team needs to share the benefit of their experience and perspective in the interest of parental orientation. The challenge is to prepare a family for the possibility of death without extinguishing hope. It requires sharing with the parents our confidence in neonatal medicine while recognizing its limitations: in other words, honestly telling a family that the best efforts possible might not be enough. Parents need as much time as possible to prepare for the loss of their infant. It is the first essential step in the long and arduous process of grieving. It is not unusual for some initial anger at the thought of losing their infant to be displaced to the health care team. It is essential that staff recognize this displacement and resist a defensive reaction. In addition, staff must often deal with their own sense of failure and loss of control when an infant dies, making it doubly hard to work supportively with the parents.

When a baby is dying, opportunities for the parents to participate in the infant's care can be offered. Separated from their baby by machines and tubes and monitors, most parents have been unable to hold or be alone with their newborn. They are apprehensive but grateful to be with their dying baby.

The circumstances of an infant's death need to be coordinated by health team members and choices for parent interaction with their infant need to be offered. The presence of extended family or clergy needs to be considered, as does the gathering of keepsakes and mementos. When death is precipitous, parents need to know they still can see and hold their infant.

> *Freed in death from the intravenous lines, endotracheal tube and monitoring systems, the final image of the baby is often one of relative or restored peace, comfort, and tranquility. The calmer memory lasts forever and possibly helps start the parents' huge, long-term effort to cope and eventually to adapt their lives to their loss. (Gorski, 1988)*

FOLLOW-UP AFTER DEATH

Bringing the family back to meet with staff after the death of an infant is a major therapeutic step in moving the parents toward resolution of their grief. While the timing of the conference varies with availability of family, staff, and autopsy results, 6 to 8 weeks seems optimal. It is a time when parents are beginning to reorganize their lives, when the mother's postpartum recovery is well along, and when the numbness and anguish of the nursery experience have begun to ease. Parents want to know more about their baby's death and its implications for future pregnancies. Sometimes they have questions and misunderstandings. Often, they simply want to make contact with those who knew their child.

These follow-up conferences are also important for staff. Those who can attend are able to share with the parents their observations and have opportunities for clarification and closure. It is a chance to hear from families when they have reestablished equilibrium and order in their lives and thoughts. It is a chance to express gratitude or vent frustration. Lastly, it is a chance to reintroduce information about support resources, which range from reading lists on dying and grieving to referrals to peer support groups and mental health professionals. Families need reassurance that grieving is a long-term adaptive process that takes different forms and disrupts their lives for even a year or more. How they cope with this task depends in part on support from partners, family, and community. They need to know that it is normal that their loss may destabilize them for a time and that their lives will be disrupted after the loss of a child. Armed with opportunities for outside help and support from those around them, parents can evaluate how their lives are going and decide for themselves whether additional outside intervention will lessen their stress. Parents can control their time of grieving and the form it takes in their lives.

■ REFERENCES

Avery, M. E., and Litwack, G.: Born Early: The Story of a Premature Baby. Boston, Little, Brown & Co., 1983.

Baird, S. F.: Crisis intervention strategies. In Johnson, S. H. (Ed.): High Risk Parenting: Nursing Assessment and Strategies for Assessment. Philadelphia, J. B. Lippincott, 1979, pp. 299–311.

Ballard, R. A. (Ed.): Pediatric Care of the ICN Graduate. Philadelphia, W.B. Saunders Compnay, 1988.

Berman, S. A.: Support of the family whose infant dies. In Ballard, R. A. (Ed.): Pediatric Care of the ICN Graduate. Philadelphia, W. B. Saunders Company, 1988, pp. 218–285.

Cagan, J.: Weaning parents from intensive care unit care. Mat. Child Nurs. 13:275, 1988.

Consolvo, C. A.: Relieving parental anxiety in the Care-By-Parent Unit. J. Obstet. Gynecol. Neonatal Nurs. 15:154, 1986.

Crnic, K. A., Greenberg, M. T., Ragozin, A. S., et al.: Effects of stress and social support on mothers and premature and full-term infants. Child Dev. 54:209–217, 1983.

Cronenwett, L. R.: Network structure, social support, and psychological outcomes of pregnancy. Nurs. Res. 34:93–99, 1985.

Etzler, C. A.: Parents' reactions to pediatric critical care settings: A review of the literature. Issues in Comprehensive Pediatr. Nurs. 7:319, 1984.

Goodman, J. R., and Sauve, R. S.: High risk infant: Concerns of the mother after discharge. Birth 12:235, 1985.

Gorski, P. A.: Comment. In Ballard, R. A. (Ed.): Pediatric Care of the ICN Graduate. Philadelphia, W. B. Saunders Company, 1988, p. 282.

Green, M.: Parent care in the intensive care unit. Am. J. Dis. Child. 133:1119, 1979.

Gyves, M. T.: The psychosocial impact of high risk pregnancy. Adv. Psychosom. Med. 12:71, 1979.

Johnson, S. H.: Behavior modification strategies. In Johnson, S. H. (Ed.): High Risk Parenting: Nursing Assessment and Strategies for Assessment. Philadelphia, J. B. Lippincott, 1979, pp. 312–317.

Leander, K., and Pettett, G.: Parental response to the birth of a high-risk neonate: Dynamics and management. Phys. Occupat. Ther. Pediatr. 6:205, 1986.

Miles, M. S.: Counseling strategies. In Johnson, S. H. (Ed.): High Risk Parenting: Nursing Assessment and Strategies for Assessment. Philadelphia, J. B. Lippincott, 1979, pp. 283–298.

Miles, M. S., and Carter, M. C.: Sources of parental stress in pediatric intensive care units. Children's Health Care 11:65, 1982.

Miles, M. S., Spicher, C., and Hassanein, R. S.: Maternal and paternal stress reactions when a child is hospitalized in a pediatric intensive care unit. Issues in Comprehensive Pediatr. Nurs. 7:333, 1984.

Minde, K. K.: The impact of prematurity on the later behavior of children and their families. Clin. Perinatol. 11:227, 1984.

Petrick, J. M.: Postpartum depression: Identification of high-risk mothers. J. O. G. N. Nurs. 13:37, 1984.

Sims-Jones, N.: Back to the theories: Another way to view mothers of prematures. Matern. Child Nurs. J. 11:394, 1986.

Taeusch, H. W., and Yogman, M. W.: Follow-up Management of the High-Risk Infant. Boston, Little, Brown & Co., 1987.

Wohlreich, M. M.: Psychiatric aspects of high-risk pregnancy. Psychiatr. Clin. North Am. 10:53, 1986.

Wolterman, M. C., and Miller, M.: Caring for parents in crisis. Nurs. Forum 22:34, 1985.

Zeskind, P. S., and Iacino, R.: Effects of maternal visitation to preterm infants in the neonatal intensive care unit. Child Dev. 55:1887, 1984.

PHARMACOLOGIC 31
PRINCIPLES AND
PRACTICALITIES

Robert M. Ward

The rapid application of new drug therapy in the neonatal intensive care unit (NICU) has made pharmacology in the newborn increasingly complex. Accompanying that complexity is the realization that while drug treatment of newborns may be curative, it may also induce significant problems. Potential morbidity and mortality associated with drug treatment of newborns must be recognized and weighed against the expected benefits.

Drug therapy of newborns follows basic principles of pharmacology superimposed on dynamic, developmental changes during the newborn period. Patients cared for in the NICU are exposed to a wide variety of drugs, many of which are incompletely studied in newborns. Therapeutic drug monitoring is often an integral part of this drug exposure in the NICU. The effective use of drug concentration measurements requires a working knowledge of pharmacokinetics and thoughtful consideration of when such measurements are appropriate and helpful.

PERINATAL DRUG EXPOSURE

Repeated warnings about fetal drug exposure were issued to physicians and the public after recognition of the teratogenic effects of thalidomide in the 1960s. Despite these warnings, drug exposure of the human fetus and newborn increased during subsequent decades and remains extensive today. The average number of drugs ingested during pregnancy increased from 3 in the 1950s to 11 in the 1970s (Ward and Green, 1988). Virtually all drugs administered to the pregnant woman reach the fetus, but careful interpretation is needed since fetal drug concentrations and effects vary widely from insignificant to life-threatening (Ward et al., 1980, 1988).

For hospitalized newborns, a similar pattern of increasing drug exposure is evident. Serial observations from the same NICU reveal almost a doubling of the average number of drugs administered to newborns in less than a decade, from 3.4 per patient during 1974 to 1975 (Aranda et al., 1976) to 6.2 per patient during 1977 to 1981 (Aranda et al., 1982a). Unfortunately, drug exposure among NICU patients is disproportionately greater in the most susceptible (and least studied) patients, the most immature newborns and those with multiple organ dysfunction (Aranda, 1983).

DRUG-INDUCED ILLNESS

The extensive exposure of newborns to drugs in the NICU is not benign. During their NICU hospitalization, 30 per cent of newborns sustain one or more adverse drug reactions of which 14.7 per cent are fatal or life-threatening (Aranda et al., 1982b). The causes of this NICU "epidemic" of drug-related morbidity and mortality are complex. Pharmacologic studies in pediatric patients are difficult because of a variety of problems from ethics to study design (Ward and Green, 1988). The difficulties of studying therapeutics in the newborn has created a situation in which a plethora of drugs is administered with a paucity of pharmacologic data. The smaller and more immature newborns, who are now surviving, lack gestational age-appropriate pharmacologic data about efficacy, dose-response, and kinetics for most drugs they receive. Furthermore, drug-induced illness is seldom considered in newborns. Failure to recognize drug-induced illness in the newborn often leads to further pharmacologic treatment as the first approach to correct unrecognized, drug-induced problems. This may reflect an expectation that drug therapy is usually effective and safe. The observations of Aranda cited above suggest the opposite. Prudent management of newborns must recognize and weigh the potential benefits of unstudied drug therapy against potential drug-induced morbidity and mortality. Some examples from the history of drug-induced mortality and morbidity in newborns should serve as a reminder of how more harm than good may accrue from uncontrolled or unstudied drug therapy in the NICU.

LESSONS FROM CHLORAMPHENICOL

Chloramphenicol was released for use in the 1940s and reports of its efficacy for treatment of *Salmonella* infections included pediatric patients. The manufacturer recommended dosages of 50 to 100 mg/kg/day for patients ≤15 kg. In 1959, when Sutherland reported three cases of sudden death in newborns treated with high dosages of chloramphenicol (up to 230 mg/kg/day), the drug was considered "well tolerated and nontoxic." Later in 1959, Burns and colleagues reported the disturbing results of a controlled trial of four prophylactic treatment regimes for newborn sepsis: (1) No treatment, (2) chloramphenicol alone, (3) penicillin and streptomycin, and (4) penicillin, streptomycin, and chloramphenicol. Groups 2 and 4, which received chloramphenicol (100 to 165 mg/kg/day), had overall mortality rates of 60 and 68 per cent, respectively, while groups 1 and 3 had mortality rates of 19 and 18 per cent, respectively. The deaths of these

285

newborns demonstrated the stereotyped sequence of symptoms and signs caused by chloramphenicol, designated the "gray syndrome," which included abdominal distention with or without emesis, poor peripheral perfusion and cyanosis, vasomotor collapse, irregular respirations, and death within hours of the onset of these symptoms. One year later, Weiss and co-workers (1960) attributed the gray syndrome in newborns to high concentrations of chloramphenicol secondary to its prolonged half-life in newborns who received dosages of 100+ mg/kg/day, which are usually used in older children. They recommended maximum dosages of 50 mg/kg/day in term infants <1 month old, half that dose for premature infants, and careful monitoring of chloramphenicol blood concentrations.

The discovery and explanation of chloramphenicol toxicity in newborns illustrate several important aspects of neonatal pharmacology. Since chloramphenicol was considered well tolerated in older children and adults, it was regarded as nontoxic for newborns. Chloramphenicol was so effective in newborns that higher dosages were used without pharmacokinetic study. Higher doses were administered to newborns despite recognition that its clearance required glucuronide conjugation, which was known to be immature in newborns. The unexpected finding that chloramphenicol in doses of 100 to 165 mg/kg/day could be lethal to newborns was demonstrated because this study included appropriate control groups. In fact, since the mortality from the most effective antibiotic treatment regime was equivalent to no antibiotic treatment, Burns and associates (1959) discontinued prophylactic use of antibiotics in the nursery. Similar pharmacologic comparisons are needed today. Even more, we need to thoughtfully consider our responses to therapeutic failure. Fewer drugs and lower dosages may be safer and more effective than additional drugs in higher dosages.

■ PRINCIPLES OF NEONATAL THERAPEUTICS

A thorough understanding of factors that affect drug concentrations helps in planning accurate therapy and in identification of the causes of therapeutic failure. Many of these factors are not chosen consciously in a therapeutic plan but have tremendous impact upon its effectiveness. Pharmacokinetics and pharmacodynamics in newborns follow the same general principles that govern drug actions in patients of any age: diagnosis, absorption, distribution, metabolism, and excretion. When applied to the newborn, these principles must accommodate several unique physiologic and pharmacologic features of the newborn, as outlined in Table 31–1.

Diagnosis. Effective treatment obviously begins with an accurate diagnosis and accurate assessment of symptoms. Although this applies to all areas of therapeutics, newborns present special diagnostic challenges since their small size and fragility may preclude useful, but inordinately invasive, diagnostic procedures. For example, many small immature newborns with chronic lung disease are treated for "bronchospasm" after decreased air entry associated with desaturation and abnormal breath sounds is observed. Relief of these symptoms with aerosolized

TABLE 31–1. Pharmacologic Principles and Pitfalls in Management of the Very-Low-Birth-Weight Infant

I. *Diagnosis*
  A. Limited diagnostic procedures
II. *Absorption*
  A. Intravenous
    1. Drug injection away from patient
    2. Uneven mixing of drugs and IV fluids
    3. Delayed administration due to *very* low flow
    4. Part of the dose discarded with tubing changes
  B. Intramuscular
    1. Poor perfusion limits absorption
    2. Danger of sclerosis or abscess formation
    3. Depot effect
  C. Oral
    1. Poorly studied
    2. Affected by delayed gastric emptying
    3. Potentially affected by reflux
    4. Passive venous congestion may occur with chronic lung disease, decreasing absorption
III. *Distribution* (affected by:)
  A. Higher (85 per cent) total body water (versus 65 per cent in adults)
  B. Lower body fat, i.e., about 1 per cent body weight (versus 15 per cent in term infants)
  C. Low protein concentration
  D. Decreased protein affinity for drugs
IV. *Metabolism*
  A. Half-life prolonged and unpredictable
  B. Total body clearance decreased
  C. Affected by nutrition, illness, and drug interaction
  D. Affected by maturational changes
V. *Excretion*
  A. Decreased renal function, both glomerular filtration rate and tubular secretion

bronchodilators may be interpreted as confirmation of the diagnosis. Although this may be correct, increased humidity, chest physiotherapy, or movement of the endotracheal tube bevel away from a pliable tracheal wall during an aerosol treatment may account for the improvement. Evaluation of ineffective therapy should include reconsideration of the diagnosis.

Absorption. Although most types of drug therapy of acute problems include *intravenous administration* to insure drug delivery to the site of action, this may *not* be reliable in newborns (Roberts, 1984). Drugs are often injected away from newborns "up the IV line" through a Y-site injection port with the expectation that the preset flow rate will deliver the drug over an appropriate infusion time. Intravenous infusion rates for very-low-birth-weight infants may be less than 2 ml/hour, sometimes divided between two infusion sites. Consequently, a drug injected away from the infant may infuse so slowly that it does not reach the circulation for several hours and then enters over a prolonged period. Gould and Roberts (1979) estimated that as much as 36 per cent of the total daily dose may be discarded when the IV solution tubing is changed. Infusion solution filters may also prevent drug delivery by direct adsorption of the drug or by allowing a heavier drug to settle in the filtration chamber and mix slowly with the infusion solution. For drug therapy in which the driving force for tissue entry is a concentration gradient between the circulation and the tissue (e.g., meningitis), sustained low drug concentrations may provide suboptimal therapy.

Intramuscular administration of drugs to newborns is

suboptimal and generally used when there is difficulty maintaining intravenous access. Absorption of drugs from an intramuscular injection site is directly related to muscle perfusion. Patients with hypothermia or shock are unlikely to absorb intramuscular doses effectively. Intramuscular administration of drugs may sclerose tissue or create large intramuscular collections of drugs, which are absorbed slowly producing a "depot effect" in which serum concentrations increase slowly over a prolonged period. Intramuscular drug administration to newborns, especially for multiple doses, should be avoided since it may not deliver effective drug concentrations to the site of action and may cause disfiguring sterile abscesses in the limited muscle mass of small newborns.

While *oral administration* of drugs is preferred for treatment of chronic illnesses in newborns, this route is not well studied. In adults, less drug is usually absorbed from the stomach than from the intestinal tracts because of its smaller surface area. Delayed gastric emptying postpones reaching peak serum drug concentrations and prolongs the absorption phase while elimination continues. Many newborns experience gastroesophageal reflux associated with delayed gastric emptying which may alter drug bioavailability. Passive venous congestion of the intestinal tract from elevated right atrial pressures decreases drug absorption in adults and may do so in premature infants with severe bronchopulmonary dysplasia complicated by cor pulmonale (Peterson et al., 1980). The administration of medications to newborns in small volumes of formula or during continuous gastric feedings may also alter drug absorption. The possible effects of feeding patterns upon drug absorption and action must be considered when enteral drug therapy fails.

Distribution. In pharmacokinetics, distribution is the partitioning of drugs among various body fluids, organs, and tissues. The distribution of a drug within the body is determined by several factors including organ blood flow, pH and composition of body fluids and tissues, physical and chemical properties of the drug (e.g., lipid solubility, molecular weight, and ionization constant), and the extent of drug binding to plasma proteins and other macromolecules (Ward et al., 1980).

Important differences among premature infants, children, and adults affect the distribution of drugs. Total body water varies from 85 per cent in premature newborns to 75 per cent in term newborns to 65 per cent in adults (Boreus, 1982). Conversely, body fat content varies from ≤1 per cent in premature infants to 15 per cent in term newborns (Mirkin, 1978). This changes the distribution of many drugs, especially polar, water-soluble drugs, such as the aminoglycosides. Protein binding of drugs in the circulation is decreased in the premature newborn through a decrease in the total amount of circulating protein and through decreased binding affinity by the protein itself. With rare exception, only the free (nonprotein-bound) drug molecules are "active," i.e., cross membranes, exert pharmacologic actions, and undergo metabolism and excretion. Clinical measurements of serum or plasma drug concentrations usually reflect total circulating drug concentrations which include both free and protein-bound drug. Thus, total circulating drug concentrations in the newborn which are low by adult standards may represent free drug concentrations which are equivalent to those of the adult owing to decreased protein binding in the newborn.

Metabolism. Many drugs require metabolic conversion before elimination from the body. Biotransformation of a drug usually produces a more polar, less lipid-soluble molecule which can then be eliminated rapidly by renal, biliary, or other routes of excretion. Drug biotransformation is classified into two broad categories: (1) nonsynthetic (Phase I) reactions which include oxidation, reduction, and hydrolysis and (2) synthetic or conjugation (Phase II) reactions which include glucuronidation, sulfation, and acetylation. Although the liver is considered the major organ responsible for drug biotransformation, many other organs carry out drug metabolism.

For most drugs in the newborn, the half-life is prolonged, and total body clearance is decreased. Important variations occur, however, among drug classes and among individuals. Glucuronide conjugation of bilirubin is usually low at birth unless this enzyme has been induced in utero through maternal exposure to drugs, cigarette smoke, or other inducing agents (Ward et al., 1980). In contrast, conjugation through sulfation is usually active at birth. Various factors after birth, such as nutrition, illness, or drug interactions, may hasten or retard the maturation of enzymes and organs responsible for drug metabolism in the newborn. Maturational changes in hepatic blood flow, drug transport into hepatocytes, synthesis of serum proteins, protein binding of drugs, and biliary secretion—alone and in combination—confound accurate predictions about drug metabolism after birth, which leads to empiric dose adjustments (Morselli et al., 1980). These factors must be restudied in the very immature, very-low-birth-weight infants who survive today.

Excretion. Another major pathway for drug elimination from the body is renal excretion of metabolized and unchanged drug. Neonatal renal function is diminished both in absolute terms and when normalized to body weight or surface area. The neonatal glomerular filtration rate averages about 30 per cent of the adult rate per unit surface area. Glomerular function increases steadily after birth while tubular function matures more slowly, causing a glomerular and tubular imbalance (Aperia et al., 1981). The postnatal increase in glomerular function reflects increased cardiac output, decreased renal vascular resistance, redistribution of intrarenal blood flow, and changes in intrinsic glomerular basement membrane permeability (Morselli et al., 1980). The dynamics of neonatal renal function markedly influence drug excretion. The rate of change of renal function and its susceptibility to hypoxemia, nephrotoxic drugs, and underperfusion confound predictions of drug elimination rates, which must be measured empirically.

■ PHARMACOKINETIC PRINCIPLES

Pharmacokinetics describes the time course of changes in drug concentrations within the body. Although rates of change are often described with differential equations, concepts useful at the bedside are emphasized here. More detailed mathematical discussions of pharmacokinetics are presented elsewhere (Gibaldi and Perrier, 1982; Greenblatt and Koch-Weser, 1975a and 1975b; Notari, 1980).

Compartment. In pharmacokinetics, compartment refers to fluid and tissue spaces into which drugs penetrate. These compartments may or may not be equivalent to anatomic or physiologic fluid volumes. In the simplest case, the compartment may correspond to the vascular space and equal the volume of a real body fluid, blood. Large or quite polar molecules may be confined to this central compartment until they are eliminated by excretion or metabolism. Many drugs, however, diffuse reversibly out of the central compartment into tissues or other fluid spaces, referred to generically as peripheral or tissue compartments. Such compartments are seldom sampled directly, but their involvement in kinetic processes may be recognized from the graphic or mathematical description of a drug's kinetics.

Apparent Volume of Distribution. The apparent volume of distribution might be better termed "volume of dilution" since it is a mathematical description of the volume (l or l/kg) required for dilution of a dose (mg or mg/kg) to produce the observed circulating drug concentration (mg/l or µg/ml). (To simplify cancellation of units, concentrations are expressed here as mg/l, which is the same as µg/ml, the more conventional units for drug concentrations.)

$$\text{Concentration (mg/l)} = \frac{\text{Dose (mg/kg)}}{\text{Apparent volume of distribution (l/kg)}}$$

For many drugs, the volume of distribution does not correspond to a specific physiologic body fluid or tissue, hence the term "apparent." In fact, the volume of distribution for drugs that are bound extensively in tissues may exceed 1.00 l/kg, a physiologic impossibility that emphasizes the arithmetic, nonphysiologic nature of the apparent volume of distribution. The calculation of distribution volume is outlined later.

First-Order Kinetics. Removal of most drugs from the body can be described by first-order (exponential or proportional) kinetics, in which a constant proportion or percentage of a drug is removed over time, rather than a constant amount over time. For drugs exhibiting first-order kinetics, the higher the concentration, the greater the amount removed. The following equations describe the concentration (C) of a drug whose first-order kinetics have a rate constant, k (min^{-1}), at time (t) and an initial concentration of C_0.

In differential form, the change in C with time is:
$$\frac{dC}{dt} = -kC.$$

In exponential form, C at time t is:
$$C_t = C_0 e^{-kt}.$$

If integrated, C at time t is expressed as the natural logarithm (ln):
$$\ln C_t = \ln C_0 - kt.$$

The last equation fits the equation of a straight line so that a graph which plots lnC$_t$ versus t has an intercept of lnC$_0$

at t = 0 and a slope = −k, the rate constant for the change in concentration, which can be used to calculate the half-life and dosages. Multiple rate constants in more complex equations are distinguished with the letter k and numbered subscripts or with Greek letters (explained later).

Half-Life. The drug half-life (t$_{1/2}$) is the time required for a drug concentration to decrease by 50 per cent. Half-life is a first-order kinetic process since the same proportion, 50 per cent, of the drug is removed during equal time periods. Half-life can be determined mathematically from the elimination rate constant, k (see the previous section).

$$t_{1/2} = \frac{\text{natural logarithm } 2}{k} = \frac{0.693}{k}$$

Figure 31–1 illustrates a graphic method for determination of half-life. Drug concentrations measured serially are graphed on semilogarithmic axes, and the best fit line is determined either visually or by linear regression analysis. In this illustration of first-order kinetics, the concentration decreases by 400 (from 800 to 400) during the 1st hour and decreases by 200 (from 400 to 200) during the 2nd hour. Thus, the half-life is 1 hour. Note that more drug is removed during one half-life at higher concentrations, although the proportion removed remains constant. The exponential equation for this graph is: C = 800 e$^{-0.0116\,t}$, where k = 0.0116/minute and C$_0$ = 800, allowing a mathematical calculation of half-life using the equation described above.

$$t_{1/2} = \frac{0.693}{k(\text{minute}^{-1})} = \frac{0.693}{0.0116/\text{minute}} = 60 \text{ minutes}$$

Multicompartment, First-Order Kinetics. The rate of removal of many drugs from the circulation is biphasic. The initial rapid decrease in concentration is the distribution (α) phase, often lasting 15 to 45 minutes, which is followed by a sustained slower rate of removal, the elimination (β) phase. Such biphasic processes are best visualized from semilogarithmic graphs of concentration versus time. When such semilogarithmic graphs reveal

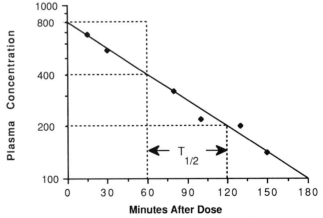

FIGURE 31–1. *Apparent single compartment, first-order plasma drug disappearance curve illustrating graphic determination of half-life from best-fit line of serial plasma concentrations.*

kinetics that best fit two straight lines, the kinetics are described as biexponential or two-compartment, first-order (Fig. 31–2). Two exponential terms are needed to describe such changes in concentration.

$$C = Ae^{-\alpha t} + Be^{-\beta t}$$

In this equation, the rate constant for distribution is designated α to discriminate it from the rate constant for elimination (β) while A and B are the time = 0 intercepts for the lines describing distribution and elimination, respectively.

After an intravenous dose, drug loss from the vascular space during the distribution phase occurs through both distribution and elimination (see Fig. 31–2). The rate constant of distribution (α) can be determined by plotting the difference between the total amount of drug lost initially and the amount of drug lost through elimination (Greenblatt et al., 1975a). This produces the line with the steeper slope (equal to α) below the serum concentration graph in Figure 31–2. The single slope of the distribution phase and of the elimination phase does not imply that distribution or elimination occurs through a single process. The observed rates usually represent the summation of several simultaneous processes, each with differing rates, occurring in various tissues.

When the time course of drug elimination is observed for prolonged periods, a third rate of elimination, or γ phase, may be observed which is usually attributed to elimination of drug that has reequilibrated from deep tissue compartments back into the plasma. Such kinetics are designated "three-compartment" and "first-order." A drug's kinetics are expressed with the smallest number of compartments that accurately describes its concentration changes over time.

Apparent Single-Compartment, First-Order Kinetics. When a semilogarithmic graph of concentration versus time reveals a single slope with no distribution phase, the kinetics are characterized as "apparent" first-order (see Fig. 31–1). This may occur when a drug remains entirely within the vascular space or central compartment or when a drug passes very rapidly back and forth between the circulation and peripheral sites until it is metabolized or excreted by first-order kinetics. The adjective "apparent"

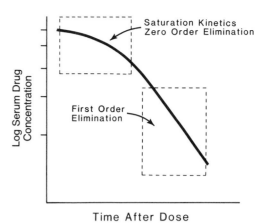

FIGURE 31–3. *Representation of saturation, or zero-order (serum concentration dependent) and first-order (serum concentration independent) pharmacokinetics.*

is used since careful study often reveals distribution does occur although the kinetic curve has only a single slope. Single-compartment kinetics implies that the drug rapidly and completely distributes homogeneously throughout the body, which rarely occurs clinically.

In many pharmacokinetic studies in newborns, blood samples are not obtained early enough to calculate the distribution phase, and the kinetics are described as single compartment. If sampling begins after the distribution phase, the concentration time points may fit a first-order, single-compartment model which determines the elimination rate constant (β). The kinetics cannot be assumed, however, to fit a single-compartment model from such a limited study. The most accurate approach to kinetic analysis, "noncompartmental analysis," makes no assumptions about the number of compartments (Gibaldi and Perrier, 1982; Notari, 1980).

Zero-Order Kinetics. Some drugs demonstrate zero-order kinetics in which a constant amount of drug is removed over time, rather than a constant proportion or percentage. This relationship can be expressed as $dC/dt = -k$. It is important to understand when zero-order kinetics occurs how to recognize it and how it affects drug concentrations. Zero-order kinetics is sometimes referred to as "saturation kinetics" since it may occur when excess amounts of drug completely saturate enzymes or transport systems so that they metabolize or transport only a constant amount of drug over time. Zero-order processes produce a curvilinear shape in a semilogarithmic graph of concentrations versus time (Fig. 31–3). When drug concentrations are high from inappropriate dosing or a drug overdose, kinetics may be zero-order, followed by first-order kinetics at lower concentrations. For drugs exhibiting zero-order kinetics, small increments in dose may cause disproportionately large increments in serum concentra-

TABLE 31–2. Drugs That Demonstrate Saturation Kinetics with Therapeutic Doses in Newborns

Caffeine
Chloramphenicol
Diazepam
Furosemide
Indomethacin
Phenytoin

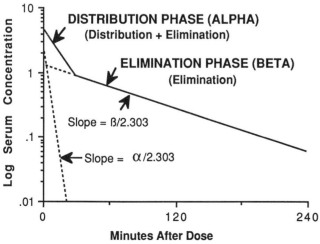

FIGURE 31–2. *Multicompartment serum drug disappearance curve.*

TABLE 31–3. Target Drug Concentration Strategy

Drug dose	→	Plasma total drug concentration	↔	Plasma unbound drug concentration	↔	Target site unbound drug concentration	→	Desired pharmacologic effect

(Data from Sheiner, L. B., and Tozer, T. N.: Clinical pharmacokinetics: The use of plasma concentrations of drugs. *In* Melmon, K. L., and Morrelli, H. F. [Eds]: Clinical Pharmacology: Basic Principles in Therapeutics. 2nd ed. New York, Macmillan, 1978, p. 71.)

tion. Certain drugs administered to newborns exhibit zero-order kinetics at therapeutic doses and concentrations and need to be recognized for their potential accumulation (Table 31–2).

Target Drug Concentration Strategy. Drug treatment of newborns frequently utilizes the target drug concentration strategy (Table 31–3) in which drug therapy corrects a specific problem by producing an effective concentration of free drug at a specific site of action (Sheiner et al., 1978). The target site of drug action is usually inaccessible for monitoring concentrations.

The requirements for effective and accurate application of the target drug concentration treatment to adults have been discussed by Spector and colleagues (1988). When applied to newborns, these requirements highlight the special problems of drug therapy in these patients and the special circumstances in which clinical drug concentration monitoring is appropriate. Some of these requirements include:

1. An available analytic procedure for accurate measurement of drug concentrations in small volumes of blood.

2. A wide variation in pharmacokinetics among individuals with the knowledge that population-based kinetics do not accurately predict individual kinetics.

3. Drug effects that are proportional to plasma drug concentrations.

4. A narrow concentration range between efficacy and toxicity (narrow therapeutic index).

5. Constant pharmacologic effect over time in which tolerance does not develop.

6. Clinical studies that have determined the therapeutic and toxic drug concentration ranges.

Therapeutic Drug Monitoring. Table 31–3 illustrates the basic assumptions of therapeutic drug monitoring: that total plasma drug concentrations correlate with dose as well as with circulating unbound drug concentrations and unbound drug concentration at the site of action. Clinical measurements of drug concentrations usually include both bound and unbound drug while the active portion is that which is unbound (see the Distribution section). There are two broad indications for monitoring drug concentrations: (1) attainment of effective concentrations and (2) avoidance of toxic concentrations. As pointed out by Kauffman (1981), drug concentration ranges are not absolute reflections of effective therapy. Patient response, not a specific drug concentration range, is the end point of therapy.

Although concentrations of aminoglycoside antibiotics, such as gentamicin, are monitored frequently in newborns, toxicity is rare in newborns compared to adults (McCracken, 1986). Because of the limited evidence of toxicity in newborns, it is more important to measure aminoglycoside concentrations in order to achieve effective concentrations for treatment of culture-proven infections than to avoid toxicity. In newborns with serious therapeutic problems, measurement of serum drug concentrations

should be used to achieve effective concentrations as well as to avoid toxicity. When the desired concentration range and kinetic parameters are known, doses may be estimated to reach that concentration with single bolus doses or bolus doses followed by continuous infusions.

Kinetic Dosing. The following equations can be used both to guide dosing and to derive kinetic parameters for individual patients.

Where C = concentration and Vd = volume of distribution:

$$\underset{\text{(mg/kg)}}{\text{Dose}} = \underset{\text{(mg/l)}}{\Delta C} \cdot \underset{\text{(l/kg)}}{\text{Vd}}$$

$$= \underset{\text{(mg/l)}}{[\text{C desired} - \text{C initial}]} \cdot \underset{\text{(l/kg)}}{\text{VD}}$$

This equation may be used to estimate dosage changes needed to increase or decrease concentration. For the first dose, the starting concentration is zero; for doses after the first, the calculation of distribution volume should use the change (Δ) in concentration from the preceding trough to the peak associated with that dose. To reach a desired concentration rapidly, a loading dose can be administered followed by a sustaining infusion. The equation for calculation of infusion doses to maintain a constant concentration is shown below.

Where C = concentration, Vd = volume of distribution, and K = rate constant of elimination:

$$\underset{\text{(mg/kg} \cdot \text{minute)}}{\text{Infusion rate}} = \underset{\text{(minute}^{-1})}{\text{K}} \cdot \underset{\text{(l/kg)}}{\text{Vd}} \cdot \underset{\text{(mg/l)}}{\text{C}}$$

Steady state is reached when tissues are in equilibrium and the amount of drug removed equals the amount of drug infused. The time to reach a steady state depends upon the elimination half-life and is *not* shortened by the administration of a loading dose.

Repetitive Dosing and the "Plateau Principle." During the typical course of drug therapy, drug doses are administered before complete elimination of the previous dose, and the kinetics are more complex (Greenblatt et al., 1975b). During repeated administration, the peak and trough levels after each dose increase for a time. Steady state, or plateau, concentrations are reached when the amount of drug eliminated equals the amount of drug administered during each dosing interval. During repetitive dosing, the steady-state concentrations achieved are related to the half-life, dose, and dosing interval relative to the half-life (Greenblatt et al., 1975b).

Figure 31–4 illustrates a hypothetical concentration time curve for a drug with a half-life of 4 hours administered orally every 4 hours, so the dosing interval corresponds to 1 half-life. Several important principles of pharmacokinetics are illustrated in this figure with the mathematics described in detail elsewhere (Greenblatt et al., 1975b). Drug concentrations rise and fall due to drug

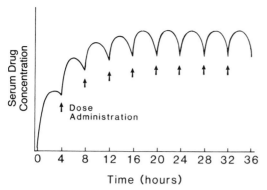

FIGURE 31–4. Representation of multiple dosing with accumulation of serum drug levels to steady-state concentration.

administration (absorption) and elimination. For dosing intervals of one half-life, accumulation is 88 per cent complete after the third dose, 94 per cent complete after the fourth dose and 97 per cent complete after the fifth dose. At steady state, the peak and trough concentrations between doses are the same after each dose. If a drug is administered with a dosing interval equal to one half-life, the steady-state peak and trough concentrations will be two times those reached after the first dose. If the dosing interval is shortened to half of a half-life, the concentration decreases less before the next dose, more total drug is administered per day, and the steady-state peak and trough concentrations are considerably higher (3.4 times the peak and trough concentrations after the first dose). Thus, the shorter the dosing interval–to–half-life ratio, the greater the degree of drug accumulation. As noted during infusions, the *length of time* required to reach steady-state concentrations depends primarily upon the elimination half-life, not the dosing interval.

If the time to reach a therapeutic concentration is excessive, a loading dose can be administered, based upon the desired concentration and estimated distribution volume. Care must be exercised with such doses since toxic concentrations may be reached if the patient has developed a decreased distribution volume or if certain tissues preferentially absorb the particular drug. Digoxin exhibits the latter problem, so the loading dose is usually divided into two or three smaller doses to decrease toxicity while shortening the time to reach a therapeutic concentration.

■ PHARMACOKINETIC PRACTICALITIES

DOSE ADJUSTMENTS

Gentamicin and phenobarbital can be used to illustrate the practical application of the principles of pharmacokinetics and therapeutic drug monitoring already outlined. The calculations may be carried out at the bedside with standard arithmetic calculators.

Gentamicin. Assume that optimal gentamicin concentrations are: 10 μg/ml ≥peak ≥6 μg/ml; 2 μg/ml ≥trough ≥0.5 μg/ml. Gentamicin peak concentration was 5.0 μg/ml, and 18 hours later the trough was 2.5 μg/ml after the fourth 2.5 mg/kg dose was administered IV to an edematous premature newborn. It is apparent that the distribution volume is greater than predicted since the peak

concentration is lower than anticipated, and the half-life is longer than anticipated since the trough is higher than expected. The times of drug infusion and blood sampling were confirmed (an important step), so the half-life is 18 hours since the concentration decreases 50 per cent from 5.0 to 2.5 μg/ml in 18 hrs. (This assumes that the kinetics are linear and first-order.)

$$\text{Volume of distribution} = \frac{\text{Dose (mg/kg)}}{\Delta\text{Concentration (μg/ml)} \cdot 1 \text{ mg/1000 μg}}$$

$$= \frac{2.5 \text{ mg/kg} \cdot 1000 \text{ μg/mg}}{(5.0 - 2.5) \text{ (μg/ml)}}$$

Volume of distribution (ml/kg) = 1000 ml/kg

To insure a trough concentration ≤2.0 μg/ml, doses are administered every two half-lives or every 36 hours. When two half-lives have passed after the fourth dose, the gentamicin concentration should be about 1.25 μg/ml (50 per cent of 2.5 μg/ml). To raise the concentration from the 1.25 μg/ml trough to >6 μg/ml requires a concentration difference of ≥4.75 μg/ml. A dose of 4.75 mg/kg is selected and estimated to produce a peak concentration of 6 μg/ml. In one half-life this concentration will decrease to 3.0 μg/ml, and in two half-lives or 36 hours, to 1.5 μg/ml. Another 4.75 mg/kg dose will increase the peak to 6.25 μg/ml, which will decrease to 3.12 μg/ml in one half-life and to 1.6 μg/ml in two half-lives. The variation between the peak and trough concentrations after the last dose is within the measurement error for gentamicin and should achieve the optimum concentrations defined above.

Phenobarbital. A 3.6 kg asphyxiated newborn developed seizures at birth which were hard to control. Seizures continued after two 20 mg/kg phenobarbital doses until an additional 10 mg/kg dose was administered. A maintenance dose of 7 mg/kg/day was started 24 hours after the loading doses were administered. At 10 days, this child was increasingly somnolent. A phenobarbital level drawn 2 hours after the oral maintenance dose was 50 μg/ml. Additional doses were held, and the phenobarbital concentration was checked daily, as follows: 24 hours = 40 μg/ml; 48 hours = 31 μg/ml; 72 hours = 25 μg/ml; 96 hrs = 21 μg/ml. The maintenance dose (7 mg/kg) was resumed immediately after the 21 μg/ml concentration was measured and produced a concentration of 30 μg/ml. These concentrations and dosages can be used to calculate the volume of distribution and a dose to maintain the phenobarbital concentration between 20 and 30 μg/ml.

$$\text{Volume of distribution (l/kg)} = \frac{\text{Dose (mg/kg)}}{\Delta\text{Concentration (μg/m)} = \text{mg/l}}$$

$$= \frac{7.0 \text{ (mg/kg)}}{(30 - 21) \text{ (mg/l)}}$$

$$= \frac{7 \text{ (mg/kg)}}{9 \text{ (mg/l)}}$$

Volume of distribution (l/kg) = 0.78 (l/kg)

Half-life can be determined from inspection since the concentration decreased from 50 to 25 μg/ml in 72 hours. Thus, it should take 72 hours for the concentration to decrease by 15 μg/ml, from 30 to 15 μg/ml. The concentration will decrease approximately 5 μg/ml every 24 hours or one-third of a half-life. Dividing the half-life into fractions is an approximation since it estimates the change in concentration as linear rather than exponential. To be more accurate, the concentration decreases 59 per cent in half of one half-life. Although this approximation violates certain principles of pharmacokinetics, it allows one to estimate the change in concentration for each third of a half-life as one-third of the change during one half-life. Thus, the concentration will decrease about 5 μg/ml in 24 hours. The following approach can be used to estimate the daily phenobarbital dose needed to return the concentration to 30 μg/ml, a change in concentration of 5 μg/ml.

$$\Delta \text{Concentration (mg/l)} = \frac{\text{Dose (mg/kg)}}{\text{Volume of distribution (l/kg)}}$$

$$5 \text{ (mg/l)} = \frac{\text{Dose (mg/kg)}}{(0.78) \text{ (l/kg)}}$$

$$3.9 \text{ mg/kg} = \text{Dose (mg/kg)}$$

■ BREAST-MILK DRUG EXCRETION

The excretion of drugs in breast milk remains a source of confusion and concern for many physicians and families. Newer analytic techniques and more thorough pharmacokinetic studies have improved the available data in this area of neonatal pharmacology. The available data regarding drug exposure of the newborn through human milk has been organized recently by decreasing levels of concern from drugs that are clearly contraindicated during nursing to those that are of concern pharmacologically to those that have not been associated with problems during nursing. The list of drugs clearly contraindicated during nursing is surprisingly short (see Appendix I).

■ SUMMARY

The extensive drug exposure of the sick newborn in the NICU is dangerous because of the frequency of adverse, sometimes fatal, drug reactions. Unfortunately, in the rapidly changing fetus and newborn, drug therapy is often empiric owing to a lack of gestational age-appropriate kinetic data. Methods appropriate for the study of therapeutics in newborns present unique difficulties, but a review by Ward and Green (1988) may provide assistance for investigators. Drug therapy of newborns requires practical application of the principles of pharmacokinetics and pharmacodynamics that describe the processes of drug absorption, distribution, metabolism, and excretion to estimate and individualize dosages.

■ REFERENCES

Aperia, A., Broberger, O., Elinder, G., et al.: Postnatal development of renal function in pre-term and full-term infants. Acta Paediatr. Scand. 70:183, 1981.

Aranda, J. V., Cohen, S., and Neims, A. H.: Drug utilization in a newborn intensive care unit. J. Pediatr. 89:315, 1976.

Aranda, J. V., Collinge, J. M., and Clarkson, S.: Epidemiologic aspects of drug utilization in a newborn intensive care unit. Semin. Perinatol. 6:148, 1982a.

Aranda, J. V., Portuguez-Malavasi, A., Collinge, J. M., et al.: Epidemiology of adverse drug reactions in the newborn. Dev. Pharmacol. Ther. 5:173, 1982b.

Aranda, J. V.: Factors associated with adverse drug reactions in the newborn. Pediatr. Pharmacol. 3:245, 1983.

Boreus, L. O.: Principles of Pediatric Pharmacology. New York, Churchill Livingstone, 1982.

Burns, L. E., Hodgman, J. E., and Cass, A. B.: Fatal circulatory collapse in premature infants receiving chloramphenicol. N. Engl. J. Med. 261:1318, 1959.

Gibaldi, M., and Perrier, D.: Pharmacokinetics, 2nd ed. New York, Marcel Dekker, 1982.

Gould, T., and Roberts, R. J.: Therapeutic problems arising from the use of the intravenous route for drug administration. J. Pediatr. 95:465, 1979.

Greenblatt, D. J., and Koch-Weser, J.: Clinical pharmacokinetics (first part). N. Engl. J. Med. 293:702, 1975a.

Greenblatt, D. J., and Koch-Weser, J.: Clinical pharmacokinetics (second part). N. Engl. J. Med. 293:964, 1975b.

Kauffman, R. E.: The clinical interpretation and application of drug concentration data. Pediatr. Clin. North Am. 28:35, 1981.

McCracken, G. H.: Aminoglycoside toxicity in infants and children. Am. J. Med. 80(Suppl. 6B):172, 1986.

Mirkin, B. L.: Pharmacodynamics and drug disposition in pregnant women, in neonates, and in children. In Melmon, K. L., and Morrelli, H. F. (Eds.): Clinical Pharmacology: Basic Principles in Therapeutics, 2nd ed. New York, Macmillan, 1978, p. 127.

Morselli, P. L., Franco-Morselli, R., and Bossi, L.: Clinical pharmacokinetics in newborns and infants: Age-related differences and therapeutic implications. Clin. Pharmacokinet. 5:485, 1980.

Notari, R. E.: Biopharmaceutics and Clinical Pharmacokinetics, 3rd ed. New York, Marcel Dekker, 1980.

Peterson, R. G., Simmons, M. A., Rumack, B. H., et al.: Pharmacology of furosemide in the premature newborn infant. J. Pediatr. 97:139, 1980.

Roberts, R. J.: Drug Therapy in Infants: Pharmacologic Principles and Clinical Experience. Philadelphia, W. B. Saunders Company, 1984, p. 3.

Sheiner, L. B., and Tozer, T. N.: Clinical pharmacokinetics: The use of plasma concentrations of drugs. In Melmon, K. L., and Morrelli, H. F. (Eds.): Clinical Pharmacology: Basic Principles in Therapeutics, 2nd ed. New York, Macmillan, 1978, p. 71.

Spector, R., Park, G. D., Johnson, G. F., et al.: Therapeutic drug monitoring. Clin. Pharmacol. Ther. 43:345, 1988.

Sutherland, J. M.: Fatal cardiovascular collapse of infants receiving large amounts of chloramphenicol. J. Dis. Child. 13:761, 1959.

Ward, R. M., Singh, S., and Mirkin, B. L.: Fetal clinical pharmacology. In Avery, G. S. (Ed.): Drug Treatment: Principles and Practice of Clinical Pharmacology and Therapeutics. 2nd ed. New York, Adis Press, 1980, p. 76.

Ward, R. M., and Green, T. P.: Developmental pharmacology and toxicology: Principles of study design and problems of methodology. Pharmacol. Ther. 36:309, 1988.

Weiss, C. F., Glazko, A. J., and Weston, J. K.: Chloramphenicol in the newborn infant: A physiologic explanation of its toxicity when given in excessive doses. N. Engl. J. Med. 262:787, 1960.

AFTERCARE OF HIGH-RISK INFANTS AND LONG-TERM OUTCOME

Victor Y. H. Yu

The success of neonatal intensive care has resulted in survival of increasing numbers of high-risk infants whose hospital discharge does not always imply resolution of the infant's problems. There has been an increased complexity of special problems in these high-risk survivors, some of whom may recover completely with no more than routine care while others may develop chronic illnesses and disabilities requiring the involvement of multiple services, frequent medical consultations, and repeated hospitalizations. The American Academy of Pediatrics (1983) has listed perinatal conditions that identify a significant number of infants at risk: very low birth weight (VLBW) <1500 g, or gestation less than 34 weeks; small for gestational age (SGA); birth asphyxia; seizures; intraventricular hemorrhage; severe hyperbilirubinemia; specific genetic, dysmorphic, or metabolic disorders; perinatal infection; and psychosocial abnormalities, such as maternal drug or alcohol addiction.

Regional centers now routinely enroll high-risk survivors in prospective follow-up programs that enable systematic monitoring of neurologic, developmental, medical, nutritional, and psychosocial status and that provide referrals for early intervention, when indicated. These multidisciplinary assessment clinics complement the primary care delivered by general pediatricians. Both neonatologists and general pediatricians have important roles in ensuring that efforts spent in the neonatal intensive care unit (NICU) are not negated by potentially preventable problems developing after discharge. Their collaboration in aftercare is vital for enhancing the quality of life for all high-risk survivors and their families.

■ AFTERCARE OF HIGH-RISK INFANTS

PRIMARY CARE PROGRAM

Primary care is best delivered by the general pediatrician who often functions as the coordinator to ensure comprehensive aftercare. Some special problems high-risk survivors bring to the primary care pediatrician include the following:

Immunization. The safety and effectiveness of immunization in high-risk infants are often questioned. Delays in immunization have been reported for NICU graduates (Vohr and Oh, 1986) especially in preterm infants (Roper and Day, 1988). The American Academy of Pediatrics' Committee on Infectious Disease (1982) recommended that diphtheria, tetanus, and pertussis (DTP) and oral poliomyelitis vaccine (OPV) be administered to preterm infants at the appropriate chronologic age. Only DTP should be given to infants who are still hospitalized at 2 months of age to avoid cross-infection with OPV in the nursery. For these infants, the OPV series can be initiated on discharge.

Vitamin and Mineral Requirements. All preterm infants should routinely receive daily multivitamin preparations with vitamins A, B, C, and D (Tsang, 1985). Supplementation with 2 mg/kg/day of elemental iron is also recommended when the infant has doubled his or her birth weight. The Committee on Nutrition of the American Academy of Pediatrics (1977) recommends that formulas designed for preterm infants provide a minimum of 0.7 IU of vitamin E per 100 kcal/day and, in addition, that the infants receive between 5 and 25 IU of vitamin E supplement per day. Preterm infants also need 35 to 60 µg/day of folate. It is important that the physician caring for an infant knows the folate content of the child's formula and that supplements are given until the daily intake is at least 300 ml/day of most formulas. Many infants with special problems, including hemolysis or gastrointestinal problems, may require folate for a much longer period of time.

Medical Disorders. Preterm infants, especially those who need mechanical ventilation, are susceptible to middle ear effusions in infancy (Gravel et al., 1988). Among extremely-low-birth-weight (ELBW) survivors (<1000g), otitis media (55 per cent of children), wheezing episodes (48 per cent), chest infections (29 per cent), and gastroenteritis (26 per cent) were the most common medical disorders (Bowman and Yu, 1988). This prevalence of wheezing was six times that in normal birth weight children. It has been reported that less than 10 per cent of children who had just one wheezing episode by 5 years continued to wheeze at 10 years, but the more attacks the child has had, the higher the risk of persistent wheezing (Park et al., 1986).

Many special problems are experienced by high-risk survivors, such as deviations from expected patterns of growth and development, hearing impairment, retinopathy of prematurity (ROP), anemia, home monitoring for apnea, bronchopulmonary dysplasia, home oxygen therapy, intracranial hemorrhage, posthemorrhagic hydrocephalus, seizures, congenital heart disease, short bowel syndrome, home parenteral nutrition, and cosmetic defects, both congenital or iatrogenically acquired. The pathogenesis of these problems, their effects on the child and family, and detailed methods for their aftercare are described in the relevant sections of this book as well as in three published monographs (Ballard, 1988; Hurt, 1984; Taeusch and Yogman, 1987).

Surgical Disorders. Following hospital discharge, 36 per cent of ELBW children were readmitted for surgery in the first 2 years, aural ventilation tube insertions (10 per cent of children) and inguinal herniorrhaphy (9 per cent) being the two most common surgical procedures (Bowman and Yu, 1988). Because inguinal hernia has a 31 per cent risk of incarceration and 9 per cent risk of bowel obstruction in early infancy, their elective repair in VLBW infants before hospital discharge has been recommended (Rescoria and Grosfeld, 1984).

Rehospitalization. Readmission rates were reported at 22 to 53 per cent for VLBW children in the first 1 to 2 years after discharge, compared with 9 to 18 per cent in comparative groups of larger infants (McCormick et al., 1980; Mutch et al., 1986). The relative risk of rehospitalization in VLBW children was therefore 2.2 to 5.5 compared with 3.4 reported in ELBW children (Bowman and Yu, 1988). Studies suggested that socioeconomic disadvantages increase the risk of morbidity and rehospitalization in high-risk survivors (Combs-Orme et al., 1988). The two most common reasons for rehospitalization were respiratory tract disorders and surgical procedures. Significant behavior disturbances in children who required hospitalization in infancy have been reported (Vernon et al., 1986), though in a modern pediatric setting, little evidence was found of such long-term sequelae (Shannon et al., 1984).

Postneonatal Mortality. NICU graduates and VLBW infants were reported to have a postneonatal and postdischarge mortality 5 to 10 times the rate for normal infants. The majority of postneonatal deaths prior to hospital discharge were caused by bronchopulmonary dysplasia (Yu et al., 1984c). Sudden and unexpected death was the predominant cause of postneonatal death after hospital discharge in NICU graduates and in VLBW infants with a relative risk of three to eight times the normal population. The pathophysiology might be different from sudden infant death syndrome (SIDS) that occurs in healthy term infants, as the majority of these deaths occur in infants with some residual illness, such as bronchopulmonary dysplasia. The proportion of deaths that occurred in the postneonatal period was found to be significantly higher in infants with a 1001 to 1500 g birth weight than in those who were ELBW. In ELBW infants, the postdischarge

mortality rate of 3.4 per cent in the first 3 years (Bowman and Yu, 1988) was similar to the 3.8 per cent reported for children of all birth weights discharged from the NICU.

HIGH-RISK FOLLOW-UP PROGRAM

Aftercare of high-risk infants should include careful evaluation of the nervous system and systematic visual, hearing, developmental, and social-behavioral assessments. This is best carried out in a specialized follow-up program established within a regional center and staffed by a multidisciplinary team that includes a developmental pediatrician, nurse coordinator, psychologist, physical therapist, and social worker. Follow-up programs are designed to meet one or more of the following objectives:

1. Monitoring long-term mortality and morbidity of NICU graduates.
2. Determining perinatal etiologic factors for major disabilities.
3. Assessing social-environmental influences that may exacerbate or diminish biological risks.
4. Providing good training programs in developmental pediatrics.
5. Participating in research studies with long-term outcome measures.
6. Contributing to the aftercare of high-risk infants, including the prediction of those likely to develop problems by school age and their selection for early intervention.

Suggestions for the organization of follow-up clinics and for improving the design, analysis, and reporting of results of follow-up studies have been published (Davies, 1984; Kiely and Paneth, 1981; Taeusch and Yogman, 1987). Guidelines have also been drawn up by national expert bodies such as the American Academy of Pediatrics (1983) and the Australian National Health and Medical Research Council (1983) (see the chapter Appendix).

The terms "impairment," "disability," and "handicap" (World Health Organization, 1980) help improve the precision used to describe the long-term outcome of high-risk infants. Impairment describes the medical category of the disorder, for example, cerebral palsy, blindness, deafness, or developmental delay. Disability results if the impairment causes restriction of ability, which may be major or minor in severity. Handicap is the disadvantage accruing to the disabled individual because certain aspects of normal life are denied to the person by society. An attempt must be made to determine the degree of interference in function that may result from any given impairment.

Neurologic Assessment. Major neurologic disabilities can be identified by 2 years of age. Caution must be exercised in labeling younger children with motor impairments and in predicting their future motor disability. In the Collaborative Perinatal Project, over half the children diagnosed to have cerebral palsy at one year of age were free of motor disorders by age 7 (Nelson and Ellenberg, 1982). It has been recommended that every effort should be made to follow children at least until age 4 and preferably age 7 (Kiely and Paneth, 1981).

Visual Assessment. All preterm infants treated with oxygen require an indirect ophthalmoscopic examination. If ROP is diagnosed, frequent follow-up examinations are indicated until the disease has reached a quiescent stage, after which yearly examinations are recommended.

Hearing Assessment. Infants at risk of hearing loss include those with a positive family history, congenital or perinatal infection, anatomic malformations of the head and neck, VLBW, hyperbilirubinemia requiring exchange transfusions, bacterial meningitis, and severe birth asphxyia (Joint Committee on Infant Hearing, 1983). Their hearing should be screened by 3 months of age and no later than 6 months. If results are equivocal, the infant should be referred for comprehensive audiologic evaluation. For the hearing-impaired infant, speech and language function should be assessed periodically.

Cognitive Assessment. Tests most widely used include the Gesell Developmental Schedules, from 1 month of age; the Bayley Scales of Infant Development, between 6 months and 2 years of age; the McCarthy Cognitive Index and Stanford-Binet Intelligence Scale, at 3 years; the Beery Visual Motor Integration and Zimmerman Receptive Expressive Language Assessment, at 4 years; the Wechsler Preschool and Primary Intelligence Scale, at 6 years; and the Wechsler Intelligence Scale for Children, at 8 years of age. The Denver Developmental Screening Test is unsatisfactory because it is not a sensitive indicator of developmental delay, particularly in preterm infants. The transactional model of child development provides insight of the importance of the environment in relation to the child's development after infancy. The instrument most commonly used to assess the home environment is the Home Observation for Measurement of the Environment (Caldwell, 1978).

For preterm infants, it has been the custom to correct test scores for prematurity during the first 2 years, though this practice has been shown to overcorrect after the first 12 months (Siegal, 1983). It is important that tests be administered by professionals who have sound knowledge of child development, training in the use of the tests and who understand the tests' strengths and limitations (Aylward, 1987). Although the benefits of early identification of intellectual impairment are great, the discontinuous nature of child development results in poor correlation between developmental scores under 2 years and later intellectual abilities (McCall, 1983).

Social-Behavioral Assessment. Social-behavioral assessment of the high-risk infant and family helps to identify behaviors that cause family disruption or are developmentally incapacitating. Abnormal behavior at 2 years has been found to identify a subgroup of VLBW children at high risk of learning disability at school age (Astbury et al., 1990). Socioeconomic status and family characteristics are important factors known to affect intellectual development (Hunt et al., 1988). Identification of family relationships at risk is important because it permits counseling and referral to mental health services and parent support groups. Factors reported to be associated with increased risk of child abuse include prematurity, prolonged hospitalization, single or adolescent mother, and infrequent visitation by the family during initial hospitalization. However, one study was unable to confirm that prematurity and low birth weight are risk factors for child abuse (Leventhal et al., 1984).

EARLY INTERVENTION PROGRAM

School problems in NICU graduates can be reliably predicted 60 per cent of the time prior to hospital discharge and, by means of a prospective follow-up program, 80 per cent of the time prior to school entry (Sell et al., 1985). Early intervention can thus be focused on those most likely to benefit from it. Intervention programs differ on location of the treatment and who is the recipient of the efforts. Hospital-based infant-focused interventions, involving tactile, auditory, or kinesthetic stimulation programs, have shown short-term benefits, such as weight gain or alertness (Field et al., 1986) but are not efficacious in altering the long-term pattern of motor development (Piper et al., 1986). Hospital-based parent-focused interventions have been shown to improve parent-infant interactions, but long-term effects were inconsistent (Minde et al., 1980). A meta-analysis of 31 parent- and infant-focused early intervention programs with a home-based component confirmed that they are effective in promoting developmental progress in children younger than 3 years old with biologically based disabilities (Shonkoff and Hauser-Cram, 1987). Those that provide a structured curriculum with a high level of parental involvement were found to be most effective. Programs were also found to be more effective in VLBW infants compared with those who weighed 1500 to 2000 g at birth. Home-based intervention programs have also been shown to enhance the quality of parent-infant interactions in preterm infants and reduce rehospitalization rates in NICU graduates (Perrault et al., 1986). Recently, in a multicenter intervention program, Gross (1990) demonstrated that a program of home visits and family support, coupled with an enriched day care experience, can result in significant improvements in cognitive outcome for LBW infants.

■ LONG-TERM OUTCOME OF HIGH-RISK INFANTS

Numerous reports have been published that describe the long-term outcome for specific high-risk categories. For example, infants have been selected for study because they have birth asphyxia, respiratory distress syndrome, neonatal apneic attacks, polycythemia-hyperviscosity syndrome, hypoglycemia, or seizures as well as if they were born of mothers with diabetes mellitus or rhesus incompatibility, if they required mechanical ventilation, or if they developed complications such as bronchopulmonary dysplasia or posthemorrhagic hydrocephalus. More recent studies with ultrasound, computed tomography, positron emission tomography, and magnetic resonance imaging provide information on actual brain injury, thus defining further specific groups at risk for neurodevelopmental disabilities. The long-term outcome of many of these high-risk categories is described in other sections of this book in which the respective neonatal disorders are reviewed. The next section reports the outcome of a group of infants who are at high risk because they are low birth weight

TABLE 32–1. Pooled Institutional Neonatal Mortality Rates for Inborn Very-Low-Birth-Weight Infants

YEAR OF BIRTH	≤1000 GRAMS	1001 TO 1500 GRAMS
1961–65	185/197 (93.9%)	142/274 (51.8%)
1966–70	381/443 (86.0%)	212/567 (37.4%)
1971–75	209/274 (76.3%)	54/253 (21.3%)
1976–80	458/818 (56.0%)	284/1611 (17.6%)
1981–85	243/467 (52.0%)	186/1879 (9.9%)

Data expressed as deaths/births (per cent mortality).
Office of Technology Assessment: Neonatal intensive care for low birthweight infants: Costs and effectiveness. Washington, D.C., Government Printing Office, 1987.

and/or preterm, infants for whom the long-term outcome has dramatically improved over the past few decades in association with rapid changes in perinatal care.

EXTREMELY LOW-BIRTH-WEIGHT AND PRETERM INFANTS

The progressive improvement in mortality rate in ELBW infants with a <1500 g birth weight is summarized in Table 32–1, based on data published by the Office of Technology Assessment (1987) of the United States Congress. When neonatal intensive care was introduced, concern was raised that infants who otherwise would have died would now survive with major disabilities.

MORTALITY

Over 15 studies reporting the mortality of ELBW infants have been reviewed, but the problems involved with the interpretation and comparison of published data are multiple (Yu, 1987). The results from three institutional-based series which include all inborn live births are shown in Table 32–2. Note that the results are very similar. Other reports describing survival in 100 g increments may exclude those with birth defects, exclude delivery room deaths, include outborn infants, or define mortality at 28 days only and thus make comparisons less meaningful.

Most studies used birth weight as a framework for reporting outcome. Outcome data based on individual gestations began to appear in the literature in 1984 (Yu

TABLE 32–2. Hospital Mortality Rates of Extremely-Low-Birth-Weight Infants

BIRTH WEIGHT	MELBOURNE* 1977 TO 1983	MEMPHIS† 1981 TO 1985	CLEVELAND‡ 1986 TO 1987
500–599	31/35 (89%)	75/79 (95%)	21/23 (91%)
600–699	27/37 (73%)	74/94 (79%)	14/21 (67%)
700–799	17/34 (50%)	54/83 (65%)	14/28 (50%)
800–899	20/56 (36%)	36/96 (38%)	9/26 (35%)
900–999	16/48 (33%)	45/124 (36%)	10/31 (32%)
Total	111/210 (53%)	284/476 (60%)	68/129 (53%)

Data expressed as deaths/births (per cent mortality).
*Yu, V. Y. H., Wong, P. Y., Bajuk, B., et al.: Outcome of extremely low birthweight infants. Brit. J. Obstet. Gynaecol. 93:162, 1986c.
†Amon, E., Sibai, B. M., Anderson, G. D., et al.: Obstetric variables predicting survival of the immature newborn (≤1000 gm): A five-year experience at a single perinatal center. Am. J. Obstet. Gynecol. 156:1380, 1987.
‡Hack, M., and Fanaroff, A. A.: How small is too small? Considerations in evaluating the outcome of the tiny infant. Clin. Perinatol. 15:775, 1988.

et al., 1984b). Pooled data of survival and disability rates of inborn cohorts from the period 1977 to 1984 showed that the hospital mortality rate was 76 per cent (76 of 100) at 24 weeks, 65 per cent (100 of 155) at 25 weeks, 45 per cent (89 of 200) at 26 weeks, 27 per cent (63 of 231) at 27 weeks, and 23 per cent (66 of 281) at 28 weeks.

Selection bias in institutional-based studies prevents their results from being extrapolated to a geographic region. Regional ELBW studies were first published in 1984 from the State of Victoria in Australia (Kitchen et al., 1984b) and the Hamilton-Wentworth County in Ontario, Canada (Saigal et al., 1984). The Canadian study showed that survival of ELBW infants has doubled over time. The Australian study showed that the mortality of infants born in tertiary perinatal centers was significantly lower than that of outborn infants. They also have shown that stillbirth rates among ELBW infants, and hence, the perinatal mortality rate, were significantly lower in perinatal center births compared to those born elsewhere (Lumley et al., 1988).

For ELBW or extremely preterm infants born in perinatal centers, risk factors associated with increased mortality include antepartum hemorrhage, multiple pregnancy, breech presentation, absence of labor prior to delivery, absence of maternal steroid therapy, perinatal asphyxia, male sex, hypothermia, hyptension, hyaline membrane disease, persistent pulmonary hypertension, infection, intraventricular hemorrhage, and delayed onset of diuresis. The optimal mode of delivery for ELBW or extremely preterm infants is controversial, and opinions vary with retrospective reports in the literature (Yu et al., 1984a). We have found no evidence to support the routine use of cesarean section in those with vertex presentation (Yu et al., 1987).

MORBIDITY

Pooled data from the literature showed a major disability in 123 (25 per cent) of 483 ELBW survivors born over the period 1965 to 1983 (Yu, 1987). Similar findings were reported by Hack and Famaroff (1989). The major disability rate among ELBW survivors has not changed even though many who previously would have died are now surviving. Extremely preterm infants born at 28 weeks or less have a major disability rate of about 20 per cent (Yu et al., 1986b). A regional-based study from Australia further emphasized the importance of place of birth. The disability rate of inborn ELBW survivors was significantly lower than that of outborn survivors at 2 years and 5 years of age (Kitchen et al., 1987). For ELBW or extremely preterm infants born in perinatal centers, risk factors associated with increased impairment included antepartum hemorrhage, absence of maternal steroid therapy, severe respiratory failure, delay in regaining birthweight, seizures, and intraventricular hemorrhage (Yu et al., 1986a). Furthermore, extremely preterm vaginal births of the nonvertex group had a significantly lower survival rate and higher disability rate compared with the vertex group (Yu et al., 1987). It was in the nonvertex group that cesarean births were associated with a significantly lower disability rate compared with vaginal births. These findings suggested that there is definite need for a randomized clinical trial to investigate the potential benefits of cesarean section in extremely preterm infants with nonvertex presentation.

Pooled data on specific impairments in 483 ELBW survivors showed a median prevalence of 12 per cent for cerebral palsy, 3 per cent for blindness, 2 per cent for sensorineural deafness, and 15 per cent for developmental delay (Yu, 1987). Spastic quadriplegia (3.8 per cent) was the most common type of cerebral palsy, followed by spastic hemiplegia (3.5 per cent), spastic diplegia (2.2 per cent), athetoid cerebral palsy (0.8 per cent), and spastic monoplegia (0.5 per cent). The reported association between spastic diplegia and prematurity is therefore not prominent in ELBW infants. A regional survey reported serious visual defects in 4.3 per cent of ELBW survivors (Alberman et al., 1982a). In the last three decades, retinopathy of prematurity has become a disease of progressively smaller and less mature infants (Hoon et al., 1988). Phelps (1981), assuming a probability that 8 per cent of ELBW survivors are blind from severe ROP, estimated that these infants are responsible for 85 per cent of all cases of blindness from ROP. As many children with severe ROP also have neurodevelopmental problems, they should be referred early to appropriate support services and intervention programs to optimize their cognitive and emotional development. Sensorineural hearing loss was reported in 9 per cent of VLBW survivors born 10 to 20 years ago (Abramovich et al., 1979) but a decrease in prevalence was observed in recent years (Kitchen et al., 1982), probably as a result of the reduction in such perinatal risk factors as hypoxia, hyperbilirubinemia, ototoxic drugs, apneic attacks, and meningitis. Hearing should nevertheless be periodically assessed in high-risk groups such as ELBW survivors, about half of whom develop otitis media.

High-prevalence, low-severity developmental disorders in school-age children have been described, leading to learning difficulties such as problems with attention, perception, sequencing, language, and organization of motor performance. The extent to which ELBW survivors experience behavioral and communication disorders and poor academic performance is currently being investigated. Between one-third to one-half of school-age ELBW children were found to have deficits in reading comprehension, speech and language development, visual-motor integration, gross and fine motor skills, and perceptual skills (Kenworthy et al., 1987). Routine, periodic screening of speech and language development and psychoeducational abilities of ELBW children is therefore required as part of a comprehensive management strategy.

SUMMARY

Calculations made from data in the Office of Technology Assessment's (OTA) 1987 report of the United States Congress indicate that, for every 1000 births, 76 disabled ELBW children would survive who would have died a decade ago. This figure is balanced against the 253 net increase in normal infants who would also survive with current intensive care (Fig. 32–1).

LARGER AND MORE MATURE PRETERM INFANTS

It is in the group of larger and more mature preterm infants with birth weights of over 1000 g where the "gains"

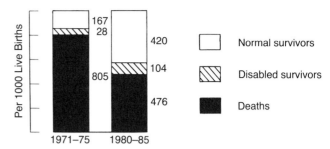

FIGURE 32–1. Gains and losses in extremely-low-birth-weight (ELBW) infants. (Data from Office of Technology Assessment Report to Congress: Neonatal intensive care for low birthweight infants: Costs and effectiveness (Health technology case study 38), OTA-HCS-38. Washington, D.C., Government Printing Office, 1987.)

with neonatal intensive care far exceed the "losses." Infants with 1000 to 1500 g birth weights currently are expected to have a mortality rate of below 10 per cent. The OTA study reported late disabilities in 100 (8 per cent) of 1215 such infants born in the period 1975 to 1985.

Clinical factors associated with adverse outcome in larger preterm infants are different from ELBW infants. Significant perinatal factors for late disability included spontaneous, uncomplicated preterm delivery, recurrent apnea, and abnormal neonatal neurologic findings (Marlow et al., 1988). Developmental delay was reported to be associated with neonatal caloric deprivation (Georgieff et al., 1985), poor head growth (Hack and Breslau, 1986), and postnatal growth failure (Astbury et al., 1986). In larger preterm infants, environmental factors appear to have a more significant impact on developmental outcome than medical factors. The strongest correlates of developmental status are not obstetric or neonatal complications but social factors. It has been suggested that environmental deficits and stresses impair early cognitive and psychosocial development in all infants, but preterm infants are more vulnerable to environmental insufficiencies than term infants. The level of parent education influences the degree of severity of the disability of VLBW survivors at 8 years of age (Hunt et al., 1988). To optimize the outcome especially for these larger preterm infants, social and environmental factors should become targets of intervention efforts.

SMALL-FOR-GESTATIONAL-AGE INFANTS

Most follow-up studies on SGA infants are in agreement about reduced growth potential but are often contradictory about neurodevelopmental outcome. The percentage of small children is higher in SGA infants than in those who are appropriate for gestational age (AGA). Preterm SGA infants may have a higher incidence of major disability than preterm AGA infants, while term SGA infants have an increased risk of speech and language problems, attention deficits, and school failures despite normal intelligence. Studies that reported SGA infants have a relatively unfavorable neurodevelopmental prognosis are primarily based on infants born before the mid-1960s or on outborn infants who were transferred to a NICU after birth—groups likely to have sustained significant perinatal insults. Nonasphyxiated SGA infants from this early era were found to have a good prognosis for neurologic and cognitive development. In cohorts from 1970 to 1976, no differences were found between SGA and AGA children in major disability, mental performance, hearing, vision, speech, or specific ill health, especially when SGA infants with congenital and genetic disorders were excluded (Ounsted et al., 1984). The improved prognosis for SGA infants coincided with rapid changes in perinatal care aimed at minimizing fetal and neonatal compromise. Indeed, it has been found that in SGA infants, there was a significant negative correlation between gestational age and developmental scores at 4 to 7 years (Ounsted et al., 1986). Those with retardation of head growth in the second trimester were noted to be at high risk of neurologic deficit, developmental delay, and perceptual-motor and gross motor disorders (Harvey et al., 1982). These findings suggest that when intrauterine growth restriction is operative, some of the SGA fetuses may have been adversely affected by remaining in utero, and elective delivery before term may enhance the chances of these children achieving their full potential in later childhood. Nevertheless, when preterm SGA infants are compared with AGA infants of similar gestational age, they have smaller body dimensions, more complications in their nursery course, and more neurologic problems at 1 year of age (Pena et al., 1988). These observations need confirmation with longer follow-up, but they suggest that intrauterine growth retardation constitutes an additional risk factor for the preterm infant.

■ REFERENCES

Abramovich, S. L., Gregory, S., Slemick, M., et al.: Hearing loss in very low birthweight infants treated with neonatal intensive care. Arch. Dis. Child. 54:421, 1979.

Alberman, E., Benson, J., and Evans, S.: Visual defects in children of low birthweight. Arch. Dis. Child. 57:818, 1982a.

American Academy of Pediatrics and American College of Obstetricians and Gynecologists. Guidelines for Perinatal Care. Evanston, Ill., AAP/ACOG, 1983, p. 97.

Amon, E., Sibai, B. M., Anderson, G. D., et al.: Obstetric variables predicting survival of the immature newborn (≤1000 gm): A five-year experience at a single perinatal center. Am. J. Obstet. Gynecol. 156:1380, 1987.

Astbury, J., Orgill, A. A., Bajuk, B., et al.: The sequelae of growth failure inappropriate for gestational age, very low birthweight children. Dev. Med. Child. Neurol. 28:472, 1986.

Astbury, J., Orgill, A. A., Bajuk, B., et al.: Neurodevelopmental outcome, growth and health of extremely-low-birthweight survivors: How soon can we tell? Dev. Med. Child Neurol. 32:582, 1990.

Aylward, G. P.: Developmental assessment: Caveats and a cry for quality control. J. Pediatr. 110:253, 1987.

Ballard, R. A. (Ed.): Pediatric care of the ICN graduate. Philadelphia, W. B. Saunders Company, 1988.

Bowman, E., and Yu, V. Y. H.: Continuing morbidity in extremely low birthweight infants. Early Hum. Dev. 18:165, 1988.

Caldwell, B. M.: Home Observation for Measurement of the Environment. Little Rock, Ark., University of Arkansas, 1978.

Child Health Committee: Long-Term Follow-Up of Small Preterm Infants. Canberra, Australian National Health and Medical Research Council, 1983.

Combs-Orme, T., Fishbein, J., Summerville, C., et al.: Rehospitalization of very-low-birth-weight infants. Am. J. Dis. Child. 142:1109, 1988.

Committee on Infectious Disease: The 1982 Red Book, 19th ed. Evanston, Ill., American Academy of Pediatrics, 1982, p. 20.

Committee on Nutrition; American Academy of Pediatrics. Nutritional needs of low-birth-weight infants. Pediatrics 60:519, 1977.

Davies, P. A.: Follow-up of low birthweight children. Arch. Dis. Child. 59:794, 1984.

Field, T. M., Schanberg, S. M., Scafidi, F., et al.: Tactile/kinesthetic stimulation effects on preterm neonates. Pediatrics 77:654, 1986.

Geogieff, M. K., Hoffman, J. S., Pereira, G. R., et al.: Effect of neonatal caloric deprivation on head growth and 1-year developmental status in preterm infants. J. Pediatr. 107:581, 1985.

Gravel, J. S., McCarton, C. M., and Ruben, R. J.: Otitis media in neonatal intensive care unit graduates: A 1-year prospective study. Pediatrics 82:44, 1988.

Gross, R. T., et al.: Enhancing the outcomes of low birth weight premature infants. J.A.M.A. 263:3035, 1990.

Hack, M., and Breslau, N.: Very low birthweight infants: Effects of brain growth during infancy on intelligence quotient at 3 years of age. Pediatrics 77:196, 1986.

Hack, M., and Fanaroff, A. A. How small is too small? Considerations in evaluating the outcome of the tiny infant. Clin. Perinatol. 15:775, 1988.

Hack, M., and Fanaroff, A. A.: Outcomes of extremely-low-birth infants between 1982 and 1988. N. Engl. J. Med. 321:1642, 1989.

Harvey, D., Prince, J., Bunton, J., et al.: Abilities of children who were small for gestational age babies. Pediatrics 69:296, 1982.

Hoon, A. H., Jan, J. E., Whitfield, M. F., et al.: Changing pattern of retinopathy of prematurity: a 37-year clinic experience. Pediatrics 82:344, 1988.

Hunt, J. V., Cooper, B. A. B., and Tooley, W. H.: Very low birth weight infants at 8 and 11 years of age: Role of neonatal illness and family status. Pediatrics 82:596, 1988.

Hurt, H. (Ed.): Continuing care of the high-risk infant. Philadelphia, W. B. Saunders Company, 1984.

Joint Committee on Infant Hearing: Position statement, 1982. Ear Hear. 4:3, 1983.

Kenworthy, O. T., Bess, F. H., Stahlman, M. T., et al.: Hearing, speech, and language outcome in infants of extreme immaturity. Am. J. Otol. 8:419, 1987.

Kiely, J. L., and Paneth, N.: Follow-up studies of low-birthweight infants: Suggestions for design, analysis and reporting. Dev. Med. Child. Neurol. 23:96, 1981.

Kitchen, W. H., Ford, G., Orgill, A. A., et al.: Outcome of infants of birthweight 500–999 grams: A continuing regional study of 5 year old survivors. J. Pediatr. 111:761, 1987.

Kitchen, W. H., Orgill, A. A., Ford, G., et al.: Outcome of infants of birthweight 500–599 g: A regional study of 1979–1980 births. J. Paediatr. 104:921, 1984.

Kitchen, W. H., Ryan, M. M., Rickards, A., et al.: Changing outcome over 13 years of very low birthweight infants. Semin. Perinatol. 6:373, 1982.

Leventhal, J. M., Egerter, S. A., and Murphy, J. M.: Reassessment of the relationship of perinatal risk factors and child abuse. Am. J. Dis. Child. 138:1034, 1984.

Lumley, J., Kitchen, W. H., Roy, R. N. D., et al.: The survival of extremely low birthweight infants in Victoria: 1982–85. Med. J. Aust. 149:242, 1988.

McCall, R. B.: Predicting developmental outcome. Resume and redirection. In Brazelton, T. B., and Lester, B. M. (Eds.). New Approaches to Developmental Screening of Infants. New York, Elsevier, 1983.

McCormick, M. C., Shapiro, S., and Starfield, B. H.: Rehospitalization in the first year of life for high-risk survivors. Pediatrics 66:991, 1980.

Marlow, N., Hunt, L. P., and Chiswick, M. L.: Clinical factors associated with adverse outcome for babies weighing 2000 g or less at birth. Arch. Dis. Child. 63:1131, 1988.

Minde, K., Shosenberg, N., Marton, P., et al.: Self-help groups in a premature nursery: A controlled evaluation. J. Pediatr. 96:933, 1980.

Mutch, L., Newdick, M., Lodwick, A., et al.: Secular changes in rehospitalization of very low birthweight infants. Pediatrics 78:164, 1986.

Nelson, K. B., and Ellenberg, J. H.: Children who 'outgrew' cerebral palsy. Pediatrics 69:529, 1982.

Office of Technology Assessment Report to Congress: Neonatal intensive care for low birthweight infants: Costs and effectiveness (Health technology case study 38), OTA-HCS-38. Washington, D.C., Government Printing Office, 1987.

Ounsted, M. K., Moar, V. A., and Scott, A.: Children of deviant birthweight at the age of 7 years: Health, handicap, size and developmental status. Early Hum. Dev. 9:323, 1984.

Ounsted, M. K., Moar, V. A., and Scott, A.: Factors affecting development: Similarities and differences among children who were small, average, and large for gestational age at birth. Acta Paediatr. Scand. 75:261, 1986.

Park, E. S., Golding, J., Carswell, F., et al.: Preschool wheezing and prognosis at 10. Arch. Dis. Child. 61:642, 1986.

Pena, I. C., Teberg, A. J., and Finello, K. M.: The premature small-for-gestational-age infant during the first year of life: Comparison by birth weight and gestational age. J. Pediatr. *113*:1066, 1988.

Perrault, C., Coates, A. L., Collinge, J., et al.: Family support system in newborn medicine: Does it work? Follow-up study of infants at risk. J. Pediatr. *108*:1025, 1986.

Phelps, D. L.: Retinopathy of prematurity: An estimate of vision loss in the United States. Pediatrics *67*:924, 1981.

Piper, M. C., Kunos, V. I., Willis, D. M., et al.: Early physical therapy effects on the high-risk infant: A randomised controlled trial. Pediatrics *78*:216, 1986.

Rescoria, F. J., and Grosfeld, J. L.: Inguinal hernia repair in the perinatal period and early infancy: Clinical considerations. J. Pediatr. Surg. *19*:832, 1984.

Roper, J., and Day, S.: Uptake of immunisation in low birthweight infants. Arch. Dis. Child. *63*:518, 1988.

Saigal, S., Rosenbaum, P., Stoskopf, B., et al.: Outcome in infants 501 to 1000gm birth weight delivered to residents of the McMaster Health Region. J. Pediatr. *105*:969, 1984.

Sell, E. J., Gaines, J. A., Gluckman, C., et al.: Early identification of learning problems in neonatal intensive care graduates. Am. J. Dis. Child. *139*:460, 1985.

Shannon, F. T., Fergusson, D. M., and Dimond, M. E.: Early hospital admissions and subsequent behaviour problems in 6 year olds. Arch. Dis. Child. *59*:815, 1984.

Shonkoff, J. P., and Hauser-Cram, P.: Early intervention for disabled infants and their families: A quantitative analysis. Pediatrics *80*:650, 1987.

Siegal, L. S.: Correction for prematurity and its consequences for the assessment of the very low birthweight infant. Child Dev. *54*:1176, 1983.

Taeusch, H. W. and Yogman, M. W. (Eds.): Follow-Up Management of the High-Risk Infant. Boston, Little, Brown & Company, 1987.

Tsang, R. C. (Ed.): Vitamin and Mineral Requirements in Preterm Infants. New York, Marcel Dekker, 1985.

Vernon, D. T., Silverman, J. L., and Foley, J. M.: Changes in children's behavior after hospitalization. Am. J. Dis. Child. *111*:581, 1986.

Vohr, B. R., and Oh, W.: Age of diphtheria, tetanus, and pertussis immunization of special care nursery graduates. Pediatrics *77*:569, 1986.

World Health Organization: International classification of impairments, disabilities and handicaps. A manual of classification relating to the consequences of disease. Geneva, World Health Organization, 1980.

Yu, V. Y. H.: Survival and neurodevelopmental outcome of preterm infants. *In* Yu, V. Y. H. and Wood, E. C. (Eds.). Prematurity. London, Churchill Livingstone, 1987, p. 223.

Yu, V. Y. H., Bajuk, B., Cutting, D., et al.: Effect of mode of delivery on outcome of very low birthweight infants. Brit. J. Obstet. Gynaecol. *9*:633, 1984a.

Yu, V. Y. H., Downe, L., Astbury, J., et al.: Perinatal factors associated with adverse outcome in extremely low birthweight infants. Arch. Dis. Child. *62*:554, 1986a.

Yu, V. Y. H., Loke, H. L., Bajuk, B., et al.: Prognosis for infants born 23 to 28 weeks' gestation. Brit. Med. J. *293*:1200, 1986b.

Yu, V. Y. H., Loke, H. L., Bajuk, B., et al.: Outcome of singleton infants delivered vaginally or by caesarean section at 23 to 28 weeks' gestation. Aust. N.Z. J. Obstet. Gynaecol. *27*:196, 1987.

Yu, V. Y. H., Orgill, A. A., Bajuk, B., et al.: Survival and 2-year outcome of extremely preterm infants. Brit. J. Obstet. Gynaecol. *9*:640, 1984b.

Yu, V. Y. H., Watkins, A., and Bajuk, B.: Neonatal and postneonatal mortality in very low birthweight infants. Arch. Dis. Child. *59*:987, 1984c.

Yu, V. Y. H., Wong, P. Y., Bajuk, B., et al.: Outcome of extremely low birthweight infants. Brit. J. Obstet. Gynaecol., *93*:162, 1986c.

▪ APPENDIX

Australian National Health and Medical Research Council Recommendations on the Long-Term Follow-Up of Small Preterm Infants (1983)*

With the improving survival rate of small preterm infants, their long-term outcome needs to be determined. This is an important part of the medical audit for neonatal intensive care services. In addition, it will help identify specific medical and psychosocial needs of these children and their families to enable the provision of special support services.

Follow-up services are a necessary part of patient care for these babies. They also enable hospitals providing care for the very-low-birth-weight infants to plan appropriately.

The Council recommends the following:

1. Very-low-birth-weight (VLBW) infants who weigh 1500 g or less at birth should receive long-term follow-up.

2. Studies should distinguish between infants who are small for gestational age and appropriate for gestational age and between those who are inborn or transferred to the neonatal intensive care unit from other hospitals; describe social class distribution; report data in 100 g intervals and two weekly periods of gestational age; and account for neonatal as well as postneonatal mortality, before and after discharge from the hospital. The attrition rate at follow-up should remain below 10 per cent.

3. Studies should report the frequency of specific defects or disabilities as well as the number of children with different grades of functional handicap according to clearly described definitions. The developmental or intellectual status should be obtained with standardized psychological assessment.

4. Follow-up should be effected by a multidisciplinary team that includes a developmental pediatrician, psychologist, nurse coordinator, and social worker. The period of follow-up should continue until primary school learning is established.

5. In addition to assessment of neurodevelopmental outcome, their medical morbidity during early childhood needs to be monitored as well as the quality of parent-child interaction and the degree of ongoing parental stress and adaptation. This is to ensure that the medical and community support services are being directed to those with special needs.

6. Funding should be allocated to long-term follow-up services for small preterm infants from the normal service budget of the respective hospitals; the need for funds for this service should be taken into consideration in the allocation of funds between hospitals.

---

*Child Health Committee: Long-Term Follow-Up of Small Preterm Infants. Canberra, Australian National Health and Medical Research Council, 1983.

33

LONG-TERM COSTS OF PERINATAL DISABILITIES

Marie C. McCormick and Douglas K. Richardson

Increasingly, economic jargon predominates in many medical discussions. We use such terms as "cost-containment," "cost-benefit analysis," "providers," and "products." In such an era, outcomes of medical care must be considered in a broader context than simple survival in order to acknowledge the broader societal implications of the consequences of clinical decisions. Thus, the concept of the long-term costs of perinatal disabilities makes explicit that, with the survival of newborns with handicapping conditions, society incurs a long-term responsibility for support, and the scope of this support may be characterized in monetary terms or costs.

Precise estimates of the long-term costs of perinatal disabilities, however, involve a conceptualization of outcomes that is not familiar to clinicians and requires information that may not be readily available. For example, the economic concept of "cost" extends beyond the hospital and doctors' visit fees familiar to health-care providers. Moreover, in our complex medical environment not all approaches to assigning dollar amounts to costs are equivalent. Much more difficult, however, is the conceptualization and valuation of (i.e., attributing dollar amounts to) human costs, or costs not directly related to the provision of medical and related services. Beyond the conceptual and measurement issues, however, are issues related to the availability and timeliness of data on outcomes. To estimate long-term costs requires information on the nature and relevance of disabilities as well as the types of services needed and the sources of payment for the services. Since interest in the economic implications of graduates from the neonatal intensive care unit (NICU) is fairly recent, the available data reflect the medical profession's traditional concerns about survival and severe morbidity, not necessarily the more comprehensive information needed for estimating economic burden. In addition, neonatal intensive care is not a static intervention but a changing package of services. Thus, the more complete data on longer-term outcome may not reflect the current technology.

A discussion of short- or longer-term costs may be part of an implicit or explicit agenda of assessing the value or worth of NICU care. Evaluation of the merits of an intervention, however, must always involve either the relative costs of two interventions that achieve similar effects (cost-effectiveness analysis) or a comparison between the costs and the benefits (both in dollars). The available methods of assigning dollar values to outcomes are even less clear than those for costs. The point is that although identification of the costs of perinatal disabilities may have great importance in estimating the implications of changes in survival and morbidity rates for both the individual family and larger social units, knowledge of the costs alone is not sufficient to assess the value of NICU care.

■ OVERVIEW OF DEFINITIONS

Several methods may be used to estimate costs, but general concerns pertain to all of them. When costs occur at different points in time, some adjustment must be made. A dollar spent immediately costs more than the same dollar spent a year later because of the interest accrued over that year. Thus, costs occurring over time are conventionally discounted to their net present value. Future benefits must be similarly discounted. This discounting is independent of inflation. Second, for many items, the best estimate of cost is simply the market price. Such estimation techniques are inadequate in cases where the item has no price or is subsidized, for example, routine newborn metabolic screening. In such instances, the costs of the whole screening program are summed and divided by the number of samples processed to provide an average cost. Third, average cost may be quite an inaccurate estimate for nonaverage cases. For example, the resources consumed in caring for a critically ill versus a growing premature newborn cannot both be described by the average per diem hospital costs. Yet such averages are often used because actual measurement of resource use is usually prohibitively expensive. Hospital charges (as distinct from hospital costs) are an important example of this distinction (Finkler, 1982). Distortions may be significant enough to change the conclusions of economic analyses. Finally, implicit in what is tabulated as a cost is the viewpoint of the analysis. A very narrow viewpoint might be taken by a single insurance company setting a premium, a hospital considering opening a disabilities clinic, or a governmental agency. The most appropriate viewpoint for this discussion is a societal perspective, which includes costs incurred by all parties.

DIRECT COSTS

To an economist, direct costs involve the resources consumed in making a product. In a medical context, this product is an outcome, such as a NICU graduate, or the provision of a particular service, such as a day of hospitalization or an outpatient visit. Direct costs therefore include not only hospital bills, physician and office visit fees, laboratory tests, rehabilitation services, and medication expenses (whether or not covered by insurance) but also parental out-of-pocket costs, such as transportation, parking, and child-care for siblings while seeking medical care for the NICU graduate. It also includes the incremental costs to society of providing specialized education services that are not routinely incurred by the average child.

Notably, this analytic perspective does not take into consideration questions of equity in the distribution of costs or the ability to pay, issues which in themselves have important implications for social policy.

INDIRECT COSTS

Indirect costs are costs of foregone opportunities ("opportunity costs"), such as wages lost when seeking medical treatment or convalescing. In the context of NICU graduates, indirect costs may be a significant or even the dominant cost if one parent fails to rejoin the work force for several years after the birth of a very premature infant. Such costs would also include the impact on other family members, multiple "opportunities" or events in terms of stress and divorce, limitations in geographic and job mobility, and activities of family members foregone that might occur because of the needs of the NICU graduate— issues for which monetary values may be difficult to assess.

BENEFITS

Two basic techniques have been employed in assigning dollar values to health benefits. The most common one is the human capital approach which views health in terms of economic productivity. The dollar value assigned to a given health state is derived from the earnings that a person with that health state would generate. For a child, this approach would involve an estimate of lifetime earnings, either as a completely healthy individual, or at some reduced rate for those with handicaps.

The second approach requires an estimate of how much an individual would be willing to pay to avoid death or some specified level of ill health. As one can imagine, a variety of methodologic questions pertain to ascertaining and validating such assessments.

Besides the specific methodologic issues pertaining to each method, both have limited applicability to either end of the human life span, i.e., children and the elderly. With the former approach, for example, one cannot assign a value to life and health beyond the market value of a livelihood. In addition, the long delay between medical investment (i.e., neonatal intensive care) and the eventual revenues (wages upon entry into the work force) make such estimates extremely sensitive to the discount rates. In applying the latter, the opinions of the child cannot be directly ascertained.

For these and other reasons, much of clinical research tends to involve cost-effectiveness rather than cost-benefit comparisons. In the former, the object is to compare the costs (or charges) of achieving comparable clinical effects

with the value of the effect assumed or established in some other context.

Warner and Luce (1982) and Doubilet and colleagues (1986) provide more detailed discussions of these issues.

■ COSTS RELATED TO PERINATAL DISABILITIES

What, then, is known about the costs related to perinatal disabilities along these dimensions? Table 33–1 compares the costs of medical care for the NICU and healthy infants.

DIRECT COSTS

HOSPITALIZATION

In the first years of life, very-low-birth-weight (VLBW) infants (<1500 g) experience higher rates of hospital use after discharge from the NICU. The percentage rehospitalized in the first year is between 30 to 50 per cent with an average of two or more hospital episodes for each child. In contrast, the rate is 8 to 10 per cent for normal-birth-weight infants who rarely have more than one admission. Close to half the admissions are for conditions that can be related specifically to perinatal and neonatal events, although others may be indirectly related to such events. The reported average length of stay for each

TABLE 33–1. Costs of Medical Care: NICU Versus Healthy Infant

DIRECT COSTS	NICU INFANT	HEALTHY INFANT
Initial hospitalization	$10,000 to >$100,000	<$200
Readmission, first 3 years	Two or more readmissions for 30 to 50 per cent of infants	One admission 8 to 10 per cent, >1 rare
Hospital cost of 1 readmission*	$6,027	$2,902
Hospital costs first 3 yrs/child†	$9,902	-0-
Ambulatory care first 3 years (professional fees, underestimate)	$3,924	$1,116
Other out-of-pocket costs (drugs, equipment, travel, special services)	?	
Special education	At least 2× customary	-0-

INDIRECT COSTS	NICU INFANT	HEALTHY INFANT
Parental delay or failure to return to work or lost wages for time off for visits & hospitalization‡	$36,088-54,132	-0-
Foregone wages for grown child's reduced earning potential‡	$162,396-472,146	-0-

*National Academy of Sciences, 1985, professional fees *not* included.
†Health care costs at Children's Hospital, Detroit, 1981–83 dollars (Shankaran, 1988).
‡Chu, 1988.

hospitalization has varied from 5 to 9 days, although the range of variation is wide (Hack et al., 1981; Kitchen, 1990; McCormick et al., 1980; Morgan, 1985).

After the first year, the risk of subsequent hospitalization falls to about 10 per cent each year through age 3 with evidence of relatively short lengths of stay for problems not necessarily related to perinatal events (Hack et al., 1985). Thus, by age 3 about 50 per cent of VLBW infants will have experienced at least one hospitalization, and some children will have accumulated a substantial number of hospital days (Hack et al., 1983; Shankaran et al., 1988).

No data have been published on hospital use specific to the VLBW population for children over age 3. For all children age 5 to 14 years, the rate of hospitalization is 34.2 per 1000 (Butler et al., 1985).

Only Shankaran and co-workers (1988) have reported total costs of postneonatal hospitalization of high-risk infants to age 3 derived from the total charges for inpatient care at Children's Hospital of Detroit, exclusive of charges for professional fees. In this study, the average inpatient daily charge from 1981 to 1983 was $635; average total charge per hospitalization, $4676; and average total charge per child hospitalized for all hospitalizations, $9902. Of the total, 4.5 per cent was not reimbursed by third-party payers, thus falling to the parents or, as is most often the case, to the hospital as a bad debt.

Other estimates of hospital costs have been developed by applying nationally derived per diem rates to the hospitalization use data previously cited. With an average daily charge of $372, the costs of hospitalization of the VLBW survivor in the first year are estimated to be $6027 for each child hospitalized, compared with $2902 for a hospitalized normal-birth-weight child (National Academy of Science, 1985).

OUTPATIENT CARE

Even fewer data are available on costs associated with outpatient care. In the Michigan study, the average monthly expenditures up to age 5 ranged from $31 ($1116 over 3 years) for children without residual disabilities to $109 ($3924 over 3 years) for those severely handicapped. These figures included primary health care, referral services (e.g., physical therapy and neurologic evaluations), and emergency room care. The extent to which these services were covered by medical insurance is not noted, but the proportion borne by the parents is likely to be greater than for inpatient care.

National estimates for preschool children reveal that children 0 to 2 years of age average 5.3 physician visits annually, and children 3 to 5 years, 3.3 visits (Butler et al., 1985). Annual costs for doctors' visits average $486 for those 0 to 2 years old and $177 for those 3 to 5 years old, of which anywhere from a third to a half may reflect out-of-pocket expenses. To compare with their data on NICU graduates in the preceding section, the Michigan investigators cite data that place the average monthly medical expenditures for children nationally at $22 to $26 (or $246 to $312 per year for the first 3 years), figures comparable to the average annual figures noted by Butler and associates (1985).

These figures, however, are likely to underestimate the costs of outpatient care for preschool NICU graduates both absolutely and relative to other children. First, the published data include only professional fees and some tests. No information is provided on equipment rental or purchase, purchase of medications or medical supplies, fees for nursing or other home help, parental transportation costs, or participation in home- or center-based therapeutic programs. While such items constitute a very small fraction of medical care for healthy children, the absolute and relative contributions of such services to the care of NICU graduates is likely to be substantial and is an area warranting further study.

Information on longer-term costs for NICU graduates, specifically those pertaining to school-age children, is not available. Estimates must be derived from data on all children with handicapping conditions, most of whom have been born at normal birth weights. National data reveal that school-age children (6 to 11 years) average 2.6 doctor visits per year, with 31 per cent having no visits. Despite the presence of handicapping conditions, the probability of visiting the doctor is less for children with such conditions (38 per cent with no doctor visit in a year), and increases to 74 per cent if the child lacks insurance coverage, a regular source of care, and a regular doctor (Butler et al., 1987; Singer et al., 1986). The annual costs for children in this age group average $2246, but the variation in costs for children with handicapping conditions is likely to be substantial and to be determined by factors other than the condition itself. Again, specific data on expenditures other than doctor visits are unavailable.

SPECIAL EDUCATION COSTS

For children, remedial services provided through the educational system can also be thought of as direct costs, although not, strictly speaking, medical costs. Information on preschool services is currently unavailable but likely to be available in the future, owing to recent legislation that mandates special services to be extended into the 0 to 3 year old group.

Once the child enters school, some of the responsibility for providing special remedial services shifts to the educational system. In a recent study, the average annual expenditures for students with special needs average about twice that of regular education students in three cities—$7026 versus $3966 (Raphael et al., 1985). Expenditures varied by classification from the low of $5000 for children with speech impairment to almost twice that amount for those with physical, sensory, and other health impairments. Substantial variation occurred within special education classifications with standard deviations of $2000 to $5000.

The proportion of NICU survivors requiring such services remains to be established. If estimates based on data from infant assessments pertain, then 10 to 20 per cent of NICU survivors may fall into the most expensive category of those with physical and sensory impairment (U.S. Congress, 1987). The proportion with less severe disabilities (e.g., speech impairments or learning disorders) is not well established but may be as high as 50 per cent (McCormick, 1989). Thus, a conservative estimate is that the educational expenditures for a third of NICU survivors may be twice as high as for children without impairments.

SUMMARY

Thus, the limited number of studies on the direct costs of medical care reveal some consistency on the proportion of children rehospitalized by age 3 (30 to 50 per cent) and the number of episodes. The cost estimates vary as a function of the severity of the child's condition and the daily charge rate. Although the reported studies place the direct parental burden as a small percentage of these amounts, the burden assumed by the individual family may be substantial for children with very high costs and/or in states with restricted public coverage through Medicaid or other programs. In this regard, it should be noted that young adults in the child-bearing age group are among those at greatest risk for lack of adequate insurance.

Data on outpatient services are more limited. Nationally, about half of the cost for doctor visits is covered by insurance, and most supplies and rentals must be paid for out-of-pocket. In one study of a serious childhood illness (cancer, which is also characterized by high first-year costs that then diminish sharply), only 11 per cent of family out-of-pocket costs were medical (i.e., physician fees and insurance copayments) (Bloom et al., 1985).

INDIRECT COSTS

If the studies are limited with regard to direct costs, they are virtually nonexistent for indirect costs of having a VLBW infant. In the study on children with cancer, in the first 3 years after diagnosis, 38 per cent of the family income was consumed by out-of-pocket expenses, and half of this was due to wages lost by the parent providing care to the child (Bloom et al., 1985). Similar estimates probably pertain to the VLBW infant with ongoing sequelae of prematurity, since frequent doctor visits for health care and participation in physical therapy and other intervention programs often require one parent (usually the mother) to stay home. Clearly, a spouse unable to return to the work force has implications for family income in an era when 50 per cent of new mothers are working by the time the child is 12 months old. Indirect evidence for this problem among the families of VLBW infants is provided by a study indicating that the nursing burden (number of the child's activities of daily living limited by health problems) is the major predictor of family impact for VLBW children under 3 years of age (McCormick et al., 1986). This measure of family impact taps many of the dimensions of indirect costs noted above including parental perceptions of need for more income, disruption of family activities, and social isolation due to the child's health problems, but it does not provide a direct estimate of the specific costs.

In the longer term, indirect costs would include lost wages because the child failed to join the work force due to postdischarge death or severe disability or the reduction in wages and job opportunities due to limited skills for children with moderate disabilities. Lost wages due to each infant death or severe handicap precluding work force participation ranges from $472,146 (4 per cent discount rate) to $254,809 (6 per cent discount). Based

on the salaries of those currently employed with disabilities, this same study estimates that disabled persons earn only 28 per cent of the nondisabled over a lifetime, or a loss in earning for each disabled child of $338,815 (4 per cent discount rate) to $162,396 (6 per cent discount). The loss in maternal salaries for these same children is estimated at $36,088 to $54,132 per child (Chu, 1988).

Clearly, these monetary losses represent only a part of the impact of the problems of VLBW infants. Moreover, these estimates are crude averages with wide variation and certainly may underestimate the costs for individual children.

■ IMPLICATIONS

Little specific information has been generated on the long-term costs of NICU graduates. What information exists may be flawed by methodologic problems (e.g., source of information, costs versus charges, or analytic perspective) or may rely on broad extrapolations requiring untested and sometimes disconcerting assumptions. Thus, perhaps the first implication of this overview is that more careful attention to these issues is needed. For the forseeable future, NICU care will be required to sustain the lives of some fraction of the births in the United States. While perhaps not the primary outcome, accurate assessment of the longer-term costs incurred by the survivors represents an important element in the ongoing examination of NICU care.

Part of that importance derives from pragmatic concerns about the short-term management of the NICU graduate. Although it can be criticized, the available information on the first few years of life indicates a continuing need for relatively high levels of care, in large part due to the sequelae of prematurity. While most of these conditions resolve satisfactorily, the ability to provide needed care may be severely constrained if parents are unable to sustain the financial burden of frequent visits, special equipment, and other medical expenses.

Whatever the short-term costs, they pale in significance to the life-long costs of total or partial disability. The extent to which such disability can be prevented or ameliorated by postdischarge interventions becomes exceedingly important in order to fully realize the gains achieved in the NICU.

Finally, the focus on costs should not obscure the fact that it is but one measure of outcome and may not even be the best. Current methods of cost-benefit analysis do better at estimating costs than benefits. Other values held by society may not be well characterized by techniques that rely on developing monetary estimates. The value of the survival of a child, even a child with special needs, is not solely an economic argument.

■ REFERENCES

Bloom, B. S., Knorr, R. S., and Evans, A. E.: The epidemiology of disease expenses. The costs of caring for children with cancer. J.A.M.A. 253:2393–2397, 1985.
Butler, J. A., Winter, W. D., Singer, J. P., et al.: Medical care use and expenditure among children and youth in the United States: Analysis of a national probability sample. Pediatrics 76:495–507, 1985.
Butler, J. A., Singer, J. D., Palfrey, J. S., et al.: Health insurance coverage and physician use among children with disabilities: Findings

from probability samples in five metropolitan areas. Pediatrics 79:89–98, 1987.

Chu, R. C.: 1985 Indirect costs of infant mortality and low birth weight. Washington, D.C., National Commission to Prevent Infant Mortality, 1988.

Doubilet, P., Weinstein, M. C., and McNeil, B. J.: Use and misuse of the term "cost effective" in medicine. N. Engl. J. Med. 314:253–256, 1986.

Finkler, S. A.: The distinction between costs and charges. Ann. Int. Med. 96:102–109, 1982.

Hack, M., DeMonterice, D., Merkatz, I. R., et al.: Rehospitalization of the very-low-birth-weight infant. Continuum of perinatal and environmental morbidity. Am. J. Dis. Child. 135:263–266, 1981.

Hack, M., Rivers, A., and Fanaroff, A. A.: The very low birth weight infant: The broader spectrum of morbidity during infancy and early childhood. J. Behav. Dev. Pediatr. 4:243–249, 1983.

Kitchen, W. H., Ford, G. W., Doyle, L. W., Rickards, A. L., and Kelly, E. A.: Health and hospital readmissions of VLBW and normal BW children. AJDC 144:2213–2218, 1990.

McCormick, M. C.: Long-term follow-up of infants discharged from neonatal intensive care units. J.A.M.A. 261:1767–1772, 1989.

McCormick, M. C., Shapiro, S., and Starfield, B. H.: Rehospitalization in the first year of life for high-risk survivors. Pediatrics 66:991–999, 1980.

McCormick, M. C., Stemmler, M. M., Bernbaum, J. C., et al.: The very low birth weight transport goes home: Impact on the family. J. Dev. Behav. Pediatr. 7:217–223, 1986.

Morgan, M. E. I.: Late morbidity of very low birth weight infants. Brit. Med. J. 291:171–173, 1985.

National Academy of Science: Preventing Low Birth Weight. Washington, D.C., National Academy Press, 1985.

Raphael, E. S., Singer, J. D., and Walker, D. K.: Per pupil expenditures on special education in three metropolitan school districts. J. Educ. Finance. 11(1):69–88, 1985.

Shankaran, S., Cohen, S. N., Lenver, M., et al.: Medical care costs of high-risk infants after neonatal intensive care: A controlled study. Pediatrics 81:372–378, 1988.

Singer, J. D., Butler, J. A., and Palfrey, J. S.: Health care access and use among handicapped students in five public school systems. Med. Care 24:1–13, 1986.

U.S. Congress, Office of Technology Assessment: Neonatal Intensive Care for Low Birth Weight Infants: Costs and Effectiveness (OTA-HCS-38). Washington, D.C., Government Printing Office, 1987.

Warner, K. E., and Luce, B. R.: Cost-Benefit and Cost-Effectiveness Analysis in Health Care. Principles, Practice and Potential. Ann Arbor, Mich., Health Administration Press, 1982.

PART VI

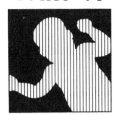

INFECTIONS AND IMMUNOLOGIC DEFENSE MECHANISMS

IMMUNOLOGY 34

F. Sessions Cole

The contrasting functions of the fetal and neonatal immunologic responses, i.e., preservation of fetal well-being as a semiallogenic graft versus adequate immunologic protection in a nonsterile, extrauterine environment, are regulated by a host of incompletely understood developmental and genetic mechanisms. The diversity and importance of these mechanisms are suggested by the heterogeneity and frequency of the infectious problems encountered in newborns. Differences in immunologic responsiveness between adults and newborn infants should not be considered defects or abnormalities: just as the ductus arteriosus, a cardiopulmonary necessity in the intrauterine environment, closes at different rates in different infants, human fetal and newborn infant immunologic response mechanisms are developmentally and genetically programmed to change from graft preservation to identification and destruction of invading pathogens at different rates.

Fortunately, systemic antimicrobial chemotherapy can control microbial invasion and permit adaptation of the infected infant's immunologic system to an extrauterine existence exposed to multiple potential pathogens. However, antibiotics coupled with advances in support technology do not insure survival of infected infants: 10 to 50 per cent of infants systemically infected with polysaccharide encapsulated organisms expire.

■ MATERNAL IMMUNOLOGY

The survival of a semiallogenic graft (the fetus) in the uterus requires multiple, poorly understood changes in maternal immunologic responses. Medawar (1953), Billingham (1964), and Simmons (1967 and 1969) have developed several hypotheses useful in understanding the mechanisms for survival of the human fetus, including:

1. The uterus is an immunologically privileged site.
2. The fetus is not antigenically mature.
3. The placenta provides a barrier to humoral and cellular maternal-fetal interaction.
4. The mother is immunosuppressed.

5. The immunologic response of the mother is altered during pregnancy to enhance fetal survival.

Since these hypotheses were developed, the first has been disproved, but experimental and clinical support for each of the others is available. Recent data suggest that maternal immunologic responsivness during pregnancy is different from the nonpregnant state and that maintenance of pregnancy and fetal/neonatal outcome are strongly linked to abnormalities in maternal immunologic responsiveness (Beer and Billingham, 1976; Hunziker and Wegmann, 1986; Jacoby et al. 1984; Lewis et al., 1986). Among the important regulators of maternal immunologic function are maternal-fetal histocompatibility, circulating blocking factors, local suppressor factors, and antipaternal leukocytotoxic antibodies (Cunningham et al., 1989).

Lack of maternal-fetal histocompatibility appears to be important in maintaining pregnancy. When couples share common alleles at the HLA-DR locus, recurrent spontaneous abortion has been observed (Coulam et al., 1987; Faulk et al., 1978; Scott et al., 1987; Thomas et al., 1985). Whether the importance of this lack of shared maternal and paternal human lymphocyte antigens (HLA) is due to the requirement for induction of specific maternal responses or the sharing of recessive, lethal alleles in parents with highly histocompatible genomes is uncertain.

Maternal blocking antibodies are IgG isotype and are directed against epitopes detectable on paternal and fetal tissue (Billington and Bell, 1983; Power et al., 1983; Raghypathy et al., 1984). Although the precise functions of these antibodies are uncertain, they may serve to mask paternal antigens whose recognition by the maternal immunologic response would result in spontaneous abortion.

Local suppressor factors are substances produced by T lymphocytes or macrophages in decidua of normal pregnancies (Papadogiannakis et al., 1985; Stankova and Roza-Pleszczynski, 1984; Wegmann, 1988). Although characterization of these factors is incomplete, prostaglandins and T-cell–derived lymphokines may act as local and systemic immunologic suppressors during pregnancy.

Antipaternal leukocytotoxic antibodies may regulate prompt clearance of fetal cells from the maternal circulation and thereby decrease immunologic response to paternal antigens displayed on the placenta or fetus (Bell and Billington, 1983; Schroder, 1974).

Abnormalities of maternal-fetal immunologic interaction can lead to spontaneous abortion or to morbidity or mortality for the fetus or newborn as seen in pregnancies complicated by rhesus (Rh) isoimmunization. Approximately 75 per cent of Rh-negative women with Rh-incompatible fetuses give birth to unaffected or mildly affected infants (Baskett et al., 1986; Berlin et al., 1985; Eklund and Nevanlinna, 1986; Mills and Napier, 1988). The regulation of the maternal immunologic response suggested by this heterogeneity is complex. The genetic immunoregulation of this response has been studied by Raum and colleagues (1984). They demonstrated that a specific complotype of genetically determined allotypic variants of the second and fourth complement proteins of the classical pathway and factor B of the alternative complement pathway, all of which are encoded by genes within the major histocompatibility complex on the short arm of human chromosome 6, is tightly linked to a single extended haplotype which is associated with fetal/neonatal morbidity and mortality. This observation suggests that maternal immunologic responsiveness to the Rh antigen is regulated by genes that are closely linked to the major histocompatibility complex. Preconceptual or antenatal determination of the complotype of Rh-negative women might supplement utilization of measurement of maternal anti-Rh titer to assess fetal risk. Genetic and developmental regulation of maternal immunologic response to polysaccharide antigens also plays a role in determining risk of individual infants for systemic bacterial infection with polysaccharide encapsulated organisms. Similar genetic markers may soon be available from studies of women whose sequential infants have developed group B streptococcal infection within the first three months of life (Christensen and Christensen, 1988).

■ PLACENTAL IMMUNOLOGY

The placenta provides a regulatory barrier between maternal immunocompetent cells and semiallogenic fetal tissue. It also regulates maternal-fetal and fetal-maternal transfer of immunologically important factors (Gitlin et al., 1964; Gurka and Rocklin, 1987; Hunziker and Wegmann, 1986; Jacoby et al., 1984). To accomplish these complex functions, the placenta has a wealth of cell populations that provide considerable regulatory diversity. The hemochorial placenta of the human is a chimeric organ. Fetal villi covered with invasive trophoblasts erode into layers of maternal epithelium, stroma, and vessel endothelium. In addition to the various cell types of the decidua, there are multiple immunologically competent cells in the placenta including lymphocytes and macrophages. The importance of these cell types has been emphasized by the finding that interleukin-1, a cytokine produced by macrophages and macrophage-like cells, is a major contributor to the initiation of parturition (Romero et al., 1989).

Besides local production of factors that regulate fetal and maternal well-being, the placenta can regulate passage of maternal immunologic effectors to the fetus (Tongio and Mayer, 1975). For example, while maternal IgG is transported efficiently beginning at 20 weeks' gestation

(Fig. 34–1), maternal antibody can also be bound and degraded by the placenta (Swinburne, 1970; Wegmann et al., 1980). On the basis of observations in rabbits and mice, there is considerable antibody-binding capacity in the placenta: radiolabeled maternal antibody is internalized and degraded by the placenta in 4 to 6 hours. Failure of this placental function may be due to elevated concentrations of maternal antibody that cannot be cleared by the placenta. Alternatively, specific antibodies may escape placental clearance and accumulate in the fetus because of a poorly understood lack of recognition of these antibodies.

In contrast to effector proteins, transplacental passage of activated effector cells from mother to fetus has not been established in normal pregnancies (Desai and Creger, 1963; Schroder, 1974). Evidence from infants with severe combined immunodeficiency (SCID) suggests that maternal T lymphocytes can cross the placenta and engraft in fetal bone marrow (Thompson et al., 1984). Whether aberrant regulation of maternal-fetal effector cell traffic plays a role in specific fetal/neonatal diseases, e.g., intrauterine growth retardation, is poorly understood (Beer and Billingham, 1973; Beer et al., 1972). As understanding of the diverse immunologic functions of the placenta increases, more specific immunoregulatory clinical information will be derived from this important organ.

■ FETAL/NEONATAL IMMUNOLOGY

HUMORAL IMMUNITY

COMPLEMENT

The complement system consists of approximately two dozen plasma and cell surface proteins (Table 34–1) that interact dynamically to regulate multiple functions of this immunologic effector system (Colten and Gitlin, in press) (Fig. 34–2). These functions include cytolysis of bacteria, nonspecific opsonization, release of anaphylatoxins, solubilization of immune complexes, and induction of B-cell proliferation and differentiation. Activation of the complement cascade can occur via the classical or alternative pathway (Muller-Eberhard, 1988; Pangburn and Muller-

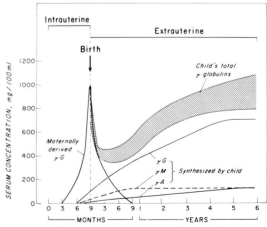

FIGURE 34–1. Schematic representation of fetal and neonatal immunoglobulin levels. (Adapted from Janeway, C. A.: Immunity, Allergy, and Infectious Diseases. In Nelson, W. E., Vaughan, V. C., and McKay, R. J. (Eds.): Textbook of Pediatrics, 9th ed. Philadelphia, W. B. Saunders Company, 1969, p. 477.)

TABLE 34–1. Proteins, Regulators, and Receptors of the Complement System

COMPLEMENT PROTEIN	MOLECULAR MASS (Daltons)	SERUM CONCENTRATION (μg/ml) Adult	Newborn Infant (term)
C1			
C1q	410	70	63
C1r	95	35	—
C1s	87	35	—
C2	110	25	18
B	93	200	110
D	24	1	0.5
C3	185	1500	700
C4	200	500	130
C5	190	75	48
C6	115	209	98
C7	115	65	—
C8	163	55	—
C9	71	60	—
C1 INH	104	150	—
P	224	25	—
C4-bp	500	150	50
I	88	35	17
H	155	500	300
S-protein	80	500	—
Membrane Regulatory Proteins			
Decay-accelerating factor (DAF)	70	—	—
Membrane cofactor protein (MCP)	58–63	—	—
Homologous restriction factor (HRF)	65	—	—
Membrane Receptors and Regulators			
Complement Receptor 1 (CR1)	190–250	—	—
Complement Receptor 2 (CR2)	140	—	—
Complement Receptor 3 (CR3)	260	—	—
C5D-R	45	—	—
C1q-R	70	—	—

(Adapted from Colten, H. R., and Gitlin, J. D.: Immunoproteins. *In* Handin, R. I., Lux, S. E., and Stossel, T. P. [Eds.]: Principles and Practice of Hematology. Philadelphia, J. B. Lippincott, in press.)

Eberhard, 1984). The activation steps in these pathways have recently been reviewed (Colten and Gitlin, in press). Several characteristics of this cascade are important for the fetal/neonatal immunologic response. First, although the specificity of classical pathway activation results from interaction of antigens with antibodies of several isotypes, activation of the alternative pathway is antibody-independent and may be initiated by structures like endotoxin and polysaccharides frequently encountered among pathogenic organisms. For the fetus or infant who lacks type-specific IgG for immunologic recognition, the alternative pathway may be critical for triggering the effector functions of the complement cascade (Cole, 1987; Cole and Colten, 1984; Edwards, 1986; Stossel et al., 1973). Secondly, the enzymatic activation of the complement cascade permits prompt amplification of its functions: deposition of a single immunoglobulin molecule or C3b fragment can generate enzymatic cleavage of thousands of later-acting components and thus multiple complement activities (Pangburn and Muller-Eberhard, 1984). In addition, the alternative pathway may be amplified via a positive feedback activation mechanism, because C3b, an activation product of the alternative pathway C3 convertase, is a component of this convertase (Volanakis, 1988). Because of the importance of antibody-independent recognition for the immunologic responsiveness of the fetus and infant, the positive amplification loop of the alternative pathway is critical for rapid generation of complement effector functions without specific immunologic recognition.

Complement activation via either pathway occurs in two distinct phases, proteolysis and assembly (see Fig. 34–2). First, early-acting components of the classical (C1, C4, and C2) or alternative (factor B, factor D, and C3) pathway are activated by highly specific, limited proteolysis. Proteolytically activated components form specific enzymatic complexes composed of classical (C2a and C4b) or alternative (C3bBb) pathway components which activate the third component of complement (C3). These two endopeptidases have identical substrate specificities: each cleaves the single peptide bond $Arginine_{77}$-$Serine_{78}$ of the alpha chain of C3 (Volanakis, 1988). The rates of formation and dissociation of both C3 convertases are regulated by multiple soluble (e.g., factor H, factor I, C4b-binding protein) and membrane associated proteins (e.g., membrane cofactor protein, delay accelerating factor) (Mollnes and Lachmann, 1988). During activation of the early acting classical components, small (8 to 10 kilodaltons) peptides are released by proteolytic cleavage from the second, third, and fourth components of complement. These fragments and an activation fragment of the fifth component of complement, C5a, have anaphylatoxin activities and modulate vascular permeability, smooth muscle reactivity, and chemotaxis of polymorphonuclear leukocytes and monocytes.

Upon activation of C3 by either convertase, the second phase of complement activation is initiated: the membrane attack complex is assembled by protein-protein interaction of terminal (C5 to C9) complement proteins (Muller-

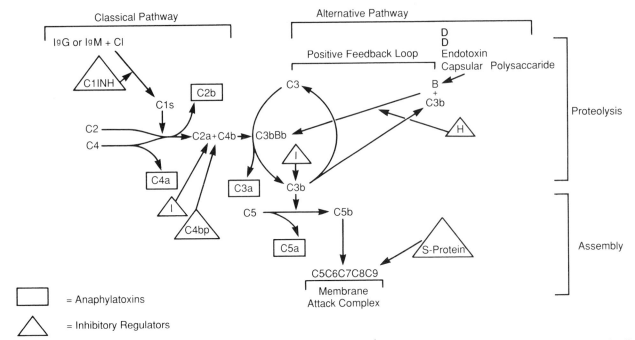

FIGURE 34–2. *Pathways of complement activation. Regulatory flexibility is afforded by multiple regulators at various steps of activation. (See Table 34–1 for definitions.)*

Eberhard, 1986). This complex alters membrane integrity via a transmembrane channel and thereby causes cytolysis of bacteria or cells.

Studies of fetal/neonatal complement have focused upon quantification of serum concentrations of individual components, determining hepatic and extrahepatic synthesis rates, examining maternal-fetal transport of these proteins, and assessing specific effector functions of the classical and alternative pathways. In the human, Gitlin and Biasucci (1969) reported detectable concentrations of C3 (1 per cent of adult levels) and C1 inhibitor (20 per cent of adult levels) by immunochemical methods as early as 5 to 6 weeks' of gestation. By 26 to 28 weeks' gestation, both C3 and C1 inhibitor concentration rise to 66 per cent of adult levels. Since these studies, multiple investigators have demonstrated that functionally and immunochemically measured complement protein concentrations in cord blood increase with advancing gestational age and that they are only 50 to 75 per cent of adult concentrations at full-term gestation (Davis et al., 1979; Fietta et al., 1987; Miyano et al., 1987; Shapiro et al., 1983; Strunk et al., 1979).

To examine the possible mechanisms of this developmental increase in serum concentrations of complement proteins, Adinolphi (1967), Gitlin and Biasucci (1969), and Colten (1972) have studied the hepatic synthesis rates of individual complement proteins in the human liver obtained at different gestational ages. They have shown that C2, C3, C4, C5, factor H, and C1 inhibitor are synthesized by the human fetal liver: C3 and C1 inhibitor synthesis can be demonstrated as early as 4 to 5 weeks of gestation. A marked increase in C4 synthesis by the fetal liver occurs at approximately 15 weeks' gestation, coincident with a rise in serum concentration. The hepatic synthesis mechanisms that regulate this increase, either a change in the amount of C4 produced by individual hepatocytes or a change in the number of hepatocytes

that produce C4, are not yet determined. Extrahepatic fetal synthesis of complement has been shown in the large and small intestines at 19 weeks of gestation (Colten et al., 1968) and in fetal monocytes obtained from cord blood (Sutton et al., 1986).

On the basis of studies of genetically determined, structurally distinct complement variants in maternal and cord serum, no transplacental passage from mother to fetus of C3, C4, factor B, or C6 has been observed (Colten et al., 1981; Propp and Alper, 1968). The presence of detectable amounts of C2 and C1 inhibitor in cord blood but not in the sera of mothers with genetic deficiencies of these proteins suggests that fetal-maternal transport of these components does not occur.

Regulation of complement effector functions in the fetus and newborn infant has not been as extensively examined. Opsonization of invading microorganisms without specific immunoglobulin recognition requires alternative pathway activation. For infants born prematurely or without organism-specific maternal IgG, alternative pathway activation provides a critical mechanism for triggering complement effector functions (Baker et al., 1986; Cole, 1987; Edwards, 1986). For example, Stossel and colleagues (1973) demonstrated opsonic deficiency in six of 40 cord sera examined due to decreased factor B concentrations despite normal C3 and IgG levels. The functional contribution of the classical pathway to neonatal effector functions has been assessed using cord blood–mediated opsonophagocytosis by adult polymorphonuclear leukocytes of group B streptococci type Ia (Edwards et al., 1983). This serotype may be opsonized by classical pathway components in the absence of specific antibodies and thus permits evaluation of the function of classical pathway activation. In eight of 20 neonatal sera examined, decreased bactericidal activity was detected and correlated with significantly lower functional activity of C1q and C4. These studies did not determine whether this decrease was mediated by an inhibitor of function or by an intrinsic change in functional activity of these components in neonatal sera.

While lower serum concentrations of classical and alternative pathway complement proteins may contribute to enhanced susceptibility of infants to systemic infection, other complement functions important for fetal/neonatal well-being but not related to antimicrobial response may require decreased classical and alternative pathway activation. For example, reduced serum concentration of C4b-binding protein (8 to 35 per cent of pooled adult plasma levels), a critical regulator of classical pathway C3 convertase activity, has been noted in fetal and neonatal sera (Fernandez et al., 1989; Malm et al., 1988; Melissari et al., 1988; Moalic et al., 1988). Lower C4b-binding protein concentration increases the functional anticoagulant activity of protein S with which it complexes and thereby contributes to decreased coagulation function of the fetus and newborn. Consideration of functions besides immunologic effector functions may be important in understanding the developmental regulation of complement component production.

Because of the low plasma concentrations of individual complement proteins, administration of purified, recombinant complement proteins has been considered as an adjunct to immunoglobulin replacement therapy and polymorphonuclear leukocyte transfusion in the treatment of neonatal systemic bacterial infection (Hill et al., 1986; Cairo et al., 1987; Krause et al., 1989). While a provocative idea, this approach must be studied thoroughly to insure that effector functions of complement activation in resting and uninfected tissues are not triggered in an unregulated fashion. Peripheral administration of one or more complement proteins might result in the unregulated activation of complement at tissue sites which would compromise rather than enhance neonatal survival.

Complement activation is the regulator of multiple effector functions of the host immunologic response. Further studies of the fetus and newborn infant will be aimed at understanding the developmental and genetic regulation of immunologic and nonimmunological functions of this important group of plasma and cell surface proteins.

IMMUNOGLOBULIN

Immunoglobulins are a heterogeneous group of proteins detectable in plasma and body fluids and on the surface of B lymphocytes. While these proteins have multiple, diverse functions, they are classified as a family of proteins because of their capacity to act as antibodies, i.e., recognize and bind specifically to antigens. The rapid advances in understanding molecular structure and regulation, genetic diversity, and differences in function of immunoglobulins have recently been reviewed (Colten and Gitlin, in press; Davey et al., 1986; Davis et al., 1981; Waldmann et al., 1983). The functions of immunoglobulins relevant to fetal/neonatal immunity are summarized in Table 34–2.

There are presently five known classes of immunoglobulins: IgG, IgM, IgA, IgE, and IgD. The prototype immunoglobulin molecule consists of a pair of identical heavy chains that determine the immunoglobulin class in combination with a pair of identical light chains (Fig. 34–3). The chains are linked by disulfide bonds and electrostatic forces. Each immunoglobulin molecule contains two identical domains with antigen-binding activity (Fab) and a third crystalizable fragment (Fc) devoid of antibody activity. The antigen-binding activity involves sites on both the heavy and light chains, while sequences in the Fc region of the heavy chain are involved in mediating immunoglobulin effector functions. Functions of individual immunoglobulin classes are different but overlapping.

IgG. IgG is the most abundant immunoglobulin class in human serum and accounts for more than 75 per cent of all antibody activity in this compartment. Its monomeric form circulates in plasma, has a molecular mass of approximately 155,000 daltons, and, in adults, approximately 45 per cent of total body IgG is in the extravascular compartment. The human conceptus is able to produce IgG by 11 weeks of gestation (Gitlin and Biasucci, 1969; Martensson and Fudenberg, 1965). The importance of its contributions to immunologic function is illustrated by the clinical problems encountered in individuals who are genetically deficient in IgG production: these patients suffer with recurrent infections if not treated with immunoglobulin replacement therapy (Sorensen and Polmar, 1987). The observations by several investigators that infants who develop group B streptococcal sepsis have low concentrations of type-specific IgG prompted attempts to treat infants acutely or prophylactically with immunoglobulin replacement therapy (Stiehm et al., 1987). Although suc-

TABLE 34–2. Immunoglobulin Classes and Functions

IMMUNOGLOBULIN	MOLECULAR MASS (Daltons)	SERUM CONCENTRATION (µg/mL) Adult	SERUM CONCENTRATION (µg/mL) Newborn Infant (term)	FUNCTIONS
IgG	155,000	1200	1200	• Neutralizes toxins. • Binds antigens. • Activates complement. • Promotes immune complex clearance or phagocytosis. • Mediates antibody-dependent cellular cytotoxicity.
IgM	>900,000	97	<20	• Activates complement. • Multivalent ligand binding. • Clearance of microorganisms.
IgA	160,000	250	ND	• Mucosal antigen recognition.
IgE	190,000	0.04	0.003	• Mediates hypersensitivity reactions.
IgD	180,000	2.2	0.1	• Identifies pre–B lymphocytes.

(Adapted from Colten, H. R., and Gitlin, J. D.: Immunoproteins. *In* Handin. R. I., Lux, S. E., and Stossel, T. P. [Eds.]: Principles and Practice of Hematology. Philadelphia, J. B. Lippincott, in press.)

cessful in some trials, replacement therapy in newborn infants has not proved as efficacious as in individuals with genetically determined hypogammaglobulinemia (Noya and Baker, 1989). This difference in part may be due to the fact that fetal/neonatal IgG synthesis is regulated by both developmental and genetic mechanisms (Cates et al., 1987).

The kinetics of IgG placental transport suggest both passive and active transport mechanisms (see Fig. 34–1). Because IgG transport begins at approximately 20 weeks' gestation, preterm infants are born with lower IgG concentrations than term infants or their mothers. The full-term infant has a complete repertoire of adult IgG antibodies. Thus, provided relevant maternal IgG has been transported to the fetus, newborn infants are not susceptible to most viral and bacterial infections (e.g., measles,

rubella, varicella, group B *Streptococcus,* and *Escherichia coli*) until transplacentally acquired antibody titers drop to biologically nonprotective concentrations. The regulation of IgG production in preterm infants has been a topic of study for four decades (Ballow et al., 1986; Cates et al., 1987; Dancis et al., 1953). Although adults with antibody deficiency syndromes have increased frequency of infections when IgG concentrations drop below 300 mg/dl, the serum IgG concentrations of many preterm infants fall below 100 mg/dl apparently without consequences. These observations suggest that preterm infants have additional immunologic protective mechanisms or that regulation of IgG function is not accurately assessed by serum IgG concentrations alone in preterm infants.

IgG functions in host defenses in several ways (Colten and Gitlin, in press). It can neutralize a variety of toxins

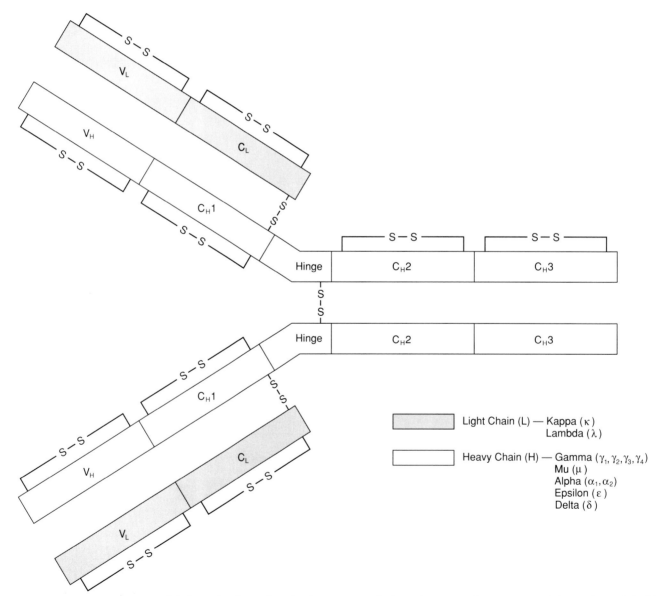

FIGURE 34–3. *Prototype immunoglobulin molecule. Each molecule is composed of two heavy (H) chains and two light (L) chains linked by disulfide (S—S) bonds. Each heavy chain and each light chain consists of constant (C) or variable (V) regions with internal disulfide bonds. Heavy chain subtype confers immunoglobulin class, i.e., gamma for IgG, Mu for IgM, alpha for IgA, epsilon for IgE, and delta for IgD. Immunoglobulin subclass specificity is conferred by heavy chain subclass, e.g., gamma, for IgG₁. Constant domains of heavy chains are designated by different numbers (C_H1, C_H2, or C_H3). (Adapted from Colten, H. R., Gitlin, J. D.: Immunoproteins. In Handin, R. I., Lux, S. E., Stossel, T. P. (Eds.): Blood: Principles and Practice of Hematology. Philadelphia, J. B. Lippincott, in press.)*

in plasma by direct binding. After antigen binding, IgG can activate the complement cascade via interaction with the early-acting complement components. The Fc portion of IgG can interact with cell surface receptors on mononuclear phagocytes and polymorphonuclear leukocytes and thereby promote clearance of immune complexes and phagocytosis of particles or microorganisms. Finally, the presence of IgG on specific target cell antigens (e.g., tumors or allogeneic transplant tissues) can mediate antibody-dependent cellular cytotoxicity, a mechanism through which lymphocyte subpopulations recognize non-self antigens.

IgM. IgM represents approximately 15 per cent of normal adult immunoglobulin. IgM circulates in serum as a pentamer of disulfide-linked immunoglobulin molecules joined by a single cross-linking peptide (Colten and Gitlin, in press). The size of IgM (molecular mass >900,000 daltons) restricts its distribution to the vascular compartment. Although the antibody-binding affinity of monomeric IgM is low, the multivalent structure of the molecule provides high pentameric antibody avidity. IgM synthesis has been detected in the human conceptus at 10 1/2 weeks' gestation (Rosen and Janeway, 1964). Because maternal-fetal transport of IgM does not occur, elevated (>20 mg/dL) concentrations of IgM in the fetus or newborn infant are suggestive of intrauterine infection or immunologic stimulation (Alford et al., 1969; Stiehm et al., 1966). However, because it is technically difficult to distinguish IgM molecules with specificity for individual organisms, diagnosis of infections by analysis for specific IgM antibody remains of limited usefulness.

IgM is important for fetal/neonatal host defenses for several reasons. First, the IgM molecule is the most efficient of any immunoglobulin isotype in activation of the classical pathway of complement. It thus can trigger multiple effector functions of this cascade. Secondly, its pentameric structure provides conformational flexibility to accomodate multivalent ligand binding. Thirdly, because of its localization in the vascular compartment and its high efficiency in complement activation, IgM plays a prominent role in clearance from serum of invading microorganisms.

IgA. Although IgA accounts for about 10 per cent of serum immunoglobulins, it is detectable in abundance in all external secretions. In serum, IgA is present as a monomer (molecular weight, 160,000 daltons), while in secretions it exists as a dimer (molecular weight, 500,000 daltons) attached to a J chain identical to that found in IgM (Colten and Gitlin, in press). In addition to the structural difference between serum and mucosal IgA, IgA found in secretions is attached to an additional protein called the secretory component (SC). This protein is a proteolytic cleavage fragment of the receptor involved in the secretion of polymeric IgA onto mucosal surfaces and into bile. Secretory IgA produced locally on mucosal surfaces by plasma cells is thus readily distinguishable from serum IgA. Although not rigorously quantified, it is estimated that the amount of IgA produced daily exceeds immunoglobulin production of all isotypes combined. Despite its relative abundance, unlike IgM and IgG, IgA cannot activate the classical pathway of complement nor effectively opsonize for phagocytosis particles or microorganisms.

Although IgA is detectable on the surface of human fetal B cells at 12 weeks' gestation, adult concentrations of serum and secretory IgA are not achieved until approximately 10 years of age. Because serum IgA is not transplacentally transferred in significant amounts, IgA is almost undetectable in cord blood. Colostrum-derived secretory IgA may provide a source of IgA in both gastrointestinal tract and other secretions for the newborn infant. Unlike other immunoglobulin isotypes, amino acid sequences of the hinge region of the IgA-2 subclass confer partial resistance to bacterial proteases. IgA is thus more resistant than other immunoglobulin isotypes to proteolytic effects of gastric acidity. Although considerable investigation suggests that passive immunization with IgA does occur with breast-feeding in humans, the overall importance of IgA in host defenses is presently not well-characterized.

IgE. The concentration of IgE is undetectable by standard immunochemical techniques and accounts for approximately 1/10,000 of the immunoglobulin in adult serum (Colten and Gitlin, in press). It circulates in the monomeric form (molecular weight, 190,000 daltons). Structurally, IgE lacks a hinge region. It is produced by most lymphoid tissues in the body but in greatest amounts in the lung and gastrointestinal tract. It is not secreted, and its appearance in body fluids generally occurs only with induction of inflammation. IgE cannot activate complement nor act as an effective opsonin. Its primary function identified to date is to mediate immediate hypersensitivity reactions. Specifically, antigen-specific IgE triggers mast cell degranulation with resultant bronchoconstriction, tissue edema, and urticaria via interactions with IgE receptors on the mast cell surface. Because of the presence of IgE in lung secretions and its potential importance in mediating allergic pulmonary and gastrointestinal reactions, considerable interest has been recently focused upon utilization of serum IgE concentrations to identify premature infants at risk for development of reactive airways disease or in the diagnosis of gastrointestinal hypersensitivity reactions (Bazaral et al., 1971; Jarrett, 1984).

IgD. Although IgD is found in trace quantities in adult human serum and has neither complement-activating activity nor the capacity to opsonize particles or microorganisms, approximately 50 per cent of cord blood lymphocytes exhibit IgD on their cell surface (Colten and Gitlin, in press). These pre–B lymphocytes express surface IgM and IgD simultaneously. Because of its wide distribution on B cells, IgD may play an important role in primary antigen recognition for the fetus and newborn infant.

IMMUNOGLOBULIN REPLACEMENT THERAPY

Klesius and co-workers (1973) suggested that lack of antibody to group B *Streptococcus* occurs in infants at risk for systemic infection with this organism. The maternal contribution to type-specific IgG was subsequently supported by the work of Hemming and associates (1976) and Baker and Kasper (1976). Animal and human studies have suggested that type-specific IgG can decrease mortality from systemic group B streptococcal infections. However, opsonization is not the sole mechanism of this protective effect (Fischer, 1988). Strain and species specific differences in protective effects of IgG have been noted. In addition, timing of administration and dosage of IgG can affect outcome. While prenatal administration has been attempted in a small number of cases (Morrell et al., 1986), postnatal administration has been studied extensively. In studies from 1981 to 1989, 261 infants were reported who received IgG replacement therapy without adverse effects (Noya et al., 1989). Pharmacokinetic studies suggest that the mean elimination half-life is approximately 23 days. While various dosages and treatment regimens have been employed, single-dose intravenous administration of 500 mg/kg or 750 mg/kg over 2 to 3 hours has been well-tolerated and results in elevation of IgG serum concentration from approximately 500 mg/dl to approximately 1400 mg/dl (Noya et al., 1989). Donors from whom IgG is isolated have sometimes been selected to insure high titer of type-specific IgG against common neonatal pathogens. IgG has been purified by various biochemical methods including ultrafiltration and ion exchange adsorption. These preparations are free of aggregated IgG and are thus unlikely to cause unregulated complement fixation and activation.

Besides prophylactic or acute treatment of systemic infection, immunoglobulin replacement therapy has been used in other clinical situations. Oral immunoglobulin administration with a preparation that contains IgG and IgA has been proposed for prevention of necrotizing enterocolitis (Eibl et al., 1988). Of 88 preterm infants who received 600 mg of an oral IgG-IgA preparation daily for 28 days, none developed necrotizing enterocolitis, while 6 of 91 concurrent control infants developed necrotizing enterocolitis confirmed by x-ray examination (pneumatosis, pneumoperitoneum, or hepatic portal vein gas) or histopathologic examination of specimens obtained during surgery or autopsy. Intravenous immunoglobulin has also been used with some success in small numbers of infants with neonatal isoimmune thrombocytopenia (Massey et al., 1987). While immunoglobulin replacement therapy may be a promising intervention in selected clinical circumstances, its role in the newborn infant in acute treatment of or prophylaxis for systemic infections, prevention of necrotizing enterocolitis, or treatment of isoimmune thrombocytopenia all warrant further study (Noya and Baker, 1989).

CELLULAR IMMUNITY

The newborn infant, especially the preterm infant, is at increased risk for development of a considerable spectrum of opportunistic infections, including *Candida albicans,* herpes simplex, and cytomegalovirus. Developmental and genetic differences between adults and infants in cell-mediated immunologic responsiveness account for this enhanced susceptibility. Considerable investigative interest has focused upon the molecular, cellular, and functional definitions of these differences (Andersson et al., 1981; Gathings et al., 1981; Hayward, 1981; Toivanen et al., 1981; Waldmann et al., 1983). This discussion focuses upon those developmental aspects of cell-mediated immunity known to be important for fetal or neonatal responsiveness to opportunistic infections.

LYMPHOCYTES

Lymphocytes play multiple critical roles in the cell-mediated immunologic response. Three lymphocytic lineages have been identified by cell surface and functional criteria: T, or thymus-dependent, lymphocytes, B, or bursa-derived, lymphocytes, and NK, or natural killer, lymphocytes (Abo et al., 1983; Balley and Schacter, 1985). T and B cells are known to differentiate from a stem cell common to other hematopoietic cells. Although not conclusively demonstrated, studies of children with severe combined immunodeficiency suggest that in some but not all of these patients defective development of all three cells is observed, and thus a common lymphoid stem cell may exist (Thompson et al., 1984).

Immunocompetent cells capable of responding to foreign lymphocytes in the mixed lymphocyte reaction are found in the fetal liver at 5 weeks' gestation. Prior to 8 weeks' gestation, lymphocytes are not detectable in the fetal thymus. After 8 weeks, lymphoid follicles, T lymphocytes, and Hassall's corpuscles can be identified. By 12 to 14 weeks, T lymphocytes can be found in the fetal spleen (Timens et al., 1987). By 15 to 20 weeks, the fetus has readily detectable numbers of peripheral T lymphocytes.

B lymphocytes with surface IgM are first found in the fetal liver at 9 weeks' gestation and in the fetal spleen at 11 weeks (Owen et al., 1977; Timens et al., 1987). Antigen-specific antibody production can be detected in the human fetus by 20 weeks' gestation. Fetal spleen cells can synthesize in vitro IgM and IgG by 11 and 13 weeks' gestation, respectively.

Multiple studies have documented differences in the proportions of fetal/neonatal T lymphocyte subpopulations and B cells at different gestational ages and in a variety of perinatal disease states (Baker et al., 1987; Lilja et al., 1984; Pittard et al., 1985). In addition, functional differences between cord blood and adult T cells and B cells have been identified (Andersson et al., 1983; Bussel et al., 1988; Hauser et al., 1985; Hayward and Mori, 1984; Hicks et al., 1983; Jacoby and Oldstone, 1983; Nelson et al., 1986; Olding and Oldstone, 1974; Oldstone et al., 1977; Papadogiannakis and Johnsen, 1988; Pittard et al., 1984 and 1989). Because of the potential importance of both of these areas to future immunologic treatment of newborns, each is reviewed here.

Although multiple functional and cell surface characteristics have been used to identify and study T lymphocytes, decreased mitogen-induced proliferation, decreased ability to induce immunoglobulin synthesis by B cells, presence of different proportions of helper and suppressor cell surface markers, and decreased capacity to produce lymphokines have all been shown to differentiate fetal/neonatal from adult T cells. While the in vivo significance of these differences has not been defined, the fetus and newborn infant can mount a cell-mediated immunologic response against certain antigens comparable to adults. Differences in the regulation of this responsiveness in the fetus and newborn are most likely the result of the necessity of preserving the fetus's immunologic role as a graft.

Availability of monoclonal antibodies directed at epitopes found upon functionally distinct T-cell subsets has permitted identification of differences in T-cell regulation in certain common perinatal medical and infectious conditions (Ryhanen et al., 1984; Wilson et al., 1985). From a therapeutic perspective, the decreased production of lymphokines has considerable potential for clinical utilization. Specifically, Wilson and colleagues (1986), Winter and associates (1983), Frenkel and Bryson (1987), and Wakasugi and Virelizier (1985) have shown that neonatal T cells produce less interferon-gamma than adult T cells, and Lewis and colleagues (1986a), have suggested that this difference results from an intrinsic characteristic of fetal/neonatal T-cell interferon-gamma production regulated at one or more pretranslational steps in interferon-gamma gene expression. These studies suggest that induction by interferon-gamma may play a major role in developmental regulation of immunologic responsiveness and may thereby provide an important reagent with which to enhance the capacity of infected infants to respond to invading microbes. Interferon-gamma might be used by systemic administration as has been done in adults with chronic granulomatous disease, leprosy, and acquired immunodeficiency syndrome (AIDS). However, an alternative in the neonatal period may be provided by in vitro activation of autologous lymphocytes, as has been used in adults with malignancies. Such an approach might avoid the unanticipatable developmental regulatory problems of systemic administration of a substance like interferon-gamma with multiple, potentially deleterious effects. Similar approaches may be considered in specific infections with individual cytokines, e.g., tumor necrosis factor–alpha and granulocyte/macrophage–colony-stimulating factor.

Considerable investigation has focused upon the ontogeny of B lymphocytes (Bofill et al., 1985; Gathings et al., 1977; Pedersen et al., 1983; Pereira et al., 1982; Tedder et al., 1985a and 1985b). In the fetus, these cells are detectable during the first trimester, but their expression of immunoglobulins differs from that observed in adults. B-cell precursors (pre–B cells) are detectable in human fetal liver at 8 weeks' gestation and in the bone marrow at 12 weeks' gestation. By the 15th week of gestation, the proportions of fetal B cells that express different immunoglobulin heavy-chain isotypes are equivalent to those in adults. These cells exhibit intracytoplasmic heavy chains. They lack stable surface immunoglobulin molecules characteristic of mature B cells but are the precursors of IgM+ B lymphocytes. Interestingly, the generation of immunoglobulin isotype diversity within the B-cell lineage occurs in the fetus without apparent stimulation by multiple foreign antigens. However, a fetal/neonatal characteristic of B lymphocytes is their concurrent expression of two or three immunoglobulin isotypes. The molecular events that regulate isotype switching and diversity are currently being investigated. (For recent review, see Colten and Gitlin, in press.)

Although the B cells of full-term and preterm infants can synthesize IgM, IgG, and IgA, the response of human infants to certain foreign antigens is qualitatively distinct from that of adults. For example, as noted in early studies of antibody responses to *Salmonella* organisms, infants

can respond vigorously to protein H antigen but are incapable of responding to polysaccharide antigenic determinants (the O antigens of the cell wall). These differences appear to be due to both intrinsic differences in B cell responsiveness and increased suppressor T-cell activity in the fetus and newborn infant. Further understanding of the mechanisms that regulate B-cell function may permit individualized immunologic manipulation of antibody responsiveness specific for the developmental stages of preterm and full-term infants. For example, systemic administration of pharmacologic agents, e.g., recombinant human cytokines, may permit enhanced B-cell or T-cell responsiveness to specific infectious agents. Alternatively, in vitro exposure of autologous T or B cells to these cytokines may also permit focused immunoenhancing therapy.

POLYMORPHONUCLEAR NEUTROPHILS

As observed for T and B lymphocytes, neonatal polymorphonuclear neutrophils (PMN) are present at early stages of gestation but have different functional capacities than adult PMNs. Progenitor cells that are committed to maturation along granulocyte or macrophage cell lineages (granulocyte/macrophage colony-forming units, or CFU-GM) are detectable in the human fetal liver between 6 and 12 weeks' gestation in proportions comparable to those observed in adult bone marrow (Christensen, 1989). Human fetal blood has detectable CFU-GM from the 12th week of gestation to term (Christensen, 1989; Liang et al., 1988). Although these progenitor cells are detectable in the fetus and newborn infant, developmental differences in mature PMNs between adult and neonatal cells in signal transduction, cell surface protein expression, cytoskeletal rigidity, microfilament contraction, oxygen metabolism, and intracellular antioxidant mechanisms have all been demonstrated (Hill, 1987; Ricevuti and Mazzone, 1987). Besides intrinsic differences in PMN function, induction of specific functions as well as maturation of these cells are developmentally regulated by the availability in the microenvironment of specific inflammatory mediators and growth factors (Christensen, 1989; Vercellotti et al., 1987). For example, an activation product of the fifth component of complement, C5a, is a chemoattractant at sites of inflammation. Low concentrations of C5 in neonatal sera may not permit establishment of chemoattractant gradients at sites of inflammation in newborn infants comparable to those in adults. Differences between adult and fetal/neonatal PMN functions may thus reflect intrinisic cellular differences required for fetal well-being and differences in the availability or activity of substances that regulate PMN function.

The recognition that systemic bacterial infection in newborns is frequently accompanied by profound neutropenia prompted investigation of neutrophil kinetics in infected infants (Christensen et al., 1980 and 1982; Santos et al., 1980). These studies have suggested diverse, developmentally specific regulatory mechanisms required for mobilization of the neutrophil response to infection. Lack of neutrophil precursors in bone marrow aspirates of infected infants and systemic neutropenia motivated several investigators to treat neutropenic, infected infants with neutrophil replacement therapy (Christensen and Rothstein, 1980). While successful in some cases, the results have not been uniformly beneficial (Cairo, 1987 and 1989; Cairo et al., 1984, 1987; Menitove and Abrams, 1987; Stegagno et al., 1985). This heterogeneity emphasizes the importance of individualizing immunologic interventions for the developmental stage of the infant and the invading microorganism being treated. In vitro treatment of neutrophil precursors in peripheral neonatal blood with recombinant cytokines as well as adjunctive therapy with immunoregulatory proteins may provide future options for this therapy (Steinbeck and Roth, 1989).

MONOCYTES/MACROPHAGES

As noted above, cells committed to phagocyte maturation (granulocyte or monocyte/macrophage) are detectable in the human fetal liver by the 6th week of gestation and in peripheral fetal blood by the 15th week. Unlike granulocytes whose tissue half-life is hours to days, macrophages migrate into tissues and reside for weeks to months. These cells regulate in a tissue-specific fashion availability of multiple factors, including proteases, antiproteases, prostaglandins, growth factors, reactive oxygen intermediates, and a considerable repertoire of monokines.

The importance of macrophages in the neonatal response to infectious agents has been documented by multiple studies. For example, increased antibody response and protection from lethal doses of Listeria monocytogenes were induced in newborn mice by administration of adult macrophages (Lu et al., 1979). Functional differences in chemotaxis and phagocytosis between adult and neonatal cells have been observed and most likely result from both intrinsic fetal/neonatal monocyte/macrophage characteristics and from nonmacrophage factors, e.g., decreased production of the lymphokine interferon gamma (English et al., 1988; Stiehm et al., 1984; Van Furth et al., 1965; Van Tol et al., 1984). Inducible expression of individual complement proteins by lipopolysaccharide (LPS), a constituent of gram-negative cell walls, has also been shown to differ between adult and neonatal monocyte/macrophages (Sutton et al., 1986). Interestingly, this difference suggests that while signal transduction mediated by LPS, LPS-induced transcription, and accumulation of mRNAs which direct the synthesis of the third component of complement and factor B are comparable in adult and neonatal cells, a translational regulatory mechanism does not permit these important inflammatory proteins to be synthesized by LPS-induced neonatal cells. This observation emphasizes the fact that fetal/neonatal monocytes/macrophages may have functions developmentally distinct from those of adult cells. For example, in utero, production of growth factors and removal of senescent cells during tissue remodeling may be critical to fetal development (Kannourakis et al., 1988). Concurrent induction of these functions and immunologic effector functions in fetal monocyte/macrophages would potentially elicit nonspecific inflammation in actively remodeling tissues.

Besides antibacterial functions, neonatal monocytes/macrophages contribute to tissue-specific regulation of the microenvironment in individual organs. For example, considerable attention has focused upon the contri-

butions of these cells to antioxidant defenses and to regulation of protease-antiprotease balance. Because of the importance in tissue injury and repair of these functions, tissue and injury-specific treatment by appropriately targeted and primed monocytes/macrophages may provide therapeutic options for treatment of a spectrum of problems from oxygen toxicity in the lung to hemorrhage in the brain.

SPECIFIC IMMUNOLOGIC DEFICIENCIES

The physician should attempt to differentiate infants with specific genetically regulated immunologic deficiencies from those with developmentally regulated, environmentally induced, or infection-related susceptibility to microbial invasion (Rosen, 1986; Rosen et al., 1984). A careful family history during an antenatal visit may be helpful in identifying relatives removed by as many as two to four generations with histories suggestive of immunodeficiency. Availability of antenatal diagnostic techniques for several of these diseases permits consideration of treatment initiation immediately following or possibly before birth (Harland et al., 1988; Holzgreve et al., 1984; Perignon et al., 1987).

When a fetus at risk for a genetic form of severe combined immunodeficiency is identified, treatment should begin in the delivery room and be coordinated with antenatal diagnostic interventions. Specifically, cord blood should be obtained for white blood cell count and differential, lymphocyte subsets, karyotype (if not performed antenatally), mitogen stimulation studies, and immunoglobulin concentrations. Because the majority of these children do not become ill within the 1st week of life, care in an incubator should be provided, and staff should observe strict hand-washing technique.

SEVERE COMBINED IMMUNODEFICIENCY

In the neonatal period, a morbilliform rash, probably the result of attenuated graft-versus-host disease from transplacental passage of maternal lymphocytes, may be the only symptom of severe combined immunodeficiency (Rosen, 1986). Over the first several months of life, failure to thrive characterized by intractable diarrhea, pneumonia, and persistent thrush, especially oral thrush, are the triad of findings most frequently seen in infants with this disease. The diagnosis is established by profound lymphopenia (<1000 lymphocytes/mm^3) and an absence of T lymphocytes. T cells detectable in peripheral blood of affected infants shortly after birth may be either maternal T cells or circulating thymocytes. The thymus gland is not seen on chest radiographs. Histologically, the gland is composed of islands of endodermal cells that have not become lymphoid and contain no identifiable Hassall's corpuscles. The pattern of inheritance of severe combined immunodeficiency can be either autosomal recessive or X-linked. Thus, 75 per cent of patients with this disorder are male. Approximately 50 per cent of the autosomal recessive cases result from a genetic deficiency of the enzyme adenosine deaminase (ADA). Although this enzyme is present in all mammalian cells, only lymphoid cells appear to be adversely affected.

If untreated, severe combined immunodeficiency is

invariably fatal in the first few years of life. In 1968, Good and colleagues performed the first successful bone marrow transplantation in a patient with this disease (Gatti et al., 1968). Progress in transplantation biology now permits successful use of parental haploidentical marrow with success for infants with all types of severe combined immunodeficiency. Besides increased susceptibility to opportunistic infections, these infants are also susceptible to development of graft-versus-host disease as a result of engraftment of maternal T lymphocytes acquired prenatally or postnatally as a result of T lymphocytes in transfused blood products (Pollack et al., 1982; Thompson et al., 1984). Thus, infants suspected of having this disorder should receive only irradiated blood products.

WISKOTT-ALDRICH SYNDROME

Another form of immunodeficiency, Wiskott-Aldrich syndrome, is characterized by severe eczema, thrombocytopenia, and susceptibility to opportunistic infection. It is inherited as a sex-linked recessive trait (Rosen, 1986). If untreated, these children survive longer than infants with severe combined immunodeficiency (median survival, 5.7 years). T lymphocytes in these patients are decreased in number and in function. Decreased platelet size and decreased thrombopoiesis are also noted. These children are potentially treatable with bone marrow transplantation. Interestingly, while transplantation corrects the T-cell defects, thrombocytopenia persists. As with children with severe combined immunodeficiency, all blood products should be irradiated prior to administration to avoid T-cell engraftment and graft-versus-host disease.

DiGEORGE SYNDROME

The embryologic anlage of the thymus gland and the parathyroid gland is the endodermal epithelium of the third and fourth pharyngeal pouches. When normal development of these structures is disturbed, thymic and parathyroid hypoplasia can occur (Rosen, 1986). Infants with this disorder may exhibit abnormalities of calcium homeostasis during the neonatal period (hypocalcemia and tetany) and variable T-cell deficits which appear to depend upon the presence and number of small, normal-appearing ectopic thymic lobes. In addition, these infants have malformations of the left ventricular outflow tract, low-set ears, midline facial clefts, hypomandibular abnormalities, and hypertelorism. Fetal thymic implants can correct the immunologic deficits (Reinherz et al., 1981).

■ IMMUNIZATION

MATERNAL IMMUNIZATION

Immunization prior to pregnancy has been effective in preventing several specific neonatal infections including diphtheria, pertussis, tetanus, hepatitis B, and rabies. For example, in developing countries, immunization during pregnancy with tetanus toxoid has been a cost-effective method of preventing neonatal tetanus (Schofield, 1986). The benefits for both mother and infant from induction during pregnancy of maternal IgG antibody that can be transferred to the fetus and protect both the fetus and mother against postpartum morbidity and mortality are substantial. However, maternal immunization, especially during pregnancy, is biologically distinct from immunization of nonpregnant individuals. Vaccine epitopes may be shared with vital fetal and/or placental tissues; therefore, vaccination may lead to unanticipated maternal or fetal morbidity. Maternal immunization may induce an antibody response in the fetus, as has been demonstrated with tetanus toxoid (Gill et al., 1983), and thereby induce potentially undesirable immunologic side effects, e.g., immunologic unresponsiveness or tolerance, in the infant. However, the increase in availability of potentially protective transplacentally transferred IgG through active maternal vaccination prompted the Institute of Medicine recently to recommend establishment of a program of active immunization to control early onset and late onset group B streptococcal disease in both infants and mothers (Institute of Medicine, 1985).

The indications for active vaccination during pregnancy rest upon assessment of maternal risk of exposure, the maternal/fetal/neonatal risk of disease, and the risk from the immunizing agent(s) (Amstey, 1989; ACOG Technical Bulletin, 1982; Immunization Practices Advisory Committee, 1985). In general, immunization with live viral vaccines during pregnancy is not recommended. Preferably, immunization with live viral vaccines should be performed before pregnancy occurs. However, rare instances may occur in which live viral vaccine administration is indicated. For example, in the event of a pregnant woman's traveling to an area of high risk for yellow fever, administration of that vaccine might be indicated due to the susceptibility of the mother and the fetus, the probability of exposure, and the risk of the mother and fetus from the disease. More common examples in the United States include influenza and polio virus vaccination. If a chronic maternal medical condition would be adversely affected by influenza, active immunization may be indicated during preg-

---

TABLE 34–3. Summary of Recommendations for Immunization During Pregnancy

Live Virus Vaccines	**Inactivated Bacterial Vaccines**	**Hyperimmune Globulin**
• Measles—contraindicated. • Mumps—contraindicated. • Poliomyelitis—not routine; increased risk exposure. • Rubella—contraindicated. • Yellow fever—travel to high-risk areas only.	• Cholera—to meet international travel requirements. • Meningococcus—same as nonpregnant. • Plague—selective vaccination of exposed persons. • Typhoid—travel to endemic areas.	• Hepatitis B—postexposure prophylaxis given along with hepatitis B vaccine initially, then vaccine alone at 1 and 6 months. • Rabies—postexposure prophylaxis. • Tetanus—postexposure prophylaxis. • Varicella—same as nonpregnant.
Inactivated Virus Vaccines	**Toxoids**	**Pooled Immune Serum Globulins**
• Influenza—serious underlying diseases. • Rabies—same as nonpregnant.	• Tetanus-Diphtheria—same as nonpregnant.	• Hepatitis A—postexposure prophylaxis. • Measles—postexposure prophylaxis.

(Adapted from American College of Obstetricians and Gynecologists: Immunization during pregnancy. [ACOG Technical Bulletin #64.] Copyright © 1982. *In* Cunningham, F. G., MacDonald, P. C., and Gant, N. F. [Eds.]: Williams' Obstetrics. 18th ed. East Norwalk, CT, Appleton and Lange, 1989, p. 269.)

TABLE 34–4. Routine Diphtheria, Tetanus, and Pertussis Immunization Schedule Summary for Children Under 7 Years Old—United States*

DOSE	AGE/INTERVAL	PRODUCT
Primary 1	6 weeks old or older	DTP†
Primary 2	4–8 weeks after first dose	DTP
Primary 3	4–8 weeks after second dose	DTP
Primary 4	6–12 months after third dose	DTP
Booster	4–6 years old, before entering kindergarten or elementary school (not necessary if fourth primary immunizing dose administered on or after fourth birthday)	DTP
Additional boosters	Every 10 years after last dose	Td

*For all products used, consult the manufacturer's package insert for instructions for storage, handling, dosage, and administration.

†DTP, Diphtheria and tetanus toxoids with pertussis vaccine; Td, adult tetanus toxoid (full dose) and diphtheria toxoid (reduced dose) for adult use.

(Adapted from Committee on Infectious Diseases, American Academy of Pediatrics: Report of the Committee on Infectious Diseases. 21st ed. Elk Grove, IL, American Academy of Pediatrics, 1988, p. 15.)

nancy. Similarly, if imminent exposure to live polio virus in an unprotected woman is anticipated, live oral polio virus vaccine may be used during pregnancy. If immunization can be completed prior to anticipated exposure, inactivated polio virus vaccine can be given. A summary of recommendations for immunizations during pregnancy is provided in Table 34–3.

For the pediatrician, maternal immunization represents an important preventive intervention. The availability of vaccines against polysaccharide encapsulated organisms (e.g., *Haemophilus influenza* type b and group B *Streptococcus*) may decrease morbidity and mortality from these diseases during the first 3 to 6 months of the infant's life (Amstey et al., 1985; Baker et al., 1988; Walsh and Hutchins, 1989). The possibility of decreasing the risks of development of hepatocellular carcinoma, cirrhosis, and chronic active hepatitis from perinatal transmission of hepatitis B through prenatal screening and active and passive immunization of the infant is substantial (Arevalho

and Washington, 1988). The implications of maternal vaccination during pregnancy for preterm infants have not been studied.

INFANT IMMUNIZATION

The recommendations of the American Academy of Pediatrics for immunization of infants are given in Tables 34–4 and 34–5. For the preterm infant, although different clinical approaches are currently used by practitioners including decreasing the dosage of immunogen, postponing the first immunization until a corrected age of 2 months, or waiting for an arbitrary weight to be achieved by the infant (e.g., 10 pounds), the American Academy of Pediatrics recommends administering full dose diphtheria, tetanus, and pertussis (DTP) immunization beginning at 2 months of age. A recent study in a group of 45 preterm infants (mean birth weight, 1460 g; mean gestational age 31 weeks; 76 per cent of whom required ventilatory support) indicated that 96 per cent of these infants who received a full dose of DTP vaccine mounted a serologic response to pertussis after the second dose, while only 45 per cent of infants who received a half-dose of DTP vaccine were able to mount a response to pertussis after the third dose (Bernbaum et al., 1989). Unfortunately, potentially confounding characteristics of these preterm infants, e.g., number of blood transfusions, maternal immunization status, and documented systemic infections, were not specified.

The recommendations by the Centers for Disease Control, the American Academy of Pediatrics, and the American Committee of Obstetricians and Gynecologists (ACOG) for universal screening of women for hepatitis B surface antigen (HBsAg) has increased the need for pediatricians to be prepared to administer adequate active and passive vaccinations shortly after birth to infants of women who carry HBsAg (Table 34–5). All infants regardless of gestational age at the time of birth whose mothers are HBsAg-positive should receive passive immunization within 12 hours of birth, and active immunization within 7 days of birth and at 1 and 6 months of

TABLE 34–5. Routine Pediatric Vaccination Schedule and HBV Prophylaxis for Infants and HBsAg-Positive Mothers*

AGE	HEPATITIS B PREVENTION SCHEDULE†	HBV MARKER SCREENING‡	ROUTINE PEDIATRIC SCHEDULE†
Birth	HBIG and HB vaccine	–	–
1 month	HB vaccine	–	–
2 months	–	–	DTP, OPV
4 months	–	–	DTP, OPV
6 months	HB vaccine	–	DTP
>9 months	–	HBsAg and anti-HBs tests	–
15 months	–	–	MMR
18 months	–	–	DTP, OPV, PRP-D

*For all products used, consult the manufacturer's package insert for instructions for storage, handling, dosage, and administration.

†HBIG, Hepatitis B immune globulin; HB vaccine, hepatitis B vaccine (for doses and schedules of these licensed HB vaccines [Heptavax-B, Recombivax HB, and Engerix-B] see Centers for Disease Control: Protection against viral hepatitis: Recommendations of the Immunization Practices Advisory Committee [ACIP]. M.M.W.R. 39[s-2]:1, 1990); DTP, diphtheria and tetanus toxoids with pertussis vaccine; OPV, oral polio vaccine containing attenuated poliovirus types 1, 2, and 3; MMR, live measles, mumps, and rubella viruses in a combined vaccine; PRP-D, *Haemophilus* b diphtheria conjugate vaccine.

‡A positive HBsAg test indicates failure of immunoprophylaxis; presence of anti-HBs indicates successful immunoprophylaxis. If both HBsAg and anti-HBs are not present, a fourth dose of vaccine should be administered, followed by repeat HBsAg and anti-HBs testing in 1 month.

(Adapted from Committee on Infectious Diseases, American Academy of Pediatrics: Report of the Committee on Infectious Diseases. 21st ed. Elk Grove, IL, American Academy of Pediatrics, 1988, p. 227.)

age. For infants whose mothers are HBsAg-negative but whose mothers have received active and/or passive immunization during pregnancy because of exposure to hepatitis B, recommendations include no treatment for the infant as long as the mother is HBsAg-negative at the time of birth. These guidelines for hepatitis immunization of infants have been developed for implementation for term and preterm infants. However, the extremely preterm infant whose mother is HBsAg-positive, a population seen with increasing frequency due to the coincidence of intravenous drug abuse and carriage of HBsAg, has not been studied.

■ REFERENCES

Abo, T., Miller, C. A., Gartland, G. L., et al.: Differentiation stages of human natural killer cells in lymphoid tissues from fetal to adult life. J. Exp. Med. *157*:273, 1983.

ACOG Technical Bulletin #64. Immunization During Pregnancy. 1982.

Adinolfi, M., and Gardner, B.: Synthesis of beta-1-E and beta-1-C components of complement in human fetuses. Acta Paediatr. Scand. *56*:450, 1967.

Alford, C. A., Blankenship, W. J., Straumfjord, J. B., et al.: The diagnostic significance of IgM globulin elevations in neonate infants with chronic intrauterine infections. Birth Defects *4*:3, 1969.

Amstey, M. S.: Immunization in pregnancy. Contemp. Ob/Gyn *34*:15, 1989.

Amstey, M. S., Insel, R. A., Munoz, J., et al.: Fetal-neonatal passive immunization against hemophilus influenzae type b. Am. J. Obstet. Gynecol. *153*:607, 1985.

Andersson, U., Bird, A. G., Britton, S., et al.: Humoral and cellular immunity in humans studied at the cell level from birth to two years of age. Immunol. Rev. *57*:5, 1981.

Andersson, U., Britton, S., De Ley, M., et al.: Evidence for the ontogenic precedence of suppressor T cell functions in the human neonate. Eur. J. Immunol. *13*:6, 1983.

Arevalho, J. A., and Washington, A. E.: Cost effectiveness of prenatal screening and immunization for hepatitis B virus. J.A.M.A. *259*:365, 1988.

Baker, C. J., and Kasper, D. L.: Correlation of maternal antibody deficiency with susceptibility to neonatal group B streptococcal infection. N. Engl. J. Med. *294*:753, 1976.

Baker, C. J., Rench, M. A., Edwards, M. S., et al.: Immunization of pregnant women with a polysaccharide vaccine of group B streptococcus. N. Engl. M. Med. *319*:1180, 1988.

Baker, C. J., Webb, B. J., Kasper, D. L., et al.: The role of complement and antibody in opsonophagocytosis of type II group B streptococci. J. Infect. Dis. *154*:47, 1986.

Baker, D. A., Hameed, C., Tejani, N., et al.: Lymphocyte subsets in the neonates of preeclamptic mothers. Am. J. Reprod. Immunol. *14*:107, 1987.

Baley, J. E., and Schacter, B. Z.: Mechanisms of diminished natural killer cell activity in pregnant women and neonates. J. Immunol. *134*:3042, 1985.

Ballow, M., Cates, K. L., Rowe, J. C., et al.: Development of the immune system in very low birth weight (less than 1500 g) premature infants: Concentrations of plasma immunoglobulins and patterns of infections. Pediatr. Res. *20*:899, 1986.

Baskett, T. F., Parsons, M. L., and Peddle, L. J.: The experience and effectiveness of the Nova Scotia Rh program, 1964–84. Can. Med. Assoc. J. *134*:1259, 1986.

Bazaral, M., Orgel, H. A., and Hamburger, R. N.: IgE levels in normal infants and mothers and an inheritance hypothesis. J. Immunol. *107*:794, 1971.

Beer, A. E., and Billingham, R. E.: Maternally acquired runt disease. Science *179*:240, 1973.

Beer, A. E., and Billingham, R. E.: The Immunobiology of Mammalian Reproduction. Englewood Cliffs, N.J., Prentice Hall, 1976.

Beer, A. E., Billingham, R. E., and Yang, S. L.: Maternally induced transplantation immunity, tolerance, and runt disease in rats. J. Exp. Med. *135*:808, 1972.

Bell, S. C., and Billington, W. D.: Humoral immune responses in murine pregnancy. III. Relationship between anti-paternal alloantibody levels in maternal serum, placenta and fetus. J. Reprod. Immunol. *5*:229, 1983.

Berlin, G., Selbing, A., and Ryden, G.: Rhesus haemolytic disease treated with high-dose intravenous immunoglobulin. Lancet *1*:1153, 1985.

Bernbaum, J., Daft, A., Samuelson, J., et al.: Half-dose immunization for diphtheria, tetanus, and pertussis: Response of preterm infants. Pediatrics *83*:471, 1989.

Billingham, R. E.: Transplantation immunity and the maternal-fetal relation. N. Engl. J. Med. *270*:667, 1964.

Billington, W. D., and Bell, S. C.: Evidence on the nature and possible function of pregnancy-induced anti-fetal alloantibody. In Isojima, S., and Billington, W. D. (Eds.): Reproductive Immunology. Amsterdam, Elsevier, 1983, p. 147.

Bofill, M., Janossy, G., Janossa, M., et al.: Human B cell development II. Subpopulations in the human fetus. J. Immunol. *134*:1343, 1985.

Bussel, J. B., Cunningham-Rundles, S., LaGamma, E. F., et al.: Analysis of lymphocyte proliferative response subpopulations in very low birth weight infants and during the first eight weeks of life. Pediatr. Res. *23*:457, 1988.

Cairo, M. S.: Granulocyte transfusions in neonates with presumed sepsis. Pediatrics *80*:738, 1987.

Cairo, M. S.: Neutrophil host defense. Am. J. Dis. Child. *143*:40, 1989.

Cairo, M. S., Rucker, R., Bennetts, G. A., et al.: Improved survival of neonates receiving leukocyte transfusions for sepsis. Pediatrics *74*:887, 1984.

Cairo, M. S., Worcester, C., Rucker, R., et al.: Role of circulating complement and polymorphonuclear leukocyte transfusion in treatment and outcome in critically ill neonates with sepsis. J. Pediatr. *110*:935, 1987.

Cates, K. L., Goetz, C., Rosenberg, N., et al.: Longitudinal development of specific and functional antibody in very low birth weight premature infants. Pediatr. Res. *23*:14, 1988.

Centers for Disease Control: Diphtheria, tetanus, and pertussis: Guidelines for vaccine prophylaxis and other measures. Recommendations of the Immunization Practices Advisory Committee (ACIP). M.M.W.R. *34*:405, 1985.

Christensen, K. K., and Christensen, P.: IgG subclasses and neonatal infections with Group B streptococci. Monogr. Allergy *23*:138, 1988.

Christensen, R. D.: Hematopoiesis in the fetus and neonate. Pediatr. Res. *26*:531, 1989.

Christensen, R. D., Anstall, H. B., and Rothstein, G.: Use of whole blood exchange transfusion to supply neutrophils to septic, neutropenic neonates. Transfusion *22*:504, 1982.

Christensen, R. D., and Rothstein, G. R.: Exhaustion of mature marrow neutrophils in neonates with sepsis. J. Pediatr. *96*:316, 1980.

Christensen, R. D., Shigeoka, A. O., Hill, H. H., et al.: Circulating and storage neutrophil changes in experimental type II group B streptococcal sepsis. Pediatr. Res. *14*:806, 1980.

Cole, F. S.: Complement function in the neonate. In Burgio, G., R., Hanson, L. A., and Ugazio, A. G. (Eds.): Immunology of the Neonate. Berlin, Springer Verlag, 1987, pp. 76–82.

Cole, F. S., and Colten, H. R.: Complement. In Ogra, P. L. (Ed.): Neonatal Infections, Nutritional and Immunologic Interactions. New York, Grune & Stratton, 1984, pp. 37–49.

Colten, H. R.: Ontogeny of the human complement system: In vitro biosynthesis of individual complement components by fetal tissues. J. Clin. Invest. *51*:725, 1972.

Colten, H. R., Alper, C. A., and Rosen, B.: Genetics and biosynthesis of complement proteins. N. Engl. J. Med. *304*:653, 1981.

Colten, H. R., and Gitlin, J. D.: Immunoproteins. In Handin, R. I., Lux, S. E., Stossel, T. P. (Eds.): Blood: Principles and Practice of Hematology. Philadelphia, J. B. Lippincott, in press.

Colten, H. R., Gordon, J. M., Borsos, T., et al.: Synthesis of the first component of human complement in vitro. J. Exp. Med. *128*:595, 1968.

Coulam, C. B., Moore, S. B., and O'Fallon, W. M.: Association between major histocompatibility antigen and reproductive performance. Am. J. Reprod. Immunol. Microbiol. *14*:54, 1987.

Cunningham, F. G., MacDonald, P. C., and Gant, N. F. (Eds.): Williams Obstetrics, 18th ed. East Norwalk, Conn., Appleton and Lang, 1989, pp. 494–495.

Dancis, J., Osborn, J. J., and Kunz, H. W.: Studies of the immunology of the neonate infants, IV. Antibody formation in the premature infant. Pediatrics *12*:151, 1953.

Davey, M. P., Bongiovanni, K. F., Kaulfersch, W., et al.: Immunoglobulin and T-cell receptor gene rearrangement and expression in human lymphoid leukemia cells at different stages of maturation. Proc. Natl. Acad. Sci. U.S.A. 83:8759, 1986.

Davis, C. A., Vallota, E. H., and Forristal, J.: Serum complement levels in infancy: Age related changes. Pediatr. Res. 13:1043, 1979.

Davis, M. M., Kim, S. R., and Hood, L.: Immunoglobulin class switching: Developmentally regulated DNA rearrangements during differentiation. Cell 22:1, 1981.

Desai, R. G., and Creger, W. P.: Maternal-fetal passage of leucocytes and platelets in man. Blood 21:665, 1963.

Edwards, M. S.: Complement in neonatal infections: an overview. Pediatr. Infect. Dis. 5:S168, 1986.

Edwards, M. S., Buffone, G. J., Fuselier, P. A., et al.: Deficient classical complement pathway activity in neonate sera. Pediatr. Res. 17:685, 1983.

Eibl, M. M., Wolf, H. M., Furnkranz, H., et al.: Prevention of necrotizing enterocolitis in low birth weight infants by IgA-IgG feeding. N. Eng. J. Med. 319:1, 1988.

Eklund, J., and Nevanlinna, H. R.: Perinatal mortality from Rh(D) hemolytic disease in Finland, 1975–1984. Acta Obstet. Gynecol. Scand. 65:187, 1986.

English, B. K., Burchett, S. K., English, J. D., et al.: Production of lymphotoxin and tumor necrosis factor by human neonatal mononuclear cells. Pediatr. Res. 24:717, 1988.

Faulk, W. P., Temple, A., Lovins, R. E., et al.: Antigens of human trophoblasts: A working hypothesis for their role in normal and abnormal pregnancies. Proc. Natl. Acad. Sci. U.S.A. 75:1947, 1978.

Fernandez, J. A., Estelles, A., Gilabert, J., et al.: Functional and immunologic protein S in normal pregnant women and in full-term neonates. Thromb. Haemost. 61:474–478, 1989.

Fietta, A., Sacchi, F., Bersani, C., et al.: Complement-dependent bactericidal activity for E. coli K12 in serum of preterm neonate infants. Acta Pediatr. Scand. 76:47, 1987.

Fischer, G. W.: Immunoglobulin therapy in neonatal group B streptococcal infections: an overview. Pediatr. Inf. Dis. 7:513, 1988.

Frenkel, L., and Bryson, Y. J.: Ontogeny of phytohemagglutinin-induced gamma interferon by leukocytes of healthy infants and children: Evidence for decreased production in infants younger than two months of age. J. Pediatr. 111:97, 1987.

Gathings, W. E., Kubagawa, K., and Cooper, M. D.: A distinctive pattern of B cell immaturity in perinatal humans. Immunol. Rev. 57:107, 1981.

Gathings, W. E., Lawton, A. R., and Cooper, M. D.: Immunofluorescent studies of the development of pre–B cells, B lymphocytes and immunoglobulin isotype diversity in humans. Eur. J. Immunol. 7:804, 1977.

Gatti, R. A., Meuwissen, H. J., Allen, H. D., et al.: Immunological reconstitution of sex-linked lymphopenic immunological deficiency. Lancet 2:1366, 1968.

Gill, T. J., Repetti, C. F., Metlay, L. A., et al.: Transplacental immunization of the human fetus to tetanus by immunization of the mother. J. Clin. Invest. 72:987, 1983.

Gitlin, D., and Biasucci, A.: Development of gamma G, gamma A, gamma M, beta1c/beta1a, C'1 esterase inhibitor, ceruloplasmin, transferrin, hemopexin, haptoglobin, fribrinogen, plasminogen, alpha-1-antitrypsin, orosomucoid beta-lipoprotein, alpha-1 macroglobulin and human prealbumin in the human conceptus. J. Clin. Invest. 48:1433, 1969.

Gitlin, D., Kumate, J., Urrusti, J., et al.: The selectivity of the human placenta in the transfer of plasma proteins from mother to fetus. J. Clin. Invest. 43:1938, 1964.

Gurka, G., Rocklin, R. E.: Reproductive immunology. J.A.M.A. 258:2983, 1987.

Harland, C., Shah, T., Webster, A. D. B., et al.: Dipeptidyl peptidase IV—subcellular localization, activity and kinetics in lymphocytes from control subjects, immunodeficient patients and cord blood. Clin. Exp. Immunol. 74:201, 1988.

Hauser, G. J., Zakuth, V., Rosenberg, H., et al.: Interleukin-2 production by cord blood lymphocytes stimulated with mitogen and in the mixed leukocyte culture. J. Clin. Lab. Immunol. 16:37, 1985.

Hayward, A. R.: Development of lymphocyte responses and interactions in the human fetus and neonates. Immunol. Rev. 57:39, 1981.

Hayward, A. R., and Mori, M.: Human neonate autologous mixed lymphocyte response: Frequency and phenotype of responders and xenoantigen specificity. J. Immunol. 133:719, 1984.

Hemming, V. G., Hall, R. T., Rhodes, P. G., et al.: Assessment of group B streptococcal opsonins in human and rabbit serum by neutrophil chemiluminescence. J. Clin. Invest. 58:1379, 1976.

Hicks, M. J., Jones, J. F., Thies, A. C., et al.: Age-related changes in mitogen-induced lymphocyte function from birth to old age. Am. J. Clin. Pathol. 80:159, 1983.

Hill, H. R.: Biochemical, structural, and functional abnormalities of polymorphonuclear leukocytes in the neonate. Pediatr. Res. 22:375, 1987.

Hill, H. R., Shigeoka, A. O., Pincus, S., et al.: Intravenous IgG in combination with other modalities in the treatment of neonatal infection. Pediatr. Infect. Dis. 5:S180, 1986.

Holzgreve, B., Goldsmith, P. C., Holzgreve, W., Golbus, M. S.: A monoclonal antibody micromethod for studying fetal lymphocytes: Potential for prenatal diagnosis of inherited immunodeficiencies. J. Reprod. Immunol. 6:341, 1984.

Hunziker, R. D., and Wegmann, T. G.: Placental immunoregulation. C.R.C. Crit. Rev. Immunol. 6:245, 1986.

Institute of Medicine, National Academy of Sciences: New vaccine development: establishing priorities. Diseases of Importance in the United States, vol. 1. Washington, D.C., National Academy Press, 1985, p. 424.

Jacoby, D. R., Olding, L. B., and Oldstone, M. B. A.: Immunologic regulation of fetal-maternal balance. Adv. Immunol. 35:157, 1984.

Jacoby, D. R., and Oldstone, M. B. A.: Delineation of suppressor and helper activity within the OKT4-defined T lymphocyte subset in human neonates. J. Immunol. 13:1765, 1983.

Jarrett, E. E. E.: Perinatal influences on IgE responses. Lancet 1:797, 1984.

Kannourakis, G., Begley, C. G., Johnson, G. R., et al.: Evidence for interactions between monocytes and natural killer cells in the regulation of in vitro hemopoiesis. J. Immunol. 140:2489, 1988.

Klesius, P. H., Zimmerman, R. A., and Matthews, J. H.: Cellular and humoral immune response to group B streptococci. J. Pediatr. 83:926, 1973.

Krause, P. J., Herson, V. C., Eisenfeld, L., et al.: Enhancement of neutrophil functions for treatment of neonatal infections. Pediatr. Inf. Dis. 8:382, 1989.

Lewis, D. B., Larsen, A., and Wilson, C. B.: Reduced interferon-gamma mRNA levels in human neonates. J. Exp. Med. 163:1018, 1986a.

Lewis, J. E., Coulam, C. B., and Moore, S. B.: Immunologic mechanisms in the maternal-fetal relationship. Mayo Clin. Proc. 61:655, 1986.

Liang, D. C., Ma, S. W., Lin-Chu, M., Lan, C. C.: Granulocyte/macrophage colony-forming units from cord blood of premature and full-term neonates: Its role in ontogeny of human hemopoiesis. Pediatr. Res. 24:701, 1988.

Lilja, G., Winbladh, B., Vedin, I., et al.: Cord blood T lymphocyte subpopulations in premature and full-term infants. Int. Arch. Allergy Appl. Immunol. 75:273, 1984.

Lu C. Y., Calamai, E. G., Unanue, E. R.: A defect in the antigen presenting function of macrophages from neonatal milk. Nature 282:327, 1979.

Malm, J., Bennhagen, R., Homberg, L., et al.: Plasma concentrations of C4b-binding protein and vitamin K–dependent protein S in term and preterm infants: Low levels of protein S-C4b–binding protein complexes. Br. J. Haematol. 68:445, 1988.

Martensson, L., and Fudenberg, H. H.: Gm genes and gamma globulin synthesis in the human fetus. J. Immunol. 94:514, 1965.

Massey, G. V., McWilliams, N. B., Mueller, D. G., et al.: Intravenous immunoglobulin in treatment of neonatal isoimmune thrombocytopenia. J. Pediatr. 111(1):133, 1987.

Medawar, P. B.: Some immunological and endocrinological problems raised by the evolution of viviparity in vertebrates. Symp. Soc. Exp. Biol. 7:320, 1953.

Melissari, P., Nicolaides, K. H., Scully, M. F., et al.: Protein S and C4b-binding protein in fetal and neonatal blood. Br. J. Haematol. 70:199, 1988.

Menitove, J. E., and Abrams, R. A.: Granulocyte transfusions in neutropenic patients. C.R.C. Crit. Rev. Onc/Hemat. 7:89, 1987.

Mills, L., and Napier, J. A. F.: Massive feto-maternal haemorrhage: Effect of passively administered anti-D in the prevention of Rh sensitization and haemolytic disease of the neonate. Br. J. Obstet. Gynecol. 45:1007, 1988.

Miyano, A., Nakayama, M., Fujita, T., et al.: Complement activation in fetuses: Assessment by the levels of complement components and split products in cord blood. Diag. Clin. Immunol. 5:86, 1987.

Miyawaki, T., Seki, H., Taga, K., et al.: Dissociated production of interleukin-2 and immune (gamma) interferon by phytohaemagglutinin stimulated lymphocytes in healthy infants. Clin. Exp. Immunol. 59:505, 1985.

Moalic, P., Gruel, Y., Body, G., et al.: Levels and plasma distribution of free and C4b-BP-bound protein S in human fetuses and full-term neonates. Thromb. Res. 49:471, 1988.

Mollnes, T. E., and Lachmann, P. J.: Regulation of complement. Scand. J. Immunol. 27:127, 1988.

Morell, A., Sidiropoulos, D., Herrmann, U., et al.: IgG subclasses and antibodies to Group B streptococci in preterm neonates after intravenous infusion of immunoglobulin to the mothers. Pediatr. Infect. Dis. 5:S195, 1986.

Muller-Eberhard, H. J.: The membrane attack complex of complement. Ann. Rev. Immunol. 4:503, 1986.

Muller-Eberhard, H. J.: Molecular organization and function of the complement system. Ann. Rev. Biochem. 57:321, 1988.

Nelson, D. L., Kurman, C. C., Fritz, M. E., et al.: The production of soluble and cellular interleukin-2 receptors by cord blood mononuclear cells following in vitro activation. Pediatr. Res. 20:136, 1986.

Noya, F. J. D., and Baker, C. J.: Intravenously administered immune globulin for premature infants: A time to wait. J. Pediatr. 115:969, 1989.

Noya, F. J. D., Rench, M. A., Garcia-Prats, J. A., et al.: Disposition of an immunoglobulin intravenous preparation in very low birth weight neonates. J. Pediatr. 112:278, 1988.

Olding, L. B., and Oldstone, M. B. A.: Lymphocytes from neonates abrogate mitosis of their mothers' lymphocytes. Nature 249:161, 1974.

Oldstone, M. B. A., Tishon, A., and Moretta, L.: Active thymus-derived suppressor lymphocytes in human cord blood. Nature 269:333, 1977.

Owen, J. J. T., Wright, D. E., Habu, S., et al.: Studies on the generation of B lymphocytes in fetal liver and bone marrow. J. Immunol. 118:2067, 1977.

Pangburn, M. D., and Muller-Eberhard, H. J.: The alternative pathway of complement. Springer Semin. Immunopathol. 7:163, 1984.

Papadogiannakis, N., and Johnsen, S. A.: Distinct mitogens reveal different mechanisms of suppressor activity in human cord blood. J. Clin. Lab. Immunol. 26:37, 1988.

Pedersen, S. A., Petersen, J., and Andersen, V.: Suppression of B lymphocytes in mature neonate infants. Acta Paediatr. Scand. 72:441, 1983.

Pereira, S., Webster, D., and Platts-Mills, T.: Immature B cells in fetal development and immunodeficiency: Studies of IgM, IgG, IgA and IgD production in vitro using Epstein-Barr virus activation. Eur. J. Immunol. 12:540, 1982.

Perignon, J. L., Durandy, A., Peter, M. O., et al.: Early prenatal diagnosis of inherited severe immunodeficiencies linked to enzyme deficiencies. J. Pediatr. 111:595, 1987.

Pittard III, W. B., Miller, K., and Sorensen, R. U.: Normal lymphocyte responses to mitogens in term and premature neonates following normal and abnormal intrauterine growth. Clin. Immunol. Immunopathol. 30:178, 1984.

Pittard III, W. B., Miller, K. M., and Sorensen, R. U.: Perinatal influences on in vitro B lymphocyte differentiation in human neonates. Pediatr. Res. 19:655, 1985.

Pittard III, W. B., Schleich, D. M., Geddes, K. M., et al.: Newborn lymphocyte subpopulations: The influence of labor. Am. J. Obstet. Gynecol. 160:151, 1989.

Pollack, M. S., Kirkpatrick, D., Kapoor, N., et al.: Identification by HLA typing of intrauterine-derived maternal T cells in four patients with severe combined immunodeficiency. N. Engl. J. Med. 307:662, 1982.

Power, D. A., Mason, R. J., Stewart, G. M., et al.: The fetus as an allograft: Evidence for protective antibodies to HLA-linked paternal antigens. Lancet 2:701, 1983.

Propp, R. P., and Alper, C. A.: C'3 Synthesis in the human fetus and lack of transplacental passage. Science 162:672, 1968.

Raghupathy, R., Singh, B., and Wegmann, T. G.: Fate of antipaternal H-2 antibodies bound to the placenta in vivo. Transplantation 37:396, 1984.

Raum, D. D., Awdeh, Z. L., Page, P. L., et al.: MHC determinants of response to Rh immunization. J. Immunol. 132:157, 1984.

Reinherz, E. L., Cooper, M. D., Schlossman, S. F., et al.: Abnormalities of T cell maturation and regulation in human beings with immunodeficiency disorders. J. Clin. Invest. 68(3):699, 1981.

Ricevuti, G., and Mazzone, A.: Clinical aspects of neutrophil locomotion disorders. Biomed. Pharmacother. 41:355, 1987.

Romero, R., Brody, D. T., Oyarzun, E., et al.: Infection and labor. III. Interleukin I: A signal for the onset of parturition. Am. J. Obstet. Gynecol. 160:1117–1123, 1989.

Rosen, F. S.: Defects in cell-mediated immunity. J. Immun. Immunopathol. 41:1, 1986.

Rosen, F. S., Cooper, M. D., and Wedgwood, R. J. P.: The primary immunodeficiencies. N. Engl. J. Med. 311:300, 1984.

Rosen, F. S., and Janeway, C. A.: Immunologic competence of the neonate infant. Pediatrics 33:159, 1964.

Ryhanen, P., Jouppila, R., Lanning, M., et al.: Effect of segmental epidural analgesia on changes in peripheral blood leucocyte counts, lymphocyte subpopulations, and in vitro transformation in healthy parturients and their neonates. Gynecol. Obstet. Invest. 17:202, 1984.

Santos, J. I., Shigeoka, A. O., and Hill, H. H.: Functional leukocyte administration in protection against experimental neonatal infection. Pediatr. Res. 14:1408, 1980.

Schofield, F.: Selective primary health care: Strategies for control of disease in the developing world. XXII. Tetanus: A Preventative Problem. Rev. Infect. Dis. 8:144, 1986.

Schroder, J.: Passage of leucocytes from mother to fetus. Scand. J. Immunol. 2:369, 1974.

Scott, J. R., Rote, N. S., and Branch, D. W.: Immunologic aspects of recurrent abortion and fetal death. Obstet. Gynecol. 70:645, 1987.

Shapiro, R., Beatty, D. W., Woods, D. L., et al.: Complement activity in the cord blood of term neonates with the amniotic fluid infection syndrome. S. Afr. Med. J. 63:86, 1983.

Simmons, R. L.: Histoincompatibility and the survival of the fetus: Current controversies. Transplant. Proc. 1:47, 1969.

Simmons, R. L., and Russell, P. S.: Immunologic interactions between mother and fetus. Adv. Obstet. Gynecol. 1:38, 1967.

Sorensen, R. U., and Polmar, S. H.: Immunoglobulin replacement therapy. Ann. Clin. Res. 19:392, 1987.

Stankova, J., and Rola-Pleszczynski, M.: Suppressor cells in the human maternal-fetal relationship. J. Reprod. Immunol. 6:49, 1984.

Stegagno, M., Pascone, R., Colarizi, P., et al.: Immunologic follow-up of infants treated with granulocyte transfusion for neonatal sepsis. Pediatrics 76:508, 1985.

Steinbeck, M. J., Roth, J. A.: Neutrophil activation by recombinant cytokines. Rev. Infect. Dis. 11:549, 1989.

Stiehm, E. R., Ammann, A. J., and Cherry, J. D.: Elevated cord macroglobulins in the diagnosis of intrauterine infections. N. Engl. J. Med. 275:971, 1966.

Stiehm, E. R., Ashida, E., Kim, K. S., et al.: Intravenous immunoglobulins as therapeutic agents. Ann. Int. Med. 107:367, 1987.

Stiehm, E. R., Sztein, M. B., Steeg, P. S., et al.: Deficient DR antigen expression on human cord blood monocytes: Reversal with lymphokines. Clin. Immunol. Immunopathol. 30:430, 1984.

Stossel, T. P., Alper, C. A., and Rosen, F. S.: Opsonic activity in neonate. Pediatrics 52:134, 1973.

Strunk, R. C., Fenton, L. J., and Gaines, J. A.: Alternative pathway of complement activation in full term and premature infants. Pediatr. Res. 13:641, 1979.

Sutton, M. B., Strunk, R. C., and Cole, F. S.: Regulation of synthesis of the third component of complement and factor B in cord blood monocytes by lipopolysaccharide. J. Immunol. 136:1366, 1986.

Swinburne, L. M.: Leucocyte antigens and placental sponge. Lancet 2:592, 1970.

Tedder, T. F., Clement, L. T., and Cooper, M. D.: Development and distribution of a human B cell subpopulation identified by the HB-4 monoclonal antibody. J. Immunol. 134:1539, 1985a.

Tedder, T. F., Clement, L. T., and Cooper, M. D.: Human lymphocyte differentiation antigens HB-10 and HB-11. I. Ontogeny of antigen expression. J. Immunol. 134:2983, 1985b.

Thomas, M. L., Harger, J. H., Wagener, D. K., et al.: HLA sharing and spontaneous abortion in humans. Am. J. Obstet. Gynecol. 151:1053, 1985.

Thompson, L. F., O'Connor, R. D., and Bastian, J. F.: Phenotype and function of engrafted maternal T cells in patients with severe combined immunodeficiency. J. Immunol. 133:2513, 1984.

Timens, W., Rozeboom, T., and Poppema, S.: Fetal and neonatal development of human spleen: An immunohistological study. Immunology 60:603, 1987.

Toivanen, P., Uksila, J., Leino, A., et al.: Development of mitogen responding T cells and natural killer cells in the human fetus. Immunol. Rev. 57:89, 1981.

Tongio, M. M., Mayer, S., and Lebel, A.: Transfer of HL-A antibodies from the mother to the child. Transplantation 20:163, 1975.

Van Furth, R., Schuitt, H. R. E., and Hijmans, W.: The immunological development of the human fetus. J. Exp. Med. 122:1173, 1965.

Van Tol, M. J. D., Zijlstra, J., Thomas, C. M. G., et al.: Distinct role of neonatal and adult monocytes in the regulation of the in vitro antigen-induced plaque-forming cell response in man. J. Immunol. 134:1902, 1984.

Vercellotti, G., Stroncek, D., Jacob, H. S.: Granulocyte oxygen radicals as potential suppressors of hemopoiesis: Potentiating roles of lactoferrin and elastase; inhibitory role of oxygen radical scavengers. Blood Cells 13:199, 1987.

Volanakis, J. E.: C3 convertases of complement. Year in Immunol. 4:218, 1988.

Wakasugi, N., and Virelizier, J-L.: Defective interferon gamma production in the human neonate. I. Dysregulation rather than intrinsic abnormality. J. Immunol. 134(1):167, 1985.

Waldmann, T. A., Korsmeyer, S. J., Hieter, P. A., et al.: Regulation of the humoral immune response from immunoglobulin genes to regulatory T cell networks. Fed. Proc 42:2498, 1983.

Walsh, J. A., and Hutchins, S.: Group B streptococcal disease: Its importance in the developing world and prospect for prevention with vaccines. Pediatr. Inf. Dis. 8:271, 1989.

Wegmann, T. G.: Maternal T cells promote placental growth and prevent spontaneous abortion. Immunol. Lett. 17:297, 1988.

Wegmann, T. G., Barrington, L. J., Carlson, G. A., et al.: Quantitation of the capacity of the mouse placenta to absorb monoclonal anti-fetal H-2K antibody. J. Reprod. Immunol. 2:53, 1980.

Wilson, C. B.: Immunologic basis for increased susceptibility of the neonate to infection. J. Pediatr. 108(1):1, 1986.

Wilson, M., Rosen, F. S., Schlossman, S. F., et al.: Ontogeny of human T and B lymphocytes during stressed and normal gestation: Phenotypic analysis of umbilical cord lymphocytes from term and preterm infants. J. Immunol. Immunopathol. 37:1, 1985.

Wilson, C. B., Westall, J., Johnston, L., et al.: Decreased production of interferon-gamma by human neonatal cells. J. Clin. Invest. 77:860, 1986.

Winter, H. S., Gard, S. E., Fischer, T. J., et al.: Deficient lymphokine production of neonate lymphocytes. Pediatr. Res. 11:573, 1983.

FETAL/NEONATAL **35** HUMAN IMMUNODEFICIENCY VIRUS INFECTION

F. Sessions Cole

Human immunodeficiency virus (HIV) infection, first described in 1981 (Gottlieb, et al., 1981; Masur et al., 1981; Siegal et al., 1981) has reached epidemic proportions in the 46 countries of the Western hemisphere, including the United States (Quinn et al., 1989). Although complicated by the prolonged incubation period of this infection and ascertainment difficulties, estimates put the number of cases of HIV infection in the Americas by 1992 at 2.5 million people and the number of cases of acquired immunodeficiency syndrome at 500,000. In the United States through September 1989, 105,990 cases of AIDS have been reported, of which 61,655 persons (58.2 per cent) have died. Recent estimates in the United States project 365,000 AIDS cases will be diagnosed by the end of 1992, and of these, 263,000 will die by the end of 1992 (Centers for Disease Control, 1989). A total of approximately 172,000 AIDS patients will require care in 1992 at an annual cost expected to range from $5 billion to $13 billion (Rogers, 1989; Winkenwerder et al., 1989). These figures significantly underestimate the true magnitude of morbidity due to HIV infection because many clinical manifestations of HIV infection are not reportable under current Centers for Disease Control (CDC) AIDS case definitions (Centers for Disease Control, 1987). A minimum of one million Americans are currently (1990) infected with HIV. The impact of new therapies (e.g., zidovudine) on survival and health-care costs cannot currently be estimated.

Because of HIV screening of donated blood products and aggressive educational programs, the risk of new infection in hemophiliacs, in persons who receive blood transfusions, and in homosexual men has declined from 1987 to 1989. However, the risk of new infections remains high in intravenous drug users and in their heterosexual or homosexual partners. These facts have resulted in an increasing net seroprevalence rate from 1988 to 1990 among child-bearing women. This observation is consistent with the increasing risk of congenitally infected newborn infants.

■ EPIDEMIOLOGY AND NATURAL HISTORY OF PERINATAL HIV INFECTION

EPIDEMIOLOGY

Since the first reported cases of HIV infection in children in 1983, more than 1600 cases of pediatric AIDS (children 13 years of age or younger) have been reported to the CDC (Centers for Disease Control, 1989; Oleske et al., 1983; Rubinstein et al., 1983). These cases represent only a fraction of the total seropositive pediatric population with the most severe clinical manifestations. Although no definitive number is available, seroprevalence estimates suggest that 3200 to 4000 total cases of HIV infection have occurred, and that pediatric patients will be one of the most rapidly increasing risk groups during the 1990s. Within the pediatric group, the majority (approximately 80 per cent) acquires HIV infection vertically from chronically infected mothers (Pizzo, 1990). With improved screening of blood products, this proportion will increase to over 95 per cent of pediatric AIDS cases from perinatal infection in the 1990s. Among women screened without knowledge of risk status, observed seroprevalence rates range from less than 1 per cent to 4.3 per cent in inner-city hospitals of the Northeast. Surveys of child-bearing women performed in nine states by anonymously testing blood routinely collected from newborns for diagnosis of hereditary metabolic disorders indicates statewide seroprevalence rates that range from 0.1 per cent in California, Colorado, Michigan, New Mexico, and Texas and 0.2 per cent in Massachusetts to 0.5 per cent in Florida and New Jersey and 0.7 per cent in New York (Centers for Disease Control, 1989; Hoff et al., 1988). Because the net seroprevalence rate among child-bearing women has been increasing, ongoing new infection of women in their child-bearing years has been occurring and will provide the most important contribution to increasing numbers of HIV seropositive children in this country (Centers for Disease Control, 1989; Katz and Wilfert, 1989). If seropositivity

321

rates derived from anonymous newborn screening are used, 6000 to 20,000 new pediatric AIDS cases can be expected between 1990 and 1995 (Pizzo, 1990).

Women at high risk for acquiring HIV infection include those who received a blood transfusion before 1985, those who share needles for intravenous drug use, and those who have unprotected sexual intercourse with an infected partner. Antenatal history-taking should include a careful transfusion history, history of intravenous drug use, and history of sexual contacts including bisexual or homosexual men, hemophiliacs, intravenous drug abusers, or males born in countries where heterosexual transmission of HIV is thought to play a major role (e.g., Haiti or Central Africa). The risk of disease acquisition from a single heterosexual encounter with an infected partner is currently undefinable. On the basis of studies of steady sexual partners of hemophiliacs or partners of patients with AIDS or AIDS-related complex, repeated sexual contact leads to a risk of 7 to 40 per cent chance of contracting HIV infection (Landesman, 1989). These studies have also suggested that HIV transmission occurs with a high degree of efficiency in some couples (after only a few sexual contacts), while in others, infection of sexual partners may not occur despite multiple contacts. It is important to note that the latency period for the virus in the adult population is 7 to 9 years (Imagawa et al., 1989).

Universal prenatal testing has been a topic of considerable discussion. Currently, the American Academy of Pediatrics and the American College of Obstetricians and Gynecologists recommend HIV screening of pregnant women who are "at increased risk of HIV infection" (American Academy of Pediatrics Task Force on Pediatric AIDS, 1988; Frigoletto and Little, 1988). Rhame and Maki (1989) advocate universal prenatal testing for HIV, while Weiss and Thier (1988) have suggested screening before blood and tissue donation only. Because of the potential inaccuracy of risk histories as demonstrated in studies of perinatal transmission of hepatitis B virus (Centers for Disease Control, 1988a), aggressive prenatal screening should continue to be considered among all pregnant women.

Because a substantial proportion of drug abuse is in inner-city areas, racial minority groups or the socioeconomically disadvantaged are most affected: of the HIV-infected children in the United States, approximately 48 per cent are black and 22 per cent are Hispanic (Pizzo, 1990). The congruence of the demographics of drug abuse and HIV infection suggests the importance of this route of infection: drug abuse is the numerically most significant high-risk group for fetal/neonatal infection. In one recent study, 76 per cent of 59 infants with vertically transmitted HIV infection had one or both parents who were intravenous drug abusers (Guinan and Hardy, 1987).

NATURAL HISTORY

Currently, no prospective data are available concerning the route or timing of HIV infection during pregnancy or during the immediate postpartum period (Table 35–1). Recovery of HIV from early gestation conceptuses, placenta, blood and amniotic fluid around the time of delivery, and breast milk suggests multiple possible perinatal routes of fetal/neonatal infection (Pizzo, 1990). In prospective studies of infants with seropositive and seronegative mothers in Zaire, Europe, and Brazil, a minimum vertical transmission rate of approximately 30 per cent has been observed, although earlier limited or retrospective surveys provide estimates of a 40 to 60 per cent transmission rate (Cortes et al., 1989; Rogers et al., 1989; Ryder et al., 1989).

Because of antenatal transfer of HIV antibody of IgG isotype from mother to fetus, serologic status of an infant at birth is not a reliable indicator of infection. In addition, cord blood T-cell subset ratios and immunoglobulin concentrations have not been helpful in predicting subsequent development of HIV infection (Pizzo, 1990). Availability of molecular diagnostic methods as well as viral isolation methods from small amounts of plasma or small numbers of peripheral blood mononuclear cells permit more accurate categorization of infected infants at birth. This categorization is especially important for prognosis and for development of prophylactic pharmacologic interventions.

In contrast to adults in whom a reversal of the ratio of inducer T cells ($CD4^+$) to suppressor T cells ($CD8^+$) is the hallmark of the disease, infants frequently have abnormalities of B-cell function (Fallon et al., 1989; Jendis et al., 1988; Katz, 1989; McNamara, 1989; Pahwa, 1988). Specifically, infected infants at 3 to 4 months of age have elevations of immunoglobulins and do not respond to specific antigen challenges with appropriate antibody increases. Elevated, but dysfunctional, immunoglobulin concentrations predispose HIV-infected infants to recurrent bacterial infections (Bernstein et al., 1985a and 1985b). In contrast to HIV-infected adults, this B-cell defect precedes the T-cell deficiency in infants. The CD4 cell count is thus not a reliable guide to disease status or response to therapeutic interventions. In addition, mononuclear cells from infected children evidence reduced proliferative responses to nonspecific or specific mitogens, and these children are anergic to delayed hypersensitivity antigens.

Children with HIV infection become symptomatic more quickly than adults and succumb to the disease sooner than adults (Pizzo, 1990). The median incubation period for children born to HIV-positive mothers is 8 months in contrast to an average 8-year incubation in adults.

There is considerable heterogeneity of disease progression among infants who are HIV-seropositive. For example, among children who contracted HIV infection after

TABLE 35–1. Perinatal Transmission of the Human Immunodeficiency Virus

INTRAUTERINE TRANSMISSION (RUBELLA MODEL)	INTRAPARTUM TRANSMISSION (HEPATITIS MODEL)	POSTPARTUM TRANSMISSION
• Virus found in 13- to 20-week fetus. • Infectivity of trophoblast cell lines. • Funisitis and chorioamnionitis of placenta. • Isolation of HIV from cord blood. • Craniofacial dysmorphic features.	• Exposure to blood during delivery (both vaginal and by cesarean). • Maternal-fetal transfusion during delivery.	• Number of definitive cases by breast-feeding is small, but transmission can occur. • No household cases reported to date.

(Adapted from Pizzo, P. A.: Pediatric AIDS: Problems within problems. J. Inf. Dis. *161*:316, 1990.)

receiving HIV-contaminated blood products at birth, disease progression has been lower than observed among HIV-seropositive infants infected via maternal-infant transmission (Albersheim et al., 1988; Ammann et al., 1983; Church and Isaacs, 1984; Saulsbury et al., 1987; Shannon et al., 1983). Approximately 5 per cent of infants HIV seropositive at birth have a rapidly deteriorating course over the first 10 to 18 months of life. These children succumb to *Pneumocystis carinii* pneumonia, encephalopathy, or recurrent bacterial infection (Pahwa, 1988). An additional 30 per cent present with nonspecific findings including failure to thrive, persistent generalized lymphadenopathy, persistent oral candidiasis, and developmental delay. These children may be seropositive or seronegative. The indolent form of the disease is also characterized by cough, arterial desaturation, digital clubbing, and immunologic abnormalities (elevated immunoglobulins, abnormal T-cell numbers, and abnormal peripheral blood mononuclear cell mitogen responses) (Pahwa, 1988). Approximately 70 per cent of newborns seropositive at birth are seronegative and free of symptoms by 18 to 24 months of age (Blanche et al., 1989). The availability of more sensitive molecular and viral isolation techniques to identify HIV-infected children will permit more accurate categorization of and assessment of prognosis for these patients (Coombs et al., 1989; Rogers et al., 1989).

The impact of maternal HIV infection on pregnancy outcome in the United States has been difficult to assess because of multiple confounding factors, including drug abuse and malnutrition. However, in a study from Zaire where none of the women reported a history of intravenous drug abuse, low birth weight, prematurity, low ratio of head circumference to length, and chorioamnionitis were all more common among infants of HIV-positive mothers with AIDS than among infants of HIV-positive, asymptomatic women or infants with seronegative mothers (Ryder et al., 1989). These problems substantially enhance the risk of death in the first year of life for infants born to seropositive mothers: 100 deaths (21 per cent) occurred among 468 children of HIV-seropositive mothers and 23 deaths (3.8 per cent) among 604 children of seronegative mothers. Based on these figures, Ryder and colleagues (1989) suggested that HIV infections will account for at least a 15 per cent increase in infant mortality in Zaire.

■ PATHOGENESIS OF HIV INFECTION

Human immunodeficiency virus type 1, previously known as lymphadenopathy-associated virus (LAV-1), human T-cell lymphotrophic virus type III (HTLV-III), or AIDS-related virus (ARV), is an RNA virus which has a lipid envelope and is approximately 100 nm in diameter (Popovic et al., 1984). It differs from other retroviruses because, in addition to the standard retroviral genes that encode core proteins *(gag)*, reverse transcriptase *(pol)*, and envelope proteins *(env)*, it has at least five additional genes *(tat, trs/art, sor, 3'ora,* and R) whose functions are unclear (Ho et al., 1987; Pahwa, 1988) (Fig. 35–1 and Table 35–2). An example of a possible pathogenetic mechanism that involves these HIV-specific genes has been suggested by Nabel and Baltimore (1987) who have demonstrated that activated T cells produce a DNA-

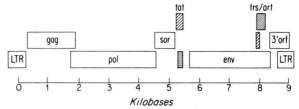

FIGURE 35–1. *The HIV genome is unique among retroviruses in that it has at least five genes in addition to the standard gag, pol, and env genes that encode the core proteins, reverse transcriptase, and envelope proteins, respectively. Tat and trs/art are thought to be essential posttranscriptional or transcriptional regulators. No virus replication occurs when either gene is inactive. LTR = long terminal repeats. (From Ho, D. D., Moudgil, T., and Alam, M.: Quantitation of human immunodeficiency virus type 1 in the blood of infected persons. N. Engl. J. Med. 321:1521, 1989.)*

binding protein structurally and functionally similar to a recognized transcription factor, nuclear factor kappa B, which binds to the enhancer sequence of HIV and permits viral replication. Nuclear factor kappa B also appears to act synergistically with the *tat* gene product.

HIV is related to a family of nontransforming, cytopathic retroviruses (lentiviruses) based upon direct comparisions of nucleotide sequence, morphologic characteristics, and in vitro comparisons (Ho et al., 1987) (Fig. 35–2). Several of these viruses cause disease in animals: visna virus and caprine arthritis encephalitis virus (CAEV) cause chronic neurodegenerative diseases in sheep and goats, equine infectious anemia virus (EIAV) causes episodic fevers and hemolytic anemia in horses, and STLV-III causes a form of simian AIDS with encephalitis. HIV-2 (also known as LAV-2 or HTLV-IV) has been isolated from humans in West Africa, is clearly associated with an immunodeficiency syndrome similar to AIDS, and has not been detected yet in natives of the Western hemisphere.

In adults, the diagnosis of HIV infection is usually predicated upon a depletion of a subpopulation of helper/inducer T lymphocytes characterized by the presence on the cell surface of an antigen called T4, or CD4. This abnormality results from the selective tropism of HIV for a CD4$^+$ subpopulation of lymphocytes. The cell surface protein CD4 functions as the receptor for HIV on lymphocytes as well as monocytes and possibly neuronal cells (Dalgleish et al., 1984; Klatzmann et al., 1984; Sattentau and Weiss, 1988) (Fig. 35–3). Viral replication

TABLE 35–2. Description of Major Gene Products of Human Immunodeficiency Virus

GENE PRODUCT*	DESCRIPTION
P17	gag protein
P24	gag protein
P31	endonuclease component of pol translate
GP41	transmembrane env glycoprotein
P51	reverse transcriptase component of pol translate
P55	precursor of gag proteins
P66	reverse transcriptase component of pol translate
GP120	outer env glycoprotein
GP160	precursor of env glycoprotein

*Number refers to molecular weight of the protein in kilodaltons; measurement of molecular weight may vary slightly in different laboratories.

Key: gag = core, pol = polymerase, env = envelope.

(From Centers for Disease Control: Update: Serologic testing for antibody to human immunodeficiency virus. M.M.W.R. 36:833, 1988.)

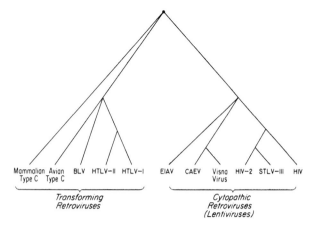

FIGURE 35–2. *Evolutionary relations among retroviruses based on comparisons of morphologic characteristics, nucleotide-sequence data, and protein cross-reactivity. BLV = bovine leukemia virus, HTLV-I and HTLV-II = human T-cell leukemia virus types I and II, EIAV = equine infectious anemia virus, and CAEV = caprine arthritis encephalitis virus. (From Ho, D. D., Pomerantz, R. J., and Kaplan, J. C.: Pathogenesis of infection with human immunodeficiency virus. N. Engl. J. Med. 317:278, 1987.)*

and cell lysis occur in CD4$^+$ lymphocytes, while in monocytes and possibly neuronal cells, the virus may replicate but is not lytic. Because of the complex and heterogeneous roles which CD4$^+$ lymphocytes and monocytes play in immunologic responsiveness, there is considerable diversity in the array of immunologic defects detected in patients infected with HIV. As might be anticipated from the developmentally distinct role which these cells play in immunologic responsiveness in infants, different immunologic abnormalities are seen in children.

Unlike adults, a clear correlation between CD4$^+$ lymphopenia and HIV disease severity does not occur in children (Mann et al., 1983; Pahwa, 1988; Pizzo, 1990). While long-term prospective indicators are currently being studied, marked polyclonal hypergammaglobulinemia with elevations in IgG and variable elevations in IgA and IgM is a common finding in infants and children even in

the early phases (ages 3 to 8 months) of the infection. Cord blood immunoglobulins have not been helpful in neonatal diagnosis. Depletion of CD4$^+$ lymphocytes with reversal of the T4/T8 ratio to <1 and decreased T-cell responsiveness to specific and nonspecific mitogens become evident later in the course of the infection. Interestingly, prematurely born HIV-infected infants appear to manifest hypogammaglobulinemia as a feature of their immunodeficiency (Pahwa et al., 1987). These children may also have intracranial calcification. Serologic diagnostic tests may be negative in children with hypogammaglobulinemia after birth, so that viral isolation is required to establish the diagnosis.

Viral coinfection may enhance HIV replication in CD4$^+$ lymphocytes through several different mechanisms (Ho et al., 1987; Pahwa, 1988). For example, cytomegalovirus (CMV), herpes simplex virus, and hepatitis B virus can directly interact with HIV long terminal repeats in the HIV genome to induce viral replication. Viral replication leads to death of CD4$^+$ lymphocytes. Loss of suppressor/cytotoxic T-cell regulation may facilitate HIV replication as well as allow latent Ebstein-Barr virus to replicate with consequent emergence of B-cell malignant lymphomas.

Syncytia formation, probably due to a lower surface density of CD4 molecules, and the relative refractoriness of HIV-induced cell death suggest that monocytes and macrophages may serve as significant reservoirs for the virus in the host and a vehicle for transport of HIV to multiple tissues including the central nervous system (Sattentau and Weiss, 1988). Among the defects observed in monocytes and macrophages from HIV-infected patients are the inability to migrate along chemotactic gradients and increased production of tumor necrosis factor. This latter abnormality may be critical in the pathogenesis of infant wasting syndrome.

The HIV envelope glycoprotein (GP120) is critical for interaction between the CD4 molecule and the virus itself as well as for syncytia formation. GP120 may also play an as yet poorly understood role in immunomediated

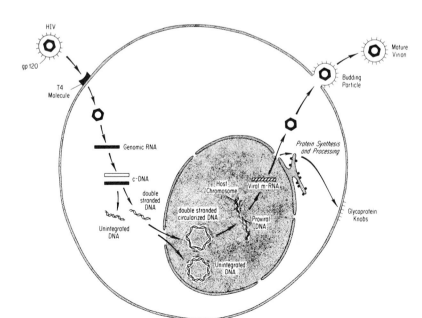

FIGURE 35–3. *HIV replication cycle. (From Ho, D. D., Pomerantz, R. J., and Kaplan, J. C.: Pathogenesis of infection with human immunodeficiency virus. N. Engl. J. Med. 317:278, 1987.)*

destruction of CD4$^+$ lymphocytes. Whether the GP120 coating of CD4$^+$ lymphocytes leads to clearance by the immune system or GP120 alters HLA class II phenotypic expression and thus enhances immune clearance has not been determined.

■ DIAGNOSIS AND CLASSIFICATION OF HIV INFECTION

In adults, the diagnosis of HIV infection is made only after the presence of HIV antibody is repeatedly documented with a licensed enzyme immunoassay by identification of multiple virus-specific proteins (e.g., P24, P31, and either GP41 or GP160) by Western blot analysis (see Table 35–2) (Centers for Disease Control, 1988c). However, the diagnosis of HIV infection in newborns is difficult because of the transplacental transport of maternal antibody to HIV, a lack of reliable tests for HIV antibody of IgM isotype produced exclusively by the fetus, and the symptomatic heterogeneity of presentation of infants with HIV infection. An additional problem in utilization of Western blot techniques results from the inability to detect the HIV-specific proteins when excess maternally derived antibody is present. Because maternally derived antibody may persist for up to 15 months, the Centers for Disease Control (CDC) recommend serologic diagnosis of HIV infection only after the infant reaches 15 months of age. However, this test may also be unreliable after 15 months of age because some infants with HIV infection become hypogammaglobulinemic and may thus not be detectable by serologic testing. These concerns have prompted efforts to develop nonserologic methods with which to identify HIV infections on small amounts of blood.

Availability of sequence data for the genes that encode P24 antigen and GP41 transmembrane glycoprotein of HIV permitted Rogers and co-workers (1989) to use the polymerase chain reaction (PCR) to identify amplified HIV proviral sequences (Fig. 35–4). The technique can be performed with DNA isolated from small numbers of peripheral blood mononuclear cells. After DNA isolation, single-stranded DNA is prepared by heating and is annealed with complementary nucleotide sequences of primers specific for HIV antigens P24 and GP41. A thermostable DNA polymerase (*Taq* DNA polymerase isolated from the thermophilic bacterium *Thermus aquaticus*) is then used to catalyse the synthesis of new DNA strands that contain HIV proviral sequences. HIV primers are removed from proviral sequences by heating. Cooling permits excess primer to reanneal to increased numbers of proviral sequences which are again copied by the thermostable DNA polymerase. By repeated cycles of heating and cooling, multiple copies of HIV-specific sequences can be synthesized. This method thus provides a means for amplification of low-abundance sequences that occur between nucleotides complementary to the HIV primers used. In their initial study, Rogers and associates (1989) demonstrated that this method can detect proviral sequences in infants in the neonatal and postneonatal periods who later develop HIV infection. Five of seven infants who later developed AIDS (mean age 9.8 months) were detected by PCR in the neonatal period. However, the sensitivity of this method may be compromised by the inability to detect HIV which is transmitted during the

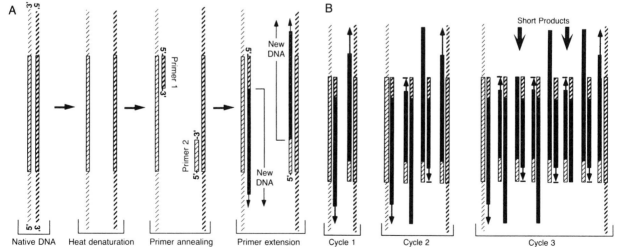

FIGURE 35–4. A, *First round of the polymerase chain reaction. The basic polymerase-chain-reaction cycle consists of three steps performed in the same closed container but at different temperatures. The elevated temperature in the first step melts the double-stranded DNA into single strands. As the temperature is lowered for the second step, the two oppositely directed oligonucleotide primers anneal to complementary sequences on the target DNA, which acts as a template. During the third step, also performed at a lower temperature, the Taq polymerase enzymatically extends the primers covalently in the presence of excess deoxyribonucleoside triphosphates, the building blocks of new DNA synthesis. The native DNA target sequences, which will be massively amplified as "short products" in the ensuing cycles, are boxed. The vector of action of the DNA polymerase is denoted by the arrows projecting from the newly synthesized DNA, indicated by the dark bars.*

B, Products at the end of the initial polymerase-chain-reaction cycles. A key element of the polymerase chain reaction is the repetitive thermocycling of the steps shown in A. At each cycle the dark bars denote the accumulated DNA that has already been synthesized, and the currently synthesized DNA is indicated by the arrows that project in the direction of active DNA polymerization. Since the synthesized products of all previous cycles act as templates for all ensuing cycles, the number of short products increases geometrically at the completion of each cycle (the first three are shown). After the completion of the 30 or so cycles typical of the method, the ratio of short products to other DNA entities becomes so large that they appear to be the only detectable DNA in the reaction mixture. (From Eisenstein, B. I.: Current concepts—the polymerase chain reaction: A new method of using molecular genetics for medical diagnosis. N. Engl. J. Med. 322:178, 1990.)

intrapartum period, by its detection of proviral sequences in maternally derived lymphocytes, or by a frequency of viral sequences too low per cell to detect in the volume of blood or white blood cells obtained. The significance of detecting proviral sequences awaits further cross-sectional and longitudinal studies.

Besides molecular amplification of proviral sequences, detection of HIV infection by viral culture of peripheral blood mononuclear cells or plasma may also provide a method for identifying HIV-infected newborns (Coombs et al., 1989; Ho et al., 1989). This method may permit greater understanding of the prognostic significance of fetal HIV infection. Although HIV has been recovered from fetuses and amniotic fluid, the prognostic implications of fetal viral recovery have not been determined. Previous anecdotal reports of monozygotic twins discordant for HIV infection (Menez-Baustista et al., 1986) and women who give birth to both HIV-infected and noninfected infants suggest the need for utilization of these sensitive methods to determine the risk of acquiring the disease.

Classification of the clinical features of HIV infections in children under 13 years old has been proposed by the Centers for Disease Control (Table 35–3). HIV-infected children are divided into three classes: asymptomatic (P1), symptomatic (P2), and indeterminant infection (P0). Class P0 is used for infants under 15 months old born to HIV-positive mothers who do not satisfy criteria for class P1 or P2. Within class P2, nonspecific features include generalized lymphadenopathy, hepatomegaly, splenomegaly, diarrhea, failure to thrive, fever, and parotitis. Lymphocytic interstitial pneumonia can be recognized radiologically in infants with bilateral reticulonodular interstitial infiltrates. Although auscultation of the lungs is usually unremarkable, clubbing and hypoxemia are frequently present. Histopathologically, the lymphocytic infiltrate can be peribronchial and/or interstitial with predominantly CD8+ lymphocytes. Other diseases (subclass F) include hepatitis, cardiomyopathy, nephropathy, dermatologic diseases, and thrombocytopenia. Of special interest is the reported craniofacial dysmorphism called AIDS embryopathy. Because of a lack of consensus concerning this embryopathy, it has not been incorporated into the CDC classification of children with HIV infection.

TABLE 35–3. Classification of HIV Infection in Children Under 13 Years Old

Class P-0. Indeterminate infection
Class P-1. Asymptomatic infection
  Subclass A. Normal immune function
  Subclass B. Abnormal immune function
  Subclass C. Immune function not tested
Class P-2. Symptomatic infection
  Subclass A. Nonspecific findings
  Subclass B. Progressive neurologic disease
  Subclass C. Lymphoid interstitial pneumonitis
  Subclass D. Secondary infectious diseases
    Category D-1. Specified secondary infectious diseases listed in the CDC surveillance definitions for AIDS
    Category D-2. Recurrent serious bacterial infections
    Category D-3. Other specified secondary infectious diseases
  Subclass E. Secondary cancers
    Category E-1. Specified secondary cancers listed in the CDC surveillance definition of AIDS
    Category E-2. Other cancers possibly secondary to HIV infection
  Subclass F. Other diseases possibly due to HIV infection

(From Centers for Disease Control: Revision of the case definition for acquired immunodeficiency syndrome. M.M.W.R. 1(Suppl.):1, 1987.)

If laboratory evidence of HIV infection is available, any of the definitively diagnosed diseases listed in Table 35–4 indicates a diagnosis of AIDS. Of special interest for physicians who care for ill newborns are the categories of recurrent bacterial infections, candidiasis, cytomegalovirus, and HIV wasting syndrome. Extremely-low-birth-weight infants who are exposed to transfusions of blood products from multiple donors often develop one or more of these symptoms. Investigating HIV infection as a primary cause for these problems rather than assigning these complications to prematurity should be considered.

■ RISK OF HIV EXPOSURE TO PERINATAL HEALTH-CARE WORKERS

As of this writing (January, 1990), there are no known instances of HIV infection acquired through exposure to infants at delivery. HIV infection among health-care workers results primarily from exposures that occur outside the health-care setting. Several prospective studies of health-care workers who have had needle-stick exposure to known HIV-positive patients suggest that the risk of seroconversion is approximately 0.4 per cent (Centers for Disease Control, 1990). The risk of mucous membrane or skin exposure to HIV-infected blood is less than 0.4 per cent (Marcus, 1988).

The CDC has made the following recommendations. First, individuals likely to be exposed to blood or body fluids should be immunized with hepatitis B vaccine. Secondly, blood and body fluid precautions should be consistently used for all patients regardless of blood-borne infection status. These universal precautions do not apply to feces, nasal secretions, sputum, sweat, tears, urine, or vomitus unless contaminated with blood. Occupational exposure to human breast milk, semen, and vaginal secretions has not been implicated in transmission of HIV infection to health-care workers. Gloves should be worn by all individuals who handle newborns or placentas immediately following birth. Hands should be washed immediately after gloves are removed and/or when skin surfaces are contaminated with blood. During resuscitation, regulated wall suction should be used. If mouth suction is necessary, traps should be installed to prevent direct aspiration. Infants of known seropositive mothers may be cared for in a normal nursery and do not require isolation. Gloves are not required for prevention of HIV transmission while changing diapers. Currently, data are insufficient to establish whether health-care workers who sustain an occupational exposure to HIV-infected blood are benefited by postexposure prophylaxis with zidovudine (Centers for Disease Control, 1990).

Counseling for the exposed individual should provide:

1. The theoretical basis for postexposure prophylaxis (primarily data from animal studies).
2. The risk of the exposure.
3. The lack of definitive information concerning efficacy of zidovudine when used as postexposure prophylaxis in humans.
4. Data concerning toxicity.
5. Emphasizing the need for postexposure serologic testing regardless of zidovudine use (Centers for Disease Control, 1990).

TABLE 35–4. Definition of Acquired Immunodeficiency Syndrome

Regardless of the presence of other causes of immunodeficiency, in the presence of laboratory evidence for HIV infection, any definitively diagnosed disease listed below indicates a diagnosis of AIDS.

1. Bacterial infections, multiple or recurrent (any combination of at least two within a 2-year period), of the following affecting a child <13 years of age: septicemia, pneumonia, meningitis, bone or joint infection, or abscess of an internal organ or body cavity (excluding otitis media or superficial skin or mucosal abscesses), caused by *Haemophilus, Streptococcus* (including pneumococcus), or other pyogenic bacteria.
2. Candidiasis of the esophagus, trachea, bronchi, or lungs.
3. Coccidioidomycosis, disseminated (at a site other than or in addition to lungs or cervical or hilar lymph nodes).
4. Cryptococcosis, extrapulmonary.
5. Cryptosporidiosis with diarrhea persisting >1 month.
6. Cytomegalovirus disease of an organ other than liver, spleen, or lymph nodes in a patient >1 month of age.
7. Herpes simplex virus infection causing a mucocutaneous ulcer that persists longer than 1 month or bronchitis, pneumonitis, or esophagitis for any duration affecting a patient >1 month of age.
8. HIV encephalopathy (also called "HIV dementia," "AIDS dementia," or "subacute encephalitis due to HIV"): clinical findings of disabling cognitive and/or motor dysfunction interfering with occupation or activities of daily living, or loss of behavioral developmental milestones affecting a child, progressing over weeks to months, in the absence of a concurrent illness or condition other than HIV infection that could explain the findings. Methods to rule out such concurrent illnesses and conditions must include cerebrospinal fluid examination and either brain imaging (computed tomography or magnetic resonance) or autopsy.
9. Histoplasmosis, disseminated (at a site other than or in addition to lungs or cervical or hilar lymph nodes).
10. Isosporiasis with diarrhea persisting >1 month.
11. Kaposi's sarcoma at any age.
12. Lymphoma of the brain (primary) at any age.
13. Other non–Hodgkin lymphoma of B-cell or unknown immunologic phenotype and the following types:
    a. Small noncleaved lymphoma (either Burkitt or non-Burkitt type).
    b. Immunoblastic sarcoma (equivalent to any of the following, although not necessarily all in combination: immunoblastic lymphoma, large-cell lymphoma, diffuse histiocytic lymphoma, diffuse undifferentiated lymphoma, or high-grade lymphoma).
    Note: Lymphomas are not included here if they are of T-cell immunologic phenotype or their histologic type is not described as "lymphocytic," "lymphoblastic," "small cleaved," or "plasmacytoid lymphocytic."
14. Lymphoid interstitial pneumonia and/or pulmonary lymphoid hyperplasia (LIP/PLH) complex affecting a child <13 years of age.
15. Any mycobacterial disease caused by mycobacteria other than *M. tuberculosis*, disseminated (at a site other than or in addition to lungs, skin, or cervical or hilar lymph nodes).
16. Disease caused by *M. tuberculosis*, extrapulmonary (involving at least one site outside the lungs, regardless of whether there is concurrent pulmonary involvement).
17. *Pneumocystis carinii* pneumonia.
18. Progressive multifocal leukoencephalopathy.
19. *Salmonella* (nontyphoid) septicemia, recurrent.
20. Toxoplasmosis of the brain affecting a patient >1 month of age.
21. HIV wasting syndrome (emaciation, "slim disease"): findings of profound involuntary weight loss >10 per cent of baseline body weight plus either chronic diarrhea (at least two loose stools per day for >30 days) or chronic weakness and documented fever (for >30 days, intermittent or constant) in the absence of a concurrent illness other than HIV infection that could explain the findings (e.g., cancer, tuberculosis, cryptosporidiosis, or other specific enteritis).

From Centers for Disease Control: Revision of the case definition for acquired immunodeficiency syndrome. M.M.W.R. 1(Suppl.):1, 1987.

While various zidovudine prophylaxis regimens have been used, 200 mg five or six times daily for 4 to 6 weeks is a generally accepted protocol (Centers for Disease Control, 1990). During all phases of follow-up, confidentiality of the worker and the source should be maintained.

■ TREATMENT AND MANAGEMENT OF HIV-INFECTED INFANTS

From a management perspective, infants seropositive for or infected with HIV are members of a family whose other members are immunocompromised and may soon die (Pizzo, 1990). Infection with HIV has been called a killer of families, not just of the infected children or adults. Thus, good therapy for this disease must begin with multidisciplinary, supportive care (Fig. 35–5). While the physician plays an important role in this care, the needs of these children and families exceed the treatment capacity of a single discipline or individual. Nurses, social workers, physical therapists, educators, internists, infectious disease and neurology specialists, obstetricians, and many other professionals must be involved with the care of these children and families.

As in other areas of pediatrics, aggressive anticipatory care must be provided. Evaluation of the mother's health, family support systems, housing, and care providers for the infant should be carried out before birth. In certain circumstances, legal guardianship or foster care plans should be formalized before birth. Medical care of the infant should also be prevention-oriented. Immunizations should be administered as in Table 35–5 (Centers for Disease Control, 1988b). Killed poliomyelitis vaccine should be used. Exposure to varicella or measles should be treated with varicella zoster immune globulin or immune serum globulin, respectively. Family members should be screened for hepatitis B surface antigen, and HIV-positive children at risk vaccinated (Wong et al.,

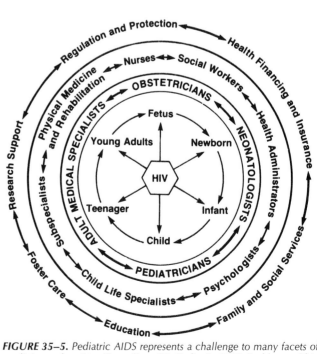

FIGURE 35–5. *Pediatric AIDS represents a challenge to many facets of medicine and society. (From Pizzo PA: Pediatric AIDS: Problems within problems. J. Inf. Dis. 161:315, 1990.)*

TABLE 35–5. Recommendations for Routine Immunization of HIV-Infected Children

VACCINE	HIV INFECTION	
	Known Asymptomatic	Symptomatic
DTP[1]	yes	yes
OPV[2]	no	no
IPV[3]	yes	yes
MMR[4]	yes	yes[5]
HbCV[6]	yes	yes
Pneumococcal	no	yes
Influenza	no	yes

[1]DTP = Diphtheria and tetanus toxoids and pertussis vaccine.
[2]OPV = Oral, attenuated poliovirus vaccine; contains poliovirus types 1, 2, and 3.
[3]IPV = Inactivated poliovirus vaccine; contains poliovirus types 1, 2, and 3.
[4]MMR = Live measles, mumps, and rubella viruses in a combined vaccine.
[5]Should be considered.
[6]HbCV = *Haemophilus influenzae* type B conjugate vaccine.
(From Centers for Disease Control: Recommendations for routine immunization of HIV infected children—United States—1988. M.M.W.R. *37*:181, 1988.)

1984). Suspected infections should be aggressively diagnosed and treated. For example, treatment of severe thrush unresponsive to nystatin should be treated with ketoconazole (5 mg/kg/day) or severe, mucocutaneous herpes infections with oral (400 mg five times per day) or intravenous (5 to 10 mg/kg every 8 hours) acyclovir (Pahwa et al., 1990). Treatment of thrombocytopenia with intravenous immunoglobulin has not produced success comparable to that seen in immune thrombocytopenia (Pizzo, 1990). Steroids have been used with limited success. Prophylactic intravenous immunoglobulin has been recommended by some investigators to increase numbers of inducer T cells, improve in vitro mitogen stimulation responses in peripheral blood mononuclear cells, and restore suppressor T cell function (Calvelli and Rubinstein, 1986). Assessment of the impact of this intervention awaits multicenter, prospective, placebo-controlled trials. Lymphocytic interstitial pneumonia has been treated with steroids (5 mg of prednisone every other day with increased dosages during times of physiologic stress) and/or acyclovir. The latter is used because Ebstein-Barr viral genome has been detected in approximately 75 per cent of the lung biopsies from children with this manifestation of HIV infection. However, evaluation of these and other treatments for lymphocytic interstitial pneumonia is difficult without a better understanding of the natural history and biology of the disease.

Specific antiretroviral chemotherapy offers several attractive treatment advantages (Pizzo, 1990). First, it might be administered antenatally to HIV-positive women to decrease fetal risk of infection. Secondly, treatment might be initiated immediately after birth to decrease further the risk of retroviral replication. Immediate postnatal, prophylactic treatment has proved effective in preventing neonatal hepatitis B infection following in utero or perinatal exposure to hepatitis B virus. Thirdly, phase I and II trials with zidovudine in children have suggested that this drug is effective (especially in children with HIV-induced neurologic disease), safe, and well tolerated (Pizzo, 1990). Zidovudine is a thymidine analogue that inhibits replication of some retroviruses, including HIV, in vitro by inhibiting

the action of reverse transcriptase and possibly by other mechanisms (Yarchoan et al., 1989).

Currently, little is known about effectiveness of antenatal therapy in humans. In several animal models, prevention of fetal infection was achieved (Sharpe et al., 1987; Tavares et al., 1987). These data plus the phase I pharmacokinetic studies in children suggest that intravenous (constant 1 hour infusion at 80, 120, or 160 mg/m^2) or oral administration (120, 180, or 240 mg/m^2) to infants is feasible (Pizzo, 1990). Preliminary data from five infants indicate that after intravenous infusion of 2.0 mg/kg of zidovudine over 1 hour, a terminal half-life of 1.5 hours was observed. Clearance of the drug ranged from 11.4 to 27.1 ml/minute/kg compared with 27.1 ml/minute/kg in adults. The mean bioavailability estimate in fasting infants following an oral dose of zidovudine (2.0 mg/kg) was 69 per cent. The major adverse effects of zidovudine in children and infants have been hematologic in nature. Specifically, a fall in hemoglobin concentration to less than 8 g/dl, a fall in platelet count to <75,000/mm^3, and a fall in neutrophil count to <750 cells/mm^3 were observed. Zidovudine and additional antiretroviral agents, including two other dideoxynucleosides 2′,3′-dideoxycytidine (DDC) and 2′,3′-dideoxyinosine (DDI) may be useful in combination with other immunoenhancing interventions, e.g., intravenous immunoglobulin, human recombinant granulocyte/macrophage colony-stimulating factor (Groopman et al., 1987), or recombinant CD4 antigen, for improved outcomes of HIV-positive infants.

■ CONCLUSION

Fetal and neonatal HIV infection will be a major health problem throughout the 1990s. Careful investigation of these infants will permit identification of improved treatment modalities and enhanced understanding of developmental and genetic immunoregulatory mechanisms. Ultimately, prevention through education of high-risk groups along with palliative and/or curative therapies will permit control of this epidemic.

■ REFERENCES

Albersheim, S. G., Smyth, J. A., Solimano, A., et al.: Passively acquired human immunodeficiency virus seropositivity in a neonate after hepatitis B immunoglobulin. J. Pediatr. 112(6):915, 1988.
American Academy of Pediatrics Task Force on Pediatric AIDS. Perinatal Human Immunodeficiency virus Infection. Pediatrics 82:941, 1988.
Ammann, A. J., Wara, D. W., Dritz, S., et al.: Acquired immunodeficiency in an infant: Possible transmission by means of blood products. Lancet 1:956, 1983.
Bernstein, L. J., Krieger, B. Z., Novick, B., et al.: Bacterial infection in the acquired immunodeficiency syndrome of children. Pediatr. Infect. Dis. 4:472, 1985a.
Bernstein, L. J., Wedgewood, R. J., Ochs, H. D., et al.: Defective humoral immunity in pediatric acquired immune deficiency syndrome. J. Pediatr. 107:352, 1985b.
Blanche, S., Rouzioux, C., Moscato, M-L. G., et al.: A prospective study of infants born to women seropositive for human immunodeficiency virus type 1. N. Engl. J. Med. 320:1643, 1989.
Calvelli, T. A., and Rubinstein, A.: Intravenous gamma-globulin in infant acquired immunodeficiency syndrome. Pediatr. Inf. Dis. 5:S207, 1986.
Centers for Disease Control: Revision of the case definition for acquired immunodeficiency syndrome. 1(Suppl.):1, 1987.
Centers for Disease Control: Prevention of perinatal transmission of hepatitis B virus: Prenatal screening of all pregnant women for hepatitis B surface antigen. M.M.W.R. 37:341, 1988a.

Centers for Disease Control: Recommendations for routine immunization of HIV infected children—United States—1988. *37*:181, 1988b.

Centers for Disease Control: Update: Serologic testing for antibody to human immunodeficiency virus. *36*:833, 1988c.

Centers for Disease Control: Morbidity and Mortality Weekly Report. AIDS and human immunodeficiency virus infection in the United States: 1988 update. *38*(S-4):1, 1989.

Centers for Disease Control: Public health service statement on management of occupational exposure to human immunodeficiency virus, including considerations regarding zidovudine postexposure use. *39*:1, 1990.

Church, J. A., and Isaacs, H.: Transfusion-associated acquired immune deficiency syndrome in infants. J. Pediatr. *105*:731, 1984.

Connor, E., Gupta, S., Joshi, V., et al.: Acquired immunodeficiency syndrome-associated renal disease in children. J. Ped. *113*:39, 1988.

Coombs, R. W., Collier, A. C., Allain, J. P., et al.: Plasma viremia in human immunodeficiency virus infection. N. Engl. J. Med. *320*:1626, 1989.

Cortes, E., Detels, R., Aboulafia, D., et al.: HIV-1, HIV-2, and HTLV-I infection in high-risk groups in Brazil. N. Engl. J. Med. *320*:953, 1989.

Dalgleish, A. G., Beverley, P. C., Clapham, P. R., et al.: The CD4 (T4) antigen is an essential component of the receptor for the AIDS retrovirus. Nature *312*:763, 1984.

Eisenstein, B. I.: Current concepts—the polymerase chain reaction: A new method of using molecular genetics for medical diagnosis. N. Engl. J. Med. *322*:178, 1990.

Fallon, J., Eddy, J., Weiner, L., et al.: Human immunodeficiency virus infection in children. J. Pediatr. *114*:1, 1989.

Frigoletto, F. D., and Little, G. A. (Eds.): Guideline for Perinatal Care. 2nd ed. Elk Grove, Il., American Academy of Pediatrics, 1988.

Gottlieb, M. S., Schroff, R., Schanker, H. M., et al.: *Pneumocystis carinii* pneumonia and mucosal candidiasis in previously healthy homosexual men: Evidence of a new acquired cellular immunodeficiency. N. Engl. J. Med. *305*:1425, 1981.

Groopman, J. E., Mitzuyasu, R. T., DeLeo, M. J., et al.: Effect of recombinant human granulocyte-macrophage colony-stimulating factor on myelopoiesis in the acquired immunodeficiency syndrome. N. Engl. J. Med. *317*:593, 1987.

Guinan, M. E., and Hardy, A.: Epidemiology of AIDS in women in the United States: 1981 through 1986. J.A.M.A. *257*:2039, 1987.

Ho, D. D., Moudgil, T., and Alam, M.: Quantitation of human immunodeficiency virus type 1 in the blood of infected persons. N. Engl. J. Med. *321*:1621, 1989.

Ho, D. D., Pomerantz, R. J., and Kaplan, J. C.: Pathogenesis of infection with human immunodeficiency virus. N. Engl. J. Med. *317*:278, 1987.

Hoff, R., Berardi, V. P., Weiblen, B. J., et al.: Seroprevalence of human immunodeficiency virus among child-bearing women: Estimation by testing samples of blood from newborns. N. Engl. J. Med. *318*:525, 1988.

Imagawa, D. T., Lee, M. H., Wolinsky, S. M., et al.: Human immunodeficiency virus type 1 infection in homosexual men who remain seronegative for prolonged periods. N. Engl. J. Med. *320*:1458, 1989.

Jendis, J. B., Tomasik, Z., Hunziker, J., et al.: Evaluation of diagnostic tests for HIV infection in infants born to HIV-infected mothers in Switzerland. AIDS 1988 *2*:273, 1988.

Katz, B. Z.: Natural history and clinical management of the infant born to a mother infected with human immunodeficiency virus. Semin. Perinatol. *13*:27, 1989.

Katz, S. L., and Wilfert, C. M.: Human immunodeficiency virus infection of newborns. N. Engl. J. Med. *320*:1687, 1989.

Klatzmann, D., Champagne, E., Chamaret, S., et al.: T-Lymphocyte T4 molecule behaves as the receptor for human retrovirus LAV. Nature *312*:767, 1984.

Landesman, S. H.: Human immunodeficiency virus infection in women: An overview. Semin. Perinatol. *13*:2, 1989.

LaPointe, N., Michaud, J., Pekovic, D., et al.: Transplacental transmission of HTLV-III virus. N. Engl. J. Med. *312*:1325, 1985.

Maayan, S., Wormser, G. P., Hewlett, D., et al.: Acquired immunodeficiency syndrome (AIDS) in an economically disadvantaged population. Arch. Intern. Med. *145*:1607, 1985.

McClure, H. M., Anderson, D. C., Fulz, P., et al.: Prophylactic effects of AZT following exposure of Macaques to an acutely lethal variant of SIV. Fifth International Conference on AIDS, June 4–9, 1989, Montreal, Canada (abstract). Veter. Immunol. Immunopath. *21*:13, 1989.

McNamara, J. G.: Immunologic abnormalities in infants infected with human immunodeficiency virus. Semin. Perinatol. *13*:35, 1989.

McNeil, J. G., Brundage, J. F., Wann, Z. F., et al.: Direct measurement of human immunodeficiency virus seroconversions in a serially tested population of young adults in the United States Army, October 1985 to October 1987: N. Engl. J. Med. *320*:1581, 1989.

Mann, D. L., Popovic, M., Murray, C., et al.: Cell surface antigen expression in newborn cord blood lymphocytes infected with HTLV. J. Immunol. *131*:2021, 1983.

Marcus, R.: CDC cooperative needlestick study group. Surveillance of health care workers exposed to blood from patients infected with human immunodeficiency virus. N. Engl. J. Med. *319*:1118, 1988.

Masur, H., Michelis, M. A., Green, J. B., et al.: An outbreak of community acquired *Pneumocystis carinii* pneumonia: An initial manifestation of cellular immune dysfunction. N. Engl. J. Med. *305*:1431, 1981.

Menez-Bautista, R., Fikrig, S. M., Pahwa, S., et al.: Monozygotic twins discordant for the acquired immunodeficiency syndrome. Am. J. Dis. Child. *140*:678, 1986.

Nabel, G., and Baltimore, D.: An inducible transcription factor activates expression of human immunodeficiency virus in T cells. Nature *326*:711, 1987.

Oleske, J., Minneror, A. B., Cooper, B., et al.: Immune deficiency syndrome in children. J.A.M.A. *249*:2345, 1983.

Pahwa, S.: Human immunodeficiency virus infection in children: Nature of immunodeficiency, clinical spectrum and management. Pediatr. Infect. Dis. *7*:S61, 1988.

Pahwa, R., Good, R., and Pahwa, S.: Prematurity, hypogammaglobulinemia, and neuropathy with human immunodeficiency virus (HIV) infection. Proc. Nat. Acad. Sci. U.S.A. *84*:3826, 1987.

Pahwa, S., Chirmule, N., Oyaizu, N.: Clinical and immunologic spectrum of HIV infection in infants and children and disease pathogenesis. Prog. Clin. Biol. Res. *325*:393, 1990.

Pizzo, P. A.: Pediatric AIDs: Problems within problems. J. Infect. Dis. *161*:316, 1990.

Pizzo, P. A., Eddy, J., Falloon, J., et al.: Effect of continuous intravenous infusion of zidovudine (AZT) in children with symptomatic HIV infection. N. Engl. J. Med. *319*:889, 1988.

Popovic, M., Sarngadharan, M. G., Read, E., Gallo, R. C.: Detection, isolation, and continuous production of cytopathic retroviruses (HTLV-III) from patients with AIDS and pre-AIDS. Science *224*:497, 1984.

Quinn, T. C., Zacarias, F. R. K., and St. John, R. K.: AIDS in the Americas: An emerging public health crisis. N. Engl. J. Med. *320*:1005, 1989.

Rhame, F. S., and Maki, D. G.: The case for wider use of testing for HIV infection. N. Engl. J. Med. *320*:1248, 1989.

Rogers, D. E.: Federal spending on AIDS—How much is enough? N. Engl. J. Med. *320*:1623, 1989.

Rogers, M. F., Ou, C. Y., Rayfield, M., et al.: Use of the polymerase chain reaction for early detection of the proviral sequences of human immunodeficiency virus in infants born to seropositive mothers. N. Engl. J. Med. *320*:1649, 1989.

Rubinstein, A.: Pediatric AIDS. Curr. Probl. Pediatr. *16*:361, 1986.

Rubenstein, A., Sicklick, M., Gupta, A., et al.: Acquired immunodeficiency with reversed T4/T8 ratios in infants born to promiscuous and drug addicted mothers. J.A.M.A. *249*:2350, 1983.

Ruprecht, R. M., O'Brien, L. G., Rossoni, L. D., et al.: Suppression of mouse viraemia and retroviral disease by 3′-azido-3′-deoxythymidine. Nature *323*:467, 1986.

Ryder, R. W., Nsa, W., Hassig, S. E., et al.: Perinatal transmission of the human immunodeficiency virus type 1 to infants of seropositive women in Zaire. N. Engl. J. Med. *320*:525, 1989.

Sattentau, Q. J., and Weiss, R. A.: The CD4 antigen: Physiological ligand and HIV receptor. Cell *52*:631, 1988.

Saulsbury, F. T., Wykoff, R. F., and Boyle, R. J.: Transfusion-acquired human immunodeficiency virus infection in twelve neonates: Epidemiologic, clinical and immunologic features. Pediatr. Infect. Dis. *6*:544, 1987.

Shannon, K., Ball, E., Wasserman, R. L., et al.: Transfusion-associated cytomegalovirus infection and acquired immune deficiency syndrome in an infant. J. Pediatr. *103*:859, 1983.

Sharpe, A. H., Jaenisch, R., and Ruprecht, R. M.: Retroviruses and mouse embryos: A rapid model for neurovirulence and transplacental antiviral therapy. Science *236*:1671, 1987.

Siegal, F. P., Lopez, C., Hammer, G. S., et al.: Severe acquired immunodeficiency in male homosexuals, manifested by chronic perianal ulcerative herpes simplex lesions. N. Engl. J. Med. *305*:1439, 1981.

Tavares, L., Roneker, C., Johnston, K., et al.: 3′-azido-3′-deoxythymidine in feline leukemia virus infected cats: A model for therapy and prophylaxis of AIDS. Cancer Res. *47*:3190, 1987.

Thomas, P. A., Lubin, K., Milberg, J., et al.: Cohort comparison study of children whose mothers have acquired immunodeficiency syndrome and children of well inner city mothers. Pediatr. Infect. Dis. *6*:247, 1987.

Weiss, R., and Thier, S. O.: HIV testing is the answer—what's the question? N. Engl. J. Med. *319*:1010, 1988.

Winkenwerder, W., Kessler, A. R., and Stolec, R. M.: Federal spending for illness caused by the human immunodeficiency virus. N. Engl. J. Med. *320*:1598, 1989.

Wong, V. C., Reesink, H. W. Reerink-Brongers, E. F., et al.: Prevention of the HBsAg carrier state in newborn infants of mothers who are chronic carriers of HBsAg by administration of hepatitis-B vaccine and hepatitis-B immunoglobulin. Lancet *1*:921, 1984.

Yarchoan, R., Mitsuya, H., Myers, C., et al.: Clinical pharmacology A²3¹-azido-2¹,3¹-dideoxythymidine (Zidovudine) and related dideoxynucleosides. N. Engl. J. Med. *321*:726, 1989.

VIRAL INFECTIONS OF THE FETUS AND NEWBORN

36

F. Sessions Cole

The infant who is born with an infection acquired transplacentally during the first, second, or early third trimester may have what is termed "congenital infection." Although in rare instances these infections are due to herpes simplex virus, varicella-zoster virus, *Mycobacterium tuberculosis,* and *Listeria monocytogenes,* the most common causes are rubella virus, cytomegalovirus (CMV), *Toxoplasma gondii, Treponema pallidum,* human immunodeficiency virus (HIV), human parvovirus B19, and Epstein-Barr virus (EBV) (Kinney and Kumar, 1988). The first four organisms are the so-called and somewhat misnamed "TORCH" group. The confusion generated by this acronym arises because "H," or herpes simplex, so rarely belongs to the group and because syphilis and other infections are omitted. Because of the increasing frequency and interest in HIV, parvovirus, and EBV, Kinney and Kumar (1988) have recommended their inclusion in the "other" category of TORCH infections. Certain other organisms may cause intrauterine infection but are usually transmitted just before delivery. This pattern is characteristic of herpes simplex virus, enteroviruses, group B streptococci, *Listeria,* and others, but these intrauterine infections differ little from those caused by the same organisms when acquired either just after delivery or during the 1st week or so of extrauterine life. For this reason, they are usually classified as "perinatal" rather than "congenital" infections.

Despite the extraordinary biologic heterogeneity of the four TORCH organisms responsible for congenital infections, the syndromes they produce are remarkably similar. The literature was carefully reviewed by Kinney and Kumar in 1988 and Alpert and Plotkin in 1986 (Tables 36–1 and 36–2). The most common manifestations include hepatomegaly, splenomegaly, pneumonia, bone lesions, and anemia. Differentiating features of individual infections are discussed below.

The rational approach to the diagnosis of congenital infection includes information on the biology, epidemiology, and disease manifestations of each infection. Once the suspicion is raised, therefore, the differences rather than similarities among these diseases should be the object of our own analysis.

Diagnostic Approach. Because the incidence of congenital infection in the fetus and newborn infant is high (0.5 to 2.5 per cent) (Alpert and Plotkin, 1986), and a significant number of congenitally infected infants are asymptomatic, a high index of suspicion plus a sensitive, specific, and cost-effective approach to diagnosis is used. Evaluation begins with complete family and maternal history, including information on birth weights and medical problems of siblings, drug utilization, sexual orientation of sexual partners, maternal travel history, and blood transfusion history. Common neonatal clinical features associated with congenital infection are listed in Table 36–3. No data are currently available to determine whether isolated findings or combinations of signs should prompt further evaluation. For example, whether the children born with a birth weight less than the third percentile for

TABLE 36–1. Incidence of Maternal and Fetal Infections Due to Selected Organisms

MICROORGANISM	MOTHER (PER 1000 PREGNANCIES)	FETUS (PER 1000 LIVE BIRTHS)
Cytomegalovirus	40 to 150	5 to 25
Rubella		
Epidemic	20 to 40	4 to 30
Interepidemic	0.1	0.5
Toxoplasma gondii	1.5 to 6.4	0.5 to 1
Herpes simplex	10 to 15	Rare
Treponema pallidum	0.2	0.1

(From Alpert, G., and Plotkin, S. A.: A practical guide to the diagnosis of congenital infections in the newborn infant. Pediatr. Clin. North Am. *33:*465, 1986.)

TABLE 36–2. Clinical Findings in Congenitally Infected Infants that Suggest a Specific Diagnosis

CONGENITAL		FINDINGS
Rubella	Eye:	cataracts, cloudy cornea, pigmented retina
	Skin:	"blueberry muffin" syndrome
	Bone:	vertical striation
	Heart:	malformation (ductus, pulmonary artery stenosis)
CMV		Microcephaly with periventricular calcifications; inguinal hernias in males; petechiae with thrombocytopenia
Toxoplasmosis		Hydrocephalus with generalized calcifications; chorioretinitis
Syphilis		Osteochondritis and periostitis, eczematoid skin rash, mucocutaneous lesions (snuffles)
Herpes		Skin vesicles, keratoconjunctivitis; acute central nervous system findings

(Modified from Stagno, S., Pass, R. F., and Alford, C. A.: Perinatal infections and maldevelopment. *In* Bloom, A. D., and James, L. S. [Eds.]: The Fetus and the Newborn. Vol. 17, Series 1. New York, Alan R. Liss, Inc., 1981. Copyright © 1981, Alan R. Liss, Inc. Reprinted by permission of Wiley-Liss, a division of John Wiley and Sons, Inc.)

331

TABLE 36–3. Common Neonatal Clinical Features Associated with TORCH Agents

Growth retardation (hydrocephalus)
Hepatosplenomegaly
Jaundice (greater than 20% direct reacting)
Hemolytic anemia
Petechiae and ecchymoses
Microcephaly and hydrocephaly
Intracranial calcification
Pneumonitis
Myocarditis
Cardiac abnormalities (especially peripheral pulmonic
  stenosis [Rubella])
Chorioretinitis
Keratoconjunctivitis
Cataracts
Glaucoma
Nonimmune hydrops

(From Kinney, J. S., and Kumar, M. L.: Should we expand the TORCH complex? Clin. Perinatol. 15:727, 1988.)

gestational age (small for gestational age [SGA]) without other signs should be evaluated is unclear. Studies from Sweden and Canada suggest that isolated growth retardation is not associated with congenital infection, but these studies had some methodological flaws (Andersson et al., 1981; Primhak and Simpson, 1982). However, growth retardation has been described as the only manifestation of congenital infection with CMV, rubella, and toxoplasmosis (Alpert and Plotkin, 1986). The clinician must rely on the history and the physical examination to identify infants for further evaluation.

If an infant is suspected of having a congenital infection, the infection may be confirmed through total cord IgM determination, although its efficacy is the subject of debate (Alpert and Plotkin, 1986; Kinney and Kumar, 1988). Approximately 4 per cent of newborn infants have elevated(>18 to 20 mg/dl) IgM in cord blood (Kinney and Kumar, 1988). Alford and associates (1969) showed that 42 of 123 infants with elevated IgM (> 19.5 mg/dl) had identifiable infections. Although a normal IgM does not exclude perinatal or congenital infection, an elevated cord blood level of total IgM provides an indication for pursuing further diagnostic studies in the context of an unclear clinical picture. The nonspecific and specific diagnostic tests are outlined in Table 36–4. Establishment of the specific agent is important for prognostic evaluation and for possible treatment. An approach to the laboratory diagnosis is outlined in Figure 36–1. It is important to remember that serologic tests not specific for IgM antibody require maternal serum for interpretation.

■ CONGENITAL RUBELLA

Since 1941, when Gregg first made the association of maternal rubella and cataracts in infants, physicians have been aware of the teratogenicity of the rubella virus. Not until the epidemic of 1964 and 1965 in North America, however, were the multiple manifestations of the rubella syndrome fully appreciated and the later consequences well delineated. Since that time, the capacity to grow the virus in tissue culture has led rapidly to the development of vaccines and a reduction in incidence of congenital disease, at least in the United States. Availability of vaccine has lowered the reported cases of congenital rubella

syndrome in the United States to only 3 in 1989 (MMWR, 1990). In other parts of the world, unfortunately, the disease retains more than merely historic interest.

Etiology. Maternal rubella infection that occurs within a month before conception and through the second trimester may be associated with disease in the infant. The classic findings of congenital rubella predominate when the onset of maternal infection occurs during the first 8 weeks of gestation. Cataracts occur with maternal rubella before the 60th day after the 1st day of the last menstrual period; heart disease is found almost exclusively when maternal infection is before the 80th day (i.e., first trimester). Deafness, the most common manifestation, occurs, along with retinopathy as a consequence of both first and second trimester maternal infections (Ueda et al., 1979). The incidence of congenital rubella defects following maternal rubella varies widely between series but is probably from 15 to 25 per cent throughout the first trimester, 5 to 7 per cent in the 4th month, and 1 to 2 per cent in the 5th month. The infant may excrete the virus for many months after birth despite the pressure of neutralizing antibody and, thus, pose a hazard to susceptible individuals in the environment. Only rarely can the virus be recovered by 1 year of age. An exception to this rule is the cataract, in which the virus may remain for as long as 3 years.

Diagnosis. The infected infants are usually born at term but are of low birth weight. They may show only a few manifestations of the disease, such as glaucoma or cataracts, or they may have a systemic illness characterized by purpuric lesions, hepatosplenomegaly, cardiac defects, pneumonia, and meningoencephalitis. Table 36–5 outlines the salient findings. The skin lesions have been described as resembling a "blueberry muffin." These

TABLE 36–4. Diagnostic Approach to the Newborn Suspected of Being Congenitally Infected

NONSPECIFIC TESTS	SPECIFIC TESTS
Complete blood and platelet counts	Viral culture*
Lumbar puncture	Oropharynx, urine, rectum
Roentgenogram of long bones	Blood for HIV
Computed tomography scan of head	Optional: cerebrospinal fluid, conjunctiva
Ophthalmologic evaluation	Smears of skin lesions:
Audiologic evaluation	FA stain
	Dark-field examination
	Tzanck smear
	Serology
	Rubella: HAI, PHA, LA or Elisa screen for IgG antibody
	Toxoplasma: SF or IFA for IgG antibody
	Syphilis: VDRL or RPR
	Hepatitis B: HB$_s$Ag test
	Polymerase chain reaction: HIV test
	ELISA or Western blot: HIV test

*African green monkey kidney cell line must be inoculated.

HAI = hemagglutination inhibition; PHA = passive hemagglutination; LA = latex agglutination; SF = Sabin-Feldman dye test; IFA = immunofluorescence test; FA = fluorescent antibody.

(From Alpert, G., and Plotkin, S. A.: A practical guide to the diagnosis of congenital infections in the newborn infant. Pediatr. Clin. North Am. 33:465, 1986.)

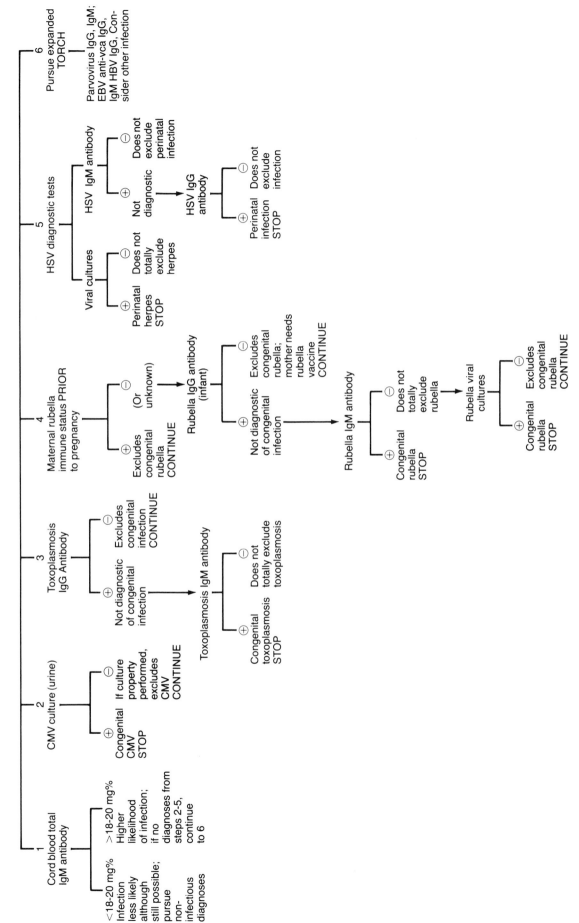

FIGURE 36–1. An approach to the laboratory diagnosis of suspected TORCH infection in the newborn. (From Kinney, J. S., and Kumar, M. L.: Should we expand the TORCH complex? Clin. Perinatol. 15:727, 1988.)

TABLE 36–5. Clinical Findings in 81 Infants with Congenital Rubella Syndrome

	GROUP 1: EXPANDED RUBELLA SYNDROME	GROUP 2: CLASSIC RUBELLA SYNDROME	GROUP 3: HISTORY OF MATERNAL RUBELLA, PRESUMABLY NORMAL BABY
Number of Infants	34	37	10
Sex { Male	26	23	7
Sex { Female	8	14	3
Mean gestational age (weeks)	40.1	39.8	39.8
Mean birth weight (g)	2178	2533	3327
Purpura	78%	0	0
Thrombocytopenia (<140,000)	100%	0	0
Hepatomegaly	85%	81%	20%
Splenomegaly	76%	62%	10%
Cardiac defects	78%	86%	0
Eye defects	41%	54%	0
Full fontanel	69%	43%	0
Positive virus isolation	66%	25%	50%
Mortality	32%	8%	0

(From Rudolph, A. J., et al.: Osseous manifestations of congenital rubella syndrome. Am. J. Dis. Child. *110*:416, 1965. Copyright 1965, American Medical Association.)

represent extramedullary hematopoietic tissue within the skin (Brough et al., 1967). Thrombocytopenia is commonly seen (Cooper et al., 1965). Osseous lesions include a large anterior fontanel and striking lesions in the long bones. Linear areas of radiolucency and increased density are found in the metaphyses. The provisional zones of calcification are also irregular. The changes in rubella are not pathognomonic of the disease but resemble those of other congenital infections, such as cytomegalic inclusion disease.

The cardiac lesions include patent ductus arteriosus, septal defects, and stenosis of the peripheral pulmonary arteries. In one recent study of 18 patients with simple pulmonary artery stenosis, an association with rubella was found in 11 (Hodgson and Morgan-Capner, 1984). Myocardial necrosis has been observed (Cooper et al., 1969).

Among the manifestations that may occur after the newborn period (late-onset disease) are a generalized rash with seborrheic features that may persist for weeks, interstitial pneumonia (either acute or chronic) such as described by Phelan and Campbell (1969), defective hearing from involvement of the organ of Corti, central auditory imperception, or even complete autism. Infants with late-onset disease sometimes have immunologic abnormalities, with elevated total IgM and depressed total IgG (Soothill et al., 1966). The principal immunologic perturbation in late-onset disease may be defective cytotoxic effector cell function that leads to defective virus elimination and immune complex disease (Verder et al., 1986). These patients may be susceptible to infection with unusual organisms such as *Pneumocystis carinii* or to development of histiocytosis (Claman et al., 1970).

Longitudinal studies of somatic growth reveal that most infants remain smaller than average throughout infancy but grow at a normal rate. Stunting of growth was more common after rubella in the first 8 weeks of pregnancy than after later infection. A higher than expected incidence of diabetes mellitus has been reported after congenital rubella.

Laboratory Findings. The laboratory diagnosis of con-

genital rubella must be made during the 1st year of life, unless one is fortunate enough to recover virus from an affected site such as the lens after that time. Both serology and virus isolation may be helpful. If IgM antirubella titers are elevated at birth or shortly thereafter or if IgG antirubella titers remain high during the first year, the diagnosis of intrauterine infection is ensured (Alpert and Plotkin, 1986). Antirubella IgM can be determined with one of several immunofluorescence or enzyme immunoassays (Alpert and Plotkin, 1986). It is important to note that not all congenitally infected infants have detectable IgM antirubella antibody in the 1st month of life (Alpert and Plotkin, 1986). If suspicion is high, repeat serology examination and culture should be performed.

The virus is most often isolated from throat swabs but may also be found in the spinal fluid or urine. In late-onset disease, the virus is found in affected skin and lung.

Treatment. There is no specific therapy for congenital rubella. The infant may need a blood transfusion for anemia or active bleeding and general supportive measures. The best therapy is to ensure that women who are considering pregnancy are immune to rubella. Vaccination of nonimmune women during the postpartum period has become an established medical practice, although prolonged polyarticular arthritis; acute neurologic sequelae, including carpal tunnel syndrome and multiple paresthesias; and chronic rubella viremia have been reported in these women (Tingle et al., 1985).

The problem of management of the pregnant woman who is exposed to or who contracts the disease should be resolved after weighing the known risks. If, at the time of exposure, serum antibody is detectable, the fetus probably is protected completely. If the level is either undetectable or borderline, then a large dose of immune serum globulin (0.3 to 0.4 ml/kg) is advised, although the protective effect of this maneuver is questionable. Decisions about the interruption of pregnancy must be made only after maternal infection has been proved. A rise in antibody must be measured in two or more sera in the same laboratory on the same day; test variation may account for apparent antibody "rises" measured on different days.

Decisions concerning elective termination of pregnancy should also take into account the risk of rubella-associated damage to the fetus. This is highest when maternal infection occurs during the first 8 weeks of pregnancy.

Prognosis. The consequences of fetal rubella infection may not be evident at birth but instead may become apparent in subsequent months. Hardy and co-workers (1966) followed 123 infants with documented congenital rubella and found that 85 per cent of them were not clinically suspect until after discharge from the nursery. Communication disorders, hearing defects, some mental or motor retardation, and microcephaly by 1 to 3 years of age were among the major problems that were discovered after the newborn period. A predisposition to inguinal hernias was also noted.

It is important to note that, even in the absence of mental retardation, neuromuscular development is frequently abnormal. Desmond and co-workers (1978) followed 29 children in this category and found that 25 of them were abnormal. Hearing loss, difficulties with balance and gait, learning deficits, and behavioral disturbances were found in more than one half the affected children.

Weil and co-workers (1975) described an alarming report of chronic progressive panencephalitis with onset at age 11 years in a child who had congenital rubella. The patient was small for his age, with sensorineural hearing loss of 60 decibels at age 4 years. At age 11 years, he had the insidious onset of motor incoordination, ataxia, and myoclonic jerks, with progressive deterioration. Although this complication of congenital rubella must be rare, it emphasizes that the cause of subacute sclerosing panencephalitis need not be restricted to the measles virus.

Prevention. Live attenuated rubella virus vaccine is now available, safe, and effective (Lepow et al., 1968), although the duration of immunity is uncertain. Given as a single subcutaneous injection, it is recommended for children between ages 15 months of age and puberty and for women of childbearing age with negative findings on both a hemagglutination inhibition antibody test and a pregnancy test. It should be given only if the physician is assured that there is no likelihood of pregnancy for the next two months, because of the potential hazard to the fetus.

Fortunately, follow-up studies of a large number of women inadvertently immunized during or just before pregnancy have indicated that although the fetus is sometimes infected there appear to be no or, at most, very rare adverse consequences (Hayden et al., 1980; MMWR, 1989). Despite this, it appears advisable to administer vaccine only in the immediate postpartum period or when pregnancy can be avoided. A mild rubella-like illness is sometimes seen after immunization, with arthralgia occurring 10 days to 3 weeks after injection. Immunization in the postpartum period has infrequently led to polyarticular arthritis, neurologic symptoms, and chronic rubella viremia (Tingle et al., 1985).

■ CYTOMEGALOVIRUS

Although all aspects of CMV infections in utero and in the newborn period are not known at present, much has been learned about this ubiquitous and often confusing virus since its first cultivation in vitro in 1955 and since the recognition that it caused the devastating syndrome called *cytomegalic inclusion disease* (Weller, 1971; Weller and Macauley, 1957). CMV infection at any age is usually asymptomatic. After a period of active replication, the virus usually becomes latent but retains the capability of reactivation under special circumstances. Such reactivation appears to occur frequently during pregnancy.

The fetus can be infected by either a newly acquired maternal infection (Davis et al., 1971) or a reactivated maternal infection (Stagno et al., 1982). The newly acquired maternal infection, although less common than the reactivated maternal infection, appears to carry a much higher risk of severe disease in the fetus. Indeed, in reactivated infections, newborns are normal on examination, and if defects appear, they do not apparently do so until some time later in childhood. At the present time, however, follow-up studies of congenitally infected infants whose mothers were proved to be antibody positive before

pregnancy are incomplete, and the prognosis of such infections, although clearly better than that of primary infections, is uncertain.

A newborn infant without congenital infection can be infected by his or her mother at the time of delivery, through breast milk, by acquisition from the nursery or home environment, or by transfusion of blood from a donor who is antibody positive (i.e., latently infected). Perinatal or postnatal acquisition from the mother appears to be entirely benign and very common. Postnatal acquisition from the environment is probably less common and may be benign, although lower respiratory illness may occur under these circumstances (Stagno et al., 1981). Acquisition from blood transfusion often results in severe, sometimes fatal, generalized disease in a setting in which maternal antibody is lacking (Yeager et al., 1981). Although neonatal intensive care units in the United States are providing CMV-negative blood for transfusion, antibody-negative women who require transfusion during pregnancy should also be considered for transfusion with CMV-negative blood (Onorato et al., 1985).

Incidence. Approximately 33,000 infants are born with congenital CMV infection annually in the United States (Stagno and Whitley, 1985). Twenty to thirty per cent of congenitally infected infants die, and more than 90 per cent have late complications (Stagno and Whitley, 1985), the most important of which is sensorineural hearing loss. Approximately 90 per cent of congenitally infected infants are asymptomatic at birth (Kinney et al., 1985). Characteristics of CMV infection in pregnancy are given in Figure 36–2. The proportion of children and adults with detectable CMV antibody varies with age, geographic location, and socioeconomic status. In the United States, about 60 per cent of adult women have complement-fixing antibody. The incidence of excretion in the cervix or urine appears to rise during pregnancy from 3 per cent in the first trimester to as much as 12 per cent at term, although such findings are extremely variable. The overall incidence of congenital infection is 1.0 to 1.5 per cent of live births (Starr et al., 1970). It is higher than this (3.4 per cent) among babies of mothers who were antibody positive before pregnancy (Stagno et al., 1977), a finding that implies either that most intrauterine infections result from reactivated maternal infections or that primary infections with different serotypes can occur in sequential pregnancies. Indeed, two babies infected in sequential pregnancies from a single mother were found to be excreting viruses that were identical by restriction endonuclease mapping (Stagno et al., 1977). The first of these infants had severe cytomegalic inclusion disease; the second, although excreting virus at birth, was clinically normal. Accumulating evidence suggests that a primary maternal CMV infection is more likely to cause congenital infection than a recurrent infection (Stagno et al., 1982).

The incidence of neonatal and postnatal infection is still higher than that of intrauterine infection. Approximately half the babies of mothers excreting virus at term acquire infection in the first weeks of life (Reynolds et al., 1973). Many of these babies are infected through breast milk (Hayes et al., 1972). None, apparently, is affected adversely by the infection. All infants, regardless of the route of infection, excrete virus for a prolonged period, usually 1 year or more (Emanuel and Kenny, 1966).

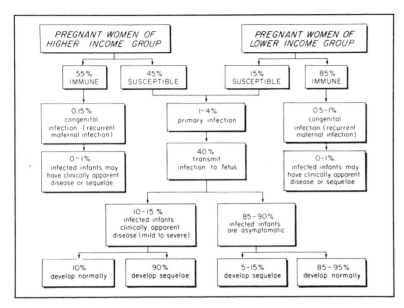

FIGURE 36–2. Characteristics of cytomegalovirus infection in pregnancy. (From Stagno, S., and Whitley, R. T.: Herpesvirus infections of pregnancy. Part I: Cytomegalovirus and Epstein-Barr virus infections. N. Engl. J. Med., 313:1270, 1985. Reprinted by permission of the New England Journal of Medicine.)

Although nosocomial infant-to-infant transmission of CMV has been reported, it most likely occurs infrequently (Spector, 1983; Adler et al., 1986; Yeager et al., 1983). However, nosocomial acquisition does occur: McCracken and associates (1969) first reported the association between exchange blood transfusion and symptomatic CMV infection in the neonatal intensive care unit, and in the same year, King-Lewis and Gardner reported primary CMV disease following intrauterine transfusion. Luthardt and co-workers (1971) first suggested the connection between seropositive blood used for exchange transfusion and CMV acquisition by CMV seronegative recipients. These authors also suggested that such infections could be prevented by selection of CMV seronegative donors. Yeager and co-workers (1972) first pointed out the connection between blood transfusions and acquired CMV infection in newborn infants. Subsequently, Yeager and colleagues (1981) found that exclusive use of CMV seronegative blood eliminated CMV infection in seronegative infants. These observations were confirmed by other investigators (Adler, 1986). Frozen deglycerolized red blood cells may provide an alternative to blood taken from CMV seronegative donors but appears not as effective in preventing CMV acquisition as blood from seronegative donors (Adler, 1986). Another useful approach is the use of filtration to remove leukocytes, the site of latent CMV infection. Although the frequency of postnatal transfusion-acquired CMV has decreased with use of CMV-negative donors, a high index of suspicion must be maintained when multiply transfused infants develop pneumonia, hepatosplenomegaly, leukopenia and thrombocytopenia, and abnormal findings on liver function tests after 6 to 8 weeks of age.

Etiology. CMV is a member of the herpes virus family and has the largest DNA genome of any known virus (Adler, 1986). Although all strains are serologically related, there appear to be some variations in antigenicity, and it is not clear at present whether this heterogeneity affects the incidence of exogenous reinfections. The virus differs from herpes simplex and varicella viruses in that it lacks

the enzyme thymidine kinase. This renders it resistant to those antiviral agents that depend on this enzyme for their action, such as acyclovir.

As with rubella, it seems likely that the virus first infects the placenta and then the fetus and that the placenta functions as a relative barrier in this sequence.

Pathology. Characteristic multinuclear giant cells with both cytoplasmic and intranuclear inclusion bodies are found in many organs. Liver, lungs, brain, pancreas, and kidneys contain them in large numbers. Mononuclear cell infiltration and diffuse fibrosis may be intense. The brain contains areas of necrosis, often subependymal and periventricular, and glial overgrowth, containing heavy deposits of calcium. Petechiae and larger hemorrhages involve skin and serous surfaces.

Diagnosis. Infants infected with the virus are often prematurely delivered. In the classic form of the infection, cytomegalic inclusion disease, newborn infants have acute progressive disseminated disease. They show petechiae and ecchymoses and are jaundiced at birth, or jaundice appears within a few hours and becomes intense. The liver and spleen are enlarged and firm from the start and may increase in size for a number of days. Skull radiographs usually demonstrate periventricular calcifications. Fever as high as 39° C (102° to 103° F) may be found. Tachypnea and moderate dyspnea suggesting pulmonary involvement may appear. Pallor may or may not be striking. Puncture wounds bleed for many minutes, and hemorrhage from internal organs may cause death.

It is clear from prospective studies that most infants with congenital CMV infections are asymptomatic at birth and that milder manifestations of infections are more common than the aforementioned classic syndrome. A chart describing the frequency of various clinical findings in 34 infants who were symptomatic by 2 weeks of age is shown in Table 36–6 (Pass et al., 1980). Petechiae, hepatosplenomegaly, and jaundice were the most common signs at this age. Ten of the thirty-four infants died of their disease, most of them before 3 months of age,

TABLE 36–6. Newborn Clinical Findings in 34 Patients with Congenital CMV Infection, All of Whom Were Symptomatic by 2 Weeks of Age

ABNORMALITY	POSITIVE/TOTAL EXAMINED (%)	
Petechiae	27/34	(79)
Hepatosplenomegaly	25/34	(74)
Jaundice	20/32	(63)
Microcephaly*	17/34	(50)
Small for gestational age†	14/34	(41)
Prematurity‡	11/32	(34)
Inguinal hernia	5/19§	(26)
Chorioretinitis	4/34	(12)

*Less than tenth percentile based upon Colorado Intrauterine Growth Charts, for premature newborns (Lubchenco et al.) or more than 2 SD below mean for term babies based upon data of Nellhaus.
†Weight less than tenth percentile for gestational age.
‡Gestational age less than 38 weeks.
§Boys.

(From Pass, R. F., et al.: Outcome of symptomatic congenital cytomegalovirus infection: Results of long-term longitudinal follow-up. Pediatrics 66:758, 1980. Reproduced by permission of Pediatrics.)

and all primarily because of severe neurologic impairment. Although microcephaly was seen in only half the infants at birth, a number of additional children became microcephalic as they grew older. Still others developed hearing or visual impairment, so that the proportion of surviving infants with sensorineural handicaps was increased to 91 per cent at the time the study was performed.

Uncommon findings at birth are cardiac defects and a number of gastrointestinal malformations. None of these has been systematically associated with CMV infection, however. Musculoskeletal abnormalities also occur, with indirect inguinal hernia being the most common.

Laboratory Investigations. The laboratory diagnosis of congenital CMV infection can be made with absolute certainty only through detection of the virus in organs or culture specimens at birth or within the first 3 weeks of life. The most sensitive detection system is growth of the virus from urine in tissue culture (Kinney and Kumar, 1988). Serologic tests are often difficult to interpret, because at the time of delivery, 50 to 75 per cent of women have anti-CMV IgG, which is transplacentally transmitted to the infant, and even serial antibody titers cannot differentiate between congenital infection and perinatally acquired infection. No reliable CMV IgM assay is currently available (Kinney and Kumar, 1988). Molecular probes may permit rapid and specific diagnosis in the future (Chou and Merigan, 1983; Schrier et al., 1985). Careful consideration should be given to obtaining urine CMV cultures immediately after birth from those infants likely to receive blood transfusions or those who are at risk for enhanced immunosusceptibility. Such cultures would permit identification of infants who are congenitally infected and those who are postnatally infected.

A presumptive diagnosis may sometimes be made after several months of age if virus is found and the clinical syndrome is classic. Other causes of congenital infection must, of course, be ruled out, since there is such extensive overlap in the symptoms of several types of infections.

The principal types of abnormalities found on laboratory tests in infants with symptomatic CMV infection at birth are shown in Table 36–7. In addition to those

features shown in this table, anemia (usually hemolytic) is common.

The urine usually contains bile but no urobilin. Albumin is commonly present, as are some red and white blood cells. Sediment that has been dried, fixed, and stained with hematoxylin and eosin often demonstrates the characteristic inclusion bodies within desquamated renal epithelial cells (Fig. 36–3), so-called "owl's eye cells." Virus may be cultivated from the urine for an extended length of time.

Treatment. Attempts to treat CMV infection with idoxuridine, cytosine arabinoside, adenine arabinoside, and interferon inducers have failed. Transient reduction in the titer of virus excretion in the urine may be seen, but no clinical benefit has been detected. Corticosteroids and cytotoxic agents have been used without success. Transfusion is indicated for anemia. Trials are underway to examine the potential efficacy of gancyclovir (9-[2-hydroxy-1-(hydroxymethyl)ethoxymethyl]guanine), an acyclic nucleoside structurally related to acyclovir but with increased potency against CMV in vitro (Shepp et al., 1985). In addition, alpha interferon (Hirsch et al., 1983) and CMV immune globulin (Bowden et al., 1988) are currently being studied.

Prognosis. Of infants who are symptomatic at birth, approximately 25 per cent die within the first 3 months (Pass et al., 1980; Weller and Hanshaw, 1962). Of the remainder, 60 to 75 per cent have intellectual or developmental impairment (Berenberg and Nankervis, 1970), about one third have hearing loss, one third have neuromuscular disorders (spasticity or seizures), and a smaller proportion have visual impairment due to chorioretinitis. Only 10 to 25 per cent are normal late in childhood, and those who demonstrated minimal abnormalities at birth have the greatest chance of being normal at long-term follow-up.

The fate of the congenitally infected infant who was normal at birth is still not entirely clear. Two published series (Hanshaw et al., 1976; Reynolds et al., 1974)

TABLE 36–7. Laboratory Abnormalities in Newborns with Symptomatic Congenital CMV Infection

TEST	ABNORMAL/TOTAL EXAMINED (%)
Increased cord serum IgM (>20 mg/100 ml); range, 22–170	21/25 (84)
Atypical lymphocytosis (≥5%)*; range, 5%–42%	8/10 (80)
Elevated SGOT (>80 μU/ml)*; range, 85–495	14/18 (79)
Thrombocytopenia (<100,000 platelets/mm³)†; range, 3000–66,000	17/28 (61)
Conjugated hyperbilirubinemia (direct serum bilirubin >2 mg/100 ml)†; range, 3–21	19‡/31 (61)
Increased CSF protein (>120 mg/100 ml)†; range, 130–198	9/19 (47)

*Determinations during first month of life.
†Determinations during first week of life.
‡One patient with jaundice had a maximum direct bilirubin of 1.2 mg/100 ml but was icteric within 24 hours of birth.

(From Pass, R. F., et al.: Outcome of symptomatic congenital cytomegalovirus infection: Results of long-term longitudinal follow-up. Pediatrics 66:758, 1980. Reproduced by permission of Pediatrics.)

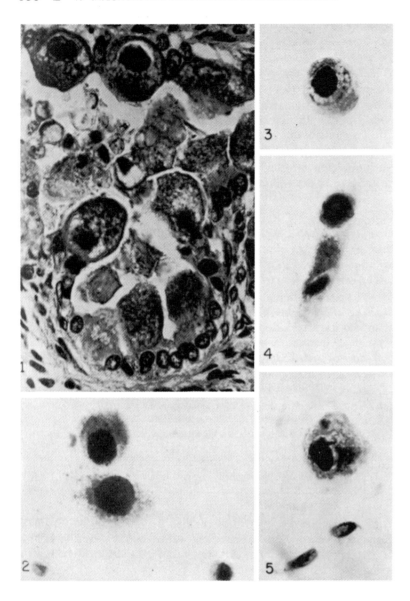

FIGURE 36–3. *1, Renal tubule from a patient who died with cytomegalic inclusion disease. Note the intranuclear and intracytoplasmic inclusion bodies, with associated degeneration and desquamation of cells. Some of the necrotic cells appear as large masses of cytoplasm. 2, 3, 4, Various types of cytomegalic cells observed in the urinary sediment from this infant. The shape of the cell in 3 suggests that it originated in the lower part of the collecting tubules or in the pelvis. In 4, note the two small desquamated cells whose size corresponds to that of normal tubular cells. 5, Cytomegalic cell and two normal cells from the gastric mucosa, observed in the sediment from a gastric washing. Hematoxylin and eosin, × 782. (From Blanc, W. A.: Am. J. Clin. Pathol. 28:46, 1957.)*

indicate variable risks of deafness and reduction of I.Q. scores. In both instances, however, the case finding method was measurement of cord IgM level; an increase in this value might be found only in more severely affected infants (possibly reflecting primary infection in the mother). In one other follow-up study (Kumar et al., 1973), the children were found to be normal at 4 years, but audiometric screening was not performed.

■ ENTEROVIRUS DISEASES

The enteroviruses of humans include polioviruses, coxsackieviruses A and B, and the echoviruses. Fortunately, poliovirus infection of newborn infants is now rare. According to early accounts, however, infants infected in the perinatal period developed severe, often fatal diseases, with a high incidence of paralysis occurring in the survivors. Readers are referred to the review by Bates (1955) and to the chapter by Cherry (1990) for further information.

Since Coxsackie A virus infections have been described only rarely, we limit this review to a consideration of only those diseases associated with Coxsackie B virus and echoviruses.

Incidence. All enterovirus infections are seasonal, occurring most frequently during the late summer and early autumn in temperate climates. The incidence varies from year to year, with outbreaks sometimes caused by a single Coxsackie or echo serotype and sometimes by several. Disease in newborn infants is uncommon but reflects the frequency of infections in the population at large (Krajden and Middleton, 1983). It seems likely that severe disease in infants is seen with a frequency equal to or greater than that of perinatal herpes virus infection.

Etiology. It appears that any of the nonpolio enteroviruses can cause disease in the newborn infant. In a recent retrospective chart review of 24 newborn infant enteroviral infections in Toronto, ten infants died, 12 had aseptic meningitis, and five had myocarditis (Krajden and Middleton, 1983). Of the 24 isolates, seven were echovirus, 15 were Coxsackie B virus, one was Coxsackie A virus, and one was nontypable. Types of Coxsackie B virus are associated primarily with myocarditis and aseptic meningitis or combinations of the two (Kibrick and Benirschke, 1958). Echoviruses, however, are seen more often with severe nonspecific febrile illnesses with disseminated intravascular coagulation (Nagington et al., 1978), aseptic meningitis (Cramblett et al., 1973; Linnemann et al., 1974), or hepatitis (Modlin, 1980). With both groups of viruses, nonspecific febrile illnesses, with or without the presence of a rash, are commonly seen.

Infection takes place either just before or just after birth. Because infected infants have been delivered by cesarean section with intact membranes, it seems likely that transplacental infection has occurred. Regardless of whether the mother, a family member, or some other caretaker is the source of the infection, severe disease may result when the baby lacks antibody to the infecting strain. It is not clear at present why the newborn infant is so highly susceptible to overwhelming illness. Nursery outbreaks of both Coxsackie B virus (Javett et al., 1956) and echovirus infections (Cramblett et al., 1973; Nagington et al., 1978) have been reported in which severe, and sometimes fatal, illnesses have occurred.

Pathology. In Coxsackie B virus infections, myocardial necrosis and inflammation may be seen that is patchy or diffuse, with extensive infiltration by lymphocytes, mononuclear cells, histiocytes, and some polymorphonuclear leukocytes. Similar infiltrates are seen in the meninges in both Coxsackie virus and echovirus infections. When liver or adrenal glands are involved, there is usually extensive hemorrhage as well as inflammation and necrosis.

Diagnosis. When disease is acquired from the mother, an infant is characteristically well at birth, although premature delivery is more frequent in this group. The mother, however, may be febrile at this time. The baby develops fever, anorexia, and vomiting after an incubation period of 1 to 5 days. The onset of illness occurs in the 1st week of life in more than 50 per cent of affected infants (Krajden and Middleton, 1983). At that point, the clinical evolution depends on the infecting virus and the extent of involvement.

In most instances, the disease is mild and self-limited. A rash may appear in some infants and aseptic meningitis in others. If myocarditis is present, the liver rapidly enlarges, the heart dilates, and the heart sounds become muffled. The echocardiogram and electrocardiogram show diffuse myocardial inflammation. Not infrequently, disseminated intravascular coagulation, refractory hypotension, and death follow rapidly. However, in many infants, myocardial involvement is temporary and recovery occurs over the course of several weeks.

The severity of central nervous system infection is also variable. Enteroviruses can produce overwhelming meningoencephalitis, sometimes with cranial nerve signs. It is more common, however, to see a moderate or mild meningitis characterized by only temporary irritability, lethargy, fever, and feeding difficulty. In a series of nine children with enteroviral meningitis and nine matched controls evaluated for sequelae at approximately 4 years of age, no differences in mean I.Q. level, head circumference, detectable sensorineuronal hearing loss, or intellectual functioning were detected (Wilfert et al., 1981).

Receptive language functioning of the meningitis group was significantly less than controls. Some infections, particularly those with echoviruses, are characterized by a rampant and overwhelming hepatitis (Modlin, 1980). Others are exhibited primarily in the form of pulmonary disease, and still others indicated by diarrhea and even necrotizing enterocolitis (Lake et al., 1976). Disseminated intravascular coagulation develops in virtually all instances of widespread, fulminant involvement.

Treatment. The symptoms of myocarditis and heart failure must be treated by slow digitalization, diuretics, and other supportive measures. Both plasma infusions and exchange transfusions have been attempted in overwhelming enterovirus infections with little evidence of beneficial effect. The use of steroids should be discouraged unless there is a clear rationale.

Prognosis. By the time disseminated intravascular coagulation has developed, the prognosis is grave. On the other hand, many infants with Coxsackie B virus myocarditis survive and the prognosis in such instances is probably closely related to early detection of the infection through electrocardiogram and viral diagnostic measures. Few long-term follow-up studies have been published, but the available information suggests that recovery is complete in most instances.

The prognosis following central nervous system involvement is also not clear. Most patients do well. However, a number of studies of infants under 3 months of age with aseptic meningitis have suggested that there may be some impairment of intellectual development when compared with carefully selected control groups (Farmer et al., 1975; Sells et al., 1975; Wilfert et al., 1981).

The following case illustrates the fulminant disease caused by Coxsackie B-2 virus.

CASE 36–1

A white male infant was born at term to a 35-year-old multiparous woman and weighed 3500 g. He did well at birth. On the 7th postnatal day, his mother became febrile. Four days later, the infant's temperature rose to 101.8° F, and he developed tachypnea with cyanosis and grunting respiration. His heart rate rose to 198 per minute. Besides an ill-appearing child, physical examination did not identify an etiology for his illness. He was treated with ampicillin (200 mg/kg/day) and gentamicin (7.5 mg/kg/day) parenterally. Fever, tachypnea, and tachycardia persisted and hepatomegaly developed. Chest x-ray study and two-dimensional echocardiogram suggested biventricular cardiac failure, and digoxin was given at 5 mg/kg/day. Lumbar puncture revealed cerebrospinal fluid, which contained 2500 red blood cells and 1200 white blood cells/mm³ as well as an increased protein concentration (>120 mg/100 mils). Within 3 days, the child developed diarrhea, which was blood tinged. Bacterial cultures of blood, cerebrospinal fluid, stool, urine, and nasopharynx revealed no pathogen. On the 13th day after presentation, the child developed intractable hypotension and hypothermia (95.6° F). Increasing hepatomegaly was noted. The child died within 24 hours thereafter. Antemortem and postmortem viral studies confirmed infection with Coxsackie virus B-2, which was grown from cerebrospinal fluid, blood, throat washings, and brain.

Comment. The onset of a febrile illness in this 11-day-old infant followed a similar illness in his mother. Tachycardia and heart failure developing in a previously normal heart suggested primary myocarditis, and cerebrospinal fluid alterations suggested encephalomyelitis. The combination of these two indicated generalized infection, with either a virus or *Toxoplasma* the most likely pathogen. A virus appeared more probable in view of the simultaneous maternal illness and the absence of jaundice, hepatosplenomegaly, and thrombocytopenia.

■ HERPES SIMPLEX INFECTIONS

Herpes simplex viruses are classified into two types: Type 1 causes about 98 per cent of oral infections (gingivostomatitis and pharyngitis), 7 to 50 per cent of primary genital herpes, and almost 100 per cent of encephalitis outside of the newborn period; type 2 causes 90 per cent of primary genital herpes, 99 per cent of recurrent genital infections, and most cases of aseptic meningitis (Freij and Sever, 1988; Nahmias and Roizman, 1973). Seventy to eighty-five per cent of neonatal herpes simplex infections are due to herpes type 2 (Whitley, 1990; Whitley et al., 1980). It is likely that most infections are acquired from the mother shortly before or at the time of delivery. Some, perhaps accounting for the slight excess of cases due to type 1 that are above the percentage found in the adult genital tract, must be acquired from other sources. Considering the frequency of labial herpes in the adult population, however, acquisition of herpes simplex from such lesions must be an extremely rare event.

Incidence. Genital herpes infections have been increasing in incidence steadily since the 1970s. The frequency of neonatal disease has probably also increased although fortunately it remains low (Prober et al., 1988). Nahmias estimates that one detected case is found in every 7500 deliveries among an indigent population, whereas others estimate an incidence of one in 2500 to one in 10,000 deliveries (Stagno and Whitley, 1985; Whitley, 1990; Whitley and Hutto, 1985). Primary infections result in an estimated attack rate of neonatal herpes of 50 per cent, whereas recurrent maternal infection results in less than an 8 per cent attack rate (Prober et al., 1987).

Etiology and Pathogenesis. Most infants acquire the virus from the maternal genital tract at the time of delivery. Lesions have been reported to develop at the site of intrapartum monitoring electrodes on the infant's scalp. A smaller number of infants are infected several days before delivery and are born with clinically evident disease. There are some cases described of infants with a syndrome more closely resembling congenital viral infection who were probably infected in utero during the first or second trimester (Florman et al., 1973; Freij and Sever, 1988; South et al., 1969). Primary herpes simplex virus infections that occur during the first half of pregnancy are associated with an increased frequency of spontaneous abortions and stillbirths (Freij and Sever, 1988; Stagno and Whitley, 1985). Cases proved to have been acquired from individuals other than the mother, or even from the mother at any time other than during delivery, are rare (Linnemann et al., 1978; Yeager et al., 1983).

The pathogenic mechanisms responsible for the newborn infant's susceptibility to herpes infection are not dependent on a single key difference between adult and infant but are the result of a spectrum of immunologic deficiencies (Kohl, 1985). Among the currently identified cellular deficits are the inability of the neonatal macrophage to mediate early viral containment, the fact that unstimulated neonatal lymphocytes are permissive for herpes simplex virus infection, and a profound defect in natural killer cell cytotoxicity (Kohl, 1985). The contribution of transplacentally acquired antibody is unresolved and controversial (Kohl, 1985). Antibody-dependent effector mechanisms, including antibody-dependent cellular cytotoxicity, which may rely upon lymphocytes, macrophages, and polymorphonuclear leukocytes, may be responsible in different infants for the conflicting data concerning anti–herpes simplex virus antibody titers and protection from infection (Kohl, 1985). The genetic and developmental regulatory mechanisms of these varied immunologic defects suggest different immunoregulatory interventions that are individualized for specific infants.

Pathology. Macroscopically, many viscera, but chiefly the liver, lungs, and adrenal glands, are riddled with pale yellow, firm, necrotic nodules, measuring 1 to 6 mm in diameter. Under the microscope, massive coagulation necrosis is seen to involve the parenchyma, stroma, and vessels in these areas. Necrotizing, calcifying lesions of the brain may also be found. Intranuclear eosinophilic inclusions as well as multinucleated giant cells, which represent the individual cell's response to viral infection, may be seen.

Diagnosis. Most infants are normal at birth and develop the illness at 5 to 10 days of age. Approximately 40 per cent of affected infants are less than 36 weeks gestational age (Whitley and Hutto, 1985). Overt herpetic disease in the maternal genital tract is evident in only about one-third of patients (Whitley et al., 1980; Yeager and Arvin, 1984). In most of the remainder, the virus probably originates from an asymptomatic maternal genital infection.

The clinical manifestations of disease have been classified into two broad groups: disseminated and localized (Whitley, 1990). Within the disseminated group, two categories are recognized—those with and those without central nervous system involvement. Localized infections include those involving the central nervous system, with or without skin, eye, or mouth lesions, and those with isolated skin, eye, or oral cavity disease. Localized infections without central nervous system involvement represent approximately 20 per cent of all cases of neonatal herpes (Whitley and Hutto, 1985). Despite undetectable central nervous system disease, 25 per cent of this group will develop neurologic abnormalities. Localized central nervous system disease with or without skin, eye, or oral cavity involvement is seen in approximately 33 per cent of infants with neonatal herpes. The mortality rate in this group is from 17 to 50 per cent, and 40 per cent will have long-term neurologic sequelae. Infants with disseminated disease represent approximately 50 per cent of all neonatal herpes patients. Without antiviral therapy, 80 per cent will die and survivors will have serious neurologic sequelae (Whitley and Hutto, 1985). With therapy, 15 to 20 per cent will die but 40 to 55 per cent will suffer neurologic sequelae (Freij and Sever, 1988).

Disseminated disease usually begins toward the end of the 1st week of life. Skin vesicles may be the first or a later sign but do not appear at all in more than half of patients. Systemic symptoms, although insidious in onset, progress rapidly. Poor feeding, lethargy, and fever may be accompanied by irritability or convulsions if the central nervous system is involved. These symptoms are followed rapidly by jaundice, hypotension, disseminated intravascular coagulation, apnea, and shock. This form of disease is indistinguishable at its onset from both neonatal enterovirus infection and bacterial sepsis.

Localized disease may begin somewhat later, with most cases appearing in the 2nd week of life. When the central nervous system is the primary site of infection, the skin or eyes may or may not be involved; if not, then brain biopsy may be the only mode of diagnosis, as with encephalitis in older subjects. The infants are lethargic, irritable, and tremulous, and seizures are frequent and difficult to control.

Eye infections usually take the form of keratoconjunctivitis or chorioretinitis. On the neonatal skin, herpes simplex virus produces the characteristic grouped vesicles seen in later life, although individual lesions may be large and even bullous and late lesions are typically eroded, flat, irregular ulcers with an erythematous base.

In disseminated disease, there is usually chemical evidence of hepatocellular injury. If the central nervous system is involved, the spinal fluid usually contains white cells (mostly lymphocytes) and sometimes demonstrates erythrocytes and the protein level is usually elevated. Except when encephalitis is the only manifestation of disease, as already mentioned, herpes simplex virus is readily recovered from clinical samples. In the disseminated form, virus is present in blood, cerebrospinal fluid, conjunctivae, respiratory secretions, and urine. In the localized form, the virus can be found at the site of disease. Scrapings of skin vesicles show giant, multinucleated cells when stained with Wright or Giesma stain (the Tzanck smear), typical of either herpes or varicella virus infection. Demonstration of viral antigens in cytologic smears using monoclonal or polyclonal antibodies is a more sensitive tool than Tzanck smear (Alpert and Plotkin, 1986). Definitive microbiologic diagnosis, however, requires growth of the virus in tissue culture. Fortunately, herpes simplex virus can be detected by its cytopathic effect in 24 to 48 hours in most instances. When herpes neonatorum is suspected, viral cultures of the throat, conjunctival and cerebrospinal fluids, blood, and urine should all be obtained as well as scrapings of any suspicious skin lesions. Moreover, the mother's genital and respiratory tracts should also be sampled. Serologic assays are rarely helpful and are difficult to interpret in view of the cross-reactions between the two herpes serotypes.

Treatment and Prevention. If a mother has active genital herpes simplex infection at the time of delivery and if the membranes are either intact or have been ruptured for less than 4 hours, strong consideration should be given

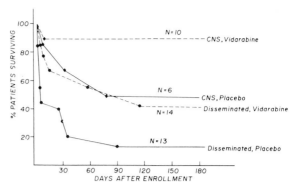

FIGURE 36–4. Outcome of herpes simplex virus infection in newborns according to type of disease and therapy. Points represent last death(s). (From Whitley, R. J., Nahmias, A. J., Visintine, A. M., et al.: The natural history of herpes simplex virus infection of mother and newborn. Pediatrics 66:489, 1980. Reproduced by permission of Pediatrics.)

to delivery by cesarean section. The risk to the child is greatest if maternal infection is primary (i.e., if the mother has previously had no infection with either type 1 or type 2 virus). Recurrences, however, with infectious virus recoverable from the genital area at the time of delivery also pose a hazard.

When neonatal disease is suspected, every effort to establish a definitive diagnosis must be made as rapidly as possible. As soon as this diagnosis is ascertained, the infant should receive adenine arabinoside (Vidarabine), 20 to 30 mg/kg/day administered intravenously over a 12 hour period for 10 days, or acyclovir, 10 to 30 mg/kg/day intravenously in every 8 to 12 hours, depending on the degree of renal impairment, for 10 to 14 days. This treatment has been shown to be effective in all forms of the disease, reducing (but by no means eliminating) both mortality and sequelae. The survival results of the Collaborative Antiviral Study Group trials for infants with central nervous system or disseminated disease are shown in Figure 36–4 (Whitley et al., 1980). The mortality rate in infants with localized disease outside the central nervous system has always been close to zero. If cultures are negative, breast-feeding is safe (Grossman et al., 1981).

Prognosis. Even with antiviral treatment, the prognosis for survivors is not good. More than half develop microcephaly, spasticity, paralysis, seizures, deafness, or blindness. Those with skin involvement often have recurrent crops of skin vesicles for several years.

The following case illustrates a typical severe generalized herpes virus infection in an infant with disseminated disease.

CASE 36–2

After an uncomplicated pregnancy and delivery, a 5-day-old full-term female infant was admitted because of fever, anorexia, and lethargy. Immediately after the delivery, the mother had noted the onset of intense vaginal pain and itching. Physical examination revealed herpetic lesions about the genitalia. The child had done well during the first 4 days of life but then developed a temperature of 102° F and anorexia. On physical examination, her temperature was 100.8° F, a large pustular lesion was noted on the left cheek, the liver was palpated 1.5 cm below the right costal margin, and the spleen was not palpable. The remainder of the physical examination was unre-

markable. Her white blood cell count was 5600/mm³ with 73 per cent polymorphonuclear leukocytes. Her hemoglobin was 16.9 g/100 ml. Cultures of blood, urine, cerebrospinal fluid, and stool showed no bacterial pathogens. She was started on ampicillin and gentamicin.

Her fever persisted, and additional skin lesions were observed over the subsequent 3 days. A repeat lumbar puncture revealed 500 white blood cells/mm³ in her cerebrospinal fluid, consisting of 50 per cent polymorphonuclear leukocytes and 50 per cent mononuclear cells. Thrombocytopenia (<100,000 platelets/ mm³) developed, and evidence of hepatocellular inflammation was noted. Hepatosplenomegaly increased. Generalized convulsions were noted on the 6th hospital day, as well as hematologic manifestations of disseminated intervascular coagulation. The infant died on the 17th day of life.

Autopsy showed extensive necrobiotic lesions characteristic of generalized herpes simplex infection in the liver, lungs, and adrenals. Herpes simplex virus was grown from the liver, lungs, and brain. Virus was also isolated from persistent vesicular lesions of the skin.

Comment. The infant was undoubtedly infected during parturition by contact with the mother's genital herpes. Skin lesions appeared on the fourth day, and new vesicles developed during the course. Unlike most instances of the disease, jaundice was never prominent. The liver and spleen were enlarged, and thrombocytopenia with bleeding and evidence of brain damage appeared. The virus was identified. Neutralizing antibodies were not found in appreciable quantities in the mother or child.

This case illustrates the course of herpes simplex infection before the advent of antiviral agents.

■ VARICELLA

There is some confusion about the term "congenital varicella" that would probably be best resolved by our reserving this term for the very rare cases transmitted to the fetus in the first or second trimester of pregnancy (Laforet and Lynch, 1947; Srabstein et al., 1974). Also called "congenital varicella" in the literature but probably better termed "neonatal varicella" are those cases of perinatal varicella beginning before or on the 10th day of life and, therefore, because of the incubation period of the disease, acquired in utero. The two syndromes are thoroughly discussed by Brunell (1983) and Feldman (1986). Some cases (e.g., that described by Bai and John in 1979) fall somewhere in between.

Incidence. Varicella-zoster virus infections occur during pregnancy with a frequency of 1 to 5 per 10,000 pregnancies (Brunell, 1983). Approximately 24 cases of congenital varicella are reported in the literature (Paryani and Arvin, 1986). On the basis of three carefully performed studies of varicella during pregnancy, the risk of symptomatic intrauterine varicella-zoster virus infection after maternal varicella during the first trimester is 4.9 per cent (3 of 61 infants) (Enders, 1984; Paryani and Arvin, 1986; Siegel, 1973). Unlike mumps and rubella infection during the first trimester, first trimester varicella does not result in a detectable increase in fetal wastage (Brunell, 1983; Siegel and Fuerst, 1966). Paryani and Arvin (1986) report that one of 11 infants with maternal varicella during the second trimester developed herpes zoster during infancy,

and two of 16 infants with maternal varicella during the third trimester had varicella at birth. For infants whose mothers contract varicella 5 days or less before delivery or up to two days after delivery, the infant attack rate is 17 to 31 per cent (Brunell, 1983; Feldman, 1986; Meyers, 1974). Two of three infants whose mothers contracted the infection less than 10 days before delivery reported by Paryani and Arvin (1986) developed varicella despite the administration of varicella zoster immune globulin at birth.

Etiology and Pathogenesis. The congenital varicella syndrome is acquired from a maternal varicella infection that occurs during the first or second trimester. The virus must be transmitted transplacentally during the viremia that precedes or accompanies the rash. Clearly, however, in most situations the fetus either is not infected at all or recovers fully in utero, since the syndrome itself is so rare and because varicella during pregnancy is not uncommon.

Neonatal varicella is also probably transplacentally acquired in most cases. Since the incubation period for varicella is between 10 and 21 days, those cases beginning in the first 10 days of life are considered to have been acquired in utero. The prognosis, however, differs markedly between those cases in which maternal illness began 5 or more days from delivery and those in which maternal illness occurred from 4 days before to 1 day after delivery. In the first group, neonatal disease usually begins with the first 4 days of life, and the prognosis is good. Of 27 cases cited by Gershon in her reviews (1975), all survived. Presumably, maternal immunity has appeared before delivery and has been transferred to the baby before birth. In the second group, neonatal disease begins between 5 and 10 days after delivery (Brunell, 1966). Of the 23 cases described, seven (30 per cent) died of overwhelming varicella and two barely survived after severe disease. In those instances in which the infant's pre-illness antibody has been measured in severe disease, none has been found.

Presumably, the placenta acts as a partial barrier to infection at term as well as earlier during pregnancy. Only about one in six such maternal infections results in neonatal disease (Meyers, 1974).

Diagnosis. The rare cases of congenital varicella syndrome are characterized by the presence of unusual cicatrices, asymmetric muscular atrophy and limb hypoplasia, low birth weight, chronic encephalitis with cortical atrophy, and ophthalmitis (chorioretinitis, microphthalmia, atrophy, and cataracts) (Brunell, 1983; Feldman, 1986).

Neonatal varicella follows typical maternal varicella and thus can usually be anticipated. When the disease appears in the infant during the danger period (from 5 to 10 days of age), it resembles closely varicella in the immunodeficient or immunosuppressed host. Recurrent crops of skin vesicles develop over a prolonged period of time, reflecting the newborn infant's inability to control the infection. Visceral dissemination is common, with involvement of the liver, lung, and brain. Secondary bacterial infection may occur.

Disease that is evident at birth or that appears in the first 4 days of life is usually mild, presumably owing to modification of the illness by maternal immunity.

The laboratory may be helpful in confirming the diagnosis. Prenatal diagnosis has been performed on blood obtained by funicentesis by quantifying varicella-specific IgM with an immunofluorescent antibody assay (Cuthbertson et al., 1987). Similar serologic studies can be performed on infants (Paryani and Arvin, 1986). Scrapings of skin lesions, as with herpes simplex infections, show large multinucleated cells when stained with Wright or Giemsa stain (Tzanck smears). The virus can be grown in tissue culture from skin and visceral lesions.

Prevention and Treatment. Infants of mothers who develop varicella from 5 days before to 2 days after delivery should receive high-titered immune globulin as soon as possible (MMWR, 1984). Such preparations (zoster immune globulin, or varicella-zoster immune globulin) have been shown to prevent chicken pox in exposed older children (Brunell et al., 1969) and are available from regional blood centers of the American Red Cross Services. If special globulin preparations are not available, then standard immune serum globulin (0.5 to 1.0 ml/kg) should be given. Administration of varicella-zoster immune globulin is not 100 per cent effective in preventing perinatal varicella. Infants at risk may develop attenuated disease, may have prolonged incubation periods, and may still require antiviral therapy.

In the event of a significant exposure in a nursery situation, as defined by prolonged contact (greater than 20 minutes) with an infectious staff member, patient, or visitor, infants who have no maternal history of varicella and who have undetectable anti-varicella titers should be considered candidates for varicella-zoster immune globulin. All infants less than 28 weeks' gestational age regardless of maternal history should be considered (MMWR, 1984). The recommended dosage is 125 units/10 kg (MMWR, 1984). Fractional doses are not recommended. However, little experience is available to guide treatment of extremely preterm infants. Currently, all infants should receive 125 units.

If severe disease develops, antiviral chemotherapy might be considered. Drugs that might be effective are adenine arabinoside (15 mg/kg/day) and acycloguanosine (acyclovir) (10 to 30 mg/kg/day).

■ VIRAL HEPATITIS

Owing to the alliance between molecular biology and virology and clinical medicine, dramatic advances have been made during the 1980s in understanding the pathogenesis of viral hepatitis (Balistreri, 1988). The known forms of acute and chronic viral hepatitis and antigens and antibodies associated with them are given in Tables 36–8 and 36–9. Although hepatitis A virus has been nosocomially transmitted in the setting of a neonatal intensive care unit, and multiply transfused infants are at increased risk for non-A, non-B hepatitis, understanding of hepatitis B is currently of greatest importance for the pediatrician (Balistreri, 1988). This discussion, therefore, focuses on perinatal hepatitis B infection.

The findings that perhaps are the most important to neonatologists pertain to the frequency with which hepatitis B is transmitted to infants at the time of birth, the short- and long-term consequences of these infections, the

TABLE 36–8. Known Forms of Acute and Chronic Viral Hepatitis

ACUTE VIRAL HEPATITIS

Type A—due to the hepatitis A virus, a 27-nm RNA virus

Type B—due to the hepatitis B virus, a 42-nm double-shelled DNA virus

Type D (delta)—due to the hepatitis delta virus, a defective 35- to 37-nm virus consisting of RNA nucleoprotein; found only in association with hepatitis B virus infection

Parenteral or post-transfusion non-A, non-B hepatitis ("classic form")—due to unidentified viral agent(s)*

"Epidemic" non-A, non-B hepatitis ("enteric form")—due to a picornavirus similar to hepatitis A virus

CHRONIC VIRAL HEPATITIS

Chronic type B hepatitis

Chronic delta hepatitis

Chronic non-A, non-B hepatitis*

*At least two separate viruses.

(From Balistreri, W. F.: Viral hepatitis. Pediatr. Clin. North Am. 35:637, 1988.)

importance of increased surveillance for maternal hepatitis B carriage, and the availability of effective hepatitis B virus immunoprophylaxis (Krugman, 1988). The frequency of transmission depends primarily on the prevalence of the hepatitis B carrier state among women of child-bearing age.

In certain parts of the world and among certain ethnic groups, as many as 7 to 10 per cent of all infants acquire hepatitis B infections at the time of birth, and a high proportion of these infections is chronic. The relationship of these infections to chronic liver failure and hepatic carcinoma in adult life has been noted (Balistreri, 1988; Beasley et al., 1981).

Incidence. The incidence of neonatal hepatitis B infection depends on a number of factors. Women with acute hepatitis B infection during the first or second trimester rarely transmit the virus to their infants (Krugman, 1988). Besides the timing of the infection, the hepatitis B surface antigen (HB_sAg) carriage rate varies from 0.1 per cent in the United States and Europe to 15 per cent in Taiwan and parts of Africa, with intermediate rates in Japan, South America, and Southeast Asia. Transmission rates among immigrant women in Western countries appear to parallel the rates in their country of origin (Krugman, 1988). Another factor is the potential of the infection to be transmitted from the mother at the time of delivery. This potential is great if symptomatic acute disease is present (60 to 70 per cent transmission) (Gerety and Schweitzer, 1977). Infants of hepatitis B e antigen (HB_eAg)–positive mothers have an 80 to 90 per cent chance of becoming HB_sAg carriers (Okada et al., 1976). Chronic neonatal infection occurs in less than 10 per cent of infants of e antigen–negative mothers (Krugman, 1988). Transplacental leakage of HB_sAg-positive maternal blood is the most likely source of intrauterine infection (Lin et al., 1987). The serologic and biochemical course of subclinical infection is outlined in Figure 36–5. Although Hb_sAg has been found in breast milk, breast-feeding does not appear to have any influence, either positive or negative, on the rate of transmission (Beasley et al., 1975).

Etiology and Pathogenesis. Hepatitis B virus is the

TABLE 36–9. The Hepatitis Viruses: Characteristics of Associated Antigens and Antibodies

	DEFINITIONS	SIGNIFICANCE
Serologic Markers of Hepatitis A Virus (HAV)*		
Anti-HAV	Total antibody (IgM and IgG subclasses) directed against HAV	Indicates recent acute (IgM) or past HAV infection (Ig) Confirms past exposure and immunity towards HAV
Anti-HAV-IgM	IgM antibody to HAV	Indicates recent acute infection
Serologic Markers of Hepatitis B Virus (HBV)*		
HB$_s$Ag	Hepatitis B surface antigen—found on the surface of the intact virus and in serum as unattached particles (spherical or tubular)	Indicates infection with HBV (either acute or chronic)
HB$_c$Ag	Hepatitis B core antigen—found within the core of the intact virus	Not detectable in serum (found only in liver tissue)
HB$_e$Ag	Hepatitis B core antigen—(soluble antigen produced during self-cleavage of HB$_c$Ag)	Indicates active HBV infection Signifies high infectivity Persistence for 6–8 months suggests chronic carrier and/or chronic liver disease
Anti-HB$_s$	Antibody to HBV surface antigen (HB$_s$Ag); subclasses	Indicates clinical recovery from HBV infection and immunity
	IgM (early and IgG)	Protective
Anti-HB$_c$	Total antibody to HBV core antigen (HB$_c$Ag)	Indicates active HBV infection (acute and chronic)
Anti-HB$_c$-IgM	IgM antibody to HB$_c$Ag	Early index of acute HBV infection Rises during acute phase then declines Not present in chronic HBV
Anti-HB$_e$	Antibody to HBV e antigen (HB$_e$Ag)	Seroconversion (HB$_e$Ag to anti-HB$_e$) indicates resolution
Serologic Markers of Hepatitis Delta (δ) Virus (HDV)*		
Anti-HDV	Total antibody to the hepatitis D (delta) virus	Indicates exposure to the δ agent (HDV) Patient may transmit HDV infection
HDV RNA	RNA of the hepatitis D (delta) virus	Present in serum

*These are detectable using sensitive and specific commercial serologic assays.

(From Balistreri, W. F.: Viral hepatitis. Pediatr. Clin. North Am. *35*:637, 1988.)

only representative of a unique group of DNA-containing viruses that infects the human host. The virus localizes primarily in hepatic parenchymal cells but circulates in the bloodstream, along with several subviral antigens, for periods of time ranging from a few days to many years. It seems clear that, despite either acute or persistent viremia in the mother, the virus rarely crosses the placenta and that infection in the neonatal period occurs at or shortly after birth, probably by means of virus carried in maternal blood. Most infants born to mothers infected with hepatitis B virus have negative test results at birth and become HB$_s$Ag positive during the first 3 months of life (Krugman, 1988).

Diagnosis. Infants with hepatitis B infection do not show clinical or chemical signs of disease at birth. The usual pattern is the development of chronic antigenemia with mild and often persistent enzyme elevations, beginning at 2 to 6 months of age. Occasionally, the antigenemia is entirely missed, and the child is merely found to have antibody to the surface antigen at 6 to 12 months of age. Sometimes, the infection becomes clinically manifest, with jaundice, fever, hepatomegaly, and anorexia, followed by either recovery or chronic active hepatitis. Very rarely, fulminant hepatitis is seen (Delaplane et al., 1983).

Laboratory tests are essential in the diagnosis of hepatitis B infection. Evaluations of serum enzymes and of bilirubin reflect the extent of liver damage. There are several helpful serologic tests that identify the virus involved (Krugman, 1988) (Figure 36–6). HB$_s$Ag appears early, usually before liver disease is found, and may disappear or persist. Antibody to the hepatitis B core antigen (anti-HB$_c$) usually appears during or shortly after the acute disease and lasts for years. Hepatitis B e antigen appears concurrently with HB$_s$Ag and is indicative of an increased potential to transmit the infection. Antibody to hepatitis B e antigen appears approximately 2 to 4 weeks after the disappearance of e antigen. The last factor to appear, usually several weeks or even months after the illness (and never if HB$_s$Ag persists), is antibody to the surface antigen, or anti-HB$_s$. It is very unusual for all three of these tests to yield negative results in the presence of hepatitis B infection.

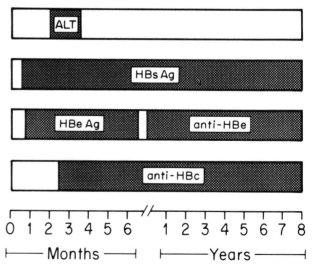

FIGURE 36–5. Serologic and biochemical course of subclinical hepatitis B infection progressing to asymptomatic chronic carrier state. (From Krugman, S.: Hepatitis B virus and the neonate. Ann. N. Y. Acad. Sci. 549:129, 1988.)

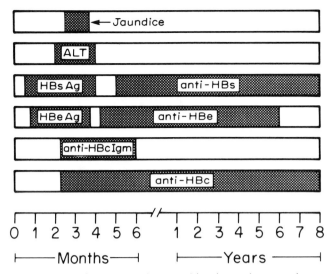

FIGURE 36–6. Chemical, serologic, and biochemical course of acute hepatitis B infection followed by recovery. (From Krugman, S.: Hepatitis B virus and the neonate. Ann. N. Y. Acad. Sci. 549:129, 1988.)

Prevention and Treatment. Important preventive measures include passive immunization with high-titered human immune serum globulin (HBIG) and use of hepatitis B vaccine. These measures are effective because of the low frequency of intrauterine infection (about 5 per cent), the occurrence of the infection at birth in most infants, and the 6-week to 6-month incubation period of hepatitis B (Krugman, 1988). Passive immunization protects against hepatitis B infection during the first 6 weeks of life, whereas active immunization provides long-term protection. Several studies have confirmed the 85 to 90 per cent efficacy of preventing chronic infections in infants of mothers who are HB_sAg positive and HB_eAg positive with the following regimen: Hepatitis B immune globulin, 0.5 ml, administered intramuscularly within the first few hours of birth; hepatitis B vaccine (0.5 ml or 10 μg of HB_sAg) administered intramuscularly by 7 days of age, a second dose of 0.5 ml at 1 month, and a third dose at 6 months (Beasley et al., 1983; Krugman, 1988; Stevens et al., 1985; Stevens et al., 1987). Passive and active immunization may be administered simultaneously to the newborn infant at different sites. Blood should be obtained at 6 months for HB_sAg detection and at 15 months for HB_sAg and anti-HB_s. If HB_sAg is detected at 6 months, immunization failure has occurred and, at 15 months, the infant is a chronic carrier (Krugman, 1988). At 15 months, if HB_sAg is not detected and anti-HB_s is detected, the infant is protected. A recent study of immunization of infants of HB_eAg-positive mothers suggests a failure rate in this group of 14 per cent (3 of 21 infants were HB_sAg positive at 1 year of age) (Farmer et al., 1987).

For immunoprophylaxis to be successful, maternal screening is important (Cruz et al., 1987; Summers et al., 1987). The United States Public Health Service Immunization Practices Advisory Committee has recently recommended routine screening of all pregnant women (MMWR, 1988). In developing countries, such a strategy is neither feasible nor affordable. In areas where hepatitis B virus infection is hyperendemic, all newborn infants should be routinely immunized (Hsu et al., 1988; Krugman, 1988).

▪ HUMAN PARVOVIRUS B19

Considerable interest in the role of human parvovirus B19 infection in neonatal hydrops fetalis (nonimmune) and fetal aplastic crisis has developed since two cases of fetal deaths in humans associated with maternal B19 infection were reported (Kinney and Kumar, 1988).

Incidence, Etiology, and Pathogenesis. Approximately 30 to 60 per cent of adults in the United States are seropositive for human parvovirus B19. A significant proportion of child-bearing women is thus presumably susceptible to human parvovirus B19 infection. To date, approximately 36 fetal deaths associated with maternal human parvovirus B19 infection have been reported as well as approximately 130 cases in which the fetus survived and was normal at birth (Kinney and Kumar, 1988). No assessment of fetal risk can be made on the basis of current information (Kinney and Kumar, 1988).

Two potential pathogenic mechanisms involve the recognized affinity of B19 for progenitor erythroid cells of bone marrow and the finding of nonimmune hydrops in several of the affected fetuses. The pathologic findings suggest bone marrow aplasia that might lead to progressive congestive heart failure and hydrops (Kinney and Kumar, 1988).

Two studies undertaken to examine the association between human parvovirus B19 infection and congenital anomalies have failed to reveal any connection (Kinney et al., 1988; Mortimer et al., 1983).

Diagnosis. The diagnosis can be made serologically or by viral culture. Both radioimmunoassays and enzyme-linked immunosorbent assays are available for detection of human parvovirus B19–specific IgG and IgM (Kinney and Kumar, 1988). Unfortunately, preliminary observations suggest that human parvovirus B19 IgM antibodies may have a shortened half-life (Anderson and Pattison, 1984). Virus can be cultured from tissue in suspension cultures of bone marrow cells from persons with hemolytic anemias. Electron microscopy has permitted visualization of parvovirus-like particles in peripheral blood. Finally, molecular probes can detect human parvovirus B19 DNA in tissues, serum, and urine (Kinney and Kumar, 1988).

Elevated maternal alpha-fetoprotein concentration may be a marker for an adverse outcome (Carrington et al., 1987). In the context of a human parvovirus B19 infection in a symptomatic, pregnant women, rising weekly measurements of maternal serum alpha-fetoprotein may indicate that the fetus is infected.

Treatment. No studies of antenatal or neonatal treatment of human parvovirus B19 have been reported. Only symptomatic, supportive care is available.

▪ NOSOCOMIAL VIRAL INFECTIONS

Previous reference has been made to nursery outbreaks of enterovirus infections that cause diseases ranging from mild, benign febrile illness to aseptic meningitis, myocarditis, and overwhelming generalized infections with disseminated intravascular coagulation (Cramblett et al., 1973; Javett et al., 1956; Nagington et al., 1978). As was also mentioned, nursery-acquired herpes simplex infections fortunately are rare and symptomatic nosocomial CMV infections appear to be largely confined to recipients of latently infected blood who themselves lack antibody. Two other groups of viruses, however, previously unrecognized as important pathogens in the newborn period, appear to be responsible for a significant proportion of nursery-acquired viral infections. These are the respiratory viruses and the viruses that cause diarrhea.

RESPIRATORY VIRUSES

It seems likely that any one of the large number of respiratory viruses can cause symptomatic respiratory disease in newborn infants. The association has been described for rhinoviruses, adenoviruses, parainfluenza viruses, influenza virus, and respiratory syncytial virus. Adenovirus, rhinovirus, and parainfluenza virus infections are characterized by mild rhinorrhea under these conditions. Influenza virus infections are usually mild, but in the absence of maternally transmitted antibody they can be life threatening, with extensive pneumonia and hypoxia and a prolonged course. The most extensive nursery outbreaks, however, have been caused by respiratory syncytial virus (Berkovich and Taranko, 1964; Hall et al., 1979). Simultaneous outbreaks of respiratory syncytial virus and parainfluenza virus type B have also been reported (Meissner et al., 1984).

Respiratory syncytial virus is the major cause of viral pneumonia and bronchiolitis in infants and children. In temperate climates, it causes large annual epidemics during the cold months. Nosocomial infections are frequent during these times, with illness in the hospital staff probably being a major factor in its spread from infant to infant. Several nursery outbreaks have been described. In one of these outbreaks, cultures were obtained prospectively so that a full picture of the viral pathogenicity and epidemiology could be drawn (Hall et al., 1979). Twenty-three of sixty-six infants hospitalized for 6 or more days, and therefore at risk of nosocomial infection, were infected. Only one was asymptomatic. Six had pneumonia, eight presented with upper respiratory infection, four had predominantly apneic spells, and four demonstrated nonspecific signs. Pneumonia and apnea were seen almost exclusively in infants over 3 weeks of age, and nonspecific signs were most commonly observed in those under that age. Four (17 per cent) infants died, two unexpectedly, during the course of their infections. Infants in isolettes did not seem to be protected against acquiring infection. Eighteen of the fifty-three nursery personnel were infected during the outbreak. Eighty-three per cent of these patients were symptomatic. Respiratory syncytial virus infection in preterm infants frequently appears to be associated with a new onset of apnea (Bruhn et al., 1977).

VIRUSES CAUSING DIARRHEA

The best studied of the viruses that cause diarrhea are the rotaviruses. This important group of viruses, with at least four serotypes, is responsible for a large proportion of significant and sometimes severe diarrhea in infants 6 to 24 months of age (Steinhoff, 1980). Nursery-acquired infections are frequent in parts of the world where they

have been sought; surprisingly, however, they appear to be benign in the great majority of infected infants. In certain nurseries in Sydney, Australia, and in London, 30 to 50 per cent of 5-day-old babies excreted the virus (Chrystie et al., 1978; Murphy et al., 1977). However, more than 90 per cent of these infected infants were asymptomatic. The remainder had loose stools and vomiting, but this proportion was only slightly greater than that found among uninfected infants.

A study from France suggested that over the first 2 years of life, 20 per cent of children develop rotaviral disease, 10 per cent have asymptomatic infection, 20 per cent are virus carriers, and 50 per cent are not infected (Champsaur et al., 1984). Rotavirus vaccine has considerable promise for stimulating protective local and systemic immunity (Anderson et al., 1986; Vesikary et al., 1986).

■ REFERENCES

Adler, S. P.: Nosocomial transmission of cytomegalovirus. Pediatr. Infect. Dis. 5:239, 1986.
Adler, S. P., Bagett, J., Wilson, M., et al.: Molecular epidemiology of cytomegalovirus in a nursery: Lack of evidence for nosocomial transmission. J. Pediatr. 108:117, 1986.
Alford, C. A., Schaefer, J., Blankenship, W. J., et al.: Subclinical central nervous system disease of neonates: A prospective study of infants born with increased levels of IgM. J. Pediatr. 75:1169, 1969.
Alpert, G., and Plotkin, S. A.: A practical guide to the diagnosis of congenital infections in the newborn infant. Pediatr. Clin. North Am. 33:465, 1986.
Anderson, E. L., Belshe, R. B., Bartram, J., et al.: Evaluation of rhesus rotavirus vaccine (MMU 18006) in infants and young children. J. Infect. Dis. 153:823, 1986.
Anderson, M. J., and Pattison, J. R.: The human parvovirus: A brief review. Arch. Virol. 82:137, 1984.
Andersson, B., Svenningsen, N. W., and Nordenfelt, E.: Screening for viral infections in infants with poor intrauterine growth. Acta Paediatr. Scand. 70:673, 1981.
Bai, P. V. A., and John, T. J.: Congenital skin ulcers following varicella in late pregnancy. J. Pediatr. 94:65, 1979.
Balistreri, W. F.: Viral hepatitis. Pediatr. Clin. North Am. 35:637, 1988.
Bates, T.: Poliomyelitis in pregnancy, fetus and newborn. Am. J. Dis. Child. 90:189, 1955.
Beasley, R. P., Stevens, C. E., Shiao, I. -S., and Meng, H. -C.: Evidence against breast-feeding as a mechanism for vertical transmission of hepatitis B. Lancet 2:740, 1975.
Beasley, R. P., Hwang, L. -Y., Lee, G. C. -Y., et al.: Prevention of perinatally transmitted hepatitis B virus infections with hepatitis B immune globulin and hepatitis B vaccine. Lancet 2:1099, 1983.
Beasley, R. P., Lin, C. -C., Hwang, L. -Y., and Chien, C. -S.: Hepatocellular carcinoma and hepatitis B virus. Lancet 2:1129, 1981.
Berenberg, W., and Nankervis, G.: Long-term follow-up of cytomegalic inclusion disease of infancy. Pediatrics 46:403, 1970.
Berkovich, S., and Taranko, L.: Acute respiratory illness in the premature nursery associated with respiratory syncytial virus infections. Pediatrics 34:753, 1964.
Bowden, R. A., Sayers, M., Flournoy, N., et al.: Cytomegalovirus immune globulin and seronegative blood products to prevent primary cytomegalovirus infection after marrow transplantation. N. Engl. J. Med. 314:1006, 1988.
Brough, A. J., Jones, D., Page, R. H., and Mizukami, I.: Dermal erythropoiesis in neonatal infants. Pediatrics 40:627, 1967.
Bruhn, F. W., Mokrohisky, S. T., and McIntosh, K.: Apnea associated with respiratory syncytial virus infection in young infants. J. Pediatr. 90:382, 1977.
Brunell, P. A.: Placental transfer of varicella zoster antibody. Pediatrics 38:1034, 1966.
Brunell, P. A.: Fetal and neonatal varicella-zoster infections. Semin. Perinatol. 7:47, 1983.
Brunell, P. A., Ross, A., Miller, L. H., et al.: Prevention of varicella by zoster immune globulin. N. Engl. J. Med. 280:1191, 1969.
Carrington, D., Gilmore, D. H., Whittle, M. J., et al.: Maternal serum

alpha-fetoprotein: A marker of fetal aplastic crisis during intrauterine human parvovirus infection. Lancet 1:433, 1987.

Champsaur, H., Henry-Amar, M., Goldszmidt, D., et al.: Rotavirus carriage, asymptomatic infection, and disease in the first two years of life. II. Serologic response. J. Infect. Dis. 149:675, 1984.

Cherry, J. D.: Enterovirus. In Remington, J. S., and Klein, J. O. (Eds.): Infectious Diseases of the Fetus and Newborn Infant. Philadelphia, W. B. Saunders Co., 1990, pp. 325–366.

Chou, S., and Merigan, T. C.: Rapid detection and quantitation of human cytomegalovirus in urine through DNA hybridization. N. Engl. J. Med. 308:921, 1983.

Chrystie, I. L., Totterdell, B. M., and Banatvala, J. E.: Asymptomatic endemic rotavirus infections in the newborn. Lancet 1:1176, 1978.

Claman, H. N., Savatte, V., Githens, J. H., and Hathaway, W. E.: Histiocytic reaction in dysgammaglobulinemia and congenital rubella. Pediatrics 46:89, 1970.

Cooper, L. Z., Green, R. H., et al.: Neonatal thrombocytopenic purpura and other manifestations of rubella contracted in utero. Am. J. Dis. Child. 110:416, 1965.

Cooper, L. Z., Ziring, P. R., Ockerse, A. R., et al.: Rubella: Clinical manifestation and management. Am. J. Dis. Child. 118:18, 1969.

Cramblett, H. G., Haynes, R. E., Azimi, P. H., et al.: Nosocomial infection with echovirus type II in handicapped and premature infants. Pediatrics 51:603, 1973.

Cruz, A. C., Frentzen, B. H., and Behnke, M.: Hepatitis B: A case for prenatal screening of all patients. Am. J. Obstet. Gynecol. 156:1180, 1987.

Cuthbertson, G., Weiner, C. P., Giller, R. H., and Grose, C.: Prenatal diagnosis of second-trimester congenital varicella syndrome by virus-specific immunoglobulin M. J. Pediatr. 111:592, 1987.

Davis, L. E., Tweed, G. V., Stewart, J. A., et al.: Cytomegalovirus mononucleosis in a first trimester pregnant female with transmission to the fetus. Pediatrics 48:200, 1971.

Delaplane, D., Yogev, R., Crussi, F., et al.: Fetal hepatitis B in early infancy: The importance of identifying HB$_s$Ag-positive pregnant women and providing immunoprophylaxis to their newborns. Pediatrics 72:176, 1983.

Desmond, M. M., Fisher, E. S., Vorderman, A. L., et al.: The longitudinal course of congenital rubella encephalitis in nonretarded children. J. Pediatr. 93:584, 1978.

Dudgeon, J. A.: Congenital rubella. J. Pediatr. 87:1078, 1975.

Emanuel, I., and Kenny, G. E.: Cytomegalic inclusion disease of infancy. Pediatrics 38:957, 1966.

Enders, G.: Varicella-Zoster virus infection in pregnancy. Prog. Med. Virol. 29:166, 1984.

Farmer, K., Gunn, T., and Woodfield, D. G.: A combination of hepatitis B vaccine and immunoglobulin does not protect all infants born to hepatitis B e antigen positive mothers. N. Z. Med. J. 100:412, 1987.

Farmer, K., MacArthur, B. A., and Clay, M. M.: A follow-up study of 15 cases of neonatal meningoencephalitis due to coxsackie virus B5. J. Pediatr. 87:568, 1975.

Feldman, S.: Varicella zoster infections of the fetus, neonate, and immunocompromised child. Curr. Prob. Pediatr. 16:99, 1986.

Florman, A. L., Gershon, A. A., Blackett, P. R., and Nahmias, A. J.: Intrauterine infection with herpes simplex virus: Resultant congenital malformations. J.A.M.A. 225:129, 1973.

Freij, B. J., and Sever, J. L.: Herpesvirus infections in pregnancy: Risks to embryo, fetus, and neonate. Clin. Perinatol. 15:203, 1988.

Gerety, R. J., and Schweitzer, I. L.: Viral hepatitis type B during pregnancy, the neonatal period, and infancy. J. Pediatr. 90:368, 1977.

Gershon, A. A.: Varicella in mother and infant: Problems old and new. In Krugman, S., and Gershon, A. A. (Eds.): Infections of the Fetus and the Newborn Infant. New York, Alan R. Liss, Inc., 1975, pp. 79–95.

Gilbert, G. L., Hayes, K., Hudson, I. L., et al.: Prevention of transfusion-acquired cytomegalovirus infection in infants by blood filtration to remove leucocytes. Lancet i:1228, 1989.

Gregg, N. M.: Congenital cataract following German measles in the mother. Trans. Ophthal. Soc. Austr. 3:35, 1941.

Grossman, J. H., Wallen, U. C., and Sever, J. L.: Management of genital herpes simplex virus infection during pregnancy. Obstet. Gynecol. 58:1, 1981.

Hall, C. B., Kopelman, A. E., Douglas, R. G., Jr., et al.: Neonatal respiratory syncytial virus infection. N. Engl. J. Med. 300:393, 1979.

Hanshaw, J. B., Scheiner, A. P., Moxley, A. W., et al.: School failure and deafness after "silent" congenital cytomegalovirus infection. N. Engl. J. Med. 295:468, 1976.

Hardy, J. B., Monif, G. R. G., and Sever, J. L.: Studies in congenital rubella. Baltimore 1964–65, II. Clin. Virol. Bull. Hopkins Hosp. 118:97, 1966.

Hayden, G. F., Herrmann, K. L., Buimovici-Klein, E., et al.: Subclinical congenital rubella infection associated with maternal rubella vaccination in early pregnancy. J. Pediatr. 96:869, 1980.

Hayes, K., Danks, D. M., Gibas, H., and Jack, I.: Cytomegalovirus in human milk. N. Engl. J. Med. 287:177, 1972.

Hirsch, M. S., Schooley, R. T., Cosimi, A. B., et al.: Effects of interferon-α on cytomegalovirus reactivation syndromes in renal-transplant recipients. N. Engl. J. Med. 308:1489, 1983.

Hodgson, J., Morgan-Capner, P.: Evaluation of a commercial antibody capture enzyme immunoassay for the detection of rubella specific IgM. J. Clin. Pathol. 37:573, 1984.

Hsu, H. -M., Chen, D. -S., Chuang, C. -H., et al.: Efficacy of a mass hepatitis B vaccination program in Taiwan. J.A.M.A. 260:2231, 1988.

Javett, S. N., Heymann, S., Mundel, B., et al.: Myocarditis in the newborn infant. J. Pediatr. 48:1, 1956.

Kaplan, K. M., Cochi, S. L., Edmonds, L. D., et al.: A profile of mothers giving birth to infants with congenital rubella syndrome. Am. J. Dis. Child. 144:118, 1990.

Kibrick, S., and Benirschke, K.: Severe generalized disease (encephalo-hepatomyocarditis) occurring in the newborn period due to infection with coxsackie virus, Group B. Pediatrics 22:857, 1958.

King-Lewis, P. A., and Gardner, S. D.: Congenital cytomegalic inclusion disease following intrauterine transfusion. Br. Med. J. 2:603, 1969.

Kinney, J. S., Anderson, L. J., Farrar, J., et al.: Risk of adverse outcomes of pregnancy following human parvovirus B19 infection. J. Infect. Dis. 157:663, 1988.

Kinney, J. S., and Kumar, M. L.: Should we expand the TORCH complex? Clin. Perinatol. 15:727, 1988.

Kinney, J. S., Onorato, I. M., Stewart, J. A., et al.: Cytomegaloviral infection and disease. J. Infect. Dis. 151:772, 1985.

Kohl, S.: Herpes simplex virus immunology: Problems, progress, and promises. J. Infect. Dis. 152:435, 1985.

Krajden, S., and Middleton, P. J.: Enterovirus infections in the neonate. Clin. Pediatr. 22:88, 1983.

Krugman, S.: Hepatitis B virus and the neonate. Ann. N. Y. Acad. Sci. 549:129, 1988.

Kumar, M. L., Nankervis, G. A., and Gold, E.: Inapparent congenital cytomegalovirus infection: A follow-up study. N. Engl. J. Med. 288:1370, 1973.

Laforet, E. G., and Lynch, C. C.: Multiple congenital defects following maternal varicella. N. Engl. J. Med. 236:534, 1947.

Lake, A. M., Lauer, B. A., Clark, J. C., et al.: Enterovirus infection in neonates. J. Pediatr. 89:787, 1976.

Lepow, M. L., Veronelli, J. A., Hostetler, D. D., et al.: A trial with live attenuated rubella vaccine. Am. J. Dis. Child. 115:639, 1968.

Lin, H. -H., Lee, T. -Y., Chen, D. -S., et al.: Transplacental leakage of HBeAg-positive maternal blood as the most likely route in causing intrauterine infection with hepatitis B virus. J. Pediatr. 111:877, 1987.

Linnemann, C. C., Jr., Buchman, T. G., Light, I. J., et al.: Transmission of herpes simplex type 1 in a newborn nursery: Identification of viral isolates by DNA "fingerprinting." Lancet 1:964, 1978.

Linnemann, C. C., Steichen, J., Sherman, W. G., and Schiff, G. M.: Febrile illness in early infancy associated with ECHO virus infection. J. Pediatr. 84:49, 1974.

Luthardt, T. H., Siebert, H., Losel, I., et al.: Cytomegalievirus-infektionen bei Kindern mit Blutaustauschtransfusion in Neugeborenenalter. Klin. Wochenschr. 49:81, 1971.

Maupas, P., Chiron, J. P., Barin, F., et al.: Efficacy of hepatitis B vaccine in prevention of early HB$_s$Ag carrier state in children: Controlled trial in an endemic area (Senegal). Lancet 1:289, 1981.

McCracken, G. H., Hardy, J. B., Chen, T. C., et al.: Serum immunoglobulin levels in newborn infants. II. Survey of cord and follow up sera from 123 infants with congenital rubella. J. Pediatr. 74:383, 1969.

McCracken, G. H., Shinefield, H. R., Cobb, K., et al.: Congenital cytomegalic inclusion disease. Am. J. Dis. Child. 117:522, 1969.

Meissner, H. C., Murray, S. A., Kiernan, M. A., et al.: A simultaneous outbreak of respiratory syncytial virus and parainfluenza virus type 3 in a newborn nursery. J. Pediatr. 104:680, 1984.

Meyers, J. D.: Congenital varicella in term infants: Risk reconsidered. J. Infect. Dis. *129*:215, 1974.

Modlin, J. F.: Fatal echovirus II disease in premature neonates. Pediatrics *66*:775, 1980.

MMWR: Varicella-zoster immune globulin distribution—United States and other countries, 1981–1983. MMWR *33*:81, 1984.

MMWR: Rubella and congenital rubella—United States, 1984–1986. MMWR *36*:664, 1987.

MMWR: Prevention of perinatal transmission of hepatitis B virus. MMWR *37*:341, 1988.

MMWR: Rubella vaccination during pregnancy—United States, 1971–1988. MMWR *38*:289, 1989.

MMWR: Summary of Notifiable Diseases, United States. MMWR *38*:8, 1989.

Mortimer, P. P., Cohen, B. J., Buckley, M. M., et al.: Human parvovirus and the fetus. Lancet *2*:1012, 1985.

Murphy, A. M., Albrey, M. B., and Crewe, E. B.: Rotavirus infections in neonates. Lancet *2*:1149, 1977.

Nagington, J., Wreghitt, T. C., Gandy, G., et al.: Fatal echovirus II infections in outbreak in special-care baby unit. Lancet *2*:725, 1978.

Nahmias, A. J., Josey, W. E., Naib, Z. M., et al.: Perinatal risk associated with maternal genital herpes simplex virus infection. Am. J. Obstet. Gynecol. *110*:825, 1971.

Nahmias, A. J., and Roizman, B.: Infection with herpes-simplex viruses 1 and 2. N. Engl. J. Med. *289*:667, 719, 781, 1973.

Okada, K., Kamiyama, I., Inomata, M., et al.: e Antigen and anti-e in the serum of asymptomatic carrier mothers as indicators of positive and negative transmission of hepatitis B virus to their infants. N. Engl. J. Med. *294*:746, 1976.

Onorato, I. M., Morens, D. M., Martone, W. J., and Stansfield, S. K.: Epidemiology of cytomegaloviral infections: Recommendations for prevention and control. Rev. Infect. Dis. *7*:479, 1985.

Overall, J. C., and Glasgow, L. A.: Virus infections of the fetus and newborn infant. J. Pediatr. *77*:315, 1970.

Paryani, S. G., and Arvin, A. M.: Intrauterine infection with varicella-zoster virus after maternal varicella. N. Engl. J. Med. *314*:1542, 1986.

Pass, R. F., Stagno, S., Myers, G. J., and Alford, C. A.: Outcome of symptomatic congenital cytomegalovirus infection: Results of long-term longitudinal follow-up. Pediatrics *66*:758, 1980.

Phelan, P., and Campbell, P.: Pulmonary complications of rubella embryopathy. J. Pediatr. *75*:202, 1969.

Primhak, R. A., and Simpson, R. M. D.: Screening small for gestational age babies for congenital infection. Clin. Pediatr. *21*:417, 1982.

Prober, C. G., Hensleigh, P. A., Boucher, F. D., et al.: Use of routine viral cultures at delivery to identify neonates exposed to herpes simplex virus. N. Engl. J. Med. *318*:887, 1988.

Prober, C. G., Sullender, W. M., Yasukawa, I. L., et al.: Low risk of herpes simplex virus infections in neonates exposed to the virus at the time of vaginal delivery to mothers with recurrent genital herpes simplex virus infections. N. Engl. J. Med. *316*:240, 1987.

Reynolds, D. W., Stagno, S., Hosty, T. S., et al.: Maternal cytomegalovirus excretion and perinatal infection. N. Engl. J. Med. *289*:1, 1973.

Reynolds, D. W., Stagno, S., Stubbs, K. G., et al.: Inapparent congenital cytomegalovirus infection with elevated cord IgM levels: Causal relation with auditory and mental deficiency. N. Engl. J. Med. *290*:291, 1974.

Robino, G., Perlman, A., Togo, Y., et al.: Fatal neonatal infection due to coxsackie B2 virus. J. Pediatr. *61*:911, 1962.

Rudolph, A. J., Singleton, E. B., et al.: Osseous manifestations of congenital rubella syndrome. Am. J. Dis. Child. *110*:428, 1965.

Schrier, R. D., Nelson, J. A., and Oldstone, M. B. A.: Detection of human cytomegalovirus in peripheral blood lymphocytes in a natural infection. Science *230*:1048, 1985.

Sells, C. J., Carpenter, R. L., and Ray, G. C.: Sequelae of central nervous system enterovirus infections. N. Engl. J. Med. *293*:1, 1975.

Shepp, D. H., Dandliker, P. S., de Miranda, P., et al.: Activity of 9-[2-hydroxy-1-(hydroxymethyl)ethoxymethyl]guanine in the treatment of cytomegalovirus pneumonia. Ann. Intern. Med. *103*:368, 1985.

Siegel, M., and Fuerst, H. T.: Low birth weight and maternal virus diseases. J.A.M.A. *197*:680, 1966.

Siegel, M.: Congenital malformations following chicken pox, measles, mumps, and hepatitis: Results of a cohort study. J.A.M.A. *276*:1521, 1973.

Skoldenberg, B., Alestig, K., Burman, L., et al.: Acyclovir versus vidarabine in herpes simplex encephalitis. Lancet *2*:707, 1984.

Soothill, J. E., Hayes, K., and Dudgeon, J. A.: The immunoglobulins in congenital rubella. Lancet *1*:1385, 1966.

South, M. A., Thompkins, W. A. F., Morris, C. R., et al.: Congenital malformation of the central nervous system associated with genital type (type 2) herpes virus. J. Pediatr. *75*:13, 1969.

Spector, S. A.: Transmission of cytomegalovirus among infants in hospital documented by restriction-endonuclease analyses. Lancet *2*:378, 1983.

Srabstein, J. C., Morris, N., Larke, R. P. B., et al.: Is there a congenital varicella syndrome? J. Pediatr. *84*:239, 1974.

Stagno, S., Brasfield, D. M., Brown, M. B., et al.: Infant pneumonitis associated with cytomegalovirus, *Chlamydia, Pneumocystis* and *Ureaplasma:* A prospective study. Pediatrics *68*:322, 1981.

Stagno, S., Pass, R. F., Dworsky, M. E., et al.: Congenital cytomegalovirus infection: The relative importance of primary and recurrent maternal infection. N. Engl. J. Med. *306*:945, 1982.

Stagno, S., Reynolds, D. W., Huang, E. S., et al.: Congenital cytomegalovirus infection: Occurrence in an immune population. N. Engl. J. Med. *296*:1254, 1977.

Stagno, S., and Whitley, R. J.: Herpesvirus infections of pregnancy. Part I: Cytomegalovirus and Epstein-Barr virus infections. N. Engl. J. Med. *313*:1270, 1985.

Stagno, S., and Whitley, R. J.: Herpes-virus infections of pregnancy: II. Herpes simplex virus and varicella-zoster virus infections. N. Engl. J. Med. *313*:1327, 1985.

Starr, J. G., Bart, R. D., Jr., and Gold, E.: Inapparent congenital cytomegalovirus infection: Clinical and epidemiological characteristics in early infancy. N. Engl. J. Med. *282*:1075, 1970.

Steinhoff, M. C.: Rotavirus: The first five years. J. Pediatr. *96*:611, 1980.

Stevens, C. E., Toy, P. J., Tong, M. W., et al.: Perinatal hepatitis B virus transmission in the United States. J.A.M.A. *253*:1740, 1985.

Stevens, C. E., Taylor, P. E., Tong, M. J., et al.: Yeast recombinant hepatitis B vaccine: Efficacy with perinatal hepatitis B virus transmission. J.A.M.A. *257*:2612, 1987.

Summers, P. R., Biswas, M. K., Pastorek, J. G., et al.: The pregnant hepatitis B carrier: Evidence favoring comprehensive antepartum screening. Obstet. Gynecol. *69*:701, 1987.

Tingle, A. J., Chantler, J. K., Pot, K. H., et al.: Postpartum rubella immunization: Association with development of prolonged arthritis, neurologic sequelae, and chronic rubella viremia. J. Infect. Dis. *152*:606, 1985.

Ueda, K., Nishida, Y., Oshina, K., and Shepard, T. H.: Congenital rubella syndrome: Correlation of gestational age at time of maternal rubella with type of defect. J. Pediatr. *94*:763, 1979.

Verder, H., Dickmeiss, E., Haahr, S., et al.: Late-onset rubella syndrome: Coexistence of immune complex disease and defective cytotoxic effector cell function. Clin. Exp. Immunol. *63*:367, 1986.

Vesikari, T., Kapikian, A. Z., Delem, A., and Zissis, G.: A comparative trial of rhesus monkey (RRV-1) and bovine (RIT 4237) oral rotavirus vaccines in young children. J. Infect. Dis. *153*:832, 1986.

Visintine, A. M., Nahmias, A. J., and Josey, W. E.: Genital herpes. Perinatal Care *2*:32, 1978.

Weil, M. L., et al.: Chronic progressive panencephalitis due to rubella virus simulating subacute sclerosing panencephalitis. N. Engl. J. Med. *292*:994, 1975.

Weller, T. H.: The cytomegaloviruses: Ubiquitous agents with protean clinical manifestations. Part I. N. Engl. J. Med. *285*:203, 267, 1971.

Weller, T. H.: The cytomegaloviruses: Ubiquitous agents with protean clinical manifestations. Part II. N. Engl. J. Med. *266*:1233, 1962.

Weller, T. H., and Hanshaw, J. B.: Virologic and clinical observations on cytomegalic inclusion disease. N. Engl. J. Med. *266*:1233, 1962.

Weller, T. H., Macauley, J. C., et al.: Isolation of intranuclear inclusion-producing agents from infants with illnesses resembling cytomegalic inclusion disease. Proc. Soc. Exp. Biol. Med. *94*:4, 1957.

Whitley, R. J.: Herpes simplex virus infections. *In* Remington, J. A., and Klein, J. O. (Eds.): Infectious Diseases of the Fetus and Newborn Infant. Philadelphia, W. B. Saunders Company, 1990, pp. 282–305.

Whitley, R. J., and Hutto, C.: Neonatal herpes simplex virus infections. Pediatr. Rev. *7*:119, 1985.

Whitley, R. J., Nahmias, A. J., Soong, S. -J., et al.: Vidarabine therapy of neonatal herpes simplex virus infections. Pediatrics *66*:495, 1980.

Whitley, R. J., Nahmias, A. J., Visintine, A. M., et al.: The natural history of herpes simplex virus infection of mother and newborn. Pediatrics *66*:489, 1980.

Wilfert, C. M., Thompson, R. J., Sunder, T. R., et al.: Longitudinal assessment of children with enteroviral meningitis during the first three months of life. Pediatrics 67:811, 1981.

Yeager, A. S., and Arvin, A. M.: Reasons for the absence of a history of recurrent genital infections in mothers of neonates infected with herpes simplex virus. Pediatrics 73:188, 1984.

Yeager, A. S., Arvin, A. M., Urbani, L. J., and Kemp, J. A.: The relationship of antibody to outcome in neonatal herpes simplex infections. Infect. Immunol. 29:532, 1980.

Yeager, A. S., Ashley, R. L., and Corey, L.: Transmission of herpes simplex virus from father to neonate. J. Pediatr. 103:905, 1983.

Yeager, A. S., Grumet, F. C., Hafleigh, E. B., et al.: Prevention of transfusion-acquired cytomegalovirus infections in newborn infants. J. Pediatr. 98:281, 1981.

Yeager, A. S., Jacobs, H., and Clark, J.: Nursery-acquired cytomegalovirus infection in two premature infants. J. Pediatr. 81:332, 1972.

Yeager, A. S., Palumbo, P., Malachowski, B., et al.: Sequelae of maternally derived cytomegalovirus infections in premature infants. J. Pediatr. 102:918, 1983.

BACTERIAL 37 INFECTIONS OF THE NEWBORN

F. Sessions Cole*

Changes during the fetal and neonatal period affect the cause of bacterial infections, an infant's response to infection, the agents used for treatment, and the pharmacology of antimicrobial agents. For example, absorption, distribution, metabolism, and excretion of drugs depend in part on the maturity and age of the infant. The administration of a particular drug is determined by the gestational and chronologic age of the infant and cannot be extrapolated from studies of normal adults. Failure to take these physiologic and metabolic factors into account when treating infants with bacterial infection may result in ineffective or toxic drug therapy.

■ USE OF ANTIBIOTICS IN NEWBORNS

The selection of antibiotic therapy in newborn infants depends on (1) general historical experience with infections in the nursery, (2) the susceptibility of commonly encountered bacterial pathogens, (3) the physician's familiarity with antibiotic pharmacokinetics in newborn infants, and (4) the physician's knowledge of maternal infections, course of labor, and antibiotic treatment administered to the mother. Pediatricians must know which are the most common organisms that cause disease in the nurseries and the current antimicrobial susceptibilities of these organisms. Moreover, it has been shown in many instances that the judicious use of antibiotics in nurseries limits the emergence and spread of resistant bacteria. Vertical transmission of organisms from the mother to the fetus must also be taken into account in the selection of antibiotics.

Generally, as few antibiotics as possible should be used to treat individual infections and, whenever possible, single-drug therapy should be employed. Frequently, however, combining two drugs is good medical practice. This is true at the initiation of treatment, before culture and sensitivity data are available, in covering wide range of likely bacterial species that cause newborn sepsis, or, sometimes, after the organism has been identified to take advantage of antibiotic synergy in widespread and severe infections by bacteria that are difficult to eliminate with a single drug.

Bacterial sepsis is frequently suspected in newborn infants because of nonspecific symptoms and signs. Usually, cultures are taken and antibiotics are administered only to reveal that, after 48 to 72 hours, the cultures are sterile. Not infrequently, the child improves during this interval. At this time, the pediatrician must use clinical judgment. If the cultures were obtained from the proper sites in the proper way and if the particular microbiology laboratory used is reliable, it is usually wise to discontinue antibiotics at this point and re-evaluate the child at frequent intervals thereafter. However, if an infant's mother was treated with antibiotics and the infant has persuasive evidence of infection, then it is prudent to continue the antibiotics for at least 7 days. Sometimes, culture results are difficult to interpret (for example, *Staphylococcus epidermidis* from a blood culture; gram-negative organisms from a tracheal aspirate in a long-term occupant of the nursery). In these instances, a knowledge of the pathogenicity of these organisms in newborn infants should be combined with information on the clinical appearance of the infant and other laboratory data so that a plan that minimizes the use of antibiotics can be developed.

Although antibiotics are commonly used in an attempt to prevent infection of newborn infants, the efficacy of this approach is limited to a few well-defined circumstances. A good example of one such circumstance is the use of topical 1 per cent silver nitrate, tetracycline, or erythromycin to prevent ophthalmia neonatorum. However, when antibiotics are used as "broad coverage" against many potential pathogens for extended intervals, they are rarely effective. This type of chemoprophylaxis encourages the emergence of resistant strains among previously susceptible bacteria and causes the alteration of the normal bacterial flora of the gastrointestinal and respiratory tracts.

Table 37–1 is a guide for treating neonatal bacterial diseases. Modification of these schedules is necessary to take into account the gestational and chronologic age of the infant, the specific infectious agent(s) that is suspected or documented, the tissue site(s) being treated, the status of excretory (hepatic or renal) function of the infant, and the cardiopulmonary stability of the infant.

■ PATHOGENESIS OF NEONATAL INFECTIONS

Throughout pregnancy, the infant is usually protected from bacterial infections by the chorioamniotic mem-

---

*This chapter includes some contributions from previous authors, Drs. Alexander Schaffer, George H. McCracken, Jr., Jorge B. Howard, and Kenneth McIntosh.

350

TABLE 37–1. Dosage Recommendations for Antibiotics Commonly Used in Newborn Infants*

DRUG	ROUTE	INFANTS < 7 DAYS OF AGE			INFANTS > 7 DAYS OF AGE†
		< 30 Weeks' Gestation†	30–37 Weeks' Gestation†	> 37 Weeks' Gestation†	
Amikacin‡	IV, IM	7.5 q 24 hr	10.0 q 24 hr	7.5 q 12 hr	7.5–10.0 q 8–q 12 hr
Ampicillin§	IV, IM	50 q 12 hr	75 q 12 hr	100 q 12 hr	100 q 8 hr
Cefotaxime	IV, IM	50 q 12 hr	50 q 12 hr	50 q 8 hr	50 q 6 hr
Ceftazidime	IV, IM	30 q 12 hr	50 q 12 hr	50 q 8 hr	50 q 6 hr
Ceftriaxone	IV, IM	50 q 24 hr	75 q 24 hr	75 q 12 hr	75 q 12 hr
Chloramphenicol‡	IV	2.5 q 6 hr	5.0 q 6 hr	5.0 q 6 hr	12.5 q 6 hr
Clindamycin‡	IV	5.0 q 8 hr	7.5 q 8 hr	10 mg q 6 hr	10 mg q 6 hr
Erythromycin	IV	10 q 12 hr	15 q 12 hr	20 q 12 hr	20 q 12 hr
Gentamicin‡	IV, IM	2.5 q 24 hr	3.0 q 24 hr	2.5 q 12 hr	2.5 q 8–q 12 hr
Methicillin	IV	25 q 12 hr	35 q 12 hr	50 q 8 hr	50 q 6–q 8 hr
Nafcillin	IV	25 q 12 hr	35 q 12 hr	50 q 8 hr	50 q 6–q 8 hr
Oxacillin	IV	25 q 12 hr	35 q 12 hr	50 q 8 hr	50 q 6–18 hr
Penicillin G§	IV, IM	25,000 IU IV q 12 hr	50,000 IU IV q 12 hr	50,000 IU IV q 8 hr	50,000 IU IV q am
Piperacillin	IV, IM	50 q 12 hr	75 q 12 hr	100 q 8 hr	100 q 6 hr
Tobramycin‡	IV	2.5 q 24 hr	3.0 q 24 hr	2.5 q 12 hr	2.5 q 8–q 12 hr
Vancomycin‡	IV	18 q 24 hr	15 q 12 hr	10 q 8 hr	10 q 6 hr

*All dosages given represent approximate schedule for initiation of therapy. These dosages should be individualized for specific clinical situations.
†mg/kg/dose
‡Dosage should be individually adjusted for each infant by monitoring serum drug concentrations
§For meningitis, double recommended dosage

branes, the placenta, and poorly understood antibacterial factors in amniotic fluid. Most viruses, especially herpes simplex, cytomegalovirus, human immunodeficiency virus-1, and rubella can infect the fetus prior to membrane rupture. Under normal circumstances, at delivery and during the immediate neonatal period, the infant is exposed to many organisms, including aerobic and anaerobic bacteria, viruses, fungi, and protozoa. This encounter initiates colonization of the respiratory and gastrointestinal tracts (Sprunt, 1985). Most newborns establish their microbial flora without incident; however, an occasional infant develops disease caused by one of these organisms. The factors contributing to conversion from colonization to disease are not completely understood (Goldmann et al., 1983; Sprunt, 1985).

There appear to be four separate mechanisms by which bacteria reach the fetus or newborn to cause infection. First, certain bacteria (particularly *Treponema pallidum*, *Listeria monocytogenes*, and *Mycobacterium tuberculosis*) can reach the fetus through the maternal bloodstream, despite placental protective mechanisms, causing transplacental infection. This process is an uncommon event, but it leads either to congenital infection not unlike infections caused by certain viruses or *Toxoplasma* or to stillbirth resulting from overwhelming infection. Second, it seems likely that many early-onset group B streptococcal diseases are the result of infection that occurs immediately before delivery (Baker, 1978). The bacteria appear to be acquired from the vagina or cervix through either ruptured or intact membranes, leading to amnionitis, pneumonitis, and premature delivery. The role of the cytokine interleukin 1 (IL-1) in the induction of preterm labor resulting from bacterial infection has recently been suggested by Romero and colleagues (1989). Third, infection may occur during passage through the birth canal at the time of delivery. Gonococcal ophthalmia and most infections of *Escherichia coli* appear to develop in this manner. In some instances (e.g., late-onset group B streptococcal infection), coloni-

zation may occur at the time of birth. The mechanisms by which colonization contributes to late-onset (occurring weeks to months later) infection are poorly understood. Genetic and developmental immunoregulatory mechanisms are most likely involved. Finally, bacteria can be introduced after birth from the environment surrounding the baby, either in the nursery or at home.

The two most common bacterial pathogens in term infants in the first 28 days of life are the group B streptococcus and *E. coli*. These two organisms account for approximately 70 per cent of systemic neonatal bacterial diseases. Either organism may be acquired from the mother during the intrapartum period, from the father, or from nosocomial acquisition. The acute (early-onset [occurring within the first 7 days of life]) septicemic form of group B streptococcal disease may be caused by any of the group B serotypes (Ia, Ib, Ic, II, or III). The frequency of recovery of individual group B streptococcal serotypes that cause disease approximates the frequency of serotypes usually found in the maternal genitourinary tract. Epidemiologic studies have shown that from 5 to 30 per cent of pregnant women are vaginally or rectally colonized with group B streptococci. Approximately one-half the infants of colonized mothers are themselves asymptomatically colonized at birth, and a similar number acquire the organism without disease from the environment (Siegel et al., 1980; Yow et al., 1979). The major colonization sites in the infant are the skin, the nasopharynx, and the rectum. The group B streptococcus persists in the nasopharynx and rectum for weeks to months. It has been estimated that for every 100 infants colonized with group B streptococci, one infant develops disease caused by this organism (Baker and Barrett, 1973). Therefore, colonization is not a sole indication for systemic antibiotic treatment (Evans et al., 1988).

Group B streptococcal meningitis is caused almost exclusively by organisms of serotype III. These organisms may be acquired from sources other than the mother.

Clusters of three or four cases of meningitis caused by group B streptococci have occurred in nurseries during short time periods, suggesting nosocomial acquisition.

Certain studies have shown that approximately 80 per cent of *E. coli* strains that cause neonatal meningitis possess a single, specific capsular polysaccharide antigen, which has been designated as K1 (Robbins et al., 1974). This is remarkable when one considers that there are over 100 recognized K antigens associated with *E. coli* strains. In contrast, approximately 40 per cent of *E. coli* strains that cause neonatal septicemia possess K1 and only 10 to 15 per cent of strains that cause septicemia and urinary tract infections in adults contain this antigen.

The reason for this association between K1 antigen and *E. coli* strains that cause neonatal meningitis and, to a lesser degree, septicemia is unknown. The K1 polysaccharide is chemically identical to that found in the capsule of group B meningococci. Animal studies have demonstrated that *E. coli* possessing K1 are highly virulent for mice and that this lethal effect can be completely prevented by the pretreatment of mice with minute amounts of specific K1 antibody (Robbins et al., 1974). Furthermore, the outcome of neonatal meningitis is directly correlated with the presence, concentration, and persistence of K1 antigen in the cerebrospinal fluid and blood of these infants (McCracken et al., 1974). Work by Edwards and associates (1982) with group B streptococci has suggested that a specific polysaccharide (sialic acid) found in the outer capsules of both K1 *E. coli* and group B streptococcus prevents the activation of the alternative complement pathway and thereby may account for the virulence of these organisms.

Extensive epidemiologic studies have shown that approximately 20 to 30 per cent of newborn babies are colonized rectally with *E. coli* (Sarff et al., 1975). This percentage may rise to 50 per cent during the 2nd and 3rd weeks of life (Peter and Nelson, 1978). Thirty to forty per cent of normal infants and children demonstrate K1 organisms on rectal swab culture, as do nearly 50 per cent of women at the time of delivery. Approximately two-thirds of babies born to K1-positive mothers are colonized with the identical serotypes of *E. coli* K1. Vertical transmission of these organisms has been documented in 70 per cent of newborns with *E. coli* K1 meningitis and is the major route of neonatal gastrointestinal colonization. The colonization to disease ratio for *E. coli* K1 is similar to that observed for group B streptococci; that is, approximately 100 to 200:1. Nosocomial infection with *E. coli* K1 has also been noted.

Although the pathogenesis of neonatal group B streptococcal and *E. coli* K1 disease has not been completely elucidated, a reasonable hypothesis can be proposed. Studies in children and adults have clearly demonstrated that protection from disease caused by pneumococci, meningococci, and *Hemophilus influenzae* type B is afforded by specific antibodies directed against the capsular polysaccharides possessed by these organisms. A lack of type-specific antibody in sera from infants and their mothers with neonatal streptococcal disease due to serotype III has been documented (Baker and Kasper, 1976). A lack of K1 antibody in the sera of neonates predisposes them to *E. coli* K1 disease as well. Mouse protection studies lend credence to this hypothesis.

Although this discussion has centered on only two organisms that cause neonatal disease, there are considerable data supporting the importance of vertical transmission of other microorganisms during the intrapartum period. These include *Listeria monocytogenes*, anaerobic bacteria (Chow et al., 1974), *Chlamydia* (Frommell et al., 1979), *Candida albicans* (Kozinn et al., 1958), and viruses such as cytomegalovirus and *Herpesvirus hominis*.

■ SEPTICEMIA

Neonatal sepsis (Siegel and McCracken, 1981) is a disease of infants who are less than 1 month of age, are clinically ill, and have positive blood cultures. The presence of clinical manifestations distinguishes this condition from the transient bacteremia observed in some healthy newborns.

The incidence of neonatal sepsis is between 1 and 4 cases per 1000 live births for full-term and premature infants, respectively. Among very-low-birth-weight infants who are undergoing prolonged hospitalization, the incidence increases dramatically to 300 per 1000 very-low-birth-weight infants. These incidence rates vary from nursery to nursery and depend on the presence of conditions that predispose infants to infection.

Diagnosis of Sepsis: Predisposing Factors. Although multiple factors have been associated with increased risk of bacterial infection within the first 7 days of life, the most important factors are the degree of prematurity of the infant and maternal medical conditions that may predispose the infant to fetal or neonatal infection, e.g., preterm labor, maternal genitourinary tract infection, or chorioamnionitis (Ferguson et al., 1985; Hillier et al., 1988; Hollander, 1986; St. Geme et al., 1984; Sperling et al., 1988). The more premature the infant, the higher the risk of infection. Maternal or fetal infection probably contributes to initiation of preterm labor and a significant proportion of preterm births. The considerable rates of morbidity and mortality associated with bacterial infection in the newborn infant have prompted multiple investigations to develop risk evaluation methods that use information on maternal infection, fetal problems, and the initial evaluation of the infant (Philip and Hewitt, 1980). Unfortunately, the spectrum of variables requires individualized decision-making for each patient. For example, duration of rupture of membranes before onset of labor, the latent period, or time before delivery has been investigated by several authors (Blackmon et al., 1986). None was able to demonstrate a significant difference in culture-proven sepsis with prolongation of the interval from rupture to delivery (Garite and Freeman, 1982). However, maternal medical risk factors should prompt suspicion of infection, more intense monitoring of vital signs, and active consideration of the need for cultures and antimicrobial therapy. Risk factors that should be considered in judging the probability that a child is infected are listed in Table 37–2.

Antenatal treatment of fetuses at risk for infection has improved infant outcome by decreasing the frequency of bacteremia (Baker, 1986). Boyer and Gotoff (1986) reported that none of 85 infants whose high-risk mothers received ampicillin developed bacteremia, whereas 5 of

TABLE 37–2. Conditions That Increase the Risk of Systemic Bacterial Infection in Newborn Infants During the First 7 Days of Life

Family history of sibling with systemic bacterial disease under 3 months of age
Maternal Conditions
  Premature or prolonged time between rupture of membranes and delivery
  Chorioamnionitis
  Urinary tract infection
Labor Characteristics
  Preterm labor
  Fetal tachycardia without maternal fever, blood loss, hypotension, or tachycardia-inducing medication
Infant Characteristics
  Apgar < 6 at 5 minutes
  Meconium-stained amniotic fluid
  Oxygen requirement
  Fever
  Neutropenia
  Male sex
  Congenital anomalies that cause breakdown of anatomic barriers to infection
  Polymorphonuclear leukocytes and intracellular organisms in gastric aspirate

79 controls did develop the disease (P = 0.024). They suggested that selective intrapartum chemoprophylaxis can prevent early-onset neonatal group B streptococcal disease.

Among infants older than 7 days of age who require neonatal intensive care, maternal risk factors become less important in predicting the risk of sepsis than the degree of prematurity, the presence of central venous or arterial catheters, poor skin integrity, and malnutrition. Attempts at preventing infection in these high-risk infants through the use of systemic prophylactic antibiotics only serve to increase the risk of selecting multiply resistant organisms and systemic opportunistic infection, especially with *Candida* species. As discussed later, the most common systemic isolate in this group is *Staphylococcus epidermidis*.

Diagnosis of Sepsis: Clinical Manifestations. The early signs and symptoms of septicemia in term or preterm infants younger than and older than 7 days of age are usually nonspecific. Early temperature imbalance with transient hyper- or hypothermia occurs in approximately 66 per cent of septic infants (Table 37–3) (Bonadio, 1988). Respiratory distress or apnea occurs in 55 per cent of septic infants. Other symptoms include tachycardia, lethargy, vomiting, or diarrhea, and unwillingness to breast-feed may be noted. Conjugated hyperbilirubinemia, petechiae, seizures, and hepatosplenomegaly are late signs that usually denote a poor prognosis.

Although it is tempting to recommend a work-up for septicemia in all infants with nonspecific clinical manifestations, this approach is both impractical and unnecessary in many instances. A complete history and physical examination, longitudinal and regular (q 1 hour to q 4 hour) assessment of symptoms and vital signs, and clinical experience are the best guides in determining the timing and extent of evaluation. Infants who are deteriorating on the basis of clinical manifestations should be strongly considered for evaluation and treatment. For example, full-term infants who require increased ambient oxygen shortly after birth should be considered for evaluation and

treatment if their respiratory distress is not improving or is getting worse by 6 hours of age.

Making the Diagnosis of Sepsis. The diagnosis of systemic bacterial infection must start with a careful evaluation of the infant's signs and symptoms, physical examination, information on longitudinal changes in vital signs and laboratory indicators, and history including maternal history and relevant recent nursery history. The diagnosis is predicated on recovery of the organism(s) from the blood or other sites. Blood (usually a minimum of 0.5 ml) may be obtained from a peripheral vein or from the umbilical vessels immediately following sterile umbilical vessel catheterization. Femoral vein aspiration should be avoided because of both potential contamination with coliform organisms from the perineum and the danger of inadvertent penetration of the hip joint capsule. It is frequently helpful to obtain cultures from other sites (e.g., cerebrospinal fluid or urine) prior to initiating antimicrobial therapy. For example, using percutaneous bladder aspiration of urine for culture is frequently helpful in identifying the urinary tract as the focus of infection or in recovering antigens as evidence of bacteremia (e.g., latex agglutination test for group B streptococcus) (Hamoudi et al., 1983). In contrast, surface cultures or urine collected in urine bags do not provide useful information for determination of which antibiotic agent should be used, the duration of therapy, or the prognosis (Evans et al., 1988). Microscopic examination of material obtained from gastric aspiration for leukocytes and bacteria has been advocated as a means of identifying infants who are at risk of developing systemic bacterial disease (Hamoudi et al., 1983). The presence of amniotic fluid infection increases the risk of systemic infection in a full-term infant from 1 to 5 per 1000 live births to 5 per 100 live births (Siegel and McCracken, 1981).

Measuring the peripheral white blood cell count and differential is a useful and rapid test, but it is nonspecific (Philip and Hewitt, 1980). If the total count is under 5000 or if the band-to-neutrophil ratio exceeds or is equal to 0.2, bacterial sepsis should be strongly considered. The

TABLE 37–3. Clinical Signs of Bacterial Sepsis and Meningitis*

CLINICAL SIGN	PER CENT OF INFANTS WITH SIGN	
	Sepsis	Meningitis
Hyperthermia	51	61
Hypothermia	15	—
Respiratory distress	33	47
Apnea	22	7
Cyanosis	24	—
Jaundice	35	28
Hepatomegaly	33	32
Anorexia	28	49
Vomiting	25	—
Abdominal distention	17	—
Diarrhea	11	17
Convulsions	—	40
Building or full fontanel	—	28
Nuchal rigidity	—	15

*Data from 455 infants studied at four medical centers.

(From Klein, J. O.: Current concepts of infectious diseases in the newborn infant. Curr. Prob. Pediatr. *31*:405–446, 1984.)

normal range of white blood cell counts in newborn infants is wide, and this wide range should be taken into account in interpreting the values (Manroe et al., 1979). Other tests, such as sedimentation rate, C-reactive protein, haptoglobin concentration, and nitroblue tetrazolium have been extensively evaluated but are rarely more useful than the history, the physical examination, and careful longitudinal evaluation of the infant's status.

Etiology. Through the years, there has been a shift in the microorganisms responsible for neonatal septicemia and meningitis. This is clearly illustrated by the experience at Yale–New Haven Hospital (Freedman et al., 1981; Kumar and Delivoria-Papadopoulos, 1985; Spigelblatt et al., 1985). During the 1930s, group A streptococci were the predominant organisms. In the 1950s, staphylococci (largely of phage group I) became a major cause of nursery outbreaks throughout the world. *Pseudomonas* was prominent during the same decade, perhaps because of the introduction of respiratory support systems. From the late 1950s to the present, *E. coli* has been an important cause of neonatal sepsis. The dramatic rise in incidence of group B streptococcal infections is notable and has been reflected in other centers as well. Both group D streptococci and *Klebsiella* are pathogens that have been found relatively recently, the latter accounting for a high proportion of antibiotic-resistant organisms that colonize and infect babies in neonatal intensive care units (Goldmann et al., 1978). During the 1980s, *Staphylococcus epidermidis* has been recovered from systemic cultures with increasing frequency (Battisti et al., 1981; Kumar and Delivoria-Papadopoulos, 1985). This organism is most commonly seen in infants who are premature and who have required prolonged maintenance with central vascular catheters, peritoneal dialysis, or thoracostomy tubes. In most intensive care nurseries, this organism is the most common nosocomial systemic isolate. The prevalence rates for a specific bacterial pathogen vary from nursery to nursery and may change rather abruptly. Knowledge of the most commonly isolated bacteria in a nursery or intensive care unit, coupled with the antimicrobial susceptibilities of these organisms, is invaluable in treating suspected neonatal sepsis.

Streptococcal Disease. The group B streptococcus is the most common gram-positive organism that causes septicemia and meningitis during the 1st month of life in infants older than 37 weeks' gestational age. Vertical transmission of this organism from mother to infant is one route of infection. Nosocomial acquisition of infection has been implicated in some nurseries and may be more common than was thought previously. The incidence of group B streptococcal disease has varied widely. However, despite this variability, group B streptococcus has been noted as an important neonatal pathogen since 1938 (Broughton et al., 1981; Eisenfeld et al., 1983; Freedman et al., 1981; Fry, 1938; Siegel et al., 1980; Spigelblatt et al., 1985).

The most common clinical manifestations of group B streptococcal infections are septicemia, pneumonia, and meningitis, but other more localized syndromes also occur, including osteomyelitis and septic arthritis, otitis media, cellulitis, and conjunctivitis as well as asymptomatic bacteremia. Generalized disease takes two clinically and epidemiologically distinct forms, early- and late-onset infection (Ferrieri, 1985). By definition the early form occurs in the first 7 days of life, usually within hours of delivery (mean age 20 hours) and up to 50 per cent of affected infants are symptomatic at birth. Infants with the early form of the disease usually deteriorate within hours of delivery and may exhibit unexplained apnea or tachypnea, respiratory distress with hypoxia, and shock (Christensen et al., 1983). Chest roentgenograms reveal a diffuse pulmonary infiltrate that may be indistinguishable from the pathologic findings characteristic of hyaline membrane disease. In some instances, disease that occurs in utero may precipitate premature delivery. The mortality rate is 20 to 25 per cent. Pneumonitis is the primary finding on pathologic examination, and post-mortem cultures of the lung, blood, cerebrospinal fluid yield group B organisms. Approximately 30 per cent of infants have concomitant meningitis (Baker, 1986).

The late onset meningitic form of disease is exhibited at 1 to 12 weeks of age and is indistinguishable from the other forms of purulent meningitis. Group B streptococci are grown from cultures of blood and cerebrospinal fluid, and the mortality rate is 20 to 40 per cent. The principal organism appears to be serotype III. The pathogenesis is uncertain.

Group A Streptococcal Disease. Group A streptococcal disease is not as common now as in previous decades (Dillon, 1966; Eisenfeld et al., 1983). The severity of disease caused by this organism varies from a low-grade, chronic omphalitis to fulminant septicemia and meningitis. Because of the explosive nature of outbreaks in nursery settings, surveillance for colonized infants is probably indicated at the time the organism is found or when infant infections are recognized (see the discussion of nosocomial infections).

Group D Streptococcal Disease. Group D streptococci include the enterococci and several other species, particularly *S. bovis*, which have been found in neonatal infection. Enterococci tend to be resistant to penicillin, and therefore ampicillin, with or without an aminoglycoside such as kanamycin or gentamicin, should be used. For nonenterococcal strains, penicillin may be adequate. The incidence of these infections appears to have increased in many centers, and they are recognized as often as, or more often than, those caused by *E. coli* (Siegel and McCracken, 1978). The clinical pattern of the disease is remarkably similar to that seen with group B streptococci (Alexander and Giacoia, 1978) and is frequently associated with complicated deliveries. With prompt and appropriate antibiotic therapy, however, prognosis appears to be somewhat better.

Infection with Streptococcus Viridans. Two reports (Broughton et al., 1981; Spigelblatt et al., 1985) have discussed the emergence of *Streptococcus viridans* as an important neonatal pathogen. In contrast to infants with systemic group B streptococcal infection, infants with *Streptococcus viridans* disease present later (mean age 3.5 days), exhibit leukopenia less frequently, and are less likely to have respiratory distress (Spigelblatt et al., 1985).

Staphylococcal Disease. In the 1950s, phage group I *Staphylococcus aureus* was the most common bacterial agent that caused septicemia in neonatal units. Its unique invasive properties caused disseminated disease with widespread manifestations, including neonatal mastitis, furunculosis, septic arthritis, osteomyelitis, and septicemia. Because infection of the bloodstream is usually secondary to local invasion, a careful search for the primary focus must be made in all septic babies. Microbial surveillance, intensified infection control measures, and increased local skin care have reduced colonization and disease rates caused by the group I organism.

In the 1970s, coagulase-positive staphylococcal disease in nurseries was caused by organisms of the phage II group (Melish and Glasgow, 1971). These organisms produce an exotoxin (exfoliatin) that causes intraepidermal cleavage through the granular cell layer due to disruption of desmosomes (Melish et al., 1972). Clinical disease may take one of several forms, which include bullous impetigo, toxic epidermal necrolysis, Riter disease, and nonstreptococcal scarlatina. The initial findings in Ritter disease are intense, painful erythema that is similar to a severe sunburn. Over the next few hours, bullae may form that, when ruptured, leave a tender, weeping erythematous area. The characteristic desquamation of large epidermal sheets occurs approximately 3 to 5 days after the onset of the illness. A fine desquamation is commonly seen in the perioral region. Bullous impetigo has been the most common disease associated with nursery outbreaks of phage group II staphylococcal infections.

In the 1980s, two additional kinds of staphylococcal infections have been recognized as major contributors to nursery infections, namely methicillin-resistant *Staphylococcus aureus* (MRSA) and *Staphylococcus epidermidis.* Since the early 1980s, adult surgical and medical intensive care units in the United States and other countries have noted an increase in nosocomially acquired and community-acquired MRSA (Bartokas et al., 1984; Saravolatz et al., 1982; Thompson and Wenzel, 1982; Wenzel, 1982). Similarly, MRSA outbreaks have been reported with increasing frequency in neonatal intensive care units (Battisti et al., 1981; Gilbert et al., 1982; Reboli et al., 1989). Although standard infection control measures including contact isolation, hand-washing with chlorhexidine, and cohorting are frequently used to control outbreaks, eradication of MRSA may require hand-washing with hexachlorophene (Reboli et al., 1989). The population at highest risk for colonization or infection include infants under 1500 g with long-standing central vascular catheters, thoracostomy tubes, or central nervous system shunts, or those infants undergoing prolonged hospitalization after surgical procedures (Storch and Rajagopazan, 1986). When colonization with MRSA is noted and clinical deterioration suggestive of systemic infection occurs, some authors have strongly suggested the inclusion of vancomycin in the initial antibiotic administration. Vancomycin has been shown to be effective therapy for systemic MRSA infection in both adults and children (Myers and Linnemann, 1982; Schaad et al., 1980). However, regular use of vancomycin may cause the development of vancomycin-resistant organisms. Decisions concerning the use of antibiotics must be individualized and predicated on the clinical condition and history of the infant, the microbiologic history of the nursery, and the contribution of indwelling catheters. Routine surveillance for MRSA in individual nurseries may be necessary if outbreaks or endemic colonization and infection are observed.

In conjunction with the emergence of MRSA as a major neonatal pathogen during the decade of the 1980s, coagulase-negative staphylococci, collectively known as *S. epidermidis,* have assumed considerable importance as troublesome nosocomial pathogens in the neonatal intensive care unit (Fleer et al., 1986; Kumar and Delivoria-Papadopoulos, 1985). Similar to MRSA, these organisms are most frequently isolated from the smallest and sickest infants, many of whom have indwelling central vascular catheters, thoracostomy tubes or central nervous system shunts (Battisti et al., 1981; Donowitz et al., 1987; Fleer et al., 1983; Noel and Edelson, 1984; Verhoef and Fleer, 1983). In contrast to MRSA infection, infants infected with coagulase-negative staphylococci have indolent presentations and infrequently develop metastatic focal infection. Although central venous catheters and contaminated hyperalimentation solutions have both been associated with *S. epidermidis* bacteremia, the surface hydrophobicity of the organism as well as opsonic differences in neonatal sera are more likely pathogenic mechanisms (Fleer et al., 1983; Fleer et al., 1985; Pascual et al., 1988). In addition, after adherence to a hydrophobic polymer used in biomaterials, e.g., teflon, these organisms produce a thick layer of amorphous material called extracellular slime (Marrie and Costerton, 1984). This substance may permit the organism to escape phagocytosis by polymorphonuclear leukocytes (Johnson et al., 1986). Treatment of these infections is also complicated by the high frequency of penicillin- and gentamicin-resistant strains. Most strains remain sensitive to vancomycin. In some cases, removal of all vascular catheters in conjunction with the administration of a penicillin and aminoglycoside is sufficient for sterilizing the bloodstream. Use of vancomycin should be reserved for those infections that involve a catheter or anatomic site that cannot be readily removed or surgically approached (e.g., a heart valve) (Bryant, 1982), or that does not respond to initial antibiotic therapy. Epidemiologic studies of *S. epidermidis* in individual nurseries have had to take into account multiple epidemiologic markers (Parisi and Hecht, 1980; Renaud et al., 1988). The recent development of restriction endonuclease analysis of DNA from clinical isolates provides a single epidemiologic marker that has both stability and discriminating capacity and can thus be used to analyze outbreaks of systemic infection (Renaud et al., 1988). Specifically, restriction endonuclease analysis permits characterization of plasmids within strains by size and provides the opportunity to identify specific resistance characteristics encoded on these plasmids. This epidemiologic marker should be used if outbreaks of *S. epidermidis* infection occur.

Infection with *Listeria monocytogenes.* *Listeria* is a small, motile gram-positive rod that grows slowly in the laboratory and that can be mistaken for either corynebacteria or streptococci in Gram stains. It is a facultative intracellular parasite that is found widely in the animal kingdom, and infections in humans are sometimes seen as a result of contact with domestic animals or contaminated food (Schlech et al., 1983). As with group B streptococcal infections, there are two forms, early- and late-onset infection. Early-onset infections are acquired transplacentally or during passage through the vaginal canal. In such instances, fetal death and abortion may result or the child may be born with hepatosplenomegaly, disseminated disease, and granulomatous papules on the trunk and oral mucous membranes. This form of the disease has been called "granulomatosis infantisepticum." Perinatal complications are common in this group, and the prognosis is often grave (Teberg et al., 1987). A mortality rate of up to 60 per cent has been reported in newborn infants with *Listeria* sepsis (Ahlfors et al., 1977; Barresi, 1980). Although precise incidence figures are not available, early-onset disease caused by *Listeria* occurs much less frequently (1.5 cases per 10,000 deliveries) than group B streptococcal disease (10 to 40 cases per 10,000 deliveries) (Boucher and Yonekora, 1986). The contribution of *Listeria* to perinatal morbidity and mortality is similarly poorly defined, but *Listeria* is estimated to be involved in 0.5 to 3.0 per cent of perinatal deaths. In the United States, for children under 1 year of age, a rate of 7.2 per million population has been reported. Late-onset disease takes the form of meningitis (Visintine et al., 1977), which occurs usually in the 2nd week of life but also may occur as late as the 4th or 5th week. The cerebrospinal fluid is highly cellular, the glucose is almost always markedly depressed, and monocytes are often seen on the smear, although they are usually not the predominant cell type. Diagnosis is predicated on isolation of the organism, because serologic tests do not provide adequate sensitivity (Hudak et al., 1984). Interestingly, the early-onset type of listeriosis, as with group B streptococcal disease, reflects the genital colonization of the mother and can be one of several serotypes. Meningitis, on the other hand, is almost always caused by type IV B and is usually acquired from the environment (Albritton et al., 1976). The prognosis of the meningitic form is relatively good with regard to both survival and sequelae. Ampicillin plus gentamicin or kanamycin should be given for the first 5 to 7 days, followed by ampicillin alone to complete a 2-week course. The combination of ampicillin and an aminoglycoside has been shown to kill listeria more rapidly than either drug alone (Gordon et al., 1972). Interestingly, follow-up studies suggest that newborn infants infected with *Listeria* at birth evidence little or no immunologic response to *Listeria* (opsonizing activity, anti-*Listeria* antibody titer, or lymphocyte proliferation in response to *Listeria*) at one year of age (Issekutz et al., 1984).

Infection with *Escherichia coli.* *E. coli* is the most common gram-negative bacteria that causes septicemia during the neonatal period. Approximately 40 per cent of *E. coli* strains that cause septicemia possess K1 capsular antigen, and strains identical with that in blood can usually be identified in the patient's nasopharynx or rectal cultures (see previous discussion of pathogenesis of neonatal infections). The clinical features of *E. coli* septicemia are generally similar to those observed in infants with disease caused by other pathogens. Recent advances in understanding the role of regular antibiotic usage in the selection of specific resistance plasmids, the efficacy of immunoglobulin replacement therapy in the treatment of *E. coli* and other gram-negative infections, the development of specific molecular probes for identification and characterization of plasmids that encode resistance factors, and

enhanced recognition of the importance of prevention through the use of vaccines and, in developing countries, through the provision of clear water, safe waste disposal, and hygiene education may act in concert over the decade of the 1990s to reduce the incidence of neonatal disease caused by *E. coli* (Bortolussi, 1986; Cates et al., 1988; Rennels and Levine, 1986; Shaio et al., 1989; Tullus and Berman, 1989).

***Pseudomonas* Septicemia.** *Pseudomonas* septicemia may present with one or several characteristic violaceous papular lesions that, after several days, develop central necrosis. Although this condition is most commonly observed in *Pseudomonas* infection, it may also be associated with other pathogens. The newborn who receives broad-spectrum antibiotics while in an environment that is potentially contaminated by bacteria from respirators or moist oxygen is likely to develop disease caused by *Pseudomonas* species or other fastidious organisms.

Infection with Nontypable *Haemophilus influenzae.* Although fewer than 50 cases of neonatal sepsis due to nontypeable *Haemophilus influenzae* were reported between 1909 and 1981, during the decade of the 1980s this organism has become a well-recognized neonatal pathogen that accounts in some centers for up to 7.9 per cent of all cases of neonatal sepsis (Campognone and Singer, 1986; Eisenfeld et al., 1983; Wallace et al., 1983). Infants infected with this organism generally present with fulminant infection, exhibit neutropenia, and are born prematurely. The most common biotypes recovered are biotype II and III (Campognone and Singer, 1986). Approximately 20 per cent of *H. influenzae* isolates recovered from the newborns are encapsulated (Biotype I) (Wallace et al., 1983). The increasing frequency of this organism should prompt consideration of ampicillin as one of the antibiotics included in the initial treatment of potentially septic newborn infants.

Prevention. Reports that there are surprisingly low rates of early-onset group B streptococcal disease in institutions in which infants receive an intramuscular dose of penicillin G at birth prompted considerable interest in this approach as a method of prevention (Siegel et al., 1980; Steigman et al., 1978). Others have screened women toward the end of pregnancy and have treated carriers of group B streptococci with one or two intravenous doses of ampicillin to prevent transmission to the newborn (Yow et al., 1979). However, the possibility exists that penicillin-resistant infections might increase and might obliterate the benefit provided by a reduction in group B streptococcal disease (Siegel et al., 1980). Use of selective intrapartum chemoprophylaxis is a useful preventive approach (Boyer and Gotoff, 1986). Identification of women at risk for delivering infected infants because of premature rupture of the membranes, preterm labor, or colonization of group B streptococci close to the time of delivery should prompt consideration of the initiation of antibiotic therapy prior to delivery. For a review of the use of maternal immunization as a method of prevention, see Chapter 34 (Immunology).

Therapy. Before the definitive diagnosis of septicemia is made and prior to the availability of microbial susceptibility studies, antibiotic therapy should be initiated using a combination that includes a penicillin and an aminoglycoside. The choice of antibiotics must be based on the historical experience of the nursery, the antimicrobial susceptibilities of bacteria recently isolated from both sick and healthy newborns, and the maternal history. For initial therapy, ampicillin in combination with gentamicin is a reasonable choice. Ampicillin is active in vitro against *Listeria monocytogenes* and enterococci as well as against many strains of *E. coli*. When the historical experience of the nursery or the physical findings suggest *Pseudomonas* infection, carbenicillin in combination with gentamicin should be used. Once the pathogen is identified and its antimicrobial susceptibilities are known, the most effective and least toxic drug or combination of drugs should be used. The aminoglycosides tobramycin and amikacin should not be used except in therapy of disease caused by kanamycin- and gentamicin-resistant gram-negative organisms to minimize the risk of aminoglycoside-resistant bacteria.

Additional immunoregulatory interventions including immunoglobulin replacement therapy, polymorphonuclear leukocyte transfusion, exchange transfusion, and treatment with recombinant cytokines have been used in specific clinical studies. They are reviewed in Chapter 34.

■ BACTERIAL MENINGITIS

The incidence of purulent meningitis of the newborn infant varies among institutions and is higher in those city hospitals in which prenatal care is suboptimal and in which complicated pregnancies and deliveries often result in high-risk premature births. Incidence rates are approximately two to four cases per 10,000 live births and may be as high as one case per 1000 live births in some nurseries. Within the 1st week of life, group B streptococci and *E. coli* strains account for about 70 per cent of all cases and *Listeria monocytogenes* is seen in an additional 5 per cent of infants. Among infants that are hospitalized for longer than a week in neonatal intensive care units, *S. epidermidis* represents the most frequent isolate. Occasionally, in *S. epidermidis* meningitis, biochemical and cellular indicators of infection in cerebrospinal fluid are absent, but cultures are positive (Gruskay et al., 1989).

Infants with group B streptococcal meningitis usually present after the first several days of life, and the principal organism encountered in these infants is serotype III. The mortality rate is 20 to 40 per cent. Streptococcal disease that occurs in the first 48 hours after delivery usually becomes manifest as acute respiratory distress with or without shock. Although the organism is frequently isolated from postmortem cerebrospinal fluid cultures taken from these infants, histologic evidence of meningeal inflammation may be lacking (Franciosi et al., 1973).

Approximately 80 per cent of all types of *E. coli* that cause meningitis possess K1 antigen. The 018 and 07 somatic types and H6 and H7 flagellar types are most commonly associated with K1 strains cultured from cerebrospinal fluid (Sarff et al., 1975). The presence, concentration, and persistence of this capsular polysaccharide antigen in cerebrospinal fluid and blood of infants with meningitis correlate directly with the outcome of the disease. The concentration and persistence of interleukin

1 beta, a macrophage-derived mediator of inflammation, correlate with an adverse outcome (McCracken et al., 1989; Mustafa et al., 1989). The mortality rates for neonatal *E. coli* meningitis vary from 20 to 30 per cent in some centers to 50 to 60 per cent in others. These figures have been relatively constant during the 1970s and 1980s despite improvements in overall perinatal mortality (Bell et al., 1989). This lack of improvement in outcome among infants with meningitis probably reflects the decrease in size and gestational age of infants who are receiving medical interventions in neonatal intensive care units and the emergence of different organisms with increased antibiotic resistance. In Sweden, where premature birth is less frequent than in other European countries and in the United States, neonatal bacterial meningitis occurs at a rate of 1.9 per 10,000 live births in 1983 (Bennhagen et al., 1987). In this report, a significant improvement in combined mortality and handicap rates from meningitis was observed between 1976 (34 per cent) and 1983 (15 per cent).

The epidemiology and clinical manifestations of *Listeria* meningitis have been described previously in the discussion of septicemia. Very rare cases of meningitis due to *Campylobacter* have also been described, with onset at 1 to 22 days of age (Goossens et al., 1986; Torphy and Bond, 1979). In these reported cases, the disease closely resembled neonatal bacterial meningitis due to other organisms.

Pathology. The pathologic findings are similar regardless of the bacterial etiology. The most consistent findings at necropsy of babies who die of meningitis are purulent exudate of the meninges and of the ependymal surfaces of the ventricles associated with vascular inflammation. The inflammatory response of newborns is similar to that observed in adults with meningitis, with the exception that babies have a sparsity of plasma cells and lymphocytes during the subacute stage of meningeal reaction. Hydrocephalus and a noninfectious encephalopathy can be demonstrated in approximately 50 per cent of infants who die of meningitis. Subdural effusions occur rarely in newborns. In contrast, this complication of meningitis is common in infants 3 to 12 months of age. Varying degrees of phlebitis and arteritis of intracranial vessels can be found in all infants who die of meningitis. Thrombophlebitis with occlusion of veins may occur in the subependymal zones. K1 antigen has been demonstrated in brain tissue of infants who succumb to *E. coli* K1 infection.

Clinical Manifestations. The early signs and symptoms of neonatal meningitis are frequently indistinguishable from those of septicemia (Table 37–3). Specific findings such as stiff neck and Kernig and Brudzinski signs are rarely found. Lethargy, feeding problems, and altered temperature are the most frequent presenting complaints, and respiratory distress, vomiting, diarrhea, and abdominal distention are common findings. A bulging fontanel may be a late sign of meningitis. Seizures are observed frequently and may be caused by direct central nervous system inflammation or may occur in association with hypoglycemia, hyponatremia, or hypocalcemia.

Diagnosis. The interpretation of cerebrospinal fluid cell counts in newborn infants may be difficult (Bonadio, 1988; Gruskay et al., 1989; Polk and Steele, 1988; Sarff et al., 1976). During the first several days of life, as many as 32 white blood cells/mm³ (mean, eight cells/mm³) may be found in cerebrospinal fluid of healthy or high-risk, uninfected babies. Approximately 60 per cent of these cells are polymorphonuclear leukocytes. During the 1st week, the cell count slowly diminishes in full-term infants but may remain high or even increase in premature babies. Cell counts in the range of 0 to 10 cells/mm³ are observed at 1 month of age. The cerebrospinal fluid protein concentration may be as high as 170 mg/100 ml, and the cerebrospinal fluid glucose to blood glucose percentage ratio is 44 per cent to greater than 100 per cent in both preterm and term infants. Thus, it is apparent that total evaluation of the cerebrospinal fluid examination is necessary in order to make an early diagnosis of neonatal meningitis. Although the cerebrospinal fluid cell counts and protein and sugar concentrations from normal infants overlap with those from infants with meningitis, less than 1 per cent of babies with proven meningitis have totally normal results from a cerebrospinal fluid study on the initial lumbar tap (Sarff et al., 1976).

Stained smears of cerebrospinal fluid must be examined carefully from every infant with suspected meningitis. Grossly clear fluid may contain few white blood cells and many bacteria. The stained smears from approximately 20 per cent of newborns with proven meningitis are interpreted as showing no bacteria. As its name implies, *Listeria monocytogenes* commonly evokes a mononuclear cellular response in the cerebrospinal fluid.

Latex agglutination assays can also be helpful in the early identification of infants with meningitis and in infants with abnormal cerebrospinal fluid findings who have received systemic antibiotics prior to culture of cerebrospinal fluid. The disadvantage of these tests is the lack of the availability of antibiotic susceptibility testing to direct antimicrobial therapy. Blood and urine cultures should be obtained from every infant with suspected meningitis.

Therapy. Infants with meningitis require multisystem, aggressive management in the setting of an intensive care unit (Roos and Scheld, 1989). Besides antibiotic administration, these infants frequently require mechanical ventilation, compulsive fluid management to minimize the effects of cerebral edema, seizure control, pressor support, and cardiopulmonary monitoring. Selection of appropriate antibiotic therapy is based in part on the achievable cerebrospinal fluid levels of these drugs in relation to the susceptibility of the organisms that cause the disease. The highest kanamycin and gentamicin concentrations in cerebrospinal fluid are approximately 40 per cent of the peak serum levels and are only equal to or slightly greater than the minimal inhibitory concentrations for disease-causing coliform bacteria. In contrast, cerebrospinal fluid penicillin and ampicillin concentrations may be only 10 per cent of the corresponding peak serum levels, but these values are usually 10- to 100-fold higher than the greatest minimal inhibitory concentrations for group B streptococci and *L. monocytogenes*. The ability to attain spinal fluid antimicrobial activity that is many times greater than is necessary to inhibit the pathogen may explain the rapid sterilization of spinal fluid cultures from infants with gram-positive

meningitis. Delayed sterilization of cerebrospinal fluid cultures from newborns with gram-negative meningitis may likewise be due to the low inhibitory and bactericidal spinal fluid concentrations. As a result of these considerations, the physician may find it necessary, in some infants with coliform meningitis, to alter the therapeutic regimens by adding a second antibiotic, selecting a different aminoglycoside, using one of the newer cephalosporin derivatives, or changing the route of administration. In addition, dosage and timing should be guided by renal, hepatic, and cardiopulmonary function. When possible, individualizing drug regimens based on regular measurement of serum drug concentrations permits the attainment of therapeutic antibiotic effects and the avoidance of toxicity. The Committee on Infectious Diseases of the American Academy of Pediatrics has recently recommended that if facilities for monitoring aminoglycoside or chloramphenicol pharmacokinetics are not available, these drugs should be avoided and cephalosporins (cefotaxine or ceftazidime) should be considered (Committee on Infectious Diseases, 1988).

In 1990 in the United States, ampicillin and either gentamicin or kanamycin are recommended as the initial therapy for neonatal meningitis. The dosages of ampicillin are 100 mg/kg/day in two divided doses during the 1st week of life and 200 mg/kg/day in three divided doses thereafter. The dosages for gentamicin and kanamycin are the same as those used for septicemia (see Table 37–1). All infants should have a repeated spinal fluid examination and culture at 24 to 36 hours after initiation of therapy. If organisms are seen on methylene blue or Gram-stained smears of the fluid, modification of the therapeutic regimen should be considered.

The Neonatal Meningitis Cooperative Study Group was unable to demonstrate a significant improvement in morbidity and mortality rates for infants with gram-negative bacillary meningitis treated with intrathecal gentamicin (1 mg daily) compared with those treated with parenteral therapy only (McCracken and Mize, 1976). Most infants with delayed sterilization of spinal fluid have ventriculitis, and cultures of ventricular fluid yield the pathogen. Intravenous and even intrathecal antibiotics often fail to achieve high concentrations in the ventricles. For these reasons, the Neonatal Meningitis Cooperative Study Group next undertook a large controlled study of intraventricular gentamicin (McCracken et al., 1980). As with intrathecal therapy, however, no advantage was gained by the direct daily instillation of gentamicin into the ventricles. In fact, the study was terminated early because infants receiving intraventricular drug had a higher mortality rate (43 per cent) than the control group (13 per cent). Despite this, there are those who believe that delivery of aminoglycosides to the ventricle, using a surgically placed reservoir, is a helpful addition to intravenous therapy in cases in which ventriculitis has been documented by ventricular tap on the 2nd or 3rd day of illness (Wright et al., 1980).

If intrathecal or intraventricular gentamicin is used, it is advisable to monitor cerebrospinal or ventricular fluid levels in order to be certain that the drug is present in therapeutic and safe concentrations. Intrathecal or intraventricular therapy is continued until the fluid is sterile. Several newer cephalosporins (cefuroxime, moxalactam, cefotaxime, ceftriaxone, and ceftazidime) have been evaluated in controlled, prospective trials (Committee on Infectious Diseases, 1988). Although cefotaxime, aztreonam, and ceftazidime have superior activity in vitro against common meningeal pathogens, no clinically detectable advantages in sterilization of cerebrospinal fluid or outcome have been observed with these drugs (Committee on Infectious Diseases, 1988; Jacobs and Kearns, 1989; Lebel and McCracken, 1988). In older children, ceftriaxone has been more effective and produced less ototoxicity than cefuroxime (Schaad et al., 1990). Chloramphenicol, because of its capacity to diffuse readily into the cerebrospinal fluid, has also been used in neonatal meningitis, and with frequent measurement of blood levels it is relatively safe (Krasinski et al., 1982).

Once the pathogen has been identified and the susceptibility studies are available, the single drug or combination of drugs that is most effective should be used. In general, penicillin or ampicillin is preferred for group B streptococcal infection, ampicillin with or without kanamycin or gentamicin for infection with *L. monocytogenes* and *Enterococcus,* ampicillin plus gentamicin or kanamycin for infection with coliform bacteria, and carbenicillin plus gentamicin for *Pseudomonas* infections. There is no precise method for determining the duration of antimicrobial therapy. A useful guide is to continue therapy for approximately 2 weeks after sterilization of cerebrospinal fluid cultures or for a minimum of 2 weeks for gram-positive meningitis and 3 weeks for gram-negative meningitis, whichever is longer (Committee on Infectious Diseases, 1988).

Prognosis. The mortality in neonatal meningitis is high. The overall mortality rate is approximately 20 to 50 per cent, depending on the etiologic agent, the high-risk factors predisposing the infant to illness, and the ability of nursery personnel and physicians to provide general supportive care. Short- and long-term sequelae of neonatal meningitis occur frequently (Bell et al., 1989; Edwards et al., 1985). The complications include communicating or noncommunicating hydrocephalus, subdural effusions, ventriculitis, deafness, and blindness. Gross retardation may be obvious at discharge. However, many infants appear relatively normal at time of discharge, and only after prolonged and careful follow-up will perceptual difficulties, reading problems, or signs of minimal brain damage become apparent. Approximately 40 to 50 per cent of survivors have some evidence of neurologic damage. Infants who survive neonatal meningitis should have regular audiology, language and neurologic evaluations until matriculation into the school system (Edwards et al., 1985).

■ OTITIS MEDIA

Otitis media is infrequently diagnosed in newborn infants because of the paucity of clinical findings and the difficulty in examining the infant's tympanic membrane (Warren and Stool, 1971). The external canal is narrow and often filled with cheesy debris. Because the healthy baby's membrane may appear thickened and dull, mobility of the drum by pneumoscopy should be used as the single most reliable indicator of middle ear infection.

Neonatal otitis media occurs most often in premature infants and in bottle-fed babies. The exact incidence of this disease is unknown, but it has been estimated to occur in approximately 1 to 5 per cent of infants from birth to 6 weeks of age. The onset of illness is insidious, and the most common complaints are rhinorrhea, irritability, and failure to thrive. The presence of a fever greater than 38° C (100.4° F) and tugging of the affected ear are unusual.

It has been suggested that all newborn infants with suspected otitis media have needle aspiration of middle ear contents, because the pathogens associated with disease may be different from those encountered in infants after the first several months of life (Bland, 1972). Of special importance is the examination of the infant who has required prolonged oral or nasotracheal intubation (Derkay et al., 1989). These children are at high risk for the development of eustachian tube dysfunction. The bacteriology of their infections is more likely to reflect the hospital environment (Derkay et al., 1989). Recent preliminary data from children not born prematurely suggest that *S. epidermidis* is as important as *H. influenzae, S. pneumoniae,* and *Branhamella catarrhalis* in otitis media of early infancy (Casselbrant, 1989). Perinatal problems, especially prematurity, appear to increase the risk of otitis media in the first 6 months of life (Harma et al., 1989). The material obtained from aspiration is cultured in suitable media, and a stained smear is prepared for direct visualization of bacteria. *E. coli, S. aureus, Klebsiella pneumoniae* and *S. epidermidis* cause approximately one-half of the cases of otitis media outside of neonatal intensive care units. *Diplococcus pneumoniae* and *H. influenzae* are the most frequently encountered pathogens during the first 6 weeks of life, as they are during the entire period of infancy (Giebink, 1989). Selection of initial therapy is based on results of the Gram-stained smear, nursery history, and previous organisms taken from the affected infant. If organisms are not observed, oxacillin and gentamicin should be started and continued until results of cultures and susceptibility studies are available.

The importance of establishing the diagnosis and cause of otitis media in newborn infants and of employing appropriate therapy cannot be overemphasized. A missed diagnosis and improper therapy may result in a chronic course of middle ear disease throughout infancy and, occasionally, extension of the infection to adjacent structures such as the mastoid or central nervous system.

■ DIARRHEAL DISEASE

Diarrheal disease during the neonatal period is usually brief and self-limited. Brief episodes of loose stools secondary to alterations of diet and feeding patterns, are common in young infants. Many infants have loose stools during an upper respiratory tract infection, or as a systemic response to infection elsewhere. Modern sterilization practices and increased emphasis on infection control measures have significantly reduced the incidence of bacterial diarrhea in nurseries in developed countries.

Etiology and Pathogenesis. Infectious diarrhea in newborns may be caused by bacteria, yeast *(Candida),* and viruses, but the most frequent of these agents are several species of bacteria. The pathogenesis of bacterial diarrhea appears to be complex and to depend on the particular species involved. In recently reported nursery outbreaks of bacterial diarrhea, enteropathogenic *E. coli, Campylobacter jejuni,* and, much less commonly, *Shigella* and *Salmonella* have all been recognized (Guerrant et al., 1986). Although five types of *E. coli* can cause gastrointestinal infections, including enteropathogenic (EPEC), enterotoxigenic (ETEC), enteroinvasive (EIEC), enterohemorrhagic (EHEC), and enteroadherent (EAEC), ETEC and EPEC are important causes in nursery outbreaks (Gorbach, 1987; Robins-Browne, 1987). ETEC strains produce well characterized heat labile or heat stable enterotoxins (Robins-Browne, 1987). Enteropathogenic strains have been identified by serotype and display characteristic adhesive histology in cultured epithelial cells (Robins-Browne, 1987). The adherence factor(s) are probably encoded on a 55 to 70 megadalton plasmid. The enteropathogenic strain may also express its pathogenicity through the production of at least one shiga-like enterotoxin.

Salmonellae produce diarrhea by mechanisms that are even less clearly understood (Rubin and Weinstein, 1977). Many species invade the mucosa without destroying it and set up an inflammatory reaction in the lamina propria. From here, particularly in newborn infants, the bloodstream may be invaded. Finally, *Campylobacter fetus* species *jejuni* (the form that most often causes diarrhea in older individuals) may sometimes be present in newborn infants and produce bloody diarrhea. The outcome is usually favorable (Anders et al., 1981; Karmali et al., 1984; Sartor and Anday, 1987). Both *Clostridium difficile* and *S. epidermidis* have been associated with a syndrome that resembles necrotizing enterocolitis (Grusky et al., 1986; Han et al., 1983; Mollitt et al., 1988). The specific pathogenic mechanisms of these agents have not been identified.

Clinical Manifestations. It is difficult to differentiate the causes of diarrhea in newborn infants on the basis of clinical findings only. As a general rule, diarrhea caused by enteropathogenic strains of *E. coli* is insidious in onset and is associated with seven to ten green, watery stools a day, but does not contain blood or mucus. The infants do not appear acutely ill. Complications are rare and are related primarily to dehydration and electrolyte disturbances. *Salmonella* gastroenteritis is usually associated with five to ten foul-smelling loose green stools a day that rarely contain mucus or blood. Complications, which are unusual, include extraintestinal foci of infection such as septicemia, osteomyelitis, and septic arthritis. Shigellosis is rare in neonates, but when encountered, it is an acute illness associated with a profuse, watery, nonodorous diarrhea frequently containing blood and mucus. The infants may be very toxic, and illness in a small number of patients initially mimics meningitis or gram-negative shock. Suppurative complications are rare, but dehydration and electrolyte disturbances are common and need immediate and constant attention.

A useful procedure for differentiating enteropathogenic from enterotoxigenic diarrhea is examination of fecal material for polymorphonuclear cells. Feces from patients with dysentery have significant numbers of polymorphonuclear cells, whereas those from patients with enterotox-

igenic disease have very few neutrophils. This test may be helpful in the selection of appropriate antimicrobial therapy.

Therapy. The single most important aspect of therapy for infantile diarrhea is maintenance of hydration and electrolyte balance. As a rule, oral electrolyte solutions with a carbohydrate-to-sodium ratio < 2:1 should be administered during the time of active diarrhea, and the infant should be examined and weighed frequently to ensure proper rehydration and to prevent complications (Williams et al., 1986). In the event of suspected sepsis or shock, intravenous fluids are needed. Estimation of fluid loss from diarrhea and vomiting should be carefully recorded and used as a basis for replacement therapy.

The selection of an antimicrobial agent depends in part on the mechanism of diarrhea (Edelman, 1985; Gorbach, 1987; Williams et al., 1986). An absorbable antibiotic such as ampicillin or chloramphenicol is indicated for disease caused by invasive bacteria, whereas orally administered nonabsorbable drugs such as neomycin or colistin sulfate should be used for noninvasive organisms that produce enterotoxin.

In the context of a nursery outbreak of bacterial diarrhea, all nursery infants with enteropathogenic *E. coli* should be considered for treatment with neomycin or colistin sulfate administered orally, whether or not they are symptomatic. Neomycin is administered orally in a dosage of 100 mg/kg/day in three or four divided doses. Colistin sulfate is administered in a dosage of 15 to 17 mg/kg/day orally in four divided doses. The duration of therapy is 3 to 5 days. Longer periods of therapy are unnecessary and may result in neomycin-induced steatorrhea (Nelson, 1971b). If enteropathogenic *E. coli* are isolated from stools of nonhospitalized, asymptomatic infants, it is usually not necessary to treat these infants with antimicrobial agents; however, they should be followed carefully.

All infants with *Salmonella* gastroenteritis should have blood cultures performed and be examined to determine whether or not the disease has developed at other sites, such as bones and joints. Newborn infants with symptomatic *Salmonella* infections should receive antimicrobial therapy if they are febrile or toxic or if their diarrhea is severe because of the greater potential for systemic infection in these patients. Older infants and children with *Salmonella* gastroenteritis and asymptomatic or minimally symptomatic newborn infants with positive stool cultures for *Salmonella* species should not receive antibiotics. In these patients, antimicrobial therapy may prolong gastrointestinal *Salmonella* carriage and does not significantly affect the clinical course of disease. When therapy is indicated in the newborn infant, ampicillin is the drug of choice and should be administered parenterally in a dosage of 50 to 100 mg/kg/day, divided into two or three doses. Therapy is continued for approximately 5 to 7 days.

Although shigellosis in the newborn infant is rare, it may be associated with high rates of morbidity and mortality. All newborns with symptomatic shigellosis should be treated with ampicillin in a dosage of 50 to 100 mg/kg/day, administered parenterally in two or three divided doses. The duration of therapy is approximately 5 days. In some hospitals, a significant percentage of ampicillin-resistant *Shigella* strains have been encountered. In these centers, trimethoprim-sulfamethoxazole is the initial drug of choice. The dosage is 10 mg trimethoprim and 50 mg sulfamethoxazole/kg/day in two divided doses for 5 days.

Any infant with diarrhea must be isolated from the other babies in the nursery. Surveillance of other infants in the unit and institution of infection control measures are also indicated (see discussion of nosocomial bacterial disease).

■ URINARY TRACT INFECTION

Improved methods of obtaining sterile specimens have made it possible to define more accurately the incidence of neonatal urinary tract infection. With bladder aspiration technique, bacteriuria may be demonstrated in approximately 1 per cent of full-term infants and 3 per cent of premature infants. Urinary tract infections are more common in babies born to bacteriuric mothers and in males during the neonatal period. After this period, these infections are more common in females and also in uncircumcised males (Wiswell and Roscelli, 1986).

Etiology. *E. coli* is the most common etiologic agent of urinary tract infections. Approximately 70 per cent of *E. coli* strains belong to one of eight common somatic antigenic groups similar to those found in older patients. Renal parenchymal disease may be associated with one of several *E. coli* capsular types: K1, K2ac, K12, or K13 (Kaijser, 1972). *Klebsiella* and *Pseudomonas* species are encountered less frequently. *Proteus* species commonly cause urinary tract disease in infants with meningomyeloceles, and gram-positive bacteria, primarily *S. epidermidis*, are increasingly frequent causes of urinary tract infection.

The higher frequency of urinary tract infections in male infants suggests that the predominant pathogenesis at this age may differ from that in the older child or adult. Bacteremia, with seeding in a kidney that is in some way abnormal, may be responsible for at least some cases.

Clinical Manifestations. The majority of infants with significant bacteriuria are asymptomatic. In a prospective study of 1460 consecutive newborn infants in New Zealand in 1972, 9 of 14 bacteriuric infants were asymptomatic (Abbott, 1972). Similar findings have been reported in Sweden (Bergstrom et al., 1972). When symptoms are present, they are usually nonspecific and include poor weight gain, altered temperature, cyanosis or gray skin color, abdominal distention with or without vomiting, and loose stools. Conjugated hyperbilirubinemia, hepatomegaly, and thrombocytopenia may be observed in a few infants with urinary tract infection, and these findings are associated with septicemia or cholestatic hepatitis or both in some babies. Localizing signs suggesting urinary tract involvement are unusual; when present, they usually consist of a weak urinary stream on voiding or an abdominal mass from bladder distention or hydronephrosis.

The diagnosis of urinary tract infection is made by examination and culture of a properly obtained specimen of urine. At any age but particularly in the neonatal period,

during which diagnosis of urinary tract infection brings with it suggestions of renal or collecting system anomalies and bacteremia, the diagnosis is never made on the basis of urinalysis alone. A culture collected from a urine bag is not useful. The presence of bacteria, even in high numbers and in pure culture, may always be accounted for by contamination from the perineum.

At all ages, urinary tract infection may be present in the absence of leukocytes in the urine. The converse is also true, particularly when the urine is collected in a sterile plastic bag. Leukocytes or round epithelial cells (easily confused with leukocytes) are often found in urine samples collected in a urine bag, particularly after circumcision, in the absence of urinary tract infection. For these reasons, culture (or, for rapid screening, Gram stain) of a suprapubic bladder aspiration is the only certain means to diagnose urinary tract infection. In newborns, in whom restriction of fluid intake is not appropriate, greater than 10,000 organisms/mm^3 of a single species (rather than greater than 100,000 as is often thought) are diagnostic if the specimen is obtained by bladder puncture or catheterization. Moreover, concern about whether an infection is in the upper or lower urinary tract is rarely justified in the newborn infant, since either one carries with it concerns about urinary tract anomalies and bacteremia. Latex agglutination assays (e.g., for group B *Streptococcus*) are sensitive and specific indicators of the presence of bacterial antigens but may not necessarily indicate a urinary tract infection. Consideration of a urinary tract infection in light of a positive latex agglutination test in the urine should include a urinalysis, urine culture, and physical examination of the genitourinary system.

Therapy. All infants with suspected or proved urinary tract infections should have blood and urine cultures obtained prior to initiation of therapy. In general, antimicrobial agents should initially be given parenterally because septicemia may occur in association with urinary tract infection and antibiotic absorption after oral administration may be erratic in newborn infants. Ampicillin plus kanamycin or gentamicin should be administered to symptomatic infants with bacteriuria prior to the receipt of results of cultures and susceptibility studies. Final antibiotic selection is based on these studies.

A repeat urine culture taken 48 to 72 hours after initiation of appropriate therapy should be sterile or show a substantial reduction in the bacterial count. Infants with persistent bacteriuria should be evaluated for resistant organisms, obstruction, or possible abscess formation. In the patient without complications, therapy is usually continued for a period of 10 to 14 days. Blood urea nitrogen and serum creatinine levels as well as blood pressure should be determined at the initiation and completion of therapy. If there is evidence of renal failure, dosage and frequency of administration of these drugs, particularly the aminoglycosides, may need to be altered. Approximately 1 week after discontinuing therapy, a repeat urine culture is obtained. If the culture is positive, therapy is reinstated and a thorough investigation of the urinary tract is made to exclude obstruction or abscess formation.

All infants with culture-documented urinary tract infections should have radiologic or ultrasonic evaluation of the urinary tract. An excretory urogram or renal ultrasound is obtained at the onset of therapy to rule out the possibility of gross congenital abnormalities of the urinary system. If obstruction is demonstrated, urologic procedures to ensure proper drainage are mandatory if therapy is to be successful. Voiding cystourethrography can be obtained within 2 weeks of the end of antibiotic therapy if reflux is suspected. Results are affected by previous bladder inflammation.

Prognosis. It is the physician's responsibility to be certain that newborn infants with culture-documented urinary tract infections do not have congenital abnormalities of the urinary system. In such patients, recurrent urinary tract infections are common, and physical growth may be retarded until definitive surgery has been performed. One must conduct careful, long-term follow-up studies in every patient to detect recurrent infections, many of which are asymptomatic (Smellie et al., 1983).

■ SEPTIC ARTHRITIS AND OSTEOMYELITIS

During the neonatal period and throughout infancy, the epiphyseal plate is traversed by multiple small trans-epiphyseal vessels that provide a direct communication between the articular space and the metaphysis of the long bones (Ogden and Lister, 1975). Thus, infection of a metaphyseal site can spread across the growth plate to penetrate the epiphysis. Because these perforating vessels disappear at approximately 1 year of age, osteomyelitis is usually not associated with septic arthritis in older infants and children. There are two possible exceptions to this rule: osteomyelitis of the proximal femur and humerus, respectively. Infection of the epiphyseal cartilage may rupture through the periosteum and enter the joint space, producing purulent arthritis. Because the capsular articulations of the hip and shoulder are permanent, osteomyelitis and septic arthritis may coexist, making the origin of infection difficult to establish. Becuase the inflammatory process of osteomyelitis or of septic arthritis can occupy the epiphyseal and metaphyseal sides of the growth plate, ischemia and necrosis of the plate may occur, resulting in permanent damage.

Etiology. Group B streptococcus, *S. aureus,* and coliform bacteria are the most common etiologic agent (Baxter and Finnegan, 1988; Dich et al., 1975; Edwards et al., 1978; Fox and Sprunt, 1978; Morrissy, 1989; Nelson, 1972; Weissberg et al., 1974). Antecedent trauma (most commonly originating from a heel stick for blood sampling, umbilical vessel catheterization, respiratory tract disease, and femoral venipunctures) have been implicated in the pathogenesis of these infections in some infants.

Clinical Manifestations. Initial signs and symptoms are usually nonspecific. Most infants are not brought to medical attention until local signs such as swelling, irritability, and decreased motion of an extremity become apparent. Fever may be observed, but normal temperature is found in over half the cases (Morrissy, 1989). Physical examination reveals swelling, localized pain on palpation, and resistance to movement of the affected extremity. These signs may be obscured in the term infant by subcutaneous fat and normal joint contractions soon after birth (Morrissy, 1989). Localized heat and fluctuation are late findings.

Although blood cultures are frequently positive, clinically the infants usually do not appear septic. An exception is group A beta-hemolytic streptococcal infection, in which the infant appears gravely ill.

Diagnosis. Blood cultures should be obtained from all infants with suspected osteomyelitis or septic arthritis. Latex agglutination assays on urine or joint fluid for group B *Streptococcus* or other pathogens should be obtained. In infants with septic arthritis, a percutaneous needle aspiration of intra-articular pus should be performed; in osteomyelitis, direct needle aspiration of the affected periosteum and bone is attempted. If pus is obtained, the material should be examined with Gram stain and cultured. Preliminary identification of the pathogen from stained smears is helpful in the selection of initial antimicrobial therapy.

In patients with suspected septic arthritis, radiographs may be normal or may show widening of the arterial space and capsular swelling. Later in the course of the disease, subluxation and destruction of the joint are common. Early in the course of osteomyelitis, the normal radiographic water markings of the deep tissues adjacent to the affected bone are obliterated, indicating inflammation (Mok et al., 1982). Lifting of the periosteum from the bone may also be observed, but cortical destruction is unusual before the 2nd week of illness, and new bone formation is a late finding. Resolution of bone changes is considerably slower than clinical improvement (Weissberg et al., 1974). Because of the multifocal nature of musculoskeletal sepsis in the newborn infants, compulsive, sequential examinations of other joints and bones must be undertaken in the affected child (Morrissy, 1989). Two types of bone scan may be useful, technetium phosphate and gallium scans (Morrissy, 1989). Technetium scans reveal areas of increased blood flow and new bone formation, whereas gallium scans identify areas of white blood cell accumulation. Because of the higher radiation dose to the patient from gallium scans, technetium scans are recommended for aiding in the identification of silent sites of infection despite their lack of specificity in the newborn infant due to normally high epiphyseal blood flow, small imaging window, and motion artifact (Morrissy, 1989).

Therapy. Selection of initial antimicrobial therapy is based on results of the examination of stained smears of aspirated purulent material and on the presence of associated clinical findings such as furuncles or cellulitis. If Gram-positive cocci are observed, the administration of oxacillin should be started. Either kanamycin or gentamicin is indicated if Gram-negative organisms are noted. If no organisms are seen or if doubt exists regarding their identification, oxacillin plus gentamicin or kanamycin should be administered until results of the cultures are available. Direct instillation of an antibiotic into the joint space is unnecessary because most drugs penetrate the inflamed synovium, and adequate concentrations are achieved in purulent material (Nelson, 1971). This also applies to treatment of osteomyelitis; direct instillation of antibiotics into acutely inflamed bone is unwarranted.

As a general rule, infection of the joint space and bone should be drained either by repeated aspiration or by surgery. Septic arthritis of the hip and shoulder is treated best with incision and drainage in order to prevent vascular compromise or extension of infection into the metaphysis. Orthopedic consultation should be obtained for all patients.

Parenteral antimicrobial therapy of neonatal musculoskeletal bacterial infections is continued for a minimum of 3 weeks. The use of oral antibiotics as a substitute for parenteral therapy during the 2nd and 3rd weeks of therapy is unwise because of the lack of experience with this route of administration in newborns. In general, systemic symptoms appear within several days of initiating therapy, although local signs such as heat, erythema, and swelling may persist for 4 to 7 days. The decision to discontinue therapy should be predicated on lack of systemic symptoms, sterile blood and joint fluid cultures, and improvement in the affected bone or joint. Full range of motion may not return to the involved limb for several months. Because of this problem, physical therapy should be instituted early in illness to prevent contractures. Complete resolution of the radiographic changes may take several months.

Prognosis. Mortality from these diseases is rare. However, morbidity due to growth plate damage may be considerable, particularly when a weight-bearing joint such as the hip or knee is involved. Contractures, muscle damage, limb-shortening, and angular deformity may be permanent.

■ OPHTHALMIA NEONATORUM

(See Chapter 105)

High prevalence rates of sexually transmitted diseases among women in labor have been observed to correlate with a high incidence of gonococcal and chlamydial ophthalmia neonatorum. In a prospective study in Nairobi in 1984, *Neisseria gonorrhoeae* was present in 3.6 per cent of infants and *Chlamydia trachomatis* was present in 8.1 per cent (Laga et al., 1988). *N. gonorrhoeae* is acquired during passage through the infected birth canal when the mucous membranes come in contact with infected secretions. Infection usually becomes apparent within the first 5 days of life and is initially characterized by a clear, watery discharge, which rapidly becomes purulent. This is associated with marked conjunctival hyperemia and chemosis. Both eyes are usually involved but not necessarily to the same degree. Untreated gonococcal ophthalmia may extend to involve the cornea (keratitis) and the anterior chamber of the eye. This extension may result in corneal perforation and blindness. Until the introduction of adequate prophylactic measures, ophthalmia neonatorum was the most frequent cause of acquired blindness in the United States. Any infant presenting with a conjunctival discharge should have the material stained and cultured for gonococcus and other bacterial agents. Demonstration of Gram-negative intracellular diplococci on a stained smear is an indication for immediate penicillin therapy prior to definitive laboratory diagnosis.

Differential Diagnosis. Conjunctivitis occurring in the 1st days of life can be either chemical or bacterial in nature. Chemical irritants such as 1 per cent silver nitrate cause transient conjunctival hyperemia and a watery discharge, but this is not associated with a purulent discharge. Common bacterial agents associated with conjunctivitis in newborns are *Haemophilus* species, *C. trachomatis, S. aureus, N. gonorrhoeae,* and *S. pneumoniae* (Armstrong et al., 1976; Pierce et al., 1982; Sandstrom et al., 1984). It is important to determine the specific cause in order to select appropriate therapy and to prevent permanent sequelae of the eye. Viral conjunctivitis in a single nursery infant is unusual.

Conjunctivitis that occurs during the 2nd or 3rd week of life may be caused by viral or bacterial agents. Viral conjunctivitis is frequently associated with other symptoms of respiratory tract disease, such as rhinorrhea, cough, and sore throat, and several individuals in the family unit may have simultaneous disease. In general, the discharge in viral conjunctivitis is watery or mucopurulent but rarely purulent. Preauricular adenopathy is common. Staphylococci, streptococci, and occasionally, gonococci cause conjunctivitis in this age group. Study of a smear of the purulent material is helpful in differentiating these etiologic agents. However, the presence of bacteria on a Gram-stained smear of material is not necessarily related etiologically to the conjunctivitis. Normal inhabitants of the skin and mucous membranes, such as staphylococci, diphtheroids, and *Neisseria catarrhalis* may be observed.

Conjunctivitis caused by *Chlamydia* (inclusion blennorrhea) is a venereally transmitted disease that is observed in infants 5 to 14 days of age (Alexander and Harrison, 1983; Goscienski, 1970). Clinical manifestations vary from mild conjunctivitis to intense inflammation and swelling of the lids associated with copious purulent discharge. Pseudomembrane formation and a diffuse "matte" injection of the tarsal conjunctiva are common. The cornea is rarely affected, and preauricular adenopathy is unusual. In the early stages of the disease, one eye may appear more swollen and infected than the other, but both eyes are almost invariably involved. Diagnosis is made by scraping the tarsal conjunctiva and culturing the material (Sandstrom et al., 1984). In addition, the conjunctival scraping should also be examined for typical cytoplasmic inclusions within epithelial cells, using Giemsa stain (Sandstrom et al., 1984). These inclusions are seen on smears of purulent discharge, and cultures of the discharge yield various bacteria that are not related etiologically to the clinical disease. Without treatment, the acute inflammation continues for several weeks, merging into a subacute phase of slight conjunctival injection with scant purulent material. Occasionally, chronicity develops, and some cases persist for over a year.

Therapy. Ophthalmia neonatorum due to *N. gonorrhoeae* should be treated with parenteral antimicrobial therapy. Crystalline penicillin G should be administered intravenously or intramuscularly in a dose of 50,000 to 75,000 units/kg/day in two divided doses for infants younger than 1 week and in three divided doses for infants older than 1 week of age. The duration of parenteral therapy is 7 to 10 days. In addition to systemic antibiotic therapy, the eyes should be washed immediately and at frequent intervals with saline solution followed by topical administration of chloramphenicol or tetracycline. Initially, local saline irrigations are given every 1 to 2 hours, and gradually the interval is increased to every 6 to 12 hours as clinical improvement is noted. Patients with ophthalmia neonatorum should be isolated, and strict hand-washing techniques should be employed because of the highly contagious nature of the exudate. Conjunctivitis caused by other bacterial agents should be treated parenterally with the single most appropriate agent as judged by susceptibility testing of the organism.

Inclusion blennorrhea is treated with the topical administration of 10 per cent sulfacetamide or 1 per cent tetracycline ointment applied every 3 to 4 hours for approximately 14 days. Marked reduction in swelling and discharge is observed within 24 hours of therapy.

Ophthalmia neonatorum is a preventable disease. One per cent silver nitrate or tetracycline ointment instilled in both eyes immediately after delivery is 90 to 95 per cent effective in preventing gonococcal ophthalmia (Laga et al., 1988). Neither silver nitrate nor tetracycline should be irrigated with saline because this may reduce efficacy. Ophthalmic ointments containing chloramphenicol or erythromycin are also effective prophylactic agents. Bacitracin ophthalmic ointment is not effective. Penicillin drops are effective and produce less conjunctivitis than does silver nitrate, but we do not recommend their routine use because of the remote but possible risk of sensitization to the drug (Hammerschlag, 1988).

■ CUTANEOUS INFECTIONS

The most common bacteria that cause skin infections during the neonatal period are *S. aureus* and groups A and B streptococci. Disease caused by *S. aureus* can assume several clinical forms, the most common of which are pustular lesions. These tend to concentrate in the periumbilical and diaper areas and rarely become invasive except when extensive areas are involved or when the use of monitoring devices, catheters, or other invasive procedures are necessary in gravely ill infants. The study of a stained smear and a culture of an intact lesion are usually helpful in identifying the pathogen. The organisms should be phage-typed (they usually belong to group I) so that if additional cases are encountered in the same nursery, these infants and others in the unit can be evaluated for the possibility of a nosocomial staphylococcal outbreak. If these infections are caused by the same phage type of staphylococcus, prompt measures should be instituted to determine the source of infection and to prevent further colonization and disease.

Therapy of cutaneous staphylococcal disease depends on the extent of the lesions and the general clinical condition of the infant. The physician can manage small, isolated pustules through local care using a mild cleansing agent or an antiseptic such as hexachlorophene or povidone iodine. Infants with more extensive cutaneous involvement or systemic signs of infection or both should be treated with parenteral antimicrobial agents. A penicillinase-resistant penicillin should be used initially; continuation of this drug depends on the results of sensitivity testing.

The second form of neonatal staphylococcal disease has been previously described (see discussion of septicemia) and is referred to as the expanded scalded-skin syndrome.

Group A and group B beta-hemolytic streptococci occasionally cause disease in the nursery (Dillon, 1966). The most common manifestation is a low-grade omphalitis characterized by a wet, malodorous umbilical stump with minimal inflammation. Disseminated disease occurs secondary to invasion of the bloodstream or by direct extension to the peritoneal cavity by way of the umbilical vessels. Identification of one infant with group A streptococcal disease in a nursery necessitates surveillance by culture of the other infants and of the personnel in the unit. The organism is usually introduced into the nursery by personnel or parents who have an asymptomatic nasopharyngeal infection. When a nursery outbreak is suspected, specific M- and T-typing of the organism is useful in defining the source and spread of infection. Group B streptococci have been associated with cellulitis, impetiginous lesions, and small abscesses in a few newborn infants. Penicillin is the drug of choice for streptococcal infections.

Necrotizing fasciitis is an unusual disease of newborn infants. This disease is frequently associated with surgical procedures, birth trauma, or cutaneous infection (Wilson and Haltalin, 1973). Staphylococci, either alone or associated with streptococci, are usually causative, but other bacteria, including Gram-negative enteric bacilli, can be cultured. In this condition, subcutaneous tissues, including muscle layers, are invaded and the organism spreads along the fascial planes. Overlying skin may appear violaceous and is edematous, which imparts a thick "woody" sensation on palpation. The borders of the lesion are usually indistinct when compared with those seen with erysipelas, which are raised and easily palpated. Extensive surgery involving resection of destroyed tissue is imperative in treating necrotizing fasciitis. Blood and tissue cultures should be obtained, and oxacillin and gentamicin are the drugs of choice for initial therapy. Necrotic, fatty tissue may combine with calcium, resulting in tetany and convulsions.

Breast Abscess. Breast abscesses are most frequently encountered during the 2nd or 3rd weeks of life and occur more commonly in females. The disease does not occur in premature infants, presumably because of underdevelopment of the mammary gland in these infants. Bilateral disease is rare.

The major presentation of neonatal breast abscess is localized swelling with or without accompanying erythema and warmth. Systemic manifestations are uncommon, and only 25 per cent of these infants have low-grade fever. *S. aureus* is the major pathogen; coliform bacteria and group B streptococci are also encountered. The diagnosis of breast abscess is best made by needle aspiration of the affected site. The single most important aspect of management is prompt incision and drainage by a skilled surgeon. Oxacillin should be administered for approximately 5 days, during the period of drainage. Experience with this condition in Dallas indicates that antimicrobial therapy plays a secondary role to adequate drainage (Rudoy and Nelson, 1975). Long-term follow-up studies suggest that some girls have diminished breast tissue on the affected side.

■ NOSOCOMIAL BACTERIAL INFECTIONS

Hospital-acquired (nosocomial) infections have become a significant problem in most hospitals and may affect 2 to 5 per cent of all hospitalized patients (Goldmann et al., 1983; Milliken et al., 1988). In nurseries, nosocomial bacterial infections are of particular importance because of the unusual susceptibility of small infants to severe illness. This applies both to routine, short-stay nurseries and to intensive care nurseries, in which babies are frequently intubated and placed on respirators and require monitoring or hyperalimentation by means of central catheters. In short-stay nurseries, problems are most frequently due to Gram-positive organisms, such as S. aureus and streptococci (groups A and B). In intensive care nurseries, many organisms may pose a threat: S. aureus, especially strains that are resistant to several antibiotics, are important; S. epidermidis is the most frequently encountered organism; Gram-negative enteric bacilli are frequently a hazard and are similarly often resistant to antibiotics. Fungi, particularly Candida albicans, are also seen.

In neonatal intensive care units, surveys have shown that as many as 15 per cent of infants hospitalized over 48 hours acquire nosocomial infections from their environment, many of them more than once (Hemming et al., 1976). In one such survey, surface conditions accounted for 40 per cent of the total of nosocomial infections; pneumonia for 29 per cent; bacteremia for 14 per cent; and surgical, urinary tract, and central nervous system infections for many of the remainder. Staphylococci and Gram-negative enteric bacilli were responsible for more than 90 per cent of these infections (Hemming et al., 1976). It has been shown that scrupulous attention to such matters as staff-to-patient ratios, nursery design, and containment principles can assist in minimizing the infection rate (Goldmann et al., 1981, 1983). The American Hospital Association urges every hospital to establish an Infection Control Committee, the functions of which are principally twofold: (1) routine surveillance and education of personnel in principles of infection control, and (2) prompt recognition and control of a nosocomial infection when it occurs. All hospitals should appoint an infection control practitioner to supervise and coordinate the infection control and surveillance programs (Garner et al., 1988; Sprunt, 1988).

When an infectious disease caused by the same organism appears in several infants from the same nursery over a short period of time, a nosocomial outbreak should be suspected. The sick infants must be isolated and cultured in order to identify the pathogen. If a specific, single pathogen is responsible for the outbreak, epidemiologic investigations facilitate the process of determining the source and mode of transmission of the infection. Specialized bacteriologic methods are frequently available to identify markers, such as characterization of plasmid size, serotyping, or identification of a specific exotoxin. Such techniques allow the systematic tracing of the spread of an organism. It is probably best for the infection control practitioner and the nursery director to obtain expert microbiologic assistance in these instances. The investigation of each outbreak and the control procedures that are consequently recommended are often matters that require multidisciplinary planning and coordination.

The following discussions of specific bacterial infections are intended to familiarize the reader with some of the more common nosocomial infections encountered in nurseries. This section is not designed to be an exhaustive review of each or all nosocomial bacterial infections.

Staphylococcal Infection. Phage group I S. aureus (phage types 29, 52, 52A, 79, and 80) caused significant hospital disease in the late 1950s and early 1960s. Disease ranging from pustules and omphalitis to pneumonia, septicemia, and meningitis occurred in newborns during this period. Although the majority of infants are colonized with the epidemic strain during a staphylococcal outbreak, disease occurs in only a small percentage of these infants. Epidemic disease caused by phage group I organisms is still an important problem in many nurseries. In some nurseries, the disease re-emerged after 3 per cent hexachlorophene bathing was discontinued. Disease is apparently milder than it was in the 1960s, but it is still widespread.

Disease caused by phage group II S. aureus (phage types 3A, 3B, 3C, 55, and 71) in newborn and young infants has been encountered. Clinical manifestations caused by this organism have been broadly classified into the expanded scalded-skin syndrome (Melish and Glasgow, 1971). Nursery epidemics of bullous impetigo caused by group II staphylococci have been reported (Anthony et al., 1972). The source of one outbreak was a member of the nursery staff, who was a carrier of the organism, whereas an infant reservoir of infection and a change in bathing technique may have contributed to the other outbreaks. Contamination of the circumcision site may be an additional source of such infections.

When staphylococcal disease occurs in a nursery, the extent of infection must first be determined. All infants and personnel associated with the index patient are cultured, and a random sampling is taken of the other infants. Personnel in the labor and delivery areas should not be omitted from the survey. The nares and umbilicus of the infant and the anterior nares and skin of personnel should be cultured. Active skin lesions are cultured also. All staphylococcal isolates are tested for coagulase production and phage type. A change in the percentage of infants colonized with S. aureus and an increase in the carriage of the specific virulent strain (phage type) are usually observed during nursery staphylococcal epidemics. As a general rule, fomites play a relatively minor role in nosocomial staphylococcal disease. Organisms carried on the hands of personnel have been implicated in outbreaks in several nursery epidemics.

Personnel who are carriers in an epidemic situation and are implicated in spread should be treated. Bacitracin ointment is smeared on the mucosa of the anterior nares three times a day and hexachlorophene showers and shampoos should be taken daily for 3 days. If possible, carriers should be kept away from work until they are free of the organism.

It should be remembered that in short-stay nurseries, staphylococcal infections are often clinically apparent only several days after the infants are discharged. For this reason, some reporting system that includes infants requiring care after discharge is essential.

It is often necessary for the physician to take certain

precautionary measures before the results of the cultures and phage-typing are available. Selection of one or several measures necessary to control a nursery epidemic must be individualized (Sutherland, 1973). The measures commonly employed are as follows:

1. Isolation of all infants colonized with virulent *Staphylococcus*. It is advisable to form a cohort system in the nursery for exposed but as yet noncolonized infants and for all new admissions to the nursery. These separate cohorts are cared for by separate nursery staff and are maintained until discharge of the infants. Infected infants are removed from the cohort and placed in isolation.

2. Enforcement of infection control techniques, such as gowning, limited access to the unit, and thorough hand-washing before and after handling each patient.

3. Use of antimicrobial agents. Topical antimicrobial therapy may be used for minor skin infections (pustules); parenteral antistaphylococcal therapy should be used for systemic staphylococcal diseases.

4. Initiation of routine bathing with antistaphylococcal cleaning agents such as 3 per cent hexachlorophene (diluted 1:2 to 1:5) or application of triple dye to the umbilicus of all new admissions to the nursery.

5. If all else fails, closing of the nursery to further admissions until the problem either has been solved or spontaneously disappears.

After an outbreak is controlled, it is sometimes helpful to monitor the activity of staphylococci for a limited period of time by routine culturing of umbilical stumps and noses of infants on discharge from the nursery. Surveillance for clinical infections after discharge by sending postcards to families of affected infants is also helpful.

Bacterial Diarrhea. The infection control practitioners should be aware of the limitation of designating *E. coli* strains as enteropathogenic on the basis of serotyping alone. However, if *Shigella*, *Salmonella*, or an enteropathogenic strain of *E. coli* is identified in a nursery infant, proper measures should be taken to prevent spread of this agent to other babies. The mother is frequently the source of infection for the index case; subsequent cases are usually transmitted from infant to infant by nursery personnel.

Any nursery infant with diarrhea should be suspected of having a potentially communicable disease and be treated accordingly. Hand-washing and other routine infection control procedures should be strongly enforced, and bacterial stool cultures should be taken. If a bacterial pathogen is isolated, the baby in whom it is found should be moved to a special isolation area, if one is available, and treated with appropriate antimicrobial therapy. If other infants develop watery stools, they should be cultured, placed in the same isolation room as the index infant, and appropriately treated. Culturing of asymptomatic babies and personnel is not always indicated but is appropriate if it is clear that simple isolation and treatment of symptomatic cases is not controlling an outbreak.

Group A Streptococcal Infection. Group A beta-hemolytic *Streptococcus* was a common cause of puerperal and neonatal sepsis in the 1930s and early 1940s. With the advent of penicillin and its frequent use in maternity and nursery units, neonatal infections caused by this organism have become relatively uncommon. The primary source of group A streptococci in nursery outbreaks is either an attendant (nurse or physician) working in the unit or the mother. Once group A streptococci are introduced into a nursery, many infants become colonized but few develop clinical disease. The most common clinical manifestation is a low-grade, granulating omphalitis that fails to heal despite the administration of therapy. However, more significant disease may occur, including extensive cellulitis, septicemia, and meningitis.

Identification of one newborn with group A streptococcal infection is enough to warrant epidemiologic investigations of the nursery. All infants in close contact with the index case, a random sampling of other infants, and all nursery personnel should be cultured. Nasopharyngeal and umbilical cultures from infants and nasopharyngeal and rectal cultures from personnel should be obtained. Because nursery and maternity personnel are frequently interchangeable, the epidemiologic work-up should be coordinated with the obstetric service in the hospital.

Infants with streptococcal disease should be treated with aqueous or procaine penicillin G. During nosocomial outbreaks, all asymptomatic infants colonized with group A streptococci should receive penicillin. The prophylactic use of penicillin for all new admissions to the nursery may also be indicated. Benzathine penicillin G has been used effectively as prophylaxis against group A streptococcal infection in several nursery outbreaks.

Gram-Negative Infections. Since the early 1970s, a number of nursery outbreaks caused by specific Gram-negative bacteria have been described, and virtually all have occurred in long-stay intensive care nurseries. Among the causative organisms were *K. pneumoniae*, *Flavobacterium meningosepticum*, *Pseudomonas aeruginosa*, *Proteus mirabilis*, *Serratia marcescens*, and *E. coli*. A common feature of these outbreaks is that the majority of colonized infants are asymptomatic; those who develop disease usually have pneumonia, septicemia, or meningitis.

Infected fomites represent a common source of nursery outbreaks caused by Gram-negative bacteria. Contaminated faucet aerators, sink traps and drains, suction equipment, bottled distilled water, cleansing solutions, humidification apparatus, and incubators have been incriminated (Javett et al., 1956). In addition, healthy colonized infants or nursery personnel may act as a source of infection because the organism is transmitted among infants by way of the hands or gowns of personnel. During epidemics, asymptomatic colonization of infants with the specific pathogen is variable, ranging from 0 to 90 per cent.

The general approach to nursery outbreaks caused by Gram-negative organisms is similar to that for epidemics of *S. aureus*. It is often helpful to use selective antibiotic-containing media for isolation of the organisms involved from carriers. In addition to the steps outlined in the discussion of staphylococcal outbreaks, the limitation or even prohibition of certain broad-spectrum antibiotics can contribute to long-term control of the problem.

■ REFERENCES

Abbott, G. D.: Neonatal bacteriuria: A prospective study in 1,460 infants. Br. Med. J. *1*:267–269, 1972.

Ahlfors, C. E., Gaetzman, B. W., Halstead, C. C., et al.: Neonatal listeriosis. Am. J. Dis. Child. *131*:405, 1977.

Albritton, W. L., Wiggins, G. L., and Feeley, J. C.: Neonatal listeriosis: Distribution of serotypes in relation to age at onset of disease. J. Pediatr. *88*:481, 1976.

Alexander, E. R., and Harrison, E. R.: Role of *Chlamydia trachomatis* in perinatal infection. Rev. Infect. Dis. *5*:713, 1983.

Alexander, J. B., and Giacoia, G. P.: Early onset non-enterococcal group D streptococcal infection in the newborn infant. J. Pediatr. *92*:489, 1978.

Anders, J. B., Lauer, B. A., and Paisley, J. W.: Campylobacter gastroenteritis in neonates. Am. J. Dis. Child. *135*:900, 1981.

Anthony, B., Giuliano, D., and Oh, W.: Nursery outbreak of staphylococcal scalded skin syndrome. Am. J. Dis. Child. *124*:41, 1972.

Armstrong, J. H., Zacarias, F., and Rein, M. F.: Ophthalmia neonatorum: A chart review. Pediatrics *57*:884–892, 1976.

Baker, C. J.: Early onset group B streptococcal disease. J. Pediatr. *93*:124, 1978.

Baker, C. J.: Group B streptococcal infection in newborns: Prevention at last? N. Engl. J. Med. *314*:1702–1704, 1986.

Baker, C. J., and Barrett, F. F.: Transmission of group B streptococci to parturient women and their neonates. J. Pediatr. *83*:919, 1973.

Baker, C. J., and Kasper, D. L.: Correlation of maternal antibody deficiency with susceptibility to neonatal group B streptococcal infection. N. Engl. J. Med. *294*:753, 1976.

Barresi, J. A.: *Listeria monocytogenes:* A cause of premature labor and neonatal sepsis. Am. J. Obstet. Gynecol. *136*:410, 1980.

Bartzokas, C. A., Paton, J. H., Gibson, M. F., et al.: Control and eradication of methicillin-resistant staphylococcus aureus on a surgical unit. N. Engl. J. Med. *311*:1422–1424, 1984.

Battisti, O., Mitchson, R., and Davies, P. A.: Changing blood culture isolates in a referral neonatal intensive care unit. Arch. Dis. Child. *56*:775, 1981.

Baxter, M. P., and Finnegan, M. A.: Skeletal infection by group B beta-haemolytic streptococci in neonates. A case report and review of the literature. J. Bone Joint Surg. *70*:812–814, 1988.

Bell, A. H., Brown, D., Halliday, H. L., et al.: Meningitis in the newborn—A 14 year review. Arch. Dis. Child. *64*:873, 1989.

Bennhagen, R., Svenningsen, N. W., and Biekiassy, A. N.: Changing pattern of neonatal meningitis in Sweden. A comparative study 1976 vs. 1983. Scand. J. Infect. Dis. *19*:587, 1987.

Bergstrom, T., Larson, J., Lincoln, K., and Winberg, J.: Studies of urinary tract infections in infancy and childhood. J. Pediatr. *80*:858–866, 1972.

Blackmon, L. R., Alger, L. S., and Crenshaw, C., Jr.: Fetal and neonatal outcomes associated with premature rupture of the membranes. Clin. Obstet. Gynecol. *29*:779–815, 1986.

Bland, R. D.: Otitis media in the first six weeks of life: Diagnosis, bacteriology and management. Pediatrics *49*:187, 1972.

Bonadio, W. A.: Acute bacterial meningitis. Cerebrospinal fluid differential count. Clin. Pediatr. *27*:445, 1988.

Boucher, M., and Yonekura, M. L.: Perinatal listeriosis (early onset): Correlation of antenatal manifestations and neonatal outcome. Obstet. Gynecol. *68*:593–597, 1986.

Boyer, K. M., and Gotoff, S. P.: Prevention of early-onset neonatal group B streptococcal disease with selective intrapartum chemoprophylaxis. N. Engl. J. Med. *314*:1665–1669, 1986.

Broughton, R. A., Krafka, R., and Baker, C. J.: Non-group D alpha-hemolytic streptococci, new neonatal pathogens. Pediatrics *99*:450, 1981.

Bryant, R. E.: Endocarditis and valve-ring abscess caused by staphylococcus epidermidis—an opportunistic pathogen keeping pace with progress. Medical Grand Rounds *1*:245–251, 1982.

Campognone, P., and Singer, D. B.: Neonatal sepsis due to nontypeable *Haemophilus influenza*. Am. J. Dis. Child. *140*:117, 1986.

Casselbrant, M. L.: Epidemiology of otitis media in infants and preschool children. Pediatr. Infect. Dis. J. *8*:510, 1989.

Cates, K. L., Goetz, C., Rosenberg, N., et al.: Longitudinal development of specific and functional antibody in very low birth weight premature infants. Pediatr. Res. *23*:14, 1988.

Chow, A. W., Leake, R. D., Yamauchi, T., et al.: The significance of anaerobes in neonatal bacteremia, analysis of 23 cases and review of the literature. Pediatrics *54*:736, 1974.

Christensen, K. K., Christensen, P., Dahlander, K., et al.: The significance of group B streptococci in neonatal pneumonia. Eur. J. Pediatr. *140*:118–122, 1983.

Committee on Infectious Diseases: Treatment of bacterial meningitis. Pediatrics *81*:904, 1988.

Derkay, C. S., Bluestone, C. D., Thompson, A. E., and Katzdatske, D.: Otitis media in the pediatric intensive care unit: A prospective study. Otolaryngol. Head Neck Surg. *100*:292, 1989.

Dich, V. Q., Nelson, J. D., and Haltalin, K. C.: Osteomyelitis in infants and children. A review of 163 cases. Am. J. Dis. Child. *129*:1273, 1975.

Dillon, H. C.: Group A streptococcal infection in a newborn nursery. Am. J. Dis. Child. *112*:177, 1966.

Donowitz, L. G., Haley, C. E., Gregory, W. W., and Wenzel, R. P.: Neonatal intensive care unit bacteremia: Emergence of gram-positive bacteria as major pathogens. Am. J. Infect. Control *15*:141–147, 1987.

Edelman, R.: Prevention and treatment of infectious diarrhea. Speculations on the next 10 years. Am. J. Med. *78*:99–106, 1985.

Edwards, M. S., Baker, C. J., Wagner, M. L., et al.: An etiologic shift in infantile osteomyelitis: The emergence of the group B streptococcus. J. Pediatr. *93*:578, 1978.

Edwards, M. S., Rench, M. A., Haffar, A. A. M., et al.: Long-term sequelae of group B streptococcal meningitis in infants. J. Pediatr. *106*:717, 1985.

Edwards, M. S., Kasper, D. L., Jennings, J. H., et al.: Capsular sialic acid prevents activation of the alternative complement pathway by Type III, group B streptococci. J. Immunol. *128*:1278, 1982.

Eisenfeld, L., Etamocilla, R., Wirtschafter, D., et al.: Systemic bacterial infections in neonatal deaths. Am. J. Dis. Child. *137*:645, 1983.

Evans, M. E., Schaffner, W., Federspiel, C. F., et al.: Sensitivity, specificity, and pediatric value of body surface cultures in a neonatal intensive care unit. J.A.M.A. *259*:748, 1988.

Ferguson, M. G., Rhodes, P. G., Morrison, J. C., and Puckett, C. M.: Clinical amniotic fluid infection and its effect on the neonate. Am. J. Obstet. Gynecol. *151*:1058–1061, 1985.

Ferrieri, P.: GBS infections in the newborn infant: Diagnosis and treatment. Antibiot. Chemother. *35*:211–224, 1985.

Fleer, A., Gerards, L. J., Aerts, P., et al.: Opsonic defense to staphylococcus epidermidis in the premature neonate. J. Infect. Dis. *152*:930–937, 1985.

Fleer, A., Senders, R. C., Visser, M. R., et al.: Septicemia due to coagulase-negative staphylococci in a neonatal intensive care unit: Clinical and bacteriological features and contaminated parenteral fluids as a source of sepsis. Pediatr. Infect. Dis. *2*:426–431, 1983.

Fleer, A., Verhoef, J., and Hernandez, A. P.: Coagulase-negative staphylococci as nosocomial pathogens in neonates. The role of host defense, artificial devices and bacterial hydrophobicity. Am. J. Med. *80*:161–165, 1986.

Fox, L., and Sprunt, K.: Neonatal osteomyelitis. Pediatrics *62*:535, 1978.

Freedman, R. M., Ingram, D. L., Gross, I., et al.: A half century of neonatal sepsis at Yale. Am. J. Dis. Child. *135*:140, 1981.

Franciosi, R. A., Knostman, J. D., and Zimmerman, R. A.: Group B streptococcal neonatal and infant infections. J. Pediatr. *83*:707, 1973.

Frommell, G. T., Rothenberg, R., Wang, S. P., and McIntosh, K.: Chlamydial infections of mothers and infants. J. Pediatr. *95*:28, 1979.

Fry, R. M.: Fatal infections by haemolytic streptococcus group B. Lancet *1*:199, 1938.

Garite, T. J., and Freeman, R. K.: Chorioamnionitis in the preterm gestation. Obstet. Gynecol. *59*:539, 1982.

Garner, J. S., Jarvis, W. R., Emori, T. G., et al.: CDC definitions for nosocomial infections, 1988. Am. J. Infect. Control *16*:128–140, 1988.

Giebink, G. S.: The microbiology of otitis media. Pediatr. Infect. Dis. J. *8*:518, 1989.

Gilbert, G. L., Asche, V., Hewstone, A. R., and Mathiesen, J. L.: Methicillin-resistant staphylococcus aureus in neonatal nurseries. Two years' experience in special-care nurseries in Melbourne. Med. J. Aust. *1*:455–459, 1982.

Goldmann, D. A., Durbin, W. A., Jr., and Freeman, J.: Nosocomial infections in a neonatal intensive care unit. J. Infect. Dis. *144*:449, 1981.

Goldmann, D. A., Freeman, J., and Durbin, W. A., Jr.: Nosocomial infection and death in a neonatal intensive care unit. J. Infect. Dis. *147*:635–641, 1983.

Goldmann, D. A., Leclair, J., and Macone, A.: Bacterial colonization of neonates admitted to an intensive care environment. J. Pediatr. *93*:288, 1978.

Goossens, H., Kremp, L., Boury, R., et al.: Nosocomial outbreak of campylobacter jejuni meningitis in newborn infants. Lancet *2*:146, 1986.

Gorbach, S. L.: Bacterial diarrhoea and its treatment. Lancet *2*:1378–1382, 1987.

Gordon, R. C., Barrett, F. F., and Clark, D. J.: Influence of several antibiotics, singly and in combination, on the growth of Listeria monocytogenes. J. Pediatr. 80:667, 1972.

Goscienski, P.: Inclusion conjunctivitis in the newborn infant. J. Pediatr. 77:19, 1970.

Gruskay, J. A., Abbasi, S., Anday, E., et al.: Staphylococcus epidermidis–associated enterocolitis. J. Pediatr. 109:520–524, 1986.

Gruskay, J., Harris, M. C., Costarino, A. T., et al.: Neonatal Staphylococcus epidermidis meningitis with unremarkable CSF examination results. Am. J. Dis. Child. 143:580, 1989.

Guerrant, R. L., Lohr, J. A., and Williams, E. K.: Acute infectious diarrhea. I. Epidemiology, etiology and pathogenesis. Pediatr. Infect. Dis. 5:353–359, 1986.

Hammerschlag, M. R.: Neonatal ocular prophylaxis. Pediatr. Infect. Dis. J. 7:81, 1988.

Hamoudi, A. C., Marcon, M. J., Cannon, H. J., and McClead, R. E.: Comparison of three major antigen detection methods for the diagnosis of group B streptococcal sepsis in neonates. Pediatr. Infect. Dis. 2:432–435, 1983.

Han, V. K. M., Sayed, H., Chance, G. W., et al.: An outbreak of clostridium difficile necrotizing enterocolitis: A case for oral vancomycin therapy? Pediatrics 71:935–941, 1983.

Hargiss, C., and Larson, E.: The epidemiology of Staphylococcus aureus in a newborn nursery from 1970 through 1976. Pediatrics 61:348, 1978.

Harma, P., Pericia, M., and Kuusela, A. L.: Morbidity of very young infants with and without acute otitis media. Acta Otolaryngol. 107:460, 1989.

Hemming, V. G., Overall, J. C., Jr., and Britt, M. R.: Nosocomial infections in a newborn intensive-care unit: Results of forty-one months of surveillance. N. Engl. J. Med. 294:1310, 1976.

Hillier, S. L., Martius, J., Krohn, M., et al.: A case-control study of chorioamniotic infection and histologic chorioamnionitis in prematurity. N. Engl. J. Med. 319:972–978, 1988.

Hollander, D.: Diagnosis of chorioamnionitis. Clin. Obstet. Gynecol. 29:816–825, 1986.

Hudak, A. P., Lee, S. H., Issekutz, A. C., and Bortolussi, R.: Comparison of three serological methods—enzyme-linked immunosorbent assay, complement fixation, and microagglutination—in the diagnosis of human perinatal Listeria monocytogenes infection. Clin. Invest. Med. 7:349–354, 1984.

Issekutz, T. B., Evans, J., and Bortolussi, R.: The immune response of human neonates to Listeria monocytogenes infection. Clin. Invest. Med. 7:281–286, 1984.

Jacobs, R. F., and Kearns, G. L.: Cefotaxime pharmacokinetics and treatment of meningitis in neonates. Infection 17:338, 1989.

Javett, S. N., Heymann, S., Mundel, B., et al.: Myocarditis in the newborn infant. J. Pediatr. 48:1, 1956.

Johnson, G. M., Lee, D. A., Regelmann, W. E., et al.: Interference with granulocyte function by Staphylococcus epidermidis slime. Infect. Immun. 54:12, 1986.

Kaijser, B.: E. coli O and K Antigens and Protective Antibodies in Relation to Urinary Tract Infection. Goteborg, Sweden, University of Goteborg Press, 1972.

Karmali, J. A., Norrish, B., Lior, H., et al.: Campylobacter enterocolitis in a neonatal nursery. J. Infect. Dis. 149:874–877, 1984.

Klein, J. O.: Current concepts of infectious diseases in the newborn infant. Curr. Probl. Pediatr. 31:405–446, 1984.

Klein, J. O., Feigin, R. D., and McCracken, G. H.: Report of the Task Force on Diagnosis and Management of Meningitis. Pediatr. 78(Suppl.):959, 1986.

Kozinn, P. J., Taschdjian, C. L., Wiener, H., et al.: Neonatal candidiasis. Pediatr. Clin. North Am. 5:803, 1958.

Krasinski, K., Kumiesz, H., and Nelson, J. D.: Pharmacologic interactions among chloramphenicol, phenytoin, and phenobarbital. Pediatr. Infect. Dis. 1:232, 1982.

Kumar, S. P., and Delivoria-Papadopoulos, M.: Infections in newborn infants in a special care unit. A changing pattern of infection. Ann. Clin. Lab. Sci. 15:351–356, 1985.

Laga, J., Plummer, F. A., Piot, P., et al.: Prophylaxis of gonococcal and chlamydial ophthalmia neonatorum. A comparison of silver nitrate and tetracycline. N. Engl. J. Med. 318:653–657, 1988.

Lebel, M. H., and McCracken, G. H.: Aztreonam: Review of the clinical experience and potential uses in pediatrics. Pediatr. Infect. Dis. J. 7:331, 1988.

Lee, E. L., Robinson, M. J., Thopng, M. L., et al.: Intraventricular chemotherapy in neonatal meningitis. J. Pediatr. 91:991, 1977.

Manroe, B. L., Weinberg, A. G., Rosenfeld, C. R., and Browne, R.: The neonatal blood count in health and disease. I. Reference values for neutrophilic cells. J. Pediatr. 95(1):89–98, 1979.

Marrie, T. J., and Costerton, J. W.: Scanning and transmission electron microscopy of in situ bacterial colonization of intravenous and intraarterial catheters. J. Clin. Microbiol. 19:687, 1984.

McCracken, G. H., and Mize, S. G.: A controlled study of intrathecal antibiotic therapy in gram-negative enteric meningitis of infancy. Report of the Neonatal Meningitis Cooperative Study Group. J. Pediatr. 89:66, 1976.

McCracken, G. H., Sarff, L. D., Glode, M. P., et al.: Relation between Escherichia coli K1 capsular polysaccharide antigen and clinical outcome of neonatal meningitis. Lancet 2:246, 1974.

McCracken, G. H., Jr., Mize, S. G., and Threlkeld, N.: Intraventricular gentamicin therapy in gram-negative bacillary meningitis of infancy: Report of the Second Neonatal Meningitis Cooperative Study Group. Lancet 1:787, 1980.

McCracken, G. H., Mustafa, M. M., Ramilo, O., et al.: Cerebrospinal fluid interleukin 1–beta and tumor necrosis factor concentrations and outcome from neonatal gram-negative enteric bacillary meningitis. Pediatr. Infect. Dis. J. 8:155, 1989.

Melish, M., and Glasgow, L.: Staphylococcus scalded skin syndrome: The expanded clinical syndrome. J. Pediatr. 78:958, 1971.

Melish, M., Glasgow, L., and Turner, M.: The staphylococcal scalded-skin syndrome: Isolation and partial characterization of the exfoliatin toxin. J. Infect. Dis. 125:129, 1972.

Milliken, J., Tait, G. A., Ford-Jones, L., et al.: Nosocomial infections in a pediatric intensive care unit. Crit. Care Med. 16:233–237, 1988.

Mok, P. M., Reilly, B. J., and Ash, J. M.: Osteomyelitis in the neonate. Clinical aspects and the role of radiography and scintigraphy in diagnosis and management. Radiology 145:677–682, 1982.

Molitt, D. L., Tepas, J. J., and Talbert, J. L.: The role of coagulase-negative staphylococcus in neonatal necrotizing enterocolitis. J. Pediatr. Surg. 23:60–63, 1988.

Morrissy, R. T.: Bone and joint infection in the neonate. Pediatr. Ann. 18:33–44, 1989.

Mustafa, M. M., Mertsola, J., Ramko, O., et al.: Increased endotoxin and interleukin-1–beta concentrations in cerebrospinal fluid of infants with coliform meningitis and ventriculitis associated with intraventricular gentamicin therapy. J. Infect. Dis. 160:891, 1989.

Myers, J. P., and Linnemann, C. C.: Bacteremia due to methicillin-resistant Staphylococcus aureus. J. Infect. Dis. 145:532, 1982.

Nelson, J.: Antibiotic concentrations in septic joint effusions. N. Engl. J. Med. 284:349, 1971a.

Nelson, J.: The bacterial etiology and antibiotic management of septic arthritis in infants and children. Pediatrics 40:437, 1972.

Nelson, J. D.: Duration of neomycin therapy for enteropathogenic Escherichia coli diarrheal disease. Pediatrics 48:248, 1971b.

Noel, G. J., and Edelson, P. J.: Staphylococcus epidermidis bacteremia in neonates: Further observations and the occurrence of focal infection. Pediatrics 74:832–837, 1984.

Ogden, J. A., and Lister, G.: The pathology of neonatal osteomyelitis. Pediatrics 55:474, 1975.

Parisi, J. T., and Hecht, D. W.: Plasmid profiles in epidemiologic studies of infections by Staphylococcus epidermidis. J. Infect. Dis. 141:637–643, 1980.

Pascual, A., Fleer, A., Westerdaal, N. A. C., et al.: Surface hydrophobicity and opsonic requirements of coagulase-negative staphylococci in suspension and adhering to a polymer substratum. Eur. J. Clin. Microbiol. Infect. Dis. 7:161–166, 1988.

Peter, G., and Nelson, J. S.: Factors affecting neonatal E. coli K1 rectal colonization. J. Pediatr. 93:866, 1978.

Philip, A. G. S., and Hewitt, J. R.: Early diagnosis of neonatal sepsis. Pediatrics 65:1036, 1980.

Pierce, J. M., Ward, M. E., and Seal, D. V.: Ophthalmia neonatorum in the 1980s: Incidence, aetiology and treatment. Br. J. Ophthal. 66:728–731, 1982.

Polk, D. B., and Steele, R. W.: Bacterial meningitis progressing with normal cerebrospinal fluid. Pediatr. Infect. Dis. J. 6:1040, 1987.

Reboli, A. C., John, J. F., Jr., and Levkoff, A. H.: Epidemic methicillin-gentamicin-resistant staphylococcus aureus in a neonatal intensive care unit. Am. J. Dis. Child. 143:34–39, 1989.

Renaud, F., Freney, J., Etienne, J., et al.: Restriction endonuclease analysis of staphylococcus epidermidis DNA may be a useful epidemiological marker. J. Clin. Microbiol. 26:1729–1734, 1988.

Rennels, M. B., and Levine, M. M.: Classical bacterial diarrhea: Perspectives and update—Salmonella, Shigella, Escherichia coli, Aero-

monas, and *Pseudomonas.* Pediatr. Infect. Dis. J. (1 Suppl.):S91, 1986.

Robbins, J. B., McCracken, G. H., Gotschlich, E. C., et al.: *Escherichia coli* K1 capsular polysaccharide associated with neonatal meningitis. N. Engl. J. Med. *290*:1216, 1974.

Robins-Browne, R. M.: Traditional enteropathogenic *Escherichia coli* of infantile diarrhea. Rev. Infect. Dis. *9*:28–53, 1987.

Romero, R., Brody, D. T., Oyarzun, E., et al.: Infection and labor. III. Interleukin 1: A signal for the onset of parturation. Am. J. Obstet. Gynecol. *160*:1117, 1989.

Roos, K. L., and Scheld, W. M.: The management of fulminant meningitis in the intensive care unit. Infect. Dis. Clin. North Am. *3*:137, 1989.

Rubin, R. H., and Weinstein, L.: Salmonellosis, Microbiologic, Pathologic and Clinical Features. New York, Stratton Intercontinental Medical Book, 1977.

Rudoy, R. C., and Nelson, J. D.: Breast abscess during the neonatal period: A review. Am. J. Dis. Child. *129*:1931, 1975.

St. Geme, J. W., Jr., Murray, D. L., Carter, J., et al.: Perinatal bacterial infection after prolonged rupture of amniotic membranes: An analysis of risk and management. J. Pediatr. *104*:608–613, 1984.

Sandstrom, K. I., Bell, T. A., Chandler, J. W., et al.: Microbial causes of neonatal conjunctivitis. J. Pediatr. *105*:706–711, 1984.

Saravolatz, L. D., Markowitz, N., Arking, L.: Methicillin-resistant *Staphylococcus aureus.* Epidemiologic observations during a community-acquired outbreak. Ann. Intern. Med. *96*:11–16, 1982.

Sarff, L. D., McCracken, G. H., Schiffer, M. S., et al.: Epidemiology of *Escherichia coli* K1 in healthy and diseased newborns. Lancet *1*:1099, 1975.

Sarff, L. D., Platt, L. H., and McCracken, G. H.: Cerebrospinal fluid evaluation in neonates: Comparison of high-risk infants with and without meningitis. J. Pediatr. *88*:473, 1976.

Sartor, O., and Anday, E.: *Campylobacter jejuni* enteritis in a premature neonate. South. Med. J. *80*:1593–1594, 1987.

Schaad, U. B., McCracken, G. H., Jr., and Nelson, J. D.: Clinical pharmacology and efficacy of vancomycin in pediatric patients. J. Pediatr. *96*:119, 1980.

Schaad, U. B., Suter, S., Gianella-Borradori, A., et al.: A comparison of ceftriaxone and cefuroxime for the treatment of bacterial meningitis in children. N. Engl. J. Med. *322*:141, 1990.

Schlech, W. F., III, Lavigne, P. M., Bortolussi, R. A., et al.: Epidemic listeriosis—evidence for transmission by food. N. Engl. J. Med. *308*:202–206, 1982.

Shaio, M. F., Yang, K. D., Bohnsack, J. F., and Hill, H. R.: Effect of immune globulin intravenous on opsonization of bacterial by classic and alternative complement pathways in premature sepsis. Pediatr. Res. *25*:634, 1989.

Siegel, J. D., and McCracken, G. H., Jr.: Group D streptococcal infections. J. Pediatr. *93*:542, 1978.

Siegel, J. D., and McCracken, G. H., Jr.: Sepsis neonatorum. N. Engl. J. Med. *304*:642, 1981.

Siegel, J. D., McCracken, G. H., Jr., Threlkeld, N., et al.: Single-dose penicillin prophylaxis against neonatal group B streptococcal infections: A controlled trial in 18,738 newborn infants. N. Engl. J. Med. *303*:769, 1980.

Smellie, J. M., Edwards, D., Normand, I. C. S., et al.: Effect of VUR on renal growth in children with urinary tract infection. Arch. Dis. Child. *56*:593, 1981.

Snowe, R., and Wilfert, C.: Epidemic reappearance of gonococcal ophthalmia neonatorum. Pediatrics *51*:110, 1973.

Sperling, R. S., Newton, E., and Gibbs, R. S.: Intraamniotic infection in low-birth-weight infants. J. Infect. Dis. *157*:113–117, 1988.

Spigelblatt, L., Saintonge, J., Chicoine, R., and Laverdiere, M.: Changing pattern of neonatal streptococcal septicemia. Pediatr. Infect. Dis. *4*:56–58, 1985.

Sprunt, K.: Practical use of surveillance for prevention of nosocomial infection. Semin. Perinatol. *9*:47–50, 1985.

Steigman, A. J., Bottone, E. J., and Hanna, B. A.: Intramuscular penicillin administration at birth: Prevention of early-onset group B streptococcal disease. Pediatrics *62*:842, 1978.

Storch, G. A., and Rajagopalan, L.: Methicillin-resistant *Staphylococcus aureus* bacteremia in children. Pediatr. Infect. Dis. *5*:59, 1986.

Sutherland, J.: Comment. Pediatrics *51*:(suppl.):351, 1973.

Teberg, A. J., Yonekura, M. L., Salminen, C., and Pavlova, I.: Clinical manifestations of epidemic neonatal listeriosis. Pediatr. Infect. Dis. J. *6*:817–820, 1987.

Thompson, R. L., and Wenzel, R. P.: International recognition of methicillin-resistant strains of *Staphylococcus aureus.* Ann. Intern. Med. *97*:925–926, 1982.

Torphy, D. E., and Bond, W. W.: *Campylobacter fetus* infections in children. Pediatrics *64*:898, 1979.

Tullus, K., and Burman, L. G.: Ecological impact of ampicillin and ceforoxime in neonatal units. Lancet *1*:1405, 1989.

Verhoef, J., and Fleer, A.: *Staphylococcus epidermidis* endocarditis and *staphylococcus epidermidis* infection in an intensive care unit. Scand. J. Infect. Dis. *41*:56–63, 1983.

Visintine, A. M., Oleske, J. M., and Nahmias, A. J.: *Listeria monocytogenes* infection in infants and children. Am. J. Dis. Child. *131*:393, 1977.

Wallace, R. J., Baker, C. J., Quinones, F. J., et al.: Non-typeable *Haemophilus influenzae* (Biotype 4) as a neonatal, maternal, and genital pathogen. Rev. Infect. Dis. *5*:123, 1983.

Warren, W. S., and Stool, S. E.: Otitis media in low-birth-weight infants. J. Pediatr. *79*:740, 1971.

Weissberg, E. D., Smith, A. L., and Smith, D. H.: Clinical features of neonatal osteomyelitis. Pediatrics *53*:505, 1974.

Wenzel, R. P.: The emergence of methicillin-resistant *Staphylococcus aureus.* Ann. Intern. Med. *97*:440–441, 1982.

Williams, E. K., Lohr, J. A., and Guerrant, R. L.: Acute infectious diarrhea. II. Diagnosis, treatment and prevention. Pediatr. Infect. Dis. *5*:458–465, 1986.

Wilson, H. D., and Haltalin, K.: Acute necrotizing fascitis in childhood. Am. J. Dis. Child. *125*:591, 1973.

Wiswell, T. E., and Roscelli, J. D.: Corroborative evidence for the decreased incidence of urinary tract infections in circumcised male infants. Pediatrics *78*:96, 1986.

Wright, P. F., Kaiser, A. B., Bowman, C. M., et al.: The pharmacokinetics and efficacy of an aminoglycoside administered into the cerebral ventricles in neonates: Implications for further evaluation of this route of therapy in meningitis. J. Infect. Dis. *143*:141, 1981.

Yow, M. D., Mason, E. D., Leeds, L. J., et al.: Ampicillin prevents intrapartum transmission of group B streptococci. J.A.M.A. *241*:1245, 1979.

OTHER SPECIFIC 38 BACTERIAL INFECTIONS

F. Sessions Cole

The bacterial infections discussed in this chapter have been chosen chiefly because their manifestations in the neonatal period differ in some respects from those of later life.

■ TUBERCULOSIS

In 1925, Debre and LeLong demonstrated convincingly that tuberculosis is, in most instances at least, not inherited but acquired by contact. They separated newborn infants from their tuberculous mothers immediately and in a large series found that none of the offspring had been infected. Similarly, Ratner and coworkers (1951), carefully reviewing 260 infants born to mothers with tuberculosis, found not one case of congenital tuberculosis, even though 39 of the mothers died of the disease shortly after delivery. There are nevertheless several examples of newborns dying of tuberculosis so early that intrauterine infection must be accepted as the only possible mode of origin. In others, in whom evidence of illness became manifest somewhat later, even though mother and child had been separated promptly after delivery, it appears likely that infection was acquired during birth by inhalation of infected amniotic fluid or vaginal secretions.

Incidence. Despite vaccination and availability of effective chemotherapy, tuberculosis continues to be an important problem in industrialized and developing countries (Nemir and Krasinski, 1988; Snider et al., 1989). Beitzke (1948) laid down certain criteria for congenital tuberculosis infection. *Mycobacterium tuberculosis* must be grown from the infant's tissues. A primary complex must be demonstrated in the liver, indicating that bacilli were carried to it by the umbilical vein, or tuberculous lesions must be discovered at birth or within a few days thereafter. Considering the great frequency of the disease among young adults within the past century, prenatal hematogenous transmission must be extremely rare. In 1980, Hageman and co-workers reviewed 26 cases of neonatal tuberculosis acquired either in utero or perinatally, all dating from after the time isoniazid was first introduced.

Pathology. Hematogenous infection is manifested by enlargement and caseation of the glands at the porta hepatis plus disseminated tubercles throughout the liver, comprising the primary complex. In addition, tubercles are scattered through the lungs and spleen and other viscera; the serous surfaces often are studded with them, and their cavities contain clear yellow fluid. Brain and meninges may be similarly involved. When lesions are most prominent in the lungs and a primary complex cannot be found

in and about the liver, it is possible that the disease originated from inhalation of infected amniotic fluid or vaginal secretions at or shortly before delivery. The tubercles belong to Rich's category of soft tubercles showing local necrosis with little cellular reaction, indicating overwhelming infection with little host resistance. Almost 50 per cent of the placentae of tuberculous mothers contain acid-fast bacilli, while congenital, i.e., antenatal, infection is rare (Bate et al., 1986).

Diagnosis. Suspicion and recognition are imperative in this disease: over 50 per cent of cases of progressive primary and acute miliary tuberculosis in infants without proper treatment are fatal (Raucher and Gribetz, 1986). Infants whose disease was acquired in utero may be ill at birth or may develop normally until fever, lethargy, hepatomegaly, and other signs or symptoms occur at several days to several weeks of life. At the time, the infection may be sudden and overwhelming or insidious and prolonged. Symptoms are typically nonspecific: poor feeding, listlessness, fever, hepatosplenomegaly, lymphadenopathy, and later, respiratory distress. Because the liver is the primary site of bacterial replication, the chest radiograph is often normal until late in the disease at which time the pattern of involvement is often miliary. Skin lesions (erythematous papules) may be seen.

To determine the specific diagnosis, one must find organisms either in biopsy tissue—liver, lymph nodes, bone marrow (usually not skin lesions)—or in tracheal or gastric aspirates. Acid-fast stains of such materials, even of gastric aspirates, are very helpful. The cerebrospinal fluid, although often abnormal, infrequently yields organisms on culture. The presence of granulomas in microscopic sections of biopsy material is also a useful finding, but they are also seen in other neonatal diseases, such as listeriosis. The tuberculin test is rarely positive early in the disease, but may become so later. Presence of demonstrated infection and disease in the mother is often the clue that leads one to the correct diagnosis of tuberculosis in the child.

Management. Modern management of neonatal tuberculosis must begin with identification and treatment of the pregnant woman with tuberculosis (Raucher and Gribetz, 1986). The first priority must be prevention of transmission to the fetus and newborn. First, all pregnant women with a history of tuberculosis or with a positive tuberculin skin test should be thoroughly evaluated. In addition, all regular household contacts should be evaluated. The evaluation should include: history of exposure to tuberculosis, results of previous skin tests and chest radiographs, previous antituberculous chemotherapy (including agents used, dosage, and duration), prior vaccination with bacille Calmette-Guérin (BCG), results of a recent intradermal Mantoux test, a recent chest radiograph (taken with proper shielding), and results of sputum and/or gastric aspirate with acid-fast stains and cultures (Raucher and Gribetz, 1986).

THE PREGNANT WOMAN WITH TUBERCULOUS DISEASE

Once cultures have been obtained, the pregnant woman with active tuberculosis should be started immediately on antituberculous chemotherapy, regardless of stage of pregnancy (Raucher and Gribetz, 1986). The agents to be considered include isoniazid (INH), rifampin, and ethambutal. Although concern about fetal effects of the drugs restricted their use during pregnancy in the past, considerable experience now suggests their safety. Women with adequately treated tuberculosis are unlikely to infect their infants; however, any clinical suggestion of active disease should prompt acquisition of smears and cultures and reinstitution of therapy. The infant should have a Mantoux test at 2 and 6 months of age.

Conversion of skin reactivity from negative to positive within the past 2 years should prompt initiation of chemotherapy. If the chest radiograph is normal, unchanged, or shows a healed primary complex, INH can be used alone. If the radiograph is abnormal or progressive disease is evident, INH plus ethambutal or rifampin should be started.

Women whose skin tests were positive in the distant past and who are under 35 years of age, are asymptomatic, and have never received antituberculous therapy should be treated with INH prior to delivery (Raucher and Gribetz, 1986). Regardless of age, women who have a positive skin test, an abnormal chest radiograph (other than a healed Ghon complex or calcifications), or who have close contact with individuals who have active tuberculosis should receive INH preventive therapy.

CONGENITAL TUBERCULOSIS

If the mother has *miliary disease,* untreated in the last part of pregnancy, the infant is at greatest risk of having congenital tuberculosis. Such an infant deserves careful clinical evaluation, including a chest film, smear and culture of gastric washings and urine, examination and culture of the spinal fluid, and drug sensitivities determined on any organism recovered (Bate et al., 1986). The tuberculin test may not become positive for approximately 3 to 5 weeks or longer in such an infant, so reliance on a negative test is unwarranted. The necessity of separating the infant from the mother, who would be hospitalized, is obvious, and institution of INH, 10 mg/kg/day, is appropriate in the absence of manifest disease. If the infant has manifest disease, whether acquired before or at birth, two-drug therapy is indicated. Isoniazid, 15 to 20 mg/kg/day in two divided doses, should be combined with rifampin (15 to 20 mg/kg/day, orally, in a single dose). Rifampin appears to have no unusual toxicities in this age group other than the well-recognized occasional problems of hepatotoxicity and allergy. Rifampin should be continued

for 9 months to 1 year and isoniazid for 1 year or more. If the infant has tuberculous meningitis, triple-drug therapy is indicated: isoniazid 20 mg/kg/day, rifampin 20 mg/kg/day, and streptomycin 40 to 50 mg/kg/day.

A study by Escobar and associates (1975) from Cali, Colombia, demonstrates the efficacy of prednisone at 1 mg/kg/day in infants with tuberculous meningitis for the first 30 days of illness. Prednisone therapy should not be initiated until adequate blood levels of antituberculous drugs are achieved, presumably after about 48 hours of initiating treatment.

INFANT OF A MOTHER ON THERAPY FOR PULMONARY TUBERCULOSIS

If the mother is sputum-positive, the risk to the infant is greater than it is if she has been on treatment for at least 2 weeks and is sputum-negative. It would seem reasonable to separate the infant from the mother and other family contacts with active tuberculosis as long as they remain sputum-positive. Once her sputum and sputum of family contacts have converted to negative, and all are known to be taking medication regularly, separation from the infant is not necessary. Such an infant remains at greater risk than normal, in part because of the likelihood of other unidentified cases of tuberculosis in the environment. The infant should be treated prophylactically with INH for 3 months after a chest radiograph and Mantoux test. If the results of the infant's skin test are negative at 3 months of age, therapy may be discontinued. When compliance with INH administration and follow-up appointments is uncertain, BCG vaccine should be given to the infant (Raucher and Gribetz, 1986). Because of the low frequency of INH-resistant strains in the United States and the concern that INH may decrease efficacy of standard BCG vaccines, separation of the infant from infected family members is recommended until the infant's Mantoux test becomes positive. In hyperendemic areas of developing countries, BCG vaccination is a reasonable intervention. Breast-feeding may be initiated when the need for isolation has passed.

INFANT OF A MOTHER WITH TREATED TUBERCULOSIS

The possibility of relapse in the mother is greatest if her disease were arrested for less than 5 years. Since the risk to the infant of a mother with inactive tuberculosis depends on her likelihood of reactivation, careful and frequent examinations of the mother are essential. Indeed, a tuberculin test in all women during pregnancy and at the time of delivery is desirable. A postpartum chest film and one 3 months and another 6 months later are indicated in tuberculin-positive mothers. The infant should have a tuberculin test with 5 T.U. (0.1 ml intermediate PPD, or 0.0001 mg) at birth and a chest radiograph. The infant should receive INH prophylaxis until the Mantoux test is negative at 3 months of age and there are no clinical signs of disease (Nakajo et al., 1989). Two drugs (INH and rifampin) should be used if active disease is observed in the infant.

ROLE OF BACILLE CALMETTE-GUÉRIN VACCINE

The arguments for using BCG vaccine are based in part on the experience gained from its wide use in many countries with a very low incidence of subsequent tuberculosis and minimal complications (Morbidity and Mortality Weekly Report, 1988). One study relevant to its role in newborns from tuberculosis households included 231 vaccinated by multiple puncture techniques and 220 control infants studied over a period of 19 years (Rosenthal et al., 1961). The infants were returned to their respective homes only if the source case was "closed." Even so, the infectivity rate in the nonvaccinated controls was 36.5 per cent at 1 year, suggesting that the state of infectiousness of an adult cannot always be ascertained with accuracy. The results of the Rosenthal study showed that there were three cases of tuberculosis among the 231 vaccinated infants, and 11 cases among the 220 controls. The controls included four deaths and four cases of miliary disease or meningitis; no deaths or disseminated disease occurred among the vaccinated. More recent studies in Thailand and Canada have confirmed the benefits of BCG immunization (Chavalittamrong et al., 1986; Young and Hershfield, 1986). The strongest argument for BCG vaccination is the advantage gained from it being given at one time instead of daily, as with chemoprophylaxis. However, because protection against tuberculous infection after BCG immunization requires development of delayed hypersensitivity over approximately 6 weeks, separation from individuals with active disease has been advocated (Raucher and Gribetz, 1986). Kendig and Chernick (1977) advocate the two-site method of BCG immunization, giving the material in two sites of the deltoid at the same time.

Not all trials have demonstrated the protective effect found in Rosenthal's study, and there are many who doubt the usefulness of BCG (Morbidity and Mortality Weekly Report, 1988). Its efficacy varies in part because of different potencies of the antigen and variations in the physiologic state of the host, especially perinatal nutritional state and feeding method (formula versus breast) (Grindulis et al., 1984; Morbidity and Mortality Weekly Report, 1988; Ormerod and Garnett, 1988; Pabst et al., 1989). The problem of differing reactions to the vaccine has been lessened by the development of freeze-dried preparation (manufactured by Glaxo Laboratories, Ltd., Middlesex, England, and distributed by Eli Lilly and Co., Indianapolis, Indiana), which has been found to be comparable to the liquid Danish vaccine in testing on newborns (Griffiths and Gaisford, 1956). The immunizing dose is 0.1 ml by intradermal injection. A small red papule appears at the site of injection within 7 to 10 days and may increase in size over the next few weeks (Cundall et al., 1988). It leaves a smooth or pitted white scar in approximately 6 months. A tuberculin test should be performed in 2 or 3 months, and the immunization repeated if it is negative. Occasionally, local granulomas and regional adenitis ensue. Another problem is the possibility that vaccination with BCG could negate the value of subsequent tuberculin testing. The reaction becomes small 1 year after BCG immunization, and thus an increase in reactivity or a large reaction indicates *Mycobacterium tuberculosis* infection. Individual differences in tuberculin sensitivity, however,

make this distinction often unreliable (Morbidity and Mortality Weekly Report, 1988; Snider, 1985). The World Health Organization has recommended that if the risk of tuberculosis is high, infants of HIV seropositive women should receive BCG vaccine at birth or as soon as possible thereafter (Morbidity and Mortality Weekly Report, 1988).

Nursery Exposure to Tuberculosis. Experiences with controlling the possible spread of infection from nursery personnel to infants led Light and co-workers (1974) to propose 3 months of oral INH prophylaxis for all exposed infants. The arguments are that the acquisition of fulminant disease may occur rapidly and in the absence of a tuberculin conversion. The time lag before effective immunity can be achieved with BCG vaccine makes this form of protection less desirable.

■ DIPHTHERIA

The virtual disappearance of diphtheria from the scene in many metropolitan areas inevitably decreases the consideration this disease receives in differential diagnosis. In view of the recent resurgence of other presumed eliminated infections, we must be careful lest a new generation of physicians who have had no experience with it forget its characteristics and its hazards.

Incidence. In 1921, more than 200,000 cases of diphtheria were reported in the United States (Morbidity and Mortality Weekly Report, 1985). Approximately 5 to 10 per cent of the cases were fatal. From 1980 to 1983, 15 cases of respiratory diphtheria were reported, 11 of which occurred in persons 20 years of age or older.

Etiology and Epidemiology. *Corynebacterium diphtheriae*, generally of the gravis type, is the responsible organism. Its soluble toxin produces antitoxin in the host during the course of natural infection and may be used, modified to toxoid, as a potent antigen to stimulate the formation of antitoxin in inoculated persons. The antitoxic titer from either source persists for a variable number of years and is capable of being boosted by reinfection or by subsequent doses of toxoid. Many newborns receive no antitoxin from a mother whose natural or artificial antitoxin titer had diminished to the vanishing point over the course of years devoid of reexposure either to *C. diphtheriae* or to stimulating injections. These infants are susceptible to diphtheria, and contact with an infected person or a healthy carrier may cause the disease. Prevention continues to be the best treatment: an exposed or unimmunized pregnant woman should receive two properly spaced disks of tetanus and diphtheria toxoids, preferably during the last two trimesters (Morbidity and Mortality Weekly Report, 1985).

Diagnosis. The diagnosis of diphtheria in the newborn differs in no respect from that in the older child. Faucial diphtheria is recognized by the characteristic membrane, nasal diphtheria by persistent discharge (often sanguineous), and the laryngeal form by slowly progressive hoarseness and aphonia and laryngotracheal obstruction. All are without sharp constitutional reaction. In all forms, diagnosis depends on bacteriologic identification of *C. diph-*

theriae. Complications, chiefly myocarditis and post-diphtheritic paralysis, have been similarly encountered in the newborn.

Treatment. Diphtheria antitoxin must be given, intravenously when the condition appears serious, intramuscularly if the situation is less urgent. Doses of 20,000 to 50,000 units on 2 or 3 successive days is sufficient. Preliminary testing for sensitivity must be carried out. Since penicillin has a bactericidal effect upon *C. diphtheriae,* it should be given in doses approximating 300,000 units every 8 to 12 hours. Erythromycin is also effective in the event of penicillin sensitivity. Treatment of complications are carried out as for those in older infants. As discussed in Chapter 34 preterm infants should be immunized on the basis of their chronologic age.

▪ TETANUS NEONATORUM

If public health interventions that emphasize hygiene and immunization were provided in developing countries, neonatal tetanus would decrease worldwide as it has in the United States. During 1980, only 2 of 95 reported cases in the United States occurred in patients under 1 year of age. In contrast, a review of 202 neonatal cases that occurred in El Salvador from 1973 to 1980 indicated that one hundred twenty-six (62.4 per cent) of the infants were male, and all 202 exhibited trismus, risus sardonicus, muscle spasms, and opisthotonos (Dowell, 1984). If the incubation period is less than 7 days, >90 per cent mortality has been reported (Dowell, 1984). Hypothermia and bronchopneumonia are the commonest events that lead to death (Salimpour, 1977).

Etiology and Pathogenesis. The causative agent is the bacterium *Clostridium tetani.* This gram-positive, anaerobic spore-bearer produces a protein neurotoxin (tetanospasmin) that is responsible for this paralysis (Dowell, 1984). This protoplasmic protein is released after the cells of *C. tetani* autolyze. This protein is encoded within a plasmid not directly related to a bacteriophage (Laird et al., 1980). Like the botulinal toxins, tetanospasmin acts at myoneural junctions by inhibiting the release of acetylcholine. Competition experiments have suggested that tetanospasmin and botulinal toxin are bound to different sites. *C. tetani* usually gains entrance into the newborn's body by way of the stump of the umbilical cord that is cut by an unsterile instrument or covered with an unclean dressing. Rarely, a vaccination wound produced by an unclean instrument or upon contaminated skin imperfectly cleansed constitutes a portal of entry. The organism is long-lived by virtue of its spore formation, is a normal inhabitant of the intestinal tract of many domestic animals, and hence abounds in the soil of many localities.

Immunity to tetanus depends on the presence in the blood of an adequate concentration of antibody to the toxin. Antibody is efficiently stimulated by immunization with toxoid. The blood of the newborn contains roughly the amount of tetanus antitoxin that is present in the mother's blood. Peterson and colleagues (1955) believe that concentrations as low as 0.01 antitoxin unit/ml may be protective against the disease, and levels higher than this may persist for years in actively immunized persons.

Transplacental immunization of the fetus has also been reported (Gill et al., 1983).

Diagnosis. Signs appear between the 6th and 14th days after birth, most often at the beginning of the 2nd week. Restlessness, irritability, and difficulty in sucking are followed within a day or two by fever, muscle stiffness, and finally, convulsions. The temperature often rises to between 40° and 41° C (104° and 106° F). Physical examination at this stage shows the characteristic trismus and risus sardonicus and the tenseness and rigidity of all muscles, including those of the abdomen. The fists are held tightly clenched and the toes rigidly fanned. Characteristic are the opisthotonic spasms plus clonic jerkings that follow sudden stimulation by touch or by loud noise.

Laboratory investigations are best held to a minimum, since any manipulation produces painful spasms. Diagnosis is clear from the clinical evidence alone, and studies of blood, urine, and cerebrospinal fluid, in all respects normal, add nothing of value. Attempts should be made to cultivate the organism from the presumed portal of entry.

Tetany of the newborn should never be confused with tetanus. Infants with tetany appear well between their convulsive episodes. The infant who is hypertonic from hypoxic-ischemic injury has usually shown evidence of brain injury from birth, before the first sign of tetanus could possibly appear. Extraocular palsies commonly are present and abdominal rigidity absent. Response to stimulation is depressed rather than increased.

Course. The infant may die within a week after onset from respiratory arrest during a convulsive episode. If not, improvement becomes manifest within 3 to 7 days by gradual decline of temperature, decrease in the number of episodes of spasm, and slow resolution of rigidity. Complete disappearance of all signs of illness may take as long as 6 weeks.

Treatment. The first requirement is for tetanus antitoxin to neutralize the circulating toxin not already bound to nerve tissue. Tetanus immune globulin (human) should be given intramuscularly, in a dose of 500 units (McCracken et al., 1971). If this is not available, 10,000 units of equine or bovine tetanus antitoxin should be given intramuscularly. In addition, débridement of the infection site to remove devitalized tissue is imperative (Dowell, 1984). Penicillin, which kills the vegetative form of the bacterium, should be given in a dose of 100,000 to 200,000 units/kg every 12 hours. Tetracycline may be of value as an alternative drug.

Every known sedative has been used to control spasm, and there is no general agreement as to which one or ones should be chosen. Diazepam (Valium) has become the mainstay of treatment of older children with tetanus, and it is probably also of great value in newborns (1 to 2 mg/kg/day in divided doses). The ideal result is to control spasm without depressing respiration. Drug administration is important. When intensive care and respirators are available, neuromuscular blockade with pancuronium bromide (Pavulon), 0.05 to 0.1 mg/kg administered every 2 to 3 hours for the duration of the spasms (up to 6 weeks), has proved successful (Adams et al., 1979). Endotracheal tubes have largely replaced tracheostomy under these circumstances. Howard and de Vere (1962) have used intramuscular administration of meprobamate with no diminution of mortality but with significant reduction in the number of days of spasms and of hospitalization.

Fluids are best given through an indwelling intravenous catheter at first, later through an indwelling gastric tube. The infant should be under close observation in a darkened room and disturbed and stimulated as infrequently as possible. Active immunization with alum-precipitated or fluid toxoid should be begun as soon as the infant improves, since the disease itself immunizes poorly, if at all.

■ INFANT BOTULISM

Although *Clostridium botulinum* is widely distributed in soil and water, reports of infant botulism were rare before 1976, when Pickett and co-workers described an outbreak in California. The incidence is unknown. Most of the cases described have been in California and Utah.

Etiology. Seven types (A, B, C, D, E, F, G) of *C. botulinum*, a heterologous group of obligatory anaerobic, spore-forming, gram-positive, rod-shaped bacteria are distinguished by antigenically distinct toxins (Dowell, 1984). Investigation of 81 cases by the Centers for Disease Control identified a potential source in opened jars of honey that had been added to baby food or used to coat pacifiers. Vacuum cleaner dust was found to contain spores of *C. botulinum* in the household of one infected infant. In the study from Utah (Thompson et al., 1980), it was noted that digging or construction was common in the neighborhoods in which cases were reported. However, food exposures accounted for only a minority of the 68 infant botulism cases reviewed, and preexisting host factors, especially those related to intestinal flora, may be the most important risk indicators (Spika et al., 1989). Of the 121 cases reported to the Centers for Disease Control from 1975 to 1979, 65 (54 per cent) involved *C. botulinum* type A, 55 (45 per cent) type B, and one, type F. Three of the patients died (Dowell, 1984). The frequency of infant botulism in the United States contrasts with the experience in the United Kingdom where a single case was reported in 1986 (Lancet Editorial, 1986).

Clinical Course. Infant botulism has been described in patients as young as 3 weeks of age, but the peak incidence occurs at the usual time of weaning, from 6 weeks to 6 months of age. The infants have usually been born at term and described as normal. Constipation is frequently noted. The infants may seem lethargic and slow to feed. Some have a more acute onset of feeding difficulties, pooling of secretions, diminished gag reflex, loss of head control, and generalized weakness. If the diagnosis is not made and appropriate supportive treatment initiated, death from respiratory arrest may occur. Some infants diagnosed as victims of sudden infant death syndrome may have died from unrecognized botulism (Sonnabend et al., 1985).

Diagnosis. The diagnosis depends on recovery of *C. botulinum* with or without its toxin from the stool in the presence of a compatible clinical picture (Dowell, 1984). Stool and serum specimens should be sent to a laboratory equipped to identify the organism and its toxin. Electromyography has been helpful in the clinical diagnosis. Brief small-amplitude motor reaction potentials have been described. Both *C. botulinum* and toxin have been found in the stools of normal infants (Thompson et al., 1980).

Treatment. Botulinal antitoxin has not been useful in infant botulism, perhaps because of the absence of demonstrable toxin in the serum. Ampicillin has been used, although its value in eliminating the organism is uncertain. Aminoglycoside antibiotics are contraindicated because of possible potentiation of neuromuscular weakness (L'Hommedieu et al., 1979).

■ TYPHOID FEVER

J. P. Crozer Griffith before the beginning of the twentieth century recognized not only that infants could acquire typhoid fever after birth but also that babies born of mothers suffering from the disease acquired the infection in utero.

Incidence. Typhoid fever attained epidemic proportions in the summer and fall of every year throughout most of the United States until the end of the 1920s. By 1902, Griffith was able to report in some detail on 18 patients under 2 1/2 years of age whom he had observed personally and on 325 certain cases plus 92 somewhat doubtful ones that he had collected from the literature. Since the early 1920s, typhoid fever among infants has declined in frequency. Griffith and Ostheimer (1902) found 23 examples of congenital typhoid fever among their collected cases. We have not seen one in a pediatric experience that dates from 1923.

Diagnosis. The following case history, first reported by Weech and Chen in 1929, illustrates the course and diagnosis of an infant with typhoid fever.

CASE 38–1

A male infant was born prematurely after an uncomplicated pregnancy. Five days postpartum, his mother had fever that proved later to be severe typhoid. The infant became febrile at the age of 26 days, but fever dropped to normal after 24 hours. The spleen was enlarged. White blood cell count was 11,000/mm³. Culture of the blood revealed B. typhosus (Salmonella typhi in modern terminology). The next day a bright-red papular eruption appeared over the entire body and lasted 2 days. The white cell count was now 17,000, of which 37 per cent were polymorphonuclears. He had no more fever for 3 weeks, and then low-grade elevation reappeared for a few days. Blood culture was still positive. Two weeks later it was negative. The only other symptom or sign was failure to gain. All other cultures, from stool and urine, remained consistently negative. Eleven Widal tests were performed throughout the course, and none was positive.

Comment. The authors note the extreme youth of their patient, the mildness of the disease and the lack of gastrointestinal symptoms, the generalized exanthem that bore no resemblance to rose spots, the leukocytosis so unlike the leukopenic response of older persons, and the total failure of agglutinins to develop.

Treatment. First chloramphenicol, then ampicillin, were found to be highly effective against *S. typhi*. In the first weeks of the infant's life, ampicillin is the preferred antibiotic.

Schaffer (unpublished data) observed an epidemic of typhoid in northern Mexico in the early 1970s that was caused by a strain of *S. typhi* that was refractory to both chloramphenicol and ampicillin. Presumably, this strain developed because of the availability of these antibiotics without prescriptions.

Prognosis. Nineteen of the 23 infants with congenital cases collected by Griffith and Ostheimer in 1902 died, three recovered, and the fate of one was not stated. More recently, all three infants in a small series treated with parenteral antibiotics (ampicillin, chloramphenicol, or trimethoprim) survived (Chin et al., 1986).

■ REFERENCES

Adams, J. M., Kenny, J. D., and Rudolph, A. J.: Modern management of tetanus neonatorum. Pediatrics 64:472, 1979.

Bailey, W. C., Albert, R. K., Davidson, P. T., et al.: Treatment of tuberculosis and other mycobacterial diseases. Am. Rev. Resp. Dis. 127:790–796, 1983.

Bate, T. W. P., Sinclair, R. E. and Robinson, M. J.: Neonatal tuberculosis. Arch. Dis. Child. 61:512–514, 1986.

Beitzke, H., cited by Harris, E. A., McCullough, G. C., Stone, J. J., et al.: Congenital tuberculosis: A review of the disease with report of a case. J. Pediatr. 32:311, 1948.

Chavalittamrong, B., Chearskul, S., and Tuchinda, M.: Protective value of BCG vaccination in children in Bangkok, Thailand. Pediatr. Pulmon. 2:202, 1986.

Chin, K. C., Simmonds, E. J., and Tarlow, M. J.: Neonatal typhoid fever. Arch. Dis. Child. 61:1228–1230, 1986.

Cundall, D. B., Ashelford, D. J., and Pearson, S. B.: BCG immunisation of infants by percutaneous multiple puncture. Brit. Med. J. 297:1173, 1988.

Debre, R., and LeLong, M.: The infant born of tuberculous parents, separated before contamination: Its growth and resistance to disease. Ann. Med. 18:317, 1925.

de Pape, A. J.: Multiple pseudocystic tuberculosis of bone. J. Bone Joint Surg. 36B:637, 1954.

Dowell, V. R., Jr.: Botulism and tetanus: Selected epidemiologic and microbiologic aspects. Rev. Infect. Dis. 6:S202–S207, 1984.

Editorial: Infant Botulism. Lancet 2:1256–1257, 1986.

Escobar, J. A., Belsey, M. A., Duenas, A., et al.: Mortality from tuberculous meningitis reduced by steroid therapy. Pediatrics 56:1050, 1975.

Gill, T. J., III, Repetti, C. F., Metlay, L. A., et al.: Transplacental immunization of the human fetus to tetanus by immunization of the mother. J. Clin. Invest. 72:987–996, 1983.

Griffith, J. P. C., and Ostheimer, M.: Typhoid fever in children under two and a half years of age. Am. J. Med. Sci. 124:868, 1902.

Griffiths, M. I., and Gaisford, W.: Freeze-dried BCG. Vaccination of newborn infants with a British vaccine. Br. Med. J., 2:565, 1956.

Grindulis, H., Baynham, M. I. D., Scott, P. H., et al.: Tuberculin response two years after BCG vaccination at birth. Arch. Dis. Child. 59:614–619, 1984.

Hageman, J., Shulman, S., Schreiber, M., et al.: Congenital tuberculosis:

Critical reappraisal of clinical findings and diagnostic procedures. Pediatrics 66:980, 1980.

Howard, F. H., and de Vere, W.: Intramuscular meprobamate in the treatment of tetanus in infants and children. J. Pediatr. 60:421, 1962.

Inselman, L. S., and Kendig, E. L.: Tuberculosis. In Chernick, V. (Ed.): Kendig's Disorders of the Respiratory Tract in Children. 5th ed. Philadelphia, W. B. Saunders Company, 1990.

Laird, W. J., Aaronson, W., Silver, R. P., et al.: Plasmid-associated toxigenicity in Clostridium tetani. J. Infect. Dis. 142:623, 1980.

L'Hommedieu, L., Stough, R., Brown, L., et al.: Potentiation of neuromuscular weakness in infant botulism by aminoglycosides. J. Pediatr. 95:1065, 1979.

Light, I. J., Saideman, M., and Sutherland, J. M.: Management of newborns after nursery exposure to tuberculosis. Am. Rev. Resp. Dis. 109:415, 1974.

McCracken, G. H., Jr., Dowell, D. L., and Marshall, F. N.: Double-blind trial of equine antitoxin and human immune globulin in tetanus neonatorum. Lancet 1:1146, 1971.

Morbidity and Mortality Weekly Report: Immunization practices advisory committee statement on diphtheria, tetanus, and pertussis. 34:405, 419, 1985.

Morbidity and Mortality Weekly Report: Use of BCG vaccines in the control of tuberculosis: A joint statement by ACIP and the Advisory Committee for Elimination of Tuberculosis. 37:663, 1988.

Nakajo, M. M., Rao, M., and Steiner, P.: Incidence of hepatotoxicity in children receiving isoniazid chemoprophylaxis. Pediatr. Infect. Dis. J. 8:649, 1989.

Nemir, R. L., and Krasinski, K.: Tuberculosis in children and adolescents in the 1980s. Pediatr. Infect. Dis. J. 7:375, 1988.

Ormerod, L. P., and Garnett, J. M.: Tuberculin response after neonatal BCG vaccination. Arch. Dis. Child. 63:1491, 1988.

Pabst, H. F., Godel, J., Grace, M., et al.: Effect of breast-feeding on immune response to BCG vaccination. Lancet 1:295–297, 1989.

Peterson, J. C., Christie, A., and Williams, W. C.: Tetanus immunization. XI. Study of the duration of primary immunity and the response to late stimulating doses of tetanus toxoid. Am. J. Dis. Child. 89:295, 1955.

Pickett, J., Berg, B., Chaplin, E., et al.: Syndrome of botulism in infancy: Clinical and electrophysiologic study. N. Engl. J. Med. 295:770, 1976.

Ratner, B., Rostler, A. E., and Salgado, P. S.: Care, feeding and fate of premature and full-term infants born of tuberculosis mothers. Am. J. Dis. Child. 81:471, 1951.

Raucher, H. S., and Gribetz, I.: Care of the pregnant woman with tuberculosis and her newborn infant: A pediatrician's perspective. Mt. Sinai J. Med. 53:70–76, 1986.

Rosenthal, S. R., Loewinsohn, E., Graham, M. L., et al.: BCG vaccination against tuberculosis in Chicago. Pediatrics 28:622, 1961.

Salimpour, R.: Cause of death in tetanus neonatorum: Study of 233 cases with 54 necropsies. Arch. Dis. Child. 52:587–594, 1977.

Snider, D. E., Salinas, L., and Kelly, G. D.: Tuberculosis: An increasing problem among minorities in the United States. Public Health Rep. 104:646, 1989.

Snider, D. E.: Bacille Calmette-Guérin vaccinations and tuberculin skin tests. J.A.M.A. 253:3438, 1985.

Sonnabend, O. A. R., Sonnabend, W. F. F., Krech, U., et al.: Continuous microbiological and pathological study of 70 sudden and unexpected infant deaths: Toxigenic intestinal clostridium botulinum infection in 9 cases of sudden infant death syndrome. Lancet 2:237–241, 1985.

Spika, J. S., Shaffer, N., Hargrett-Bean, N., et al.: Risk factors for infant botulism in the United States. Am. J. Dis. Child. 143:828–832, 1989.

Thompson, J. A., Glasgow, L. A., Warpinski, J. R., et al.: Infant botulism: Clinical spectrum and epidemiology. Pediatrics 66:936, 1980.

Weech, A. A., and Chen, K. T.: Typhoid fever: Report of a case in an infant less than one month of age. Am. J. Dis. Child. 38:1044, 1929.

Weinstein, L.: Current concepts: Tetanus. N. Engl. J. Med. 289:1293, 1973.

Young, T. K., and Hershfield, E. S.: A case-controlled study to evaluate the effectiveness of mass neonatal BCG vaccination among Canadian Indians. Am. J. Public Health 76:783, 1986.

Zalma, V. M., Older, J. J., and Brooks, G. F.: The Austin, Texas, diphtheria outbreak: Clinical and epidemiological aspects. J.A.M.A. 211:2125, 1970.

FUNGUS INFECTIONS 39

F. Sessions Cole

▪ COCCIDIOIDOMYCOSIS

Coccidioidomycosis is very rare in newborns but has been reported, especially from endemic areas of the southwestern United States and northern Mexico. *Coccidioides immitis* is a dimorphic soil fungus that causes a mild, self-limiting respiratory illness in immunocompetent children and adults. However, in infants and newborns, the untreated disease is devastating and usually lethal (Child et al., 1985). Transplacental spread has been suggested (Shafai, 1978; Spark, 1981). An increasing number of patients have been reported during the 1980s (Child et al., 1985; Shehab et al., 1988). In 1964, Ziering and Rockas described a 3-month-old infant whose initial symptoms appeared within the 1st month. In addition to the rate adult-to-infant transmission of coccidioidomycosis, it also appears that infants can be infected by porous fomites brought from an endemic area to one in which the disease is rare (Rothman et al., 1962). This brief summary of a case described by Townsend and McKey (1953) illustrates the problems of diagnosis and treatment.

CASE 39–1

A 3-week-old white female infant had been well until 2 days before admission. The only pertinent fact in the family history was that the father had lived in the San Joaquin Valley for 12 years. The infant exhibited high fever, irritability, and anorexia. She was acutely ill, with a temperature of 104°F, respirations 132/minute. She was pale, and her neck was slightly stiff. Her fontanel was full but not tense. Hemoglobin was 12.3 g/dl and fell to 8.2 g/dl after 1 week. White blood cells numbered 71,800 cells/mm³ and fell gradually to 19,800 with normal differential counts. Cerebrospinal fluid showed 700 cells/mm³, 80 per cent polymorphonuclear, 195 mg% of protein, and 15 mg% of sugar on admission. Cell count within the next month varied from 5 to 98, protein from 46 to 64 mg, and sugar from 34 to 49 mg. Cerebrospinal fluid cultures, negative on four occasions, finally became positive for C. immitis 1 month after admission. The organism never could be grown from urine, blood, bone marrow, or gastric washings. Complement fixation was positive for C. immitis in the first dilution.

The patient seemed better 5 days after multiple antibiotic therapy had been started, but then her temperature began to spike. Radiographs showed patchy infiltration of both lungs. The spleen gradually became larger; infiltration of lungs spread. Isoniazid, streptomycin, and para-aminosalicylic acid were given. Despite this therapy, the cervical nodes and spleen grew larger, a papular rash appeared over the trunk, and the infant grew steadily weaker and died 2 months after admission. Autopsy showed disseminated coccidioidomycosis.

Interesting and disturbing is the fact that repeated coccidioidin skin test results never were positive.

This chapter includes some contributions from the previous authors, Dr. Arnold Smith and Dr. Kenneth McIntosh.

Comment. This 3-week-old infant did not live in, but was exposed to a father who had lived in, the circumscribed desert region in the U.S. Southwest in which coccidioidomycosis is endemic. The infection manifested itself first as meningoencephalitis, followed by progressive pneumonitis and disseminated lesions, producing splenomegaly, glandular enlargement, and an exanthem. No thrombocytopenia or purpura ever appeared. The skin test result was never positive. Cerebrospinal fluid cultures did not become positive for the fungus until 1 month after the onset. The complement fixation test gave the earliest confirmation of the diagnosis.

Ziering and Rockas (1964) achieved a notable success in treating their very ill patient, who had extensive pulmonary lesions plus subcutaneous abscesses, osteitis, periostitis, and iridocyclitis. The infant was given courses of amphotericin B over a period of 18 months without toxic effects. His complement fixation titer diminished, and his skin test became positive, indications of marked improvement.

The first report of maternal-infant transmission was a fatal case found by Bernstein and co-workers in 1981. Their patient, born at 36 to 37 weeks' gestation to a mother who had cervical coccidioidomycosis and membranes that had been ruptured for 24 hours, was febrile at 5 days of age and had extensive pneumonia by 6 days. The organisms were seen on gram stain of the tracheal aspirate and confirmed in postmortem cultures. The course was fulminant, with death at 10 days of age.

Treatment. Prior to the introduction of amphotericin B, coccidioidomycosis was a uniformly fatal disease (Drutz and Catanzaro, 1978). Mortality has decreased with the availability of amphotericin B and, more recently, imidazole therapy (ketoconazole and miconazole), but significant morbidity is still associated with the disease and its treatments (Harrison et al., 1983; Shehab et al., 1988). Amphotericin B is administered intravenously (test dose: 0.1 mg/kg; if tolerated, 0.75 to 1.0 mg/kg/day up to 30 to 50 mg/kg total dose). Imidazole therapy has been shown to be useful as a single agent in coccidioidal meningitis (Shehab et al., 1988). Oral ketoconazole (14 to 23 mg/kg/day as a single daily dose) as well as intraventricular miconazole (3 to 5 mg diluted in 1 ml of 5 per cent dextrose in water or normal saline daily, then once weekly between 2 and 6 months) have been shown to sterilize cerebrospinal fluid within 1 month of therapy (Shehab et al., 1988). It is important to note that imidazole therapy may require prolonged and repeated treatment courses. Although no relapses up to 10 months of therapy were reported in one study (Shehab et al., 1988), systemic infection may recur up to 10 years after initial presentation (Kafka and Catanzaro, 1981; Westley, 1982). Duration of initial therapy ranges from 30 to 90 months. It is important to note that ketoconazole suppresses adrenal steroid production, both cortisol and aldosterone, by partially blocking the 11-beta-hydroxylase step of steroid hormone synthesis (Britton et al., 1988). While no studies are available in infants, none of 10 prepubertal children required adrenal steroid replacement therapy during acute illness or surgery (Britton et al., 1988).

■ CRYPTOCOCCOSIS

Cryptococcosis is caused by infection with *Cryptococcus neoformans* (former name, *Torula histolytica*) and is important in the newborn because it invades the central nervous system, where it sets up a meningoencephalitis that closely resembles that produced by *Toxoplasma* and cytomegalovirus. Some of the earliest examples were reported by Neuhauser and Tucker in 1948. Emanuel and colleagues (1961) were able to find 23 affected children reported in the literature. Three definite and three almost certain cases involved illness within the 1st month of life. The increasing frequency of human immunodeficiency virus (HIV) infection among pregnant women will lead to increasing exposure of fetuses and newborns to this pathogen, as a case report suggests (Kida et al., 1989).

Pathogenesis. *Cryptococcus* is an occasional inhabitant of the female genital tract, and the infant probably acquires infection during passage through the birth canal. Symptoms begin so promptly after birth in some cases that one is forced to consider that infection may be transmitted transplacentally. It is, however, of interest that strains of *C. neoformans* pathogenic for humans have been isolated from cow's milk, with or without concomitant bovine mastitis (Emmons, 1953; Pounder et al., 1952).

Diagnosis. The diagnosis and course of three patients with cryptococcosis who were reported by Neuhauser and Tucker (1948) are illustrated in the following case histories.

CASE 39–2

A 7-week-old male infant was admitted to the hospital. He had experienced a precipitous delivery and was cyanotic after birth, requiring resuscitation. Twitchings and rigidity followed on the 2nd day and did not entirely disappear for several weeks. He never ate well and, despite tube-feeding, did not gain weight. Upon admission he was emaciated and chronically ill. The head was a bit large, there were cataracts in both eyes, and the spleen and liver were large. Opisthotonos, ankle clonus, and positive Babinski reflex marked his neurologic examination. Cerebrospinal and subdural fluid contained an excess of protein and many red blood cells. Blood cell count was unremarkable, but no mention was made of platelets. He died suddenly after having been in the hospital for three weeks. In this case, it is difficult to date the onset, since many of the early symptoms might easily have stemmed from intracranial damage sustained at the time of birth.

CASE 39–3

The course of Neuhauser and Tucker's second patient began quite differently, the reason for admission on the 19th day of life being persistent, severe jaundice from birth. Abdominal enlargement was noted at 1 week; the urine was dark, and the stools were light. The spleen and liver were huge. Temperature never exceeded 100°F. He died 4 days after admission. No cause other than the patient's cryptococcal infection was found for the jaundice. Platelets were not mentioned. In this example, one wonders whether infection may not have begun before birth.

CASE 39–4

The third case of Neuhauser and Tucker differed from the other two in mode of onset. The infant began to have convulsions and incessant crying at 2 weeks of age and was admitted to the hospital 4 days later. He was well at birth and until he was 2 weeks old. The head, heart, and lungs seemed normal on examination. The liver and spleen were very large. Neurologic examinations showed only hyperactive reflexes. The platelets numbered only 66,000/mm³. Otherwise, the blood was normal, as was the urine. On the 9th hospital day, the infant had gross hematuria. Death occurred the following day.

Comment. Radiographs of the skull in all three cases showed spotty calcifications within the substance of the brain. In Case 39–4, interstitial pneumonitis, focal atelectasis, and a large granulomatous lesion in the right upper lobe were noted on the chest radiograph. Two infants showed chorioretinitis, and two showed physical signs of central nervous system involvement. All had hepatosplenomegaly. Fever was almost nonexistent in all. All showed hydrocephalus and diffuse areas of focal degeneration throughout their brains.

It is clear that Cases 39–2 and 39–4 are virtually indistinguishable from toxoplasmosis in early life on the basis of history and physical findings alone, whereas Case 39–3, with the principal involvement in the liver, is highly suggestive of either cytomegalic inclusion disease or viral hepatitis. Diagnosis will depend on (1) exclusion of toxoplasmosis by the Sabin dye test and complement fixation studies, (2) exclusion of cytomegalic inclusion disease by the inability to demonstrate inclusion bodies in the cells of urinary sediment or of gastric washings and by virus culture, (3) exclusion of congenital infection with rubella virus or *Treponema pallidum* by appropriate serologic tests. *Cryptococcus* has been seen in and cultivated from the cerebrospinal fluid of newborns five times, twice antemortem and three times postmortem.

Treatment. Reported untreated infants have died within days to weeks of onset of disease. Amphotericin B in a total intravenous dose of 30 mg/kg over a 3-week period may be adequate therapy for disseminated disease with meningoencephalitis. In treating serious systemic fungal diseases in infants and children, we first administer a test dose of amphotericin B (0.1 mg/kg) intravenously over a half-hour. If this is tolerated without rash, fever, or fall in blood pressure over the next 3 hours, the maintenance dose is immediately begun (0.75 to 1.0 mg/kg/day in a single infusion over several hours intravenously). Gradually increasing the dose by increments over several days has, in our experience, not been necessary. In cases that progressively deteriorate or relapse, intrathecal therapy, in addition to the intravenous route, often produces a cure, particularly in the absence of underlying disease (Edwards et al., 1970; Sarosi et al., 1969). Since intrathecal therapy is often necessary over a protracted course, an intraventricular reservoir can facilitate this route if used with knowledge of the potential hazards (Diamond and Bennett, 1972). 5-Fluorocytosine (5-FC) should not be used alone, as the emergence of 5-FC–resistant strains has been a major cause of treatment failure with this drug (Block et al., 1973). This drug has a role when used with amphotericin B because the combination is synergistic in vitro and in vivo (Medoff et al., 1971). Although clinical trials with this combination are not available in adults or in children, successful treatment of a preterm infant with a different disseminated fungal infection (candidiasis) has been reported with a dose of 25 mg/kg (Hill et al., 1974).

■ DISSEMINATED HISTOPLASMOSIS

Approximately 67 cases of disseminated histoplasmosis in children under 2 years of age were reported by Leggiadro and associates (1988). The mean age at the time of presentation was 6 months. The increasing frequency of pregnant women with HIV infection will increase the number of infants exposed to opportunistic pathogens (McGregor et al., 1986).

Incidence. The disease is widespread in the United States and elsewhere, but certain areas seem to be heavily contaminated and their populations infected in large numbers. In a recent review of two large urban outbreaks, an estimated 100,000 individuals were infected, while fewer than 0.5 per cent presented with clinical infections (Wheat et al., 1984). Cases are by no means confined to the broad central belt of high infection rate of which Tennessee appears to be the center. In the eastern United States, the shore counties of Maryland are the source of an appreciable number of histoplasmosis cases. Children under 2 years of age seem to be highly susceptible, and when they become infected, they almost always have the disseminated form. Cases developing within the 1st month of life are extremely uncommon, but many examples have been reported in the 3rd month and later.

Etiology. The invading organism is a fungus, *Histoplasma capsulatum*. Depending on environmental conditions, the fungus may grow in a yeast-like phase or in a mycelial phase. It is found in the soil in the mycelial phase, and it is from the soil that most human infection appears to be derived (Leggiadro et al., 1988).

Diagnosis. Infected infants become ill with fever that often spikes to high levels once a day accompanied by rapid enlargement of the spleen and liver, bronchopneumonic pulmonary infiltrations of a nonspecific nature, and progressive pancytopenia (Leggiadro et al., 1988). The disease resembles disseminated tuberculosis in some respects but differs from it in that histoplasmosis is associated with a greater degree of hepatosplenomegaly, has no miliary pulmonary involvement, and fails to invade the meninges. Its later appearance, the usual but not invariable absence of jaundice, and again its lack of tropism for the central nervous system distinguish it from cytomegalic inclusion disease and toxoplasmosis. Differentiation from coccidioidomycosis and cryptococcosis, which make their appearance toward the end of the 1st month or later, may

be impossible on clinical grounds alone. One will be influenced somewhat by geographic and epidemiologic considerations, but the final diagnosis depends on laboratory investigations.

A positive histoplasmin skin test is of little use, because the result may be negative in as many as half the early acute cases as well as in those patients who are severely ill with the disease. Histoplasmin reactions are frequently positive when other fungi are the responsible etiologic agents. By far the most reliable laboratory indication of the disease is growth of *Histoplasma capsulatum* from peripheral blood, liver biopsy, or bone marrow samples, especially the latter. However, in adults, individuals with known cavitary pulmonary disease may have negative cultures in up to 40 per cent of cases (Wheat et al., 1984). The chief objection to this test is the length of time one must wait for the answer. Quick and reliable confirmation can be obtained from the demonstration of specific histoplasmosis (H) and mycelia (M) precipitin bands by the Ouchterlony immunodiffusion technique (Holland and Holland, 1966; Wheat et al., 1984). Unfortunately, while serologic tests are 95 per cent sensitive and specific, these tests cannot differentiate disseminated from focal infection and can be positive in patients with chronic pulmonary infection caused by other fungi (Wheat et al., 1984). Immunoregulatory lymphocyte populations have been shown to be quantitatively and functionally abnormal in a 1-month-old child with disseminated histoplasmosis, but additional immunoregulatory data in infants are lacking (Clapp et al., 1987).

Treatment. Amphotericin B is the only effective therapy. Little and co-workers (1959) reported four cures in children, three of whom were three, five, and eight months of age at the time treatment was begun. The drug is given intravenously, in a daily dosage of 0.25 to 1.0 mg/kg, dissolved in 5 per cent dextrose to a concentration not exceeding 1.0 mg/10 ml of infusate. The infusion must be given slowly over a period of several hours. Infusions are continued for 4 to 8 weeks, daily at first, then every alternate day. A standard treatment course for infants with disseminated histoplasmosis is approximately 35 mg/kg over 6 weeks (Leggiadro et al., 1988). Vomiting and, in some babies, anaphylactoid reactions are not uncommon side effects, but they need not contraindicate continuation of therapy. The author achieved a notable success by this method in a nearly moribund 4-month-old baby. Triple sulfonamide and sulfadiazine have also been used successfully (Leggiadro et al., 1988).

■ CANDIDIASIS

Oral and cutaneous candidiasis (moniliasis) are discussed in Chapter 112 and will not be considered in detail here. Instead, a brief review of several complications of thrush that are of interest to the neonatologist is presented.

Note that gentian violet in 1 per cent aqueous solution commonly used to treat thrush can cause mucous membrane lesions (Slotkowsky, 1957).

DISSEMINATED CANDIDIASIS

This once rare disease is now a common problem in many nurseries, probably as a result of the intensive use

TABLE 39–1. *Candida* Species Associated with Human Disease and the Sites Involved in Candidiasis

SPECIES	MOUTH	VAGINA	ENDOCARDIUM	NERVOUS SYSTEM	BONE AND JOINT	MULTIORGAN INVOLVEMENT
C. albicans	+ + +	+ + +	+ + +	+ + +	+ + +	+ + +
C. glabrata	+	+	+	+	−	+ +
C. guilliermondi	+	+	+ +	−	+ + +	+ +
C. krusei	+	+	+ +	−	+	+
C. parapsilosis	+	+	+ + +	+	+	+ +
C. tropicalis	+	+	+ +	+ + +	+ + +	+ + +

Key: + + + = major cause; + + = cause; + = rare cause; − = no cases known.
(Reprinted with permission from Odds, F. C.: Candida infections: An overview. C.R.C. Crit. Rev. Microbiol. *15*:1, 1987. Copyright CRC Press, Inc. Boca Raton, FL.)

of broad-spectrum antibiotics in premature (and more vulnerable) infants, developmental, suboptimal leukocytic phagocytosis and killing of *Candida albicans* (Xanthou et al., 1975) and other immunoregulatory characteristics of premature or chronically ill infants. This population frequently requires hyperalimentation through central venous catheters. While compulsive attention must be given to aseptic technique in the management of these catheters, it is not clear from currently available data whether these catheters cause infection, whether fluids administered through them (notably hyperalimentation fluid) causes infection, or whether they represent a marker for infants with increased susceptibility to candidiasis (Eppes et al., 1989; Knox et al., 1987; Lacey et al., 1988). *Candida albicans* grows in all alimentation solutions in use, but the rate depends on the composition and temperature (Goldmann and Maki, 1973). The organisms can reach densities of approximately 100,000/ml, and yet the solution appears clear to the eye; further infection due to contaminated intravenous fluids produces an insidious infection. Several *Candida* species are known to cause disease in humans (Table 39–1), and Odds (1987) has identified virulence determinants in different species (Table 39–2). A description of a typical case, reported by Hill and co-workers (1974), follows.

CASE 39–5

The patient was a 1928 g infant born to a 33-year-old primigravida at approximately 32 weeks' gestation. The infant, who was delivered by cesarean section because of placenta previa, required intubation and resuscitation in the delivery room. Because of persistent respiratory distress and periods of apnea, the patient was transferred to the University of Minnesota Neonatal Intensive Care Unit at approximately 12 hours of age. Severe hyaline membrane disease necessitated the use of res-

piratory therapy, and an umbilical artery catheter was inserted to monitor blood gases.

On the 5th hospital day, apnea, acidosis, and questionable pneumatosis intestinalis observed on an abdominal radiograph prompted the institution and continuance of penicillin and kanamycin therapy, although blood, urine, and cerebrospinal fluid cultures remained sterile. Hyperalimentation through the umbilical arterial catheter was started on the 6th hospital day. On the 9th hospital day, a recurrence of apnea and acidosis prompted repeat cultures, and the antibiotic therapy was changed to ampicillin and gentamicin. The patient improved clinically, but after 4 days Candida albicans grew out of the blood culture drawn on the 9th day. The catheter in the umbilical artery was removed and replaced 12 hours later with an internal jugular venous catheter, and amphotericin B therapy was initiated. Four days later, after three negative blood cultures and a negative cerebrospinal fluid culture were obtained, the amphotericin B was discontinued. Urine cultures continued to yield 7000 to 50,000 colonies of C. albicans/ml. On the 26th hospital day, 17 days after the initial positive blood cultures, edema of the feet, ankles, and knees was observed. This was considered to have a vascular etiology, and the extremities were elevated.

On the 29th hospital day, bilateral knee and ankle effusions developed and were accompanied by warmth and erythema. Synovial fluid contained numerous polymorphonuclear leukocytes (PMLs), but no organisms were seen on direct examination. C. albicans subsequently grew from fluid obtained from both knees and the left ankle. Repeat urine cultures yielded 100,000 colonies of C. albicans/ml, although blood cultures remained sterile. A cerebrospinal fluid specimen obtained on the 29th hospital day contained 6 PMNs and 22 monocytes with a glucose of 29 mg/dl and protein of 84 mg/dl. This specimen also yielded C. albicans on culture.

Comment. This case illustrates several important principles in the diagnosis of disseminated candidiasis. The infection is septicemic, with blood cultures yielding the

TABLE 39–2. Possible Virulence Determinants of *Candida* Species

SPECIES	ABLE TO FORM TRUE HYPHAE	ABLE TO RESIST PHAGOCYTOSIS	ABLE TO ADHERE TO HOST SURFACES	ABLE TO SECRETE PROTEINASE
C. albicans	+ +	+ +	+ +	+ +
C. tropicalis	±	+ +	+	+
C. parapsilosis	−	+	+	±
C. pseudotropicalis	−	+	±	−
C. krusei	−	+	−	−
C. guilliermondi	−	−	−	−
C. glabrata	−	−	−	−

Species are listed in their known rank order of pathogenicity.
Key: + + = Strong/high ability; + = able; ± = little ability; − = very weak or no ability.
(Reprinted with permission from Odds, F. C.: Candida infections: An overview. C.R.C. Crit. Rev. Microbiol. *15*:1, 1987. Copyright CRC Press, Inc. Boca Raton, FL.)

organism and the urine containing the organisms cleared by the kidney. Blood cultures obtained through the hyperalimentation catheter sample infected thrombi adjacent to the tip but do not aid in differentiating between diseases that will resolve after catheter removal (Ellis and Spivack, 1967) and life-threatening illness. Peripheral blood cultures obtained by venipuncture are a more reliable indicator of ongoing candidemia. In overwhelming infections the organisms can be seen in stained smears of buffy coat preparations (Silverman et al., 1973). Skin lesions can be seen (Bodey and Luna, 1974) that yield the organism on aspiration. Candidal ophthalmitis is an occasional complication of candidemia (Fishman et al., 1972) and can serve as a focus for continued candidemia (Haring et al., 1973). Every infant in whom the diagnosis of candidal sepsis is suspected should have indirect funduscopic examination (McDonnell et al., 1985). Among common presenting symptoms usually at 1 to 2 months of age, are respiratory deterioration, hyperglycemia, and temperature instability (Baley et al., 1984). Fungal colonization represents a significant risk factor in infants <1500 g (Baley et al., 1986). A substantial proportion of infants with persistent signs and symptoms of infection has central nervous system involvement (Faix, 1984). Other manifestations of candidal sepsis in newborn infants are osteomyelitis (Adler et al., 1972; Freeman et al., 1974; Klein et al., 1972), meningitis, endocarditis (Joshi and Wang, 1973; Shapira et al., 1974), and arthritis.

Because of the importance of host factors, the course of disseminated candidiasis is unpredictable, making therapeutic generalizations impossible. If the infection is catheter-related, careful consideration should be given to removing the catheter (Eppes et al., 1989; Knox et al., 1987; Lacey et al., 1988). In most instances, amphotericin B is administered until it is clear that there are no occult foci. In patients with meningitis or progressive clinical deterioration, 5-fluorocytosine is used in combination with amphotericin B (Lilien et al., 1978).

CONGENITAL CANDIDIASIS

Many examples of candidal infection acquired in utero have been reported. Dvorak and Gavaller's patient, reported in 1966, had a diffuse macular rash and respiratory distress at birth and died at 34 hours of age. Autopsy showed extensive bronchopneumonia, the sections filled with hyphae and spores. The placenta was also heavily infected with the fungus.

In these instances, ascending infection produces chorioamnionitis with dissemination to the fetus, which can lead to spontaneous abortion (Ho and Aterman, 1970). In most instances, the severity of disseminated candidiasis acquired in utero is such that the infant expires before therapy can be considered (Schirar et al., 1974).

On the one hand, cutaneous candidiasis, evident at the time of birth, can be seen in the absence of systemic involvement (Aterman, 1968; Chapel et al., 1982; Rhatigan, 1968). On the other hand, cases of systemic candidiasis, probably acquired in utero, have been described in the absence of rash (Johnson et al., 1981; Mamlok et al., 1985; Whyte et al., 1982). The rash, when it does occur, evolves from maculopapular to vesicular to pustular.

It thus appears that *Candida,* like bacteria, may infect the fetus by hematogenous dissemination from the umbilical vessels, leading to systemic infection, or may be limited to cutaneous candidiasis.

PNEUMONIA COMPLICATING ORAL CANDIDIASIS

Adams (1944) reported that five of eight infants who had thrush showed respiratory distress, cyanosis, and leukocytosis. They all had signs of pneumonitis. In one who died, *Candida* had invaded the pulmonary parenchyma, and the author believed this to have been an example of true thrush pneumonitis. Winter (1955) cannot accept Adams' autopsied case as one of mycotic pneumonia but believes that this complication has been demonstrated beyond doubt in a 1 year old and in several older persons.

Mycotic pneumonia has also been reported as an unexpected finding at autopsies of newborns (Koenig, 1971). The course was not always fulminant, and there is little specificity to the roentgenographic picture. Infants with thrush and pneumonia should be suspected of having *Candida* as the infecting agent, particularly if they have been pretreated with broad-spectrum antibiotics. Isolation of *Candida albicans* from the blood of such infants is strongly suggestive of bronchopulmonary candidiasis, but demonstration of hyphae in tracheal aspirates obtained at bronchoscopy or pulmonary tissue obtained by open lung biopsy is the best evidence of infection. Although these procedures are hazardous, the possibility of identifying a potentially treatable disease should be strongly considered.

Beckmann and Navarro (1955) recorded the following case history.

CASE 39–6

A 2125 g infant was discharged from the nursery on the 10th day of life, well except for thick deposits of thrush upon the tongue. Gentian violet and 2 per cent ferric chloride solution were used locally, but the lesion became ulcerative and spread to involve all the oral and buccal mucous membranes. Cyanosis during feeding appeared, and rales were heard throughout both lungs. At 3 months of age, the infant was admitted to the hospital, weighing 2435 g. His temperature was 98.6°F, and never rose during his stay. He was malnourished, cyanotic, and critically ill. There were mucopurulent nasal and oral discharges. Radiographs showed patches of pneumonia, atelectasis, and emphysema. Attempted feedings caused choking and cyanosis. Intravenous fluid therapy, transfusion, penicillin, and Gantrisin failed to improve his condition. Mycostatin, 175,000 units orally every 6 hours, was begun, and within 48 hours his mouth was practically healed! The respiratory difficulty improved more slowly and was not gone until the 2nd week.

Comment. The authors admit that the diagnosis of *C. albicans* pneumonitis was far from proved but believe that the response to the fungicidal antibiotic was striking enough to be highly suggestive.

THRUSH ESOPHAGITIS

Several cases have been reported in which oral candidiasis has advanced to involve the nasopharynx and esophagus. When this occurs, swallowing becomes almost impossible, and during the attempts to swallow, much liquid appears to be aspirated into the tracheobronchial tree. Choking spells with cyanosis result.

Wolff and co-workers (1955) reported two examples from Birmingham, England. The first is described in the following case history.

CASE 39–7

A female infant weighed 2720 g at birth and seemed well until her 16th day, when anorexia and vomiting began. When she was admitted the next day, her general condition seemed good, but the tongue and buccal mucous membranes were covered with a white membrane from which C. albicans was identified by smear. After 3 days of treatment with 1 per cent gentian violet locally and 0.01 per cent solution (4 ml, three times a day orally), there was no improvement. It did not respond to sulfonamide or, later, to penicillin. Profuse viscid discharge from the mouth and nose appeared. At this stage the infant could not swallow, and attempts led to repeated bouts of cyanosis. On the 8th day, hydroxystilbamidine was begun, 15 mg (5 mg/kg) in 0.75 ml of water injected slowly into the intravenous infusion tubing. This was repeated every 12 hours. A coagulase-positive Staphylococcus was grown from the blood. Streptomycin was given in addition to the other drug. Improvement began while the infant was on hydroxystilbamidine alone. After 6 days, the intravenous drip was removed, and oral feedings were started. On the 18th day, barium swallow showed that incoordination of swallowing was still present, with much iodized oil entering the trachea during the act of deglutition. Gavage feedings were begun again and were able to be discontinued 1 week later.

Comment. Such contiguous spread should be suspected in infants with thrush when swallowing becomes difficult and aspiration seems to be taking place. Not surprisingly, the contiguous spread can be more anterior and produce signs and symptoms of congenital stridor (Perrone, 1970).

ENTERIC CANDIDIASIS

Kozinn and Taschdjian (1962) deplore the tendency to forget the possibility of enteric candidiasis in the differential diagnosis of diarrhea in the young infant. The gastrointestinal tract is believed to be the principal habitat of commensal *Candida* species (Odds, 1987). They stress that it is a not uncommon complication of thrush and that it may lead to systemic invasion and death.

The diagnosis should be suspected whenever diarrhea complicates thrush or cutaneous candidiasis, especially if the infant has been on antimicrobial therapy. Direct examination of stools reveals in many cases the mycelial form of the fungus, a finding that is much more significant than visualization of yeast forms.

Good clinical response and disappearance of the organisms can be attained with nystatin in 80 per cent of cases. Amphotericin B may be helpful in severe cases.

■ REFERENCES

Adams, J. M.: A reevaluation of the pneumonias of infancy. J. Pediatr. 25:369, 1944.

Adler, S., Randall, J., and Plotkin, S. A.: Candidal osteomyelitis and arthritis in a neonate. Am. J. Dis. Child. 123:595, 1972.

Ashcraft, K. W., and Leape, L. L.: Candida sepsis complicating parenteral feeding. J.A.M.A. 212:454, 1970.

Aterman, K.: Pathology of candida infection of the umbilical cord. Am. J. Clin. Pathol. 49:798, 1968.

Baley, J. E., Kliegman, R. M., and Fanaroff, A. A.: Disseminated fungal infections in very low-birth-weight infants: Clinical manifestations and epidemiology. Pediatrics 73:144, 1984.

Baley, J. E., Kliegman, R. M., Boxerbaum, B., et al.: Fungal colonization in the very low birth weight infant. Pediatrics 78:225, 1986.

Beckmann, A. J., and Navarro, J. E.: Pneumonia complicating oral thrush treated with mycostatin, a new antifungal antibiotic. J. Pediatr. 46:587, 1955.

Bernstein, D. I., Tipton, J. R., Schott, S. F., et al.: Coccidioidomycosis in a neonate: Maternal-infant transmission. J. Pediatr. 99:752, 1981.

Block, E. R., Jennings, A. E., and Bennett, J. E.: 5-Fluorocytosine resistance in Cryptococcus neoformans. Antimicrob. Agents Chemother. 3:649, 1973.

Bodey, G. P., and Luna, M.: Skin lesions associated with disseminated candidiasis. J.A.M.A. 229:1466, 1974.

Britton, H., Shehab, Z., Lightner, E., et al.: Adrenal response in children receiving high doses of ketoconazole for systemic coccidioidomycosis. J. Pediatr. 112:488, 1988.

Burry, A. F.: Hydrocephalus after intrauterine fungal infection. Arch. Dis. Child. 32:161, 1957.

Chapel, T. A., Gagliardi, C., and Nichols, W.: Congenital cutaneous candidiasis. J. Am. Acad. Dermatol. 6:926, 1982.

Child, D. D., Newell, J. D., Bjelland, J. C., et al.: Radiographic findings of pulmonary coccidioidomycosis in neonates and infants. Amer. J. Radiol. 145:216, 1985.

Clapp, D. W., Kleiman, M. B., and Brahmi, Z.: Immunoregulatory lymphocyte populations in disseminated histoplasmosis of infancy. J. Inf. Dis. 156:687, 1987.

Diamond, R. D., and Bennett, J. E.: A subcutaneous reservoir for intrathecal therapy of fungal meningitis. N. Engl. J. Med. 288:186, 1972.

Drutz, D. J., and Catanzaro, D.: Coccidioidomycosis. Am. Rev. Resp. Dis. 117:559, 727, 1978.

Dvorak, A. M., and Gavaller, B.: Congenital systemic candidiasis: Report of a case. N. Engl. J. Med. 274:540, 1966.

Edwards, V. E., Sutherland, J. M., and Tyner, J. H.: Cryptococcosis of the central nervous system. J. Neurol. Neurosurg. Psychiatry 33:415, 1970.

Ellis, C. A., and Spivack, M. L.: The significance of candidemia. Ann. Intern. Med. 67:511, 1967.

Emanuel, B., Ching, E., Lieberman, A. D., et al.: Cryptococcus meningitis in a child successfully treated with amphotericin B, with a review of the literature. J. Pediatr. 59:577, 1961.

Emmons, C. W.: Cryptococcus neoformans, strains from an outbreak of bovine mastitis. Mycopathol. Mycol. Appl. 6:231, 1953.

Eppes, S. C., Troutman, J. L., and Gutman, L. T.: Outcome of treatment of candidemia in children whose central catheters were removed or retained. Pediatr. Inf. Dis. 8:99, 1989.

Faix, R. G.: Systemic Candida infections in infants in intensive care nurseries: High incidence of central nervous system involvement. J. Pediatr. 105:616, 1984.

Fishman, L. S., Griffin, J. R., and Sapico, F. L.: Hematogenous candida endophthalmitis: A complication of candidemia. N. Engl. J. Med. 286:675, 1972.

Freeman, J. B., Weinke, J. W., and Soper, R. T.: Candida osteomyelitis associated with intravenous alimentation. J. Pediatr. Surg. 9:783, 1974.

Goldmann, D. A., and Maki, D. G.: Infection control in total parenteral nutrition. J.A.M.A. 223:1360, 1973.

Haring, H., Johnston, R., and Touloukian, R.: Successfully treated candida endophthalmitis. Pediatrics 51:1027, 1973.

Harrison, H. R., Galgiani, J. N., Reynolds, A. F., et al.: Amphotericin B and imidazole therapy for coccidioidal meningitis in children. Pediatr. Inf. Dis. 2:216, 1983.

Heiner, D. C.: Diagnosis of histoplasmosis. Pediatrics 22:616, 1958.

Henderson, J. L.: Infection in the newborn. Edinburgh Med. J. 50:535, 1943.

Hill, H. R., Mitchell, T. G., Matsen, J. M., et al.: Recovery from disseminated candidiasis in a premature neonate. Pediatrics 53:748, 1974.

Ho, C. Y., and Aterman, K.: Infection of the fetus by candida in a spontaneous abortion. Am. J. Obstet. Gynecol. 106:705, 1970.

Holland, P., and Holland, N. H.: Histoplasmosis in early infancy: Hematologic, histochemical and immunologic observations. Am. J. Dis. Child. 112:412, 1966.

Johnson, D. E., Thompson, T. R., and Ferrieri, P.: Congenital candidiasis. Am. J. Dis. Child 135:273, 1981.

Joshi, W., and Wang, N. S.: Repeated pulmonary embolism in an infant with subacute candida endocarditis of the right side of the heart. Am. J. Dis. Child. 125:257, 1973.

Kafka, J. A., and Catanzaro, P.: Disseminated coccidioidomycosis in children. J. Pediatr. 98:355, 1981.

Kida, M., Abromowsky, C. R., Santoscoy, C.: Cryptococcosis of the placenta in a woman with acquired immunodeficiency syndrome. Hum. Pathol. 20:920, 1989.

Klein, J. D., Yamauchi, T., and Horlick, S. P.: Neonatal candidiasis meningitis and arthritis: Observations and review of literature. J. Pediatr. 81:31, 1972.

Knox, W. F., Hooton, V. N., and Barson, A. J.: Pulmonary vascular candidiasis and use of central venous catheters in neonates. J. Clin. Pathol. 40:559, 1987.

Koenig, N. D.: Candida pneumonia in newborn infants. Dtsch. Med. Wochenschr. 96:818, 1971.

Kozinn, P., and Taschdjian, C. L.: Enteric candidiasis: Diagnosis and clinical considerations. Pediatrics 30:71, 1962.

Lacey, S. R., Zaritsky, A. L., and Azizkhan, R. G.: Successful treatment of candida-infected caval thrombosis in critically ill infants by low-dose streptokinase infusion. J. Pediatr. Surg. 23:1204, 1988.

Leggiadro, R. J., Barrett, F. F., and Hughes, W. T.: Disseminated histoplasmosis of infancy. Pediatr. Infect. Dis. 7:799, 1988.

Lilien, L. D., Ramamurhy, R. S., and Pildes, R. S.: Candida albicans meningitis in a premature neonate successfully treated with 5-fluorocytosine and amphotericin B: A case report and review of the literature. Pediatrics 61:57, 1978.

Little, J., Bruce, J., Andrews, H., et al.: Treatment of disseminated infantile histoplasmosis with amphotericin B. Pediatrics 24:1, 1959.

Mamlock, R. J., Richardson, C. J., Mamlok, V., et al.: A case of intrauterine pulmonary candidiasis. Pediatr. Inf. Dis. 4:692, 1985.

McDonnell, P. J., McDonnell, J. M., Brown, R. H., et al.: Ocular involvement in patients with fungal infections. Ophthalmology 92:706, 1985.

McGregor, J. A., Kleinschmidt-DeMasters, B. K., and Ogle, J.: Meningoencephalitis caused by Histoplasma capsulatum complicating pregnancy. Am. J. Obstet. Gynecol. 154:925, 1986.

Medoff, F., Comfort, M., and Kobayoshi, G. S.: Synergistic action of amphotericin B and 5-fluorocytosine against yeast-like organisms. Proc. Soc. Exp. Biol. Med. 138:571, 1971.

Neuhauser, E. B. D., and Tucker, A.: The roentgen changes produced by diffuse torulosis in the newborn. Am. J. Roentgenol. 59:805, 1948.

Odds, F. C.: Candida infections: An overview. C.R.C. Crit. Rev. Microbiol. 15:1, 1987.

Perrone, J. A.: Laryngeal obstruction due to Monilia albicans in a newborn. Laryngoscope 80:288, 1970.

Peterson, J. C., and Christie, A.: Histoplasmosis. Pediatr. Clin. North Am. 2:127, 1955.

Pounder, W. D., Amberson, J. M., and Jaeger, R. F.: A severe mastitis problem associated with Cryptococcus neoformans in a large dairy herd. Am. J. Vet. Res. 13:121, 1952.

Rhatigan, R. M.: Congenital cutaneous candidiasis. Am. J. Dis. Child. 116:545, 1968.

Rothman, P. E., Graw, R. G., and Harria, J. C.: Coccidioidomycosis—possible fomite transmission. Am. J. Dis. Child. 118:792, 1962.

Sarosi, G. A., Parker, J. D., Doto, I. L., et al.: Amphotericin B in cryptococcal meningitis. Ann. Intern. Med. 71:1079, 1969.

Schirar, A., Rendu, C., Vielk, J. P., et al.: Congenital mycosis (Candida albicans). Biol. Neonate 24:273, 1974.

Shapira, Y., Drucker, M., Russell, A., et al.: Candida endocarditis and encephalitis in an infant. Clin. Pediatr. 13:542, 1974.

Shafai, T.: Neonatal coccidioidomycosis in premature twins. Am. J. Dis. Child. 132:634, 1978.

Shehab, Z. M., Britton, H., and Dunn, J. H.: Imidazole therapy of coccidioidal meningitis in children. Pediatr. Infect. Dis. 7:40, 1988.

Silverman, E. M., Norman, L. F., and Goldman, R. T.: Diagnosis of systemic candidiasis in smears of venous blood stained with Wright's stain. Am. J. Clin. Pathol. 60:473, 1973.

Slotkowsky, E. L.: Formation of mucous membrane lesions secondary to prolonged use of one per cent aqueous gentian violet. J. Pediatr. 51:652, 1957.

Spark, R. P.: Does transplacental spread of coccidioidomycosis occur? Arch. Pathol. Lab. Med. 105:347, 1981.

Townsend, T. E., and McKey, R. W.: Coccidioidomycosis in infants. Am. J. Dis. Child. 86:51, 1953.

Westley, C. R.: Disseminated coccidioidomycosis in children. J. Pediatr. 101:154, 1982.

Wheat, L. J., French, M. C. V., Kohler, R. B., et al.: The diagnostic laboratory tests for histoplasmosis: Analysis of experience in a large urban outbreak. Ann. Intern. Med. 97:680, 1982.

Wheat, L. J., Wass, J., Norton, J., et al.: Cavitary histoplasmosis occurring during two large urban outbreaks. Medicine 63:201, 1984.

Whyte, R. K., Hussain, Z., and deSa, D.: Antenatal infections with Candida species. Arch. Dis. Child. 57:258, 1982.

Winter, W. G., Jr.: Candida (Monilia) infections in children. Pediatr. Clin. North Am. 2:151, 1955.

Wolff, O. H., Petty, B. W., Astley, R., et al.: Thrush oesophagitis with pharyngeal incoordination treated with hydroxystilbamidine. Lancet 1:991, 1955.

Xanthou, M., Valassi-Adawn, E., Kintzonidou, E., et al.: Phagocytosis and killing ability of Candida albicans by blood leukocytes of healthy term and preterm babies. Arch. Dis. Child. 50:72, 1975.

Ziering, W. H., and Rockas, H. R.: Coccidioidomycosis: Long-term treatment with amphotericin B of disseminated disease in a three-month-old baby. Am. J. Dis. Child. 108:454, 1964.

PROTOZOAL INFECTIONS: CONGENITAL TOXOPLASMOSIS AND MALARIA

40

F. Sessions Cole

■ CONGENITAL TOXOPLASMOSIS

One of the organisms that causes congenital infection of the human fetus, often presenting in the newborn period as a local or generalized disease, is *Toxoplasma gondii.* It is obscure why this agent, so different in its biology from cytomegalovirus, rubella, and *Treponema pallidum,* should present so similar a clinical picture. Differentiation from these other syndromes on clinical and laboratory grounds is essential to treatment and prognosis and depends on the extensive knowledge of its epidemiology, clinical behavior, and microbiology gained since the 1960s.

Incidence. Inapparent infection with the protozoan is widespread throughout the world. Population samples indicate that the percentage of adults with antibody is increased at lower geographical latitudes. Feldman (1953) found approximately 10 per cent of his sample positive by complement fixation test in Iceland, 30 per cent in New Orleans, and 65 per cent in Tahiti. However, latitude is by no means the only determining factor. The number of positive reactors in Paris, for instance, is unusually high at 2.3% of all pregnant women seroconverting during pregnancy and has been attributed to Parisians' fondness for raw or undercooked meat. With regard to congenital toxoplasmosis, Eichenwald (1957) was able to comment on the clinical findings in 75 infants and children, and Feldman in 103, observations that suggest the disease cannot be considered rare.

Serum specimens from 22,845 pregnant women in the Collaborative Perinatal Project were studied by Sever (1988) for evidence of infection with *Toxoplasma,* and 38 per cent of the women showed evidence of toxoplasmosis (detectable antibody at titers of ≥32) at some time in the past. Five infants among the group had confirmed congenital toxoplasmosis. The most recent estimates of frequency of congenital infection in the United States range from 1 to 4 per 1000 livebirths. A recent study from Malmö, Sweden, revealed that the incidence of primary maternal infection in that city is 4 to 6 per 1000 deliveries (Ahlfors et al., 1989).

Desmonts and Couvreur (1974) reporting from Paris, found 183 women considered to have been infected during pregnancy. The overall rate of infection in their survey was 6.3 per 100 pregnancies. There were 11 abortions, seven stillbirths, and 59 patients with congenital toxoplasmosis. In this latter group, two infants died, seven had severe disease, 11 had mild disease, and 39 had no symptoms or signs at the time of the surgery.

Etiology. The disease is caused by infestation with a protozoan, *Toxoplasma gondii,* so named because it was first isolated in 1909 from a North African rodent called the "gondi." In addition to the large number of human beings who are infected, many domestic and wild animals and birds harbor the organism. The domestic cat is the only definitive host and is the reservoir of the infective oocysts that are passed in the feces. Congenital toxoplasmosis is caused by invasion of the fetal blood stream by parasites during a stage of maternal parasitemia. It is likely that the parasitemia occurs only with initial infection and often in the absence of any maternal symptoms. Mothers whose infections become chronic and inapparent do not transmit the disease to subsequent fetuses. Desmonts and Couvreur describe infection of the fetus in 33 per cent of all maternal infections. This figure should, however, be considered only an estimate because many mothers in the study were treated. Recent data from the Collaborative Perinatal Project (5 of 15 infants, or 33 per cent), and from Sweden (6 of 29 infants, or 21 per cent) indicate that this estimate is reasonable (Ahlfors et al., 1989; Sever et al., 1988). The proportion infected is high throughout pregnancy, although severe disease in the newborn is usually seen only with first- and second-trimester infections.

Postnatal infections also occur in children, but the youngest patient we have encountered in the literature is a 7-month infant who became ill with diarrhea at 3 months

This chapter includes some contributions from the previous authors, Dr. Arnold Smith and Dr. Kenneth McIntosh.

of age. The disease occurred 1 month after the institution of unpasteurized goat's milk feeding and was almost surely the result of that form of alimentation (Riemann et al., 1975).

Pathology. The *Toxoplasma* is a crescent-shaped oval organism, 4 to 7 microns long, with a single, approximately central nucleus. In tissues it is intracellular, and small or large agglomerates are often seen. In later stages, the organism is often seen lying within a cystic space, especially in the brain and skeletal and heart muscle.

In the newborn, the principal locus of infection is the central nervous system. Lesions consist of areas of necrosis in which calcium is ultimately deposited and throughout which cysts or the naked parasite may be sparsely scattered. Similar lesions are less abundant in the liver, lungs, myocardium, skeletal muscle, spleen, and other tissues. There is little cellular inflammatory reaction, consisting mostly of lymphocytes, monocytes, and plasma cells. The pathologic picture is not specific unless organisms or cysts can be demonstrated.

Diagnosis. The majority of infants with congenital toxoplasmosis have no symptoms or apparent abnormalities at birth. In Desmonts and Couvreur's series, there were two subclinical cases for each clinical one. Such infants, however, usually develop disease as they grow older. The natural history of the disease described by these authors may be different in the 1990s due to antenatal diagnosis and treatment. In a 1988 study by Daffos and co-workers, all 15 infants whose mothers had acute infection between the 17th and 25th week of pregnancy were found to be asymptomatic at birth with normal fundoscopic examinations and normal cerebrospinal fluid findings. Four had cerebral calcifications, and two of the 15 infants developed chorioretinitis (at 4 months and 18 months of age). It is important to note that all mothers and infants received treatment.

The so-called classic triad of congenital toxoplasmosis is present in only a small proportion of symptomatic cases. Chorioretinitis, hydrocephalus, and intracranial calcifications were present in 86, 20, and 37 per cent, respectively, of the large series of Eichenwald (1957). Fever, hepatosplenomegaly, and jaundice are frequent signs, even in the absence of central nervous system or ocular findings. Rash and pneumonitis occasionally occur. The spinal fluid is often abnormal. Anemia is frequent, and thrombocytopenia and eosinophilia are occasionally seen. Cataracts, microphthalmia, and glaucoma, so common in rubella, are rare. Microcephaly is less common than hydrocephalus. Diarrhea is occasionally a prominent symptom. More recent data from a study of 210 congenitally infected infants by Couvreur and associates (1984) adapted by Remington and Desmonts (1990) indicate lower frequencies for these signs and symptoms (Table 40–1). These differences may be due to antenatal therapy or to detection of primary maternal infections and subsequent termination.

Neurologic and ocular involvement frequently appear later if they are absent at birth. Convulsions, mental retardation, and spasticity are all common sequelae. A morphologically characteristic relapsing chorioretinitis is the commonest sequela of congenital toxoplasmosis, al-

though involvement of the anterior uveal tract also occurs (O'Connor, 1974). It is also clear that most, if not all cases of *Toxoplasma* chorioretinitis represent the sequelae of congenital infection. Treatment has probably changed the rather grim prognosis of congenital disease, as discussed further on.

Although some infants are highly symptomatic at birth, the disease may also be insidious in onset.

In 1953, Beckett and Flynn reported two infants with toxoplasmosis. The first is described in the following case history.

CASE 40–1

An infant born at term seemed normal until the 5th day, when ptosis of one lid was noted. In the 4th week, vomiting and pallor developed; in the 5th week, high-pitched cry, enlargement of the head, and opisthotonos were noted. Examination at 6 weeks showed dehydration, pallor, sluggishness, hydrocephalus, bulging fontanel, separated sutures, and right facial nerve palsy. The liver and spleen were not large, purpura was absent, and platelets were normal. Cerebrospinal fluid was grossly abnormal and xanthochromic, containing 200 red blood cells/mm³ and 2900 mg of protein/dl. Skull radiographs showed fine scattered calcifications.

The epidemiology in this example was noteworthy. The antibody titer of the mother against Toxoplasma registered 1:4906, whereas that of a pet dachshund that had had "brain fever" with residual paralysis of one leg at the time of the infant's conception was 1:256!

Other more bizarre forms of the disease have been described. Silver and Dixon's case (1954), described in the following paragraph, is one of the more remarkable ones, demonstrating how protean the manifestations of congenital toxoplasmosis can be.

CASE 40–2

This infant's course was one of increasing lethargy, poor appetite, and bleeding manifestations until hospital admission in his 6th week. Facial nerve palsy, hepatosplenomegaly, lethargy, pupillary membranes, and cataracts were found. Cerebrospinal fluid was xanthochromic and contained a few white and red blood cells and 1000 mg of protein/dl. Radiographs of the skull showed flaky calcific densities. This patient's course in the hospital was characterized by hypothermia, persistent hypernatremia, and inability to concentrate urine except when treated with posterior pituitary extract. He also showed eosinophilia of the peripheral blood (30 per cent) and of the bone marrow.

Laboratory Findings. Since culture of the organism is tedious and expensive, laboratory diagnosis depends heavily on interpretation of various serologic tests. There are several valuable tests for antibody to *Toxoplasma gondii*. Although the Sabin-Feldman dye test (lysis of *Toxoplasma* organisms by various dilutions of maternal or infant serum after incubation for 1 hour at 37°C) used to be the standard method, several newer tests easier to perform and of equal reliability have supplanted it in many laboratories, particularly the indirect fluorescent antibody (IFA) test and the enzyme-linked immunosorbent assay (ELISA). Both tests can be adapted to measure IgM

TABLE 40–1. Prospective Study of Infants Born to Women Who Acquired *Toxoplasma* Infection During Pregnancy: Signs and Symptoms in 210 Infants with Proved Congenital Infection

FINDING		NUMBER EXAMINED	NUMBER POSITIVE (%)
Prematurity	Birth weight below 2500 g	210	8 (3.8)
	Birth weight of 2500–3000 g		5 (7.1)
Dysmaturity (intrauterine growth retardation)			13 (6.2)
Postmaturity		108	9 (8.3)
Icterus		201	20 (10)
Hepatosplenomegaly		210	9 (4.2)
Thrombocytopenic purpura		210	3 (1.4)
Abnormal blood count (anemia, eosinophilia)		102	9 (4.4)
Microcephaly		210	11 (5.2)
Hydrocephalus		210	8 (3.8)
Hypotonia		210	2 (5.7)
Convulsions		210	8 (3.8)
Psychomotor retardation		210	11 (5.2)
Intracranial calcifications on x-ray		210	24 (11.4)
Abnormal ultrasound examination		49	5 (10)
Abnormal computer tomographic scan of brain		13	11 (84)
Abnormal electroencephalographic result		191	16 (8.3)
Abnormal cerebrospinal fluid		163	56 (34.2)
Microphthalmia		210	6 (2.8)
Strabismus		210	11 (5.2)
Chorioretinitis	Unilateral	210	34 (16.1)
	Bilateral		12 (5.7)

(From Remington, J. S., and Desmonts, G.: Toxoplasmosis. *In* Remington, J. S., and Klein, J. O. (Eds.): Infectious Diseases of the Fetus and Newborn Infant. Philadelphia, W. B. Saunders Company, 1990, p. 132.)

antibody. As with other congenital infections, false-positive IgM antibody titers may be caused by rheumatoid factor. Complement fixation and indirect hemagglutination tests may also be performed but are somewhat more difficult to interpret. Detection of IgA antibodies against P30, a major surface protein of *Toxoplasma gondii,* has recently been reported to be more sensitive than detection of anti-P30 IgM antibodies in identification of congenitally infected infants (DeCoster et al., 1988). All eight congenitally infected infants from 26 mothers infected during pregnancy were identified by the presence of anti-P30 IgA antibodies, while anti-P30 IgM antibodies were found in three of the eight infected infants.

Antibody develops during acute infection in the mother and remains high or drops slowly over time. A single high antibody titer implies, but does not prove, recent infection. In the infant, the titer at birth equals or exceeds the mother's, regardless of whether or not the baby is congenitally infected. Over the 1st year in the uninfected infant, the titer drops with a half-life of about 30 days. In the infected infant, although the titer may drop somewhat for the first few months, it rises again to a high level by the first birthday. IgM anti-*Toxoplasma* antibody may be present at birth or at any time for the next few months. A negative *Toxoplasma* antibody titer in the infant's serum at 6 months to 1 year of age essentially excludes the diagnosis.

When symptomatic and/or serologic evidence of *Toxoplasma* infection is detected during pregnancy, fetal infection can be diagnosed (Daffos et al., 1988; Desmonts et al., 1985). Specific fetal diagnosis is predicated upon detection of IgM anti-*Toxoplasma* antibodies and upon isolation (by mouse inoculation) of the parasite from fetal blood or amniotic fluid obtained between 20 and 26 weeks of gestation. In the study by Daffos and colleagues (1988), fetal *Toxoplasma* infection was documented by parasite isolation from fetal blood or amniotic fluid in 34

of 746 pregnancies. An additional five pregnancies had serologic fetal biochemical and ultrasonographic evidence of fetal *Toxoplasma* infection. *Toxoplasma*-specific IgM antibodies were identified in fetal blood in only nine cases. Ultrasound examination was helpful in antenatal diagnosis by detecting ascites in two cases and ventricular dilation in 17 cases. Important to note is the fact that 10 of the 17 cases of ventricular dilation were noted in the third trimester after positive results were obtained by blood or amniotic fluid sampling. Ultrasound findings consistent with *Toxoplasma* infection in the context of maternal seroconversion permits consideration of maternal treatment prior to availability of culture results and findings with which to monitor fetal progress (Daffos et al., 1988). Finally, besides the 34 infected fetuses, an additional three pregnancies resulted in congenital infection. These infections occurred despite antenatal maternal therapy and most likely represent parasite transmission to the fetus after the time of fetal blood sampling (Daffos et al., 1988).

Treatment. Maternal treatment for women who acquire *Toxoplasma* infection during pregnancy reduces the likelihood of congenital transmission by as much as 70 per cent (Daffos et al., 1988; McCabe and Remington, 1988). Because 85 to 95 per cent of women of child-bearing age in the United States are at risk and only 10 per cent of immunocompetent women are symptomatic if infected, serologic screening as described by Daffos and co-workers (1988) prior to or early in pregnancy should be strongly considered to identify women at risk for infection. Seroconversion should prompt institution of maternal therapy (spiramycin, 3 g/day). This treatment should be continued throughout pregnancy. If fetal infection is diagnosed, 3 weeks of spiramycin therapy should be alternated with 3 weeks of pyrimethamine, 50 mg/day, and sulfadiazine, 3 g/day after the 24th week of gestation (Daffos et al., 1988). Careful hematologic monitoring should be

TABLE 40–2. Guidelines for the Treatment of Congenital Toxoplasmosis[a, b]

Drugs

1. *Pyrimethamine + sulfadiazine:*
   Pyrimethamine: 15 mg/m² per day or 1 mg/kg per day (maximum daily dose is 25 mg) by the oral route. Although the half-life of the drug is 4 to 5 days, it should be given on a daily basis unless breaking of the tablets is grossly inaccurate during preparation of the smaller doses. In such cases, as for very small infants (e.g., when a daily dose of 3 mg is indicated), breaking of a tablet may result in a slightly higher dose, which could be administered every 2 days.
   Sulfadiazine or trisulfapyrimidines: 85 mg/kg per day by the oral route in two divided doses daily.
2. *Spiramycin*[c]: 100 mg/kg per day by the oral route in two divided doses.
3. *Corticosteroids: (prednisone or methylprednisolone):* 1.5 mg/kg per day by the oral route in two divided doses daily. The drug is continued until the inflammatory process (e.g., high level of cerebrospinal fluid protein [≥100 mg/dl before the age of 1 month], chorioretinitis) has subsided; dosage should then be tapered progressively and discontinued.
4. *Folinic acid:* 5 mg every 3 days (intramuscularly in young infants) during treatment with pyrimethamine. If bone marrow toxicity occurs at this dose, increase to 10 mg every 3 days. If bone marrow toxicity is severe, discontinue pyrimethamine until the abnormality is corrected and then begin pyrimethamine again using 10 mg folinic acid every 3 days. In some infants, it may be necessary to administer folinic acid more frequently.

Indications

1. *Overt congenital toxoplasmosis:* The course of treatment is for 1 year in all cases. For infants in whom clinical signs of the infection are present, treatment during the first 6 months is with pyrimethamine + sulfadiazine. During the following 6 months, 1 month of pyrimethamine + sulfadiazine is alternated with 1 month of spiramycin. Folinic acid should be started as soon as possible. No treatment is usually given after 12 months of age except when there is evidence of evolution of the infection, such as a flare-up of chorioretinitis.
2. *Overt congenital toxoplasmosis with evidence of inflammatory process* (chorioretinitis, high level of cerebrospinal fluid protein, generalized infection, jaundice): as in no. 1 above + corticosteroids.
3. *Subclinical congenital Toxoplasma infection:* Pyrimethamine + sulfadiazine for 6 weeks; thereafter, alternate with spiramycin. Spiramycin is given for 6 weeks and alternated with 4 weeks of pyrimethamine + sulfadiazine to complete a treatment course of 1 year.
4. *Healthy newborn in whom serologic testing has not provided definitive results but maternal infection was proved to have been acquired during pregnancy:* One course of pyrimethamine + sulfadiazine for 1 month. Obtain consultation with appropriate authority to determine necessity for continued therapy and drug and dosage regimen. This decision must be made on an individual basis and depends on multiple factors, including serologic test titers, immune load and clinical findings in the infant.
5. *Healthy newborn born to a mother with high Sabin-Feldman dye test titer—date of maternal infection undetermined:* Spiramycin for 1 month. Then as in no. 4 above. It must be borne in mind that in certain cases the indication for treatment is difficult to define because of a lack of information about the pregnancy and lack of isolation attempts from the corresponding placenta.

[a]Recommendations of Dr. Jacques Couvreur, Laboratoire de Sérologie Néonatale et de Recherche sur la Toxoplasmose, Institut de Puériculture, Paris.
[b]See under Therapy section for qualifications to the treatment recommended here.
[c]Available in the United States only by request to the U.S. Food and Drug Administration.
(From Remington, J. S., and Desmonts, G.: Toxoplasmosis. In Remington, J. S., and Klein, J. O. (Eds.): Infectious Diseases of the Fetus and Newborn Infant. Philadelphia, W. B. Saunders Company, 1990.)

performed along with concurrent treatment with folinic acid. Because of the lack of data, it is currently impossible to estimate the teratogenic and toxic risks to the fetus from antenatal therapy with pyrimethamine and sulfadiazine. Before initiation of therapy, fetal diagnosis should be attempted to permit evaluation of risk and benefit of these drugs.

Treatment is recommended for all cases of congenital toxoplasmosis or congenital *Toxoplasma* infection. Guidelines for treatment are given in Table 40–2.

Prognosis. It has been known for some time that the prognosis in untreated infants with overt disease at birth is poor (Eichenwald, 1960). Cerebral calcifications were thought to be a particularly ominous finding. Prospective follow-up studies in the 1960s and 1970s of congenitally infected infants asymptomatic at birth have shown that, even in this group, chorioretinitis is frequent and central nervous system involvement is not uncommon. In 1980, Wilson and co-workers found that 11 of 13 such infants developed chorioretinitis and that one developed, in addition, seizures and severe psychomotor retardation. In the same study, 11 other children were identified and followed because they presented with symptoms. All 11 had been asymptomatic at birth. In this group, three developed major neurologic sequelae, five were blind in both eyes, and three were blind in one eye. Ocular involvement may not begin until the end of the first decade.

More recently, the impact of antenatal diagnosis, antenatal treatment, and treatment during infancy has decreased the frequency of major neurologic sequelae (Daffos et al., 1988). The overall risk of fetal infection in symptomatic or asymptomatic women who become seropositive is dependent upon the time in gestation when maternal infection occurs: the later the stage in gestation, the more likely the transmission of parasites (Hohlfeld et al., 1989). The overall risk of fetal infection in Hohlfeld's study was 7 per cent, most likely a reflection of antenatal spiramycin treatment. Fifty-four infants from this study have been followed for periods from 6 months to 4 years. The infants' condition at birth is indicated in Table 40–3. Forty-seven of the 54 infants followed received treatment consisting of pyrimethamine and sulfonamides alternating with spiramycin. The overall rate of subclinical infections was 76 per cent. Fifty-three infants had normal development and neurologic status at follow-up. Five of the 53 had peripheral chorioretinitis, as demonstrated by a scar noted between 5 and 17 months of life. One infant who did not receive prenatal treatment because of a false-

TABLE 40–3. Condition of Live Neonates and Positive Findings at Birth

OBSERVATIONS	NUMBER	PER CENT
Subclinical infection	44/54	81
Multiple cranial calcifications	5/54	9
Single intracranial calcification	2/54	4
Chorioretinitis scar	3/54	6
Abnormal lumbar puncture	1/54	2
Positive findings on inoculation of placenta	23/46	50
Positive cord blood IgM	8/53	15

(From Hohlfeld, P., Daggos, F., Thulliez, P., et al: Fetal toxoplasmosis: Outcome of pregnancy and infant follow-up after in utero treatment. J. Pediatr. *115*:765, 1989.)

TABLE 40–4. Comparison of Different Outcomes of Liveborn Infants with Congenital *Toxoplasma* Infection

	TRIMESTER											
	First				Second				Third			
	1972–1981		1982–1988		1972–1981		1982–1988		1972–1981		1982–1988	
Outcome	No.	%	No.	%	No.	%	No.	%	No.	%	No.	
Subclinical	1	10	6	67	23	37	33	77	74	68	2	
Benign	5	50	2	22	28	45	10	23	31	29	0	
Severe	4	40	1	11	11	18	0		3	3	0	
TOTAL	10		9		62		43		108		2	

(From Hohlfeld, P., Daggos, F., Thulliez, P., et al.: Fetal toxoplasmosis: Outcome of pregnancy and infant follow-up after in utero treatment. J. Pediatr. *115*:765, 1989.)

negative prenatal diagnosis developed bilateral chorioretinitis and ventricular dilation that necessitated a ventriculoperitoneal shunt at 1 month of age. The improving outcome of infants with congenital *Toxoplasma* infection are indicated in Table 40–4.

■ CONGENITAL MALARIA

Despite the high prevalence of malaria in many parts of the world, congenital malaria, that is, malaria acquired either in utero or in the perinatal period, is a relatively uncommon disease. Maternal parasitemia is presumably frequent, but transmission to the fetus appears to be effectively prevented in the great majority of instances by the placental barrier. Disease acquired in utero is, consequently, rare. Transmission at the time of birth is somewhat more common and is probably a consequence of placental leak of infected erythrocytes during delivery combined with inadequate immunity at the time of transmission (Randall and Seidel, 1985).

Etiology and Incidence. The incidence of malaria in the United States and North America has risen during the 1980s due to increasing overseas travel, immigration, and the spread of drug-resistant parasites (Lynk and Gold, 1989). Infections have involved all four species of *Plasmodium* infecting humans. The incidence in endemic areas has been estimated to be 0.3 per cent, with disease more likely when a mother acquires malaria for the first time during pregnancy and in primigravidas (Randall and Seidel, 1985). The risk of transfusion malaria in the United States from 1972 to 1981 was 0.25 per million donor units (Guerro et al., 1983). Transfusion has been infrequently associated with malaria infection in neonatal intensive care units (Bove, 1986; Piccoli et al., 1983; Randall and Seidel, 1985; Shulman et al., 1984).

Diagnosis. The mother may or may not have symptomatic malaria during pregnancy, and cases have been described in which maternal disease was acquired not in an endemic area but through intravenous drug use or transfusion. In most instances, however, the history of exposure to malaria is clear. The child is usually normal at birth. Symptoms appear at 3 to 12 weeks of age. Fever is followed by hepatosplenomegaly, loss of appetite, listlessness, progressive hemolytic anemia, diarrhea, and jaundice.

The diagnosis is normally confirmed by demonstration of characteristic parasites on a thin or thick blood smear, and the particular species is determined by the morphology of the stained forms. Serologic studies can be used to confirm the diagnosis. If intrauterine transmission occurred, IgM antibody may be present in cord blood (Hindi and Azimi, 1980; Thomas and Chit, 1980). A rapid diagnostic test based on acridine orange staining of centrifuged parasites in a microhematocrit tube has been reported by Rickman and associates (1989). While not a substitute for the thick blood smear, it may provide easy, prompt diagnosis.

Treatment and Prognosis. Congenital malaria, like transfusion-acquired malaria, has no exoerythrocytic (liver) stage. When the organism is chloroquine-sensitive, therefore, chloroquine alone (5 mg/kg of the base by mouth or gavage daily for 5 days) is adequate for treatment, and primaquine is not required. Chloroquine pharmacokinetics has been studied in children, and the drug can be used in infants who do not tolerate enteral treatment. Parenteral chloroquine (0.83 mg of base per kg per hour for 30 hours intravenously, or 3.5 mg/kg every 6 hours by intramuscular or subcutaneous injection) provided an acceptable therapeutic ratio (White et al., 1988). When chloroquine resistance is suspected, multiple drugs may be necessary, including parenteral quinidine gluconate or alternatively, exchange transfusion (Miller et al., 1989).

Not every child of every mother with malaria requires treatment at birth, since most will not acquire the disease. When maternal malaria is recognized at parturition, the infant should be followed carefully, and treatment instituted, if necessary. Blood transfusion is frequently necessary in affected children, and in areas with a high frequency of human immunodeficiency virus (HIV) infection, these transfusions put congenitally infected children at increased risk for HIV infection (Greenberg et al., 1988).

Follow-up blood smears should confirm that treatment has been successful. In such instances, the prognosis is excellent.

■ REFERENCES

Ahlfors, K., Borjeson, M., Huldt, G., et al.: Incidence of toxoplasmosis in pregnant women in the city of Malmö. Scand. J. Inf. Dis. *21*:315, 1989.

Beckett, R. S., and Flynn, F. J., Jr.: Toxoplasmosis: Report of two new cases with a classification and with a demonstration of the organisms in the human placenta. N. Engl. J. Med. *249*:345, 1953.

Bove, J. R.: Transfusion transmitted diseases: Current problems and challenges. Prog. Hematol. *14*:123, 1986.

Couvreur, J., Desmonts, G., Tournier, G., et al.: A homogeneous series of 20 cases of congenital toxoplasmosis in 0 to 11 month old infants detected prospectively. Ann. Pediatr. *31*:815, 1984.

Daffos, F., Forestier, F., Capola-Pavlovsky, M., et al.: Prenatal management of 746 pregnancies at risk for congenital toxoplasmosis. N. Engl. J. Med. *318*:271, 1988.

Decoster, A., Darcy, F., Caron, A., et al.: IgA antibodies against P30 as markers of congenital acute toxoplasmosis. Lancet *2*:1104, 1988.

Desmonts, G., and Couvreur, J.: Cerebral toxoplasmosis, a prospective study of 378 pregnancies. N. Engl. J. Med. *270*:1110, 1974.

Desmonts, G., Forestier, F., Thulliez, P., et al.: Prenatal diagnosis of congenital toxoplasmosis. Lancet *1*:500, 1985.

Eichenwald, H.: Congenital toxoplasmosis. A study of one hundred fifty cases. Am. J. Dis. Child. *94*:411, 1957.

Eichenwald, H.: A study of congenital toxoplasmosis. *In* Slim, J. D. (Ed.): Human Toxoplasmosis. Copenhagen, Munksgaard, 1960.

Feldman, H. A.: The clinical manifestations and laboratory diagnosis of toxoplasmosis. Am. J. Trop. Med. *2*:420, 1953.

Feldman, H. A.: Toxoplasmosis. N. Engl. J. Med. *279*:1370, 1431, 1968.

Greenberg, A. E., Nguyen-Dinh, P., Mann, J. M., et al.: The association between malaria, blood transfusions, and HIV seropositivity in a pediatric population in Kinshasa, Zaire. J.A.M.A. *259*:545, 1988.

Guero, I. C., Weniger, B. C., and Schultz, M. G.: Transfusion malaria in the United States, 1972–1981. Ann. Intern. Med. *99*:21, 1983.

Hindi, R. D., and Azimi, P. H.: Congenital malaria due to *Plasmodium falciparum*. Pediatrics *66*:977, 1980.

Hohlfeld, P., Daffos, F., Thulliez, P., et al.: Fetal toxoplasmosis: Outcome of pregnancy and infant follow-up after in utero treatment. J. Pediatr. *115*:765, 1989.

Lynk, A., and Gold, R.: Review of 40 children with imported malaria. Pediatr. Infect. Dis. J. *8*:745, 1989.

McCabe, R., and Remington, J. S.: Toxoplasmosis: The time has come. N. Engl. J. Med. *318*:313, 1988.

Miller, K. D., Greenberg, A. E., and Campbell, C. C.: Treatment of severe malaria in the United States with a continuous infusion of quinidine gluconate and exchange transfusion. N. Engl. J. Med. *321*:65, 1989.

O'Connor, G. R.: Manifestations and management of ocular toxoplasmosis. Bull. N.Y. Acad. Med. *50*:192, 1974.

Piccoli, D. A., Perlman, S., and Ephros, M.: Transfusion-acquired *Plasmodium malariae* infection in two premature infants. Pediatrics *72*:560, 1983.

Randall, G., and Seidel, J. S.: Malaria. Pediatr. Clin. North Am. *32*:893, 1985.

Remington, J. S., and Desmonts, G.: Toxoplasmosis. *In* Remington, J. S., and Klein, J. O. (Eds.): Infectious Diseases of the Fetus and Newborn Infant. Philadelphia, W. B. Saunders Company, 1990, pp. 89–195.

Rickman, L. S., Long, G. W., Oberst, R., et al.: Rapid diagnosis of malaria by acridine orange staining of centrifuged parasites. Lancet *1*:68, 1989.

Riemann, H. P., Meyer, M. E., Theis, J. H., et al.: Toxoplasmosis in an infant fed unpasteurized goat milk. J. Pediatr. *87*:573, 1975.

Sabin, A. B., and Feldman, H. A.: Dyes as microchemical indicators of a new immunity phenomenon affecting a protozoon parasite *(Toxoplasma)*. Science *108*:660, 1948.

Sever, J. L., Ellenberg, J. H., Ley, A. C., et al.: Toxoplasmosis: Maternal and pediatric findings in 23,000 pregnancies. Pediatrics *82*:181, 1988.

Shabin, B., Papadopoulou, Z. L., and Jenis, H.: Congenital nephrotic syndrome associated with congenital toxoplasmosis. J. Pediatr. *85*:366, 1974.

Shulman, I. A., Saxena, S., Nelson, J. M., et al.: Neonatal exchange transfusions complicated by transfusion-induced malaria. Pediatrics *73*:330, 1984.

Silver, H. K., and Dixon, M. S., Jr.: Congenital toxoplasmosis: Report of case with cataract, "atypical" vasopressin-sensitive diabetes insipidus, and marked eosinophilia. J. Dis. Child. *88*:84, 1954.

Thomas, V., and Chit, C. W.: A case of congenital malaria in Malaysia with IgM malaria antibodies. Trans. Roy. Soc. Trop. Med. Hyg. *74*:73, 1980.

White, N. J., Miller, K. D., Churchill, F. C., et al.: Choroquine treatment of severe malaria in children. Pharmacokinetics, toxicity, and new dosage recommendations. N. Engl. J. Med. *319*:1493, 1988.

Wilson, C. B., Remington, J. S., Stagno, S., et al.: Development of adverse sequelae in children born with subclinical congenital *Toxoplasma* infection. Pediatrics *66*:767, 1980.

INFECTIONS WITH **41** SPIROCHETAL AND PARASITIC ORGANISMS

F. Sessions Cole

■ CONGENITAL SYPHILIS

Prior to 1945, a chapter on congenital syphilis in a textbook devoted to diseases of the newborn would have been the most important one in the infectious disease section because of the great number of newborns affected and the broad variety of clinical syndromes produced. If this chapter had been omitted in the 1950s and 1960s, it would have been scarcely missed. In many parts of the United States, a young pediatrician might have completed 3 years of residency in a large urban hospital without ever having encountered one case, but now the situation has changed. The disease is staging a modest comeback.

Incidence. During the 1930s and 1940s, in the congenital syphilis clinic of the Harriet Lane Home in Baltimore, Maryland, 60 to 80 infants and children showed up each week for arsenical therapy. A great many more were lost to view before completing their 2- to 3-year course of treatment. It was an unusual week if three or four new examples in the general outpatient department were not discovered. Then for several decades the frequency of the disease fell. The curve of incidence has been rising since the 1970s, however (Fig. 41–1). From 1980 to 1986, the number of cases of congenital syphilis rose from 111 cases to 365 cases per year in the United States. Over 600 cases were reported in 1989. Of note are the recent roles of inadequate or no prenatal care (48 per cent of cases) and treatment failure (19 per cent of total cases and 35 per cent of women who had prenatal care) in the rising frequency of congenital syphilis (MMWR, 1986).

Etiology and Pathogenesis. The organism responsible for syphilis is *Treponema pallidum*. This delicate, corkscrew-shaped, flagellated, highly motile spirochete is almost identical in appearance with *T. pertenue,* which causes yaws. These two diseases, like smallpox and cowpox, produce a cross-immunity for one another. This fact was established for Alexander Schaffer, the first editor of this textbook, when, after having spent 2 years on yaws-infested Fiji without encountering one case of syphilis, he was transferred to yaws-free India, where syphilis became one of his main medical preoccupations.

Syphilis can be acquired by introduction of *Treponema*

through an abrasion in the skin or mucous membrane or by transplacental transmission. While adults and some children become infected percutaneously, young infants almost invariably receive the organism from their mothers via the placenta and the umbilical vein. Transplacental transmission may take place at any time during gestation but ordinarily occurs during the second half of pregnancy. Fetuses infected early may die in utero or are at high risk for significant neurodevelopmental morbidity. The usual outcome of a third-trimester infection is the birth of an apparently normal infant who becomes ill within the first few weeks of life. While virtually all infants born to women with primary or secondary infection have congenital infection, only 50 per cent are clinically symptomatic. Early latent infection results in a 40 per cent infant infection rate, and late latent infection in a 6 to 14 per cent infant infection rate (Wendel, 1988).

Pathology. Since *Treponema* enters the fetal bloodstream directly, the primary stage of infection is completely bypassed. There is no chancre and no local lymphadenopathy. Instead, the liver, the immediate target of the

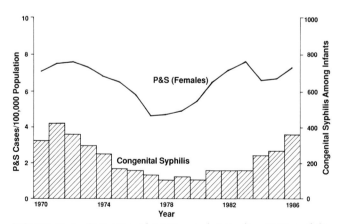

FIGURE 41–1. *Case rates of primary and secondary (P&S) syphilis among females and congenital syphilis among infants less than 1 year of age in the United States, 1970 to 1986. Unpublished observations, Statistical Branch, Sexually Transmitted Diseases, Centers for Disease Control. (From Ingall, D., Dobson, S. R. M., and Musher, D.: Syphilis. In Remington, J. S., and Klein, J. O. [Eds.]: Infectious Diseases of the Fetus and Newborn Infant. Philadelphia, W. B. Saunders Company, 1990, pp. 367–394.)*

TABLE 41–1. Clinical Features of Early Congenital Syphilis

FEATURE	AGE <4 WEEKS (%)	AGE >4 WEEKS (%)
Hepatosplenomegaly	91	87
Joint swellings	3	34
Skin rash	31	55
Anemia	64	89
Jaundice	49	7
Snuffles	12	50
Metaphyseal dystrophy	95	91
Periostitis	37	80
Cerebrospinal fluid changes	44	37

(From Hira, S. K., Bhat, G. J., Patel, J. B., et al.: Early congenital syphilis: Clinicoradiologic features in 202 patients. Sex. Transm. Dis. *12*:177, 1985.)

invasion, is flooded with organisms, which then penetrate all the other organs and tissues of the body to a lesser degree. Exactly where they take root and arouse local pathologic response, which in turn produces the presenting signs and symptoms, is unpredictable. Principal sites of predilection are the liver, skin, mucous membranes of the lips and anus, bones, and the central nervous system. If fetal invasion has taken place early, the lungs may be heavily involved in a characteristic *pneumonia alba,* but this condition is seldom compatible with life. *Treponema* may be found in almost any other organ or tissue of the body but seldom causes inflammatory and destructive changes in loci other than the ones named previously.

Under the microscope, the tissue alterations consist of nonspecific interstitial fibrosis with or without evidences of low-grade inflammatory response in the form of round cell inflammation. Necrosis follows fairly regularly in bone but only rarely in other tissues. Localization and gumma formation are not common in the neonate. Noteworthy is extensive extramedullary hematopoiesis in the liver, spleen, kidneys, and other organs.

Diagnosis. The most common signs and symptoms of congenital infection in the neonatal period are listed in Table 41–1. Additional diagnoses associated with congenital syphilis are nonimmune hydrops, nephrosis, and myocarditis (Wendel, 1988). The earliest sign of congenital syphilis may be snuffles. The nose becomes obstructed and begins to discharge clear fluid at first then purulent or even sanguineous material later.

Cutaneous lesions appear at any time from the 2nd week on. They are sparse or numerous and are copper-colored, round, oval, iris-shaped, circinate, or desquamative. Even more characteristic than their appearance is

their distribution which most frequently includes perioral, perinasal, and diaper regions. Palms and soles are also involved, but the rash is soon replaced there by diffuse reddening, thickening, and wrinkling. In heavily infected infants, the rash may become generalized. Mucocutaneous junctions become involved in typical fashion. The lips become thickened and roughened and tend to weep. Radial cracks appear that traverse the vermilion zone up to and a bit beyond the mucocutaneous margins of the lips. These are the beginnings of the radiating scars that may persist for many years as rhagades. Similar mucocutaneous lesions involve the anus and vulva, but in these locations one also encounters, though less frequently, the white, flat, moist, raised plaques known as "condylomata."

Radiographs of the bones reveal characteristic osteochondritis and periostitis in 80 to 90 per cent of infants with congenital syphilis. In most, the bone lesions are asymptomatic, but in a few, severe enough to lead to subepiphyseal fracture and epiphyseal dislocation, extremely painful pseudoparalysis of one or more extremities may supervene. Radiographic alterations include an unusually dense band at the epiphyseal ends, below which is a band of translucency whose margins are at first sharp but that later become serrated, jagged, and irregular. The shafts become generally more opaque, but spotty areas of translucency throughout them may give them a moth-eaten look. The periosteum of the long bones becomes more and more thickened. Epiphyses separate because the dense end plate breaks away from the shaft by fracture through the subepiphyseal zone of decalcification. This is exactly what happens in the pseudoparalysis of scurvy, although the reason for the weakening of the subepiphyseal bone is quite different. In syphilis, pseudoparalysis appears within the first 3 months; in scurvy, it seldom presents before 5 months.

Signs of visceral involvement include hepatomegaly, splenomegaly, and general glandular enlargement. Palpable epitrochlear nodes are not pathognomonic but are highly suggestive of congenital syphilis. The liver may be greatly enlarged, firm, and nontender. Associated with this may be jaundice, which appears in the 2nd or 3rd week, is seldom intense, and does not persist for many days. Anemia, probably indicative of bone marrow infection and hematopoietic suppression, may become severe. Lesions in the gastrointestinal tract and pancreas may occur and produce distention and delay in passage of meconium.

Clinical signs of central nervous system involvement seldom appear in the newborn infant, even though one-third to one-half of those infected suffer such involvement.

TABLE 41–2. Cerebrospinal Fluid Findings in 108 Patients with Congenital Syphilis*

	% OF TOTAL NO. OF INFANTS IN AGE GROUP FOR INFANTS AGED			CEREBROSPINAL FLUID		
	91–180 Days (47)†	181–365 Days (31)	366–731 Days (30)	Cells/ml	Protein (mg/100 ml)	VDRL Titer
Asymptomatic (normal)	28	45	63	0–5	15–30	Negative
Minimal involvement	30	32	27	5–30	30–75	Negative
Intermediate involvement	36	20	10	0–100	Moderate increase	Positive
Paretic formula	6	3	0	10–200	50–200	Positive

*Infants with congenital syphilis are defined by clinical status, repeated serologic testing, or dark-field microscopic examination.
†Figure in parentheses refers to number of infants in each age group.
(Modified from Moore, J. F.: The Modern Treatment of Syphilis. 2nd ed. Springfield, IL, Charles C Thomas, 1943. Courtesy of Charles C Thomas, Publisher, Springfield, Illinois; and Platou, R. V. Adv. Pediatr. *4*:35, 1949.)

This is demonstrated by CSF changes of increased protein content, by a mononuclear pleocytosis of up to 200 or 300 cells/mm³, or by positive Venereal Disease Research Laboratories (VDRL) test (Table 41–2).

Diagnosis is confirmed by dark-field visualization of *Treponema* in scrapings from any lesion or from any body fluid, by charcteristic bone changes on radiographs, and by positive serologic tests for syphilis. These tests must be interpreted with caution, however. Since the IgG portion of reagin is transmitted across the placenta, its finding in the baby's serum means no more than that the mother has or has had syphilis. She may have been cured during pregnancy and yet still have quantities of reagin in her blood or she may not have been treated at all and still not have passed the disease on to her fetus. A higher titer in the infant's blood than in the mother's is not evidence of fetal infection, nor is an elevated concentration of total IgM in the cord serum.

The most helpful specific test is a positive finding in the newborn's blood of IgM antibody against *T. pallidum*, IgM-FTA-ABS (fluorescent treponemal antibody absorption). This is fluorescent *Treponema* antibody from which antibodies from treponemes other than *T. pallidum* have been removed by absorption. If positive, this finding is usually an indicator of congenital syphilis, although in the

TABLE 41–3. Recommended Treatment of Pregnant Patients with Syphilis

STAGES OF SYPHILIS	DRUG	DOSE
Early (<1 yr duration) Primary, secondary, or early latent	**Recommended**	
HIV antibody negative	Benzathine penicillin G	2.4 million units IM single dose; possibly repeat in 1 week
	Procaine penicillin G	600,000 units IM daily × 10–15 days
HIV antibody positive	Procaine penicillin G	1.2 million units IM daily × 15 days
	Aqueous penicillin G	4 million units every 4 hr × 15 days
	Alternative	
	Erythromycin[a]	500 mg QID × 15 days orally
	Penicillin desensitization[b]	
Latent (>1 yr duration)	**Recommended** Benzathine penicillin G	2.4 million units IM weekly × 3 weeks
	Procaine penicillin G	600,000 units IM daily × 15 days
	Alternative Erythromycin[c]	500 mg QID × 30 days orally
	Penicillin desensitization[b]	

[a]Use currently discouraged: offspring should be treated with penicillin.
[b]For details, see M.M.W.R. 37:S1, 1988.
[c]After neurosyphilis is excluded.
(From Ingall, D., Dobson, S. R. M., and Musher, D.: Syphilis. In Remington, J. S., and Klein, J. O. (Eds.): Infectious Diseases of the Fetus and Newborn Infant. Philadelphia, W. B. Saunders Company, 1990, p. 387.)

TABLE 41–4. Recommended Treatment of the Newborn with Syphilis

MATERNAL Rx	CLINICAL FINDINGS	DRUG (Penicillin G)	DOSE (50,000 units/kg)
None or inadequate	Present or absent	Aqueous	IM or IV daily × 10 days in 2 divided doses
		or procaine	IM daily × 10 days
Adequate	Absent	Benzathine (only if follow-up cannot be ensured)	IM single dose

(From Ingall, D., Dobson, S. R. M., and Musher, D.: Syphilis. In Remington, J. S., and Klein, J. O. (Eds.): Infectious Diseases of the Fetus and Newborn Infant. Philadelphia, W. B. Saunders Company, 1990, p. 388.)

presence of rheumatoid factor, false-positive tests are occasionally seen. However, this test is not always positive at first, even when infection is present in the infant, possibly because, if the infection is acquired late in pregnancy, specific antibodies do not have time to form.

Thus, when an infant's blood VDRL is positive at birth, one is not justified in making the diagnosis of congenital syphilis unless pathognomonic signs are also present. If they are not, serial determinations of reagin titer must be performed. If passively acquired, the titer falls to zero within 4 to 12 weeks; it will rise if the disease is actually present. If the IgM-FTA-ABS test is also positive at birth, treatment may be initiated. If the test is negative, however, it should be repeated several times at 3- or 4-week intervals.

Treatment. Treatment is recommended for all pregnant women regardless of the stage of pregnancy (Table 41–3). Recent recommendations from the Centers for Disease Control (Morbidity and Mortality Weekly Report, 1988) for treatment of symptomatic or asymptomatic infants are shown in Table 41–4. Long-term follow-up recommendations are outlined in Table 41–5.

Hardy and coworkers (1970) reported a case, rare in their and our experience, of a male infant who died of congenital syphilis. His mother had received penicillin G 10 days before delivery, and he was given massive doses for 17 days after birth. Despite all this, *T. pallidum* was recovered from the infant's eyes after his death.

■ LEPTOSPIROSIS

Lindsay and Luke (1949) reported the only case of congenital leptospirosis (Weil syndrome) on record. It is briefly abstracted here because of its similarity to several of the other transplacentally transmitted infections.

CASE 41–1

A male infant's mother had been a waitress in a restaurant known to be infested with rats, but she had never become ill. The infant was born at term, weighing 3540 g; vernix and amniotic fluid were brown, but the infant seemed well. Icterus appeared at 34 hours, and listlessness, cyanosis, dyspnea, and convulsions followed rapidly. The liver enlarged slightly. The blood was essentially normal, although platelets were not

TABLE 41–5. Follow-Up After Treatment or Prophylaxis for Congenital Syphilis

PATIENT CATEGORY	FOLLOW-UP PROCEDURES
Patients diagnosed as having congenital syphilis	1. Reagin testing every 3 months for the first 15 months then every 6 months until negative or stable at low titer 2. Treponemal antibody test after 15 months of age 3. Repeat cerebrospinal fluid evaluation 12 months after treatment if patient was treated for or showed any signs of central nervous system disease 4. Careful developmental evaluation, vision testing, and hearing testing before 3 years of age or at time of diagnosis
Patients treated in utero or at birth because of maternal syphilis	1. Reagin testing at birth and then every 3 months until at least 6 months of age and test is negative 2. Treponemal antibody test after 15 months of age
Women treated for syphilis during pregnancy	1. Reagin testing monthly until delivery, then every 3 months until negative 2. Retreatment anytime there is a fourfold rise in reagin titer

(Modified from Rathbun, K. C.: Congenital syphilis: A proposal for improved surveillance, diagnosis and treatment. Sex. Transm. Dis. *10*:102, 1983.)

counted or mentioned. The urine contained bile. Cerebrospinal fluid was normal. The infant died at 48 hours.

Autopsy revealed heavy lungs with bloody, frothy fluid in the trachea and bronchi. There were numerous subpleural hemorrhages, and the parenchyma was congested, edematous, and hemorrhagic, but there was no inflammatory reaction. The enlarged liver showed extensive degenerative and necrotic changes with no evidence of bile stasis or regeneration. There were equally striking degenerative alterations of renal tubular epithelium, with protein and cellular casts within the tubules. Rare leptospirae were seen scattered throughout the liver sections prepared with Dieterle and Levaditi stains. The mother's blood showed a high titer of agglutinins to Leptospira icterohaemorrhagiae *and* L. canicola, *which disappeared after a few months.*

Comment. Weil syndrome is contracted through contact with feces of infected rats. One cannot doubt that the mother acquired infection in this way but that the disease remained asymptomatic. Leptospirae crossed the placenta and produced disease in the fetus that became apparent on the 2nd day of extrauterine life and quickly caused death. Such transplacental transmission has been observed in animals.

A more recent case suggested human-to-human transmission through breast milk (Boli and Koellner, 1988). The infant became ill at 21 days of age and was being breast-fed by her mother, who as a veterinarian performed an autopsy on a pregnant cow infected with *Leptospira interrogans* serovar *Hardjo.* The same organism was cultured from the infant's urine. The infant was treated with high-dose intravenous penicillin for 3 days and subsequently a 10-day course of oral amoxicillin. A Jarisch-Herxheimer reaction was noted after antibiotic therapy was begun.

■ NEONATAL HELMINTHIASIS*

HOOKWORM

Definition. Hookworm is a common infection in tropical and subtropical areas caused by *Ancylostoma duodenale* or *Necator americanus.* These nematodes live in the human intestine, feed on blood, and expel ova into the feces.

---

*This section was written by Mary Ellen Avery.

Epidemiology. It is estimated that perhaps as many as one billion people are infected with hookworm, particularly in the developing world. The most common mode of larval transmission is through penetration of the skin, often the soles of the feet, with the larvae entering the venulas from which they are delivered by the circulation into the lungs and gastrointestinal tract. In some regions of China, the practice of putting sand in diapers to absorb urine has led to infection in infancy.

Other modes of transmission include infection of the infant via colostrum and breast milk. The evidence for this is convincing in animals but is indirect in humans since soiled bedding and infant clothing may also be sources of infective larvae. Transplacental infection is probably very rare; however, lactogenic transfer can be fatal.

Natural History. With heavy infection, pulmonary lesions may be evident, and cough and dyspnea may occur. The affected child suffers mostly from the consequence of intestinal blood loss, which leads to iron deficiency anemia and hypoalbuminemia.

The diagnosis depends on demonstration of ova in fecal smears. Occult blood in stools is also common.

Treatment. Mebendazole is effective for hookworm disease, ascariasis, enterobiasis, and trichuriasis. The experience with this drug is extensive in children but not in newborns. Pyrantel pamoate (120 mg/kg/day) given orally in three divided doses for 3 days is the most effective drug against *A. duodenale* (Wang, 1988).

Prevention. If a mother is known to have hookworm disease, she should be treated and breast-feeding should be deferred until maternal disease has been eradicated. The wisdom of this depends on individual circumstances, since the risk of lactogenic infection is not known. Meticulous attention to personal hygiene is essential in a mother who may be shedding ova in the stool.

ASCARIS

Chu and co-workers (1972) encountered an infant of 8 months' gestational age, delivered by cesarean section because of prolonged labor and fetal distress, whose mother vaginally passed a mature worm. The infant was well on the 2nd day but rectally passed a 30 cm mature

Ascaris lumbricoides and another on the 6th day. The worms almost certainly had penetrated the fetus's intestinal tract after migration into the uterus and across the placenta.

The authors point out that similar migrations have been reported for *Schistosoma (Bilharzia)*, *Taenia*, and *Enterobius* helminths.

■ AMERICAN TRYPANOSOMIASIS

Infection with *Trypanosoma cruzi* (Chagas disease) affects several million individuals in Central and South America. Although 226 of 2651 pregnant women recently surveyed in Brazil were seropositive, and 28.3 per cent had parasitemia, congenital infections occur in only 1 to 4 per cent of women with serologic evidence of having Chagas disease (Bittencourt, 1976; Bittencourt et al., 1985). Infected infants are usually of low birth weight (Azogue et al., 1985) and may present at birth or during the first weeks of life with jaundice, anemia, petecchiae, hepatosplenomegaly, cardiomegaly, and congestive heart failure. Of congenitally infected infants, 57.8 per cent die before 2 years of age. The diagnosis can be made by examining the placenta or with thin and thick blood smears. Serologic tests are also available (Arvin and Yeager, 1990; Bruckner 1985). Treatment has been attempted with nitrofurans, 8-aminoquinones, and metronidazole with some success in controlling blood-borne infection (Arvin and Yeager, 1990). Nifurtimox has also been used, but no experience is available in congenitally infected infants. Information concerning treatment should be sought from the Parasitic Disease Drug Service, Centers for Disease Control, Atlanta, Georgia.

■ REFERENCES

Alford, C. A., Polt, S. S., Cassady, G. E., et al.: Gamma-M-fluorescent treponemal antibody in the diagnosis of congenital syphilis. N. Engl. J. Med. *280*:1086, 1969.

Arvin, A. M., and Yeager, A. S.: Other viral infections of the fetus and newborn. *In* Remington, J. S., and Klein, J. O. (Eds.) Infectious Diseases of the Fetus and Newborn Infant. Philadelphia, W. B. Saunders Company, 1990, pp. 516–527.

Azogue, E., LaFuente, C., and Darras, C.: Congenital Chagas' disease in Boliva: Epidemiological aspects and pathological findings. Trans. R. Soc. Trop. Med. Hyg. *79*:176, 1985.

Bittencourt, A. L.: Congenital Chagas' disease. Am. J. Dis. Child. *130*:97, 1976.

Bittencourt, A. L., Mota, E., Filho, R. R., et al.: Incidence of congenital Chagas' disease in Bahaia, Brazil. J. Trop. Pediatr. *31*:242, 1985.

Boli, C. A., and Koellner, P.: Human-to-human transmission of *Leptospira interrogans* by milk. J. Infect. Dis. *158*:246, 1988.

Bruckner, D. A.: Serologic and intradermal tests for parasitic infections. Ped. Clin. North Am. *32*:1063, 1985.

Cheng-I, W.: Parasitic diarrhoeas in China. Parasitology Today *4*:284, 1988.

Chu, W.-G., Chen, P.-M., Huang, L. C., et al.: Neonatal ascariasis. J. Pediatr. *81*:783, 1972.

Hardy, J. B., Hardy, P. H., et al.: Failure of penicillin in a newborn with congenital syphilis. J.A.M.A. *212*:1345, 1970.

Hotez, P. J.: Hookworm disease in children. Pediatr. Infect. Dis. J. *8*:516, 1989.

Ingall, D., Dobson, S. R. M., and Musher, D.: Syphilis. *In* Remington, J. S., and Klein, J. O. (Eds.): Infectious Diseases of the Fetus and Newborn Infant. Philadelphia, W. B. Saunders Company, 1990, pp. 367–394.

Lindsay, S., and Luke, J. W.: Fatal leptospirosis (Weil's disease) in a newborn infant. J. Pediatr. *34*:90, 1949.

McCracken, G. H., and Kaplan, M.: Penicillin treatment for congenital syphilis: A critical reappraisal. J.A.M.A. *228*:855, 1974.

Morbidity and Mortality Weekly Report: Congenital syphilis, United States, 1983–1985. M.M.W.R. *35*:625, 1986.

Morbidity and Mortality Weekly Report: Guidelines for the prevention and control of congenital syphilis. M.M.W.R. *37*:S1, 1988.

Morbidity and Mortality Weekly Report: Summary of notifiable diseases, United States, 1989. M.M.W.R. *38*(54), 1989.

Nelson, N. A., and Struve, V. R.: Prevention of congenital syphilis by treatment of syphilis in pregnancy. J.A.M.A. *161*:869, 1956.

Oppenheimer, E. H., and Hardy, J. B. H.: Congenital syphilis in the newborn: Clinical and pathological observations in recent cases. Johns Hopkins Med. J. *129*:63, 1971.

Rosen, E. U., and Richardson, N. J.: A reappraisal of the value of the IgM fluorescent treponemal antibody absorption test in the diagnosis of congenital syphilis. J. Pediatr. *87*:38, 1975.

Scotti, A. T., and Logan, L.: A specific IgM antibody test in neonatal congenital syphilis. J. Pediatr. *73*:242, 1968.

Wendel, G. D.: Gestational and congenital syphilis. Clin. Perinatol. *15*:287, 1988.

Wilkinson, R. H., and Heller, R. H.: Congenital syphilis: Resurgence of an old problem. Pediatrics *47*:27, 1971.

Zimmerman, H. M.: Fatal hookworm disease in infancy and children on Guam. Am. J. Pathol. *22*:1081, 1946.

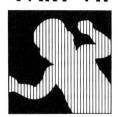
NEUROLOGIC 42 EVALUATION OF THE NEWBORN INFANT

John H. Menkes

The ontogenesis of the human nervous system can be divided into four stages. The initial stage is one of embryogenesis and induction and occurs during the first 54 to 60 days following ovulation. During this period, the neural plate and groove and, subsequently, the neural tube are formed, the vascular primordia are elaborated, and the anlagen for the facial structures are laid down, the latter process being activated by the rostral neural tube. Interference with ontogenesis during this period results in such dysraphic or facial-forebrain anomalies as anencephaly and myelomeningocele (O'Rahilly, 1986).

The second ontogenetic stage is one of neuronal proliferation and outward migration from the area surrounding the neural tube. As a rule, earlier cells form the deeper layers, and later arrivals pass through these to form the more superficial regions of the cerebral and cerebellar cortex. The peak period for neuronal proliferation is 2 to 4 months' gestation; for neuronal migration it is 3 to 5 months. In the cerebral cortex, the process continues for as long as the 6th month of postnatal life. In the cerebellum, cellular proliferation begins later and lasts longer, with migration continuing well into the 2nd postnatal year.

By 25 weeks' gestation, the cerebral cortex has reached its full neuronal complement, neuronal proliferation has probably ceased, and electrical activity has become recognizable. Insults to morphogenesis during this period give rise to the various disorders of cellular proliferation and migration, such as the microcephalies, schizencephaly, and polymicrogyria.

At the beginning of the last trimester of gestation, a rapid multiplication of glial cells commences. This event is accompanied by an elaboration of neural processes, the formation of synapses, and the ultimate alignment and orientation of the cortical neurons. These events continue throughout the neonatal period into the first few years of postnatal life. A number of disorders, including perinatal insults, may affect this developmental stage.

Myelination occurs over a long time span. It commences during the second trimester of gestation, is maximal during the first year of postnatal life, and may continue into the third decade.

The brain of the term newborn infant weighs 325 to 435 g, only one-fourth the weight of the average adult brain, but accounts for approximately 10 per cent of the total body weight at birth. All primary and secondary fissures and sulci are present, but the tertiary sulci are only partly developed. The four major lobes are clearly distinguishable, although the frontal and temporal poles are relatively shorter than those of the older child, and the demarcation between cortical gray matter and underlying white matter is not yet distinct. On microscopic examination, the cerebral cortex of the term newborn exhibits lamination similar to that of the adult brain. Nissl bodies (ribosomal material) are not yet present in cortical neurons, except in certain large pyramidal (Betz) cells in the motor cortex. The cerebellum in the newborn is notable for its prominent external granular cell layer, composed of 8 to 12 rows of densely packed cells, which gradually disappear during the first postnatal year. Myelin, elaborated from proliferating oligodendrocytes, appears, generally speaking, in a caudocranial order. At birth, all cranial nerves except the optic are myelinated, as are the spinal roots, the olivary and cerebellar connections, and the tracts of the spinal cord posterior columns. Myelination of the corticospinal tract, the corticocerebellar fibers, and the optic nerve commences just prior to birth (Sarnat, 1989).

The rapid brain growth that occurs during the first postnatal year is largely the result of continued myelination and tremendous elaboration of dendritic processes, events that establish the neuronal connections necessary for the complex behavior that is characteristic of the older infant and child.

■ NEUROLOGIC EXAMINATION

Neurologic examination of the newborn infant is an observational art that requires a certain degree of knowledge of the variations of neonatal behavior, a considerable degree of patience, and a conservative attitude regarding the significance and the predictive value of certain deviations of performance that can be influenced by many systemic and environmental factors. A single examination may suffice to document the presence of neurologic integrity in a newborn and may be adequate when signs of disease are obvious and definite. When signs are marginal or only suggestively abnormal, however, a second examination or even daily evaluations will yield more reliable information regarding the nature of the problem. Many of our present concepts of neurologic and behavioral function of the newborn infant are derived from the detailed and astute observations of André-Thomas and co-workers (1960), and others.

OBSERVATION

Neurologic examination of the newborn should begin with an adequate period of observation before removal of the clothing and then in more detail with the infant completely undressed. Attention should be paid to the state of the baby, as reviewed in Chapter 24. General aspects to be noted because of their possible association with neurologic function include the respiratory rate and rhythm, cutaneous abnormalities such as plethora, jaundice, or evidence of sepsis, and the presence of external minor anomalies, especially of the hands, feet, external ears, eyes, or genitalia.

Important components of the infant's behavior to be observed include the state of alertness, the resting posture the child assumes in the supine and prone positions, the capability of the child to perform similar but not necessarily symmetric movements of the limbs on the two sides, and the character of the cry. These are covered in greater detail in Chapter 24.

Several factors influence the normal infant's state of alertness. These include time of last feeding, environmental stimuli, and gestational age. By 28 weeks' gestation, an infant may be aroused by persistent stimulation or may alert spontaneously. Sleep-wake cycles are apparent by 32 weeks.

The neurologic examination of the neonate can be divided into three parts:
1. Evaluation of posture and muscle tone.
2. Evaluation of primitive reflexes.
3. Examination of relatively age-invariable items.

EVALUATION OF POSTURE AND MUSCLE TONE

Evaluation of muscle tone is a fundamental part of the neurologic examination of infants. It involves examination of the resting posture, passive tone, and active tone of each of the major muscle groups.

The posture of the normal term infant in the prone position is one of partial flexion of the arms and legs, with legs adducted so that the thighs are maintained under the abdomen. When awake, the baby on his abdomen is able to rotate the head from side to side and temporarily elevate it from the surface of the crib. The awake infant lying on his back will exhibit purposeless, poorly coordinated limb movements, usually consisting of alternating flexion and extension in reciprocal fashion on the two sides. Minimal or absent motor activity, or strikingly asymmetric motor activity in which one arm or one side of the body is little moved, is clearly suggestive of neurologic dysfunction. The cry of an intact newborn is a vigorous and reasonably sustained one, easily elicited by flicking the bottom of the foot or sometimes by eliciting the Moro response. A high-pitched shrill cry, a cry that on repeated observations on different examinations is weak and unsustained, or an inability to provoke a cry are indicators of probable neurologic abnormalities.

Muscle tone is also evaluated by passive movement of various parts of the body, ideally with the infant awake and not crying. Since limb tone, like various reflexes, is influenced or altered by tonic neck reflexes, it is important to have the child's head in a neutral position when these assessments are made. In the infant of 28 weeks' gestation, there is minimal resistance to passive movements of the limbs. By 32 weeks, flexor tone appears in the lower extremities and is prominent by 36 weeks. The normal term infant assumes a flexed posture of both upper and lower extremities with a certain degree of resistance being present at the elbows and knees. Muscle tone should be symmetric when one side is compared with the other. A reduction in muscle tone is an important diagnostic sign but by itself is without localizing value.

In the upper extremities the scarf sign is a valuable maneuver. The infant is sustained in a semireclining position; by taking the infant's hand, the arm is pulled across his chest toward the opposite shoulder. The position of the elbow in relationship to the midline is noted. Hypotonia is present if the elbow passes the midline. In the lower extremity, the fall-away response serves a similar purpose. The infant is suspended by the feet, upside down, and each lower extremity is released in turn. The rapidity with which the lower extremity drops when released is noted. Normally the extremity maintains its position for a few moments, then drops. In hypotonia the drop occurs immediately; in hypertonia the released lower extremity remains hung up. Flaccidity is most often encountered in the comatose infant but can also result from traumatic insults to the upper portion of the spinal cord, disease of the spinal anterior horn cells, and abnormalities of the muscles or neuromuscular junction.

The traction response is an excellent means of ascertaining active tone. The examiner, who should be sitting down and facing the child, places his thumbs in the infant's palms, and his fingers around the wrists, and gently pulls the infant from the supine position. In the normal infant under 3 months of age, the palmar grasp reflex becomes operative, the elbows tend to flex, and the flexor muscles of the neck are stimulated to raise the head so that even in the full-term newborn the extensor and flexor tone are balanced, and the head will be briefly maintained in the axis of the trunk. The test is abnormal if the head is pulled passively and drops forward or if the head is maintained backward. In the former case, there is abnormal hypotonia of the neck and trunk muscles; in the latter case, there is abnormal hypertonia of the neck extensors. With abnormal hypertonia one may also note the infant's head to be rotated laterally and extended when he is in the resting prone position.

EVALUATION OF PRIMITIVE REFLEXES

The evaluation of various primitive reflexes represents an integral part of the neurologic examination of the neonate. Many of the reflexes exhibited by the newborn are also observed in a "spinal animal"—one in which the spinal cord has been permanently transected. With progressive maturation, some of these reflexes disappear (Paine and Oppe, 1966). This should not be construed as meaning that they are actually lost, for a reflex once acquired in the course of development is retained permanently. Rather, these reflexes are suppressed by the higher centers as they become functional. Reflexes develop during intrauterine life and are gradually suppressed as the higher cortical centers become functional.

A number of segmental medullary reflexes become functional during the last trimester of gestation, including:

1. Respiratory activity.
2. Cardiovascular reflexes.
3. Coughing reflex mediated by the vagus nerve.
4. Sneezing reflex evoked by afferent fibers of the trigeminal nerve.
5. Swallowing reflex mediated by the trigeminal and glossopharyngeal nerves.
6. Sucking reflex evoked by the afferent fibers of the trigeminal and glossopharyngeal nerves and executed by the efferent fibers of the facial, glossopharyngeal, and hypoglossal nerves.

Another reflex demonstrable in the isolated spinal cord is the flexion reflex. This response is elicited by the noxious stimulation of the skin of the lower extremity and consists of dorsiflexion of the great toe and flexion of the ankle, knee, and hip. This reflex has been elicited in very immature fetuses, and may persist as a fragment, the extensor plantar response, for the first 2 years of life. Reflex stepping, which is at least partly a function of the flexion response, is present in the normal newborn when he is supported in the standing position; it disappears in the 4th or 5th month of life.

The Moro reflex is best elicited by a sudden dropping of the baby's head in relation to its trunk. Moro however elicited this reflex by hitting the infant's pillow with both hands (Moro, 1918). The infant will open his or her hands, extend and abduct the upper extremities, and then draw them together. The reflex first appears between 28 and 32 weeks' gestation and is present in all newborns. It fades out between 3 and 5 months of age. Its persistence beyond that time, or its absence or diminution during the first few weeks of life, indicates neurologic dysfunction.

The tonic neck response is obtained by rotating the infant's head to the side with the chest being maintained in a flat position. A positive response is extension of the arm and leg on the side toward which the face is rotated, and flexion of the limbs on the opposite side. An asymmetric tonic neck response is abnormal, that is, responses are different when the face is turned to the right than when it is turned to the left. Also, an obligatory and sustained pattern, that is, one from which the infant is unable to extricate himself, is abnormal. Inconstant tonic neck responses can be elicited for as long as 6 months, and may even be momentarily present during sleep in the normal 2- to 3-year old (Table 42–1).

The righting reflex is elicited with the infant in the supine position. When the examiner turns the head to one side, the normal infant rotates the shoulder in the same direction, followed by the trunk, and finally by the pelvis. An obligate neck-righting reflex, in which the shoulders, trunk, and pelvis rotate simultaneously and the infant can be rolled over and over like a log, is always abnormal. Normally, the reflex can be imposed briefly in newborns, but the infant is soon able to break through it.

Palmar and plantar grasp reflexes are elicited by pressure on the palm or on the sole of the foot. As a rule, the plantar grasp reflex is weaker than the palmar reflex. The palmar grasp reflex appears at 28 weeks' gestation, is well established by 32 weeks, and becomes weak and inconsistent between 2 and 3 months of age, when it is covered up by voluntary activity. Absence of the reflex prior to then, persistence beyond that age, or a consistent asymmetry are abnormal. The reappearance of the grasp reflex in frontal lobe lesions reflects the unopposed parietal lobe activity.

For vertical suspension, the examiner suspends the child with his hands under the axillae, and notes the position of the lower extremities. Marked extension or scissoring are indications of spasticity.

The Landau reflex is elicited by lifting the infant with one hand under the trunk, face downward. Normally, there is a reflex extension of the vertebral column, causing the newborn infant to lift the head to slightly below the horizontal, which results in a slightly convex upward curvature of the spine. With hypotonia the infant's body tends to collapse into an inverted U-shape.

Reflex placing and stepping responses are of lesser value. The former is elicited by stimulating the dorsum of the foot against the edge of the examining table. Reflex stepping, which is at least partly a function of the flexion response to noxious stimuli, is present in the normal newborn when he is supported in the standing position. The response disappears by 4 to 5 months of age.

A number of other primitive reflexes have been discovered, including the curious bowing reflex, first described in 1926 by Gamper. This reflex, which can occasionally be demonstrated in normal premature infants of 7 months' gestation, is invariably present in anencephalics. It can be elicited by placing the infant into the supine position and extending the thighs at the hip joints. The head will then lift itself slowly, followed by the trunk, so that the infant ultimately achieves the sitting position.

Other primitive reflexes add little to the neurologic examination of the infant; I believe the physician should gather experience in a few selected tests, rather than try to elicit the entire gamut of responses.

EXAMINATION OF RELATIVELY AGE-INVARIABLE ITEMS

The last part of the neurologic examination involves items similar to those performed in older children or adults, as for instance the funduscopic examination, and the deep tendon reflexes. A variety of deep tendon reflexes can be elicited in the infant, but are of limited value except when they are clearly asymmetric. The triceps and brachioradialis reflexes are usually difficult to elicit during the period of neonatal flexion hypertonia. The patellar reflex is accompanied by adduction of the opposite thigh, the crossed

TABLE 42–1. Percentage of Normal Babies Showing Various Infantile Reflexes with Increasing Age

| | SIGNS THAT DISAPPEAR WITH AGE | | | SIGNS THAT APPEAR WITH AGE | | | | |
	Moro	Tonic Neck-Reflex	Crossed Adduction to KJ	Neck-Righting Reflex	Supporting Reaction	Landau	Parachute	Hand Grasp
	Extension Even Without Flexor Phase	Imposable Even for 30 Degrees or Inconstant	Strong or Slight	Imposable but Transient	Fair or Good	Head Above Horizontal and Back Arched	Complete	Thumb to Forefinger Alone
Age (months)								
1	93	67	?*	13	50	0	0	0
2	89	90	?*	23	43	0	0	0
3	70	50	41	25	52	0	0	0
4	59	34	41	26	40	0	0	0
5	22	31	41	38	61	29	0	0
6	0	11	21	40	66	42	3	0
7	0	0	12	43	74	42	29	16
8	0	0	15	54	81	44	40	53
9	0	0	6	67	96	97	76	63
10	0	0	3	100	100	100	79	84
11	0	0	3	100	100	100	90	95
12	0	0	2	100	100	100	100	100

*Divergence of experience and opinion between different examiners.
(From Paine, R. S., and Oppe, T. E.: Neurological examination of children. Clin. Dev. Med. 20:1, 1966.)

adductor reflex. Unsustained ankle clonus is common in the normal neonate.

The plantar response to stimulation of the lateral surface of the sole of the foot is a much discussed phenomenon but of limited usefulness in the clinical assessment of the newborn. The claim that all newborn and young infants have Babinski signs is an overstatement in need of qualification. Although it is true that extension of the great toe is often part of the response to plantar stimulation in early infancy, this normal response is usually quite different from the slow, tonic extension associated with fanning of the other toes seen in the 3- or 4-month-old with spastic lower limbs. The normal response to plantar stimulation is frequently a quick withdrawal with flexion of the knee and prompt but unsustained extension of the great toe. The first, and most important, response to stroking of the sole of the newborn's foot is a flexor reaction of the great toe, which may then be followed by other movements.

CRANIAL NERVES

Visual responses can first be demonstrated at 28 weeks' gestation. At that time, the infant will blink consistently when confronted by a bright light (Table 42–2). By 32 weeks, light induces persistent closure of the lids. The pupillary light reflex appears at 29 weeks and is consistently present at 32 weeks. An optokinetic nystagmus is elicitable at term. Although more complex visual behavior is demonstrable with special techniques, these tests have little value in the routine neurologic examination. In contrast, the funduscopic examination is of considerable importance. The examiner must keep in mind the fact that the newborn's optic disc has a grayish-white appearance and that the macular light reflex is normally absent.

Eye movements are difficult to assess during the first few weeks of life. Discrete following movements are not expected at that time, but an alert infant often appears to fixate on the examiner's face, and some degree of conjugate ocular activity is usually seen. Abrupt, transient horizontal nystagmus is commonly present in the new-

born, especially on movement of the child, and should not be judged to be abnormal. The response to the doll's head maneuver is first noted at 30 weeks' gestation and usually is elicitable in the full-term infant. Oculovestibular responses can best be elicited by spinning the infant while he is held in the upright position, facing the examiner.

The amplitude and symmetry of facial movements are noted with the infant at rest and when he is crying or sucking.

After 28 weeks' gestation, an infant will blink or startle to sudden loud noises. In the full-term infant, the sound of a bell may elicit more complex responses, such as cessation of sucking and opening of eyes.

Examination of the head of a newborn should include observation and description of its shape, measurement in centimeters of the occipitofrontal circumference, palpation and estimation of degree of separation of sutures, and palpation and measurement of the size of the anterior fontanel. Care must be used in determining the head circumference, and the same landmarks should be used with each estimate. A disposable paper tape is preferred to a metal one and should extend around the head from

TABLE 42–2. Tests Designed to Assess Cranial Nerve Function

CRANIAL NERVE	TEST
I	Smell (rarely tested).
II	Vision, blink to light; fixing; following; opticokinetic nystagmus; retinal exam.
III, IV, VI	Ocular movement; pupillary size; doll's eyes movements; nystagmoid movements on vertical spin; caloric stimulation.
V	Facial muscle tone; Bell's palsy.
VIII	Hearing; clap; attend to tuning fork or bell; hearing-evoked potentials.
V, VII, XII	Sucking.
IX, X	Swallowing; pharyngeal incoordination.
VII, IX	Taste (rarely tested).
XII	Tongue function.

(Data from Volpe, J. Neurology of the Newborn, 2nd ed. Philadelphia, W. B. Saunders Company, 1987.)

a point approximately 1 cm above the supraorbital margin anteriorly to the farthest point on the occiput posteriorly. In some instances, auscultation, transillumination, and ultrasonography of the head are useful additional procedures. The status of the cranial sutures and anterior fontanel, especially on serial examinations over the course of weeks or months, is one of the most reliable indicators of conditions that induce increased intracranial pressure or those that have interfered with continued normal brain growth. The anterior fontanel is best evaluated with the infant quiet and held in the sitting position. The range of normal fontanel size and the conditions that retard fontanel closure have been reviewed by Popich and Smith (1972). In addition to indicating primary neurologic conditions in which increased intracranial pressure is present, a tense fontanel in infancy occurs in some cases with cardiac failure. An unusual finding on examination of the head is a parietal bony defect along the sagittal suture, located approximately 2 cm anterior to the posterior fontanel. This is referred to as a third fontanel but is in fact not a fontanel because it is not located at the junction of the parietal and adjacent bones. This bony defect results from failure of completion of ossification in the parasagittal parietal region and has been identified especially in infants with Down syndrome and the congenital rubella syndrome.

The neurologic examination, when performed in the aforementioned manner, can be interpreted as normal, abnormal, or suspect. The predictive value of the examination in terms of subsequent neurologic deficits is considerable. In the Collaborative Perinatal Project of the National Institutes of Health, 16 per cent of neonates who had an abnormal neurologic examination were subsequently found to have cerebral palsy. Conversely, a suspect or abnormal examination was seen in only 11 per cent and 0.5 per cent, respectively, of subsequently normal children but in 34 per cent and 23 per cent, respectively, of children with cerebral palsy (Nelson and Ellenberg, 1979).

Every physician examining infants suspected of having sustained a cerebral birth injury has encountered a group of patients who appear to have clear-cut neurologic deficits during the neonatal period but who on subsequent examinations have lost all signs of motor dysfunction. Some of these infants may show delayed milestones and ultimately are found to be grossly retarded, whereas others may only demonstrate visual perceptual handicaps, speech defects, nonfebrile seizures, or hyperkinetic behavior (Nelson and Ellenberg, 1982).

■ ASSESSMENT OF NEUROLOGIC MATURITY

For many years it has been recognized that the gestational age of the newborn can be approximated by the assessment of various physical characteristics—notably those of the skin and CNS. However, these characteristics can be affected by factors other than the length of gestation, as can length and weight. Judging gestational age is discussed in Chapter 43. In general, neurologic assessment is more reliable than skin characteristics, but clearly, maternal illness, in utero fetal stress, maternal drugs (licit and illicit), the degree of sickness of the

newborn, state, and postnatal age are all factors that affect neurologic maturity. Robinson (1966) and Dubowitz and associates (1970), among others, have devised an assessment of neurologic maturity (Table 42–3). This scheme utilizes five reflex responses, including pupillary reaction, traction response, glabellar tap, neck-righting, and head-turning to diffuse light. Neurologic maturity can be roughly estimated by these observations, since pupillary reaction to light develops from 29 to 31 weeks of gestation, glabellar tap reflex from 32 to 34 weeks, traction response from 33 to 36 weeks, neck-righting reflex from 34 to 37 weeks, and head-turning to diffuse light from 32 to 36 weeks. The method developed by Amiel-Tison (1968) is largely dependent on the gradual increase of muscle tone that occurs progressively with increasing gestational age (Fig. 42–1). This scheme is sensitive to a variety of exogenous factors, notably maternal sedation, method of delivery, and the position of the fetus in utero.

Additional methods of assessing neurologic maturity include the ulnar nerve conduction velocity. The mean conduction velocity for the ulnar nerve of the term newborn infant is approximately 30 meters per second and is progressively slower with shorter gestational ages. Electroencephalographic methods have also been used to judge neurologic maturity by determination of the latency of photoevoked responses from the occipital cortex. Infants of a conceptual age of 40 weeks were found to have a mean latency of the response to photic stimulation of approximately 153 milliseconds. At 38 weeks the latency was 169 milliseconds, at 36 weeks 203 milliseconds, at 32 weeks 221 milliseconds, and at 29 weeks 230 milliseconds. More recently, the detection of sulci by cranial ultrasound has been shown to be reliable.

■ NEURODIAGNOSTIC PROCEDURES

TRANSILLUMINATION

Transillumination of the head is a valuable technique that is inexpensive and entirely safe, but it requires the examiner to recognize and to be familiar with normal variations, especially in the low-birth-weight infant. The examiner should use the same flashlight powered with two D batteries for all examinations so that the intensity of illumination remains constant. The room must be entirely darkened, and one should wait briefly before making the evaluation to permit adaptation to the dark. The light, with a soft rubber adapter, must be placed flush with the head of the child. The glow of light extends 2 to 2.5 cm from the rim of the light source in the frontal region of the term infant and about 1 cm farther in the premature child. Transillumination in the occipital region is significantly less and changes little with gestational age. High-intensity fiberoptic light sources can be used in the neonatal intensive care unit (NICU) where transport of a sick newborn to a completely dark room is not possible.

Abnormally increased transillumination can result from various extracranial factors such as the infiltration of intravenous solutions into the scalp. Reduced transillumination is normally encountered in black children or in the presence of a subgaleal hematoma. Enhanced transillumination is seen in a variety of conditions that cause increased fluid collection in the subdural space, the sub-

TABLE 42–3. Reflexes of Value in Assessing Gestational Age

| REFLEX | STIMULUS | POSITIVE RESPONSE | GESTATION (wk.) IF REFLEX IS: | |
			Absent	Present
Pupil reaction	Light	Pupil contraction	<31	29 or more
Traction	Pull up by wrists from supine	Flexion of neck or arms	<36	33 or more
Glabellar tap	Tap on glabella	Blink	<34	32 or more
Neck-righting	Rotation of head	Trunk follows	<37	34 or more
Head-turning	Diffuse light from one side	Head-turning to light	Doubtful	32 or more

Note: Twenty-nine weeks means 203 days after the first day of the last menstrual period. If there is a conflict between two results, the reflex placed higher in the table is more likely to give the true gestational age.

(From Robinson, R. J.: Assessment of gestational age by neurological examination. Arch. Dis. Child. *41*:437, 1966.)

arachnoid space, and the ventricular system. In the Dandy-Walker syndrome, increased transillumination may be localized to the region over the posterior fossa. In addition, transillumination increases with decreasing gestational age.

LUMBAR PUNCTURE

In the newborn or small infant, a lumbar puncture is best performed with the baby in the sitting position. A small pillow placed against the abdomen will keep the spine flexed, while an assistant maintains the head in a perfect anterior-posterior alignment. Following cleaning of the back with an antibacterial solution, the tap is performed. I purposely omit local anesthesia in that it entails twice as much struggling than a tap performed without it. A 22- or 23-gauge needle without a stylet is optimal for the newborn. Since the spinal cord in the newborn

terminates at approximately the level of the second lumbar vertebral body, the needle is inserted into the L4-L5 interspace (one interspace below the top of the iliac crest), with the bevel being maintained parallel to the longitudinal dural fibers in order to decrease the size of the dural tear. The needle is then pushed forward as slowly as possible. Entry into the subarachnoid space can be felt by a sudden pop. As a rule, a bloody tap results from the needle going too deep, and penetrating the dorsal epidural venous plexus overlying the vertebral bodies. Less often it is caused by injury to the vessels along the cauda equina.

Concern has been raised that a penetrating needle without a stylet might possibly introduce epithelial fragments into the subarachnoid space that later might give rise to intraspinal epidermoid tumors. This remains speculative and is more applicable to the child who requires multiple spinal taps and the injection of intrathecal medi-

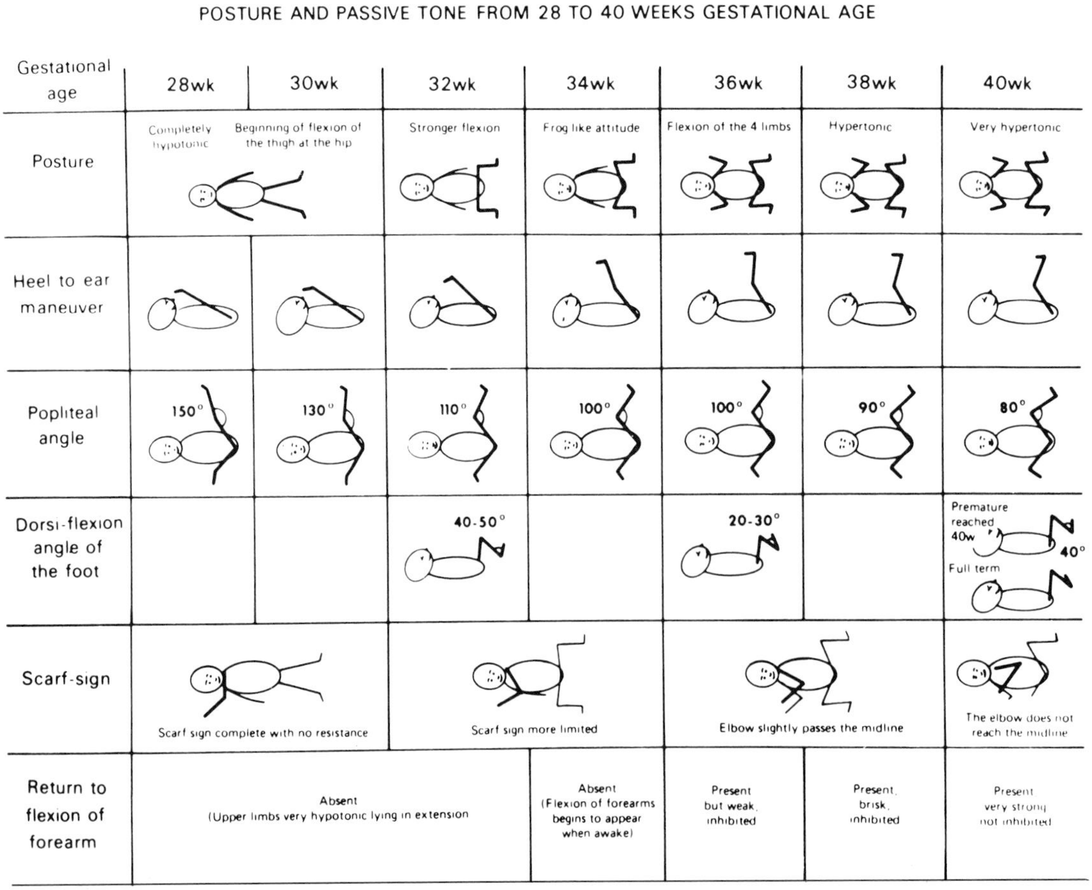

FIGURE 42–1. Posture and passive tone from 28 to 40 weeks' gestation, indicating increasing muscle tone in upper and lower extremities, which develops with increasing gestational age. (Adapted from Amiel-Tison, C., and Davis, S. W.: Newborn neurologic examination. In Rudolph, A. M., and Hoffman, J. I. E. [Eds.]: Pediatrics. 19th ed. Norwalk, CT, Appleton and Lange, 1991.)

cation. Points to remember in the performance of the procedure are the short distance from the skin surface to the subarachnoid space, especially in the premature child, and the absolute requirement to maintain the tip of the needle in the midline as it is directed through the soft tissues toward the subarachnoid space. The slightest deviation of the plane of the needle is likely to result in an unsuccessful tap.

Measurement of the pressure of cerebrospinal fluid is unreliable in the crying, struggling infant and is best not attempted when these circumstances prevail. The time required and the manipulation of the needle incurred by attaching the manometer increase the risk of dislodging the tip from the subarachnoid space, thus eliminating the opportunity to obtain a CSF specimen uncontaminated by blood. When coma or lack of response to needle penetration prevails, an opening pressure may be obtained, but only after a small quantity of fluid has been secured for cell count culture.

Postnatal water loss includes a decrease in cerebrospinal fluid. Head circumference usually decreases in the first days after birth so that the fontanelles are depressed. In some infants, the sutures override. Cerebrospinal fluid pressure is at its lowest when body weight is at its nadir.

In the normal term infant, the cerebrospinal fluid is usually crystal clear, whereas variable degrees of xanthochromia are more often seen in the premature baby. Xanthochromia can be due to the presence of approximately 400 to 500 red blood cells per cubic millimeter or may be secondary to hyperbilirubinemia. Studies have shown that there is no direct relationship between the levels of serum and spinal fluid bilirubin in the newborn child, probably reflecting the individual variations in the blood-CSF and blood-brain barriers. A number of red blood cells and up to 10 white blood cells/mm^3 can be accepted as insignificant in the first few days after birth. White cells are largely mononuclear, although two or three neutrophils/mm^3 can be present in the absence of infection. The range of values for cerebrospinal fluid protein is far greater in the intact newborn infant than in the older child. In the full-term infant, levels between 45 and 100 mg/dl can be considered normal, whereas in the premature baby, a protein content of up to 180 mg/dl can occur without evident neurologic disease (Bauer et al., 1965). The CSF protein concentration bears a roughly inverse relationship to weight of the premature child and thus either is a function of degree of maturity of vascular permeability and the blood-CSF barrier or reflects the frequency of intracranial hemorrhages in the smaller preterm infant.

Up to the last few years, a carefully performed lumbar puncture was one of the principal diagnostic procedures for establishing the presence of an intracranial hemorrhage in the newborn, and judicious evaluation of whether or not the tap was traumatic was usually required. For that purpose, the physician had to pay particular attention to the red cell count in the first and last specimen of fluid. It is now clear that traumatic lumbar punctures are less common than had been appreciated, and, conversely, in some 30 per cent of infants the presence of clear CSF is compatible with an intracranial hemorrhage of considerable proportions.

By far, the most important reason for cerebrospinal fluid examination in the newborn is to ascertain the presence or absence of an infection.

The cerebrospinal fluid alterations associated with bacterial meningitis in the newborn period are generally similar to those at any other age. The protein value is commonly much higher than the usual value in the older child with meningitis, probably indicative of the greater necrotizing effect of bacterial infection on the immature brain. It is important to recognize that it is possible, although unusual, for a child to have meningitis even though the cerebrospinal fluid is clear to gross observation, contains few cells, and has a normal glucose content (Sarff et al., 1976). For this reason, gram stain and appropriate cultures should be made on every spinal fluid specimen obtained from the neonate, regardless of the other findings.

SUBDURAL TAPS

In the past, a transfontanel subdural tap was used primarily for the diagnosis of a convexity subdural hematoma. For this procedure, the hair should be shaved well beyond the site of the needle penetration, and the scalp should be properly cleansed with the appropriate substances. After application of a sterilizing agent to the skin, it should be allowed to dry, or it can be wiped dry before insertion of the needle. The site chosen for the tap should be as close as possible to the junction of the fontanel with the coronal suture in order to avoid injury to the midline superior sagittal sinus.

For ascertaining the presence of blood in the subdural space, a CT scan is a preferable procedure, and in most instances subdural taps have been relegated to a therapeutic role in the treatment of empyema complicating bacterial meningitis.

ELECTROENCEPHALOGRAPHY

In the older infant or child, the electroencephalogram, when interpreted by a competent individual, is a valuable diagnostic tool in confirming a convulsive disorder. Even in the patient with a mature nervous system, however, one must recognize the limitations of electroencephalography, namely, that minor deviations from normal need not be of clinical significance and that the results of an electroencephalogram must be used in conjunction with the historical data, the physical findings, and the information accumulated from other studies.

In the newborn period, the electroencephalogram has even greater restrictions of its clinical applicability, in part because of the limited ability of the immature cerebral cortex to produce recordable electrical potentials. As a consequence, there is considerable controversy as to whether neonatal seizures should be diagnosed on the basis of behavioral or EEG criteria. The electroencephalogram of the premature infant is characterized by discontinuous and disorganized activity that gradually becomes synergistic over the two hemispheres with increasing gestational age. Before the 26th week of gestational age, the recording is irregular, with bursts of up to 1-per-second waves alternating with periods of near electrical silence lasting several seconds. Beyond 28 weeks, bursts become more regular, and some intermittent fast activity begins to emerge. By about 37 weeks, the tracing becomes continuous. In the full-term infant, the electroencephalogram reveals low-voltage activity, generally less than 50 microvolts, with occasional 3- to 5-per-second waves of slightly higher voltage than the general background (Engel, 1975).

The value of the electroencephalogram in assessing the neonate lies in its prognostic rather than its diagnostic applications. This is because the tracing reflects the state of functional impairment of the brain, and consequently, identical abnormalities can be seen regardless of the nature of the infant's encephalopathy. The prognostic value of the electroencephalogram is considerable, however, and has been placed on firm footing by the longitudinal studies of Rose and Lombroso (1970) and of Sarnat and Sarnat (1976). In the former study, a normal interictal tracing in a neonate with seizures was followed by normal development in 86 per cent of the cases, whereas 88 per cent of infants whose electroencephalogram demonstrated multifocal abnormalities either died or were left with major neurologic deficits. Unifocal electroencephalographic abnormalities were associated with a good prognosis, whereas a flat electroencephalogram, or one that showed bursts of high-voltage discharges, was almost invariably indicative of a poor clinical outcome.

The interpretation of the electroencephalogram in the premature infant is difficult because electrical bursts are a normal phenomenon prior to 37 weeks' gestation, and, consequently, a paroxysmal electroencephalogram in an early premature infant does not carry the certainty of a poor prognosis, as it would in a term infant.

SKULL RADIOGRAPHS

With the availability of neuroimaging studies and ultrasonography, the role of the skull radiograph in the evaluation of the newborn has become of relatively small importance. As a rule, this study is obtained when there are abnormalities in the shape of the head not explained by molding secondary to the delivery process or when the possibility of a fracture exists on the basis of a cephalhematoma or a traumatic delivery.

COMPUTED TOMOGRAPHY

Computed tomography (CT scan) has a wide spectrum of application to the diagnostic evaluation of the newborn with neurologic disease. The procedure is useful not only in the evaluation of infants suspected of harboring an intracranial hemorrhage but also in the diagnosis of a wide variety of congenital malformations of the nervous system.

Whereas certain pathologic appearances (e.g., those of hemorrhage) are readily interpreted, difficulties are encountered in the CT analysis of parenchymal changes. This occurs because of the frequent presence of alternating areas of high and low densities within the cerebral substance that do not have adult equivalents. However, both gray and white matter have lower attenuation coefficients in newborns than in older children, and the difference in density between gray and white matter is greater than in adults. Sulci and subarachnoid spaces are often quite prominent and should not be interpreted as cerebral atrophy.

In the preterm infant, interpretation of the CT scan is even further complicated by the poor visualization of the ventricular system. This is due to its small volume in relationship to brain parenchyma and to the similarity of its density to that of the parenchyma. Localized areas of low density in the periventricular region have little significance, as do hypodense parenchymal areas. In most instances, these changes are transient and may reflect a developmental stage.

MAGNETIC RESONANCE IMAGING

Magnetic resonance imaging (MRI) is a versatile and noninvasive procedure that provides information on brain structure without exposure to ionizing radiation. As a rule, T1-weighted images provide a better view of structural anatomy, while T2-weighted images are preferred for the detection of structural abnormalities.

When T2-weighted spin-echo pulse sequences are used, white matter is lighter (higher signal intensity) than gray matter for the first 6 to 7 months of life. Between 8 and 12 months of age, the signal intensities from white and gray matter are about equal. Thereafter, one observes the adult appearance, with gray matter lighter than white matter. This orderly progression may be disturbed in developmentally delayed youngsters, and MRI can provide valuable information with respect to the status of myelination in the various neuronal systems (Dietrich et al., 1988).

For the evaluation of an infant suspected of harboring anomalies of cortical architecture, MRI is far superior to CT scanning because it can depict areas of micropolygyria, lissencephaly, or heterotopic gray matter. In addition, the quality of images is, as a rule, superior to that offered by CT scans.

In choosing between CT scans and MRI studies, the physician should not forget that the critically ill patient requiring a variety of infusions and respiratory support cannot be managed properly in most MRI units and that the procedure costs 20 to 300 per cent more than CT scans.

ULTRASONOGRAPHY

Ultrasonography of the brain has emerged as the major tool for evaluating neonatal brain anatomy and for attempting to predict long-term outcome of the sick premature infant (Levene et al., 1985). Because of the infant's wide-open fontanelle, ultrasound studies that include sector scanning provide remarkable examinations of the brain, with excellent visualization of the ventricular system, basal ganglia, choroid plexus, and corpus callosum.

Emerging evidence suggests that both the immediate prognosis for an infant and the long-term developmental outcome are related to the severity of intracranial ischemia and hemorrhage. Therefore, efforts have been made to develop grading systems to categorize the extent of hemorrhage and, thus, provide a basis for clinical decisions during the neonatal hospitalization and care needs after discharge (Table 42–4).

INTRACRANIAL HEMORRHAGE IN SMALL PRETERM INFANTS

Subependymal hemorrhages (Grade I) (Fig. 42–2A) usually resolve in the great majority of infants without any

TABLE 42–4. Grading System for Assessment of Intracranial Hemorrhage

GRADE	ASSESSMENT
I	Subependymal hemorrhage, alone.
II	Subependymal hemorrhage or choroid plexus hemorrhage *with* intraventricular hemorrhage but *without* intraventricular dilatation.
III	Subependymal hemorrhage or choroid plexus hemorrhage *with* intraventricular hemorrhage and *with* intraventricular dilatation.
IV	Subependymal hemorrhage or choroid plexus hemorrhage *with* intraventricular hemorrhage and *with* intraparenchymal hemorrhage.

(Adapted from Papile, L., Burstein, J., Burstein, J., et al.: Incidence and evolution of subependymal and intraventricular hemorrhage: A study of infants with birth weight less than 1500 grams. J. Pediatr. 92:529, 1978.)

apparent influence on long-term growth and development. Grade II includes subependymal hemorrhages complicated by intraventricular hemorrhage (Fig. 42–2B), and in general, these infants have also ultimately had good outcomes. However, this score also illustrates echodensities, which have been associated with later development of periventricular leukomalacia and a more ominous long-term outcome. Figure 42–2C shows intraventricular hemorrhage with some degree of intraventricular dilatation (Grade III), with a clot that is retracting. The prognosis for infants with these findings is more guarded and depends upon the degree of periventricular ischemia that the infant has experienced. Grade IV hemorrhage represents a germinal matrix hemorrhage with extension into the adjacent white matter and is associated with intraventricular hemorrhage and ventricular enlargement (Guzetta et al., 1986). The most ominous finding with respect to outcome, i.e., the extensive cystic necrosis of periventricular leukomalacia, involves almost the entire periventricular white matter in this infant (Fig. 42–2D).

In most cases, *periventricular leukomalacia* presents initially as some periventricular echo-dense areas that subsequently become echo-lucent cystic areas. These findings are associated with an ominous prognosis, particularly when present bilaterally. Ordinarily, the lesions are seen in proximity to the lateral ventricles, either in front of the anterior horns in the corona radiata or posterior to the occipital horns. Areas of increased echogenicity may also be seen in the parenchyma, an entity termed "subcortical leukomalacia."

Ultrasonography does not give the precision or detail of computerized tomography or magnetic resonance imaging; therefore, before major decisions are made based on review of ultrasound scans, it is important that CT and/or MR scanning be done to confirm the extensiveness of the damage.

BRAIN-STEM AUDITORY-EVOKED RESPONSE

No physiologic test available can yield the equivalent of a pure-tone audiogram or indicate exactly what a subject hears. The brain-stem auditory-evoked response (BAER) is a diagnostic test that permits evaluation of both auditory and brain-stem functions. Briefly stated, the BAER is a computerized test that averages and records electrical changes that occur at the eighth cranial nerve

and brain stem in response to auditory stimuli. These electrical events consist of six waves in the first 10 milliseconds after the acoustic stimulus and can be recorded from scalp electrodes of the infant. It is generally agreed that wave I with a latency of 1.5 milliseconds is generated by the auditory nerve activity, wave II by the cochlear nucleus, wave III by the superior olive, wave IV by the lateral lemniscus, and wave V by the inferior colliculus. The shape of the BAER and the latencies of its various peaks depend on several factors: the stimulus intensity, the repetition rate of the stimulus, and the maturity of the infant. The latency of these waves systematically shortens as the baby develops during the first year of life. Neonates with hearing deficits deviate from the normal latency in ways characteristic of the type of deafness, either conductive or sensorineural (Hecox and Cone, 1981).

Even though the BAER has some limitations, it is recordable from neonates as young as 25 weeks' gestation (Cox, 1984). Neonates who deserve close attention and follow-up are those who are at risk for sensorineural hearing loss and include: (1) infants with hypoxic ischemic encephalopathy, (2) those with a family history of sensorineural hearing loss, (3) those exposed in utero to maternal rubella or other viral illness, (4) those with congenital anomalies of the head and neck, including cleft palate, microtia, and so forth, (5) those who weigh less than 1500 g at birth, (6) those with bilirubin levels greater than 20 mg, and (7) those with neonatal meningitis. (Bergman et al., 1985). Some infants with hypoxic ischemic encephalopathy have an initially normal BAER, which subsequently becomes abnormal. Likewise, some premature infants may initially have a normal BAER, which subsequently becomes abnormal. The sensitivity and specificity of BAER for infants with different conditions and ages have not yet been well described.

Patients identified as having a negative response to these basic acoustic stimuli should be seen by an otolaryngologist and speech and hearing pathologist who can perform behavioral audiometry under soundproof environmental conditions.

OTHER PROCEDURES

The concentration of adenosine triphosphate (ATP), and some of the other high-energy phosphates involved in cellular energetics of brain and muscle, can be measured by nuclear magnetic resonance (NMR) spectroscopy. In addition, the method can be used to determine intracellular pH, lactate production, and the flux through the glycolytic pathway.

Most of these studies have utilized the P^{31} NMR signal which is normally present in sufficiently high concentrations to be detectable. Spectra can be recorded within 10 seconds to 5 minutes, and changes in intracellular pH and metabolites can be followed. The procedure will undoubtedly play an increasingly important role in evaluating the extent, timing, and prognosis of perinatal hypoxic-ischemic encephalopathy (Corbett et al., 1987; Hope et al., 1984).

Positron emission tomography (PET) is a technique that enables one to detect localized functional abnormalities of the brain. It is based on the emission by certain unstable isotopes of positrons, positive-charged electrons, which, after a short path in tissue, collide with negatively

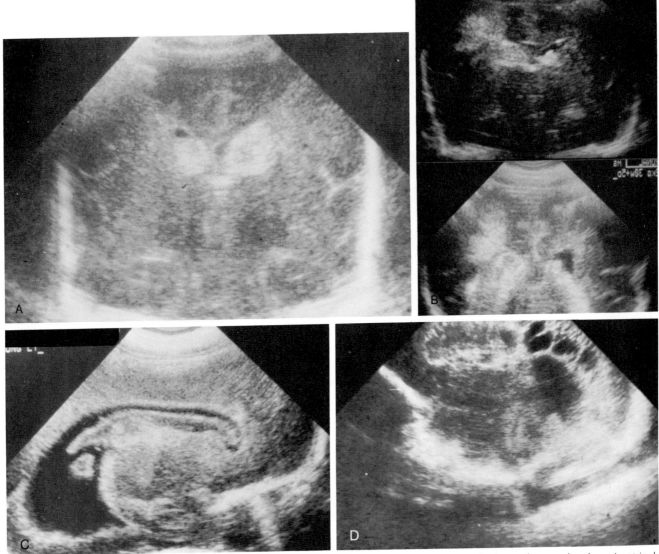

FIGURE 42–2. *A, Bilateral subependymal hemorrhages. B, Subependymal hemorrhage plus intraventricular hemorrhage and early periventricular leukomalacia in a 1200 g, 30-week-gestation infant at 5 days of age. C, Intraventricular hemorrhage in evolution in 970 g, 27-week-gestation infant. Note somewhat retracted and hypoechoic clot. D, Extensive cystic necrosis of periventricular leukomalacia, which involves nearly the entire periventricular white matter. (Courtesy of Ruth Goldstein, M.D., Assistant Professor of Radiology, University of California, San Francisco.)*

charged electrons and emit energy that can be localized by tomography. Isotopes of carbon, nitrogen, oxygen, and fluorine have been utilized for PET scanning. All have short half-lives, and are generally prepared by an on-site cyclotron. F[18] labeled 2-fluorodeoxyglucose (FDG) is particularly useful for measuring transport and phosphorylation of glucose in that it is not metabolized beyond deoxyglucose-6-phosphate and therefore remains within brain. FDG enables accurate measurements of cerebral blood flow, and of local oxygen and glucose metabolism. Although the PET scan is mainly an investigational procedure, and is only available in a few university centers, it promises to be invaluable in the study of the functional development of normal and diseased brains (Chugani et al., 1987).

Abnormalities of the visually evoked responses have been described in hypoxic infants and in those with posthemorrhagic hydrocephalus. The clinical value of this procedure is, however, not of the magnitude of the auditory-evoked responses.

■ REFERENCES

Ahmann, P. A., Lazzara, A., Dykes, F. D., et al.: Intraventricular hemorrhage in the high-risk preterm infant: Incidence and outcome. Ann. Neurol. 7:118, 1980.

Amiel-Tison, C.: Neurological evaluation of the maturity of newborn infants. Arch. Dis. Child. 43:89, 1968.

André-Thomas, C. Y., Chesni, Y., and Saint-Anne Dargassies, S.: The neurological examination of the infant. Little Club Clinics in Developmental Medicine, No. 1, 1960.

Bauer, C. H., New, M. I., and Miller, J. H.: Cerebrospinal fluid protein values of premature infants. J. Pediatr. 66:1017, 1965.

Bergman, I., Hirsch, R. P., Fria, T. J., et al: Cause of hearing loss in the high-risk preterm infant. J. Pediatr. 106:95, 1985.

Chugani, H. T., Phelps, M. E., and Massiotta, J. C.: Positron emission tomography study of human brain functional development. Ann. Neurol. 22:487, 1987.

Corbett, R. J. T., Laptook, A. R., and Nunally, R. L.: The use of the chemical shift of the phosphomonoester P-31 magnetic resonance peak for the determination of intracellular pH in the brain of neonates. Neurology 37:1771, 1987.

Cox, L.: The current status of auditory brainstem response testing in neonatal populations. Pediatr. Res. 18:780, 1984.

Dietrich, R. B., Bradley, W. G., Zaragoza, E. J., et al.: MR evaluation of early myelination patterns in normal and developmentally delayed infants. Am. J. Neuroradiol. 9:69, 1988.

Dubowitz, L. M. S., Dubowitz, V., and Goldberg, C.: Clinical assessment of gestational age in the newborn infant. J. Pediatr. 77:1, 1970.

Engel, R.: Abnormal Electroencephalograms in the Neonatal Period. Springfield, Ill., Charles C Thomas, 1975.

Friede, R. L.: Developmental Neuropathology. New York: Springer Verlag, 1975.

Gamper, E, cited by Peiper, A.: Cerebral Function in Infancy and Childhood. New York, Consultants Bureau, 1963, pp. 171–174.

Guzzetta, F., Shackelford, G. D., Volpe, S., et al.: Periventricular intraparenchymal echodensities in the premature newborn: Critical determinant of neurologic outcome. Pediatrics 78:995, 1986.

Hecox, K. E., and Cone, B.: Prognostic importance of brainstem auditory evoked responses after asphyxia. Neurology 31:1429, 1981.

Hope, P. L., et al.: Cerebral energy metabolism studied with phosphorus NMR spectroscopy in normal and birth-asphyxiated infants. Lancet 2:366, 1984.

Levene, M. I., Williams, J. L., and Fawer, C-L.: Ultrasound of the Infant Brain. Oxford, Blackwell Scientific Publications, 1985.

Moro, E.: Das erste Trimenon. München Med. Wchschr. p. 1147, 1918.

Nelson, K. B., and Ellenberg, J. H.: Children who "outgrew" cerebral palsy. Pediatrics 69:529, 1982.

O'Rahilly, R.: The embryonic period. Teratology 34:119, 1986.

Paine, R. S., and Oppe, T. E.: Neurological examination of children. Clin. Dev. Med. 20:1, 1966.

Papile, L., Burstein, J., Burstein, R., et al.: Incidence and evolution of subependymal and intraventricular hemorrhage: A study of infants with birthweight less than 1500 grams. J. Pediatr. 92:529, 1978.

Picard, L., et al.: Cerebral computed tomography in premature infants, with an attempt at staging developmental features. J. Comput. Assist. Tomogr. 4:435, 1980.

Popich, G. A., and Smith, D. W.: Fontanels: Range of normal size. J. Pediatr. 80:749, 1972.

Robinson, R.: Cerebral function in the newborn. Dev. Med. Child Neurol. 8:561, 1966.

Robinson, R. J.: Assessment of gestational age by neurological examination. Arch. Dis. Child. 41:437, 1966.

Rose, A. L., and Lombroso, C. T.: Neonatal seizure states. A study of clinical, pathological, and electroencephalographic features in 137 full-term babies with a long-term follow-up. Pediatrics 45:404, 1970.

Saint-Anne Dargassies, S.: Neurodevelopmental symptoms during the first year of life. Dev. Med. Child Neurol. 14:235, 1972.

Sarff, L. D., Platt, L. H., and McCracken, G. H., Jr.: Cerebrospinal fluid evaluation in neonates. Comparison of high risk infants with and without meningitis. J. Pediatr. 88:473, 1976.

Sarnat, H. B.: Do the corticospinal and corticobulbar tracts mediate functions in the human newborn? Can. J. Neurol. Sci. 16:157, 1989.

Sarnat, H. B., and Sarnat, M. S.: Neonatal encephalopathy following fetal distress. Arch. Neurol. 33:696, 1976.

Shewmon, D. A.: What is a neonatal seizure? Problems in definition and quantification for investigative and clinical purposes. J. Clin. Neurophysiol. 7:315, 1990.

Volpe, J. A.: Neurology of the Newborn, 2nd ed. Philadelphia: W. B. Saunders Company, 1987.

PERINATAL CENTRAL NERVOUS SYSTEM ASPHYXIA AND TRAUMA

John H. Menkes

The immediate and delayed consequences of perinatal asphyxia and trauma constitute the most important neurologic problems of the neonatal period. Several factors, acting solely or in concert, may traumatize the infant brain in utero, in the course of the birth process, or in the immediate postnatal period. Mechanical trauma to the central or peripheral nervous system is probably the insult that is understood best. A focal or generalized disorder of cerebral circulation occurring during the prenatal or early postnatal period and acting in isolation is probably an uncommon cause of brain damage. When present, the occlusion usually is in the distribution of the middle cerebral artery and is presumed to result from embolization due to placental infarcts or from thrombosis caused by vascular maldevelopment, sepsis, or (in the case of a twin to a macerated fetus) the exchange of thromboplastic material from the dead infant (Friede, 1989).

■ MECHANICAL TRAUMA AND ITS CONSEQUENCES

Mechanical trauma to the fetal head may produce extracranial lesions, notably molding of the head, caput succedaneum, and cephalhematoma.

MOLDING OF THE HEAD AND CAPUT SUCCEDANEUM

The fetal head is frequently asymmetrically shaped as a consequence of pressure while it is still within the uterus or in the birth canal. The sutures override one another, the fontanelles are small or obliterated, and the soft tissues overlying the skull may be soft and boggy because of caput succedaneum. When molding of the fetal head is extreme, tears of the tentorium or cerebral falx may ensue. These can be accompanied by lacerations of the venous structures and thus give rise to a subdural hematoma or other varieties of intracranial hemorrhage.

A caput usually appears at the vertex, and it is commonly accompanied by marked molding of the head. The hemorrhage and edema are situated beneath the skin and may extend under the aponeurosis (subgaleal hemorrhage) but are still external to the periosteum (Fig. 43–1A). In rare instances, sufficient blood is sequestered to produce a significant anemia. Massive scalp hemorrhages may indicate an underlying coagulation defect such as hemophilia or hemorrhagic disease of the newborn.

CEPHALHEMATOMA

Cephalhematoma refers to a usually benign traumatic subperiosteal hemorrhage in the parietal region of the newborn skull (Fig. 43–1B). Bleeding is characteristically restricted in its location by the suture lines, across which it cannot extend. The incidence of neonatal cephalhematoma has been found to range from 1.5 to 2.5 per cent of deliveries. It is twice as common in males, and approximately 15 per cent occur bilaterally. Vaginal delivery is not necessarily a prerequisite for occurrence of this lesion, since it has been encountered in infants born by cesarean section. Linear skull fractures are found in the underlying parietal bones in about 18 per cent of infants with bilateral cephalhematomas. When the cephalhematoma is unilateral, the incidence of linear fractures is much less, probably about 5 per cent. Rarely, a cephalhematoma is found in the occipital region, where its midline location may cause it to be confused with an encephalocele.

The cephalhematoma in the newborn appears in the form of a firm, localized mass that does not transilluminate. Within a few days after birth, change in the consistency of the clotted blood gives rise to a sharp, palpable ridge, or "crater edge," near the periphery that can be confused with a fracture by the inexperienced examiner. Depending on the size of the lesion, a cephalhematoma is usually gradually absorbed by 2 to 8 weeks.

In many patients, neuroimaging studies will reveal hyperostosis of the outer table of the skull that persists for several months after clinical evidence of the lesion has disappeared. Much less often there is persistent thickening of the parietal calvarium at the site of the original lesion, at times with widening of the diploic space, or cystic defects in the region. In some cases, calcium deposition within the clot occurs in a surprisingly short period of time and can be visualized by skull x-rays or CT scans.

Cephalhematomas of large volume can be associated with anemia or, more often, hyperbilirubinemia, as a consequence of absorption of the blood products. An infrequent but dangerous complication is abscess forma-

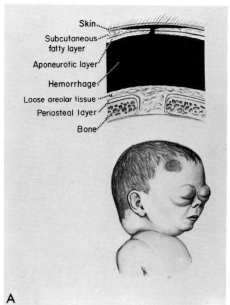

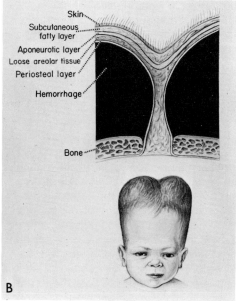

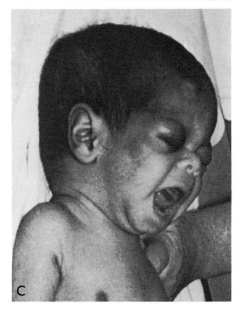

FIGURE 43–1. A, Location of edema and hemorrhage in caput succedaneum. B, Location of hemorrhage in cephalhematoma. C, Patient with massive hemorrhagic caput succedaneum, whose hemoglobin level fell to 2.2 g/dl by the age of 48 hours. (Reprinted with the permission of Daniel J. Pachman, M.D., of the University of Illinois Pediatric Department. The photograph, but not the sketches, appeared in Pediatrics 29:907, 1962. Reproduced by permission of Pediatrics.)

tion within a cephalhematoma in a septic newborn or secondary to contamination during attempted needle aspiration of the lesion. Suppuration within a cephalhematoma may be associated with obvious signs of localized infection or can remain surprisingly silent during progression of the lesion. It should be suspected whenever there is rapid enlargement of the mass several days after birth, the development of cutaneous erythema over the lesion, or otherwise unexplained fever and leukocytosis. An infected cephalhematoma may be complicated by osteomyelitis of the underlying skull or by meningitis, either associated with sepsis or secondary to intracranial extension through an adjacent skull fracture or a cranial suture (Ellis et al., 1974). Diagnosis is established by needle aspiration whenever an infected cephalhematoma is suspected.

Management of a cephalhematoma in the newborn is fundamentally conservative but should include the obtaining of imaging studies to determine the presence or absence of an underlying fracture as well as periodic checks of the hemoglobin and serum bilirubin, especially the latter if the child becomes jaundiced. Needle aspiration of the uncomplicated cephalhematoma is not indicated, since spontaneous resolution is expected and because of the hazard of bacterial contamination by needle penetration. Underlying skull fractures do not create a management problem and need no specific therapy unless there is significant depression of bone fragments.

SKULL FRACTURES IN THE NEWBORN INFANT

The skull of the infant at birth is less mineralized than it is later in childhood and also is more pliable because of the patency of the cranial sutures. For these reasons, there can be considerable distortion of the infant's head shape in utero and during the birth process without injury to the skull itself. Fractures can occur, however, and may be acquired in utero, during labor, or secondary to the application of forceps. Intrauterine fracture of the infant's skull is usually the result of compression of the skull against the promontory of the sacrum and can complicate a traumatic event to the mother's abdomen or pelvis or can occur secondary to the forces of uterine contraction.

Most skull fractures identified in the neonate are parietal or frontal in location and linear in type. Some are associated with an overlying cephalhematoma. Simple linear fractures are radiographically visible as lines of decreased density and may be seen only in one view. Such nondisplaced fractures are considered to be benign lesions that are expected to heal spontaneously and that need no therapeutic measures. A depressed skull fracture may result from pressure of the head against the pelvis or may be induced by incorrect application of the obstetric forceps. It is associated with inward buckling of the parietal bone, much like the indentation in a ping-pong ball (Fig. 43–2). A break in the continuity of the bone may not be present or may be evident over only a short length at the margin of the depression. This form of depressed skull injury is best seen in the anteroposterior or posteroanterior views of the skull and sometimes is not apparent at all on the lateral skull views. Compound depressed skull fractures acquired before or during the birth process should usually be corrected. Nonsurgical methods of elevation of simple depressed fractures appear to have the same outcome as surgically treated cases (Steinbok et al., 1987). However, in view of the simplicity of the surgical procedure and the possibility that an uncorrected fracture may act as a seizure focus, this author opts for early operative intervention in all depressed fractures.

SUBDURAL HEMORRHAGE

Mechanical trauma to the infant's brain during delivery may induce lacerations in the tentorium or falx with subsequent subdural hemorrhage. With improved obstetric techniques, these injuries have become relatively uncommon, and they are now generally restricted to large full-term infants delivered through a birth canal that is too small (cephalopelvic disproportion) or to premature infants whose skulls are unusually compliant (Wigglesworth and Husemeyer, 1977). Compression of the head along its occipitofrontal diameter, resulting in vertical molding, may occur with vertex presentations, whereas compression of the skull between the vault and the base, resulting in an anterior-posterior elongation, is likely to be the outcome of face and brow presentations. Tears of the falx and of the tentorium can be caused by both forms of overstretch. The damage is usually located in the region in which the falx joins the anterior edge of the tentorium. Tears and thromboses of the dural sinuses and of the larger cerebral veins, including the vein of Galen, are commonly accompanied by subdural hemorrhages. These may be either major and potentially fatal or minor and clinically unrecognizable. The hemorrhages are mainly localized to the base of the brain, but when the tears extend to involve the straight sinus and the vein of Galen, they can expand into the posterior fossa.

Overriding of the parietal bones occasionally produces a laceration of the superior sagittal sinus and a major fatal hemorrhage. Another uncommon traumatic lesion is a laceration of the occipital sinus associated with occipital osteodiastasis, a separation of the cartilaginous joint between the squamous and lateral portions of the occipital bone (Wigglesworth and Husemeyer, 1977). This injury is most often seen in infants delivered in the breech position.

Tearing of the superficial cerebral veins is probably a relatively common phenomenon. The subsequent hemorrhage results in a thin layer of blood over the cerebral convexity. Bleeding is often unilateral and is usually accompanied by a subarachnoid hemorrhage. Because the superficial cerebral veins of the premature infant are still underdeveloped, this type of hemorrhage is limited to full-term infants.

Subdural hemorrhage over the cerebral convexities usually results in minimal or no clinical signs. When these do occur, they are variable and nonspecific. Volpe (1987) has stressed the presence of focal cerebral signs, including

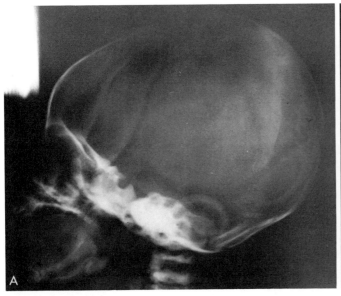
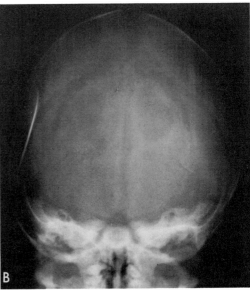

FIGURE 43–2. A and B, Lateral and anteroposterior (AP) skull x-ray films of a 1-day-old infant. Depressed skull injury is visualized clearly on the AP view as a linear streak of increased density. Such injuries are the result of inward buckling of the poorly mineralized skull of the newborn. The actual break in the continuity of the bone is present over a short distance only.

hemiparesis, deviation of the eyes, and a nonreactive or poorly reactive pupil. In addition, nonspecific signs indicative of acute subdural collections of blood include pallor, lethargy, irritability, vomiting, a poor Moro response, and bulging of the anterior fontanel (Deonna and Oberson, 1974). In some instances, a clinically inapparent subdural hematoma of the neonatal period may not be identified until a few months after birth, when it presents with progressive heart enlargement, seizures, developmental delay, and anemia (Matson, 1969).

Subdural hemorrhage within the posterior fossa is being increasingly recognized by CT scanning. Typically, symptoms appear following a lag period of 12 hours to 4 days. They include decreased responsiveness, apnea, bradycardia, opisthotonos, and seizures. As the subdural hematoma enlarges, the fourth ventricle is displaced forward and soon becomes obstructed, producing signs of increased intracranial pressure, including a bulging fontanel and progressive enlargement of the head circumference. Posterior fossa hemorrhage may be accompanied by intraventricular hemorrhage or an intracerebellar hematoma.

The diagnosis of neonatal subdural hemorrhage rests mainly on demonstration of the lesion by CT scan. This procedure is indicated in infants who have had a traumatic delivery and who develop nonspecific neurologic signs. Ultrasonography is not as adequate a procedure to detect this lesion as the CT scan.

Treatment is usually inadequate for the neonate who has sustained major subdural hemorrhage, although rapid surgical evacuation of the clot has saved some infants with extensive posterior fossa bleeding. Subdural taps are indicated solely to reduce increased intracranial pressure and should not be performed when the infant is asymptomatic. A subdural hematoma that produces a persistent increase in intracranial pressure may require a subdural-peritoneal or other shunting procedure. As in the other forms of intracranial hemorrhage, hydrocephalus may ensue and may require neurosurgical intervention.

In some instances, mechanical trauma may induce a hemorrhage that is primarily within the subarachnoid space, with the bleeding presumed to be of venous or subpial origin (Friede, 1989). Rarely, the hemorrhage is localized to the epidural space.

SCALP LESIONS DUE TO FETAL ASSESSMENT

In the past 20 years, bleeding or infection from use of scalp electrodes for fetal heart rate monitoring or lesions due to sampling of fetal blood from scalp incisions have become evident. For the most part, these problems are minor, requiring only pressure for bleeding or local care for inflammation at the incision site. In premature infants it is impossible to know to what degree these scalp wounds lead to significant infection since congenital infections with the same infecting organisms are common. The incidence of infections has been reported as 1 per cent for fetal blood sampling. Presumably, the same rate pertains for fetal scalp electrode usage. Serious bleeding from these traumas is extremely rare, but one fatality has been reported, and the author has observed an infant bleed sufficiently to cause hypotension. It has been suggested that asphyxia or hypotension at birth may prevent bleed-

ing from the affected site, which can then bleed an hour or so later when blood pressure is restored and peripheral vasoconstriction alleviated.

PERINATAL TRAUMA TO THE SPINAL CORD

Although spinal birth injuries were first described during the nineteenth century, much of our understanding of perinatal spinal trauma can be attributed to the classic papers of Crothers (1923) and Ford (1925). Relatively common several decades ago, this type of birth injury has become less frequent with improved obstetric practice, and it accounted for only 0.6 per cent of the series of patients with cerebral palsy encountered by Crothers and Paine (1959). The apparent rarity of this lesion may in part reflect the fact that few infants with major spinal cord damage survive the neonatal period, and in those who do survive, mild injuries to the lower cervical and upper thoracic spinal cord with attendant spastic paraparesis can easily be confused with the similar constellation of findings characteristic of the cerebral diplegic form of cerebral palsy occurring in the premature infant.

Perinatal traumatic lesions of the spinal cord result more commonly from stretching of the cord than from compression or transection. Longitudinal or lateral traction to the infant's neck or excessive torsion, particularly during a difficult breech delivery, stretches the cord, its covering meninges, the surface vessels, and the nerve roots. Lesions are most frequent in the lower cervical and upper thoracic regions. The most common gross pathologic findings are epidural hemorrhage, dural laceration with subdural hemorrhage, tears of the nerve roots, laceration and distortion of the cord, and focal hemorrhage and malacia within the cord. Ischemic lesions of the cord are less common. Gross or petechial hemorrhages may also be seen within the substance of the cord, and myelination of the tracts may be impaired above the transection.

A difficult breech delivery can be recorded in 75 per cent of infants who have suffered a spinal birth injury (Stern and Rand, 1959). When damage to the cord is severe, death of the neonate occurs during labor or soon after. With a less extensive injury, infants show respiratory depression and generalized hypotonia, or flaccid paraplegia (Bucher et al., 1979). An associated urinary retention and abdominal distention with paradoxical respirations occur. In addition to impaired motor function, there is absence of sensation and perspiration below the level of injury. The deep tendon reflexes are usually unelicitable during the neonatal period, and mass reflex movements do not become apparent until later.

In about 20 per cent of cases, damage to the brachial plexus can also be documented. In others, the lower brain stem is involved as well, with consequent bulbar signs.

Aside from being caused by trauma, hemorrhage within the vertebral canal may result from an extension of an intracranial hemorrhage due to prematurity or asphyxia. This complication has received relatively little attention in the United States. Both epidural and subdural bleeding have been encountered, the former being by far more common (Volbert and Schweitzer, 1954). Although these hemorrhages are either asymptomatic or induce deficits that are obscured by the more obvious symptoms of an intracranial hemorrhage, diagnosis by magnetic resonance imaging (MRI) of the spinal cord is now possible.

The clinical picture following complete transection of the cord evolves from the stage of spinal shock seen during the neonatal period to the appearance of reflex flexion withdrawal movements and a final picture of pure reflex activity of the isolated cord. A great number of survivors have normal intelligence.

The presence of poor muscle tone and flaccid weakness involving all extremities or only the legs following a breech delivery should suggest a cord injury. A sensory deficit in the neonate or young infant is best demonstrated by finding abnormalities in autonomic function, notably reduced skin temperature and perspiration.

Neuromuscular disorders, notably spinal muscular atrophy, are not associated with loss of either sensory function or sphincter control. Of the other neuromuscular disorders, congenital myasthenia gravis is diagnosed by reversibility of symptoms following injection of anticholinesterase drugs. Occasionally, an infant with a congenital tumor of the cervical or lumbar cord may present a clinical picture similar to that of a spinal cord injury. Abnormalities of the skin along the posterior lumbosacral midline, including dimpling, hemangiomata, or tufts of hair are commonly seen in the latter.

In some cases, the immediate problem is respiratory support. Fractures or fracture dislocations of the spine are generally absent, and there is no specific treatment for the injured spinal cord. Although the majority of clinically apparent spinal birth injuries are severe and irreversible, milder degrees of injury are potentially reversible.

BIRTH INJURIES TO THE CRANIAL NERVES

FACIAL NERVE

The most common cranial nerve to be injured during birth is the facial nerve. It is generally believed that unilateral facial weakness noted at birth is the result of compression of the facial nerve, although the precise site of injury and time of occurrence have been a subject of debate. Trauma to the nerve distal to its emergence from the stylomastoid foramen by forceps application has been regarded as one important cause, but the incidence of facial palsy is the same in infants born with and without the use of forceps. It is therefore likely that pressure on the maternal sacrum during labor is responsible for most cases of unilateral facial paralysis in the newborn. Parmelee (1931) proposed that some cases were the result of intrauterine posture of the fetal head in which marked flexion and rotation of the head resulted in compression of the mandible and lateral neck against the shoulder with associated compression of the peripheral portion of the facial nerve. Involvement of the seventh nerve as it traverses the facial canal within the mastoid is probably unusual but has been reported.

The degree of facial paresis ranges from complete loss of function in all three main branches to weakness limited to a small group of muscles. Unilateral facial weakness is most obvious when the infant cries, at which time there is lack of complete eyelid closure along with lack of normal lower facial muscle contraction on the paretic side. Experience with electrodiagnostic tests is limited in infants with congenital facial paresis as compared to older children and adults with acquired facial nerve deficits. The facial nerve excitability test in some instances can, however, distinguish complete from partial denervation, thus providing information concerning the extent of nerve damage. The ability to produce contraction of the muscle by stimulating the nerve implies that the conductivity of the nerve is only partially interrupted and suggests a favorable prognosis. However, good recovery is possible even when electric reactions are completely absent. It is important to wait at least 3 to 4 days before undertaking these studies to allow any injured fibers to regenerate.

The prognosis for recovery is good. In most instances, the facial nerve palsy is mild, and some improvement becomes evident within a week. In the more severe cases, the start of recovery may be delayed for several months. If improvement is not noted within a couple of weeks or if the facial palsy is severe, the infant should be evaluated by a neurologist.

Treatment of facial nerve palsy is limited to protection of the eye by application of methylcellulose drops and taping of the paralytic lid. Electric stimulation of the nerve does not hasten recovery. Neurosurgical repair of the nerve should be considered only when there is evidence that the nerve is severed.

Congenital Hypoplasia of the Depressor Anguli Oris Muscle. This well-described syndrome with localized facial weakness in which the lower lip on one side fails to be depressed on crying results in an "asymmetric crying facies" (Nelson and Eng, 1972). This localized muscle deficit is the result of congenital hypoplasia of the depressor anguli oris muscle, whose normal function is to draw the lower corner of the lip downward and evert it. The resulting facial asymmetry when the child cries is often misinterpreted by the parents, who may assume the normal side of the face is the abnormal one because they observe the lower lip on the intact side to be pulled down. The abnormal side is, in fact, the side on which the lower lip remains unaltered in position when crying occurs. The cosmetic significance of this minor anomaly lessens as the child gets older, probably largely because the older child is engaged in crying far less than in infancy.

Localized facial paresis causing an asymmetric crying facies can occur in isolation; however, observations have revealed a variable association with other anomalies. Of 44 infants with this syndrome, Pape and Pickering (1972) found 27 to have major anomalies of the skeletal, genitourinary, respiratory, or cardiovascular systems. A much lower incidence of associated defects was reported by Perlman and Reisner (1973), who found two patients with significant anomalies among 41 with the localized facial defect. The disorder most strongly associated with this facial defect is congenital cardiac disease, with the most common defect being ventricular septal defect, but other cardiac lesions have also been described.

OTHER CRANIAL NERVES

Conjunctival and retinal hemorrhages are common in the newborn, but birth injury involving the optic nerve exclusively is relatively rare. Unilateral and bilateral optic atrophy have been reported, the result of direct injury to the nerve through fracture of the orbit or, less often, of the base of the skull.

A transient postnatal paralysis of the abducens and oculomotor nerves is occasionally encountered. Paralysis of the latter may take the form of a transient postnatal ptosis. Congenital weakness of the musculature of the face, tongue, and palate unassociated with atrophy has been termed "congenital suprabulbar paresis." This condition may appear in isolation or may be accompanied by bilateral cerebral lesions, as in spastic quadriplegia, or extrapyramidal cerebral palsy. Although Worster-Drought in 1974 postulated a developmental defect of the corticobulbar tract, pathologic studies supporting this suggestion are lacking.

BIRTH INJURIES TO THE PERIPHERAL NERVES

BRACHIAL PLEXUS PALSY

Traction, stretch, or avulsion injuries during birth to part or all of the brachial plexus are potentially serious from the functional standpoint. In most instances, the injury and resulting limb weakness are unilateral, with the right arm being affected approximately twice as often as the left. Rarely, the disorder is bilateral, giving rise to serious disabilities if recovery does not occur. The incidence of this type of birth injury has not been well documented, but it is generally agreed that it has decreased considerably in recent decades with improved obstetric techniques.

Etiology. The two factors most consistently associated with birth injury to the brachial plexus are excessive weight of the child and complications of the labor and delivery process. Prolonged and difficult labor accompanied by heavy sedation of the mother resulting in a relaxed, large infant represent a combination of factors that increase the vulnerability of the child to this lesion.

The most common form of brachial plexus injury is one involving the fifth and sixth cervical roots. In most instances, this is the consequence of stretching of the plexus resulting from traction of the shoulder in the course of delivering the aftercoming head in a breech presentation or of turning the head away from the shoulder in a difficult cephalic presentation. In most instances, the brachial plexus is compressed by hemorrhage and edema within the nerve sheath. Less often, there is an actual tear of the nerves or avulsion of the roots from the spinal cord with segmental damage to the gray matter of the spinal cord. With traction, the fifth cervical root gives way first, then the sixth, and so on down the plexus. Thus, the mildest plexus injuries only involve C_5 and C_6, and the more severe involve the entire plexus.

Clinical Features. In about 80 per cent of infants, the paralysis is confined to the upper brachial plexus (Erb-Duchenne paralysis). In about 90 per cent, involvement is unilateral, more often on the right. The weakness is recognized soon after delivery. It affects the deltoid, serratus anterior, biceps, teres major, brachioradialis, and supinator muscles. Weakness of these muscles, which are innervated by the fifth and sixth cervical roots, results in

the characteristic clinical picture in which the affected arm is in a position of tight adduction and internal rotation at the shoulder, in addition to extension and pronation at the elbow. Added involvement of the seventh cervical root causes weakness of the extensors of the wrist and fingers leading to a flexion deformity of the hand due to sustained contraction of the flexor muscles supplied by the median nerve. Denervation of the serratus anterior, rhomboids, and other periscapular muscles adds to the motor disability around the shoulder and produces winging of the scapula.

In addition to the characteristic posture of the affected arm, there is an absent or diminished Moro reflex on the denervated side but an intact grasp reflex. The biceps reflex is absent or less active than the triceps reflex, a picture that is the converse of normal. In most instances, one is unable to demonstrate a sensory loss, although occasionally the examiner can convince himself of a loss of cutaneous sensation over the deltoid region and the adjacent radial surface of the upper arm. This is evidenced by reduced temperature and reduced perspiration over the affected area. Fractures of the clavicle or of the humerus, slippage of the capital head of the radius, and subluxation of the shoulder and the cervical spine often accompany an Erb-Duchenne injury. When a significant degree of injury to the fourth cervical root is present, phrenic nerve paralysis may accompany injury to the upper brachial plexus. Such an infant may show signs of respiratory distress, including tachypnea, cyanosis, and decreased movement of the affected hemithorax. When phrenic nerve palsy is unaccompanied by injury to the brachial plexus, as occurs occasionally, the condition may mimic congenital pulmonary or heart disease (Smith, 1972).

Klumpke's paralysis, or birth injury to the lower brachial plexus, is relatively uncommon (2.5 per cent of brachial plexus birth palsies). In this lesion, the paralysis involves the intrinsic muscles of the hand, with weakness of the flexors of the wrist and fingers. The grasp reflex is absent, and there is often a unilateral Horner's syndrome caused by involvement of the cervical sympathetic nerves. Loss of sensation and sudomotor function over the hand may also be found. Interference with the sympathetic innervation of the eye results in a delay or failure in pigmentation of the iris.

More commonly, the entire brachial plexus is damaged, resulting in a complete paralysis of the arm (Fig. 43–3).

Diagnosis. The diagnosis of brachial plexus injuries is usually readily apparent from the posture of the affected arm and from the absence of voluntary and reflex movements. Congenital Horner's syndrome may occur in the absence of trauma and may be associated with anomalies of the cervical vertebrae, enterogenous cysts, or congenital nerve deafness. Radiographic examinations to detect associated fractures and fluoroscopy to ascertain any limitation of diaphragmatic movement are indicated. Somatosensory-evoked potentials may be used to distinguish between an avulsed root ruptured at the entry to the spinal cord and a more distal lesion (Jones, 1979). In severe injuries causing avulsion of the spinal roots and bleeding into the subarachnoid space, the cerebrospinal fluid may be bloody. Magnetic resonance imaging can be

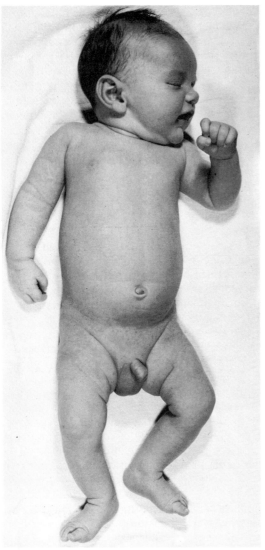

FIGURE 43–3. Brachial plexus stretch paralysis affecting the right arm. Child was the result of a difficult vertex delivery, birth weight was 4350 g. In addition to the paresis of the right arm, the Horner syndrome occurred on the infant's right side. The right arm is virtually immobile and is held in a position of adduction and partial internal rotation.

used to demonstrate root avulsion. Electromyography performed 2 to 3 weeks after the injury may confirm the extent of denervation.

Management. Treatment is directed primarily toward prevention of contractures. Gentle passive exercises of the affected arm should be begun about 1 week after birth. The infant's sleeve should be pinned in a natural position, rather than in abduction and external rotation as was recommended in the past. Follow-up studies indicate that overimmobilization of the affected arm is conducive to contractures and deformities that can persist despite spontaneous recovery of nerve function.

Reconstructive orthopedic surgery is indicated in certain instances to improve function of the permanently affected arm and hand, but it is not usually performed until 4 years of age or later.

Prognosis. Probability of recovery is difficult to predict in the immediate newborn period, although the child with a partial plexus lesion who shows definite improvement of motor function by 1 to 2 weeks after birth will probably recover completely or with only minor deficits. For some children with Erb-Duchenne palsy, recovery may be complete within a few weeks; for others, the maximum recovery is achieved within 1 to 18 months. In complete brachial plexus injury and in Klumpke's paralysis, the outlook is less optimistic, and the majority of children are left with serious difficulties (Eng, 1987). Permanent lesions are accompanied by muscle atrophy, contractures, and impaired limb growth. Some infants have an apparently good return of neuromuscular function and sensation yet are unable to use the affected arm (Eng, 1987). It is likely that transitory sensory motor deprivation in early life impairs the development of normal movement patterns and the organization of cortical body image.

SCIATIC NERVE PALSY

The sciatic nerve is ordinarily not susceptible to birth injury; however, it can be damaged in the infant by injection of materials or drugs into the umbilical artery or by misplaced gluteal injections. Injuries to the sciatic nerve can result in either temporary or permanent deficits and may be of variable degrees of severity. In some cases, weakness of dorsiflexion of the foot along with sensory loss on the dorsal surface of the foot are the only obvious deficits. More severe injuries are associated with extensive weakness and eventual atrophy of all muscle groups below the knee, in addition to weakness of the hamstring muscles on the affected side.

Ischemic sciatic neuropathy in the infant has been described following injections into the umbilical artery and secondary to accidental intra-arterial injection of drugs administered to the region of the buttocks. Sciatic nerve involvement in such cases has been attributed to spasm or occlusion of the inferior gluteal artery. Motor and sensory deficits corresponding to the innervation supplied by the sciatic nerve are accompanied by signs of vascular insufficiency in the region of the buttocks and throughout the affected lower limb. Improvement usually follows the insult, but permanent sequelae, including weakness and atrophy, are not uncommon.

Direct trauma to the sciatic nerve can result from misplaced gluteal injections of antibiotics or other substances. The young infant, and especially the premature one, is particularly susceptible to this type of nerve injury, mainly because of the much smaller size of the gluteal musculature. Early recognition of this complication of intramuscular injection is important to allow one to institute physical therapy and other measures promptly to minimize joint contractures. Surgical resection of the damaged nerve segment has been advocated if clinical improvement does not occur within 6 months following the injury.

Birth injuries to the other peripheral nerves are relatively uncommon. Injury to the lumbosacral plexus may occur after a frank breech delivery. Palsies of the radial nerve, laryngeal nerve, and obturator nerve have also been recorded.

■ PERINATAL HYPOXIC-ISCHEMIC ENCEPHALOPATHY AND ITS CONSEQUENCES

In recent years it has become clear that in the majority of instances brain damage, or cerebral palsy, is not attributable to birth trauma or perinatal asphyxia, and that in fact, permanent neurologic residua are infrequently the consequence of perinatal asphyxia. The current epidemic of malpractice lawsuits requires that the physician establish a diagnosis of perinatal asphyxia with considerable care rather than use the term indiscriminately, and that he keep in mind that in many instances conditions that follow fetal distress are not necessarily their consequence. In a relatively recent study, the incidence of hypoxic-ischemic encephalopathy (HIE) in Leicester, England was 6 in 1000 term infants, with 1 in 1000 dying or suffering severe neurologic deficits as a consequence of the asphyxial insult (Levene et al., 1985).

Of all the criteria for the diagnosis of HIE, the clinical condition of the infant following birth is the most important. The pediatrician must therefore detail the presence or absence of encephalopathy and its severity. Most infants with mild to moderate HIE do well, most infants with severe HIE die or do poorly (Robertson et al., 1989).

Criteria for the diagnosis of HIE include the following:

1. History of significant fetal distress, including evidence of acute or chronic placental insufficiency, fetal heart rate or pH abnormalities, clinical evidence of fetal malpositioning, protracted or difficult delivery, extensive meconium in amniotic fluid, or maternal hypotension.

2. Evidence of CNS insult after birth, such as low Apgar scores, sustained blood gas and pH abnormalities, seizures, abnormalities of CNS state, hypoventilation (ventilator support is usually required), and tone abnormalities. Other organ dysfunction is frequently present, such as persistent fetal circulation or renal and cardiac dysfunction. For the diagnosis of severe encephalopathy, many of these findings persist over the 1st week of life.

3. Laboratory studies that may reveal increased CSF protein, elevation of CSF lactate and pyruvate, and increased creatine kinase–BB isoenzyme (Walsh, 1982). Cord blood or CSF hypoxanthine levels have also been reported to be helpful. Most infants with even mild degrees of HIE have evidence of inappropriate ADH secretion.

4. Neuroimaging studies and electroencephalography on the 3rd to 6th day may show evidence of diffuse CNS injury.

5. Absence of other major CNS metabolic, infectious, or structural abnormality.

Pathogenesis and Pathology. Asphyxia is a condition in which the brain is subjected not only to hypoxia but also to ischemia and hypercarbia, which in turn may lead to cerebral edema and various circulatory disturbances (Volpe, 1987). Asphyxia may occur at one or more points during intrauterine and extrauterine life. In the large series of asphyxiated infants studied by Brown and associates (1974), the insult was believed to have occurred primarily antepartum in 51 per cent of the cases, intrapartum in 40 per cent, and postpartum in 9 per cent. With protracted hospital stays in the neonatal intensive care unit (NICU)

for extremely premature infants, the incidence of postpartum asphyxia has probably increased since then.

The biochemical and physiologic changes attending acute asphyxia have been studied extensively (Volpe, 1987).

Within seconds after its induction, NAD converts to NADH, and the ion permeability of neuronal membranes increases. This increase in permeability results in a marked increase in extracellular potassium and an influx into cells of sodium, chloride, and calcium. These ionic changes result in depolarization of neurons and loss of spontaneous electrical activity. The increased concentration of extracellular potassium may also be responsible for astrocytic swelling.

An acceleration of glycolysis accompanies these alterations and causes a rapid increase in brain lactate (Vannucci and Duffy, 1977). At the same time, the concentration of tricarboxylic acid cycle intermediates falls, and the production of high-energy phosphates diminishes. These changes result in a rapid fall in phosphocreatine and a slower reduction in brain ATP concentrations. Brain glucose and glycogen also decrease rapidly. The water content of brain increases, and within 15 minutes after induction of asphyxia, some brain swelling may already be evident.

In asphyxiated neonates, the fall in phosphocreatine, as measured by phosphorus nuclear magnetic spectroscopy, is less rapid, and for unknown reasons, intracellular pH and other indices of cellular energy status frequently remain normal for the 1st day of life.

Alterations in cerebral blood flow induced by asphyxia are equally important in understanding the genesis of birth injuries (Volpe, 1987) (Fig. 43–4). Initially, there is a redistribution of cardiac output so that a large proportion enters the brain. This results in a 30 to 175 per cent increase in cerebral blood flow. At the same time, there is a loss of cerebral vascular autoregulation (Lou et al., 1979a). As a consequence, cerebral arterioles fail to respond to changes in perfusion pressure and carbon dioxide concentrations, resulting in a pressure-passive cerebral blood flow. As asphyxia persists, cardiac output drops and hypotension follows. Since cerebral autoregulation is no longer functional, the arteriolar system is unable to respond to the decreased perfusion pressure with vasodilation, and the result is a striking reduction of cerebral blood flow (Lou et al., 1979b). Cerebral blood flow may be further compromised by the development of localized or generalized brain edema.

After an undetermined period, a point of irreversibility is reached. The exact mechanism of tissue damage is still unclear. The studies of Brann and Myers (1975) have stressed the role of intracellular and generalized brain edema induced by the combination of hypoxia, acidosis, hypocarbia, and hypotension. Volpe (1987), on the other hand, believes that the loss of vascular autoregulation coupled with hypotension reduces cerebral blood flow to a degree sufficient to produce tissue necrosis and subsequent cerebral edema. Combined clinical and imaging studies by Lupton and associates (1988), in which intracranial pressure of asphyxiated term infants was correlated with their CT scans, corroborate Volpe's view that tissue necrosis precedes cerebral edema, rather than vice versa, with maximum abnormalities being seen between 36 and

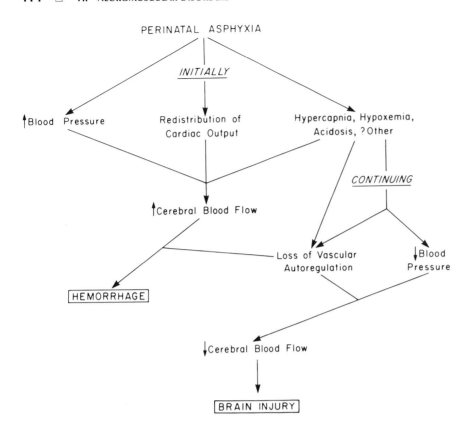

FIGURE 43–4. Interrelationships between perinatal asphyxia, alterations in cerebral blood flow, and brain damage. In addition to the mechanisms depicted, acidosis may induce focal or generalized cerebral edema, which reduces cerebral blood flow. (From Volpe, J. J.: Neurology of the Newborn. Philadelphia, W. B. Saunders Company, 1981.)

72 hours following the insult. From these studies it is also evident that increased intracranial pressure is a relatively uncommon complication, being encountered in 22 per cent of asphyxiated infants. The role of postischemic impairment of microvascular perfusion ("No-reflow phenomenon") in the genesis of tissue damage in the asphyxiated human neonate is still unclear.

On a cellular level, the ability of excitotoxic neurotransmitters to mediate hypoxic brain damage has received a considerable amount of attention. The reader is referred to reviews by Vannucci (1990a) and Auer and Siesjö (1988). In hypoxia, reuptake of glutamate, the natural-occurring excitatory neurotransmitter, is interfered with, resulting in excessive stimulation of neuronal excitatory receptors. Rothman and Olney (1986) propose that prolonged neuronal depolarization induces both a rapid and a slowly evolving cell death. Rapid cell death is due to the entry of chloride into neurons. The increased intracellular chloride induces further cation influx to maintain electroneutrality, and finally, the chloride and cation entry draws water into cells with ultimate osmotic lysis. A variety of chemicals, all sharing the property of being antagonists to N-methyl-D-aspartate (NMDA), a synthetic excitatory neurotransmitter, are able to protect neurons from asphyxial damage (Park et al., 1988).

Calcium influx appears to have an additive function, in that it induces a slower neuronal death in the absence of cell swelling. The actual mechanism of calcium-induced cell death is still a matter of speculation. It may involve the activation of phospholipases or proteases and the consequent disruption of membrane phospholipids. In addition, the release of polyunsaturated fatty acids, notably arachidonic acid, results in the formation of free radicals and ensuing tissue injury.

In the neonate, hypoglycemia, by hastening the depletion of energy stores under anoxic conditions, contributes to asphyxial brain damage (Vannucci, 1990a).

Whatever the biochemical and physiologic mechanisms for brain damage, the relative resistance of the newborn brain to oxygen lack has been known for some time. It is likely that this phenomenon reflects a reduction in overall cerebral metabolism and decreased energy demands by the newborn brain in comparison with the adult organ. Total metabolism of the newborn mouse brain is about one-tenth that of the adult, and glycolysis also proceeds at a much slower rate. A relative resistance of the cardiovascular system to hypoxic injury may also be operative.

Small-for-gestational-age infants are at increased risk for neurologic deficits caused by perinatal asphyxia. In part, this appears to be the result of a reduced cerebral tolerance to asphyxia in these subjects (Thordstein and Kjellmer, 1988).

In addition to the aforementioned biochemical and physiologic alterations, the type and density of the various neuronal receptors and their changes with maturation may determine selective cellular vulnerability and thus explain the remarkable regional variations in the pathology in the brains of asphyxiated infants (Silverstein et al., 1990). For many years, several distinct pathologic lesions have been known to occur singly or jointly.

When the primate fetus is subjected to acute total asphyxia, a reproducible pattern of brain pathology ensues (Auer and Sjesjö, 1988). This includes bilaterally symmetric lesions in the thalamus and in a number of brainstem nuclei, notably those of the inferior colliculi, the superior olive, and the lateral lemniscus. The neurons of the cerebral cortex, particularly the hippocampus, are especially vulnerable, as are the Purkinje cells of the cerebellum (Norman, 1978). On electron microscopy, the first changes are observed in the neuronal mitochondria, whose internal structure becomes swollen and disrupted (Brown and Brierley, 1973). These pathologic changes, seen soon after the initial insult, are followed by the gradual appearance of widespread transneuronal degeneration. With progressively longer periods of total asphyxia, the destructive changes in the thalamus become more extensive, and damage appears in the putamen and in the deeper layers of the cortex. In its extreme form, the brain of asphyxiated animals shows an extensive cystic degeneration of both cortex and white matter with connective tissue replacement of the damaged areas in the forebrain but a relative lack of cellular reaction in the central nuclear areas.

This experimentally produced picture resembles cystic degeneration of the infant brain (cystic encephalomalacia), a condition characterized by the formation of cystic cavities in white matter (Fig. 43–5). When small, the cysts are trabeculated and do not communicate with the ventricular system. In their most extensive form, they may involve both hemispheres, leaving only small remains of cortical tissue. The cavities are generally believed to be the products of insufficient glial reaction, perhaps the result of cerebral immaturity, or reflections of the sudden and massive tissue damage from circulatory or anoxic events. Infants surviving this type of insult usually go on to develop a severe form of spastic quadriparesis.

The distribution of cerebral lesions induced by acute total asphyxia rarely reproduces the lesions found in infants who have survived partial but prolonged asphyxia. When these conditions are induced experimentally, primates develop high P_{CO_2} levels and mixed metabolic and respiratory acidosis (Brann and Myers, 1975). This usually is accompanied by marked brain swelling, which compresses the small blood vessels of the cerebral parenchyma. The resultant increase in vascular resistance superimposed on the aforementioned systemic alterations

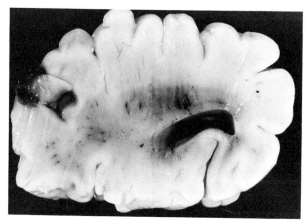

FIGURE 43–6. *Periventricular leukomalacia (PVL) in a prematurely born child with perinatal asphyxia. There is hemorrhagic softening of the cerebral white matter adjacent to the lateral ventricle.*

leads to various focal cerebral circulatory lesions whose location is governed in part by vascular patterns and in part by the gestational age of the fetus at the time of the asphyxial insult (Skov et al., 1984).

Cystic encephalomalacia is distinct from periventricular leukomalacia (PVL), which may also become cystic, and which occurs in premature infants (Fig. 43–6) (Banker and Larroche, 1962). Essentially, PVL consists of a bilateral (but not necessarily symmetric) necrosis having a periventricular distribution. Tissue destruction is accompanied by proliferation of astrocytes and microglia, a loss of ependyma, and areas of subcortical degeneration. In about 25 per cent of infants, there is hemorrhage into the lesion. This complication is the consequence of a hemorrhage into the ischemic area, the outcome of subsequent reperfusion (Volpe, 1989). The distribution of PVL suggests inadequate circulatory perfusion with subsequent infarction of the vascular border zones between the branches of the middle cerebral and posterior cerebral arteries (deReuck et al., 1972; Leviton and Gilles, 1984). Volpe (1987) considers PVL as the principal ischemic lesion of the premature infant and proposes that its predilection to the periventricular area reflects the immaturity of the vasculature in this particular region. A number of adverse perinatal events correlate with the development of PVL, including perinatal asphyxia, recurrent apnea, a patent ductus arteriosus, septicemia, hypocarbia, seizures, and prolonged mechanical ventilation. Even though it appears likely that all these events are accompanied by hypotension (Young et al., 1982), this cannot be documented consistently. In part, this may reflect the lack of direct and continuous blood pressure recordings, or it may indicate that PVL results from a discrepancy between the metabolic requirements of periventricular white matter and its perfusion (Ment et al., 1985). As a rule, the more mature the periventricular vasculature, the more significant the clinical complications accompanying the evolution of PVL. The incidence of this complication, as obtained from autopsy series, varies considerably. In a series of ventilated infants weighing less than 1500 g, 38 per cent were found to have PVL (Volpe, 1987). Gilles and associates (1977) found that exposure to *Escherichia coli* endotoxin produces white matter destruction in neonatal experimental animals and suggested that transient bacteremia may at

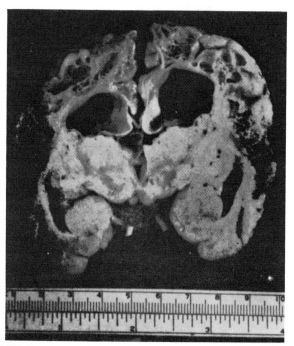

FIGURE 43–5. *Cystic degeneration of dorsal parts of the hemispheres. Coronal section of brain. (From Malamud, N.: Sequelae of perinatal trauma. Neuropathol. Exp. Neurol. 18:146, 1959.)*

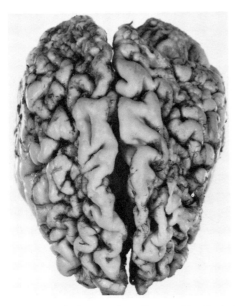

FIGURE 43–7. Watershed pattern in a 10-year-old patient with history of prolonged labor, subsequent spastic quadriparesis. Symmetric atrophy in border zones of anterior, middle, and posterior cerebral arteries. (Courtesy of Dr. Richard Lindenberg, Towson, Md.)

least contribute to this pathologic picture. The usual condition in the older child commensurate with this cerebral lesion is spastic diplegia.

Newer imaging techniques, such as ultrasound and MR, have permitted better diagnosis of the presence of PVL and understanding of its evolution.

Usually within 2 to 4 weeks, the lesions become gliotic, or if sufficiently extensive, they are replaced by cystic lesions (cystic leukomalacia). These may be confined to the periventricular region or may also involve the subcortical white matter (DeVries et al., 1987). In some instances, gliosis persists and becomes interspersed with areas of microcalcification. The clinical picture of the infant who has survived PVL is dependent on its severity and any other associated cerebral lesions. Spastic diplegia is the usual outcome, although the author has seen several youngsters who evolved into a fairly symmetric spastic quadriplegia.

Although PVL has been seen in term infants with a difficult postnatal course, the most common site of brain damage in the full-term newborn is the cortex. Infarctions in this area are secondary to arterial or venous stasis and thromboses. One common pattern for the distribution of lesions (arterial "border zone," or "watershed") is usually the direct result of a sudden fall in systolic blood pressure. The lesions characteristically involve the territory supplied by the most peripheral branches of the three large cerebral arteries (Fig. 43–7) (Freytag and Lindenberg, 1967). Damage is maximal in the posterior parietal-occipital region, becoming less marked in the more anterior portions of the cortex. This distribution may reflect the distribution of receptors for glutamate and other excitatory neurotransmitters (Silverstein et al., 1990). Lesions in the affected area may be located preferentially in the cortex or in the white matter. When gray matter is affected, the brunt of the damage involves the portions around the depths of the sulci. In part, this distribution may reflect the effect of cerebral edema on the drainage of the cortical veins, and

in part, it may be the consequence of the impoverished vascular supply of this area in the normal human newborn (Takashima et al., 1978).

This type of lesion has been termed *ulegyria* (mantle sclerosis) (Friede, 1989). It is a common abnormality, accounting for about one-third of clinical defects caused by circulatory disorders during the neonatal period (Freytag and Lindenberg, 1967). Ulegyria may be extensive or so restricted that the appearance of the brain is grossly normal. When ulegyria is widespread, an associated cystic defect in the subcortical white matter (porencephalic cyst) and dilation of the lateral ventricles often occur. Less often, ulegyria involves the cerebellum. This neuropathologic picture accounts for many cases of both spastic quadriparesis and congenital spastic hemiparesis.

Abnormalities within the basal ganglia are seen in the majority of infants subjected to perinatal asphyxia (84 per cent in the series of Christensen and Melchior, 1967). One common lesion seen in this area has been termed *status marmoratus*. This picture is characterized by gross shrinkage of the striatum, particularly the globus pallidus, associated with defects in myelination. In some cases myelinated nerve fibers may be found in coarse networks resembling the veining of marble, hence the name of the condition (Fig. 43–8); in other cases, the principal pattern is one of a symmetric demyelination. It is clear that both hypermyelination and demyelination represent different

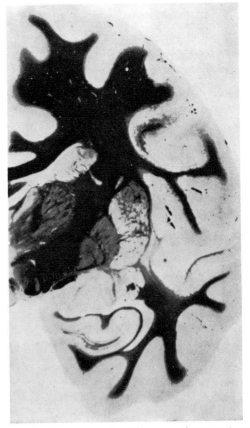

FIGURE 43–8. Status marmoratus. This coronal section is stained for myelin fibers and demonstrates aggregations of myelinated fibers throughout the basal ganglia. (Courtesy of Dr. E. P. Richardson, Harvard Medical School, Boston. From Cooke, R. E.: The Biologic Basis of Pediatric Practice, 1968. Courtesy of McGraw-Hill Book Co., New York.)

responses to the same insult. Nerve cells in the affected areas are usually conspicuously reduced in number, with the smaller neurons in the putamen and caudate appearing to be more vulnerable. Although the abnormalities within the basal ganglia are the most striking, a variety of associated cortical lesions can be demonstrated in most instances.

This condition is believed to result from damage to the basal ganglia incurred before the onset of myelination. This deranges the subsequent deposition of myelin and the course, density, and caliber of fibers passing through the affected area. These pathologic alterations are seen in the vast majority of children suffering from extrapyramidal cerebral palsy.

Rarely, the major structural alterations resulting from perinatal asphyxia are localized to the cerebellum. In the majority of instances, the involvement is diffuse with widespread disappearance of the cellular elements of the cerebellar cortex and dentate nucleus (Friede, 1989).

Circulatory lesions of the brain stem secondary to perinatal asphyxia have received relatively little attention. Neuronal necrosis of the ventral portion of the pons has been observed in premature and term infants, particularly those having a history of respiratory distress. This picture may occur as a selective brain-stem lesion or may be accompanied by widespread cerebral damage. In addition, transient compression of the vertebral arteries in the course of rotation or hyperextension of the infant's head during delivery may also be a cause for circulatory lesions of the brain stem.

Clinical Aspects of Hypoxic-Ischemic Encephalopathy. The degree of functional abnormality of the newborn secondary to asphyxia incurred during labor and delivery depends on the severity, timing, and duration of the insult.

After birth, the infant suffering from significant hypoxic-ischemic encephalopathy can be expected to show certain alterations of alertness, muscle tone, and respirations whose severity depends on the extent of oxygen deprivation (Brown et al., 1974; Volpe, 1987). The mildly affected infant may have essentially normal muscle tone but may be jittery with tactile stimulation and exhibit irritability as well as some degree of feeding difficulty. A greater hypoxic insult gives rise to more definite signs, including irritability, vomiting, increased muscle tone, excessive clonus, and a high-pitched, poorly sustained cry. Tremulousness, especially when provoked by abrupt changes of limb position or tactile stimulation, can closely resemble clonic seizures. The severely affected newborn is either deeply stuporous or in coma. He has marked hypotonia or flaccidity and exhibits little spontaneous limb movements. Periodic breathing or other respiratory irregularities are prominent, and they are often complicated by episodes of apnea with bradycardia. These episodes can sometimes be triggered by handling the infant. The severely asphyxiated infant does not cry on painful stimulation and has minimal, if any, Moro or grasp reactions and absent sucking and swallowing responses. The pupils tend to be the size of a pinpoint, and the blink response to light is absent. Seizures occur in approximately 50 per cent of the infants by 6 to 12 hours following birth.

The Apgar score has been used to quantitate the severity of the initial intrauterine insult. Although a depressed score at 1 and 5 minutes implies the possibility of a hypoxic insult, the value of the score becomes significant in terms of measuring neurologic deficits only when it is obtained at 10 minutes or even later (Nelson and Ellenberg, 1979), and it is evident that 1- and 5-minute scores do not usually reflect the degree of the infant's acidosis (Sykes et al., 1982). The scores are influenced by the infant's level of maturity and do not necessarily reflect well-being in low-birth-weight infants (Catlin et al., 1986).

After 12 to 48 hours of age, there may be a change in the clinical picture of the previously hypotonic infant. He becomes jittery, his cry is shrill and monotonous, the Moro reflex becomes exaggerated, there is an increased startle response to sound, and the face assumes a staring or "worried" appearance. The deep tendon reflexes become hyperactive, and an increased extensor tone develops. Seizures may make their first appearance at this time. These signs of cerebral irritation are particularly common in the infant who has experienced a major intracranial hemorrhage. In the series of Brown and co-workers (1974) 24 per cent of infants who were subjected to perinatal hypoxia demonstrated hypotonia progressing to extensor hypertonus. In the experience of De Souza and Richards (1978), this clinical course has an ominous prognosis, and none of the infants following it were ultimately free of neurologic deficits.

In other instances (24 per cent in the series of Brown and co-workers), an infant who has sustained perinatal hypoxia exhibits hypertonia and rigidity during the neonatal period. The clinical picture of spasticity in the neonate is modified by the immaturity of some of the higher centers. In the spastic infant, the deep tendon reflexes are not exaggerated and in fact may even be depressed as a result of muscular rigidity. Hyperreflexia becomes evident only during the second half of the first year of life. More reliable physical signs indicating spasticity include the presence of a sustained tonic neck response. The presence of a spastic hemiparesis is manifest during the neonatal period in only 10 per cent of infants, usually by a unilateral reduction of spontaneous movements or excessive fisting in one extremity. Obvious paralyses during the neonatal period are rarely caused by cerebral damage; rather, they should suggest a peripheral nerve or spinal cord lesion.

Seizures associated with hypoxic-ischemic encephalopathy usually occur after 12 hours of age. However, when asphyxia is profound, as occurs in a prolapsed cord, their onset may be as soon as 2 to 3 hours following the insult. The characterization and classification of seizures is covered in a subsequent section.

Infants surviving a major asphyxial insult begin to improve toward the end of the 1st week of life. Seizures usually come under control, and there is a gradual change from the generalized hypotonia of the newborn period to the spasticity of later life. As a rule, the longer the duration of hypotonia, the more severely handicapped the child will be. Feeding disturbances are frequent, and the infant may require tube feeding.

CT scans performed in asphyxiated infants 1 to 2 weeks after birth demonstrate local areas of hyperperfusion, with a dense network of proliferating capillaries that almost completely replace the parenchyma. This alteration is most commonly observed in the basal ganglia but may also occur in the brain stem and cerebellum, the periventricular area, the depth of the cortical sulci, and the hippocampus. Shewmon and co-workers (1981) consider this hypervascularity a response to the antecedent hypoxia and reduced cerebral blood flow.

The ultimate manifestations of hypoxic-ischemic encephalopathy and mechanical birth trauma to the brain are so varied that their full description and the relationship between the clinical and neuropathologic pictures are outside the scope of this chapter. The interested reader is referred to several texts of child neurology (e.g., Menkes, 1990).

Diagnosis. As already indicated, the diagnosis of the neurologic disorder hypoxic-ischemic encephalopathy (HIE) depends on the following:

1. A history of intrauterine distress. This may include evidence in alteration of fetal heart rate, the passage of meconium, abnormalities in fetal acid-base status (as determined by scalp blood sampling), and a second stage of labor lasting more than 30 minutes, often accompanied by sufficient maternal or fetal distress to require blood transfusion or administration of oxygen. Breech presentation and the application of midforceps are both significantly associated with both mechanical and asphyxial birth injury.

2. A history of an abnormal neonatal course. This includes delayed or impaired respiration requiring such resuscitative measures as endotracheal intubation and assisted ventilation. Other abnormalities observed during the neonatal period include seizures, hypotonia, and a bulging fontanelle, or less obviously, irritability, feeding difficulties, excessive jitteriness, or an abnormal cry. Conversely, it has become evident that the infant whose birth was complicated but whose neonatal period was normal, that is to say, activity after the 1st day of life was normal and that he did not need incubator care beyond 3 days of age, did not develop HIE. Further, if there are no feeding problems, impaired sucking, respiratory difficulties, or neonatal seizures, the infant is not at increased risk for neurologic damage (Nelson and Ellenberg, 1987).

3. Laboratory studies suggesting hypoxic-ischemic encephalopathy. All of the available tests, including scalp pH, umbilical artery pH, and cord blood hypoxanthine levels, can provide only inferential evidence for hypoxic-ischemic encephalopathy or its severity. CSF protein may be elevated following perinatal asphyxia. In the term neonate, the mean protein concentration is 90 mg/dl; values above 150 mg/dl are considered abnormal. In the premature neonate, the mean CSF protein is 115 mg/dl (Volpe, 1987). An elevation in the ratio of CSF lactate to pyruvate has been found to persist in asphyxiated infants for several hours after normal oxygenation has been reestablished, as does a striking elevation of the blood creatine kinase-BB isoenzyme (Walsh et al., 1982). The clinical staging of hypoxic-ischemic encephalopathy is shown in Table 43–1.

Treatment. The prevention of perinatal asphyxia is largely the task of the obstetrician and therefore is outside the scope of this text.

The immediate and long-term supportive care of the infant with HIE is a matter of considerable debate. Besides

TABLE 43–1. Clinical Staging of Hypoxic-Ischemic Encephalopathy

FACTOR	STAGE I	STAGE II	STAGE III
Level of consciousness	Alert	Lethargy	Coma
Muscle tone	Normal	Hypotonia	Flaccidity
Tendon reflexes	Increased	Increased	Depressed or absent
Myoclonus	Present	Present	Absent
Complex reflexes			
Sucking	Active	Weak	Absent
Moro response	Exaggerated	Incomplete	Absent
Grasping	Normal to exaggerated	Exaggerated	Absent
Oculocephalic (doll's eyes)	Normal	Overreactive	Reduced to absent

(Adapted from Sarnat, N. B., and Sarnat, M. S.: Neonatal encephalopathy following distress. Arch. Neurol. 33:696–705, 1975. Copyright 1975, American Medical Association.)

providing an appropriate airway and maintaining circulation, there is controversy with respect to whether or not fluid should be restricted and whether or not treatment of cerebral edema with corticosteroids and other agents affects outcome. I do not advise the use of steroids in the asphyxiated infant, nor do I think that high-dose barbiturates are of any benefit. Vannucci (1990b) is of the same opinion. However, controlled hyperventilation ($PaCO_2$ 20 to 25 mm Hg), and hyperosmolar and diuretic agents (mannitol, furosemide) are generally employed when cerebral edema is observed clinically or by neuroimaging studies. The experimental studies of Mujsce and colleagues (1990), however, suggest that reducing cerebral edema does not improve cerebral blood flow and thus should not alter the ultimate severity of brain damage.

There is no unanimity with respect to the importance of cerebral edema in producing the sequelae of neonatal asphyxia. Accordingly, the value of treating this complication with the accepted methods—avoiding fluid overload and using hypertonic solutions (e.g., mannitol), glucocorticoids, and high doses of barbiturates—is a matter of considerable controversy. The use of glutamate antagonists is still in the experimental stages (Park et al., 1988).

The control of neonatal seizures is discussed in the section on Paroxysmal Disorders (Chapter 45).

Occasionally, porencephaly resulting from focal brain necrosis or a periventricular-intracerebral hemorrhage may expand, producing increased intracranial pressure or increasing head size. Under these circumstances, surgical drainage of the cyst is indicated (Tardieu et al., 1981).

Prognosis. Underlying the prognosis of the infant with HIE is the question whether asphyxia produces a continuum of brain damage, that is to say, whether mild asphyxia causes a small amount of damage and more severe asphyxia causes more severe damage or whether there is a threshold beyond which the brain is damaged in an all-or-nothing manner. Evidence for both views has been presented (Low et al., 1988; Robertson and Finer, 1985), but their resolution will have to await studies in which a continuous and accurate assessment of perinatal asphyxia is combined with complete and individualized neurologic and neuropsychologic evaluations of asphyxiated and control subjects performed at an age when subtle cognitive deficits can be detected. Until such time, my opinion is that there is a threshold of asphyxia beyond which there is a continuum of brain injury.

It is clear, however, that there is no single sign or symptom that accurately predicts subsequent brain damage and that both severity and duration of asphyxia are only two of many factors that influence the ultimate outcome (Freeman and Nelson, 1988). Others include preexisting cerebral anomalies, fetal maturity, cerebral energy stores at the time of asphyxia, and the adequacy of uteroplacental blood flow. Finally, experimental data indicate that asphyxial injury may not only cause neuronal loss but may also interfere with the normal subtractive processes including axon retraction and programmed cell death which may have been in progress at the time of injury (Janovsky and Finlay, 1986).

In view of the interaction of these several factors, it should come as no surprise that many infants with severe and prolonged asphyxia recover without any neurodevelopmental deficits.

Several methods have been used to identify infants with a poor prognosis. The most traditional of these has been the Apgar score, even though it is now evident that a low Apgar score does not indicate the presence of asphyxia in either term or premature infants (Nelson and Ellenberg, 1981, 1986; Sykes et al., 1982). Even though the predictive value of the 1- and 5-minute Apgar scores in terms of subsequent neurologic deficits is limited, term infants with 5-minute Apgar scores of 6 or less are three times as likely to be neurologically abnormal at 1 year of age than are those with scores of 6 to 10. The likelihood of permanent brain damage increases even more significantly when depressed Apgar scores persist. Of infants with scores of 3 or less at 10 minutes of age, 68 per cent die during the 1st year of life, and 12.5 per cent of the survivors are neurologically damaged. The prognosis is even worse when an Apgar score of 3 or less persists for 20 minutes. Of those infants, 87 per cent die, and 36 per cent of the survivors are found to have cerebral palsy (Nelson and Ellenberg, 1979). Conversely, several studies have shown that if an asphyxiated infant fails to show neurologic or behavioral abnormalities during his neonatal period on repeated careful examinations, he is unlikely to develop neurologic or intellectual sequelae. Even if there is mild HIE, that is to say, when the infant is in a hyperalert and hyperexcitable state, the outcome appears to be excellent. In the experience of Robertson and coworkers (1985, 1989), the presence of neonatal convulsions did not appear to affect the prognosis in the mildly asphyxiated group (Table 43–2). When the infant is hypotonic with suppressed primitive reflexes, the outcome is less favorable. The outcome is almost invariably poor when after 24 hours the infant is still stuporous and flaccid with absent primitive reflexes and experiences recurrent apnea (Low et al., 1988; Robertson and Finer, 1985).

Neonatal seizures in the small-for-gestational-age infant are ominous, and the smaller the term infant with neonatal seizures, the worse his outlook.

Fetal blood sampling may provide better prognostic information, but it must be stressed that there are no absolute values of blood Po_2, Pco_2, or pH beyond which irreparable brain damage is certain to ensue. Since most of the asphyxial insults occur in utero, electronic monitoring of the fetal heart rate was considered to be of

TABLE 43–2. Outcome 3 to 5 Years After Hypoxic-Ischemic Encephalopathy (HIE) (Using the Classification System of Sarnat and Sarnat)

SEVERITY OF HIE	n	INFORMATION AVAILABLE 3 TO 5 YEARS	DEATHS	SURVIVORS AT 3 TO 5 YEARS	
				Normal	Handicapped
Mild	79	69	0	69	0
Moderate	119	103	6*	75	22
Severe†	28	28	21	0	7
Total	226	200	27	144	29
Percentage	100	88.5	13.5	83.2	16.8

*One due to unrelated accident.
†All infants died or handicapped.
(Adapted from Robertson, C., and Finer, N.: Term infants with hypoxic-ischemic encephalopathy: Outcome at 3.5 years. Dev. Med. Child Neurol. 27:473, 1985.)

prognostic value. Prospective studies indicate that although one-fourth of high-risk infants whose fetal heart rate pattern showed severe variable decelerations or late decelerations were neurologically abnormal at 1 year of age, these abnormalities have not persisted into later childhood (Painter et al., 1978).

CT scanning and ultrasonography have also been used for prognostic purposes. The presence after the 1st week of life of areas of decreased density in brain parenchyma indicates a poor outlook in terms of a major neurologic handicap. This is particularly true when there are two or more focal areas of hypodensity, or when there is reduced density of the basal ganglia. Infants with mild to moderate HIE and normal CT findings rarely exhibit major neurologic residua. The presence of small ventricles (implying brain swelling) does not correlate with ultimate outcome.

Ultrasonography may provide evidence for injury to the basal ganglia and the presence of focal or multifocal ischemic parenchymal lesions and, thus, suggest ultimate major neurologic deficits. The presence of periventricular echodensities is a particularly poor prognostic sign. Small ventricles are not predictive of neurologic damage and may be seen in a large proportion of control infants during the 1st week of life.

The electroencephalogram may be of prognostic significance. Recovery is more likely to occur if the tracing is normal, or demonstrates a single focus, rather than showing multifocal paroxysmal discharges or a burst suppression pattern.

Renal injury, particularly prolonged oliguria when associated with asphyxia, presages a poor neurologic outcome (Perlman and Tack, 1988).

From an epidemiologic point of view, it has become evident that severe mental retardation in the absence of other neurologic sequelae is only rarely due to asphyxia. In the experience of Hagberg, a perinatal cause could only be assigned to 18 per cent of children with moderately severe mental retardation (IQ 50 to 70), and to 15 per cent of children with mild mental retardation (Hagberg et al., 1981). Perinatal HIE could not be implicated in any of the children whose IQs fell between 70 and 75. Nelson and Ellenberg (1986) have calculated that in the National Collaborative Perinatal Project the proportion of cerebral palsy due to intrapartum asphyxia ranged between 3 and 13 per cent and did not exceed 21 per cent. In a more recent Australian study intrapartum asphyxia produced cerebral palsy in 4.9 to 8.2 per cent (Blair and Stanley, 1988).

In this respect, it is important to note that Nelson and Ellenberg failed to find a statistically significant increase in mental retardation in children with low Apgar scores who did not also have cerebral palsy. They concluded that when mental retardation is a consequence of perinatal HIE, it is usually severe and accompanied by evidence of neurologic damage, notably spastic quadriparesis or athetosis, or both.

■ REFERENCES

Aver, R. N., and Siesjö, B. K.: Biological differences between ischemia, hypoglycemia and epilepsy. Ann. Neurol. 24:699, 1988.

Banker, B. Q., and Larroche, J. C.: Periventricular leukomalacia of infancy. Arch. Neurol. 7:386, 1962.

Blair, E., and Stanley, F. J.: Intrapartum asphyxia: A rare cause of cerebral palsy. J. Pediatr. 112:515, 1988.

Brann, A. W., and Myers, R. E.: Central nervous system findings in the newborn monkey following severe in utero partial asphyxia. Neurology 25:327, 1975.

Brown, A. W., and Brierley, J. B.: The earliest alterations in rat neurones and astrocytes after anoxia-ischaemia. Acta Neuropathol. 23:9, 1973.

Brown, J. K., Purvis, R. J., Forfar, J. O., and Cockburn, F.: Neurologic aspects of perinatal asphyxia. Dev. Med. Child Neurol. 16:567, 1974.

Bucher, H. U., Boltshauser, E., Friderich, J., and Isler, W.: Birth injury to the spinal cord. Helv. Paediatr. Acta 34:517, 1979.

Catlin, E. A., Carpenter, M. W., Brann, B. S., et al.: The Apgar score revisited: Influence of gestational age. J. Pediatr. 109:865, 1986.

Christensen, E., and Melchior, J.: Cerebral palsy—a clinical and neuropathological study. Clin. Dev. Med. 25:1, 1967.

Crothers, B.: Injuries of the spinal cord in breech extraction as an important cause of fetal death and paraplegia in childhood. Am. J. Med. Sci. 165:94, 1923.

Crothers, B., and Paine, R. S.: The Natural History of Cerebral Palsy. Cambridge, Harvard University Press, 1959.

Deonna, T., and Oberson, R.: Acute subdural hematoma in the newborn. Neuropaediatrie 5:181, 1974.

deReuck, J., Chattha, A. S., and Richardson, E. P.: Pathogenesis and evolution of periventricular leukomalacia in infancy. Arch. Neurol. 27:229, 1972.

DeSouza, S. W., and Richards, B.: Neurological sequelae in newborn babies after perinatal asphyxia. Arch. Dis. Child. 53:564, 1978.

DeVries, L. S., et al.: Neurological, electrophysiological and MRI abnormalities in infants with extensive cystic leukomalacia. Neuropediatrics 18:61, 1987.

Ellis, S. S., Montgomery, J. R., Wagner, M., and Hill, R. M.: Osteomyelitis complicating neonatal cephalhematoma. Am. J. Dis. Child. 127:100, 1974.

Eng, G. D.: Neuromuscular disease. In Avery, G. B. (Ed.): Neonatology: Pathophysiology and Management of the Newborn, 3rd ed. Philadelphia, J. B. Lippincott, 1987, pp. 1158–1162.

Ford, F. R.: Breech delivery in its possible relation to injury of the spinal cord, with special reference to infantile paraplegia. Arch. Neurol. Psychiatry 14:742, 1925.

Freeman, J. M., and Nelson, K. B.: Intrapartum asphyxia and cerebral palsy. Pediatrics 82:240, 1988.

Freytag, E., and Lindenberg, R.: Neuropathological findings in patients of a hospital for the mentally deficient: a survey of 359 cases. Johns Hopkins Med. J. 121:379, 1967.

Friede, R. L.: Developmental Neuropathology, 2nd ed. Berlin, New York, Springer Verlag, 1989.

Gilles, F. H., Averill, D. R., and Kerr, C. S.: Neonatal endotoxin encephalopathy. Ann. Neurol. 2:49, 1977.

Hagberg, B., Hagberg, G., Lewerth, A., et al.: Mild mental retardation in Swedish school children. II. Etiologic and pathogenetic aspects. Acta Paediatr. Scand. 70:445, 1981.

Janowsky, J. S., and Finlay, B. L.: The outcome of perinatal brain damage: The role of normal neuron loss and axon retraction. Dev. Med. Child Neurol. 28:375, 1984.

Jones, S. J.: Investigations of brachial plexus traction lesions by peripheral and spinal somatosensory evoked potentials. J. Neurol. Neurosurg. Psychiatry 42:107, 1979.

Levene, M. I., Kornberg, J., and Williams, T. H. C.: The incidence and severity of post-asphyxial encephalopathy in full-term infants. Early Human Development 11:21, 1985.

Leviton, A., and Gilles, F. H.: Acquired perinatal leukoencephalopathy. Ann. Neurol. 16:1, 1984.

Lou, H. C., Skov, H., and Pedersen, H.: Low cerebral blood flow as a risk factor in the neonate. J. Pediatr. 95:606, 1979b.

Lou, H. C., Lassen, N. A., Tweed, W. A., et al.: Pressure passive cerebral blood flow and breakdown of the blood-brain barrier in experimental fetal asphyxia. Acta Paediatr. Scand. 68:57, 1979a.

Low, J. A., et al.: Motor and cognitive deficits after intrapartum asphyxia in the mature fetus. Am. J. Obstet. Gynecol. 158:356, 1988.

Lupton, B. A., Hill, A., Roland, E. H., et al.: Brain swelling in the asphyxiated term newborn: Pathogenesis and outcome. Pediatrics 82:139, 1988.

Menkes, J. H.: Textbook of Child Neurology. 4th ed. Philadelphia, Lea and Febiger, 1990.

Ment, L. R., Duncan, C. C., Ehrenkranz, R. A., et al.: Intraventricular hemorrhage in preterm neonate: Timing and cerebral blood flow changes. J. Pediatr. 104:419, 1984.

Mujsce, D. J., Christensen, M. A., Vannucci, R. C.: Cerebral blood flow and edema in perinatal hypoxic-ischemic brain damage. Pediatr. Res. 27:450, 1990.

Nelson, K. B., and Ellenberg, J. H.: Neonatal signs as predictors of cerebral palsy. Pediatrics 64:225, 1979.

Nelson, K. B., and Ellenberg, J. H.: Apgar scores as predictors of chronic neurologic disability. Pediatrics 68:36, 1981.

Nelson, K. B., and Ellenberg, J. H.: Antecedents of cerebral palsy. N. Engl. J. Med. 315:81, 1986.

Nelson, K. B., and Ellenberg, J. H.: The asymptomatic newborn and risk of cerebral palsy. Am. J. Dis. Child. 141:1333, 1987.

Nelson, K. B., and Eng, G. C.: Congenital hypoplasia of the depressor anguli oris muscle: Differentiation from congenital facial palsy. J. Pediatr. 81:16, 1972.

Norman, M. G.: Perinatal brain damage. Perspect. Pediatr. Pathol. 4:41, 1978.

Painter, M. J., Depp, R., and O'Donoghue, M. N.: Fetal heart rate patterns and development in the first year of life. Am. J. Obstet. Gynecol. 132:271, 1978.

Pape, K. E., and Pickering, D.: Asymmetric crying facies: An index of other congenital anomalies. J. Pediatr. 81:21, 1972.

Park, C. K., Nehls, D. G., Graham, D. I., et al.: The glutamate antagonist MK-801 reduces focal ischemic brain damage in the rat. Ann. Neurol. 24:543, 1988.

Parmelee, A. H.: Molding due to intra-uterine posture. Facial paralysis probably due to such molding. Am. J. Dis. Child. 42:1155, 1931.

Perlman, M., and Reisner, S. H.: Asymmetric crying facies and congenital anomalies. Arch. Dis. Child. 48:627, 1973.

Perlman, J. L., and Tack, E. D.: Renal injury in the asphyxiated newborn: Relationship to neurologic outcome. J. Pediatr. 113:875, 1988.

Robertson, C., and Finer, N.: Term infants with hypoxic-ischemic encephalopathy: Outcome at 3.5 years. Dev. Med. Child Neurol. 27:473, 1985.

Robertson, C. M. T., Finer, N. N., and Grace, M. G. A.: School performance of survivors of neonatal encephalopathy associated with birth asphyxia at term. J. Pediatr. 114:753, 1989.

Rothman, S. M., and Olney, J. W.: Glutamate and the pathophysiology of hypoxic-ischemic brain damage. Ann. Neurol 19:105, 1986.

Sarnat, H., and Sarnat, M.: Neonatal encephalopathy following fetal distress: A clinical and electroencephalographic study. Arch. Neurol. 33:696, 1976.

Shewmon, D. A., Fine, M., Masdeu, J. C., et al.: Postischemic hypervascularity of infancy: A stage in the evolution of ischemic brain damage with characteristic CT scan. Ann. Neurol. 9:358, 1981.

Silverstein, F. S., McDonald, J. W., Bommarito, M., et al.: Effects of hypoxia-ischemia and MK-801 treatment on the binding of a phencyclidine analogue in the developing rat brain. Stroke 21:310, 1990.

Silverstein, F. S., et al.: Hypoxia-ischemia produces focal disruption of glutamate receptors in developing brain. Dev. Brain Res. 34:33, 1987.

Skov, H., Lou, H., and Pederson, H.: Perinatal brain ischaemia: Impact at four years of age. Dev. Med. Child Neurol. 26:353, 1984.

Smith, B. T.: Isolated phrenic nerve palsy in the newborn. Pediatrics 49:449, 1972.

Steinbok, P., Flodmark, O., Markers, D.; et al.: Management of simple depressed skull fractures in children. J. Neurosurg. 66:506, 1987.

Stern, W. E., and Rand, R. W.: Birth injuries to the spinal cord. Am. J. Obstet. Gynecol. 78:498, 1959.

Sykes, G. S., et al.: Do Apgar scores indicate asphyxia? Lancet 1:494, 1982.

Takashima, S., Armstrong, D. L., and Becker, L. E.: Subcortical leukomalacia, relationship to development of the cerebral sulcus and its vascular supply. Arch. Neurol. 35:470, 1978.

Tardieu, M., Evrard, P., and Lyon, G.: Progressive expanding congenital porencephalies: A treatable cause of progressive encephalopathy. Pediatrics 68:198, 1981.

Thordstein, M., and Kjellmer, I.: Cerebral tolerance of hypoxia in growth-retarded and appropriately grown newborn guinea pigs. Pediatr. Res. 24:633, 1988.

Vannucci, R. C.: Experimental biology of cerebral hypoxia-ischemia. Relationship to perinatal brain damage. Pediatr. Res. 27:317, 1990a.

Vannucci, R. C., Current and potentially new management strategies for perinatal hypoxic-ischemic encephalopathy. Pediatrics 85:961, 1990b.

Vannucci, R. C., and Duffy, T. E.: Cerebral metabolism in newborn dogs during reversible asphyxia. Ann. Neurol. 1:528, 1977.

Volbert, H., and Schweitzer, H.: Über Häufigkeit, Lokalization und Aetiologie von Blutungen im Wirbelkanal bei unreifen Früchten und Frühgeburten. Geburtshilfe Frauenheilkd. 11:1041, 1954.

Volpe, J. J.: Neonatal neurology. Semin. Perinatol. 16:435, 1989.

Volpe, J. J.: Neurology of the Newborn. 2nd ed. Philadelphia, W. B. Saunders Company, 1987.

Walsh, P., et al.: Assessment of neurologic outcome in asphyxiated infants by use of several CK-BB isoenzyme measurements. J. Pediatr. 101:988, 1982.

Wigglesworth, J. S., and Husemeyer, R. P.: Intracranial birth trauma in vaginal breech delivery: The continued importance of injury to the occipital bone. Br. J. Obstet. Gynaecol. 84:684, 1977.

Worcester-Drought, C.: Suprabulbar paresis. Dev. Med. Child Neurol. 16:1(suppl. 30), 1974.

Young, R. S. K., Hernandez, M. J., and Yagel, S. K.: Selective reduction of blood flow to white matter during hypotension in newborn dogs: a possible mechanism of periventricular leukomalacia. Ann. Neurol. 12:445, 1982.

INTRACRANIAL 44 HEMORRHAGE: PATHOGENESIS AND PATHOLOGY

John H. Menkes

Intracranial hemorrhage can result from factors other than mechanical trauma to the brain. Whereas subdural hemorrhage and, to a lesser extent, primary subarachnoid hemorrhage are related to mechanical trauma, the relationship of periventricular-intraventricular hemorrhage (PVH/IVH), the most common form of neonatal intracranial hemorrhage, to prematurity and, most likely, to complications of superimposed asphyxia appears well substantiated (Dykes et al., 1980; Hill and Volpe, 1981b; Pape and Wigglesworth, 1979) (Table 44–1).

The site of the bleeding is determined by the maturity of the infant. In the premature infant it originates in the capillaries of the germinal matrix, usually over the body of the caudate nucleus. With increasing maturation the germinal matrix involutes, so that in the term infant the choroid plexus becomes the principal site of the hemorrhage (Hambleton and Wigglesworth, 1976; Pape and Wigglesworth, 1979). The predisposition of the premature infant to PVH/IVH may in part be due to the presence of a highly vascularized subependymal germinal matrix, to which a major portion of the blood supply of the immature cerebrum is directed. Furthermore, the capillaries of the premature infant have less basement membrane than those of the mature brain. Finally, abnormalities in the autoregulation of arterioles in premature infants and distressed term infants impair their response to hypoxia and hypercarbia and thus permit the transmission of arterial pressure fluctuations to the fragile periventricular capillary bed. Elevations in venous pressure, although less well studied, may also contribute to the evolution of PVH/IVH by altering the hemodynamics at the confluence of the terminal, choroid, and thalamostriate veins, the most

common site of germinal matrix hemorrhage (Perlman and Volpe, 1987).

In the premature infant, the hemorrhage does not occur at the time of the delivery but tends to commence later, most commonly about 24 to 48 hours after a major asphyxial insult, usually either at the time of birth or subsequently (Tsiantos et al., 1974). In the experience of Ment and associates (1984), 74 per cent of hemorrhages were detected by ultrasound within 30 hours of age. In some infants, however, bleeding may be a slow process, rather than a sudden event. The extent of the hemorrhage ranges from slight oozing to a massive intraventricular bleed with extension into the cerebral parenchyma, and the subarachnoid space of the posterior fossa (Figs. 44–1 and 44–2) (Babcock and Han, 1981).

The pathogenesis of this lesion is not completely understood. Although Hayden and co-workers (1985) encountered it in 4.6 per cent of full-term newborns, PVH/IVH may even develop in utero. It is clear that its incidence increases markedly with decreasing maturity, so that when ultrasonography is performed on infants with birth weights under 1500 g, a hemorrhage can be documented in as many as 50 per cent of infants (Trounce et al., 1986).

In addition to prematurity, other contributing factors include respiratory distress, pneumothorax, and various complications of superimposed asphyxia. All these factors share the propensity to increase the normal fluctuations

TABLE 44–1. Major Types of Neonatal Intracranial Hemorrhage and Usual Clinical Setting

TYPE OF HEMORRHAGE	USUAL CLINICAL SETTING
Subdural	Full-term > premature; trauma
Primary subarachnoid	Premature > full-term; trauma or "hypoxic" event(s)
Intracerebellar	Premature; "hypoxic" event(s); trauma(?)
Periventricular-intraventricular	Premature > full-term; "hypoxic" event(s)

(From Volpe, J. J.: Neurology of the Newborn. 2nd ed. Philadelphia, W. B. Saunders Co., 1987.)

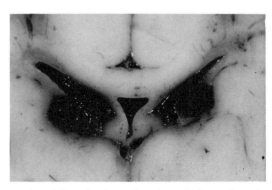

FIGURE 44–1. Bilateral subependymal matrix hemorrhage in a premature newborn. Note extensive intraventricular spread of bleeding in addition to periventricular leukomalacia in the form of hemorrhagic softening extending out from the angles of the lateral ventricles.

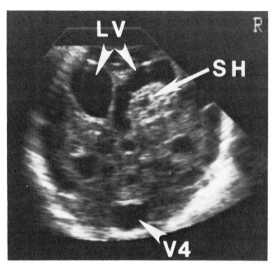

FIGURE 44–2. Coronal ultrasonographic scan of an intraventricular hemorrhage in a 1400 g infant of 30 weeks' gestation who suffered birth asphyxia. There is moderate hydrocephalus and a large subependymal hemorrhage (SH) in the wall of the right lateral ventricle. LV = lateral ventricles; V4 = fourth ventricle. (From Babcock, D.S., and Han, B. K.: The accuracy of high resolution, real-time ultrasonography of the head in infancy. Radiology 139:665, 1981.)

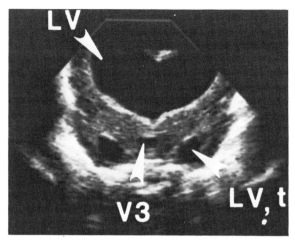

FIGURE 44–3. Coronal ultrasonographic scan of hydrocephalus in a 2-day-old infant with lumbosacral meningomyelocele. There is marked dilatation of the lateral ventricles (LV) and their temporal horns (LV,t). The third ventricle (V3) is also enlarged but to a lesser degree. (From Babcock, D.S., and Han, B. K.: The accuracy of high resolution, real-time ultrasonography of the head in infancy. Radiology 139:665, 1981.)

in cerebral blood flow velocity (Perlman et al., 1985). Other risk factors that play a role in the development of PVH/IVH include increased venous pressure secondary to myocardial failure, hypothermia, and hyperosmolarity induced by administration of excess sodium bicarbonate (Volpe, 1987). Clotting disorders, in particular, may predispose the infant to an extensive hemorrhage.

Blood usually clears rapidly from the intraventricular and subarachnoid spaces. Nevertheless, brain injury is a relatively common result of intraventricular hemorrhage. In part, this relates to the antecedent asphyxial injury that predisposes the infant to the bleed. Other factors are also operative. As demonstrated by positron emission tomography (PET) cerebral blood flow is abolished in the area of an intraparenchymal hematoma and is reduced twofold to threefold over the entire affected hemisphere (Volpe et al., 1983). In addition, metabolic alterations are also responsible for subsequent neurologic abnormalities. Cerebral glucose metabolism is markedly reduced (Altman and Volpe, 1987), and as determined by nuclear magnetic resonance spectroscopy, the brain phosphocreatine concentration is reduced for several weeks (Younkin et al., 1988).

A hemorrhagic infarct, visualized by ultrasonography as an intracerebral periventricular, echo-dense lesion, is not unusual, and a major intracerebral hematoma is seen in a third of the infants with severe hemorrhages (Fig. 44–3) (Volpe, 1987). The latter is commonly preceded by PVH, an indication that it is the result of bleeding into infarcted brain tissue, rather than being due to physical extension of a germinal matrix hemorrhage (Schellinger et al., 1988). An intraparenchymal hemorrhage goes on to tissue destruction and formation of cystic cavities, perhaps as a consequence of the aforementioned reduction of cerebral blood flow, and is associated with a poor outcome. Porencephalic cysts may develop in survivors and can be visualized within 10 days to 8 weeks after the event.

A progressive ventricular dilation is a common sequel

to intraventricular hemorrhage (Fig. 44–4). It evolves 1 to 3 weeks after the hemorrhage and is due to a fibrotic reaction that obliterates the subarachnoid spaces and induces ventricular dilatation with or without increased intracranial pressure (Hill and Volpe, 1981a).

Clinical Aspects. The evolution of PVH/IVH may go clinically unnoted in more than half of the infants affected (Dubowitz et al., 1981). In the remainder, there may be a sudden, sometimes catastrophic deterioration, highlighted by alterations in consciousness, abnormal eye movements, and respiratory irregularities. Deterioration may continue over several hours then stop, only to resume hours or days later (Volpe, 1987). The presence of a full fontanel, which is noted in a significant proportion of infants, may be the consequence of a massive intracranial hemorrhage, cerebral edema, or less often, an acute subdural hemorrhage (Brown, et al., 1974).

Rarely, an intraventricular hemorrhage may result from a congenital arteriovenous malformation or a ruptured

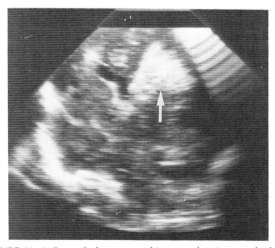

FIGURE 44–4. Coronal ultrasonographic scan of an intracerebral hemorrhage in newborn. The arrow indicates the presence of the hematoma. There is displacement of the ventricular system. (Courtesy of Dr. Eric E. Sauerbrei, Kingston General Hospital, Kingston, Ontario.)

aneurysm (Schum, et al., 1979). Intraventricular hemorrhage can also arise from small hemangiomas of the choroid plexus. Clinical signs of aneurysms of the vein of Galen in the newborn sometimes include bleeding but are usually caused by obstructive hydrocephalus or high-output cardiac failure. Intraventricular bleeding in newborns or early infancy can also arise from a papilloma of the choroid plexus, but the customary picture produced by this unusual tumor is a rapidly progressive enlargement of the head.

Ultrasonography and, to a lesser extent, CT scanning are the sine qua non for diagnosing the presence and the extent of an intracranial hemorrhage (see Figs. 44–2 and 44–3). On the basis of ultrasonography, periventricular and intraventricular hemorrhages have been classified into four grades of severity:

1. Subependymal (germinal matrix) hemorrhage with minimal or no intraventricular hemorrhage.
2. Definite intraventricular hemorrhage but with neither lateral ventricle being filled with blood.
3. Intraventricular hemorrhage that completely fills and distends at least one lateral ventricle.
4. A germinal matrix hemorrhage with extension into the adjacent white matter and associated with intraventricular hemorrhage and ventricular enlargement (Guzetta et al., 1986).

Treatment. Volpe (1987) has suggested that muscle paralysis can correct the fluctuating cerebral blood velocity and thus reduce the incidence of severe PVH/IVH. However, as of this writing no well-controlled clinical trial has shown reduction of PVH/IVH with this approach. Phenobarbital given to the infant, or antenatally to the mother is ineffective in preventing PVH/IVH (Kuban, 1989). Ethamsylate may be able to reduce the incidence of the smaller hemorrhages but has no effect on the larger ones (Benson, et al., 1986). The value of early administration of indomethacin to low-birth-weight infants has been shown to reduce PVH/IVH in several recent studies (Bandstra et al., 1988).

Our nurseries currently do not rely on any pharmacologic therapy; rather, we believe that maintaining the airway with a good cardiovascular support system and trying to prevent excessive swings in blood pressure and cardiac output reduce the likelihood of a large PVH/IVH. In addition, allowing the Pco_2 to rise, but maintaining it below 55 torr, appears to reduce the incidence of pneumothorax, which contributes to the evolution of PVH/IVH. In addition such factors as hypoxemia, acidemia, and rapid-volume expansion all may lead to extension of the hemorrhage and should therefore be avoided.

The question of whether surfactant, by reducing the severity of respiratory distress syndrome, may affect risk and severity of PVH/IVH has been reviewed by Leviton and colleagues (1989). While questions of dose and timing of treatment still need to be resolved, the trend is toward a reduction in severe PVH/IVH in some but not most of the studies.

When progressive ventricular dilation ensues after intraventricular hemorrhage, surgical decompression is indicated. Generally, this takes the form of a ventriculoperitoneal shunt. However, the decision when to temporize

and when to proceed with surgery and risk the associated high morbidity is difficult, especially in the small premature infant who also has suffered significant asphyxia. Repeated ultrasound examinations are essential in arriving at a decision. Volpe (1987) suggests that slowly progressive ventricular dilatation be treated medically with serial lumbar punctures, and drugs that reduce CSF production. When there is a rapidly progressive ventricular dilation, shunting is unavoidable.

Prognosis. The outcome of a periventricular-intraventricular hemorrhage is a function of its severity. According to data compiled by Volpe (1987), infants with a grade IV hemorrhage have a 60 per cent mortality rate, and 80 per cent of the survivors have progressive ventricular dilation. Conversely, infants with grades I and II hemorrhage have a mortality of 15 and 20 per cent, respectively, and progressive ventricular dilation is seen in 5 and 25 per cent of the survivors, respectively.

The outcome in terms of neurologic and intellectual function is poor in infants with persistent ventricular dilation, whether or not they have been shunted. The prognosis reflects the extent of the antecedent hemorrhage and the amount of parenchymal involvement. In addition, alterations in brain perfusion and metabolism resulting from the hemorrhage and the ensuing ventriculomegaly contribute to the poor outcome.

■ REFERENCES

Altman, D. I., and Volpe, J. J.: Cerebral blood flow in the newborn infant: Measurement and role in the pathogenesis of periventricular and intraventricular hemorrhage. Adv. Pediatr. 34:111, 1987.

Babcock, D. S., and Han, B. K.: The accuracy of high-resolution real-time ultrasonography of the head in infancy. Radiology 139:665, 1981.

Bandstra, E. S., Montalvo, B., Goldberg, R., et al.: Prophylactic indomethacin for prevention of intraventricular hemorrhage in premature infants. Pediatrics 82:533, 1988.

Benson, J. W. T., Drayton, M. R., Hayward, C., et al.: Multicentre trial of ethamsylate for prevention of periventricular haemorrhage in very low birth weight infants. Lancet 2:1297, 1986.

Brown, J. K., Purvis, R. J., Forfar, J. O., et al.: Neurologic aspects of perinatal asphyxia. Dev. Med. Child Neurol. 16:567, 1974.

Dubowitz, L. M. S., Levene, M. I., Morante, A., et al.: Neurologic signs in neonatal intraventricular hemorrhage: A correlation with real-time ultrasound. J. Pediatr. 99:127, 1981.

Dykes, F. D., Lazzara, A., Ahmann, P., et al.: Intraventricular hemorrhage—a prospective evaluation of etiopathogenesis. Pediatrics 66:42, 1980.

Hambleton, G., and Wigglesworth, J. S.: Origin of intraventricular haemorrhage in the preterm infant. Arch. Dis. Child. 51:651, 1976.

Hayden, C. K., Shattuck, K. E., Richardson, C. J., et al.: Subependymal germinal matrix hemorrhage in full-term neonates. Pediatrics 75:714, 1985.

Hill, A., and Volpe, J. J.: Normal pressure hydrocephalus in the newborn. Pediatrics 68:623, 1981a.

Hill, A., and Volpe, J. J.: Seizures, hypoxic-ischemic brain injury, and intraventricular hemorrhage in the newborn. Ann. Neurol. 10:109, 1981b.

Kuban, K. C. K., Leviton, A., Krishnamoorthy, K. S., et al.: Neonatal intracranial hemorrhage and phenobarbital. Pediatrics 77:443, 1986.

Leviton, A., VanMarter, L., and Kuban, K.: Respiratory distress syndrome and intracranial hemorrhage: Cause or association? Inferences from surfactant clinical trials. Pediatrics 84:915, 1989.

Ment, L. R., Duncan, C. C., Ehrenkranz, R. A., et al.: Intraventricular hemorrhage in preterm neonates: Timing and cerebral blood flow changes. J. Pediatr. 104:419, 1984.

Pape, K. E., and Wigglesworth, J. S.: Haemorrhage, Ischaemia, and the Perinatal Brain. Philadelphia, J. B. Lippincott, 1979.

Perlman, J. M., and Volpe, J. J.: Are venous circulatory abnormalities important in the pathogenesis of hemorrhagic and ischemic cerebral injury? Pediatrics 80:705, 1987.

Schellinger, D., Grant, E. G., Manz, H. J., et al.: Intraparenchymal hemorrhage in preterm neonates: A broadening spectrum. Am. J. Neuroradiology 9:327, 1988.

Schum, T. R., Meyer, G. A., Grausz, J. P., et al.: Neonatal intraventricular hemorrhage due to an intracranial arteriovenous malformation: A case report. Pediatrics 64:242, 1979.

Speer, M. E., Blifeld, C., Rudolph, A. J., et al.: Intraventricular hemorrhage and vitamin E in the very-low-birth-weight infant: Evidence for efficacy of early intramuscular vitamin E administration. Pediatrics 74:1107, 1984.

Trounce, J. Q., Rutter, N., and Levene, M.: Periventricular leucomalacia and intraventricular hemorrhage in the preterm neonate. Arch. Dis. Child. 61:1196, 1986.

Tsiantos, A., Victorin, A., Relier, J. P., et al.: Intracranial hemorrhage in the prematurely born infant: Timing of clots and evaluation of clinical signs and symptoms. J. Pediatr. 85:854, 1974.

Volpe, J. J.: Neurology of the Newborn. 2nd ed. Philadelphia, W. B. Saunders Company, 1987.

Volpe, J. J., et al.: Positron emission tomography in the newborn: Extensive impairment of regional cerebral blood flow with intraventricular hemorrhage and hemorrhagic intracerebral involvement. Pediatrics 72:589, 1983.

Younkin, D., et al.: In vivo ^{31}P nuclear magnetic resonance measurement of chronic changes in cerebral metabolites following neonatal intraventricular hemorrhage. Pediatrics 82:331, 1988.

MALFORMATIONS OF 45
THE CENTRAL
NERVOUS SYSTEM

John H. Menkes*

Only those congenital malformations of the nervous system that are apparent in the newborn are discussed in this chapter. They will be subdivided into disorders of induction and of cellular migration and proliferation.

■ EMBRYOGENIC INDUCTION DISORDERS

These disorders represent a failure in the mutual induction of mesoderm and neuroectoderm. The primary defect is a failure of the neural folds to fuse and form the neural tube, with secondary maldevelopment of skeletal structures enclosing the CNS. The defects range from anencephaly to sacral meningomyelocele in the cephalic to caudal direction of the neural tube and from holoprosencephaly to craniospinal rachischisis (midline posterior splitting of skull and vertebral column) in the anterior to posterior direction.

ANENCEPHALY

Anencephaly is a lethal malformation in which the vault of the skull is absent and the exposed brain is amorphous. The insult responsible for this defect is believed to occur after the onset of neural fold development (16 days) but before closure of the anterior neuropore (24 to 26 days). Between 75 and 80 per cent of infants are stillborn, and the remainder succumb within hours or a few weeks after birth. The *etiology* of this grotesque anomaly is unknown, although epidemiologic studies suggest a familial predisposition. The malformation is stimulus nonspecific because a variety of genetic, infectious, and chemical insults have been implicated in its formation. In the United States, anencephaly has been found in 0.5 to 2 per 1000 births, whereas in Ireland the prevalence rate has been as high as 5.9 per 1000 births (Alter, 1962; Nakano, 1973). The incidence of this malformation has declined over the last decade or two. In part, this reflects the widespread use of antenatal screening with subsequent elective abortion, but other factors, notably the correction of maternal vitamin deficiency, may also be responsible (Stone, 1987). Factors such as decreased prenatal care, decreased screening, and poor prenatal nutrition contribute to the fact that women who are poor and who live in inner cities have infants with a higher frequency of neural tube defects. Most

investigators have favored nonclosure of the neural tube in early embryonic life as the cause of this defect.

Anencephaly occurs two to four times more often in girls than in boys. Associated polyhydramnios and onset of labor after 40 weeks' gestation are common. The cranial defect is associated with open spinal cord anomalies in as many as half the cases (Friede, 1989). In addition to the grossly anomalous character of the cerebral hemispheres, the hypothalamus is malformed, and the cerebellum is usually rudimentary or absent. Brain-stem tissue is identifiable. The internal carotid arteries are hypoplastic, a condition probably secondary to the lack of normal brain formation (Vogel, 1961). The anterior lobe of the pituitary gland is present in the anencephalic infant, but the adrenal glands are abnormally small. Major defects in the cardiovascular system occur in 4 to 15 per cent of live-born infants with anencephaly.

Diagnosis of anencephaly is obvious at birth. Live-born subjects do not survive infancy. During their few weeks of life, they exhibit slow, sterotyped movements and frequent decerebrate posturing. Head, facial, and limb movements may be spontaneous or pain-induced. Some brain-stem functions and automatisms, such as sucking, rooting, and righting responses and the Moro reflex, are present and are more readily and more reproducibly elicited than in normal infants. The "bowing reflex," which occasionally can be demonstrated in normal premature infants of 7 months' gestation, is invariably present in anencephalics. It can be elicited by placing the infant into the supine position and extending the thighs at the hip joints. The head then lifts itself slowly, followed by the trunk, so that the infant ultimately achieves the sitting position. The presence of reflexes such as these reflects the absence of cortical inhibitory influences on subcortical and brain-stem function. Asking parents to consent to allowing their infant with anencephaly serve as an organ donor or for clinical research is currently widely debated (see Chapter 2, and Medical Task Force on Anencephaly, 1990).

Most infants die within the first few days after birth. It is not clear what the longest survival could be if all aspects of neonatal intensive care were used to prolong life. Survival as long as 3 months has been reported (Pomerantz and Schifrin, 1987).

The presence of anencephaly and other organ neural tube defects may be predicted by measuring alpha-fetoprotein (AFP) in maternal serum. AFP is the major serum protein in early embryonic life, representing 90 per cent of total serum globulins. It is a fetus-specific alpha-1-

---

*This chapter includes portions written by Dr. William E. Bell that appeared in previous editions.

globulin probably involved in preventing fetal immune rejection, and it is produced first by the yolk sac and later by the fetal liver and the gastrointestinal tract. Normally, it passes from fetal serum into fetal urine and then into amniotic fluid. Because of a substantial leak of fetal blood components directly into amniotic fluid, AFP concentrations and maternal serum AFP levels are elevated in anencephaly and open spina bifida or cranium bifidum.

Mothers who have borne one or more children with neural tube defects, spinal dysraphism, or multiple vertebral anomalies, or who have a pedigree history of any of these disorders, or who have themselves survived with spina bifida are at risk to bear children with neural tube defects. Measurements of maternal AFP levels at 14 weeks' gestation serve as a preliminary screen. Normal AFP in adult serum is less than 10 nanograms (ng) per ml, and in normal maternal serum and amniotic fluid it ranges from 15 to 500 ng/ml. During 15 to 20 weeks' gestation, an AFP concentration of 1000 ng/ml or greater strongly suggests an open neural tube defect. A positive test on maternal serum is followed-up by measurement of amniotic fluid AFP or sonography for anatomic configuration of the fetus or both (Milunsky, 1980; Nicolaides et al., 1986).

With all diagnostic techniques now available, the efficiency of detection of anencephaly approaches 100 per cent. Of the neural tube defects, 4.9 per cent are closed and are undetected. False-positive results are obtained in a variety of unrelated conditions, including omphalocele, duodenal atresia, Turner syndrome, and several other fetal defects (Milunsky, 1980).

CRANIUM BIFIDUM AND SPINA BIFIDA

These defects are caused by a failure in fusion of the posterior midline of the skull (cranium bifidum) or the vertebral column (spina bifida). The result is a bony cleft through which varying quantities of brain or spinal cord tissue protrude.

Like anencephaly, these defects are time specific and stimulus nonspecific. The insult must occur before 26 to 28 days' gestation—the time of closure of the posterior neuropore. Several genetic and environmental factors are believed to act in conjunction, with the genetic factors accounting for about 20 per cent of cases. In the majority of instances (65 to 70 per cent) the cause is unknown and may be multifactorial (Matson, 1969).

CRANIUM BIFIDUM WITH ENCEPHALOCELE

In cranium bifidum, the neural herniation is termed *encephalocele* and may consist of brain parenchyma and meninges or only meninges. These cranial defects were classified by Emery and Kalhan in 1970. A practical and simple way of classifying these defects is to consider those lesions containing only meningeal tissue or meningeal tissue and glial elements to be cranial meningoceles and those harboring components of brain to be cranial encephaloceles. The incidence of the latter significantly exceeds that of the former. Approximately 60 per cent occur in the occipital region, and the remainder are in the parietal, frontonasal, intranasal, or nasopharyngeal region (Diebler and Dulac, 1987).

Clinical Aspects. Cranium bifidum with occipital encephalocele affects girls more than boys. Although the cranial lesion may be the only abnormality, a significant number of cases are associated with other defects, such as meningomyelocele, midline facial clefts, deformities of the extremities, or congenital heart disease. Unless the encephalocele is small and covered by hair, it is readily apparent at birth in the form of a soft, round, midline mass that is usually partially or totally covered by skin and that varies in size from a centimeter in diameter to up to two or three times the circumference of the infant's head (Fig. 45–1). The head size of the newborn with occipital encephalocele is normal in some cases; in others, microcephaly is present initially, and hydrocephalus subsequently develops.

A frontonasal encephalocele presents as a rounded mass at the base of the nose, usually associated with widening of the nasal root and separation of the eyes. Basal encephaloceles, including the intranasal and nasopharyngeal types, differ from the aforementioned, more common, types in that there is no visible external mass, and thus diagnosis is not usually established until later in childhood or even until adulthood. The intranasal (transethmoidal) encephalocele is accompanied by a widened nasal root and increased intraocular distance but does not ordinarily become symptomatic until the occurrence of nasal obstruction, epistaxis, or recurrent episodes of bacterial meningitis. Less common types of basal encephaloceles are located in the nasopharynx, sphenoid sinus, or posterior orbit, and they likewise are not usually identified in the infant age group.

Diagnosis. Occipital and parietal encephaloceles are identified in the newborn infant by the character of the lesion and the common but not invariable roentgenographic demonstration of the associated skull defect (Fig. 45–2). Transillumination of the lesion is of some diagnostic value in certain cases, and CT scans, magnetic resonance imaging (MRI) studies, and ultrasonographic studies before and after surgical repair provide information about associated cerebral anomalies and the presence and degree of hydrocephalus.

Frontonasal encephalocele must be differentiated from the so-called nasal "glioma" and dermoids or teratomas in the same region. Pulsation of the mass or bulging with brief bilateral jugular vein compression suggests that it communicates with the subarachnoid space and therefore indicates that it is an encephalocele. In many instances, a precise diagnosis is not available until histologic examination is performed following surgical removal. Intranasal encephalocele should be suspected when an intranasal mass is identified in the child or adult who has a broad nasal bridge and wide-set eyes. It should also be considered in any child who has unexplained recurrent meningitis. This lesion is occasionally biopsied, the preoperative assumption being that it represents a polyp. Specimens obtained from the nasal cavity by biopsy should be submitted for histologic examination because, if not diagnosed, a biopsied encephalocele is likely to lead to cerebrospinal fluid rhinorrhea and subsequent meningitis. Imaging studies are of great importance in the diagnosis of basal encephaloceles, regardless of their location (Diebler and Dulac, 1987).

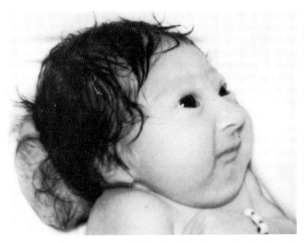
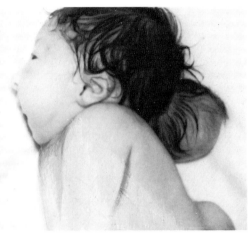

FIGURE 45–1. Occipital meningoencephalocele. The sloping forehead and small head circumference are evident, although progressive ventricular enlargement often subsequently occurs in such children.

Treatment. Whenever possible, an encephalocele should be surgically removed early in life. Hydrocephalus complicates surgical repair in a significant number of cases and is handled by some form of shunt procedure when it occurs. Certain cases must be managed conservatively when the head is distinctly small and the sac contains large amounts of brain tissue, especially if the contained brain includes brain-stem or cervical spinal cord elements. Prognosis in terms of survival and intellectual development is far better for infants with meningoceles and considerably worse for those whose lesions contain brain tissue.

SPINA BIFIDA CYSTICA (MENINGOCELE, MENINGOMYELOCELE, AND LIPOMENINGOCELE)

The newborn infant with a meningomyelocele complicated by the usual motor and sensory defects of the lower extremities, the associated intracranial abnormalities, and neurogenic sphincter dysfunction represents a great tragedy for the family as well as an extremely difficult multidisciplinary management problem for the physician. Probably no other problem in the category of neurologic diseases in infancy has been the source of greater dispute than that of the optimal management of the defective child who is afflicted with spina bifida cystica (McLaughlin et al., 1985; Menzies et al., 1985).

Pathology. Of the defects collectively termed *spina bifida cystica*, 75 per cent are meningomyeloceles and 25 per cent are meningoceles. A lumbar or lumbosacral defect is most common, and it is found in 69 per cent of infants with spina bifida cystica (Matson, 1969).

In 95 per cent of children with lumbar or lumbosacral meningomyelocele, the brain demonstrates abnormalities generally referred to as the Arnold-Chiari II malformation (Fig. 45–3). This consists of a caudal displacement of the cerebellar vermis, pons, and medulla through the foramen magnum into the cervical canal. In addition, hydromyelia is seen in 40 per cent of cases, and in 20 per cent there is syringomyelia, diplomyelia, or other malformations (Mackenzie and Emery, 1971). A variety of gross and microscopic anomalies are also seen in the spinal cord and in the cerebral hemispheres (Yakovlev and Wads-

worth, 1946). The most likely explanation for these anomalies is the presence of a teratogenic influence that accounts not only for the induction anomaly but also for the later malformations of cellular proliferation, migration, and architectonics.

Most authors have accepted the concept that these defects are produced by an undetermined insult that prevents normal fusion and closure.

A number of mesodermal lesions accompany these ectodermal defects. These lesions include splitting of the vertebral arches and other dysplasias of bone, such as double ribs and defects in the base of the skull, notably the posterior arch of the atlas (Blaauw, 1971).

Clinical Manifestations. The most common and clinically least significant form of spina bifida is spina bifida occulta, a mesodermal abnormality in which the vertebral laminar arches are not fused and the meninges do not protrude externally. As isolated defects, most lesions are located at the first sacral or fifth lumbar vertebra. Occasionally, spina bifida occulta is accompanied by other congenital defects of the neuraxis. The most common are dermal sinuses and dimples (35 per cent), lipoid tumors

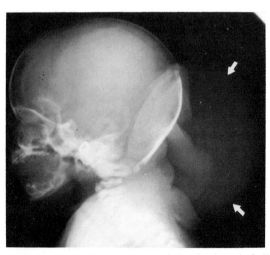

FIGURE 45–2. Occipital meningoencephalocele, lateral skull x-ray film. The large extracranial sac containing meningeal and brain tissue is outlined by white arrows. Surgical excision of the lesion was followed by progressive hydrocephalus, which required a shunting procedure.

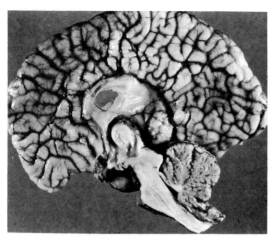

FIGURE 45–3. *Arnold-Chiari malformation. Child with a thoracolumbar meningomyelocele. The Arnold-Chiari malformation consists of elongation of the lower brain stem with downward displacement of the inferior part of the vermis of the cerebellum. The tectal plate is "beaked," and the massa intermedia is enlarged. Polymicrogyria is present.*

(29 per cent), and abnormalities of the filum terminale (24 per cent) (Anderson, 1975).

Spina bifida cystica is one of the most common anomalies of the nervous system, with an incidence that ranges from 0.2 per 1000 live births in Japan to 4.2 per 1000 in Ireland (Laurence and Tew, 1971). These prevalence rates, which were obtained during the 1960s, probably represent peak values. Since then there has been a steady decline in both the United States and the United Kingdom. Thus, between 1971 and 1984 the incidence of the various forms of spina bifida fell from 2 per 1000 live births to 0.6 per 1000 (Stone, 1987). A recurrence rate of 10 per cent is seen in affected families. At birth, the defect may assume any one of a variety of appearances. These range from complete exposure of neural tissue to a flat, partially epithelialized membrane. In all instances, there is a laminar arch defect through which either meninges or meninges and neural elements protrude. Herniation of dura and arachnoid alone without neural components in the sac is called a "meningocele." The soft, rounded mass on the back is usually skin-covered, although, infrequently, associated failure of ectodermal closure produces a sac covered by a delicate membrane that is susceptible to infection. Motor function in the legs is expected to be normal with this lesion unless there are other dysplastic changes of the spinal cord or brain. Meningomyeloceles (myeloceles, localized rachischisis) are 10 to 20 times more frequent than meningoceles and are of far greater consequence. The herniated sac contains meninges as well as neural tissue (Fig. 45–4). Only infrequently does skin cover the lesion except in those patients in whom an associated lipoma overlies the defect, the so-called lipomeningomyelocele (Fig. 45–5). In most cases, the defect at birth is flat, consisting of poorly organized cord tissue lying exposed on the surface at the midline and surrounded by a pink or bluish, delicate, semitransparent membrane (Fig. 45–6). With the passage of time, the accumulation of fluid results in elevation of the lesion, giving rise to its cystlike appearance of variable size (Fig. 45–7). The spinal cord superior to the surface lesion is frequently malformed, most commonly with hydromyelia.

The type and degree of neurologic deficit in a child with a meningomyelocele are determined by the location and size of the lesion, a matter succinctly reviewed by Stark in 1971. A large myelocele with the upper level extending to T8 vertebral level creates denervation of the abdominal muscles bilaterally and of all muscle groups in the lower extremities. The abdomen bulges in the flank regions, and the legs are motionless and flaccid, without significant joint deformity if the entire spinal cord below the upper level is affected. The anal sphincter is patulous, and sensation is absent to the upper limits of the midline lesion. A low lumbar meningomyelocele with sparing of function down to L4 results in sustained contraction of the hip flexors, quadriceps, and tibialis anterior muscles but paralysis of the hamstrings, gastrocnemius, and intrinsic musculature of the feet. The result is a striking deformity in which the lower limbs are held in flexion at the hips. The deformity includes extension of the knees and a calcaneovarus position of the feet. Several types of foot deformity may result with lumbosacral and sacral myeloceles, the position and posture being determined by which muscles retain innervation and which are paralyzed. Regardless of the upper level of the lesion, infants with clinical evidence of denervation of muscles supplied by S2,3,4 can be expected to have neurogenic bladder dysfunction.

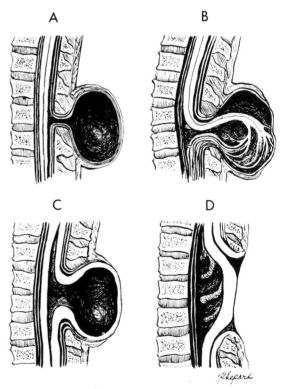

FIGURE 45–4. *Diagram of meningoceles. A, Meningocele: Through the bony defect (spina bifida), the meninges herniate and form a cystic sac filled with spinal fluid. The spinal cord does not participate in the herniation and may or may not be abnormal. B, Myelomeningocele: Spina bifida with meningocele; the spinal cord is herniated into the sac and ends there or may continue in an abnormal way farther downward. C, Myelocystocele or syringomyelocele: The spinal cord shows hydromyelia; the posterior wall of the spinal cord is attached to the ectoderm and undifferentiated. D, Myelocele: The spinal cord is araphic; a cystic cavity is in front of the anterior wall of the spinal cord. (From Benda, C. E.: Developmental Disorders of Mentation and Cerebral Palsies. New York, Grune & Stratton, Inc., 1952. Reprinted by permission.)*

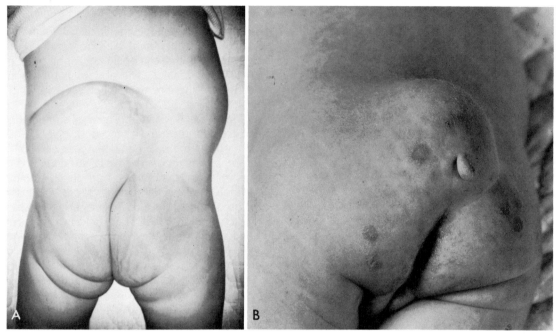

FIGURE 45–5. Two examples of lipomeningocele. Each presents in the left buttock as a firm, well-circumscribed, lobulated tumor that became tense when the infant cried. Over the surface of B are some macular erosions and a congenital skin tag and dimple. This last feature may be the pilonidal dimple displaced by the tumor.

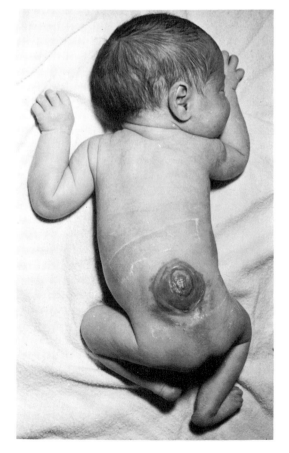

FIGURE 45–6. Lumbar meningomyelocele in a 3-day-old infant. There is moderate weakness of the proximal muscle groups and more extensive weakness of the distal musculature in the lower extremities. The lesion was flat at birth but began to elevate in the next 2 days.

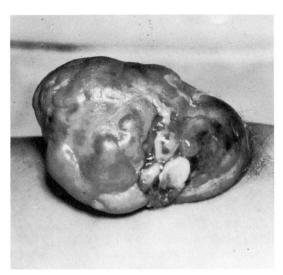

FIGURE 45–7. *Close-up view of a lumbosacral myelomeningocele. The mass is covered with a thin, transparent membrane. No well-differentiated nervous tissue can be distinguished with assurance.*

Hydrocephalus only infrequently complicates spinal meningoceles but is a common complicating problem in the child with a meningomyelocele. In the large series reported by Lorber (1961), it was seen in approximately 90 per cent of infants with lumbar myelomeningocele. This complication results from an associated Arnold-Chiari II malformation, which is found in virtually every case of myelomeningocele, aqueductal stenosis, or both. MRI studies reveal the downward displacement of the stretched brain stem, a link between the medulla and the cervical spinal cord, and herniation of the cerebellar vermis. These findings are best seen on sagittal views. As a consequence, blockage of cerebrospinal fluid circulation occurs at the level of the foramen magnum. In addition, there is a significant incidence of hydromyelia of the cervical or thoracic spinal cord (El Gammal et al., 1987). MRI studies can also be used to display the aqueduct, and aqueductal stenosis was found in 40 per cent of patients with myelomeningocele surveyed by El Gammal and co-workers.

Other cerebral anomalies have also been described. These include microgyria and other types of cortical dysgenesis. These are frequently visualized by MRI studies.

An interesting but somewhat unusual clinical disturbance in the infant with a meningomyelocele and the Arnold-Chiari malformation is vocal cord paralysis with respiratory stridor. Apnea, dysphagia, and cyanotic spells may also be present. Most reported patients have developed stridor a few weeks after birth, at a time when hydrocephalus was notably progressive. In some, stridor disappeared following shunt therapy or suboccipital craniectomy, but in others, relief of hydrocephalus had little influence on the respiratory difficulty. Caudal displacement of the medulla, secondary to increased pressure above, resulting in traction on the vagus nerves, has been suggested as an explanation for infants whose symptoms resolve with surgery. In others, there is brain-stem hemorrhage or ischemia or even an underlying neuronal dysgenesis.

Diagnosis. The presence of a meningomyelocele in the newborn infant is obvious in most instances. The small, skin-covered lesion accompanied by minimal motor deficits in the legs can present some initial diagnostic difficulties and definition of the defect requires MR imaging studies. More practical diagnostic issues in the infant with a meningomyelocele are whether or not hydrocephalus coexists or hydronephrosis is present. Measurement of head size, transillumination, ultrasonography, or MRI, and CT scanning indicate the presence of hydrocephalus and other associated malformations. Increased intracranial pressure is seen in only about 15 per cent of infants with myelomeningocele, and its absence, consequently, does not correlate with the absence of ventricular enlargement.

On roentgenographic examination of the skull, most infants with myelomeningocele exhibit a characteristic defect, referred to as "lückenschädel," or "craniolacunia" (Fig. 45–8). This peculiar, honeycombed appearance of the skull is seen in approximately 85 per cent of patients with the Arnold-Chiari II malformation (Peach, 1965). The malformation is transient and disappears in the first 3 months after birth. It probably is the result of a defect in membranous bone formation and not secondary to in utero intracranial hypertension, as is often stated.

Treatment. Management of the child with a neural tube closure defect of the spinal region requires a multi-disciplinary approach that involves several medical and surgical specialties. The spinal meningocele, which is covered only by a delicate membrane, is surgically corrected as early as possible because of the excellent potential outcome and the danger of infection until the lesion is removed. Those meningoceles that are skin covered are also surgically excised, although the timing of the procedure is much less critical. Even when the meningocele appears to be uncomplicated, the child should be evaluated periodically following surgery to be certain that hydrocephalus is not developing and that bladder function remains normal.

Selection of methods of treatment for the child with an "open" meningomyelocele with neurologic bladder dysfunction, weakness of the legs, and hydrocephalus is far more controversial (Guthkelch, 1986). In 1971, Lorber proposed the principle of selective surgery, and suggested that there were four indicators that predicted an adverse

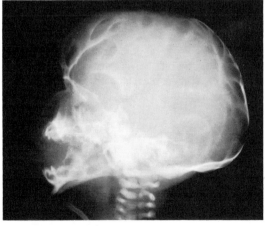

FIGURE 45–8. *Lückenschädel, or craniolacunia. Honeycombed pattern of the skull in the newborn infant with meningomyelocele, usually associated with hydrocephalus.*

outcome: (1) a high level of paraplegia, (2) clinically evident hydrocephalus present at birth, (3) congenital lumbar kyphosis, and (4) other major malformations. Other workers, however, have obtained a relatively good outcome in about one-half of infants who would have fared badly according to Lorber's criteria (Soare and Raimondi, 1977). A further hindrance to the prediction of the future neurologic status of an infant with myelomeningocele is the subsequent progressive cavitation of the cervical and thoracic spinal cord, which produces increasing weakness and spasticity of the upper extremities, and progressive scoliosis (Park et al., 1985).

The question of whether or not all infants with myelomeningocele should be subjected to immediate surgery remains unresolved. The author's personal view is that if major malformations of other organ systems are present or if MRI studies demonstrate major abnormalities of the cerebral cortical architecture, parents should be advised of these malformations and of the likelihood of a poor functional outcome. This combination of an aggressive but selective approach is also favored by McLaughlin and associates (1985) and Volpe (1987).

There is also much controversy as to whether surgery should be immediate or whether it can be delayed for a few days. Generally, it appears that surgery within the first 48 hours of birth does not improve functional outcome nor does it reduce the incidence of infection, as long as infants are given broad-spectrum antibiotics (Guthkelch, 1986). However, if surgery is decided on after all appropriate diagnostic studies have been completed and presented to the parents, it should not be delayed until the infant is older than 1 week of age.

The current outlook of infants who were deemed suitable candidates for surgery and operated on within the neonatal period is fairly good. In the series presented by McLaughlin and co-workers, 72 per cent were ambulatory and 79 per cent had normal intellectual capacity.

A discussion of the various long-term complications of the child with a surgically corrected myelomeningocele is beyond the scope of this text. They include the various complications of hydrocephalus and syringomyelia and deterioration of urologic function (Spindel et al., 1987).

OTHER DYSRAPHIC STATES

DIASTEMATOMYELIA

The term *diastematomyelia* designates a split, or cleft, in a segment of the spinal cord; conventionally, however, it refers to a congenital anomaly in which the cord is transected by a bony or cartilaginous septum that extends from the posterior surface of a vertebral body to the dura or laminar arch dorsally. The etiology of this unusual malformation is unknown; however, it occurs more frequently in girls than in boys and is usually associated with other defects that allow identification of its presence. In almost all cases, the lesion is in the lower thoracic or lumbar region and is associated with an overlying cutaneous abnormality in the form of a tuft of hair, a hemangioma, or a visible and palpable lipoma. The absence of such overlying cutaneous abnormalities has been described with diastematomyelia but is rare. Except for the associated cutaneous lesions, detectable abnormalities in the newborn or early infant period are not common, but, when present, they consist of a unilateral foot deformity such as talipes varus or pes cavus or atrophy of one lower extremity, usually with a foot deformity. Two distinct clinical syndromes occur. The first is a unilateral nonprogressive neural and mesodermal hypoplasia in which one hypoplastic lower extremity is enervated by the relevant hypoplastic segment of cord. The second, seen more commonly, is a progressive condition that either appears de novo or is superimposed on the first syndrome. Neurologic signs are not noted until after the child begins to ambulate, when a disturbance of gait becomes evident.

With suspicion aroused by cutaneous anomalies and hypoplasia of one extremity, one can establish the diagnosis with MRI studies or CT of the lumbosacral spine following contrast infusion (Brunberg et al., 1988).

Treatment consists of laminectomy with removal of the median septum, which traverses the cord. Past experience has indicated that surgical treatment is not followed by recovery of limb atrophy or foot deformity but that it can usually be expected to arrest further progression of neurologic deficits.

SACRAL AGENESIS

Agenesis of the sacrum and coccyx is usually associated with anomalous development of the lumbosacral cord and other major or minor dysraphisms. The defect is seen in approximately 1 per cent of offspring of diabetic mothers (Sarnat et al., 1976).

NEURODERMAL SINUS (CONGENITAL DERMAL SINUS)

The majority of dermal sinuses (e.g., the pilonidal sinus) do not connect with the central nervous system and are therefore of limited neurologic importance. Neurodermal sinuses are one of the most common occult spinal dysraphisms. They represent a communication lined by stratified squamous epithelium between skin and any portion of the neuraxis. Most commonly, the defects are in the lumbosacral and occipital regions. These two points represent the posterior and anterior neuropores, respectively.

The sinus is often surrounded by a small mound of skin, a dimple, or by other cutaneous lesions, such as tufts of hair or angiomas. It often overlies a spina bifida occulta. It may expand into an epidermoid or dermoid cyst at its proximal end, thus causing segmental neurologic deficits. The presence of an open sinus tract may allow drainage of cerebrospinal fluid or provide a portal of entry for bacterial infection. A neurodermal sinus is one of the most common causes of recurrent meningitis.

These lesions require neurosurgical exploration with complete excision of the sinus (Matson, 1969).

CONGENITAL SCALP DEFECT

Congenital scalp defect, also known as aplasia cutis congenita, is an uncommon anomaly that occurs in either sex. It may occur in an otherwise normal child or may be associated with a wide variety of other cerebral or extracranial anomalies (Fowler and Dumars, 1973), including trisomy 13–15. Rarely, congenital scalp defects are associated with similar cutaneous lesions elsewhere on the body. In many cases, congenital scalp defect occurs in a sporadic fashion. It has also been observed in siblings and in both a parent and offspring.

The disorder may be inherited as a dominant trait, although recessive transmission and sporadic cases also have been recorded. Posterior midline scalp defects may be accompanied by the Johanson-Blizzard syndrome, which includes mental retardation, congenital deafness, and hypothyroidism, and are seen in infants with deletion of the short arm of chromosome 4. Holoprosencephaly has been reported with a variety of other chromosomal abnormalities as well (Munke et al., 1988).

The most common location of the defect is at the vertex, but, occasionally, paired lesions are found in the parietal regions. At birth, a congenital scalp defect is often ulcerated or crusted and may appear to be infected. Over the following weeks or months, the lesion becomes covered by a layer of epithelium and subsequently resembles a scarred area. The region of the defect remains devoid of hair thereafter.

In most cases, the underlying skull is intact; however, in some infants there are underlying skull defects of variable size that close spontaneously during the first few months after birth. Still others have associated oval or circular defects in the skull that persist into adulthood.

Treatment is conservative for most patients, especially for those with cerebral anomalies resulting in severe functional defects. Plastic repair has been recommended in certain instances.

ANTERIOR MIDLINE DEFECTS

HOLOPROSENCEPHALY

Whereas anencephaly is the most catastrophic dysraphism, holoprosencephaly is the most devastating of the anterior anomalies. It is caused by induction failure of three germ layers: cephalic mesoderm, adjacent neuroectoderm, and the entodermal anlage for facial structures. Like anencephaly, it is time specific and stimulus nonspecific. Associated chromosomal abnormalities are frequent, including nondisjunction leading most commonly to trisomy 13. In addition, 18p⁻ and 13p⁻ have also been encountered (Cohen, 1982). The malformation also is over-represented in infants of diabetic mothers. It is likely that an environmental toxic stimulus accounts for both the embryonic failure and the chromosomal defects.

In essence, the defect is one of failure of the primary cerebral vesicle to cleave and expand bilaterally resulting in associated midline facial defects (DeMyer, 1971). Various degrees of severity are recognized. In its most complete expression, the brain is characterized by a single large ventricular cavity. The thalamus remains undivided, the inferior frontal and temporal regions are often absent, and the remainder of the isocortex is rudimentary. In the less severe forms, partial or complete division of the hemispheres is evident, but the olfactory bulbs and tracts are absent or hypoplastic (arhinencephaly) (DeMyer, 1971; Kobori et al., 1987).

In the most extreme form, the infant's face is overwhelmed by cyclopia, a single median orbital fossa and eye with protruding noselike appendage above the orbit.

Other constitutional dysplastic features include polydactyly, ventricular septal defect, and cardiac and digestive tract anomalies.

The less extensively malformed infant demonstrates hypotelorism, a median cleft lip, and a nose that lacks its bridge, columella, or septum.

The neurologic picture in these anomalies is highlighted by severe developmental retardation, seizures, rigidity, apnea, temperature imbalance, and rarely, hydrocephalus. The condition can be diagnosed by CT or MRI studies. When the patient has many extracephalic anomalies, a chromosomal defect is likely, whereas in their absence the karyotype is usually normal. A minority of cases are familial. In terms of intellectual function, the prognosis depends on the extent of the cortical malformations.

OTHER FACIOTELENCEPHALOPATHIES

A number of disorders are included in this group, all sharing the characteristics of median cleft lip and palate and various degrees of induction anomalies of the brain (DeMyer, 1971), which result in developmental defects of varying severity. CT or MRI studies often delineate the nature and extent of the cerebral maldevelopment.

■ DISORDERS OF CELLULAR MIGRATION AND PROLIFERATION

Although it is recognized that disorders of induction produce secondary migration or proliferation anomalies, this discussion is confined to those disorders of cellular migration that are unassociated with defects of embryogenesis.

MICROCEPHALY

Inasmuch as several of these developmental anomalies become manifest by microcephaly, this condition is considered first.

Microcephaly is defined by a head circumference, as measured around the glabella and the occipital protuberance, that is more than two standard deviations below the mean for age, sex, race, and gestation. The expected normal head circumferences at birth and in the first few weeks can be obtained for term infants from the graphs compiled by Nellhaus (1968), and those for premature infants from the data collected by Lubchenco and colleagues (1966). Except for cases in which there is premature closure of the sutures (craniosynostosis), the small size of the skull reflects a small brain. However, not all children with head circumferences below two standard deviations are mentally retarded. A child with "measurement microcephaly" who is of small stature because of familial factors or growth retardation secondary to malabsorption or cardiac disease is, therefore, not necessarily in the same category from the standpoint of CNS function as one with microcephaly resulting from organic brain disease. The most common conditions associated with primary microcephaly are listed in Table 45–1.

An abnormally small brain either is caused by anomalous development during the first 7 months of gestation (primary microcephaly) or is the result of an insult incurred

TABLE 45–1. Most Common Conditions Associated with Primary Microcephaly

Gross chromosomal abnormalities
  Trisomy 18
  Trisomy 13
  Partial deletion short arm of 4 (Wolf-Hirschhorn syndrome)
  Partial deletion short arm of 5 (Cri du Chat syndrome)
  Partial deletion of long arm of 13

Contiguous gene syndromes
  Miller-Dieker syndrome (Defect on short arm of chromosome 17)
  Langer-Giedion syndrome (Defect on long arm of chromosome 8)
  Prader-Willi syndrome (Partial deletion of long arm of chromosome 15)
  Aniridia-Wilms tumor syndrome (Partial deletion of short arm of chromosome 11)

Autosomal recessive disorders
  Johanson-Blizzard syndrome
  Seckel syndrome
  Smith-Lemli-Opitz syndrome
  ? Coffin-Siris syndrome

Rubinstein-Taybi syndrome

Maternal phenylketonuria

during the last 2 months of gestation or during the perinatal period (secondary microcephaly).

Primary microcephaly includes a variety of insults that cause anomalies of induction and migration. The condition may be transmitted as an autosomal recessive disorder or may accompany a variety of chromosomal disorders. Most infants with this condition are obviously abnormal at birth. They have not only a distinctly small head but also characteristic facial and cranial configurations. Their rounded heads, with small or absent anterior fontanel and recessed or sloped forehead indicative of the shallow anterior cranial fossa, readily identify them as infants with severe morphologic cerebral abnormalities. Some demonstrate immediate signs of neurologic dysfunction such as hypotonicity, hypertonicity, or an abnormal cry, whereas others function surprisingly normally for the first few months after birth. The type of pathology found in infants of this sort varies, but abnormalities of the gross configuration of the brain are usual.

Lissencephaly is near total or total absence of cerebral convolutions (agyria), reminiscent of the fetal brain during the second to fourth months of gestation. This condition is a feature of several syndromes, including the Miller-Dieker syndrome, which is associated with a defect in the short arm of chromosome 17 (17p3) (Dobyns et al., 1984). The clinical picture includes microcephaly, hypotonia, and seizures, most commonly, infantile spasms (Gastaut et al., 1987).

Pachygyria is characterized by relatively few broad gyria and shallow sulci. It appears to represent a developmental arrest of maturation and cell migration at a slightly later stage, with the result being abnormally broad, flat cerebral convolutions with a thick cerebral cortex. The ventricular system is usually mildly enlarged, and other anomalies, such as areas of gray matter heterotopia, are usually present in these types of malformed brains (Barkovich et al., 1987).

Polymicrogyria is more often associated with hydrocephalus than microcephaly and is characterized by either localized or generalized excessive and small cerebral convolutions. Whether microgyria is associated with an arrest of neuronal migration or is a result of an insult to the postmigratory cortex has not been entirely clarified. The clinical picture is generally one of mental retardation and spasticity, or hypotonia with active deep tendon reflexes ("atonic cerebral palsy").

Microcephaly is present in infants with various chromosomal disturbances, such as trisomy 13p and trisomy 18. There are also at least 45 well-defined dysmorphic syndromes with apparently normal karyotypes that are associated with microcephaly.

The best known intrauterine acquired causes for microcephaly include transplacentally transmitted infections such as rubella, cytomegalovirus disease, and toxoplasmosis. Maternal phenylketonuria with serum phenylalanine levels over 15 mg/100 ml during pregnancy is another cause of microcephaly and intrauterine growth failure. Maternal irradiation exposure and certain drugs can possibly lead to brain damage and microcephaly.

A variety of insults—infectious, traumatic, metabolic, and anoxic—during the last part of the third trimester and/or the perinatal period cause destruction of brain with reduced brain growth and early closure of sutures. As a rule, when the injury has occurred in the perinatal period, the head circumference at birth is normal, and microcephaly only becomes apparent months later.

CRANIOSYNOSTOSIS

Craniosynostosis (craniostenosis) is a disorder in which premature closure of one or more cranial sutures results in a disturbance of the shape and configuration of the skull (David et al., 1982). In many instances, premature fusion of the sutures is the only evident abnormality the child exhibits; in others, craniosynostosis and other associated anomalies represent an identifiable syndrome that is often genetically determined. These "primary" forms of premature cranial suture closure contrast with conditions in which early suture closure is a passive process resulting from lack of normal brain growth. This is observed in the infant with microcephaly and can occur subsequent to successful shunt procedures for advanced hydrocephalus. Abnormally rapid suture closure in early infancy can also occur in association with certain metabolic disturbances, the most notable being hyperthyroidism, Hurler syndrome, the rachitic disorders, and idiopathic hypercalcemia (Cohen, 1988).

The cause of primary craniosynostosis is not known. Most cases unassociated with other anomalies are sporadic, although repeated occurrence within a family has been described. Craniosynostoses consistently associated with certain other anomalies, such as Crouzon disease or Apert syndrome, may appear in sporadic fashion but are generally regarded to be inherited disorders (Cohen, 1988). An explanation for the type of deformity of the head resulting from premature closure of one or other cranial sutures was proposed by Virchow in 1851. He observed that inhibition of normal growth of the skull occurred in a direction perpendicular to the suture that is prematurely fused, resulting in compensatory enlargement in a direction parallel to the unyielding suture. The time at which cranial sutures normally achieve functional closure is variable, but abnormal sutural diastasis is commonly observed in children up to 10 or 12 years of age suffering increased intracranial pressure. The metopic su-

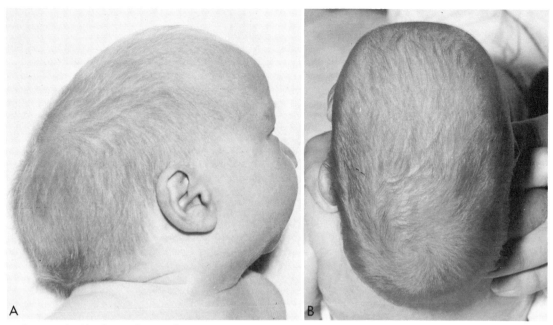

FIGURE 45–9. Three-week-old infant with sagittal craniosynostosis. A, Lateral view demonstrates the elongated head shape with tapering in the occipital region. Except for the abnormal configuration of the head, the child is developmentally normal for age. B, Vertex view reveals the characteristic long, narrow shape of the calvarium with premature closure of the sagittal suture.

ture differs from the other major sutures in that closure normally occurs in the 1st year of life. Trigonocephaly, therefore, occurs only when fusion of the metopic suture takes place in fetal or very early postnatal life. In general, the most overt cranial deformities are the result of prenatal suture closure, regardless of which suture or sutures are affected. Since the brain reaches approximately 80 per cent of the adult weight by 3 to 4 years of age, individual suture closure at this time is a matter of little consequence.

Clinical Aspects. Certain types of craniosynostosis, such as sagittal suture synostosis (scaphocephaly), are more common in males than in females. Isolated closure of the sagittal suture, the most common variety of the disease, accounts for approximately 40 to 70 per cent of craniosynostoses. It is the type least often associated with other defects. Premature closure of the coronal sutures can likewise occur as the only apparent abnormality but

is more often associated with other congenital anomalies. Oxycephaly secondary to multiple cranial suture fusion represents the least common form of the condition and is the most severe type because of the resulting restriction of cerebral growth and subsequent increased intracranial pressure.

The newborn infant with sagittal craniosynostosis presents with an elongated but narrow head, often with a small or absent anterior fontanel (Figs. 45–9 and 45–10). The forehead is usually considerably broader than the occipital region. A palpable ridge is present, especially over the posterior portion of the fused suture. Although the sagittal suture may be closed along its total length, it is important to recognize that suture closure over even a short segment will effectively limit growth of the skull perpendicular to the entire length of that suture. In the absence of the other anomalies, the infant with scaphocephaly secondary to sagittal synostosis is not expected to

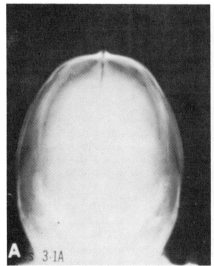
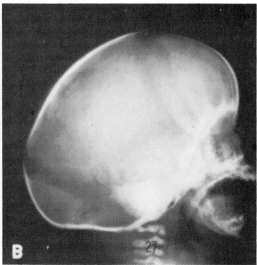

FIGURE 45–10. Roentgenographic findings in a 3-week-old child with sagittal craniosynostosis. A, Occipital view reveals the narrow configuration of the skull with "heaping up" of bone along the fused sagittal suture. B, Lateral view demonstrates the scaphocephalic shape of the skull with hyperostosis of the closed sagittal suture. The coronal and lambdoidal sutures are more separated than is normal. (Hope, J. W., Spitz, E. B., and Slade, H. W.: Radiology 65:183, 1955.)

have abnormal neurologic signs or signs of increased pressure. The signs are only those of distortion of head shape, since compensatory growth through other sutures permits normal brain growth. The problem is generally considered to be primarily cosmetic; however, examples are not rare of older children with uncorrected sagittal synostosis who subsequently developed visual disturbances or increased intracranial pressure.

Bilateral coronal synostosis results in a brachycephalic head shape in which the skull is broad anteriorly but shortened in the anteroposterior direction and elevated in the region anterior to the fontanel (Fig. 45–11). The forehead is broad and flattened, usually with a "pinched" appearance just above and lateral to the eyebrows. The eyes appear wide-set, and, in some cases, proptosis is present. Palpable ridges are sometimes present over fused coronal sutures but are rarely as definite as the ridging over a closed sagittal suture. Bilateral coronal craniosynostosis is frequently associated with other anomalies and is the most common type of suture closure in children with familial craniosynostosis, including Crouzon disease and Apert syndrome. Unilateral coronal synostosis gives rise to an asymmetric cranial deformity called *plagiocephaly*. The forehead adjacent to the fused coronal suture is flattened or indented, the eyebrow is elevated, and the homolateral eye appears prominent. The ocular prominence results from the associated involvement of the orbit, which is shallower and more oblique than is normally the case.

Prenatal or early postnatal fusion of the metopic suture results in a narrow, triangularly shaped forehead, which has a palpable and visible ridge betraying the underlying closed suture. The orbits are oval shaped and the eyes are abnormally closely approximated, a condition referred to as *hypotelorism*. The keel-shaped, angulated forehead of the infant with trigonocephaly is best observed by viewing the head from the vertex angle. Metopic suture synostosis occurs either in isolated fashion without other defects or is associated with other, often significant, anomalies (Anderson et al., 1962). One associated pattern is the presence of midline facial clefts and arhinencephaly, or absence of the olfactory nerves and other parts of the rhinencephalon, in addition to a single anterior lateral ventricle with hypoplasia or absence of the corpus callosum. The child with trigonocephaly and associated cerebral defects is expected to reveal early developmental retardation and eventual mental retardation.

Premature closure of the lambdoid sutures alone is very rare but can occur on occasion with sagittal synostosis or with total cranial suture fusion. Oxycephaly, or total suture synostosis, is an infrequent but severe form of craniosynostosis and is the only type of the disease in which the head circumference of the child may be significantly reduced. Inability of the brain to expand causes both clinical and roentgenographic signs and symptoms of increased pressure. Growth of the skull in such infants occurs in regions of least resistance, with the result being bilateral bulging of the temporal squama about the ears and striking prominence at the bregma. Thinning of the calvarium and deeply convolutional markings are seen on radiographs in such cases. Visual loss, retardation, and seizures may later complicate this disorder, owing to the effects of chronic increased pressure on the immature brain.

In certain cases, premature cranial suture closure is part of a spectrum of anomalies giving rise to identifiable syndromes with eponymic designations. Crouzon disease, or craniofacial dysostosis, is transmitted as a dominant trait with variable penetrance, although some cases occur in the absence of a family history. Clinical features include cranial deformity, usually due to coronal synostosis, but other sutures may also be affected. In rare instances, all cranial sutures are fused at birth in the child with Crouzon disease, leading to gross disturbances of the face and head and severe effects of increased pressure. Facial abnormalities that are constantly present include a "parrot's beak" deformity of the nose, maxillary hypoplasia, protrusion of the mandible, and exophthalmos, often

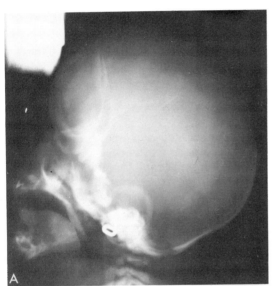
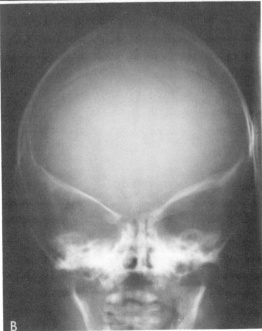

FIGURE 45–11. Roentgenographic findings in a newborn infant with a bilateral coronal craniosynostosis. A, Lateral view of the skull shows the short anteroposterior diameter and hyperostosis along both fused coronal sutures. B, The PA view of the skull demonstrates the elevated and oblique position of the sphenoid ridge on either side.

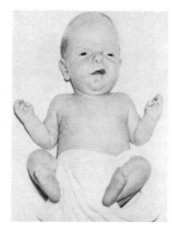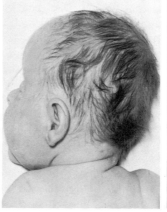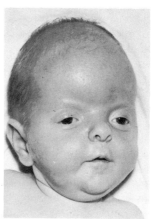

FIGURE 45–12. Apert syndrome (acrocephalosyndactyly). Bilateral coronal synostosis results in a brachycephalic head shape with "high" forehead and shortened AP diameter of the skull. Note the bilateral syndactyly.

associated with divergent strabismus. Untreated patients are susceptible to a variety of problems secondary to intracranial hypertension or compression of the orbital contents and optic nerves. A bizarre but rare disorder with features somewhat similar to those of Crouzon disease is referred to as kleeblattschädel, or cloverleaf skull. Intrauterine synostosis of multiple or all cranial sutures in concert with hydrocephalus accounts for the grotesque characteristics of the child with this severe malformation. At birth, the infant exhibits advanced exophthalmos, hypertelorism, bulging in the areas of the closed anterior fontanel and the squamosal sutures, and downward displacement of the ears. In some cases, facial bone deformities are similar to those of Crouzon disease, suggesting a possible relationship of kleeblattschädel to hereditary craniofacial dysostosis. The anomaly has also been associated with the skeletal changes of thanatophoric dwarfism and with other anomalies.

Apert syndrome, or acrocephalosyndactyly, is usually a sporadic condition, although there have been families

TABLE 45–2. Classification of Premature Cranial Suture Closure

I. "Simple" craniosynostosis
   A. Scaphocephaly—premature closure of the sagittal suture.
   B. Brachycephaly—premature closure of the coronal sutures.
   C. Oxycephaly—premature closure of all cranial sutures.
   D. Trigonocephaly—premature closure of the metopic suture.
   E. Plagiocephaly—premature closure of one coronal or lambdoidal suture.
II. Craniosynostosis with associated anomalies
   A. Crouzon disease (craniofacial dysotosis). Premature closure of coronal or other sutures, beaked nose, maxillary hypoplasia, prognathism, exophthalmos.
   B. Kleeblattschädel (cloverleaf skull). Multiple cranial suture synostosis with hydrocephalus. Facial dysostosis and long bone anomalies in some cases.
   C. Apert syndrome (acrocephalosyndactyly). Premature closure of coronal or other sutures, syndactylism.
   D. Carpenter syndrome (acrocephalopolysyndactyly). Acrocephaly, peculiar facies, brachysyndactyly of fingers, polysyndactyly of toes, mental retardation, other anomalies.
   E. Chotzen syndrome. Acrocephalosyndactyly with hypertelorism, ptosis, mental retardation.
   F. Pfeiffer syndrome. Acrocephalosyndactyly with broad thumbs and great toes, normal intellect.
   G. Trigonocephaly with hypotelorism, arhinencephaly.
III. Secondary craniosynostosis
   A. Following shunts for hydrocephalus.
   B. Early, passive sutural closure with microcephaly.
   C. Associated with metabolic disease (rickets, idiopathic hypercalcemia of infancy, hypophosphatasia).

in whom the defect was transmitted in a dominant manner. The pattern of suture closure varies to some degree, but bilateral coronal synostosis is by far the most common (Fig. 45–12). Syndactylism of the hands and feet is the distinguishing feature of this disorder, although other anomalies may also be found. Choanal atresia or stenosis has been observed in some infants and can create airway problems during certain diagnostic studies unless recognized. Related syndromes have received a variety of designations, such as Carpenter syndrome, and Chotzen syndrome depending on the associated anomalies (Table 45–2).

Diagnosis. Craniosynostosis in the newborn or young infant is usually suspected on the basis of an abnormality of the shape of the head. The distinctive palpable and sometimes visible ridge over the prematurely closed suture is an additional aid in identification of the condition. Roentgenographic or CT examinations are confirmatory in most instances but can be misleading unless one is familiar with the possible radiographic variations. For example, trigonocephaly may be obvious from the appearance of the child and the presence of a distinctive ridge, even though the metopic suture may appear patent on radiographic examination. The metopic suture is best observed by an x-ray examination in which a modified Water view or the submental-vertex view is used. Hyperostosis and "heaping up" of a synostosed suture, in addition to a generally abnormal configuration of the skull, are the most dependable x-ray findings indicative of craniosynostosis. Unaffected sutures are often disproportionately separated, reflecting compensatory effects allowing brain growth.

Several conditions must be differentiated from craniosynostosis in the newborn and young infant. The infant's head is frequently asymmetric because of postural effects, a condition especially likely to occur when the child lies with his head turned in one direction. This is seen with torticollis and also in developmentally retarded children who remain relatively immobile for a longer period than normal. The result is unilateral occipital flattening, usually with some degree of flattening of the forehead on the opposite side. A small or absent anterior fontanel in the first few weeks after birth raises concern regarding either the rate of brain growth or the patency of sutures. This anomaly can occur as a normal variation or can be the result of an accessory bone arising from a separate ossification center in the anterior fontanel. This is called an anterior fontanel bone (Girdany and Blank, 1965) and is of no clinical significance. The size and shape of the head are normal in such infants, and sutures are patent radiographically. Microcephaly is the most commonly discussed differential diagnostic consideration with craniosynostosis but is usually easily differentiated on the basis of physical examination of the child and x-ray or CT scan examination of the skull. Although the size of the head is abnormally small in the microcephalic child, it is the configuration that is disturbed in most cases of craniosynostosis. Microcephaly is characterized on skull radiographs by a relatively thick calvarium in many instances, without convolutional markings and with sutures that are approximated or overlapped but without bony fusion, at least in the newborn period.

Treatment. There are two reasons for surgical treatment: (1) in cases with multiple suture closure, to limit the extent of brain damage resulting from chronic increased intracranial pressure; (2) in children with synostosis of only one suture, to effect a good cosmetic result.

There is a consensus regarding the need for an operation in the presence of raised intracranial pressure. There has been considerable debate, however, regarding the need of surgery for cosmetic reasons, particularly in scaphocephaly, and some clinicians believe that scaphocephaly is rarely complicated by intellectual or neurologic dysfunction and that skull surgery is not justified for cosmetic reasons alone.

The author believes that surgery for craniosynostosis should be viewed as a corrective rather than a cosmetic procedure, because a child with uncorrected synostosis and a significant skull deformity is fated to a lifetime of being considered and treated as abnormal.

It is fortunate that premature closure of the sagittal suture (scaphocephaly) occurs in the bulk of patients with synostosis; the technical procedure to correct this condition is straightforward and produces excellent results. The most common method of treating sagittal synostosis is to remove a midline strip of bone several centimeters in width from anterior to the coronal suture to posterior to the lambdoidal sutures. This is followed by the placement of interpositional material on the bony edges to prevent early refusion. A much wider removal of bone without interpositional material can serve the same purpose. The application of a fixative such as Zenker solution to the dura mater for this or any form of synostosis, with the intent to retard reossification, is definitely not recommended because the solution can penetrate the dura and injure the underlying brain or it may destroy the ossifying potential of the dura, necessitating subsequent cranioplasty. Several techniques are currently advocated for the correction of the other synostoses (Marsh and Schwartz, 1983).

Morbidity consists of local hematoma, wound infection, or rarely, the development of a leptomeningeal cyst. At centers where operative procedures for craniosynostosis are performed frequently, the operative mortality rate is virtually nil, and prolonged morbidity is less than 1 per cent (Shillito and Matson, 1968).

MEGALENCEPHALY

Megalencephaly is a disorder in which the head is enlarged because of abnormal enlargement of the brain. It occurs under a wide variety of circumstances, sometimes being present at birth but often not becoming evident until later in infancy. Megalencephaly is familial in some instances and can occur with or without other associated anomalies. Although it is frequently accompanied by developmental and mental retardation, hypotonia, or convulsions, it can occur in the absence of any evident neurologic deficit. In the newborn or young infant, megalencephaly is often difficult to differentiate from hydrocephalus by the clinical findings. However, in megalencephaly signs of increased intracranial pressure are absent, cranial sutures are not abnormally separated, and the anterior fontanel, although frequently large, is soft. Demonstration of normal or only slightly enlarged ventricles by CT scan or ultrasonographic studies will establish the diagnosis. Megalencephaly occurs in several recognized syndromes, most of which are diagnosed more readily in the older infant or child than in the newborn. In the newborn infant, megalencephaly may be associated with achondroplasia, cerebral gigantism (Sotos syndrome), Hallermann-Streiff syndrome, or the Beckwith-Wiedemann syndrome. The Russell-Silver syndrome is a form of intrauterine growth retardation in which an abnormally large head is notably associated with a low birth weight (Fig. 45–13). The striking discrepancy between head size and body size of children with this disorder raises the consideration of hydrocephalus, but the large head is the result of a relatively large brain. Other features often observed with the Russell-Silver syndrome include limb asymmetry, triangular shape of the face, and elevated urinary gonadotropins.

CONGENITAL HYDROCEPHALUS

The term *hydrocephalus* includes a group of conditions associated with ventricular enlargement. The amount of cerebrospinal fluid (CSF) is increased and in most cases is under increased pressure. Hydrocephalus is usually the consequence of obstructed CSF drainage. The variation in the pathologic picture, including the nature and the extent of CSF pathway dilatation and the amount of brain damage, depends primarily on the site of obstruction, whereas the clinical evolution depends on the time at which obstruction develops.

An account of the embryology, physiology, and anatomy of CSF dynamics and ventricular and subarachnoid spaces is outside the scope of this text. The interested reader is referred to the 1980 review by Fishman.

Etiology and Pathology. Hydrocephalus occurs whenever there is a disequilibrium between production and absorption of CSF. Any block in the CSF pathway from the foramina of Monro to the tubular arachnoid villi of the subarachnoid space results in CSF under increased pressure and dilation of ventricular and subarachnoid spaces. Therefore, with one possible exception, all hydrocephalic conditions are obstructive. Obstructive hydrocephalus is conventionally divided into noncommunicating and communicating types. In the former, the obstruction site is

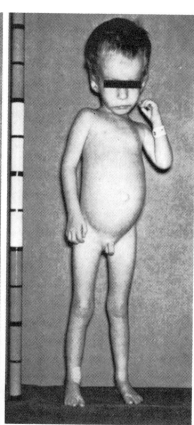

FIGURE 45–13. *Abnormally large head compared with body size in a child with the Russell-Silver syndrome. Such children are often erroneously suspected of having hydrocephalus but can be identified appropriately by the low birth weight for gestational age and the characteristic facial features. Striking limb asymmetry is often present. (Szalay, G. C.: Pseudohydrocephalus in dwarfs. The Russell dwarf. J. Pediatr. 63:622, 1963.)*

within the ventricular cavity, including the outlet foramina of the fourth ventricle. In the latter, the obstruction occurs distally to the fourth ventricle foramina (Magendie and Luschka), in the cisterns or cerebral subarachnoid spaces.

Regardless of the site of the obstruction, it is the arterial pulse thrust of the choroid plexus that is responsible for compressing the ventricular wall, enlarging the ventricular cavity, and producing parenchymal disruption. The pulse thrust increases with increasing mean CSF pressure and splits the ventricular ependymal lining. This allows free and continuing transependymal flow of CSF into white matter, producing a spongy, atrophic, and edematous dissolution of nerve fibers and swelling of gray matter neurons and astrocytes. It is still unclear to what extent normally nonfunctioning CSF drainage routes, including the choroid plexuses and the periventricular capillaries, become operative with increased CSF pressure and contribute to stabilization of pressure in the human hydrocephalic. In the newborn, particularly the premature infant, the paucity of cerebral myelin and any preexisting asphyxial tissue damage frequently allow ventricular dilation to occur at normal CSF pressures (Hill and Volpe, 1981).

Noncommunicating hydrocephalus is most likely caused by abnormalities in which the pathways are most narrow, notably the aqueduct of Sylvius, the fourth ventricle, or the foramina of Monro (Table 45–3).

The most common site of intraventricular obstruction in infants with congenital hydrocephalus is within the aqueduct. In the series compiled by Volpe (1987), this accounted for 33 per cent of cases of hydrocephalus apparent at birth. The underlying pathology may be one of several types, separable in most instances only by histologic examination. Forking ("atresia") of the aque-

duct represents a nonpatent system in which the aqueduct at various levels consists of multiple channels lined by ependyma that may or may not communicate with one another and that are separated by neural tissue. This lesion may occur as an isolated abnormality or may be associated with other anomalies, especially meningomyelocele and the Arnold-Chiari malformation. Hydrocephalus due to the Arnold-Chiari malformation accounted for 28 per cent of neonatal cases (Volpe, 1987).

In stenosis of the aqueduct, the aqueduct is histologically normal but abnormally small in caliber. There is an absence of excessive subependymal glia and of other evidence of an inflammatory reaction. Little is known of the origin of this disorder. It may represent a form of hydrocephalus that is slowly progressive or may even

TABLE 45–3. Classification and Types of Hydrocephalus

Noncommunicating (intraventricular obstructive)
1. Maldevelopments of the aqueduct (stenosis, forking ["atresia"], septal defects, gliosis).
2. Obstruction due to mass lesions (neoplasm, cyst, hematoma, aneurysm of the vein of Galen).
3. Obstruction secondary to exudate, hemorrhage, or parasites.
4. Obstruction of the fourth ventricle outlet foramina (Dandy-Walker syndrome, arachnoiditis).

Communicating (extraventricular obstructive)
1. Postinfectious, posthemorrhagic, or developmental adhesions of basilar cisterns or surface subarachnoid space.
2. Arachnoid villi obstruction by erythrocytes.
3. Communicating hydrocephalus with the Arnold-Chiari malformation.
4. Developmental failure of arachnoid villi (presumptive).
5. Hypovitaminosis A (experimental animals).

Communicating hydrocephalus due to excessive cerebrospinal fluid formation (choroid plexus papilloma)

remain silent until later in childhood. Gliosis of the aqueduct is generally considered a postinflammatory process, perhaps secondary to an intrauterine viral infection. A variety of experimental viral infections have been shown to produce structural abnormalities of the aqueduct. In particular, Johnson and Johnson in 1968 were able to induce hydrocephalus due to aqueductal stenosis in hamsters by intracerebral injection of mumps virus. Fluorescent antibody staining indicated virus growth to be limited to the ependymal cells. That this observation may have applicability to the clinical situation was shown by the presence of a cell-mediated immune response to mumps virus in two infants with aqueductal stenosis and in one-third of newborns with myelomeningoceles (Thompson and Glasgow, 1980).

In a small percentage of infants, aqueductal stenosis is inherited as a sex-linked condition (Edwards et al., 1961). Except for the clustering of affected males within a family, and flexed, adducted thumbs that are present in about one-half of cases, this form of hydrocephalus is indistinguishable from the other forms of aqueductal stenosis.

The Dandy-Walker syndrome includes a hugely dilated fourth ventricle that behaves like a cyst and is roofed by a neuroglial-vascular membrane lined with ependyma. This cyst herniates caudally and separates the cerebellar hemispheres posteriorly. The vermis and choroid plexi are rudimentary. The foramina of the fourth ventricle are often occluded by membranes or are atretic. Occasionally, hydrocephalus fails to develop, either because the foramina are small but patent or because CSF is absorbed through their membranes. Most authorities consider the Dandy-Walker syndrome to be a defect of neural tube closure at the cerebellar level. A variety of other neural and systemic anomalies are frequently associated (Friede, 1989; Hirsch, et al., 1984). This condition accounts for 7 per cent of cases of hydrocephalus apparent at birth (Volpe, 1987).

Clinically, the Dandy-Walker syndrome is characterized by a bulging occiput, nystagmus, ataxia, and cranial nerve deficits. In some infants, there are recurrent attacks of pallor, ataxia, and abnormal respirations. A significant proportion succumb to sudden respiratory arrest, which is probably the result of pressure on the pons. Although head enlargement may be obvious at birth, in some cases it does not become apparent until the infant is several months of age. The diagnosis is confirmed by CT or MRI scans.

A variety of other lesions may cause noncommunicating hydrocephalus in the newborn or small infant (see Table 45-3). These include neoplasms within the posterior fossa or of the choroid plexus, arachnoid cysts (Gandy and Heier, 1987), aneurysms of the vein of Galen, and a posterior fossa subdural hematoma secondary to mechanical trauma of the infant (see Chapter 46).

Communicating hydrocephalus accounted for 22 per cent of cases of neonatal hydrocephalus (Volpe, 1987). Despite the terminology, these conditions are the consequence of an obstruction in CSF circulation. Once the CSF leaves the foramina of the fourth ventricle and enters the cisterns, it must progress into the cerebral and cerebellar subarachnoid spaces where it is reabsorbed. Drainage is jeopardized if the cisterns or the arachnoid villi over the cerebral cortex are obstructed by thickened arachnoid or meninges. Such a process may be the result of a variety of infections or an intracranial hemorrhage. Among the infections that may be involved are toxoplasmosis and cytomegalovirus. Intrauterine intraventricular hemorrhage has been reported; in the majority of cases, intraventricular hemorrhage is seen in premature infants, particularly those weighing less than 1500 g. Subarachnoid hemorrhage may develop as a consequence of asphyxia or mechanical trauma in term infants. The pathogenesis and pathology of these conditions are discussed more fully in Chapter 46.

The genetic factors operative in the etiology of hydrocephalus have not been clarified.

Among siblings of patients with primary congenital hydrocephalus without spinal defects, the prevalence of anencephaly and spina bifida cystica has been estimated to be five times higher than the expected incidence in the general population (Lorber and De, 1970). The empiric risk of a major congenital malformation in subsequent offspring following the birth of a child with congenital hydrocephalus is approximately one in 25 (Lorber and De, 1970).

The only recognized exception to the rule that hydrocephalus results from obstruction either within or without the ventricular system occurs with a case of the rare choroid plexus papilloma. Ventricular enlargement in infants with this tumor has been attributed to cerebrospinal fluid secretion from the lesion in excess of the system's absorptive capabilities. Indeed, Eisenberg and co-workers found that the preoperative rate of CSF production in a child with such a tumor was about four times the normal rate, a value known to exceed the normal absorptive capacity of the subarachnoid space (Eisenberg et al., 1974). However, it has also been argued that hydrocephalus in this condition occurs as a consequence of arachnoidal adhesions, obstruction of the subarachnoid spaces secondary to an elevated CSF protein, and frequent bleeding from the tumor (Laurence et al., 1961).

Clinical Aspects. Symptoms and signs observed vary, depending on the age of the child, the acuteness of onset of hydrocephalus, and the rapidity of its progression. In the newborn period and in early infancy, the head grows at an abnormal rate, so that the infant is macrocephalic within 1 to 2 months, if not at birth. Occasionally, the head is so large at term that normal birth is impossible unless the head is decompressed by insertion of a needle into the ventricle. As a rule, infants with intraventricular obstructive hydrocephalus show more rapid progression of head enlargement and other clinical signs than do those with communicating hydrocephalus. In some instances, the baby shows no abnormality of behavior, feeds well, and progresses adequately in motor skills, and the only sign that a medical problem exists is the abnormally rapid rate of growth of the head. More often, the infant with congenital hydrocephalus is irritable, feeds poorly, has recurrent vomiting, and shows inadequate weight gain. Seizures are not common in infants with hydrocephalus, and papilledema is infrequent, even in those with marked head enlargement. If the condition proceeds unarrested, optic atrophy may eventually develop. The infant with hydrocephalus resulting from aqueductal obstruction from compression by an aneurysm of the great vein of Galen may show signs of high-output cardiac failure. Heart failure in the absence of evidence of internal cardiac anomalies plus a loud bruit over the scalp suggests this unusual condition.

Developmental motor skills are occasionally delayed, but some hydrocephalic infants progress in a remarkably normal fashion during the 1st year. Hydrocephalus of mild degree does not account for profound developmental delay by 6 to 12 months of age unless the retardation is due to the disorder that caused the hydrocephalus. As hydrocephalus progresses, the disproportion between head size and size of the facial structures becomes more apparent. Distention of scalp veins and enlargement and bulging of the anterior fontanel reflect elevated intracranial pressure. Increased muscle tone and hyperreflexia in the lower limbs have been attributed to stretching of fibers arising in the parasagittal area that must project around the angle of the lateral ventricle to enter the internal capsule en route to supply the legs (Yakovlev, 1947). These fibers could be affected earlier, with progressive ventricular enlargement, than the descending fibers to the upper limbs, which arise more laterally on the motor strip. Late signs in hydrocephalic infants include the "setting-sun" sign and the "cerebral cry," the latter being characterized by its brevity and high-pitched, shrill quality. The "setting-sun" sign is believed to be due to pressure of the suprapineal recess of the third ventricle upon the mesencephalic tectum. The phenomenon may, however, also be elicited in normal infants under 4 weeks of age by a sudden change in the position of the head and in infants up to 20 or even 40 weeks of age by removal of a bright light that has been placed in front of their eyes. A variety of other ocular signs may occur in the infant with congenital hydrocephalus, although lack of cooperation and irritability make analysis difficult. Internal strabismus is occasionally observed, and limited vertical gaze may be present. Horizontal nystagmus also may be evident.

Diagnosis. The most important aspect of the physical examination of an infant who is believed to have hydrocephalus is accurate measurement of the occipitofrontal circumference of the head. A single measurement is useful and may strongly suggest the existence of some form of disease state; however, serial determinations at periodic intervals with results plotted on a graph are of greater value. Attention should be paid to any change in the rate of growth, especially any precipitous increase in head size.

Transillumination of the skull is a simple and inexpensive procedure that should be performed whenever hydrocephalus is suspected. Abnormalities of transillumination in hydrocephalus indicate that the cerebral mantle is less than 1 cm in depth. In addition to indicating advanced hydrocephalus or "hydranencephaly," abnormal transillumination may be observed in infants with subdural effusions, scalp edema, or porencephaly. Arachnoid cysts over the convexity of the brain may also be demonstrable by transillumination. An infant with the Dandy-Walker syndrome may exhibit abnormal transillumination adjacent to the dilated fourth ventricle. Care must be taken not to overinterpret the findings with small premature infants because of the extreme thinness of the skull overlying the subarachnoid space characteristic of such infants.

Ultrasonography and neuroimaging have enormously simplified the evaluation of the hydrocephalic infant and are unassociated with patient morbidity and study failures inherent in air encephalography and angiography. CT and MRI scans demonstrate not only the size and position of the ventricles but also the width of the subarachnoid spaces at the base of the brain and over its convexity. Aqueductal stenosis can be demonstrated by the dilation of the lateral and third ventricles and the presence of a normal-sized or small fourth ventricle. One can diagnose the Dandy-Walker syndrome by observing an enlarged fourth ventricle and a large posterior fossa cyst. Communicating hydrocephalus becomes manifest by dilation of the entire ventricular system and the subarachnoid spaces at the base of the brain and over the lower portion of the convexity. In contrast to diffuse cerebral atrophy (hydrocephalus ex vacuo), communicating hydrocephalus is usually associated with an absence or narrowing of the subarachnoid spaces over the higher portions of the convexity of the brain. The possibility of the presence of tumors or larger arteriovenous malformations can be excluded by CT and MRI scans supplemented by intravenous injection of contrast material (Fig. 45–14).

Treatment. Two issues must be addressed: (1) which infant to treat, and (2) how to treat the infant. As a rule, every infant with neonatal hydrocephalus should be treated surgically, with an exception being made for those with major associated congenital defects. Even an extremely thin cortical mantle may not be a contraindication for surgery; all of us have encountered children in whom there was a remarkable return to normal following the placement of a shunt. In the experience of McCullough and Balzer-Martin (1982), 86 per cent of infants survived

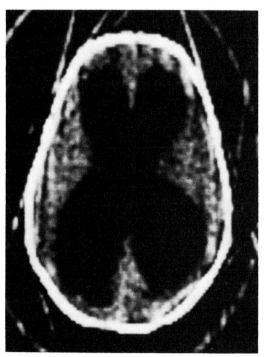

FIGURE 45–14. *Computerized axial tomography. Advanced hydrocephalus in a 2-month-old infant. Horizontal plane with frontal portion of the skull at the top.*

following their shunt placement. Of these infants, 46 per cent were reported as normal on follow-up.

The decision about whether or not to place a shunt in the premature infant who develops hydrocephalus following an intraventricular hemorrhage is discussed in the section on intracranial hemorrhage (Chapter 44).

When surgical treatment of the infant or child with progressive hydrocephalus is necessary, the method selected depends on many factors, including the site of the obstruction, certain characteristics of the ventricular fluid, and the experience with different surgical procedures. In some cases, procedures of a temporary nature are indicated when it is suspected that the more conventional shunt operations will be unsuccessful. The ventriculoperitoneal shunt is currently the preferred procedure. It is technically easier to insert and is associated with less severe complications than the other extracranial shunts.

The advent of high-resolution ultrasonography has facilitated the diagnosis of fetal hydrocephalus and has permitted surgery in the form of a ventriculoamniotic fluid shunt, which, at birth, is converted into a ventriculoperitoneal bypass. The majority of shunted fetuses have had aqueductal stenosis. Although the mortality rate for this procedure is acceptable, the outlook for the infant in terms of normal intellectual and neurologic function is not good. This reflects our inability to distinguish, by ultrasound alone, between ventriculomegaly due to high CSF pressure from that which reflects underdevelopment of the brain. Until this becomes possible, fetal shunting will remain an experimental procedure.

Shunt-induced infections, such as meningitis and ventriculitis, occur in approximately 5 per cent of patients. Revisions may be required periodically with somatic growth. All shunts are subject to obstruction, disconnection, and infection. The frequency and location of obstruction and disconnection depend to a fair degree on the shunting hardware. In general, the most frequent malfunction is that of occlusion of the ventricular catheter by choroid plexus or glial tissue that actually grows into the lumen of the catheter. Disconnection can occur at any point within the system, but most commonly it occurs where the various components are joined. Pressure-regulated valves in the shunting system can cause obstruction, drain CSF at higher or lower pressures than intended, and rarely, allow retrograde flow. Retrograde flow is of concern only in ventriculovascular shunts.

Although considerable apprehension has centered on the fact that an elevated CSF protein content may obstruct the valves, this has never been confirmed. It is the author's experience, however, that increased CSF protein is commonly associated with a higher incidence of ventricular catheter obstruction.

Ultrasonography or imaging techniques can be used to determine the patency of the shunt. Each type of shunting system has its own peculiarities that determine how to evaluate the adequacy of its function. It is unfortunate that most shunting systems contain a pumping mechanism in either the valve or the reservoir that is designed to test whether or not the shunt is functioning properly; the correlation between the response to pumping and functioning of the shunt is poor. Many functioning shunts do not pump normally, whereas other shunts that pump well are malfunctioning. Therefore, the author strongly advocates that the response to pumping of the shunt not be used to establish its adequacy. In a shunt-dependent infant, malfunction results in a progressive rise in intracranial pressure, which may be acute or chronic, depending on the rate at which intracranial pressure becomes elevated. The symptoms differ little from those seen prior to the insertion of the shunt.

The use of implanted foreign material is always associated with a risk of infection. The primary goal is to prevent infection rather than to treat it. The vast majority of shunt infections occur at the time of insertion, revision, or improper tapping. The use of meticulous aseptic surgical technique and prophylactic antibiotics have steadily reduced the risk of infection so that an infection rate of 1 to 5 per cent is now standard. Shunt infection may become manifest by swelling and redness over a portion or all of the shunting tract, and by such generalized symptoms as peritonitis with a ventriculoperitoneal shunt. Infections can also occur as a result of breakdown of the skin over the hardware. In some instances, the infection is confined to the ventricular system and the shunt, without any external evidence of infection.

The most reliable way to confirm a shunt infection is to obtain multiple CSF samples from the shunting system. Approximately 50 per cent of infecting organisms are *Staphylococcus epidermidis,* and 25 per cent are *Staphylococcus aureus.* The remainder represent a wide variety of pathogens.

The management of shunt infections is still a matter of considerable debate. All would advocate the use of appropriate intraventricular and systemic antibiotics. Some authorities attempt to clear the infection without replacement of the shunting system, whereas others favor removal with immediate or delayed replacement. We advocate complete removal of the infected system with delayed replacement; this approach has the highest chance of success with the lowest rate of morbidity. Delayed replacement usually necessitates intermittent CSF drainage via a reservoir or continuous drainage by establishing an external ventricular drainage system.

In considering the prognosis of the shunted child in terms of mental development and neurologic sequelae, the primary pathology, the degree of hydrocephalus prior to shunting, and the shunt course after placement of the shunt must all be borne in mind.

The issue of whether or not a shunt, once placed, can ever be removed has been considered by Hemmer and Böhm (1976). In their series, only 9 per cent of shunts could be removed in children with communicating hydrocephalus or hydrocephalus associated with myelomeningoceles. The author believes that no asymptomatic shunting device should ever be removed because, in many instances, it is impossible to establish beyond doubt whether or not the shunt is totally nonfunctional.

HYDRANENCEPHALY

Hydranencephaly is a purely descriptive term referring to a condition in which the greater portion of both the cerebral hemispheres and the corpus striatum are reduced to membranous sacs composed of glial tissue covered by intact meninges, encompassing a cavity filled with clear, protein-rich CSF (Fig. 45–15). The basal ganglia, brain

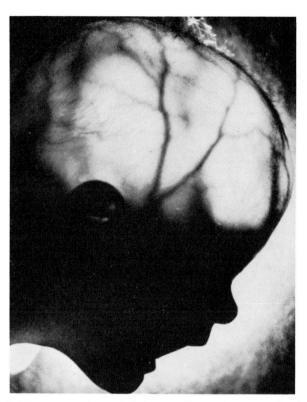

FIGURE 45–15. Hydranencephaly. Transillumination causes the skull to light up and to show the blood vessels in sharp relief. In this infant, the vault of the skull is not unduly enlarged. (From Laurence, K. M.: Congenital Abnormalities in Infancy. Oxford, Blackwell Scientific Publications, 1963.)

stem, and cerebellum are preserved but may reveal a variety of morphologic abnormalities.

At least four different pathogenic mechanisms have been postulated to produce hydranencephaly. First, it has been argued that hydranencephaly is a type of hydrocephalus that has run its course in utero. The presence of preserved ependyma and aqueductal stenosis in some cases supports this as one possible mechanism. In other instances, hydranencephaly has been the consequence of intrauterine infections or other gestational insults. The condition may also develop as a genetically determined defect in vascular ontogenesis or as the outcome of vascular occlusion of both internal carotid arteries or their main branches. A small number of cases probably result from a severe developmental anomaly in which normal formation of the cerebral mantle has not occurred (Yakovlev and Wadsworth, 1946). Thus, hydranencephaly should not be considered a diagnostic entity but the end result of one of many destructive processes in the cerebrum occurring during the prenatal period or the birth process or even postnatally.

The clinical manifestations observed in infants with hydranencephaly are variable. Although children with these disorders may appear intact to the mother, careful examination by one familiar with neurologic activity of the newborn reveals abnormalities in most. These include excessive sleepiness and irritability that is manifested by continuous crying during the waking state. Feeding problems are usual, often because of lethargy and poor sucking ability. Tremulousness of limbs and increased muscle tone are frequently observed along with enhanced deep tendon

reflexes. Nystagmus may be excessive, and optic atrophy is common. The normal neonatal reflexes, such as the grasp, Moro, and stepping reflexes, can usually be elicited but become abnormal because of their persistence beyond the expected time of disappearance (Halsey et al., 1968). If the child survives beyond 2 or 3 months, expected developmental landmarks are not achieved and the evidence of spasticity becomes more apparent. Autonomic dysfunction sometimes is manifested by wide swings in body temperature, in part related to the environmental temperature. In most of these infants, electroencephalography reveals markedly depressed voltages or even a virtually flat tracing. Ventricular fluid may be clear and have a normal protein content, or it may be xanthochromic and show a marked increase in protein, again depending on the cause of the process. Many infants with these disorders characterized by severe cerebral destruction die early in infancy, whereas a few survive for remarkably long periods of time.

MÖBIUS SYNDROME

This condition is characterized by congenital paralysis of the facial muscles and impairment of lateral gaze. The syndrome results from diverse causes. Pathologic lesions include complete or partial absence of the facial nuclei, dysplasia of the facial musculature, and hypoplasia of the facial nerve. The entity has also been seen in a variety of conditions in which there is progressive disease of muscle, anterior horn cell, or peripheral neurons. In other instances, there has been an absence, faulty attachment, or fibrosis of the extraocular muscles; electromyographic studies have suggested the added presence of a supranuclear lesion.

Although it has been described as an autosomal dominant trait, most cases occur at random, with a risk of recurrence of about 2 per cent.

Most cases of Möbius syndrome show a variable degree of unilateral or asymmetric or symmetric bilateral facial paralysis, with an inability to abduct the eyes beyond the midline. Occasionally, the weakness may be restricted to portions (e.g., quadrants) of the face. Atrophy of the tongue, paralysis of the soft palate or masseters, congenital clubfoot, deafness, or a mild spastic diplegia may also be present. Because of bulbar deficits, the disorder in language communication is far greater than general intelligence would suggest. The condition is nonprogressive but must be distinguished from myotonic dystrophy, or congenital muscular dystrophy (see Chapter 47).

■ REFERENCES

Alter, M.: Anencephalus, hydrocephalus, and spina bifida. Arch. Neurol. 7:411, 1962.

Anderson, F. M.: Occult spinal dysraphism. A series of 73 cases. Pediatrics 55:826, 1975.

Anderson, F. M., Gwinn, J. L., and Todt, J. C.: Trigonocephaly. Identity and surgical treatment. J. Neurosurg. 19:723, 1962.

Barkovich, A. J., Chuang, S. H., and Norman, D.: MR of neuronal migration anomalies. Am. J. Neuroradiol. 8:1009, 1987.

Blaauw, G.: Defect in posterior arch of atlas in myelomeningocele. Dev. Med. Child. Neurol. 25(Suppl.):113, 1971.

Brunberg, J. A., Latchaw, R. E., Kanal, E., et al.: Magnetic resonance imaging of spinal dysraphism. Radiol. Clin. North Am. 26:181, 1988.

Cohen, M. M.: An update on the holoprosencephalic disorders. J. Pediatr. *101*:865, 1982.

Cohen, M. M.: Craniosynostosis update 1987. Amer. J. Med. Genet. (Suppl. 4):99, 1988.

David, J. D., Poswillo, D., and Simpson, D.: The Craniosynostoses. Berlin, Springer Verlag, 1982.

DeMyer, W.: Classification of cerebral malformations. Birth Defects Original Article Series 7:78, 1971.

Diebler, C., and Dulac, O.: Pediatric Neurology and Neuroradiology. Berlin, Springer Verlag, 1987, pp. 51–59.

Dobyns, W. B., Stratton, R. F., and Greenberg, F.: Syndromes with lissencephaly. Miller-Dieker and Norman-Roberts syndrome and isolated lissencephaly. Am. J. Med. Genet. *18*:509, 1984.

Edwards, J. H., Norman, R. M., and Roberts, J. M.: Sex-linked hydrocephalus: Report of a family with 15 affected members. Arch. Dis. Child *36*:481, 1961.

Eisenberg, H. M., McComb, J. G., and Lorenzo, A. V.: Cerebrospinal fluid overproduction and hydrocephalus associated with choroid plexus papilloma. J. Neurosurg. *40*:381, 1974.

El Gammal, T., Mark, E. K., and Brooks, B. S.: MR imaging of Chiari II malformation. Am. J. Neuroradiol. *8*:1037, 1987.

Emery, J. L., and Kalhan, S. C.: The pathology of exencephalus. Dev. Med. Child Neurol. *12*(suppl.):51, 1970.

Fishman, R. A.: Cerebrospinal Fluid in Diseases of the Nervous System. Philadelphia, W. B. Saunders Co., 1980.

Fowler, G. W., and Dumars, K. W.: Cutis aplasia and cerebral malformation. Pediatrics *52*:861, 1973.

Friede, R. L.: Developmental Neuropathology. 2nd ed., Berlin, Springer-Verlag, 1989.

Gandy, S. E., and Heier, L. A.: Clinical and magnetic resonance features of primary intracranial arachnoid cysts. Ann. Neurol. *21*:342, 1987.

Gastaut, H., Pinsard, N., Raybaud, C., et al.: Lissencephaly (agyria-pachygyria). Clinical findings and serial EEG studies. Devel. Med. Child. Neurol. *29*:167, 1987.

Girdany, B. R., and Blank, E.: Anterior fontanel bone. Am. J. Roentgenol. *95*:148, 1965.

Guthkelch, A. N.: Aspects of the surgical management of myelomeningocele: A review. Dev. Med. Child Neurol. *28*:525, 1986.

Halsey, J. H., Jr., Allen, N., and Chamberlin, H. R.: Chronic decerebrate state in infancy. Neurologic observations in long surviving cases of hydranencephaly. Arch. Neurol. *19*:339, 1968.

Hemmer, R., and Böhm, B.: Once a shunt, always a shunt? Dev. Med. Child. Neurol. *37*(suppl.):69, 1976.

Hill, A., and Volpe, J. J.: Normal pressure hydrocephalus in the newborn. Pediatrics *68*:623, 1981.

Hirsch, J. F., Pierre-Kahn, A., Renier, D., et al.: The Dandy-Walker malformation. A review of 40 cases. J. Neurosurg. *61*:515, 1984.

Johnson, R. T., and Johnson, K. P.: Hydrocephalus following viral infection. The pathology of aqueductal stenosis developing after experimental mumps virus infection. J. Neuropathol. Exper. Neurol. *27*:591, 1968.

Kobori, J., Herrick, M. K., and Urich, H.: Arhinencephaly. The spectrum of associated malformations. Brain *110*:237, 1987.

Laurence, K. M., Hoare, R. D., and Till, K.: The diagnosis of the choroid plexus papilloma of the lateral ventricle. Brain *84*:628, 1961.

Laurence, K. M., and Tew, B. J.: Natural history of spina bifida cystica and cranium bifidum cysticum. Arch. Dis. Child. *46*:127, 1971.

Lorber, J.: Systematic ventriculographic studies in infants born with meningomyelocele and encephalocele. Arch. Dis. Child. *36*:381, 1961.

Lorber, J.: Results of treatment of myelomeningocele: Analysis of 524 unselected cases, with special reference to possible selection for treatment. Dev. Med. Child Neurol. *13*:279, 1971.

Lorber, J., and De, N. C.: Family history of congenital hydrocephalus. Dev. Med. Child Neurol. *12*(suppl. 22):94, 1970.

Lubchenco, L. O., Hansman, C., and Boyd, E.: Intrauterine growth in length and head circumference as estimated from live births at gestational ages from 26 to 42 weeks. Pediatrics *37*:403, 1966.

Mackenzie, N. G., and Emery, J. L.: Deformities of the cervical cord in children with neurospinal dysraphism. Dev. Med. Child. Neurol. *25*(suppl.):58, 1971.

Marsh, J. L., and Schwartz, H. G.: The surgical correction of coronal and metopic craniosynostoses. J. Neurosurg. *59*:245, 1983.

Matson, D. D.: Neurosurgery of Infancy and Childhood. 2nd ed. Springfield, Ill., Charles C Thomas, 1969.

McCullough, D. C., and Balzer-Martin, L. A.: Current prognosis in overt neonatal hydrocephalus. J. Neurosurg. *57*:378, 1982.

McLaughlin, J. F., Shurtleff, D. B., Lamers, J. Y., et al.: Influence of prognosis on decisions regarding the care of newborns with myelinodysplasia. N. Engl. J. Med. *312*:1589, 1985.

Medical Task Force on Anencephaly: The infant with anencephaly. N. Engl. J. Med. *322*:669, 1990.

Menzies, R. G., Parkin, J. M., and Hey, E. N.: Prognosis for babies with meningomyelocele and high lumbar paraplegia at birth. Lancet *2*:993, 1985.

Milunsky, A.: Prenatal detection of neural tube defects. J.A.M.A. *244*:2731, 1980.

Munke, M., Emanuel, B., and Zackai, E.: Holoprosencephaly: Association with interstitial deletion of 2p and review of cytogenetic literature. Am. J. Med. Gen. *30*:929, 1988.

Nakano, K. K.: Anencephaly: A review. Dev. Med. Child Neurol. *15*:383, 1973.

Nellhaus, G.: Head circumference from birth to eighteen years. Pediatrics *41*:106, 1968.

Nicolaides, K. H., Campbell, S., Gabbe, S. G., et al.: Ultrasound screening for spina bifida: Cranial and cerebellar signs. Lancet *2*:72, 1986.

Park, T. S., Cail, W. S., Maggio, W. M., et al.: Progressive spasticity and scoliosis in children with myelomeningocele. J. Neurosurg. *62*:367, 1985.

Peabody, J. L., Emery, J. R., and Ashwal, S.: Experience with anencephalic infants as prospective organ donors. N. Engl. J. Med. *321*:344, 1989.

Peach, B.: Arnold-Chiari malformation. Anatomic features of 20 cases. Arch. Neurol. *12*:613, 1965.

Pomerantz, J., and Schifrin, B. S.: Anencephaly and "Baby Doe" regulations. Pediatr. Res. *21*:373A, 1987.

Sarnat, H. B., Case, M. E., and Graviss, R.: Sacral agenesis: Neurologic and neuropathologic features. Neurology *26*:1124, 1976.

Shillito, J., Jr., and Matson, D. D.: Craniostenosis: a review of 519 surgical patients. Pediatrics *41*:229, 1968.

Soare, P. L., and Raimondi, A. J.: Intellectual and perceptual motor characteristics of treated myelomeningocele children. Am. J. Dis. Child. *131*:199, 1977.

Spindel, M. R., Bauer, S. B., Dyro, F. M., et al.: The changing neurourologic lesion in myelodysplasia. J. Am. Med. Assoc. *258*:1630, 1987.

Stark, G. D.: Neonatal assessment of the child with a myelomeningocele. Arch. Dis. Child. *46*:539, 1971.

Stone, D. H.: The declining prevalence of anencephalus and spina bifida: Its nature, causes and implications. Dev. Med. Child. Neurol. *29*:541, 1987.

Thompson, J. A., and Glasgow, L. A.: Intrauterine viral infection and the cell-mediated immune response. Neurology *30*:212, 1980.

Virchow, R.: Ueber den Cretinismus, namentlich in Franken, und üeber pathologische Schädelformen. Verh. Phys-med. Ges. Würzburg *2*:230, 1851.

Vogel, F. S.: The anatomic character of the vascular anomalies associated with anencephaly, with consideration of the role of abnormal angiogenesis in the pathogenesis of cerebral malformation. Am. J. Pathol. *39*:163, 1961.

Volpe, J. J.: Neurology of the Newborn. Second Edition. Philadelphia, W. B. Saunders Co., 1987.

Yakovlev, P. I.: Paraplegias of hydrocephalus (clinical note and interpretation). Am. J. Ment. Defic. *51*:561, 1947.

Yakovlev, P., and Wadsworth, R. C.: Schizencephalies. A study of the congenital clefts in the cerebral mantle. Part I. J. Neuropathol. Exper. Neurol. *5*:116, 1946.

PAROXYSMAL 46 DISORDERS

John H. Menkes

Seizures occur with a relatively high frequency during the neonatal period and present special problems in terms of their diagnosis and treatment. The basic mechanisms underlying seizures will not be discussed in this chapter. Instead, the interested reader is referred to a volume by Engel (1989) that covers the genetic, biochemical, electrophysiologic, and neuropathologic factors involved in seizures.

Etiology. The various causes for seizures during the newborn period and their relative frequency as determined by autopsy are presented in Table 46–1 (Mizrahi, 1987). Currently, the most common identifiable causes are hypoxic-ischemic encephalopathy and infections. Trauma, resulting in intracerebral and intraventricular hemorrhage, is less common. Developmental anomalies of the brain are probably more common than would appear from the data of Mizrahi (1987) and the autopsy series of Volpe (1987 and 1989), since a large proportion of infants with these conditions do not succumb to them. Characteristically, seizures due to perinatal asphyxia and its complications start within the first 24 hours of life. According to Volpe, 60 per cent of asphyxiated infants experience their first seizure within 12 hours of birth. Neonatal seizures due to developmental defects also start in the first 3 days of life; in fact, when seizures are first noted within 2 hours of birth, they are unlikely to be caused by perinatal asphyxia, and a developmental defect, pyridoxine dependency, or drug withdrawal should be suspected (Brann and Dykes, 1977). The reason for the delay in the onset of seizures in hypoxic-ischemic encephalopathy is still not fully understood (Williams et al., 1990).

Hypoglycemic and hypocalcemic seizures used to be relatively common during the neonatal period. According to Keen (1969), they account for 6 per cent and 34 per cent of neonatal seizures, respectively. Hypocalcemia of "early onset," occurring during the first 2 or 3 days after birth, is observed in the infant of low birth weight for gestational age, associated with perinatal complications, in infants of diabetic mothers, and in a variety of other stress situations. The reduced serum calcium in such infants may cause or contribute to the occurrence of convulsions; however, in some infants, correction of the calcium deficit does not alleviate the neurologic abnormalities. Hypocalcemia of "late onset" occurs late in the 1st week or early in the 2nd week after birth and is usually attributed to the phosphate load in feedings in the presence of relative parathyroid and renal immaturity. Seizures due to this are rapidly abolished by elevation of the serum calcium level. It is important to remember that neonatal hypocalcemia that proves to be resistant to therapy may be secondary to maternal hyperparathyroidism (Hartenstein and Gardner, 1966); idiopathic neonatal hypoparathyroidism (Smith and Zike, 1963), or the DiGeorge syndrome, in which congenital absence of the parathyroid and thymus glands is associated with other anomalies (Kretschmer et al., 1968). A curious and poorly understood disorder is a form of neonatal hypocalcemia that responds poorly to supplemental calcium: the reduction of the ion is secondary to primary hypomagnesemia (Vainsel et al., 1970). Tetany, convulsions, and hypocalcemia characterize this condition; however, the reduced serum calcium cannot be corrected until the deficiency of serum magnesium is eliminated (Davis et al., 1973). In this disorder, the onset of seizures generally occurs in the neonatal period but can be delayed for several months after birth.

Neonatal hypoglycemia is another important metabolic cause of seizures as well as other abnormal neurologic signs. Hypoglycemia in the newborn is diagnosed when glucose levels are less than 30 mg/dl in the full-term infant and less than 20 mg/dl in the premature child. The infant of a diabetic mother, the infant stressed during parturition or in the newborn period, and the newborn infant with hyperviscosity are all susceptible to hypoglycemia, which may precipitate convulsions. Rarely, hyperinsulinism is caused by such lesions as islet cell hyperplasia and islet cell tumors. Symptoms may appear as early as 1 to 2 hours following birth, particularly in infants who are small for gestational age, but as a rule, they are delayed until 3 to 24 hours. In about 25 per cent of such infants, hypoglycemia does not become symptomatic until after 24 hours. The clinical picture of symptomatic hypoglycemia is highlighted by tremors, apnea or tachypnea, cyanosis, convulsions, and lethargy (Raivio, 1968). Addi-

TABLE 46–1. Etiology of Neonatal Seizures

ETIOLOGY	PER CENT 1986	PER CENT 1971
Hypoxic-ischemic encephalopathy	46	36
Infection	17	4
Intracerebral hemorrhage	7	—
Intraventricular hemorrhage	6	—
Infarction	6	—
Hypoglycemia	5	5
Congenital anomaly of CNS	4	6
Inborn errors of metabolism	4	—
Subarachnoid hemorrhage	2	—
Unknown	2	23
Hypocalcemia	0	31

(Data from Mizrahi, E. M.: Neonatal seizures: Problems in diagnosis and classification. Epilepsia 28(Suppl):546, 1987.)

445

tional metabolic causes of neonatal seizures include hyponatremia, hypernatremia, and polycythemia with hyperviscosity (Gross et al., 1973). Hyponatremia in the newborn infant can be caused by excessive administration of salt-free fluids to the mother during labor or to the child after birth. It may also occur as the result of inappropriate secretion of antidiuretic hormone, resulting in water retention, or increased salt loss secondary to diarrhea. Neonatal hypernatremia has followed accidental substitution of salt for sugar in infant feedings and has occurred with severe diarrhea. In exceptional circumstances, inborn errors of metabolism may be responsible for neonatal convulsions (Table 46–2).

Although vitamin B$_6$ or pyridoxine dependency is an even more unusual metabolic defect that causes neonatal or even intrauterine seizures (Bankier et al., 1983), it is important because of the availability of treatment. Infants with this familial inborn metabolic error require far more pyridoxine than the normal child and exhibit neonatal difficulties when it is not provided (Waldinger and Berg, 1963). Respiratory dysfunction, neuromuscular hyperirritability, and convulsions that can lead to death unless treatment is instituted are the clinical hallmarks of this disorder.

Seizures are common events in newborn infants who have infections of various types, the most important being bacterial meningitis. Because of this possibility, lumbar puncture and cerebrospinal fluid examination are warranted whenever unexplained seizures occur in the young infant. Other infectious illnesses that may be associated with neonatal seizures are congenital rubella, cytomegalovirus encephalitis, toxoplasmosis, and disseminated infection with herpes simplex or Coxsackie B viruses.

The narcotic withdrawal syndrome in newborns of mothers who are narcotic addicts has been recognized with increased frequency in recent years. Although convulsions are not common among these infants, they have been observed in those severely affected (Herzlinger et al., 1977; Zelson et al., 1971). The seizure incidence is somewhat higher in infants born to methadone-addicted mothers. Seizures are even more likely to be encountered in infants of mothers taking barbiturates, particularly the shorter acting type, and in newborns passively addicted to alcohol (Pierog et al., 1977). Signs of neonatal withdrawal usually appear during the 1st or 2nd day after birth but in exceptional cases can be delayed for several days (Kandall and Gartner, 1974). The offspring of addicted mothers are usually prematurely born or small for gestational age. The usual withdrawal signs include irritability, tremulousness, tachypnea, vomiting or diarrhea, and fever. The more severely affected infant may have sufficient fluid loss to become dehydrated, develop hypocalcemia, or exhibit frank generalized convulsions. Diagnosis might be anticipated when the mother admits to drug intake, has withdrawal symptoms herself, or attempts to leave the hospital with the infant against medical advice within 1 day after birth. Currently, cocaine is the most common drug causing withdrawal in newborns. Seizures as a part of neonatal cocaine withdrawal are rare (see Chapter 26).

Intoxication of the infant by accidental injection of a local anesthetic, such as mepivacaine, into the scalp during caudal anesthesia of the mother is an additional possible cause of seizures soon after birth (Kim et al., 1979). Bradycardia is associated with respiratory depression, limpness, dilated pupils, and convulsions within the first 6 hours of birth (Hillman et al., 1979). The puncture wound, identifying the site of the injection into the fetal scalp, is visible in some cases. Gastric lavage and exchange transfusion have been recommended for this condition because of its life-threatening characteristics.

Lastly, one may also encounter an autosomal dominant syndrome of benign neonatal seizures (Quattlebaum, 1979). In this condition, seizures begin at about 48 hours after birth and may last up to 8 months of age.

Clinical Findings. Only a small percentage of newborns experience classic tonic-clonic convulsions, and neither petit mal nor psychomotor attacks have been encountered in that age range (Mizrahi and Kellaway, 1987). More commonly, they are difficult to recognize, and their appearance reflects the immature nervous system of the newborn and its inability to propagate epileptic discharges. Volpe (1989) has delineated these various seizure types in order of decreasing frequency: subtle, tonic, multifocal clonic, focal clonic, and myoclonic seizures. Subtle seizures, or motor automatisms are characterized by rhythmic eye movements, chewing, or unusual rowing, swimming, or pedaling movements of the arms and legs. Tonic seizures may be generalized or focal. The former are more common, and are marked by sustained hyperextension of the upper and lower extremities or of the trunk and neck. Another common seizure takes the form of focal or multifocal clonic movements of the extremities. These are usually at 1 to 3 jerks per second, and can be distinguished from a tremor in that the latter is faster, usually five to six jerks per second, and can be stopped by restraining or repositioning the limb. Other seizure forms include symmetric posturing of the limbs or trunk, and atonic attacks characterized by the arrest of movement with the infant becoming limp and unresponsive. In the experience of Mizrahi and Kellaway (1987) apnea is not seen as the sole seizure manifestation. When seizures are correlated with a simultaneously recorded electroencephalogram (EEG), it becomes evident that not all of these seizure types are accompanied by cortical seizure activity. In particular, motor automatisms, and generalized tonic seizures can be seen without associated EEG seizure activity. This implies that either seizures originate from subcortical gray matter or they represent brain stem release phenomena. Mizrahi and Kellaway favor the latter alternative and argue against treatment of

TABLE 46–2. Time of First Seizures in Various Inborn Errors of Metabolism

CONDITION	ONSET OF SEIZURES
Phenylketonuria	1 to 18 months
Maple syrup urine disease	1 to 2 weeks
Urea cycle disorders	2 days to 2½ years
Organic acidemias	
Propionic acidemia	First week
Methylmalonic acidemia	First week to 1st month
Pyruvic dehydrogenase defects	1 day or later
Isovaleric acidemia	First week
Galactosemia	First week
Pyridoxine dependency	3 hours to 7 days
Congenital amaurotic idiocy	2 weeks or later

these phenomena with anticonvulsants for fear of further depression of the higher centers.

Although these various seizure forms cannot yet be related to gestational age, or etiology, seizures without corresponding EEG abnormalities are more likely to be seen following hypoxic-ischemic encephalopathy and are a poor prognostic sign. Newborns with focal clonic seizures tend to have a better outcome.

The occasional infant with electrocortical paroxysmal discharges but no apparent clinical seizures presents a therapeutic dilemma (Shewmon, 1990). On the one hand, there is considerable evidence that uncontrolled seizures have a deleterious effect on the developing brain; on the other hand, so does chronic administration of phenobarbital. Not wishing to treat an EEG, I prefer to delay the use of anticonvulsants under such circumstances until there is clinical evidence for seizures.

Diagnosis. Episodic disturbances in the newborn that must be differentiated from convulsive activity include "jitteriness," which differs from seizures in its tendency to be provoked or aggravated by tactile stimulation and in its precipitation by placement of the body parts into certain positions. This author has encountered a familial syndrome of excessive jitteriness. It may well be related to familial quivering of the chin as described by Grossman (1957). This condition must be distinguished from the excessive jitteriness induced by the sequelae of neonatal asphyxia.

The intensely spastic infant may erroneously be assumed to be convulsing when clonus is provoked by certain exogenous stimuli. Such movements in the hypertonic child can usually be stopped promptly by altering the limb position.

The primary concern of the physician treating the newborn with seizures is the immediate identification of those causes that are amenable to some specific form of treatment. Therefore, the appropriate studies must be performed to exclude hypocalcemia, hypoglycemia, hypomagnesemia, hyponatremia, sepsis, and meningitis. Pyridoxine dependency can be added to this list, although it is a rare disorder. Diagnosis of seizures secondary to perinatal complications or congenital malformations of the brain can be accepted only after the aforementioned possibilities have been eliminated by the results of the laboratory examinations. In most cases, the infant who is convulsing because of hypoxic-ischemic injuries acquired during birth can be diagnosed on the basis of the history of perinatal distress, the presence of other abnormal neurologic signs, and the presence of an abnormal ultrasonographic, CT, or magnetic resonance imaging (MRI) studies.

The diagnostic assessment should include a complete blood count and urinalysis, serum glucose, calcium, phosphorus, magnesium, and electrolytes. A rapid estimate of the blood sugar range can be made by a Dextrostix test. If the test indicates a low serum glucose, it is advisable to administer 25 per cent glucose intravenously, after blood is obtained for glucose determination.

Other indicated studies may include determinations of blood pH, serum ammonia, and serum amino acids. Serologic tests for rubella, cytomegalovirus, toxoplasmosis, and other infections may also be advisable, depending on the other laboratory findings. Blood culture and lumbar puncture for cerebrospinal fluid examination, as well as ultrasonographic, CT or MRI studies, are additional valuable procedures.

An electroencephalogram is best obtained in the interictal period. This procedure, however, is a minor factor in the diagnosis and management of the patient. It is more valuable in helping one determine the prognosis for the newborn with a seizure disorder and, less often, in verifying whether a clinical phenomenon represents a seizure equivalent.

Treatment. When the underlying cause for seizures cannot be treated specifically, physicians will have to content themselves with symptomatic therapy.

Phenobarbital is the best anticonvulsant for use during the neonatal period. The drug is administered in an intramuscular loading dose of 15 to 30 mg/kg (Donn et al., 1985; Lockman et al., 1979; Painter et al., 1986). It is clear that this dosage is required in order to achieve adequate anticonvulsant blood levels (15 to 30 μg/ml). Peak concentrations are reached within 1½ to 6 hours following the injection, and maintenance doses of 3 to 4 mg/kg/day are initiated once the blood barbiturate level drops below 15 to 20 μg/ml. Because of the very long half-life of the drug in the newborn (greater than 6 days), this usually does not occur until 5 to 7 days of age (Lockman et al., 1979). These dosages are not influenced by gestational age. Nevertheless, it is imperative that for optimal seizure control daily or twice daily barbiturate levels be secured.

We have not had much success in the control of neonatal convulsions using oral or parenteral phenytoin, but we have seen a number of toxic reactions when the latter route has been used. This may be due to the immaturity of the hepatic hydroxylating system responsible for phenytoin detoxification.

Diazepam has also been suggested as an anticonvulsant in the newborn. The drug, however, is no better than phenobarbital for the treatment of neonatal seizures (Volpe, 1989). However, its short duration of action makes it a poor drug for maintenance. Furthermore, one of the principal side effects of diazepam is respiratory depression, which is most likely to occur in infants receiving a combination of diazepam and phenobarbital.

Koren and co-workers (1986) have suggested the use of intravenous paraldehyde. A 5 per cent solution in 5 per cent dextrose and water is given at a rate of 200 mg/kg over the course of 1 hour, followed by a continuous infusion of 16 mg/kg/hour for the subsequent 12 hours. Alternatively, 400 mg/kg can be infused over the course of 2 hours with no subsequent dose. The author has no experience with this anticonvulsant in newborns but has found that, if seizures are not controlled by phenobarbital, they are usually poorly controlled by other drugs. The ultimate prognosis of such infants, most of whom have congenital cerebral malformations, is poor with respect to intellectual development.

Prognosis. The prognosis of neonatal seizures depends on their cause. In other words, the eventual outcome is heavily determined by the nature of the underlying brain disease or systemic disorder that triggers the convulsions.

Seizures due to hypocalcemia starting 5 to 10 days after birth in an otherwise normal infant are generally associated with an excellent prognosis. Conversely, the majority of infants who experience seizures as a result of cardiopulmonary disease die within a few months of birth. Those having convulsions as a consequence of perinatal asphyxia or malformations of the central nervous system have a better prognosis with respect to survival but not with respect to normal intellectual development and freedom from subsequent seizures (Dennis, 1978). In the series of Watanabe et al. (1982), about one-third of infants who experienced seizures during the neonatal period as a consequence of perinatal asphyxia or perinatal trauma go on to develop a chronic seizure disorder. Follow-up studies on infants with neonatal seizures are summarized in Table 46–3. These results, reported in 1964, are not significantly different from those recorded in more current publications (Bergman et al., 1983; Volpe, 1987). In a significant proportion of children, seizures recur during the first 2 years of life, and some of these patients go on to suffer from infantile spasms.

The results from the National Institutes of Health Collaborative Project are somewhat more optimistic in that 70 per cent of 7-year-old children who experienced seizures during the neonatal period were neurologically and intellectually normal (Holden et al., 1982).

An infant with neonatal convulsions has a relatively good prognosis with respect to normal development in the presence of the following findings:

1. Seizures subside within 24 hours.
2. The neurologic examination is normal and no abnormalities of eye movements can be observed.
3. The child returns to a routine feeding schedule within 5 days.
4. The electroencephalogram, probably the most useful prognostic indicator, is normal. In the 1970 experience of Rose and Lombroso, newborns with seizures but a normal interictal electroencephalogram have an 86 per cent chance of normal development at age 4 years. The presence of multifocal spikes, or sharp waves, is a particularly ominous finding, and only 12 per cent of infants showing such a pattern achieve normal development.
5. In the experience of Painter and co-worker (1986), only 6 per cent of newborns who had experienced a seizure, but who were seizure-free at the time of hospital discharge, had a recurrence.

Factors that indicate a poor prognosis include a 5-minute Apgar score of less than 7, seizures lasting more than 30 minutes, and the need for prolonged resuscitation (Mellits et al., 1982).

When prognosis is classified according to causation of the seizures, one finds that 50 per cent of infants whose convulsions are due to an underlying asphyxial injury will develop normally. By contrast, less than 10 per cent of infants with intraventricular hemorrhage and none of those with congenital anomalies of the brain will escape intellectual deficits (Volpe, 1987).

There is much controversy but little data with respect to how long anticonvulsants should be given to an infant who has suffered seizures during the neonatal period.

Although experimental data derived from rats suggest an adverse effect of phenobarbital on the developing nervous system, the applicability of these results to the human whose brain is more mature at birth has not been demonstrated.

Nevertheless, we have made it a practice to maintain adequate phenobarbital blood levels for the first 3 months of life. Thereafter, in the face of normal development, continued freedom from seizures, and a normal electroencephalogram, we allow the infant to outgrow his phenobarbital dosage, so that when blood levels drop below 15 µg/ml the drug can be discontinued.

■ REFERENCES

Bankier, A., Turner, M., and Hopkins, I.: Pyridoxine dependent seizures—A wider clinical spectrum. Arch. Dis. Child. 58:415, 1983.

Bergman, I., Painter, M. J., Hirsch, R. P., et al.: Outcome in neonates with convulsions treated in an intensive care unit. Ann. Neurol. 14:642, 1983.

Brann, A. W., and Dykes, F. D.: The effects of intrauterine asphyxia on the full-term neonate. Clin. Perinatol. 4:149, 1977.

Craig, W. S. Convulsive movements occurring in first 10 days of life. Arch. Dis. Child. 35:336, 1960.

Davis, J. A., Harvey, D. R., and Yu, J. S.: Neonatal fits associated with hypomagnesaemia. Arch. Dis. Child. 40:286, 1973.

Dennis, J.: Neonatal convulsions: aetiology, late neonatal status and long-term outcome. Dev. Med. Child Neurol. 20:143, 1978.

Donn, S. M., Grasela, T. H., and Goldstein, G. W.: Safety of a higher loading dose of phenobarbital in the term newborn. Pediatrics 75:1061, 1985.

Engel, J.: Seizures and Epilepsy. F. A. Davis Co., Philadelphia, 1989.

Freeman, J. M.: Neonatal seizures—diagnosis and management. J. Pediatr. 77:701, 1970.

Gross, G. P., Hathaway, W. E., and McGaughey, H. R.: Hyperviscosity in the neonate. J. Pediatr. 82:1004, 1973.

Grossman, B. J.: Trembling of chin. Pediatrics 19:453, 1957.

Hartenstein, H., and Gardner, L. I.: Tetany of the newborn associated with maternal parathyroid adenoma. N. Engl. J. Med. 274:266, 1966.

Herzlinger, R. A., Kandall, S. R., and Vaughan, H. G.: Neonatal seizures associated with narcotic withdrawal. J. Pediatr. 91:638, 1977.

Hillman, L. S., Hillman, R. E., and Dodson, W. E: Diagnosis, treatment, and follow-up of neonatal mepivacaine intoxication secondary to paracervical and pudendal blocks during labor. J. Pediatr. 95:472, 1979.

Holden, K. R., Mellits, E. D., and Freeman, J. M.: Neonatal seizures. I. Correlation of prenatal and perinatal events with outcomes. Pediatrics 70:165, 1982.

Hopkins, I. J.: Seizures in the first week of life. A study of aetiological factors. Med. J. Aust. 2:647, 1972.

Kandall, S. R., and Gartner, L. M.: Later presentation of drug withdrawal symptoms in newborns. Am. J. Dis. Child. 127:58, 1974.

TABLE 46–3. Follow-up of 278 Infants with Neonatal Seizures*

	NUMBER OF PATIENTS	
Normal	140	–
Died within 3 months	63	–
Cerebral hemorrhage	–	26
Cerebral edema	–	16
Malformation of CNS	–	3
Abnormal	75	
Mental retardation	–	17
Mental retardation and seizures	–	14
Seizures	–	5
"Cerebral palsy"	–	37

*After Prichard, J. S.: The character and significance of epileptic seizures in infancy. *In* Kellaway, P., and Petersen, I. (Eds.): Neurological and Electroencephalographic Correlative Studies in Infancy. New York, Grune & Stratton, 1964.

(From Menkes, J. H.: Textbook of Child Neurology. 4th ed. Philadelphia, Lea & Febiger, 1990.)

Keen, J. H.: Significance of hypocalcemia in neonatal convulsions. Arch. Dis. Child. 44:356, 1969.

Kim, W. Y., Pomerance, J. J., and Miller, A. A.: Lidocaine intoxication in a newborn following local anesthesia for episiotomy. Pediatrics 64:643, 1979.

Koren, G., Butt, W., Rajchgot, P., et al.: Intravenous paraldehyde for seizure control in newborn infants. Neurology 36:108, 1986.

Kretschmer, R., Say, B., Brown, D., and Rosen, F. S.: Congenital aplasia of the thymus gland (DiGeorge's syndrome). N. Engl. J. Med. 279:1295, 1968.

Lockman, L. A., et al.: Phenobarbital dosage for control of neonatal seizures. Neurology 29:1445, 1979.

Mellits, E. D., Holden, K. R., and Freeman, J. M.: Neonatal seizures. II. A multivariate analysis of factors associated with outcome. Pediatrics 70:177, 1982.

Mizrahi, E. M.: Neonatal seizures: Problems in diagnosis and classification. Epilepsia 28(Suppl. 1):S46, 1987.

Mizrahi, E. M., and Kellaway, P.: Characterization and classification of neonatal seizures. Neurology 37:1837, 1987.

Painter, M. J., Bergman, I., and Crumrine, P.: Neonatal seizures. Pediatr. Clin. North Am. 33:91, 1986.

Pierog, S., Chandavasu, O., and Wexler, I.: Withdrawal symptoms in infants with the fetal alcohol syndrome. J. Pediatr. 90:630, 1977.

Prichard, J. S.: The character and significance of epileptic seizures in infancy. In Kellaway, P., and Petersen, I. (Eds.): Neurological and Electroencephalographic Correlative Studies in Infancy. New York, Grune & Stratton, 1964.

Quattlebaum, T. G.: Benign familial convulsions in the neonatal period and early infancy. J. Pediatr. 95:257, 1979.

Raivio, K. O.: Neonatal hypoglycemia. II. A clinical study of 44 idiopathic cases with special reference to corticosteroid hormones. Acta Paediatr. Scand. 57:540, 1968.

Rose, A. L., and Lombroso, C. T.: Neonatal seizure states. A study of clinical, pathological, and electroencephalographic features in 137 full-term babies with a long-term follow-up. Pediatrics 45:404, 1970.

Shewmon, D. A.: What is a neonatal seizure? Problems in definition and quantification for investigative and clinical purposes. J. Clin. Neurophysiol. 7:315, 1990.

Smith, F. G., Jr., and Zike, K.: Idiopathic hypoparathyroidism in neonatal period. Am. J. Dis. Child. 105:182, 1963.

Vainsel, M., Vandervelde, G., Smulders, J., et al.: Tetany due to hypomagnesaemia with secondary hypocalcemia. Arch. Dis. Child. 45:254, 1970.

Volpe, J. J.: Neonatal seizures: Current concepts and revised classification. Pediatrics 84:422, 1989.

Volpe, J. J.: Neurology of the Newborn. 2nd ed. Philadelphia, W. B. Saunders Company, 1987.

Waldinger, C., and Berg, R. B.: Signs of pyridoxine dependency manifest at birth in siblings. Pediatrics 32:161, 1963.

Watanabe, K., Kuroyanagi, M., Hara, K., et al.: Neonatal seizures and subsequent epilepsy. Brain Dev. 4:341, 1982.

Williams, C. E., Gunn, A. J., Synek, B., et al.: Delayed seizures occurring with hypoxic-ischemic encephalopathy in the fetal sheep. Pediatr. Res. 27:561, 1990.

Zelson, C., Rubio, E., and Wasserman, E.: Neonatal narcotic addiction: 10 year observation. Pediatrics 48:178, 1971.

DISEASES OF THE MOTOR UNIT 47

John H. Menkes

Because of the relative simplicity of the motor unit, the disorders discussed in this chapter have a limited means of clinical expression, and their diagnosis rests to a great extent on the proper application of laboratory techniques. An approach to the diagnostic evaluation of the hypotonic infant follows:

1. Establish whether hypotonia is due to central nervous system involvement, a systemic or metabolic disease, or a neuromuscular disorder. No details need to be given at this point, but there has been a recent tendency to underestimate the importance of a careful history and a good physical examination. One of the chief distinguishing features of a neuromuscular disorder is the appearance of alertness and responsiveness in the flaccid child with muscle disease as opposed to the lethargy and stupor that accompany cerebral birth insults.
2. Once the infant's difficulties have been shown to be the consequence of a neuromuscular disorder, perform laboratory studies to obtain further information.
   a. Evaluate serum enzymes. The most widely used enzyme assay in the assessment of muscle disease is serum creatine phosphokinase (CPK). An elevation in its level is seen in some infants with congenital muscular dystrophy but is also found in normal newborns for the first few days of life.
   b. Examine the cerebrospinal fluid. An elevated CSF protein is the hallmark of neonatal polyneuropathy.
   c. Obtain an electrocardiogram. The ECG is abnormal in glycogen storage disease, Type II (Pompe disease), in some cases of congenital muscular dystrophy, and, less often, in congenital myotonic dystrophy. It is normal in spinal muscular atrophy (Werdnig-Hoffmann disease).
   d. Obtain an electromyogram. In the newborn, the quadriceps and deltoid muscles are best suited for this procedure. The EMG will provide information as to whether hypotonia is neurogenic—due to involvement of the anterior horn cells (e.g., in infantile spinal muscular atrophy) or the peripheral nerve—or myopathic. In most instances, the EMG will not provide an answer regarding the type of denervation or the nature of the myopathy. However, in myasthenia gravis and infantile botulism, special electrodiagnostic techniques will be diagnostic (Aminoff, 1986). Little additional information can be gathered from nerve conduction studies.
3. Perform a muscle biopsy. This procedure is essential to the diagnosis of most infants with neuromuscular diseases. The biopsy is performed on a muscle that has not been previously subjected to EMG, and the specimen is prepared for histology, histochemistry, and electron microscopy. Open and needle biopsy both have their proponents, and the interested reader is referred to Dubowitz (1985) for further discussion.

■ DISEASES OF THE MOTONEURON

SPINAL MUSCULAR ATROPHY (WERDNIG-HOFFMANN DISEASE)

In infants, spinal muscular atrophy is the principal disease affecting the motoneuron. This is a disease or group of diseases transmitted by an autosomal recessive gene located on the long arm of chromosome 5 (5q 11.2–13.3) and manifested by widespread muscular atrophy.

Although initial pathologic descriptions of the disease pointed to the conspicuous loss of anterior horn cells from spinal cord and brain stem (Byers and Banker, 1961), it is becoming evident that when carefully searched for, other areas of the central nervous system, notably the dorsal root ganglia, posterior columns, optic nerves, and cranial nerve nuclei, are also involved (Probst et al., 1981). In the usual infant coming to necropsy, anterior horn cells are absent from the entire length of the spinal cord. Of the residual cells, some are in the process of degenerating or are being phagocytized by satellite cells. An unusual finding that may reflect the basic defect in this puzzling disease is the prominent glial proliferation at the proximal portion of the anterior spinal roots, changes that are believed to start during fetal life.

In about one-third of cases, the disease is present at birth. The infants present a classic picture of a neuromuscular disease. They are hypotonic or floppy, with a symmetric muscle weakness that is more extensive in the proximal part of the limbs. What little spontaneous movements are left can be found in the small muscles of the hands and feet. The affected muscles are atrophied, although this is concealed by the normal amounts of subcutaneous fat seen in the newborn. Muscles of the trunk, neck, and thorax are equally affected, and the infant assumes a characteristic "frog posture." Muscles of the face and diaphragm are commonly spared during the initial phases. Bulbar musculature is affected with consequent impairment of sucking and swallowing. Fasciculation may be noted in the tongue, but this finding is often difficult to obtain in the crying youngster. Deep tendon reflexes are nearly always reduced or absent. There are no sensory loss, no intellectual retardation, and no sphincter disturbances.

In most instances, the disease progresses rapidly, so that infants who are affected at birth rarely survive the first year of life. In some, neonatal respiratory distress may be fatal.

Electromyographic findings help confirm the clinical impression of motoneuron disease. The finding most specific for this condition—and not observed in any other—is the presence of spontaneous, rhythmic muscle activity at a frequency of 5 to 15 contractions per second, which can be activated by voluntary effort. Still, muscle biopsy is the only certain way of determining the diagnosis (Dubowitz, 1985).

Neither the cause of this disease nor its treatment is known.

ARTHROGRYPOSIS

Arthrogryposis refers to multiple congenital contractures of limbs fixed in flexion or, less commonly, in extension accompanied by diminution and wasting of skeletal muscle. Other congenital malformations, particularly clubfoot and cerebral maldevelopment, are often part of the syndrome. The condition is due to a variety of causes, all having in common reduced fetal mobility (Hageman et al., 1987a). In one group of infants, the neuromuscular apparatus is normal, and arthrogryposis results from restricted intrauterine muscle movements. This can result from either a malformed uterus or oligohydramnios (e.g., Potter syndrome). In another group of infants, the condition is due to one of at least three distinct neuromuscular syndromes. Probably the most common is one in which the anterior horn cells are markedly reduced, and the EMG findings are consistent with denervation. About 10 to 20 per cent of infants with spinal muscular atrophy will demonstrate contractures, especially of the distal portion of the limbs (Byers and Banker, 1961). In other instances, there are changes compatible with congenital muscular dystrophy, congenital myotonic dystrophy, fibrosis of the anterior spinal roots, or evidence of embryonic denervation and maturation arrest of the muscle.

In the Pena-Shokeir syndrome, a heterogeneous condition, arthrogryposis is accompanied by facial anomalies, intrauterine growth retardation, and a variety of cerebral malformations (Hageman, et al., 1987b). Some restrict the use of "Pena-Shokeir syndrome" to those with an autosomal recessive disorder (one per 12,000 livebirths), and term the nongenetic condition "fetal akinesia sequence." Several other malformation syndromes, some with chromosomal disorders, may be accompanied by arthrogryposis. These are reviewed by Hageman and co-workers (1987a) and by Hall (1986).

The reduced fetal movements permit an in utero diagnosis by ultrasound and, if necessary, by fetoscopy.

Treatment of arthrogryposis should commence immediately after birth, with passive motion exercises, braces, and casts. Subsequently, surgery is usually necessary, particularly for contractions of the lower extremities and hips. In the presence of considerable weakness and amyoplasia, these procedures are contraindicated. As a rule, functional improvement of extension contractures is better than that of flexion contractures, and arthrogryposis secondary to maternal factors has a better outlook than that due to neuromuscular disorders (Hall, 1986).

An early and vigorous orthopedic program has been advocated. This is often of considerable benefit to infants with arthrogryposis of non-neuromuscular origin.

Of the various other conditions affecting the motoneuron of the newborn, only type II glycogen storage disease (Pompe disease) and neonatal poliomyelitis occur with sufficient frequency to be mentioned at this point.

■ DISEASES OF THE AXON

Both acute and chronic polyneuropathies have been documented in newborns (Goebel et al., 1976; Kasman et al., 1976). We have seen two such cases in hypotonic infants in whom an elevated CSF protein in the absence of pleocytosis suggested the diagnosis. Occasionally, the polyneuropathy appears to be transmitted as a dominant trait with partial expressivity in one parent (Kasman et al., 1976).

■ DISEASES OF THE NEUROMUSCULAR JUNCTION

The disorders to be considered under this heading include myasthenia gravis, infantile botulism, and neonatal tetanus. The venoms of several reptiles and insects also affect the neuromuscular junction, but these conditions need not be considered in this text.

MYASTHENIA GRAVIS

Seven forms of myasthenia gravis have been encountered in the neonatal period (Misulis and Fenichel, 1989). All demonstrate muscular weakness responsive to anticholinesterase medication and display a decremental response to repetitive motor nerve stimulation. Neonatal myasthenia gravis is the most common of these disorders. It is seen in 10 to 15 per cent of infants born to myasthenic mothers. "Congenital myasthenia gravis" is the term used to designate children with myasthenia born to mothers without the disease. As a rule, antibodies against the acetylcholine receptor (AChR) protein are undetectable. Several syndromes have been recognized. These include a sporadic form associated with a congenital deficiency of acetylcholinesterase; at least two autosomal recessive conditions, possibly due to a defect in acetylcholine resynthesis or mobilization; a defect in AChR ligand binding affinity, and an autosomal dominant condition, believed to be the consequence of an abnormally prolonged open-time of the acetylcholine-ion channels. In another group of patients presenting with a familial, congenital myasthenic syndrome, the number of receptors is reduced, and endplate morphology is distorted.

Clinically, the picture is also heterogeneous. In about half of the instances, symptoms commence before 2 years of age, and more than one sibling may be affected. In many instances, fetal movements are reduced, and during the neonatal period, one may note feeding difficulties, ptosis, limitation of eye movements, and a weak cry. The initial symptoms in congenital myasthenia gravis are not as severe as in the neonatal variety, and the diagnosis is therefore more difficult to establish. A few patients with congenital myasthenia have spontaneous remissions, but the course of the disease is usually protracted with mild symptoms that are refractory to both medical and surgical therapy.

Juvenile myasthenia gravis designates a disorder that is similar to the one seen in adults. However, onset of this condition prior to 1 year of age has not yet been documented. In this condition, as in adult myasthenia, the pathophysiology has now been fairly well delineated. For as yet unknown reasons an autoimmune response, stimulated, possibly, by an infectious agent and selectively enhanced by thymus cells, is mounted against the postsynaptic acetylcholine receptors. The ensuing antibodies induce an increased degradation of these receptors, so that the number of functional receptors may be reduced to as little as 10 per cent of normal.

Neonatal myasthenia presumably results from the passive transfer of anti-acetylcholine receptor antibodies across the placenta (Keesey et al., 1977). In this form of myasthenia, symptoms usually appear during the first 24 hours or, at the latest, by the third day of life. In all instances, there is a paresis of the lower bulbar muscles that results in a weak cry and difficulty in sucking or swallowing. Generalized hypotonia is found in about one half the infants. It may be severe enough to produce respiratory difficulty (Misulis and Fenichel, 1989).

The clinical diagnosis is confirmed by administration of 0.1 mg of edrophonium chloride (Tensilon). In some infants, a positive response may be obscured by the response to the injection, and the longer acting neostigmine (Prostigmin) should be used. The latency of Prostigmin is greater than that of Tensilon, but it is sufficiently long-acting for one to determine muscle strength accurately. The diagnosis is further documented by repetitive nerve stimulation at 10 to 50 Hz, which produces transmission fatigue. Serum anti-acetylcholine receptor antibody levels are elevated in some asymptomatic newborns of myasthenic mothers.

Myasthenic symptoms usually respond promptly to anticholinesterase medication, and even if the illness is untreated, its duration is generally less than 5 weeks.

INFANT BOTULISM

Botulism is a toxic condition induced by the ingestion of food in which Clostridium botulinum has grown and produced toxin.

Over the past 10 years, a syndrome of infantile botulism has been delineated. This condition has its onset between 3 and 18 weeks of age and is characterized by hypotonia, hyporeflexia, and weakness of the cranial musculature. Infants often have a history of constipation and poor feeding, and a large proportion (44 per cent) have been fed honey (Arnon, 1980).

The severity of symptoms ranges from a mild disorder to one that resembles sudden infant death syndrome (SIDS). Bulbar signs predominate. These include a poor cry, poor suck, impaired pupillary light response, and external ophthalmoplegia. With progression of the illness a flaccid paralysis develops. Autonomic dysfunction may be present; cardiovascular symptoms are absent, however, and the ECG remains normal. Almost all infants recover completely, with the illness lasting between 3 and 20 weeks.

On electromyography, the motor unit action potentials are brief, of small amplitude, and excessive in number—a picture consistent with that observed in botulism in older individuals. Fibrillation potentials, consistent with functional denervation are observed in about half of the patients. Stimulation at 50 Hz results in a marked incremental response. This finding is essentially diagnostic. This facilitation is generally not observed in older children and adults with botulism, probably because of the large amounts of toxin present.

Whereas botulism in older children and adults is generally, but not invariably due to the ingestion of preformed toxin, infant botulism results from the colonization of the gut with type A and type B spores of C. botulinum, and the subsequent release of the toxin, which has been demonstrated in feces (Arnon, 1986). Since spores of C. botulinum are ubiquitous and most individuals ingest C. botulinum without adverse effects, the cause for the illness is still obscure. A number of host factors, possibly constipation, immune deficiency, or an unusual gut flora, must also be present to permit germination of the spores and production of the toxin within the gastrointestinal tract.

The diagnosis of infantile botulism is difficult to establish because the condition mimics septicemia, viral encephalitis, neonatal myasthenia gravis, and infectious polyneuritis. The predominance of bulbar symptoms in an infant who appears fairly aware of the surroundings should alert the clinician to the diagnosis, and prompt the performance of an EMG. The diagnosis is confirmed by isolation of C. botulinum and botulinal toxin from the feces.

Symptomatic therapy, including respiratory support and nasogastric feeding, must suffice.

NEONATAL TETANUS

This condition is caused by a clostridial infection of the umbilical stump. Although extremely rare in this country and limited to home-delivered infants (Adams et al., 1979), the condition is a major health hazard in some underdeveloped countries (Pinheiro, 1964). The manifestations of tetanus result from the action of the toxin within the spinal cord and brain stem. The toxin prevents the release of the neurotransmitters gamma-aminobutyric acid (GABA) and glycine from the presynaptic terminals of the inhibitory polysynaptic circuits surrounding the motor neurons. Abolition of the inhibitory influence of afferent fibers on the motor neurons produces the uncontrolled firing that results in the paroxysmal muscle spasms. At high concentrations, excitatory transmission is also reduced, and the toxin prevents release of acetylcholine from the neuromuscular junction, thereby producing a flaccid paralysis. In addition, elevation of serum creatine phosphokinase (CPK) and fluorescent binding techniques provide evidence that tetanospasmin produces direct injury to skeletal muscles. The molecular pharmacology of tetanus and botulinal toxins is reviewed by Simpson (1986).

This condition is a major cause of neonatal mortality in those underdeveloped countries where cord sepsis and lack of maternal immunity contribute to its high incidence.

It develops between the 5th to 10th day of life, with the more severe cases having a shorter incubation period. Irritability and trismus, with consequent inability to suck, are usually the earliest signs. As the disease progresses, infants develop opisthotonos and generalized tetanic spasms. These can be induced by stimulation or, in more severe cases, appear spontaneously. In the most severe cases, the spasms become continuous and are accompanied by apneic episodes.

Treatment of neonatal tetanus is difficult even in the technically more advanced countries. In their series of five patients, Adams and associates (1979) used nasotracheal intubation, mechanical ventilation, and neuromuscular blockade with pancuronium bromide to permit ventilatory control. When such facilities are not available, the infant is placed in a dark room, and penicillin is administered intravenously for 7 to 10 days together with other antibiotics, as indicated by the culture of the umbilical stump. Tetanus antiserum (30,000 to 40,000 U) is administered subcutaneously around the umbilicus and 1500 U are given intravenously. A variety of sedatives have been advocated, but the choice of sedative does not appear to influence the outcome. Rather, early tracheostomy and ventilator support may be responsible for the overall reduction in mortality in a series by Udwadia et al. (1987) in India.

Symptoms gradually abate after 25 to 45 days, and survivors appear neurologically and developmentally normal at 12 months of age.

■ DISEASES OF MUSCLE

THE MUSCULAR DYSTROPHIES

Of the various forms of muscular dystrophy only one group of conditions, termed "congenital muscular dystrophy," is evident at birth. Duchenne muscular dystrophy, which is sex-linked and the most common of these conditions, does not produce obvious clinical symptoms until after the child begins walking.

The cause of congenital muscular dystrophy is unknown. In one variant, first described by Fukuyama and co-workers (1981), severe mental retardation and seizures accompany muscular weakness. Although rare outside of Japan, this condition is only second in frequency to Duchenne muscular dystrophy in that country. It is transmitted as an autosomal recessive disorder. Muscle weakness is present from birth on, with contractures appearing early. In addition to generalized limb and trunk weakness, there is also facial involvement. Creatine kinase (CK) levels are generally elevated, and may reach 10 to 50 times normal after 6 months of age. The CT scan is often spectacular with massive decrease in the density of white matter in about one-third of these infants. The electroencephalogram (EEG) may show paroxysmal discharges, and the visual evoked potentials may also be abnormal. An inflammatory cell infiltration of muscle can be quite striking, and has led some authors to postulate that the condition is the consequence of an intrauterine infection. Within the brain there is micropolygyria, and hypoplasia of myelin. The condition is progressive and generally fatal by the end of the first decade.

Another variant, Ullrich disease, is an autosomal recessive condition characterized by a nonprogressive or slowly advancing congenital muscle weakness, striking congenital contractures of the proximal joints, hyperextensibility of the distal joints, and normal intelligence (Nonaka et al., 1981).

In most of the other congenital muscular dystrophies, serum CK levels are mildly to moderately elevated (McMenamin et al., 1982), and ECG abnormalities are found in about 20 per cent of patients (Donner et al., 1975). Electromyography usually elicits a myopathic pattern, although neurogenic changes have been recorded (McMenamin et al., 1982). Muscle biopsy demonstrates pathologic changes consistent with a dystrophic process (Dubowitz, 1985). As is the case for Duchenne muscular dystrophy, treatment is entirely supportive. Nevertheless, the clinical course is not inexorably downhill but remains more or less static.

MYOTONIC DISORDERS

A number of genetically distinct conditions share the clinical feature of myotonia of the voluntary muscles. Of these, congenital myotonic dystrophy is the only one liable to be encountered in the newborn.

The main features of the disease, as it expresses itself in infancy, are generalized hypotonia (involving principally the neck muscles), difficulty with sucking and swallowing, and, occasionally, severe respiratory difficulties (Harper, 1975). Arthrogryposis may be present at birth, and there may be a history of recurrent hydramnios. Myotonia is not demonstrable on clinical examination or by electromyography (Dubowitz, 1980).

The disease is transmitted as an autosomal dominant trait, but for unknown reasons, the mother is the affected parent in some 90 per cent of infants (Dyken and Harper, 1973). Inasmuch as serum CPK values and electromyographic findings are usually normal during the neonatal period and muscle biopsy demonstrates only arrested maturation of fibers (Sarnat and Silbert, 1976), the diagnosis is best determined by eliciting myotonia on the electromyogram of the affected parent.

About one-half of the infants whose myotonic dystrophy is symptomatic during the neonatal period die before 1 year of age. The survivors show gradual improvement of their hypotonia and respiratory and feeding difficulties; in fact, many of them will learn to walk. However, mental retardation becomes apparent in some 80 to 90 per cent (Harper, 1975).

Only supportive treatment is available for the myotonic infant. Linkage of the locus for myotonic dystrophy with those of apolipoprotein C2, and several anonymous genomic clones have allowed the gene to be localized to the proximal long arm of chromosome 19 (19q 13.2). The combined use of these probes will facilitate carrier detection and prenatal diagnosis.

CONGENITAL MYOPATHIES ("BENIGN CONGENITAL HYPOTONIAS")

For several years, the term "benign congenital hypotonia" has designated muscular weakness in an infant who, rather than getting progressively worse and finally dying of his condition (as is usually the case in infantile spinal muscular atrophy), may either improve with progressive muscular maturation or at least hold his own. Oppenheim's (1900) poorly described patients with amyotonia congenita would probably belong to this group, along with a number of those with new and pathologically

TABLE 47–1. Some Congenital Myopathies

DISEASE	CHARACTERISTIC CLINICAL FEATURES	MUSCLE BIOPSY ABNORMALITIES
Nemaline myopathy	Dominant or sporadic transmission; associated skeletal dysmorphism; respiratory problems	Rod-like expansions of Z band
Central core disease	Dominant or sporadic transmission; associated congenital dislocation of hip	Central area of fiber devoid of mitochondria; myofibril disruption variable
Myotubular myopathies	Ptosis; weak external ocular muscles; autosomal dominant and sex-linked forms	Small fibers, mostly type I, with central nuclei in chains
Mitochondrial myopathies	Extremely variable	Increased size or numbers of mitochondria, "ragged-red" fibers
Multicore (Minicore) disease	Nonprogressive proximal weakness; neck muscle weakness	Multiple small areas of severe filament disruption devoid of mitochondrial enzymes
Congenital fiber type disproportion	Muscle contractures; congenital dislocation of hips	Type I fibers smaller than type II; increased variability in fiber diameter
Fingerprint myopathy	Tremors; mental retardation	Subsarcolemmal; inclusions resembling fingerprints
Sarcotubular myopathy	None	Dilated and fragmented sarcotubules in type II fibers
Zebra-body myopathy	None	Unique bodies on electron microscopy
Reducing body myopathy	None	Inclusions rich in SH groups and ribonucleic acid
Trilaminar myopathy	Rigidity of muscle tone gradually disappearing with age; increased serum CPK	Distinctive 3-zone fibers by histochemistry and electron microscopy
Cytoplasmic body myopathy	None	Cytoplasmic bodies in myofibrils
Central nuclei myopathy	X-linked transmission; fatal during neonatal period	Small muscle fibers with central nuclei
Cylindrical spiral	Cramps, percussion myotonia, autosomal dominant	Cylindrical spirals
Myopathy with excessive autophagy	Early onset, affecting proximal muscles, slow progression, marked CK elevation, sex-linked	Increased number autophagic vacuoles
Polysaccharide storage myopathy	Proximal myopathy, no demonstrable abnormality of glycogen pathway	Branched-chain polysaccharides and mucoprotein storage

(From Menkes, J. H.: Textbook of Child Neurology. 4th ed. Philadelphia, Lea & Febiger, 1990.)

well-defined muscular disorders (Brooke et al., 1979). Clinical features characteristic of each entity are listed in Table 47–1.

MUSCULAR HYPERTROPHY

Congenital muscular hypertrophy can be associated with several distinct conditions. A syndrome of generalized muscular enlargement, severe mental retardation with widespread porencephaly, was first described by de Lange in 1934. It is probably not too uncommon, for we have seen several such infants in whom severe developmental retardation was the consequence of perinatal asphyxia.

Hypothyroidism (Debré-Sémélaigne syndrome) and myotonic dystrophy are two rare causes of congenital muscular hypertrophy (Wilson and Walton, 1959). Finally, a syndrome (Beckwith-Wiedemann) of muscular hypertrophy, macroglossia, omphalocele or umbilical hernia, transient neonatal hypoglycemia, mental retardation, and microcephaly has been described by a number of authors (Sotelo-Avila et al., 1980).

OTHER MUSCULAR DISEASES

In addition to the disorders listed in Table 47–1, several disorders of glycogen metabolism can present during the neonatal period. Of these, glycogen storage disease, type II (Pompe disease) is probably the most common. This condition presents with severe weakness and hypotonia and impaired swallowing and sucking. It can be distinguished clinically from the other muscular disorders by the associated presence of cardiomegaly, ECG abnormalities, and, occasionally, hepatomegaly. An excess of glycogen is apparent on muscle biopsy (Dubowitz, 1980).

Glycogen storage diseases, type III (debrancher deficiency) and type V (McArdle disease), have also been

reported in early infancy (Dubowitz, 1980; DiMauro and Hartlage, 1978).

■ REFERENCES

Adams, J. M., Kenny, J. D., and Rudolph, A. J.: Modern management of tetanus neonatorum. Pediatrics 64:472, 1979.

Aminoff, M. J.: Electrodiagnosis in Clinical Neurology. New York, Churchill-Livingstone, 1986.

Arnon, S. S.: Infant botulism. Ann. Rev. Med. 31:541, 1980.

Arnon, S. S.: Infant botulism: Anticipating the second decade. J. Infect. Dis. 154:201, 1986.

Brooke, M. H.: A Clinician's View of Neuromuscular Diseases. 2nd ed. Baltimore, Williams and Wilkins, 1986.

Brooke, M. H., Carroll, J. E., and Ringel, S. P.: Congenital hypotonia revisited. Muscle and Nerve 2:84, 1979.

Byers, R. K., and Banker, B. Q.: Infantile muscular atrophy. Arch. Neurol. 5:140, 1961.

de Lange, C.: Congenital hypertrophy of the muscles, extrapyramidal motor disturbances and mental deficiency. Am. J. Dis. Child. 48:243, 1934.

DiMauro, S., and Hartlage, P. L.: Fatal infantile form of muscle phosphorylase deficiency. Neurology 28:1124, 1978.

Donner, M., Rapola, J., and Somer, H.: Congenital muscular dystrophy: A clinico-pathological and follow-up study of 15 patients. Neuropädiatrie 6:239, 1975.

Dubowitz, V.: The Floppy Infant. Clin. Dev. Med. No. 76, London, William Heinemann, 1980.

Dubowitz, V.: Muscle Biopsy. A Practical Approach. 2nd ed. London, Baillière Tindall, 1985.

Dyken, P. R., and Harper, P. S.: Congenital dysmorphica myotonica. Neurology 24:465, 1973.

Fukuyama, Y., Osawa, M., Suzuki, H.: Congenital progressive muscular dystrophy of the Fukuyama Type—Clinical, genetic and pathological considerations. Brain Dev 3:1, 1981.

Goebel, H. H., Zeman, W., and DeMyer, W.: Peripheral motor and sensory neuropathy of early childhood simulating Werdnig-Hoffmann disease. Neuropädiatrie 7:182, 1976.

Hageman, G., et al.: The pathogenesis of fetal hypokinesia. A neurological study of 75 cases of congenital contractures with emphasis on cerebral lesions. Neuropediatrics 18:22, 1987a.

Hageman, G., et al.: The heterogeneity of the Pena-Shokeir syndrome. Neuropediatrics 18:45, 1987b.

Hall, J. G.: Arthrogryposis and the other neuromuscular and motor neuron disorders. *In* Hoffman, H. J., and Epstein, F. (Eds.): Disorders of the Developing Nervous System. Boston, Blackwell Scientific Publications, 1986, pp. 289–300.

Harper, P. S.: Congenital myotonic dystrophy in Britain. I. Clinical aspects. Arch. Dis. Child. *50*:505, 1975.

Kasman, M., Bernstein, L., and Schulman, S.: Chronic polyradiculoneuropathy of infancy. Neurology *26*:565, 1976.

Keesey, J., et al.: Anti-acetylcholine receptor antibody in neonatal myasthenia gravis. N. Engl. J. Med. *296*:55, 1977.

McMenamin, J. B., Becker, L. E., and Murphy, E. G.: Congenital muscular dystrophy: a clinicopathological report of 24 cases. J. Pediatr. *100*:692, 1982.

Misulis, K. E., Fenichel, G. M.: Genetic forms of myasthenia gravis. Pediatr Neurol 5:205, 1989.

Nonaka, I., Une, Y., Ishihara, T., et al.: A clinical and histological study of Ullrich's disease (congenital atonic-sclerotic muscular dystrophy). Neuropediatrics 12:197, 1981.

Oppenheim, H.: Über allgemeine und lokalisierte Atonie der Muskulatur (Myotonia) im frühen Kindesalter. Monatsschr. Psychiat. Neurol. *8*:232, 1900.

Péña, C. E., et al.: Arthrogryposis multiplex congenita: Report of two cases of a radicular type with familial incidence. Neurology *18*:926, 1968.

Pinheiro, D.: Tetanus of the newborn infant. Pediatrics *34*:32, 1964.

Probst, A., et al.: Sensory ganglioneuropathy in infantile spinal muscular atrophy. Neuropediatrics *12*:215, 1981.

Sarnat, H. B., and Silbert, S. W.: Maturational arrest of fetal muscle in neonatal myotonic dystrophy. Arch. Neurol. *33*:466, 1976.

Simpson, L. L.: Molecular pharmacology of botulinus toxin and tetanus toxin. Ann. Rev. Pharmacol. Toxicol. *26*:427, 1986.

Sotelo-Avila, C., Gonzalez-Crussi, F., and Fowler, J. W.: Complete and incomplete forms of Beckwith-Wiedemann syndrome: Their oncogenic potential. J. Pediatr. *96*:47, 1980.

Udwadia, F. E., Lall, A., Udwadia, Z. F., et al.: Tetanus and its complications: Intensive care and management experience in 150 Indian patients. Epidemiol. Infect. 99:675, 1987.

Wilson, J., and Walton, J. N.: Some muscular manifestations of hypothyroidism. J. Neurol. Neurosurg. Psychiat. *22*:320, 1959.

MISCELLANEOUS NEUROLOGIC DISORDERS PRESENTING IN THE NEWBORN

48

John H. Menkes*

■ FOCAL INTRACRANIAL SUPPURATIVE LESIONS

Despite the frequent occurrence of bacterial sepsis and meningitis in the newborn and young infant, brain abscesses as well as other focal suppurative infections are unusual in this age group. When abscess within the cerebrum does occur in early infancy, it is usually secondary to septicemia. Because of its rarity and the nonspecific character of its clinical manifestations, the condition often goes unsuspected.

Vomiting, lethargy, convulsions, and signs of increased intracranial pressure are the most common features of brain abscess in the young infant. Tenseness of the anterior fontanel and rapidly progressive head enlargement have been present in most reported cases in early infancy (Hoffman et al., 1970). Fever is frequently absent, but peripheral blood leukocytosis is customary. Cerebral abscess formation in the infant is multiple in some cases but when solitary is likely to reach enormous proportions before causing death or until the lesion is identified by neuroimaging studies or ultrasonography. Treatment consists of appropriate antibiotic therapy and proper drainage of the lesion. The mortality rate is high in this age group. Progressive hydrocephalus requiring shunting is a common complication among survivors.

Subdural empyema is a more common intracranial suppurative lesion than brain abscess in early infancy (Farmer and Wise, 1973). Suppuration may be either unilateral or bilateral, and most cases complicate gram-negative or staphylococcal meningitis. Either subdural empyema, epidural emphyema, or meningitis may also complicate an infected cephalhematoma in the newborn child. Pus in the subdural space is poorly tolerated by the young infant and sometimes leads to cortical vein or venous sinus thrombosis. Signs due to the lesion are usually obscured by those of meningitis, and diagnosis is made by neuroimaging studies. Subdural empyema rep-

resents a serious complication of meningitis in the infant and is associated with a high incidence of lasting sequelae.

■ SPINAL EPIDURAL ABSCESS

Spinal epidural suppuration is uncommon at any age but is especially rare in early infancy. Of the few reported cases in the young infant, most have been caused by *Staphylococcus aureus* and have resulted from hematogenous spread in the septic child. Congenital dermal sinus in the low back can be complicated by epidural abscess formation, although this is infrequent, particularly in infancy.

Although symptoms are usually nonspecific, this condition should always be considered in an irritable infant who screams when moved or handled and in whom tenderness of the spine can be elicited.

The diagnosis is best made by magnetic resonance imaging of the spinal canal.

Treatment of the condition includes intravenously administered antibiotics and surgical drainage of the lesion. The prognosis is far better in early recognized cases, and the greater the neurologic deficits, and the longer they persist before surgical drainage, the less the extent of expected recovery (Aicardi and Lepintre, 1967).

■ REYE SYNDROME

Reye syndrome is characterized by an acute, usually severe noninflammatory encephalopathy and impaired liver function with hypoglycemia and elevated glutamic oxalacetic transaminase and ammonia levels. It often follows a viral illness by several days. The pathogenesis remains obscure. In essence, the condition represents a generalized impairment of mitochondrial function. It accompanies a large number of viral illnesses, notably varicella; in addition, the association between Reye syndrome and administration of salicylates has been established by epidemiological studies.

Although Reye syndrome is unusual in infancy, it has been described in at least three infants in the first month

---

*This chapter includes portions written by Dr. William E. Bell that appeared in the 4th edition of this book.

of life (Huttenlocher and Trauner, 1978). In 1980, Sullivan-Bolyai and co-workers noted a high percentage of affected black males in their series and a more severe outcome when the disorder occurred in the first months of life.

■ INTRACRANIAL DURAL VENOUS SINUS AND CEREBRAL VEIN THROMBOSIS

Once a common entity, thrombosis of the dural sinuses or cerebral veins has become a relatively infrequent condition as a consequence of the use of fluid therapy and antibiotics. At present, its clinical picture is seen in infants with severe and usually cyanotic congenital heart disease and in various other conditions associated with a hypercoagulable state (Vomberg, et al., 1987).

Purulent venous thrombosis is also now rarely seen. In infants with cyanotic congenital heart disease, the thrombus generally involves the dural sinus, most often the superior longitudinal (sagittal) sinus, and the tributary cerebral veins. The clinical picture is protean and nonspecific, and the entity must be kept in mind whenever neurologic symptoms complicate a febrile illness in an infant with cyanotic congenital heart disease or some other debilitating condition (Banker, 1961; Yang et al., 1969). Most commonly, one sees changes in consciousness, focal or generalized seizures, focal motor deficits, and evidence of increased intracranial pressure in the form of papilledema or a full fontanel. Dilatation of the scalp veins is quite rare. Abnormalities in the CSF depend on when in the course of the illness the specimen is secured. Soon after thrombosis, the CSF is clear and under slightly increased pressure. Later on, increased pressure is seen in about 50 per cent of instances. The fluid may be xanthochromic or grossly bloody, and there may be a striking increase of protein content. Pleocytosis in the absence of an infection is not unusual.

The diagnosis of sinus or cortical vein thrombosis by neuroimaging studies is difficult and full of pitfalls, even in the most expert hands. Whenever cerebral angiography is used, it is imperative that the venous phase be adequately visualized, and that venous subtraction films be obtained. In some instances, the diagnosis is not possible without jugular venography. On CT scans evaluation of the noncontrast portion of the study is always necessary, and the distinction between filling defects and artifacts is not at all clear-cut. Magnetic resonance imaging (MRI) may be superior in that it can demonstrate sinus or venous thromboses not visualized on CT (Hanigan et al., 1986).

Aside from maintaining an adequate state of hydration and the usual supportive measures, little can be done to help the infant with dural sinus or cerebral vein thrombosis once this process has begun. Heparin has been used in the hope that its early administration may prevent the spread of the thrombus. At present there is no randomized study to document its effectiveness, and it is contraindicated when there is evidence of cortical vein infarction and, thus, a significant likelihood for cerebral hemorrhage.

■ CONGENITAL INTRACRANIAL ANEURYSMS AND VASCULAR MALFORMATIONS

Saccular, or berry, aneurysms, generally considered to be the result of localized congenital defects of the media of the arterial wall, rarely give rise to clinical illness in infancy or childhood. They are usually located on major vessels at the base of the brain, and they give rise to symptoms and signs either by rupture with subarachnoid hemorrhage or by a mass effect with compression on adjacent structures. Clinical manifestations in the newborn period or in early infancy caused by aneurysms of this type are extremely rare but have been described (Lee et al., 1978). In the few neonatal cases described, spontaneous intracranial bleeding is characterized by an abrupt onset, irritability, vomiting, decreased alertness or coma, and findings indicative of sudden increase in intracranial pressure. Diagnosis before death depends on imaging studies, and if necessary, angiographic examination.

A better known type of congenital aneurysm that can produce signs in the newborn is aneurysmal malformation of the great vein of Galen (Fig. 48–1).

This lesion actually represents an arteriovenous shunt of large volume. When signs of a vein of Galen arteriovenous malformation (AVM) appear during the neonatal period, initial manifestations take the form of hydrocephalus (42 per cent), seizures (26 per cent), or distention and tortuosity of scalp veins (26 per cent) (Gold et al., 1964). Congestive heart failure with cardiomegaly is sometimes the presenting finding. Hydrocephalus is caused by aqueductal obstruction by the vein of Galen or aqueductal ependymitis and subarachnoid adhesions associated with intracranial hemorrhage. A loud intracranial bruit, often heard without auscultation, a palpable thrill, and engorged scalp veins are other notable features (Gomez et al., 1963; So, 1978). Diagnosis of this type of vascular malformation is made on the basis of imaging studies. Treatment is by embolization or by ligation of the afferent vessels.

Arteriovenous malformations in the cerebral parenchyma only rarely produce clinical signs in the newborn or young infant but can be a source of spontaneous bleeding or seizures. Intraventricular hemorrhage, sometimes fatal, can occur in early infancy as well as in older persons from a cryptic hemangioma of the choroid plexus (Doe et al., 1972). Most described cases have been identified at necropsy.

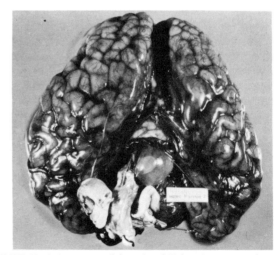

FIGURE 48–1. *Aneurysm of the vein of Galen: Large, saccular mass is located just dorsal to the upper brain stem and, thus, in close proximity to the aqueduct of Sylvius. Initial clinical manifestations are caused by either aqueductal obstruction or high-output cardiac failure.*

■ CONGENITAL BRAIN TUMORS

Although certain types of intracranial tumors are believed to arise from congenital "rests," it is decidedly unusual for abnormal signs to be present in the neonatal period. Chordomas originate from notochord remnants but rarely become symptomatic until adulthood. It has been postulated that craniopharyngiomas develop from remains of the embryonic Rathke pouch but only infrequently cause abnormal signs in the young infant (Azar-Kia et al., 1975).

Congenital brain tumors that do give rise to neurologic abnormalities in the newborn period are more often supratentorial (75 to 80 per cent of cases) and tend to present with increased intracranial pressure, enlarging head size, and less often, intracerebral hemorrhage (Tellinger and Sunder-Plassmann, 1973). Their histologic characteristics are generally unusual. A number of cases with cerebral teratomas have been described in newborns, sometimes with massive involvement of the brain by the neoplasm (Oberman, 1964). Meningiomas, medulloblastomas, and pontine gliomas have also been reported in the newborn but have no characteristic clinical features that will aid in their recognition.

Papilloma of the choroid plexus sometimes will cause abnormal head enlargement in the early weeks of life and is an important lesion because of the possibility of its surgical removal. Infants with this tumor are usually considered to have hydrocephalus due to the more common causes until an intraventricular mass is demonstrated by imaging studies or ultrasonography.

Nasal glioma is a congenital tumor composed of connective tissue and neural elements. The lesion may present extranasally, as a firm nonpulsatile mass at the base of the nose or intranasally, in which case it is easily confused with a nasal polyp (Strauss et al., 1966). The mass is benign and is generally regarded to be a glial heterotopia and not a brain tumor in the usual sense. Differential diagnosis includes dermoid cyst, nasal polyp, and nasal encephalocele.

Although more properly a concern of the physician dealing with neurologic problems of late infancy and childhood, the phakomatoses (neurocutaneous syndromes) occasionally are evident at birth.

Approximately 43 per cent of infants with neurofibromatosis exhibit physical signs at birth, usually multiple café-au-lait spots (Fienman and Yakovac, 1970). Symptoms of tuberous sclerosis can be present at birth or in early infancy (Thibault and Manuelides, 1970). The characteristic depigmented nevi are sometimes visible at birth; in the experience of Pampiglione and Moynahan, reported in 1976, 12 per cent of their patients developed adenoma sebaceum prior to 1 year of age. Seizures may also be present during the neonatal period, and the CT scan demonstrates the multiple scattered calcium deposits at a time when plain radiographs of the skull are still negative (Gomez, 1987).

Sturge-Weber syndrome is readily diagnosable in the newborn by observation of the presence of a port-wine vascular nevus on the upper part of the face involving at least one eyelid and the supraorbital region. CT scans or even plain skull films may show intracranial calcifications (Nellhaus et al., 1967).

■ CONGENITAL INTRASPINAL TUMORS

Intraspinal tumors, which are infrequent in early infancy, are less likely to be intramedullary in infants than they are in older children. Because of the rare occurrence of intraspinal masses in this age group, the difficulty in recognizing the progressive nature of the neurologic deficits and the relatively poor diagnostic value of neurogenic bladder and sensory disturbances, early identification of such lesions is often delayed. They are easily confused with, and erroneously diagnosed as, cerebral palsy, cervical cord birth injury, or brachial plexus stretch palsy.

Intraspinal lesions above the second lumbar vertebra cause signs of spinal cord dysfunction. The character of signs of cord involvement or compression is less predictable in infants than in older children. Although spastic signs are expected, the infant with a cervical or thoracic cord lesion can present with hypotonic limbs that exhibit enhanced deep stretch reflexes. Spinal rigidity, although not always present, is a finding that should suggest the possibility of some form of intraspinal mass, regardless of the age of the child. Intraspinal lesions below the second lumbar vertebra give rise to manifestations of cauda equina compression or to a combination of signs indicative of involvement of the conus medullaris and the cauda equina. Compression of the cauda equina results in hypotonic or flaccid legs, often asymmetrically so, with reflex loss and muscular atrophy in affected regions. A sensory level to pin stimulation usually indicates a spinal cord lesion but can also occur with intraspinal lesions below the termination of the spinal cord.

Although astrocytomas or ependymomas of the spinal cord can occur in infancy, they are unusual in the newborn period (Tachdjian and Matson, 1965.) Signs of congenital neuroblastoma are usually those of metastatic disease and include hepatomegaly and cutaneous nodules (Schneider et al., 1965), but direct invasion to the intraspinal epidural space can also complicate these lesions. Direct extension from a primary adrenal tumor is likely to affect the mid-to-low thoracic cord, whereas that from a mediastinal neuroblastoma will involve the low cervical or upper thoracic portion of the spinal cord. Sarcomatous lesions of various types can either invade the epidural space from the retroperitoneal region or arise primarily within the spinal canal. Extramedullary compression of the spinal cord can also result from a variety of benign or malignant tumors of the vertebrae.

Probably the most frequently identified intraspinal tumor in the young infant is the intradural lipoma (Dubowitz et al., 1965). Most are found in the lumbar or lumbosacral region, although they can occur elsewhere. The presence of a lumbar intradural lipoma is usually signaled by the presence of an associated extradural lipomatous mass, which presents as a soft painless swelling on the midline of the low back. A cutaneous dermal sinus or hemangioma is frequently observed in the region of the superficial mass. Radiographs of the spine are diagnostically revealing in most cases because of the presence of widening of the pedicles with pedicular erosion. When the intradural mass extends into the lower part of the spinal canal, hypoplasia or destructive changes of the sacrum are often visualized. Neurologic signs caused by an intradural lipoma usually do not develop until the child is a few years of age.

In the infant with intradural lipoma, signs of denervation, when present, are usually in the form of a foot deformity and wasting of one lower limb, with associated deep reflex asymmetry. The advisability of surgical excision of the intradural lipoma is a controversial matter. Complete removal can usually not be accomplished because of the intimate relationship between the mass and the neural elements. Partial excision is recommended when there is evidence of progressive neurologic dysfunction, although every effort must be made not to produce additional deficits from the surgical procedure itself.

Diagnosis of an intraspinal tumor of any type is on the basis of the clinical findings and appropriate imaging studies of the cord. MRI with gadolinium enhancement has become the study of choice, almost completely replacing the need for myelography and intrathecal contrast-enhanced CT (Hyman and Gorey, 1988). MRI provides a direct image of the spinal cord, and following gadolinium enhancement, which offers better delineation of tumor tissue from the low signal of CSF, demonstrates both extramedullary and intramedullary tumors, readily distinguishing the latter from hydromyelia. In these studies it is essential to obtain midsagittal views. Should MRI be negative, a CT scan with intrathecal metrizamide can be considered, since this procedure is preferable for the detection of extramedullary, intradural infiltrates. For the delineation of vascular tumors of the cord, MRI can be followed by CT scanning in combination with digital subtraction angiography, with intravenous injection of contrast material.

■ HEREDODEGENERATIVE DISEASES

Only a few of the heredodegenerative diseases affecting the nervous system occur in the newborn (Table 48–1).

TABLE 48–1. Heredodegenerative Diseases Apparent During the First Month of Life

CONDITION
Diffuse cerebral degenerative diseases
White matter degenerations
Globoid cell leukodystrophy (Krabbe's disease)
Spongy degeneration of white matter (Canavan's disease)
Metachromatic leukodystrophy
Pelizaeus-Merzbacher disease
Infantile neuroaxonal dystrophy
Alexander's disease
Gray matter degenerations
"Alper's disease" (lactic acidoses, mitochondrial myopathies)
Kinky hair disease (Menkes syndrome)
Heredodegenerative diseases of the basal ganglia
None
Heredodegenerative diseases of cerebellum, brain stem, spinal cord, and peripheral nerve
Hypertrophic interstitial polyneuropathy (Dejerine-Sottas disease)
White matter hypoplasia
Giant axonal neuropathy
Familial dysautonomia
Lipid storage diseases
Congenital amaurotic idiocy
GM₁ gangliosidosis
GM₃ gangliosidosis
Lipogranulomatosis (Farber's disease)
I-cell disease
Peroxisomal disorders
Infantile Refsum disease
Zellweger syndrome
Neonatal adrenoleukodystrophy

TABLE 48–2. Clinical Pointers to the Presence of Heredodegenerative Diseases

Cutaneous Abnormalities
Erythema becoming ichthyosis: Sjögren-Larsson (spasticity and seizures)
Hair Abnormalities
Kinky hair: Kinky hair disease
Argininosuccinic aciduria
Multiple carboxylase deficiency
Giant axonal neuropathy
Pollitt syndrome (mental retardation, seizures)
Unusual Facies
Coarse: I-cell disease (Mucolipidosis II)
GM₁ gangliosidosis (infantile)
Slight coarsening (difficult to pick up without other family members): Sialidosis II
Cataracts
Galactosemia
Cherry-Red Spot
Tay-Sachs and Sandhoff disease (GM₂ gangliosidosis)
GM₁ gangliosidosis (infantile)
Niemann-Pick disease (Types A and C)
Infantile Gaucher (Type II)

As a rule, these diseases are difficult to diagnose during the neonatal period. Their clinical manifestations (i.e., spasticity, hypotonia, seizures, unusual eye movements) are far more commonly the consequence of perinatal asphyxia or cerebral malformations. Thus, it is only when the infant's progressive deterioration becomes evident that their presence begins to be suspected.

A few clues, however, have been established. The presence of combined upper and lower motor neuron signs—the most common of which are seizures, hypotonia, and absent deep tendon reflexes—should alert the physician to a white matter degenerative disease. One can confirm the diagnosis by finding a striking elevation of CSF protein and characteristic pathologic alterations on a sural nerve biopsy. Some of the clues disclosed on physical examination that suggest a heredodegenerative disease are summarized in Table 48–2.

The presence of kinky, poorly pigmented hair points to kinky hair disease (Menkes disease) or giant axonal neuropathy, whereas a hoarse cry suggests lipogranulomatosis, cretinism, or Cornelia de Lange syndrome. Coarse facies is an early feature of I-cell disease and generalized GM₁ and GM₃ gangliosidoses. Macroglossia occurs in the newborn not only with cretinism but also with Beckwith-Wiedemann syndrome, GM₁ gangliosidosis, and GM₃ gangliosidosis. The diagnosis of the last two disorders depends on a biopsy of bone marrow or skin.

For a fuller discussion of these disorders, the reader is referred to texts of child neurology (e.g., Menkes, 1990).

FAMILIAL DYSAUTONOMIA (RILEY-DAY SYNDROME)

Although its name suggests that the disease is exclusively a disorder of the autonomic nervous system, peripheral sensory neurons, peripheral motor neurons, and other neuronal populations are also affected. The condition is transmitted as an autosomal recessive trait, and is confined to Jews of Eastern European descent. In the United States, the frequency of the carrier state in this ethnic group is 1:50 (Mahloudji et al., 1970).

No consistent structural abnormality has been found

within the CNS. The sympathetic ganglia are hypoplastic, and there is a reduction in the number of neurons in the spinal ganglia, with hypoplasia of the dorsal root entry zones and the Lissauer tract (Pearson, 1979). In peripheral nerves, the number of myelinated and nonmyelinated axons is reduced, and the transverse fascicular area is diminished. Most importantly, it appears as if the catecholamine endings are absent. The primary metabolic lesion is still unknown, and no consistent abnormality in blood levels, urinary excretion, or tissue concentration of catecholamines or their metabolites has been found. Most clinical and pathologic alterations can best be explained by a deficit of a trophic factor essential to antenatal development, which also continues to have a minor postnatal sustaining function.

Familial dysautonomia is characterized by symptoms referable to the sensory and autonomic nervous system. No single feature, but rather their association, points to the diagnosis.

Nervous system dysfunction is usually evident in the neonatal period as a poor or absent sucking reflex, hypotonia, and hypothermia. Nursing difficulties result in frequent regurgitation (Axelrod et al., 1987). A high incidence of breech presentation (31 per cent) is unrelated to the birth weight but reflects intrauterine hypotonia. Many infants have serious feeding difficulties, including cyclic vomiting and recurrent pneumonia. In part, these may be attributed to absent or decreased lower esophageal peristalsis, a dilated esophagus, and impaired gastric motility.

Prognosis. Many patients succumb to the disease during infancy as a consequence of respiratory arrest during sleep, aspiration or infectious pneumonia, or cardiac and respiratory arrest precipitated by hypotension. More patients now survive to adulthood and many achieve independent function. Several women have had normal offspring.

The diagnosis of dysautonomia depends on the patient's history and genetic background and on the clinical features of the condition. Of the various tests designed to elicit autonomic dysfunction, the intradermal histamine test has been the most reliable in our experience. In normal subjects, intradermal injection of histamine phosphate (0.03 to 0.05 ml of a 1:1000 solution) produces a local wheal and a red erythematous flare extending 1 to 3 cm beyond the wheal. In dysautonomic patients, the flare response is absent. A similar response may be produced in atopic dermatitis and in some disorders of the spinal cord or peripheral nerves (e.g., progressive sensory neuropathy).

Treatment of the condition is purely symptomatic. Impaired swallowing as well as vomiting and abdominal distention may be relieved with bethanechol (Urecholine), a parasympathomimetic agent (Axelrod and Bloom, 1975).

REFERENCES

Aicardi, J., and Lepintre, J.: Spinal epidural abscess in a 1-month old child. Am. J. Dis. Child. *114*:665, 1967.

Axelrod, F. B., and Bloom, J.: Caring for the Child with Familial Dysautonomia (A Handbook for Patients). New York, Dysautonomic Foundation, 1975.

Axelrod, F. B., Porges, R. F. and Sein, M. E.: Neonatal recognition of familial dysautonomia. J. Pediatr. *110*:946, 1987.

Azar-Kia, B., Krishnan, U. R., and Schechter, M. M.: Neonatal craniopharyngioma. J. Neurosurg. *42*:91, 1975.

Banker, B. Q.: Cerebral vascular disease in infancy and childhood. I. Occlusive vascular disease. J. Neuropathol. Exp. Neurol. *20*:127, 1961.

Doe, F. D., Shuangshoti, S., and Netsky, M. G.: Cryptic hemangioma of the choroid plexus. Neurology *22*:1232, 1972.

Dubowitz, V., Lorber, J., and Zachary, R. B.: Lipoma of the cauda equina. Arch. Dis. Child. *40*:207, 1965.

Farmer, T. W., and Wise, G. R.: Subdural empyema in infants, children and adults. Neurology *23*:254, 1973.

Fienman, N. L., and Yakovac, W. C.: Neurofibromatosis in childhood. J. Pediatr. *76*:339, 1970.

Gold, A. P., Ransohoff, J., and Carter S.: Vein of Galen malformation. Acta Neurol. Scand. *40*(Suppl.11):1, 1964.

Gomez, M. R.: Tuberous sclerosis. *In* Gomez, M. R. (ed.): Neurocutaneous Diseases; A Practical Approach. Boston, Butterworths, 1987, pp. 30–52.

Gomez, M. R., Whitten, C. F., Nolke, A., et al.: Aneurysmal malformation of the great vein of Galen causing heart failure in early infancy. Pediatrics *31*:400, 1963.

Hanigan, W. C., Rossi, L. J., McLean, J. M., et al.: MRI of cerebral vein thrombosis in infancy: A case report. Neurology *36*:1354, 1986.

Hoffman, H. J., Hendrick, E. B., and Hiscox, J. L.: Cerebral abscess in early infancy. J. Neurosurg. *33*:172, 1970.

Huttenlocher, P. R., and Trauner, D. A.: Reye's syndrome in infancy. Pediatrics *62*:84, 1978.

Hyman, R. A., and Gorey, M. T.: Imaging strategies for MR of the spine. Radiol. Clin. North Am. *26*:505, 1988.

Jellinger, K., and Sunder-Plassmann, M.: Connatal intracranial tumors. Neuropädiatrie *4*:46, 1973.

Lee, Y. J., Kandall, S. R., and Ghali, V. S.: Intracerebral arterial aneurysm in a newborn. Arch. Neurol. *35*:171, 1978.

Mahloudji, M., Brunt, P. W., and McKusick, V. A.: Clinical neurological aspects of familial dysautonomia. J. Neurol. Sci. *11*:383, 1970.

Menkes, J. H.: Textbook of Child Neurology. 4th ed. Philadelphia, Lea & Febiger, 1990.

Nellhaus, G., Haberland, C., and Hill, B. J.: Sturge-Weber disease with bilateral intracranial calcification at birth and unusual pathologic findings. Acta Neurol. Scand. *43*:314, 1967.

Pampiglione, G., and Moynahan, E. J.: The tuberous sclerosis syndrome: Clinical and EEG studies in 100 children. J. Neurol. Neurosurg. Psychiat. *39*:666, 1976.

Pearson, J.: Familial dysautonomia. J. Auton. Nerv. Syst. *1*:119, 1979.

Schneider, K. M., Becker, J. M., and Krasna, I. H.: Neonatal neuroblastoma. Pediatrics *36*:359, 1965.

So, S. C.: Cerebral arteriovenous malformations in children. Childs Brain *2*:242, 1978.

Strauss, R. B., Callicott, J. H., and Hargett, I. R.: Intranasal neuroglial heterotopia. Am. J. Dis. Child. *111*:317, 1966.

Sullivan-Bolyai, J., Nielson, D. B., Morens, D. M., et al.: Reye syndrome in children less than 1 year old: Some epidemiological observations. Pediatrics *65*:627, 1980.

Tachdjian, M. O., and Matson, D. D.: Orthopaedic aspects of intraspinal tumors in infants and children. J. Bone Joint Surg. *47A*:223, 1965.

Thibault, J. H., and Manuelidis, E. E.: Tuberous sclerosis in a premature infant. Report of a case and review of the literature. Neurology *20*:139, 1970.

Vomberg, P. P., et al.: Cerebral thromboembolism due to antithrombin III deficiency in two children. Neuropediatrics *18*:42, 1987.

Yang, D. C., Sohn, D., and Anand, H.: K.: Thrombosis of the superior longitudinal sinus during infancy. J. Pediatr. *74*:570, 1969.

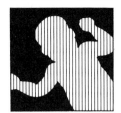

PART VIII

LUNG DEVELOPMENT AND FUNCTION **49**

Thomas Hansen and Anthony Corbet

■ LUNG DEVELOPMENT

The primordial lung bud appears on Day 26 of gestation as a ventral epithelial outgrowth from the foregut, with progressive caudal penetration of the primitive lung mesenchyme by continuous dichotomous branching. The mesenchyme exerts an inductive interaction with the epithelium. Lung development may be divided into five phases:

1. *Embryonic period, formation of proximal airways, 4 to 6 weeks.* The right and left main bronchi appear at 4 weeks, the five lobar bronchi at 5 weeks, and the 10 segmental bronchi on each side at 6 weeks.

2. *Glandular period, formation of conducting airways, 7 to 16 weeks.* By the end of this phase a total of about 20 generations of conducting airways have developed, the last eight generations being called bronchioles, because they are not destined to develop cartilage like the preceding bronchi. These conducting airways, lined by columnar epithelium, are nourished by capillaries from the bronchial circulation. Cartilage appears at 7 weeks in the trachea and develops peripherally, reaching the last bronchi at term. The pleural membranes and pulmonary lymphatics develop between 8 and 10 weeks.

3. *Canalicular period, formation of acini, 17 to 24 weeks.* At 17 weeks the first intra-acinar respiratory bronchioles develop by dichotomous branching, perhaps two to three generations, marking the birth of the acinus or gas-exchange part of the lung. An increasing number of capillaries appear in the prominent mesoderm, and connect with the pulmonary rather than the bronchial arteries. From 18 weeks multiple saccules arise from the last generation of respiratory bronchioles. The saccule is a wide channel with sparsely cellular mesoderm and a double capillary network. As the acini grow the saccules elongate, and the distance between the terminal bronchiole and pleura increases. Initially, the saccules have a smooth contour and are lined by cuboidal epithelium (Fig. 49–1) (Weibel, 1984). Granular pneumocytes, the site of

synthesis of surfactants, are usually distinguished at 20 weeks by the appearance of lamellar inclusions, but lamellar bodies may not be seen until later (Spear et al., 1969). Flattened membranous pneumocytes first appear at 24 weeks. This occurrence and a progressive decrease of mesoderm with development of more saccules allow the capillaries to approach closely and bulge into the

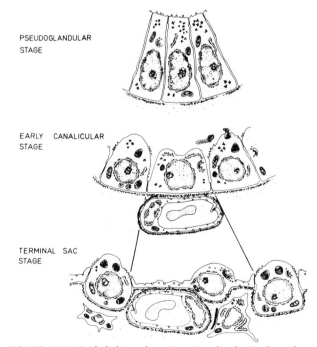

FIGURE 49–1. *Epithelial transformation in a developing lung, from a high columnar epithelium of uniform cell population in the glandular phase, to a cuboidal epithelium with two distinct cell types in the canalicular phase. In the saccular phase the prospective lining cells (type I) become flattened and broadened so that a thin barrier to the capillary is formed. Note that secretory type II cells with lamellar bodies occur as in the canalicular phase. (From Burri, P.H., and Weibel, E. R.: Ultrastructure and Morphometry of the Developing Lung. In Hodson, W. A. [Ed.]: Development of the Lung. New York, Marcel Dekker Inc., 1977, p. 215.)*

461

lumen, at which point the saccules assume a more irregular contour. Gas exchange requires close proximity of capillaries and air space. At 19 to 20 weeks, apposition of the capillary endothelial cells and alveolar lining cells occurs with sporadic points of fusion of the respective basement membranes. From that time, the total area of the alveolar-blood barrier increases exponentially. This structural development is one of the factors that determines preterm viability (Dimaio et al., 1989). Clinical observations are consistent with an insufficient alveolar-blood barrier before 23 to 24 weeks or even later in some infants.

4. *Saccular period, expansion of gas-exchange sites, 27 to 35 weeks.* At about 27 to 28 weeks there is an important change. The appearance of secondary crests begins the division of primary saccules into subsaccules or primitive alveoli, which have a flattened epithelium and a double capillary network. The interstitium becomes noticeably less prominent, and saccular development accelerates with a sudden increase of lung volume and surface area.

5. *Alveolar period, expansion of surface area, 36 weeks to 3 years post-term.* Starting as early as 30 weeks, but nearly always before 36 weeks, the subsaccules become alveoli. Before the first breath of air, the configuration is mostly saccular. Alveolation is accomplished by thinning of the interstitium and the appearance of a single capillary network, in which one capillary bulges into both the alveoli with which it is associated. The alveolus has a very thin wall, very thin interstitium, a single capillary network, and is polyhedral rather than rounded in contour. The process of alveolation starts distally in the saccules and proceeds proximally. At term gestation about 50 million alveoli are present, comprising the majority of terminal air spaces. After birth there is a comparative slowing in the development of alveoli during the first 3 months. But later, there is a rapid increase in alveolar number during the first year of life, reaching approximately the adult number of 300 million by 3 years of age (Fig. 49-2) (Weibel, 1984).

■ LUNG LIQUID

The potential airways of the fetus are in contact with amniotic fluid when the glottis is open. The possibility that the lung could contribute to amniotic fluid was first proposed by Jost and Policard (1948), when they demonstrated an increase in lung volume in the rabbit fetus after ligation of the trachea. Secretions from the nasopharyngeal and buccal cavities as well as the lung itself contribute to the tracheal effluent. Rarely does amniotic fluid itself enter the developing lung, except in circumstances of fetal distress. When the fetus is stimulated to gasp, sufficient pressure is applied across the lung to allow entry of amniotic fluid and sometimes its squamous debris and even meconium. The rapid, irregular respiratory movements described as fetal breathing do not, in effect, move much fluid, since fluid is approximately 100 times as viscous as air, and the rapid, small respiratory movements of the fetus are not associated with high transpulmonary pressures.

The lung liquid that fills the potential air spaces of the lung (20 to 30 ml/kg of body weight) is quite distinct from amniotic fluid or plasma (Table 49–1) (Adams, 1963; Adamson, 1969; Humphreys, 1967). Evidence for active secretion of lung liquid was provided by Strang (1967), who measured the ratios of cations and anions between lung liquid and plasma. He and co-workers later demonstrated that lung liquid required active transport of chloride ions from plasma in excess of the bicarbonate movement in the opposite direction (Olver and Strang, 1974). This liquid contains large amounts of chloride, relatively small amounts of bicarbonate, and almost no protein. Its potassium concentration is similar to that of plasma until near term, when it increases in response to surfactant secretion. Fetal lung liquid is secreted by the lung at approximately 4 to 6 ml/kg/hour along an electrochemical gradient that is produced by the active pumping of chloride from the interstitium into the air space. Although the site of the "chloride pump" is unknown, it can be inhibited by a variety of mediators that include beta-agonists, arginine vasopressin, and prostaglandin E_2 (Bland, 1988; Walters and Olver, 1978).

In order for the fetus to complete the transition from intrauterine to extrauterine life, the lung must clear this liquid soon after birth. The process of clearing liquid from the lung actually begins 2 to 3 days before birth with a decrease in the rate of secretion of fetal lung liquid, but lung liquid begins to clear in earnest only with the onset of labor. Recent data obtained from experiments using fetal lambs show that nearly two-thirds of the total clearance of liquid that occurs during the transition from intrauterine to extrauterine life occurs during labor (Bland, 1983 and 1988; Bland et al., 1982). Presumably, with the onset of labor, the active secretion of chloride ceases; hence, the secretion of fetal lung liquid ceases. Since this liquid contains very little protein, oncotic pressure favors the movement of water from the air space back into the

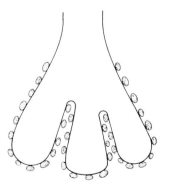

SACCULAR

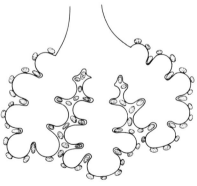

ALVEOLAR

FIGURE 49–2. Simplified model to show how a saccular lung is transformed postnatally into an alveolar lung. (From Weibel, E.R.: The Pathway for Oxygen: Structure and Function in the Mammalian Respiratory System. Cambridge, Mass., Harvard University Press, 1984.)

interstitium and then favors the movement of water from the interstitium back into the vascular compartment. Recent data also suggest that sodium may be transported actively from the air space to the interstitium, which would further facilitate the reabsorption of liquid (Berthiaume et al., 1987; Bland, 1988).

When the lungs expand after birth, water moves rapidly from the air spaces to the loose connective tissue of the extra-alveolar interstitium. It is then gradually removed from the lung by lymphatics and pulmonary blood vessels (Bland et al., 1982; Humphreys et al., 1967). The concomitant increase in pulmonary blood flow that occurs with air breathing facilitates water reabsorption into the vascular compartment. It has long been known that some infants delivered by cesarean section have transient respiratory distress related to delayed clearance of lung water. A small amount of liquid is expelled from the upper airways by vaginal compression of the chest at the time of birth. However, although lung water content in fetal rabbits delivered vaginally with labor is less than the lung water of rabbits delivered by cesarean section without labor, there is no difference in lung water if labor occurs in either vaginal or cesarean deliveries.

■ FETAL BREATHING

After many years of controversy, it is now established that the fetus breathes (Dawes, 1973). This breathing activity, which is essentially diaphragmatic, is present for 30 to 35 per cent of the time in mothers examined with a real-time ultrasonic scanner (Patrick, 1978). It is irregular in rate and amplitude; recorded rates in the human fetus range between 30 to 70 bpm. The tidal volume of liquid is small, quite insufficient to clear the dead space. Owing to active lung liquid secretion, the net flow is out of the lung. Periods of apnea may last as long as 1 hour in the normal human fetus. In the lamb, breathing occurs during active sleep, associated with low-voltage electrocortical activity, and is inhibited during quiet sleep, associated with high-voltage activity. There appears to be a circadian rhythm, breathing activity being lowest in the early morning and rising during the afternoon to peak in the early evening (Dawes, 1974). Fetal breathing has been detected as early as 10 weeks' gestation. However, it is suppressed as labor approaches, probably due to a progressive rise of plasma prostaglandins (Kitterman et al., 1983), and remains suppressed during active labor (Boylan and Lewis, 1980).

Fetal breathing is increased by drugs that stimulate the central nervous system, such as caffeine and isoproterenol, and it is inhibited by anesthetics, narcotics, barbiturates, ethanol, and smoking (Manning, 1977). Hypoglycemia or maternal fasting is associated with decreased fetal breathing, whereas it is stimulated after maternal meals and by hyperglycemia. Mild fetal hypoxemia severely depresses fetal breathing, but more severe fetal hypoxemia induces primitive deep gasping. It is thought that the hypoxia-sensitive carotid body chemoreceptors are active in the fetus, and provide a constant stimulus to breathing (Murai et al., 1985), but their effect on the central respiratory neurons is easily overridden by high-voltage electrocortical activity, or under certain conditions, by endogenous depressants such as prostaglandins, endorphins, or adeno-

TABLE 49–1. Interstitial Fluid Estimated from Measurements in Lung Lymph

COMPONENT	LUNG LIQUID	INTERSTITIAL FLUID	PLASMA	AMNIOTIC FLUID
Sodium (mEq/l)	150	147	150	113
Potassium (mEq/l)	6.3	4.8	4.8	7.6
Chloride (mEq/l)	157	107	107	87
Bicarbonate (mEq/l)	3	25	24	19
pH	6.27	7.31	7.34	7.02
Protein (g/dl)	0.03	3.27	4.09	0.10

sine (Jansen and Chernick, 1988). Hypercarbia has a rapid stimulatory effect on fetal breathing. A similar stimulation occurs with production of metabolic acidemia, but only after a latent interval to allow diffusion into the nervous system (Harding, 1984). The purpose of fetal breathing appears at least two-fold. To many physiologists, it is inconceivable that efficient postnatal breathing could be accomplished without prenatal practice. In addition, it appears that growth and development of the lungs is highly dependent on the distensive forces produced by fetal breathing.

ONSET OF BREATHING

Prior to birth, fetal breathing is episodic and dependent on the electrocortical state, but after birth breathing becomes continuous and independent of the electrocortical state. Experimentally in fetal lambs, breathing becomes continuous and independent of electrocortical state when the brain stem is sectioned just below the midbrain level (Dawes et al., 1983). Continuous breathing after birth may be due to suppression of this midbrain inhibitory influence. The somatic sensory stimulation associated with delivery can be a powerful stimulus to continuous breathing (Condorelli and Scarpelli, 1975). Similarly, cooling the skin without change of core temperature has been shown to stimulate continuous breathing in fetuses with normal blood gases (Gluckman et al., 1983). By increasing neuronal traffic in the brain stem, this may suppress the midbrain inhibition of breathing during the high-voltage electrocortical state.

After birth, the arterial P_{O_2} is much higher than before birth, increasing from 30 mm Hg to 70 mm Hg, and the arterial P_{CO_2} decreases from 45 mm Hg in the fetus to 35 mm Hg. Therefore, continuous postnatal breathing must be associated with a resetting of the threshold for both peripheral and central chemoreceptors. Without such a phenomenon, mild hypoxemia and hypercarbia could not be considered cause for continuous breathing in the newborn. In fact, mild fetal asphyxia, produced by clamping the umbilical cord, always induces continuous fetal breathing, and it does this without cooling or somatic sensory stimulation (Adamson et al., 1987). Because fetal hypoxemia causes respiratory depression and because the onset of breathing is not abolished by carotid body denervation (Jansen et al., 1981), it seems unlikely that hypoxemia is important. Hypercarbia, on the other hand, induced with CO_2 breathing by the mother, is a powerful stimulus to fetal breathing (Dawes et al., 1982), but not during the high-voltage electrocortical state. Even if hypercarbia is given the prime responsibility for continuous breathing at birth, there must still be an adjustment to the central chemoreceptor threshold, and there must still be a suppression of the inhibition during the high-voltage electrocortical state. In addition, the cord clamp that induced asphyxia may cut off the supply of a placental inhibitor and so facilitate the onset of breathing. It has been demonstrated in the fetal lamb that when the cord is unclamped, breathing soon becomes inhibited (Adamson et al., 1987). The conclusion must be that no single factor is responsible, but that multiple factors provide insurance for this important transition to be accomplished without incident (Jansen and Chernick, 1988).

■ SURFACTANT

Composition. Preparations of lung surfactant have been derived from lung lavage fluid and mature animals have the composition indicated in Table 49–2. During fetal life phosphatidylinositol predominates over phosphatidylglycerol, which replaces it after birth (Hallman and Gluck, 1977). The backbone of phosphatidylcholine is three carbon glycerol molecules. At the first two positions fatty acid tails are added, while at the head of the molecule, a phosphocholine moiety is added in the third position.

Function. The insoluble phospholipids of the alveolar lining layer have at least four major functions: (1) to stabilize the lung during deflation, (2) to prevent high surface tension pulmonary edema, (3) to protect the lung against epithelial damage, and (4) to provide a defense against infection.

Because they have a hydrophilic head and a hydrophobic fatty acid tail, phospholipid molecules aggregate at the surface of the alveolar lining liquid, thereby displacing water molecules and reducing the surface tension (Possmayer, 1982). As the fatty acid chains in saturated phosphatidylcholine are straight, rather than bent at each unsaturated bond, more molecules of disaturated phosphatidylcholine can be packed into the surface, displacing more water molecules and reducing the surface tension to much lower levels. The surface tension of water is 72 dynes/cm. If the surface is occupied by saturated phosphatidylcholine molecules, packed side by side, the surface tension falls to an equilibrium value of about 25 dynes/cm. If the phospholipid film is compressed, as happens during deflation, more water molecules are excluded and the surface tension falls to near zero (Notter and Morrow, 1975). On expansion of the film, as happens during inflation, respreading may be too slow, allowing too many water molecules to re-enter the surface. Respreading may

TABLE 49–2. Composition of Surfactant in Mature Animals

COMPONENT	PERCENTAGE	
Lipid	90	
Saturated phosphatidylcholine		45
Unsaturated phosphatidylcholine		25
Phosphatidylglycerol		5
Other phospholipids		5
Neutral lipids		10
Protein	8	
Carbohydrate	2	

(From King, R. J.: Pulmonary surface active material: Basic concepts. *In* Bloom, R. S., Sinclair, J. C., and Warshaw, J. B. (Eds.): The Surfactant and the Neonatal Lung. Evansville, IN, Mead Johnson and Co., 1979.)

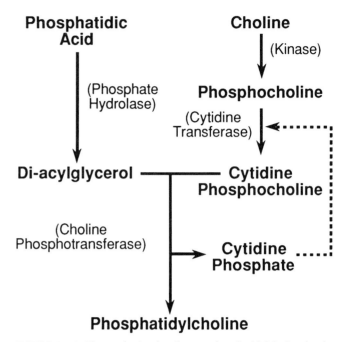

FIGURE 49–3. *The synthesis of surfactant phosphatidylcholine by the choline incorporation pathway, using phosphatidic acid as substrate.*

be facilitated by the addition of unsaturated phosphatidylcholine (Hawko et al., 1981) and phosphatidylglycerol (Bangham et al., 1979), which make the mixture more fluid.

The pressure required to prevent collapse of spherical air spaces is given by the LaPlace equation: $P = 2.\gamma.10/r$, where P = pressure in cm H_2O, γ = surface tension in dynes/cm, r = radius in μm, and the factor 10 corrects for the units. At the end of deflation the transpulmonary pressure may be as low as 2 cm H_2O. If γ is as high as 10 dynes/cm, air spaces larger than 100 μm radius will remain open, but those that are smaller will collapse at a pressure of 2 cm H_2O. On the other hand, if the surface tension is 1 dyne/cm, then only units smaller than 10 μm radius will collapse at a pressure of 2 cm H_2O. By reducing surface tension to near zero, surfactant guarantees the stability of even the smallest air spaces. This maximizes the surface area at the end of expiration, and thus the gas-exchange capabilities of the lung.

Synthesis. Surfactant phospholipids are synthesized in the smooth endoplasmic reticulum of granular pneumocytes (VanGolde et al., 1988), cells that line the air spaces and constitute about 10 per cent of the internal surface area of the lung. The glucose substrate may be derived from glycogen stores or directly from the plasma. In addition, fatty acids may be derived from the plasma pool, from triglycerides following the action of lipoprotein lipase, or from glucose metabolism. The initial phase involves the synthesis of phosphatidic acid, which is similar to phosphatidylcholine but without the choline head. The major pathway for the synthesis of phosphatidylcholine is the choline incorporation pathway for phosphatidic acid (Fig. 49–3). Most phosphatidylcholine produced is initially unsaturated at the second position. By a process involving phospholipase and acyltransferase enzymes, the unsaturated fatty acid is removed and replaced with saturated palmitic acid, thus remodeling phosphatidylcholine to pro-

Phosphatidic Acid

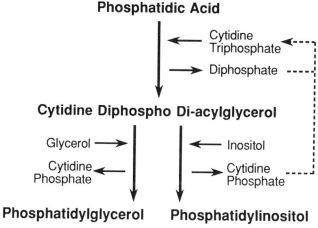

FIGURE 49–4. *The synthesis of surfactant phosphatidylglycerol and phosphatidylinositol, using phosphatidic acid as substrate.*

duce a more surface active molecule (Engle et al., 1980). Other surfactant phospholipids are also produced from phosphatidic acid (Fig. 49–4).

Packaging, Transport, Secretion, and Reutilization. After synthesis in the endoplasmic reticulum, surfactant phospholipids are packaged for export in the Golgi apparatus (VanGolde et al., 1988). They emerge as small lamellar bodies coalescing into mature lamellar bodies, which are stored near the apical plasma membrane prior to secretion by exocytosis. Once in the alveolar lining liquid, lamellar bodies are converted into tubular myelin, a specialized form of surfactant that rapidly donates a phospholipid monolayer to the surface (Goerke, 1974) (Fig. 49–5). After secretion, surfactant phospholipid is also taken back into the granular pneumocytes by endocytosis, forming multivesicular bodies, which are rapidly incorpo-

rated into lamellar bodies before being secreted again (VanGolde et al., 1988). Thus, there is constant cycling of lamellar bodies, tubular myelin, and multivesicular bodies (Fig. 49–6). A turnover time of 10 hours has been estimated in the newborn rabbit (Jacobs et al., 1982).

Surfactant Development. During the glandular phase of lung development epithelial cells are columnar, but during the canalicular phase, they become cuboidal in shape. At about 24 weeks' gestation in the human, many cuboidal cells differentiate into granular pneumocytes, developing an abundant apparatus for synthesis, packaging, and storage of surfactant. Saturated phosphatidylcholine is present early in whole lung extracts and increases after about 24 weeks (Ballard, 1989). Based upon the analysis of amniotic fluid samples, the appearance of surfactant in the alveolar fluid is considerably delayed in relation to its appearance in the tissue (Fig. 49–7).

Control of Synthesis. The synthesis of the fully developed surfactant package is under control of genetic material in chromosomes. The information is transcribed from encoded DNA to messenger RNA, and translated at the polyribosomes of rough endoplasmic reticulum, where proteins controlling the process are synthesized. This includes enzymes, receptors, transporters and other proteins. Corticosteroid (Rooney et al., 1979) and thyroid (Ballard et al., 1980) hormones have a well-established regulatory role in accelerating the development of mature surfactant packages as well as having an effect on lung structure. There is evidence that some glucocorticoid effects may be mediated by fibroblast-pneumocyte factor,

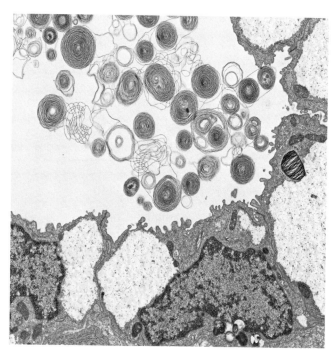

FIGURE 49–5. *Fetal rat lung (low magnification), day 20 (term day 22), showing developing type II cells, stored glycogen (pale areas), secreted lamellar bodies, and tubular myelin. (Courtesy of Mary Williams, M.D., University of California, San Francisco.)*

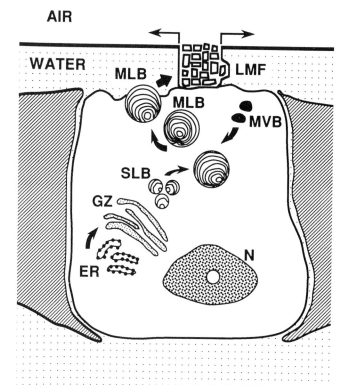

FIGURE 49–6. *Possible pathway for transport, secretion and reuptake of surfactant. N, nucleus; ER, endoplasmic reticulum; G2, Golgi zone; SLB, small lamellar body; MLB, mature lamellar body; LMF, lattice (tubular) myelin figure; MVB, multivesicular body.*

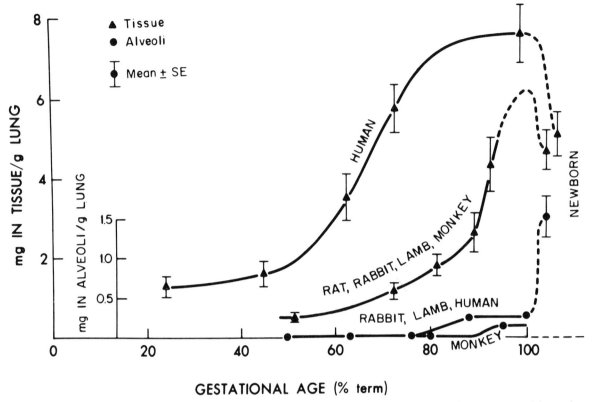

FIGURE 49–7. Concentration of saturated PC in lung tissue and alveoli plotted against relative gestational age. (Reprinted from Clements, J. A., and Tooley, W. H.: Kinetics of surface active material in the fetal lung. In Hodson, W. A. (Ed.): Development of the Lung. New York, Marcel Dekker, 1977, by courtesy of Marcel Dekker Inc.)

synthesized by fibroblasts in the lung interstitium (Smith, 1984). Glucocorticoid and thyroid hormones first bind to their receptors and the hormone-receptor complexes then exert their effects on specific genes in the DNA material. The amount of gene expression is also regulated by catecholamines and cyclic adenosine monophosphate (AMP) (Mettler et al., 1981), which facilitate the transcription process (Martin, 1981).

Control of Secretion. In mature animals a single deep breath completely replenishes the exhausted alveolar surfactant pool (Hildebran et al., 1981). Catecholamines and cyclic AMP play an important role (Mettler et al., 1981). During labor and at birth, the levels of circulating catecholamines increase enormously and stimulate surfactant secretion (Marino and Rooney, 1981). Other agents that increase cyclic AMP stimulate secretion, e.g., thyroxine, thyrotropin-releasing hormone, adrenocorticotropic hormone, and prostaglandin E (Hollingsworth and Gilfillan, 1984). Drugs, such as theophylline, which decrease the degradation of cyclic AMP, increase surfactant secretion (Corbet et al., 1978). During the latter part of gestation, there is an increase of lung adrenergic receptors (Cheng et al., 1980), which increase the response to catecholamines. The density of adrenergic receptors is increased by corticosteroids, thyroid hormone, and estrogen, presumably by their regulation of protein synthesis. In addition, surfactant secretion is regulated by protein kinase C (Sano et al., 1985), and stimulation of purine receptors by ATP (Rice and Singleton, 1986).

Surfactant Protein. There are at least three types of surfactant protein (SP) recognized: SP-A, SP-B, and SP-C.

SP-A is hydrophilic; it has a relative molecular weight of 28,000 but is glycosylated to about 35,000 and then linked by disulphide bonds to form large oligomers greater than 300,000 (Phelps et al., 1986; Whitsett et al., 1985). It is synthesized in the alveolar type II cell and secreted with phospholipid. It forms an integral part of tubular myelin, and while it inhibits surfactant secretion, it stimulates the reutilization process in isolated cells (Wright et al., 1987). SP-B and SP-C are smaller, with relative molecular weights of 8000 and 5000, respectively. They are hydrophobic and greatly accelerate the adsorption of phospholipid to the surface (Phelps et al., 1987; Suzuki et al., 1986). They too are synthesized in type II cells, as well as in bronchiolar cells known as Clara cells (Phelps and Harding, 1987). Glucocorticords increase synthesis of all three surfactant proteins in cultured lung, and cyclic AMP stimulates SP-A and SP-B. Other hormones (e.g., insulin and transforming growth factor B) are reported to inhibit production of SP-A (Ballard, 1989).

Surfactant Clearance. Although surfactant is recycled continuously, the conservation is not complete. Surfactant, excluded from the monolayer during deflation, forms heaps on the air side and micelles on the liquid side of the monolayer. The heaps may possibly be consumed by alveolar macrophages, whereas the micelles are eliminated from the lung by membranous pneumocytes (Wright and Clements, 1987).

■ PULMONARY CIRCULATION

The lung has a dual circulation—pulmonary and bronchial. The pulmonary circulation transports poorly oxygenated systemic venous blood to the lung via a branching network of pulmonary arteries. These arteries may be conventional arteries that course through the interstitium and branch with major airways, or they may be supernumerary arteries that branch independently of the airways and supply peribronchial alveolar regions. Both types of arteries ultimately enter the acinus (the gas exchanging unit of the lung) and branch into a meshwork of capillaries within the alveolar septa. The converging capillaries form venules and pulmonary veins that course through the intralobular and intersegmental septa and then return oxygenated blood to the left atrium (Hoffman, 1975).

The bronchial arteries arise from the systemic circulation. They branch with airways and deliver oxygenated blood to the airways, pulmonary blood vessels, visceral pleura, and connective tissue. Two-thirds of this blood returns to the pulmonary veins while one-third returns via the bronchial veins to the azygous vein (Hoffman, 1975).

The pulmonary arteries arise from the sixth branchial arch during the 5th week of gestation. They branch along with the developing airways until the 16th week. After the 16th week, preacinar arteries increase only in diameter and length rather than in number (Hislop and Reid, 1972). Intra-acinar development, however, continues such that the total number of arteries increases ten-fold from 20 to 40 weeks' gestation (Levin et al., 1976). During this period capillaries also proliferate in the acinus. The alveolar-capillary membrane thins, and the lung becomes capable of gas exchange with the circulation.

The large fetal pulmonary arteries (>1700 μm in diameter) are elastic and resemble the aorta. Arteries measuring between 180 and 1700 μm in diameter are muscular, while those measuring between 100 and 180 μm are surrounded only by a spiral coat of muscle. Arteries measuring <100 μm in diameter are nonmuscular (Rabinovitch, 1985). For any given diameter of muscular artery, wall thickness as a percentage of diameter is greater in the fetus than in the adult (Hislop and Reid, 1972). For any given vessel diameter, however, the percentage of wall thickness remains constant throughout the second half of gestation (Levin et al., 1976).

Pulmonary veins grow from the atrium with the airways as far as the secondary bronchi and then course through the connective tissue between pulmonary segments. The pulmonary veins of the fetus are less muscular than those of the adult (Hislop and Reid, 1973). Bronchial arteries develop from the first segmental dorsal aortic arch between the 9th and 12th weeks of gestation.

In the fetus, blood is diverted from the lungs by the relatively high pulmonary vascular resistance and is shunted across the patent ductus arteriosus to the placenta, where gas exchange occurs (Rudolph and Heymann, 1974; Teitel, 1988). Because pulmonary blood flow (hence, venous return) to the left atrium is low, left atrial pressure is less than right atrial pressure and oxygenated umbilical venous blood is shunted across the foramen ovale to the left ventricle and to the coronary and cerebral circulations. Midway through gestation, the lung receives only 3.5 per cent of the combined ventricular output. Late in gestation, blood flow to the lung increases out of proportion to lung mass and constitutes 7 per cent of the combined ventricular output. This increase can be best accounted for by the marked increase in the number of pulmonary arteries that occurs during the same interval. Recent data show that during this period of increased vascularization, the pulmonary arteries of the fetus begin to constrict in response to their relatively hypoxic milieu. If this increase in vascular tone did not occur, pulmonary blood flow would increase even more during this period (Morin et al., 1988).

With air breathing at birth, pulmonary vascular resistance decreases dramatically and the systemic resistance increases. As a result, the gradient favoring right-to-left shunting of blood at the ductus arteriosus is reversed, and the pulmonary blood flow increases. In fact, a small left-to-right shunt may occur across the ductus arteriosus until ductal closure occurs. In addition, pulmonary venous return increases, left atrial pressure increases, and the right-to-left shunt at the foramen ovale ceases. The net result of these circulatory changes is that the lung replaces the placenta as the organ of gas exchange.

The decrease in pulmonary vascular resistance that occurs with air breathing results from an increase in alveolar oxygen tension and from mechanical distention of the lung. Oxygen tension in the fetal lung is similar to pulmonary arterial blood and is sufficiently low to constrict the pulmonary arteries. With air breathing, hypoxic constriction is relieved and vascular resistance decreases. The mechanism that causes this decrease to occur is unknown. Increased production of bradykinin (Heymann et al., 1969) and inhibition of leukotriene synthesis (Soifer et al., 1985) have both been implicated as possible mediators. Recent data show that the inflation of the lungs, even in the absence of oxygen, can decrease pulmonary vascular resistance (Teitel, 1988). Some of this decrease may result from mechanical distention of pulmonary vessels, but a large part of this decrease appears to result from a release of prostacyclin—a potent pulmonary vasodilator (Leffler et al., 1984).

Postnatal lung development is characterized by remodeling of pulmonary arteries with a thinning of the medial musculature, and a further reduction in pulmonary vascular resistance. Arterioles continue to proliferate in the acinus, and the muscularization extends into the acinus so that by adulthood, muscular arteries can be found at the level of the alveolus (Rabinovitch, 1985). Alveoli and alveolar capillaries continue to develop until approximately 3 years of age.

■ REFERENCES

Adams, F. H., Fujiwara, T., and Rowshan, G.: The nature and origin of the fluid in the fetal lamb lung. J. Pediatr. 63:881, 1963.

Adamson, S. L., Richardson, B. S., and Homan, J.: Initiation of pulmonary gas exchange by fetal sheep in utero. J. Appl. Physiol. 62:989, 1987.

Adamson, T. M., Boyd, R. D. H., Platt, H. S., et al.: Composition of alveolar liquid in the foetal lamb. J. Physiol. 204:159, 1969.

Ballard, P. L.: Hormonal regulation of pulmonary surfactant. Endocr. Rev. 10:165, 1989.

Ballard, P. L., Benson, B. J., Brehier, A., et al.: Transplacental stimulation of lung development in the fetal rabbit by 3,5-dimethyl-3-isopropyl-L-thyronine. J. Clin. Invest. 65:1407, 1980.

Bangham, A. D., Morley, C. J., and Phillips, M. C.: The physical properties of an effective lung surfactant. Biochim. Biophys. Acta 573:552, 1979.

Berthiaume, Y., Staub, N. C., and Matthay, M. A.: Beta-adrenergic agonists increase lung liquid clearance in anesthetized sheep. J. Clin. Invest. 79:335, 1987.

Bland, R. D.: Dynamics of pulmonary water before and after birth. Acta Paediatr. Scand. 305(Suppl):12, 1983.

Bland, R. D.: Lung liquid clearance before and after birth. Semin. Perinatol. 12:124, 1988.

Bland, R. D., Bressack, M. A., and McMillan, D. D.: Labor decreases the lung water content of newborn rabbits. Am. J. Obstet. Gynecol. 35:364, 1979.

Bland, R. D., Hansen, T. N., Haberkern, C. M., et al.: Lung fluid balance in lambs before and after birth. J. Appl. Physiol. 53:992, 1982.

Boylan, P., and Lewis, P. J.: Fetal breathing in labor. Obstet. Gynecol. 56:35, 1980.

Cheng, J. B., Goldfein, A., Ballard, P. L., et al.: Glucocorticoids increase pulmonary beta-adrenergic receptors in fetal rabbit. Endocrinology 107:1646, 1980.

Clements, J. A., and Tooley, W. H.: Kinetics of surface active material in the fetal lung. In Hodson, W. A. (Ed.): Development of the Lung. New York, Marcel Dekker, 1977.

Condorelli, S., and Scarpelli, E. M.: Somatic-respiratory reflex and onset of regular breathing movements in the lamb fetus in utero. Pediatr. Res. 9:879, 1975.

Corbet, A. J. S., Flax, P., Alston, C., et al.: Effect of aminophyllin and dexamethasone on secretion of pulmonary surfactant in fetal rabbits. Pediatr. Res. 12:797, 1978.

Dawes, G. S.: Revolutions and cyclical rhythms in prenatal life: Fetal respiratory movements rediscovered. Pediatrics 51:965, 1973.

Dawes, G. S.: Breathing before birth in animals and man. N. Engl. J. Med. 290:557, 1974.

Dawes, G. S., Gardner, W. N., Johnston, B. M., et al.: Effects of hypercapnia on tracheal pressure, diaphragm and intercostal electromyograms in unanesthetized sheep J. Physiol. (Lond.) 326:461, 1982.

Dawes, G. S., Gardner, W. N., Johnston, B. M., et al.: Breathing in fetal lambs: The effect of brainstem section. J. Physiol. (Lond.) 335:535, 1983.

DiMaio, M., Gil, J., Ciurea, D., et al.: Structural maturation of the human fetal lung: A morphometric study of the development of air-blood barriers. Pediatr. Res. 26:88, 1989.

Engle, M. J., Sanders, R. L., and Longmore, W. J.: Evidence for the synthesis of lung surfactant dipalmitoyl phosphatidylcholine by a "remodelling" mechanism. Biochem. Biophys. Res. Commun. 94:23, 1980.

Gluck, L., and Kulovich, M. V.: Lecithin-sphingomyelin ratios in amniotic fluid in normal and abnormal pregnancy. Am. J. Obstet. Gynecol. 115:539, 1973.

Gluckman, P. D., Gunn, T. R., and Johnston, B. M.: The effect of cooling on breathing and shivering in unanesthetized fetal lambs in utero. J. Physiol. (Lond.) 343:495, 1983.

Goerke, J.: Lung surfactant. Biochim. Biophys. Acta 344:241, 1974.

Hallman, M., and Gluck, L.: Development of the fetal lung. J. Perinat. Med. 5:3, 1977.

Harding, R.: Fetal breathing. In Beard, R. W., and Nathanielsz, P. W. (Eds.), Fetal Physiology and Medicine. New York, Marcel Dekker, 1984.

Hawko, M. W., Davis, P. J., and Keough, K. M. W.: Lipid fluidity in lung surfactant.: Monolayers of saturated and unsaturated lecithins. J. Appl. Physiol. 51:509, 1981.

Heymann, M. A., Rudolph, A. M., Nies, A. S., et al.: Bradykinin production associated with oxygenation of the fetal lamb. Circ. Res. 25:521, 1969.

Hildebran, J. N., Goerke, J., and Clements, J. A.: Surfactant release in excised rat lung is stimulated by air inflation. J. Appl. Physiol. 51:905, 1981.

Hislop, A., and Reid, L.: Intra-pulmonary arterial development during fetal life—branching pattern and structure. J. Anat. 113:35, 1972.

Hislop, A., and Reid, L.: Fetal and childhood development of the intrapulmonary veins in man—branching pattern and structure. Thorax 28:313, 1973.

Hislop, A., and Reid, L.: Development of the acinus in the human lung. Thorax 29:90, 1974.

Hoffman, J. I. E.: The normal pulmonary circulation. In Scarpelli, E. M. (Ed.): Pulmonary Physiology of the Fetus and Newborn and Child. Philadelphia, Lea & Febiger, 1975, p. 258.

Hollingsworth, M., and Gilfillan, A. M.: The pharmacology of lung surfactant secretion. Pharmacol. Rev. 36:69, 1984.

Humphreys, P. W., Normand, I. C. S., Reynolds, E. O. R., et al.: Pulmonary lymph flow and the uptake of liquid from the lungs of the lamb at the start of breathing. J. Physiol. 193:1, 1967.

Jacobs, H., Jobe, A., Ikegami, M., et al.: Surfactant phosphatidylcholine source, fluxes and turnover times in 3 day old, 10 day old, and adult rabbits. J. Biol. Chem. 257:1805, 1982.

Jansen, A. H., and Chernick, V.: Onset of breathing and control of respiration. Semin. Perinatol. 12:104, 1988.

Jansen, A. H., Ioffe, S., Russell, B. J., et al.: Effect of carotid chemoreceptor denervation on breathing in utero and after birth. J. Appl. Physiol. 51:630, 1981.

Jost, A., and Policard, A.: Contribution expérimentale a l'étude du développement du poumon chez le lapin. Arch. Anat. Microsc. 37:323, 1948.

King, R. J.: Pulmonary surface active material: Basic concepts. In Bloom, R. S., Sinclair, J. C., and Warshaw, J. B. (Eds.): The Surfactant and the Neonatal Lung. Evansville, IN, Mead Johnson and Co., 1979.

Kitterman, J. A., Liggins, G. C., Fewell, J. E., et al.: Inhibition of breathing movements in fetal sheep by prostaglandins. J. Appl. Physiol. 54:687, 1983.

Langston, C., Kida, K., Reed, M., et al.: Human lung growth in late gestation and in the neonate. Am. Rev. Respir. Dis. 129:607, 1984.

Leffler, C. W., Hessler, J. R., and Green, R. S.: The onset of breathing at birth stimulates pulmonary vascular prostacyclin synthesis. Pediatr. Res. 18:938, 1984.

Levin, D. L., Rudolph, A. M., Heymann, M. A., et al.: Morphological development of the pulmonary vascular bed in fetal lambs. Circulation 53:144, 1976.

Manning, F. A.: Fetal breathing movements as a reflection of fetal status. Postgrad. Med. 61:116, 1977.

Marino, P. A., and Rooney, S. A.: The effect of labor on surfactant secretion in newborn rabbit lung slices. Biochim. Biophys. Acta 664:389, 1981.

Martin, D. W.: Regulation of gene expression. In Martin, D. W., Mayes, P. A., and Rodwell, V. W. (Eds.): Harpers Review of Biochemistry. Los Altos, Calif., Lange Medical Publications, 1981.

Mettler, N. R., Gray, M. E., Schuffman, S., et al.: Beta-adrenergic induced synthesis and secretion of phosphatidylcholine by isolated alveolar type 2 cells. Lab. Invest. 45:575, 1981.

Morin, F. C., III, Egan, E. A., Ferguson, W., et al.: Development of pulmonary vascular response to oxygen. Am. J. Physiol. 254:H542, 1988.

Murai, D. T., Lee, C. H., Wallen, L. D., et al.: Denervation of peripheral chemoreceptors decreases breathing movements in fetal sheep. J. Appl. Physiol. 59:575, 1985.

Notter, R. H., and Morrow, P. E.: Pulmonary surfactant: A surface chemistry viewpoint. Ann. Biomed. Engin. 3:119, 1975.

Olver, R. E., and Strang, L. B.: Ion fluxes across the pulmonary epithelium and secretion of lung liquid in the foetal lamb. J. Physiol. 241:327, 1974.

Patrick, J., Fetherston, W., Vick, H., et al.: Human fetal breathing movements at weeks 34 to 35 of gestation. Am. J. Obstet. Gynecol. 130:693, 1978.

Phelps, D. S., Floros, J., and Taeusch, H. W.: Post-translational modification of the major surfactant-associated proteins. Biochem. J. 237:373, 1986.

Phelps, D. S., and Harding, H.: Immunohistochemical localization of a low molecular weight surfactant-associated protein in human lung. J. Histochem. Cytochem. 35:1139, 1987.

Phelps, D. S., Smith, L. W., and Taeusch, H. W.: Characterization and partial amino acid sequence of a low molecular weight surfactant protein. Am. Rev. Resp. Dis. 135:1112, 1987.

Possmayer, F.: The perinatal lung. In Jones, C. T. (Ed.): Biochemical Development of the Fetus and Neonate. New York, Elsevier Press, 1982.

Rabinovitch, M.: Morphology of the developing pulmonary bed: Pharmacologic implications. Pediatr. Pharmacol. 5:31, 1985.

Rice, W. R., and Singleton, F. M.: P_2—purinoceptors regulate surfactant secretion from rat isolated alveolar type 2 cells. Brit. J. Pharmacol. 89:485, 1986

Rooney, S. A., Gobran, L. I., Marino, P. A., et al.: Effects of betamethasone on phospholipid content, composition and biosynthesis in the fetal rabbit lung. Biochim. Biophys. Acta 572:64, 1979.

Rudolph, A. M., and Heymann, M. A.: Fetal and neonatal circulation and respiration. Ann. Rev. Physiol. 36:187, 1974.

Sano, K., Voelker, D. R., and Mason, R. J.: Involvement of protein kinase C in pulmonary surfactant secretion from alveolar type 2 cells. J. Biol. Chem. 260:12725, 1985.

Smith, B. T.: Pulmonary surfactant during fetal development and neonatal adaption: Hormonal control. In Robertson, B., VanGolde, L. M.

G., and Batenburg, J. J. (Eds.): Pulmonary Surfactant. Amsterdam, Elsevier Press, 1984.

Soifer, S. D., Loitz, R. D., Roman, C., et al.: Leukotriene end organ antagonists increase pulmonary blood flow in fetal lambs. Am. J. Physiol. 249:H570, 1985.

Spear, G. S., Vaeusorn, O., Avery, M. E., et al.: Inclusions in terminal air spaces of fetal and neonatal lung. Biol. Neonate 14:344, 1969.

Strang, L. B.: Uptake of liquid from the lungs at the start of breathing. In DeReuch, A. V. S., and Porter, R. (Eds.): CIBA Foundation Symposium: Development of the Lung. London, J. & A. Churchill, 1967.

Suzuki, Y., Curstedt, T., Grossman, G., et al.: The role of the low molecular weight apoproteins of pulmonary surfactant. Eur. J. Respir. Dis. 69:336, 1986.

Teitel, D. F.: Circulatory adjustments to postnatal life. Semin. Perinatol. 12:96, 1988.

VanGolde, L. M. G., Batenburg, J. J., and Robertson, B.: The pulmonary surfactant system: Biochemical aspects and functional significance. Physiol. Rev. 68:374, 1988.

Walters, D. V., and Olver, R. W.: The role of catecholamines in lung liquid absorption at birth. Pediatr. Res. 12:239, 1978.

Weibel, E. R.: The Pathway for Oxygen Structure and Function in the Mammalian Respiratory System. Cambridge, Mass., Harvard University Press, 1984.

Whitsett, J. A., Hull, W., Ross, G., et al.: Characteristics of human surfactant associated glycoproteins A. Pediatr. Res. 19:501, 1985.

Wright, J. R., and Clements, J. A.: Metabolism and turnover of lung surfactant. Am. Rev. Resp. Dis. 135:426, 1987.

Wright, J. R., Wager, R. E., Hawgood, S., et al.: Surfactant apoprotein 26000–36000 enhances uptake of liposomes by type 2 cells. J. Biol. Chem. 262:2888, 1987.

CONTROL OF 50 BREATHING

Thomas Hansen and Anthony Corbet

■ CONTROL OF BREATHING

Rhythmic breathing is maintained by alternating discharges of inspiratory and expiratory neurons, located diffusely in the medulla oblongata, and is activated by nonspecific neuronal traffic. One concept is that expiratory neurons discharge continuously under the influence of the reticular activating system, but rhythmical breathing is produced by the central inspiratory activator (CIA), which intermittently discharges and temporarily inhibits expiratory neurons (Cohen, 1979). Some of the inspiratory neurons are organized into the nucleus para-gigantocellularis lateralis, thought to be the CIA, and located close to the central chemoreceptors on the ventral surface of the medulla (Von Euler, 1983).

In adults inspiration is active and expiration is passive. Expiration is divided into two phases. In the first phase a group of inspiratory neurons apply postinspiratory "braking" to slow exhalation. In the second phase exhalation continues passively, or it is accelerated by contraction of expiratory muscles. The main inspiratory muscles are the diaphragm, intercostals, and upper airway abductors. The main expiratory muscles are intercostal and abdominal groups, which accelerate expiration, and upper airway adductors, which retard expiration.

Inspiration is controlled by an "off-switch" (Fig. 50–1). During inspiration, the augmenting discharge of the CIA to inspiratory motor neurons and specialized R_b neurons suddenly causes the off-switch neurons to discharge, transiently inhibiting the CIA and allowing passive exhalation. The off-switch is also controlled by the pulmonary volume sensors and the rostral pontine pneumotaxic center, which together decrease the depth and increase the rate of breathing (Kosch et al., 1986). The threshold of the off-switch, and thus the depth and rate of breathing, is modulated up or down from a number of sources—peripheral chemoreceptors, central chemoreceptors, chest wall propriosensors, hypothalamus, and cerebral cortex (Von Euler, 1983). The respiratory control mechanisms develop progressively throughout gestation and infancy, so the system does not attain maturity until late in the first year of life. During quiet sleep, modulation of breathing is metabolic, through central and peripheral chemoreceptors, which sense PCO_2 and PO_2, respectively. During active sleep and wakefulness, there are additional behavioral controls, e.g., crying, sucking, and gross body motions (Schulte, 1977; Thach et al., 1978).

CONTROL OF BREATHING IN THE PREMATURE INFANT

Sensitivity of the central chemosensor to CO_2 is reduced in premature infants and increases progressively with gestational age to adult levels by term (Rigatto, 1977).

Higher oxygen concentrations increase sensitivity, and hypoxemia decreases sensitivity to CO_2. In small premature infants adult levels of sensitivity are reached by 4 weeks' postnatal age (Fig. 50–2).

The newborn responds to decreased oxygen by a transient hyperpnea, followed by a relative ventilatory depression of quite variable magnitude (Brady and Ceruti, 1966). This suggests rapid exhaustion of the peripheral chemoreceptor in the face of moderate hypoxic respiratory center depression. On the other hand, if the infant is given 100 per cent oxygen to breathe, there is a transient depression followed by a sustained stimulation of ventilation (Rigatto and Brady, 1972). This suggests persistent activity of the peripheral chemoreceptors under normal circumstances. Thus, the main problem may be that the peripheral chemoreceptor function is relatively weak. The hypoxic depression disappears about 2 to 3 weeks after birth, when the mature response of sustained hypoxic stimulation becomes dominant (Rigatto et al., 1975a).

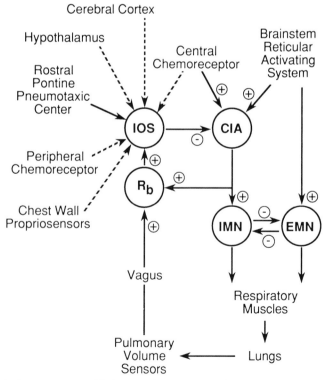

FIGURE 50–1. Possible functional organization of the central respiratory pattern generator. CIA = central inspiratory activator; IOS = inspiratory "off-switch"; IMN = inspiratory motor neurons; EMN = expiratory motor neurons. Solid arrows indicate direct effects. Interrupted arrows indicate modulatory effects. Effects are stimulatory (+) or inhibitory (–). (From Von Euler, C.: On the central pattern generator for the basic breathing rhythmicity. J. Appl. Physiol. 55:1647, 1983.)

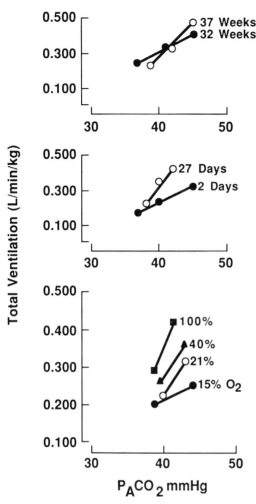

FIGURE 50–2. *The relationship between ventilatory sensitivity to carbon dioxide and gestational age, postnatal age, and the concentration of inspired oxygen. (From Rigatto, H., Brady, J., and Verduzco, R. T.: Chemoreceptor reflexes in preterm infants. The effect of gestational and postnatal age on the ventilatory response to inhaled carbon dioxide. Pediatrics 55:614, 1975, and Rigatto, H., Verduzco, R. T., and Cates, D. B.: Effects of O_2 on the ventilatory response to CO_2 in preterm infants. J. Appl. Physiol. 39:896, 1975. Reproduced by permission of Pediatrics.)*

Evidence for the presence of a Hering-Breuer reflex has been obtained, and the strength of the reflex increases with gestational age until term (Gerhardt and Bancalari, 1981) but declines after birth (Bodegard et al., 1969). The Hering-Breuer reflex is mediated by stretch and irritant receptors. The function of stretch receptors is to increase inspiratory flow and tidal volume without changing inspiration time (Haddad and Mellins, 1977). This means that stretch receptors increase the output of the respiratory center. The function of irritant receptors is to shorten inspiration and expiration time, and to reduce tidal volume without changing inspiratory flow. These receptors must operate the off-switch neurons (see Fig. 50–1) but have no effect on respiratory center output. The combined activity of stretch and irritant receptors, the volume sensor, shortens both inspiration and expiration, reduces tidal volume, and increases the inspiratory flow. Thus, increasing activity of the Hering-Breuer reflex throughout gestation is consistent with a maturational increase of respiratory drive induced by the stretch receptors.

PERIODIC BREATHING

This pattern consists of breathing for 10 to 15 seconds, followed by apnea for 5 to 10 seconds without change of heart rate or skin color. The net effect may be hypoventilation (Rigatto and Brady, 1972). It is very common at high altitude and is abolished by supplemental oxygen (Graham et al., 1950) and by continuous positive airway pressure. The more premature the infant, the more frequent its occurrence, but to a lesser extent, it persists in term infants and during early infancy (Hoppenbrouwers et al., 1977). It is not common during the first days of life and is more frequent during active sleep. The prognosis is excellent, so no treatment is required, except there is a high risk it will be associated with apnea of prematurity (Daily et al., 1969).

■ APNEA OF PREMATURITY

Apneic spells usually seen in infants are episodic and random (Daily et al., 1969). Episodes prolonged for 20 seconds or more, or those accompanied by bradycardia or color change, are considered significant. This diagnosis can be made only after exclusion of all other causes of recurrent apnea. In some infants only bradycardia is recognized, but polygraphic recordings indicate that bradycardia is always preceded by apnea (Dransfield et al., 1983). It is thought that 40 per cent of the episodes are central or diaphragmatic, 10 per cent are obstructive, and 50 per cent are mixed, which may indicate either obstructive followed by central apnea (Martin et al., 1986) or central followed by obstructive apnea (Butcher-Puech et al., 1985). In an individual infant, one type tends to dominate. Central apneas tend to be shorter, whereas obstruction tends to prolong the episode and accelerate the onset of bradycardia. The bradycardia is not related to hypoxemia (Hiatt et al., 1981), but presumably it has a central origin (Schulte, 1977).

Pathogenesis. The cause is unknown, but a number of theories have been considered for central, diaphragmatic, and obstructive apnea. The neurons of the central pattern generator are poorly myelinated, and have a reduced number of dendrites and synaptic connections, thus impairing the capability for sustained ventilatory drive. Prolonged auditory conduction times have been demonstrated in infants with apnea, a problem assumed to reflect the function of the medulla in general (Henderson-Smart et al., 1983). Along similar lines, since infants with apnea of prematurity have a deficiency of catecholamine excretion in the urine, others have suggested a neurotransmitter deficiency (Kattwinkel et al., 1976b).

The chest wall of premature infants is highly compliant, so considerably more work is performed to generate adequate tidal ventilation. This results in substrate depletion and diaphragmatic failure from fatigue. Evidence for fatigue has been shown by examination of the diaphragmatic electromyogram (Muller et al., 1979).

There is some evidence that the diaphragm may activate before the upper airway abductors, which would predispose to upper airway closure during inspiration. The same problem may occur if abductor activation is insufficient (Mathew, 1985). Since airway obstruction imposes a load on the inspiratory muscles, the ability to load-compensate is important. It has been shown that load compensation is poor in small prematures and increases as term is approached (Gerhardt and Bancalari, 1982). The poor load compensation is due to the highly compliant chest wall and the presence of an intercostal phrenic inhibitory reflex, which is activated by chest distortion, and which shortens the duration of inspiration (Gerhardt and Bancalari, 1984). This predisposes to obstructive apnea, especially under conditions of excessive neck flexion, when the upper airway tends to narrow, and in the supine position, when the tongue falls backward.

Relation to Sleep State. Most apneas occur during active sleep (Schulte, 1977) and are less common during states of quiet sleep or wakefulness. During active sleep, there is a low-voltage electrocortical state, decreased arousal from sleep, decreased muscular tone, absence of upper airway adductor activity, decreased respiratory drive, irregular breathing, and inspiratory chest wall distortion. The loss of chest wall muscle tone and airway adductor activity causes a 30 per cent reduction in lung volume and a decreased arterial P_{O_2} (Henderson-Smart and Read, 1979). Reduced ventilatory drive causes a slight elevation in arterial P_{CO_2}. The ventilatory response to hypoxia is depressed during active sleep, much more than in quiet sleep. The ventilatory sensitivity to CO_2 is also thought to be more depressed in active sleep (Rigatto, 1982). The newborn and premature infant is asleep 80 per cent of the time, compared with the adult who is asleep for 30 per cent of the time. More than 50 per cent of sleep is active in the small premature infant, and the mature amount of 20 per cent is not reached until 6 months of age (Bryan and Bryan, 1986).

Treatment. All infants at risk for apnea should have a heart rate monitor, which should be continued until the infant is at least 32 weeks' postconceptional age, or after that time until the infant has been free of bradycardia for 1 week. Heart rate monitors are preferred because apnea without bradycardia is not as significant, obstructive apnea with bradycardia is detected reliably, and false alarms are infrequent. The principal objections to the usual apnea monitor are that it misses obstructive apnea and may confuse bradycardia with breathing.

Since respiratory center output is dependent on general neuronal traffic, cutaneous stimulation is effective (Kattwinkel et al., 1975). The use of oscillation water beds has been helpful sometimes (Korner et al., 1975). Because diaphragmatic fatigue has been implicated, it is essential to maintain the circulation and a general state of good nutrition.

Most infants are treated with methylxanthines, which have been demonstrated effective in controlled trials (Murat et al., 1981). Because caffeine produces less tachycardia, has a more favorable therapeutic index, and blood level fluctuations are less erratic, it may be preferred over theophylline (Aranda and Turmen, 1979). The drug may be given for 2 weeks and then stopped to observe whether apnea has ceased, or it may be continued until 32 to 34 weeks' postconceptional age, by which time the problem has frequently resolved. Infants should not be discharged before caffeine has been eliminated. There is

reason to believe that methylxanthines increase CO_2 sensitivity, decrease diaphragmatic fatigue, and improve load compensation (Gerhardt et al., 1983).

The other mainstay of treatment is nasal continuous positive airway pressure (CPAP) (Kattwinkel, 1975). Although the effect of 5 cm H_2O should be tried, frequently as much as 8 to 10 cm H_2O is necessary for satisfactory control. Infants may be fed by continuous gastric infusion during this procedure. It has been postulated that CPAP provides increased ventilatory drive by directly stimulating the pulmonary stretch receptors (Speidel and Dunn, 1976). Others consider that obstructive and mixed apneas are selectively relieved by CPAP (Miller et al., 1985), which suggests that CPAP may also work by supporting the pharynx. In addition, CPAP prevents chest distortion during inspiration. Improved load compensation in small premature infants on CPAP has been demonstrated (Martin et al., 1977).

Another drug that has proved useful is doxapram (Barrington et al., 1987). At low doses it stimulates the peripheral chemoreceptors, while at higher doses it stimulates the respiratory center directly. It should be reserved for those infants failing to respond to optimal xanthine and CPAP therapy.

Symptomatic Apnea. Apnea is a frequent manifestation of general problems in newborn and premature infants (Kattwinkel, 1977). The more common ones are as follows: (1) local infection, (2) septicemia, (3) necrotizing enterocolitis, (4) hypoxic-ischemic encephalopathy, (5) intracranial hemorrhage, (6) patent ductus arteriosus, (7) hypoglycemia, (8) anemia, (9) any condition causing hypoxemia or hypovolemia, and (10) upper airway obstructions. These should be excluded and appropriately treated before a diagnosis of apnea of prematurity is made.

■ APNEA OF INFANCY

Isolated apneas of 5 to 15 seconds, with or without periodic breathing, occur commonly in term infants during the first 6 months of life (Richards et al., 1984). There is no associated bradycardia or color change, and the episodes resolve spontaneously. Certain infants have prolonged apneas, usually more than 20 seconds' duration but shorter if associated with bradycardia or color change. These too usually resolve spontaneously. The diagnosis is reserved for those with onset after 38 weeks' gestation, to distinguish them from infants with apnea of prematurity persisting until 42 weeks' postconceptional age (Consensus Statement, 1987).

Usually after discharge from the nursery, some infants with apnea of infancy have an acute life-threatening event (ALTE), requiring resuscitation by vigorous stimulation or positive-pressure ventilation (Consensus Statement, 1987). Apnea of infancy is just one cause of an ALTE, perhaps representing 50 per cent of the cases. Other causes include: (1) gastroesophageal reflux, (2) pharyngeal incoordination, (3) convulsions, (4) infection, (5) heart disease, (6) breath-holding spells, (7) central hypoventilation syndrome, (8) CNS abnormality, and (9) accidental or intentional smothering by the mother. Many infants with an ALTE, after appropriate investigation to exclude other causes, are considered to have "near-miss SIDS." Investigation of these infants, by a 24-hour recording of their breathing, reveals that they have an increased incidence of periodic breathing, brief apneas and prolonged apneas, when compared with control infants (Guilleminault et al., 1979). Infants with idiopathic ALTE have been shown to have abnormalities in their control of breathing, including slow brain stem conduction, reduced ventilatory sensitivity to CO_2, blunted arousal response to hypoxia, and hypoventilation during sleep (Hunt and Brouillete, 1987). It is not certain whether these abnormalities were present before their ALTE or only appeared afterward. Nevertheless, a significant number of these infants later die suddenly.

■ SUDDEN INFANT DEATH SYNDROME

Sudden infant death syndrome (SIDS) describes the sudden death of an infant, which is unexplained by history and an adequate autopsy (Consensus Statement, 1987). Death occurs during sleep, most commonly during the night. The incidence in the United States is generally 2 per 1000 live births. It is a major cause of infant mortality, with a peak incidence between 2 to 4 months. One hypothesis is that these infants die from obstructive apnea and that they have apnea of infancy before their demise.

In fact, infants with apnea of infancy, diagnosed by pneumogram, have only a slightly increased risk of SIDS over that in the general population, except if they experience an ALTE, when the risk increases to 4 per cent. If they have several ALTEs, then the risk is enormous. However, only 7 per cent of infants with SIDS have a preceding ALTE. Nonselected infants destined to die of SIDS do not have a breathing pattern, based on 24-hour recordings, that is significantly different from the breathing pattern of closely matched infants who do not die of SIDS (Southall et al., 1986). Infants with SIDS seldom have a prior diagnosis of apnea of infancy. It seems reasonable to conclude that the apnea hypothesis for SIDS remains unproved, that SIDS and apnea of infancy should be considered separate problems.

Home Monitoring Programs. There is considerable controversy about which infants should have apnea monitoring at home. Parents must be skilled in the use of the monitor, in the interpretation of frequent false alarms, and in cardiopulmonary resuscitation. There is no evidence that home apnea monitoring reduces the number of deaths, but to many physicians and parents this approach is sensible. If it is necessary to discharge an infant from the hospital, it is reasonable to monitor at home those with persisting apnea of prematurity as well as those with diagnosed apnea of infancy. In both cases the purpose is to prevent the consequences of an ALTE. Any infant with a history of an ALTE should be monitored, unless the cause has been removed, e.g., infection. There are a number of situations in which there is a slight increase in the risk of SIDS, e.g., premature infants without apnea, siblings of SIDS victims, infants of drug-abusing mothers. While some may favor home monitoring, especially if the parents are insistent, unless apnea is demonstrable, there seems little point in view of the unproven nature of the apnea hypothesis for SIDS. The pneumogram appears to be of little help in deciding who to monitor and should not be used for this purpose. In one British study, 4 per cent of 1157 premature infants discharged from the hospital had unrecognized prolonged infantile apnea by pneumogram. None of the babies with later SIDS had prolonged apnea at discharge, and none with prolonged apnea had SIDS (Southall et al., 1982).

■ FEEDING HYPOXEMIA

This problem is frequent in premature infants given nipple feeds too soon, but sometimes occurs in term infants (Rosen et al., 1984). While sucking and swallowing, ventilation is severely interrupted. The associated bradycardia is thought to be reflex in origin because of its rapid onset. Feeding hypoxemia resolves with maturation, usually by 44 weeks but occasionally as late as 54 weeks' postconceptional age. Infants are treated by frequent interruptions during a feed, supplemental oxygen while feeding, and in extreme cases by gavage. Sometimes atropine before feeds may be helpful, but more for bradycardia than for hypoventilation (Kattwinkel et al., 1976a).

■ REFERENCES

Aranda, J. V., and Turmen, T.: Methylxanthines in apnea of prematurity. Clin. Perinatol. 6:87, 1979.

Barrington, K. J., Finer, N. M., Torok-Both, G., et al.: Dose-response relationship of doxapram in the therapy for refractory idiopathic apnea of prematurity. Pediatrics 80:22, 1987.

Bodegard, G., Schweiler, G. H., Skoglund, S., et al.: Control of respiration in newborn babies. The development of the Hering-Breuer inflation reflex. Acta Paediatr. Scand. 58:567, 1969.

Brady, J. P., and Ceruti, E.: Chemoreceptor reflexes in the newborn infant: Effects of varying degrees of hypoxia on heart rate and ventilation in a warm environment. J. Physiol. (Lond.) 184:631, 1966.

Bryan, A. C., and Bryan, M. H.: Control of respiration in the newborn. In Thibeault, D. W., and Gregory, G. A. (Eds.): Neonatal Pulmonary Care. Norwalk, Conn., Appleton-Century-Crofts, 1986.

Butcher-Puech, M. C., Henderson-Smart, D. J., Holley, D., et al.: Relation between apnea duration and type and neurological status of preterm infants. Arch. Dis. Child. 60:953, 1985.

Cohen, M. I.: Neurogenesis of respiratory rhythm in the mammal. Physiol. Rev. 59:1105, 1979.

Consensus Statement, National Institutes of Health Consensus Development Conference on Infantile Apnea and Home Monitoring. Pediatrics 79:292, 1987.

Daily, W. J. R., Klaus, M., and Meyer, H. B.: Apnea in premature infants: Monitoring, incidence, heart rate changes and an effect of environmental temperature. Pediatrics 43:510, 1969.

Dransfield, D. A., Spitzer, A. R., and Fox, W. W.: Episodic airway obstruction in premature infants. Am. J. Dis. Child. 137:441, 1983.

Gerhardt, T., and Bancalari, E.: Maturational changes of reflexes influencing inspiratory timing in newborns. J. Appl. Physiol. 50:1282, 1981.

Gerhardt, T., and Bancalari, E.: Components of effective elastance and their maturational changes in human newborns. J. Appl. Physiol. 53:766, 1982

Gerhardt, T., and Bancalari, E.: Apnea of prematurity. II. Respiratory reflexes. Pediatrics 74:63, 1984.

Gerhardt, T., McCarthy, J., and Bancalari, E.: Effects of aminophylline on respiratory center and reflex activity in premature infants with apnea. Pediatr. Res. 17:188, 1983.

Graham, B. D., Reardon, H. S., Wilson, J. L., et al.: Physiologic and chemical response of premature infants to oxygen enriched atmosphere. Pediatrics 6:55, 1950.

Guilleminault, C., Ariagno, R., Korobkin, R., et al.: Mixed and obstructive sleep apnea and near-miss for sudden infant death syndrome: 2. Comparison of near-miss and normal control infants by age. Pediatrics 64:882, 1979.

Haddad, G. G., and Mellins, R. B.: The role of airway receptors in the control of respiration in infants: A review. J. Pediatr. 91:281, 1977.

Henderson-Smart, D. J., and Read, D. J. C.: Reduced lung volume during behavioral active sleep in the newborn. J. Appl. Physiol. 46:1081, 1979.

Henderson-Smart, D. J., Pettigrew, A. G., and Campbell, D. J.: Clinical apnea and brain-stem neural function in preterm infants. N. Engl. J. Med. 308:353, 1983.

Hiatt, I. M., Hegyi, T., Indyk, L., et al.: Continuous monitoring of P_{O_2} during apnea of prematurity. J. Pediatr. 98:288, 1981.

Hoppenbrouwers, T., Hodgman, J. E., Harper, R. M., et al.: Polygraphic studies of normal infants during the first six months of life. III. Incidence of apnea and periodic breathing. Pediatrics 60:418, 1977.

Hunt, C. E., and Brouillete, R. T.: Sudden infant death syndrome: 1987 perspective. J. Pediatr. 110:669, 1987.

Kattwinkel, J.: Neonatal apnea: Pathogenesis and therapy. J. Pediatr. 90:342, 1977.

Kattwinkel, J., Fanaroff, A. A., and Klaus, M. H.: Bradycardia in preterm infants: Indications and hazards of atropine therapy. Pediatrics 58:494, 1976a.

Kattwinkel, J., Mars, H., Fanaroff, A., et al.: Urinary biogenic amines in idiopathic apnea of prematurity. J. Pediatr. 88:1003, 1976b.

Kattwinkel J., Nearman, H. S., Fanaroff, A. A., Katona, P. G., and Klaus, M. H.: Apnea of prematurity: Comparative therapeutic effects of cutaneous stimulation and nasal continuous positive airway pressure. J. Pediatr.: 86:588, 1975.

Korner, A. F., Kraemer, H. C., Hoffner, M. E., et al.: Effects of waterbed flotation on premature infants: A pilot study. Pediatrics 56:361, 1975.

Kosch, P. C., Davenport, P. W., Wozniak, J. A., et al.: Reflex control of inspiratory duration in breathing. J. Appl. Physiol. 60:2007, 1986.

Martin, R. J., Miller, M. J., and Carlo, W. A.: Pathogenesis of apnea in preterm infants. J. Pediatr. 109:733, 1986.

Martin, R. J., Nearman, H. S., Katona, P. G., et al.: The effect of a low continuous positive airway pressure on the reflex control of respiration in the preterm infant. J. Pediatr. 90:976, 1977.

Mathew, O. P.: Maintenance of upper airway patency. J. Pediatr. 106:863, 1985.

Miller, M. J., Carlo W. A., and Martin, R. J.: Continuous positive airway pressure selectively reduces obstructive apnea in preterm infants. J. Pediatr. 106:91, 1985.

Muller, N., Volgyesi, G., Eng, P., et al.: The consequences of diaphragmatic muscle fatigue in the newborn infant. J. Pediatr. 95:793, 1979.

Murat, I., Morriette, G., Blin, M. C., et al.: The efficacy of caffeine in the treatment of recurrent idiopathic apnea in premature infants. J. Pediatr. 99:984, 1981.

Richards, J. M., Alexander, J. R., Shinebourne, E. A., et al.: Sequential 22-hour profiles of breathing patterns and heart rate in 110 full-term infants during their first 6 months of life. Pediatrics 74:763, 1984.

Rigatto, H.: Ventilatory response to hypercapnia. Semin. Perinatol. 1:363, 1977.

Rigatto, H.: Apnea. Pediatr. Clin. North Am. 29:1105, 1982.

Rigatto, H., and Brady, J. P.: Periodic breathing and apnea in preterm infants. Evidence for hypoventilation possibly due to central respiratory depression. Pediatrics 50:202, 1972.

Rigatto, H., Brady, J. P., and Verduzco, R. T.: Chemoreceptor reflexes in preterm infants: The effect of gestational and postnatal age on the ventilatory response to inhalation of 100% and 15% oxygen. Pediatrics 55:604, 1975a.

Rigatto, H., Brady, J., and Verduzco, R. T.: Chemoreceptor reflexes in preterm infants. The effect of gestational and postnatal age on the ventilatory response to inhaled carbon dioxide. Pediatrics 55:614, 1975b.

Rigatto, H., Verduzco, R. T., and Cates, D. B.: Effects of O_2 on the ventilatory response to CO_2 in preterm infants. J. Appl. Physiol. 39:896, 1975c.

Rosen, C. L., Glaze, D. G., and Frost, J. D.: Hypoxemia associated with feeding in the preterm infant and full-term neonate. Am. J. Dis. Child. 138:623, 1984.

Schulte, F. J.: Apnea. Clin. Perinatol. 4:65, 1977.

Southall, D. P., Richards, J. M., Rhoden, K. J., et al.: Prolonged apnea and cardiac arrhythmias in infants discharged from neonatal intensive care units: Failure to predict an increased risk for sudden infant death syndrome. Pediatrics 70:844, 1982.

Southall, D. P., Richards, J. M., Stebbens, V., et al.: Cardiorespiratory function in 16 full-term infants with sudden infant death syndrome. Pediatrics 78:787, 1986.

Speidel, B. D., and Dunn, P. M.: Use of nasal continuous positive airway pressure to treat severe recurrent apnea in very preterm infants. Lancet 2:658, 1976.

Thach, B. T., Frantz, I. D., Adler, S., et al.: Maturation of reflexes influencing inspiratory duration in human infants. J. Appl. Physiol. 45:203, 1978.

Von Euler, C: On the central pattern generator for the basic breathing rhythmicity. J. Appl. Physiol. 55:1647, 1983.

PULMONARY **51** PHYSIOLOGY OF THE NEWBORN

Thomas Hansen and Anthony Corbet

■ LUNG MECHANICS AND LUNG VOLUMES

The lungs possess physical, or mechanical, properties that resist inflation, such as elastic recoil, resistance, and inertance. The dynamic interaction between these properties determines the effort that must be exerted during spontaneous breathing and the resting and extreme values for the volume of gas in the lung.

ELASTIC RECOIL

The lung contains elastic tissues that must be stretched in order for lung inflation to occur. The Hooke law requires that the pressure needed to inflate the lung must be proportional to the volume of inflation (Fig. 51–1). Conventionally, volume of inflation is plotted on the y-axis, and the distending pressure is plotted on the x-axis. In this way, the constant of proportionality is volume divided by pressure, or *lung compliance*. Throughout the range of tidal ventilation, the relationship between pressure and volume is linear. At higher lung volumes, as the lung reaches its elastic limit *(total lung capacity)*, this relationship plateaus.

The lungs and the chest wall function as a unit (the respiratory system) coupled by the interface between the parietal and visceral pleura. The tendency for the lung to collapse at rest is balanced by the outward recoil of the chest wall resulting in a negative (subatmospheric) intrapleural pressure. In the infant, the chest wall is almost infinitely compliant so that pleural pressure is only slightly subatmospheric. The volume at which this balance occurs is the functional residual capacity (FRC). Deflation below FRC requires an active expiratory maneuver.

Residual volume (RV) is defined as the volume of air that cannot be expired with a forced deflation. Inflation of the respiratory system above FRC requires a positive distending pressure which, at higher lung volumes, must overcome the elastic recoil of both the lung and the chest wall.

As depicted in Figure 51–1, the relative compliance of the lung of the newborn is similar to that of the adult (Krieger, 1963); however, the infant's chest wall compliance (Table 51–1) is greater than the adult's (Fig. 51–1). Measurements of lung and chest wall compliance suggest that the newborn should have a lower per cent RV and a lower per cent FRC than the adult. In fact, the per cent FRC in the newborn is equal to the adult's, and the

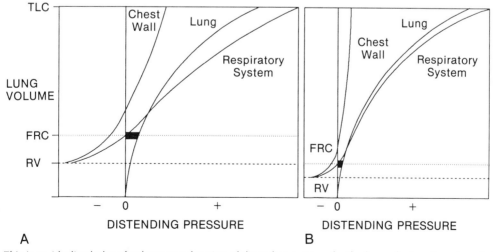

FIGURE 51–1. *This is an idealized plot of volume as a function of distending pressure for the lung, chest wall, and respiratory system (lung plus chest wall) of an adult (A) and an infant (B). These curves are derived by instilling or removing a measured volume of gas, allowing the respiratory system to come to rest, and then measuring the distending pressure for the lung (airway pressure minus intrapleural pressure), for the chest wall (intrapleural pressure minus atmospheric pressure), and for the respiratory system (airway pressure minus atmospheric pressure). Compliance is the change in volume divided by the change in distending pressure. The shaded area is the resting intrapleural pressure at functional residual capacity. Lung volumes depicted include residual volume (RV), functional residual capacity (FRC), and total lung capacity (TLC).*

TABLE 51–1. Lung Volumes and Mechanics in the Normal Newborn

Lung Volumes	ml/kg
Total lung capacity	63
Functional residual capacity	30
Residual volume	23
Tidal volume	6

Compliance	ml/cm H_2O
Total respiratory system	3
Chest wall	20
Lung	4

Resistance	cm H_2O/ml/sec
Total pulmonary resistance	0.03–0.04

(Data from Cook et al., 1957; Gerhardt and Bancalari, 1980; Polgar and Promadhat, 1971; Polgar and String, 1966; Reynolds and Etsten, 1966.)

infant's per cent RV is slightly greater. This seeming paradox exists because FRC and RV are measured while the infant is breathing, and predictions from the pressure volume curves assume that there is no air movement and passive relaxation of all respiratory muscles (Bryan, 1984). Recent data suggests two mechanisms by which the newborn can maintain a normal FRC during spontaneous breathing: (1) by maintaining inspiratory muscle activity throughout expiration and splinting the chest wall, or (2) by increasing expiratory resistance by glottic narrowing. In fact, FRC decreases when intercostal muscle activity is inhibited during active sleep (Moriette et al., 1983). This is especially true in the preterm infant with a highly compliant chest wall and is implicated as the cause of chronic pulmonary insufficiency of prematurity (CPIP). The reason for the elevated RV is not entirely clear, but it could result from airway closure during an active expiration as part of a crying vital capacity maneuver.

RESISTANCE

Resistance to gas flow arises because of friction between gas molecules and the walls of airways (*airway resistance*) and also because of friction between the tissues of the lung and the chest wall (*viscous tissue resistance*). Airway resistance represents approximately 80 per cent of the total resistance of the respiratory system (Polgar and String, 1966). In the newborn, nasal resistance represents nearly half the total airway resistance; in the adult, it accounts for about 65 per cent of the airway resistance (Polgar and Kong, 1965).

Gas flows only in response to a pressure gradient (Fig. 51–2). During laminar flow, the pressure difference needed to force gas through the airway is directly related to the flow rate times a constant—airway resistance. During turbulent flow, however, this pressure is directly proportional to a constant times the flow rate squared. Gas flow becomes turbulent at branch points in airways, at sites of obstruction and at high flow rates. Turbulence occurs whenever flow increases to a point that the Reynold number exceeds 2000. This dimensionless number is directly proportional to the volumetric flow rate and gas density, and it is inversely proportional to the radius of the tube and gas viscosity. Obviously, turbulent flow is most likely to occur in the central airways where volumetric

flow is high, rather than in lung periphery where flow is distributed across a large number of airways. Both types of flow exist in the lung so the net pressure drop is calculated as follows (Pedley et al., 1977):

$$\Delta P = (K_1 \times \dot{V}) + (K_2 \times \dot{V}^2). \qquad (1)$$

It is possible to take advantage of the differences between laminar and turbulent flow to determine the site of airway obstruction in the lung. If obstruction to gas flow is in the central airways, turbulent flow is affected the most. Since turbulent gas flow is density-dependent, allowing the patient to breathe a less dense gas (such as helium mixed with oxygen) reduces the resistance to gas flow. If the site of obstruction is peripheral, the mixture of helium and oxygen does not appreciably affect resistance.

Inflation of the lung increases the length of airways and might therefore be expected to increase airway resistance. However, lung inflation also increases airway diameter. Since airway resistance varies with the fourth to fifth power of the radius of the airway, the effects of changes in airway diameter dominate, and resistance is inversely proportional to lung volume (Rodarte and Rehder, 1986). Thus, airway resistance is lower during inspiration than during expiration because of the effects of changes in intrapleural pressure on airway diameter. During inspiration, pleural pressure becomes negative, and a distending pressure is applied across the lung. This distending pressure increases airway diameter as well as alveolar diameter and decreases the resistance to gas flow. During expiration, pleural pressure increases and airways are compressed. Collapse of airways is opposed by their cartilaginous support and

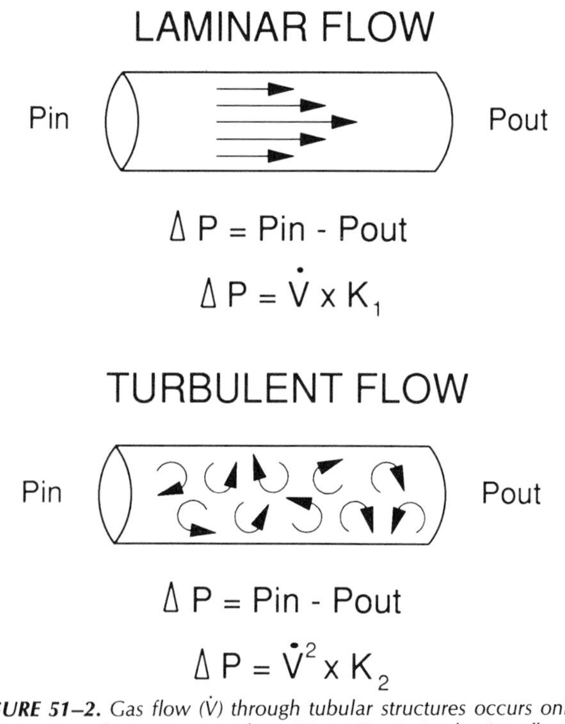

LAMINAR FLOW

Pin   Pout

$\Delta P = Pin - Pout$

$\Delta P = \dot{V} \times K_1$

TURBULENT FLOW

Pin   Pout

$\Delta P = Pin - Pout$

$\Delta P = \dot{V}^2 \times K_2$

FIGURE 51–2. Gas flow ($\dot{V}$) through tubular structures occurs only in the presence of a pressure gradient (Pin > Pout). For laminar flow, ΔP is directly proportional to $\dot{V}$, while for turbulent flow ΔP is proportional to $\dot{V}^2$. For laminar flow, $\Delta P = \dot{V} \times K_1$, where $K_1 = 8 \times L \times \eta/(\pi \times r^4)$ (L = length, η = gas viscosity, r = radius). For turbulent flow, $\Delta P = \dot{V}^2 \times K_2$, where $K_2 = 0.32 \times Re^{-1/4} \times \rho \times L/4 \times \pi^2 \times r^5$. ($R_e$ = Reynold's number, ρ = gas density.)

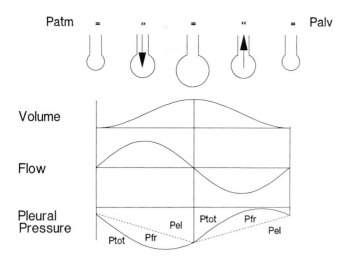

FIGURE 51–3. *Gas flows from the atmosphere into the lung only if atmospheric pressure (Patm) is greater than alveolar pressure (Palv). At end exhalation, when Patm equals Palv, there is no gas movement in or out of the lung. During a spontaneous inspiration, the diaphragm contracts, the chest wall expands, and the volume in the intrathoracic space increases. As a result, pleural pressure (Ppl) decreases relative to Patm, and a gradient is created between Ppl and alveolar pressure (Palv), distending the lung, increasing alveolar volume, and decreasing Palv. A gradient is created between Patm and Palv, and gas flows from the atmosphere into the alveolar space. The rate of gas flow increases rapidly, reaches a maximum (peak flow), and then decreases as the alveolus fills with gas and Palv approaches Patm. At peak inspiration, Palv equals Patm, and lung volume is at its maximum, as is Ppl. The curved solid line connecting end-expiration to end-inspiration is the total driving pressure for inspiration (Ptot). The dotted line represents the pressure needed to overcome elastic forces alone (Pel). The difference between the two lines is the pressure dissipated overcoming flow resistive forces (Pfr). During exhalation, this cycle is reversed.*

by the pressure exerted by gas in their lumina. During passive expiration, these defenses are sufficient to prevent airway closure. When intrapleural pressure is high during active expiration, airways may collapse and gas may be trapped in the lung. This problem may be accentuated in the small preterm infant with poorly supported central airways.

INERTANCE

Gas and tissues in the respiratory system also resist accelerations in flow. Inertance is a property that is negligible during quiet breathing and physiologically significant only at very rapid respiratory rates.

DYNAMIC INTERACTION

Compliance, resistance, and inertance all interact during spontaneous breathing (Fig. 51–3). This interaction is described by the equation of motion for the respiratory system:

$$P(t) = (V[t] \times 1/C) + (\dot{V}[t] \times R) + (\ddot{V}[t] \times I), \quad (2)$$

where $P(t)$ is the driving pressure at time, t, $V[t]$ is the lung volume above FRC, C is the respiratory system compliance, $\dot{V}[t]$ is the rate of gas flow, R is the resistance of the respiratory system, $\ddot{V}[t]$ is the rate of acceleration of gas in the airways, and I is the inertance of the respiratory system. If I is neglected, the equation simplifies to:

$$P(t) = (V[t] \times 1/C) + (\dot{V}[t] \times R). \quad (3)$$

At times of zero gas flow (end-expiration and end-inspiration), the equation further simplifies to:

$$P(t) = (V[t] \times 1/C) \text{ and } C = V(t)/P(t). \quad (4)$$

This series of equations and Figure 51–3 demonstrate that at points of no gas flow (end-expiration and end-inspiration) only elastic forces are operating on the lung. During inflation or deflation of the lung, however, both elastic and resistive forces are important.

Although the solution to the equation of motion for the respiratory system is beyond the scope of this discussion, the behavior of the respiratory system during passive exhalation is a special situation for which a solution can be obtained relatively easily (McIlroy et al., 1963; LeSouef et al., 1984). Before a passive exhalation maneuver, the infant is given a positive-pressure breath, and the airway is occluded—invoking the Hering-Breuer reflex and a brief apnea. Airway pressure is measured and the occlusion is released. Expired gas flow is measured using a pneumotachometer and integrated to volume; flow is then plotted as a function of volume (Fig. 51–4A). During a passive exhalation, there are no external forces acting on the respiratory system (P[t] = 0) so the equation of motion simplifies to:

$$(V[t] \times 1/C) + (\dot{V}[t] \times R) = 0$$

$$\text{Rearranging: } \dot{V}(t) = (-1/[RC]) \times V(t) \quad (5)$$

This equation states that during passive exhalation, flow plotted against volume is a straight line with slope −1/(RC). The quantity RC has the units of time and is termed the "respiratory time constant" (Trs). Trs defines the rate at which the lung deflates during a passive exhalation (Fig. 51–4).

Time constants affect the rate of lung inflation in the same manner that they affect lung deflation (see Chapter 52).

MEASUREMENTS OF LUNG MECHANICS

A true measurement of static lung compliance requires instilling a known volume of gas into the lung and then measuring airway pressure at equilibrium in the absence of respiratory muscle activity (see Fig. 51–1) (McCann et al., 1987). This technique is used to measure compliance during the passive exhalation maneuver described above (see Fig. 51–4). Another technique for measuring compliance takes advantage of the fact that gas flow is transiently equal to zero at end-inspiration and end-expiration (see Fig. 51–3). Compliance is calculated by dividing the change in volume between these two points by the concomitant change in distending pressure. Because the measurement is made while the infant is breathing, it is termed "dynamic compliance." In the normal infant, dynamic compliance should be equal to static compliance.

As was alluded to earlier, measurements of compliance are affected by lung size. For example, if a 5 cm H_2O distending pressure results in a 25 ml increase in lung volume in a newborn, calculated lung compliance is 5 ml/cm H_2O. In an adult, the same 5 cm H_2O distending

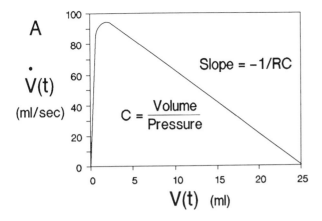

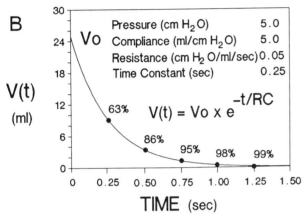

FIGURE 51–4. *A, Plot of flow [V̇(t)] versus volume [V(t)] for a passive exhalation. After an initial sharp increase, flow decreases linearly as the lung empties. Static compliance of the respiratory system is obtained by dividing the exhaled volume by the airway pressure at the beginning of the passive exhalation. Resistance is calculated from the slope of the flow volume plot (− 1/RC) and the compliance. This technique has the advantage of not requiring measurements of pleural pressure and being relatively unaffected by chest wall distortion.*

B, V(t) is plotted as a function of time for a passive exhalation. The graph is an exponential with the equation: V(t) = Vo × e⁻ᵗ/ᴿᶜ. Vo is the starting volume, and e is a mathematical constant (roughly 2.72). For this example, the time constant is roughly 0.25 second. Calculations show that when exhalation has persisted for a time equal to one time constant (t = 0.25 sec = 1 × Trs), 63 per cent of the gas in the lung will have been exhaled. For t = 2 Trs, 86 per cent of the gas will be exhaled; for 3 Trs, 95 per cent; 4 Trs, 98 per cent; and 5 Trs, 99 per cent. If expiration is interrupted before a time t = 3 Trs, gas will be trapped in the lung.

pressure increases the lung volume by roughly 500 ml, and calculated compliance is 100 ml/cm H_2O. While the calculated lung compliances are very different, the forces needed to carry out tidal ventilation are similar, i.e., lung function is normal in both circumstances. This example points out that if lung compliances are to be compared, they must be corrected for size. This is usually done by dividing compliance by resting lung volume to get *specific compliance*. For the newborn, resting lung volume is roughly 100 ml, so specific compliance is 0.05 ml/cm H_2O/ml lung volume. For the adult, resting lung volume is nearly 2000 ml, so specific compliance is 0.05 ml/cm H_2O/ml lung volume—identical to that of the newborn.

Lung compliance changes with volume history, meaning that it decreases with fixed tidal volumes and increases after deep breaths that recruit air spaces that may have been poorly ventilated or atelectatic. The periodic sigh in spontaneous breathing is associated with an increase in lung compliance and in oxygenation.

Many respiratory disorders result in nonhomogeneous increases in small-airway resistance in the lung. Therefore, if lung compliance remains relatively uniform, the product of resistance and compliance (Trs) will vary throughout the lung. During lung inflation, units with normal resistance have the lowest Trs and fill rapidly. Units with high resistance have a longer Trs and fill more slowly. At rapid respiratory rates when the duration of inspiration is short, only those lung units with a short Trs are ventilated. In effect, the ventilated lung becomes smaller. As discussed above, as the lung becomes smaller, its measured compliance decreases. Therefore, in infants with ventilation inhomogeneities, dynamic lung compliance decreases as respiratory rate increases. This decrease in lung compliance with increasing respiratory rate is termed "frequency dependence of compliance," and it is suggestive of inhomogeneous small-airway obstruction.

Resistance of the total respiratory system can be measured using the passive exhalation technique described previously (see Fig. 51–4), or it can be calculated from measurements of distending pressure, volume and flow (see Fig. 51–3). Points of equal volume are chosen during inspiration and expiration. The gas flow and the distending pressure are measured at each point. The pressure needed to overcome elastic forces should be the same for inspiration and expiration and therefore cancel out. Total resistance, consequently, is equal to distending pressure at the inspiratory point minus distending pressure at the expiratory point, divided by the sum of the respective inspiratory and expiratory point gas flows. Investigators have calculated compliance and resistance by measuring distending pressure, gas flow, and volume (see Fig. 51–3), then fitting these measurements to the equation of motion (equation 3 above), using multiple linear regression techniques, and solving for the coefficients 1/C and R (Bhutani et al., 1988).

Functional residual capacity is measured by inert gas dilution techniques (helium dilution) or inert gas displacement (nitrogen washout) (Fig. 51–5). Both of these techniques measure gas that communicates with the airways. The total volume of gas in the thorax at end-expiration (thoracic gas volume, or TGV) can be measured using a body plethysmograph and applying the Boyle law. This technique measures all gas in the thorax—even trapped gas that is not in contact with the airways. Obviously, FRC measured by inert gas dilution is less than TGV if significant volumes of trapped gas are present.

■ ALVEOLAR VENTILATION

The tissues of the body continuously consume O_2 and produce CO_2 (Fig. 51–6). The primary function of the circulation is to pick up O_2 from the lungs and deliver it to the tissues, and then to pick up CO_2 from the tissues and deliver it to the lungs. The exchange of O_2 and CO_2 with the blood occurs within the alveolar volume of the lungs. The alveolar volume acts as a "large sink" from which O_2 is continuously extracted by the blood, and to which CO_2 is continuously added. This mechanism for acquiring O_2 from the atmosphere and excreting CO_2 into

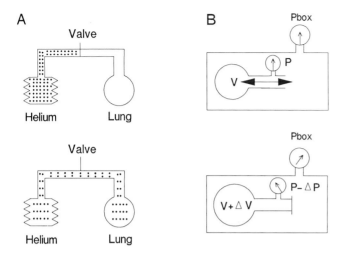

FIGURE 51–5. A, Measurement of functional residual capacity (FRC) by helium dilution. At end exhalation, the infant breathes from a bag containing a known volume (V_{bag}) and concentration of helium (He_i) in oxygen. The gas in the infant's lungs dilutes the helium-oxygen mixture to a new concentration (He_f): $FRC = Bag\ volume \times (He_i - He_f)/He_f$.

B, Measurement of thoracic gas volume (TGV) using a plethysmograph. The infant breathes spontaneously in a sealed body plethysmograph. At end exhalation, the airway is closed with a shutter. As the infant attempts to inspire against the shutter, the volume of the thorax increases and airway pressure decreases. The increase in volume of the thorax can be measured from the change in the pressure inside of the plethysmograph (Pbox). By Boyle's law: $P \times TGV = (P - \Delta P) \times (TGV + \Delta V)$, where P is atmospheric pressure, $(P - \Delta P)$ is airway pressure during occlusion, and $(TGV + \Delta V)$ is thoracic volume during occlusion. Therefore, $TGV = (P - \Delta P) \times \Delta V/\Delta P$. Since ΔP is very small compared with P, this can be simplified to: $TGV = P \times \Delta V/\Delta P$.

the atmosphere is the *alveolar ventilation* (Slonim and Hamilton, 1987).

The alveolar volume of the lung includes all lung units capable of exchanging gas with mixed venous blood: respiratory bronchioles, alveolar ducts, and alveoli. Since the conducting airways do not participate in gas exchange, they constitute the *anatomic dead space*. At end-exhalation, the functional residual capacity is the sum of the volume of gas in the alveolar volume and in the anatomic dead space. During normal breathing, the amount of gas entering and leaving the lung with each breath is the tidal volume (V_T): $V_T \times$ respiratory rate (RR) = minute ventilation ($\dot{V}$). Part of each tidal volume is wasted ventilation because it moves gas in and out of the dead space (V_D). Therefore, alveolar ventilation ($\dot{V}_A$) can be expressed as:

$$\dot{V}_A = (V_T - V_D) \times RR. \qquad (6)$$

Alveolar ventilation is an intermittent process while gas exchange between the alveolar space and the blood occurs continuously. Because arterial O_2 and CO_2 tensions (PaO_2 and $PaCO_2$, respectively) are roughly equal to the O_2 and CO_2 tensions within the alveolar space, these fluctuations in breathing could result in intermittent hypoxemia and hypercarbia. Fortunately, the lung has a very large buffer—the functional residual capacity. The functional residual capacity is four to five times as large as the tidal volume; therefore, only a fraction of the total gas in the lung is exchanged during normal breathing. This large buffer continues to supply O_2 to the blood during expiration and acts as a sump to accept CO_2 from the blood, so alveolar O_2 and CO_2 tensions (PaO_2 and

$PaCO_2$, respectively) change very little throughout the ventilatory cycle.

Alveolar ventilation is linked tightly to metabolism. When alveolar ventilation is uncoupled from the body's metabolic rate, hypoventilation or hyperventilation results. During hypoventilation, less O_2 is added to the alveolar space than is removed by the blood, and less CO_2 is removed from the alveolar space than is added by the blood. As a result, PaO_2 decreases and $PaCO_2$ increases. The net result of hypoventilation is hypoxemia and hypercapnia. Administering supplemental O_2 increases the quantity of O_2 in each breath delivered to the alveolar space, and it may prevent arterial hypoxemia. For example, suppose a 1 kg male infant has a tidal volume of 6 ml, an anatomic dead space of 2 ml, and a respiratory rate of 40 breaths/minute. His alveolar ventilation is 160 ml/minute ([6 ml − 2 ml] × 40/minute). If he breathes room air (21 per cent O_2), he will deliver 33.6 ml of O_2 to the alveolar space every minute (160 ml/minute × 0.21). If he maintains the same tidal volume but breathes only 20 times/minute, his alveolar ventilation will decrease to 80 ml/minute, only 16.8 ml of O_2 (80 ml/minute × 0.21) will be delivered to the alveolar space each minute, and his PaO_2 and PaO_2 will decrease. If he is allowed to breathe 50 per cent O_2, O_2 delivery to the alveolar space will increase to 40 ml/minute (80 ml/minute × 0.50), and both his PaO_2 and PaO_2 will increase. Since O_2 administration has no effect upon the accumulation of CO_2, it does not prevent hypercapnia.

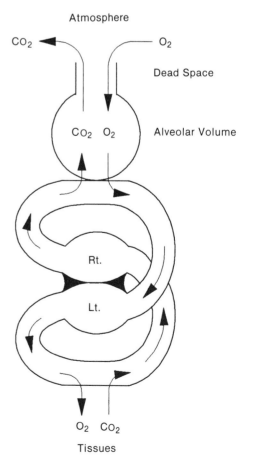

FIGURE 51–6. Schematic showing coupling of alveolar ventilation to tissue oxygen consumption.

Hyperventilation delivers more O_2 to the alveolar space than can be removed by the blood and also removes more CO_2 than can be added by the blood. As a result, PA_{O_2} increases and PA_{CO_2} decreases.

Measurements of alveolar ventilation and anatomic dead space in the infant rely upon the relationship between CO_2 production ($\dot{V}_{CO_2}$), $\dot{V}_A$ and PA_{CO_2}. The mathematical expression of this relationship states (Cook et al., 1955):

$$FA_{CO_2} = \dot{V}_{CO_2} / \dot{V}_A. \quad (7)$$

FA_{CO_2} is the ratio of CO_2 to total alveolar gas, or

$$FA_{CO_2} = PA_{CO_2} / (P_B - 47). \quad (8)$$

P_B is the barometric pressure, and 47 mm Hg is the vapor pressure of water at body temperature. Therefore,

$$\dot{V}_A = (\dot{V}_{CO_2} \times [P_B - 47]) / PA_{CO_2}. \quad (9)$$

If minute ventilation ($\dot{V}$) is measured, then dead space ventilation ($\dot{V}_D$) is calculated as:

$$\dot{V}_D = \dot{V} - \dot{V}_A. \quad (10)$$

Dead space volume is calculated by dividing by the respiratory rate.

This method measures the anatomic dead space in the lung. As will be seen in the next section, portions of some gas exchanging units in the lung can also function as dead space; therefore, the total dead space, or the physiologic dead space, may be greater than the anatomic dead space. Physiologic dead space is calculated by substituting Pa_{CO_2} into equation 9. When $Pa_{CO_2} = PA_{CO_2}$, all the dead space is anatomic dead space, and the gas exchanging units are all functioning normally. As physiologic dead space increases, however, Pa_{CO_2} will increase relative to PA_{CO_2}. Therefore, the difference between Pa_{CO_2} and PA_{CO_2} (the $aA.D_{CO_2}$) is a measure of efficiency of gas exchange in the lung.

For clinical purposes, $\dot{V}_{CO_2}$ in equation 9 is assumed to be a constant so that $\dot{V}_A$ is proportional to $1/Pa_{CO_2}$. Thus, increased Pa_{CO_2} means that alveolar ventilation has decreased; decreased Pa_{CO_2} means that alveolar ventilation has increased.

■ VENTILATION-PERFUSION RELATIONSHIPS

Under ideal circumstances ventilation and perfusion of the lung are evenly matched ($\dot{V}/\dot{Q} = 1$), both in the lung as a whole and in each individual air space. The air spaces receive O_2 from the inspired gas and CO_2 from the blood. Oxygen is transported into the blood, while CO_2 is transported to the atmosphere. Even though $\dot{V}/\dot{Q}$ is 1, CO_2 and O_2 are exchanged in the lung at the same ratio at which they are exchanged in the tissues, a little less CO_2 is transported out than O_2 is transported in, so the respiratory exchange ratio R equals 0.8. If there is no diffusion defect, the gas composition of the air spaces and the blood comes into equilibrium. Nitrogen makes up the balance of dry gas. The sum of partial pressures of all gases in the air spaces is equal to the atmospheric pressure. The "ideal" alveolar gas composition is: P_{O_2} equals 100, P_{CO_2} equals 40, P_{N_2} equals 573, and P_{H_2O} equals 47 mm

Hg at an atmospheric pressure of 760 mm Hg. The ideal arterial blood composition is the same. Therefore, differences between alveolar and arterial gas composition under ideal circumstances are all zero.

Knowing the values for PA_{CO_2} and inspired gas, ideal alveolar gas composition can be calculated from the alveolar gas equations (Farhi, 1966):

$$PA_{O_2} = PI_{O_2} - PA_{CO_2} \times (FI_{O_2} + [1 - FI_{O_2}]/R) \quad (11)$$

$$PA_{N_2} = FI_{N_2} \times (PA_{CO_2} \times [1 - R]/R + [P_B - P_{H_2O}]) \quad (12)$$

Under normal circumstances and certainly in the presence of lung disease, this ideal situation is not the case, some air spaces receive more ventilation than perfusion, while others receive more perfusion than ventilation. A reduction of ventilation may occur because of atelectasis, alveolar fluid, or airway narrowing. Reduced ventilation in one part of the lung may cause increased ventilation elsewhere. A reduction of perfusion may occur if air spaces are collapsed or overdistended or because of gravitational effects, while increased perfusion may occur in congenital heart disease. As with ventilation, reduced perfusion in one part of the lung may cause increased perfusion in other regions. If an air space is relatively overventilated (high $\dot{V}/\dot{Q}$), its gas composition tends toward that of inspired gas, which in the case of room air is $P_{O_2} = 150$ and $P_{CO_2} = 0$ mm Hg. If an air space is relatively underventilated (low $\dot{V}/\dot{Q}$), its gas composition tends toward that of mixed venous blood, which is $P_{O_2} = 40$, $P_{CO_2} = 46$ mm Hg. What counts is the $\dot{V}/\dot{Q}$ ratio, not absolute values of $\dot{V}$ or $\dot{Q}$ (West, 1986).

To understand $\dot{V}/\dot{Q}$ imbalance it is common to view the lung as a three compartment model (Fig. 51–7), namely $\dot{V}/\dot{Q} = 0$ (A), $\dot{V}/\dot{Q} = 1$ (B), and $\dot{V}/\dot{Q} = $ infinity (C). The oxygen saturation of blood in each compartment depends on the P_{O_2} and the oxygen dissociation curve. For illustrative purposes, in a badly diseased lung, 50 per cent of ventilation goes to $\dot{V}/\dot{Q} = 1$ and 50 per cent to $\dot{V}/\dot{Q} = $ infinity, while 50 per cent of perfusion goes to $\dot{V}/\dot{Q} = 1$ and 50 per cent to $\dot{V}/\dot{Q} = 0$. Perfusion of $\dot{V}/\dot{Q} = 0$ causes venous admixture, while ventilation of $\dot{V}/\dot{Q} = $ infinity causes alveolar dead space. The mixed alveolar gas composition is easily calculated as the mean. For mixed arterial blood the P_{O_2} must be read from the oxygen dissociation curve, but since the CO_2 dissociation curve is fairly linear, the values for CO_2 are easily calculated as the mean. The abnormalities in distribution of $\dot{V}$ and $\dot{Q}$ have created an $Aa.D_{O_2} = 70$, $aA.D_{CO_2} = 23$, and $aA.D_{N_2} = 32$ mm Hg (see Fig. 51–7). The $Aa.D_{O_2}$ is greater than the sum of the other two because the O_2 dissociation curve is not linear. Of course, the situation in most lungs is not as extreme as the one illustrated. But from this illustration it can be seen that:

1. Open low $\dot{V}/\dot{Q}$ units produce increased $Aa.D_{O_2}$, significant hypoxemia, and increased $aA.D_{N_2}$, but since they are poorly ventilated and have a P_{CO_2} close to the ideal value, they do not change the $aA.D_{CO_2}$ significantly.

2. High $\dot{V}/\dot{Q}$ units produce increased $Aa.D_{O_2}$ without hypoxemia and increased $aA.D_{CO_2}$, but since they are poorly perfused and have a P_{N_2} close to the ideal value, they do not change the $aA.D_{N_2}$ significantly.

For the calculation of $Aa.D_{O_2}$ and $aA.D_{N_2}$ it is customary to calculate the ideal alveolar gas composition for O_2 and N_2 from the alveolar gas equations, and use these values with those measured for arterial P_{O_2} and P_{N_2}. This emphasizes that part of the $Aa.D_{O_2}$ and $aA.D_{N_2}$ responsible for hypoxemia. For $aA.D_{CO_2}$, both an arterial and mixed alveolar sample are required.

In the newborn, a fourth compartment in the model is important. A significant part of the venous return may be shunted from right to left at the foramen ovale, ductus arteriosus, pulmonary A-V vessels, or lung mesenchyme without airway development, thus adding mixed venous to mixed arterial blood. This substantially increases the $Aa.D_{O_2}$ but has little effect on $aA.D_{CO_2}$ and no effect on $aA.D_{N_2}$. The latter is because there is no significant exchange of N_2 in the body, so venous and arterial P_{N_2} are the same. The effect on $aA.D_{CO_2}$ is small because venous P_{CO_2} is only slightly higher than arterial.

From this analysis it can be seen that hypoxemia is produced by a true right-to-left shunt and open low $\dot{V}/\dot{Q}$ units. Diffusional problems are not thought to be important in the newborn. Hypoxemia may be modeled as a venous admixture, the part of mixed venous blood, expressed as a fraction of cardiac output, that when added to blood equilibrated with an ideal lung would produce the measured arterial oxygen saturation. It is calculated as follows:

$$\dot{Q}va/\dot{Q}t = C\dot{c}O_2 - CaO_2/C\dot{c}O_2 - C\bar{v}O_2 \quad (13)$$

where $\dot{Q}va/\dot{Q}t$ = venous admixture, CO_2 = oxygen

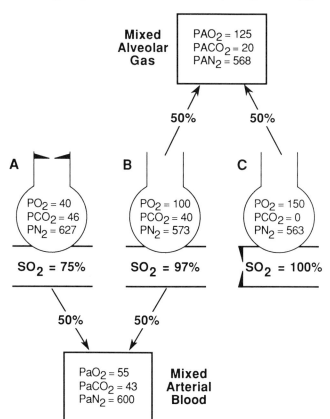

Mixed Alveolar Gas
$PA_{O_2} = 125$
$PA_{CO_2} = 20$
$PA_{N_2} = 568$

50%   50%

A
$P_{O_2} = 40$
$P_{CO_2} = 46$
$P_{N_2} = 627$
$S_{O_2} = 75\%$

B
$P_{O_2} = 100$
$P_{CO_2} = 40$
$P_{N_2} = 573$
$S_{O_2} = 97\%$

C
$P_{O_2} = 150$
$P_{CO_2} = 0$
$P_{N_2} = 563$
$S_{O_2} = 100\%$

50%   50%

$Pa_{O_2} = 55$
$Pa_{CO_2} = 43$
$Pa_{N_2} = 600$
Mixed Arterial Blood

FIGURE 51–7. *Three-compartment model of the lung with $\dot{V}/\dot{Q} = 0$ (A), $\dot{V}/\dot{Q} = 1$ (B), and $\dot{V}/\dot{Q} = $ infinity (C). The inspired gas is room air, and B is the ideal compartment. The sum of alveolar gas partial pressures is always 713 mm Hg. S_{O_2} is oxygen saturation in capillary blood. Pa_{O_2} is read from the oxygen dissociation curve for a saturation of 86%. By calculated differences, $Aa.D_{O_2}$ is 70 mm Hg, $aA.D_{CO_2}$ is 23 mm Hg, and $aA.D_{N_2}$ is 32 mm Hg.*

TABLE 51–2. Indices of Ventilation-Perfusion Imbalance in the Normal Newborn Breathing Room Air.

	$Aa.D_{O_2}$ mm Hg	$\dot{Q}va/\dot{Q}t$	$aA.D_{N_2}$ mm Hg	$\dot{Q}o/\dot{Q}t$	$\dot{Q}s/\dot{Q}t$	$aA.D_{CO_2}$ mm Hg
Newborn	25	0.25	10	0.10	0.15	1
Adult	10	0.07	7	0.05	0.02	1

(Adapted from Nelson, N. M.: Respiration and circulation after birth. *In* Smith, C. A., and Nelson, N. M. (Eds.): The Physiology of the Newborn Infant. Springfield, Ill., Charles C Thomas, 1976.)

content, $\dot{c}$ = pulmonary capillary, a = arterial, and $\bar{v}$ = mixed venous blood. For practical application $C\bar{v}O_2$ is calculated from a constant $a\bar{v}.O_2$ difference, which does introduce an error.

If an infant breathes 100 per cent oxygen for 15 minutes, most nitrogen is washed out of the lung, and the P_{O_2} in open low $\dot{V}/\dot{Q}$ units becomes so high that associated blood is 100 per cent saturated with oxygen. The remaining venous admixture is attributed to true right-to-left shunt ($\dot{Q}s/\dot{Q}t$). If an infant has the total venous admixture ($\dot{Q}va/\dot{Q}t$) measured while breathing room air, and then true shunt ($\dot{Q}s/\dot{Q}t$) measured while breathing 100 per cent oxygen, the venous admixture due to open low $\dot{V}/\dot{Q}$ units ($\dot{Q}o/\dot{Q}t$) can be calculated as the difference. The venous admixture due to open low $\dot{V}/\dot{Q}$ units can also be calculated from the $aA.D_{N_2}$ (Markello et al., 1972):

$$\dot{Q}o/\dot{Q}t = Pa_{N_2} - PA_{N_2}/Po_{N_2} - Pa_{N_2}, \quad (14)$$

where Po_{N_2} is the P_{N_2} in the $\dot{V}/\dot{Q}$-0 units (see Fig. 51–7), Pa_{N_2} is measured and PA_{N_2} is the ideal value calculated from the alveolar gas equation. Unfortunately, in newborns with a significant value for true shunt, this value really represents venous admixture as a fraction of effective pulmonary blood flow ($\dot{Q}o/\dot{Q}c$). A better estimate for $\dot{Q}o/\dot{Q}t$ can be obtained from simple arithmetic (Corbet et al., 1974):

$$\dot{Q}o/\dot{Q}t = \dot{Q}o/\dot{Q}\dot{c} \cdot (1 - \dot{Q}va/\dot{Q}t)/(1 - \dot{Q}o/\dot{Q}\dot{c}) \quad (15)$$

The true right-to-left shunt can then be estimated without 100 per cent oxygen breathing using the equation:

$$\dot{Q}s/\dot{Q}t = \dot{Q}va/\dot{Q}t - \dot{Q}o/\dot{Q}t. \quad (16)$$

The normal values for the various indices of ventilation-perfusion imbalance in normal newborn infants are shown in Table 51–2.

■ HEART-LUNG INTERACTION

EFFECTS OF THE LUNG ON THE HEART

There exists considerable potential for the lung to affect the heart. Because they share the thoracic cavity, changes in intrathoracic pressure accompanying lung inflation are transmitted directly to the heart. In addition, all of the blood leaving the right ventricle must traverse the pulmonary vascular bed, so changes in pulmonary vascular resistance may greatly affect right ventricular function.

EFFECTS OF CHANGES IN INTRATHORACIC PRESSURE ON THE HEART

Negative Intrathoracic Pressure. During spontaneous inspiratory efforts, the chest wall and diaphragm move outward, intrathoracic volume increases and intrathoracic pressure decreases (Fig. 51–8A). The heart also resides within the thoracic cavity and is subject to the same negative intrathoracic pressure during inspiration. With a decrease in intrathoracic pressure, the heart increases in volume, and the pressure within its chambers decreases relative to atmospheric pressure. Analogous to the lung, when the pressure within the heart decreases, blood is literally sucked back into the heart from systemic veins and arteries. On the right side of the heart, the phenomenon serves to increase the flow of blood from systemic veins into the right atrium, increasing right ventricular preload and ventricular output. On the left side of the heart, however, ventricular ejection is impaired. During systole, the left ventricle must overcome not only the load imposed by the systemic vascular resistance but it must also overcome the additional load imposed by the negative intrathoracic pressure (McGregor, 1979).

In infants with normal lungs, spontaneous respiratory efforts result in relatively small swings in pleural pressure (−2 to −3 torr) that have little effect on the pressure within the heart. With airway obstruction or parenchymal lung disease, however, swings in pleural pressure can be much greater (−5 to −20 torr), and systemic arterial pressure may fluctuate as much as 5 to 20 torr depending on where in the respiratory cycle ventricular systole occurs. In older children with asthma or some other form of airway obstruction, these fluctuations in blood pressure constitute pulsus paradoxus and are indicative of severe airway obstruction.

Positive Intrathoracic Pressure. During positive-pressure ventilation the lung inflates and pushes the chest wall and diaphragm outward (Fig. 51–8B). This outward push generates a pressure in the thoracic space that is greater than atmospheric pressure. The magnitude of the increase (relative transmission of airway pressure to the pleural space) is determined by the volume of lung inflation (which in turn is determined by the airway pressure and

lung compliance) and by the compliance of the chest wall and diaphragm. If the lung is very compliant and the chest wall rigid, little airway pressure is lost inflating the lung, but considerable pressure is generated in the thoracic cavity as the lung attempts to push the rigid chest wall outward. In this instance intrathoracic pressure (intrapleural pressure) is much greater than atmospheric and in fact nearly equal to airway pressure. On the other hand, if the lung is poorly compliant and the chest wall highly compliant, most of the airway pressure is dissipated trying to inflate the lungs and very little is transmitted to the thoracic cavity.

The effects of positive intrathoracic pressure on the heart are opposite to those of negative intrathoracic pressure. The heart is compressed by the lungs and chest wall, and blood is squeezed out of the heart and the thoracic cavity. Return of blood from systemic veins is impaired, and right ventricular preload and output decrease. On the other hand, if the increase in intrathoracic pressure coincides with ventricular systole, the effect is to augment left ventricular ejection and reduce the load on the left ventricle.

In the infant undergoing positive-pressure ventilation, the degree to which lung inflation compromises venous return is related to the relative compliances of the lung and chest wall. If the infant's lung is poorly compliant and the chest wall is very compliant, as in hyaline membrane disease, there is little effect of lung inflation on venous return. On the other hand, if the infant's lung is normally compliant but tight abdominal distention prevents descent of the diaphragm, intrathoracic pressure increases dramatically during positive-pressure ventilation and venous return and cardiac output can be impaired. This mechanism may help explain the circulatory instability of infants after repair of gastroschisis or omphalocele. A similar situation may arise in the preterm infant with pulmonary interstitial emphysema and massive lung overinflation. In these infants the heart is tightly compressed between the hyperinflated lungs, the other structures of the mediastinum and the diaphragm. Venous return may be severely limited and venous pressures so increased that massive peripheral edema often accompanies the reduction in cardiac output.

Whereas the effects of increased pleural pressure on the right atrium are detrimental, the effects on the left ventricle may be extremely beneficial (Niemann et al., 1980). During cardiopulmonary resuscitation, the chest wall is compressed against the lung and intrathoracic pressure increases. Since the left ventricle is in the thorax, left ventricular pressure increases as well. A gradient is created favoring flow of blood out of the ventricle and thorax and into the extrathoracic systemic circulation. Between chest compressions, elastic recoil causes the chest wall to pull away from the lung and heart, decreasing pleural pressure and favoring return of venous blood and priming the heart for the next chest compression. A similar phenomenon may result in augmentation of systemic pressure when ventilator breaths coincide with ventricular systole.

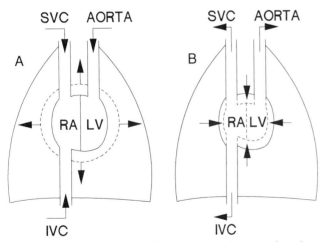

FIGURE 51–8. A, Negative intrathoracic pressure increases the volume of the heart and decreases the pressure within the chambers. This facilitates return of blood from the superior vena cava (SVC) and inferior vena cava (IVC) to the right atrium (RA) and impedes ejection of blood from the left ventricle (LV) into the extrathoracic aorta.

B, Positive intrathoracic pressure decreases the volume of the heart and increases pressure within its chambers. This impedes blood return to the right atrium and augments ejection of blood from the left ventricle.

Effect of Lung Inflation on Pulmonary Vascular Resistance. The pulmonary interstitium comprises three different interconnected connective tissue compartments, each containing a different element of the pulmonary circulation (Fishman, 1986). The first—the perivascular cuffs—consists of a sheath of fibers that contain the preacinar pulmonary arteries, lymphatics, and bronchi. The second consists of the intersegmental and interlobular septa and contains pulmonary veins and additional lymphatics. The third connects these two within the alveolar septa and contains the majority of the pulmonary capillaries. The first and second compartments represent the extra-alveolar interstitium while the third represents the alveolar interstitium. The perivascular cuffs are surrounded by alveoli and expand during lung inflation (Fig. 51–9A). As a result pressure within each cuff decreases, distending extra-alveolar blood vessels and decreasing their resistance to blood flow. The alveolar interstitium lies between adjacent alveoli and contains the majority of gas-exchanging vessels in the lung. These vessels are exposed to alveolar pressure on both sides and during lung inflation (Fig. 51–9B) are compressed so that their resistance to blood flow increases.

Therefore, during lung inflation (Fig. 51–9C), the resistance in extra-alveolar vessels (dotted line) decreases while resistance in alveolar vessels (dashed line) increases. As a result, the overall pulmonary vascular resistance (solid line) decreases initially, with lung inflation reaching its nadir at functional residual capacity, and then increases with further inflation.

If transition from intrauterine life to extrauterine life is to be successful, after birth all of the right ventricular output must traverse the pulmonary vascular bed. To some extent this adaptation is facilitated by a reduction in pulmonary vascular resistance that occurs with inflation of the lungs (Fig. 51–9) to a stable functional residual capacity. Inflation of the lung beyond functional residual capacity increases pulmonary vascular resistance. If care is not taken during positive-pressure ventilation, it is possible to inflate the lung to the point that alveolar vessels close and blood flow through the lung is impaired. When this occurs either cardiac output will decrease or the blood will bypass the lung via the foramen ovale or ductus arteriosus. Clinically this will be manifest as circulatory insufficiency from impaired right ventricular output or hypoxemia from right-to-left shunting of blood or both.

EFFECTS OF THE HEART ON THE LUNG—PULMONARY EDEMA

Pulmonary edema is the abnormal accumulation of water and solute in the interstitial and alveolar spaces of the lung (Staub, 1974; Bland and Hansen, 1985). In the lung, fluid is filtered from capillaries in the alveolar septa into the alveolar interstitium (Fig. 51–10A) and then siphoned into the lower pressure extra-alveolar interstitium. The extra-alveolar interstitium contains the pulmonary lymphatics, and under normal conditions, they remove fluid from the lung so that there is no net accumulation in the interstitium (see Chapter 49). Pulmonary edema results only when the rate of fluid filtration exceeds the rate of lymphatic removal. There are only three mechanisms by which this can occur (Fig. 51–10B): (1) the driving pressure for fluid filtration (filtration pressure) increases, (2) the permeability of the vascular bed (hence, the filtration coefficient K_f) increases, or (3) lymphatic drainage decreases.

Increased Driving Pressure. Filtration pressure can be increased by increased intravascular hydrostatic pressure, decreased interstitial hydrostatic pressure, decreased intravascular oncotic pressure, or increased interstitial oncotic pressure (Fig. 51–10C and 51–10D). By far the most common cause of increased filtration pressure is increased intravascular hydrostatic pressure (Table 51–3). In the newborn, intravascular hydrostatic pressure increases with increased left atrial pressure from volume overload or a number of congenital and acquired heart defects. In the preterm and term newborn, evidence suggests that alterations in pulmonary blood flow that are independent of any change in left atrial pressure may also influence fluid filtration in the lung. Preterm infants with patent ductus arteriosus and left-to-right shunts exhibit signs of respiratory insufficiency before they develop any evidence of heart failure, and experiments performed in newborn lambs show that fluid filtration in the lung can be increased by increasing pulmonary blood flow without increasing left atrial pressure (Feltes and Hansen, 1986). In the newborn with a reduced pulmonary vascular bed, either from lung injury or from hypoplasia, cardiac output appropriate for body size may represent a relative overperfusion to the lung and can result in increased fluid filtration. This phenomenon has been invoked to explain the lung edema that often complicates the course of the infant with bronchopulmonary dysplasia.

The exact cause of pulmonary edema that accompanies severe hypoxia or asphyxia in the newborn is still a controversial issue. Data suggest that it is the result of increased filtration pressure and not the result of any alteration in permeability. Heart failure accounts for some of the increased filtration pressure following severe asphyxia. In addition, there may be some element of pulmonary venous constriction. Finally, there is evidence that hypoxia and acidosis may redistribute pulmonary blood flow to a smaller portion of the lung and result in relative overperfusion and edema, much like that seen with anatomic loss of vascular bed (Hansen et al., 1984).

Several investigators have suggested that upper airway obstruction may cause pulmonary edema by decreasing interstitial hydrostatic pressure relative to intravascular

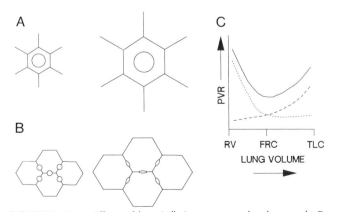

FIGURE 51–9. A, *Effects of lung inflation on extra-alveolar vessels.* B, *Effects of lung inflation on alveolar vessels.* C, *Effect of lung volume on pulmonary vascular resistance (PVR) (solid line). Inflation is from residual volume (RV) to functional residual capacity (FRC) to total lung capacity (TLC). Dashed line represents alveolar vessels; dotted line represents extra-alveolar vessels.*

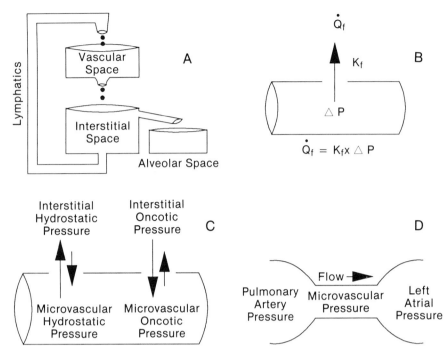

FIGURE 51–10. A, In the lung, fluid is continuously filtered out of vessels in the microcirculation into the interstitium and then returned to the intravascular compartment by the lymphatics. Only when the rate of filtration exceeds the rate of lymphatic removal can fluid accumulate in the interstitium. Spillover of fluid into the alveolar space occurs only when the interstitial space fills, or when the alveolar membrane is damaged.

B, Fluid flows out of vessels at a flow rate ($\dot{Q}_f$) that is equal to the driving pressure for fluid flow (ΔP) times the filtration coefficient (K_f): $\dot{Q}_f = K_f \times \Delta P$. K_f can be thought of as the relative permeability of the vascular bed to fluid flux. K_f in the normal lung is a very small number so that despite a driving pressure of roughly 5 torr the net rate of fluid filtration is approximately 1 to 2 ml/kg/hour.

C, The driving pressure for fluid flow out of the microvascular bed represents a balance of 2 sets of pressures. Within the blood vessel hydrostatic pressure tends to push fluid out of the vessel into the interstitium. This pressure is partially opposed by a smaller hydrostatic pressure within the interstitium pushing fluid back into the blood vessel. Within the blood vessel there also exists a discrete oncotic pressure that results predominantly from intravascular albumin that tends to draw fluid from the interstitium back into the blood vessel. This pressure is opposed by an interstitial oncotic pressure tending to draw fluid from the blood vessel into the interstitium.

D, The intravascular hydrostatic pressure must be less than pulmonary artery pressure (Ppa) in order for blood to flow into the microvascular bed and greater than left atrial pressure (Pla) in order for blood to flow out. Intravascular pressure is roughly equal to 0.4 (Ppa − Pla) + Pla. The interstitial hydrostatic pressure is roughly equal to alveolar pressure. The intravascular oncotic pressure can be calculated from the plasma albumin concentration. The interstitial oncotic pressure is roughly 2/3 of the intravascular oncotic pressure. The balance of these pressures favors filtration out of the vessel (in the normal lamb this pressure equals 5 torr).

hydrostatic pressure. Other data suggest, however, that with airway obstruction vascular pressures decrease with intrapleural pressure in such a way that filtration pressure remains unchanged (Hansen et al., 1985).

Hypoproteinemia in infants results in a decrease in intravascular oncotic pressure. Its effects upon filtration pressure, however, are blunted by the simultaneous decrease in protein concentration in the interstitial space of the lung. As a result edema is unlikely to occur unless hydrostatic pressure also increases (Hazinski et al., 1986).

Increased Permeability. Another possible mechanism for increased fluid filtration in the lung is a change in the permeability of the microvascular membrane to protein—permeability pulmonary edema. In this form of edema, the sieving properties of the microvascular endothelium are altered so that K_f increases and patients may develop pulmonary edema despite relatively normal vascular pressures (Albertine, 1985). Furthermore, even small changes in vascular pressures can result in a dramatic worsening of their pulmonary status. Permeability pulmonary edema usually implies either direct or indirect injury to the capillary endothelium of the lung. Direct injuries result from local effects of an inhaled toxin such as oxygen. Indirect injuries imply that the initial insult occurs elsewhere in the body and that the lung injury occurs secondarily. An example of indirect lung injury is sepsis: neutrophils activated by bacterial toxins attack endothelial cells in the lung and increase permeability to water and protein (Brigham et al., 1974). Indirect injuries usually involve blood-borne mediators, such as leukocytes, leukotrienes, histamine, or bradykinin.

TABLE 51–3. Increased Intravascular Hydrostatic Pressure

Increased Left Atrial Pressure
Intravascular Volume Overload
    Overzealous fluid administration
    Overtransfusion
    Renal insufficiency
Heart Failure
    Left sided obstructive lesions
    Left to right shunts
    Myocardiopathies
Increased Pulmonary Blood Flow
Normal Pulmonary Vascular Bed
    Patent ductus arteriosus
    Increased cardiac output
Reduced Pulmonary Vascular Bed
    Bronchopulmonary dysplasia
    Pulmonary hypoplasia

Decreased Lymphatic Drainage. In the normal lung, the rate of lung lymph flow is equal to the net rate of fluid filtration, and as long as lymphatic function can keep up with the rate of fluid filtration, water does not accumulate in the lung. While lymphatics can actively pump fluid against a pressure gradient, recent studies show that this ability is limited and that lung lymph flow varies inversely with the outflow pressure (pressure in the superior vena cava). Several groups of investigators have demonstrated that, in the presence of an increased rate of transvascular fluid filtration, the rate of fluid accumulation in the lung is substantially greater if systemic venous pressure is increased (Drake et al., 1985). This theory explains why pulmonary edema often complicates the course of infants with bronchopulmonary dysplasia and cor pulmonale and also explains the particular problem of edema with pleural effusions complicating the course of superior vena cava syndrome.

Symptoms. As discussed previously, fluid filtered into the alveolar interstitium ordinarily moves rapidly along pressure gradients into the extra-alveolar interstitium where it is removed by the lymphatics. A delay in this process at birth can result in clinical transient respiratory distress (see Chapter 52). The extra-alveolar interstitium has a large storage capacity. Fluid does not begin to spill over into the alveoli and airways until total lung water is increased more than 50 per cent, unless the alveolar membrane is damaged. Therefore, the first signs and symptoms of pulmonary edema are related to the presence of extra fluid in the interstitial cuffs of tissue that surround airways. As fluid builds up in these cuffs, airways are compressed and the infants develop signs of obstructive lung disease. The chest may appear hyperinflated and auscultation reveals rales, rhonchi, and a prolonged expiration. Early in the course, chest radiographs reveal lung overinflation and an accumulation of fluid in the extra-alveolar interstitium—linear densities of fluid that extend from the hilum to the periphery of the lung (the so-called sunburst appearance) and fluid in the fissures. With more severe edema, fluffy densities appear throughout the lung as alveoli fill with fluid (Fig. 51–11). Heart size may be increased in infants with edema from increased intravascular pressure. Initially, infants present with increased $PaCO_2$ secondary to impaired ventilation. Later PaO_2 decreases secondary to ventilation-perfusion mismatching and alveolar flooding. In adults, a ratio of protein concentration in tracheal aspirate to that in plasma greater than 0.5 may help to differentiate permeability pulmonary edema from high-pressure pulmonary edema (Fein, 1979).

Treatment. Treatment of pulmonary edema is directed at relieving hypoxemia and lowering vascular pressures. Hypoxemia should be treated with the administration of oxygen and, if necessary, positive-pressure ventilation. Positive end-expiratory pressure frequently improves oxygenation in individuals with pulmonary edema by improving ventilation-perfusion matching within the lung. Available evidence suggests that positive-pressure ventilation *does not* reduce the rate of transvascular fluid filtration in the lung (Woolverton et al., 1978). Optimal treatment of pulmonary edema requires correction of the underlying cause. In infants with patent ductus arteriosus (see Fig. 51–11) or other heart disease amenable to surgery, this is often easily accomplished. In cases of permeability edema or edema from nonsurgical heart defects, correction of the underlying cause may not be possible. In these instances the only remaining option is to lower vascular pressures (even in permeability edema, lowering vascular pressures lowers the rate of fluid filtration). This can be accomplished by lowering circulating blood volume by use of diuretics and fluid restriction, by improving myocardial function with the use of digitalis or other inotropic agents, or in severe cases by the use of a drug such as nitroprusside to reduce afterload and lower vascular pressures directly. Whether theophylline reduces airway obstruction in infants with pulmonary edema is not known.

PULMONARY HEMORRHAGE

Landing (1957) described pulmonary hemorrhage in 68 per cent of lungs of 125 consecutive infants who died in the 1st week of life; massive pulmonary hemorrhage was found in 17.8 per cent of neonatal autopsies at the Johns Hopkins Hospital (Rowe and Avery, 1966). Fedrick and Butler (1971) judged massive pulmonary hemorrhage to be the principal cause of death in about 9 per cent of neonatal autopsies.

Etiology and Pathogenesis. Pulmonary hemorrhage usually occurs between the 2nd and 4th days of life in infants who are being treated with mechanical ventilation. It has been associated with a wide variety of predisposing factors, including prematurity, asphyxia, overwhelming sepsis, intrauterine growth retardation, massive aspiration, severe hypothermia, severe Rh-hemolytic disease, congenital heart disease, and coagulopathies. It is often as-

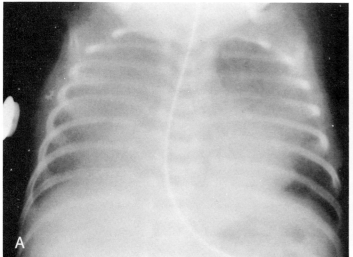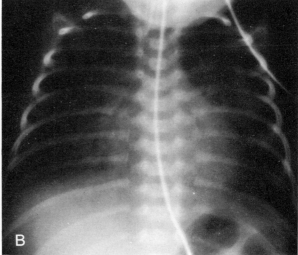

FIGURE 51–11. Preterm infant with a large patent ductus arteriosus and pulmonary edema (A). The same infant 24 hours after the ductus arteriosus was closed by administration of indomethacin (B).

sociated with central nervous system injury, such as asphyxia or intracranial hemorrhage. Cole and associates (1973) studied a group of infants with pulmonary hemorrhage to determine the clinical circumstances under which the illness occurred, as well as the hematocrit and protein composition of fluid obtained from lung effluent and arterial or venous blood. Their results indicated that the lung effluent was, in most cases, hemorrhagic edema fluid and not whole blood, i.e., as indicated by hematocrit values significantly lower than those of whole blood. In addition, they did not find that coagulation disorders initiated the condition but probably served to exacerbate it in some cases. They postulated that the important precipitating factor was acute left ventricular failure caused by asphyxia or other events that might increase filtration of lung liquid from pulmonary capillaries or cause lung damage.

Pulmonary edema following central nervous system (CNS) injury probably results from increased hydrostatic pressure and some increase in vascular permeability (Malik, 1985). With the massive sympathetic discharge that accompanies CNS injury, left atrial pressure increases, and pulmonary arteries and veins constrict. As a result, microvascular pressure increases dramatically and causes dramatic damage to the microvascular endothelium, increasing its permeability to proteins and red blood cells. In infants with overwhelming sepsis and endotoxin production, increased microvascular permeability is apparent in the pulmonary circulation as well, undoubtedly contributing to the massive pulmonary hemorrhage sometimes seen in this group of infants. Pulmonary hemorrhage also has been described occasionally in the presence of a very large patent ductus arteriosus, with a left-to-right shunt that results in high flow and high pressure injurious to the vascular bed.

Pulmonary hemorrhage has occurred within hours of surfactant replacement therapy. The number of instances recorded has been too small to substantiate that a cause-and-effect relationship exists. Nonetheless, it may be that improved oxygenation of pulmonary blood may cause hemorrhagic pulmonary edema.

Diagnosis. Infants with any of the conditions mentioned above should be observed carefully for possible pulmonary hemorrhage. Particular note should be made of any occurrence of blood-stained fluid from endotracheal tube aspirates, especially if repeated suctioning shows an increase in the amount of hemorrhagic fluid. The infant's chest radiograph may show the fluffy appearance of pulmonary edema in addition to the underlying pathology, and the infant may have increased respiratory distress. Frank pulmonary hemorrhage, when it occurs, is an acute emergency, and the fluid has the appearance of fresh blood being pumped directly from the vascular system, although hematocrit values of the fluid will be at least 15 to 20 points lower than the hematocrit of circulating blood, in keeping with hemorrhagic pulmonary edema.

Treatment. Effective treatment of pulmonary hemorrhage requires (1) Clearing the airway of blood to allow ventilation. (2) Use of adequate mean airway pressure, particularly end-expiratory pressure. (3) Resisting the temptation to administer large volumes of blood, since in most cases the infant will not have had a large loss of volume, and thus, administration of excessive volume will exacerbate the increase in left atrial pressure and hemorrhagic pulmonary edema. Rather, red cell replacement should be done as a very slow administration of packed cells after the infant's pulmonary status has been stabilized. (4) Evaluation of the possibility of coagulopathy and administration of vitamin K and platelets, if appropriate.

■ REFERENCES

Albertine, K. H.: Ultrastructural abnormalities in increased-permeability pulmonary edema. Clin. Chest Med. 6:345, 1985.

Bhutani, V. K., Sivieri, E. M., Abbasi, S., and Shaffer, T. H.: Evaluation of neonatal pulmonary mechanics and energetics: A two factor least mean square analysis. Pediatr. Pulmonol. 4:150, 1988.

Bland, R. D., and Hansen, T. N.: Neonatal lung edema. In Said, S. I. (Ed.): The Pulmonary Circulation and Acute Lung Injury. Mount Kisco, N. Y., Futura Publishing Co., 1985, p. 225.

Brigham, K. L., Woolverton, W., Blake, L., et al.: Increased sheep lung vascular permeability caused by Pseudomonas bacteremia. J. Clin. Invest. 54:792, 1974.

Bryan, A. C., and England, S. J.: Maintenance of an elevated FRC in the newborn: Paradox of REM sleep. Am. Rev. Respir. Dis. 129:209, 1984.

Cole, V. A., Normand, I. C. S., Reynolds, E. O. R., et al.: Pathogenesis of hemorrhagic pulmonary edema and massive pulmonary hemorrhage in the newborn. Pediatrics 51:175, 1973.

Cook, C. D., Cherry, R. B., O'Brien, D., et al.: Studies of respiratory physiology in the newborn infant. I. Observations on normal premature and full-term infants. J. Clin. Invest. 34:975, 1955.

Cook, C. D., Sutherland, J. M., Segal, S., et al.: Studies of respiratory physiology in the newborn infant. III. Measurements of mechanics of respiration. J. Clin. Invest. 36:440, 1957.

Corbet, A. J. S., Ross, J. A., Beaudry, P. H., et al.: Ventilation-perfusion relationships as assessed by aADN$_2$ in hyaline membrane disease. J. Appl. Physiol., 36:74–81, 1974.

Drake, R., Giesler, M., Laine, G., et al.: Effect of outflow pressure on lung lymph flow in unanesthetized sheep. J. Appl. Physiol. 58:70, 1985.

Farhi, L. E.: Ventilation-perfusion relationship and its role in alveolar gas exchange. In Caro, C. G. (Ed.): Advances in Respiratory Physiology. Baltimore, Williams & Wilkins, 1966.

Fedrick, J., and Butler, N. R.: Certain causes of neonatal death. IV. Massive pulmonary hemorrhage. Biol. Neonate 18:243, 1971.

Fein, A., Grossman, R. F., Jones, J. G., et al.: The value of edema fluid protein measurement in patients with pulmonary edema. Am. J. Med. 67:32, 1979.

Feltes, T. F., and Hansen, T. N.: Effects of a large aorticopulmonary shunt on lung fluid balance in newborn lambs. Pediatr. Res. 20:368A, 1986.

Fishman, A. P.: Pulmonary circulation. In Fishman, A. P., Fisher, A. B., and Geiger, S. R. (Eds.): Handbook of Physiology. Bethesda, Md., American Physiological Society, 1986, p. 131.

Gerhardt, T., and Bancalari, E.: Chestwall compliance in full-term and premature infants. Acta Paediatr. Scand. 69:359, 1980.

Hansen, T. N., Gest, A. L., and Landers, S.: Inspiratory airway obstruction does not affect lung fluid balance in lambs. J. Appl. Physiol. 58:1314, 1985.

Hansen, T. N., Hazinski, T. A., and Bland, R. D.: Effects of asphyxia on lung fluid balance in baby lambs. J. Clin. Invest. 741:370, 1984.

Hazinski, T. A., Bland, R. D., Hansen, T. N., et al.: Effect of hypoproteinemia on lung fluid balance in awake newborn lambs. J. Appl. Physiol. 61:1139, 1986.

Krieger, I.: Studies on mechanics of respiration in infancy. Am. J. Dis. Child. 105:439, 1963.

Landing, B. H.: Pulmonary lesions in newborn infants: A statistical study. Pediatrics 19:217, 1957

Lesouef, P. N., England, S. J., and Bryan, A. C.: Passive respiratory mechanics in newborns and children. Am. Rev. Respir. Dis. 129:552, 1984.

McCann, E. M., Goldman, S. L., and Brady, J. P.: Pulmonary function in the sick newborn infant. Pediatr. Res. 21:313, 1987.

McGregor, M.: Pulsus paradoxus. N. Engl. J. Med. 301:480, 1979.

McIlroy, M. B., Tierney, D. F., and Nadel, J. A.: A new method for measurement of compliance and resistance of lungs and thorax. J. Appl. Physiol. *18*:424, 1963.

Malik, A. B.: Mechanisms of neurogenic pulmonary edema. Circ. Res. *57*:1, 1985.

Markello, R., Winter, P., and Olszowka, A.: Assessment of ventilation-perfusion inequalities by arterial-alveolar nitrogen differences in intensive care patients. Anesthesiology *37*:4, 1972.

Moriette, G., Chaussain, M., Radvanyi-Bouvet, M., et al.: Functional residual capacity and sleep states in the premature newborn. Biol. Neonate. *43*:125, 1983.

Nelson, N. M.: Neonatal pulmonary function. Pediatr. Clin. North Am. *13*:769, 1966.

Nelson, N. M.: Respiration and circulation after birth. *In* Smith, C. A., and Nelson, N. M. (Eds.): The Physiology of the Newborn Infant. Springfield, Ill., Charles C Thomas, 1976.

Nelson, N. M., Prod'hom, L. S., Cherry, R. B., et al.: Pulmonary function in the newborn infant. V. Trapped gas in the normal infant's lung. J. Clin. Invest. *42*:1850, 1963.

Niemann, J. T., Rosborough, J., Hausknect, M., et al.: Documentation of systemic perfusion in man and in an experimental model: A "window" to the mechanism of blood flow in external CPR. Crit. Care Med. *8*:141, 1980.

Pedley, T. J., Sudlow, M. F., and Schroter, R. C.: Gas flow and mixing in the airways. *In* West, J. B. (Ed.): Bioengineering Aspects of the Lung. New York, Marcel Dekker, 1977, p. 163.

Perlman, J., and Thach, B.: Respiratory origin of fluctuations in arterial blood pressure in premature infants with respiratory distress syndrome. Pediatrics *81*:399, 1988.

Polgar, G., and Kong, G. P.: The Nasal Resistance of Newborn Infants. J. Pediatr. *67*:557, 1965.

Polgar, G., and Promadhat, V.: Pulmonary function testing in children: Techniques and standards. Philadelphia, W. B. Saunders Company, 1971, p. 273.

Polgar, G., and String, S. T.: The viscous resistance of the lung tissues in newborn infants. J. Pediatr. *69*:787, 1966.

Reynolds, R. N., and Etsten, B. E.: Mechanics of respiration in apneic anesthetized infants. Anesthesiology *27*:13, 1966.

Rodarte, J. R., and Rehder, K.: Dynamics of respiration. *In* Fishman, A. P., Macklem, P. T., Mead, J., and Geiger, S. R. (Eds.): Handbook of Physiology, vol. III. Bethesda, Md., American Physiological Society, 1986, p. 131.

Rowe, S., and Avery, M. E.: Massive pulmonary hemorrhage in the newborn. II. Clinical considerations. J. Pediatr. *69*:12, 1966.

Slonim, N. B., and Hamilton, L. H.: Respiratory physiology, 5th ed. St. Louis, C. V. Mosby, 1987, p. 52.

Staub, N. C.: Pulmonary edema. Physiol. Rev. *54*:678, 1974.

West, J. B.: Ventilation: Blood Flow and Gas Exchange, 4th ed. St. Louis, C. V. Mosby, 1986.

Woolverton, N. C., Brigham, K. L., and Staub, N. C.: Effect of positive pressure breathing on lung lymph flow and water content in sheep. Circ. Res. *42*:550, 1978.

PRINCIPLES OF 52
RESPIRATORY MONITORING AND THERAPY

Thomas Hansen and Anthony Corbet

■ OXYGEN THERAPY

In an emergency, high concentrations of oxygen may be administered by face mask, head hood, or endotracheal tube for the relief of cyanosis. If oxygen must be continued beyond the emergency, it should be warmed, humidified, and delivered by a flow proportioner connected to compressed sources of air and oxygen. The concentration of oxygen should be analyzed continuously or at least every hour, using an oxygen analyzer that is calibrated with air and oxygen every 8 hours. The use of oxygen therapy beyond the emergency period should be monitored by means of regular estimates of arterial oxygen pressure. When this is not possible, oxygen should be given in a concentration just sufficient to abolish central cyanosis; but within a few hours, arrangements should be made for appropriate measurements.

MONITORING OXYGEN THERAPY

ARTERIAL CATHETERS

In infants with significant respiratory distress, it is common to monitor oxygen therapy during the first few days of life using an umbilical artery catheter. In most infants, the arterial oxygen pressure should be maintained between 50 and 70 mm Hg, but in some patients with labile pulmonary hypertension, it is frequently recommended to keep the arterial oxygen pressure as high as 80 to 100 mm Hg. However, in infants requiring high ventilator pressures, levels between 30 and 40 mm Hg may be accepted, provided that the circulatory status is well maintained and metabolic acidosis does not occur.

The reported complications of umbilical arterial (UA) catheters include perforation, vasospasm, thrombosis, embolism, and infection. The most obvious sign of vasospasm is ischemia to the ipsilateral leg, and if this persists after a brief period of warming the contralateral leg, the catheter should be removed. During a difficult insertion procedure, it is possible (although this rarely occurs) to perforate the umbilical artery and enter the peritoneum, with consequent hemoperitoneum and hemorrhagic shock. By far, the most feared complication is thrombosis, and small thrombi, as documented by contrast aortography, may develop around the catheter in up to 95 per cent of infants

(Neal et al., 1972). Minute emboli may explain transient episodes of ischemia that later result in bluish discoloration of the toes. Clinical evidence of obstruction to a mesenteric, renal, pelvic, or femoral artery, or to the aorta itself, is comparatively uncommon but has been found in 13 per cent of autopsy cases (Cochran, 1976). The evidence that this complication is correlated with the duration of catheterization is unconvincing (Symanski and Fox, 1972), but suggestive evidence was found serendipitously by Jackson and co-workers (1987) that aortic thrombosis, detected by ultrasound, is more common after 11 days than after 4 days of catheterization. Infants with thrombosis can usually be managed conservatively with removal of the catheter and supportive care. Renovascular hypertension may occur and require antihypertensive therapy. The condition usually resolves in time (Caplan et al., 1989). Another significant complication of UA catheterization is infection, with sepsis occurring in 5 per cent of cases (Moise et al., 1986). However, the incidence is clearly higher (13 per cent) if the catheter remains in place more than 14 days.

The problem for clinicians is that the umbilical arterial catheter has become the easiest and most reliable way to monitor oxygen therapy. The need for arterial access should always be weighed against the inherent risks of an indwelling line when a decision is made to leave a catheter in place for more than a few days.

As an alternative to the umbilical artery catheter, wide use is now made of short catheters inserted percutaneously or by the cut-down procedure into the radial, posterior tibial, or dorsalis pedis arteries. Unfortunately, these catheters usually last only a few days to a week, but the rates of infection and other complications are quite low (Adams et al., 1980).

INTERMITTENT ARTERIAL PUNCTURE

Arterial samples for blood gas analysis may be obtained by percutaneous needle aspiration of brachial, radial, or temporal arteries. The problem with this procedure is that unless the sample is obtained immediately on penetration, or with the use of effective local anesthesia, the infant is disturbed, and this changes the actual oxygen tension,

488

usually in a downward direction. Spasm or thrombosis with local ischemia is, however, comparatively rare.

NONINVASIVE MONITORS

The first noninvasive technique to gain widespread clinical acceptance was the skin-surface oxygen (PsO_2) electrode (Huch, 1976; Landers, 1986) (Fig. 52–1). The PsO_2 electrode does not measure PaO_2 directly; it simply measures the PO_2 on the surface of the skin. If certain conditions are met, namely, an appropriate electrode temperature for a given skin thickness (Fig. 52–2) and normal circulation, the two measurements are highly related, and the PsO_2 provides a reasonable estimate of the PaO_2 for values between 15 and 150 torr.

Problems arise when the PsO_2 differs from the PaO_2 (Table 52–1). Skin thickness, skin blood flow, oxygen consumption and electrode temperature all affect the correlation (see Fig. 52–2). The PsO_2 electrode itself may also interfere with the correlation between PsO_2 and PaO_2. The electrode consumes oxygen at a rate limited by the membrane permeability. If membrane permeability increases, oxygen consumption by the electrode can lower the PsO_2. Since an infinite supply of oxygen exists at the time of calibration, the electrode calibrates normally.

The skin surface carbon dioxide ($PsCO_2$) electrode is a glass pH electrode modified so that it can be heated and mounted upon the skin (Hansen and Tooley, 1979; Brunstler et al., 1982). CO_2 diffuses into the electrode and produces a change in pH. The $PsCO_2$ electrode measures the concentration of carbon dioxide on the surface of the skin and is little affected by skin thickness or membrane

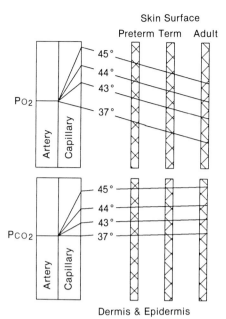

FIGURE 52–2. *In unheated skin, as oxygen diffuses from the capillary bed across the dermis and epidermis, PO_2 decreases relative to PaO_2 because of skin consumption of oxygen (top). As skin thickness increases (preterm infant versus term infant versus adult), this discrepancy increases. To counteract this effect, PsO_2 electrodes are heated. Heating increases capillary and tissue PO_2 by producing vasodilatation, thereby increasing oxygen delivery to the skin, and by shifting the oxygen hemoglobin dissociation curve to the right. The subsequent fall in PO_2 as oxygen diffuses to the skin surface counterbalances effect of heating and lowers PO_2 at the skin surface to a value approaching PaO_2. Optimal correlation between PaO_2 and PsO_2 requires that electrode temperature be appropriate for skin thickness. On the other hand, because of local carbon dioxide production the $PsCO_2$ of even unheated skin is greater than $PaCO_2$ (bottom). Heating the electrode increases $PsCO_2$ further. The effect of electrode temperature on $PsCO_2$ is constant and predictable so that correction factors can be built into the calibration procedure.*

permeability. It is affected by blood flow to the skin and must be heated to 42 to 44°C to produce vasodilatation. Heating increases $PsCO_2$ relative to $PaCO_2$ and correction factors must be incorporated into the calibration procedure so that the digital or graphic readout of $PsCO_2$ equals $PaCO_2$ (see Fig. 52–2).

Continuous noninvasive estimates of arterial oxygen saturation (SaO_2) by pulse oximetry represent an innovative noninvasive monitoring technique (Fig. 52–3) (Pologe, 1987; Wukitsch, 1987). In the red region of the spectrum, reduced hemoglobin absorbs more light than oxyhemoglobin. In the infrared region (IR), oxyhemoglobin absorbs more light than reduced hemoglobin. Total light absorption (at any wavelength) is the sum of the independent absorptions. For whole blood the ratio of

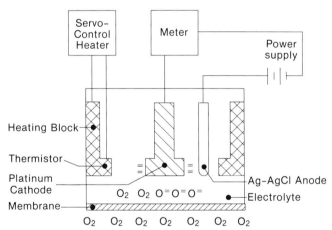

FIGURE 52–1. *The PsO_2 electrode consists of a servo-controlled heater, a platinum cathode, and a silver–silver chloride anode that is immersed in an electrolyte solution and covered with semipermeable membrane. An external voltage maintains the cathode negative with respect to the anode. Oxygen diffuses across the membrane to the negatively charged cathode, and since it is extremely electrophilic, it readily accepts electrons from the cathode. The reduced oxygen species react with KCl in the electrolyte to form KOH while liberated Cl^- ions are deposited on the anode. As electrons are removed from the cathode, electrons flow from the anode and generate an electrical current that can be measured in the external circuit. This current is proportional to the rate of diffusion of oxygen molecules across the membrane into the electrode. The rate of diffusion, in turn, is proportional to the PsO_2 and the permeability of the membrane to oxygen. Oxygen electrodes must be "zeroed" to compensate for the current produced by the external voltage, and a gain must be set to adjust the output for a given membrane permeability.*

TABLE 52–1. Factors Affecting Skin Surface O₂ and CO₂ Tensions

Increase PsO_2	Increase $PsCO_2$
• Increased PaO_2	• Increased $PaCO_2$
• Increased temperature	• Increased temperature
Decrease PsO_2	• Increased skin CO_2 production
• Decreased PaO_2	• Decreased perfusion
• Decreased skin perfusion	**Decrease $PsCO_2$**
• Increased skin thickness (age-related)	• Decreased $PaCO_2$
• Edema	• Decreased temperature
• Damaged membrane	

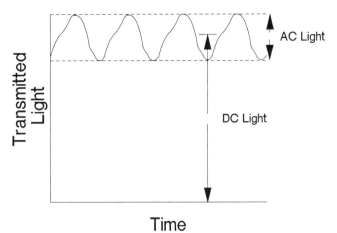

Time

FIGURE 52–3. The pulse oximeter uses light-emitting diodes (LED) to send pulses of light of two different wavelengths through tissue containing a peripheral artery. A photodiode located opposite from the LEDs measures the intensity of the transmitted light. At each wavelength, the light transmitted to the diode consists of two components: (1) an AC component where the intensity of transmitted light changes with the volume of blood (light absorber) in the artery, and (2) a DC or constant component that results from light being transmitted through the tissues without being absorbed or scattered.

The pulse oximeter measures the intensity of transmitted light as it illuminates one LED, then the other, and then switches both off. With both LEDs off, the oximeter can measure and correct for the effects of external light incident on the photodiode. These cycles occur 480 times/ second. The pulse oximeter focuses on the pulse added component of the transmitted light by dividing the AC component by the DC component at each wavelength and creating the ratio: $R = [AC_{RED}/DC_{RED}]/[AC_{IR}/DC_{IR}]$. In this way, it ignores absorbances of venous blood, tissue, and pigmentation.

absorption in the red region to that in the IR region decreases as SaO_2 increases.

The pulse oximeter is not affected by skin thickness, but it is affected by the circulatory status of the patient. The AC signal detected by the pulse oximeter is only 1 per cent of the DC level, so if changes in tissue perfusion reduce arterial pulsations further, the pulse oximeter cannot function. Although the pulse oximeter assumes that there are only two types of hemoglobin present in arterial blood, a consistent effect of fetal hemoglobin on the relationship has not been demonstrated (Jennis and Peabody, 1987; Ramanathan et al., 1987).

Each of these techniques allows continuous noninvasive monitoring of arterial blood gas tensions. The pulse oximeter's advantages are (1) it does not require heat, (2) it has a very rapid response time, and (3) it is not affected by skin thickness. This latter property makes the pulse oximeter useful in assessing oxygenation in the older infant with chronic lung disease. The chief disadvantage is its rapid (and sometimes inaccurate) response to small changes in oxygenation induced by movement or even brief physiologic changes in the infant. The PsO_2 electrode, on the other hand, must be heated and may result in burns to the skin—especially in the preterm infant. Therefore, it must be moved to a new site at least every 4 hours. In addition, it is more affected by changes in skin thickness and skin blood flow. The advantages of the PsO_2 electrode are that it estimates PaO_2 rather than SaO_2 and is not subject to wide swings with minor changes in the infant. Although PaO_2 can be roughly calculated from SaO_2, particularly at higher ranges of saturation, the range

of PaO_2 values for any given confidence interval of saturations can be broad.

■ MECHANICAL VENTILATION

Continuous Distending Airway Pressure. Continuous distending airway pressure may be applied with positive pressure through nasal prongs or an endotracheal tube or by continuous negative pressure applied to the chest. By stabilizing the poorly supported small airways of the premature infant and preventing the generalized atelectasis of the surfactant-deficient lung, continuous distending pressure improves ventilation in the low $\dot{V}/\dot{Q}$ air spaces, converting them to high $\dot{V}/\dot{Q}$ air spaces, with relief of local vasoconstriction, decreased right-to-left shunting, and improved arterial oxygen saturation (Hansen et al., 1979). In addition, a new, open low $\dot{V}/\dot{Q}$ compartment is formed by recruitment of collapsed air spaces. The physiologic consequences of continuous positive airway pressure (CPAP) in hyaline membrane disease (HMD) may include decreased tidal volume, decreased minute ventilation, increased lung volume, reduced lung compliance, increased work of breathing, increased arterial oxygen pressure, decreased $Aa.DO_2$, $aA.DN_2$, and $aA.DO_2$ and reduced true right-to-left shunt (Corbet et al., 1975).

Intermittent Positive Pressure Ventilation. Advances in techniques for intermittent positive pressure ventilation (IPPV) have dramatically altered the outcomes of infants with a variety of lung diseases. To use these techniques effectively, one must have a thorough understanding of how the various components of IPPV affect the lung of the newborn.

Positive Pressure Inflation of the Lung. During a positive pressure breath, gas flows into the lung because airway pressure is greater than alveolar pressure. The volume of gas entering the lung over time is a function of the peak inflation pressure (PIP), duration of inspiration (Ti), and respiratory system compliance (Crs) and resistance (Rrs) (Figs. 52–4 and 52–5). For purposes of this discussion, exhalation is considered to be passive (see Chapter 51).

Most ventilators that are currently in use in neonatal intensive care units are time-cycled and pressure-limited (Fig. 52–6). PIP, positive end-expiratory pressure (PEEP), Ti, and expiratory time (Te) are adjusted independently (Table 52–2). The rate is altered by changing Ti or Te or both. Mean airway pressure (MAP) is the average pressure at the proximal airway over time. If the inspiratory pressure wave form resembles a square wave (see Fig. 52–6), then

$$MAP = (PIP - PEEP) \times (Ti/[Ti + Te]) + PEEP.$$

EFFECTS OF POSITIVE PRESSURE VENTILATION ON GAS EXCHANGE

In infants with parenchymal lung disease, hypoxemia is related to the presence of open but severely underventilated lung units (see Chapter 51). In these units, alveolar ventilation is not sufficient to maintain the alveolar oxygen tension (PaO_2) much above mixed venous PO_2. These lung units can cause arterial hypoxemia by two different mechanisms.

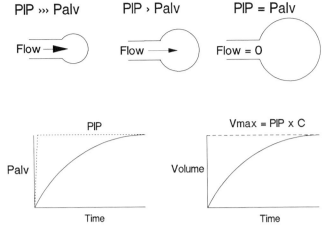

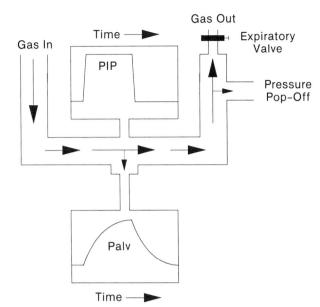

FIGURE 52–4. *Positive pressure inflation of the lung. In this example, airway pressure increases rapidly to a plateau (peak inflation pressure, PIP) (dashed line). Initially, alveolar pressure (Palv) is equal to atmospheric pressure and is much less than airway pressure (PIP >>> Palv). As a result of this large driving pressure, gas flows into the lung and the volume of gas in the lung increases as a function of time. Obviously, since Palv is directly related to lung volume (Palv = Volume/compliance), it also increases as a function of time. Therefore, the driving pressure for gas flow, PIP − Palv, and the rate of gas flow into the lung both decrease over time. Ultimately, Palv becomes equal to PIP, and flow ceases. Therefore, the maximum volume of gas that can enter the lung (Vmax) during any positive-pressure breath is ultimately determined by PIP and compliance (C) (Vmax = PIP × C).*

FIGURE 52–6. *Time-cycled, pressure-limited ventilator. Gas flows continuously through the ventilator circuit while a flow resistor on the exhalation limb of the circuit provides PEEP. During inspiration, the expiratory valve is closed and pressure builds up in the circuit for a preset time (Ti). The rate of the pressure build up is determined to a large extent by the system flow. In this example, flow is high and the pressure wave form is a square wave. PIP is limited by venting excessive pressure to the atmosphere. Airway pressure increases rapidly and is held at a plateau. Alveolar pressure increases gradually as gas flows into the lung from the ventilator. The rate of gas flow to the patient is determined by the driving pressure (PIP − Palv) and the resistance (R): Flow = (PIP − Palv)/R, not by the rate of gas flow through the ventilator circuit.*

Ventilation-Perfusion Mismatch. In term infants with meconium aspiration pneumonia or older infants with bronchopulmonary dysplasia, blood continues to flow past the poorly ventilated lung units and remains poorly oxygenated. When it mixes with the remainder of the pulmonary venous return, it decreases overall systemic oxygen saturation. The severity of the resultant hypoxemia is directly related to the severity of the hypoxia in the poorly ventilated lung units and to the quantity of blood flowing past them.

Right-to-Left Shunt. In infants with hyaline membrane disease, the cause of hypoxemia is right-to-left shunt. In these infants intense vasoconstriction occurs in blood vessels supplying severely underventilated lung units causing blood to be directed away from these lung units through intrapulmonary and extrapulmonary shunts (Hansen et al., 1979). The magnitude of the right-to-left shunt, hence the severity of the arterial hypoxemia, is related to the severity of the hypoxia in the open underventilated

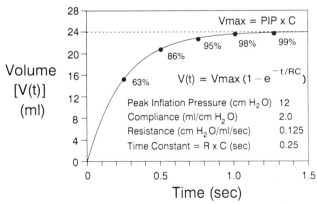

FIGURE 52–5. *Lung inflation over time: as in Figure 52–4, airway pressure is rapidly increased to 25 cm H_2O and then maintained at a plateau. The volume of gas in the lung [V(t)] increases over time according to the relationship: V(t) = Vmax × (1 − e$^{-t/RC}$), where R is the resistance of the respiratory system and C is the compliance. The maximum volume of gas that can flow into the lung (Vmax) is limited by the peak airway pressure (PIP) and C, i.e., Vmax = PIP × C. The rate of lung inflation, like the rate of deflation is described by an exponential equation involving the respiratory time constant (Trs). As described in Chapter 51, Trs = RC. For an inspiratory time equal to one time constant (Ti = 1 × Trs), the lung will inflate to 63 per cent of its maximum volume (Vmax). For Ti = 2 × Trs it will reach 86 per cent of Vmax; for 3 × Trs, 95 per cent; for 4 × Trs 98 per cent; and for 5 × Trs 99 per cent. Therefore, the volume of gas entering the lung during a positive-pressure breath is determined by the peak inflation pressure (PIP), the duration of inspiration (Ti), and respiratory system compliance (Crs) and resistance (Rrs).*

TABLE 52–2. Initial and Subsequent Settings for Mechanical Ventilation

Initial Settings		
FIO_2	As indicated	
System flow	10 l/minute	
Rate	60 breaths/minute	
Ti/Te	1/4	
PIP	Good breath sounds	
PEEP	5 cm H_2O	
Subsequent Settings	**PEEP**	**PIP**
Low Pao_2,* low $Paco_2$	Increase	
Low Pao_2, high $Paco_2$		Increase
High Pao_2, high $Paco_2$	Decrease	
High Pao_2, low $Paco_2$		Decrease

*This may indicate poor pulmonary blood flow.

lung units and to the number of these units present in the lung.

Therefore, regardless of the underlying parenchymal disease, the degree of arterial hypoxemia is determined by the P_{AO_2} in open but severely underventilated units of the lung; the only way to increase arterial oxygen tension (Pa_{O_2}) is to increase the P_{AO_2} in these lung units.

Several studies have shown that increasing the MAP increases Pa_{O_2} in infants with lung disease suggesting that increases in MAP must somehow increase the Pa_{O_2} in poorly ventilated units of the lung (Herman and Reynolds, 1973; Stewart et al., 1981). As discussed previously, MAP is really a function of PIP, PEEP, and Ti. Increasing MAP by increasing PIP increases the driving pressure for gas flow into poorly ventilated lung units (Fig. 52–7). Increasing MAP by increasing Ti allows more time for gas to distribute to these units. Finally, increasing MAP by increasing PEEP splints small airways open, decreases airway resistance, decreases the time constant for inspiration and allows more gas to enter the lung unit for any given PIP or Ti. All three techniques improve ventilation to the poorly ventilated lung units and increase their Pa_{O_2}. For a given increase in MAP, increasing PEEP or PIP results in a greater increase in Pa_{O_2} than increasing Ti (Stewart et al., 1981). The reason for this discrepancy lies in the effects of mechanical ventilation on the normal parts of the lung.

None of the parenchymal lung diseases are homogeneous. Relatively normal lung units coexist with severely underventilated lung units. Since all are connected, however, all are exposed to the same airway pressures during mechanical ventilation. Relatively normal units may have a low airway resistance and high compliance and may be subject to overdistention with increases in MAP. The risk of overdistention is greatest when MAP is increased by increasing Ti, less with increases in PIP, and least with increases in PEEP (Fig. 52–7). As discussed in Chapter 51, overdistended lung units compress intra-alveolar vessels and redirect blood flow past poorly ventilated lung units or through shunt pathways. This increase in ventilation-perfusion mismatching tends to offset any increase in Pa_{O_2} that occurs because of increased oxygenation in poorly ventilated lung units. This phenomenon probably explains why Pa_{O_2} increases less when MAP is increased by increasing Ti than when it is increased by increasing PEEP or PIP.

Besides its effects on oxygenation, alveolar overdistention carries the risk of alveolar rupture and PIE (see Chapter 54). The propensity for increases in Ti to result in alveolar overdistention is supported by its high association with pulmonary air leaks in one study that explored the antecedents of alveolar rupture (Primhak, 1983). It is also supported by the results of a single controlled trial showing a higher incidence of pneumothorax in infants ventilated with a long Ti than in those ventilated with a short Ti (Heicher et al., 1981).

The other important function of mechanical ventilation is to ventilate adequately, and the Pa_{CO_2} is an indication of this. Pa_{CO_2} is equal to the rate of CO_2 production divided by the alveolar ventilation ($\dot{V}_A$). $\dot{V}_A$ equals ($V_T - V_D$) × RR, where V_T and V_D are the tidal volume and dead space volume, respectively. If V_D and CO_2 production are relatively constant, then Pa_{CO_2} is proportional to

$1 \div (RR \times V_T)$. Pa_{CO_2} decreases if either RR or V_T is increased and Pa_{CO_2} increases if RR or V_T is decreased. On a pressure-limited respirator at a constant inspiratory time, the V_T is determined by the lung compliance and by PIP and PEEP (Fig. 52–8). (If Ti is less than 3 time constants, then increasing Ti increases tidal volume but at the expense of overdistention of more normal lung units.) To summarize, Pa_{CO_2} can be decreased by increasing RR, by increasing PIP, or by decreased PEEP. Conversely, Pa_{CO_2} can be increased by decreasing RR, by decreasing PIP, or by increasing PEEP.

Although it is attractive to try to lower the Pa_{CO_2} by increasing the respirator rate, rather than by adjusting ventilatory pressures, recent data suggest that this may not be entirely without risk. As the respirator rate increases, the absolute time allotted for expiration decreases. If expiratory time decreases to less than 3 time constants for expiration, gas trapping and alveolar overdistention may occur.

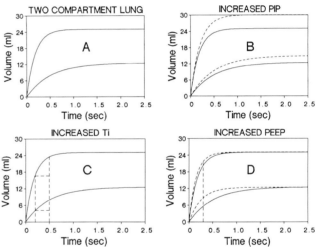

FIGURE 52–7. Effects of ventilatory manipulations on each compartment of a two-compartment lung: A, Plot of lung volume over time during a positive pressure inflation of the lung (PIP = 25 cm H_2O). The top curve represents normal lung units (compliance = 1 ml/cm H_2O, resistance = 0.150 cm H_2O/ml/second and time constant = 0.15 second). These lung units inflate to a greater maximum volume (Vmax = PIP × C = 25 ml) and reach Vmax quickly (5 time constants = 0.75 second). The lower curve represents poorly ventilated lung units (compliance = 0.5 ml/cm H_2O, resistance = 1.0 cm H_2O/ml/second, and time constant = 0.5 second). Obviously, these units will have a lower Vmax (12.5 ml) and will take longer to reach Vmax (5 time constants = 2.5 seconds). As stated previously, unless there is poor pulmonary blood flow, which can be corrected, the only ventilatory way to increase the patient's Pa_{O_2} is to increase the volume of gas entering poorly ventilated lung units.

B, Increasing peak inflation pressure (dashed curves) increases the volume of gas entering each group of lung units. The increase is greater in normal lung units than in poorly ventilated lung units for any value of Ti. The net result is overdistention of normal parts of the lung in an attempt to ventilate the poorly ventilated lung units.

C, Increasing inspiratory time (Ti) from 0.2 to 0.5 second increases the volume of gas entering each group of lung units. As in B, the increase, hence tendency for overdistention, is much more pronounced in the normal parts of the lung.

D, Increasing positive end-expiratory pressure (PEEP) decreases the time constant in each group of lung units. The net effect is to allow more gas to enter each part of the lung for any given PIP or Ti. In this case, the effect is more pronounced in the poorly ventilated lung units. As a result, the likelihood of overdistention of normal lung units is less.

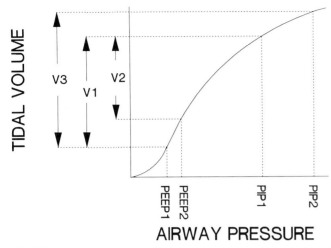

FIGURE 52–8. Determinants of tidal volume: Lung volume is plotted as a function of inflation pressure. As the ventilator cycles between positive end-expiratory pressure (PEEP1) and peak inflation pressure (PIP1), the lung volume changes, generating tidal volume (V1). Increasing positive end-expiratory pressure to PEEP2 forces the ventilator to cycle between PEEP2 and PIP1 and results in a lower tidal volume, V2. On the other hand, leaving positive end-expiratory pressure at PEEP1 and increasing peak inflation pressure to PIP2 increases the tidal volume to V3.

APPLICATIONS

Because tiny premature infants characteristically have structurally immature lungs and weak chest walls, many centers have a standard practice of providing some form of respiratory support (i.e., nasal CPAP or mechanical ventilation) for all infants who weigh less than 1250 g. For all infants who weigh between 1250 g and 1500 g and have hyaline membrane disease, ventilatory assistance is also necessary, as well as for larger infants with apneic episodes or those who cannot maintain a PaO_2 of more than 50 torr on a continuous distending pressure of 10 to 12 cm H_2O and 100 per cent oxygen. Infants usually are intubated orally with an endotracheal tube that allows an audible air leak in order to prevent later development of subglottic stenosis. A 2.5 mm I.D. tube is appropriate for infants weighing less than 1 kg, 3.0 mm for those between 1 and 2 kg, and a 3.5 mm for those weighing more than 2 kg. Orotracheal intubation is preferred over nasotracheal, because nasotracheal intubation has been found to cause nasal deformities (McMillan et al., 1986), and with orotracheal intubation, the tip of the tube is thought to be less likely to move with changes in head position (Donn and Blane, 1975).

During intubation, infants often require a fractional inspired oxygen (FIO_2) that is 10 per cent greater than they were receiving before the initiation of mechanical ventilation. It is always valuable to hand-ventilate an infant initially to determine the minimal PIP necessary to achieve good chest wall excursion and good bilateral breath sounds. A rate of 60 breaths per minute (which approximates the normal rate for a premature infant) and PEEP of 5 are used. In general, oxygenation can be improved by increasing MAP by increasing PEEP or PIP (see Table 52–1). Ti should rarely be prolonged, because of the risk of alveolar overdistention. Hypercarbia is treated by increasing PIP or decreasing PEEP. To allow sufficient time for exhalation, the respirator rate should not ordinarily

exceed 100 breaths per minute (Simbruner, 1986). The entire cardiopulmonary status of the infant must be kept in mind. An infant with poor pulmonary blood flow, because of hypotension, hypovolemia, cardiac failure, or high pulmonary vascular resistance, may also have a low PaO_2, and treatment should be directed to improving blood pressure and volume and cardiac output.

Weaning can be accomplished, as shown in Table 52–2. For larger infants, weaning to endotracheal CPAP may begin when PIP has been stable at <25 cm H_2O and FIO_2 is <0.40, and then to an oxygen hood when they require <5 cm H_2O of end-expiratory pressure. For infants weighing <1750 g, when PIP is <20 cm H_2O and FIO_2 <0.30, it is possible to decrease gradually the respiratory rate to 15 to 20 breaths per minute and then to wean directly to nasal CPAP (Wung et al., 1975). For this group of infants, the resistance of the endotracheal tube is such that periods of endotracheal CPAP or ventilatory rates less than 15 breaths per minute cannot be tolerated (Lesouef et al., 1984). For infants who cannot be weaned from the ventilator because of apnea or chronic lung disease, a respiratory rate of 20 to 30 breaths per minute and a slightly prolonged Ti allow the best distribution of ventilation through damaged airways.

Ventilator gas should be warmed to 32°C and humidified to 80 to 90 per cent to prevent excessive water loss from the respiratory tract and injury to the lung from exposure to cold dry air. This is most easily accomplished by using a heated nebulizer with heated ventilator circuits to prevent condensation of water in the ventilator tubing. Tracheal suctioning and chest physiotherapy should be minimized in the infant with hyaline membrane disease (HMD) in the first few days after birth since their secretions are scant and there is little evidence that suctioning and chest physiotherapy are of benefit. On the other hand, concern has been expressed that these interventions might increase the risk of intracranial hemorrhage (Griesen et al., 1985). Infants with secretions (e.g., meconium aspiration or pneumonia) and older infants with HMD may require suctioning of the trachea as often as every 2 to 4 hours. Even then, suctioning is often associated with acute side effects of hypoxia, hypertension, and bradycardia (Simbruner et al., 1981) and, with deep suctioning, the risk of airway injury (Miller et al., 1981) (see Chapter 29). If hand ventilation accompanies suctioning, a manometer must be attached to the bag to prevent delivery of excessive PIP.

The use of neuromuscular blockade to facilitate mechanical ventilation in the neonate remains controversial. Available data suggest that paralysis may shorten the course of HMD and reduce the periods of nonoptimal oxygenation and increased intracranial pressure associated with mechanical ventilation (Crone and Favorito, 1980; Finer and Tomney, 1981; Henry et al., 1979; Pollitzer et al., 1981). However, paralysis may result in decreased dynamic lung compliance and increased airway resistance and will remove any contribution of the infant's own respiratory effort from tidal breathing (Bhutani et al., 1988). Therefore, it is often necessary to increase ventilator pressures after initiation of neuromuscular blockade. Venous return is also impaired by lack of movement and decreased muscle tone; therefore, generalized edema develops with this treatment.

COMPLICATIONS OF THERAPY

Prolonged orotracheal intubation may cause palatal grooving and may interfere with dentition (Duke et al., 1976; Moylan et al., 1980), whereas nasotracheal intubation may result in cosmetic deformities of the nose (Jung and Thomas, 1974) and even nasal obstruction (see Chapter 54). Subglottic stenosis, although rare, can be a disastrous complication of intubation. A too snugly fitting endotracheal tube, duration of intubation, and number of reintubations all correlate with subsequent subglottic stenosis (Fan et al., 1983; Sherman et al., 1986). Some infants have required tracheostomy.

Necrotizing tracheobronchitis (Pietsch, 1985) is a necrotic inflammatory process involving the trachea and mainstem bronchi that has been described in neonates requiring mechanical ventilation. Sloughing of the tracheal epithelium results in occlusion of the distal trachea. Infants present with acute respiratory deterioration with symptoms of airway obstruction, hyperexpansion on chest radiograph, and poor chest movement. Emergency bronchoscopy may be necessary to relieve airway obstruction. The lesion is thought to result from drying of the tracheal mucosa secondary to inadequate humidification in the presence of high rates of gas flow and high concentrations of oxygen.

Atelectasis occasionally occurs following extubation from mechanical ventilation, with the right upper lobe most commonly affected. In some instances, atelectasis may reflect injury to the bronchi from suction catheters. In small preterm infants, postextubation atelectasis may result from chest wall instability and may be prevented by weaning to nasal CPAP.

HIGH-FREQUENCY VENTILATION

Respiratory rates on the ventilator between 60 and 80 breaths per minute represent conventional ventilation while high-frequency ventilation (HFV) refers to respirator rates between 150 and 3000 breaths per minute. Three types of ventilators have been used for HFV in the neonate (Slutsky, 1988): the high-frequency jet ventilator (HFJV) with rates up to 600 breaths per minute, the high-frequency flow interrupter (HFFI) with rates up to 1200 breaths per minute, and the high-frequency oscillator (HFO) with rates up to 3000 breaths per minute.

The HFJV delivers a high-pressure puff of gas through a small-bore cannula usually positioned in the airway at the proximal end of the endotracheal tube. The actual volume of gas delivered cannot be known because the volume delivered by the jet may be augmented by gas from the auxiliary circuit that is dragged along with the high-pressure puff. Exhalation is passive.

The HFFI uses a circuit similar to a conventional ventilator. Gas flow through the circuit is interrupted by a motorized rotating ball to produce oscillations. Constant end-expiratory pressure is adjusted by a valve on the expiratory limb of the circuit. As it is for the HFJV, exhalation is passive.

The HFO uses a piston or moving diaphragm to actively pump gas in and out of the lung. The oscillator uses very small tidal volumes (usually less than dead space) and relies on a bias flow of gas to flush CO_2 out of the system and maintain a supply of fresh gas at the proximal end of the endotracheal tube.

Mechanisms of Gas Exchange. The mechanism responsible for oxygenation with HFV is the same as for conventional ventilation—it depends on increasing the Pa_{O_2} in the poorly ventilated part of the lung (Froese and Bryan, 1987; Slutsky, 1988). Like the conventional ventilator the high-frequency ventilator accomplishes this by increasing mean airway pressure. Whether or not HFV results in comparable levels of oxygenation with lower mean airway pressures is still controversial.

The difference between HFV and conventional ventilation lies in the methods of removing CO_2. HFV seemingly defies conventional pulmonary physiology by removing CO_2 by rapid ventilation of the lung with tidal volumes less than the anatomic dead space. There are five mechanisms by which HFV might accomplish CO_2 removal:

1. Some alveoli are located near enough to central airways that bulk convection of gas can play a role in CO_2 exchange.

2. Like conventional ventilation, HFV relies on molecular diffusion for gas exchange within the terminal lung units.

3. At the high frequencies employed with HFV, gas exchange between lung units with uneven time constants (pendelluft) can set up circulating currents that enhance gas mixing in the lung and CO_2 exchange.

4. The velocity profile of gas in the airways is asymmetric, i.e., in the center of the parabolic gas stream, forward transport is slightly greater than backward transport of gas, and at the edge of the stream, backward transport is greater than forward. At high frequencies, this results in a net forward flow of fresh gas down the center of the airway and a net backward flow of alveolar-airway gas up the airway.

5. At very high frequencies, a form of facilitated diffusion occurs secondary to enhanced dispersion of both turbulent and laminar streams of gas flow (Taylor dispersion). During HFV these mechanisms combine so that the rate of CO_2 elimination is proportional to the respiratory frequency times the tidal volume squared.

Potential Problems. One of the major problems associated with HFV is related to humidification of inspired gas. This is a particular problem with the HFJV where inadequate humidification combined with the high-pressure pulses of gas has resulted in cases of necrotizing tracheitis. It is much less of a problem with the HFFI and HFO ventilators where the bias flow can be adequately humidified. The other concern with the use of HFV is that of gas trapping. At very high frequencies, expiration may be shortened to the point that Te is less than 3 time constants and gas trapping may occur. This may be a particular problem with ventilators that use a fixed Ti/Te of 1/1.

Clinical Experience. High-frequency jet ventilation has been used for short periods of time in infants with hyaline membrane disease (Carlo et al., 1984). In these patients HFJV provides adequate oxygenation with low MAP and PIP. A single study in which HFJV was used for longer periods of time in infants with intractable respiratory failure suggested that HFJV may be useful in managing patients with air leaks or diaphragmatic hernia (Boros et al., 1985). In infants with pulmonary hypertension, HFJV results in a reduction in $PaCO_2$ and required ventilatory pressures, but it has no effect on ultimate outcome (Carlo et al., 1989). One study comparing HFJV to conventional ventilation in an experimental model of meconium aspiration pneumonia found HFJV to be superior, while another found conventional ventilation to be superior (Mammel et al., 1983; Trindade et al., 1985). Ongoing trials are using this technique to try to avoid the need for extracorporeal membrane oxygenation (ECMO).

In two uncontrolled trials, HFFI appeared to provide some benefit in management of low-birth-weight infants with pulmonary interstitial emphysema (Frantz et al., 1983; Gaylord et al., 1987), and several promising studies of this group of infants are now underway. In another trial, HFFI was successful in reducing $PaCO_2$ in infants with congenital diaphragmatic hernia and hypercarbia. Despite improved ventilation, however, all four infants in the study eventually died (Karl et al., 1983).

In a multicenter trial of HFO in infants with hyaline membrane disease (birth weights between 750 g and 2000 g), no advantage over conventional ventilation techniques could be demonstrated (HiFi Study Group, 1989). In addition, the incidence of Grade III to IV intraventricular hemorrhage was greater in the HFO group than in the conventionally ventilated group. However, there may have been significant differences among the centers in their experience in management of this technique in tiny infants. Further evaluation of different forms of high-frequency ventilation seems warranted (Fredberg et al., 1987).

■ EXTRACORPOREAL MEMBRANE OXYGENATION

A group of infants with respiratory failure, who do not respond to maximal ventilatory support, may be considered for extracorporeal membrane oxygenation (ECMO). Physicians using ECMO must review their own experience and find criteria for selecting infants who have at least an 80 per cent chance of dying. Most centers report that results at the present time suggest that 80 per cent of such infants survive when treated with ECMO. The system consists of a roller pump, membrane oxygenator, and heat exchanger connected in series and primed with heparinized blood (Short and Pearson, 1986) (Fig. 52–9). A catheter is inserted in the right internal jugular vein with its tip in the right atrium, and another catheter is inserted in the right common carotid artery with its tip in the arch of the aorta. The infant is given a bolus dose of heparin and connected to the system, fully oxygenated blood being infused at the aorta. Over 30 minutes, the flow is slowly increased to about 200 ml/kg/minute, after which the mechanical ventilator can be reduced to 30 per cent oxygen, 20 cm H_2O peak pressure, and a rate of 10 breaths per minute (Bartlett et al., 1985), settings designed to allow the lung comparative rest. The arterial oxygen pressure can be maintained between 50 and 70 mm Hg by adjusting the ECMO flow. Heparinization is continued in order to maintain the clotting time two to three times

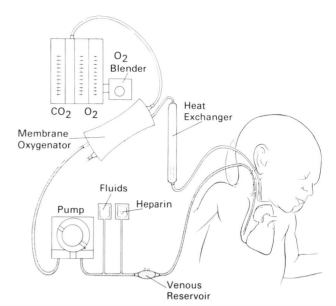

FIGURE 52–9. *Extracorporeal membrane oxygenation (ECMO) system. (From Short, B. L., Miller, M. K., and Anderson, K. D.: Extracorporeal membrane oxygenation in the management of respiratory failure in the newborn. Clin. Perinatol. 14:737–748, 1987.)*

slower than normal, and platelets are transfused to maintain the platelet count above 50,000/mm³. After 4 to 5 days of ECMO, the flow is gradually reduced to allow the still ventilated lung to again assume responsibility for gas exchange. After a brief period at very low flow to ensure adequate pulmonary function, the infant can be decannulated and the vessels ligated. There is evidence that not only is mortality decreased but also both the length and cost of treatment can be reduced (Short and Pearson, 1986).

Patients with meconium aspiration pneumonia, early onset pneumonia, or persistent pulmonary hypertension and certain infants with congenital diaphragmatic hernia and severe pulmonary air leaks are prime candidates for this therapy. Because of systemic heparinization, infants under 2000 g and 34 weeks' gestation have a high incidence of cerebral hemorrhage (Cilley et al., 1986) and should be excluded, as should larger infants if they already have evidence for hemorrhage. Those who are older than 7 days and have been exposed to prolonged mechanical ventilation with oxygen, are not good candidates, since their lung disease may not be reversible. Obviously, those with severe malformations should also usually be excluded.

Although the definition of maximal ventilatory support may vary, it appears that an arterial oxygen pressure under 40 mm Hg for 4 hours during maximal support (usually an FIO_2 of 1.0 and a MAP >18) is a reasonable index of suitability, providing a positive test predictive accuracy of 94 per cent (Marsh et al., 1988). Others have suggested using an a/A ratio of 0.04 or less (Ortega et al., 1988), which corresponds to an arterial PO_2 of <30 mm Hg in 100 per cent oxygen. There is concern that this treatment has not been adequately evaluated by randomized controlled trials.

The ability to manage infants with severe pulmonary disease has been significantly improved in the past few years (Wung et al., 1985). Dworetz and co-workers (1989) reviewed the experience at Yale with infants who met ECMO criteria; they found that, although in 1980–81 only one of every six such infants survived, in 1986–88, nine out of 10 such infants survived in their unit. This raises serious concerns about the appropriateness of using 1980 criteria for treatment.

There has been much concern about the long-term outcomes of these infants. Currently, most centers report approximately 70 per cent of infants doing well at 1 year (Glass et al., 1989), but the later effects of ligation of the common carotid artery may be significant, and long-term follow-up is essential.

■ REFERENCES

Adams, J. M., Speer, M. E., and Rudolph, A. J.: Bacterial colonization of radial artery catheters. Pediatrics 65:94, 1980.

Bartlett, R. H., Roloff, D. W., Cornell, R. G., et al.: Extracorporeal circulation in neonatal respiratory failure: A prospective randomized study. Pediatrics 76:479, 1985.

Bhutani, V. K., Abbasi, S., and Silvieri, E. M.: Continuous skeletal muscle paralysis: Effect on neonatal pulmonary mechanics. Pediatrics 81:419, 1988.

Bland, R. D., Kim, M. H., Light, M. J., et al: High-frequency mechanical ventilation in severe hyaline membrane disease. Crit. Care Med. 8:275, 1980.

Boros, S. J., Mammel, M. D., and Coleman, J. M.: Neonatal high-frequency jet ventilation: Four years' experience. Pediatrics 75:657, 1985.

Boros, S. J., Matalon, S. V., Ewald, R., et al.: The effect of independent variations in inspiratory-expiratory ratio and end-expiratory pressure during mechanical ventilation in hyaline membrane disease: The significance of mean airway pressure. J. Pediatr. 91:794, 1977.

Brunstler, I., Enders, A., and Versmold, H. T.: Skin surface PCO_2 monitoring in newborn infants in shock: Effect of hypotension and electrode temperature. J. Pediatr. 100:454, 1982.

Caplan, M. S., Cohn, R. A., Langman, C. B., et al.: Favorable outcome of neonatal aortic thrombosis and renovascular hypertension. Pediatrics 115:291, 1989.

Carlo, W. A., Beoglos, A., Chatburn, R. L., et al.: High-frequency jet ventilation in neonatal pulmonary hypertension. Am. J. Dis. Child. 143:233, 1989.

Carlo, W. A., Chatburn, R. L., Martin, R. J., et al.: Decrease in airway pressure during high-frequency jet ventilation in infants with respiratory distress syndrome. J. Pediatr. 104:11, 1984.

Cilley, R. E., Zwischenberger, J. B., Andrews, A. F., et al.: Intracranial hemorrhage during extracorporeal membrane oxygenation in neonates. Pediatrics 78:699, 1986.

Cochran, W. D.: Umbilical artery catheterization. In Moore, T. D. (Ed.): Iatrogenic Problems in Neonatal Intensive Care. Proceedings of the 69th Ross Conference on Pediatric Research. Columbus, Ohio, Ross Laboratories, 1976, p. 28.

Corbet, A. J. S., Ross, J. A., Beaudry, P. H., and Stern, L.: Effect of positive pressure breathing on aA.DN_2 in hyaline membrane disease. J. Appl. Physiol. 38:33, 1975.

Crone, R. K., and Favorito, J.: The effects of pancuronium bromide on infants with hyaline membrane disease. J. Pediatr. 97:991, 1980.

Donn, S. M., and Blane, C. E.: Endotracheal tube movement in the preterm neonate: Oral versus nasal intubation. Ann. Otol. Rhinol. Laryngol. 84:18, 1985.

Duke, P. M., Coulson, J. D., Santos, J. I., et al.: Cleft palate associated with prolonged orotracheal intubation in infancy. J. Pediatr. 89:990, 1976.

Dworetz, A. R., Moya, F. R., Sabo, B., et al.: Survival of infants with persistent pulmonary hypertension without extracorporeal membrane oxygenation. Pediatrics 84:1, 1989.

Emmrich, P., Stechele, U., Duc, G., et al.: Transcutaneous PO_2 monitoring in routine management of infants and children with cardiorespiratory problems. Pediatrics 57:681, 1976.

Fan, L. L., Flynn, J. W., and Pathak, D. R.: Risk factors predicting laryngeal injury in intubated neonates. Crit. Care Med. 11:431, 1983.

Finer, N. N., and Tomney, P. M.: Controlled evaluation of muscle relaxation in the ventilated neonate. Pediatrics 67:641, 1981.

Frantz, I. D.: Newer methods for treatment of respiratory distress. In Cowett, R. M., and Hay, W. W. (Eds.): The Micropremie: The Next Frontier. Report of the 99th Ross Conference on Pediatric Research. Columbus, Ohio, Ross Laboratories, 1990, p. 29.

Frantz, I. D., Werthammer, J., and Stark, A. R.: High-frequency ventilation in premature infants with lung disease: Adequate gas exchange at low tracheal pressure. Pediatrics 71:483, 1983.

Fredberg, J. J., Glass, G. M., Boynton, B. R., et al.: Factors influencing mechanical performances of neonatal high-frequency ventilators. J. Appl. Physiol. 62:2485, 1987.

Froese, A. B., and Bryan, A. D.: High-frequency ventilation. Am. Rev. Respir. Dis. 135:1363, 1987.

Gaylord, M. S., Quissell, B. J., and Lair, M. E.: High-frequency ventilation in the treatment of infants weighing less than 1,500 grams with pulmonary interstitial emphysema: A pilot study. Pediatrics 79:915, 1987.

Glass, P., Miller, M., and Short, B.: Morbidity for survivors of ECMO. Neurodevelopmental outcome at one year of age. Pediatrics 83:72, 1989.

Greisen, G., Frederiksen, P. S., Hertel, J., et al.: Catecholamine response to chest physiotherapy and endotracheal suctioning in preterm infants. Acta Paediatr. Scan. 74:525, 1985.

Hansen, T. N., Corbet, A. J. S., Kenny, J. D., et al.: Effects of oxygen and constant positive pressure breathing on aA.DCO_2 in hyaline membrane disease. Pediatr. Res. 13:1167, 1979.

Hansen, T. N., and Tooley, W. H.: Skin surface carbon dioxide tension in sick infants. Pediatrics 64:942, 1979.

Heicher, D. A., Kasting, D. S., and Harrod, J. R.: Prospective clinical comparison of two methods for mechanical ventilation of neonates: Rapid rate and short inspiratory time versus slow rate and long inspiratory time. J. Pediatr. 98:957, 1981.

Henry, G. W., Stevens, D. C., Schreiner, R. L., et al.: Respiratory paralysis to improve oxygenation and mortality in large newborn infants with respiratory distress. J. Pediatr. Surg. 14:761, 1979.

Herman, S., and Reynolds, E. O. R.: Methods for improving oxygenation in infants mechanically ventilated for severe hyaline membrane disease. Arch. Dis. Child. 48:612, 1973.

HiFi Study Group: High-frequency oscillatory ventilation compared with conventional mechanical ventilation in the treatment of respiratory failure in preterm infants. N. Engl. J. Med. 320:88, 1989.

Jackson, J. C., Truog, W. E., Watchko, J. F., et al.: Efficacy of thromboresistant umbilical artery catheters in reducing aortic thrombosis and related complications. J. Pediatr. 110:102, 1987.

Jennis, M. S., and Peabody, J. L.: Pulse oximetry: An alternative method for the assessment of oxygenation in newborn infants. Pediatrics 79:524, 1987.

Jonzon, A., Oberg, P. A., Sedin, G., et al.: High-frequency positive-pressure ventilation by endotracheal insufflation. Acta Anaesthesiol. Scand. 15:(Suppl 43), 1971.

Jung, A. L., and Thomas, G. K.: Stricture of the nasal vestibule: A complication of nasotracheal intubation in newborn infants. J. Pediatr. 85:412, 1974.

Karl, S. R., Ballantine, R. V. N., and Snider, M. T.: High-frequency ventilation at rates of 375 to 1800 cycles per minute in four neonates with congenital diaphragmatic hernia. J. Pediatr. Surg. 18:822, 1983.

Landers, S., and Hansen, T. N.: Skin surface oxygen monitoring. Perinatol. Neonatol. 8:39, 1984.

Lesouef, P. N., England, S. J., and Bryan, A. C.: Total resistance of the respiratory system in preterm infants with and without an endotracheal tube. J. Pediatr. 104:108, 1984.

McMillan, D. D., Rademaker, A. W., Buchan, K. A., et al.: Benefits of orotracheal and nasotracheal intubation in neonates requiring ventilatory assistance. Pediatrics 77:39, 1986.

Mammel, M. C., Gordon, M. J., Connett, J. E., et al.: Comparison of high-frequency jet ventilation and conventional mechanical ventilation in a meconium aspiration model. J. Pediatr. 103:630, 1983.

Marsh, T. D., Wilkerson, S. A., and Cook, L. N.: Extracorporeal membrane oxygenation selection criteria: Partial pressure of arterial oxygen versus alveolar-arterial oxygen gradient. Pediatrics 82:162, 1988.

Miller, K. E., Edwards, D. K., Hilton, S., et al.: Acquired lobar emphysema in premature infants with bronchopulmonary dysplasia: An iatrogenic disease? Pediatr. Radiol. 138:589, 1981.

Moise, A., Landers, S., and Fraley, K.: Colonization and infection of umbilical catheters in newborn infants. Pediatr. Res. 20:400A, 1986.

Moylan, F. M. B., Seldin, E. B., Shannon, D. C., et al.: Defective primary dentition in survivors of neonatal mechanical ventilation. J. Pediatr. 96:106, 1980.

Neal, W. A., Reynolds, J. W., Jarvis, C. W., et al.: Umbilical artery catheterization: Demonstration of arterial thrombosis by aortography. Pediatrics 50:6, 1972.

Norsted, T., Jonzon, A., and Sedin, G.: Pancuronium bromide does not lower airway pressures during intermittent positive pressure ventilation in young cats. Acta Anaesthesiol. Scand. 33:21, 1985.

O'Rourke, P. P., Crone, R. K., Vacanti, J. P., et al.: Extracorporeal membrane oxygenation and conventional medical therapy in neonates with persistent pulmonary hypertension of the newborn: A prospective randomized study. Pediatrics 84(6):957–963, 1989.

Ortega, M., Ramos, A. D., Platzker, A. C. G., et al.: Early prediction of ultimate outcome in newborn infants with severe respiratory failure. J. Pediatr. 113:744, 1988.

Pietsch, J. G., Nagaraj, H. S., Groff, D. B., et al.: Necrotizing tracheo-bronchitis: A new indication for emergency bronchoscopy in the neonate. J. Pediatr. Surg. 20:391, 1985.

Pollitzer, M. J., Reynolds, E. O. R., Shaw, D. G., et al.: Pancuronium during mechanical ventilation speeds recovery of lungs of infants with hyaline membrane disease. Lancet 1:346, 1981.

Pologe, J. A.: Pulse oximetry: Technical aspects of machine design. Int. Anesthesiol. Clin. 25:137, 1987.

Primhak, R. A.: Factors associated with pulmonary air leak in premature infants receiving mechanical ventilation. J. Pediatr. 102:764, 1983.

Ramanathan, R., Durand, M., and Larazabal, C.: Pulse oximetry in very low birthweight infants with acute and chronic lung disease. Pediatrics 79:612, 1987.

Sherman, J. M., Lowitt, S., Stephenson, C., et al.: Factors influencing acquired subglottic stenosis in infants. J. Pediatr. 109:322, 1986.

Short, B. L., and Pearson, G. D.: Neonatal extracorporeal membrane oxygenation: A review. J. Intens. Care Med. 1:47, 1986.

Simbruner, G.: Inadvertent positive end-expiratory pressure in mechanically ventilated newborn infants: Detection and effect on lung mechanics and gas exchange. J. Pediatr. 108:589, 1986.

Simbruner, G., Coradello, H., Fodor, M., et al.: Effect of tracheal suction on oxygenation, circulation, and lung mechanics in newborn infants. 0Arch. Dis. Child. 56:326, 1981.

Slutsky, A. S.: Nonconventional methods of ventilation. Am. Rev. Respir. Dis. 138:175, 1988.

Stewart, A. R., Finer, N. N., and Peters, K. L.: Effects of alteration of inspiratory and expiratory pressures and inspiratory/expiratory ratios on mean airway pressure, blood gases, and intracranial pressure. Pediatrics 67:474, 1981.

Symanski, M. R., and Fox, H. A.: Umbilical vessel catheterization: Indications, management, and evaluation of the technique. J. Pediatr. 80:820, 1972.

Trindade, W., Goldberg, R. N., Bancalari, E., et al.: Conventional versus high-frequency jet ventilation in a piglet model of meconium aspiration: Comparison of pulmonary and hemodynamic effects. Pediatrics 107:115, 1985.

Wukitsch, M. W.: Pulse oximetry: Historical review and Ohmeda functional analysis. Int. J. Clin. Monit. Comput. 4:161, 1987.

Wung, J. T., Driscoll, J. M., Epstein, R. A., et al.: A new device for CPAP by nasal route. Crit. Care Med. 3:76, 1975.

DISORDERS OF THE 53 TRANSITION

Thomas Hansen and Anthony Corbet

■ HYALINE MEMBRANE DISEASE

Hyaline membrane disease (HMD), frequently referred to as the respiratory distress syndrome (RDS), occurs after the onset of breathing in infants with insufficiency of the pulmonary surfactant system.

Epidemiology. There are an estimated 40,000 cases of HMD annually in the United States (Farrell and Wood, 1976), about 14 per cent of all low-birth-weight infants (Farrell and Avery, 1975). The incidence is 60 per cent at 29 weeks' gestation but declines with maturation to near zero by 39 weeks (Usher et al., 1971). The condition is more common in male than in female infants (Miller and Futrakul, 1968) and in white than in nonwhite infants. At any given gestational age, the incidence is higher for cesarean section without labor than for vaginal delivery (Fedrick and Butler, 1972). When corrected for the important effect of gestational age, the occurrence of HMD is significantly increased in gestational diabetes and in insulin-dependent mothers without vascular disease (Robert et al., 1976). Most such infants are large for gestational age, and similarly overnourished infants in the absence of maternal diabetes are also at increased risk (Naeye et al., 1974). Early reports suggested that the risk is decreased in infants who are small for gestational age (Gluck and Kulovich, 1973); however, recent comparisons of both birth weight–matched and gestational age–matched average-for-gestational-age (AGA) infants with small-for-gestational age (SGA) infants suggest that SGA infants do not have this advantage (Pena et al., 1988). Maternal conditions that compromise fetal growth and produce this effect include pregnancy-induced hypertension (Yoon et al., 1980), chronic hypertension, subacute placental abruption, and narcotic addiction (Glass et al., 1971).

There has been controversy as to whether prolonged rupture of membranes may protect against HMD (Jones et al., 1975). When gestational age is carefully controlled, however, there is a significant reduction in the incidence of HMD after prolonged rupture of membranes for more than 24 hours and a still greater reduction after 48 hours (Chiswick, 1976).

Suggestions that birth asphyxia predisposes to HMD are based on lower Apgar scores (James, 1975), but most affected infants are not more acidemic at birth (Kenny et al., 1976), and the lower Apgar scores associated with HMD are better explained by relative immaturity and defective lung function. Nevertheless, in studies in lambs, asphyxia in association with relative pulmonary immaturity produces HMD. The same degree of asphyxia does not produce lung disease in term lambs (Orzalesi et al., 1965) (Table 53–1).

Pathology. The gross findings at autopsy include diffuse lung atelectasis and congestion; if the lungs are inflated at postmortem examination, distensibility is greatly reduced and the lungs collapse more readily with deflation (Gribetz et al., 1959). On histologic examination the peripheral air spaces are collapsed, but more proximal respiratory bronchioles, lined with necrotic epithelium and hyaline membranes, have an overdistended appearance (Finlay-Jones et al., 1974) (Figs. 53–1 and 53–2). There is obvious pulmonary edema with congested capillaries, and the lymphatic and interstitial spaces are distended with fluid. The epithelial damage appears within 30 minutes of the onset of breathing, while the hyaline membranes, composed of plasma exudation products and associated with damaged capillaries, appear within 3 hours of birth (Gandy et al., 1970). In experimental animals, the bronchiolar lesions may be completely prevented by the administration of exogenous surfactant at birth (Nilsson et al., 1978). This has led to the conclusion that the bronchiolar lesions are secondary to atelectasis in terminal air spaces and disruptive overdistention of more proximal airways.

Pathophysiology. In HMD the respiratory rate is elevated, so despite a reduction in each tidal volume the minute ventilation initially is increased. The functional residual capacity, analyzed by nitrogen washout, is reduced; the greater the need for oxygen (Richardson et al., 1986), the smaller the measured value. In keeping with the reduced static lung compliance found at autopsy (Gribetz et al., 1959), the compliance measured by multiple airway occlusions during exhalation is also markedly reduced, the average value being only 0.5 ml/kg/cm H_2O (Dreizzen et al., 1988). As a result, the work of breathing is greatly increased. Measurements of airway resistance suggest values in the normal range, but there is a tendency toward an increase. In one study the average value was 69 cm H_2O/l/sec compared with a reference value of 42 cm H_2O/l/sec (Hjalmarson and Olsson, 1974). From these data, it can be approximated that the overall time constant in HMD would be less than 0.05 second (see p. 477). Because the patency of small peripheral airways depends on proximal spread of surfactant (Macklem et al., 1970), in some regions of lung the local time constants may be more prolonged. The curvature of nitrogen washout traces is better represented by a two-space mathematical model than by a one-space assumption (Richardson and Jung,

TABLE 53–1. Hyaline Membrane Disease*

EPIDEMIOLOGY

Worldwide	Second-born twin at greater risk
Prematurity predisposes	PROM spares
Cesarean section without labor predisposes	IUGR spares
	Maternal "stress" spares
Perinatal asphyxia predisposes	Maternal diabetes predisposes if
Male > female	< 37 weeks
Caucasian > black	Maternal hemorrage predisposes

CLINICAL SIGNS

Onset near the time of birth	Fine inspiratory rales
Retractions and tachypnea	Hypothermia
Expiratory grunt	Peripheral edema
Cyanosis	Pulmonary edema
Systemic hypotension	
Characteristic chest film	
Course to death or improvement 3 to 5 days	

PATHOPHYSIOLOGY

Reduced lung compliance	If hypotensive and hypoxic,
Reduced FRC	poor peripheral perfusion,
Poor lung distensibility	poor renal perfusion,
Poor alveolar stability	myocardial malfunction
Right-to-left shunts	Patent ductus arteriosus contributes
Reduced effective pulmonary blood flow	

PATHOBIOCHEMISTRY

Respiratory acidosis	Decreased total serum proteins
Decreased saturated phospholipids	Decreased fibrinolysins
	Low thyroxine levels
Low AF L/S ratio	
Low surfactant associated proteins	

PATHOLOGY

Atelectasis	Osmiophilic lamellar bodies decreased early, increased later
Injury to epithelial cells, edema	
Membrane contains fibrin and cellular products	
No tubular myelin	

ETIOLOGY

Surfactant deficiency during disease	Probable inadequate hormonal (corticoid) stimulus in utero
	DPL synthesis impaired and/or destruction increased
	Autonomic dysfunction

PREVENTION

Prenatal glucocorticoids for > 24 hours
Surfactant replacement before 1–2 hours

*Abbreviations: PROM, prolonged rupture of membranes (> 16 hours); IUGR, intrauterine growth retardation; FRC, functional residual capacity; AF, amniotic fluid; L/S, lecithin/sphingomyelin ratio; DPL, dipalmitoyl lecithin.

1978). The postulated "slow" space may represent those parts of the lung with more prolonged time constants.

The $Aa.Do_2$ and right-to-left shunt while breathing 100 per cent oxygen are greatly increased, many infants having values for shunt in the range of 50 to 90 per cent of cardiac output (Strang and MacLeish, 1961). As there is no evidence for a diffusion limitation, it is commonly stated that large shunts at the foramen ovale and ductus arteriosus and in atelectatic lung constitute the only cause of severe hypoxemia in HMD (Krauss et al., 1976). If this were true and the shunt were 50 per cent, it can be seen from Figure 53–3 that changing inspired oxygen would have little effect on arterial oxygen pressure, and oxygen

therapy would be relatively ineffective. In fact, precipitous changes of arterial oxygen tension and calculated venous admixture occur if inspired oxygen is reduced. This indicates the presence of an open, poorly ventilated lung compartment with extremely low V/Q, representing a significant portion of the lung and producing variable hypoxic vasoconstriction and alterations in right-to-left shunt as the inspired oxygen changes (Corbet et al., 1974). Therefore, in infants with HMD the severity of arterial hypoxemia is directly related to the size of the open, poorly ventilated compartment. The relationship among V/Q, alveolar oxygen tension, and changing inspired oxygen (Fig. 53–4) indicates how oxygen as high as 90 per cent is required before the oxygen pressure in very low V/Q units will rise significantly (West, 1969). (See also Chapter 51.) Because perfusion of the open, extremely low V/Q compartment is greatly reduced by hypoxic vasoconstriction, it makes only a small contribution to cardiac output, and measurements of $aA.DN_2$ are not increased in HMD (Corbet et al., 1974). It should not be overlooked that this lung compartment makes a significant contribution to the oxygenation defect in HMD.

Measurements of $aA.Dco_2$ and alveolar dead space are markedly increased in HMD (Nelson et al., 1962). Although minute ventilation is increased, the alveolar ventilation is actually decreased, as reflected by the elevated values for arterial CO_2 tension. Because a large part of the lung is collapsed or poorly ventilated, most alveolar ventilation is diverted to a relatively small part of the lung, represented by the reduced functional residual capacity. Because this compartment is small, it is relatively overventilated, so the V/Q and the measured $aA.Dco_2$ are high (Hansen et al., 1979). Measurements of pulmonary blood

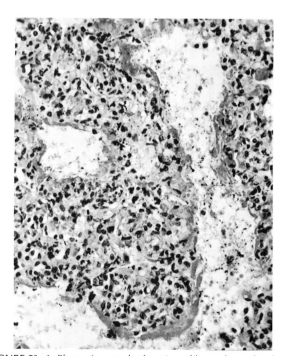

FIGURE 53–1. *Photomicrograph of section of lung of an infant born in the thirty-second week of gestation weighing 1640 g. He seemed well for one hour; then dyspnea appeared and gradually increased with deepening sternal and costal retraction. He died at 22 hours of age. One sees unexpanded lung, with dilated air spaces lined with thick, homogeneously staining membrane.*

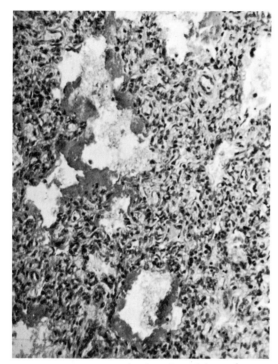

FIGURE 53–2. *Photomicrograph of section of lung of a premature infant weighing 2270 g at birth whose dyspnea was first noticed at eight hours and who died after steadily increasing respiratory difficulty at 27 hours. The appearance of the section of lung is in all respects similar to that in Figure 53–1. The pattern of aeration and atelectasis has been described as Swiss cheese–like in contrast to lace-like aeration.*

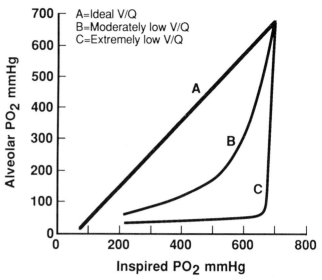

FIGURE 53–4. *The relationship between inspired PO_2 and alveolar PO_2. In a lung compartment with extremely low V/Q, the alveolar PO_2 rises very slowly until over 90 per cent inspired oxygen is reached, when it rises rapidly. (From West, J. B.: Ventilation perfusion inequality and overall gas exchange in computer models of the lung. Respir. Physiol. 7:88, 1969.)*

flow, utilizing the disappearance of gases that enter ventilated parts of the lung, confirm that perfusion of ventilated lung is very low (Chu et al., 1967). Based on the foregoing considerations, an idealized model of the lung in HMD is shown in Figure 53–5 representing the three lung compartments: shunt, open low V/Q, and high V/Q. There is a close correspondence between predicted and measured values for aA.DCO_2, suggesting the validity of this model (Hansen et al., 1979; Landers et al., 1986).

Clinical Diagnosis. The infant with HMD is almost always premature and is cyanotic in room air. There is rapid or labored breathing, beginning at or immediately after birth. The severity of respiratory distress can be represented by the Silverman score (Fig. 53–6). Infants usually have a characteristic grunt during expiration, caused by closure of the glottis, the effect of which is to maintain lung volume and gas exchange during exhalation. Frequently, the unventilated infant requires 40 to 50 per cent oxygen after birth for relief of central cyanosis but then develops an increasing oxygen requirement over

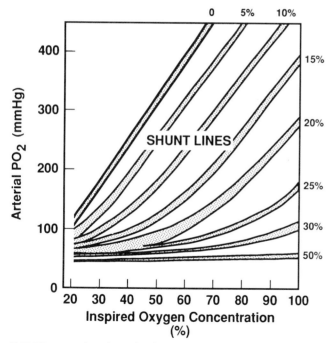

FIGURE 53–3. *The relationship between inspired oxygen concentration and arterial oxygen tension as it is affected by true right-to-left shunting. The assumptions are hemoglobin, 10 to 14 g/dl; arterial PCO_2, 25 to 40 mm Hg; and av·O_2 difference, 5 ml/100 ml. (From Benatar, S. R., Hewlett, A. M., and Nunn, J. F.: The use of iso-shunt lines for control of oxygen therapy. Br. J. Anesthesiol. 45:711, 1973.)*

	V/Q>1	V/Q<<1	V/Q=O
Ventilation	0.999	0.001	0.000
Perfusion	0.330	0.030	0.640
	V/Q=3	Qo/Qt	Qs/Qt

FIGURE 53–5. *Three-compartment lung model of HMD. The high V/Q compartment receives nearly all the ventilation. The calculated venous admixture is 0.67. If a value of 0.03 is assumed for Qo/Qt, then the calculated value for Qs/Qt is 0.64. Thus, perfusion of the high V/Q compartment is 0.33 and the value for V/Q is 3. From the latter value, a predicted value of aA.DCO_2 can be calculated and compared with the measured value. (From Hansen, T. N., Corbet, A. J. S., Kenny, J. D., et al.: Effects of oxygen and constant positive pressure breathing on aA.DCO_2 in hyaline membrane disease. Pediatr. Res. 13:1167, 1979.)*

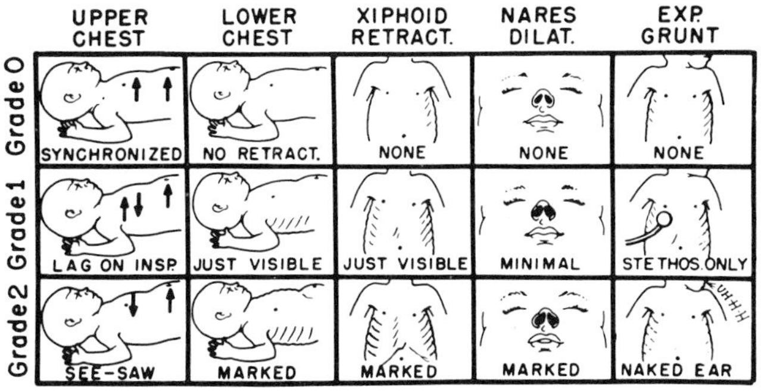

	UPPER CHEST	LOWER CHEST	XIPHOID RETRACT.	NARES DILAT.	EXP. GRUNT
Grade 0	SYNCHRONIZED	NO RETRACT.	NONE	NONE	NONE
Grade 1	LAG ON INSP.	JUST VISIBLE	JUST VISIBLE	MINIMAL	STETHOS. ONLY
Grade 2	SEE-SAW	MARKED	MARKED	MARKED	NAKED EAR

FIGURE 53–6. The Silverman score for assessing the magnitude of respiratory distress. (From Avery, M. E., and Fletcher, B. D.: The Lung and Its Disorders in the Newborn. Philadelphia, W. B. Saunders Company, 1974.) (Courtesy of W. A. Silverman.)

24 to 48 hours; this may reach as high as 100 per cent. In other infants, the oxygen requirement transiently decreases as acidosis or hypothermia is corrected or fetal lung fluid is cleared; it begins to increase only after 3 to 6 hours. More severely affected infants have an immediate high-oxygen requirement that progresses rapidly to 100 per cent; without mechanical ventilation, they may die within 24 hours. Another group of larger infants need less oxygen initially and manifest a slowly progressive course of generalized atelectasis over 48 to 72 hours. The urine output is low for the first 24 to 48 hours, but soon after this time a diuresis ensues. If HMD is uncomplicated, recovery starts after 48 hours. The decline in oxygen requirement is relatively rapid after 72 hours, and usually oxygen can be discontinued after 1 week. The very-low-birth-weight infant (< 1500 g) will usually require mechanical ventilation and have a more prolonged course.

Laboratory Diagnosis. Based upon arterial blood gas values, infants with HMD have a moderate to severe oxygenation defect, significant hypercarbia, and a mild metabolic acidosis with only slight elevation of blood lactate (Sinclair, 1973).

Radiographic Diagnosis. Diffuse, fine granular densities that develop during the first 6 hours of life are seen on the chest radiograph (Fig. 53–7); these densities are influenced by size of the infant, severity of disease, and degree of ventilatory support. The appearance may be more marked at the lung bases than at the apices. The lung volume may appear normal early, especially if the infant is strong enough to overdistend less affected regions, but ultimately the lung volume is decreased. Positive airway pressure frequently obliterates these diagnostic findings.

Etiology. HMD is primarily a developmental deficiency in the amount of surface-active material at the air-liquid interface of the lung, as demonstrated by pressure-volume curves with air and saline in infants who died from HMD (Avery and Fletcher, 1974). Saline extracts of minced lung have higher surface tension than do controls (Avery and Mead, 1959), which is associated with lower levels of total tissue phospholipid (Brumley et al., 1967) and saturated phosphatidylcholine (PC) (Adams et al., 1970). Although, based on theoretical considerations of the amount required, there appear to be more adequate

amounts of phospholipid present in total lung (Clements and Tooley, 1977), only a small proportion of lung phospholipid is surface-active material (Rieutort et al., 1986). Infants with HMD may synthesize adequate amounts of saturated PC but cannot package and export it to the alveolar surface in a way that makes it function as surfactant.

It has been suggested that surfactant function in infants with HMD is inhibited by plasma proteins (Ikegami et al., 1986), which leak into the respiratory bronchioles at the sites of overdistention and epithelial damage. In particular, a plasma protein of relative molecular weight 110,000 has been implicated. It is of critical importance to the lungs to have adequate surfactant at the gas-liquid interface from the earliest possible moment after birth; otherwise, acute lung injury and surfactant inhibition will supervene and contribute, with hypoxia and acidosis, to a cycle of worsening disease.

Prevention. Since HMD is a problem of insufficient lung maturity, the best way to prevent it would be to prevent premature birth. At the present time, however, the two major approaches to the problem are (1) prediction of the risk for HMD by antenatal testing of amniotic fluid samples, and (2) antenatal treatment of women in preterm labor with glucocorticoid hormones to accelerate fetal lung maturation.

Prenatal Prediction. Before birth, the surfactant system can be assessed in amniotic fluid because some fetal lung fluid enters the amniotic cavity. The most common material measured is lecithin or PC, in particular, saturated PC. Because changes in amniotic fluid volume may alter the concentration of PC, it is standardized to the concentration of sphingomyelin, which remains relatively constant throughout gestation; it is expressed as the lecithin/sphingomyelin ratio (L/S).

In normal pregnancy, the L/S ratio displays a remarkably stable pattern, increasing slowly to 1 at 32 weeks, rising more rapidly to 2 at 35 weeks, and accelerating

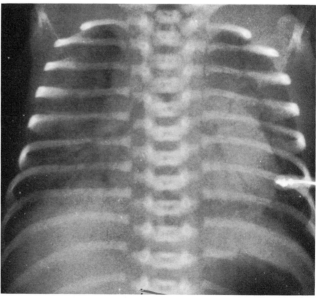

FIGURE 53–7. Typical chest radiograph from an infant with HMD.

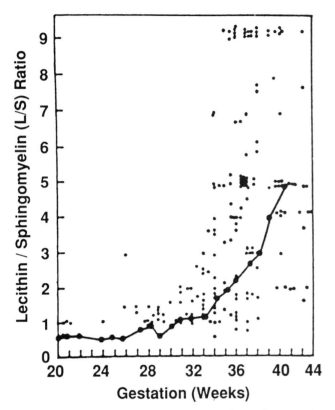

FIGURE 53–8. The L/S ratio in normal and abnormal pregnancies, indicating wide biologic scatter. (From Gluck, L., and Kulovich, M. V.: The evaluation of functional maturity in the human fetus. In Gluck, L. [Ed.]: Modern Perinatal Medicine. Chicago, Year Book Medical Publishers, 1974.)

very rapidly thereafter (Gluck and Kulovich, 1973) (Fig. 53–8). In abnormal pregnancy, there is much wider scatter, reflecting conditions that accelerate or decelerate lung maturation. The ratio may reach 2 as early as 28 weeks or remain at 1 until close to term. The incidence of HMD is only 0.5 per cent for an L/S ratio of 2 or more but 100 per cent for an L/S below 1; between 1 and 2 the risk of HMD decreases progressively. The L/S ratio represents the secretory activity of the lung, which is greatly accelerated at 35 weeks. During labor, there is a substantial increase in the L/S ratio (Whittle and Hill, 1977). Elective cesarean section delivery of infants having a low L/S ratio carries an unnecessary risk of HMD (Hack et al., 1976).

Phosphatidylinositol (PI) in amniotic fluid progressively increases until 36 weeks and then decreases (Hallman et al., 1976). At about this time, phosphatidylglycerol (PG) appears and increases until term (Fig. 53–9). The appearance time of PG may be accelerated or delayed in the same way as the L/S ratio. The presence of PG indicates a remarkably low risk of HMD, less than 0.5 per cent. If a patient has both an L/S ratio of less than 2 and an absence of PG, the risk for HMD is over 80 per cent (Hallman and Teramo, 1981). Besides an L/S ratio below 1, this combination is the best predictor of HMD available to the clinician. In certain pregnancies characterized by diabetes and Rh isoimmunization, the L/S ratio has proved less reliable, the risk of HMD at a value between 2 and 3 still being approximately 13 per cent (Hallman and Teramo, 1981). However, in those with both an L/S ratio

above 2 and PG present, the risk has been reduced to zero.

Prophylaxis with Glucocorticoid Hormones. Since 1972, when Liggins and Howie described decreased mortality, decreased incidence of RDS, and less severe RDS in a prospective, blinded study done in New Zealand, more than 23 studies have been published worldwide that demonstrate the efficacy of prenatal glucocorticoid therapy. Twelve of the 23 studies report decreased mortality; 21 report significantly less RDS with the use of glucocorticoids; the remaining two show a trend toward less RDS. The efficacy of glucocorticoids with preterm rupture of membranes (PROM) has remained controversial; however, Morales and co-workers (1986) found decreased RDS, intraventricular hemorrhage, and hospital stay among infants born to mothers with PROM who received prenatal glucocorticoids. Meta-analysis of prospective, randomized studies reviewing the effect of steroids versus no steroids in women with PROM shows a significant decrease in RDS with steroids in this group. The decreased incidence of RDS with PROM has not been accompanied by any problems with infection in either mothers or infants.

Another area of controversy has been the influence of gender on corticosteroid therapy. Although some investigators have described decreased efficacy of glucocorticoids in the male (Ballard et al., 1979; Papageorgiou et al., 1981; Collaborative Group Study, 1981), others have found that glucocorticoids are effective in preventing RDS in males (Kuhn, 1982; Howie, 1984). In addition, prenatal glucocorticoids appear to have several other beneficial effects on the small preterm infant (Ballard, 1986). These include lower incidence of patent ductus arteriosus requiring therapy, less necrotizing enterocolitis (Bauer et al., 1984), and decreased intracranial hemorrhage. Other effects observed in animal models include decreased pulmonary protein leaks (Rider et al., 1989), stimulation of rat lung antioxidant (Frank et al., 1985), and acceleration of renal function in the fetal lamb (Stonestreet et al., 1983; Scholle and Braunlich, 1989). Because of concern that

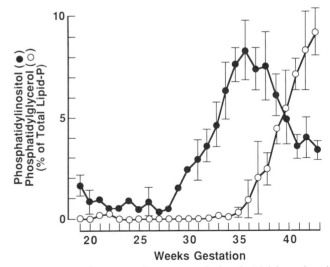

FIGURE 53–9. Changes in the content of phosphatidylglycerol and phosphatidylinositol in amniotic fluid, plotted against gestational age. (From Hallman, M., Merritt, T. A., Jarvenpaa, A. L., et al.: Effects of oxygen and constant positive positive pressure breathing on aA·DCO₂ in hyaline membrane disease. Pediatr. Res. 13:1167, 1979.)

prenatal administration of glucocorticoids might have an adverse effect on fetal development, extensive outcome studies have been done on infants whose mothers received this therapy (for review, see Ballard [1986]). Long-term outcome in treated infants has shown no disadvantages associated with prenatal glucocorticoid therapy, in spite of the improved survival of smaller infants. Table 53–2 presents the known risks versus the benefits of glucocorticoid administration.

An effort is under way to improve prevention of RDS with prenatal hormonal administration. Several other hormones, particularly thyroid hormone, are known to have a positive effect on lung development in tissue culture and animal models. It is hoped, therefore, that a combination of glucocorticoid and thyroid hormone (administered as thyrotropin-releasing hormone to the mother) will promote improvement in outcome for these infants. Since thyrotropin-releasing hormone also stimulates prolactin production—and prolactin appears to have a permissive effect on lung development—it is possible that a combination of glucocorticoid and thyroid hormone will further the prevention of chronic lung disease in the small premature infant (Ballard, 1990).

Treatment

Resuscitation. The mortality among all infants, including those with HMD, is increased by asphyxia. Therefore, the presence of a skilled resuscitation team at delivery of high-risk infants can reduce the morbidity and mortality of the disease (see Chapter 22).

Lung Expansion. Since secretion of surfactant is impaired by inadequate expansion of the lungs at birth (Lawson et al., 1979), many believe that it is appropriate to intubate all infants under 1000 to 1250 g at birth and to initiate mechanical ventilation with PEEP in the delivery room. Similar treatment may be used for larger premature infants if they are having respiratory distress or are not

TABLE 53–2. Risk-versus-Benefit Analysis of Prenatal Glucocorticoid Therapy

RISKS

Possible increased risk of infection in mothers with prolonged rupture of membranes
Disturbs glucose homeostasis in diabetic mothers
Possible impact on T-cell development (with postnatal treatment)
Questionable effect on visual perception in boys

NO DIFFERENCE

Infection in infants
Growth: Height, weight, head circumference; neurologic development; cognitive development
Development of very-low-birth-weight infants
Lung mechanics and growth
Retrolental fibroplasia or vision

BENEFIT

Improved survival
Decreased incidence of RDS
Decreased severity of RDS
Decreased incidence of significant patent ductus arteriosus
Decreased incidence of intracranial hemorrhage
Decreased incidence of necrotizing enterocolitis
Decreased hospital costs
Decreased hospital stay

RDS, respiratory distress syndrome.

vigorous. The administration of artificial replacement surfactant may greatly improve the course of the disease (see Surfactant Replacement).

Thermal Neutrality. Infants should be nursed in a warm environment so that oxygen consumption is maintained at minimal levels. This usually means servo-controlling anterior abdominal skin temperature to 36.5° C.

Blood Gas Monitoring. Infants with HMD require monitoring of blood pressure, blood gases, electrolytes, and glucose, which may be obtained via an umbilical arterial catheter (see Chapter 52).

Oxygen. As previously discussed (see Chapter 51), oxygen therapy is beneficial, despite the presence of large right-to-left shunts. Increased inspired oxygen produces (1) a rise of alveolar oxygen pressure in open low $\dot{V}/\dot{Q}$ units (see Fig. 53–4); (2) relief of regional hypoxic vasoconstriction in this compartment; (3) a reduction in true right-to-left shunt; and (4) an increase of arterial oxygen saturation (Hansen et al., 1979).

Fluid Restriction. Since HMD is characterized by high-surface-tension pulmonary edema (Boughton et al., 1970) and high-permeability pulmonary edema (Jefferies et al., 1984), fluid restriction to 50 ml/kg/day is indicated for many infants with HMD for the first 48 hours or until the onset of diuresis. Close attention should be paid to fluid intake, urine output, urine concentration, and serum electrolytes. Premature infants have an excess of extracellular fluid and are expected to lose at least 10 per cent of body weight by the end of the first week of life. However, in the very immature infant (25 to 26 weeks' gestation) with very permeable skin, there may be excessive evaporative losses and much higher amounts of fluid may be required (see Chapter 28). If the serum sodium rises sharply, especially if it approaches 150 mEq/l, it can be assumed that insensible water losses through the skin are excessive, and the fluid intake should be liberalized accordingly.

Minimal Stimulation. Manipulations, such as heel sticks, tracheal suctioning, diaper changes, and even weighing, should be kept to a minimum, as these procedures have been shown to reduce arterial oxygen tension (Lucey, 1981); they probably also increase oxygen consumption and may contribute to the genesis of cerebral hemorrhage by rapidly raising arterial blood pressure. It is not appropriate to give enteral feedings to infants with HMD, because these infants have an ileus as part of their disease.

Blood Pressure Support. Premature infants frequently have a low arterial blood pressure in the first 12 hours of life, as defined by normative data (Versmold et al., 1981). In infants with a low hematocrit, poor peripheral perfusion, and metabolic acidosis, the hypotension is usually due to hypovolemia and will respond to a cautious infusion of 10 to 20 ml/kg of saline or blood. If there are no signs of hypovolemia, the infusion of dopamine at 2 to 8 μg/kg/min is usually effective. Serial echocardiographic data have shown dose-dependent increases in cardiac output and stroke volume without significant changes in heart rate or systemic vascular resistance (Padbury et al., 1986).

Alkali Therapy. Severe metabolic acidosis may increase pulmonary vascular resistance, impair surfactant synthesis, reduce cardiac output, and, ultimately, reduce ventilation. An early trial showed that continuous infusion of glucose-bicarbonate solutions reduced the mortality of

HMD (Usher, 1963). With the introduction of better methods for oxygenating infants, however, bicarbonate therapy no longer appears to have much benefit (Corbet et al., 1977), and it may be harmful in infants who are not being ventilated adequately and thus have a high $PaCO_2$.

Constant Positive Airway Pressure (CPAP). Since it was first described (Gregory et al., 1971), CPAP has been shown to reduce mortality in infants who weigh > 1500 g (Rhodes and Hall, 1973) and to reduce requirements for oxygen and mechanical ventilation (Fanaroff et al., 1973). CPAP increased survival when applied early with an oxygen requirement of 50 per cent, in contrast to later intervention with CPAP and oxygen at 100 per cent (Allen et al., 1977). CPAP alone can be used in larger infants (> 1500 to 1750 g) and should be started when the oxygen requirement reaches 50 per cent; nasal CPAP may be started earlier. The initial level of CPAP used is 5 cm H_2O, and the pressure is increased by 2 cm–H_2O steps until the oxygen requirement decreases. Infants who require an FIO_2 > 0.8 with CPAP of 10 cm H_2O will usually need mechanical ventilation and should receive surfactant replacement. The incidence of pulmonary air leak is no higher than the spontaneous rate with this regimen (Corbet and Adams, 1978). Because CPAP may overdistend the lung and impair the pulmonary circulation, attempts have been made to identify optimal levels. As CPAP is increased and approaches optimum, the aA.DCO_2 falls significantly; but as the optimal level is exceeded, both the aA.DCO_2 and the arterial CO_2 rise significantly (Landers et al., 1986). Under clinical conditions, increased hypercarbia may indicate excessive CPAP, particularly in association with a falling PaO_2.

Mechanical Ventilation. Infants with HMD who weigh < 1500 g will usually require mechanical ventilation. Otherwise, the indications are apnea, hypercarbia with pH < 7.20, and arterial oxygen pressure under 50 mm Hg in 80 to 100 per cent oxygen, particularly early in the infant's course (see Chapter 52 for a discussion of mechanical ventilation and respiratory therapy).

Closure of the Patent Ductus Arteriosus. Especially in infants under 1000 g, a patent ductus arteriosus may contribute significantly to the overall problem of HMD. If the ductus can be demonstrated to be patent on the third day of life by two-dimensional echocardiography and pulsed Doppler ultrasonography, the evidence suggests that it is unlikely to close spontaneously within a reasonable time (Dudell and Gersony, 1984); therefore, it should be closed either with indomethacin therapy or with surgery (see Chapter 61).

Surfactant Replacement. Recent results of clinical trials of surfactant replacement have resulted in the Federal Drug Administration's release of some materials for clinical use. Two broad strategies are being investigated: (1) prophylaxis at birth in small premature infants at high risk for HMD, and (2) treatment of infants with established HMD. Replacement surfactant should be given by direct tracheal instillation under conditions of adequate PEEP to ensure distribution to poorly ventilated regions of the lung. The dose should be 75 to 100 mg/kg, high enough to overcome destruction by macrophages and inhibition by plasma proteins. Surfactants are currently prepared from lung lavage material, lung mince extracts, or amniotic fluid

sediment; there are also synthetic mixtures of saturated PC and a fluidizing additive, such as PG or hexadecanol. The prophylactic approach under controlled conditions has shown a reduction in the severity of HMD (Enhorning et al., 1985), and controlled trials have suggested that there may be a reduction in the incidence of both mortality and bronchopulmonary dysplasia. Single-dose surfactant in established HMD may produce a significant improvement in oxygen and ventilatory requirements and a reduced incidence of pulmonary air leaks (Hallman et al., 1985). It is apparent that the effect is often short-lived, presumably owing to inhibition by plasma proteins, and that in some patients multiple doses will be required. A reduction in chronic lung disease and death has been shown with up to four doses in the first 48 hours of life. In addition, there is evidence in animal models (Ikegami et al., 1986) that replacement surfactant is much more effective in those that have been treated prenatally with glucocorticoids.

Prognosis. The chances of survival in HMD are directly related to birth weight and are affected by prenatal treatment with glucocorticoids, surfactant replacement, and the severity and complications of the disease. (See Chapter 55 for a discussion of pulmonary residua, and Chapter 32 for a discussion of outcome in these infants.)

■ TRANSIENT TACHYPNEA OF THE NEWBORN (TTN)

Transient tachypnea of the newborn is also known as *wet lung disease* or *delayed clearance of lung water*. In 1966, Avery and co-workers reported on eight near-term infants with early onset of respiratory distress whose chest radiographs showed hyperaeration of the lungs, prominent pulmonary vascular markings, and mild cardiomegaly (Fig. 53–10). The respiratory symptoms were transient and relatively mild, and most infants improved within 24 hours. The investigators named the disorder "transient tachypnea of the newborn" (TTN) and speculated that it was the result of delayed clearance of fetal lung liquid.

Pathophysiology. Most authors agree with Avery and her co-workers that TTN represents a transient pulmonary edema resulting from delayed clearance of fetal lung liquid. This may result from any condition that elevates central venous pressure and delays the clearance of lung liquid by the lymphatics. Delayed cord clamping or milking of the cord can promote a transfusion of blood from placenta to infant, with transient elevation of central venous pressure (Saigal et al., 1977). (See Chapter 49 and Chapter 51 for a discussion of normal clearance of lung water.) Infants born prematurely or without labor have not had an opportunity for early lung liquid clearance, and they begin their extrauterine life with excess water in their lungs. After birth, in the term infant, water in the air spaces normally moves rapidly to the extra-alveolar interstitium, where it pools in perivascular cuffs of tissue and in the interlobar fissures. It is then cleared by lung lymphatics or by absorption directly into the small blood vessels.

The symptoms of TTN result from compression of the compliant airways by water that has accumulated in the

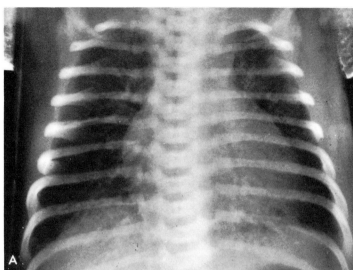

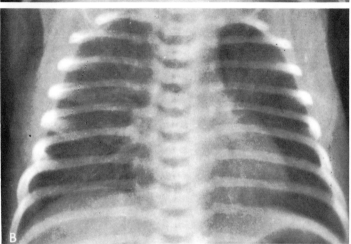

FIGURE 53–10. The large cardiovascular silhouette, air bronchogram, and streaky lung fields were seen at 2 hours of age (A) but had cleared by 24 hours of age (B), typical of transient tachypnea of the newborn or delayed clearance of lung liquid.

perivascular cuffs of the extra-alveolar interstitium. This compression results in airway obstruction and hyperaeration of the lungs secondary to gas trapping. Hypoxia results from the continued perfusion of poorly ventilated lung units; hypercarbia results from mechanical interference with alveolar ventilation and from central nervous system depression. Lung function measurements in infants with TTN are compatible with airway obstruction and gas trapping. The functional residual capacity measured by gas dilution is normal or reduced, whereas measurements of thoracic gas volume by plethysmography are increased, suggesting that some of the gas in the lungs is not in communication with the airways (Krauss and Auld, 1971).

Clinical Signs. It was initially thought that TTN was limited to term or larger preterm infants, but it is now clear that very small infants also may present with pulmonary edema from retained fetal lung liquid; this may complicate their surfactant deficiency and account for some of their need for supplemental oxygen and ventilation. There is often a history of heavy maternal sedation, maternal diabetes, or delivery by elective cesarean section. Affected infants may be mildly depressed at birth, and this may mask many of their early symptoms. They are often very tachypneic with respiratory rates ranging from 60 to 120 breaths/minute and may have hyperinflation with grunting, chest wall retractions, and nasal flaring.

Arterial blood gas tensions often reveal a respiratory acidosis, which resolves within 8 to 24 hours, and mild to moderate hypoxemia. These infants seldom require more than 40 per cent oxygen to maintain an adequate PaO_2 and usually are in room air by 24 hours of age. They have no evidence to indicate right-to-left shunting of blood at the ductus arteriosus or foramen ovale.

Chest radiographs reveal hyperaeration, which is often accompanied by mild cardiomegaly (Fig. 53–11). Water contained in the perivascular cuffs produces prominent vascular markings in a "sunburst pattern" emanating from the hilum. The interlobar fissures are widened, and pleural effusions may be present. Occasionally, coarse fluffy densities may be present, indicating alveolar edema. The radiographic abnormalities resolve over the first 2 to 3 days after birth.

Clinical Course and Treatment. As its name implies, TTN is a benign, self-limited disease. The infant's need for supplemental oxygen is usually highest at the onset of the disease and then progressively decreases. Infants with uncomplicated disease usually recover rapidly without any residual pulmonary disability. While the symptoms of TTN relate to pulmonary edema, one controlled trial that assessed therapy with diuretics found no evidence for their efficacy (Wiswell et al., 1985).

TABLE 53–3. Causes of Persistent Pulmonary Hypertension

TRANSIENT PULMONARY HYPERTENSION
    Hypoxia with or without acidosis
    Hypothermia
    Hypoglycemia
    Polycythemia
PERSISTENT PULMONARY HYPERTENSION
    Active Vasoconstriction
        Bacterial sepsis and/or pneumonia
        Perinatal aspiration syndromes
    Underdevelopment of the Lung
        Diaphragmatic hernia
        Potter syndrome
        Other causes of pulmonary hypoplasia
    Maldevelopment of Pulmonary Vessels
        Idiopathic
        Chronic intrauterine asphyxia
        Meconium aspiration pneumonitis
        Premature closure of the fetal ductus arteriosus

■ PERSISTENT PULMONARY HYPERTENSION OF THE NEWBORN (PPHN)

Gersony and co-workers (1969) described a group of term infants without structural heart disease who became cyanotic shortly after birth and had only mild respiratory distress. These infants all had suprasystemic pulmonary arterial pressures and evidence of right-to-left shunting of blood across persistent fetal pathways (the foramen ovale and ductus arteriosus). The nature of these shunts led to the name "persistence of the fetal circulation." Subsequently the name was changed to "persistent pulmonary hypertension of the newborn" (PPHN) to more accurately describe the pathophysiology of the disorder.

Pathogenesis. Successful transition from intrauterine to extrauterine life requires that the pulmonary vascular resistance decrease precipitously at birth. In infants with PPHN, this decrease does not occur: Pulmonary arterial pressure remains elevated, and blood is shunted right to left across the ductus arteriosus and foramen ovale. In addition, the persistently high pulmonary vascular resistance increases right ventricular afterload and oxygen demand and impairs oxygen delivery to the right ventricle, the posterior wall of the left ventricle, and the subendocardial regions of the right ventricle. Ischemic damage resulting from this reduction in oxygen delivery may cause both right and left ventricular failure, papillary muscle necrosis, and tricuspid insufficiency (Setzer et al., 1980). Finally, increased right ventricular afterload results in displacement of the septum into the left ventricle, impaired left ventricular filling, and reduced cardiac output.

There are instances in which pulmonary vascular resistance remains only transiently elevated at birth (Table 53–3) and decreases rapidly once the underlying condition is corrected. However, there are also a number of other conditions in which the pulmonary vascular resistance remains persistently elevated either because of active constriction of pulmonary vessels or because of some anatomic abnormality.

Active constriction of pulmonary vessels can complicate the course of bacterial sepsis or pneumonia in the newborn (Shankaran et al., 1982). Experiments in animals show that this increase in pulmonary vascular resistance is temporally related to increased plasma thromboxane concentrations (Hammerman et al., 1988); it can be blocked by the administration of inhibitors of prostaglandin synthesis (Rojas et al., 1983). Active constriction of pulmonary vessels can also complicate the course of meconium aspiration pneumonia. Some studies suggest that vasoactive substances present in meconium or amniotic fluid diffuse through the lung and either constrict pulmonary vessels directly or induce platelet aggregation in the microcirculation with the subsequent release of thrombox-

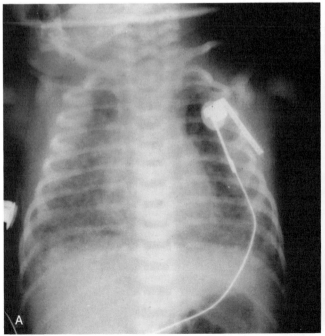 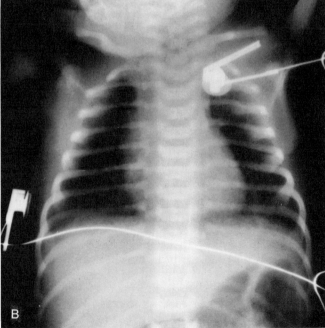

FIGURE 53–11. Chest radiographs from an infant with TTN. Initially the x-ray study is compatible with massive interstitial and alveolar edema (A). The x-ray study is clear 48 hours later (B).

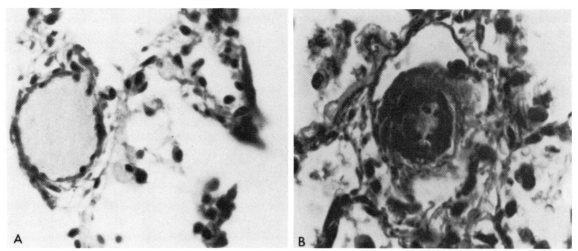

FIGURE 53–12. *Photomicrographs of alveolar wall arteries distended with the barium gelatin suspension from A, a 3-day-old infant with normal lungs and B, a 3-day-old infant with persistent hypertension. The normal artery (A) is nonmuscular with a single endothelial cell lining surrounded by a thin layer of connective tissue. In section (B), the artery wall is composed of smooth muscle (darkly stained) two-cell-layers thick surrounded by a thick connective tissue sheath enclosing a dilated lymphatic (located superiorly). (Elastin-van Gieson stain ×250.) (Courtesy Dr. John Murphy.)*

ane. Clinical data support this hypothesis and show an association among perinatal aspiration syndromes, transient thrombocytopenia, and PPHN (Segall et al., 1980). Moreover, pathologic data demonstrate platelet plugging in the microcirculation of the lung of infants dying of PPHN associated with meconium aspiration pneumonia (Levin et al., 1983).

Anatomic abnormalities of the pulmonary vascular bed fall into two general categories: those associated with underdevelopment of the lung, and those that result from maldevelopment of the vessels. In the case of pulmonary hypoplasia, lung mass is reduced; yet cardiac output is

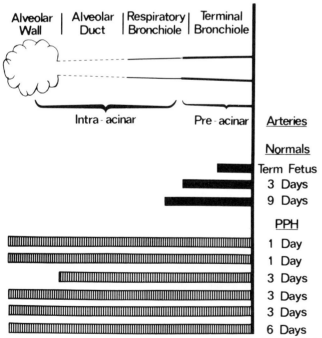

FIGURE 53–13. *Vascular maldevelopment in infants with PPHN. In normal infants, no muscular arteries are found within the acinus. All patients with pulmonary hypertension had extension of muscle into intra-acinar arteries. (From Murphy, J.D., Rabinovitch, M., Goldstein, J.D., and Reid, L.M.: The structural basis of persistent pulmonary hypertension of the newborn infant. J. Pediatr. 98:962, 1981.)*

appropriate for body size. As a result, the volume of blood flowing through the existing pulmonary vessels is relatively high, pulmonary arterial pressures are high, and relative pulmonary vascular resistance is increased. In addition to this anatomic impediment to flow, infants with pulmonary hypoplasia are likely to have maldevelopment of the pulmonary vessels and an increased pulmonary vascular resistance from anatomic obstruction of existing vessels (Naeye et al., 1976; Geggel et al., 1985).

Maldevelopment of pulmonary vessels refers predominantly to abnormalities of vascular smooth muscle found in lungs of infants dying from PPHN (Murphy et al., 1981) (Fig. 53–12). In these infants, pulmonary arterial smooth muscle hypertrophies and extends from preacinar arteries into normally nonmuscular intra-acinar arteries—even to the level of the alveolus (Fig. 53–13). This thickened muscle encroaches upon the vessel lumen and results in mechanical obstruction to blood flow. In extreme cases, vascular maldevelopment can cause a reduction in number of arteries per cross-sectional area of the lung. A review of the associated clinical entities and the available data from experiments in animals suggests that this vascular maldevelopment is the result of sustained pulmonary hypertension in utero. PPHN is strongly associated with low-grade chronic intrauterine hypoxia. In fact, it is likely that unrecognized asphyxia or ductal closure may account for a large proportion of those cases labeled as idiopathic. In chronically asphyxiated fetuses, pulmonary arterial pressure can be increased by active constriction of pulmonary arterioles secondary to hypoxia. However, since the pulmonary circulation is parallel to the systemic circulation, it also can be increased secondary to asphyxia-induced increases in systemic arterial pressure. Experimental data from fetal rats and lambs support both these hypotheses (Soifer et al., 1987); however, while systemic hypertension (even by itself) consistently results in vascular maldevelopment (Levin et al., 1978b), intrauterine hypoxia does not consistently result in vascular maldevelopment (Geggel et al., 1986). Premature closure of the ductus arteriosus secondary to maternal ingestion of inhibitors of prostaglandin synthesis has been associated with PPHN. Two infants whose mothers chronically took prostaglandin synthetase inhibitors during pregnancy presented with severe PPHN but had no evidence of a ductal shunt at birth, suggesting early ductal closure. Furthermore, in two groups of infants with idiopathic PPHN, those without ductal level shunting had higher salicylate levels than those with ductal level shunting (Perkin et al., 1980). Experiments in animals show that premature closure of the ductus (Morin, 1989; Wild et al., 1989) results in maldevelopment of pulmonary vessels, presumably by forcing a greater portion of the combined ventricular output through the lungs at a significantly higher pressure (Levin et al., 1978a). The association between meconium aspiration pneumonia and vascular maldevelopment is interesting. Of 11 infants dying of meconium aspiration pneumonia, 10 were found to have significant vascular smooth muscle hypertrophy with extension of muscle into intra-acinar arteries (Murphy et al., 1984). This maldevelopment could be secondary to chronic intrauterine asphyxia, the release of vasoactive substances by meconium in the trachea, or a circulating intestinal peptide stimulating both pulmonary vasoconstriction and intestinal motility. Finally, since disorders associated with underdevelopment of the lung also result in intrauterine pulmonary hypertension, it is not too surprising that they also frequently are associated with maldevelopment of existing vessels. This is particularly true in infants with congenital diaphragmatic hernia and accounts for much of the respiratory instability of these infants (Geggel et al., 1985, Naeye et al., 1976).

Clinical Manifestations. Affected infants are usually delivered at term or post term and frequently are born through meconium-stained fluid. They are often thought to be normal after brief distress at birth. Then, within the first 12 hours after birth they are recognized as having cyanosis and tachypnea without apnea and retractions or grunting. They frequently have a cardiac murmur that is compatible with tricuspid insufficiency, but systemic blood pressure is normal. Hypoglycemia frequently complicates many of the associated conditions, such as sepsis and meconium aspiration, and hypocalcemia also occurs often.

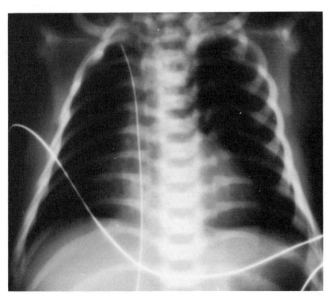

FIGURE 53–14. *Chest radiograph from infant with idiopathic PPHN. Lung fields appear hyperlucent with decreased vascularity.*

Arterial blood gas tensions reveal severe arterial oxygen desaturation with relatively normal carbon dioxide tensions. In infants with significant ductal level shunting, the oxygen saturation measured from the right brachial or radial artery will be greater than that obtained from the umbilical artery. Chest radiographs reveal cardiomegaly in about half the infants. For infants with idiopathic PPHN, the lung fields are clear and appear undervascularized (Fig. 53–14). For the remainder of the associated entities, chest radiographs reflect the underlying parenchymal disease. Electrocardiograms reveal ventricular hypertrophy appropriate for age; in more severe cases, they also reveal S-T segment depression in the precordial leads, suggestive of ischemia. All infants suspected of having PPHN should undergo ultrasound examination of the heart to rule out cyanotic congenital heart disease, to document right-to-left shunting of blood at the foramen ovale and ductus arteriosus, and to measure systolic time intervals. Prolonged systolic time intervals support a diagnosis of pulmonary hypertension, but they are not definitive since they also can be prolonged by right ventricular dysfunction. Infants in whom cyanotic congenital heart disease cannot be ruled out by echocardiogram should undergo cardiac catheterization. At some point in the course of their disease, most infants with PPHN will increase their SaO_2, at least transiently, in response to some therapeutic intervention. Infants who can never be oxygenated should be considered for cardiac catheterization.

Therapy. The objectives of therapy for infants with PPHN are to lower the pulmonary vascular resistance, to maintain the systemic blood pressure, to reverse the right-to-left shunts, and to improve arterial oxygen saturation and oxygen delivery to the tissues without producing severe damage to the lungs. All these infants should be nursed in a neutral thermal environment. Cold stress raises the metabolic rate, increases oxygen consumption, and causes the infant to release norepinephrine, a pulmonary vasoconstrictor. Fluids should be restricted and hypoglycemia and hypocalcemia corrected. Systemic hypotension and acidosis should be corrected by judicious use of blood and alkali. Calcium, blood products, and hyperosmolar solutions are potentially vasoactive and should be infused with caution. Infusion of dopamine at low doses (2 to 10 μg/kg/min) may increase cardiac output without affecting systemic or pulmonary vascular resistance. At higher doses, dopamine exhibits considerable alpha-adrenergic activity and may result in systemic vasoconstriction and increased blood pressure along with an actual reduction in cardiac output (Feltes et al., 1987). In addition, higher doses of dopamine can constrict both pulmonary and systemic vessels. If the central hematocrit is greater than 60 to 65 per cent, a partial exchange transfusion should be performed to lower the hematocrit and to reduce the effects of hyperviscosity on the pulmonary arterial pressure.

In infants with PPHN, the pulmonary circulation seems to be exceptionally sensitive to changes in oxygen tension. Therefore, it is advisable when possible, to try to maintain their PaO_2 between 80 and 100 mm Hg. There is no evidence that maintaining PaO_2 in excess of 100 mm Hg improves the outcome, and prolonged exposure to excessively high PaO_2 can injure other organs such as the brain and the eye (Hansen and Gest, 1984), besides often requiring high pressures on the ventilator. Oxygen should be given by hood, up to 100 per cent if necessary, and PaO_2 values of ≥ 40 should be accepted (Wung et al., 1985). If oxygen alone does not lower the pulmonary vascular resistance and improve arterial oxygen saturation, the next step is to induce alkalosis. Several studies in animals have shown that both respiratory and metabolic alkalosis effectively lower pulmonary vascular resistance (Schreiber et al., 1986; Fike and Hansen, 1989). In an infant with a $PaCO_2$ in the low normal range, administration of $NaHCO_3$ or THAM may improve oxygenation.

It is clear that mechanical ventilation sufficient to lower the $PaCO_2$ to the point at which pH exceeds 7.55 to 7.60 will often result in a dramatic increase in arterial oxygen saturation (Peckham and Fox, 1978; Drummond et al., 1981). However, this hyperventilation usually requires excessive pressures that lead to barotrauma and worsening lung disease. There is some controversy about the use of neuromuscular blockers in this group of infants. Clinicians at some centers routinely use paralytic agents such as pancuronium bromide, whereas others believe that with careful ventilator management, paralysis is not necessary (Wung et al., 1985). In addition, since these infants are extremely sensitive to external stimuli, it has been recommended that they be sedated with either morphine or fentanyl and that they be handled as little as possible (Hickey et al., 1985). To avoid alveolar overdistention, the inspiratory time is kept short, i.e., 0.15 to 0.20 sec. The lungs of infants with PPHN frequently have normal to prolonged expiratory time constants, so expiratory time must be kept relatively long to prevent gas trapping. Therefore, the respirator rate is set at 60 to 80 breaths/min. Inspiratory pressure is adjusted to control the $PaCO_2$. Prolonged hyperventilation is inappropriate, however. Positive end-expiratory pressure is useful only in patients with parenchymal lung disease. Treatment of PPHN by hyperventilation is associated with a high incidence of pneumothorax. Moreover, there is concern that chronic hyperventilation may impair cerebral blood flow and, hence, oxygen delivery to the brain of these already compromised infants (Bruce, 1984).

After several days of ventilation with high concentrations of oxygen and high airway pressures, infants with PPHN develop pulmonary parenchymal abnormalities that are characterized by decreased lung compliance, which may be due to impaired surfactant metabolism; infiltrates compatible with pulmonary edema may be seen on the chest radiograph. At this point, the pulmonary vascular bed is no longer sensitive to changes in pH and much less sensitive to changes in FIO_2 (Sosulski and Fox, 1985). It is imperative that this transition phase be recognized, so that FIO_2 and airway pressure can be reduced to prevent further lung injury (Hansen and Gest, 1984).

For the infant in whom ventilation with oxygen and circulatory support with vasoactive agents do not result in acceptable PaO_2, an alternative is attempting to lower the pulmonary vascular resistance by pharmacologic means. Tolazoline is the drug most commonly used to dilate the pulmonary vascular bed (Peckham and Fox, 1978; Drummond et al., 1981), but it has multiple drawbacks. It is an alpha-adrenergic blocker with some mild cholinergic properties, and it is also a potent histamine-releasing agent,

which results in pulmonary vasodilation in the newborn. Unfortunately, its effects are not specific for the lung. In most studies, the effects of tolazoline on the systemic circulation are at least as great as those on the pulmonary circulation. Its administration usually requires circulatory support with volume expansion or further use of pressor agents. The dose remains controversial, but a bolus of 1 to 2 mg/kg may be given slowly over several minutes. Clinicians at some centers then administer 0.15 to 0.30 mg/kg/hour through a scalp vein. Tolazoline has a plasma half-life of between 2 and 8 hours and is excreted mostly in the urine. Therefore, if urine output is less than 1 ml/kg/min, excretion is reduced markedly (Ward et al., 1986). The dose should be decreased in infants with oliguria, since there is no way to reverse the effects of the drug. In one review of 314 patients, 59 per cent improved after receiving tolazoline, while only 54 per cent survived. Complications referable to tolazoline therapy occurred in 70 per cent of the patients—42 per cent had increased gastrointestinal secretions, 31 per cent had gastrointestinal bleeding, 32 per cent developed hypotension, and 36 per cent became oliguric (Peckham, 1982).

Sodium nitroprusside is another vasodilator used to treat infants with PPHN (Benitz et al., 1985). It is a balanced arterial and venous dilator that affects both the pulmonary and the systemic circulations and, like tolazoline, requires that the systemic circulation be supported. It is administered by constant infusion at 1 to 5 μg/kg/min. One advantage of nitroprusside over tolazoline is that it is rapidly cleared from the circulation (2 to 4 sec) so that any complications are rapidly reversible. Thiocyanate and cyanide are metabolic products of nitroprusside, and levels must be monitored in order to avoid toxicity.

Despite their early promise, other pharmacologic agents, such as prostacyclin and prostaglandin D_2, have not proved to be efficacious in the treatment of PPHN (Soifer et al., 1982; Kaapa et al., 1985).

The failure of some infants to respond to maximal therapy has led to the use of extracorporeal membrane oxygenation (ECMO) in some centers. Because other centers show comparable results with conservative medical management of patients who meet the criteria for ECMO, this form of treatment remains controversial (Wung et al., 1985; Dworetz et al., 1989). Infants with PaO_2 as low as 40 mm Hg can be managed medically if careful attention is paid to other determinants of oxygen delivery. In these infants, repeated measurements of blood lactate may be useful to assess tissue oxygenation.

Outcome. In most studies, the mortality for infants with PPHN ranges from 20 to 40 per cent while the incidence of neurologic handicap ranges from 12 to 25 per cent (Ballard and Leonard, 1984). Sell and co-workers (1985), however, found that only 40 per cent of 40 infants with PPHN in their institution were developmentally normal at 1 to 4 years: 32 per cent had an abnormal or suspect neurologic examination, and 20 per cent had neurosensory hearing loss. It is not clear what the relative contributions of the underlying disease (chronic hypoxia in utero, sepsis), asphyxia at birth or during the course of the disease, or therapies such as hyperventilation and use of vasodilator agents are to the outcome of these infants.

■ MECONIUM ASPIRATION PNEUMONIA (MAP)

Meconium, an odorless, thick, blackish green material, is first demonstrable in the fetal intestine during the third month of gestation. It is an accumulation of debris that consists of desquamated cells from the alimentary tract and skin, lanugo hairs, fatty material from the vernix caseosa, amniotic fluid, and various intestinal secretions. Meconium is biochemically composed of a mucopolysaccharide of high blood group specificity, a small amount of lipid, and a small amount of protein that decreases throughout gestation. Its blackish green color is the result of bile pigments.

Pathogenesis. Meconium staining of amniotic fluid occurs in roughly 10 per cent of all deliveries (Desmond et al., 1957). It has a strong correlation with gestational age. The risk of meconium staining before 37 weeks of gestation is less than 2 per cent (Matthews and Warshaw, 1979), whereas after 42 weeks it is nearly 44 per cent (Miller and Read, 1981). Although the passage of meconium in utero is generally thought to be synonymous with fetal asphyxia, the relationship has not yet been established. Multiple studies have failed to show any consistent effects of meconium staining on Apgar score, fetal scalp pH, or the incidence of fetal heart rate abnormalities (Fenton and Steer, 1962; Abramovici et al., 1974; Miller et al., 1975). These studies have led to speculation that asphyxial episodes too brief to decrease pH or Apgar scores may cause the passage of meconium in utero. The strong correlation between meconium staining and gestational age, however, also supports two additional theories: (1) It is possible that the passage of meconium in utero is the result of transient parasympathetic stimulation from cord compression in a neurologically mature fetus; or (2) it is a natural phenomenon that reflects the maturity of the gastrointestinal tract. Despite these theories, most physicians agree that meconium staining of the amniotic fluid in connection with fetal heart rate abnormalities is a marker for fetal distress and is associated with an increased perinatal morbidity.

Meconium may enter the trachea and airways in utero. In one study, meconium was recovered from the tracheas of 56 per cent of meconium-stained infants in the delivery room (Gregory et al., 1970). Another recent study (Davis et al., 1985) described 12 infants who died with MAP even though their tracheas were suctioned vigorously in the delivery room. These findings suggest that in some instances, particularly with distressed infants who are gasping, considerable peripheral migration of meconium can occur while the fetus is still in utero (Davis et al., 1985). Autopsy data that show meconium in the terminal airways of stillborn fetuses support this theory (Brown and Gleicher, 1981). It is highly unlikely, however, that significant intrauterine aspiration of meconium is the result of normal fetal breathing, since the rate of production of fetal lung fluid is such that the net movement of fluid is out of the lung. It is more likely that meconium is aspirated into the tracheobronchial tree when the fetus begins to gasp deeply in response to hypoxia and acidosis. It is unknown whether the reduced rate of production of fetal lung fluid that accompanies labor contributes to the movement of meconium into the trachea or to its migration peripherally.

If meconium is not removed from the trachea after delivery, with the onset of respiration it will migrate from the central airways to the periphery of the lung. Initially, particles of meconium produce mechanical obstruction of the small airways that results in hyperinflation with patchy atelectasis. Later, small airway obstruction is the result of chemical pneumonitis and interstitial edema (Tyler et al., 1978). During this later stage, hyperinflation persists and areas of atelectasis become more extensive. In addition, there is infiltration of the alveolar septa by neutrophils, necrosis of alveolar and airway epithelia, and accumulation of proteinaceous debris within the alveolus.

Infants who die of MAP complicated by pulmonary hypertension frequently have evidence of injury to the vascular bed of the lung that dates back several weeks prior to birth (Murphy et al., 1984). In these infants, vascular smooth muscle extends into the walls of normally nonmuscular intra-acinar arterioles and reduces their luminal diameter, which subsequently interferes with the normal postnatal drop in pulmonary vascular resistance. In addition, these infants may demonstrate plugs of platelets in their small vessels that reduce the overall cross-sectional area of the pulmonary vascular bed (Levin et al., 1983).

Airway resistance is increased in newborn infants and experimental animals with MAP (Tran et al., 1980; Yeh et al., 1982). In addition, dynamic lung compliance is reduced while static lung compliance is unchanged, suggesting that airway obstruction is patchy and is located in peripheral airways. Functional residual capacity is increased in animals with MAP but not in humans. There is also some evidence that meconium interferes with surfactant function, further contributing to atelectasis. Hypoxia is the result of continued perfusion of poorly ventilated lung units, whereas hypercarbia is the result of a decrease in minute ventilation and an increase in respiratory dead space.

Some infants with MAP have elevated pulmonary arterial pressures with shunting of blood right to left across the foramen ovale and ductus arteriosus (Fox et al., 1977). While this is in part a consequence of the anatomic abnormalities described above, active constriction of pulmonary vessels may also complicate MAP or may be caused by the same perinatal insult that caused passage of meconium. Vasoactive substances in meconium may constrict pulmonary vessels directly or may cause platelet aggregation in the lung with the release of thromboxane— a potent pulmonary vasoconstrictor. Data that support the latter hypothesis show that pulmonary vascular resistance increases in experimental MAP before any anatomic change can occur (Tyler et al., 1978) and that thrombocytopenia and intrapulmonary platelet aggregation accompany MAP in infants (Segall et al., 1980; Levin et al., 1983).

Clinical Manifestations. Infants with meconium aspiration are often postmature and have visible meconium staining of the nails, the skin, and the umbilical cord. Many infants with MAP have been asphyxiated, and much of the early distress may relate more to asphyxia and retained fetal lung fluid complicated by elevated pulmo-

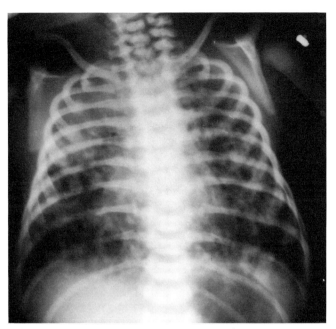

FIGURE 53–15. Chest x-ray study of an infant with meconium aspiration pneumonia.

nary vascular resistance than to the presence of meconium in the airways. Infants with MAP have clinical evidence of lung overinflation, with a barrel chest. Auscultation of the chest reveals diffuse rales and rhonchi. The chest radiograph shows patchy areas of atelectasis and areas of overinflation (Fig. 53–15). Pneumothorax and pneumomediastinum are common. The clinical symptoms progress over 12 to 24 hours as meconium migrates to the periphery of the lung. Because meconium must ultimately be removed by phagocytes, respiratory distress and requirements for supplemental oxygen may persist for days or even weeks after birth. Infants who present with a shorter course and with rapid resolution of symptoms are more likely to have had retained fetal lung fluid than MAP.

Therapy. Symptomatic infants with meconium suctioned from their tracheas should be given chest physiotherapy and warmed humidified oxygen to breathe. Lung lavage may result in deterioration of lung function. Because of the high incidence of air leaks, positive-pressure ventilation should be avoided, if possible. Judicious use of constant positive airway pressure (4 to 7 cm H_2O) via nasal or endotracheal CPAP may improve oxygenation in the patient who is unresponsive to oxygen administration alone. This improvement in oxygenation is achieved presumably by stabilizing the small airways and improving the ventilation of poorly ventilated lung units. High airway pressures may impair oxygenation by impeding blood flow to well-ventilated lung units. Mechanical ventilation should be reserved for infants with apnea from birth asphyxia or for those who cannot maintain their PaO_2 greater than 50 mm Hg in 100 per cent oxygen. These infants are often large and vigorous and tend to fight mechanical ventilation, which makes oxygenation difficult and increases the chances of air leak. If this occurs, the patient may require neuromuscular blockade. Moderate amounts of PEEP may aid in oxygenation (Fox et al., 1975). Because MAP is an obstructive lung disease, the time constant for

expiration is prolonged in severely involved areas of the lung. Careful attention must be paid to expiratory time (ventilatory rate) to prevent inadvertent PEEP, further gas trapping, and alveolar rupture (see p. 490).

Therapy for the infant with MAP and PPHN is covered in the discussion of the use of ECMO on p. 495.

The role of antibiotics in the treatment of MAP is controversial. Meconium enhances bacterial growth by reducing host resistance, but no studies have shown that infection plays a role in the pathogenesis of MAP. The use of corticosteroids is not recommended (Yeh et al., 1977; Frantz et al., 1975).

Outcome. Once established, MAP carries a significant risk of pneumothorax and pneumomediastinum. The overall mortality for meconium-stained infants is 3 to 5 per cent (Desmond et al., 1957), while the mortality for infants who require mechanical ventilation may be as high as 30 per cent (Vidyasagar et al., 1975). Infants who do not respond to conventional therapy may respond to ECMO.

Prevention. Several studies show that by clearing the airway of meconium at the time of birth, MAP can be virtually eliminated (Gregory et al., 1970; Ting and Brady, 1975). Current recommendations are for a combined obstetric and pediatric approach to the infant born through thick, or "pea soup," meconium. This approach calls for DeLee suctioning of the nasopharynx by the obstetrician at the time of delivery of the head, and it requires visualization and direct suctioning of the trachea by the pediatrician immediately after birth. Universal precautions now preclude the use of one's mouth as a means to apply suction to the endotracheal tube. However, several commercial devices are available that can be interposed between the endotracheal tube and a vacuum source. Intubation and suction are required even when meconium is not visible in the posterior pharynx, since one study found that 10 per cent of meconium-stained infants had meconium in their tracheas even when there was no meconium visible at the vocal cords (Gregory, 1974). One recent study questions the need for intubation and suctioning of nondistressed term infants who are meconium-stained. This study suggests that in the absence of asphyxia these infants are unlikely to have significant amounts of meconium in their tracheas and that the complications of intubation may outweigh any benefit (Linder et al., 1988).

■ REFERENCES

Abramovici, J., Brandes, J.M., Fuchs, K., and Timor-Tritsch, I.: Meconium during delivery: A sign of compensated fetal distress. Am. J. Obstet. Gynecol. *118*:251, 1974.

Adams, F.H., Fujiwara, T., Emmanouilides, G.C., and Raiha, N.: Lung phospholipids of human fetuses and infants with and without hyaline membrane disease. Pediatrics 77:833, 1970.

Allen, L.P., Reynolds, E.O.R., Rivers, R.P.A., et al.: Controlled trial of continuous positive airway pressure given by face mask for hyaline membrane disease. Arch. Dis. Child. *52*:373, 1977.

Avery, M.E., and Fletcher, B.D.: The Lung and Its Disorders in the Newborn Infant. Philadelphia, W.B. Saunders Company, 1974.

Avery, M.E., and Mead, J.: Surface properties in relation to atelectasis and hyaline membrane disease. Am. J. Dis. Child. *97*:517, 1959.

Avery, M.E., Gatewood, O.B., and Brumley, G.: Transient tachypnea of newborn: Possible delayed resorption of fluid at birth. Am. J. Dis. Child. *111*:380, 1966.

Ballard, P.L.: Hormones and Lung Maturation. New York, Springer-Verlag, 1986.

Ballard, R.A., Ballard, P.L., Creasy, R., et al.: Prenatal thyrotropin-releasing hormone plus corticosteroid decreases chronic lung disease in very low birth weight infants. Clin. Res. 38:192A, 1990.

Ballard, R.A., and Leonard, C.H.: Development follow-up of infants with persistent pulmonary hypertension of the newborn. Clin. Perinatol. 11:737, 1984.

Ballard, R.A., Ballard, P.L., Granberg, J.P., and Sniderman, S.: Prenatal administration of betamethasone for prevention of respiratory distress syndrome. J. Pediatr. 94:97, 1979.

Bancalari, E., Garcia, O.L., and Jesse, M.J.: Effects of continuous negative pressure on lung mechanics in idiopathic respiratory distress syndrome. Pediatrics 51:485, 1973.

Bartlett, R.H., Roloff, D.W., Cornell, R.G., et al.: Extracorporeal circulation in neonatal respiratory failure: a prospective randomized study. Pediatrics 76:479, 1985.

Bauer, C.R., Morrison, J.C., Poole, W.K., et al.: Decreased incidence of necrotizing enterocolitis after prenatal glucocorticoid therapy. Pediatrics 73:682, 1984.

Benatar, S.R., Hewlett, A.M., and Nunn, J.F.: The use of iso-shunt lines for control of oxygen therapy. Br. J. Anaesthesiol. 45:711, 1973.

Benitz, W.E., Malachowski, N., Cohen, R.S., et al.: Use of sodium nitroprusside in neonates: efficacy and safety. J. Pediatr. 106:102, 1985.

Bolton, D.P.G., and Cross, K.W.: Further observations on cost of preventing retrolental fibroplasia. Lancet 1:445, 1974.

Boughton, K., Gandy, G., and Gairdner, D.: Hyaline membrane disease II. Lung lecithin. Arch. Dis. Child. 45:311, 1970.

Brown, B.L., and Gleicher, N.: Intrauterine meconium aspiration. Obstet. Gynecol. 57:26, 1981.

Bruce, D.A.: Effects of hyperventilation on cerebral blood flow and metabolism. Clin. Perinatol. 11:673, 1984.

Brumley, G.W., Hodson, W.A., and Avery, M.E.: Lung phospholipids and surface tension correlations in infants with and without hyaline membrane disease. Pediatrics 40:13, 1967.

Chiswick, M.L.: Prolonged rupture of membranes, pre-eclamptic toxemia and respiratory distress syndrome. Arch. Dis. Child. 51:674, 1976.

Chu, J., Clements, J.A., Cotton, E.K., et al.: Neonatal pulmonary ischemia: clinical and physiological studies. Pediatrics 40:709, 1967.

Clements, J.A., and Tooley, W.H.: Kinetics of surface active material in the fetal lung. In Hodson, W.A. (Ed.): Development of the Lung. New York, Marcel Dekker, 1977.

Collaborative Group on Antenatal Steroid Treatment: Effect of antenatal dexamethasone administration on the prevention of respiratory distress syndrome. Am. J. Obstet. Gynecol. 141:276, 1981.

Corbet, A., and Adams, J.: Current therapy in hyaline membrane disease. Clin. Perinatol. 5:299, 1978.

Corbet, A.J.S., Adams, J.M., Kenny, J.D., et al.: Controlled trial of bicarbonate therapy in high risk premature newborn infants. J. Pediatr. 91:771, 1977.

Corbet, A.J.S., Ross, J.A., Beaudry, P.H., and Stern, L.: Effect of positive pressure breathing on aA·DN$_2$ in hyaline membrane disease. J. Appl. Physiol. 38:33, 1975.

Corbet, A.J.S., Ross, J.A., Beaudry, P.H., and Stern, L.: Ventilation perfusion relationships as assessed by aA·DN$_2$ in hyaline membrane disease. J. Appl. Physiol. 36:74, 1974.

Davis, R.O., Philips, J.B., Harris, B.A., et al.: Fatal meconium aspiration syndrome occurring despite airway management considered appropriate. Am. J. Obstet. Gynecol. 151:731, 1985.

deMello, D.E., Chi, E.Y., Doo, E., and Lagunoff, D.: Absence of tubular myelin in lungs of infants dying with hyaline membrane disease. Am. J. Pathol. 127:131, 1987.

Desmond, M.M., Moore, J., Lindley, J.E., and Brown, C.A.: Meconium staining of the amniotic fluid: A marker of fetal hypoxia. Obstet. Gynecol. 9:91, 1957.

Dreizzen, E., Migdal, M., Praud, J.P., et al.: Passive compliance of total respiratory system in preterm newborn infants with respiratory distress syndrome. J. Pediatr. 112:778, 1988.

Drew, J.H.: Immediate intubation at birth of the very low birthweight infant. Am. J. Dis. Child. 136:207, 1982.

Drummond, W.H., Gregory, G.A., Heymann, M.A., and Phibbs, R.H.: The independent effects of hyperventilation, tolazoline and dopamine on infants with persistent pulmonary hypertension. J. Pediatr. 98:603, 1981.

Dudell, G.G., and Gersony, W.M.: Patent ductus arteriosus in neonates with severe respiratory disease. J. Pediatr. 104:915, 1984.

Dworetz, A.R., Moya, F.R., Sabo, B., et al.: Survival of infants with persistent pulmonary hypertension without extracorporeal membrane oxygenation. Pediatrics 84:1, 1989.

Enhorning, G., Shennan, A., Possmayer, F., et al.: Prevention of neonatal respiratory distress syndrome by tracheal instillation of surfactant: a randomized clinical trial. Pediatrics 76:145, 1985.

Fanaroff, A.A., Cha, C.C., Sosa, R., et al.: Controlled trial of continuous negative external pressure in the treatment of severe respiratory distress syndrome. J. Pediatr. 82:921, 1973.

Farrell, P.M., and Avery, M.E.: State of the art: hyaline membrane disease. Am. Rev. Respir. Dis. 111:657, 1975.

Farrell, P.M., and Wood, R.E.: Epidemiology of hyaline membrane disease in the United States: analysis of national mortality statistics. Pediatrics 58:167, 1976.

Fedrick, J., and Butler, N.R.: Hyaline membrane disease. Lancet 2:768, 1972.

Feltes, T.F., Hansen, T.N., Martin, C.G., et al.: The effects of dopamine infusion on regional blood flow in newborn lambs. Pediatr. Res. 21:131, 1987.

Fenton, A.N., and Steer, C.M.: Fetal distress. Am. J. Obstet. Gynecol. 83:354, 1962.

Fike, C., and Hansen, T.N.: Effects of alkalosis on hypoxic pulmonary vasoconstriction in newborn rabbit lungs. Pediatr. Res. 25:383, 1989.

Finlay-Jones, J.M., Papadimitriou, J.M., and Barter, R.A.: Pulmonary hyaline membrane: light and election microscopic study of the early stage. J. Pathol. 112:117, 1974.

Fox, W.W., Berman, L.S., Downes, J.J., and Peckham, G.J.: The therapeutic application of end-expiratory pressure in the meconium aspiration syndrome. Pediatrics 56:214, 1975.

Fox, W.W., Gewitz, M.H., Dinwiddie, R., et al.: Pulmonary hypertension in the perinatal aspiration syndromes. Pediatrics 59:205, 1977.

Frank, L., Lewis, P.L., and Sosenko, I.R.S.: Dexamethasone-stimulated fetal rat lung antioxidant enzyme activity in parallel with surfactant stimulation. Pediatrics 75:569–574, 1985.

Frantz, I.D., Wang, N.S., and Thach, B.T.: Experimental meconium aspiration: effects of glucocorticoid treatment. J. Pediatr. 86:438, 1975.

Gandy, G., Jacobson, W., and Gairdner, D.: Hyaline membrane disease: cellular changes. Arch. Dis. Child. 45:289, 1970.

Geggel, R.L., Aronovitz, M.J., and Reid, L.M.: Effects of chronic in utero hypoxemia on rat neonatal pulmonary arterial structure. J. Pediatr. 108:756, 1986.

Geggel, R.L., Murphy, J.D., Langleben, D., et al.: Congenital diaphragmatic hernia: arterial structural changes and persistent pulmonary hypertension after surgical repair. J. Pediatr. 107:457, 1985.

Gersony, W.M., Duc, G.V., and Sinclair, J.C.: "PFC" syndrome (persistence of the fetal circulation). Circulation (Suppl.) 39:III–87, 1969.

Glass, L., Rajegowda, B.K., and Evans, H.E.: Absence of respiratory distress syndrome in premature infants of heroin addicted mothers. Lancet 2:685, 1971.

Gluck, L., and Kulovich, M.V.: Lecithin-sphingomyelin ratios in amniotic fluid in normal and abnormal pregnancy. Am. J. Obstet. Gynecol. 115:539, 1973.

Gluck, L., and Kulovich, M.V.: The evaluation of functional maturity in the human fetus. In Gluck, L. (Ed.): Modern Perinatal Medicine. Chicago, Yearbook Medical Publishers, 1974.

Gregory, G.A., Gooding, C.A., Phibbs, R.H., and Tooley, W.H.: Meconium aspiration in infants—a prospective study. J. Pediatr. 85:848, 1970.

Gregory, G.A., Kitterman, J.A., Phibbs, R.H., et al.: Treatment of idiopathic respiratory distress syndrome with continuous positive airway pressure. N. Engl. J. Med. 284: 1333, 1971.

Gribetz, I., Frank, N.R., and Avery, M.E.: Static volume pressure relations of excised lungs of infants with hyaline membrane disease, newborn and stillborn infants. J. Clin. Invest. 38:2168, 1959.

Hack, M., Fanaroff, A., and Klaus, M.: Neonatal respiratory distress following elective delivery: a preventable disease? Am. J. Obstet. Gynecol. 126:43, 1976.

Halliday, H.L., McClure, G., and McCreid, M.: Transient tachypnoea of the newborn: two distinct clinical entities? Arch. Dis. Child. 56:322, 1981.

Hallman, M., and Teramo, K.: Measurement of the lecithin sphingomyelin ratio and phosphatidylglycerol in amniotic fluid: an accurate method for the assessment of fetal lung maturity. Br. J. Obstet. Gynaecol. 88:806, 1981.

Hallman, M., Kulovich, M.V., Kirkpatrick, E., et al.: Phosphatidylinositol and phosphatidylglycerol in amniotic fluid: indices of lung maturity. Am. J. Obstet. Gynecol. 125:613, 1976.

Hallman, M., Merritt, T.A., Jarvenpaa, A.L., et al.: Exogenous human surfactant for treatment of severe respiratory distress syndrome: a randomized prospective clinical trial. J. Pediatr. *106:*963, 1985.

Hammerman, C., Komar, K., and Abu-Khudair, H.: Hypoxic vs septic pulmonary hypertension. Am. J. Dis. Child. *142:*319, 1988.

Hansen, T.N., and Gest, A.L.: Oxygen toxicity and other ventilatory complications of treatment of infants with persistent pulmonary hypertension. Clin. Perinatol. *11:*653, 1984.

Hansen, T.N., Corbet, A.J.S., Kenny, J.D., et al.: Effects of oxygen and constant positive pressure breathing on aA·Dco₂ in hyaline membrane disease. Pediatr. Res. *13:*1167, 1979.

Hickey, P.R., Hansen, D.D., Wessel, D.L., et al.: Blunting of stress responses in the pulmonary circulation of infants by fentanyl. Anesth. Analg. *64:*1137, 1985.

Hjalmarson, O., and Olsson, T.: Mechanical and ventilatory parameters in healthy and diseased newborn infants. Acta Paediatr. Scand. (Suppl.) *247:*26, 1974.

Horbar, J.D., Sutherland, J., Philip, A.G.S., et al.: Multicenter trial of single dose surfactant-TA for treatment of respiratory distress syndrome (Abstract). Pediatr. Res. *23:*410A, 1988.

Howie, R.N.: Pharmacological acceleration of lung maturation. *In* Raivio, K.O., Hallman, N., Kouvalainen, K., and Valimaki, I. (Eds.): Respiratory Distress Syndrome. New York, Academic Press, 1984, pp. 385–396.

Ikegami, M., Jobe, A., and Berry, D.: A protein that inhibits surfactant in respiratory distress syndrome. Biol. Neonate *50:*121, 1986.

Jacob, J., Gluck, L., DiSessa, T., et al.: The contribution of PDA in the neonate with severe RDS. J. Pediatr. *96:*79, 1980.

James, L.S.: Perinatal events and respiratory distress syndrome. N. Engl. J. Med. *292:*1291, 1975.

Jefferies, A.L., Coates, G., and O'Brodovich, H.: Pulmonary epithelial permeability in hyaline membrane disease. N. Engl. J. Med. *311:*1075, 1984.

Jones, M.D., Burd, L.I., Bowes, W.A., et al.: Failure of association of premature rupture of membranes with respiratory distress syndrome. N. Engl. J. Med. *292:*1253, 1975.

Kaapa, P., Koivisto, M., Ylikorkala, O., and Koiuvalainen, K.: Prostacyclin in the treatment of neonatal pulmonary hypertension. J. Pediatr. *107:*951, 1985.

Kenny, J.D., Adams, J.M., Corbet, A.J.S., and Rudolph, A.J.: The role of acidosis at birth in the development of hyaline membrane disease. Pediatrics *58:*184, 1976.

Krauss, A.N., and Auld, P.A.M.: Pulmonary gas trapping in premature infants. Pediatr. Res. *5:*10, 1971.

Krauss, A.N., Klain, D.B., and Auld, P.A.M.: Carbon monoxide diffusing capacity in newborn infants. Pediatr. Res. *10:*771, 1976.

Landers, S., Hansen, T.N., Corbet, A.J.S., et al.: Optimal constant positive airway pressure assessed by arterial alveolar difference for CO₂ in hyaline membrane disease. Pediatr. Res. *20:*884, 1986.

Lawson, E.E., Birdwell, R.L., Huang, P.S., and Taeusch, H.W.: Augmentation of pulmonary surfactant secretion by lung expansion at birth. Pediatr. Res. *13:*611, 1979.

Levin, D.L., Fixler, D.E., Morriss, F.C., and Tyson, J.: Morphologic analysis of the pulmonary vascular bed in infants exposed in utero to prostaglandin synthetase inhibitors. J. Pediatr. *92:*478, 1978a.

Levin, D.L., Heymann, M.A., Kitterman, J.A., et al.: Persistent pulmonary hypertension of the newborn infant. J. Pediatr. *89:*626, 1976.

Levin, D.L., Hyman, A.I., Heymann, M.A., and Rudolph, A.M.: Fetal hypertension and the development of increased pulmonary vascular smooth muscle: a possible mechanism for persistent pulmonary hypertension of the newborn infant. J. Pediatr. *92:*265, 1978b.

Levin, D.L., Weinberg, A.G., and Perkin, R.M.: Pulmonary microthrombi syndrome in newborn infants with unresponsive persistent pulmonary hypertension. J. Pediatr. *102:*299, 1983.

Liggins, G.C., and Howie, R.N.: A controlled trial of antepartum glucocorticoid treatment for prevention of the respiratory distress syndrome in premature infants. Pediatrics *50:*515, 1972.

Linder, N., Aranda, J.V., Tsur, M., et al.: Need for endotracheal intubation and suction in meconium-stained neonates. J. Pediatr. *112:*613, 1988.

Lucey, J.F.: Clinical uses of transcutaneous oxygen monitoring. Adv. Pediatr. *28:*27, 1981.

MacArthur, B.A., Howie, R.N., Dezoete, J.A., and Elkins, J.: School progress and cognitive development of 6 year old children whose mothers were treated antenatally with betamethasone. Pediatrics *70:*99, 1982.

Macklem, P.T., Proctor, D.F., and Hogg, J.C.: The stability of peripheral airways. Respir. Physiol. *8:*191, 1970.

Matthews, T.G., and Warshaw, J.B.: Relevance of the gestational age distribution of meconium passage in utero. Pediatrics *64:*30, 1979.

Merritt, T.A., Harris, J.P., Roghmann, K., et al.: Early closure of the patent ductus arteriosus in very low birth weight infants: a controlled trial. J. Pediatr. *99:*281, 1981.

Miller, F.C., and Read, J.A.: Intrapartum assessment of the postdate fetus. Am. J. Obstet. Gynecol. *141:*516, 1981.

Miller, F.C., Sacks, D.A., Yeh, S.Y., et al.: Significance of meconium during labor. Am. J. Obstet. Gynecol. *122:*573, 1975.

Miller, H.C., and Futrakul, P.: Birth weight, gestational age and sex as determining factors in the incidence of respiratory distress syndrome of prematurely born infants. J. Pediatr. *72:*628, 1968.

Morales, W.J., Diebel, D., Lazar, A.J., et al.: The effect of antenatal dexamethasone administration on the prevention of respiratory distress syndrome in preterm gestations with premature rupture of membranes. Am. J. Obstet. Gynecol. *154:*591, 1986.

Morin, F.C., III: Ligating the ductus arteriosus before birth causes persistent pulmonary hypertension in the newborn lamb. Pediatr. Res. *25:*245, 1989.

Murphy, J.D., Rabinovitch, M., Goldstein, J.D., and Reid, L.M.: The structural basis of persistent pulmonary hypertension of the newborn infant. J. Pediatr. *98:*962, 1981.

Murphy, J.D., Vawter, G.F., and Reid, L.M.: Pulmonary vascular disease in fetal meconium aspiration. J. Pediatr. *104:*758, 1984.

Naeye, R.L., Freeman, R.K., and Blanc, W.A.: Nutrition, sex, and fetal lung maturation. Pediatr. Res. *8:*200, 1974.

Naeye, R.L., Schochat, S.J., Whitman, V., and Maisels, M.J.: Unsuspected pulmonary vascular abnormalities associated with diaphragmatic hernia. Pediatrics *58:*902, 1976.

Nelson, N.M., Prod'hom, L.S., Cherry, R.B., et al.: Pulmonary function in the newborn infant. Perfusion, estimation by analysis of the arterial-alveolar carbon dioxide difference. Pediatrics *30:*975, 1962.

Nilsson, R., Grossman, G., and Robertson, B.: Lung surfactant and the pathogenesis of neonatal bronchiolar lesions induced by artificial ventilation. Pediatr. Res. *12:*249, 1978.

Orzalesi, M.M., Motoyama, E.K., Jacobson, H.N., et al.: The development of the lungs of lambs. Pediatrics *35:*373, 1965.

Padbury, J.F., Agata, Y., Baylen, B.G., et al.: Dopamine pharmacokinetics in critically ill newborn infants. J. Pediatr. *110:*293, 1986.

Papageorgiou, A.N., Colle, E., Farri-Kostopoulos, E., and Gelfand, M.M.: Incidence of respiratory distress syndrome following antenatal betamethasone: role of sex, type of delivery and prolonged rupture of membranes. Pediatrics *67:*614, 1981.

Papageorgiou, A.N., Doray, J.-L., Ardilia, R., et al.: Reduction of mortality, morbidity and respiratory distress syndrome in infants weighing less than 1,000 grams by treatment with betamethasone and ritodrine. Pediatrics *83:*493, 1989.

Peckham, G.J.: Risk-benefit relationships of current therapeutic approaches. Proceedings of the 83rd Ross Conference on Cardiovascular Sequelae of Asphyxia in the Newborn 110, 1982.

Peckham, G.J., and Fox, W.W.: Physiologic factors affecting pulmonary artery pressure in infants with persistent pulmonary hypertension. J. Pediatr. *93:*1005, 1978.

Pena, I.C., Teberg, A.J. and Finella, K.M.: The premature small for gestational age infant during the first year of life: Comparison by birth weight and gestational age. J. Pediatr. *113:*1066, 1988.

Perkin, R.M., Levin, D.L., and Clark, R.: Serum salicylate levels and right-to-left ductus shunts in newborn infants with persistent pulmonary hypertension. J. Pediatr. *96:*721, 1980.

Rhodes, P.G., and Hall, R.T.: Continuous positive airway pressure delivered by face mask in infants with the idiopathic respiratory distress syndrome: a controlled study. Pediatrics *52:*1, 1973.

Richardson, C.P., and Jung, A.L.: Effects of continuous positive airway pressure on pulmonary function and blood gases of infants with respiratory distress syndrome. Pediatr. Res. *12:*771, 1978.

Richardson, P., Bose, C.L., and Carlstrom, J.R.: The functional residual capacity of infants with respiratory distress syndrome. Acta Paediatr. Scand. *75:*267, 1986.

Rider, E., Jobe, A., Ikegami, M., et al.: Effects of maternal corticosteroid dose on surfactant pool sizes, protein leaks and SPC precursor incorporation in preterm rabbits. Clin. Res. *37:*207A, 1989.

Rieutort, M., Farrell, P.M., Engle, M.J., et al.: Changes in surfactant phospholipids in fetal rat lungs from normal and diabetic pregnancies. Pediatr. Res. *20:*650, 1986.

Robert, M.F., Neff, R.K., Hubbell, J.P., et al.: Association between maternal diabetes and the respiratory distress syndrome in the newborn. N. Engl. J. Med. *294:*357, 1976.

Rojas, J., Larsson, L.E., Ogletree, M.L., et al.: Effects of cyclooxygenase inhibition on the response to group B streptococcal toxin in sheep. Pediatr. Res. *17*:107, 1983.

Saigal, S., Wilson, R., and Usher, R.: Radiological findings in symptomatic neonatal plethora resulting from placental transfusion. Radiology *125*:1851, 1977.

Scholle, S., and Braunlich, H.: Effects of prenatally administered thyroid hormones or glucocorticoids on maturation of kidney function in newborn rats. Dev. Pharmacol. Ther. *112*:162, 1989.

Schreiber, M.E., Heymann, M.A., and Soifer, S.J.: Increased arterial pH, not decreased PACO$_2$, attenuates hypoxia-induced pulmonary vasoconstriction in newborn lambs. Pediatr. Res. *20*:113, 1986.

Segall, M.L., Goetzman, B.W., and Schick, J.B.: Thrombocytopenia and pulmonary hypertension in the perinatal aspiration syndromes. J. Pediatr. *96*:727, 1980.

Sell, E.J., Gaines, J.A., Gluckman, C., and Williams, E.: Persistent fetal circulation. Am. J. Dis. Child. *139*:25, 1985.

Setzer, E., Ermocilla, R., Tonkin, I., et al.: Papillary muscle necrosis in a neonatal autopsy population: incidence and associated clinical manifestations. J. Pediatr. *96*:289, 1980.

Shankaran, S., Farooki, Q., and Desai, R.: Beta-hemolytic streptococcal infection appearing as persistent fetal circulation. Am. J. Dis. Child. *136*:725, 1982.

Sinclair, J.C.: Pathophysiology of hyaline membrane disease. *In* Winter, R.W. (Ed.): The Body Fluids in Pediatrics. Boston, Little, Brown, 1973.

Sinclair, J.C., Engel, K., and Silverman, W.A.: Early correction of hypoxemia and acidemia in infants of low birthweight: a controlled trial of oxygen breathing, rapid alkali infusion and assisted ventilation. Pediatrics *42*:565, 1968.

Soifer, S.J., Kaslow, D., Roman, C., and Heymann, M.A.: Umbilical cord compression produces pulmonary hypertension in newborn lambs: a model to study the pathophysiology of persistent pulmonary hypertension in the newborn. J. Dev. Physiol. *9*:239, 1987.

Soifer, S.J., Morin, F.C., III, and Heymann, M.A.: Prostaglandin D$_2$ reverses induced pulmonary hypertension in the newborn lamb. J. Pediatr. *100*:458, 1982.

Sosulski, R., and Fox, W.W.: Transition phase during hyperventilation therapy for persistent pulmonary hypertension of the neonate. Crit. Care Med. *13*:715, 1985.

Stonestreet, B.S., Hansen, M.B., Laptock, A.R., et al.: Glucocorticoids accelerate renal function maturation in fetal lambs. Early Hum. Dev. *8*:331, 1983.

Strang, L.B., and MacLeish, M.H.: Ventilatory failure and right to left shunt in newborn infants with respiratory distress. Pediatrics *28*:17, 1961.

Sundell, H., Garrott, J., Blankenship, W.J., et al.: Studies on infants with type II respiratory distress syndrome. J. Pediatr. *78*:754, 1971.

Ting, P., and Brady, J.P.: Tracheal suction in meconium aspiration. Am. J. Obstet. Gynecol. *122*:767, 1975.

Tran, N., Lowe, C., Sivieri, E.M., and Shaffer, T.H.: Sequential effects of acute meconium obstruction on pulmonary function. Pediatr. Res. *14*:34, 1980.

Tyler, D.C., Murphy, J., and Cheney, F.W.: Mechanical and chemical damage to lung tissue caused by meconium aspiration. Pediatrics *62*:454, 1978.

Usher, R.: Reduction in mortality from respiratory distress syndrome and prematurity with early administration of intravenous glucose and sodium bicarbonate. Pediatrics *32*:966, 1963.

Usher, R.H., Allen, A.C., and McLean, F.H.: Risk of respiratory distress syndrome related to gestational age, route of delivery and maternal diabetes. Am. J. Obstet. Gynecol. *111*:826, 1971.

Versmold, H.T., Kitterman, J.A., Phibbs, R.H., et al.: Aortic blood pressure during the first 12 hours of life in infants with birthweight 610–4220 grams. Pediatrics *67*:607, 1981.

Vidyasagar, D., Yeh, T.F., Harris, V., and Pildes, R.S.: Assisted ventilation in infants with meconium aspiration syndrome. Pediatrics *56*:208, 1975.

Ward, R.M., Daniel, C.H., Kendig, J.W., and Wood, M.A.: Oliguria and tolazoline pharmacokinetics in the newborn. Pediatrics *77*:307, 1986.

West, J.B.: Ventilation perfusion inequality and overall gas exchange in computer models of the lung. Respir. Physiol. *7*:88, 1969.

Whittle, M.J., and Hill, C.M.: Effect of labour on the lecithin sphingomyelin ratio in serial samples of amniotic fluid. Br. J. Obstet. Gynaecol. *84*:500, 1977.

Wild, L.M., Nickerson, P.A., and Morin, F.C., III: Ligating the ductus arteriosus before birth remodels the pulmonary vasculature of the lamb. Pediatr. Res. *25*:251, 1989.

Wiswell, T.E., Rawlings, J.S., Smith, F.R., and Goo, E.D.: Effect of furosemide on the clinical course of transient tachypnea of the newborn. Pediatrics *75*:908, 1985.

Wung, J.-T., James, L.S., Kichevsky, E., and James, E.: Management of infants with severe respiratory failure and persistence of the fetal circulation, without hyperventilation. Pediatrics *76*:488, 1985.

Yeh, T.F., Scrinivasan, G., Harris, V., and Pildes, R.S.: Hydrocortisone therapy in meconium aspiration syndrome: a controlled study. J. Pediatr. *90*:140, 1977.

Yeh, T.F., Lilien, L.D., Aiyanadar, B., and Pildes, R.S.: Lung volume, dynamic lung compliance, and blood gases during the first 3 days of postnatal life in infants with meconium aspiration syndrome. Crit. Care Med. *10*:588, 1982.

Yoder, P.R., Gibbs, R.S., Blanco, J.D., et al.: A prospective controlled study of maternal and perinatal outcome after intra-amniotic infection at term. Am. J. Obstet. Gynecol. *145*(6):695, 1983.

Yoon, J.J., Kohl, S., and Harper, R.G.: The relationship between maternal hypertensive disease of pregnancy and the incidence of idiopathic respiratory distress syndrome. Pediatrics *65*:735, 1980.

Zachman, R.D.: The NIH multicenter study and miscellaneous clinical trials of antenatal corticosteroid administration. *In* Farrell, P.M. (Ed.): Lung Development: Biological and Clinical Perspectives. II. Neonatal Respiratory Distress. New York, Academic Press, 1982.

AIRBLOCK 54 SYNDROMES

Thomas Hansen and Anthony Corbet

Pulmonary interstitial emphysema, pneumomediastinum, subcutaneous emphysema, pneumothorax, pneumopericardium, pneumoperitoneum, and intravascular air are all manifestations of the airblock syndrome and all begin with some degree of pulmonary interstitial emphysema (PIE) (Kirkpatrick et al., 1974; Macklin and Macklin, 1944).

■ PULMONARY INTERSTITIAL EMPHYSEMA (PIE)

Pathophysiology. PIE is the result of alveolar rupture from overdistention of alveoli abutting against nonalveolar structures and marginal alveoli (Figs. 54–1 and 54–2) (Caldwell et al., 1970; Hansen and Gest, 1984). It occurs most commonly in preterm or term infants undergoing mechanical ventilation for some form of parenchymal lung disease. In these infants, distribution of inspired gas is nonuniform, with the bulk of each breath being distributed to the more normal lung units. As a result, these lung units may become overdistended and rupture. Gas trapping from an insufficient expiratory time can also result in alveolar overdistention and rupture. Once alveolar rupture occurs, air is forced from the alveolus into the loose connective tissue sheaths surrounding airways and pulmonary arterioles and into the interlobular septa containing pulmonary veins. The air follows a track along these sheaths to the hilum of the lung, producing the characteristic radiographic appearance of PIE (Fig. 54–3).

PIE increases the volume of gas within the lung parenchyma and splints the lung in full inflation, thereby decreasing lung compliance. Air trapped within the interstitial cuffs compresses airways and increases airway resistance. In addition, air in the interstitial space impairs lymphatic function, allowing fluid to accumulate in the interstitial cuffs and in alveoli (Leonidas et al., 1979). $PaCO_2$ increases and PaO_2 decreases. The increase in $PaCO_2$ occurs early and is the result of increased respiratory dead space and reduced minute ventilation. The decrease in PaO_2 results in part from reduction in alveolar ventilation and in part from ventilation-perfusion mismatch secondary to mechanical obstruction of airways by interstitial air and edema fluid. It also results from compression of pulmonary arterioles by air in the perivascular cuffs with increased pulmonary vascular resistance (Brazy and Blackmon, 1977) and right-to-left shunting of blood.

Once interstitial air reaches the hilum of the lung, it coalesces to form large hilar blebs or it tracks beneath the visceral pleura to form large subpleural pockets of air. In both instances, these accumulations of air can be large enough to compress normal lung and impair ventilation or cause circulatory embarrassment by encroaching on mediastinal structures (Plenat et al., 1978).

Treatment. Since the site of the air leak behaves like a check valve, gas trapping occurs and results in further alveolar overdistention and rupture. Therefore, the first step in treatment must be to interrupt this cycle by putting the more severely involved areas in the lung to rest. If PIE is unilateral, this can be done by positioning the infant with the involved side down (Swingle et al., 1984) or by selectively intubating the mainstem bronchus on the uninvolved side (Brooks et al., 1977). If PIE is bilateral, the involved areas can be put to rest by taking advantage of

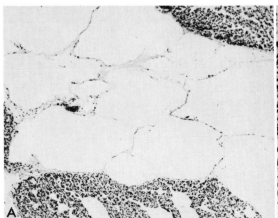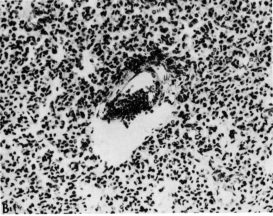

FIGURE 54–1. A, *Photomicrograph of the lung of an infant who died of emphysema and bilateral pneumothorax. The alveoli in the center show much distention, their septa thinned. Some of the septa have ruptured. In the periphery, the lung is atelectatic. B, Higher-power view showing a blood vessel in cross section. The vessel is compressed by a surrounding collar of air that has filled and ballooned the perivascular space.*

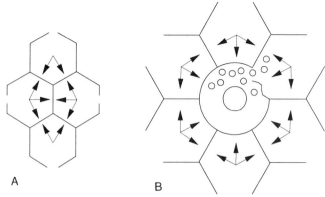

FIGURE 54–2. *Mechanism of alveolar rupture. Partitional alveoli (A) have their bases lying against other alveoli, while marginal alveoli (B) abut against bronchi, blood vessels, or pleura. During lung inflation these two different types of alveoli behave quite differently. Partitional alveoli are free to expand equally in all directions, since they abut on the equally distensible walls of adjacent alveoli. In addition, the pressure within each alveolus is balanced by an equal pressure inside surrounding alveoli so no unbalanced forces across the alveolar wall occur. Marginal alveoli, especially those surrounding blood vessels, are tethered at the base to a less distensible structure and are not as free to expand in all directions. During lung inflation, the connective tissue sheaths surrounding pulmonary blood vessels attempt to expand with the alveoli while the vessels themselves increase in size only slightly. As a result, unbalanced forces develop across the wall at the base of the alveolus and air ruptures into the adjacent connective tissue sheath.*

regional differences in time constants in the lung. Areas with PIE have airway compression and long time constants for inspiration and expiration. Mechanical ventilation using short inspiratory times (0.1 second), low inflation pressures, and small tidal volumes are ineffective in inflating these areas of the lung and should not contribute to further gas trapping (Meadow and Cheromcha, 1985). Over time, these areas deflate and collapse. Unfortunately, it may be difficult to maintain oxygenation and ventilation while selectively underventilating the areas of the lung with PIE. If this happens, it may be necessary to increase the respirator rate to 80 to 100 breaths/min. The advantage of rapid-rate ventilation is that it makes maximal use of the less severely involved lung units and may compensate for the respiratory deterioration associated with selective underventilation of areas with extensive PIE. High-frequency ventilation has shown some promise in treatment of severe PIE.

Prognoses. PIE is a serious complication of mechanical ventilation (Gaylord et al., 1985). Infants with PIE who weigh less than 1500 g have a significant mortality rate. If the infant survives the initial episode of PIE, recovery is slow and the incidence of chronic lung disease may exceed 50 per cent. Prevention of PIE by minimizing alveolar overdistention has been discussed in detail in Chapter 52.

■ PNEUMOMEDIASTINUM AND PNEUMOTHORAX

Epidemiology. The incidence of spontaneous pneumomediastinum and pneumothorax in term infants is 1 to 2 per cent, presumably because high transpulmonary pressures exerted at birth, when coupled with some degree of ventilation inhomogeneity, result in alveolar overdistention and rupture (Chernick and Avery, 1963; Lubchenco

1959). In the presence of underlying lung disease, the incidence of pneumothorax increases dramatically. Ten per cent of infants with retained fetal lung fluid develop pneumothorax, as do 5 to 10 per cent of spontaneously breathing infants with hyaline membrane disease. Interestingly, continuous positive airway pressure does not appear to increase the incidence of pneumothorax in infants with hyaline membrane disease, but positive pressure ventilation does produce an increase (incidence between 20 and 50 per cent of ventilated infants). Positive pressure ventilation of term infants with meconium aspiration pneumonia or persistent pulmonary hypertension is associated with an incidence of pneumothorax of roughly 40 per cent.

Natural History. Pneumomediastinum occurs when air that has tracked through the perivascular and peribronchial cuffs to the hilum ruptures into the mediastinum. From there air can rupture through the mediastinum into the pleural space and produce tension pneumothorax. Available evidence suggests that air in the mediastinum seldom achieves enough tension to cause circulatory embarrassment, because as the tension increases, air can dissect into the soft tissues of the neck to produce subcutaneous emphysema or rupture into the intrapleural space. On the other hand, tension pneumothorax can result in very high pressures within the pleural space, collapsing the lung on the involved side and resulting in immediate hypoxia and hypercapnia. In addition, by compressing mediastinal structures and impeding venous return, pneumothorax may result in circulatory collapse.

Diagnosis. Pneumomediastinum is usually asymptomatic or associated with mild tachypnea. In the spontaneously breathing infant, however, pneumothorax usually results in clinically significant tachypnea, grunting, irritability, pallor, and cyanosis. The cardiac point of maximum

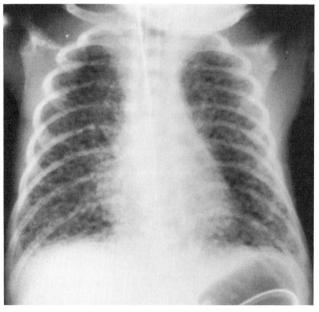

FIGURE 54–3. *Pulmonary interstitial emphysema. The lung is grossly hyperinflated with coarse radiolucencies extending from the pleura to the hilum. These radiolucencies represent bubbles of air in the perivascular and peribronchial interstitial cuffs.*

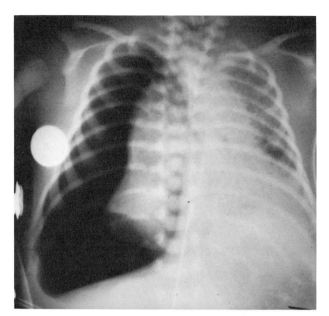

FIGURE 54–4. Tension pneumothorax. The lung on the involved side is collapsed and the mediastinum is shifted to the opposite side. Pleura can be seen bulging into the intercostal spaces.

impulse may be shifted away from the pneumothorax, and often the affected hemithorax appears to bulge. Differential breath sounds are unreliable markers of pneumothorax in the infant. Arterial pressure tracings may reveal a reduction in pulse pressure. In the infant on the mechanical ventilator, signs may be more dramatic with sudden onset of hypoxemia and cardiovascular collapse (Ogata et al., 1976). Transillumination of the chest is increased over the affected side. Pneumothorax should be confirmed by chest radiograph (Fig. 54–4), if at all possible. Needle aspiration of the chest to diagnose pneumothorax relieves acute distress but should be discouraged. If needle aspiration is performed, it should ordinarily be followed by tube thoracostomy.

Treatment. Asymptomatic or mildly symptomatic spontaneously breathing infants may simply be observed closely until spontaneous resolution occurs. Although allowing infants to breathe 100 per cent oxygen hastens reabsorption of intrapleural air (Chernick and Avery, 1963), the risk associated with prolonged hyperoxia limits usefulness of this therapy in preterm infants. Infants with moderate to severe symptoms and all infants receiving positive pressure ventilation must be treated with tube thoracostomy. Since most mechanically ventilated infants are nursed supine and since gas rises, the tube is usually placed in the second intercostal space in the midclavicular line and directed toward the diaphragm so that the tip lies between the lung and the anterior chest wall (Allen et al., 1981). Alternatively, the tube may be inserted at the midaxillary line and directed anteriorly. When placing the tube, one must take care to avoid impaling the lung, especially if a trocar is used to direct the tube rather than curved hemostats. Care must also be taken to avoid placing the tube too far into the chest and compressing mediastinal structures (Gooding et al., 1981). The thoracostomy tube usually is connected to water seal with 10 to 20 cm H_2O negative pressure and is left in place until it ceases to drain. The negative pressure should be dis-

continued, and the tube should be left under the water seal for 12 to 24 hours prior to removal. Infant chest tubes should never be clamped.

■ PNEUMOPERICARDIUM

Pneumopericardium results from direct tracking of interstitial air along the great vessels into the pericardial sac (Varano and Maisels, 1974). Gas under tension in the pericardium impairs atrial and ventricular filling, decreases stroke volume, and ultimately decreases cardiac output and systemic blood pressure. Infants present with increasing cyanosis, muffled heart sounds, and decreased systemic blood pressure. The chest radiograph is diagnostic (Fig. 54–5). Needle aspiration alleviates the acute symptoms, but since recurrence rate is high (53 per cent), continuous tube drainage is frequently necessary (Reppert et al., 1977). The mortality rate associated with pneumopericardium has been reported to be as high as 75 per cent.

■ PNEUMOPERITONEUM

Pneumoperitoneum results from dissection of air from the mediastinum along the sheaths of the aorta and vena cava, with subsequent rupture into the peritoneal cavity. Infants with this condition present with sudden abdominal distention and a typical abdominal radiograph. Occasionally, the pneumoperitoneum may be large enough to cause respiratory embarrassment by compromising descent of the diaphragm and may require drainage. A more common problem, however, is the difficulty of distinguishing this cause of peritoneal air from a primary gastrointestinal catastrophe, such as perforated ulcer or necrotizing enterocolitis (Knight and Abdenour, 1981). Obtaining more than 0.5 ml of green or brown fluid on paracentesis is suggestive of primary bowel disease, especially if bacteria are present on Gram stain. Measurement of the Po_2 of the gas aspirated from the abdomen may also be of some help, since it is likely to be very high if the gas is of

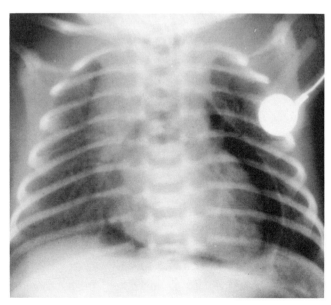

FIGURE 54–5. Pneumopericardium. A thin rim of pericardium is visible and clearly separated from the heart by air within the pericardial sac.

pulmonary origin. Finally, a careful upper GI series performed with water-soluble contrast may be of use in distinguishing the cause of intraperitoneal air (Cohen et al., 1982).

■ INTRAVASCULAR AIR

Intravascular air results from air being pumped directly into the pulmonary venous system and occurs only when airway pressure is extremely high (70 cm H_2O). It results in immediate cardiovascular collapse and is often diagnosed when air is withdrawn from the umbilical arterial catheter. Although intravascular air is usually fatal, placing the infant head down on the left side may favor displacement of cerebral emboli.

■ REFERENCES

Allen, R. W., Jung, A. L., and Lester, P. D.: Effectiveness of chest tube evacuation of pneumothorax in neonates. J. Pediatr. 99:629, 1981.

Brazy, J. E., and Blackmon, L. R.: Hypotension and bradycardia associated with airblock in the neonate. J. Pediatr. 90:796, 1977.

Brooks, J. G., Bustamante, S. A., Koops, B. L., et al.: Selective bronchial intubation for the treatment of severe localized pulmonary interstitial emphysema in newborn infants. Pediatrics 91:648, 1977.

Caldwell, E. J., Powell, R. D., and Mullooly, J. P.: Interstitial emphysema: A study of physiologic factors involved in experimental induction of the lesion. Am. Rev. Respir. Dis. 102:516, 1970.

Chernick, V., and Avery, M. E.: Spontaneous alveolar rupture at birth. Pediatrics 32:816, 1963.

Cohen, M. D., Schreiner, R., and Lemons, J.: Neonatal pneumoperitoneum without significant adventitious pulmonary air: Use of metrizamide to rule out perforation of the bowel. Pediatrics 69:587, 1982.

Gaylord, M. S., Thieme, R. E., Woodall, D. L., and Quissell, B. J.: Predicting mortality in low-birth-weight infants with pulmonary interstitial emphysema. Pediatrics 76:219, 1985.

Gooding, C. A., Kerlan, R. K., and Brasch, R. C.: Partial aortic obstruction produced by a thoracostomy tube. J. Pediatr. 98:471, 1981.

Hansen, T. N., and Gest, A. L.: Oxygen toxicity and other ventilatory complications of treatment of infants with persistent pulmonary hypertension. Clin. Perinatol. 11:653, 1984.

Kirkpatrick, B. V., Felman, A. H., and Eitzman, D. V.: Complications of ventilator therapy in respiratory distress syndrome. Am. J. Dis. Child. 128:496, 1974.

Knight, P. J., and Abdenour, G.: Pneumoperitoneum in the ventilated neonate: Respiratory or gastrointestinal origin? J. Pediatr. 98:972, 1981.

Leonidas, J. C., Bhan, I., and McCauley, G. K.: Persistent localized pulmonary interstitial emphysema and lymphangiectasia: A causal relationship? Pediatrics 64:165, 1979.

Lubchenco, L. O.: Recognition of spontaneous pneumothorax in premature infants. Pediatrics 24:996, 1959.

Macklin, M. T., and Macklin, C. C.: Malignant interstitial emphysema of the lungs and mediastinum as an important occult complication in many respiratory diseases and other conditions: An interpretation of the clinical literature in the light of laboratory experiment. Medicine 23:281, 1944.

Meadow, W. L., and Cheromcha, D.: Successful therapy of unilateral pulmonary emphysema: Mechanical ventilation with extremely short inspiratory time. Am. J. Perinatol. 2:194, 1985.

Ogata, E., Gregory, G. A., Kitterman, J. A., et al.: Pneumothorax in respiratory distress syndrome: Incidence and effect on vital signs, blood gases and pH. Pediatrics 58:177, 1976.

Plenat, F., Vert, P., Didier, F., and Andre, M.: Pulmonary interstitial emphysema. Clin. Perinatol. 5:351, 1978.

Reppert, S. M., Ment, L. R., and Todres, I. D.: The treatment of pneumopericardium in the newborn infant. J. Pediatr. 905:115, 1977.

Swingle, H. M., Eggert, L. D., and Bucciarelli, R. L.: New approach to management of unilateral tension pulmonary interstitial emphysema in premature infants. Pediatrics 74:354, 1984.

Varano, L. A., and Maisels, M. J.: Pneumopericardium in the newborn: Diagnosis and pathogenesis. Pediatrics 53:941, 1974.

CHRONIC LUNG 55 DISEASE— BRONCHOPULMONARY DYSPLASIA

Thomas Hansen and Anthony Corbet

■ BRONCHOPULMONARY DYSPLASIA

DEFINITION

Bronchopulmonary dysplasia (BPD) was first described by Northway and associates in 1967 in a report on 32 infants. They described the severe chronic lung disease (CLD) that occurs in very sick, small infants with severe hyaline membrane disease who require treatment with mechanical ventilation and oxygen. They suggested it might result from several different causes, such as pulmonary healing, a residual toxic effect of oxygen itself, barotrauma of intermittent positive pressure ventilation, the problems of endotracheal intubation, or a combination of these.

Since then, much has been learned about BPD, and an appreciation has emerged that CLD may also occur in a whole group of infants who have not previously had hyaline membrane disease. Consequently, the spectrum of patients affected by CLD includes tiny preterm infants who require ventilatory support because of pulmonary structural immaturity as well as infants with severe initial surfactant deficiency. For purposes of uniform reporting, however, the definition of CLD has been changed to *respiratory sequelae in an infant requiring oxygen at more than 28 days after birth*. Many physicians have questioned this definition, however, because it includes such a wide range of infants, i.e., from those who ultimately appear to have no residual problems at one extreme to those with severe BPD, as described by Northway and associates, at the other. A proposed, more practical definition would be *respiratory sequelae in an infant who reaches term age but cannot be discharged from the hospital because of continued oxygen or mechanical ventilatory requirement, or an infant who is discharged home on oxygen or ventilatory support.*

INCIDENCE

Merritt and co-workers (1988) have reviewed the epidemiology of bronchopulmonary dysplasia. The incidence is clearly highest in very-low-birth-weight infants who require mechanical ventilation for severe respiratory distress. The incidence is inversely related to birth weight (75 per cent for survivors weighing 700 to 800 g, and 13 per cent for those weighing 1250 to 1500 g) (Avery et al., 1987).

Bancalari (1985) has estimated that 1300 new cases of BPD occur in the United States each year, and it is believed that this figure is probably conservative. Based on expected survival and estimating that full resolution takes 3 years, one would expect that there are at least 3000 infants suffering from BPD in the United States at any given time.

PATHOLOGIC STAGES OF BPD

There are four distinctive clinical and pathologic stages to BPD, as described by Northway and associates (1967). Postmortem examination of the lung during stage 1 (at 1 to 3 days of age) reveals marked alveolar and interstitial edema with hyaline membranes, atelectasis, and necrosis of bronchial mucosa. The chest radiograph is consistent with hyaline membrane disease (Fig. 55–1A).

During stage 2 (at 4 to 10 days of age), atelectasis becomes more extensive, alternating with areas of emphysema. There is widespread necrosis and repair of bronchial mucosa. Cellular debris fills the airways. On chest x-ray study, the lung fields are opaque with air bronchograms (Fig. 55–1B). Interstitial air is commonly evident.

During stage 3 (at 11 to 30 days of age), extensive bronchial and bronchiolar metaplasia and hyperplasia evolve. Areas of emphysema are surrounded by areas of atelectasis, accompanied by massive interstitial edema with thickening of the basement membranes. On chest x-ray study, the lung now appears cystic with areas of hyperinflation and areas of atelectasis (Fig. 55–1C).

During stage 4 (after 30 days of age), there is massive fibrosis of the lung with destruction of alveoli and airways. In addition, there is hypertrophy of bronchial smooth muscle and metaplasia of airway mucosa. Finally, there is actual loss of pulmonary arterioles and capillaries and medial muscular hypertrophy of remaining vessels. The chest x-ray study reveals massive fibrosis and edema with areas of consolidation and areas of overinflation (Fig. 55–1D).

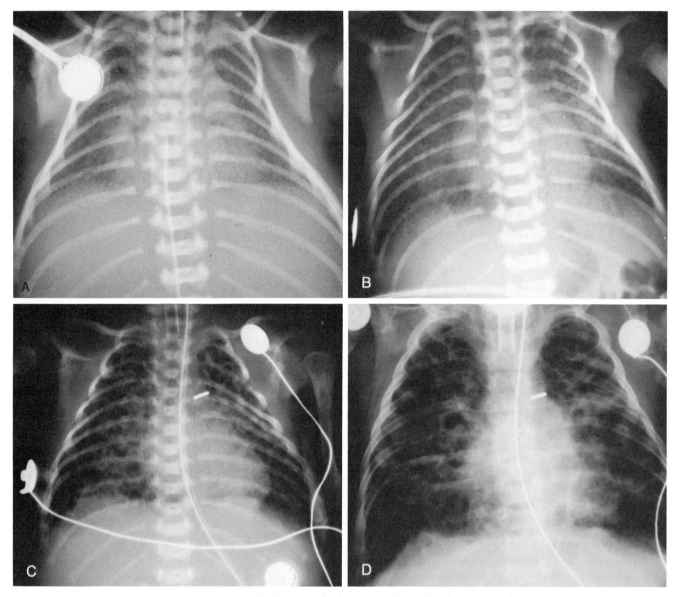

FIGURE 55—1. Radiographs illustrating the four stages of bronchopulmonary dysplasia.

ETIOLOGY AND PATHOGENESIS

Current theories on the cause of BPD include those originally suggested by Northway and co-workers expanded by further knowledge that suggests additional causal components. Most workers in the field today believe that the cause is multifactorial. Probable contributing factors are discussed in the following sections.

Genetic Predisposition. Even for infants of early gestational age, there is clearly a difference in the maturational level of the lung in infants of certain families compared with those of others. It is also clear that a familial history of asthma and reactive airway disease puts the infant at an additional disadvantage (Bertrand et al., 1985; Nickerson and Taussig, 1980).

Immaturity of the Lung. As demonstrated by the high incidence (70 to 75 per cent) of BPD in very premature infants, immaturity is clearly a major etiologic factor, whether it is surfactant deficiency that leads to severe hyaline membrane disease, or immaturity of the parenchymal structure of the lung or chest wall that contributes to chronic pulmonary insufficiency of the premature.

Oxygen Toxicity. As noted previously, many infants who develop BPD have had prolonged exposure to high, potentially toxic levels of oxygen (Hansen and Gest, 1984). BPD was first described as a form of chronic lung disease that occurred only in survivors of hyaline membrane disease who were ventilated with 80 to 100 per cent oxygen for more than 150 hours. Subsequent reports have continued to show an association between oxygen exposure and lung damage in ventilated and nonventilated infants and, in fact, have suggested that even prolonged exposure to 60 per cent oxygen can be toxic to the lungs of newborn infants (Philip, 1975).

Data obtained from experiments in animals and human volunteers and information gleaned from reports of patients inadvertently exposed to high concentrations of oxygen provide support for the theory that oxygen is a causative agent in BPD (Deneke 1980); also in ventilated animals, oxygen damages the lung independent of the ventilator (DeLemos et al., 1988). In experimental animals, oxygen toxicity follows a course similar to BPD and has similar postmortem findings. Oxygen toxicity has an initial exudative phase that lasts up to 7 days, which is characterized by damage to airway and alveolar epithelium and capillary endothelium. With loss of endothelial and epithelial integrity, there is massive interstitial and alveolar edema with formation of hyaline membranes. Finally, there is a marked infiltration of the lung by neutrophils— the significance of which is still unclear. Animals surviving this phase enter the proliferative phase, which is characterized by proliferation of alveolar type 2 cells and interstitial fibrosis. The amount of fibrosis is related to the length of the exposure to oxygen in the proliferative phase.

Experimental and clinical data has shown that humans are also susceptible to oxygen toxicity and that the course is similar to that seen in experimental animals. Short-term exposure to high concentrations of oxygen results in tracheitis and damage to airway epithelium, impaired mucociliary clearance, atelectasis, and eventually a significant alveolar-capillary leak. Long-term exposure results in pulmonary edema and impaired gas exchange.

Damage to the lung by oxygen toxicity is mediated by oxygen radicals produced during the univalent reduction of molecular oxygen (Roberts and Frank, 1984). These radical species include superoxide anion (O_2^-) hydrogen peroxide (H_2O_2), hydroxyl radical (OH•), and singlet oxygen ($^1O_2$). Oxygen radicals damage the lung by initiating lipid peroxidation, inactivating sulfhydryl enzymes, and damaging nucleic acids. The lung is equipped with antioxidant enzymes to protect it from injury by oxygen radicals. Superoxide dismutase catalyzes the conversion of superoxide anion to hydrogen peroxide, whereas catalase and glutathione peroxidase help convert hydrogen peroxide to water. Glutathione acts as a donor of hydrogen atoms in the detoxification of hydrogen peroxide and is converted to the disulfide. Glutathione disulfide is converted back to glutathione in a reaction with reduced nicotinamide adenine dinucleotide phosphate (NADPH) catalyzed by glutathione reductase. NADPH is supplied by the pentose shunt. Finally, because of its lipid solubility and ability to donate hydrogen atoms, vitamin E is important in stopping the chain reaction of lipid peroxidation in cell membranes. These defense mechanisms develop roughly in parallel with the surfactant system and may be inadequate at birth in preterm infants, especially in those with hyaline membrane disease (Frank, 1985) (Fig. 55–2).

Barotrauma. Follow-up studies of some of the early survivors with CLD have suggested that persistent abnormalities of airway function seem to be related only to whether or not infants were mechanically ventilated rather than to the duration of oxygen exposure (Stocks, 1979). It is now clear from numerous studies that barotrauma, particularly that associated with high inspiratory pressure, is a major factor in the evolution of CLD. Currently, there is no evidence that appropriate levels of end-expiratory pressure contribute to BPD (Kraybill et al., 1989). Overdistention of lung with high inspiratory pressure can result in both alveolar disruption and interstitial or alveolar edema similar to that seen in experimental oxygen toxicity and in infants with BPD. Certainly, pulmonary interstitial

emphysema is a frequent precursor. On the other hand, it is becoming increasingly clear that diffuse atelectasis may also be a contributing factor (Jarriel et al., 1989; Johnson et al., 1989). In addition, particulate water-spilling into the airway from the ventilator and ventilation with cold, dry gas result in lung injury similar to that seen in BPD (John et al., 1980).

Pulmonary Edema. Some studies have stressed the importance of pulmonary edema due to either excessive fluid administration or patent ductus arteriosus in the genesis of BPD (Brown et al., 1978).

Infection. Recent reports (Holtzman et al., 1989; Sanchez and Regan, 1988; Wang et al., 1988) suggest that organisms such as *Ureaplasma, Chlamydia,* or cytomegalovirus may produce chronic infection and thereby contribute to the pathogenesis of BPD.

Other Factors. Nutritional factors may well play a role in the development of BPD (Frank and Sosenko, 1988), as may deficiencies of vitamins, such as vitamin A (Shenai et al., 1987; Stahlman et al., 1988).

In summary, bronchopulmonary dysplasia is a multifactorial disease in which oxygen toxicity, mechanical ventilation, endotracheal intubation, airleak, atelectasis, and other factors such as infection and nutritional state play a role.

CLINICAL COURSE OF BPD

Stage 4 BPD is a type of chronic obstructive lung disease. The infants have a barrel chest, prolonged expiration time, expiratory wheezing, and evidence of lung overinflation on chest radiograph (see Fig. 55–1.) (Merritt et al., 1988). Pulmonary function tests demonstrate increased airway resistance and functional residual capacity and decreased tidal volume (Heldt, 1988). Increased airway resistance is in part the result of damage and destruction of airways, in part the result of increased airway reactivity, and in part a manifestation of the interstitial edema that invariably accompanies BPD. Infants with BPD have bronchial smooth muscle hypertrophy, and cold air provocation tests and trials of bronchodilators have demonstrated that bronchospasm may contribute to their increased airway resistance (Greenspan et al., 1989), even when they are as young as 14 days old. In addition, infants with BPD have radiographic and clinical evidence of pulmonary edema. Presumably, the loss of arterioles and capillaries in the lung results in increased blood flow through remaining vessels and increased filtration of fluid from these vessels. In infants with cor pulmonale, systemic venous pressure is high and the ability of the lymphatics to clear this filtered fluid is impaired. Fluid in perivascular cuffs compresses airways and increases airway resistance.

In infants with BPD, static lung compliance is usually decreased but may be increased if damage to the lung is sufficient to result in loss of elastic recoil. Dynamic compliance is invariably decreased and nitrogen washout is delayed (Watts et al., 1977), indicating a severe maldistribution of ventilation. Maldistribution of ventilation results in mismatch of ventilation and perfusion, which leads to hypoxemia. While the respiratory rate is usually increased,

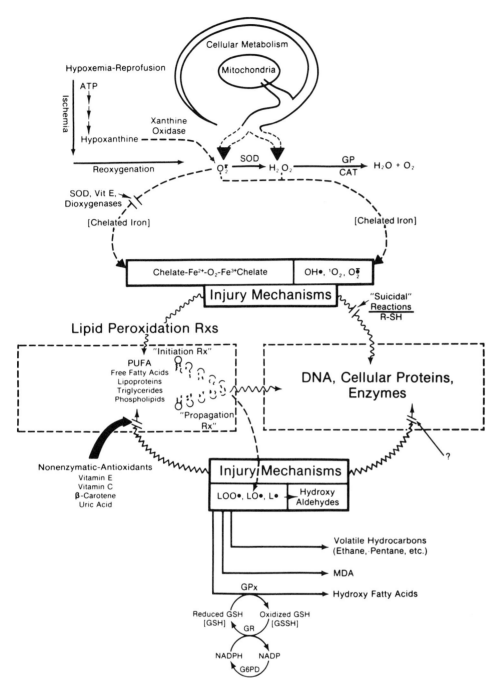

FIGURE 55–2. *The source and generation of free radicals and reactive intermediates, and the enzymatic and nonenzymatic protective systems available to the cell. (From Roberts, R. J., and Frank, L.: Developmental consequences of oxygen toxicity. In Kacew, S., and Reasor, M. J. (Eds.): Toxicology and the Newborn. Amsterdam, Elsevier Science Publishers, 1984.)*

physiologic dead space is also increased so that alveolar ventilation is decreased and $PaCO_2$ is increased.

Obliteration of arterioles and capillaries results in a reduction in available surface area for gas exchange and may contribute to arterial hypoxemia, especially during exercise. The loss of vessels, coupled with smooth muscle hypertrophy from chronic alveolar hypoxia, may also result in pulmonary hypertension and cor pulmonale. With cor pulmonale, cardiac output falls and oxygen delivery may be impaired.

MANAGEMENT AND TREATMENT OF BPD

Issues that have been raised in the management of infants with BPD include preventive measures as well as therapeutic regimens.

Management of Mechanical Ventilation to Prevent Barotrauma. Clearly, excessive inspiratory pressure is harmful, but much controversy surrounds the definition of optimal ventilation (also see Chapter 52). One uncontrolled study has suggested that the incidence of BPD could be reduced by reducing ventilator pressures and accepting lower values for PaO_2 and higher values for $PaCO_2$ (Rhodes et al., 1983). A collaborative study on the incidence of BPD in various institutions suggested that early introduction of nasal continuous positive airway pressure and avoidance of hyperventilation might shorten the time an infant is maintained on mechanical ventilation and thus reduce the incidence of BPD (Avery et al., 1987).

Prevention of Oxygen Toxicity. Maintenance of low

inspired oxygen concentrations is important in preventing oxygen toxicity. This can be accomplished to some degree by the use of continuous distending pressure.

Behavioral Issues. The management of infants with minimal handling and disruption of their clinical course is now believed to contribute to more rapid recovery and, hence, reduced rates of morbidity.

Nutrition. Since infants with BPD usually outgrow their chronic lug disease, a major aim of therapy is provision of adequate nutritional support for growth and prevention of complications. Nutritional support is complicated by an increased resting metabolic rate (Kurzner et al., 1988; Weinstein and Oh, 1981; Yeh et al., 1989), with a caloric need for as much as 140 to 160 kcal/Kg/day in the face of a relative inability to tolerate fluid loads. Thus, these infants must often be fed high-caloric-density formulas supplemented with calcium and potassium to replace losses resulting from concomitant diuretic therapy.

Supplemental oxygen should be administered to maintain the infant's PaO_2 between 55 and 70 mm Hg in order to prevent hypoxic airway constriction (Tay-Uyboco et al., 1989) and alveolar hypoxemia as well as cor pulmonale, which is the most devastating complication of BPD (Abman et al., 1985). This approach may require prolonged mechanical ventilation but eventually can be accomplished by the administration of oxygen by nasal cannula or hood. In the past, chronic oxygen administration usually required prolonged hospitalization; however, several neonatal programs have reported successful management of these infants at home (Campbell et al., 1983; Goldberg and Monahan, 1989; Hudak et al., 1989; Pinney and Cotton, 1976).

Booster transfusions of blood to maintain the hematocrit above 40 per cent have been shown to reduce resting oxygen consumption and to increase systemic oxygen transport in infants with BPD (Alverson et al., 1988). Fluid restriction and judicious use of diuretics may reduce interstitial edema in the lung and improve pulmonary function. Furosemide alone (Englehardt et al., 1986; Kao et al., 1983) and chlorothiazide in combination with spironolactone (Kao et al., 1984) have been shown to be effective in improving lung function in infants with BPD. However, chronic diuretic therapy may result in excessive urinary losses of calcium, potassium, and chloride. Calcium loss may compromise bone mineralization and exacerbate osteopenia of prematurity. In addition, prolonged administration of furosemide has been associated with nephrocalcinosis in infants with BPD (Ezzedeen et al., 1988; Hufnagle et al., 1982). Although it has been suggested that substitution of chlorothiazide for furosemide may reduce calcium wasting, a recent study has questioned this effect (Atkinson et al., 1988); and Englehardt and associates (1989) were unable to demonstrate improvement in lung mechanics with spirolactone thiazide treatment. In addition, chloride loss can result in metabolic alkalosis, decreased ventilatory drive, and hypercapnia and may also contribute to an erroneous conclusion that furosemide therapy is ineffective (Hazinski, 1985).

Bronchospasm often contributes to the increased airway resistance associated with BPD. Treatment with a variety of bronchodilators has been shown to be effective

in relieving bronchoconstriction and improving lung function (Cabal et al., 1987; Wilkie et al., 1987). It is useful to assess the response to a single dose of terbutaline administered subcutaneously and continue bronchodilator therapy only if significant improvement in lung function is observed. Chronic therapy consists of theophylline alone or theophylline in combination with a selective beta₂ agonist.

There is some evidence that the administration of corticosteroids improves lung function in some infants with BPD and facilitates weaning from the ventilator (Avery et al., 1985; Cummings et al., 1989). Unfortunately, corticosteroid administration also increases the incidence of sepsis and frequently results in systemic hypertension. The status of adrenal function in these infants has not been studied adequately and is not well understood.

The most severe complication of BPD is cor pulmonale with pulmonary hypertension. Infants whose disease has reached this stage may require cardiovascular assessment to determine their response to increased oxygen or to agents that might reduce pulmonary vascular resistance.

PREVENTION OF BPD

Prevention of preterm birth is, of course, the most effective means of preventing this disorder; short of that, acceleration of lung maturation with prenatal glucocorticoid treatment (see Chapters 49 and 53) is the optimal approach. Preventive management of the newborn now includes administration of artificial surfactant at birth as well as avoidance of barotrauma and oxygen toxicity. Since this is not always possible, some investigators have tried to prevent oxygen toxicity and development of BPD by administering various antioxidants (Roberts and Frank, 1984). Unfortunately, neither vitamin E nor superoxide dismutase has proved effective in reducing the incidence of BPD. Some studies suggest that malnutrition potentiates oxygen toxicity and that dietary supplementation with unsaturated fats protects the infant from oxygen-induced lung injury (Sosenko et al., 1988). Nutritional management may indeed play an important role in the prevention of BPD in the future.

VITAMIN A AND CHRONIC LUNG DISEASE

Shenai and colleagues (1981, 1985a, 1985b 1990) have suggested that vitamin A deficiency may play an important role in chronic lung disease. Most very-low-birth-weight infants are born with low plasma concentrations of vitamin A and retinol-binding protein. The liver reserves of vitamin A are also low in most of these infants, indicating a potential inability to adjust to inadequate vitamin A intake during the postnatal period. In addition, these infants are at risk for developing vitamin A deficiency because they often have difficulty with enteral feeding and require intravenous feeding. Substantial losses of vitamin A occur in the intravenous delivery system from photodegradation and adsorption (Shenai et al., 1981).

Very-low-birth-weight infants who develop bronchopulmonary dysplasia (BPD), in contrast to those without lung disease, often exhibit clinical, biochemical, and histopathologic evidence of vitamin A deficiency (Shenai et al., 1985a). Vitamin A supplementation during the early postnatal life appears to decrease the incidence of BPD and to promote regenerative healing from lung injury (Shenai et al., 1985b). Shenai and co-workers (1990) have developed a protocol for routine vitamin A supplementation in very-low-birth-weight infants and are continuing to investigate this important aspect of preventive care.

OUTCOME

The mortality rate among infants with BPD after discharge from the hospital is roughly 10 per cent. Survivors have an increased incidence of lower respiratory infections and of increased airway reactivity in the 1st year after discharge (Smyth et al., 1981). Although pulmonary function studies may indicate increased small airway resistance among infants with BPD, the exercise tolerance of these infants is comparable to their normal peers (Bader et al., 1987; Heldt et al., 1980). Growth may be delayed initially, but catch-up growth occurs with resolution of pulmonary symptoms.

Neurodevelopmental Outcome. In general, when discharged to a good home and provided with appropriate nutrition, these infants also demonstrate significant catch-up growth in their neurodevelopmental status if they have not sustained a significant intracranial insult. However, Campbell and co-workers (1988) have recently reported a progressive neurologic syndrome in some infants with BPD and have raised concerns that this syndrome may be caused by some of the therapies being used in the clinical management of these infants.

■ CHRONIC PULMONARY INSUFFICIENCY OF PREMATURITY (CPIP)

This condition, which occurs usually in premature infants weighing less than 1200 g at birth, is also known as *late-onset respiratory distress,* characterized by the development of serious respiratory difficulty and recurrent apnea after the first few days of life. Recovery generally occurs during the 2nd month of life (Krauss et al., 1975). During the 1st month, these infants exhibit a substantially reduced lung volume that is manifested clinically by an oxygen requirement of 25 to 40 per cent, the presence of modest hypercapnia, and poorly defined, diffuse density without cystic changes on the chest radiograph. The $Aa.D_{O_2}$, $aA.D_{CO_2}$, and $aA.D_{N_2}$ are all increased. The very compliant chest wall of these infants probably contributes to the atelectasis associated with this condition. This common problem responds well to prolonged management with nasal continuous positive airway pressure.

■ WILSON-MIKITY SYNDROME

This eponym describes a form of late-developing respiratory distress in small premature infants, which was described in 1960 by Wilson and Mikity. It is characterized by the onset of tachypnea, chest retractions, and cyanosis at 1 to 4 weeks of age in infants who were free of respiratory distress at birth. Their respiratory distress progresses for about 2 months and then slowly regresses until recovery is achieved over a period of 1 to 2 years

(Hodgman et al., 1969). As the condition develops, on the chest radiograph, the lung has a "bubbly" appearance, with diffuse streaks of infiltrate and widespread cystic change; during the recovery phase, hyperinflation is present at the lung bases, with flattening of the diaphragm, and streaky atelectasis at the apices.

Dynamic lung compliance is reduced, and airway resistance is increased (Burnard et al., 1965). Measurements of lung volume initially appear normal and tend to increase as the condition progresses. Pathologically, the lung shows alternating areas of atelectasis and hyperinflation, accounting for the "normal" measurements of lung volume. The $Aa.D_{O_2}$, $aA.D_{CO_2}$, and $aA.D_{N_2}$ are all increased, suggesting severe ventilation-perfusion imbalance (Krauss et al., 1970), and most patients require 35 to 50 per cent oxygen.

The cause of Wilson-Mikity syndrome is unknown. The airways of premature infants are very compliant (Burnard, 1966), and if compliance values are unevenly distributed, this might cause airway closure and gas trapping in certain regions of the lung and adjacent compression atelectasis in other regions. This condition has rarely been diagnosed since the advent of continuous positive airway pressure. It is possible that higher mean airway pressures stabilize the peripheral airways and prevent widespread closure.

■ REFERENCES

Abman, S. H., Wolfe, R. R., Accurso, F. J., et al.: Pulmonary vascular response to oxygen in infants with severe bronchopulmonary dysplasia. Pediatrics 75:90, 1985.

Alverson, D. C., Isken, V. H., and Cohen, R. S.: Effect of booster blood transfusions on oxygen utilization in infants with bronchopulmonary dysplasia. J. Pediatr. 113:722, 1988.

Atkinson, S. A., Shah, J. K., McGee, C., et al.: Mineral excretion in premature infants receiving various diuretic therapies. J. Pediatr. 113:540, 1988.

Avery, G. B., Fletcher, A. B., Kaplan, M., et al.: Controlled trial of dexamethasone in respirator-dependent infants with bronchopulmonary dysplasia. Pediatrics 75:106, 1985.

Avery, M. E., Tooley, W. H., Keller, J. B., et al.: Is chronic lung disease in low-birth-weight infants preventable? A survey of eight centers. Pediatrics 79:26, 1987.

Bader, D., Ramos, A. D., Lew, C. D., et al.: Childhood sequelae of infant lung disease: Exercise and pulmonary function abnormalities after bronchopulmonary dysplasia. J. Pediatr. 110:693, 1987.

Bancalari, E.: Bronchopulmonary dysplasia. In Milner, A. D., and Martin, R. J. (Eds.): Neonatal and Pediatric Respiratory Medicine. London, Butterworths, 1985.

Berman, W., Jr., Katz, R., Yabek, et al.: Long-term follow-up of bronchopulmonary dysplasia. J. Pediatr. 109:45, 1986.

Bertrand, J. M., Riley, S. P., Popkin, J., et al.: The long-term pulmonary sequelae of prematurity. The role of familial airway hyperreactivity and the respiratory distress syndrome. N. Engl. J. Med. 312:742, 1985.

Brown, E. R., Stark, A., Sosenko, I., et al.: Bronchopulmonary dysplasia: Possible relationship to pulmonary edema. Pediatrics 92:982, 1978.

Burnard, E. D.: The pulmonary syndrome of Wilson and Mikity, and respiratory function in very small premature infants. Pediatr. Clin. North Am. 13:999, 1966.

Burnard, E. D., Grattan-Smith, P., Picton-Warlow, C. G., and Grauaug, A.: Pulmonary insufficiency in prematurity. Aust Paediatr. J 1:12, 1965.

Cabal, L. A., Larrazabalo, C., Ramanathan, R., et al.: Effects of metaproterenol on pulmonary mechanics, oxygenation, and ventilation in infants with chronic lung disease. J. Pediatr. 110:116, 1987.

Campbell, A. N., Zarfin, Y., Groenveld, M., et al.: Low-flow oxygen therapy in infants. Arch. Dis. Child. 58:795, 1983.

Campbell, R. L., McAlister, W., and Volpe, J. J.: Neurologic aspects of bronchopulmonary dysplasia. Clin. Pediatr. 27:7, 1988.

Clement, A., Chadelat, K., Sardet, A., et al.: Alveolar macrophage status in bronchopulmonary dysplasia. Pediatr. Res. *23*:470, 1988.

Cummings, J. J., D'Eugenio, D. B., and Gross, S. J.: A controlled trial of dexamethasone in preterm infants at high risk for bronchopulmonary dysplasia. N. Engl. J. Med. *320*:1505, 1989.

DeLemos, R. A., Coalson, J. J., Gerstmann, D. R., et al.: Oxygen toxicity in the premature baboon with hyaline membrane disease. Am. Rev. Respir. Dis. *136*:677, 1988.

Deneke, S. M., and Fanburg, B. L.: Normobaric oxygen toxicity of the lung. N. Engl. J. Med. *303*:76, 1980.

Engelhardt, B., Blalock, W. A., Donlevy, S., et al.: Effect of spironolactone-hydrochlorothiazide on lung function in infants with chronic bronchopulmonary dysplasia. J. Pediatr. *114*:619, 1989.

Englehardt, B., Elliott, S., and Hazinski, T. A.: Short- and long-term effects of furosemide on lung function in infants with bronchopulmonary dysplasia. J. Pediatr. *109*:1034, 1986.

Ezzedeen, R., Adelman, R. D., and Ahlfors, C. E.: Renal calcification in preterm infants: Pathophysiology and long-term sequelae. J. Pediatr. *113*:532, 1988.

Fiascone, J. M., Rhodes, R. G., Grandgeorge, S. R., et al.: Bronchopulmonary dysplasia: A review for the pediatrician. Curr. Prob. Pediatr. *19*:169, 1989.

Frank, L.: Effects of oxygen on the newborn. Fed. Proc. *44*:2328, 1985.

Frank, L., and Sosenko, I. R.: Undernutrition as a major contributing factor in the pathogenesis of bronchopulmonary dysplasia. Am. Rev. Respir. Dis. *138*:725, 1988.

Gerdes, J. S., Harris, M. C., and Polin, R. A.: Effects of dexamethasone and indomethacin on elastase, a₁-proteinase inhibitor, and fibronectin in bronchoalveolar lavage fluid from neonates. J. Pediatr. *113*:727, 1988.

Gerhardt, T., Hehre, D., Feller, R., et al.: Serial determination of pulmonary function in infants with chronic lung disease. J. Pediatr. *110*:446, 1987.

Goldberg, A. I., and Monahan, C. A.: Home health care for children assisted by mechanical ventilation: The physician's perspective. J. Pediatr. *114*:378, 1989.

Goodman, G., Perkin, R. M., Anas, N. G., et al.: Pulmonary hypertension in infants with bronchopulmonary dysplasia. J. Pediatr. *112*:67, 1988.

Goodwin, S. F., Graves, S. A., and Haberkern, C. M.: Aspiration in intubated premature infants. Pediatrics *75*:85, 1985.

Greenspan, J. S., DeGiulio, P. A., and Bhutani, V. K.: Airway reactivity as determined by a cold air challenge in infants with bronchopulmonary dysplasia. J. Pediatr. *114*:452, 1989.

Hansen, T. N., and Gest, A. L.: Oxygen toxicity and other ventilatory complications of treatment of infants with persistent pulmonary hypertension. Clin. Perinatol. *11*:6653, 1984.

Hazinski, T. A.: Furosemide decreases ventilation in young rabbits. J. Pediatr. *106*:81, 1985.

Heldt, G. P.: Pulmonary status of infants and children with bronchopulmonary dysplasia. *In* Merritt, T. A., Northway, W. J., Jr., and Boynton, B. R. (Eds.): Bronchopulmonary Dysplasia. Boston, Blackwell Scientific Publications, 1988, p. 421.

Heldt, G. P., McIlroy, M. B., Hansen, T. N., et al.: Exercise performance of the survivors of hyaline membrane disease. Pediatrics. *96*:995, 1980.

Hodgman, J. E., Mikity, V. G., Tatter, D. and Cleland, R. S.: Chronic respiratory distress in the premature infant: Wilson-Mikity syndrome. Pediatrics *44*:179, 1969.

Holtzman, R. B., Hageman, J. R., and Yogev, R.: Role of *Ureaplasma urealyticum* in bronchopulmonary dysplasia. J. Pediatr. *114*:1061, 1989.

Hudak, B. B., Allen, M. D., Hudak, M. L., et al.: Home oxygen therapy for chronic lung disease in extremely low-birth-weight infants. Am. J. Dis. Child. *143*:357, 1989.

Hufnagle, K. G., Khan, S. N., Penn, D., et al.: Renal calcifications: a complication of long-term furosemide therapy in preterm infants. Pediatrics *70*:360, 1982.

Jarriel, S., Richardon, P., Pace, R., et al.: Positive end-expiratory pressure (PEEP) reduces ventilation inhomogeneities in hyaline membrane disease in lambs. Pediatr. Res. *25*:314A, 1989.

John, E., Ermocilla, R., Golden, J., et al.: Effects of gas temperature and particulate water on rabbit lungs during ventilation. Pediatr. Res. *14*:1186, 1980.

Johnson, W. H., Jr., Young, J. A., Hernandes, L. A., et al.: Positive end-expiratory pressure (PEEP) prevents barotrauma-induced microvascular injury due to high peak inspiratory pressure (PIP). Pediatr. Res. *25*:369A, 1989.

Kao, L. C., Warburton, D., Cheng, M. H., et al.: Effect of oral diuretics on pulmonary mechanics in infants with chronic bronchopulmonary dysplasia: Results of a double-blind crossover sequential trial. Pediatrics *74*:37, 1984.

Kao, L. C., Warburton, D., Sargent, C. S., et al.: Furosemide acutely decreases airways resistance in chronic pulmonary dysplasia. J. Pediatrics *103*:624, 1983.

Krauss, A. N., Levin, A. R., Grossman, H., and Auld, P. A. M.: Physiologic studies on infants with Wilson-Mikity syndrome. J. Pediatr. *77*:27, 1970.

Krauss, A. N., Klain, D. B., and Auld, P. A. M.: Chronic pulmonary insufficiency of prematurity (CPIP). Pediatrics *55*:55, 1975.

Kraybill, E. N., Runyan, D. K., Bose, C. L., et al.: Risk factors for chronic lung disease in infants with birth weights of 751 to 1000 grams. J. Pediatr. *115*:115, 1989.

Kurzner, S. I., Garg, M., Bautista, D. B., et al.: Growth failure in bronchopulmonary dysplasia: Elevated metabolic rates and pulmonary mechanics. J. Pediatr. *112*:73, 1988.

Merritt, T. A., and Boynton, B. R.: Clinical presentation of bronchopulmonary dysplasia. In Merritt, T. A., Northway, W. H., Jr., Boynton, B. R. (Eds.): Contemporary Issues in Fetal and Neonatal Medicine. Vol. 4, Bronchopulmonary Dysplasia. Boston, Blackwell Scientific Publications, 1988, p. 179.

Merritt, T. A., Northway, W. H., Jr., and Boynton, B. R., (Eds.): Contemporary Issues in Fetal and Neonatal Medicine. Vol. 4, Bronchopulmonary Dysplasia. Boston, Blackwell Scientific Publications, 1988.

Moshini, K., and Tanswell, K.: Resolution of acquired lobar emphysema with dexamethasone therapy. J. Pediatr. *11*:901, 1987.

Nickerson, B. G., and Taussig, L. M.: Family history of asthma in infants with bronchopulmonary dysplasia. Pediatrics *65*:1140, 1980.

Northway, W. H., Rosan, R. C., and Porter, D. Y.: Pulmonary disease following therapy of hyaline membrane disease. N. Engl. J. Med. *276*:357. 1967.

O'Brodovich, H. M., and Mellins, R. B.: Bronchopulmonary dysplasia—unresolved neonatal acute lung injury. Am. Rev. Respir. Dis. *132*:694, 1985.

Philip, A. G. S.: Oxygen plus pressure plus time: The etiology of bronchopulmonary dysplasia. Pediatrics *55*:44, 1975.

Pinney, M. A., and Cotton, E. K.: Home management of bronchopulmonary dysplasia. Pediatrics *58*:856, 1976.

Rhodes, P. G., Graves, G. R., Patel, D. M., et al.: Minimizing pneumothorax and bronchopulmonary dysplasia in ventilated infants with hyaline membrane disease. J. Pediatr. *103*:634, 1983.

Roberts, R. J., and Frank, L.: Developmental consequences of oxygen toxicity. *In* Kacew, S., and Reasor, M. J. (Eds.): Toxicology and the Newborn. Amsterdam, Elsevier Science Publishers, 1984, p. 143.

Sanchez, P. J., and Regan, U. A.: Ureaplasma urealyticum colonization and chronic lung disease in low-birth weight infants. Pediatr. Infect. Dis. *7*:542, 1988.

Sauve, R. S., and Singhai, N.: Long-term morbidity of infants with bronchopulmonary dysplasia. Pediatrics *76*:725, 1985.

Shenai, J. P., Chytil, F., Jhaveri, A., et al.: Plasma vitamin A and retinol-binding protein in premature and term neonates. J. Pediatr *99*:302, 1981.

Shenai, J. P., Chytil, F., and Stahlman, M. T.: Vitamin A status of neonates with bronchopulmonary dysplasia. Pediatr. Res. *19*:185, 1985a.

Shenai, J. P., Chytil, F., and Stahlman, M. T.: Liver vitamin A reserves of very low birth weight neonates. Pediatr. Res. *19*:892, 1985b.

Shenai, J. P., Rush, M. B., Stahlman, M. T., et al.: Plasma retinol-binding protein response to vitamin A administration in infants susceptible to bronchopulmonary dysplasia. J. Pediatr. *116*:607, 1990.

Shenai, J. P., Stahlman, M. T., and Chytil, F.: Vitamin A delivery from parenteral alimentation solution. J. Pediatr. *99*:661, 1981.

Smyth, J. A., Tabachnik, E., Duncan, W. J., et al.: Pulmonary function and bronchial hyperreactivity in long-term survivors of bronchopulmonary dysplasia. Pediatrics *68*:336, 1981.

Sosenko, I. R., Innis, S. M., and Frank, L.: Polyunsaturated fatty acids and protection of newborn rats from oxygen toxicity. J. Pediatr. *112*:630, 1988.

Stahlman, M. T., Gray, M. E., Chytil, F., et al.: Effect of retinol on fetal lamb tracheal epithelium with and without epidermal growth factor. Lab. Invest. *59*:25, 1988.

Stern, L. (Ed.): The respiratory system in the newborn. Clin. Perinatol. *14*:3, 1987.

Stocks, J., Godfrey, S., and Reynolds, E. O. R.: Airway resistance in infants after various treatments for hyaline membrane disease: Special emphasis on prolonged high levels of inspired oxygen. Pediatrics 61:178, 1979.

Tay-Uyboco, J. S., Kwiatkowski, K., Cates, D. B., et al.: Hypoxic airway constriction in infants of very low birth weight recovering from moderate to severe bronchopulmonary dysplasia. J. Pediatr. 115:456, 1989.

U.S. Congress, Office of Technology Assessment: Technology-Dependent Children: Hospital v. Home Care. Washington, D. C.: U.S. Government Printing Office, OTA-TM-H–38, May, 1987.

Wang, E. E. L., Frayha, H., Watts, J., et al.: Role of *Ureaplasma urealyticum* and other pathogens in the development of CLD of prematurity. Pediatr. Infect. Dis. 7:547, 1988.

Watts, J. L., Ariagno, R. L., and Brady, J. P.: Chronic pulmonary disease in neonates after artificial ventilation: Distribution of ventilation and pulmonary interstitial emphysema. Pediatrics 60:273, 1977.

Weinstein, M. R., and Oh, W.: Oxygen consumption in infants with bronchopulmonary dysplasia. Pediatrics 99:958. 1981.

Wilkie, R. A., and Bryan, M. H.: Effect of bronchodilators on airway resistance in ventilator-dependent neonates with chronic lung disease. J. Pediatr. 114:448, 1989.

Wilson M. G., and Mikity V. C. A new form of respiratory disease in premature infants. Am J Dis Child 99:489, 1960.

Yeh, T. F., McClenan, D. A., and Ajayl, O. A.: Metabolic rate and energy balance in infants with bronchopulmonary dysplasia. J. Pediatr. 114:448, 1989.

NEONATAL 56 PNEUMONIAS

Thomas Hansen and Anthony Corbet

■ PNEUMONIA ACQUIRED FROM THE MOTHER

Most pneumonias acquired from the mother have an onset within the first 3 days after birth. It is estimated that the incidence of early onset pneumonia is 0.5 per cent of all live births. Two types of pneumonia appear to be acquired from the mother: (1) *congenital,* and (2) *transnatal.* In transnatal pneumonias, however, the onset may be delayed well beyond 3 days with certain types of pathogens, such as Chlamydia.

CONGENITAL PNEUMONIA

Infections with onset in the fetus, called "congenital pneumonias," present as either transplacental or postamnionitis pneumonia.

Transplacental Pneumonia. In transplacental pneumonia, bacteria cross the placenta and invade the fetal lungs by the hematogenous route, as in congenital syphilis and some cases of listeriosis with maternal septicemia. Pneumonia may be well established in utero, causing fetal death or immediate, severe disease at birth. Most cases of transplacental pneumonia have evidence of preceding maternal infection with inflammatory lesions of the placenta.

Postamnionitis Pneumonia. Amnionitis can be explained by invasion of bacteria (Lauweryns et al., 1973), or other infective agents, such as viruses, mycoplasmas, or fungi. This is believed to be an ascending infection, arising from vaginal flora and beginning in the amnion at the cervical os and then spreading by the membranes to the chorionic plate (Blanc, 1961) (Fig. 56–1). For aspiration into the lung, significant fetal asphyxia with gasping is thought to be necessary. This is evidenced by the presence of aspirated amniotic squames in the lungs.

Most cases of amnionitis, however, are not associated with pneumonia in the newborn. In some infants, aspiration of infected amniotic fluid occurs, but the lung parenchyma is not invaded by pathogens. As a result, neutrophils of maternal origin are confined to the air spaces, fetal neutrophils do not infiltrate the septal walls, and fibrinous exudate does not occur. Blood culture in these infants is negative, and the clinical picture is that of fetal asphyxia. Thus, in the presence of amnionitis, a true pneumonia is frequently absent for two reasons: (1) there may be no significant fetal asphyxia (i.e., gasping does not occur), and (2) some bacteria may not produce lung inflammation even if aspiration does occur. This may be partly due to the anti-infective properties of surface-active material.

When an active pneumonia does occur, the usual organisms are group B streptococcis, *Escherichia coli,* and, sometimes, enterococcus, *Haemophilus influenzae, Streptococcus viridans, Listeria,* or anaerobes. These cases are characterized by lung inflammation, fetal neutrophils in the septal walls and saccules, fibrinous exudate, and usually a positive blood culture.

Factors Predisposing to Amnionitis and Pneumonia. The conditions associated with amniotic fluid infection are:

1. Premature labor
2. Rupture of membranes prior to the onset of labor
3. Prolonged membrane rupture (≥24 hours) before delivery
4. Prolonged active labor with cervical dilatation
5. Frequent obstetric digital examinations.

The strong association with premature birth may be due to a developmental deficiency of bacteriostatic factors in amniotic fluid (Schlievert, 1975) or to the infection per se as the precipitating factor for preterm labor. With an increasing latent interval between rupture of membranes and labor, the incidence of clinical amnionitis also increases (Burchell, 1964) as well as the frequency of bacteremia in cord blood samples collected at birth (Tyler and Albers, 1966). However, if gestational age is adequately controlled, there is no evidence for increased perinatal mortality (Daikoku et al., 1981; Schutte et al., 1983). A prolonged interval between rupture of membranes and labor is a significant, independent factor only in amnionitis for gestations of 37 weeks or more (Johnson et al., 1981). In preterm gestations, a prolonged interval between rupture and labor does not necessarily increase the risk of amnionitis because preterm gestations are more prone to amnionitis for reasons quite independent of membrane rupture. In fact, infection may be one of the *causes* of premature labor, since amnionitis may occur in the presence of intact membranes (Naeye and Peters, 1978). Thus, in assessing the risk of neonatal infection, the important thing to consider is not the length of membrane rupture but whether amnionitis is actually established.

Active labor with cervical dilatation has a considerable effect on the incidence of amnionitis. As the duration of labor increases, more women have bacteria in the amniotic fluid. The absence of labor, and delivery by cesarean section, is associated with a greatly reduced risk of congenital pneumonia (Avery, 1984). There are also data suggesting that obstetric digital examinations after rupture

527

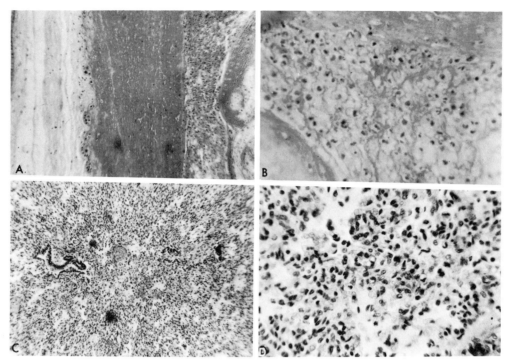

FIGURE 56–1. A, Microscopic section of placenta showing ascending fetal infection leading to intrauterine pneumonia. B, High-power view of the subchorionic region. C, Low-power view of section of lung to show dense homogeneous exudation and leukocytic infiltration. No amniotic debris is visible. D, Higher-power view of same. The infant was one whose mother's labor was induced, because of Rh incompatibility, two weeks before term. Manual stripping of the membranes did not succeed on one day and was repeated the following day. The infant was promptly exchange-transfused but died, for unknown reasons, in the midst of the procedure. The findings of placentitis and pneumonitis were unexpected. (This case was presented by Dr. Peter Gruenwald at a Johns Hopkins Fetal Mortality Clinic. The photographs are reprinted with his kind permission.)

of membranes significantly increase the chance of amniotic infection (Schutte et al., 1983). Amnionitis is more common in undernourished populations, perhaps because bacteriostatic factors may be lacking in the amniotic fluid (Naeye and Blanc, 1970). At comparable levels of family income, however, amnionitis is more frequent among black than white women. Infants of mothers with active urinary tract infection in the 2 weeks prior to birth are at increased risk for amnionitis (Naeye, 1979).

Yoder and associates (1983) has estimated that in the presence of amnionitis term infants are subject to an 8 per cent risk of infection with positive blood culture and a 4 per cent risk of congenital pneumonia. Other estimates for term infants have been lower (Koh et al., 1979), but the risk of infection is clearly greater in premature infants.

TRANSNATAL PNEUMONIA

In transnatal pneumonia, there is no evidence of either preceding amnionitis or maternal infection, although the infant is believed to acquire vaginal flora during the birth process. The onset of clinical signs of pneumonia is delayed for a few hours or days or even longer. A true inflammatory process is always present.

DIAGNOSIS OF EARLY-ONSET PNEUMONIA

Clinical Findings. Some infants have a history of fetal tachycardia and loss of beat-to-beat variability. It is not uncommon for the Apgar score to be low and the first breath delayed, or for the cord pH to reflect significant fetal asphyxia. The usual clinical picture is that of respiratory distress with onset at or soon after birth. Sometimes,

however, the onset of respiratory distress is delayed, preceded by increasing tachypnea during the first day of life. Infants with infection often have poor peripheral perfusion and tachycardia. Larger infants who are not on mechanical ventilation may have brief or prolonged apneas with bradycardia, significant lethargy, and poor feeding. Other signs are abdominal distention, temperature instability, unexplained metabolic acidosis, or excessive jaundice. Some infants progress to a state of septic shock, with or without pulmonary hypertension. Pulmonary hemorrhage may occur, as may disseminated intravascular coagulation.

Laboratory Findings. Analysis of the *gastric aspirate*, collected at or soon after birth, is a useful screening test (Ramos and Stern, 1969). The presence of white cells of maternal origin can be interpreted as indicating inflammation of the amnion and, therefore, increased risk of pneumonia in the infant. The presence of bacteria on Gram stain may reflect swallowed vaginal flora, but if they are identified as group B streptococci or *Escherichia coli*, organisms with high pathogenicity, the level of suspicion for pneumonia should be great—especially in the face of prematurity or asphyxia (Figs. 56–2 and 56–3).

Culture and Gram stain of *tracheal aspirate*, collected within 8 hours of delivery, is also helpful (Sherman et al., 1984), since the trachea is normally sterile and, hopefully, colonization after intubation has not occurred. The presence of bacteria on Gram stain has a 47 per cent positive test-predictive accuracy (Sherman et al., 1980), and a 79 per cent negative test-predictive accuracy. Brook and co-workers (1980) worried about the high number of false

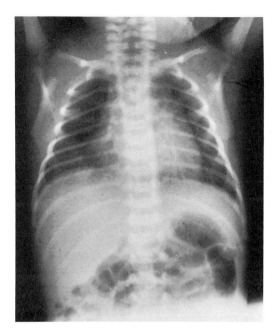

FIGURE 56–2. Film of an infant, age 4 hours, with moderate tachypnea, born of a mother with group B streptococcal urinary tract infection. Although the infiltrates appear only moderate, the infant died of septicemia and pneumonia at 20 hours of age.

positives, tested tracheal aspirate for white cells by Wright stain and found white cells present only in cases of proven pneumonia. Patients with both bacteria and white cells in early tracheal aspirate samples are highly likely to have pneumonia.

Blood culture should be done in all cases of suspected pneumonia as well as *cerebrospinal fluid (CSF) analysis*, since meningitis may also be present. However, lumbar puncture may be postponed if the infant's condition is extremely unstable. *Surface cultures* are of little value because they indicate only the state of colonization and are never diagnostic of bacterial infection (Evans et al., 1988).

Radiographic Findings. In the most severe cases of congenital pneumonia, the chest radiograph shows diffuse homogeneous density (Figs. 56–4 and 56–5). In other cases, the picture is one of diffuse reticulogranular density (similar to that in hyaline membrane disease), or it may have a somewhat more coarse reticulonodular density. Occasionally, the picture is more like that expected in older infants, with linear radiating densities (similar to those found in bronchopneumonia or, less commonly, lobar consolidation) (Fig. 56–6). Pleural effusions may be present. Sometimes the radiograph initially is normal, but later films show abnormalities developing over the first few days. This course is suggestive of transnatal pneumonia (Fig. 56–7). The diffuse pattern is consistent with intrauterine acquisition, whereas the bronchopneumonia pattern suggests infection via aspiration at birth.

Treatment. Antibiotic treatment with a broad-spectrum penicillin and an aminoglycoside is indicated, pending culture results. Without CSF findings, it is usual to double the customary dose of ampicillin to ensure adequate CSF levels. Plasma aminoglycoside levels should be monitored because of unpredictable and prolonged elimination half-

life. When the results of appropriate cultures are available, treatment with the single most effective antibiotic may be the treatment of choice for gram-positive bacterial infections. It is often wise to repeat the blood culture at 48 to 72 hours to document effectiveness of the antibiotic regimen. Regardless of the antibiotic used, treatment should be continued for 10 to 14 days.

SPECIFIC PNEUMONIAS ACQUIRED FROM THE MOTHER

GROUP B STREPTOCOCCAL PNEUMONIA OF EARLY ONSET

Pneumonia due to group B streptococcal infections may be of either of the postamnionitis or transnatal form.

Epidemiology. Group B streptococcal disease with onset before 3 days of life is manifested by (1) septicemia without diagnosed pneumonia in 30 per cent of the cases, (2) pneumonia with bacteremia in 40 per cent, and (3) septicemia or pneumonia with meningitis in 30 per cent (Baker, 1979). The distribution of bacterial strains causing disease is the same as that in vaginal flora. Mothers are reported to have vaginal colonization rates as high as 28 per cent, and similar rates of colonization are seen in the newborn (Paredes et al., 1977). The attack rate is estimated to be 3 per 1000 live births, but is higher with preterm delivery and with evidence of maternal amnionitis.

Diagnosis. Over 80 per cent of infants with pneumonia develop respiratory distress at birth or within a few hours. *Blood and CSF cultures* are most important for determining the diagnosis. In addition, the *rapid latex agglutination test* for capsular polysaccharide antigen has proved useful

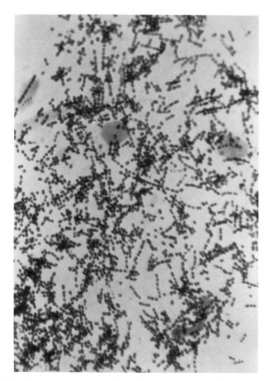

FIGURE 56–3. Gram stain of gastric aspirate of infant described in legend of Figure 56–2. Note the myriad of streptococci evident on this smear. (Courtesy of Dr. William Cochran, Boston Hospital for Women.)

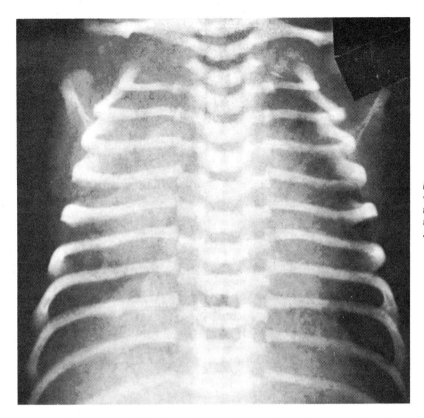

FIGURE 56–4. Congenital pneumonia. Anteroposterior view of chest taken at 16 hours of age. The lungs appear to be almost completely consolidated, the periphery of the left lung and the extreme right base alone containing air. The opacification is homogeneous and dense.

(Hamoudi et al., 1983). It is frequently performed on urine collected by bag, after thorough cleansing of the perineum to remove colonizing bacteria. Properly performed, the negative test-predictive accuracy is 100 per cent, and the positive test-predictive accuracy is 80 per cent. This test also diagnoses infection after antibiotics have been given to the mother or infant.

Treatment. The synergistic combination of ampicillin and gentamicin is recommended for 3 days, followed by penicillin alone for a total of 10 to 14 days. The dose of penicillin should be higher than usually recommended because the minimal inhibitory concentration is high and recurrence has been reported after use of lower doses (Baker, 1979).

PNEUMONIA DUE TO LISTERIA MONOCYTOGENES

Listeria monocytogenes is a gram-positive, beta-hemolytic bacillus, sometimes confused with diphtheroids. It may cause a febrile illness in the mother, but asymptomatic rectal and vaginal colonization is common. The pneumonia occurring in infants infected with *L. monocytogenes* may be transplacental, postamnionitis, or transnatal in type. In transplacental pneumonia, granulomatous disease of the placenta is present. The amniotic fluid in listeria amnionitis has a greenish or chocolate-brown appearance. The chest radiograph shows a diffuse reticulonodular pattern of pneumonia if the onset is intrauterine. In transnatal pneumonia, the chest radiograph shows a bronchopneumonia pattern.

The recommended treatment for *L. monocytogenes* pneumonia is ampicillin and gentamicin for 3 days, followed by ampicillin alone for a total of 10 to 14 days

(Gordon et al., 1970). The earlier the onset, the worse the prognosis; the mortality rate is close to 100 per cent in transplacental pneumonia, despite adequate antibiotic therapy, but quite low in transnatal pneumonia.

PNEUMONIA ALBA DUE TO SYPHILIS

Pneumonia alba, a classic transplacental pneumonia, occurs in infants with syphilis. This diagnosis should be

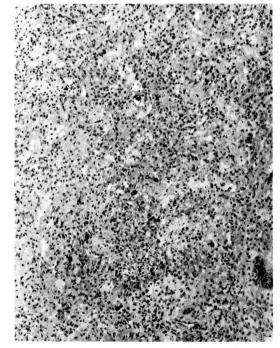

FIGURE 56–5. Microscopic section of lung shows widespread homogeneous exudation and leukocytic infiltration. Alveoli, bronchi, and interstitial tissue are all equally involved.

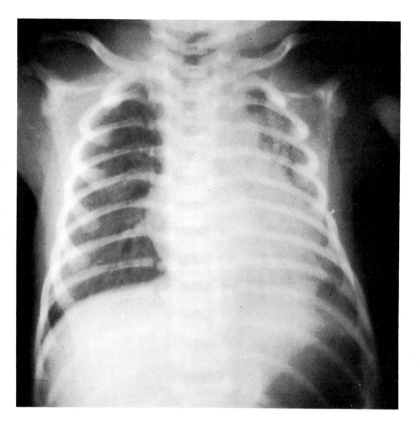

FIGURE 56–6. There is soft linear infiltration spreading outward fanwise from the right hilus. The left lung is almost entirely opacified by confluent areas of homogeneous density. This infant, whose weight was 4 pounds 5 ounces (1956 g), was born 11½ hours after membranes had been ruptured. Amniotic fluid was meconium-stained; Apgar score was 2 at one minute. Tachypnea and dyspnea were followed by apneic spells and then convulsions; he died at 25 hours of age.

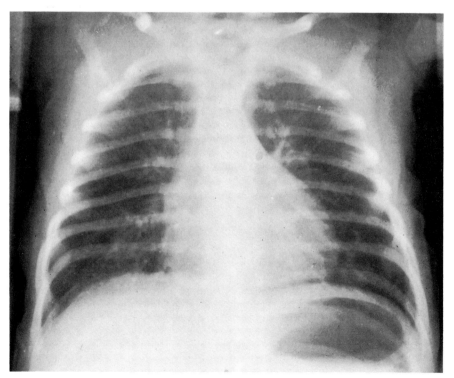

FIGURE 56–7. Anteroposterior view of chest of an infant who was born 36 hours after membrane rupture and demonstrated fever and tachypnea with mild retraction for five days. He undoubtedly had intrauterine pneumonia.

suspected when infants with congenital pneumonia have other signs of congenital syphilis, such as desquamation of the palms and soles, macular rash, hepatosplenomegaly, metaphysitis, thrombocytopenia, obstructive hepatitis, hydrops, or meningoencephalitis (Mascola et al., 1985). The treatment of choice is crystalline penicillin for 10 days.

HERPES SIMPLEX PNEUMONIA

Herpes simplex pneumonia is acquired by aspiration of the virus from the vaginal canal during delivery and is consequently a typical transnatal pneumonia. The infection is disseminated in about a third of the cases, and pneumonia is present in most of these. In 30 per cent, a maternal genital lesion has been documented, but usually shedding of the virus is asymptomatic (Whitley, 1980). The onset in the infant typically occurs at 5 to 7 days after birth, and the mortality rate is at least 85 per cent. Infected infants manifest respiratory distress similar to those of bacterial septicemia. Diffuse densities and lobar consolidation are apparent on the chest radiograph. Often, the diagnosis can be confirmed within 1 to 3 days by viral growth in tissue cultures of tracheal aspirate. Controlled trials have shown that treatment with acyclovir (30 mg/kg/day) for 10 to 14 days is superior to vidarabine therapy (Whitley, 1986). Prevention consists of delivery by cesarean section if virus shedding can be identified in the mother; however, for most infants with this disease, the mothers are apparently asymptomatic.

VARICELLA PNEUMONIA

An infant, delivered vaginally, whose mother develops chicken pox within 5 days of delivery is at risk for transnatal pneumonia, as a result of aspiration of infected secretions from the vaginal canal. The onset for varicella pneumonia is between 5 and 10 days after birth. The disease is severe, with skin rash, coagulopathy, and liver disease, and it is associated with a mortality rate of 30 per cent (Meyers, 1974). The recommended treatment is intravenous vidarabine (15 mg/kg/day) for 10 to 14 days.

SYSTEMIC CANDIDIASIS WITH PNEUMONIA

About 25 per cent of infants weighing less than 1500 g at birth are colonized by Candida, probably during the birth process. This is usually evident by 1 week of age, but it may take 2 to 3 weeks before multiplication is sufficient for cultures to be positive (Baley et al., 1986). The common sites for colonization are the rectum, groin, and throat, but systemic disease occurs only in infants who are colonized. About 70 per cent of infants with systemic candidiasis have pneumonia. These infants are usually small premature infants, about 1 month of age, who have required mechanical ventilation, prolonged use of intravascular catheters, and multiple courses of antibiotics. The signs resemble those of bacterial septicemia. There may be respiratory deterioration with increased oxygen requirements, apnea and bradycardia, temperature instability, glucose intolerance, hypotension, or abdominal distention. Recovery of Candida from the tracheal aspirate cannot differentiate colonization from infection, and the only way to prove pneumonia is by open lung biopsy. However, if the fungus can be recovered from the blood, CSF, urine, or other body fluids, or if eye disease is present, then infection of the lung is very likely. The radiographic signs of Candida pneumonia are nonspecific against the usual background of chronic lung disease. The recommended treatment is amphotericin (1 mg/kg/day) for 30 days (Butler and Baker, 1988).

CHLAMYDIAL PNEUMONIA

Although the onset of pneumonia caused by Chlamydia trachomatis is usually delayed until 1 to 3 months of age, it is considered to be a transnatal pneumonia, the pathogen being acquired from the mother's vagina at delivery (Gilbert, 1986). About 10 per cent of pregnant women have vaginal colonization with chlamydia. The pneumonia is characterized by insidious respiratory distress, cough, wheezing, absence of fever, and bilateral diffuse densities and hyperinflation on the chest radiograph. Significant eosinophilia and elevated serum IgM levels are frequently observed. Infants with chronic lung disease are particularly susceptible (Stagno et al., 1981). To confirm the diagnosis, nasopharyngeal or tracheal secretions should be plated in specific tissue culture cells (Harrison et al., 1978). Alternatively, secretions should be examined for antigen, using rapid direct slide immunofluorescence with monoclonal antibodies (Bell et al., 1984). The recommended treatment is oral erythromycin (50 mg/kg/day) for 14 days.

■ NOSOCOMIAL PNEUMONIA

Pathogenesis. Although hospital-acquired pneumonia is a problem for all newborn and premature infants, in recent years it has become a particular problem for those requiring mechanical ventilatory support. These infections are a major determinant of late morbidity and mortality.

Endotracheal intubation is the single most important factor predisposing to nosocomial pneumonia. The risk for intubated patients is about four times higher than in nonintubated patients (Cross and Roup, 1981), and even higher with tracheostomy. The endotracheal tube eliminates the upper airway as a bacterial filter, tracheal mucosal damage encourages colonization, and ventilator equipment may be contaminated.

Predisposing factors in the occurrence of nosocomial infection are:

1. Birth weight under 1500 g
2. Prolonged hospitalization
3. Severe underlying disease
4. Multiple invasive procedures
5. Overcrowding
6. Low nurse-patient ratio
7. Contaminated ventilator equipment
8. Insufficiently washed hands of health care personnel
(Hemming et al., 1976).

The nose, throat, and rectum are colonized with bacteria during the first 3 days of life. Normally, the predominant bacteria in the nose are Staphylococus aureus, in the throat hemolytic streptococci, and in the rectum Escherichia coli and lactobacillus.

Colonization is somewhat delayed in those admitted to the neonatal intensive care unit (NICU) immediately after birth, especially those treated with antibiotics. The colonizing bacteria are often different, e.g., *Staphylococcus aureus, Staphylococcus epidermidis,* or *Klebsiella* in the throat, or *Klebsiella, Enterobacter,* or *Citrobacter* in the rectum, presumably a reflection of exposure to antibiotics. It is thought that colonization with so-called normal flora provides protection against infection, but that colonization with unusual flora is associated with increased risk of infection (Sprunt et al., 1978).

The trachea and bronchi are normally sterile, despite heavy colonization in the nose and throat. Placement of an endotracheal tube soon leads to colonization of the trachea (Harris et al., 1976). This is especially true if the patient is intubated after 12 hours of age, for more than 72 hours, or more than once. The presence of colonization in the trachea and bronchi does not mean infection in the absence of clinical signs, but it substantially increases the risk (Johanson et al., 1972). Nosocomial pneumonia may also result from the inhalation of aerosols containing bacteria (Simmons and Wong, 1982) and requires routine daily decontamination procedures and periodic surveillance cultures.

Diagnosis. The clinical diagnosis of nosocomial pneumonia depends on the appearance of new infiltrates on the chest radiograph, increased oxygen and ventilator requirements, abnormal white cell count, and the finding of purulent tracheal secretions. Bacteriologic diagnosis depends on the results of blood cultures, tracheal aspirate, and pleural fluid, if available. A good correlation has been shown between tracheal aspirate bacteria and bacteria grown from blood in cases of bacterial pneumonia (Schwartz et al., 1984). However, tracheal aspirates, as performed in the NICU, are subject to contamination from the upper airway. It has been suggested that this problem can be overcome by passing a long sterile catheter with stylet through the endotracheal tube into a peripheral bronchus, and aspirating a sample for culture after brief saline lavage (Frankel et al., 1988).

Treatment. The choice of antibiotics depends on the recent history of infection in the NICU. In the past ampicillin and gentamicin have frequently been chosen. Once sensitivities are known, this choice can be changed for the individual patient.

SPECIFIC NOSOCOMIAL PNEUMONIAS

Staphylococcus aureus Pneumonia. *Staphylococcus aureus* colonize the nose frequently but may also colonize the throat and trachea of debilitated infants. The chest radiograph suggests a nonspecific bronchopneumonia, frequently superimposed over chronic lung disease. However, in more severe cases, ultimately leading to death, there are multiple small lung abscesses. These infants have lethargy, poor circulation, increased oxygen and ventilator requirements, and changes in the white blood cell count. The treatment of choice is vancomycin in most cases, but in a few, methicillin for 14 days is appropriate.

Pneumonia from Staphylococcus epidermidis. A normal inhabitant of the skin, *Staphylococcus epidermidis* may also colonize the throat and trachea of small debilitated infants. Although it more frequently causes a generalized infection, about a fifth of the cases have lung involvement, with the chest radiograph suggesting a nonspecific bronchopneumonia (LaGamma et al., 1983). Because it is usually resistant to methicillin, the treatment is vancomycin for 14 days, with monitoring of plasma levels.

Pseudomonas Pneumonia. *Pseudomonas* is not part of the normal flora at any site, and its isolation from throat or tracheal aspirate is cause for considerable concern. It is sometimes isolated from moist equipment such as nebulizers, humidifiers, incubators, faucets, and disinfectant and respiratory therapy solutions, which act as dangerous sources of infection. The signs are nonspecific, but necrotic skin ulcerations are characteristic, if present. The chest radiograph suggests bronchopneumonia. Small premature infants with a tracheal tube in place are very susceptible (Barson, 1971). The mortality is high because of antibiotic resistance. Treatment consists of an anti-*Pseudomonas* penicillin, such as ticarcillin, and an aminoglycoside, such as gentamicin, tobramycin, or amikacin. Synergistic activity is thought to be important. Ceftazidime may be the best treatment, in combination with an aminoglycoside.

Klebsiella Pneumonia. *Klebsiella* is not part of the normal flora at any site, and its isolation from the throat, tracheal aspirate, or rectum is cause for alarm. Its transmission is usually by the hands of attendants from one baby to another. On the chest radiograph there is a nonspecific bronchopneumonia, but since this is a necrotizing pneumonia, lung abscesses and pneumatoceles may also be evident (Papageorgiou et al., 1973). The mortality is high. Since *Klebsiella* is frequently ampicillin-resistant, the treatment is currently cefotaxime and amikacin for 14 days.

Cytomegalovirus Pneumonia. Very small premature infants may acquire cytomegalovirus (CMV) infection around the age of 1 to 3 months. About a third of such infants have pneumonia, which may contribute to the development of bronchopulmonary dysplasia (Sawyer et al., 1987), or otherwise complicate its course (Ballard et al., 1979). Characteristically, there is increased respiratory distress, greater oxygen or ventilator requirements, hepatosplenomegaly, a peculiar gray color suggestive of sepsis, thrombocytopenia, and both an atypical and absolute lymphocytosis. It is thought that most of these infants acquire this infection from multiple seropositive blood transfusions, although it may be acquired perinatally from a positive mother. The lung infection lasts about 2 weeks, but some cases are more prolonged. Deaths have generally been related to systemic infection beyond the lungs. The diagnosis is made by identifying CMV in tissue culture or by plating urine, throat washings, or tracheal secretions. Although the culture is frequently positive within 7 days, it may take up to 4 weeks. Preventative measures include limiting the number of blood transfusions, limiting the number of blood donors, or using only seronegative blood.

Respiratory Syncytial Virus Pneumonia. The respiratory syncytial virus causes broncholitis and pneumonia, and frequently apnea as well, and has been seen in small premature infants, usually those with chronic lung disease, especially during the winter months. It may be acquired in the community after discharge, but is sometimes acquired from visitors or health-care personnel in the hospital. The characteristic finding on the chest radiograph is hyperinflation, with or without lobar densities suggesting pneumonia. Identification of the virus in tissue culture takes 3 to 8 days or longer. The most rapid way of diagnosis is antigen detection by enzyme-linked immunosorbent assay performed on tracheal aspirate secretions. The virus is transmitted by aerosol droplets, carried by the hands of attendants to the mucous membranes of susceptible hosts. Patients should be isolated. Adequate handwashing diminishes noscomial spread.

The treatment recommended is aerosol administration of the antiviral drug ribavirin (Taber et al., 1983) by hood, mask, or ventilator for 3 to 7 days. Although controlled trials showed that ribavirin-treated infants recovered faster than untreated infants and had significantly improved arterial oxygenation (Hall et al., 1983), there is some evidence that ribavirin may be toxic, especially as a teratogen. Special precautions must be taken with ventilators to prevent obstruction of mechanical valves (Outwater et al., 1988).

***Pneumocystis carinii* Pneumonia.** *Pneumocystis carinii* pneumonia has been seen in epidemic form in European premature nurseries, but has been identified only sporadically in North America in immunocompetent infants under 3 months of age (Stagno et al., 1980) as well as in older immunocompromised patients. It may have been overlooked in the past. The parasite causes a diffuse interstitial mononuclear pneumonia without fever (Fig. 56–7). In small prematures, the onset is insidious during the 3rd month of life, with tachypnea, retractions, cyanosis, crepitant rales, cough, eosinophilia, and a diffuse granular infiltrate on the chest radiograph. Epidemics represent baby-to-baby spread and can be terminated by isolation techniques. The diagnosis may be made by examination of tracheal secretions for the encapsulated cyst or may require lung aspirate, using a Gomori methenamine silver stain. Alternatively, the antigen may be detected by counterimmunoelectrophoresis (Pifer, 1983). The treatment is administration of trimethoprim-sulfamethoxazole for 14 days.

■ REFERENCES

Avery, M. E.: Pneumonia. *In* Avery, M. E., and Taeusch, H. W. (Eds.): Diseases of the Newborn, 5th ed. Philadelphia, W. B. Saunders Company, 1984.

Baker, C. J.: Group B streptococcal infections in neonates. Pediatr. Rev. 1:5, 1979.

Baker, C. J., Webb, B. J., Jackson, C. V., et al.: Countercurrent electrophoresis in the evaluation of infants with group B streptococcal disease. Pediatrics 65:1110, 1980.

Baley, J. E., Kliegman, R. M., Boxerbaum, B., et al.: Fungal colonization in the very low birth weight infant. Pediatrics 78:225, 1986.

Ballard, R. A., Drew, L., Hufnagle, K. G., et al.: Acquired cytomegalovirus infection in preterm infants. Am. J. Dis. Child. 133:482, 1979.

Barson, A. J.: Fatal *Pseudomonas aeruginosa* bronchopneumonia in a children's hospital. Arch. Dis. Child. 46:55, 1971.

Bell, T. A., Kuo, C., Stamm, W. E., et al.: Direct fluorescent monoclonal antibody stain for rapid detection of infant *Chlamydia trachomatis* infections. Pediatrics 74:224, 1984.

Blanc, W. A.: Pathways of fetal and early neonatal infection. J. Pediatr. 59:473, 1961.

Brook, I., Martin, W. J., and Finegold, S. M.: Bacteriology of tracheal aspirates in intubated newborn. Chest 78:875, 1980.

Burchell, R. C.: Premature spontaneous rupture of the membranes. Am. J. Obstet. Gynecol. 88:251, 1964.

Butler, K. M., and Baker, C. J.: *Candida:* An increasingly important pathogen in the nursery. Pediatr. Clin. North Am. 35:543, 1988.

Cross, A. S., and Roup, B.: Role of respiratory assistance devices in endemic nosocomial pneumonia. Am. J. Med. 70:681, 1981.

Daikoku, N. H., Kaltreider, D. F., Johnson, T. R. B., et al.: Premature rupture of membranes and preterm labor: Neonatal infection and perinatal mortality risks. Obstet. Gynecol. 58:417, 1981.

Evans, M. E., Schaffner, W., Federspiel, C. F., et al.: Sensitivity, specificity, and predictive value of body surface cultures in a neonatal intensive care unit. J.A.M.A. 259:248, 1988.

Frankel, L. R., Smith, D. W., and Lewiston, N. J.: Bronchoalveolar lavage for diagnosis of pneumonia in the immunocompromised child. Pediatrics 81:785, 1988.

Gilbert, G. L.: Chlamydial infections in infancy. Aust. Paediatr. J. 22::13, 1986.

Goldmann, D. A., Leclair, J. and Macone, A.: Bacterial colonization of neonates admitted to an intensive care environment. J. Pediatr. 93:288, 1978.

Gordon, R. C., Barrett, F. F., and Yow, M. D.: Ampicillin treatment of listeriosis. J. Pediatr. 77:1067, 1970.

Hall, C. B., McBride, J. T., Walsh, E. E., et al.: Aerosolized ribavirin treatment of infants with respiratory syncytial viral infection. N. Engl. J. Med. 308:1443, 1983.

Hamoudi, A. C., Marcon, M. J., Cannon, H. J., et al.: Comparison of three major antigen detection methods for the diagnosis of group B streptococci in a newborn nursery. Pediatrics 58:679, 1983.

Harris, H., Wirtschafter, D., and Cassady, G.: Endotracheal intubation and its relationship to bacterial colonization and systemic infection of newborn infants. Pediatrics 58:816, 1976.

Harrison, H. R., English, M. G., Lee, C. K., et al.: *Chlamydia trachomatis* infant pneumonitis. N. Engl. J. Med. 298:702, 1978.

Hemming, V. G., Overall, J. C., and Britt, M. R.: Nosocomial infections in a newborn intensive-care unit. N. Engl. J. Med. 294:1310, 1976.

Johanson, W. G., Pierce, A. K., Sanford, J. P., et al.: Nosocomial respiratory infections with gram-negative bacilli. Ann. Intern. Med. 77:701, 1972.

Johnson, J. W. C., Daikoku, N. H., Neibyl, J. R., et al.: Premature rupture of the membranes and prolonged latency. Obstet. Gynecol. 57:547, 1981.

Koh, K. S., Chan, F. H., Monfared, A. H., et al.: The changing perinatal and maternal outcome in chorioamnionitis. Obstet. Gynecol. 53::730, 1979.

LaGamma, E. F., Drusin, L. M., Mackles, A. W., et al.: Neonatal infections. An important determinant of late NICU mortality in infants less than 1000 g at birth. Am. J. Dis. Child. 137:838, 1983.

Lauweryns, J., Bernat, R., Lerut, A., et al.: Intrauterine pneumonia. Biol. Neonate 22:301, 1973.

Maki, D. G., Alvarado, C. J., Hassemer, C. A., et al.: Relation of the inanimate hospital environment to endemic nosocomial infection. N. Engl. J. Med. 307:1562, 1982.

Mascola, L., Pelosi, R., Blount, J. H., et al.: Congenital syphilis revisited. Am. J. Dis. Child. 139:575, 1985.

Meyers, J. D.: Congenital varicella in term infants: Risk reconsidered. J. Infect. Dis. 129:215, 1974.

Naeye, R. L.: Causes of the excessive rates of perinatal mortality and prematurity in pregnancies complicated by maternal urinary-tract infections. N. Engl. J. Med. 300:819, 1979.

Naeye, R. L.: Coitus and associated amniotic-fluid infections. N. Engl. J. Med. 301:1198, 1979.

Naeye, R. L., and Blanc, W. A.: Relation of poverty and race to antenatal infection. N. Engl. J. Med. 283:555, 1970.

Naeye, R. L., and Peters, E. C.: Amniotic fluid infections with intact membranes leading to perinatal death: A prospective study. Pediatrics 61:171, 1978.

Outwater, K. M., Meissner, H. C., and Peterson, M. B.: Ribavirin administration to infants receiving mechanical ventilation. Am. J. Dis. Child. 142:512, 1988.

Papageorgiou, A., Bauer, C. R., Fletcher, B. D., et al.: *Klebsiella* pneumonia with pneumatocele formation in a newborn infant. Can. Med. Assoc. J. 109:1217, 1973.

Paredes, A., Wong, P., Mason, E. O., et al.: Nosocomial transmission of group B streptococci in a newborn nursery. Pediatrics 59:679, 1977.

Pennington, J. E.: Community-acquired and hospital-acquired pneumonia in adults. *In* Simmons, D. H. (Ed.), Current Pulmonology, vol. 7. Chicago, Year Book Medical Publishers, 1986.

Phillip, A. G. S., and Hewitt, J. R.: Early diagnosis of neonatal sepsis. Pediatrics 65:1036, 1980.

Pierce, A. K., and Sanford, J. P.: Bacterial contamination of aerosols. Arch. Intern. Med. 131:156, 1973.

Pifer, L. L.: *Pneumocystis carinii:* A diagnostic dilemma. Pediatr. Infect. Dis. 2:177, 1983.

Ramos, A., and Stern, L.: Relationship of premature rupture of the membranes to gastric fluid aspirate in the newborn. Am. J. Obstet. Gynecol. 105:1247, 1969.

Sawyer, M. H., Edwards, D. K., and Spector, S. A.: Cytomegalovirus infection and bronchopulmonary dysplasia in premature infants. Am. J. Dis. Child. 141:303, 1988.

Schlievert, P., Larsen, B., Johnson, W., et al.: Bacterial growth inhibition by amniotic fluid. Am. J. Obstet. Gynecol. 122:809, 1975.

Schutte, M. F., Treffers, P. E., Kloosterman, G. J., et al.: Management of premature rupture of membranes: The risk of vaginal examination to the infant. Am. J. Obstet. Gynecol. 146:395, 1983.

Schwartz, D. B., Oslon, D. E., and Kauffman, C. A.: The utility of pharyngeal and tracheal cultures during endotracheal intubation. Chest 86:335, 1984.

Selden, R., Lee, S., Wang, W. L. L., et al.: Nosocomial *Klebsiella* infections: Intestinal colonization as a reservoir: Ann. Intern. Med. 74:657, 1971.

Sherman, M. P., Chance, K. H., and Goetzman, B. W.: Gram's stains of tracheal secretions predict neonatal bacteremia. Am. J. Dis. Child. 138:848, 1984.

Sherman, M. P., Goetzman, B. W., Ahlfors, C. E., et al.: Tracheal aspiration and its clinical correlates in the diagnosis of congenital pneumonia. Pediatrics 65:258, 1980.

Shurin, P. A., Alpert, S., Rosner, B., et al.: Chorioamnionitis and colonization of the newborn infant with genital mycoplasmas. N. Engl. J. Med. 293:5, 1975.

Simmons, B. P., and Wong, E. S.: Guidelines for prevention of nosocomial pneumonia. Infect. Control 3:327, 1982.

Sprunt, K., Leidy, G., and Redman, W.: Abnormal colonization of neonates in an intensive care unit: Means of identifying neonates at risk of infection. Pediatr. Res. 12:998, 1978.

Stagno, S., Pifer, L. L., Hughes, W. T., et al.: *Pneumocystis carinii* pneumonitis in young immunocompetent infants. Pediatrics 66:56, 1980.

Stagno, S., Brasfield, D. M., Brown, M. B., et al.: Infant pneumonitis associated with cytomegalovirus, *Chlamydia, Pneumocystis* and *Ureaplasma:* A prospective study. Pediatrics 68:322, 1981.

Taber, L. H., Knight, V., Gilbert, B. E., et al.: Ribavirin aerosol treatment of bronchiolitis associated with respiratory syncytial virus infection in infants. Pediatrics 72:613, 1983.

Tyler, C. W., and Albers, W. H.: Obstetric factors related to bacteremia in the newborn infant. Am. J. Obstet. Gynecol. 94:970, 1966.

Whitley, R. J., Alford, C. A., Hirsch, M. S., et al.: Vidarabine versus acyclovir therapy in herpes simplex encephalitis. N. Engl. J. Med. 314:144, 1986.

Whitley, R. J., Nahmias, A. J., Visintine, A. M., et al.: The natural history of herpes simplex virus infection of mother and newborn. Pediatrics 66:489, 1980.

DISEASES OF THE 57 AIRWAYS

Thomas Hansen and Anthony Corbet

Respiratory distress due to partial or complete obstruction of the nares or upper airway may present a serious, or even life-threatening, event shortly after birth. Infants who have no apparent respiratory distress when crying but who develop cyanosis and severe retractions when quiet or attempting to feed should be evaluated immediately for choanal atresia. The diagnosis may be more complex in the infant with inspiratory stridor or wheezing.

■ CHOANAL ATRESIA

Epidemiology. This malformation, due to persistence of the bucconasal membrane, occurs one in 10,000 births and has a significant female preponderance. About half the occurrences are bilateral, in which case there may be an immediate neonatal emergency. Associated anomalies are present in 50 per cent of the cases (Hall, 1979), including the Treacher Collins syndrome. The most common collection of anomalies can be called the "CHARGE association," consisting of some combination of Colobomas of the eyes, congenital Heart disease, choanal Atresia, Retardation of physical and mental Growth, and Ear anomalies associated with deafness (Pagon et al., 1981).

Diagnosis. Because newborns are preferential "nose breathers" for the first 2 to 3 weeks of life, bilateral choanal atresia is associated with chest retractions and severe cyanosis, particularly during feedings and only relieved when the mouth is opened to cry. A catheter cannot be passed through the nose, and nasal instillation of radiopaque dye demonstrates obstruction. The use of computed tomography (CT) is now the method of choice in making a definitive diagnosis.

Treatment. Emergency prophylaxis consists of endotracheal intubation. Although 90 per cent of cases are bony, rather than membranous, in some the bone is soft and easily penetrated. Correction can be accomplished using the transnasal approach with either Hegar dilators (Stahl and Jurkiewicz, 1985) or a carbon dioxide surgical laser (Healy et al., 1978). After creating the appropriate airway, polyvinyl tubes are sutured in place to prevent subsequent closure. The tubes are lavaged with saline and suctioned, and after 6 weeks, they can be removed. This procedure is often definitive, or it can be followed by a transpalatal operation when the infant is much larger. If CT scan demonstrates a thick bony component, transpalatal surgery during the newborn period is probably the best method of correction.

■ PHARYNGEAL DEFORMITIES

PIERRE ROBIN SYNDROME

The Pierre Robin syndrome has an incidence of one per 2000 births. The major feature is micrognathia with posterior displacement of the tongue into the pharynx, but 60 per cent of the patients also have a cleft palate. Hereditary transmission may be through a dominant gene with variable expressivity. Because the pharyngeal airway is narrowed, obstructive respiratory distress and cyanosis are common during the newborn period; these episodes may progress to dangerous spells of apnea (Cozzi and Pierro, 1985). Obstruction is common when the infant is in the supine position, during feeding, and in active sleep, when pharyngeal muscle tone is absent. Excessive air swallowing, followed by gastric distention, vomiting, and tracheal aspiration are frequent problems. The pharyngeal obstruction is maintained by the generation of large negative pressures in the lower pharynx during inspiration and swallowing (Fletcher et al., 1969). Chronic obstruction leads to carbon-dioxide retention, failure to thrive, and development of pulmonary hypertension with right ventricular failure (Johnson and Todd, 1980).

Treatment. In an emergency, tracheal intubation should be performed. However, it is now customary to pass a 3.5 mm tube through the nose and into the hypopharynx (Heaf et al., 1982). This prevents the generation of negative pressure and greatly relieves the respiratory difficulty. The nasopharyngeal tube may be left in place for weeks or even months with adequate lavage and suctioning. The infant should be placed in the prone position to prevent the tongue from falling backward. If a nasopharyngeal tube is not adequately relieving the obstruction, then tracheotomy is indicated to prevent progression to cor pulmonale. Nutrition can be maintained with a hypercaloric formula fed by nasogastric tube or gastrostomy. With the passage of time, the problem becomes less threatening, especially after a few months, when the infant gains better control of the tongue (Mallory and Paradise, 1979). Oral feedings can be introduced, usually with a long lamb's nipple to help hold the tongue forward. With adequate nutrition and growth of the mandible, the problem usually resolves by 6 to 12 months of age.

GLOSSOPTOSIS-APNEA SYNDROME

The Pierre Robin syndrome is not the only condition characterized by the tongue obstructing the airway. Infants with unilateral choanal atresia, choanal stenosis, or swelling of the nasal mucosa may generate large negative pressures in the pharynx and, in the absence of adequate muscular control over the tongue, may develop pharyngeal obstruction that causes respiratory distress, cyanosis, and severe episodes of apnea (Cozzi and Pierro, 1985).

PHARYNGEAL INCOORDINATION

Pharyngeal incoordination causes choking and cyanosis with feedings and may be complicated by aspiration pneumonia (Avery and Fletcher, 1974). It may be seen in infants with severe hypoxic-ischemic encephalopathy and pseudobulbar palsy, in infants with Arnold-Chiari malformation, and in those with Möbius syndrome. Although some infants may gradually improve, the long-term management includes tube feedings or even gastrostomy.

■ LARYNGEAL DEFORMITIES

CONGENITAL LARYNGEAL STRIDOR

A relatively common condition, congenital laryngeal stridor (laryngomalacia) is due to the prolapse of poorly supported supraglottic structures, namely the arytenoids, aryepiglottic folds, and the epiglottis into the airway during inspiration. Despite loud inspiratory stridor and significant chest retractions, usually from birth or the first month of life, the infant seldom has cyanosis, hypercarbia, notable feeding difficulty or growth failure, or abnormal cry (Richardson and Cotton, 1984). Congenital stridor is worse in the supine position with the neck flexed, and better in the prone position with the neck extended (Cotton and Richardson, 1981a). Obstruction is worse during episodes of agitation, better when the infant is calmed. Radiographic demonstration of prolapse of the aryepiglottic folds supports the diagnosis. Confirmation may be obtained at laryngoscopy, but care must be taken not to fixate the supraglottic structures with the instrument. Some practitioners prefer to pass a flexible fiberoptic bronchoscope through the nose. In some cases, gastroesophageal reflux or episodes of obstructive apnea may be associated with this condition (Belmont and Grundfast, 1984). About 18 per cent of the infants with a congenital lesion of the airway have a second lesion of some kind. Thus, the evaluation of stridor must include the examination of the entire upper aerodigestive tract (Friedman et al., 1984). The treatment is conservative, tracheostomy rarely being required, and the condition spontaneously improves over about 18 months (Smith and Catlin, 1984).

VOCAL CORD PARALYSIS

Unilateral cord paralysis is usually left-sided; stridor and retractions are not marked, and the voice is weak and hoarse. The infant may cough and choke during feedings. The condition is due to a lesion involving the recurrent laryngeal nerve, perhaps caused by excessive stretching of the neck during delivery. Other possible causes include trauma from ligation of a patent ductus arteriosus (Davis et al., 1988). Stridor may be less if the infant lies on the paralyzed side, when the affected cord can fall away from

the midline (Cotton and Richardson, 1981a). The condition often tends to improve over a period of several weeks or months.

Bilateral cord paralysis is a much more serious condition, accompanied by serious inspiratory stridor. Frequently, however, the cry is normal. Associated problems may include pharyngeal incoordination with swallowing difficulty, recurrent apnea, and tracheal aspiration. Usually, severe central nervous system problems are also present, such as hypoxic-ischemic encephalopathy, cerebral hemorrhage, Arnold-Chiari malformation, hydrocephalus, or brain-stem dysgenesis. The stridor may improve slowly if brain swelling subsides after birth. Tracheostomy is frequently required (Smith and Catlin, 1984), and the prognosis is usually very poor.

CONGENITAL LARYNGEAL STENOSIS

The larynx may be partially obstructed by a web or cyst that causes inspiratory stridor from birth and a hoarse cry. The diagnosis of congenital laryngeal stenosis is made by laryngoscopy. Treatment consists of endoscopic lysis with microlaryngeal surgery or a carbon dioxide laser (Smith and Catlin, 1984). Usually, one application is sufficient to correct this difficulty, and the prognosis is excellent.

LARYNGEAL ATRESIA

In laryngeal atresia, the larynx may be completely obstructed by a web, seen in the delivery room during attempts to intubate the cyanotic infant. An endotracheal tube can sometimes be forced beyond the obstruction into the trachea. Otherwise, a large-bore needle should be inserted percutaneously into the trachea to maintain marginal gas exchange while preparations for emergency tracheostomy are made. Unfortunately, most infants with laryngeal atresia have other lethal malformations (Smith and Catlin, 1984).

CONGENITAL SUBGLOTTIC STENOSIS

Congenital subglottic stenosis is secondary to malformation of the cricoid cartilage. In severe cases, stridor is present from birth, and respiratory distress is obvious. In milder cases, excessive "croup" may indicate the presence of this malformation (McGill, 1984; Healy et al., 1988).

SUBGLOTTIC HEMANGIOMA

Subglottic hemangioma, often in association with cutaneous hemangioma, may cause biphasic stridor, which progresses with slow enlargement of the tumor (Cotton and Richardson, 1981a). Although some have advocated high-dose corticosteroid therapy (Brown et al., 1972), intubation or tracheostomy is usually required. Results of removal by carbon dioxide laser have been encouraging (Healy and McGill, 1984), and have enabled treatment without tracheostomy in many cases.

ACQUIRED SUBGLOTTIC STENOSIS

Extubation after prolonged endotracheal intubation is sometimes followed by biphasic stridor, produced by subglottic edema and fibrosis. The risk is greatest in infants who have had tightly fitting endotracheal tubes, frequent intubations, and prolonged mechanical ventilation (Sherman et al., 1986). Adequate humidification of inspired gas and nebulization of racemic epinephrine have proved useful, and in cases with no response to these measures, reintubation with a smaller endotracheal tube for a short period, while growth occurs, may be helpful. Treatment with dexamethasone before extubation is often suggested and occasionally may be successful. Difficult cases should be evaluated by rigid endoscopy. In some infants, a cricoid split procedure may be successful (Seid and Canty, 1985), while more severely affected infants may require tracheostomy, followed by a formal surgical procedure to reconstruct the subglottic space.

LARYNGO-TRACHEO-ESOPHAGEAL CLEFT

In laryngo-tracheo-esophageal cleft, a longitudinal communication is present between the airway and esophagus, stretching from the larynx into the upper trachea or sometimes as far as the carina. Such infants have respiratory distress and cyanosis, associated with tracheal aspiration of saliva and feedings. The chest radiograph may show evidence of aspiration pneumonia, while the cine-esophogram shows contrast material spilling into the trachea. The airway must be adequately secured with an endotracheal tube or tracheostomy (Richardson and Cotton, 1984); an esophagostomy diverts saliva, and feedings should be accomplished by gastric division and gastrostomy. Attempts at operative repair through a lateral pharyngotomy, and thoracotomy if necessary, have been successful in a few infants (Burroughs and Leape, 1974; Cotton and Schreiber, 1981b).

■ TRACHEAL DEFORMITIES

TRACHEAL AGENESIS SYNDROME

In this rare condition, the trachea is atretic just below the vocal cords, or it is absent all the way down to the carina (Altman et al., 1972). These infants usually have a tracheo-esophageal (TE) fistula, as well as severe cardiac malformations. Despite the presence of a larynx, intubation cannot be accomplished; however, if the tracheal tube is positioned in the esophagus and connected to a mechanical ventilator, reasonable gas exchange can be obtained through the TE fistula. When the atresia is high, a tracheostomy can be done. If survival seems possible, gastric division and a gastrostomy for feeding should be performed. However, reconstructive surgery is not likely to be successful, and the prognosis is extremely poor.

CONGENITAL TRACHEAL STENOSIS

In congenital tracheal stenosis, a segment of the trachea is narrowed, producing inspiratory stridor, expiratory wheezing, and often cyanotic episodes. The segment may be short or long; occasionally, the entire trachea is hypoplastic, and the bronchi may be involved. In many cases, other congenital malformations are also present, such as vascular ring anomalies, congenital heart defects, tracheoesophageal fistula, or hemivertebrae (Benjamin et al.,

1981). A series of cases without accompanying defects has been reported in premature infants, who presented with difficulties at tracheal intubation (Hauft et al., 1988). Sometimes, the diagnosis can be made by chest radiograph, with air as the contrast medium, but flexible fiberoptic bronchoscopy is usually required. To examine the lower limits of the stenosis, it is sometimes necessary to proceed with tracheobronchography. Cine-CT scan is also being developed as a useful diagnostic technique. In most cases, the stenosis requires treatment of some kind: simple dilation, segmental excision, or tracheoplasty. The use of cardiopulmonary bypass has improved treatment in many cases.

TRACHEOBRONCHOMALACIA

Rarely, development of tracheal cartilage support may be delayed, resulting in tracheobronchomalacia, a condition characterized by wheezing and respiratory distress. The chest radiograph shows diffuse overinflation. At bronchoscopy, the anterior and posterior walls of the trachea are approximated during expiration (Salzberg, 1983). The respiratory distress may be alleviated by passage of a bronchoscope to the carina. Many affected infants improve by 6 to 12 months of age. Severe cases may benefit from treatment with constant positive airway pressure, but prolonged treatment for 1 to 2 years may be required (Wiseman et al., 1985). A strong association with tracheoesophageal fistula has been reported, and some authors have resorted to tracheopexy to treat severe cases (Benjamin et al., 1976). Prolonged tracheostomy may be useful, with the tube acting as a stent for the compliant trachea (Cogbill et al., 1983), but this is less useful when the bronchi are also involved. In recent years, this condition has been seen in respirator-dependent infants with bronchopulmonary dysplasia (Sotomayor et al., 1986). Such infants may have significant, dynamic compression of the trachea from reactive lower-airway disease and thus gain some improvement from bronchodilator therapy.

VASCULAR RINGS

The trachea may be compressed by (1) a double aortic arch, (2) a right aortic arch, (3) left-sided origin of the innominate artery or right-sided origin of the left common carotid artery, or (4) an anomalous origin of the left pulmonary artery from the right pulmonary artery (Hendren and Kim, 1978). With a right aortic arch, the trachea is compressed by the main pulmonary trunk, aortic arch, and ligamentum arteriosus. The anomalous innominate or carotid arteries form a tight crotch, which impinges on the anterior trachea. The anomalous left pulmonary artery returns to the left by passing between the esophagus and trachea, compressing the trachea between the right and left pulmonary arteries. Infants with tracheal compression have inspiratory stridor and expiratory wheezing. The onset of symptoms is usually later in the neonatal period. These infants often lie with the head and neck hyperextended to stretch the trachea and make it less compressible. If the esophagus is compressed, feeding is associated with regurgitation. The chest radiograph may show mild overinflation, a right-sided aorta, and with appropriate technique, evidence of tracheal narrowing. A barium-swallow examination may show indentation of the esophagus. Magnetic resonance imaging (MRI) has proved to be accurate in defining most vascular malformations compressing the airway. Bronchoscopy should reveal a pulsatile mass at the carina while echocardiography confirms the diagnosis. After surgical relief, the respiratory distress may persist for weeks because of localized tracheal deformity.

■ REFERENCES

Altman, R. P., Randolph, J. G., and Shearin, R. B.: Tracheal agenesis: Recognition and management. J. Pediatr. Surg. 7:112, 1972.

Avery, M. E., and Fletcher, B. D.: The Lung and Its Disorders in the Newborn Infant. Philadelphia, W. B. Saunders Company, 1974, p. 238.

Belmont, J. R. and Grundfast, K.: Congenital laryngeal stridor (laryngomalacia): Etiologic factors and associated disorders. Ann. Otol. Rhinol. Laryngol. 93:430, 1984.

Benjamin B., Cohen, D., and Glasson, M.: Tracheomalacia in association with congenital tracheo-esophageal fistula. Surgery 79, 504, 1976.

Benjamin, B., Pitkin, J., and Cohen, D.: Congenital tracheal stenosis. Ann. Otol. Rhinol. Laryngol. 90:364, 1981.

Brown, S. H., Neerhout, R. C., and Fonkalsrud, E. W.: Prednisone therapy in the management of large hemangiomas in infants and children. Surgery 71:168, 1972.

Burroughs, N., and Leape, L. L.: Laryngotracheoesophageal cleft: Report of a case successfully treated and review of the literature. Pediatrics 53:516, 1974.

Cogbill, T. H., Moore, F. A., Accurso, F. J., et al.: Primary tracheomalacia. Ann. Thorac. Surg. 35:538, 1983.

Cohn, R. C., Kercsmar, C., and Dearborn, D.: Safety and flexibility of flexible endoscopy in children with bronchopulmonary dysplasia. Am. J. Dis. Child. 142:1225, 1988.

Cotton, R. T. and Richardson, M. A.: Congenital laryngeal anomalies. Otolaryngol. Clin. North Am. 14:203, 1981a.

Cotton, R. T. and Schreiber, J. H.: Management of laryngotracheoesophageal cleft. Ann. Otol. 90:401, 1981b.

Cozzi, F., and Pierro, A.: Glossoptosis-apnea syndrome in infancy. Pediatrics 75:836, 1985.

Crockett, D. M., Healy, G. B., McGill, T. J., et al.: Computed tomography in the evaluation of choanal atresia in infants and children. Laryngoscope 97:174, 1987.

Davis, J. T., Baciewicz, F. A., Suriyapa, S., et al.: Vocal cord paralysis in premature infants undergoing ductal closure. Ann. Thorac. Surg. 46:214, 1988.

Douglas, B.: The treatment of micrognathia associated with obstruction by a plastic procedure. Plast. Reconstruct. Surg. 1:300, 1946.

Fletcher, M. M., Blum, S. L., and Blanchard, C. L.: Pierre-Robin syndrome: Pathophysiology of obstructive episodes. Laryngoscope 79:547, 1969.

Friedman, E. M., Williams, M., Healy G. B., et al.: Pediatric endoscopy: A review of 616 cases. Ann. Otol. 93:517, 1984.

Friedman, E. M., Vastola, A. D., McGill, T. J., et al.: Chronic pediatric stridor: Etiology and outcome. Laryngoscope 100:277, 1990.

Hall, B. D.: Choanal atresia and associated multiple anomalies. J. Pediatr. 95:395, 1979.

Hauft, S. M., Perlman, J. M., Siegel, M. J., et al.: Tracheal stenosis in the sick premature infant: Clinical and radiologic features. Am. J. Dis. Child. 142:206, 1988.

Heaf, D. P., Helms, P. J., Dimwiddie, R., et al.: Nasopharyngeal airways in Pierre Robin syndrome. J. Pediatr 100:698, 1982.

Healy, G. B.: Subglottic stenosis. Otolaryngol. Clin. North Am. 22:599, 1989.

Healy, G. B., and McGill, T.: CO_2 laser in subglottic hemangioma—an update. Ann. Otol. Rhinol. Laryngol. 93:270, 1984.

Healy, G. B., McTill, T., Jako, G. J., et al.: Management of choanal atresia with the carbon-dioxide laser. Ann. Otol. Rhinol. Laryngol. 87:658, 1978.

Healy, G. B., Schuster, S. R., Jonas, R. A., et al.: Correction of segmental tracheal stenosis in children. Ann. Otol. Rhinol. Laryngol. 97:444, 1988.

Hendren, W. H., and Kim, S. H.: Pediatric thoracic surgery. In Scarpelli, E. M., Auld, P. A. M., and Goldman, H. S. (Eds.): Pulmonary Disease of the Fetus and Newborn and Child. Philadelphia, Lea & Febiger, 1978, p. 166.

Johnson, G. M., and Todd, D. W.: Cor pulmonale in severe Pierre Robin syndrome. Pediatrics 65:152, 1980.

McGill, T.: Congenital diseases of the larynx. Otolaryngol. Clin. North Am. 17:57, 1984.

McGovern, F. H.: Bilateral choanal atresia: A new method of management. Laryngoscope 71:480, 1961.

Mallory, S. F., and Paradise, J. L.: Glossoptosis revisited: On the development and resolution of airway obstruction in the Pierre Robin syndrome. Pediatrics 64:946, 1979.

Nakayama, D. K., Harrison, M. R., deLorimier, A. A., et al.: Reconstructive surgery of obstructing lesions of the intrathoracic trachea in infants and small children. J. Pediatr. Surg. 17:854, 1982.

Pagon, R. A., Graham, J. M., Zonana, J., et al.: Coloboma, congenital heart disease, and choanal atresia with multiple anomalies: CHARGE association. J. Pediatr. 99:223, 1981.

Richardson, M. A. and Cotton, R. T.: Anatomic abnormalities of the pediatric airway. Pediatr. Clin. North Am. 31:821, 1984.

Saltzberg, A. M.: Congenital malformations of the lower respiratory tract. In Kendig, E. L., and Chernick, V. (Eds.): Disorders of the Respiratory Tract in Children. Philadelphia, W. B. Saunders Company, 1983, p. 169.

Seid, A. B., and Canty, T. G.: The anterior cricoid split procedure for the management of subglottic stenosis in infants and children. J. Pediatr. Surg. 20:388, 1985.

Sherman, J. M., Lowitt, S., Stephenson, C., et al.: Factors influencing acquired subglottic stenosis in infants. J. Pediatr 109:322,1986.

Smith, R. J. H. and Catlin, F. I.: Congenital anomalies of the larynx. Am. J. Dis. Child. 138:35, 1984.

Sotomayor, J. L., Godinez, R. I., Borden, S., et al.: Large airway collapse due to acquired tracheobronchomalacia in infancy. Am. J. Dis. Child. 140:367, 1986.

Stahl, R. S., and Jurkiewicz, M. J.: Congenital posterior choanal atresia. Pediatrics 76:429, 1985.

Stern, L. M., Fonkalsrud, E. W., Hassakis, P., et al.: Management of Pierre Robin syndrome in infancy by prolonged naso-esophageal intubation. Am. J. Dis. Child. 124:79, 1972.

Wiseman, N. E., Duncan, P. G., and Cameron, C. B.: Management of tracheobroncomalacia with continous positive airway pressure. J. Pediatr. Surg. 20:489, 1985.

MALFORMATIONS OF THE MEDIASTINUM AND LUNG PARENCHYMA

Thomas Hansen, Anthony Corbet, and Mary Ellen Avery

■ PARENCHYMAL ABNORMALITIES

LUNG INJURY FROM ASPIRATION

Aspiration of small amounts of amniotic fluid is probably a normal physiologic event for the fetus, particularly when a gasp occurs. It is only during fetal distress, however, that meconium is passed and the aspiration of meconium-stained amniotic fluid takes place, with sequential gasping by a compromised fetus. The lung of stillborn infants may thus contain squamous cells from the skin and other particulate matter as well as bacteria in the potential airspaces when infection is involved (Fig. 58–1).

The risk of meconium aspiration increases with gestational age. It is rare in preterm infants and increasingly common in postmature infants. Infection may accompany aspiration or even cause it. Thus, there are situations where the differential diagnosis between intrauterine pneumonia and meconium aspiration pneumonia is difficult.

The diagnosis of meconium aspiration depends on inspection of the larynx during intubation. In severe cases, the chest radiographs will show wide-spread infiltrates. Hyperinflation alternating with atelectasis is the rule. Occasionally, loculated air can produce pneumatoceles or pneumothorax. If the meconium can be removed by suction, the infant may have a very mild course. If there

has been extensive aspiration, prolonged oxygen dependency and severe pulmonary hypertension may result. However, pulmonary hypertension may have been caused by the same insult that caused the infant to pass meconium in utero. The tachypnea may persist for weeks. (For a discussion of pathogenesis and treatment, see Chapter 509.)

Newborn infants are handicapped with respect to some of the defenses against aspiration. They may have a degree of pharyngeal incoordination in the 1st day of life and aspirate normal upper airway secretions. Furthermore, cough is less easily provoked in infants during the first days of life. Less than half of all newborns cough spontaneously, even on direct laryngeal stimulation. The presence of an endotracheal tube inhibits the normal clearance of mucus from the airways. Not only does the tube itself obstruct the mucus flow, but infants who are intubated are unable to cough. Furthermore, when an endotracheal tube is in place, upper airway secretions may be aspirated.

Premature babies, in particular, are frequently found to have gastric contents in the oral pharynx. If they have swallowed air during oral feedings, they may demonstrate significant gastroesophageal reflux with aspiration. This is one of the reasons for giving premature infants frequent, small feedings and for the preference for intravenous

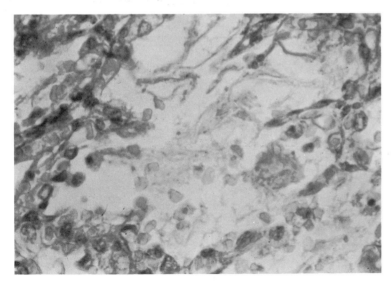

FIGURE 58–1. *Section of lung of a full-term infant weighing 3400 g, who died 15 minutes after birth, having gasped only a few times. Prolonged labor, uterine inertia, stimulation of labor by Pitocin, and, finally, midforceps extraction characterized his delivery. The microscopic section shows much fluid and debris, and many squames within dilated terminal air spaces. Virtually every section from both lungs looked like this one.*

alimentation in infants who are neurologically depressed and at risk for aspiration-induced apnea. It should be noted that almost all preterm infants have significant gastroesophageal reflux as well as many term infants during the first months of life. Although almost all children who later are diagnosed as having reflux present by 6 weeks of age, the condition is so common in the first months of life that it should always be treated conservatively. Conservative management includes frequent, small feedings, routine burping, and placing the infant in a prone position on a 30-degree plane after meals to facilitate retention of feedings. These measures are so likely to be successful in most circumstances that drugs are not required.

Abnormal communications between the trachea and esophagus, as in laryngo-tracheo-esophageal cleft or tracheoesophageal fistula, are recognized by repeated bouts of choking after feeding and the development of aspiration pneumonia. Early recognition, prevention of aspiration by insertion of a nasogastric tube, and prompt surgical intervention are essential to prevent lung injury.

■ CONGENITAL PULMONARY CYSTS

Most pulmonary cysts in the newborn are pneumatoceles, acquired after pneumonia or during the course of pulmonary interstitial emphysema, or bronchopulmonary dysplasia. Congenital cysts are much less common; they may be single or multiple but are always confined to one lobe of the lung. Although acquired cysts tend to disappear with time, congenital cysts are persistent. All cysts have a communication with peripheral airways and, hence, are filled with air. The diagnosis is easily made from the chest radiograph. In the newborn, the most common presentation is with air trapping, tension cyst or pneumothorax, and severe respiratory distress that requires lobectomy (Gwinn et al., 1970). Otherwise, pulmonary cysts present later with recurring bouts of infection.

Diagnosis. Newborns who become ill with cystic disease of the lungs usually suffer from the effects of rapid expansion of the cysts. Tachypnea or dyspnea may begin at birth or at any time thereafter. Dyspnea may progress rapidly or slowly. In the first instance, the infant's condition can become critical within hours; in the latter, it may remain almost static for weeks or months.

A minority of neonates demonstrate the effects of infection rather than of increased tension. In these, persistent or repeated exacerbations of pneumonitis are the presenting symptom. When this is so, it is often difficult to decide whether infection came first and produced emphysematous bullae and subpleural blebs or whether the cystic areas were true congenital cysts that became secondarily infected.

When cysts are solitary and large, they are discoverable by flatness of the percussion note if pus-filled, or, if they are air-filled (as is more commonly the case), they are indicated by hyperresonance or tympany. Breath sounds are diminished to absent over them. The heart is shifted away from the affected side, unless a cyst lying adjacent to a bronchus has completely occluded it and has produced atelectasis of the distal segment of lung. Rales may be heard, owing to compression of contiguous lobes. Even when multiple cysts are present, the physical signs may be exactly the same, since the condition of the largest of the cysts dominates the clinical picture. (Figs. 58–2 to 58–6).

Radiographic Findings. Large balloon cysts filled with air under tension are often mistaken for tension pneumothorax. One hemithorax is overfilled, the diaphragm flattened or even concave, the mediastinum and heart pushed to or beyond the midline. Points that may distinguish balloon cysts from pneumothorax are (1) a delicate linear pattern within the translucent area denoting their fine trabeculation, (2) the presence of compressed lung at the apex and at the costophrenic and cardiohepatic angles, often demarcated from the cyst by a curving line visible in one or another projection, and (3) the absence of all hilar shadows. In pneumothorax, the collapsed lung is often visible as a dense shadow projecting from the hilar region or upward from the diaphragm.

Multiple cysts are visualized as a collection of round or oval translucent areas within the hemithorax. If similar shadows are present in both sides of the chest, they are more likely to represent emphysematous bullae or blebs, but unilaterality does not rule out the latter possibility.

The round or oval areas of translucency produced by intrathoracic bowel may offer difficulty at times. When one is in doubt about the possibility of diaphragmatic hernia, a barium meal gastrointestinal series must be performed.

Large cysts containing both air and fluid are hard to differentiate from hydropneumothorax or pyopneumothorax. Here again, visualization of a curved concave border between the cyst and compressed lung at the apex or base is the important differentiating feature.

Prognosis. Since many cystic lesions of the lung are completely asymptomatic and are discovered accidentally on chest films, it is safe to assume that a good many of those that might be discovered in this way in the neonatal period will never cause trouble. Once symptoms have developed, whether of increasing tension or of infection, the outlook becomes more serious. It is nevertheless true that most cystic-appearing lung lesions disappear with no surgical treatment.

Treatment. The absolute indication for immediate surgical treatment is increasing air tension within the cyst. This indication is unequivocal, and, what is more, radical intervention is called for. Repeated aspirations of air by needle and syringe or constant suction through an introduced catheter gives no more than temporary relief. They should be used, if at all, only for that reason, to tide the infant over a critical period until definitive operative measures can be taken. Operation should then consist of removal of as small a portion of the lung as is necessary, either a segment of a lobe or one or two lobes or the entire lung.

Infection within the cyst cavity constitutes the second indication for lobectomy or pneumonectomy. When there is pus, with or without air, within the cyst cavity, operation may be delayed until antibiotic and supportive therapy has improved the infant's general condition.

Cystic lesions that cause obstruction or infection are

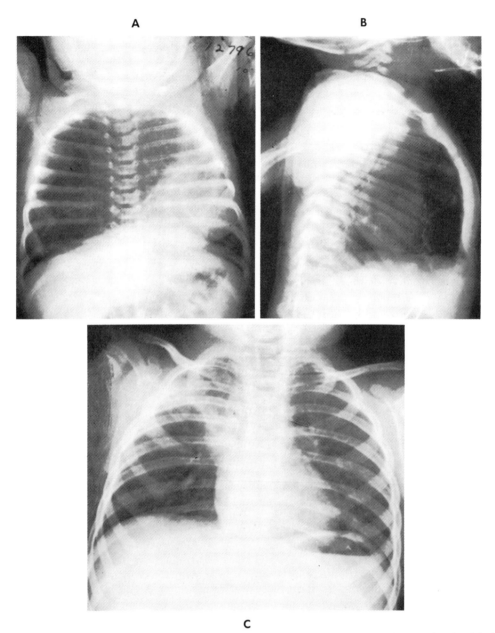

FIGURE 58–2. A, *Anteroposterior chest film taken at 1 month of age. Several cystic shadows can be made out within the right lung field. The right lung herniates across the midline to half fill the left upper part of the chest. The heart is displaced far to the left. B, Lateral view, same time. The sternum is thrust forward, and the heart is dislocated posteriorly by the herniated lung in the anterior mediastinum. Rounded cystic shadows can again be seen. C, Two years after operation: aside from pleural thickening at the right upper lobe and overaeration of the right lower lobe, the lungs appear quite normal. (Fischer, C. C., Tropea, F., Jr., and Bailey, C. P.: J. Pediatr. 23:219, 1943.)*

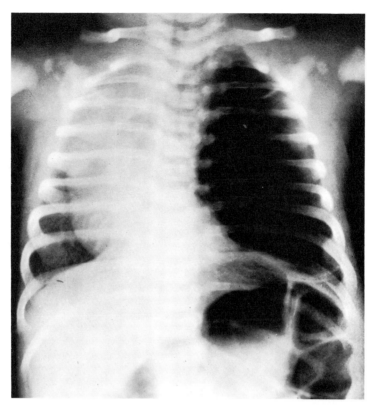

FIGURE 58–3. Anteroposterior chest film made at 8 weeks of age. Note the shift of heart and mediastinum far to the right, herniation of left lung into right hemithorax, and deviation of trachea to the right. The overfilled, overaerated left hemithorax suggests the appearance of tension cyst rather than pneumothorax because the left hilus is empty and the lower border is curved. No collapsed lung can be seen. (From Hill, L. F.: Conference at Raymond Blank Memorial Hospital for Children, Des Moines, Iowa. J. Pediatr. 38:511, 1951.)

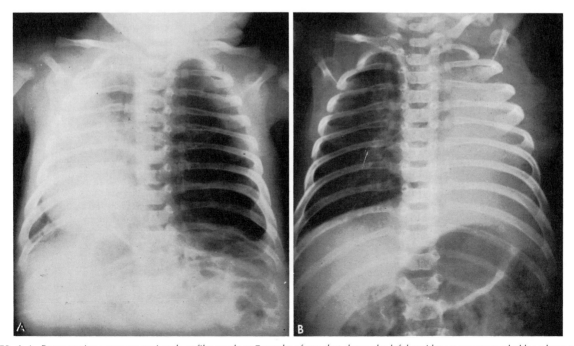

FIGURE 58–4. A, Preoperative anteroposterior chest film made at 7 weeks of age that shows the left hemithorax overexpanded by a huge translucent mass. Pneumothorax can be ruled out because the lower border is rounded, there is no shadow of collapsed lung, and fine trabecular markings are visible throughout most of the translucent area. The left upper lobe is herniated into the right upper hemithorax, and the heart and mediastinum are dislocated far to the right. B, Postoperative film shows the heart now displaced to the left, homogeneous opacification of the entire left hemithorax, probably due to thickened pleura, and compensatory emphysema of the right lung. (Leahy, L. J., and Butsch, W. L.: Surgical management of respiratory emergencies during the first few weeks of life. Arch. Surg. 59:466, 1949. Copyright 1949, American Medical Association.)

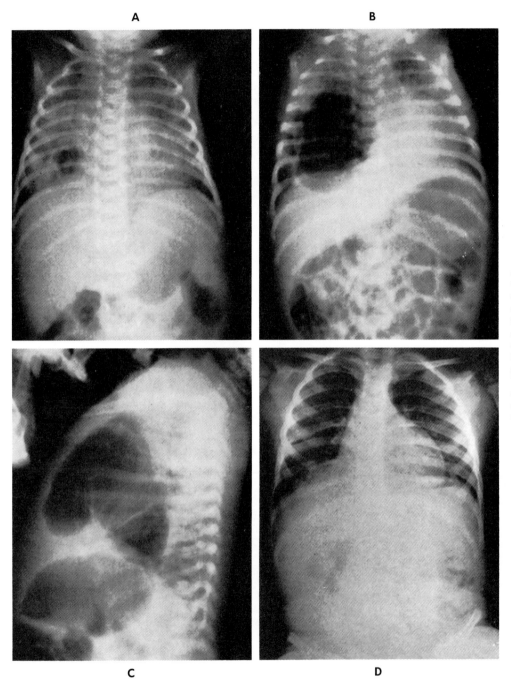

A

B

C

D

FIGURE 58–5. A, *Anteroposterior view of the chest taken on the 21st day of life. An air-filled cyst can be seen in the right lower part of the chest. B and C, Thirty days later, showing great increase in size of cyst and dislocation of heart toward the left axilla. D, Anteroposterior view at the age of 3 years. The lungs appear essentially normal. (Swan, H., and Aragon, G. E.: Pediatrics 14:651, 1954. Reproduced by permission of Pediatrics.)*

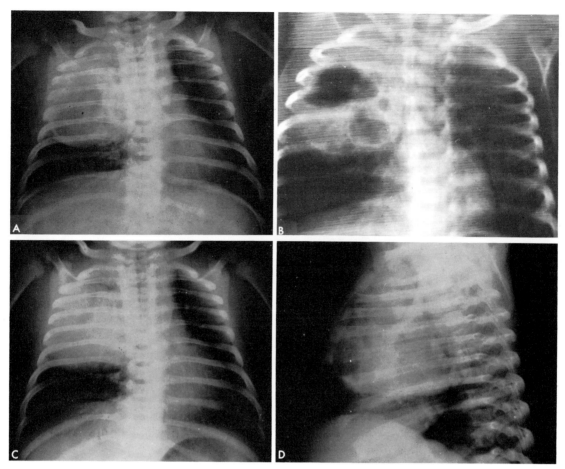

FIGURE 58–6. A to C, Anteroposterior views of the chest of an infant at different times showing the great variability in appearance of the same cystic lung. Differences in appearance depend upon whether one or all the component cysts are air-filled or fluid-filled at that particular time. D, Lateral view made on the same day that C was taken.

seldom lethal in themselves, and only treatment directed toward the underlying condition is indicated. If, after a waiting period of months, improvement has not occurred or if growth and development are retarded by persistent or repeated respiratory infection, it may be necessary to perform lobectomy or pneumonectomy.

CONGENITAL CYSTIC ADENOMATOID MALFORMATION

This condition may affect any single lobe of the lung, causing a great increase in mass from multiple cystic proliferation (Merenstein, 1969). The lesion is a type of hamartoma with cystic structures. Many of the infants are stillborn or premature or both. Associated malformations are present in about 20 per cent of affected infants. Owing to its great mass, this malformation displaces the mediastinum and impedes venous return to the heart, accounting for a 50 per cent incidence of hydrops fetalis. Because the cysts communicate with the airway and secrete fluid actively, polyhydramnios may occur prior to birth. After birth, for the same reason, the multiple cysts fill with air and produce further compression of the adjacent lung. If born alive, these infants have an early onset of respiratory distress, and the diagnosis is made by chest radiograph (Fig. 58–7). This condition may be confused with congenital diaphragmatic hernia, but in cystic malformation, the abdominal gas pattern is normal and a feeding catheter

follows the normal path. Prenatal diagnosis by ultrasonography can allow plans to be made for resection of the tumor immediately after delivery (Adzick et al., 1985).

■ INTRATHORACIC TUMORS AND FLUID-FILLED CYSTS

A large variety of solid tumors and fluid-filled cysts, in addition to the air-filled cysts just described, are encountered in the thoraces of adults. Many of these have already been observed in newborns, and we have no doubt that others will be recorded. Those that result from congenital maldevelopment, such as intrathoracic cysts of gastrointestinal origin and dermoid cysts, or teratomatous tumors, are more common in the neonatal period than are neoplasms and lymphomas. This last group, so common in adults as to account for up to 40 per cent of most series of mediastinal tumors, is of small numerical importance in the young infant. Too few neonatal cases have accumulated up to the present to warrant detailed classification.

Hope and Koop (1959) believe that intrathoracic mass lesions are best subdivided into those that arise in the posterior, middle, and anterior mediastinal spaces. A few others arise within the substance of the lung itself. In the posterior space, neurogenic tumors, duplications of the foregut, and neurenteric and bronchogenic cysts are most commonly encountered in the neonate. The middle mediastinum is the site almost exclusively of vascular lesions,

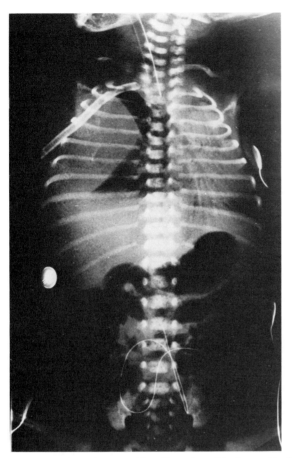

FIGURE 58–7. *Cystic adenomatoid malformation of the lung, with chest tube on the right.*

while enlarged thymus and teratomas are masses most often seen in the anterior mediastinal space.

THYMUS

The thymus occupies the upper anterior mediastinum, and it is more prominent in the newborn period than at any time of life. It may be so large as to reach the diaphragm or obscure both cardiac borders on radiographs. The normal thymus can be distinguished from an abnormal mass by the absence of tracheal deviation or compression. It changes in position with respiration and is less prominent with deep inspiration. It also involutes with stress as well as with corticosteroid therapy. Absence of the thymic shadow in an infant should alert one to the possibility of thymic agenesis and subacute combined immunodeficiency.

The cardiothymic-thoracic ratio provides an index of thymic size. Fletcher and associates (1979) as well as Gewolb and colleagues (1979) noted that a large ratio is present on the 1st day in infants at risk for hyaline membrane disease, presumably because of less than normal levels of glucocorticoids before birth.

Thymic cysts have been reported in infants but rarely in newborns. Thompson and Love (1972) described a persistent cervical thymoma in a newborn infant that presented as an outpouch in the sternal notch with crying.

MEDIASTINAL NEUROBLASTOMA

Neuroblastoma, the most common solid tumor in the mediastinum of infants, arises from neural tissue, either intercostal or sympathetic nerves for the most part. Because it typically lies in the thoracic gutter, it is almost always posterior in location, and it may involve superior, middle, or inferior mediastinum. From here it may extend to either side and invade one or both lungs. Extension through a vertebral foramen may result in neurologic manifestations.

Diagnosis is suggested by the discovery of an intrathoracic mass. It may follow roentgenography of the chest because of lower respiratory tract infection. Such infections afflict these infants more commonly than others because the growing tumor compresses bronchi. Alternatively, radiographs may be taken because of increasing dyspnea coupled with the physical signs of a solid intrathoracic mass.

Differentiation from other posterior mediastinal masses may be impossible before exploration. Neuroblastoma is not likely to be so sharply demarcated or to have so smooth and round a lower border as does a mediastinal cyst. Invasion of neighboring lung parenchyma strongly supports a diagnosis of neuroblastoma. Elevated urinary vanillylmandelic acid may be present. Its absence does not rule out neuroblastoma. (Fig. 58–8 and 58–9).

Treatment. Exploration is indicated for any intrathoracic mass. If the tumor proves to be neuroblastoma, as much of it should be excised as is feasible surgically. The tumor should be staged according to the system of Evans, and subsequent therapy should be dictated by the stage.

Prognosis. The outlook for neuroblastomas in extra-adrenal locations is better than that for their suprarenal counterparts (Young et al., 1970). If the lesion can be completely removed and if no distant metastases are present, the probable survival rate is better than 75 per cent.

BRONCHOGENIC CYSTS

Fluid-filled cysts of tracheobronchogenous origin are distinguished with difficulty from those of gastroenterogenous origin.

Incidence. In several series of cases of neoplasms and cysts of the mediastinum among patients of all ages reported from various clinics, bronchogenic cysts outnumber those of gastric or enteric derivation. Most observers comment upon the fact that the distribution differs in young infants and children, so that gastroenterogenous and enterogenous ones outnumber the bronchogenic. In a 20-year experience and review of the literature, de Paredes and associates (1970) found 68 cases and added 12 of their own. In the neonate, bronchogenic cysts are encountered infrequently.

Pathology. Bronchogenic cysts seldom attain large size. They contain clear fluid and are lined with columnar, cuboidal, or pseudostratified epithelium, and their walls generally contain smooth muscle and cartilage. They may, but do not always, communicate with the tracheobronchial tree. They tend to lie in the posterior mediastinum, but some have been found in the anterior space.

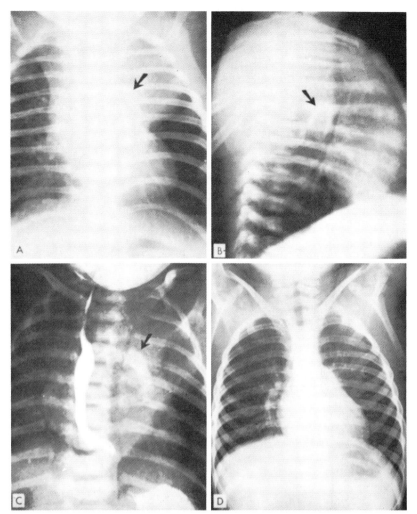

FIGURE 58–8. A 7-week-old male infant entered the hospital for repair of an inguinal hernia and was found to have an enlarged lymph node in the left cervical region. This finding prompted an x-ray examination of the chest. A, Anteroposterior roentgenogram showing a large area of density in the left upper hemithorax. Within the homogeneous density, a curvilinear calcification is present (arrow). B, Lateral roentgenogram showing the mass lesion to be in the posterior mediastinum with some anterior deviation of the trachea. The calcification appears to be in the shape of a horseshoe (arrow). C, Anteroposterior view of barium-filled esophagus showing the large size of the mass lesion more graphically. The calcification is more clearly visualized (arrow). At operation, the lesion proved to be a neuroblastoma. It was entirely excised. D, Posteroanterior roentgenogram 5 years later showing a normal chest. (From Hope, J. W., and Koop, C. E.: Differential diagnosis of mediastinal masses. Pediatr. Clin. North Am. 6:379, 1959.)

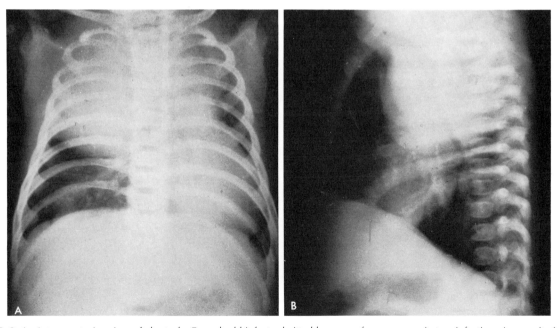

FIGURE 58–9. A, Anteroposterior view of chest of a 7-week-old infant admitted because of a severe respiratory infection. An opacity is seen filling the upper half of the right hemithorax and extending beyond the midline halfway to the left axilla. Its lower and left borders are rounded. The heart is displaced to the left and downward. The opacity gives the appearance of a solid tumor. B, Lateral view shows an opaque mass jutting forward from the posterior chest wall from the clavicle halfway down the chest to abut on the heart. Its outline is round.

At operation, a tumor was seen in the mediastinum that invaded all adjacent structures, including the left upper lobe. Biopsy revealed neuroblastoma. No excision was attempted. Radiotherapy was ineffective. Aminopterin was begun 2 months later and was followed by rapid improvement. Two years later, the patient appeared perfectly well, and no tumor was visualized on x-ray films. (Case 7 of Dr. Gladys Boyd, abstracted with her kind permission.)

Diagnosis. Lying as they do, near the carina, these cysts commonly produce signs of respiratory embarrassment from birth or soon after. Generally, their size is not such that they can be discovered by percussion or auscultation, but physical signs are likely to reveal their secondary effects, emphysema or atelectasis, rather than the tumor itself. Opsahl and Berman (1962) reported a case that showed emphysema on the left, followed by clearing, then equally notable emphysema on the right.

Radiographic examination often shows a mass projecting forward from the superior mediastinal shadow, not large and not necessarily rounded (Fig. 58–10 and 58–11). Ultrasonography can help localize the lesion.

Barium swallow may reveal indentation of the esophagus from an anterior direction.

Bronchoscopy reveals compression of the trachea and often of one major bronchus.

Treatment. Immediate excision should be performed.

ESOPHAGEAL, GASTROGENIC, AND ENTEROGENOUS CYSTS

These three varieties of intrathoracic fluid-filled cysts are discussed together, since they are indistinguishable on clinical grounds.

Incidence. Together they constitute a large group of mediastinal masses found in the neonatal period. Although they are not encountered frequently, they are far from uncommon.

Pathology and Etiology. These cysts are duplicated segments of gut that have become partially or completely detached from the parent viscus. They lie in or near the posterior mediastinum but, with increasing size, may project far into one or the other hemithorax. Their walls are composed of a mucosal layer, characteristic of that of their site of origin, and of one or more muscular layers. They contain fluid that is also similar to the secretion normally manufactured in their parent locus. The material within gastrogenic cysts contains pepsin, protein, and inorganic salts in roughly the same concentrations as are present in gastric juice.

The foregut becomes duplicated in the course of embryonic development by failure of complete resorption of occluding epithelium, resulting in the formation of a supernumerary wall. The high percentage of vertebral malformations coincident with gastroenterogenous cysts led Veeneklaas (1952) to suggest that the primary embryonic defect lies in abnormal persistence of the primitive adherence of notochord to foregut. When foregut descends from its early position in the region of the neck, this adhesion causes anomalies in vertebral bodies derived from notochord and pinches off a portion of the foregut and prevents its descent.

Diagnosis. Symptoms depend upon the size and location of the cyst. Since the cysts are all posterior and lie close to the trachea, esophagus, and great vessels, they are seldom symptomless. Cyanosis, tachypnea, and dyspnea are often present from birth. Swallowing difficulty and vomiting are less frequent. Recurrent lower respiratory tract infections characterize a few. Hemorrhage, from either the mouth or nose, from lungs or stomach, or in the form of melena, is not at all uncommon. In most instances, hemorrhage indicates that the cyst is of gastrogenic origin, since the fluid within these cysts contains pepsin and is capable of eroding through the cyst wall to break down adjacent blood vessels. Technetium scans should be useful in delineating cysts lined with gastric mucosa.

Radiographs of the chest show abnormal shadows that are often difficult to distinguish from unusual cardiac contours (Fig. 58–12). Lateral and oblique films may be needed in order to make the differentiation with certainty. In one or another projection, the rounded border of the cyst contiguous to the heart should be able to be visualized. Barium swallow commonly shows displacement of the esophagus. Gastroenterogenous cysts may either partially or totally compress the bronchus, with consequent overdistention or atelectasis. Sometimes, the symptoms are intermittent as the cyst enlarges or empties.

Bronchoscopy and esophagoscopy are not ordinarily required in order to clinch the diagnosis. When performed, they may show compression of one or both structures from without. Cyst puncture should not be performed.

Superina and colleagues (1984) reviewed 25 years' experience with neurenteric cysts at the Hospital for Sick Children in Toronto and noted that a spinal component may accompany the mediastinal cyst in as many as 20 per cent of the children. They recommend careful radiographic evaluation of the spinal canal with CT scan and excision of the cyst if possible.

Treatment. Operation is indicated as soon as the diagnosis of mediastinal mass is made. It is neither necessary nor wise to delay exploration until a specific diagnosis has been made.

MEDIASTINAL TERATOMAS

The shadow of the enlarged thymus is the most common radiopaque mass visualized in the anterior mediastinum of the newborn. The enlarged thymus, however, appears to cause little if any trouble in the neonatal period. Thymoma has not been reported. When an anterior mediastinal mass is associated with respiratory distress in the newborn, the strong likelihood is that the lesion is a teratoma (Fig. 58–13). Seibert and co-workers (1976) reported one infant with tracheal compression from a teratoma. Normal thymus should not compress the trachea or great vessels. All other anterior masses (lymphomas, lymphangiomas, substernal thyroids, etc.) occur with the utmost infrequency in this age period.

FIBROSARCOMA OF THE LUNG

An unusual solid tumor of the lung in a newborn was reported to us in a personal communication from Sir Douglas Robb, of Auckland, New Zealand. As far as we can determine, this is the only fibrosarcoma of the lung thus far identified in a newborn.

HAMARTOMA OF LUNG

Hamartoma is not a true neoplasm. It is a mass composed of the normal elements that make up an organ,

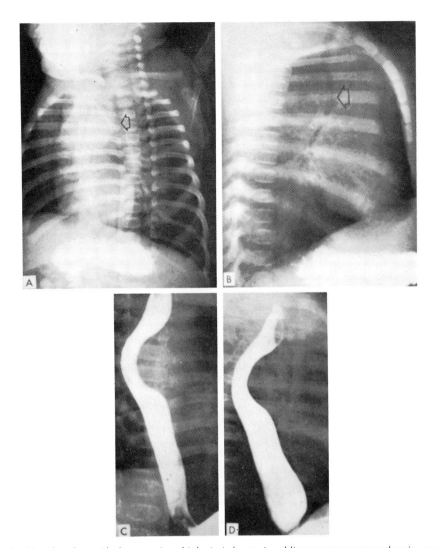

FIGURE 58–10. *A 10-week-old male infant with dyspnea since birth. A, Left anterior oblique roentgenogram showing a mass lesion just below the carina (arrow). B, Lateral roentgenogram showing anterior deviation of the trachea (arrow). C, Anteroposterior view of barium-filled esophagus showing extreme deviation of the esophagus to the right just above the level of the carina. D, Lateral view of barium-filled esophagus showing posterior deviation of the esophagus just above the level of the carina. A bronchogenic cyst was removed at operation. (From Hope, J. W., and Koop, C. E.: Differential diagnosis of mediastinal masses. Pediatr. Clin. North Am. 6:379, 1959.)*

FIGURE 58–11. *Air within the stomach shows the level of the left hemidiaphragm. The ribs on the left are separated, and the mediastinal structures are displaced slightly to the right. At thoracotomy, the left lung was large and engorged. During operation, the lung became aerated, presumably as bronchial obstruction was relieved, and a bronchogenic cyst was removed. (From Griscom, N. T., Harris, G. B. C., Wohl, M. E. B., Vawter, G. F., Eraklis, A. J.: Fluid filled lung due to airway obstruction in the newborn. Pediatrics 43:383, 1969. Reproduced by permission of Pediatrics.)*

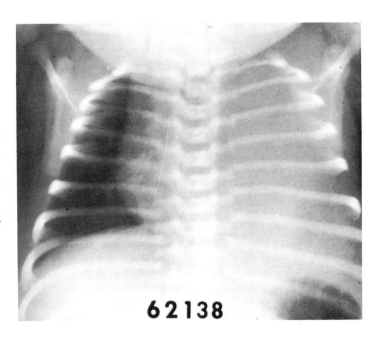

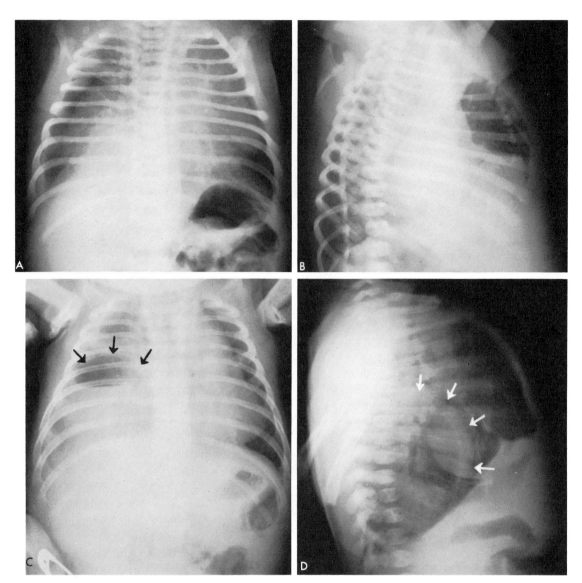

FIGURE 58–12. ENTEROGENOUS CYST. A, Anteroposterior view of the chest taken within the first week of life, interpreted as showing atelectasis of right upper and lower lobes. The left border of the heart almost touches the left axillary wall, while its right border appears to be almost as far in the right hemithorax. It is difficult to tell whether this shadow is that of a hugely enlarged heart or whether it is composed of more than one element. B, Lateral view showing the opacity filling the lower half of the chest, which is also difficult to diagnose, but it almost surely is not all heart. C, Anteroposterior view taken 4 weeks later. In the interim, fluid had been withdrawn six times, and in the process air had been introduced into the right hemithorax. Now one can see a mass in the right middle and lower hemithorax containing a bubble of air that delineates its rounded upper border. Removal of fluid has permitted the heart to return to a position more nearly normal. D, Lateral view, same day. Here the rounded margin of almost the entire cyst can be visualized. (From Leahy, L. J., and Butsch, W. L.: Surgical management of respiratory emergencies during the first few weeks of life. Arch. Surg. 59:466, 1949. Copyright 1949, American Medical Association.)

combined in an abnormal manner. In the lung it is usually encapsulated and firm and ordinarily does not attain a great size. Under the microscope, varying amounts of mesenchymal and epithelial elements are seen, often surrounding bits of cartilage.

■ PULMONARY SEQUESTRATION

More than 300 cases of pulmonary sequestration have been reported in the literature; these were reviewed by Carter in 1969 and by Landing in 1979. They have rarely produced symptoms in newborn infants and have usually been detected on chest films taken for other reasons. A sequestered lobe sometimes manifests itself in children or young adults by repeated infections in a fluid-filled cyst. The lesion should be suspected in infants with cystic lesions, especially in the lower lobes (Fig. 58–14).

The malformation is slightly more common in males and is distinctly more likely on the left side. Approximately two-thirds of the cases involve the left lower lobe. Sequestration is a term for lung tissue that does not communicate with the tracheobronchial tree and that derives its blood supply from the aorta. Anomalous arteries from above or below the diaphragm supply the sequestered lobe. The venous drainage may be pulmonary or systemic. In over 80 per cent of the cases, a communication with the foregut can be demonstrated by contrast studies (Heithoff et al., 1976). The usual location is the lower esophagus or gastric fundus. The affected lung is highly abnormal, consisting of atelectatic areas interspersed with fluid-filled cysts. There is an increased incidence of associated malformations, e.g., diaphragmatic hernia, congenital heart disease, eventration of the diaphragm, enterogenous cysts, and vertebral or rib anomalies. Pulmonary

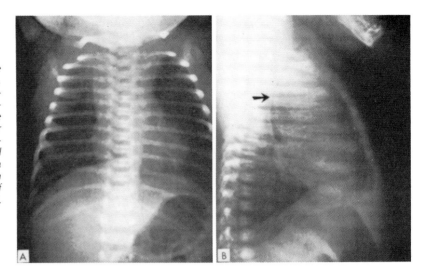

FIGURE 58–13. An 11-day-old male infant with severe respiratory distress and cyanosis since 2 days of age. A, Anteroposterior roentgenogram showing extreme hyper-aeration of both lung fields and a wide superior mediastinum. B, Lateral roentgenogram showing extreme hyperaeration of the lungs and a mass filling the anterior mediastinum producing posterior deviation and compression of the trachea (arrow). The tumor was excised and proved to be a benign teratoma lying behind a normal thymus gland and in front of the trachea. (From Hope, J. W., and Koop, C. E.: Differential diagnosis of mediastinal masses. Pediatr. Clin. North Am. 6:379, 1959.)

sequestration is thought to be caused by an accessory lung bud originating lower down in the primitive foregut. If the bud originates early, the normal and sequestered lung have a common pleural covering, whereas if the supernumerary bud originates later, the sequestered lung has its own pleura. If the sequestered lobe is found to obtain its blood supply from the pulmonary system, it may be called an accessory lobe.

Most infants with pulmonary sequestration are not symptomatic in the neonatal period, but if the sequestration is large, there may be persistent respiratory distress (Pearl, 1972). Later, frequent bouts of pneumonia may occur. On the chest radiograph, the classic appearance consists of a triangular or oval-shaped basal lung mass on one side of the chest. Ultrasound examination confirms the presence of a thoracic mass. The barium swallow frequently demonstrates contrast entering the sequestered lung. Treatment consists of surgical resection, because repeated infections are the rule. It is helpful to have an angiographic study preoperatively to alert the surgeon to the position of anomalous vessels.

■ CONGENITAL PULMONARY LYMPHANGIECTASIS

Congenital pulmonary lymphangiectasis is a congenital abnormality of the pulmonary lymphatic vessels and has been characterized into two principal groups: (1) cases associated with congenital heart disease, and (2) cases not associated with congenital heart disease. The cardiac anomalies may include hypoplastic left heart syndrome, total anomalous pulmonary venous drainage, and pul-

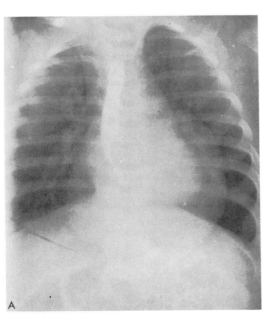
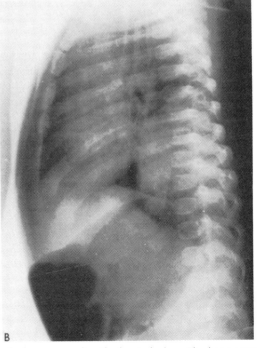

FIGURE 58–14. A, Anteroposterior view shows a homogeneous circular shadow surrounding the heart shadow. The heart appears normal, the lungs clear. B, In the lateral view, the disc-shaped mass lies in the posterior mediastinum, and proved to be an accessory lobe, a variant of pulmonary sequestration which derives its blood supply from the pulmonary, instead of the systemic, system.

monary stenosis, including Noonan syndrome. The group that does not include associated cardiac anomalies may be of early or late onset and has a wide spectrum of severity. In some individuals the lesion is asymptomatic, while in others it can lead to severe respiratory failure, usually in the first hours after birth, but sometimes during the first weeks or months of life. Most infants with this condition die early in the neonatal period. Pulmonary lymphangiectasis has been reported twice as often in males and has been seen in families (Scott-Emuakpor et al., 1981).

Usually, the radiologist is the first to suggest the diagnosis after observing dilated lymphatic vessels and sometimes small accumulations of pleural fluid on the chest film. The older infant may have no symptoms or mild to moderate tachypnea with various degrees of hypoxemia. If pleural fluid has accumulated, examination of the fluid is important. If the infant has received milk feedings, it will be chylous, and if not, there will be an elevation in mononuclear cells and moderate protein of up to about 4 per cent. These findings in the absence of fever or other signs of systemic illness are diagnostic of impaired lymphatic drainage.

Lung biopsy is probably not indicated and can be hazardous because, once the distended lymphatic channels are severed, they can leak fluid for weeks. Only if the diagnosis is in doubt is open lung biopsy appropriate.

In non–cardiac-associated diffuse lymphangiectasis only supportive treatment is available. The long-term prognosis depends on the severity of the lesion, but this form of pulmonary lymphangiectasis is compatible with asymptomatic life as an adult (Wohl, 1989).

■ CONGENITAL LOBAR EMPHYSEMA

Congenital lobar emphysema describes a condition with respiratory distress caused by overinflation of one lobe of the lung, usually the left upper, right upper, or right middle lobe. Onset may be anytime in the first 6 months of life, but frequently in the newborn period. The respiratory distress may be severe, but in many cases it is mild, without cyanosis in room air. The chest radiograph shows overdistension of one lobe, compression of the adjacent lung, herniation across the mediastinum, and diaphragmatic depression. About 15 per cent of the cases are associated with congenital heart disease. Before making this diagnosis, a mucus plug obstruction should be excluded by vigorous physical therapy or sometimes bronchoscopy.

Some authors contend that most cases are caused by local bronchial cartilage deficiency, with airway closure and gas trapping in exhalation (Campbell, 1969). Other causes have been suggested, e.g., redundant bronchial mucosal fold, stenosis of the bronchial wall, or external compression by an anomalous pulmonary artery. It is possible for a lobe to be rotated on its pedicle with resultant obstruction (Hislop and Reid, 1971). Sometimes the condition represents a polyalveolar lobe in which, despite a normal number of airways, there is a five-fold increase in the number of alveoli in each acinus (Hislop and Reid, 1970).

In those with severe respiratory distress, the treatment is surgical lobectomy, the results of which have been excellent. In those infants with mild tachypnea and no significant oxygen requirement, the treatment may be expectant (Shannon et al., 1977). The mild symptoms frequently subside by the age of 1 year. No matter whether treated medically or surgically, at age 10 all such children have evidence of mild airway obstruction, suggesting a more generalized abnormality (McBride et al., 1980).

■ PULMONARY HYPOPLASIA

Pulmonary hypoplasia is a pathologic condition in which the combined lung weight is less than 1.2 per cent of body weight, the standardized autopsy lung volume is less than 60 per cent of predicted lung volume, lung DNA is less than 100 mg/kg of body weight, or the radial alveolar count is less than 4 (Langston and Thurlbeck, 1986). On the chest radiograph, the lungs appear small and clear, unless another condition is superimposed. These infants have hypercarbia, which responds poorly to mechanical ventilation, and the risk of pneumothorax is high. They often have persistent pulmonary hypertension, due to a reduced vascular bed and secondary arterial muscle hypertrophy (Hislop et al., 1979).

Normal lung growth is dependent on lung distention (Wigglesworth and Desai, 1982), which in turn is dependent on space to occupy, and expansion caused by lung fluid secretion and fetal breathing. Conditions causing oligohydramnios and fetal compression are associated with pulmonary hypoplasia. These include renal agenesis, renal dysplasia, obstructive uropathy (Thomas and Smith, 1974), and chronic amnion rupture (Thibeault et al., 1985). Lung compression may also be due to congenital diaphragmatic hernia, eventration of the diaphragm, ascites, or pleural effusion, all of which may cause pulmonary hypoplasia. Effective fetal breathing may be impaired by chest cage insufficiency as in congenital thoracic dystrophy, by neuromuscular problems such as motor neuron disease or myotonic dystrophy, and by brain malformations that affect the brain stem, such as iniencephaly. Patients with giant omphalocele may have pulmonary hypoplasia because the lower chest cage is not adequately supported by abdominal contents (Hershenson et al., 1985). Finally, in a significant number of infants, no cause for primary pulmonary hypoplasia can be found (Swischuk et al., 1979), although suppression of fetal breathing caused by maternal use of tobacco, barbiturates, or ethanol may be implicated (Collins et al., 1985).

In many cases of hypoplasia, the number of bronchial generations is reduced, suggesting an insult occurring between 10 and 14 weeks' gestation, as in diaphragmatic hernia or renal dysplasia. Although the total number of acini is reduced, the number of alveoli per acinus is relatively well preserved (Hislop et al., 1979). In many cases of chronic amnion rupture, the onset is much later, the bronchial number is normal, and the number of alveoli per acinus is reduced.

The possibilities for treatment are limited. A major objective of fetal surgery today is the relief of fetal lung compression, such as that caused by diaphragmatic hernia.

■ PULMONARY HEMANGIOMATOSIS

Pulmonary hemangiomatosis is a proliferation of small blood vessels that may be peribronchovascular, septal, or pleural in location. If the lesions also involve the airways, hemoptysis may occur.

Natural History. Pulmonary hemangiomatosis may be a part of a disseminated hemangiomatosis that can involve the liver, gastrointestinal tract, central nervous system, and skin. Cutaneous lesions may be present at birth or develop within the first few weeks of life. In some instances, the hemangiomas may be confined to the lung and remain asymptomatic until childhood. Since the flow through the hemangiomas in the lung is right to left, there is significant venous admixture and associated clubbing of all digits. In some instances, clubbing may take place even in the absence of arterial desaturation. The major symptom is dyspnea, which is progressive. The most likely cause of death is from bleeding or in adults from pulmonary hypertension.

Diagnosis. The diagnosis is suggested by the chest film, which may resemble an interstitial infiltrate or thickened fissures. Pulmonary angiography or magnetic resonance imaging are useful in diagnosis.

Treatment. In at least one instance, a 12-year old boy had a good response to treatment with interferon alfa–2a administered subcutaneously. He received daily interferon therapy for 14 months during which his dyspnea remitted, his digital clubbing resolved, and his pulmonary function tests were restored to normal. Abnormal vessels were still evident in the angiogram, but their density had been substantially reduced (White et al., 1989). This therapy seems to be less toxic than long-term corticosteroids or cyclophosphamides, which have been used in the past.

Prognosis. Experience with interferon is too recent to know whether all visceral hemangiomas will respond.

■ PULMONARY ARTERIOVENOUS FISTULA OR ANGIOMA

Although rare, pulmonary arteriovenous fistula or angioma is characterized by persistent cyanosis in the newborn, but unless the fistula is large and compresses the surrounding lung, it does not cause respiratory difficulty (Hodgson et al., 1959). Lesions may be single or multiple and aneurysmal or microscopic in size. About 50 per cent of the cases are associated with hereditary hemorrhagic telangiectasia. The chest radiograph most commonly shows a small mass lesion, usually in the lower lobes; the electrocardiogram may suggest unusual left-ventricular dominance. The diagnosis is made by radionuclide perfusion study or digital subtraction angiography, and the treatment is surgical excision if possible. For large lesions, embolotherapy is useful. Multiple hemangiomas may respond to glucocorticoid therapy or newer inhibitors of angiogenesis. The mortality and morbidity in untreated cases is considerable (Dines et al., 1983). Fewer than 10 per cent are diagnosed in infancy (Adzick et al., 1985).

■ REFERENCES

Abell, M. R.: Mediastinal cysts. A.M.A. Arch. Pathol. 61:360, 1956.

Adzick, N. S., Harrison, M. R., and Glick, P. C.: Fetal cystic adenomatoid malformation: Prenatal diagnosis and natural history. J. Pediatr. Surg. 20:483, 1985.

Anspach, W. E., and Wolman, I. J.: Large pulmonary air cysts of infancy, with special reference to pathogenesis and diagnosis. Surg. Gynecol. Obstet. 56:634, 1933.

Bates, M.: Total unilateral pulmonary sequestration. Thorax 23:311, 1968.

Boyd, G. L.: Solid intrathoracic masses in children. Pediatrics 19:142, 1957.

Brooks, J. W.: Tumors of the chest. In Kendig, E. L., and Chernick, V. (Eds.): Disorders of the Respiratory Tract in Children. Philadelphia, W. B. Saunders Company, 1983.

Buntain, W. L., Isaacs, H., Payne, V. C., et al.: Lobar emphysema, cystic adenomatoid malformation, pulmonary sequestration and bronchogenic cyst in infancy and childhood: A clinical group. J. Pediatr. Surg. 9:85, 1974.

Burnett, W. E., and Caswell, H. T.: Lobectomy for pulmonary cysts in a fifteen-day-old infant with recovery. Surgery 23:84, 1948.

Caffey, J.: On the natural regression of pulmonary cysts during early infancy. Pediatrics 11:48, 1953.

Campbell, P. E.: Congenital lobar emphysema: Etiological studies. Aust. Paediatr. J. 5:226, 1969.

Carter, R.: Pulmonary sequestration—collective review. Ann. Thorac. Surg. 7:68, 1969.

Clark, N. S., Nairn, R. C., and Gowar, F. J. S.: Cystic disease of the lung in the newborn treated by pneumonectomy. Arch. Dis. Child. 31:358, 1956.

Collins, M. D., Moessinger, A. C., Kleinerman, J., et al.: Fetal lung hypoplasia associated with maternal smoking: A morphometric analysis. Pediatr. Res. 19:408, 1985.

Cooke, F. N., and Blades, B. B.: Cystic disease of the lungs. J. Thorac. Surg. 23:546, 1952.

de Paredes, C. G., Pierce, W. S., Johnson, D. G., et al.: Pulmonary sequestration in infants and children. A 20-year experience and review of the literature. J. Pediatr. Surg. 5:136, 1970.

Dines, D. E., Seward, J. B., Bernatz, P. E., et al.: Pulmonary arteriovenous fistulas. Mayo Clin. Proc.58:176, 1983.

Ellis, F. H., Jr., Kirklin, J. W., Hodgson, et al.: Surgical implications of the mediastinal shadow in thoracic roentgenograms of infants and children. Surg. Gynecol. Obstet. 100:532, 1955.

Erkalis, A. J., Griscom, N. T., and McGovern, J. B.: Bronchogenic cyst of the mediastinum. N. Engl. J. Med. 281:1150, 1969.

Evans, A. E., D'Angio, G. J., and Randolph, J.: A proposed staging for children with neuroblastoma. Cancer 27:324, 1971.

Ferguson, C. C., Young, L. N., Sutherland, J. B., et al.: Intrathoracic gastrogenic cyst—preoperative diagnosis by technetium pertechnetate scan. J. Pediatr. Surg. 8:827, 1973.

Fischer, C. C., Tropea, F., Jr., and Bailey, C. P.: Congenital pulmonary cysts; report of an infant treated by lobectomy with recovery. J. Pediatr. 23:219, 1943.

Fletcher, B. D., Masson, M., Lisbona, A., et al.: Thymic response to endogenous and exogenous steroids in premature infants. J. Pediatr. 95:111, 1979.

France, N. E., and Brown, R. J. K.: Congenital pulmonary lymphagiectasis. Report of 11 examples with special reference to cardiovascular findings. Arch. Dis. Child. 46:528, 1971.

Gerle, R. D., Jaretski, A., Ashley, C. A., et al.: Congenital bronchopulmonary foregut malformation. Pulmonary sequestration communicating with the gastrointestinal tract. N. Engl. J. Med.278:1413, 1968.

Gewolb, I. H., Lebowitz, R. L., and Taeusch, H. W.: Thymic size and its relationship to the respiratory distress syndrome. J. Pediatr. 95:108, 1979.

Goodwin, S. R., Graven, S. A., and Haberkern, C. M.: Aspiration in intubated premature infants. Pediatrics 75:85, 1985.

Gottschalk, W., and Abramson, D.: Placental edema and fetal hydrops. Obstet. Gynecol. 10:626, 1957.

Graham, G. G., and Singleton, J. W.: Diffuse hamartoma of the upper lobe in an infant: Report of successful surgical removal. A.M.A. J. Dis. Child. 89:609, 1955.

Gross, R. E.: Congenital cystic lung: Successful pneumonectomy in a three-week-old baby. Ann. Surg. 123:229, 1946.

Gwinn, J. L., Lee, F. A., and Rao, P. S. Radiological case of the month. Am. J. Dis. Child. 119:341, 1970.

Heitoff, K. B., Sane, S. M., Williams, H. J., et al.: Bronchopulmonary foregut malformations: A unifying etiological concept. Am. J. Roentgenol. 126:46, 1976.

Hershenson, M. B., Brouillette, R. T., Klemka, L., et al.: Respiratory insufficiency in newborns with abdominal wall defects. J. Pediatr. Surg. *20*:348, 1985.

Hill, L. F.: Conference at Raymond Blank Memorial Hospital for Children, Des Moines, Iowa, J. Pediatr. *38*:511, 1951.

Hislop, A., Hey, E., and Reid, L.: The lungs in congenital bilateral renal agenesis and dysplasia. Arch. Dis. Child. *54*:32, 1979.

Hislop, A., and Reid, L.: New pathological findings in emphysema of childhood: Polyalveolar lobe with emphysema. Thorax *25*:682, 1970.

Hislop, A., and Reid, L.: New pathological findings in emphysema of childhood: Overinflation of a normal lobe. Thorax *26*:190, 1971.

Hodgson, C. H., Burchell, H. B., Good, C. A., et al.: Hereditary hemorrhagic telangectasia and pulmonary arteriovenous fistula. N. Engl. J. Med. *261*:625, 1959.

Holder, T. M., and Christy, M. G.: Cystic adenomatoid malformation of the lung. J. Thorac. Cardiovasc. Surg. *47*:590, 1964.

Hope, J. W., and Koop, C. E.: Differential diagnosis of mediastinal masses. Pediatr. Clin. N. Amer. *6*:379, 1959.

Izzo, C., and Rickham, P. P.: Neonatal pulmonary hamartoma. J. Pediatr. Surg. *3*:77, 1968.

Kafka, V., and Beco, V.: Simultaneous intra- and extrapulmonary sequestration. Arch. Dis. Child. *35*:51, 1960.

Kwittken, J., and Reiner, L.: Congenital cystic adenomatoid malformation of the lung. Pediatrics *30*:759, 1962.

Landing, B. H.: Congenital malformations and genetic disorders of the respiratory tract (larynx, trachea, bronchi and lungs). Am. Rev. Resp. Dis. *120*:151, 1979.

Langston, C., and Thurlbeck, W. M.: Conditions altering normal lung growth and development. *In* Thibeault, D. W., and Gregory, G. S. (Eds.): Neonatal Pulmonary Care. Norwalk, Conn., Appleton-Century-Crofts, 1986.

Leahy, L. J., and Butsch, W. L.: Surgical management of respiratory emergencies during the first few weeks of life. Arch. Surg. *59*:466, 1949.

McBride, J. T., Wohl, M. E. B., Strieder, D. J., et al.: Lung growth and airway function after lobectomy in infancy for congenital lobar emphysema. J. Clin. Invest. *66*:962, 1980.

Merenstein, G. B. Congenital cystic adenomatoid malformation of the lung. Am. J. Dis. Child. *118*:772, 1969.

Nishibayashi, S. W., Andrassy, R. J., and Woolley, M. M.: Congenital cystic adenomatoid malformation: A 30-year experience. J. Pediatr. Surg. *16*:704, 1981.

Opsahl, T., and Berman, E. J.: Bronchogenic mediastinal cysts in infants: Case report and review of the literature. Pediatrics *30*:372, 1962.

Pearl, M.: Sequestration of the lung. Am. J. Dis. Child *124*:706, 1972.

Sabiston, D. C., Jr., and Scott, H. W., Jr.: Primary neoplasms and cysts of the mediastinum. Ann. Surg. *136*:777, 1952.

Scott-Emuakpor, A. B., Warren, S. T., Kapur, S., et al.: Familial occurrence of congenital pulmonary lymphangiectasis: Genetic implications. Am. J. Dis. Child. *135*:532, 1981.

Seibert, J. J., Marvin, W. J., and Schieker, R. M.: Mediastinal teratoma: a rare cause of severe respiratory distress in the newborn. J. Pediatr. Surg. *11*:253, 1976.

Shannon, D. C., Todres, I. D., and Moylan, F. M. B.: Infantile lobar hyperinflation: Expectant treatment. Pediatrics *59*:1012, 1977.

Spock, A., Schneider, S., and Baylin, G. J.: Mediastinal gastric cysts: A case report and review of the English literature. Am. Rev. Resp. Dis. *94*:97, 1966.

Stocker, J. T., Drake, R. M., and Madewell, J. E.: Cystic and congenital lung disease in the newborn. Perspect. Pediat. Path. *4*:93, 1978.

Superina, R. A., Ein, S. H., and Humphreys, R. P.: Cystic duplications of the esophagus and neuroenteric cysts. J. Pediatr. Surg. *19*:527, 1984.

Swan, H., and Aragon, G. E.: Surgical treatment of pulmonary cysts in infancy. Pediatrics *14*:651, 1954.

Swischuk, L. E., Richarson, C. J., Nichols, M. M., et al. Primary pulmonary hypoplasia in the neonate. J. Pediatr. *95*:573, 1979.

Thibeault, D. W., Beatty, E. C., Hall, R. T., et la.: Neonatal pulmonary hypoplasia with premature rupture of fetal membranes and oligohydramnios. J. Pediatr. *107*:273, 1985.

Thomas, I. T., and Smith, D. W.: Oligohydramnios, cause of the non-renal features of Potter's syndrome, including pulmonary hypoplasia. J. Pediatr. *84*:811, 1974.

Thompson, R. E., and Love, W. G.: Persistent cervical thymoma, apparent with crying. Am. J. Dis. Child. *124*:761, 1972.

Veeneklaas, G. M. H.: Pathogenesis of intrathoracic gastrogenic cysts. Am. J. Dis. Child. *83*:500, 1952.

Wexler, H. A., and Valdes-Dapena, M.: Congenital cystic adenomatoid malformation: A report of three unusual cases. Radiology *126*:737, 1978.

White, C. W.: Treatment of hemangiomatosis with recombinant interferon alpha. Semin. Hematol. *27*:15, 1990.

White, C. W., Sondheimer, H. M., Crough, E. C., et al.: Treatment of pulmonary hemangiomatosis with recombinant interferon alfa–2a. N. Engl. J. Med. *320*:1197, 1989.

Wigglesworth, J. S., and Desai, R.: Is fetal respiratory function a major determinant of perinatal survival? Lancet *1*:264, 1982.

Wohl, M. E. B.: Case record of Massachusetts General Hospital. N. Engl. J. Med. *321*:309, 1989.

Young, L. W., Rubin, P., and Hanson, R. E.: The extra-adrenal neuroblastoma: High radiocurability and diagnostic accuracy. Am. J. Roentgenol. *108*:75, 1970.

ACCUMULATION OF FLUID IN THE PLEURAL SPACE

59

Thomas Hansen and Anthony Corbet

■ PLEURAL EFFUSION

The pleural space exists between the parietal pleura of the chest wall and the visceral pleura of the lung. Each pleural surface is comprised of a mesothelial layer that covers a layer of connective tissue containing lymphatics, blood vessels, and nerves. In the parietal pleura, lymphatic channels communicate with the pleural space to provide a direct pathway for fluid and protein reabsorption. It was initially believed that the blood supply to the parietal pleura emanated from the systemic circulation, and that the blood supply to the visceral pleura emanated from the pulmonary circulation. The capillary hydrostatic pressure in the visceral pleura was believed to be correspondingly low leading to the assumption that fluid was filtered out of the parietal pleura and reabsorbed by the visceral pleura. Recent data shows, however, that the blood supply to the visceral pleura emanates from the bronchial circulation: both pleural surfaces filter fluid into the pleural space, and the lymphatics are responsible for most of the fluid reabsorption (Wiener-Kronish et al., 1985).

Fluid accumulates in the pleural space only if the rate of filtration increases or if the rate of lymphatic clearance decreases (or if both of these processes occur). The rate of fluid filtration can be increased by increasing the filtration pressure. The parietal pleura is drained by the systemic veins while the visceral pleura is drained by the pulmonary veins. Therefore, filtration pressure increases with increases in either systemic or pulmonary venous pressure. Raised venous pressure (along with hypoproteinemia) is the most likely etiology for pleural effusions that complicate heart failure as well as for effusions that occur with hydrops fetalis. The rate of fluid filtration into the pleural space also increases if the permeability of the pleura to water and protein increases (e.g., with infection).

Any impairment of lymphatic function from direct mechanical obstruction or from raised central venous pressure has marked effects on the rate of clearance of pleural fluid (Mellins et al., 1970). Raised venous pressure contributes substantially to the problem of effusions complicating heart failure or hydrops fetalis and also accounts for the massive pleural effusions that accompany superior vena cava thrombosis (Dhande et al., 1983).

Pleural effusions should be suspected in any infant with respiratory difficulty who is hydropic or who has been receiving intravenous nutrition. Infants who receive central venous alimentation should have the glucose content of their pleural fluid checked immediately to make sure that the catheter has not perforated into the pleural space. Differential breath sounds are valuable in localizing unilateral effusions. The chest radiograph is diagnostic (Fig. 59–1). Thoracentesis is useful to identify effusions secondary to infections and to distinguish chylothorax from other causes of pleural effusions.

Infants with hydrops fetalis can occasionally have effusions that are large enough to impair ventilation and require drainage in the delivery room. Once the underlying abnormality is corrected, most effusions resolve without further need for drainage. Effusions that accompany superior vena cava syndrome can persist and require interventions similar to those described for persistent chylothorax.

■ CHYLOTHORAX

Accumulations of chyle in the pleural space may be congenital or acquired. Congenital chylothorax is probably one part of the spectrum of anomalies that result from intrauterine obstruction of the thoracic duct (Chervenak et al., 1983; Smeltzer et al., 1986). It may occur alone or

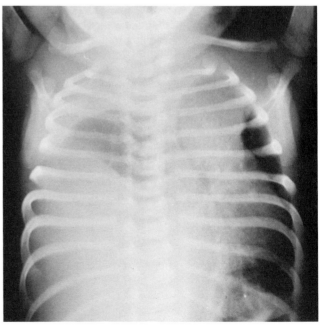

FIGURE 59–1. Chest radiograph of an infant with a right-sided chylothorax.

555

TABLE 59–1. Composition of Chyle

Measurement	Units	Mean	Range		
Total protein	g/dl	3.56	1.89	to	6.17
Albumin	g/dl	2.24	1.26	to	3.0
Total lipids	mg/dl	1,180	56	to	3,500
Cholesterol	mg/dl	81	48	to	200
Triglycerides	mg/dl	197	123	to	234
White blood cells	/mm³	15,200	0	to	29,000
Lymphocytes	%	90	70	to	100
pH	–	7.5	7.4	to	7.8
Specific gravity	–	1.013	1.008	to	1.027

(From Brodman, R. F.: Congenital chylothorax: Recommendation for treatment. N.Y. State J. Med. *75*:553, 1975.)

in combination with other lymphatic anomalies. Presumably, lymph flow obstruction results in the development of fistulas between the thoracic duct and the pleural space or in rupture of the thoracic duct. Congenital chylothorax occurs more commonly in males than in females (2:1), and it occurs more commonly on the right side (right 53 per cent, left 35 per cent, bilateral 12 per cent) (Chernick and Reed, 1970). Acquired chylothorax results from damage to the thoracic duct. It has been reported as a surgical complication of the repair of diaphragmatic hernia, tracheo-esophageal fistula, and a variety of congenital heart disorders.

Acquired chylothorax is usually diagnosed by a chest radiograph obtained because of a change in respiratory status. Congenital chylothorax has been diagnosed in utero by ultrasonography. Bilateral chylothoraces should be considered in the differential diagnosis of any infant who cannot be ventilated in the delivery room. Thoracentesis is required for a definitive diagnosis. Chyle can be distinguished from transudates by its high protein and lipid content; it can be distinguished from exudates by its high lipid content, the characteristic preponderance of lymphocytes, and its slightly alkalotic pH (Table 59–1).

Treatment of chylothorax may require repeated thoracenteses or even thoracostomy tube drainage in order to prevent respiratory failure (Brodman 1975). Recently, drainage has been performed in the fetus to try to prevent compression of the lungs and pulmonary hypoplasia (Rodeck et al., 1988; Schmidt et al., 1985). Once drainage is accomplished, these infants are placed on formulas containing medium-chain triglycerides, rather than long-chain fats, to reduce thoracic duct lymph flow and the rate of reaccumulation of chyle. However, oral intake of protein and water also stimulates thoracic duct lymph flow, so often the infant will not be allowed anything by mouth, and nutritional support must be provided intravenously.

A variety of approaches have been used with some success to treat the infant with persistent chylothorax including direct attempts at repair, patching with fibrin glue (Stenzl et al., 1983), and the obliteration of the pleural space with sclerosing agents. Chylothorax has also been managed successfully using a pleural-peritoneal shunt (Azizkhan et al., 1983). Finally, some reports suggest that ligation of the thoracic duct below the area of leakage is highly effective in stopping reaccumulation (Stringel et al., 1984). It is interesting to note that thoracic duct ligation appears to be well tolerated without accumulations of fluid in the peripheral tissues or in the peritoneum.

The prognosis for infants with chylothorax is good. In a review of 34 cases in 1975, two-thirds of the infants with chylothorax responded to thoracentesis alone, and only five infants died (15 per cent). The complications reported in this review included weight loss from malnutrition, hypoproteinemia, and lymphopenia (Brodman, 1975).

■ REFERENCES

Azizkhan, R. G., Canfield, J., Alford, B. A., et al.: Pleuroperitoneal shunts in the management of neonatal chylothorax. J. Pediatr. Surg. *18*:842, 1983.

Brodman, R. F.: Congenital chylothorax: Recommendations for treatment. N.Y. State J. Med. *75*:553, 1975.

Chernick, V., and Reed, M. H.: Pneumothorax and chylothorax in the neonatal period. J. Pediatr. *76*:624, 1970.

Chervenak, F. A., Isaacson, G., Blakemore, K. J., et al.: Fetal cystic hygroma. Cause and natural history. N. Engl. J. Med. *309*:822, 1983.

Dhande, V., Kattwinkel, J. and Alford, B.: Recurrent bilateral pleural effusions secondary to superior vena cava obstruction as a complication of central venous catheterization. Pediatrics *72*:109, 1983.

Mellins, R. B., Levine, O. R., and Fishman, A. P.: Effect of systemic and pulmonary venous hypertension on pleural and pericardial fluid accumulation. J. Appl. Physiol. *29*:564, 1970.

Rodeck, C. H., Fisk, N. M., Fraser, D. I., et al.: Long-term in utero drainage of fetal hydrothorax. N. Engl. J. Med. *319*:1135, 1988.

Schmidt, W., Harms, E., and Wolf, D.: Successful prenatal treatment of nonimmune hydrops fetalis due to congenital chylothorax. Case report. Br. J. Obstet. Gynaecol. *92*:685, 1985.

Smeltzer, D. M., Stickler, G. B., and Fleming, R. E.: Primary lymphatic dysplasia in children: Chylothorax, chylous ascites, and generalized lymphatic dysplasia. Eur. J. Pediatr. *145*:286, 1986.

Stenzl, W., Rigler, B., Tscheliessnigg, K. H., et al.: Treatment of postsurgical chylothorax with fibrin glue. Thorac. Cardiovasc. Surg. *31*:35, 1983.

Stringel, G., Mercer, S., and Bass, J.: Surgical management of persistent postoperative chylothorax in children. Can. J. Surg. *27*:543, 1984.

Wiener-Kronish, J. P., Berthiaume, Y., and Albertine, K. H.: Pleural effusions and pulmonary edema. Clin. Chest Med. *6*:509, 1985.

DISORDERS OF THE CHEST WALL AND DIAPHRAGM 60

Thomas Hansen and Anthony Corbet

■ DISORDERS OF THE CHEST WALL

Abnormalities of bone and muscle of the chest wall may be a mechanical hindrance to ventilation. Although bony abnormalities are rare, they may be recognized immediately and are sometimes amenable to operative correction.

Defects in fusion of the sternum are uncommon. *Complete separation of the sternum* allows protrusion of cardiovascular structures (ectopia cordis). Lethal malformations of the heart are commonly associated with this condition. *Upper sternal clefts* are more common. Early operation is advised in order to shield the underlying structures from injury and because of the greater ease of approximating the separated parts in the first days of life than later.

The most common of the sternal defects is *pectus excavatum,* sometimes associated with the Pierre Robin syndrome and Marfan syndrome. Rarely is it a fixed or severe deformity until several months of postnatal age. A family history of some type of anterior thoracic deformity was found in 37 per cent of patients, according to Welch (1980). The indications for operative correction are debatable. In our opinion, correction should not be undertaken until several years of age and then only in those few children in whom the deformity appears to be progressing. Serial photographs are the best way to document changes in pectus excavatum. Periodic evaluation of cardiovascular status with ultrasonography and ECG and assessment of pulmonary function is appropriate in the presence of progressive deformity. Results of operative correction are excellent in over 80 per cent of patients and almost always lead to improvement. Recurrences are possible during later active growth.

A rare deformity of the thoracic cage, *asphyxiating thoracic dystrophy,* is part of a serious generalized chondrodystrophy (Fig. 60–1). It was first described by Jeune and co-workers in 1954. The ribs are broad and short and the thorax rigid. Some degree of lung hypoplasia may be present. Renal cystic dysplasia may be present and lead to hypertension and renal failure. About 60 cases have been reported. Oberkaid and co-workers (1977) studied 10 of them and noted that only two patients were alive at the time of the report. One of the two was in excellent health at 15 years of age. The more severely affected infants had respiratory distress from birth. Three patients have been described in one family. The expectation is occurrence in one of four siblings. No parent-child occurrence has been described. The disorder is familial and is inherited as an autosomal recessive trait. Attempts at operative correction have not been successful. Prenatal diagnosis with ultrasonography is possible.

Deficiency of pectoral muscles on one side (Poland syndrome) may also be associated with abnormal ribs (2 to 4) and hypoplasia of the breast. Breathing may be paradoxical and the cardiac impulse easily observed through the soft tissues. No operative intervention is required in infancy, although mammoplasty may later be desirable in affected girls after puberty.

Other causes of thoracic dysfunction are diseases of the muscles, including myasthenia gravis, poliomyelitis, amyotonia congenita, muscular dystrophy, glycogen storage disease, and spinal cord injury or tumor. Such conditions are usually recognized in the context of the associated systemic muscular weakness or paralysis. They should be suspected in any infant in whom hypoventilation is present when the chest film shows normal heart and lungs.

■ DISORDERS OF THE DIAPHRAGM

CONGENITAL DIAPHRAGMATIC HERNIA

Most infants with this condition are mature, two-thirds are male, and in 90 per cent the hernia is left-sided. The incidence is one in 2500 live births. In the newborn, nearly all hernias pass through the posterolateral foramen of Bochdalek.

Pathogenesis. The diaphragm develops anteriorly as a septum between the heart and liver and progresses backward to close last at the left Bochdalek foramen around 8 to 10 weeks' gestation. The bowel migrates from the yolk sac at about 10 weeks, and if it arrives before the foramen has closed, a hernia results. Lung compression from an early age is associated with pulmonary hypoplasia, most severe on the ipsilateral side but also present on the contralateral side. There is a marked reduction in the number of bronchial generations, and a less marked reduction in the number of alveoli per acinus. The number of arterial vessels is proportionately reduced (Bohn et al., 1987), and there is a modest increase in the medial muscle of pulmonary arterioles, together with abnormal extension of muscle into arterioles at the acinar level. In many cases, herniation occurs comparatively late in gestation, or the hernia is small, in which case the lung hypoplasia is less marked (Adzick et al., 1985). The

557

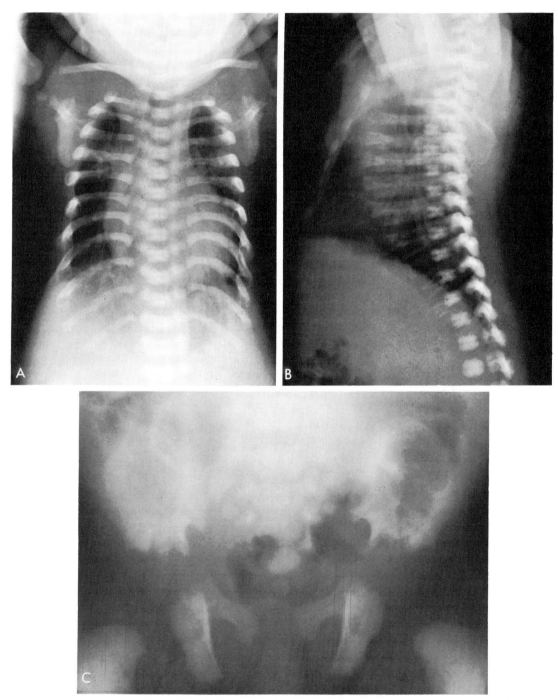

FIGURE 60–1. A, Anteroposterior film of infant with asphyxiating thoracic dystrophy. The thoracic circumference is reduced as compared with the abdominal circumference, and the liver and spleen are displaced downward. B, Lateral projection of the same infant further demonstrates the reduced thoracic volume. (A, and B, courtesy of Dr. John Kirkpatrick.) C, The film of the pelvis shows flaring of the iliac crest and irregular calcification of the triradiate cartilage with typical bony protrusions. (C from Avery, M.E., Fletcher, B.D., and Williams, R.G.: The Lung and its Disorders in the Newborn Infant. 4th ed. Philadelphia, W. B. Saunders Company, 1981.)

prognosis depends on the degree of pulmonary hypoplasia (Nguyen et al., 1983), with its associated reduction in alveolar and vascular surface area. There may be severe hypercarbia and hypoxemia with persistent pulmonary hypertension and large right-to-left shunts at the atrial and ductal levels. After birth when the hernia fills, compression of the lungs is increased, thus superimposing atelectasis on the hypoplasia.

Diagnosis. The onset of symptoms is usually respiratory distress in the first few hours or days of life. Patients with the most severe symptoms present in the delivery room with a difficult resuscitation. Breath sounds are absent on the left side, the chest is barrel-shaped, the abdomen is scaphoid, and the heart beat is displaced to the right. The diagnosis is made easily with a chest radiograph, aided by a feeding tube placed in the stomach. The left hemithorax is filled with a mass, usually incorporating air-filled bowel loops, and the stomach tube enters the chest. The heart is displaced to the right, and the abdomen is remarkably devoid of gas patterns (Fig. 60–2).

Prediction of Outcome. Infants presenting within 6 hours of birth have a high mortality, approaching 50 per cent (Marshall and Sumner, 1982). The prognosis is poor if the Aa.DO$_2$ exceeds 500 mm Hg (Raphaely and Downes, 1973), or if the arterial pH is < 7.0. But the prognosis is best assessed by the arterial Pco$_2$ and the intensity of mechanical ventilation required, reflecting the degree of pulmonary hypoplasia. Bohn and co-workers (1987) found that if mechanical ventilation could not reduce the arterial Pco$_2$ below 40 mm Hg, mortality was 77 per cent, and if Paco$_2$ < 40 could only be achieved with maximal ventilation, the mortality was still more than 50 per cent.

Treatment. Once the diagnosis is suspected, a feeding tube should be passed and suctioned continuously to reduce the amount of air in the hernia and decrease compression of the involved lung. The infant should not be ventilated by bag and mask but instead intubated and connected to a mechanical ventilator using low peak pressure, a rapid rate, and minimal PEEP. Because the danger of pneumothorax is high and substantially increases mortality, paralysis with pancuronium and sedation with morphine may be indicated. The infant should have a right radial artery catheter, if possible, because right-to-left ductal shunting may be significant (Schumacher and Farrell, 1985). Support should be given in the form of colloid and continuous dopamine infusion if hypotension is present. When respiratory acidosis is controlled, metabolic acidosis may be corrected by infusion of sodium bicarbonate.

The definitive treatment is surgical reduction of the hernia; but there is no evidence that this is an emergency, and time should be spent in adequately stabilizing the infant (Sakai et al., 1987; Langer et al., 1988). An abdominal approach to surgery is favored. Most patients have malrotation of the cecum, and this problem should be treated by adequate fixation of the restored bowel. The diaphragm may require considerable stretching to make the repair, in which case chest wall compliance may be greatly reduced. A synthetic patch graft may produce a better result. If the abdominal cavity is too poorly developed to accommodate the bowel, then closure should be accomplished with skin only, and the ventral hernia repaired at a later date. Some surgeons recommend placement of a thoracostomy tube to protect against the catastrophic development of tension pneumothorax, but the underwater seal should be at atmospheric pressure and never placed to suction, because of the hazard of a shift of mediastinal structures (Cloutier et al., 1983). Every attempt should be made to keep the mediastinum in the midline. Postoperatively, patients often require quite large volumes of colloid to overcome the effects of third-space fluid losses on systemic perfusion. All too commonly, the course is complicated by the development of pulmonary hypertension. This may be prevented by maintenance of some degree of postoperative anesthesia with frequent doses of morphine or fentanyl (Vacanti et al., 1984) and avoidance of painful stimuli, such as arterial puncture or tracheal suctioning. There is no evidence that hyperventilation is helpful in these infants. Many centers are now using extracorporeal membrane oxygenation (ECMO) as adjunctive treatment.

The left lung may take only a few days to expand and occupy the hemithorax, which means that atelectasis predominated over hypoplasia. Otherwise, the space initially filled with air becomes filled with fluid. The lung may slowly increase in size over the next few weeks, but in the most severe cases, growth may take several months. In older children, although the chest radiograph appears normal, lung volumes are slightly reduced, and there is

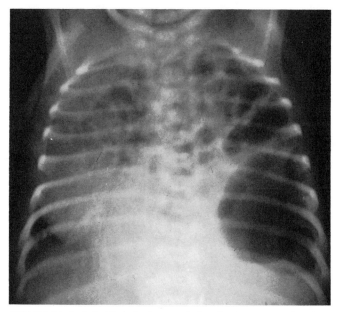

FIGURE 60–2. *Left-sided diaphragmatic hernia. Anteroposterior view of chest taken on the second day of life. The chest is overexpanded and barrel-shaped. Round translucencies of varying size fill the left hemithorax and part of the right. The heart occupies the lower lateral corner of the right hemithorax. Both diaphragms are depressed, the left more than the right. The translucency in the left lower hemithorax resembles stomach, slightly above it looks like large bowel, while the remainder appear to be loops of small bowel.*

persistent evidence of a reduced vascular bed in the left lung (Reid and Hutcherson, 1976; Wohl et al., 1977).

RIGHT-SIDED DIAPHRAGMATIC HERNIA OF DELAYED ONSET

Because the liver is a large organ, herniation into the thorax is a slow process and may only occur after birth with the onset of breathing. The lung problem reflects compression atelectasis rather than hypoplasia, and the right basal mass may present a confusing problem on the chest radiograph (Fig. 60–3). The abdominal gas pattern on the right side may appear higher than usual, and the lower edge of the liver, more horizontal. Ultrasonography or a radionuclide liver scan usually indicates that the liver is excessively high. Induction of a diagnostic pneumoperitoneum with nitrous oxide, and demonstration of a small pneumothorax on the right side, proves the existence of a defect in the diaphragm (Kenny et al., 1977) and strongly suggests that the problem is not paralysis or eventration of the diaphragm.

EVENTRATION OF THE DIAPHRAGM

Eventration of the diaphragm results from insufficient muscle development or absence of phrenic nerves so that the diaphragm is replaced by a fibrous sheet. An eventration may be localized or diffuse, and most of the latter are unilateral, frequently on the left side. Many, especially those that are localized, produce no clinical signs. When severe, however, newborns have significant respiratory distress. There may be lung hypoplasia on the affected side and, if the mediastinum is shifted, even hypoplasia on the contralateral side. In addition, basal lung compression may cause atelectasis, poor drainage, and complicating bronchopneumonia. The diagnosis is suspected from undue elevation of the diaphragm in frontal and lateral chest radiographs and may be confirmed by fluoroscopy or ultrasound examination. (Figs. 60–4 and 60–5). The

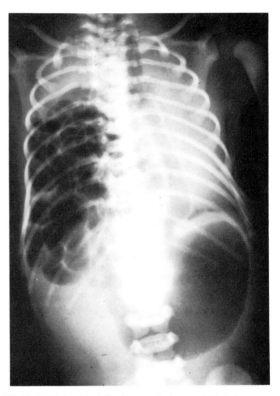

FIGURE 60–3. *Right-sided diaphragmatic hernia. This infant was resuscitated by mask and bag without intubation. The consequence was disastrous overdistention of stomach and bowel. When lungs resist insufflation, intubation is mandatory to prevent this kind of complication.*

major cause of confusion is a paralyzed diaphragm, but evidence for birth trauma or thoracotomy is absent in eventration. The diaphragm may show minimal motion while breathing, or the motion may be paradoxical, rising with inspiration and falling with expiration. In those cases where signs are persistent, the treatment of choice is surgical plication (Wayne et al., 1974; Goldstein and Reid, 1980).

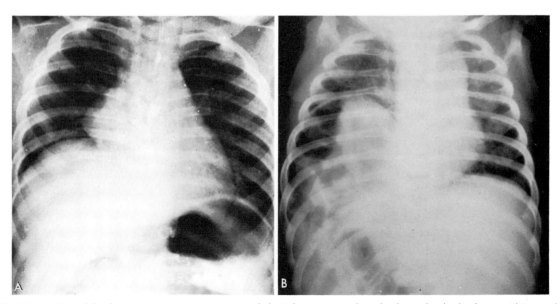

FIGURE 60–4. *Eventration of diaphragm. A, Anteroposterior view of chest showing a moderately elevated right diaphragm. This case history is not summarized in the text because the infant was completely asymptomatic, the x-ray picture having been taken because a sibling had tuberculosis. There had been no difficulty in labor and no respiratory trouble in the neonate. The probable diagnosis is eventration of the diaphragm. B, Diaphragmatic paralysis has the same appearance. On fluoroscopy, paradoxical diaphragmatic movement would indicate paralysis.*

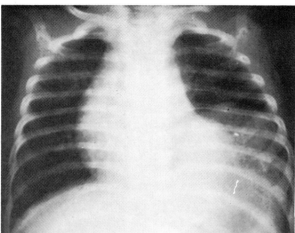

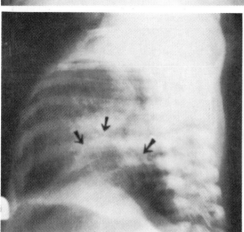

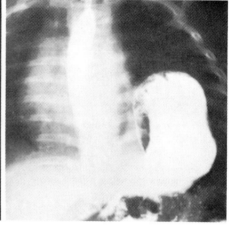

FIGURE 60–5. Eventration of diaphragm. A, Anteroposterior view of chest made at 3½ months of age. The left diaphragm is elevated to the level of the fourth rib. The heart is displaced a little to the right. B, Lateral view on same date. The left diaphragm can be seen considerably higher in the chest than the right. Arrows point to the domed diaphragm. C, With barium in the esophagus and stomach, the stomach can be seen to lie largely within the thorax. It is inverted. The esophagus is displaced toward the right.

A

B   C

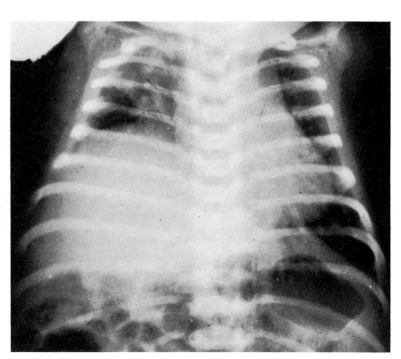

FIGURE 60–6. Paralysis of diaphragm. Anteroposterior view of chest made when patient was 3 weeks old. Labor had been difficult and prolonged because of shoulder dystocia; delivery was completed by forceps extraction. Right-sided Erb palsy, tachypnea, and dyspnea were noted, and there was one severe bout of pneumonitis at 4 weeks. All finally cleared at 2½ months of age. The right diaphragm is elevated to the level of the fourth rib. The right lung contains patches of increased density. The heart is displaced a little toward the left. The left lung is moderately emphysematous, its diaphragm flattened and depressed.

PARALYSIS OF THE DIAPHRAGM

There are two clinical situations where diaphragmatic paralysis may occur, after birth trauma or after thoracotomy.

Birth Trauma. Although sometimes bilateral, most cases of diaphragmatic paralysis are unilateral on the right side. The usual presentation is with respiratory distress, but in cases of bilateral paralysis, there is cyanosis and poor breathing effort that requires mechanical ventilation. The infants are usually large and have other signs of birth trauma. There is excessive stretching of the C3 to C5 nerve roots in the neck. The diaphragm is an especially important respiratory muscle in the newborn (Muller and Bryan, 1979). Furthermore, during active sleep the intercostals are inhibited, the supine position of the newborn pushes the paralyzed diaphragm upward, and the newborn is especially prone to muscle fatigue. The diagnosis is suggested on the chest radiograph if the right hemidiaphragm is two intercostal spaces higher than the left, or if the left hemidiaphragm is one intercostal space higher than the right (Greene et al., 1975) (Fig. 60–6). On fluoroscopy or ultrasound examination, the involved diaphragm shows either limited or paradoxical motion (Ambler et al., 1985). There may be associated basal atelectasis, which explains why some infants are markedly helped by nasal continuous positive airway pressure (CPAP) (Bucci et al., 1974). When both hemidiaphragms are paralyzed, these infants require prolonged mechanical ventilation (Aldrich et al., 1980). Although many improve over 2 weeks, further improvement is possible over a period of 2 months. Once it is felt no further improvement will occur, and the patient cannot be weaned from ventilatory support, surgical plication of the diaphragm should be performed.

Post-Thoracotomy. Diaphragmatic paralysis from phrenic nerve trauma is a common reason for failure to wean from mechanical ventilation after a thoracic operation, such as ligation of patent ductus arteriosus, creation of a systemic pulmonary shunt, or repair of a tracheoesophageal fistula. Management is similar to that for paralysis following birth trauma (Haller et al., 1979).

■ REFERENCES

Adzick, N. C., Harrison, M. R., Glick, P. L., et al.: Diaphragmatic hernia in the fetus: Prenatal detection and outcome in 94 cases. J. Pediatr. Surg. 20:357, 1985.

Aldrich, T. K., Herman, J. H., and Rochester, D. F.: Bilateral diaphragmatic paralysis in the newborn infant. J. Pediatr. 97:988, 1980.

Ambler, R., Gruenewald, S., and John, E.: Ultrasound monitoring of diaphragm activity in bilateral diaphragmatic paralysis. Arch. Dis. Child. 60:170, 1985.

Bohn, D., Tamura, M., Perrin, D., et al.: Ventilatory predictors of pulmonary hypoplasia in congenital diaphragmatic hernia, confirmed by morphologic assessment. J. Pediatr. 111:423, 1987.

Bucci, G., Marzetti, G., Picece-Bucci, S., et al.: Phrenic nerve palsy treated by continuous positive-pressure breathing by nasal cannula. Arch. Dis. Child. 49:230, 1974.

Cloutier, R., Fournier, L., and Levasseur, L.: Reversion to fetal circulation in congenital diaphragmatic hernia: A preventable postoperative complication. J. Pediatr. Surg. 18:551, 1983.

Goldstein, J. D., and Reid, L. M.: Pulmonary hypoplasia resulting from phrenic nerve agenesis and diaphragmatic amyoplasia. J. Pediatr. 97:282, 1980.

Greene, W., L'Heureux, P., and Hunt, C. E.: Paralysis of the diaphragm. Am. J. Dis. Child. 129:1402, 1975.

Gyllesward, A.: Pectus excavatum. A clinical study with long-term postoperative follow-up. Acta Pediatr. Scand. 255 (Suppl.):1, 1975.

Haller, J. A., Pickard, L. R., Tepas, J. J., et al.: Management of diaphragmatic paralysis in infants with special emphasis on selection of patients for operative plication. J. Pediatr. Surg. 14:779, 1979.

Jeune, N., Cararon, R., Berand, C., et al.: Polychondrodystrophie avec blocage thoracique d'évolution fatale. Pediatrie 9:390, 1954.

Kenny, J. D., Wagner, M. L., Harberg, F. J., et al.: Right-sided diaphragmatic hernia of delayed onset in the newborn infant. South. Med. J. 70:373, 1977.

Kohler, E., and Babbitt, D. P.: Dystrophic thoraces and infantile asphyxia. Radiology 94:55, 1970.

Langer, J. C., Filler, R. M., Bohn, D. J., et al.: Timing of surgery for congenital diaphragmatic hernia: Is emergency operation necessary? J. Pediatr. Surg. 23:731, 1988.

Maier, H. C., and Bortone, F.: Complete failure of sternal fusion with herniation of pericardium. J. Thorac. Surg. 18:851, 1949.

Marshall, A., and Sumner, E.: Improved prognosis in congenital diaphragmatic hernia: Experience of 62 cases over 2 year period. J. Royal Soc. Med. 75:607, 1982.

Muller, N. L., and Bryan, A. C.: Chest wall mechanics and respiratory muscles in infants. Pediatr. Clin. North Am. 26:503, 1979.

Nguyen, L., Guttman, F. M., DeChadarevian, J. P., et al.: The mortality of congenital diaphragmatic hernia. Is total pulmonary mass inadequate, no matter what? Ann. Surg. 198:766, 1983.

Oberkaid, F., Danks, D. M., Mayne, V., et al.: Asphyxiating thoracic dysplasia: Clinical radiological and pathological information on 10 patients. Arch. Dis. Child. 52:758, 1977.

Raphaely, R. C., and Downes, J. J.: Congenital diaphragmatic hernia: Prediction of survival. J. Pediatr. Surg. 8:815, 1973.

Ravitch, M. M.: Congenital Deformities of the Chest Wall and Their Operative Correction. Philadelphia, W. B. Saunders Company, 1977.

Reid, I. S., and Hutcherson, R. J.: Long-term follow-up of patients with congenital diaphragmatic hernia. J. Pediatr. Surg. 11:939, 1976.

Sabiston, D. C.: The surgical management of congenital bifid sternum with partial ectopia cordis. J. Thorac. Surg. 35:118, 1958.

Sakai, H., Tamura, M., Hosokawa, Y., et al.: Effect of surgical repair on respiratory mechanics in congenital diaphragmatic hernia. J. Pediatr. 111:432, 1987.

Schumacher, R. E., and Farrell, P. M.: Congenital diaphragmatic hernia. A major remaining challenge in neonatal respiratory care. Perinatology-Neonatology 9(4):29, 1985.

Vacanti, J. P., Crone, R. K., Murphy, J. D., et al.: The pulmonary hemodynamic response to peri-operative anesthesia in the treatment of high risk infants with congenital diaphragmatic hernia. J. Pediatr. Surg. 19:672, 1984.

Wayne, E. R., Campbell, J. B., Burrington, J. D., et al.: Eventration of the diaphragm. J. Pediatr. Surg. 9:643, 1974.

Welch, K. J.: Chest wall deformities. In Holder, T. M., and Ashcraft, K. W. (Eds.): Pediatric Surgery. Philadelphia, W. B. Saunders Company, 1980, p. 162.

Wohl, M. E. B., Griscou, N. T., Strieder, D. J., et al.: The lung following repair of congenital diaphragmatic hernia. J. Pediatr. 90:405, 1977.

PART IX

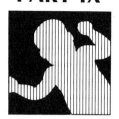

PATENT DUCTUS ARTERIOSUS

PATENT DUCTUS ARTERIOSUS IN THE PREMATURE INFANT

61

Ronald I. Clyman

The ductus arteriosus represents a persistence of the terminal portion of the left pulmonary or sixth branchial arch. More muscular than the elastic pulmonary artery and aorta at either end, the ductus arteriosus also has a looser structure with increased amounts of mucopolysaccharide in the muscle media. During fetal life, it serves to divert blood away from the fluid-filled lungs toward the descending aorta and placenta. Obliteration of the ductus arteriosus takes place after birth. In the full-term animal or human newborn, the ductus begins to constrict rapidly after delivery and initiation of air breathing. During postnatal closure of the ductus in the human, the media indents into the lumen and the intima increases in size and forms intimal mounds or cushions that partially occlude the lumen. These intimal changes are secondary to extensive constriction and shortening of the ductus as well as migration of smooth muscle cells from the media into the intima. Shortly after birth, cells in the inner part of the media appear to disintegrate, perhaps because the central part of the vessel receives no nutrients through either the ductus lumen or vasa vasorum after muscular closure of the lumen. If this is true, the precipitating cause of the histologic changes would be a lack of blood supply brought on by muscular contraction of the wall. Anatomic closure has been reported to be complete one to several months after birth.

■ REGULATION OF DUCTUS ARTERIOSUS PATENCY

Since the initial studies of Kennedy and Clark (1942), many investigators have demonstrated that oxygen is responsible for constricting the ductus arteriosus after birth. However, the biochemical basis for the oxygen response has never been fully explained (Coceani et al., 1984; Fay and Jobsis, 1972). Although neural and hormonal factors possibly contribute to ductus closure under physiologic conditions, they do not mediate oxygen-induced vessel closure. Oxygen has a greater constrictor effect in the ductus from older rather than younger fetuses. Studies in fetal animals indicate that the increased contractile response of the mature ductus arteriosus to oxygen is due to a developmental alteration in the sensitivity of the vessel to locally produced prostaglandins: ductus smooth muscle from preterm animals is more sensitive to the dilating action of prostaglandin (PGE_2) than that from animals near term (Clyman, 1987). This may account for the higher incidence of persistent patent ductus arteriosus in preterm newborns. There is some evidence to suggest that PGE_2 production by the ductus after delivery may be stimulated by reactive oxygen metabolites (Clyman et al., 1988), but the factors that alter the sensitivity of the ductus to locally produced PGE_2 are unknown. Elevated cortisol concentrations in the fetus have been found to decrease the sensitivity of the ductus to PGE_2 (Clyman et al., 1981a). Consistent with these findings, prenatal administration of glucocorticoids causes a significant reduction in the incidence of patent ductus arteriosus (PDA) in premature human and animal infants (Clyman et al., 1981b; Collaborative Group on Antenatal Steroid Therapy, 1985; Momma et al., 1981; Thibeault et al., 1978; Waffarn et al., 1983).

In normal, full-term animals, loss of responsiveness to PGE_2 shortly after birth prevents the ductus arteriosus from reopening once it has constricted. In premature infants, once the ductus has closed (either spontaneously or as a result of indomethacin administration), it may reopen at a later date, with recurrence of the left-to-right shunt (Mellander et al., 1984). The incidence of the ductus reopening is inversely related to birth weight: 33 per cent of infants with birth weights less than 1000 g experienced a reopening of the ductus after initial closure compared with only 8 per cent of infants with birth weights greater than 1500 g (Clyman et al., 1985). Premature animals' persistent responsiveness to PGE_2 after ductus constriction may account for the high rate of ductus reopening observed in preterm infants after successful indomethacin-induced closure. Of those infants whose ductus reopens after initial closure, 80 per cent apparently remain responsive to indomethacin. The factors that maintain ductus responsiveness to PGE_2 in immature animals after postnatal ductus constriction are unknown, as is the reason why the premature ductus fails to develop the normal anatomic obliteration of its lumen after birth.

■ HEMODYNAMIC AND PULMONARY ALTERATIONS

Virtually all shunting through the ductus in the preterm infant is left to right. Only in larger infants with persistent pulmonary hypertension does right-to-left shunting become a problem (see also Chapters 51 and 62). The exact consequences of a left-to-right shunt through a PDA for the preterm infant have not been elucidated clearly. The pathophysiologic features of a PDA depend both on the magnitude of the left-to-right shunt and on the cardiac and pulmonary responses to the shunt. There are important differences between immature and mature infants in the heart's ability to handle a volume load. Before term, the myocardium has more water and less contractile mass. Therefore, in the immature fetus the ventricles are less distensible than at term and also generate less force per gram of myocardium, even though they have the same ability to generate force per sarcomere as those in more mature infants (Friedman, 1972). The relative lack of left ventricular distensibility in immature infants is more a function of the ventricle's tissue constituents than of poor muscle function. As a result, left ventricular distention secondary to a large left-to-right PDA shunt may produce a higher left ventricular end-diastolic pressure at smaller ventricular volumes in the immature than in the mature infant. Elevations in left ventricular end-diastolic pressures, which increase pulmonary venous pressures and cause pulmonary congestion, occur with smaller left-to-right shunts in immature than in mature infants. In addition, several studies have demonstrated that immature infants have poorer cardiac sympathetic innervation (Friedman, 1972).

Studies in preterm lambs with a patent ductus arteriosus have shown that the lambs are able to increase left ventricular output to maintain "effective" systemic blood flow. The increase in left ventricular output is accomplished not by an increase in heart rate but by an increase in stroke volume (Clyman et al., 1987). Stroke volume increases primarily as a result of the simultaneous decrease in afterload resistance on the heart and the increase in left ventricular preload. Despite the ability of the left ventricle to increase its output with increasing amounts of ductus shunt, blood flow distribution is significantly rearranged. This redistribution of systemic blood flow occurs even with small shunts. Certain organs, such as the gastrointestinal tract and spleen, may receive decreased blood flow due to a combination of decreased perfusion pressure (related to a drop in diastolic pressure) and localized vasoconstriction. These organs may experience significant hypoperfusion before there are any signs of left ventricular compromise. This decrease in organ perfusion may explain

some of the pathophysiologic manifestations of a patent ductus arteriosus in preterm infants.

At this time, we can only guess what importance the magnitude and duration of left-to-right shunt as well as the changes in pulmonary arterial and venous pressures caused by PDA may have in preterm human infants. Alverson and co-workers (1983) observed that the left ventricular output was increased in the presence of a left-to-right ductus shunt and fell significantly after closure of the ductus. The increase in left ventricular output seen in the presence of PDA did not provide an increase in effective systemic blood flow; femoral blood flow velocity was low prior to closure of the PDA, and returned to normal after closure.

Very-low-birth-weight infants with a PDA have been found to have increased flow in the ascending aorta (with increased forearm blood flow) and decreased flow in the descending aorta with an associated metabolic acidosis (Johnson et al., 1978). Such alterations in cardiac output distribution have been implicated in the high incidence of intracranial hemorrhage (Martin et al., 1982; Perlman et al., 1981) and necrotizing enterocolitis (Cotton et al., 1978; Kitterman, 1975) associated with PDA. Significant aortic backflow has been observed over large distances in some infants with PDA, consistent with a "diastolic steal" of blood from the abdominal organs to the pulmonary artery (Spach et al., 1980). The continuous distention of the pulmonary vessels during diastole may be important in the production of pulmonary vascular disease and bronchopulmonary dysplasia.

The decreased ability of the preterm infant to maintain active pulmonary vasoconstriction (Lewis et al., 1976) may be responsible in part for the earlier presentation of a "large" left-to-right PDA shunt in the most immature infants (Gersony et al., 1983; Jacob et al., 1980). In addition, therapeutic maneuvers (e.g., surfactant replacement) that lead to decreased pulmonary vascular resistance can exacerbate the amount of left-to-right shunt in preterm infants with respiratory distress syndrome (Clyman et al., 1982; Fujiwara et al., 1980).

The factors responsible for preventing fluid and proteins from moving from the plasma to the lung interstitium (microvascular barrier) and from the interstitium to the air spaces (alveolar barrier) have been described previously in detail (Staub, 1980). Several groups have observed an improvement in lung compliance in preterm infants with a PDA of several days duration following ligation of the PDA (Gerhardt and Bancalari, 1980; Johnson et al., 1978; Naulty et al., 1978). With a wide-open PDA, the pulmonary vasculature is exposed to systemic blood pressure and increased pulmonary blood flow. Because the premature infant with respiratory distress syndrome frequently has a low plasma oncotic pressure and may have increased capillary permeability, increases in microvascular perfusion pressure that result from PDA may increase interstitial and alveolar lung fluid. Leakage of plasma proteins into the alveolar space may inhibit surfactant function and increase surface tension in the immature air sacs, which are already compromised by surfactant deficiency (Ikegami et al., 1983). The increased FIO_2 and mean airway pressures required to overcome these early changes in compliance caused by PDA may be important factors in the association of PDA with chronic lung disease (Brown, 1979; Cotton et al., 1978). However, these changes in pulmonary mechanics appear to occur only after some period of exposure to a PDA. Experiments performed in preterm animals with a PDA have shown no increase in lung water accumulation or protein leak and no change in pulmonary mechanics when the exposure to left-to-right shunt has been limited to the 1st day after delivery (Alpan et al., 1989; Pérez Fontán et al., 1987; Shimada et al., 1987).

DIAGNOSIS

Studies designed to determine how a patent ductus arteriosus contributes to an infant's morbidity or when it becomes persistent have been hampered by the lack of consistent diagnostic criteria for defining the condition. Ellison and co-workers (1983) attempted to evaluate several commonly used criteria for diagnosing a large left-to-right shunt through the ductus arteriosus by noting the occurrence of each sign both before and 36 to 48 hours after surgical ligation. No single criterion alone sufficed as an indicator of PDA. Certain signs, such as continuous murmur or hyperactive left ventricular impulse, were specific for a PDA but lacked sensitivity; conversely, M-mode echocardiography and ventilatory support criteria were very sensitive but lacked specificity.

The combination of two-dimensional echocardiographic visualization of the ductus with either pulsed, continuous wave, or color Doppler measurements appears to be not only very sensitive but also specific for identifying ductus patency (Drayton and Skidmore 1987; Stevenson et al., 1980). This combination may also be useful in determining pressure gradients across the ductus (Musewe et al., 1987). However, its usefulness in determining the magnitude of the ductus shunt has not yet been convincingly demonstrated. Attempts to correlate echocardiographic or angiographic findings with the presence of a symptomatic patent ductus arteriosus have been hampered by the lack of a gold standard for measuring symptomatic PDA (Dudell and Gersony 1984; Ellison et al., 1983). In addition, the presence of a significant ductus shunt may be required for several days before symptoms develop. Thus, we have the ability to determine whether some degree of ductus patency exists but no clear consensus on how to decide which patent ductus is a potential source of problems.

INCIDENCE

Pulsed Doppler echocardiographic assessments of full-term infants indicate that functional closure of the ductus has occurred in almost 50 per cent by 24 hours, in 90 per cent by 48 hours, and in all by 96 hours. In contrast, the ductus of many preterm infants remains open for many days or weeks, and 12 hours after delivery, ductus shunts in preterm infants can be shown to be greater than those in term infants (Drayton and Skidmore, 1987). However, not all infants with angiographic or Doppler-demonstrable ductus patency develop clinical symptomatology: the more mature the infant, the less the likelihood that ductus patency within the first 48 hours after delivery will require subsequent therapeutic intervention. In one study of 1689 infants with birth weights less than 1750 g, a large "hemodynamically significant" PDA was noted in

42 per cent of the infants with birth weights less than 1000 g, in 21 per cent of infants between 1000 and 1500 g, and in 7 per cent of those between 1500 and 1750 g (Ellison et al., 1983). The incidence of PDA is also much higher in infants with respiratory distress syndrome (Clyman et al. 1981a; Thibeault et al., 1975). Furthermore, an increased incidence of symptomatic PDA has been noted in preterm infants who experience perinatal asphyxia (Cotton et al., 1981). The rate of fluid administration during the initial several days after birth may influence the incidence of symptomatic PDA (Bell et al., 1980) or may only alter its detection (Green et al., 1980).

TREATMENT

Definitive treatment of a PDA is closure of the ductus arteriosus. Eventually, unless there is a primary defect of the ductus wall, constriction and permanent anatomic closure should occur spontaneously. In order to forestall the use of therapeutic interventions to close the PDA (indomethacin or surgical ligation), other conservative measures have been advocated, e.g., fluid restriction, diuretics, and digitalis. Although excessive fluid administration has been associated with an increased incidence of PDA, fluid restriction is unlikely to cause ductus closure. In addition, the combination of fluid restriction and diuretics frequently leads to electrolyte abnormalities, dehydration, and most important, caloric deprivation. Furthermore, furosemide, the most commonly used diuretic, has been associated with an increased incidence of PDA in one study (Green et al., 1983). One would not expect digitalis to be very useful because myocardial contractility is increased rather than reduced in infants with PDA; in infants under 1250 g, it often appears to be toxic. In fact, a controlled study by McGrath (1978) failed to show any advantage to digoxin. Finally, there may be an interaction between digoxin and indomethacin that increases the patient's susceptibility to the toxic effects of digoxin (Berman et al., 1978; Koren et al., 1984; Wilkerson and Glenn, 1977).

The addition of positive end-expiratory pressure has been found clinically useful in managing infants with a PDA. When end-expiratory pressure is added, the amount of left-to-right shunt through the ductus arteriosus decreases; as a result, effective systemic blood flow increases (Cotton et al., 1980). A low hematocrit has been shown to aggravate left-to-right shunting by lowering the resistance to blood flow through the pulmonary vascular bed (Lister et al., 1982), leading some to advocate maintaining hematocrit in the mid–40s. Higher hematocrits diminish excessive shunting through the PDA and help ensure systemic oxygen delivery when perfusion is limited. Similarly, demands on left ventricular output should be minimized in infants with PDA by maintaining adequate oxygenation and by keeping the patient in a neutral thermal environment. Nevertheless, such therapies usually only delay, rather than prevent, the ultimate need for PDA closure. Ligation of a symptomatic PDA in premature infants now can be done with low mortality and morbidity requiring only 20 to 30 minutes of surgical time and actually being done in the neonatal intensive care unit (NICU) in some hospitals (Mikhail et al., 1982; Wagner et al., 1984).

Indomethacin appears to be an effective alternative to surgery for treatment of a PDA (Gersony et al., 1983). Its efficacy and toxicity have been explored extensively, and it appears comparable to surgical ligation in preventing the complications associated with a PDA: bronchopulmonary dysplasia (BPD), necrotizing enterocolitis (NEC), intracranial hemorrhage (ICH), and intolerance of enteral feedings (Gersony et al., 1983). In most intensive care nurseries, indomethacin has replaced surgery as the preferred therapy for a persistent PDA, probably because the most frequently occurring risks associated with ligation (increased incidence of cicatricial retinopathy of prematurity and the need for thoracotomy) seem more serious than those associated with indomethacin (decreased urine output and increased bleeding other than ICH). While there may be general consensus on the efficacy of indomethacin for treatment of a PDA, questions about proper dosage, treatment duration, and optimal timing of treatment remain quite controversial.

When treating infants 8 to 10 days old with left-to-right shunts that are causing cardiovascular compromise, the response of the ductus to indomethacin depends on the size of the dose (0.3 mg/kg versus 0.1 mg/kg) as well as on the number of doses administered (one versus two or three) (Yeh et al., 1983 and 1985). Because drug clearance depends on postnatal age (Brash et al., 1981; Clyman et al., 1985; Smith et al., 1984; Thalji et al., 1980; Yaffe et al., 1980; Yeh et al., 1985), one can envision that using the same indomethacin dosage regimen recommended for infants at 8 to 10 days (when the half-life of the drug is 21 hours) in infants who are treated on Day 1 (when the half-life is 71 hours) (Smith et al., 1984) may lead to elevated and prolonged plasma concentrations. Not surprisingly therefore, Krueger and coworkers (1987) found a single loading dose of indomethacin (0.2 mg/kg), without subsequent maintenance doses, effective in preventing clinical symptoms associated with a PDA when administered to very-low-birth-weight (VLBW) infants within the first 24 hours after delivery.

The age at which infants are treated with indomethacin is another important variable in the treatment's overall effectiveness (Firth and Pickering, 1980). Several investigators have suggested that the relative ineffectiveness of indomethacin in treating infants of advanced postnatal age may be due to rapid drug clearance and a resultant inability to maintain desired plasma concentrations (Brash et al., 1981; Thalji et al., 1980). In general, however, the response of the ductus and the side effects of indomethacin do not correlate with the peak concentration of the drug (Alpert et al., 1979; Bhat et al., 1980; Bianchetti et al., 1980; Brash et al., 1981; Yeh et al., 1985). Thus, in most infants the failure of indomethacin to produce ductus constriction is not due to lowered drug concentrations alone. In addition, there has been no consistent correlation between ductus closure after treatment with indomethacin and either the area under the curve or the plasma concentrations at 6, 12, or 24 hours (Achanti et al., 1986; Ramsey et al., 1987; Rennie et al., 1986; Rheuban et al., 1987). Even when indomethacin concentrations have been maintained in the "desired" range, the drug's ability to produce ductus closure remains inversely proportional to the postnatal age at the time of treatment. This decreasing effectiveness of indomethacin to produce ductus clo-

sure with advancing postnatal age has been shown to be due to the diminishing ability of PGE_2 to maintain ductus patency (Clyman et al., 1983). Thus, patency of the ductus arteriosus becomes independent of dilator prostaglandins with advance in postnatal age (Achanti et al., 1986).

A second type of indomethacin treatment failure is found in patients whose ductus initially constricts when treated with indomethacin, only to reopen several days later. Recurrence of a symptomatic PDA after initial successful treatment is independent of initial plasma indomethacin concentrations (Brash et al., 1981; Gersony et al., 1983; Ramsey et al., 1987). Prolonged treatment with indomethacin may delay reopening of the PDA as long as the drug administration continues; however, the ultimate rate of reopening remains constant whether indomethacin treatment is administered for 5 to 7 days or only for 36 hours (Rhodes et al., 1988; Setzer et al., 1984). The rate of reopening, which is greatest among the most immature infants, may also be related to the timing and completeness of initial ductus closure after delivery (Clyman et al. 1985). Infants with spontaneous closure during the first 3 postnatal days do not have subsequent signs of a symptomatic PDA (Dudell and Gersony 1984; Ment et al., 1985). Similarly, those infants whose ductus is closed with indomethacin during the first 2 days after delivery (Kaapa et al., 1983; Mahony et al., 1982, 1985) appear to have a lower incidence of reopening when compared with those treated between 8 to 10 days (Ramsey et al., 1987; Rudd et al., 1983) or after 20 days (Ivey et al., 1979). Because of the lower incidence of indomethacin failure and ductus reopening when indomethacin is administered within the first 48 hours, there is less need for surgical ligation than when it is given after the 1st week (Gersony et al., 1983; Hammerman et al., 1986; Mahony et al., 1982 and 1985; Sola et al., 1986). In summary, indomethacin is most effective when administered within the first days after delivery; not only can the total dose be lower (although there are probably equal plasma concentrations), but the overall success rate is also greater than when indomethacin is given after the 1st week.

Indomethacin treatment may be most effective in the first 24 to 48 hours after delivery, but is that necessarily the best time to administer it? Ninety per cent of infants with severe respiratory distress have evidence of a PDA on contrast echocardiogram within the first 24 hours; however, only 40 per cent subsequently develop symptoms of a hemodynamically large left-to-right shunt that requires intervention with indomethacin or surgery. In addition, most infants will not develop the symptoms of cardiovascular compromise before 7 days. Therefore, treating infants within the first 24 to 48 hours implies that approximately 60 per cent of the infants treated would never have developed symptoms of cardiovascular compromise. Because indomethacin has been associated with several frequent as well as infrequent complications (Alpan et al., 1985; Appleton et al., 1986; Friedman et al., 1978; Gersony et al., 1983; Krueger et al., 1987; Lilien et al., 1983, Rennie et al., 1986; Yeh et al., 1985), such an aggressive approach to therapy can be justified only if early treatment can be demonstrated to significantly alter outcome in these infants.

Cotton and co-workers (1978) demonstrated that failure to close the ductus after significant clinical symptoms of cardiovascular compromise have developed (approximately 7 to 10 days) significantly increases neonatal morbidity. Similarly, treating infants after signs of a hemodynamically significant PDA develop (2 to 3 days), but before the presence of cardiovascular compromise (7 to 10 days), leads to a reduction in mortality and BPD (Kaapa et al., 1983; Merritt et al., 1981).

If infants receive indomethacin treatment at the first clinical sign of a PDA (an asymptomatic murmur) instead of after the symptoms of a hemodynamically significant shunt are apparent, they demonstrate a significant reduction in the development of large shunts and in the number of surgical ligations required as well as in the total duration of oxygen therapy and time to regain birth weight. In addition, the frequency of complications does not increase significantly with this approach (Mahony et al., 1982 and 1985). However, the effectiveness of indomethacin treatment as soon as clinical signs of a PDA become apparent, but before a major shunt has developed, can be demonstrated only among infants weighing less than 1000 g. These small premature infants with asymptomatic murmurs are at high risk (80 per cent) for developing large ductus shunts and appear to benefit from early indomethacin treatment. In contrast, only 30 per cent of infants with birth weights greater than 1000 g who have an asymptomatic murmur subsequently develop symptoms of a major shunt. These larger infants have a high rate of spontaneous closure. As a result, early treatment of an asymptomatic murmur in these infants offers no advantage over initiating therapy only after symptoms of a significant hemodynamic shunt have developed.

Even less evidence supports treating infants with indomethacin *before* clinical signs of a PDA develop. Hammerman and co-workers (1986) treated infants with birth weights less than 1000 g who had no clinical evidence of a PDA but who had evidence of left-to-right ductal flow on contrast echocardiogram (Day 2 to 3). Prophylactic closure in these infants with "silent" PDA decreased the incidence of clinically symptomatic PDA and the need for ultimate ligation; however, it did not affect the development of BPD (as was seen in the studies discussed above) nor the incidence of ICH or NEC.

To date, at least ten centers have performed controlled studies to examine the effect on the ductus of prophylactic indomethacin treatment during the first 24 hours after delivery (Bada et al., 1989; Hannigan et al., 1988; Krueger et al., 1987; Mahony et al., 1985; Ment et al., 1985 and 1988; Nystrom et al., 1985; Puckett et al., 1985; Rennie et al., 1986; Setzer et al., 1984; Setzer-Bandstra et al., 1988; Sola et al., 1986; Vincer et al., 1987). Some preliminary conclusions can be made from the results of 840 infants with birth weights less than 1500 g ($\overline{m}$ = 1100 g) and gestational age of 28.5 weeks that have been reported. More than 85 per cent had respiratory distress at the time of entry, which was between 6 and 24 hours after delivery. Only 11 per cent of the infants who received prophylactic indomethacin, compared with 40 per cent of those in the control group, developed a hemodynamically significant PDA (p $<$ 10^{-6}). There were no significant differences between the two groups in the total duration of oxygen therapy or ventilatory support nor were there significant differences in the incidence of BPD, NEC or time to regain birth weight. Five of six studies reported a

transient but significant alteration in renal function in the prophylactic treatment group (Bada et al., 1989; Krueger et al., 1987; Mahony et al., 1985; Nystrom et al., 1985; Rennie et al., 1986; Setzer-Bandstra et al., 1988). One study (Rennie et al., 1986) found a significant increase in the incidence of gastrointestinal hemorrhage in the prophylactic treatment group. Three centers have reported a significant reduction in the incidence of ICH (Bada et al., 1989; Ment et al., 1985 and 1988; Setzer-Bandstra et al., 1988). However, due to the large number of infants enrolled in those 3 centers, there was a significant reduction in the overall incidence of ICH (ICH $\geq$ grade 1: control 201/429 [47 per cent] vs indomethacin 153/423 [36 per cent], p$<$0.02) and in the incidence of bleeds $\geq$ grade III (ICH $\geq$ grade III: Control 58/299 [19 per cent] vs indomethacin = 39/299 [13 per cent], p$<$0.05) when the results from all the studies were combined. It is interesting to note that the mechanism by which indomethacin decreases the incidence of ICH appears to be independent of its effect on the ductus arteriosus (Ment et al., 1985; Bada et al., 1989; Ment et al., 1988).

These findings must be considered in light of the fact that only 40 per cent of the infants who were eligible for treatment within the first 24 hours ultimately would have developed a hemodynamically significant PDA. The chances of this occurring would be even less (14 per cent) among the infants with birth weights greater than 900 g. The findings in these ten centers are also consistent with the increasing number of animal studies that suggest that during the 1st day after birth, a PDA does not alter the course of hyaline membrane disease (Alpan et al., 1989; Pérez Fontán et al., 1987; Shimada et al., 1989).

At this time, the available information does not yet support routine indomethacin treatment on the 1st day of life in small premature infants since most of these infants never have signs of a hemodynamically significant PDA. Except for decreasing the incidence of symptomatic PDA and the need for surgical ligation, routine first-day treatment does not significantly decrease morbidity. (Its independent effects on ICH need to be evaluated more thoroughly.) Rather, in infants who weigh less than 1000 g at birth, it would seem appropriate to treat a PDA when it first becomes *clinically* apparent and before signs of a large shunt are evident. About 80 per cent of these infants develop a large shunt, and treatment at this time has been associated with both a decreased need for surgical ligation and decreased neonatal morbidity. There appears to be no advantage in treating infants with birth weights over 1000 g before they develop signs of a hemodynamically significant shunt; however, once this does occur, prompt treatment rather than conservative management significantly diminishes later morbidity.

There are many variations in dosage regimens reported in the literature. We currently recommend an initial dose of lyophilized indomethacin of 0.2 mg/kg by intravenous administration over 5 to 10 minutes. A second and third dose are given 12 and 36 hours after the first dose. Infants who weigh less than 1250 g at birth are given 0.1 mg/kg per dose for the second and third doses (unless they are older than 7 days). Infants weighing more than 1250 g or older than 7 days are given 0.2 mg/kg per dose for the second and third doses. In most instances, a single dose has not resulted in persistent constriction of the ductus arteriosus.

CONTRAINDICATIONS TO USE OF INDOMETHACIN

Most contraindications are relative, and few are beyond dispute.

Poor Renal Function. Many centers do not use indomethacin if serum creatinine is above 1.2 to 1.7 mg/dl or if urine output is below 1 ml/kg/hour. The reasoning behind this is that indomethacin may decrease urine output further and cause significant water and electrolyte problems. A critical value of serum creatinine is not available; however, not only have different upper limits been selected arbitrarily in different studies, but different laboratories may give different values for the same sample. Furthermore, the interpretation of any given serum creatinine concentration differs according to gestational and postnatal age. Whether giving indomethacin to a patient with moderate renal failure damages the kidney is uncertain; nevertheless, it is prudent to withhold indomethacin in infants who have significant renal failure, however it is defined. In some infants, indomethacin is followed by a markedly decreased urine output which must be allowed for when replacing fluid and electrolyte losses. Simultaneous administration of furosemide may prevent these renal changes (Yeh et al., 1982).

Bleeding Disorders and Low Platelets. Frank renal or gastrointestinal bleeding are contraindications to the use of indomethacin. Intracranial hemorrhage, however, is not a contraindication to the use of indomethacin (Maher et al., 1985). And as mentioned previously, indomethacin may actually decrease the incidence of ICH.

It is customary to withhold indomethacin if platelets are under 50,000/mm^3, even in the absence of overt bleeding. There seems to be no continuing reason for this ban. Indomethacin in adequate doses impairs platelet function somewhat for 7 to 9 days, no matter how many platelets there are but this has not been clinically relevant (Friedman et al., 1978).

Necrotizing Enterocolitis. If infants have signs of early NEC, indomethacin is usually contraindicated. Part of the rationale for this is that the NEC may be due to bowel ischemia secondary to the ductus arteriosus, and indomethacin may further decrease blood flow to the bowel. A more important reason is that if closing the ductus arteriosus prevents the progression of NEC, as many neonatologists believe, then surgical ligation is a more certain and rapid way of achieving ductus closure. Indomethacin may not close the ductus or may take 36 hours to do so, and such a delay may not preserve viability of the bowel.

Although indomethacin has been associated infrequently with intestinal perforation (Alpan et al., 1985), none of the controlled trials has shown an increase in the incidence of NEC in the indomethacin treatment groups. This may be due to the beneficial effects of indomethacin on ductus closure (and subsequent improvement in bowel blood flow) outweighing the negative direct effects of indomethacin on intestinal perfusion. This hypothesis has recently been supported in a controlled study using surgical ligation to treat the ductus arteriosus on the first day

after delivery. The authors found that early surgical closure of the ductus decreased the incidence of NEC in infants with birth weights less than 1000 g (Cassady et al., 1989). This is in contrast to the early indomethacin treatment studies (see above), in which no effect was seen on the incidence of NEC.

Sepsis. All anti-inflammatory agents should be withheld if there is sepsis unless no alternative is available. Thus, indomethacin should not be used if sepsis is proved or strongly suspected.

■ SUMMARY

Patent ductus arteriosus is an important problem in the small preterm infant that increases in incidence with decreasing gestational age. The clinical consequences of this problem are related chiefly to the degree of left-to-right shunting that occurs across the ductus, producing a relative increase in blood flow to the heart and pulmonary bed and decreased flow to the lower body, particularly to the kidneys and intestines. PDA contributes to the incidence of intracranial hemorrhage as well as to worsening pulmonary disease, increased incidence of necrotizing enterocolitis and to oliguria, and electrolyte disturbances. Surgical ligation of the ductus is a relatively simple procedure in the preterm infant; however, in large studies ligation has been associated with increased incidence of retinopathy of prematurity (and, of course, requires thoracotomy). Treatment with indomethacin has been demonstrated in many studies to be effective in closing a patent ductus, particularly when given within the first few days of life. In addition, it is possible that through a direct effect of indomethacin on cerebral blood flow indomethacin treatment may also contribute to decreased incidence of severe intracranial hemorrhage. Indomethacin treatment is currently recommended in preterm infants weighing less than 1000 g who develop a typical ductus murmur, unless clinical complications such as necrotizing enterocolitis or sepsis require consideration of surgical ligation. Infants appear to tolerate indomethacin, for the most part, but the occurrence of occasional side effects mitigates against the current recommendation for routine prophylactic use of indomethacin.

■ REFERENCES

Achanti, B., Yeh, T. F., and Pildes, R. S.: Indomethacin therapy in infants with advanced postnatal age and patent ductus arteriosus. Clin. Invest. Med. 9:250–253, 1986.

Alpan, G. M., Eyal, F., Vinograd, I., et al.: Localized intestinal perforations after enteral administration of indomethacin in premature infants. J. Pediatr. 106:277–281, 1985.

Alpan, G., Mauray, F., and Clyman, R. I.: Effect of patent ductus arteriosus on water accumulation and protein permeability in the premature lungs of mechanically ventilated premature lambs. Pediatr. Res. 26:520–525, 1989.

Alpert, B. S., Lewins, M. J., Rowland, D. W., et al.: Plasma indomethacin levels in preterm newborn infants with symptomatic patent ductus arteriosus—clinical and echocardiographic assessments of response. J. Pediatr. 95:578–582, 1979.

Alverson, D. C., Eldridge, M. W., Johnson, J. D., et al.: Effect of patent ductus arteriosus on left ventricular output in premature infants. J. Pediatr. 102: 754–757, 1983.

Appleton, R. S., Graham, T. P., Cotton, R. B., et al.: Abnormal diastolic cardiac function following indomethacin therapy of patent ductus arteriosus. Pediatr. Res. *20*:167A, 1986.

Bada, H. S., Green, R. S., Pourcyrous, M., et al.: Indomethacin reduces the risks of severe intraventricular hemorrhage. J. Pediatr. *115*:631–637, 1989.

Bell, E. F., Warburton, D., Stonestreet, B., et al.: Effect of fluid administration on the development of symptomatic patent ductus arteriosus and congestive heart failure in premature infants. N. Engl. J. Med. *302*:598–604, 1980.

Berman, W., Jr, Dubynsky, O., Whitman, V., et al.: Digoxin therapy in low-birth-weight infants with patent ductus arteriosus. J. Pediatr. *93*:652–655, 1978.

Bhat, R., Vidyasagar, D., Fisher, E., et al.: Pharmacokinetics of oral and intravenous indomethacin in preterm infants. Dev. Pharmacol. Ther. *1*:101–110, 1980.

Bianchetti, G., Monin, P., Marchal, F., et al.: Pharmacokinetics of indomethacin in the premature infant. Dev. Pharmacol. Ther. *1*:111–124, 1980.

Brash, A. R., Hickey, D. E., Graham, T. P., et al.: Pharmacokinetics of indomethacin in the neonate. N. Engl. J. Med. *305*:67–72, 1981.

Brown, E.: Increased risk of bronchopulmonary dysplasia in infants with patent ductus arteriosus. J. Pediatr. *95*:865–866, 1979.

Cassady, G., Crouse, D. T. Kirklin, J. W., Strange, M. J., Janier, C. H., et al.: A randomized controlled trial at very early prophylactic ligation of the ductus arteriosus in babies who weighed 1000 grams or less at birth. N. Engl. J. Med. *320*:1511–1516, 1989.

Clyman, R. I.: Ductus arteriosus: Current theories of prenatal and postnatal regulation. Semin. Perinatol. *11*:64–71, 1987.

Clyman, R. I., Ballard, P. L., Sniderman, S., et al.: Prenatal administration of betamethasone for prevention of patent ductus arteriosus. J. Pediatr. *98*:123–126, 1981b.

Clyman, R. I., Campbell, D., Heymann, M. A., et al.: Persistent responsiveness of the neonatal ductus arteriosus in immature lambs: A possible cause for reopening of patent ductus arteriosus after indomethacin induced closure. Circulation *71*:141–145, 1985.

Clyman, R. I., Jobe, A., Heymann, M. A., et al.: Increased shunt through the patent ductus arteriosus after surfactant replacement therapy. J. Pediatr. *100*:101–107, 1982.

Clyman, R. I., Mauray, F., Heymann, M. A., et al.: Cardiovascular effects of a patent ductus arteriosus in preterm lambs with respiratory distress. J. Pediatr. *111*:579–587, 1987.

Clyman, R. I., Mauray, F., Roman, C., et al.: Effects of antenatal glucocorticoid administration on the ductus arteriosus of preterm lambs. Am. J. Physiol. *241*:H415–H420, 1981a.

Clyman, R. I., Mauray, F., Roman, C., et al.: Factors determining the loss of ductus arteriosus responsiveness to prostaglandin E. Circulation *68*:433–436, 1983.

Clyman, R. I., Saugstad, O. D., and Mauray, F.: Oxygen metabolites stimulate prostaglandin E_2 production and relaxation of the ductus arteriosus. Clin. Res. *36*:228A, 1988.

Coceani, F., Hamilton, N. C., Labuc, J., et al.: Cytochrome P 450 linked menooxygenase: Involvement in the lamb ductus arteriosus. Am. J. Physiol. *246*:H640–H643, 1984.

Collaborative Group on Antenatal Steroid Therapy: Prevention of respiratory distress syndrome: Effect of antenatal dexamethasone administration (Publication No. 85–2695). Washington, D.C., National Institutes of Health, 1985, p. 44.

Cotton, R. B., Lindstrom, D. P., Kanarek, K. S., et al.: Effect of positive end-expiratory pressure on right ventricular output in lambs with hyaline membrane disease. Acta Paediatr. Scand. *69*:603–606, 1980.

Cotton, R. B., Lindstrom, D. P., and Stahlman M. T.: Early prediction of symptomatic patent ductus arteriosus from perinatal risk factors: Discriminant analysis. Acta Paediatr. Scand. *70*:723–727, 1981.

Cotton, R. B., Stahlman, M. T., Berder, H. W., et al.: Randomized trial of early closure of symptomatic patent ductus arteriosus in small preterm infants. J. Pediatr. *93*:647–651, 1978.

Drayton, M. R., and Skidmore, R.: Ductus arteriosus blood flow during first 48 hours of life. Arch. Dis. Child. *62*:1030–1034, 1987.

Dudell, G. G., and Gersony, W. M.: Patent ductus arteriosus in neonates with severe respiratory disease. J. Pediatr. *104*:915–920, 1984.

Ellison, R. C., Peckham, G. J., Lang, P., et al.: Evaluation of the preterm infant for patent ductus arteriosus. Pediatrics *71*:364–372, 1983.

Fay, F. S., and Jobsis, F. F.: Guinea pig ductus arteriosus. III. Light absorption changes during response to O_2. Am. J. Physiol. *223*:588–595, 1972.

Firth, J., and Pickering, D.: Timing of indomethacin therapy in persistent ductus. Lancet *2*:144, 1980.

Friedman, W. F.: The intrinsic physiologic properties of the developing heart. In Friedman, W. F., Lesch, M., and Sonnenblick, E. H. (Eds.): Neonatal Heart Disease. New York, Grune & Stratton, 1972, pp. 21–49.

Friedman, Z., Whitman, V., Maisels, M. J., et al.: Indomethacin disposition and indomethacin induced platelet dysfunction in premature infants. J. Clin. Pharmacol. *18*:272–279, 1978.

Fujiwara, T., Maeta, H., Morita, T., et al.: Artificial surfactant therapy in hyaline membrane disease. Lancet *1*:55–59, 1980.

Gerhardt, T., and Bancalari, E.: Lung compliance in newborns with patent ductus arteriosus before and after surgical ligation. Biol. Newborn *38*:96–105, 1980.

Gersony, W. M., Peckham, G. J., Ellison, R. C., et al.: Effects of indomethacin in premature infants with patent ductus arteriosus: Results of a national collaborative study. J. Pediatr. *102*:895–906, 1983.

Green, T. P., Thompson, T. R., Johnson, D., et al.: Fluid administration and the development of patent ductus arteriosus. N. Engl. J. Med. *303*:337–338, 1980.

Green, T. P., Thompson, T. R., Johnson, D. E., et al.: Furosemide promotes patent ductus arteriosus in premature infants with the respiratory distress syndrome. N. Engl. J. Med. *308*:743–748, 1983.

Hammerman, C., Strates, C., and Valaitis, S.: The silent ductus: Its precursors and its aftermath. Pediatr. Cardiol. *7*:121–127, 1986.

Hannigan, W. C., Kennedy, G., Roemisch, F., et al.: Administration of indomethacin for prevention of periventricular-intraventricular hemorrhage in high-risk infants. J. Pediatr. *112*:941–947, 1988.

Ikegami, M., Jacobs, H., and Jobe, A.: Surfactant function in respiratory distress syndrome. J. Pediatr. *102*:443–447, 1983.

Ivey, H. H., Kattwinkel, J., Park, T. S., et al.: Failure of indomethacin to close patent ductus arteriosus in infants weighing under 1000 g. Br. Heart J. *41*:304–307, 1979.

Jacob, J., Gluck, L., Di Sessa, T., et al.: The contribution of PDA in the neonate with severe RDS. J. Pediatr. *96*:79–87, 1980.

Johnson, D. S., Rogers, J. H., Null, D. M., et al.: The physiologic consequences of the ductus arteriosus in the extremely immature newborn. Clin. Res. *26*:826A, 1978.

Kaapa, P., Lanning, P., and Koivisto, M.: Early closure of patent ductus arteriosus with indomethacin in preterm infants with idiopathic respiratory distress syndrome. Acta Paediatr. Scand. *72*:179–184, 1983.

Kennedy, J. A., and Clark, S. L.: Observations on the physiological reactions of the ductus arteriosus. Am. J. Physiol. *136*:140–147, 1942.

Kitterman, J. A.: Effects of intestinal ischemia in necrotizing enterocolitis in the newborn infant. In Moore, T. D. (Ed.): Report of the 68th Ross Conference of Pediatric Research. Columbus, Ohio, Ross Laboratories, 1975 p. 38.

Koren, G., Zarfin, Y., Perlman, M., et al.: Effects of indomethacin on digoxin pharmacokinetics in preterm infants. Pediatr. Pharmacol. *4*:25–30, 1984.

Krueger, E., Mellander, M., Bratton, D., et al.: Prevention of symptomatic patent ductus arteriosus with a single dose of indomethacin. J. Pediatr. *111*:749–754, 1987.

Lewis, A. B., Heymann, M. A., and Rudolph, A. M.: Gestational changes in pulmonary vascular responses in fetal lambs in utero. Circ. Res. *39*:536–541, 1976.

Lilien, L. D., Srinivasan, G. M., Yeh, T. F., et al.: Decreased plasma glucose following indomethacin therapy in small prematures with PDA. Pediatr. Res. *17*:323A, 1983.

Lister, G., Hellenbrand, W. E., Kleinman, C. S., et al.: Physiologic effects of increasing hemoglobin concentration in left-to-right shunting in infants with ventricular septal defects. N. Engl. J. Med. *306*:502–506, 1982.

McGrath, R. L.: General Discussion. Session III: in Rudolph, A., Heymann, M. A. (eds.): Ross Conference on Pediatric Research: Persistent patency of ductus arteriosus in premature infants. Columbus, Ohio, Ross Laboratories, 1978.

Maher, P., Lane, B., Ballard, R., et al.: Does indomethacin cause extension of intracranial hemorrhages: A preliminary study. Pediatrics *75*:497–500, 1985.

Mahony, L., Caldwell, R. L., Girod, D. A., et al.: Indomethacin therapy on the first day of life in infants with very low birth weight. J. Pediatr. *106*:801–805, 1985.

Mahony, L., Carnero, V., Brett, C., et al.: Prophylactic indomethacin therapy for patent ductus arteriosus in very-low-birth-weight infants. N. Engl. J. Med. *306*::506–510, 1982.

Martin, C. G., Snider, A. R., Katz, S. M., et al.: Abnormal cerebral blood flow patterns in preterm infants with a large patent ductus arteriosus. J. Pediatr. *101*:587–593, 1982.

Mellander, M., Leheup, B., Lindstrom, D. P., et al.: Recurrence of symptomatic patent ductus arteriosus in extremely premature infants, treated with indomethacin. J. Pediatr. *105*:138–143, 1984.

Ment, L. R., Duncan, C. C., Ehrenkranz, R. A., et al.: Randomized indomethacin trial for prevention of intraventricular hemorrhage in very low birth weight infants. J. Pediatr. *107*:937–943, 1985.

Ment, L. R., Duncan, C. C., Ehrenkranz, R. A., et al.: Randomized low-dose indomethacin trial for prevention of intraventricular hemorrhage in very low birth weight neonates. J. Pediatr. *112*:948–955, 1988.

Merritt, T. A., Harris, J. P., Roghmann, K., et al.: Early closure of the patent ductus arteriosus in very low birthweight infants. A controlled trial. J. Pediatr. *99*:281–286, 1981.

Mikhail, M., Lei, W., Toews, W., et al.: Surgical and medical experience with 734 premature infants with patent ductus arteriosus. J. Thorac. Cardiovasc. Surg. *83*:349–357, 1982.

Momma, K., Mishihara, S., and Ota Y.: Constriction of the fetal ductus arteriosus by glucocorticoid hormones. Pediatr. Res. *15*:19–21, 1981.

Musewe, N. N., Smallhorn, J. F., Benson, L. N., et al.: Validation of Doppler derived pulmonary arterial pressure in patients with ductus arteriosus under different hemodynamic states. Circulation *76*:1081–1091, 1987.

Naulty, C. M., Horn, S., Conry, J., et al.: Improved lung compliance after ligation of patent ductus arteriosus in hyaline membrane disease. J. Pediatr. *93*:682–684, 1978.

Nystrom, G. A., Setzer, E. S., Zilleruelo, G. E., et al.: Prophylactic indomethacin: Effects on renal function. Pediatr. Res. *19*:178A, 1985.

Pérez Fontán, J. J., Clyman, R. I., Mauray, F., et al.: Respiratory effects of a patent ductus arteriosus in premature newborn lambs. J. Appl. Physiol. *63*:2315–2324, 1987.

Perlman, J. M., Hill, A., and Volpe, J. J.: The effect of patent ductus arteriosus on flow velocity in the anterior cerebral arteries: Ductal steal in the premature newborn infant. J. Pediatr. *99*:767–771, 1981.

Puckett, C. G., Cox, M. A., Haskins, K. S., et al.: Prophylactic indomethacin for the prevention of patent ductus arteriosus. Pediatr. Res. *19*:358A, 1985.

Ramsey, J. M., Murphy, D. J., Vick G. W., III, et al.: Response of the patent ductus arteriosus to indomethacin treatment. Am. J. Dis. Child. *141*:294–297, 1987.

Rennie, J. M., Doyle, J., and Cooke R. W. I.: Early administration of indomethacin to preterm infants. Arch. Dis. Child. *61*:233–238, 1986.

Rheuban, K. S., Everett, A. D., Zellers, T. M., et al.: Ductus arteriosus closure rates and indomethacin levels in premature infants. Pediatr. Res. *21*:387A, 1987.

Rhodes, P. G., Ferguson, M. G., Reddy, N. S., Joransen, J. A., Gibson, J.: Effects of prolonged versus acute indomethacin therapy in very low birth weight infants with patent ductus arteriosus. Eur. J. Pediatr. *147*:481–484, 1988.

Rudd, P., Montanez, P., Hallidie-Smith, K., et al.: Indomethacin treatment for patent ductus arteriosus in very low birthweight infants: Double blind trial. Arch. Dis. Child. *58*:267–270, 1983.

Setzer, E. S., Torres-Arraut, E., Gomez del Rio, M., et al.: Cardiopulmonary effects of prophylactic indomethacin in the very low birthweight infant. Pediatr. Res. *18*:346A, 1984.

Setzer-Bandstra, E., Montalvo, B. M., Goldberg, R. N., et al.: Prophylactic indomethacin for prevention of intraventricular hemorrhage in premature infants. Pediatrics *82*:533–542, 1988.

Shimada, S., Raju, T., Bhat, R., et al.: Treatment of patent ductus arteriosus after exogenous surfactant in baboons with hyaline membrane disease. Pediatr. Res. *26*:565–569, 1989.

Smith, M., Setzer, E. S., Garg, D. C., et al.: Pharmacokinetics of prophylactic indomethacin in very low birthweight premature infants. Pediatr. Res. *18*:161A, 1984.

Sola, A., Rogido, M., Lezama, C., et al.: Effects of "prophylactic" IV indomethacin in VLBW infants with HMD. Pediatr. Res. *20*:361A, 1986.

Spach, M. S., Serwer, G. A., Anderson, P. A. W., et al.: Pulsatile aortopulmonary pressure flow dynamics of patent ductus arteriosus in patients with various hemodynamic states. Circulation *61*:110–122, 1980.

Staub, N. C.: Pathogenesis of pulmonary edema. Prog. Cardiovasc. Dis. *23*:53–80, 1980.

Stevenson, J. G., Kawabori, I., and Guntheroth W. G.: Pulsed doppler echocardiographic diagnosis of patent ductus arteriosus: Sensitivity, limitations and technical features. Cathet. Cardiovasc. Diagn. *6*:255–263, 1980.

Thalji, A. A., Carr, I., Yeh, T. F., et al.: Pharmacokinetics of intravenously administered indomethacin in premature infants. J. Pediatr. *97*:995–1000, 1980.

Thibeault, D. W., Emmanouilides, G. C., and Dodge, M. E.: Pulmonary and circulatory function in preterm lambs treated with hydrocortisone in utero. Biol. Newborn *34*:238–247, 1978.

Thibeault, D. W., Emmanouilides, G. C. Nelson, R. J., et al.: Patent ductus arteriosus complicating the respiratory distress syndrome in preterm infants. J. Pediatr. *86*:120–126, 1975.

Vincer, M., Allen, A., Evans, J. R., et al.: Early intravenous indomethacin prolongs respiratory support in very low birthweight infants. Acta Paediatr. Scand. *76*:894–897, 1987.

Waffarn, F., Siassi, B., Cabal, L., et al.: Effect of antenatal glucocorticoids on clinical closure of the ductus arteriosus. Am. J. Dis. Child. *137*:336–338, 1983.

Wagner, H. R., Ellison, R. C., Zierler, S., et al.: Surgical closure of patent ductus arteriosus in 268 preterm infants. J. Thorac. Cardiovasc. Surg. *87*:870–875, 1984.

Wilkerson, R. D., and Glenn, T. M.: Influence of nonsteroidal anti-inflammatory drugs on ouabain toxicity. Am. Heart J. *94*:454–459, 1977.

Yaffe, S. J., Friedman, W. F., Rogers, D., et al.: The disposition of indomethacin in premature babies. J. Pediatr. *97*:1001–1006, 1980.

Yeh, T. F., Achanti, B., Jain, R., et al.: Indomethacin therapy in premature infants with PDA—determination of therapeutic plasma levels. Dev. Pharmacol. Thera. *12*:169–178, 1989.

Yeh, T. F., Luken, J. A., Raval, D., et al.: Indomethacin treatment in small versus large premature infants with ductus arteriosus—comparison of plasma indomethacin concentration and clinical response. Br. Heart J. *50*:27–30, 1983.

Yeh, T. F., Wilks, A., Betkerur, M., et al.: Furosemide prevents the renal side effects of indomethacin therapy in premature infants with patent ductus arteriosus. J. Pediatr. *101*:433–437, 1982.

PART X

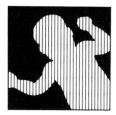

CARDIOVASCULAR SYSTEM

GENERAL 62 CONSIDERATIONS

Michael D. Freed

During the 1980s, much progress has been made in the diagnosis and treatment of neonatal cardiac conditions. A better understanding of the physiology of the neonate as well as technical improvements in angiography, echocardiography, and radionuclide imaging have allowed for a more complete diagnosis to be made without undue risk. Advances in cardiovascular surgery in the neonate, especially the introduction of deep hypothermia (20°C) with circulatory arrest, have permitted total correction of some forms of congenital heart disease (e.g., ventricular septal defect, tetralogy of Fallot, and transposition of the great arteries) during the neonatal period in some centers. Even repair of one of the most complex cardiac conditions, aortic and mitral value atresia with a hypoplastic left ventricle, has yielded to a physiologic correction (Norwood et al., 1983; Pigott et al., 1988). However, Fyler and co-workers (1980) reported that more than 50 per cent of children who presented with critical congenital heart disease in the first month of life were dead before their first birthday.

Newborns with critical heart disease rarely get better on their own and frequently deteriorate over a short period of time. Much of the recent progress results from more prompt recognition and referral to major centers with staffs skilled in cardiology and cardiovascular surgery. The chapters that follow are an attempt to describe the state-of-the-art early in 1990. The certainty that these chapters will be outdated within a few years remains one of the most exciting aspects of neonatal cardiology.

■ THE FETAL CIRCULATION

Although some research has been done with human fetuses (Lind and Wegelius, 1954; Lind et al., 1964), most of our understanding of the in utero circulation is from work on fetal lambs (Dawes, 1968; Heymann and Rudolph, 1972; Rudolph, 1970; Teitel et al., 1987).

The fetal circulation is arranged in parallel rather than in series, with mixing between the streams at the atrial and great vessel level (Fig. 62–1). These adaptations allowing diversion of blood from the immature lungs to the placenta for oxygen exchange permit fetal survival with a variety of cardiac lesions.

Normally, blood returning from the placenta passes either into the portal system of the liver and then into the inferior vena cava (IVC) or into the ductus venosus and inferior vena cava directly. In the right atrium, the IVC blood is diverted into two streams by the crista dividens. The smaller stream is diverted across the foramen ovale into the left atrium, where it mixes with pulmonary venous return and passes through the mitral valve into the left ventricle. This blood is pumped out into the ascending aorta, where it supplies the coronary, carotid, and subclavian arteries with only 10 per cent of combined ventricular output passing through the aortic arch into the descending aorta.

The majority of blood from the IVC is diverted into the right atrium, where it joins the superior vena caval (SVC) drainage and coronary sinus return before passing through the tricuspid valve into the right ventricle and pulmonary artery. Since the fluid-filled lungs and constricted pulmonary arterioles offer a high resistance to flow, most of the blood in the main pulmonary artery goes through the ductus arteriosus into the low-resistance descending aorta and placenta.

The oxygen content of blood in the fetus is considerably lower than that in the newborn or child (Fig. 62–2). Since the placenta is the organ of oxygen exchange, umbilical venous blood has the highest PO_2 (32 to 35 torr, oxygen saturation 70 per cent, with the mother breathing room air). The blood destined for the left side of the heart mixes with the less saturated inferior vena caval and pulmonary venous return, lowering the PO_2 to about 26 to 28 torr (oxygen saturation about 65 per cent) before passing into the left ventricle and ascending aorta.

The umbilical venous return for the right ventricle mixes with the SVC return (PO_2 12 to 14 torr, oxygen saturation 40 per cent), reducing the oxygen in the blood destined to go to the right ventricle, pulmonary artery, descending aorta, and placenta to 20 to 22 torr (oxygen saturation 50 to 55 per cent). Thus, the blood with the highest oxygen content is diverted to the coronary arteries and

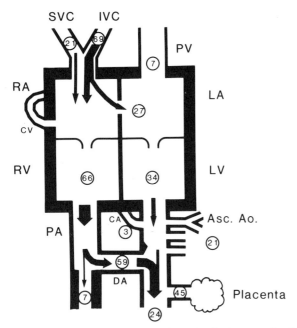

FIGURE 62–1. *The course of the circulation in the late gestation fetal lamb. The numbers within the circles represent percentage of combined ventricular output. Some of the return from the inferior vena cava (IVC) is diverted by the crista dividens in the right atrium (RA) through the foramen ovale into the left atrium (LA), where it meets the pulmonary venous (PV) return and passes into the left ventricle (LV) and is pumped into the ascending aorta (Asc Ao). Most of the aortic flow goes to the coronary artery (CA) and subclavian and carotid arteries with only 10 per cent of combined ventricular output passing through the aortic arch into the descending aorta.*

The remainder of the inferior vena cava flow mixes with return from the superior vena cava (SVC) and coronary veins (CV) and passes into the right atrium and right ventricle (RV) and is pumped into the pulmonary artery (PA). Because of the high pulmonary resistance, only 7 per cent passes into the lungs, with the rest going into the ductus arteriosus (DA) and then to the descending aorta to the placenta and lower half of the body. (Modified from Rudolph, A. M.: Congenital Disease of the Heart. Chicago, Year Book Medical Publishers, Inc., 1974.)

brain, and that with the lowest oxygen content is diverted to the placenta. An additional fetal adaptation to oxygen transport at low oxygen saturation is the presence of high levels of fetal hemoglobin, which has a high oxygen affinity and, consequently, a low P 50 (partial pressure of oxygen at 50 per cent hemoglobin saturation) of approximately 18 to 19 torr. This leftward shift of the oxygen dissociation curve facilitates oxygen uptake at the placenta.

The wide communication between the atria allows for equalization of pressures in the atrium; similarly, the patency of the ductus arteriosus results in equalization of pressures in the aorta and pulmonary artery.

The fetus has a limited ability to regulate cardiac output. Cardiac output is a function of heart rate, filling pressures (preload), resistance against which the ventricles eject (afterload), and myocardial contractility. Spontaneous changes in heart rate have been found to be associated with electrocortical activity as well as the sleep state and fetal activity. Rudolph and Heymann (1976) have shown, using continuous measurements of left and right ventricular output with electromagnetic flow probes, that spontaneous increases in heart rate were associated with increasing ventricular output while decreases in heart rate resulted in a considerable fall of both right and left

ventricular output. By electrically pacing the right atrium above the resting level of 160 to 180 beats per minute, the same changes were found.

While changes in heart rate caused significant output differences, increasing preload even to levels as high as a right atrial pressure of 20 mm Hg produced only very small increases in ventricular output (Heymann and Rudolph, 1973), suggesting that the fetal ventricle normally operates near the top of its function curve and has little functional reserve. Increasing afterload by inflating a balloon in the fetal descending aorta or by methoxamine (Gilbert, 1987) produces a dramatic fall in right ventricular output, suggesting that the fetal heart is very sensitive to increases in afterload.

An increase in quantities of sarcoplasmic reticulum (Hoerter et al., 1982; Nakanishi et al., 1984) and myofibrils (Nakanishi and Jannakani, 1984) with development provides an explanation of the mechanisms of increasing tension produced by excised strips of adult myocardium compared with the equivalent strips of fetal tissue (Friedman, 1973). Additionally, some increase in contractility perinatally may be explained by a parallel increase in myofibrillar protein function associated with changes in the molecular structure of myocin (Mahdavi et al., 1987)

All of the above data suggest that fetal myocardium is structurally and functionally quite immature compared with the older child or adult. The fetal heart appears to be working at the peak of its ventricular function curve with increases in preload causing little or no change in cardiac output, and increases in afterload resulting in a marked depression. The limited ability of the fetal heart to

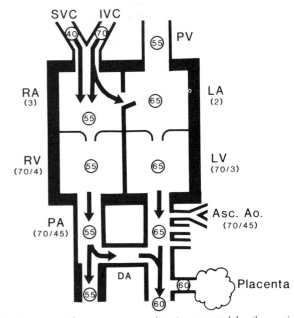

FIGURE 62–2. *The oxygen saturation (represented by the encircled numbers) and pressures (shown in parentheses) in the late gestation fetal lamb. The oxygen saturation is the highest in the inferior vena cava, representing flow that is primarily from the placenta. The saturation of the blood in the heart is slightly higher on the left side than on the right side. Since large communications between the atrium and great vessels are present, the pressures on both sides of the heart are virtually identical. The abbreviations in this diagram are the same as those in Figure 62–1. (Modified from Rudolph, A. M.: Congenital Disease of the Heart. Chicago, Year Book Medical Publishers, Inc., 1974.)*

respond to stress seems to be primarily mediated through increased heart rate.

The structure, hemodynamics, and myocardial function of the fetus have significant consequences in the neonate with congenital heart disease:

1. The parallel circulation with connections at the atrial and great vessel level allows a wide variety of structural cardiac problems to occur while still normally transporting blood to the placenta and fetal organs for gas exchange.

2. The right ventricle does approximately two-thirds of the cardiac work before birth. This is reflected in the size and thickness of the right ventricle before and after birth and may explain why left-sided heart defects are tolerated more poorly after birth than are right-sided lesions.

3. The normal flow across the preductal aortic arch is small (10 per cent of CVO), particularly when compared with the flow across the ductus arteriosus (60 per cent of CVO), with most of the descending aortic flow derived from the pulmonary artery. This makes the aortic isthmus especially vulnerable to small changes in blood flow and may explain the high incidence of coarctation of the aorta and interruption in this region in association with other congenital cardiac lesions.

4. Since pulmonary blood flow in utero accounts for a small proportion of the necessary flow after birth, anomalies that prevent normal pulmonary venous return (such as total anomalous pulmonary venous return or mitral stenosis) may be masked in utero when pulmonary venous return is minimal.

5. The low levels of circulating oxygen before birth (Po_2 26 to 28 torr in the ascending aorta and Po_2 20 to 22 torr in the descending aorta) may account for the relative postnatal comfort of infants with cyanotic congenital heart disease, who may be quite active and feed well with an arterial Po_2 of 25, a level that would lead to cerebral and cardiac anoxia, acidosis, and death within a few minutes in the older child or adult.

■ TRANSITIONAL CIRCULATION

Soon after the neonate begins to breathe air, the low-resistance placenta is removed from the circulation, and systemic resistance increases. At the same time, the onset of air breathing expands the lung and brings oxygen to the pulmonary alveoli. This drop in pulmonary resistance can be explained by simple physical expansion and by chemoreflex vasodilatation of the pulmonary arteries, which is caused by the high level of oxygen in the alveolar gas.

Both the increase in systemic vascular resistance due to clamping of the umbilical cord and the approximately 80 per cent drop in pulmonary vascular resistance that occurs with the onset of respiration cause increased pulmonary flow and decreased ductal flow. Before birth, the relative pulmonary and systemic resistances cause 90 per cent of right ventricular blood to go through the ductus to the descending aorta; by a few minutes after birth, 90 per cent goes to the pulmonary arteries.

The rapid drop in systemic venous return to the IVC as the umbilical venous flow is cut off and the increase in pulmonary venous return as the pulmonary blood flow increases cause the left atrial pressure to increase and

exceed right atrial pressure, resulting in apposition of the valve of the foramen ovale against the edge of the crista dividens with functional closure of the foramen ovale. Thus, within moments, the pulmonary and systemic circulations have changed from a parallel to a series arrangement (Fig. 62–3).

There has been much discussion about the relative contributions to the circulatory changes from the mechanical or chemoreflex lowering of the pulmonary resistance, and the sudden increase in systemic resistance. Recently, Tietel and co-workers (1987), using instrumented fetal sheep near term, found that ventilation alone caused dramatic changes in the central flow patterns attributable to a large decrease in pulmonary vascular resistance and associated increase in pulmonary blood flow. Ventilation alone increased the pulmonary venous return from approximately 8 per cent of combined ventricular output to 31 per cent of combined ventricular output, causing the right ventricle which had ejected about 90 per cent of its output through the ductus arteriosus to the placenta, to reduce this to less than 50 per cent. Oxygenation further changed the flow patterns so that more than 90 per cent of the flow from the main pulmonary artery went to the lungs rather than through the ductus arteriosus. Umbilical cord occlusion had few additional effects.

The ductus arteriosus usually remains patent for several hours or days after birth. Initially, the pulmonary vascular resistance may exceed systemic, resulting in a small right-to-left (pulmonary artery-to-aorta) shunt with some systemic desaturation in the lower half of the body (Fig. 62–4). Anything that increases pulmonary vascular resistance

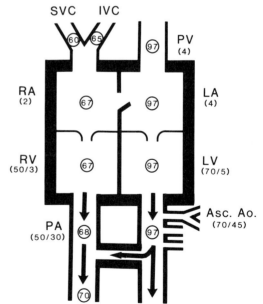

FIGURE 62–3. *The course of the circulation soon after birth. The numbers within the circles represent oxygen saturation in per cent, and the numbers within the parentheses signify pressures in mm Hg. The circulation is now arranged in series rather than in parallel with blood traversing the right side of the heart to get to the lungs for oxygenation and then the left side of the heart for delivery to the body. There is still minimal shunting from aorta to pulmonary artery through the constricting ductus arteriosus. The right-sided pressures have dropped below left-sided pressures and will drop further over the next 48 hours of life. The abbreviations in this diagram are the same as those used in Figure 62–1. (Modified from Rudolph, A. M.: Congenital Disease of the Heart. Chicago, Year Book Medical Publishers, Inc., 1974.)*

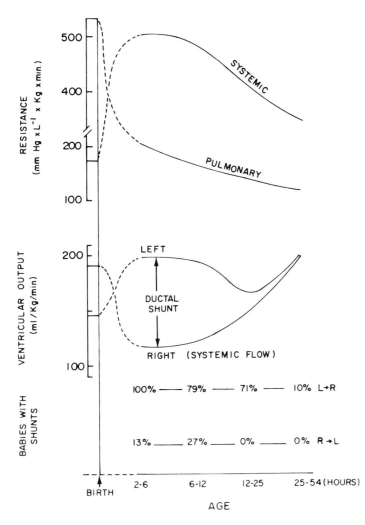

FIGURE 62–4. Hemodynamics of the cardiorespiratory conversion in the newborn. The pulmonary and systemic vascular resistance are shown on top, the ventricular outputs in the middle, and the percentage of babies with left-to-right and right-to-left shunts in the bottom panel. Before birth, the pulmonary resistance exceeds the systemic resistance, so shunting through the ductus is from the right side of the heart (pulmonary artery) to the left side of the heart (aorta).

Soon after birth, the pulmonary resistance falls secondary to arteriolar vasodilatation, and the systemic resistance increases as the low resistance placenta is excluded from the systemic circulation. When the systemic resistance exceeds pulmonary resistance within a few moments of birth, shunting through the ductus reverses, going from the higher resistance aorta (left) to the lower resistance pulmonary artery (right). By 12 to 24 hours of age, the ductus has closed. Anything that increases pulmonary resistance (e.g., hypoxemia, acidosis, or hypoglycemia) will cause the right-to-left shunt to persist or temporarily reduce left-to-right shunting. (From Nelson, N. M.: Respiration and circulation after birth. In Smith, C. A., and Nelson, N. M.: The Physiology of the Newborn Infant. 4th ed. Springfield Ill., Charles C Thomas, Publisher, 1976. Courtesy of Charles C Thomas, Publisher, Springfield, Illinois.)

or prevents postnatal decrease in it (e.g., acidosis, hypoxemia, polycythemia, lung disease, or cesarean section) may exacerbate or prolong this normally transient right-to-left shunt.

Within a few hours of life, the pulmonary vascular resistance normally falls lower than systemic resistance, resulting in a small "physiologic" left-to-right (aorta-to-pulmonary artery) shunt. Normally, within 10 to 15 hours after birth, the ductus arteriosus closes, although permanent structural closure may not take place for another 2 to 3 weeks. The mechanism of ductal closure is still not completely understood, although it has been clear for some time that oxygen plays a role. Prostaglandins (PG) of the E series seem to be responsible for maintaining patency of the ductus arteriosus during fetal life (Coceani and Olley, 1973). It has been possible to keep the ductus open for days or weeks in infants with congenital heart disease by infusion of exogenous PGE_1 or PGE_2 (Freed et al., 1981), and it has been possible to close the ductus arteriosus in about 80 per cent of preterm infants weighing less than 1750 with indomethacin, a nonselective prostaglandin-synthesis inhibitor. It remains unclear whether normal ductal closure is due to reduced synthesis or increased removal in the lung of E prostaglandins, production of another prostanoic acid (possibly thromboxane) with constrictor properties, or a lack of local responsiveness of all prostaglandin receptors that is due to an increase in oxygen with active ductal constriction (Coceani and Olley, 1980).

Although some hypoxemia is present soon after birth, the normal arterial Po_2 gradually increases (Po_2 50 at 10 minutes. 62 at 1 hour. and 75 to 83 between 3 hours and 2 days) over the first hours of life, with continued pulmonary vasodilatation and improved ventilation-perfusion ratios. In addition, the pulmonary pressure gradually falls to about 30 torr systolic within about 48 hours (Emmanouilides et al., 1964). Although the pulmonary vascular resistance will continue to decrease for several weeks, the transition to the adult circulation is virtually complete by 2 days of age.

▪ EVALUATION OF THE CARDIOVASCULAR SYSTEM IN THE NEWBORN

History. The age at which symptoms or murmurs presented may be helpful; for example, heart failure at birth suggests an intrauterine arrhythmia such as supraventricular tachycardia, or an arteriovenous fistula. Murmurs of semilunar valve obstruction or atrioventricular regurgitation are usually present soon after birth, whereas the murmur of a ventricular septal defect or patent ductus arteriosus is usually not audible until later, since the magnitude of the left-to-right shunt depends on the decline in pulmonary vascular resistance over the first days and weeks of life.

A good feeding history is essential. Neonates with congestive heart failure may tire with feeding and be able to ingest only 1 or 2 ounces before becoming exhausted and falling asleep. These infants remain quite hungry and irritable and frequently exhibit poor weight gain, partly because their caloric intake is reduced.

Infants with congestive heart failure are often tachypneic and dyspneic. Parents or nurses may report rapid respiratory rates that occur while the infant is sleeping or subcostal and intercostal retractions. Excessive perspiration, most obvious on the head while the infant is feeding, is another sign of congestive failure.

The history should include questions regarding cyanosis. Acrocyanosis of the hands and feet, a benign manifestation of increased extraction of oxygen in the peripheral capillary beds, can be quite marked in the first few days or weeks of life. It is usually most noticeable when the extremities are cold and improves or disappears with warming. True cyanosis of the mucous membranes beyond 2 to 3 hours of age is abnormal. It is highly suggestive of (but does not necessarily prove the existence of) pulmonary, central nervous system, and congenital heart disease (see further on). A history of illness during pregnancy should be obtained whenever possible because of the association of congenital heart disease with maternal diabetes, congenital heart block with maternal lupus erythematosus, and patent ductus arteriosus with maternal rubella during the first trimester. Finally, a careful family history is important because the recurrence rate for congenital heart disease is higher in affected families and approximately 5 per cent of congenital heart disease is in children with inherited syndromes.

Physical Examination. A thorough physical examination of the neonate begins with observation. The chromosomal anomalies and such syndromes as Holt-Oram and Williams have obvious stigmata and are associated with heart disease in a large number of cases.

The vital signs should be checked, preferably with the infant resting or asleep. Heart rates above 160 to 180 beats/minute may be seen with agitation but may also indicate congestive failure or a tachyarrhythmia. Bradycardia may be normal as a manifestation of increased vagal tone but may be due to complete heart block. A respiratory rate of greater than 60 per minute in the neonatal period and more than 45 thereafter is probably abnormal. While there are many causes, most of them pulmonary, congenital heart disease must be considered.

The blood pressure in both arms and a leg should be taken in all neonates suspected of having congenital heart disease. We have found the Doppler to be an excellent method for measuring blood pressures in neonates, although palpation can also be used successfully. The flush method is probably outdated. One must be sure to use a large cuff (preferably the 2-inch size), placing it over the forearm if the upper arm is too small. In coarctation of the aorta, the blood pressure is increased in both arms compared with that in the legs, although the left arm pressure may be low if the coarctation involves the origin of the left subclavian, and the right arm may be low if the right subclavian arises anomalously below the coarctation.

The infant should be weighed and measured. Normally, the newborn loses 5 to 10 per cent of the birth weight in the first few days of life but regains birth weight by 7 to 10 days. Thereafter, the infant should gain about 28 g (1

ounce) every day for the remainder of the first month. Infants who have not gained 350 to 450 g (12 to 16 ounces) by the end of the first month are failing to thrive.

The color of the skin and mucous membranes should then be evaluated, and evidence of acrocyanosis or true cyanosis should be recorded. Occasionally, the lower body is more cyanotic than the upper (differential cyanosis), which suggests right-to-left shunting of venous blood through the ductus arteriosus. This finding may be present in coarctation of the aorta, interrupted aortic arch, or the persistent fetal circulation syndrome but may be normal in the first hours of life.

Observation of the thorax can sometimes reveal anomalies in the neonate. Occasionally, the heart is hyperactive and the cardiac impulse is visible on the left side of the chest. Subcostal or intercostal retractions suggest respiratory distress. The precordium should then be palpated. Volume overload lesions such as a ventricular septal defect, atrioventricular valve regurgitation, and arteriovenous fistula will give a tapping or even rocking impulse. Rarely, stenosis of a semilunar valve, regurgitation of an atrioventricular valve, or a large left-to-right shunt through a ventricular septal defect or patent ductus arteriosus will cause a thrill.

Auscultation remains the most important part of the examination of the newborn but is in danger of being neglected with the advent of more complicated technical tools. The first heart sound (S_1) is loudest at the apex. It represents mitral and tricuspid closure and is narrowly split (phonocardiographically) but is usually heard as a single sound. A split S_1 suggests delayed tricuspid closure and is occasionally present in the Ebstein anomaly. An accentuated S_1 suggests an atrial septal defect, or a short P–R interval; a diminished S_1 suggests a prolonged P–R interval, or congestive heart failure.

The second heart sound (S_2), heard best at the left upper sternal border, has two components representing aortic and pulmonic valve closure. Normally, S_2 is split during inspiration (when increased right heart volume prolongs right ventricular ejection) and single during expiration. The rapid heart rates may make appreciation of the splitting difficult, which is unfortunate because it is one of the most helpful signs in the clinical evaluation of the newborn. Wide splitting of S_2 is seen with an atrial septal defect or anomalous pulmonary venous return or when there is a delay in right ventricular ejection because of either a conduction delay (e.g., right bundle-branch block) or an obstruction to right ventricular ejection (e.g., pulmonic stenosis).

The pulmonary component of S_2 is loud in the presence of pulmonary hypertension and soft or inaudible in the presence of pulmonic stenosis, either isolated or in association with a ventricular septal defect, single ventricle, or tricuspid atresia. Obviously, S_2 is single in the presence of pulmonary or aortic atresia.

Third and fourth heart sounds (S_3 and S_4) are infrequently heard. They may be present in infants with congestive cardiac failure, but the rapid heart rates associated with failure make appreciation on auscultation difficult.

Systolic ejection clicks, early in systole, result from dilatation of the great vessels. Aortic ejection clicks, constant through the respiratory cycle and loudest at the apex, are usually found in association with valvular aortic stenosis. Variable ejection clicks are soft or inaudible during inspiration and loudest along the left sternal border, and they are noted in association with pulmonary valve stenosis.

Heart murmurs may be audible during systole or diastole or may be continuous. A systolic murmur is classified as either an ejection or a regurgitant type.

Ejection murmurs are caused by turbulence of blood as it leaves the heart through a narrowed orifice. The murmur is crescendo-decrescendo, or diamond-shaped, and begins a fraction of a second after S_1, the delay caused by the isovolumic contraction phase between closing of the atrioventricular valves and opening of the semilunar valves. Ejection murmurs are characteristic of aortic or pulmonic valve, or subvalvular, stenosis.

Regurgitant murmurs are pansystolic; that is, they start with S_1 and last until S_2. Regurgitant murmurs are even in intensity through systole and are characteristic of atrioventricular valve regurgitation (either mitral or tricuspid) or a ventricular septal defect. The presence of a regurgitant murmur in the first day or two of life suggests A-V valve regurgitation, since the normal elevation of pulmonary vascular resistance usually prevents the murmurs of a ventricular defect from being audible until later in the first week of life.

Diastolic murmurs may represent regurgitation through one of the semilunar valves or stenosis across an atrioventricular valve. Murmurs of aortic or pulmonary regurgitation tend to occur early in diastole and are uncommon in neonates. Infants with tetralogy of Fallot with an absent pulmonary valve, however, may have loud systolic and low-pitched diastolic murmurs generated by stenosis and regurgitation at the pulmonary valve annulus. Mid- and late-diastolic murmurs usually represent murmurs across one of the atrioventricular valves. Occasionally, these are due to anatomic narrowing, either mitral or tricuspid stenosis, but they more frequently result from relative stenosis from a large flow across a structurally normal valve. For example, a large left-to-right shunt through a ventricular septal defect often causes a mid-diastolic mitral flow rumble at the apex, and total anomalous pulmonary venous return without pulmonary venous obstruction is likely to cause a tricuspid flow rumble along the left sternal border.

Continuous murmurs heard throughout systole and diastole result from flow between a high-pressure vessel and a low-pressure vessel throughout the cardiac cycle, usually the aorta and pulmonary artery with a patent ductus arteriosus. Occasionally, an arteriovenous fistula may cause a continuous murmur over the head or liver. A continuous murmur in a cyanotic newborn in the 1st week of life is almost always due to collateral vessels from aorta to pulmonary artery in infants with a ventricular septal defect and pulmonary atresia.

The liver is usually palpable 3 cm (at most) below the costal margin in the right midclavicular line. It may be larger in cases of congestive heart failure, hemolytic disease, and a variety of liver diseases, and it may be downwardly displaced without hepatomegaly with hyperexpansion of the lung. A midline or left-sided liver suggests the heterotaxia syndrome.

Peripheral edema is rarely due to heart disease, but it may be seen during the early postnatal period in infants with in utero supraventricular tachycardia.

Finally, the peripheral pulses should be evaluated. Asymmetric pulses between the arm and legs suggest coarctation of the aorta or interrupted aortic arch with a closing ductus arteriosus. Symmetrically decreased pulses suggest congestive heart failure or cardiogenic shock. Increased pulses are present when there is a diastolic "run-off" from the aorta seen in patent ductus arteriosus, aorticopulmonary window–truncus arteriosus, and arteriovenous fistula.

Electrocardiography. Although most of the methods used in the cardiac evaluation of the newborn are helpful in assessing the child's current status, electrocardiography in great part reflects the abnormal hemodynamic burdens placed on the heart in utero For example, in the normal fetus the right ventricle does most of the cardiac work before birth; therefore, the presence of left ventricular hypertrophy on the electrocardiogram in a newborn suggests either the increased left ventricular work in utero that is seen with aortic stenosis or the decreased right ventricular work in utero that appears with tricuspid atresia and a hypoplastic right ventricle.

Some electrocardiographic patterns are virtually diagnostic of specific cardiac lesions; these are discussed in more detail in Chapter 63.

Electrocardiography can be used to assess severity of disease by determining the degree of atrial or ventricular hypertrophy or by revealing changes in the S–T segments or T waves, which suggest myocardial ischemia. Electrocardiography is also the major diagnostic method of evaluating dysrhythmias (see Chapter 65) and electrolyte imbalances of potassium or calcium.

The Normal Electrocardiogram in the Term Infant. Before electrocardiography can be used successfully in the management of infants with congenital heart disease, the ranges of normal must be appreciated. The rest of this section, dealing primarily with the normal electrocardiogram, is based on the classic work of Ziegler (1951) and Cassels and Ziegler (1966) and, more recently, Davignon and co-workers (1980), and Liebman and co-workers (1982).

Heart Rate. The average resting heart rate for a neonate in the first week of life is about 125 to 130 beats per minute, but rates as low as 85 or 90 beats per minute with sleep or as high as 190 to 200 with crying or agitation may be seen. In general, the normal resting rate gradually increases over the first month of life so that the mean value at 30 days is about 150 beats per minute (Table 62–1).

Rhythm. Normal sinus rhythm with a P wave preceding each QRS complex predominates. A sinus arrhythmia with each QRS preceded by a P wave, but slight variation in the interval between P waves (P–P interval) is not uncommon, especially with careful monitoring and 24-hour recordings.

P Wave. The P wave represents atrial depolarization. The P-wave duration varies but is usually between 0.04 and 0.08 second. Although a prolonged P wave suggests left atrial hypertrophy in the older child or adult, this sign is not as helpful in diagnosis of the newborn. The amplitude of the P wave is best appreciated in lead II and

TABLE 62–1. Electrocardiographic Standards in Newborns

MEASURE	AGE IN DAYS			
	0–1	1–3	3–7	7–30
Number of patients	189	179	181	119
Heart rate (beats/minutes)	122 (99–147)	123 (97–148)	128 (100–160)	148 (114–177)
QRS axis (degrees)	135 (91–185)	134 (93–188)	133 (92–185)	108 (78–152)
P–R duration II (msec)	107 (82–138)	108 (85–132)	103 (78–130)	101 (75–128)
QRS duration V$_5$ (msec)	50 (26–69)	48 (27–61)	49 (26–63)	53 (27–75)
Q–T duration V$_5$ (msec)	290 (220–360)	280 (235–330)	272 (272–315)	258 (230–290)
P amplitude II (mvolts)	0.16 (0.07–0.25)	0.16 (0.05–0.25)	0.17 (0.08–0.27)	0.19 (0.09–0.29)
R amplitude V$_{3R}$ (mvolts)	1.05 (0.40–1.79)	1.19 (0.52–1.95)	1.02 (0.18–1.80)	0.82 (0.30–1.50)
R amplitude V$_1$ (mvolts)	1.35 (0.65–2.37)	1.48 (0.70–2.42)	1.28 (0.50–2.15)	1.05 (0.45–1.81)
R amplitude V$_5$ (mvolts)	1.0 (0.25–1.85)	1.1 (0.48–1.95)	1.3 (0.48–1.95)	1.45 (0.60–2.1)
R amplitude V$_6$ (mvolts)	0.45 (0.05–0.95)	0.48 (0.05–0.95)	0.51 (0.10–1.05)	0.76 (0.26–1.35)
S amplitude V$_{3R}$ (mvolts)	0.43 (0.07–1.18)	0.5 (0.05–1.2)	0.36 (0.05–0.8)	0.20 (0.05–0.64)
S amplitude V$_1$ (mvolts)	0.85 (0.10–1.85)	0.95 (0.15–1.90)	0.68 (0.10–1.50)	0.4 (0.05–0.97)
S amplitude V$_5$ (mvolts)	0.99 (0.38–1.79)	0.98 (0.20–1.59)	0.95 (0.38–1.63)	0.8 (0.24–1.38)
S amplitude V$_6$ (mvolts)	0.35 (0.02–0.79)	0.32 (0.02–0.76)	0.37 (0.02–0.80)	0.32 (0.02–0.82)
R/S amplitude V$_{3R}$	1.5 (0.2–4.8)	1.6 (0.2–4.2)	1.8 (0.2–5.8)	1.9 (0.2–2.5)
R/S amplitude V$_1$	2.2 (0.4–7.0)	2.0 (0.4–5.4)	2.8 (0.05–7.2)	2.9 (1.1–6.3)
R/S amplitude V$_5$	0.7 (0–7.0)	1.0 (0–5.0)	1.5 (0–5.0)	2.0 (0–5.1)
R/S amplitude V$_6$	2 (0–8)	3 (0–9)	2 (0–8)	4 (0–9)
Mean (5 and 95 per cent values)				

(From Davignon, A., Rautaharju, P., Boiselle, E., et al.: Normal ECG standards for infants and children. Pediatr. Cardiol. *1*:123, 1979–1980.)

should be less than 3 mm (0.3 mv) in height; taller P waves suggest right atrial hypertrophy. The P-wave axis is usually between 0 and +90 degrees (upright in leads I and aV$_f$), averaging +60 degrees; an abnormal P-wave axis suggests an ectopic atrial pacemaker or abnormal position of the atria.

P–R Interval. The P–R interval, the time from the onset of the P wave to the onset of the QRS, represents the time that the electrical impulse takes to traverse the atrium, the A-V node and the Purkinje system to the ventricular myocardium. The normal P–R interval is 0.08 to 0.14 second (mean = 0.10) (see Table 62–1). A short P–R interval suggests a nodal pacemaker, rapid conduction through a bypass tract (as in Wolff-Parkinson-White syndrome), or facilitated conduction in glycogen storage disease. A prolonged P–R interval (first-degree heart block) is frequently benign but may be a manifestation of conduction system disease.

QRS Complex. The QRS duration represents ventricular depolarization and is usually 0.03 to 0.07 second (see Table 62–1). A longer interval suggests an interventricular conduction delay. The QRS axis is usually +90 to +180 degrees (negative in lead I, positive in aV$_F$) with a mean of about 135 degrees during the first week of life, but it shifts leftward so that by 1 month of age the mean value is about 105 degrees (range 75 to 150). An axis that is shifted abnormally leftward (0 to 60 degrees) suggests the right ventricular hypoplasia that is seen in pulmonary atresia and an intact ventricular septum. A superior leftward axis of −30 to −90 degrees suggests either tricuspid atresia or an endocardial cushion defect.

The amplitude of the QRS complexes varies considerably (see Table 62–1). Since the right ventricle predominates in utero, is anterior in the chest, and benefits from its proximity to the electrodes, right ventricular hypertrophy is the rule.

Although there is still some controversy concerning diagnosis of right, left, and combined ventricular hypertrophy in the newborn, some guidelines based on the 1980 data of Davignon and co-workers are listed in Table 62–2.

T Wave. The T wave is from repolarization of the ventricles. There are marked shifts in the T waves on the surface electrocardiogram that represent ventricular repolarization changes over the first few minutes, hours, and days of life.

The T waves are usually upright in the right chest leads (V$_{3R}$ to V$_2$) for the first 6 to 24 hours of life. They become inverted during the 1st or 2nd day in virtually all neonates; persistently upright T waves in leads V$_{4R}$ or V$_1$ beyond 4 days suggest elevated right ventricular pressure. The T waves may be inverted in V$_6$ and V$_7$ soon after birth but are usually upright by 8 hours of age; persistence of inverted T waves beyond 48 hours is definitely abnormal and suggests left ventricular strain.

Q–T Interval. The Q–T interval usually decreases over the first month of life. At birth, it averages 0.28 to 0.30 second but may vary considerably (95th percentile values range from 0.22 to 0.36 second). By 1 day of age. the average has fallen to 0.26 second. Since the Q–T interval is closely correlated with heart rate, the corrected (Q–T$_c$) interval is usually calculated (Q–T/R–R interval). This is

TABLE 62–2. Criteria for Ventricular Overload in Newborn Infants

1. Right ventricular
   qR in V$_{4R}$ or V$_1$
   RV$_{3R}$ > 18 mm
   RV$_1$ > 25 mm
   SV$_6$ > 10 mm
   R/S ratio V$_{4R}$, V$_1$ > 7
   TV$_1$ positive after day 4
2. Left ventricular
   SV$_{3R}$ > 15 mm
   SV$_1$ > 20 mm
   RV$_6$ > 12 mm (15 at 1 month)
   R/S V$_6$ > 8 mm
   QV$_6$ > 3 mm
3. Combined
   Signs of LV and RV
   Signs of RV plus:
   a. Q > 2 mm in left chest
   b. Normal LV forces in V$_6$

quite constant over the first month, averaging 0.40 second. A prolonged Q–T$_c$ interval is associated with hypocalcemia; hypercalcemia shortens the Q–T$_c$ interval.

Electrocardiogram in the Premature Infant. Premature infants tend to have a slightly higher resting heart rate with a greater variation; rates of 70 beats per minute may be seen during sleep, and rates of up to 210 with crying are not unusual. The P waves tend to be of shorter duration, with a slight leftward shift in the P-wave axis to about +40 degrees. The P–R and QRS intervals for the premature infant are shorter than those for the term infant, averaging 0.10 and 0.04 second, respectively. The QRS amplitudes tend to be lower, and there is less right ventricular predominance and a more rapid shift to the adult pattern, with the initial R/S ratio in V$_1$ often less than 1.

Chest Radiograph. The chest radiograph provides useful and often unique information about the cardiovascular system in the newborn (Swischuk and Sapire, 1986). However, it is frequently either not helpful or frankly misleading because of variations in technique (e.g., underexposure, overexposure, and expiratory or rotated film) that make interpretation difficult. Although the hazards of excess radiation should not be underestimated, the dosage from a standard chest radiograph is minimal, about 9 mrad (approximating the radiation in Denver over a 3-week period), and thus poor studies should be repeated to obtain precise information. Data concerning the cardiac size, contour, and position as well as the status of the pulmonary vascular markings may give important clues about the differential diagnosis and hemodynamic status of the newborn with congenital heart disease. We have found that the oblique films have little diagnostic value and now use only anteroposterior and lateral projections. Fluoroscopy for cardiac diagnosis except as a part of cardiac catheterization is now used only in cases in which a vascular ring must be excluded.

Cardiac Size. Some noncardiac factors influence the size of the cardiac silhouette. The most common is radiographing the heart during the expiratory phase of respiration. Also, a large thymus in the anterior mediastinum may obscure the heart border on the anteroposterior projection, but with the stress of cardiac disease, the thymus often involutes, making evaluation of the heart size more accurate in the sick newborn. Rarely, a pericardial effusion may enlarge the cardiac silhouette when the heart is not enlarged, but an echocardiogram will usually clarify such findings. Cardiac size depends primarily on the volume of blood within the chambers rather than on the thickness of the muscle. Thus, events that tend to increase intravascular volume (e.g., stripping the umbilical cord at birth and overhydration) tend to increase the heart size.

Normally, the cardiothoracic ratio in the newborn should be less than 0.60. Cardiac enlargement may appear with left-to-right shunts, atrioventricular or semilunar valve regurgitation, or ventricular failure. Specific chamber size is often very difficult to evaluate, but occasionally, the right atrial dilatation with Ebstein disease of the tricuspid valve or with pulmonary atresia and an intact ventricular septum and tricuspid regurgitation may be evident.

Cardiac Position. The heart may be in the right or left thorax or present as a midline structure. Malpositioning may be secondary to hypoplasia of one of the lungs, atelectasis, tension pneumothorax, or diaphragmatic hernia. Primary malpositions are frequently associated with heart disease. Dextrocardia (heart in the right chest), is associated with a very high incidence of intracardiac anomalies unless there is associated situs inversus of the viscera (stomach on the right, liver on the left, etc.). Similarly, levocardia (heart in the left chest) is frequently associated with major anomalies if there is situs inversus of the viscera. Both these situations suggest the heterotaxia syndromes.

Pulmonary Vascularity. The assessment of pulmonary vascularity is one of the most important parts of the cardiac evaluation of the newborn since it may be helpful in the differential diagnosis of neonatal heart disease.

In the posteroanterior film of the normal infant, the right pulmonary artery and the primary branches are usually visible in the right hilum. The left pulmonary artery and its primary branches may be hidden behind the heart. The vessels seen gradually taper peripherally and are usually too small to be seen in the distal third of the lung fields (Fig. 62–5A).

Four abnormal patterns can be distinguished. If the pulmonary blood flow is decreased (Fig. 62–5B), as is seen with most cyanotic heart disease, the lungs appear dark, the pulmonary vessels in the hilum are decreased in size, and no vessels are seen in the middle third of the lung fields. If the pulmonary blood flow is increased, as is seen with all significant left-to-right shunts, the hilar vessels are enlarged, the middle third of the lung fields has vessels larger than normal, and vessels may often be seen out to the distal third of the lung (Fig. 62–5C).

The third pattern is associated with pulmonary venous hypertension. The hila are prominent owing to dilation of the pulmonary veins, and the peripheral pulmonary arteries are indistinct because the elevated pulmonary venous pressure causes an increase in interstitial fluid, diminishing the contrast between the air-filled alveoli and the fluid-filled arteries (Fig. 62–5D). The entire lung field may be hazy. Pulmonary redistribution with vessels that are larger in the upper lung fields than in the lower, Kerley B lines, and the butterfly pattern of pulmonary edema are characteristic of older children and adults with pulmonary venous hypertension and are not seen in the newborn. Pulmonary venous congestion may be seen with total anomalous pulmonary venous return with obstruction, the hypoplastic left heart syndrome, or any lesion causing significant left-sided heart failure.

The last pattern, infrequently seen, is pulmonary plethora in the peripheral lung fields but decreased central and hilar vessels. This pattern is occasionally seen with tetralogy of Fallot with pulmonary atresia, in which the central pulmonary arteries may be quite hypoplastic or atretic with pulmonary blood flow supplied by large collateral vessels from the aorta that enter the lung distally and anastomose to the peripheral pulmonary arteries.

Echocardiography. Echocardiography is a valuable method of diagnosing neonatal congenital heart disease. One should not underestimate the usefulness of two-dimensional echocardiography in the differentiation of congenital heart disease from other abnormalities (e.g., sepsis and persistent fetal circulation) and in the distinction

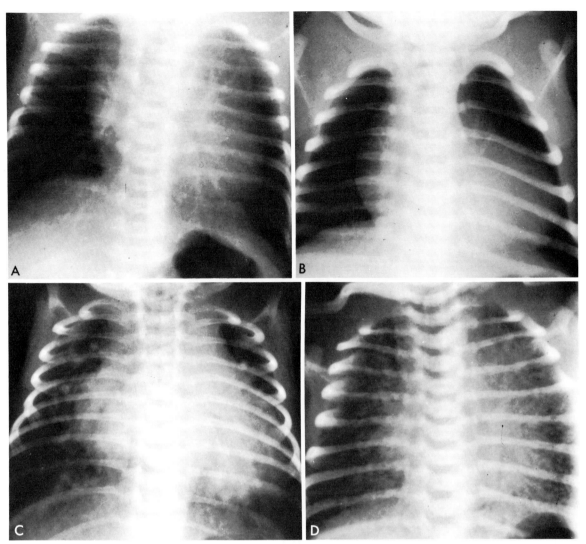

FIGURE 62–5. A, Chest radiograph in a normal newborn infant. The cardiothoracic silhouette is increased in size, especially in the superior mediastinum, probably because of an enlarged thymus. The pulmonary vascularity is visible in the middle third of the lung field, but no large vessels are seen distally. B, Chest radiograph in a child with Ebstein disease of the tricuspid valve with right-to-left shunting at the atrial level. The heart is enlarged secondary to tricuspid regurgitation. The lung fields are dark, with no pulmonary vessels visible in the middle third of the lung field, findings that reflect diminished pulmonary vascularity. C, Chest radiograph in an infant with a large ventricular septal defect. The heart is enlarged, and the distal pulmonary vessels are engorged because of the large left-to-right shunt. D, Chest radiograph in a child with total anomalous pulmonary venous return with obstruction. The pulmonary vessels are indistinct, and the lung fields are hazy, indicating increased pulmonary venous pressure.

among the various forms of congenital heart disease. Ultrasonography appeals to clinicians because it is noninvasive, painless, and with the equipment now available, associated with no adverse effects. It must be emphasized, however, that echocardiography should not be used alone but with physical examination, electrocardiography, and chest radiography, to plan effectively for future studies (often cardiac catheterization and angiography) and to make intelligent diagnostic and prognostic decisions.

While initially most echocardiographic images were obtained using single-crystal technology (M-mode) which provided a one-dimensional view of the heart, this has been almost completely supplanted by two-dimensional echocardiography. Using a phased array system and pulsing the energy at very short intervals (usually less than a microsecond), the ultrasonic beam can be directed and focused to give images on a two-dimensional plane. The advantages to this system are that since the focusing is

electronic, there is no noise, vibration, or wear, and excellent images can be obtained using a small transducer and a relatively small echo window. Several different windows are used to image the heart. In the parasternal long-axis view, the right ventricle, interventricular septum, left ventricle, mitral valve, and left atrium are viewed (Fig. 62–6). By rotating the transducer 90 degrees clockwise from this long-axis view, a short-axis view of the great vessels is described. The aorta and the three valve cusps are usually displayed in the midportion of the screen (Fig. 62–7A). By angulating the transducer superiorly, the pulmonary valve and pulmonary trunk can be seen, and by angulating the transducer inferiorly, one can see the mitral and tricuspid valves. By placing the transducer at the apex of the heart and aiming the beam toward the base with a plane parallel to the septum, one gets an apical four-chamber view of the heart showing right and left ventricles as well as the right and left atrium (Fig. 62–

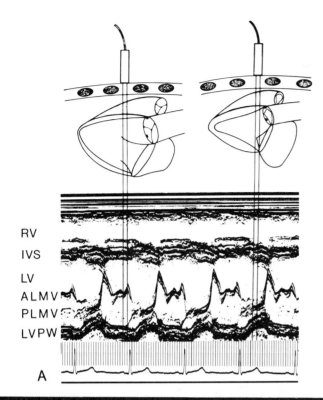

RV
IVS
LV
ALMV
PLMV
LVPW

A

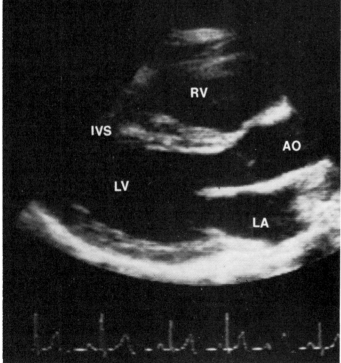

RV

IVS

AO

LV

LA

B

FIGURE 62–6. A, A normal M-mode echocardiogram with the ultrasonographic beam traversing the chest wall, right ventricle (RV), interventricular septum (IVS), left ventricular (LV) cavity, and left ventricular posterior wall (LVPW). On the left, the anterior leaflet of the mitral valve (ALMV) and posterior leaflet of the mitral valve (PLMV) are imaged in diastole when the leaflets are open. On the right side, the imaging is in systole when the valve is closed. (From Williams, R. G., and Tucker, C. R.: Echocardiographic Diagnosis of Congenital Heart Disease. Boston, Little, Brown and Company, 1977.)

B, Parasternal long axis view on the two dimensional echocardiogram similar to A. RV = right ventricle; IVS-interventricular septum; LV-left ventricle; AO-aorta; LA-left atrium. (From Williams, R. G., Bierman, F. Z, and Saunders, S. P.: Echocardiographic Diagnosis of Cardiac Malformations. Boston, Little, Brown and Company, 1986.)

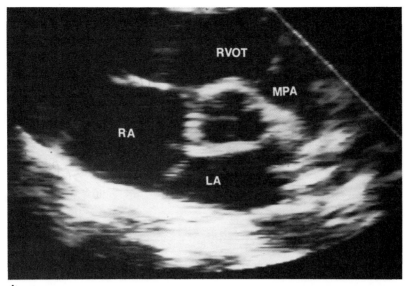

A

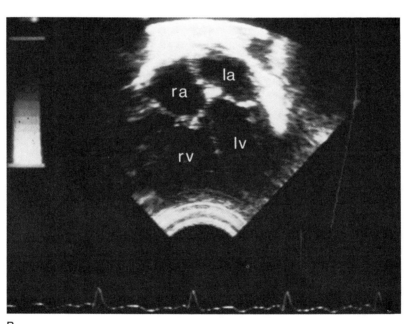

B

FIGURE 62–7. A, In the transverse parasternal view of the aortic valve, three cusps of the aortic valve are seen within the central circular structure representing the aortic root. The right ventricular outflow tract (RVOT) crosses anteriorly. A portion of the main pulmonary artery (MPA) is also seen. The right atrium (RA) lies to the right of the aorta. The linear structure between RA and RVOT is the tricuspid valve. The left atrium (LA) lies directly posterior to the aorta. The linear echoes between the RA and LA represent a portion of the interatrial septum.

B, This apical four-chamber view displays the right atrium (ra) and left atrium (la) and inflow portions of the right ventricle (rv) and left ventricle (lv), with intervening interatrial and interventricular septa and atrioventricular valves. (A and B from Williams, R. G., Bierman, F. Z., and Sanders, S. P.: Echocardiographic Diagnosis of Cardiac Malformations. Boston, Little, Brown and Company, 1986. Reproduced with permission.)

Illustration continued on following page

7B). A subxiphoid or subcostal approach is best for visualizing the atrial septum because the beam is more perpendicular to the plane of the septum (Fig. 62–7C). By rotating the transducer right along the horizontal plane, one can also see the venous structures as they enter the heart. Finally, from a suprasternal notch view, the aortic arch and ascending aorta can be visualized (Fig. 62–7D). Combining these views, plus variations, depending on

anatomic findings, specific defects can almost invariably be identified.

In addition, a spectrum analysis of the returning echo signal to quantitate the frequency components, allows qualification of the velocity of blood flow, using the Doppler principle. Gradients across valves can be quantitated since the pressure drop is approximately equal to 4 times the velocity squared. By color-coding these changes

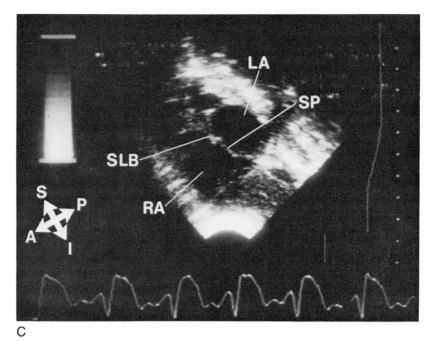

C

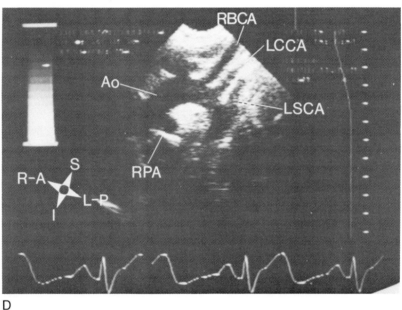

D

FIGURE 62–7 Continued C, Subxiphoid short-axis view of the atria through the midportion of the intra-atrial septum. Septum primum (SP) can be seen overlapping the SLB on the LA side. (From Sanders, S. P.: Echocardiography and related techniques in the diagnosis of congenital heart defects: Part I, veins, atria and interatrial septum. Echocardiography 1:185, 1984. Reproduced with permission.)

D, Suprasternal notch long-axis view of the aortic arch. LCCA = left common carotid artery; LSCA = left subclavian artery; RBCA = right brachiocephalic artery. (From Sanders, S. P.: Echocardiography and related techniques in the diagnosis of congenital heart defects: Part III, Conotruncus and Great Arteries. Echocardiography. 1:443, 1984. Reproduced with permission.)

RPA, right pulmonary artery; S, superior; L-P, left posterior; I, inferior; R-A, right anterior.

in frequency, relatively small disturbances in flow can be visualized and small intra- or extracardiac shunts (atrial septal defects, ventricular septal defects, patent ductus arteriosus) or small degrees of AV valve regurgitation, can be identified. A list of normal values is found in Table 62–3.

Brief descriptions of the pertinent echographic cardiographic findings in specific types of congenital heart disease are listed in the discussion of the individual lesions in Chapter 63. Those interested in more comprehensive reviews of the principles and techniques of ultrasonography, are referred to one of the standard texts (Silverman

and Snider, 1982; Williams et al., 1986; Snider and Serwer, 1990).

Cardiac Catheterization and Angiocardiography. Over the past decade, the increased use of noninvasive or semi-invasive studies such as echocardiography and radionuclide studies has improved the diagnostic acumen of the cardiologist. Although these studies have occasionally obviated the need for catheterization (as in aortic atresia or Ebstein disease of the tricuspid valve in which the diagnosis is unmistakable on echocardiogram), we

TABLE 62–3. Echocardiographic Values for Normal Newborns

WEIGHT	PREMATURE*	
	Left Atrial Dimension (cm)	Left Ventricular End Diastolic Dimension (cm)
600–900	0.60 (0.5–0.7)	1.07 (0.9–1.2)
901–1200	0.65 (0.5–0.8)	1.08 (0.9–1.3)
1201–1500	0.69 (0.5–0.9)	1.18 (1.0–1.3)
1501–1800	0.79 (0.6–1.0)	1.37 (1.2–1.5)
1801–2200	0.88 (0.7–1.1)	1.39 (1.1–1.6)
	mean (± 2 SD)	

FULL-TERM†	
Number	200
Weight (lbs)	7.6 (6–10)
Aortic root diameter (mm)	10.0 (8.1–12.0)
Left atrial diameter (mm)	7.0 (5.0–10.0)
Pulmonary artery diameter (mm)	11.1 (9.4–13.0)
Interventricular septal thickness (mm)	2.7 (1.8–4.0)
LV end systolic dimension (mm)	13.3 (8.0–18.6)
LV end diastolic dimension (mm)	18.7 (12.0–23.3)
LV end systolic wall thickness (mm)	4.3 (2.5–6.0)
LV end diastolic wall thickness (mm)	2.6 (1.6–3.7)
RV end diastolic dimension (mm)	11.4 (6.1–15.0)
Mean (± 2 SD)	

*Data from Meyer, R. A.: Pediatric Echocardiography. Philadelphia, Lea & Febiger, 1977.

†Data from Hagan, A. D., et al: Echocardiographic criteria for normal newborn infants. Circulation 48:1221, 1973.

continue to depend on catheterization for definitive anatomic and physiologic information.

At present, we catheterize all infants critically ill with cyanotic congenital heart disease, those with congestive heart failure (except the premature with an obvious patent ductus arteriosus or the newborn with paroxysmal supraventricular tachycardia), and those doing poorly after cardiac surgery if there is a possibility that a significant residual problem is present.

Infants with heart disease are often critically ill, and careful monitoring during the procedure is necessary. We continuously evaluate body temperature with a rectal probe, pulse rate and rhythm with an oscilloscope, arterial blood pressure through an umbilical artery or femoral artery cannula, and PO_2 with a transcutaneous oxygen monitor. In addition, every 15 to 30 minutes we obtain arterial blood gases and replace blood loss. Meticulous monitoring will minimize complications. We do not routinely sedate newborns, but if they remain unconsolable after receiving a pacifier dipped in glucose water, we administer morphine (0.05 mg/kg I.V.) judiciously.

Methods. The techniques of catheterization vary widely depending upon local customs. For the purpose of simplicity, only our methodology is considered here (Freed 1989; Lock et al., 1987). Those interested in other approaches should read the excellent chapters in Rudolph (1974) or Moller and Neal (1990).

In the first week of life we prefer to use the umbilical vessels when patent. If access to the heart is not possible after the umbilical vein and ductus venosus are probed, we use the femoral vein. Catheterization of the femoral vein is almost always performed percutaneously. A No. 21 needle is introduced into the vessel, and a 0.021-inch guide wire is inserted through the needle. The needle is then removed, and a dilator and sheath are advanced over the wire. Once the sheath is in place, the wire and dilator are removed and a catheter is inserted. Alternatively, the femoral vein or artery or both may be surgically isolated by cutdown, and the catheter can be inserted through a hole made with small scissors or a scalpel blade. Although many types of catheters have been used over the years, we prefer the balloon-tipped, flow-directed variety. They seem easier to use and cause less cardiac trauma, and at least in our experience, they are associated with a lower incidence of cardiac perforation with catheter manipulation or angiography. A No. 5 French catheter (external circumference 5 mm, external diameter 1.6 mm) is used almost exclusively on the venous side, since this is large enough for good pressure measurement and angiography but still small enough to be flexible and fit a newborn's femoral vein comfortably.

If the arterial study can be performed using the umbilical artery, a No. 5 umbilical artery catheter is usually used, but a No. 4 French or No. 5 French angiographic catheter may be substituted if angiography is necessary. After 1 week of age, the umbilical artery may not be accessible. We then percutaneously place a No. 21 or No. 22 Teflon cannula into the femoral artery for pressure monitoring and blood-gas sampling. If a retrograde arterial study is necessary, we exchange the cannula for a No. 4 French or, more recently, a No. 3.2 French pigtail-shaped angiographic catheter. At the end of the study, the catheters are removed unless needed for monitoring. If the vessels were entered percutaneously, pressure is applied to the site for 10 minutes. If a cutdown was performed, the vessels are repaired and the skin is closed.

Data Collection and Analysis. Information at catheterization is provided by one or more of the following: catheter course, oxygen data, pressure data, and angiography.

Catheter Course. Normally, the catheter course is predictable: the venous catheter can be advanced from the vena cava to the right atrium and ventricle and then into the pulmonary artery, and the arterial catheter can be advanced retrograde from the aorta into the left ventricle. Occasionally, the catheter will take an anomalous course. If the catheter can be passed from the right to the left atrium, it suggests a patent foramen ovale or atrial septal defect. If it passes from the pulmonary artery into the descending aorta, it suggests an aortopulmonary window or a patent ductus arteriosus. These unusual catheter positions often provide helpful information regarding the nature of the underlying anomaly.

Oxygen Data. In the normal infant, the oxygen saturation in the superior vena cava is about 70 per cent, with no changes as the venous blood goes through the right atrium, right ventricle, and the main and peripheral pulmonary arteries. Similarly, the oxygen saturation of the pulmonary veins, normally 95 to 98 per cent, should not change in the passage through the left heart to the peripheral arteries. Any significant increase in the oxygen saturation as the blood goes through the right heart chambers suggests contamination with blood from the left heart, a left-to-right shunt. This "step-up" may occur (1) at the atrial level in the presence of an atrial septal defect, a partial anomalous pulmonary venous return, endocardial cushion defect, or a ventricular septal defect with tricuspid regurgitation; (2) at the ventricular level with a ventricular septal defect or single ventricle; or (3) at the great-vessel level in aorticopulmonary window or patent ductus arteriosus. Some variation in saturation is usually present because of incomplete mixing, and the step-up should be at least 10 per cent at the atrial level, 7 per cent at the ventricular level, or 5 per cent at the great-vessel level to be considered significant if only one sample is obtained.

The oxygen saturation in the pulmonary veins should be about 95 per cent. Lung disease may reduce the pulmonary venous oxygen content, and inhomogeneous lung disease may lead to different saturations in the individual pulmonary veins. A drop in saturation between pulmonary veins and left atrium, a right-to-left shunt, suggests tricuspid atresia, pulmonary atresia, or right ventricular dysfunction. Right-to-left shunting at the ventricular level is seen with a ventricular septal defect and pulmonary stenosis or in a single ventricle. Right-to-left shunting at the great vessel level may be seen in truncus arteriosus or tetralogy of Fallot.

Pressure Data. The normal intracardiac pressures beyond 3 days of age are listed in Table 62–4. The atrial mean pressures are elevated in the presence of congestive heart failure or atrioventricular-valve stenosis. If the latter is present, the ventricular end-diastolic pressure will be normal; with heart failure, the end-diastolic pressures are increased as well. Increased V waves in the atrium suggest atrioventricular-valve regurgitation (mitral or tricuspid), and elevated A waves suggest atrioventricular-valve stenosis.

The pulmonary artery pressure is elevated for the first 8 to 72 hours of life. Persistently elevated pulmonary artery pressure may be seen with active pulmonary arteriolar vasoconstriction in the presence of lung disease and hypoxia. The pulmonary artery pressure will also be elevated when there is obstruction to the egress of pulmonary venous blood seen with mitral stenosis or atresia, or total anomalous pulmonary venous return, or when the pulmonary arteries are indirectly connected to the left ventricle in newborns with a large ventricular septal defect or single ventricle or with a large connection at the great-vessel level (e.g., a large patent ductus, aorticopulmonary window, or truncus arteriosus).

Right ventricular systolic hypertension occurs with increased pulmonary artery pressure and also, if there is obstruction to right ventricular egress secondary to pulmonic stenosis or atresia, with normal pulmonary artery pressure.

Systemic hypertension in the ascending aorta is seen in newborns with coarctation of the aorta and, rarely, in those with catastrophic renal vascular disease. In the latter, the ascending aorta and descending aorta pressures are equal. In the former, there is a gradient from obstruction at the site of the coarctation.

Left ventricular systolic pressures are increased whenever the aortic pressures are increased and in valvular aortic stenosis when the aortic pressures are normal or low.

Angiocardiography. Angiocardiography remains the mainstay of the anatomic delineation of the various forms of congenital heart disease. Over the past few years, we have switched from "all purpose" catheters to special catheters for angiocardiography in the hope of increasing the information obtained while reducing the complications. On the venous side, we use a No. 5 French balloon-tipped angiography catheter with multiple side holes proximal to the balloon. In those situations that require an arterial study, we prefer a specially designed No. 3.2 French thin-walled catheter with a pigtail at the end to minimize recoil. Nonionic and low osmolar contrast materials have become available and offer a higher margin of safety with sick newborns compared with the older materials, albeit with a much higher price. Each angiocardiogram is performed with 1 ml/kg of contrast material injected within about 1/2 second, unless a large left-to-right shunt is present, in which case 1.5 or even 2.0 ml/kg is necessary. We rarely inject more than 4 ml/kg during the entire study.

Filming is done on cine film at 64 frames/second, with simultaneous video taping of the television image so that the pictures can be reviewed immediately, before the angiocardiograms are developed. Biplane filming is usually preferred, since it gives much more information without significantly increased risks.

A major advance in angiocardiography is the recognition that the heart does not lie in the anteroposterior projection in the chest and that rotation of the x-ray beam or the patient or both reveals previously hidden anatomic details (Bargeron et al., 1977; Elliot et al., 1977; Fellows et al., 1977) (Table 62–5). It is occasionally hard to position the patient, but the advantages of these views more than compensate for difficulties encountered.

Complications. Complications of cardiac catheterization may arise from the procedure itself or from the precarious nature of these critically ill newborns. The Society for Cardiac Angiography has reviewed complications among 53,581 people, primarily adults, undergoing catheterization and angiography. The mortality rate for 457 infants under 1 year of age was 1.75 per cent (Kennedy et al., 1982).

In 1974, Stanger and co-workers reviewed their experience from 1970 to 1972 with 218 newborns in San Francisco. There were 20 deaths (9 per cent), two during the catheterization, and 18 within 24 hours of the study. Almost all the deaths were in children with irreparable heart disease and were believed to be the result of progressive clinical deterioration rather than a specific incident leading to demise. In only two infants (1 per cent) was there reason to believe that the catheterization was causally related to death.

Our review of the data from New England Regional Infant Cardiac Program for the year 1979 revealed two deaths among 300 newborns. Findings of this group support those of Stanger and colleagues (1974). With balloon-tipped catheters for manipulation and either balloon or pigtail catheters for angiography, myocardial perforation and intramyocardial injection of contrast rarely

TABLE 62–4. Normal Intracardiac Pressures in the Infant (Older Than 72 Hours)

Right atrium	a = 5–7	Left atrium	a = 3–5
	v = 3–5		v = 5–8
	m = 0–2		m = 3–6
Right ventricle	15–25 / 5–7	Left ventricle	65–80 / 3–5
Pulmonary artery	15–25 / 8–12	Aorta	65–80 / 45–60
	m = 10–16		m = 60–65

TABLE 62–5. Angled Views in the Cineangiography of Congenital Heart Disease

1. *Cranial 45°, left oblique 30°*
   ("Hepatoclavicular," or "4-chamber," view of Bargeron; with vertical (frontal) intensifier, patient's thorax is elevated 45° to sitting position and his left shoulder is rotated 45° anteriorly while his body is slanted to the right 10°–15° in the horizontal plane.)
   General advantage: Distinguishes the four chambers of the heart and demonstrates the posterior aspect of the ventricular septum.
   Specific advantage in:
   Defects in endocardial cushion, A–V canal
   LV-to-RA shunt
   VSD of 1–V canal type
   Left coronary artery distribution
   Overriding A–V valves
2. *Cranial 20°, left oblique 70°*
   ("Long axial oblique" view of Bargeron; with horizontal or lateral intensifier, the patient's right shoulder is elevated 15° to 20° and his body is slanted 15° to 20° away from the intensifier.)
   General advantage: Demonstrates left ventricular outflow tract and most of the interventricular septum.
   Specific advantage in:
   VSD (muscular and membranous)
   Subaortic stenosis
   Subpulmonic stenosis in transposition
   Asymmetric septal hypertrophy
   Prolapse, anterior leaflet of mitral valve
   Overriding tricuspid valve
3. *Cranial 45° (± right or left oblique 10° to 15°)*
   ("Sitting" view of Bargeron; with the vertical intensifier, the patient's thorax is elevated 45°.)
   General advantage: Provides superior view of extracardiac mediastinal vessels
   Specific advantage in:
   Bifurcation of pulmonry artery
   Supravalvular PS, pulmonry artery band
   Pulmonary arteries in pseudotruncus
   Pulmonary arteries in truncus
   Vascular rings and slings

Courtesy of Dr. K. Fellows, Children's Hospital Medical Center, Boston.

occur. Arrhythmias (primarily atrial tachycardia and complete atrioventricular dissociation) still occur, but the judicious use of drugs, cardioversion, and pacing have made these complications less feared than previously. Umbilical and percutaneous femoral catheterizations have made infections at the site of catheter insertion less common, and infusion of prostaglandin E₁ to maintain the ductal patency has reduced the incidence of cyanotic spells and progressive deterioration from hypoxia and acidosis.

■ MANIFESTATIONS OF CARDIAC DISEASE IN THE NEWBORN

Fortunately, there are only a limited number of ways that newborns with cardiovascular problems present to the pediatrician or neonatologist (Rowe et al., 1981). A cardiac disorder should be suspected in the presence of any one or more of the following: (1) congestive heart failure, (2) cyanosis, (3) heart murmurs, and (4) dysrhythmias. The first three of these cardinal manifestations of heart disease are reviewed here. Dysrhythmias are discussed in Chapter 65.

CONGESTIVE HEART FAILURE

Congestive heart failure (CHF) is a clinical syndrome in which the heart is unable to perform its pump function to meet the metabolic demands of the body. CHF may be the result of either increased demands on the heart, usually due to structural alterations that impose a volume or a pressure load, or a diminished ability of the heart to meet the normal metabolic demands of the tissues, usually secondary to inflammatory disease or metabolic abnormalities. Occasionally, both factors may coexist. Compared with the older child or adult, the newborn seems particularly susceptible to congestive failure. Part of this tendency is undoubtedly due to the complex structural abnormalities that affect the newborn, but other factors may also be important. For example, the ventricular myocardium has fewer contractile elements per unit mass compared with that in older children (Sheldon et al., 1976) and produces less active tension on contraction (Friedman, 1973). In addition, the heavy demands placed on the left ventricle at birth undoubtedly reduce the cardiac reserve.

In congestive failure, a number of compensatory mechanisms become operational. Chronic volume overload causes cardiac dilatation, which by the Frank-Starling mechanism permits ejection of a larger stroke volume, albeit at a higher wall tension and increased myocardial oxygen requirements. The increased wall tension, by an as yet unknown mechanism, stimulates protein synthesis, resulting in myocardial hypertrophy. There is also an increase in the release of catecholamines, especially norepinephrine, which increases both the heart rate and the velocity of ejection. As CHF progresses and cardiac output diminishes, blood is redistributed by vasoconstriction away from the periphery to other organs with greater metabolic needs. Reduction in renal blood flow stimulates release of aldosterone and renin, leading to sodium and water retention. Finally, tissue oxygenation is facilitated by release of 2,3-diphosphoglycerates, which increases the P-50 and shifts the oxygen dissociation curve to the right.

Unfortunately, the infant is less able to take advantage of many of these compensatory mechanisms than is the older child or adult. For example, heart failure develops and progresses too rapidly for RNA synthesis and myocardial hypertrophy to be of much benefit. In addition, the adrenergic receptors are only partially innervated at birth, and the norepinephrine stores are reduced, so the newborn derives less benefit than does the older child from the release of catecholamines (Friedman et al., 1968). Finally, newborns have predominantly fetal hemoglobin in the red cells, which tightly binds oxygen, negating the beneficial effects on tissue oxygenation of 2,3-diphosphoglycerate.

Clinical Manifestations. The signs and symptoms of heart failure are related to impaired myocardial performance as well as to pulmonary and systemic venous congestion and include tachycardia, tachypnea, hepatomegaly, diaphoresis, feeding difficulties, cardiomegaly, and occasionally peripheral edema or rales.

Normally, the heart rate of the newborn increases to 180 to 200 with crying as a result of adrenergic stimulation, but persistent heart rates at this level when the newborn is quiet suggest increased autonomic activity that occurs to compensate for a failing myocardium. An early sign of left-sided failure is an increase in the respiratory rate above 50 to 60 per minute, usually without an increase in depth of respiration. At first, the baby is not distressed; grunting, flaring of the alae nasi, and intercostal retractions are unusual unless there is associated pulmonary disease or frank pulmonary edema. The tachypnea is probably associated with increased stiffness of the lung secondary to increased interstitial fluid from elevated pulmonary venous pressure (Rushmer, 1976).

Although neck vein distention is usually not discernible in the newborn, elevated systemic venous pressure results in enlargement of the liver beyond 3 cm below the right costal margin in the midclavicular line. However, other signs of systemic venous congestion in the older child and adult, edema and ascites, are unusual in the newborn. Hepatomegaly is not specific for CHF and may also be present in the newborn with a blood dyscrasia or congenital infection. A palpable liver without true hepatomegaly may also be seen with hyperinflated lungs when the liver is displaced inferiorly.

A fairly constant feature of heart failure in the newborn is difficult feeding. Although the normal infant takes an appropriate volume of formula for age and size within 15 to 20 minutes, the term newborn with heart failure often takes 45 to 60 minutes to consume 1 or 2 ounces. Occasionally, the child becomes dyspneic with the exertion required, but frequently he or she tires and falls asleep after a minimal effort. Diaphoresis, especially of the head with feeding, is a common finding that is probably a manifestation of increased adrenergic activity.

Cardiac enlargement on physical examination or, more commonly, on chest radiograph is one of the most consistent signs of impaired cardiac function and congestive failure. Rales over both lung fields may occasionally be heard, a result of a pulmonary venous congestion. As left heart failure progresses, the transudate may reach the level of the bronchioles, making wheezing or rhonchi more prominent.

Heart failure may progress very rapidly, with cardiovascular collapse and cardiogenic shock being the first manifestations. These infants have no pulses, mottled and cool extremities, rapid or gasping respirations, hypothermia, indistinct heart sounds, and usually no murmurs. The liver and spleen are usually very large. This picture simulates that of the infant with septicemia or meningitis; the very large liver and cardiomegaly on radiograph should indicate heart disease as the cause.

Pharmacologic Management

Digitalis. Digitalis (see also Chapter 65) has been used to treat congestive heart failure for more than 200 years. Digoxin is the most widely used preparation in newborns, infants, and older children because of its excellent bioavailability (oral absorption is rapid, with peak levels occurring within 1 hour) and its relatively rapid excretion rate. Both factors allow for adjustments of dosage to meet individual demands. A consensus has developed suggesting that the inotropic effects result from digitalis binding to, and thereby inhibiting, Na-K ATPase—the enzyme that maintains high intracellular concentrations of sodium in myocardial cells. This inhibition alters excitation contraction coupling making more calcium available to the contractile elements resulting in increased force of contraction (Smith, 1988). In addition, digitalis increases the sensitivity of the arterial baroreceptor reflex resulting in an increase in vagal and a decrease in sympathetic efferent activity.

Digoxin may be given orally, intravenously, or, rarely, intramuscularly. Absorption from the gastrointestinal tract is relatively rapid, with peak plasma levels and onset of action occurring within 30 to 60 minutes. Oral absorption is somewhat variable, but usually 75 per cent is absorbed, with the rest lost in the feces (Wettrell and Anderson, 1977). In cases in which more rapid action is necessary, the intravenous preparation may be used, with the onset of action occurring within 5 to 30 minutes and the peak effect appearing within 2 hours. The half-life of digoxin is about 37 hours in the small full-term newborn and 57 hours in the premature (Lang and Von Bernuth, 1977), with approximately one-fourth of the body stores metabolized daily. Therefore, after digitalization to fill the body stores, the maintenance dose is about one-fourth of the total digitalizing dose and is usually given in two divided doses. Digoxin is excreted primarily by the kidney. Decreased renal function reduces the dose of digoxin required. In adults, the percentage of digoxin lost per day equals 14 + creatine clearance in ml/min/5. This probably applies to children as well. To calculate an approximate value for the daily dosage, multiply the percentage lost per day by the total digitalizing dose.

Several points should be emphasized. First, digitalization is an individual titration; there are wide variations in the responses, and each child must be watched carefully for signs of toxicity. This is especially true of infants with inflammatory disease of the myocardium, in which enhanced sensitivity to the drug is common. Secondly, the dose calculation should be done in duplicate and preferably by two physicians. Explicit instructions must then be given with the dosage in milligrams as well as milliliters to the person administering the digoxin. Although it might seem unnecessary to emphasize these details, the toxic–therapeutic range is narrow, and the author has personally seen a few tragedies because of dosage errors with digitalis in infants.

The starting dose for digitalization has been a source of controversy for many years. Although infants may tolerate higher serum concentrations before manifesting toxicity, there is little evidence that they substantially benefit from the higher level. At present, we tend to be conservative and recommend a total oral digitalizing dose of 0.02 mg/kg in the preterm infant and 0.04 mg/kg in the term infant. Parenteral administration requires only 70 per cent of the oral dose because of more complete absorption.

Digitalis toxicity is an all too frequent occurrence because of the narrow gap between therapeutic and toxic levels and frequent abnormalities of electrolytes and renal function in the critically ill infant. Serum levels greater than 3.5 mg/ml indicate toxicity. The most common manifestations of digitalis toxicity in the newborn are poor feeding and vomiting, symptoms for which there are many other causes. Dysrhythmias, especially sinus bradycardia, second and third degree heart block, and supraventricular arrhythmias are the usual manifestations, but virtually any dysrhythmia may be seen. It is probably safest to consider any arrhythmia (except possibly atrial fibrillation) a manifestation of digoxin toxicity especially if the drug is being given parenterally. Serum digoxin concentrations are especially helpful in questionable situations, but withholding digoxin while awaiting the laboratory report is prudent. Prolongation of the P–R interval, sagging S–T segments, and T-wave inversion on the electrocardiogram are signs of digoxin effect and do not imply toxicity; no dosage changes are required for these ECG changes alone.

The treatment of digitalis toxicity is to stop the drug. This is usually sufficient. If potassium levels are low, supplemental potassium should be supplied. Life-threatening ectopic arrhythmias should be suppressed; phenytoin (diphenylhydantoin) and lidocaine may be especially helpful. For serious bradyarrhythmias, a pacemaker may be required. Digitalis-specific antibody has been used in a few cases of suicidal ingestion of digoxin in adults and may play a future role in digitalis toxicity in the newborn (Smith et al., 1982).

Diuretics. Diminished renal blood flow secondary to congestive heart failure results in sodium and fluid retention. Diuretics act directly on the kidney to inhibit solute and water reabsorption and thus increase urine volume and have been found to be effective in treating neonatal heart failure (Green and Mirkin, 1982). A wide variety of diuretics have been used, but only furosemide (Lasix), ethacrynic acid (Edacrin), and, occasionally, chlorothiazide (Diuril) and spironolactone (Aldactone) are used with any frequency in infants. Furosemide and ethacrynic acid, the most potent of the diuretics, act by inhibiting chloride transport in the ascending limb of Henle and thereby moving the gradient for water movement from the medullary ducts into the renal interstitium (Grantham and Chonko, 1978). The thiazide diuretics reduce the permeability of the distal convoluted tubule to sodium, chloride, and potassium and thereby increase excretion of these ions as well as water. Spironolactone is a weak diuretic when used alone, but when it is used in conjunction with one of the other three diuretics, it contributes to an antialdosterone effect that promotes retention of potassium. We currently use furosemide (1 mg/kg I.V.) for acute diuresis with chlorothiazide (10 to 20 mg/kg/day) and spironolactone (1 to 2 mg/kg/day) as maintenance therapy. Abnormalities of electrolyte balance are not uncommon, and serum sodium, potassium, and chloride must be monitored during vigorous diuresis.

Other Inotropic Agents. Other inotropic agents may be necessary in severe congestive heart failure and cardiogenic shock (see also Chapter 31). The beta-adrenergic agonists, isoproterenol and dopamine, have been the most commonly used. Isoproterenol improves tissue perfusion primarily by its positive inotropic effects on contractility, but unfortunately, its chronotropic effects increase heart rate excessively, limiting its clinical usefulness. Dopamine, the immediate precursor of norepinephrine, appears to have much the same inotropic effects but less chronotropic effect and also selectively increases renal, mesenteric, cerebral, and myocardial blood flow without increasing flow to the skeletal muscle bed (Driscoll et al., 1978; Lang et al., 1980; Walther et al., 1985). Amrinone (Inocor), an inotropic-vasodilator derivative of the anticholinergic drug biperidonen, has been used in adults and children and occasionally infants. It probably acts by inhibiting phosphodiesterase, thereby increasing intracellular concentrations of cyclic AMP, which increases the calcium uptake in myocardial cells. Pharmacokinetic data (Lawless et al., 1988) suggests a bolus of 3.0 to 4.5 mg/kg followed by an infusion of 10 µg/kg/minute in infants and 3.5 µg/kg/minute in newborns.

Afterload Reduction. It has been recognized for some time that myocardial performance is a function of the preload (atrial filling pressures), contractility, and afterload (systemic vascular resistance). Children and adults with congestive failure have increased levels of circulating catecholamines that cause peripheral vasoconstriction, which increases the systemic vascular resistance. Although this helps maintain systemic blood pressure in the presence of a low cardiac output (blood pressure = cardiac output × systemic vascular resistance), the increased afterload adversely affects myocardial performance. It has been found that in children and adults with elevated systemic vascular resistance, the use of vasodilators to reduce afterload may result in such an improvement in cardiac output that the blood pressure remains stable. Sodium nitroprusside is the most widely used vasodilator in adults and probably in children as well. (Benitz et al., 1985). It would seem more useful in newborns with myocardial disease than in those with shunts or obstructive lesions. Arterial blood pressure and atrial pressures must be carefully monitored. The starting dose is usually 0.1 µg/kg/min, with the dose titrated up to 5 µg/kg/min, depending on the response. Hydralazine may be used as an oral preparation.

Other Therapeutic Measures. Using a modified neonatal chair or tilting the incubator or radiant heater to 15 to 45 degrees maintains the lower extremities dependent and permits some peripheral pooling, which seems to reduce pulmonary congestion and ease the work of breathing by lessening pressure on the diaphragm. Since virtually all the infants with congestive failure have some pulmonary venous desaturation secondary to ventilation perfusion imbalance, they may benefit from 30 to 35 per cent oxygen either in the incubator or by mask. An occasional child will be relatively anemic; slow transfusion of packed red blood cells should be given to increase the hematocrit to 45 to 55 per cent to improve the oxygen-carrying capacity of the blood.

If severe pulmonary edema and congestive heart failure exhaust the newborn so that he or she develops respiratory failure (e.g., $PCO_2 > 45$ torr), nasotracheal intubation with respirator-assisted ventilation may be necessary. By utilizing positive end-expiratory pressure, one may improve pulmonary congestion, facilitating further diagnostic studies and therapeutic measures.

Finally, attention should be given to a proper diet. Although breast milk and usual infant formulas may be adequate for growth of a normal newborn, they contain excessive sodium and insufficient solute for the newborn with congestive heart failure. We usually recommend a low-sodium formula (Similac PM 60/40 or SMA) and slowly increase the caloric content from 2 calories/3 ml (20 calories/ounce) to 1 calorie/ml with glucose polymers and medium-chain triglycerides if such a diet can be tolerated without diarrhea. By providing frequent small feedings of 45 to 75 ml, we are often able to maintain the newborn's caloric intake at 125 to 150 calories/kg/day, enough for normal or slightly below normal growth. We have found this far more efficacious than fluid restriction, which almost inevitably slowly deprives the newborn of necessary caloric intake.

CYANOSIS

It is now commonly accepted that the clinical perception of cyanosis is determined not by the percentage of hemoglobin attached to oxygen (percentage of oxygen saturation) but by the absolute amount of reduced hemoglobin in the arterial and capillary beds (Lees, 1970). The critical amount of reduced hemoglobin necessary for recognition depends on the clinical experience of the observer and the lighting but is probably about 4 g/dl in the newborn and slightly less in the older child. In patients with a normal hematocrit and hemoglobin, this corresponds to an arterial saturation of about 78 to 80 per cent. However, if the newborn is polycythemic (hemoglobin 25 g/dl), cyanosis may be recognized at an arterial saturation of 84 per cent; if he or she is anemic (hemoglobin 10 g/dl), it will not be noticeable until the arterial saturation is 60 per cent or less.

Central cyanosis involves the trunk and mucous membranes as well as the extremities and is caused by an increase of reduced hemoglobin in the arterial blood because of an abnormality of oxygen transport originating in the heart, lung, or blood. Central cyanosis may be caused by one of five pathophysiologic mechanisms: (1) right-to-left shunting. (2) alveolar hypoventilation. (3) diffusion impairment in the lung, (4) ventilation perfusion imbalance, and (5) abnormalities in hemoglobin transport of oxygen. Diffusion abnormalities seem not to play a role in central cyanosis of the infant.

Diagnosis. The differentiation of central cyanosis of a cardiac origin due to right-to-left shunts from central cyanosis caused by other factors can almost always be made without or prior to echocardiography.

One of the most helpful signs is the breathing pattern. Infants with cardiac cyanosis may be tachypneic but are seldom in significant distress. They rarely exhibit intercostal retractions, flaring of the alae nasi, or grunting. The latter signs suggest primary pulmonary pathology. Stridor suggests mechanical interference with ventilation and is seen with vascular rings, Pierre Robin syndrome, tracheomalacia, and other conditions in which there is obstruction of the airway during inspiration. Cyanosis due to central nervous system disease usually is episodic and associated with periodic breathing, bradypnea, or apnea.

The chest radiograph of infants with cyanotic congenital heart disease usually shows decreased pulmonary blood flow, although the flow may be normal in transposition of the great arteries. With pulmonary disease, the vascular markings of the lungs are normal. The pulmonary causes of cyanosis, including respiratory distress syndrome, pneumonia, pneumothorax, diaphragmatic hernia, and hypoplasia or agenesis of the lungs, reveal characteristic patterns on radiograph that are usually not difficult to distinguish from heart disease. However, it may be difficult to distinguish infants with severe heart failure and pulmonary edema from those with lung disease. The signs and symptoms of heart failure and the massive cardiac enlargement on radiograph should allow differentiation in difficult cases.

The arterial blood gases in room air and in 100 per cent oxygen may be helpful in differentiating the cyanosis from hypoventilation, from ventilation-perfusion ($\dot{V}/\dot{Q}$) imbalance, and from right-to-left shunting. In all three situations, the Pa_{CO_2} is decreased in room air. However, with alveolar hypoventilation the Pa_{CO_2} is usually increased to 50 torr or greater, whereas with $\dot{V}/\dot{Q}$ abnormalities or intracardiac shunts, the Pa_{CO_2} is normal. When the infant with alveolar hypoventilation or $\dot{V}/\dot{Q}$ abnormality is placed in 100 per cent oxygen for 10 minutes, the increased O_2 concentration in the alveoli will raise the pulmonary venous Po_2 and therefore the Pa_{O_2} to more than 150 torr. By contrast, those with right-to-left intracardiac shunt under similar conditions will increase the pulmonary venous Po_2, but because of the intracardiac shunting of hypoxemic blood to the aorta, the Pa_{O_2} will not change significantly. A rise of greater than 30 torr is highly suggestive of lung disease. Occasionally, however, intracardiac shunting may be present with lung disease (persistent fetal circulation syndrome), and hypoventilation and ventilation-perfusion imbalances may be found with pulmonary edema secondary to structural heart disease. One should be careful to avoid exposing the premature infants to even transient hyperoxemia. Differentiation of causes of cyanosis can be inferred from alveolar-arterial differences at any known inspired concentration.

Infants with methemoglobinemia have an alarming lavender hue to their skin but are rarely in any distress. On arterial blood gases, the Pa_{O_2} is normal and increases to greater than 200 torr in 100 per cent oxygen. Confirmation of the diagnosis is by spectroscopy and by the rapid response to IV methylene blue (1 mg/kg).

If history, physical examination, chest radiograph, and arterial blood gases do not distinguish primary pulmonary from cardiac disease, the two-dimensional echocardiogram can virtually always determine whether the heart, great vessels, and pulmonary venous return are normal.

HEART MURMURS

Heart murmurs are the auditory manifestations of turbulence within the heart or great vessels that is transmitted to the chest wall. As pointed out by others, soft murmurs are not uncommon during the transitional circulation as the branch pulmonary arteries increase their flow from 7 per cent to 50 per cent of combined ventricular output, causing physiologic peripheral pulmonary stenosis (Danilowicz et al., 1965), and the ductus arteriosus closes. In 1961, Braudo and Rowe serially examined a group of 80 newborn infants and found that 48 (60 per cent) had murmurs audible in the first 24 hours of life. Nevertheless, loud murmurs heard in the 1st day or so of life usually represent stenosis of one of the semilunar valves or regurgitation through one of the atrioventricular valves, since the high pulmonary vascular resistance in the 1st or 2nd day of life usually prevents enough shunting in the presence of communications between the left and right side of the heart to cause a loud murmur. Murmurs of a ventricular septal defect or patent ductus arteriosus may be heard on discharge from the hospital, but with the increasing tendency to discharge on the 2nd or 3rd day of life, the murmurs are often now being heard for the first time at 4- to 6-week well-baby checkup. Murmurs of pulmonic stenosis are usually loudest at the left upper sternal border and may be associated with an ejection click early in systole that diminishes in intensity or disappears during inspiration. Murmurs of aortic stenosis may be audible at the left upper sternal border, but they are usually loudest at the right upper sternal border and are associated with a constant ejection click. The murmur of a ventricular septal defect is pansystolic and loudest along the left lower sternal border. Unfortunately, wide radiation of the murmurs over the entire precordium is the rule in infancy, and it may be difficult to localize the point of maximum intensity. The minimum evaluation of a heart murmur that is loud or that persists for 24 hours consists of a chest radiograph and an electrocardiogram. If these tests are normal and there is no evidence of cyanosis or congestive heart failure, elective referral to a pediatric cardiologist is sufficient.

■ REFERENCES

Bargeron, L. M., Jr., Elliott, L. P., Soto, B., et al.: Axial cineangiography in congenital heart disease. Section 1: Concept, technical and anatomic consideration. Circulation 56:1075, 1977.

Benitz, W. E., Malachowski, N., Cohen, R. S., et al.: Use of sodium nitroprusside in neonates: Efficacy and safety. J. Pediatr. 106:102, 1985.

Braudo, M., and Rowe, R. D.: Auscultation of the heart in the early neonatal period. Am. J. Dis. Child. 101:575, 1961.

Braunwald, E., and Swan, H. J. C. (Eds.): Cooperative study on cardiac catheterization. Circulation 37–38(Suppl. III). 1968.

Cassels, D. E., and Ziegler, R. F. (Eds.): Electrocardiography in Infants and Children. New York. Grune & Stratton. 1966.

Coceani, F., and Olley, P. M.: The response of the ductus arteriosus to prostaglandins. Can. J. Physiol. Pharmacol. 51:220, 1973.

Coceani, F., and Olley, P. M.: Role of prostaglandins, prostacyclin, and thromboxanes in the control of prenatal patency and postnatal closure of the ductus arteriosus. Semin. Perinatol. 4:109, 1980.

Danilowicz, D., Rudolph, A. M., and Hoffman, J. I. E.: Vascular resistance in the large pulmonary arteries in infancy. Circulation 31–32(Suppl. II):74, 1965.

Davignon, A., Rautaharju, P., Boiselle, E., Soumis, F., Megelas, M., and Choquette, A.: Normal ECG standards for infants and children. Pediatr. Cardiol. 1: 123, 1980.

Dawes, G. S.: Foetal and Neonatal Physiology. Chicago, Year Book Medical Publishers, Inc., 1968.

Driscoll, D. J., Gillette, P. C., and McNamara, D. G.: The use of dopamine in children. J. Pediatr. 92:309, 1978.

Elliott, L. P., Bargeron, L. M., Jr., Bream, P. R., et al.: Axial cineangiography in congenital heart disease. Section II: Specific lesions. Circulation 56:1084, 1977.

Emmanouilides, G. C., Moss, A. J., Duffie, E. R., Jr., et al.: Pulmonary arterial pressure changes in human newborn infants from birth to 3 days of age. J. Pediatr. 65:327, 1964.

Fellows, K. E., Keane, J. F., and Freed, M. D.: Angled views in cineangiocardiography of congenital heart disease. Circulation 56:485, 1977.

Freed, M. D., Heymann, M. A., Lewis, A. B., et al.: Prostaglandin E–1 in infants with ductus arteriosus dependent congenital heart disease. Circulation 64:899, 1981.

Freed, M. D.: Cardiac catheterization. In Adams, F. H., Emmanouilides, G. C., and Reimenschneider, T. A. (Eds.): Moss' Heart Disease in Infants and Children and Adolescents, 4th ed. Baltimore, Williams & Wilkins, 1989.

Friedman, W. F.: The intrinsic properties of the developing heart. In Friedman, W. F., Lesch, M., and Sonnenblick, E. H. (Eds.): Neonatal Heart Disease. New York, Grune & Stratton, 1973, pp. 21–49.

Friedman, W. F., Pool, P. E., Jacobowitz, D., et al.: Sympathetic innervation of the developing rabbit heart. Circ. Res. 23:25, 1968.

Fyler, D. C., Buckley, L. P., Hellenbrand, W. E., et al.: Report of the New England Regional Infant Cardiac Program. Pediatrics 65(Suppl.):375, 1980.

Gilbert, R. D.: Effects of afterload and baroreceptors on cardiac function in fetal sheep. J. Dev. Physiol. 4:229, 1987.

Goldberg, S. J., Allen, H. D., and Sahn, D. J.: Pediatric and Adolescent Echocardiography. 2nd ed. Chicago, Year Book Medical Publishers, Inc., 1980.

Grantham, J. J., and Chonko, A. M.: The physiological basis and clinical use of diuretics. In Brenner, B. M., and Stein, J. H. (Eds.): Sodium and Water Homeostasis, vol. 1. New York, Churchill-Livingstone, 1978, p. 178.

Green, T. P., and Mirkin, B. L.: Determinants of diuretic response to furosemide in infants with congestive heart failure. Pediatr. Cardiol. 3:47, 1982.

Hagan, A. D., Deeley, W. J., Sahn, D., et al.: Echocardiographic criteria for normal newborn infants. Circulation 48:1221, 1973.

Heymann, M. A., and Rudolph, A. M.: Effects of congenital heart disease on fetal and neonatal circulations. Prog. Cardiovasc. Dis. 15:115, 1972.

Heymann, M. A., and Rudolph, A. M.: Effects of increasing preload on right ventricular output in fetal lambs in utero. Circulation 48(Suppl.):37, 1973.

Hoerter, J., Mazet, F., Vassort, G.: Perinatal growth of the rabbit cardiac cell: Possible implications for the mechanism of relaxation. J. Mol. Cell. Cardiol. 13:725, 1982.

Kennedy, J. W., and the Registry Committee of the Society for Cardiac Angiography: Complications associated with cardiac catheterization and angiography: Symposium on catheterization complications. Cathet. Cardiovasc. Diagn. 8:5, 1982.

Lang, D., and Von Bermuth, G.: Serum concentration and serum half-life of Digoxin in premature and mature newborns. Pediatrics 59:902, 1977.

Lang, P., Williams, R. G., Norwood, W. I., et al.: The hemodynamic effects of dopamine in infants after corrective cardiac surgery. J. Pediatr. 96:630, 1980.

Lawless, S., Burckart, G., Divin, W., et al.: Amrinone pharmacokinetics in neonates and infants. J. Clin. Pharmacol. 28:283, 1988.

Lees, M. H.: Cyanosis of the newborn infant. Recognition and clinical evaluation. J. Pediatr. 77:484, 1970.

Liebman, J., Plonsey, R., Gillette, P.: Pediatric Electrocardiography. Baltimore, Williams & Wilkins, 1982.

Lind, J., Stern, L., and Wegelius, C.: Human Foetal and Neonatal Circulation. Springfield, Ill., Charles C Thomas, 1964.

Lind, J., and Wegelius, C.: Human fetal circulation changes in the cardiovascular system at birth and disturbances in the post-natal closure of the foramen ovale and ductus arteriosus. Cold Spring Harbor Symp. Quant. Biol. 19:109, 1954.

Lock, J. E., Keane, J. F., and Fellows, K. E.: Diagnostic and interventional catheterization in congenital heart disease. Boston, Martinus Nijhoff Publishing, 1987.

Mahdavi, V., Izumo, S., and Nadal-Ginard, B.: Developmental hormonal regulation of the sarcomeric myocin heavy chain gene family. Circ. Res. 60:804, 1987.

Meyer, R. A.: Pediatric Echocardiography. Philadelphia, Lea & Febiger, 1977.

Moller, J. H., and Neal, W. A.: Neonatal and Infant Heart Disease. Norwalk, Conn., Appleton & Lange, 1990.

Nakanishi, T., Okunda, H., Kamata, K., et al.: Developmental myocardial contractive system in the fetal rabbit. Pediatr. Res. 22:201, 1987.

Nakanishi, T., and Jannakani, J. M.,: Developmental changes in myocardial mechanical function and subcellular organelles. Am. J. Physiol. 246:H615, 1984.

Norwood, W. I., Lang, P., and Hansen, D. D.: Physiologic repair of aortic atresia—hypoplastic left heart syndrome. N. Engl. J. Med. 308:23, 1983.

Pigott, J. E., Murphy, J. D., Barber, G., et al.: Palliative reconstructive surgery for hypoplastic left heart syndrome. Ann. Thorac. Surg. 45:122, 1988.

Rowe, R. D., Freedom, R. M., Mehrizi, A., et al.: The Neonate with Congenital Heart Disease, 2nd ed. Philadelphia, W. B. Saunders Company, 1981.

Rudolph, A. M.: The changes in the circulation after birth. Their importance in congenital heart disease. Circulation 41:343, 1970.

Rudolph, A. M.: Congenital Diseases of the Heart. Chicago, Year Book Medical Publishers, 1974.

Rudolph, A. M., and Heymann, M. A.: Cardiac output in the fetal lamb.

The effects of spontaneous and induced changes of heart rate on right and left ventricular output. J. Obstet. Gynecol. *124*:183, 1976.

Rushmer, R. F.: Cardiac compensation, hypertrophy, myopathy, and congestive heart failure. *In* Rushmer, R. F. (Ed.): Cardiovascular Dynamics. Philadelphia, W. B. Saunders Company, 1976.

Sheldon, C. A., Friedman, W. F., and Sybers, H. D.: Scanning electron microscopy of fetal and neonatal lamb cardiac cells. J. Mol. Cell Cardiol. *8*:853, 1976.

Silverman, N. H., and Snider, A. R.: Two Dimensional Echocardiography in Congenital Heart Disease. Norwalk, Conn., Appleton-Century-Crofts, 1982.

Smith, T. W.: Digitalis mechanisms of action and clinical use. N. Engl. J. Med. *318*:358, 1988.

Smith, T. W., Butler, V. P., Jr., Haber, E., et al.: Treatment of life-threatening digtalis intoxication with digoxin-specific Fab fragments: Experience in 26 cases. N. Engl. J. Med. *307*:1357, 1982.

Snider, A. R., and Serwer, G. A.: Echocardiography in Pediatric Heart Disease. Chicago, Mosby-Year Book Inc., 1990.

Stranger, P., Heymann, M. A., Tarnoff, H., et al.: Complications of cardiac catheterization of neonates, infants, and children. A three-year study. Circulation *50*:595, 1974.

Swischuk, L. E., and Sapire, D. W.: Basic Imaging in Congenital Heart Disease, 3rd ed. Baltimore, Williams & Wilkins, 1986.

Tajik, A. J., Seward, J. B., Hagler, D. J., et al.: Two-dimensional realtime ultrasonic imaging of the heart and great vessels. Technique, image orientation, structure identification, and validation. Mayo Clin. Proc. *54*:271, 1978.

Teitel, D. F., Iwamoto, H. S., and Rudolph, A. M.: Effects of birth related events on central flow patterns. Pediatr. Res. *22*:557, 1987.

Walther, F. J., Siassi, B., Ramadan, N. A., et al.: Cardiac output in newborn infants with transient myocardial dysfunction. J. Pediatr. *107*:781, 1985.

Wettrell, G., and Andersson, K. E.: Clinical pharmacokinetics of digoxin in infants. Clin. Pharmacokinet. *2*:17, 1977.

Williams, R. G., Bierman, F. Z., and Sanders, S. P.: Echocardiographic Diagnosis of Cardiac Malformation. Boston, Little, Brown & Company, 1986.

Ziegler, R. F.: Electrocardiographic Studies in Normal Infants and Children. Springfield, Ill., Charles C Thomas, 1951.

CONGENITAL CARDIAC MALFORMATIONS **63**

Michael D. Freed

In this chapter, the incidence, etiology, and embryology of congenital heart disease will be discussed, and the current status of some common cardiac problems presenting in the first month of life will subsequently be reviewed. The discussion of each cardiac malformation will understandably be brief; those readers interested in a more comprehensive consideration of this subject are encouraged to consult one of the textbooks on newborn heart disease by Rowe and coworkers (1981), Moller and Neal (1990), or Long (1990).

Incidence. Congenital malformations of the heart occur in about 8 of every 1000 live births and represent about 10 per cent of all congenital malformations. It is difficult to obtain precise incidence data for all congenital heart disease, since signs and symptoms of heart disease may be absent at birth and not be evident until years or, as in the case of a bicuspid aortic valve, decades later. In addition, some newborns with murmurs at birth do not have significant disease; the murmurs are due to normal turbulence of the closing ductus arteriosus or physiologic turbulence in the pulmonary artery.

Two large studies have provided information on the incidence of congenital heart disease in the United States. The New England Regional Infant Cardiac Program (NERICP) reviewed more than 1 million births in a 6-year period (1968–1974) and found 2251 infants with heart disease requiring cardiac catheterization or cardiac surgery, or who died, an incidence of critical heart disease of 2.08/1000 live births (Fyler et al., 1980). In the Baltimore-Washington infant study, Ferencz et al. (1985) noted a slightly higher incidence, 2.4/1000 live births when only invasive confirmation was used, and 3.7/1000 live births when noninvasive confirmation, usually echocardiography, was allowed.

The relative frequency of the different diagnoses are listed in Table 63–1. Ventricular septal defects, the most common type of heart disease in older children, are the most common type in newborns as well. In contrast, newborns with atrial defects are rarely symptomatic and thus represent a small percentage of this group, although a large proportion of older children with heart disease have atrial defects.

In the NERICP study, 58 per cent (1310/2251) of

TABLE 63–1. Diagnostic Frequency of Congenital Heart Disease

	NERICP*		BWIS**	APPROXIMATE NUMBER
	Per Cent Newborns	Number/1000 Live Births	Number/1000 Live Births	LIVE BIRTHS/AFFECTED INFANTS
Ventricular septal defect	15.7	0.345	0.345	3,000
D transposition	9.9	0.218	0.211	4,500
Tetralogy of Fallot	8.9	0.196	0.190	5,000
Coarctation of the aorta	7.5	0.165	0.200	5,500
Hypoplastic left heart	7.4	0.163	0.209	5,500
Endocardial cushion defect	5.0	0.110	0.251	5,500
Patent ductus arteriosus	6.1	0.135	0.062	10,000
Heterotaxias	4.0	0.088	*	11,500
Atrial septal defect	2.9	0.065	0.094	12,500
Pulmonary stenosis	3.3	0.073	0.080	13,000
Pulmonary atresia	3.1	0.069	0.077	14,000
Total anomalous pulmonary venous connector	2.6	0.058	0.083	14,000
Aortic stenosis	1.9	0.041	0.083	16,000
Myocardial disease	2.6	0.056	*	18,000
Single ventricle	2.4	0.054	*	18,500
Double outlet, right ventricle	1.4	0.041	0.056	20,000
Tricuspid atresia	2.6	0.056	0.034	22,000
Truncus arteriosus	0.7	0.030	0.056	23,000
Other	4.9	0.113	0.349	4,500
TOTAL		2.08	2.38	

*The New England Regional Infant Cardiac Program encompassed 1,083,083 infants younger than 1 year of age, born within the six New England states from 1969 to 1974 who were sick enough to require cardiac catheterization or surgery, or to die from their congenital heart disease. (Data from Fyler, D. C., Buckley, L. P., Hellenbrand, W., et al.: Report of the New England Regional Infant Cardiac Program. Pediatrics 65[Suppl.]: 375, 1980.)

**The Baltimore-Washington Infant Study covered births in the Maryland and Washington, D.C., metropolitan area. It involved 179,697 births during 1981 to 1982, using the same admission criteria. (Data from Ferencz, C., Rubin, J. D., McCarter, R. J., et al.: Congenital heart disease: Prevalence of live birth. The Baltimore-Washington Infant Study. Am. J. Epidemiol. *121*:31, 1985.)

infants with congenital heart disease were seen in the first 4 weeks of life and 896 (40 per cent) were seen in the first week. The most common diagnosis found in each age group (during the first, second, third, and fourth weeks of life) is listed in Table 63–2.

Transposition of the great arteries is the most common lesion seen in the first week of life, coarctation is the most common malformation seen during the second week, and ventricular septal defects are the most common abnormalities observed in the third and fourth weeks of life.

Etiology. Although it has been a topic of great interest over the past two decades, there is as yet no clear understanding of the etiology of most congenital heart disease (Pyeritz and Murphy, 1989). In about 18 per cent of children with heart disease, there are clear genetic causes (Ferencz et al., 1987). Most of these are associated with obvious chromosomal anomalies. Down syndrome (trisomy 21) is associated with congenital heart disease in 50 per cent of cases, trisomy 18 and 13 in more than 90 per cent, and the deletion syndromes of chromosomes 18, 13, 5, and 4 in 25 to 50 per cent.

Congenital heart disease is also associated with many of the single mutant gene syndromes. Autosomal dominant syndromes associated with heart disease include Holt-Oram (atrial defects), Alport (ventricular defects), leopard (pulmonary stenosis), Noonan (pulmonary stenosis), and tuberous sclerosis (myocardial rhabdomyoma). Autosomal recessive syndromes associated with heart disease include Ellis–van Creveld (single atrium) as well as Friedreich ataxia and Laurence-Moon-Biedl (ventricular defects). In total, however, the single gene syndromes account for only about 6 per cent of all cases of congenital heart disease.

Environmental factors may play an important role in the cause of congenital cardiac malformations. Maternal ingestion of drugs such as thalidomide, the antimetabolites, and warfarin have been shown to be associated with a high incidence of cardiac malformations, and recent interest has focused on congenital malformations associated with the maternal ingestion of alcohol. Several viral infections have been shown to be associated with congenital cardiac malformations, but only congenital rubella, which results in peripheral pulmonic stenosis and patent ductus arteriosus, is known to be clinically significant. In total, however, environmental factors account for no more than 2 per cent of all cases of congenital heart disease.

In more than 73 per cent of children with congenital heart disease, the cause is unclear. The best explanation seems to be a multifactorial type of inheritance in which a hereditary predisposition for cardiac anomalies in concert with an environmental "trigger" at a vulnerable period during cardiac morphogenesis causes the congenital anomaly (Nora, 1977). This model allows calculation of risk of recurrence among other children in an affected family. For most cases of congenital heart disease, the recurrence risk is between 1 and 5 per cent, with the more common abnormalities falling in the higher end of the range. Several large studies of the families of children with congenital heart disease have confirmed these approximations, although in 1982 Whittemore and co-workers found a much higher recurrence rate, 14.2 per cent, in children born of mothers with congenital heart disease, raising the possibility that other factors may be involved (Nora and Nora, 1987).

Children with congenital heart disease frequently have associated extracardiac anomalies (Fyler et al., 1980) that involve the skeletal, gastrointestinal, or genitourinary system. Such findings suggest that the environmental trigger may affect several organs undergoing morphogenesis at the same time. Recent advances in molecular biology may provide information on oncogenes, growth factors, and cell surface factors, and in conjunction with improved embryologic modeling, these advances will improve our understanding in the decade ahead (Pyeritz and Murphy, 1989).

Embryology. Although knowledge about the embryologic development of the heart is helpful in understanding diagnosis and management of children with congenital heart disease, the subject is complex, incompletely understood, and for the most part, beyond the scope of this chapter (Hamilton and Mossman, 1972; Van Mierop et al., 1978; Langman, 1981).

TABLE 63–2. Diagnosis of Infants at Selected Ages*

0–6 DAYS (n = 896)		7–13 DAYS (n = 210)		14–20 DAYS (n = 116)		21–27 DAYS (n = 88)		0–28 DAYS (n = 1310)	
(Per Cent)		(Per Cent)		(Per Cent)		(Per Cent)		(Per Cent)	
TGA	17	CoA	19	VSD	20	VSD	21	TGA	14
HLH	12	VSD	15	TGA	17	TGA	9	HLH	11
Lung	10	HLH	11	CoA	16	TOF	8	VSD	9
TOF	9	TGA	9	TOF	8	CoA	8	COA	9
CoA	7	TOF	6	ECD	6	TAPVR	8	TOF	8
PA	7	Truncus	4	Hetero	6	PDA	7	Lung	7
Hetero	6	Hetero	4	PDA	4	TA	6	PA	5
VSD	7	SV	4	Lung	4	ECD	5	Hetero	5
PDA	4	TAPVR	3	TAPVR	3	SV	3	TA	3
						Lung	3	ECD	3

*Diagnostic frequency of infants less than 4 weeks of age. *Abbreviations:* AS = aortic stenosis, CoA = coarctation of the aorta, ECD = endocardial cushion defect, Hetero = heterotaxia syndrome, HLH = hypoplastic left heart syndrome, Lung = primary lung disease, PA = pulmonary atresia with an intact ventricular septum, PDA = patent ductus arteriosus, SV = single ventricle, TA = tricuspid atresia, TAPVR = total anomalous pulmonary venous return, TGA = transposition of the great arteries, TOF = tetralogy of Fallot, Truncus = truncus arteriosus, VSD = ventricular septal defect.

(Adapted from Fyler, D. C., et al.: Report of the New England Regional Infant Cardiac Program. Pediatrics 65[Suppl.]:375, 1980. Reproduced by permission of Pediatrics.)

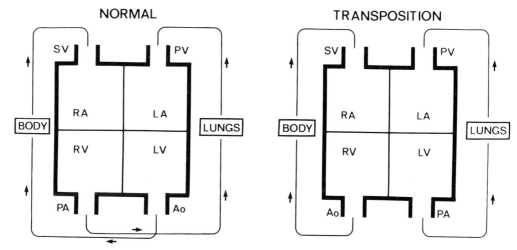

FIGURE 63–1. A schematic diagram of the circulation in the normal newborn and the newborn with transposition of the great arteries. In the normal newborn, the circulation is arranged in series; that is, venous blood goes through the right heart chambers to the lungs for oxygenation and then through the left side of the heart to be delivered to the body. In the newborn with transposition, the circulation is arranged in parallel with venous blood passing through the right side of the heart to the aorta and body and oxygenated blood passing through the left side of the heart to the lungs. Mixing between the circuits is necessary for survival after birth. Ao, aorta; LA, left atrium; LV, left ventricle; PA, pulmonary artery; PV, pulmonary vein; RA, right atrium; RV, right ventricle; SV, systemic veins.

The heart appears on the 18th day after conception and is normally complete by the 40th day, when the embryo is approximately 15 mm (3/4 in) long. Initially, the heart is a straight tube ventral to the gut and consists of, from cephalad to caudad, the truncus arteriosus, bulbus cordis (later right ventricle), primitive ventricle (later left ventricle), and atrium. Soon after the initiation of the heartbeat at 20 days, the heart tube normally loops to the right so that the bulbus cordis lies to the right of the primitive ventricle. During the 4th week after conception, the heart continues to twist and bend so that the atrium lies above the primitive ventricles. During the 5th week, the ventricular septum forms, and the aorta and pulmonary artery are septated from the truncus arteriosus, with the conus muscle under the aorta being resorbed so that the aorta comes into continuity with the left ventricle. The endocardial tissue in the central portion of the heart differentiates into separate mitral and tricuspid valves, and the ostium primum closes, separating the right and left atrium. Thus, by the end of the 5th week, the "in series" circulation of the primitive cardiac tube is exchanged for the "in parallel" circulation characteristic of later fetal life. During the 6th week after conception, the membranous septum closes and anatomic cardiac development is completed, the first organ system to do so.

The vessels leading to and exiting from the heart develop at about the same time. By the 3rd week of gestation, a total of six pairs of aortic arches have formed, although not all are present at the same time. Over the next 3 weeks the first, second, and fifth pairs disappear. The third arch becomes the right and left internal carotid artery, the left fourth arch the ascending aorta, and the right fourth becomes the innominate and part of the right subclavian artery. The pulmonary arteries arise from the sixth arch, with the sixth right becoming disconnected from the aorta to become the right pulmonary artery, and the left from the left sixth forming the ductus arteriosus and left pulmonary artery.

Congenital anomalies may be due to any one or more of the following developmental errors:

1. Aplasia or agenesis (failure of development).
2. Hypoplasia (incomplete or defective development).
3. Dysplasia (abnormal development).
4. Malposition.
5. Failure of fusion of adjoining parts.
6. Abnormal fusion.
7. Incomplete resorption.
8. Abnormal persistence of a vessel.
9. Early obliteration of a vessel.

The multitude of things that can go wrong during cardiac morphogenesis reflects the complexity of the embryogenesis of the heart.

■ CYANOTIC CONGENITAL HEART DISEASE

COMPLETE TRANSPOSITION OF THE GREAT ARTERIES

Anatomy. In transposition of the great arteries (TGA), the position of the great arteries is reversed; that is, the aorta arises anteriorly from the right ventricle and the pulmonary artery posteriorly from the left ventricle. The pulmonary and systemic circulations are therefore arranged in parallel rather than in series, with the systemic venous blood passing through the right heart chambers and then back out to the body and pulmonary venous blood traversing the left heart and returning to the lungs (Fig. 63–1). Survival after birth depends on mixing between the circuits.

The prefixes "D" and "L" are used to denote whether the aorta arises to the right (dextro) or to the left (levo) of the pulmonary artery.

TGA in the newborn is often an isolated defect, but other associated malformations involving defects of the atrial or ventricular septum, stenosis or atresia of the pulmonic valve, and anomalies of the atrioventricular valves are not uncommon and may alter the physiology considerably. Interestingly, extracardiac anomalies are unusual in newborns with TGA.

The embryology of this condition is still not completely understood. Although it was once thought that this anomaly was due to failure of spiraling of the truncal septum, Van Praagh and Van Praagh noted in 1966 that during cardiac development both great vessels are initially elevated by muscular tissue (conus), and they suggested that differential resorption of the subpulmonary rather than subaortic conus allows the pulmonic valve rather than aortic to be inferior and posterior and therefore in continuity with the left ventricle, with the aortic valve superior and anterior in continuity with the right ventricle, with the rest of the heart unaffected.

Incidence. TGA occurs in slightly more than one per 4500 live births and was the most common form of cyanotic congenital heart disease in both the NERICP and the Baltimore-Washington infant study. Of infants presenting in New England with critical heart disease in the first week of life, 17 per cent had TGA.

Hemodynamics. In TGA, the pulmonary and systemic circulations are arranged in parallel rather than in series, with the aorta arising from the right ventricle and the pulmonary artery from the left. In utero, there is little disruption in fetal hemodynamics (Fig. 63–2), since blood returning from the systemic and pulmonary veins passes unimpeded into the atrium and ventricles in the normal fashion. Blood from the right ventricle is pumped into the ascending aorta and then to the systemic arteries and placenta. Blood from the left ventricle passes into the pulmonary artery, and then, because of the high pulmonary resistance, most is diverted into the ductus arteriosus and descending aorta. The only variation from the normal fetal circulation is that the slightly less saturated blood

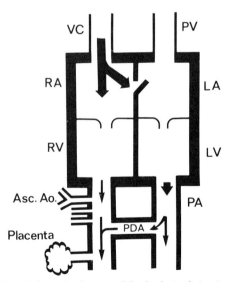

FIGURE 63–2. *Schematic diagram of the fetal circulation in transposition of the great arteries. Venous blood returning to the heart via the vena cava passes either into the right atrium, right ventricle, and aorta or through the foramen ovale to the left atrium, left ventricle, and pulmonary artery. As in the normal fetus, most of the blood entering the main pulmonary artery is diverted through the ductus arteriosus into the descending aorta and placenta because of the high pulmonary vascular resistance. Asc Ao, ascending aorta; LA, left atrium; LV, left ventricle; PA, pulmonary artery; PDA, patent ductus arteriosus; PV, pulmonary vein; RA, right atrium; RV, right ventricle; VC, vena cava.*

from the superior vena cava is preferentially shunted to the head vessels rather than through the ductus arteriosus, and the more saturated blood from the inferior vena cava is shunted to the lungs rather than to the cerebral circulation. In spite of these differences, in utero development appears normal, and thus far no major extrauterine abnormalities have been identified.

After birth, newborns completely depend on mixing between pulmonary and systemic circulations for survival. For a while the fetal pathways, the ductus arteriosus and foramen ovale, suffice. By a few hours of age, the pulmonary resistance is significantly lower than the systemic, so shunting of hypoxemic blood from the aorta to the pulmonary artery is facilitated. Since the pulmonary circuit cannot be overloaded, obligatory shunting of pulmonary venous return from left atrium to right atrium occurs. This bidirectional shunting from aorta to pulmonary artery and left atrium to right atrium improves mixing and prevents severe cyanosis. As the ductus arteriosus closes, however, the obligatory shunting is eliminated and the only site of mixing is the foramen ovale. Although some bidirectional shunting may occur allowing deoxygenated blood to get to the lungs and oxygenated blood to the systemic circulation, this is usually inadequate and severe systemic hypoxemia (PO$_2$, 15 to 40 mm Hg; O$_2$ saturation, 30 to 60) results. Occasionally, a small ventricular defect may be present, slightly ameliorating the hypoxemia.

Clinical Manifestations. There is a strong sex predilection in TGA, with males outnumbering females by almost 2:1. Infants are usually cyanotic within the first 12 to 24 hours after birth. In the NERICP, 59 per cent of infants with TGA were seen at a cardiac center within the first 2 days of life, and 79 per cent were observed by the end of the 2nd week.

The physical examination is usually unrewarding except for generalized cyanosis. Although peripheral pulses may be somewhat bounding and the right ventricular impulse slightly hyperactive, the heart sounds are usually normal, with physiologic splitting of the second sound present about half the time. Prominent heart murmurs are uncommon, although there may be a short grade 2/6 systolic murmur along the left sternal border. A loud murmur should alert one to the possibility of associated heart disease (e.g., a ventricular septal defect). Signs of congestive failure are usually absent, although tachypnea may be present, probably as a compensatory mechanism for the hypoxemia.

Since there is little disturbance in the intrauterine blood flow, the electrocardiogram is usually normal showing right axis deviation and right ventricular hypertrophy that is within the normal limits for age.

The chest radiograph is also usually normal for a newborn, although the relative anterioposterior position of the great vessels and the usual (although unexplained) absence of a thymic shadow give the narrow appearance of the superior mediastinum frequently described as an "egg-on-side" appearance (Fig. 63–3). The pulmonary blood flow is rarely increased in the first few days of life, although it may be increased in infants who present later.

With the recent development of echocardiography, the diagnosis of TGA can usually be made with certainty before cardiac catheterization. Since in D transposition the posterior great vessel arising from the left ventricle is the

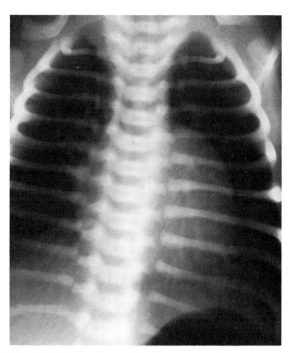

FIGURE 63–3. Chest radiograph in the anteroposterior projection in a newborn with transposition of the great arteries and an intact ventricular septum. The upper mediastinum is narrowed because of the anteroposterior relationship of the aorta and pulmonary artery. The heart is not enlarged. The pulmonary blood flow is not decreased.

pulmonary artery rather than the aorta, one can establish the diagnosis with two-dimensional echocardiography by identifying the posterior great vessel (pulmonary artery) and tracing it from the LV to the bifurcation usually using a subxiphoid long axis view, or tracing the anterior vessel from the right ventricle to the innominate, carotid, or subclavian branches using a subxiphoid short axis view (Fig. 63–4).

Cardiac catheterization and angiography confirm the diagnosis. Saturations on the right side of the heart are often very low (<40 per cent), with a slight increase between vena cava and right atrium. The saturation in the aorta is about the same as the right ventricle. Saturations in the pulmonary veins and left heart chambers are normal or slightly increased, and the pulmonary artery (when entered) often has a saturation of 92 to 95 per cent. The atrial pressures are usually normal and equal. Any difference between right and left atrial pressure suggests a significant shunt at the ventricular or ductal level. The left ventricular pressure is usually less than simultaneous systemic arterial pressure; TGA is the only heart disease in which this is true. Angiography confirms that the aorta arises from the right ventricle and the pulmonary artery arises from the left ventricle (Fig. 63–4). A balloon atrial septostomy (see discussion of treatment further on) is usually performed.

Diagnosis. Transposition of the great arteries should be strongly suspected in any cyanotic newborn showing normal-to-increased pulmonary blood flow on the radiograph and right ventricular hypertrophy on the electrocardiogram. Indeed, a severely hypoxemic infant breathing comfortably with a normal physical examination, chest radiograph, and electrocardiogram almost invariably has transposition. All other types of cyanotic congenital heart disease are associated with diminished or congested pulmonary vascular markings on the radiograph and a single second heart sound. Persistent fetal circulation can usually be distinguished by echocardiography.

Treatment. Untreated, TGA in infants is associated with a dismal prognosis, since 30 per cent die in the first week and 50 per cent succumb in the first months of life (Liebman et al., 1969). Improved survival depends on early recognition and transfer to a cardiac center. The management involves three phases: rapid correction of metabolic derangements, palliation, and later correction. If the infant is acidotic with a pH of less than 7.25 when first seen, sodium bicarbonate should be given to correct the base deficit.

In those who are severely acidotic or in whom further palliation must be delayed, prostaglandin E_1 has been employed to open the ductus arteriosus and improve mixing and oxygenation.

For those who remain severely hypoxemic or acidotic, the palliation of choice is balloon atrial septostomy, developed and described by Rashkind and Miller in 1966. A specially made balloon catheter is inserted into the

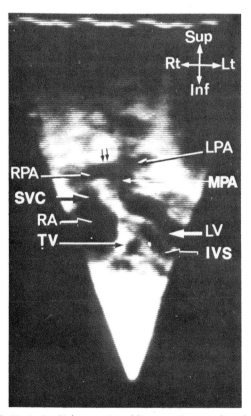

FIGURE 63–4. A, Right anterior oblique angiogram that shows d-transposition of the great arteries. B, Longitudinal subxiphoid two-dimensional echocardiogram that shows D transposition of the great arteries. The main pulmonary artery (MPA) arises from the left ventricle (LV) and bifurcates into the right pulmonary artery (RPA) and left pulmonary artery (LPA). SVC, superior vena cava; RA, right atrium; TV, tricuspid valve; IVS, interventricular septum; IVS, MPA-RPA junction. (From Bierman, F. Z., and Williams, R. G.: Prospective diagnosis of d-transposition of the great arteries in neonates by subxiphoid two-dimensional echocardiography. Circulation 60:1496, 1979. Reproduced with permission from the American Heart Association.)

femoral or umbilical vein and advanced through the foramen ovale into the left atrium and then inflated. The catheter is quickly withdrawn from left to right, tearing the fibrous tissue of the fossa ovalis. This iatrogenic atrial septal defect often increases the mixing between the systemic and pulmonary circulations to such an extent that the PaO_2 rises into the 30s and the saturation elevates into the 70s. Frequently, this improvement is sustained until corrective surgery can be undertaken. For those with a thick atrial septum, a septostomy can be performed with a cutting blade.

The conventional reparative surgical approach to TGA has been an atrial baffle operation to divert systemic venous blood through the mitral valve, left ventricle, and pulmonary arteries to the lungs and the pulmonary venous blood through the tricuspid valve and right ventricle to the aorta (Mustard et al., 1964; Senning, 1959). This corrects the circulation physiologically, although anatomically the right ventricle remains the systemic ventricle and the left ventricle pumps blood to the lungs.

Recently, many centers have abandoned this approach for an "arterial switch," in which the great vessels are divided, the coronary arteries and a button of tissue around them moved from the anterior vessel to the posterior one, and the distal arteries reversed so that the right ventricular blood goes to the pulmonary artery and the left ventricular blood to the aorta (Castaneda et al., 1984; Jatene et al., 1976; Yacoub et al., 1980; Kirklin et al., 1990). This normalizes the circulation and, if promising early results continue, will almost certainly become the procedure of choice.

Prognosis. It is difficult to assess long-term prognosis in a time of rapid advances. Recently, the Toronto group has reviewed its experience with Mustard's repair (Trusler et al., 1987). The mortality rate between 1974 and 1985 has been reduced to 0.9 per cent (2 in 223 patients), with a 10-year actuarial survival rate of 93.7 per cent. Complications included baffle obstruction, largely eliminated in those operated upon recently; arrhythmias; and right (systemic) ventricular dysfunction.

Since the arterial switch operation is newer, follow-up is necessarily shorter. An early report shows a predicted 1-year survival rate of greater than 99 per cent (Quaegenbeur et al., 1986), and our early follow-up data suggest a low incidence of late problems (Wernovsky et al., 1988). Evaluation of long-term studies will be necessary to choose between these techniques, although certainly anatomic correction with the arterial switch is conceptually more appealing.

TETRALOGY OF FALLOT

Anatomy. In 1888, Etienne Fallot described a series of cyanotic patients with a ventricular septal defect, pulmonary stenosis, right ventricular hypertrophy, and an aorta that appeared to be over the ventricular septum. For many years, it has been appreciated that the latter two manifestations are secondary to the former two lesions.

The ventricular septal defect location is predictably high in ventricular septum; additional defects are present in 15 per cent of the patients. The degree of pulmonic obstruction at the infundibulum (subvalvular) or secondarily at

the pulmonary valve or peripheral pulmonary arteries is variable, ranging from mild stenosis to complete atresia, and accounts for the variability of presentation. Associated anomalies include atrial septal defects, right aortic arch (25 per cent), and anomalies of the coronary arteries (5 per cent).

Incidence. Tetralogy of Fallot (TOF) occurred slightly less frequently than transpositions (1 of every 5000 live births) and accounted for 9 per cent of infants presenting in the 1st week of life.

Hemodynamics. In utero, there does not seem to be any major hemodynamic disturbance, and consequently, newborns with TOF are well developed at birth. During fetal life, the aorta carries an increased percentage of combined ventricular output with the exact proportion a function of the degree of pulmonic stenosis (Fig. 63–5). The ductus arteriosus is smaller than normal, since its flow is diminished, and it may be quite tortuous. Since there is no volume or pressure overload within the heart, the ventricles and atrioventricular valves usually develop normally.

After birth, the degree of shunting depends on the severity of the pulmonary stenosis and the relative pulmonary and systemic arteriolar resistance. In the newborn with severe pulmonary stenosis, the resistance to blood passing out the right ventricular outflow tract is very high, and desaturated venous blood preferentially passes through the ventricular septal defect into the aorta, resulting in arterial hypoxemia and cyanosis. If the pulmonary stenosis is mild, there may be little resistance to blood passing out the pulmonary artery; infants with this condition, may behave like those with a ventricular septal defect, with increasing left-to-right shunt and heart failure as the pulmonary arteriolar resistance drops over the first weeks

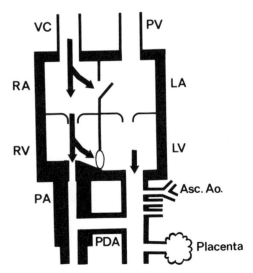

FIGURE 63–5. *Schematic diagram of the circulation in the fetus with tetralogy of Fallot. Because of the right ventricular outflow obstruction, some of the right ventricular output passes across the ventricular septal defect into the left ventricle and out the aorta. If the pulmonary stenosis is severe, pulmonary blood flow may be augmented by blood from the aorta passing through the ductus arteriosus. Blood flow to the placenta is unimpeded. The abbreviations in this diagram are the same as those used in Figure 63–2.*

of life. The usual hallmarks of TOF, arterial hypoxemia and cyanosis, may be completely absent in this group at first. Occasionally, mild-to-moderate pulmonary stenosis may occur in a balanced situation in which pulmonary and systemic resistances are equal and little shunt in either direction occurs; often these infants shunt right-to-left with crying.

Clinical Manifestations. The presentation of infants with tetralogy is a function of the degree of pulmonary stenosis. Those with severe obstruction usually present in the first days with extreme cyanosis as the ductus arteriosus closes. Those with lesser degrees of pulmonary stenosis may be only mildly cyanotic and present with a systolic ejection murmur along the left sternal border in the delivery room or in the nursery. The pulmonary component of the second heart sound is diminished or inaudible. Signs of congestive heart failure are absent except in a small group with an absent pulmonary valve who present with a to-and-fro murmur at the left upper sternal border due to pulmonary stenosis and regurgitation.

Tetralogy "spells," which are attacks of paroxysmal dyspnea associated with irritability, extreme cyanosis, and loss of the systolic murmur, are an emergency, because cerebral hypoxemia may lead to convulsions, coma, and death. Spells are fortunately unusual in the first months of life.

Since the right ventricle receives normal flow in utero, the electrocardiogram of the newborn is normal, showing right axis-deviation and right ventricular hypertrophy.

The heart size on the chest radiograph is usually normal, because neither of the atria or the ventricles is exposed to a volume overload. In those who are very hypoxemic, the pulmonary blood flow is decreased, because venous blood is being diverted away from the lungs to the systemic circuit. The main pulmonary artery segment is often diminished, giving the classic "coeur-en-sabot" appearance (Fig. 63–6). A right aortic arch is present in one-fourth of the cases.

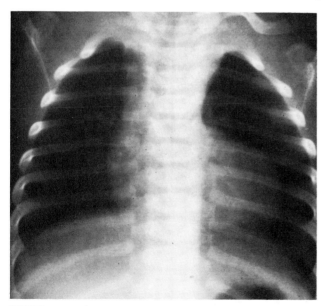

FIGURE 63–6. *Plain anteroposterior roentgenogram from a newborn with tetralogy of Fallot. Note the absent main pulmonary artery segment and uplifted apex (coeur-en-sabot). The pulmonary blood flow is decreased.*

The two-dimensional echocardiographic study shows the anatomy clearly, especially from the subxiphoid view (Sanders et al., 1982), and can usually localize the coronary arteries, occasionally precluding the need for catheterization (Fig. 63–7).

Cardiac catheterization and angiography are indicated if the two-dimensional echocardiogram is equivocal.

A right ventricular angiogram with the baby "sitting" to obtain 40 degrees of cranial angulation allows one to visualize the infundibular, valvular, and peripheral pulmonary stenosis (Fig. 63–8), and a left ventricular angiogram in the left anterior oblique with axial angulation or hepatoclavicular view outlines the ventricular septal defect(s) and the coronary arteries. Occasionally, an aortic angiogram in the left anterior oblique is necessary to outline the origin and course of the anterior descending coronary artery. This is important, because it occasionally arises as the first branch of the right rather than left coronary artery and traverses the external surface of the right ventricular infundibulum to reach the interventricular groove. Its presence prevents easy patching of the subpulmonic stenosis at surgical repair; because division of this large vessel is almost invariably fatal, a conduit to bridge over this vessel may be necessary.

Diagnosis. The cyanotic infant with decreased pulmonary blood flow and a normal heart size on the chest radiograph, right axis deviation and right ventricular hypertrophy on the electrocardiogram, and a systolic ejection murmur on examination, usually has TOF (see Differential Diagnosis).

Infants with a systolic murmur without cyanosis may be confused with patients with isolated valvular pulmonary stenosis or even those with a ventricular septal defect. More complicated lesions with a physiology similar to that of TOF, ventricular defect, and pulmonary stenosis must be differentiated by echocardiography or angiocardiography. Examples are double outlet ventricle with pulmonary stenosis, single ventricle with pulmonary stenosis, and transposition (either D or L).

Treatment. We have reserved pharmacologic treatment for those few newborns who are profoundly cyanotic, with arterial saturations of less than 75 per cent, or those who are having spells for whom surgery is either not available or contraindicated. Propranolol, 2 to 6 mg/kg/day, has been recommended in this group (Garson et al., 1981).

The surgical therapy in the past has been palliative. The Blalock-Taussig shunt connecting the subclavian artery to the pulmonary artery directly or using a 4 or 5 mm diameter Gore-Tex tube has been extensively performed and provides good palliation at low risk for several years (Ilbawi et al., 1984).

Recently one-stage repair has gained favor and is now the procedure of choice for children older than 1 year of age at most centers and at any age in some centers (Walsh et al., 1988). The ventricular septum is closed with a Dacron patch, and the right ventricular outflow obstruction is relieved by a combination of muscle resection and a patch of pericardium to widen the outlet for egress of blood from the right ventricle when necessary.

Prognosis. The risks of the Blalock-Taussig shunt are small, certainly under 10 per cent and as low as 3 per

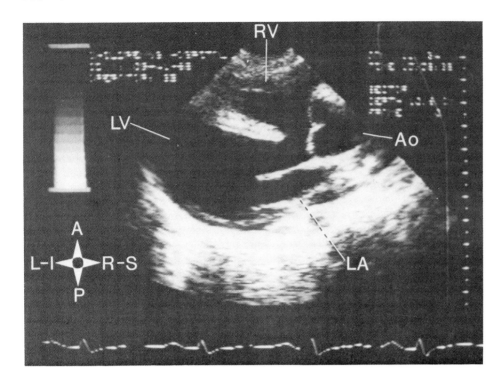

FIGURE 63–7. Parasternal long-axis view of tetralogy of Fallot showing a malalignment ventricular septal defect and an overriding aorta. RV, right ventricle; LV, left ventricle; Ao, aorta; LA, left atrium. (Reprinted from Sanders, S. P.: Echocardiography and related techniques in the diagnosis of congenital heart defects: Part III, conotruncus and great arteries. Echocardiography 1:443, 1984.)

cent in many centers (Ilbawi et al., 1984). This serves as good palliation usually for several years. Total repair in infancy also has a good prognosis, with a 5-year survival rate of at least 90 per cent (Walsh et al., 1988). Late postoperative complications have included residual cardiac defects (pulmonary stenosis, regurgitation, or ventricular defects), and arrhythmias, but these effects have been uncommon. A recent 26- to 31-year follow-up of the original patients operated on between 1954 and 1960 have shown an actuarial survival of 77 per cent at 30 years (Lillehei et al., 1986). With modern techniques, the results should be much better.

TETRALOGY OF FALLOT WITH PULMONARY ATRESIA

Anatomy. This is the severest form of TOF, with the deviated parietal band of the infundibulum completely occluding the right ventricular outflow tract. Since there is no antegrade flow through the pulmonic valve, development of the pulmonary arteries depends on flow from the ductus arteriosus and embryologic intersegmental or bronchial arteries. If the flow into the pulmonary arteries is proximal, the mediastinal portion of the right and left pulmonary arteries may be of good size. If, however, the collaterals insert well within the hilum of the lungs, the mediastinal portions may be hypoplastic or even atretic. Even when central pulmonary arteries are present, there may be incomplete arborization of the pulmonary arteries with some or most of the lung parenchyma supplied via the collateral systemic arteries rather than the mediastinal pulmonary arteries (Fig. 63–8). In a study by Shimazaki and associates (1988), 28 of 172 (16 per cent) patients with tetralogy and pulmonary atresia had congenital absence of one or both of the central and unbranched hilar portions of the left or right pulmonary arteries, and among 132 patients with confluent pulmonary arteries, 70 (53

per cent) had incomplete arborization (distribution) of one or both pulmonary arteries. Seventy-nine (60 per cent) of those with confluent pulmonary arteries had large aortopulmonary collateral arteries as did all those with nonconfluent pulmonary arteries. The postnatal presentation and prognosis of these infants are in great part a function of the intrauterine pulmonary artery development. The ventricular septal defect is invariably large.

Incidence. In the NERICP, 46 of 2251 infants seen between 1969 and 1974 had TOF with pulmonary atresia, representing an incidence of one of every 25,000 births in the region (Fyler et al., 1980).

Hemodynamics. This lesion does not seem to influence the fetal circulation adversely, because in utero pulmonary blood flow is only about 7 per cent of combined ventricular output, a minimal volume that is easily accommodated by a left-to-right shunt through the ductus arteriosus. Since there is no antegrade flow through the pulmonary valve, the combined ventricular output exits the heart through the aorta, which is usually dilated.

After birth, flow to the pulmonary arteries continues to be through the ductus arteriosus and collateral vessels. As the ductus usually closes in the first few days of life, the infant depends on flow through the collateral channels. If they are small, hypoxemia may be profound. If the collaterals are huge, pulmonary flow may be large and cyanosis minimal, with congestive heart failure from a torrential left-to-right shunt occasionally being present.

Clinical Features. In the newborn with inadequate collaterals, cyanosis is prominent and increases as the ductus arteriosus constricts. Heart murmurs are frequently absent, although a continuous murmur over the back from the aortopulmonary collaterals may be heard. The second heart sound is single, and a systolic ejection click (presumably from a large aorta) is often present. As in TOF with pulmonary stenosis, the heart is normal in size, with a concavity in the area of the main pulmonary artery apparent on the radiograph if this region is not obscured by the thymus. The pulmonary flow is usually reduced, especially when arterial hypoxemia is profound, and a right aortic arch may be present. The electrocardiogram is usually normal, with a QRS axis of +90 to 180 degrees and a normal degree of right ventricular hypertrophy. On the M-mode echocardiogram, there is overriding of the ventricular septum by the aorta with a small left atrium reflecting diminished pulmonary venous return. The two-dimensional echocardiogram shows the ventricular septal defect and the atretic right ventricular outflow tract.

In the 10 per cent of newborns with large collaterals, congestive heart failure may be the presenting symptom,

with cyanosis mild or even absent. Loud continuous murmurs over the chest and back are common. The cardiac silhouette on radiographs is increased, and the pulmonary vessels are prominent because of the increased blood flow. The cardiogram is usually normal, although some infants have more left ventricular forces than usual because of the left ventricular volume overload. On the M-mode echocardiogram, the aorta overrides the ventricular septum, and the left atrial size is normal or increased.

In all newborns with TOF with pulmonary atresia, cardiac catheterization demonstrates arterial hypoxemia due to right-to-left shunting at the ventricular level and equal systolic pressure in both ventricles. Visualization of the pulmonary arteries, necessary for treatment, is best accomplished with an aortogram with the patient positioned so that the camera is angled cranially about 40

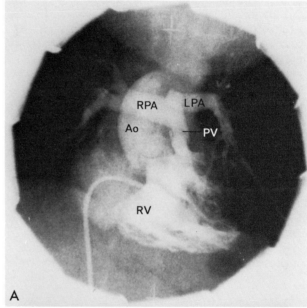

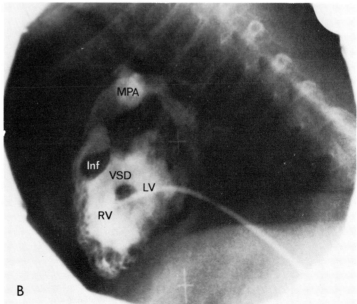

FIGURE 63–8. The cranially angulated (40 degrees) anteroposterior (A) and lateral (B) projections of a right ventricular angiogram in a newborn with tetralogy of Fallot. The subpulmonic area (infundibulum) and pulmonary valve are narrowed. The ventricular septal defect is seen on the lateral projection with filling of the left ventricle. Ao, aorta; Inf, infundibulum of the right ventricle; LV, left ventricle; LPA, left pulmonary artery; MPA, main pulmonary artery; PV, pulmonary valve; RPA, right pulmonary artery; RV, right ventricle; VSD, ventricular septal defect.

degrees to allow visualization of the pulmonary arteries filled through the ductus arteriosus or aortopulmonary collaterals (Fig. 63–9).

Diagnosis. A cyanotic infant showing decreased pulmonary blood flow on the radiograph, right ventricular hypertrophy on the electrocardiogram, and no murmur or a continuous murmur usually has TOF with pulmonary atresia (see Differential Diagnosis). Newborns with transposition and an intact ventricular septum have no murmurs and may be just as cyanotic but have normal or increased pulmonary blood flow visible on chest radiographs. Infants with total anomalous pulmonary venous return usually show a pulmonary venous congestion pattern on the chest radiographs. More complicated lesions simulating TOF with pulmonary atresia (e.g., D or L transposition with a ventricular septal defect and pulmonary atresia or single ventricle with pulmonary atresia) must be distinguished by two-dimensional echocardiogram or angiography.

Those infants with large collaterals and congestive heart failure can usually be distinguished from infants with a ventricular septal defect, patent ductus arteriosus, or aortopulmonary window on the basis of their arterial hypoxemia as well as from those with truncus arteriosus and transposition with a ventricular septal defect on the basis of the continuous murmurs.

Treatment. If the collateral vessels are adequate to ensure a systemic saturation of greater than 75 per cent, a conservative approach is warranted in the neonatal period. If the infant becomes progressively cyanotic or acidotic, prostaglandin E_1 usually improves arterial hypoxemia by maintaining patency of the ductus arteriosus (Freed et al., 1981; Olley et al., 1976). Palliative surgery to ensure patency of the ductus arteriosus by a Blalock-Taussig shunt is necessary if oxygenation is inadequate without prostaglandin E_1. Corrective surgery has not yet

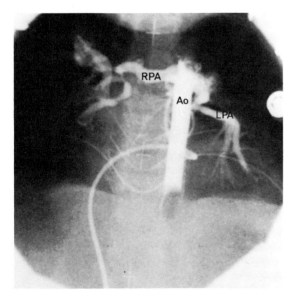

FIGURE 63–9. *Aortogram with cranial angulation in a newborn with tetralogy of Fallot with pulmonary atresia. Both right pulmonary artery (RPA) and left pulmonary artery (LPA) fill from collateral vessels arising from the aorta (Ao).*

gained favor among those treating newborns because of the need for a conduit, usually an aortic homograft from the right ventricle to the pulmonary artery and the certainty of having to replace the conduit as the infant grows. A conduit should be considered in infants with discontinuous or hypoplastic pulmonary arteries (leaving the ventricular defect open) with later balloon dilation of the hypoplastic vessels in an attempt to make the pulmonary arteries grow so a later reparative operation is possible.

Prognosis. The prognosis of these infants primarily depends on the size of the pulmonary arteries. If these structures are small, palliative and corrective surgery remain problematic. If they are near normal in size, the prognosis is improved. Of 46 infants seen in the NERICP between 1969 and 1974, the 1-year mortality rate was 44 per cent (Fyler et al., 1980). Among 139 patients with adequate-sized pulmonary arteries that were repaired when they were children, the survival rates at 1 month and at 1, 5, 10, and 20 years were 85 per cent, 82 per cent, 76 per cent, 69 per cent, and 58 per cent, respectively (Kirklin et al., 1988).

PULMONARY ATRESIA WITH AN INTACT VENTRICULAR SEPTUM

Anatomy. In pulmonary atresia (PA) with an intact ventricular septum (IVS), the pulmonary valve is an imperforate membrane. In more than 80 per cent of the newborn patients, the right ventricle is moderately or severely hypoplastic, often having a volume of only 1 or 2 ml at birth (Van Praagh et al., 1976). The tricuspid valve annulus is also hypoplastic, corresponding to the size of the right ventricle, and the valve may be stenotic owing to fusion of the chordae. The right atrium is invariably enlarged and hypertrophied and may be enormous in infants with severe tricuspid regurgitation. The high pressure within the right ventricular cavity causes dilation of the normal myocardial sinusoids, and connections are often present between the sinusoids and coronary arteries, with flow going from right ventricle to ascending aorta. Obstructions in the coronary arteries are not uncommon in this group with sinusoids, and myocardial perfusion may be via the right ventricle, the aorta, or both (Calder et al., 1987). In contrast to patients with TOF associated with pulmonary atresia, the infants with PA and an IVS almost invariably have normal pulmonary arteries.

Incidence. In the NERICP (Fyler et al., 1980), there were 75 infants with PA and an IVS (1 per 14,000 live births), 85 per cent of whom were seen by a cardiologist within the 1st week of life. They represent 7 per cent of infants presenting with heart disease in the 1st week.

Hemodynamics. Prenatally, egress of blood from the right ventricle is prevented by the pulmonary atresia (Fig. 63–10). All the venous blood returning to the right atrium must pass through the foramen ovale to the left atrium, left ventricle, and ascending aorta; these chambers are dilated compared with those in the normal fetus. Conversely, since flow to the right ventricle is minimal, this chamber is usually hypoplastic. The pulmonary blood flow in utero is derived entirely from the aorta via a small,

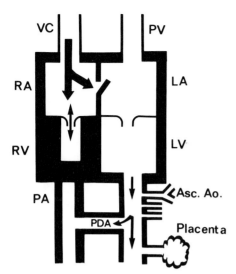

FIGURE 63–10. Schematic diagram of the circulation in the fetus with pulmonary atresia and an intact ventricular septum. All the systemic venous return from the vena cava passes across the foramen ovale into the left atrium. Pulmonary blood flow before and after birth is derived from the aorta via the ductus arteriosus. Since right ventricular flow is minimal, the chamber remains quite small. The abbreviations in this diagram are the same as those used in Figure 63–2.

usually tortuous, ductus arteriosus. This physiologic arrangement does not disrupt the normal growth and development during fetal life. After birth, there is a continuation of the fetal pattern; the pulmonary blood flow continues to be totally dependent on the small ductus arteriosus. As this closes in the first hours or days of life, the minimal pulmonary blood flow diminishes further, and severe hypoxemia and acidosis follow.

Clinical Manifestations. Infants with PA are mildly cyanotic soon after birth but are often intensely cyanotic by 24 hours of age as the ductus arteriosus constricts. On physical examination, the second heart sound is single. A continuous murmur, from left-to-right shunting through the ductus arteriosus, or a systolic regurgitant murmur along the left sternal border, secondary to tricuspid regurgitation, may be heard; however, in about 20 per cent of infants, no murmur is audible. The liver is enlarged if tricuspid regurgitation is severe and the foramen ovale is restrictive.

On chest radiographs, the cardiothoracic ratio is increased because of dilation of the right atrium and left ventricle, and the pulmonary vascular markings are invariably reduced. The aortic arch is to the left of the trachea in almost all infants.

The electrocardiogram is characteristic and extremely helpful in the differential diagnosis (Fig. 63–11). Because of the right ventricular hypoplasia and low volume of blood in the right ventricle and large left ventricle in utero, there is a left ventricular predominance in the precordial leads, with a QRS axis of +30 to +120 degrees. Right atrial hypertrophy is also often seen.

A two-dimensional echocardiogram can be used to identify the small right ventricle, usually by apical four-chamber view, and a color flow Doppler study can be used to differentiate pulmonary stenosis from atresia by turbulence and direction of flow in the main pulmonary artery.

Cardiac catheterization confirms the right-to-left shunt at the atrial level with a normal pulmonary venous saturation but marked desaturation in the left atrium, left ventricle, and aorta. The right ventricular systolic pressure

FIGURE 63–11. Electrocardiogram from a 3-day-old newborn with pulmonary atresia and an intact ventricular septum. Note the leftward QRS axis (+75 degrees) and the left ventricular predominance for age. The P waves are tall and peaked in II, suggesting right atrial hypertrophy.

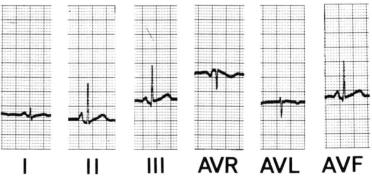

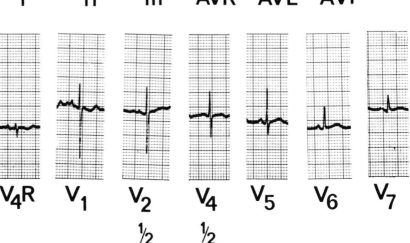

usually exceeds the left ventricular pressure. Right ventricular angiography is useful in demonstrating the size of the right ventricle, the magnitude of the tricuspid regurgitation, and any right ventricular sinusoidal–coronary artery fistulas (Fig. 63–12). An angiogram in the left ventricle or aorta allows one to visualize the ductus arteriosus and the pulmonary arteries. An aortic root injection is necessary to observe the distribution of the coronary arteries in those patients with right ventricular sinusoidal–coronary fistulas.

Diagnosis. A very cyanotic newborn with PA and an IVS can usually be distinguished from an infant with transposition of the great arteries with an IVS, since the latter child has a split second heart sound, increased pulmonary flow on the radiograph, right ventricular hypertrophy on the electrocardiogram, and a characteristic echocardiogram. Infants with tricuspid atresia and a hypoplastic right ventricle show decreased pulmonary flow on the radiograph and left ventricular predominance on electrocardiogram, but they almost invariably have a QRS axis of −30 to −90 degrees on the electrocardiogram, whereas infants with PA have a QRS axis of +30 to +120 degrees. Infants with pulmonary stenosis and a hypoplastic right ventricle may be difficult to distinguish from those with pulmonary atresia before angiography but usually have a pulmonary ejection murmur rather than a regurgitant murmur and a valve that can be seen on two-dimensional echocardiography.

Treatment. The initial treatment must be directed at correcting the metabolic acidosis with oxygen and bicarbonate. The use of prostaglandin E_1 to dilate the ductus arteriosus, increase pulmonary blood flow, and improve oxygenation has been well demonstrated (Freed et al., 1981; Olley et al., 1976) and is useful in allowing time for stabilization of the infants prior to initiation of surgery.

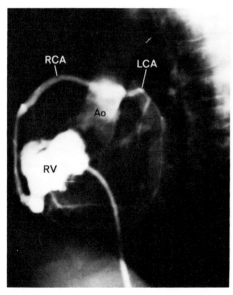

FIGURE 63–12. Right ventricular angiogram in the lateral position in a newborn with pulmonary atresia and an intact ventricular septum. The right ventricular cavity is small. The right and left coronary arteries and the aorta fill from a right ventricular sinusoid. No ventricular septal defect is present. Ao, aorta; LCA, left coronary artery; RCA, right coronary artery; RV, right ventricle.

In the few infants with mild right ventricular hypoplasia and a nonobstructive tricuspid valve, pulmonary valvotomy has been effective. Some hypoxemia almost invariably persists even after a successful valvotomy, but this usually decreases as the pulmonary vascular resistance drops over the 1st or 2nd week of life. If extreme hypoxemia persists (arterial saturation less than 60 per cent) after 2 weeks of age, a systemic-to-pulmonary artery shunt may be necessary.

In the presence of severe hypoplasia of the right ventricle and tricuspid valve, it is recognized that pulmonary valvotomy alone is insufficient. The proper initial palliation of these infants is still to be determined, with some favoring a Blalock-Taussig shunt alone, shunt plus atrial septectomy, shunt plus pulmonary valvotomy, or more recently, shunt plus righty ventricular outflow tract reconstruction and pericardial patching. The hope is that by increasing flow through the right ventricle, the cavity size will increase, allowing a two-ventricle repair. In those patients with right ventricle to coronary sinusoids, care must be taken to visualize the coronary arteries prior to decompressing the right ventricular hypertension, since with proximal narrowing in the coronaries, myocardial perfusion may be dependent on right ventricular hypertension. A corrective operation for those with a large right ventricular outflow track involves closure of the atrial defect and closure of the shunt. For those with a small tricuspid valve or right ventricle, a modified Fontan operation (Fontan and Baudet, 1971), connecting the right ventricle to the pulmonary artery, is probably the procedure of choice (Alboliras et al., 1987).

Prognosis. Unfortunately, the prognosis for patients with this lesion remains poor, with 77 per cent dying by their first birthday in the NERICP (Fyler et al., 1980). In the group of infants with a good-sized right ventricle, the mortality was 50 per cent. Lightfoot and associates (1989) have reported a median survival time of 1.43 years among 98 patients seen at the Hospital for Sick Children in Toronto.

PULMONARY STENOSIS WITH AN INTACT VENTRICULAR SEPTUM

Anatomy. In this lesion, the pulmonary valve has a narrowed orifice that is usually due to fusion of the three pulmonary commissures. The size of the right ventricular cavity can be normal but is usually somewhat hypoplastic in those infants who present with cyanosis in the 1st month of life (Freed et al., 1973). The size of the chamber is rarely, if ever, as small as that seen in infants with PA and an IVS, and abnormalities of the tricuspid valve and right ventricular sinusoidal–coronary artery fistulas are less common. The main and peripheral pulmonary arteries are usually normal.

Incidence. In the NERICP and the Boston-Washington Infant Study, the incidence was about 1 per 14,000 live births; 40 per cent presented in the 1st week of life (Fyler et al., 1980).

Hemodynamics. In utero, the obstruction at the pulmonary valve results in hypertrophy as well as a loss of compliance of the right ventricle. This leads to diversion of an increased proportion of venous return through the foramen ovale to the left side of the heart and ascending aorta. If the stenosis appears early in gestation and is severe, significant hypoplasia of the right ventricle with corresponding enlargement of the left ventricle occurs, resembling that seen in pulmonary atresia and an intact ventricular septum. If the stenosis is milder and occurs later in gestation, the right ventricle can be normal or near normal in size (Rudolph, 1974).

After birth, the degree of right-to-left shunting at the atrial level and thus arterial hypoxemia depends on the degree of pulmonary stenosis and right ventricular hypoplasia. If the stenosis is severe, right-to-left shunting at the atrial level may be massive and adequate pulmonary blood flow dependent on left-to-right shunting through the ductus arteriosus. If the stenosis is milder, with most of the pulmonary blood flow through the pulmonary valve, there may be little effect from ductal closure. As the pulmonary arteriolar resistance (in series with the pulmonary valve resistance) decreases over the first few weeks of life, the right-to-left shunt at the atrial level and, thus, the systemic hypoxemia may decrease.

Clinical Features. In mild pulmonary stenosis, a loud systolic ejection murmur at the left upper sternal border may be the only finding. In moderate or severe stenosis, the murmur is less prominent but cyanosis is present, increasing as the ductus arteriosus constricts. There is a prominent "a" wave in the jugular venous pulse reflecting reduced right ventricular compliance, and the liver is often enlarged and may even be pulsatile. The pulmonary component of the second heart sound is delayed and diminished and may be inaudible.

On chest radiographs, there is mild cardiomegaly due to an enlarged right atrium and diminished pulmonary blood flow. Poststenotic dilatation in the main pulmonary artery in the newborn is unusual.

The electrocardiogram is normal if the pulmonary stenosis is mild or moderate. With severe pulmonary stenosis and a diminutive right ventricle, the electrocardiogram usually demonstrates right atrial enlargement and left ventricular predominance with a QRS axis of +30 to +120 degrees, similar to that seen in pulmonary atresia with an intact ventricular septum (Fig. 63–10).

Two-dimensional echocardiography can be used to evaluate the tricuspid valve, right ventricle, and pulmonary arteries. Doppler study can be used to evaluate the gradient and, usually, to estimate right ventricular pressure from the velocity of the tricuspid regurgitation jet.

At cardiac catheterization, the right ventricular systolic pressure is elevated and usually exceeds left ventricular pressure. If the stenosis is severe, right-to-left shunting at the atrial level is common, with the degree of arterial hypoxemia a function of the degree of obstruction and hypoplasia of the right ventricle. On angiograms, the pulmonary valve is domed, thickened, and immobile, and the right ventricle is hypertrophied, with muscle bundles crossing and compromising the cavity size.

Diagnosis. With severe obstruction and right ventricular hypoplasia, pulmonary stenosis can be confused with PA with an IVS. Usually, an ejection rather than regurgitant murmur at the left upper sternal border allows one to differentiate these conditions, but, occasionally, echocardiography, angiography, or even surgical inspection is necessary to make the diagnosis with certainty. Newborns with tricuspid atresia usually have a superior axis (– 90 to – 30 degrees) on the electrocardiogram, and those with transposition rarely have a loud murmur and have normal or increased flow on the chest radiograph. If the right ventricle is not diminutive, the electrocardiogram has right ventricular predominance, and it may be difficult to differentiate pulmonary stenosis with an IVS from pulmonary stenosis with a ventricular septal defect (TOF). Echocardiography usually detects the latter because of the overriding aorta and absence of echoes in the area of the ventricular septum.

The murmur of mild valvular pulmonary stenosis can be confused with the murmur of a ventricular septal defect, atrial septal defect, or peripheral pulmonary stenosis.

Treatment. The treatment of the cyanotic newborn with critical pulmonary stenosis is surgical or balloon dilation. For the severely hypoxemic neonate, oxygen and prostaglandin E_1 are the initial therapy, with bicarbonate added if a metabolic acidosis is present.

Relief of the obstruction can be surgical valvotomy, usually under inflow occlusion rather than cardiopulmonary bypass (Freed et al., 1973) or, more recently at some centers, by balloon dilation (Zeevi et al., 1988 a–c). Afterward, some cyanosis is usually present for a few days or weeks but gradually diminishes, presumably as the right ventricular compliance improves and the pulmonary vascular resistance drops. An occasional infant with severe hypoplasia of the right ventricle remains cyanotic after adequate valvotomy and requires long-term prostaglandin E_1 or a systemic-to-pulmonary artery shunt.

Infants with pulmonary stenosis but no cyanosis are usually managed conservatively in the neonatal period, and if the stenosis appears severe, the insertion of a catheter is suggested at 6 to 12 months of age, with balloon dilation recommended if the right ventricular systolic pressure approaches systemic levels.

Prognosis. These infants usually do very well. In our experience, the survival rate is more than 90 per cent (Freed et al., 1973). In the NERICP, 1-year survival was 79 per cent (Fyler et al., 1980). Occasionally, a repeat valvotomy is necessary later in childhood owing to a lack of growth of the pulmonary valve or incomplete relief at the initial operation.

TRICUSPID ATRESIA

Anatomy. In tricuspid atresia, there is a failure of development of the right atrioventricular valve; therefore, an intra-atrial communication, usually a patent foramen ovale, is necessary for survival. There is usually a ventricular septal defect connecting a large left ventricular cavity with a hypoplastic chamber that represents the infundibulum or outflow portion of the right ventricle. The great arteries may be either normally related (Type I) or transposed (Type II), and there may be pulmonary atresia (a), pulmonary stenosis (b), or no pulmonary stenosis (c) (Edwards and Burchell, 1949; Keith et al., 1958). About

70 per cent of infants with tricuspid atresia have Type I, with three fourths of these having pulmonary stenosis (b). In contrast, of the 30 per cent who have Type II (transposition), more than three-fourths have no pulmonary stenosis (c) (Dick et al., 1975). The presentation of newborns with tricuspid atresia depends on the anatomy. Those with severe pulmonary stenosis or atresia present with cyanosis in the first few days of life. Infants with a large ventricular septal defect and no pulmonary stenosis present with congestive heart failure, usually late in the 1st or during the 2nd month as the pulmonary vascular resistance falls.

Incidence. In the NERICP there were 61 infants with tricuspid atresia, an incidence of 1 per 18,000 live births (Fyler et al., 1980). Slightly less (1 per 30,000 live births) were seen in the Baltimore-Washington study (Ferencz et al., 1985). They represented less than 5 per cent of infants presenting in the 1st month of life with serious congenital heart disease. Of all patients with tricuspid atresia, 57 per cent were hospitalized in the 1st week of life and 78 per cent were hospitalized by 1 month of age.

Hemodynamics. The presence of tricuspid atresia in utero must be compatible with a relatively normal intrauterine circulation, because growth and development proceed normally. Since the tricuspid valve is atretic, all systemic venous return is diverted across the foramen ovale into left atrium and left ventricle (Fig. 63–13). If the great arteries are normally related and the ventricular septum is intact or if the pulmonary valve is atretic, all the left ventricular output passes through the aorta, and pulmonary blood flow is via the ductus arteriosus. If the ventricular septal defect is large, some of the left ventricular output passes through the ventricular septal defect into the hypoplastic right ventricle, exiting the pulmonary artery if the vessels are normally related and exiting the aorta if

transposition is present. Either way, there is antegrade flow through the pulmonary artery and ductus arteriosus.

After birth, there is little change in the circulation, but the normal postnatal alterations impose significant handicaps. The newborns with pulmonary atresia or severe pulmonary stenosis continue to depend on the ductus arteriosus for pulmonary blood flow. When the ductus begins to close, severe hypoxemia, acidosis, and eventually, death follow.

In those infants with a large ventricular septal defect and no pulmonary stenosis, the pulmonary blood flow increases as the pulmonary arteriolar resistance drops and congestive heart failure ensues, usually within the 1st month of life. Infants with transposition in whom the aorta arises from the hypoplastic right ventricle may develop obstruction physiologically comparable to subaortic stenosis in the infant with normally related great arteries if the ventricular defect is small.

Clinical Features. Infants with pulmonary stenosis or atresia (a,b) are usually cyanotic soon after birth, with the cyanosis increasing as the ductus arteriosus closes. Those with pulmonary stenosis usually have a loud systolic ejection murmur along the left sternal border; those with pulmonary atresia may have no murmur at all or a continuous murmur from the ductus arteriosus. Infants with type c (no pulmonary stenosis) may have minimal cyanosis with an ejection murmur and heart failure as the major manifestations of heart disease. The heart size and the pulmonary blood flow visible on the radiographs are determined by the degree of pulmonary stenosis. Infants with pulmonary atresia or stenosis have a small heart with decreased pulmonary blood flow; those without pulmonary stenosis have a large heart with increased pulmonary flow. A right aortic arch is occasionally present.

The electrocardiogram is usually very helpful (Fig. 63–14). Because of the right ventricular hypoplasia and increased left ventricular flow in utero, left ventricular predominance with diminished right ventricular forces is almost universal. The QRS axis is almost always superior (0 to −90 degrees) in Type I (Dick et al., 1975), probably in large part owing to early origin of the left bundle of the conducting system and the resultant abnormal depolarization sequence. Right atrial hypertrophy is frequently present.

Apical and subxiphoid four-chamber views on two-dimensional echocardiography demonstrate the imperforate tricuspid membrane, the size of the right ventricle, the ventricular septal defect, and the relationship between the great arteries (Fig. 63–15).

The diagnosis can be confirmed at cardiac catheterization by the demonstration of a right-to-left shunt at the atrial level with desaturation in the left atrium and a normal saturation in the pulmonary veins and an elevated right atrial pressure (especially the "a" wave) slightly higher than left atrial pressure. Also helpful in confirming the diagnosis is the injection of contrast medium into the right atrium. Dye spills across the atrial septum and fills the left atrium and left ventricle, revealing a characteristically unopacified defect along the left border of the right atrium, where the tricuspid valve and right ventricle are usually seen. Angiocardiography in the left ventricle using 40 degrees of left anterior obliquity and 40 degrees of

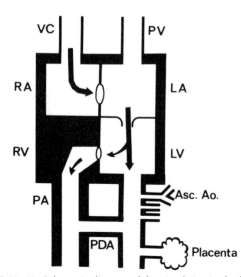

FIGURE 63–13. *Schematic diagram of the circulation in the fetus with tricuspid atresia. All the venous return from the vena cava passes across the atrial septum into the left atrium and ventricle. Pulmonary blood flow before (and after) birth is via a ventricular septal defect or through the ductus arteriosus. Blood flow to the placenta for oxygenation is unimpeded. The abbreviations in this diagram are the same as those used in Figure 63–2.*

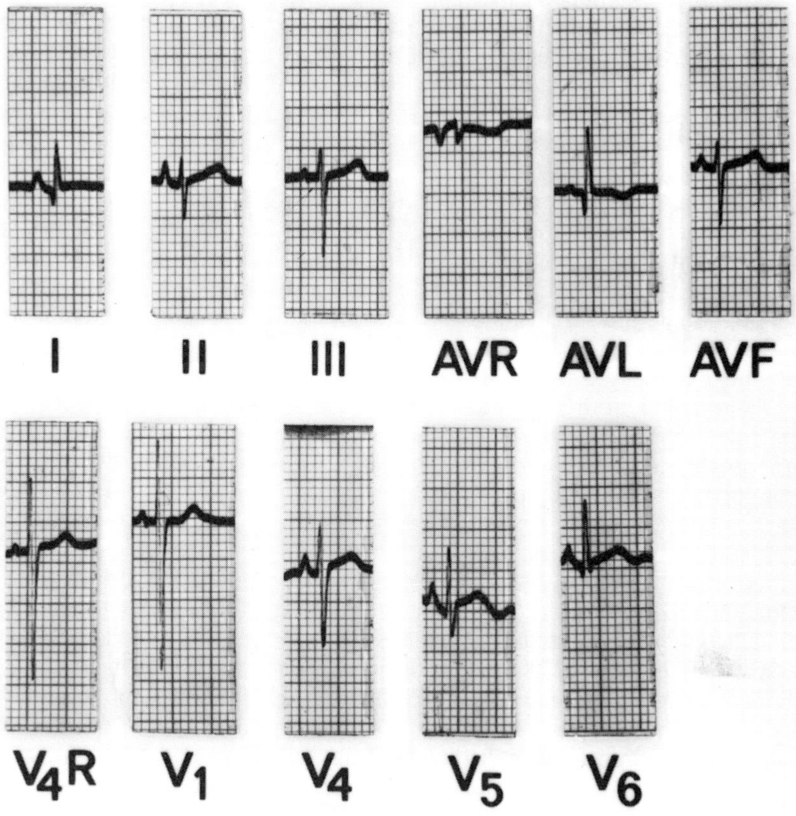

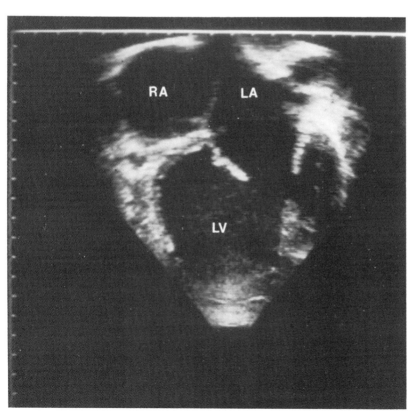

FIGURE 63–14. An electrocardiogram from a 5-day-old newborn with tricuspid atresia. The QRS axis is superior (−50 degrees). The P waves are peaked in leads II and V_4 to V_6 suggesting right atrial hypertrophy. There is left ventricular predominance for age with a predominant S wave in V_4R and V_1 and a qRS in V_6.

I   II   III   AVR   AVL   AVF

V_4R V_1 V_4 V_5 V_6

FIGURE 63–15. Apical four-chamber view of a patient with tricuspid atresia. A single atrioventricular valve, the mitral valve, is present. LA, left atrium; RA, right atrium; LV, left ventricle. (Reprinted from Williams, R. G., Bierman, F. Z., and Sanders, S. P.: Echocardiographic Diagnosis of Cardiac Malformations. Boston, Little Brown & Company, 1986.)

cranial angulation (hepatoclavicular, or four-chambered, view) outlines the ventricular defect(s) and demonstrates the size of the right ventricle as well as the degree and location of pulmonary stenosis (Fig. 63–16). Although others have advocated balloon septostomy to enlarge the atrial defect, we have rarely found this necessary.

Diagnosis. In the cyanotic infant, tricuspid atresia can be differentiated from transposition, TOF, and Ebstein disease of the tricuspid valve by the demonstration of left ventricular predominance on the electrocardiogram and from pulmonary atresia or stenosis with a diminutive right ventricle on the basis of the superior QRS axis.

In the minimally cyanotic infant, tricuspid atresia can be differentiated from the atrioventricular canal type of ventricular septal defect by electrocardiography or echocardiography and from the more complicated types of acyanotic heart disease by the presence of arterial hypoxemia, which is especially evident while the infant is crying.

Treatment. In the severely hypoxic infant, the primary treatment is oxygen, bicarbonate, and prostaglandin E_1 to maintain patency of the ductus arteriosus (Freed et al., 1981; Olley et al., 1976) followed by a systemic-to-pulmonary artery shunt, usually, a modified Blalock-Taussig shunt connecting the subclavian to pulmonary artery using a 4- or 5-mm tube graft (Ilbawi et al., 1984) or a central (ascending aorta to main pulmonary artery) or Waterston (ascending aorta to right pulmonary artery) anastomosis.

Children with a large ventricular septal defect and little pulmonary stenosis require pulmonary artery banding to restrict pulmonary blood flow so that congestive heart failure can be controlled and pulmonary vascular disease can be prevented.

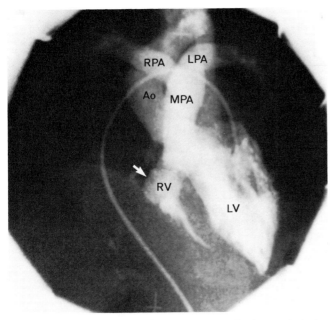

FIGURE 63–16. Left ventricular angiogram in the hepatoclavicular "four-chamber" position in a newborn with tricuspid atresia. The hypoplastic right ventricle fills through a ventricular septal defect. The arrow points to the atretic tricuspid valve. Ao, aorta; LPA, left pulmonary artery; LV, left ventricle; MPA, main pulmonary artery; RPA, right pulmonary artery; RV, right ventricle.

Prior to 1971, there was no "corrective" surgery for tricuspid atresia. Over the past decade, many have followed the suggestions of Fontan and Baudet, who recommended connecting the right atrium with either the right ventricular outflow tract or the pulmonary artery, depending on systemic venous pressure and right atrial contraction to force blood through the lungs. In selected children older than 3 years with low pulmonary artery, left ventricular end-diastolic pressure and normal pulmonary arterial anatomy, this approach has shown great promise and can be performed with a short-term survival of greater than 90 per cent (Mair et al., 1985). It seems unlikely that this approach is feasible in the newborn, because it seems to require very low pulmonary vascular resistance, normally not present until 3 to 6 months of age.

Prognosis. When Dick and co-workers reviewed the experience of children with tricuspid atresia at Children's Hospital in Boston between 1941 and 1973, the 1-year survival rate was 50 per cent, and the 20-year survival rate was 30 percent. In data from the NERICP that were collected between 1969 and 1974 (Fyler et al., 1980), the 1-year survival rate of those requiring surgery was 63 per cent. With improvement of surgical techniques on small infants and the application of the Fontan principle to older children, we expect that these rather dismal results will be improved.

EBSTEIN ANOMALY OF THE TRICUSPID VALVE

Anatomy. In 1866, Ebstein described the heart of a 19-year-old male patient with cyanosis and palpitations who died of heart failure with an anomaly of the tricuspid valve. The lesion, now known as Ebstein anomaly of the tricuspid valve, is due to redundancy and dysplasia of the tricuspid valve with adherence of a variable portion of the septal and, often, posterior leaflets to the right ventricular wall so that the free portion of the leaflets is displaced downward, away from the normal atrioventricular ring. Thus, the atrium and ventricle are divided in three segments: a normal right atrium, a portion of the atrium above the displaced valve that is partly ventricular myocardium, and the true right ventricle. The tricuspid valve is usually regurgitant and, at least in the newborn, stenotic. The right atrium is often very large, in part owing to the muscularized segment but primarily because of the tricuspid stenosis and regurgitation; the right ventricle is correspondingly small. An atrial septal defect (or patent foramen ovale) is almost always present in the newborn, and pulmonary stenosis and atresia are not uncommon. Other associated lesions such as ventricular septal defects, coarctation, and transposition are rarely seen.

Incidence. Ebstein anomaly is rare in the newborn. There were only 18 infants in the NERICP over 5 years, an incidence of 1 per 80,000 live births (Fyler et al., 1980), representing about 0.5 per cent of all children with congenital heart disease.

Hemodynamics. In utero, the incompetent or stenotic tricuspid valve diverts systemic venous return through the foramen ovale into the left side of the heart, resulting in increased left atrial and ventricular flow. The tricuspid regurgitation into the right atrium leads to severe right atrial dilatation and hypertrophy before birth and may cause in utero heart failure with edema or anasarca.

After birth, the degree of hypoxemia is a function of the right-to-left shunting at the atrial level. This depends on the degree of difficulty with which blood passes through the right ventricle and pulmonary artery into the lungs. With high pulmonary vascular resistance of the newborn increasing right ventricular afterload, the tricuspid regurgitation may be exacerbated and the right-to-left shunting at the atrial level massive. These severely hypoxic infants may depend on the ductus arteriosus for most of their pulmonary blood flow, and when the ductus closes, the hypoxemia may be very severe and acidosis may develop. If the foramen ovale is restrictive, preventing decompensation of the right atrium, right-sided heart failure with hepatomegaly may be prominent.

If the tricuspid stenosis and regurgitation are less severe, right-to-left shunting and, therefore, cyanosis may be less prominent. In either case, as the pulmonary vascular resistance drops over the first few days and weeks of life, reducing right ventricular afterload and tricuspid regurgitation, dramatic improvements in arterial saturation and congestive heart failure may be seen.

Clinical Manifestations. The infants with Ebstein anomaly who present during the neonatal period are almost invariably cyanotic (Kumar et al., 1971; Radford et al., 1985). Right-sided congestive heart failure with hepatomegaly due to severe tricuspid regurgitation is frequently present. On auscultation, there may be a quadruple rhythm composed of a loud first sound, single second sound, and loud third and fourth sounds. A pansystolic murmur of tricuspid regurgitation is often audible.

On chest radiographs, the cardiac silhouette is usually enlarged because of massive dilatation of the right atrium (Fig. 63–17). The largest hearts in infants with congenital

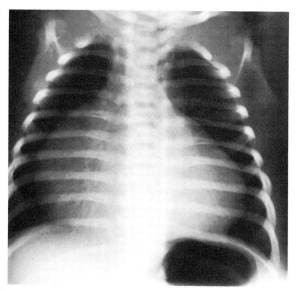

FIGURE 63–17. Chest radiograph in anteroposterior projection in a newborn with Ebstein's disease. The right atrium is markedly enlarged, and the pulmonary blood flow is reduced.

disease are seen in this condition. Often it is difficult for one to see enough lung field to note the diminished pulmonary flow.

The P waves on the electrocardiogram are often tall and peaked, suggesting right atrial hypertrophy. Right ventricular conduction abnormalities prolonging the QRS duration are common, although they are not seen as frequently in the newborn as in the older child. Wolff-Parkinson-White syndrome with a short P-R interval and a delta wave may be seen in as many as 20 per cent of children (Kumar et al., 1971), and atrial tachycardias and flutter are not uncommon.

The two-dimensional study is usually diagnostic, with the right atrial dilatation and displaced anterior leaflet visible from the apical four-chamber view (Fig. 63–18). At cardiac catheterization, demonstration of normal pulmonary venous oxygen saturation but desaturation in the left atrium, left ventricle, and aorta confirms the presence of right-to-left shunting at the atrial level. It may be difficult to pass the catheter into the right ventricle because of its small size (especially compared with that of the right atrium) and the tricuspid regurgitation. The right ventricular pressure is usually normal but may be elevated if there is associated pulmonary stenosis or atresia.

Angiography in the right ventricle in the anteroposterior projection shows a double notch, one at the site of the normal tricuspid annulus and another where the displaced anterior leaflet inserts. Atrial arrhythmias are quite common during catheterization, but the dangers of catheterization have probably been exaggerated, and catheterization in infants with this condition is probably no more hazardous than in other cyanotic newborns (Kumar et al., 1971).

Diagnosis. On chest radiographs, the hearts of children with Ebstein disease are larger than those of children with any other form of congenital heart disease. In the minimally distressed infant with cyanosis, a murmur along the left sternal border, right ventricular hypertrophy on the electrocardiogram, and massive cardiomegaly, the diagnosis is almost certain (see Differential Diagnosis).

Patients with pulmonary atresia with an intact ventricular septum or tricuspid atresia may have cyanosis and cardiac enlargement, but they usually have left rather than right ventricular hypertrophy on the electrocardiogram, and the tricuspid valve is hypoplastic or atretic on echocardiogram rather than large and redundant as in Ebstein disease. Infants with transposition of the great arteries or TOF may be just as cyanotic, but the former have increased pulmonary vascularity, and the latter rarely show cardiac enlargement on chest radiographs.

Treatment. Treatment of this condition in the newborn is based on two premises: (1) many infants improve markedly over the first weeks of life, presumably as the pulmonary vascular resistance drops, and (2) surgical approaches to treating the critically ill newborn have thus far been almost uniformly unsuccessful. Anticongestives including digoxin and diuretics may prove useful. Prostaglandin E_1 has been helpful in improving oxygenation in the severely cyanotic infant, presumably by maintaining patency of the ductus arteriosus while the pulmonary vascular resistance falls (Freed et al., 1981).

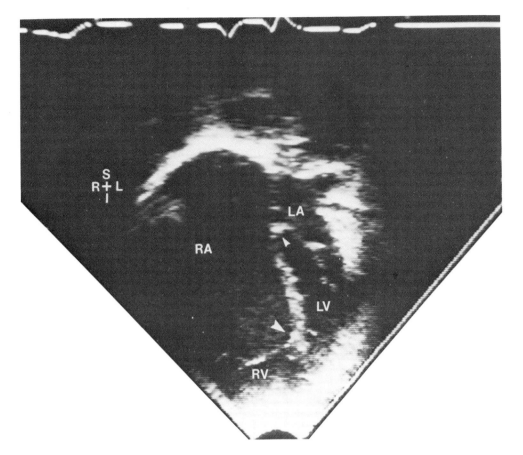

FIGURE 63–18. *Apical four-chamber view of Ebstein anomaly shows marked displacement of septal tricuspid attachment to the interventricular septum (large arrow) relative to the attachment of the mitral leaflet (small arrow). The right atrium (RA) is very large and includes the atrialized portion of the right ventricle (RV). LA, left atrium; LV, left ventricle. (Reprinted from Williams, R. G., Bierman, F. Z., and Sanders, S. P.: Echocardiographic Diagnosis of Cardiac Malformations. Boston, Little Brown and Company, 1986.)*

Tricuspid annuloplasty, or valve replacement, is occasionally successful in the older child but has not been successful in the newborn, and palliative shunts have only occasionally been successful for reasons that remain unclear. Older children have been successfully palliated by either a Glenn (superior vena cava-to-right pulmonary artery) or a Fontan (right atrium-to-main pulmonary artery) procedure, but these operations seem contraindicated in these patients because of the high pulmonary vascular resistance in newborns. A corrective operation has been successful in older children and adults but has not been reported in infants (Mair et al., 1985).

Prognosis. The prognosis is worse for patients presenting in the newborn period. In an international collaborative study (Watson, 1974), 29 of 35 infants died—15 from heart failure, eight from surgery, five from catheterization, and one suddenly, presumably from an arrhythmia. More recently, there were 12 deaths of 23 patients at the Hospital for Sick Children in Toronto (Rowe et al., 1981), and in the NERICP there were three deaths among 13 patients catheterized or operated on in the 1st year of life (Fyler et al., 1980).

TRUNCUS ARTERIOSUS

Anatomy. Truncus arteriosus has been defined as the cardiac defect in which a single great artery arises from the base of the heart supplying the coronary, pulmonary, and systemic arteries (Lev and Saphir, 1942). It was previously classified according to the site of origin of the pulmonary arteries and aortopulmonary septum (Van Praagh and Van Praagh, 1965), but this practice has largely been abandoned because it is often difficult to differentiate a single pulmonary trunk from separate but closely related left and right pulmonary arteries, even when pathologic specimens are available.

Embryologically, this defect is thought to result from failure of septation of the truncus arteriosus (Edwards, 1976), although Van Praagh and Van Praagh believe that it is closely related to TOF with atresia rather than hypoplasia of the subpulmonary infundibulum, partial or complete absence of the pulmonary valve, and an aortopulmonary septal defect. This theory is attractive, since both lesions are almost invariably associated with a ventricular septal defect and overriding of the aorta and because a right aortic arch is frequently present in both.

The truncal valve usually resembles a normal aortic valve. In the series of 79 necropsy cases reported in 1976 by Calder and co-workers, the truncal valve was tricuspid in 61 per cent, quadricuspid in 31 per cent, and bicuspid in 8 per cent. Truncal valve thickening was seen in two-thirds of the patients, with truncal stenosis in 11 per cent and truncal regurgitation in 15 per cent. Approximately one-third of patients with truncus arteriosus have DiGeorge syndrome (Van Mierop and Kutche, 1986).

Incidence. Thirty-three cases of truncus arteriosus were seen in the NERICP, representing an incidence of one per 33,000 live births (Fyler et al., 1980); they represent about 2 per cent of infants with congenital heart disease seen in the 1st year of life.

Hemodynamics. In utero, the main consequence of truncus arteriosus is complete mixing of the systemic and pulmonary venous return above the truncal valve. The truncus is usually large, and the ductus arteriosus arising from the pulmonary arteries may be smaller than normal. Since blood flow through the heart is normal, the atrium and ventricles develop normally.

After birth, the flow to the pulmonary arteries and systemic arteries is a function of the relative resistances in the two circuits. Initially, the pulmonary resistance is high, and pulmonary flow equals or slightly exceeds systemic flow. Over the first hours or days of life, however, the pulmonary arteriolar resistance decreases and pulmonary blood flow increases. As the pulmonary venous return increases, the left ventricle must eject an increasing volume load, which eventually leads to congestive failure. Since there is common mixing of systemic and pulmonary venous blood above the truncal valve, the degree of hypoxemia decreases as the pulmonary flow increases so that these infants are only mildly cyanotic until left heart failure and pulmonary edema interfere with oxygen exchange and pulmonary venous desaturation ensues.

In some infants, the pulmonary arteries are hypoplastic or stenotic at their origin; in these patients, the pulmonary blood flow is restricted, and cyanosis rather than congestive failure may be the presenting symptom.

Clinical Manifestations. Children with truncus arteriosus usually present in the 1st month (and often in the 1st week) with predominantly left-sided heart failure. Tachypnea, poor feeding, increased perspiration, and intermittent cyanosis are usually prominent, and hepatomegaly is occasionally present. On physical examination, the cardiac impulse is hyperactive and the pulses are usually bounding secondary to the diastolic run-off from the aorta. On auscultation, the second heart sound is single, although the phonocardiogram can often detect multiple components, presumably from the abnormal truncal valve cusps. Commonly, a systolic ejection click is audible. Although a continuous murmur is often thought to be characteristic of truncus, it is actually unusual, since pulmonary hypertension is the rule. Systolic ejection murmurs of moderate intensity (grade 2 or 3/6) due to relative truncal stenosis are common, and a mid-diastolic flow rumble across the mitral valve is often present.

The heart is enlarged on the chest radiograph because of dilatation of the left atrium and ventricle. The pulmonary vascular markings are increased, and pulmonary venous congestion is frequently seen. A right aortic arch is present in about one-fourth of cases. The QRS axis is usually normal, with biventricular hypertrophy present in about 60 percent of infants, left ventricular hypertrophy in 20 per cent, and pure right ventricular hypertrophy in the remainder.

On the two-dimensional echocardiogram, using a coronal suprasternal or subxiphoid or a short-axis parasternal view, the truncal valve and pulmonary arteries arising from the side of the aorta can usually be visualized.

At cardiac catheterization, the pressures in the two ventricles are identical, and the pulse pressure in the aorta is increased, usually to more than 40 mm Hg. There is often a gradient between the aorta and pulmonary arteries, presumably from the torrential pulmonary flow with relative stenosis at the origin of the pulmonary arteries.

Angiocardiography in the left ventricle in the left anterior oblique projection with some axial angulation outlines the ventricular septal defect(s), and an angiocardiogram above the truncal valve with cranial angulation outlines the truncal valve and pulmonary arteries and rules out truncal regurgitations (Fig. 63–19).

Diagnosis. A newborn with mild cyanosis, congestive heart failure, and bounding pulses probably has truncus arteriosus (see Differential Diagnosis).

Infants with a ventricular septal defect, patent ductus arteriosus, aortopulmonary window, A-V fistula, or coarctation of the aorta are not cyanotic and infants with TOF and pulmonary atresia and large collaterals who may have cyanosis and heart failure have loud continuous murmurs. In infants with tricuspid atresia and a large ventricular septal defect, the electrocardiogram shows a superior axis and left ventricular hypertrophy, and infants with transposition and a large ventricular septal defect do not usually have bounding pulses.

Treatment. For the newborn with congestive heart failure, digoxin and diuretics should be tried but they rarely suffice. Pulmonary artery banding, either single in the rare case of one pulmonary trunk or, more commonly, bilaterally for those with separate origins of the right and left pulmonary artery was formerly the procedure of choice. Unfortunately, banding of these small pulmonary arteries has been associated with a high risk (50 per cent) in most series (Poirier et al., 1975) and frequently deforms the pulmonary arteries so that later correction is impossible.

Recently, several centers have tried surgical repair in infants by removing the origin of the pulmonary arteries with a cuff of aorta, closing the aorta with a patch, attaching the cuff of the aorta to a valve-bearing conduit that is then attached to the right ventricle, and, finally,

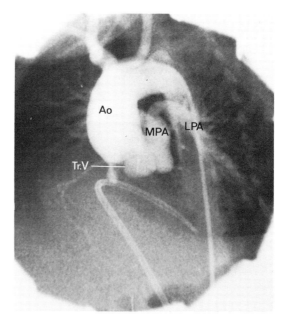

FIGURE 63–19. Hepatoclavicular view (40 degrees left anterior oblique, 40 degrees cranial angulation) in a newborn with truncus arteriosus. The aorta and main pulmonary artery arise above the truncal valve. Ao, aorta; LPA, left pulmonary artery; MPA, main pulmonary artery; TrV, truncal valve.

closing the ventricular septal defect with the left ventricle in continuity with the truncal valve. In his 1984 review, Ebert reported a series of 106 patients under 6 months of age who underwent this physiologic correction, and the mortality rate was only 11 per cent.

Prognosis. Untreated, infants with this anomaly have a dismal prognosis. In one series, the median age of death was 5 weeks (Calder et al., 1976). In the NERICP covering the early 1970s, 77 per cent of the 33 infants with this lesion died before their first birthday (Fyler et al., 1980). The current 1-year survival rate is probably close to 80 per cent. The long-term results of more innovative surgical approaches are awaited.

TOTAL ANOMALOUS PULMONARY VENOUS RETURN

Anatomy. In this anomaly, the pulmonary veins have no connection with the left atrium and drain either directly or, more commonly, indirectly into the right atrium via one of the normal embryonic channels. The embryologic defect seems to be a failure of development of the common pulmonary vein normally connecting the developing pulmonary venous plexus with the posterior aspect of the left atrium. As a consequence, one or more of the normal anastomotic channels between the pulmonary venous plexus of the lung buds and the cardinal or umbilicovitelline vein persists, allowing drainage of the pulmonary blood flow into the systemic venous atrium (Delisle et al., 1976). If the connection to the left common cardinal system persists, postnatal drainage is to the left innominate vein (35 per cent of cases) or to the coronary sinus (19 per cent). Other pathways that may persist include the right common cardinal system (drainage to right superior vena cava or azygos, 11 per cent of cases) and the umbilicovitelline system (ductus venosus or portal system, 21 per cent). Alternatively, the pulmonary veins may drain directly into the right atrium (4 per cent). In 10 per cent of cases, there is mixed drainage (Gathman and Nadas, 1970). The presence of an interatrial communication, either a patent foramen ovale or a true atrial septal defect, is necessary to sustain life after birth.

The postnatal presentation depends on the degree of obstruction to pulmonary venous drainage. If obstruction is severe (almost invariable with drainage into the umbilicovitelline system, and frequent with drainage into the right superior vena cava or innominate vein), the children present within the 1st week of life. If obstruction is mild or absent, presentation is usually during the second half of the 1st year or later. The remainder of this discussion deals only with the former group, infants with obstruction to the pulmonary venous return.

Incidence. In the NERICP, 63 among 2251 infants under 1 year with critical heart disease seen between 1969 and 1974 had total anomalous pulmonary venous return (TAPVR), representing an incidence of one per 17,000 live births.

Hemodynamics. In utero, there is little hemodynamic disruption from TAPVR, since before birth the pulmonary blood flow represents only 5 to 10 per cent of combined ventricular output, an amount that can be handled by the anomalous systemic venous connection (Fig. 63–20). The drainage of pulmonary venous blood to the right side of the heart rather than the left causes no apparent sequelae; the newborns are normal in size and development.

After birth, the fetal pathways persist. The pulmonary venous return continues to drain to the right atrium via one of the systemic venous channels, where it mixes with the normal systemic venous return. A portion of the totally mixed pulmonary and systemic venous return passes into the left atrium, left ventricle, and aorta, and the rest passes into the right ventricle and pulmonary artery. As the pulmonary arteriolar resistance drops, the pulmonary blood flow increases, and if there is obstruction to the increased pulmonary venous flow, pulmonary edema follows.

The pulmonary venous obstruction increases the pulmonary vascular resistance above systemic, diverting blood from the pulmonary artery into the descending aorta as long as the ductus arteriosus remains open. When the ductus begins to close, the increased pulmonary resistance elevates right ventricular and right atrial pressure and leads to increasing right-to-left shunting at the atrial level. The increased pulmonary resistance secondary to the obstruction reduces pulmonary flow, and the pulmonary edema reduces the oxygen content of the blood that is not obstructed, resulting in arterial hypoxemia and, eventually, acidosis and death.

Clinical Manifestations. In infants with severe pulmonary venous obstruction, the predominant finding is cyanosis. The heart is not hyperactive, and other than experiencing tachypnea, the child is usually comfortable, at least initially. The second heart sound is single or

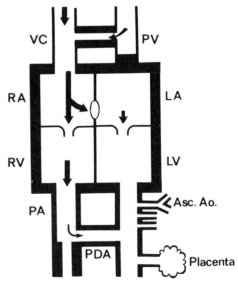

FIGURE 63–20. *Schematic diagram of the circulation in a fetus with total anomalous pulmonary venous return. The intracardiac circulation is normal. Pulmonary venous return is to the anomalous channel connecting with one of the systemic veins. In utero, there is no hemodynamic embarrassment, since pulmonary blood flow is minimal. After birth, if the anomalous channel restricts egress of blood from the pulmonary veins, pulmonary venous hypertension and pulmonary edema follow. The abbreviations are the same as those used in Figure 63–2.*

narrowly split and accentuated. Often, no murmurs are audible.

In newborns with lesser degrees of pulmonary venous obstruction, cyanosis may be less impressive and the signs and symptoms of heart failure—tachypnea, dyspnea, and feeding difficulties—may predominate. In these infants, the right ventricular impulse is hyperdynamic, and the second heart sound is widely split, with the pulmonary component increased. A systolic ejection murmur at the left upper sternal border and a mid-diastolic murmur at the left lower sternal border secondary to increased blood flow across the pulmonary and tricuspid valves may be audible.

In infants with severe obstruction, the heart is normal in size on the chest radiograph, and pulmonary venous congestion is obvious (Fig. 63–21). Those with milder obstruction have right ventricular dilatation and increased pulmonary blood flow. Occasionally, the dilated accessory venous channels to the left or right superior vena cava can be seen on the anteroposterior projection.

The electrocardiogram almost invariably shows right axis deviation and right ventricular hypertrophy (Gathman and Nadas, 1970). In the 1st week, this may be difficult to distinguish from normal, but in those who present in the 2nd week, the right ventricular hypertrophy becomes more obvious and may be associated with right atrial hypertrophy. On two-dimensional echocardiographic study, the posterior wall of the left atrium is bare, and the anomalous channel can be seen connecting the dilated common pulmonary vein behind the left atrium with the left or right superior vena cava, the coronary sinus, or the right atrium, or it may be seen dipping below the diaphragm to connect with the portal system (Chin et al., 1987). The site of obstruction can frequently be localized by turbulence detected on Doppler study.

On catheterization, the oxygen saturation is nearly identical in both atria, ventricles, and great arteries, reflect-

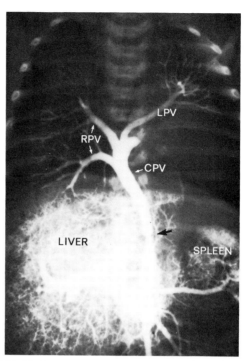

FIGURE 63–22. A postmortem angiogram in a newborn who died with total anomalous pulmonary venous return into the portal system. The right and left pulmonary veins drain into a common trunk that descends below the diaphragm to join the portal system. Note the discrete narrowing in the pulmonary vein (arrow) that probably occurs as it pierces the diaphragm. CPV, common pulmonary vein; LPV, left pulmonary vein; RPV, right pulmonary vein.

ing common mixing at the right atrial level. Occasionally, the common pulmonary vein can be entered where the oxygen saturation is higher. The pulmonary artery pressure is elevated and may be above systemic if the ductus arteriosus is closed. The pulmonary artery "wedge" pressure reflecting pulmonary venous pressure is increased, and right atrial exceeds the left atrial pressure.

Angiocardiography, either in the common pulmonary vein entered from the systemic venous connection or in the pulmonary artery with usual long filming, outlines the site or sites of pulmonary venous drainage except when the obstruction is almost complete (Fig. 63–22).

Diagnosis. In the infant with severe cyanosis that is unresponsive to oxygen and a small heart and pulmonary venous congestion visible on the radiographs, the diagnosis is usually clear. It is occasionally difficult to distinguish infants with total anomalous pulmonary venous return from those with persistent fetal circulation with or without primary lung disease because (1) both groups of patients demonstrate tachypnea, dyspnea, and cyanosis on physical examination as well as haziness of the lung fields on radiographs, and (2) both may transiently improve with 100 per cent oxygen, since a perfusion imbalance may occur in either condition. In preterm infants, lung disease is more common, but in the term infant, the index of suspicion must be high for total anomalous pulmonary venous return. Echocardiography or even catheterization may occasionally be necessary to distinguish the two with certainty.

The hypoplastic left heart syndrome may also be associated with pulmonary edema on radiographs, but there

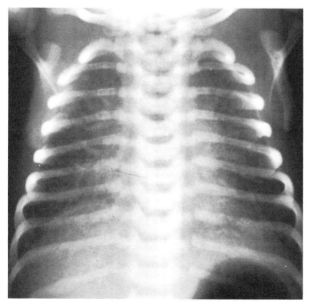

FIGURE 63–21. Chest radiograph in anteroposterior projection in a newborn with total anomalous venous return to the portal system. The pulmonary vessels are indistinct, reflecting increased interstitial fluid from pulmonary venous congestion. The heart is not enlarged.

is usually extreme cardiac enlargement with increased pulmonary blood flow visible on the films and severe circulatory collapse.

Treatment. The treatment of TAPVR with obstruction is surgical. Although some authors have advocated balloon atrial septostomy at the time of diagnostic catheterization followed by observation, we have not found this to be a safe approach and now recommend surgery soon after diagnosis.

The surgical technique consists of anastomosis of the horizontal pulmonary venous confluence to the posterior wall of the left atrium and ligation of the anomalous systemic venous channel.

Prognosis. In the 1970s, the risks of surgery were very high, with the mortality rate approaching 50 per cent. Results from the Northern Plains Registry of Congenital Heart Disease showed a mortality rate of 27 per cent from 1983 to 1987 (Lucas and Kraybill, 1989), whereas other series from single centers reveal slightly better results, with a mortality rate of 12 to 16 per cent (Norwood et al., 1980; Yee et al., 1987).

HETEROTAXIA SYNDROMES

The heterotaxia syndromes are characterized by positional abnormalities of the abdominal viscera (midline liver, stomach on the right, malrotation of the gut), splenic abnormalities (absence of spleen or multiple tiny splenules), and complex, usually cyanotic, congenital heart disease. For convenience, they have been classified as asplenia and polysplenia, although the disease associated with asplenia may be present with a normal spleen and polysplenia heart disease may exist with no spleen, many splenules, or a normal spleen.

ASPLENIA

Anatomy. The liver tends to be midline, with right and left lobes equal in size. Both lungs are trilobed with epiarterial bronchi (bronchus over the pulmonary artery) similar to the bronchus seen in the normal right lung. There is often no rotation or reverse rotation of the midgut loop, with abnormal mesenteric attachments. Often the entire small bowel is on one side of the abdomen and the large intestine on the other. Cardiac malformations usually include bilateral superior vena cava, inferior cava either to the right or left of the spine, common atrium, complete atrioventricular canal, single ventricle, and total anomalous pulmonary venous return. Transposition of the great arteries is common, and severe pulmonary stenosis or atresia is almost invariably present (Rose et al., 1975; Van Mierop et al., 1972).

A helpful pathognomonic feature of asplenia, demonstrable by echocardiography, catheter passage, or angiocardiography, is the finding of the abdominal aorta and inferior vena cava on the same side of the spine.

Incidence. In the NERICP, infants with asplenia and polysplenia were not considered separately. There was a combined incidence of one per 12,000 live births (Fyler et al., 1980). In other series, virtually all pathologic in

origin, these conditions account for about 1 per cent of all cases of congenital heart disease.

Hemodynamics. The infants are usually normal at birth, a finding that suggests relatively normal intrauterine development. This is not surprising because virtual common mixing of systemic venous and pulmonary venous blood normally occurs before birth, and the pulmonary stenosis or atresia and total anomalous pulmonary venous drainage are less important in utero, since pulmonary blood flow is minimal.

After birth, the presentation is usually similar to that of newborns with a large ventricular septal defect and severe pulmonary stenosis or atresia—profound cyanosis, especially as the ductus arteriosus closes.

Clinical Manifestations. As already noted, cyanosis is usually the presenting symptom. If the infant has pulmonary stenosis rather than atresia, a systolic murmur is audible along the left sternal border. The second heart sound is single. The asplenia syndrome may be diagnosed by the plain chest radiograph (Fig. 63–23). The liver is midline and symmetric, and the stomach is found in the midline or on the right or left side of the abdomen. If the chest film is of good quality, the bilateral epiarterial bronchi are visible. The heart may be in the right chest (dextrocardia), midline (mesocardia), or in the left chest (levocardia) and is usually normal in size with reduced pulmonary vascularity. The electrocardiogram is variable. There is often a superior QRS axis (0 to −120 degrees) with a

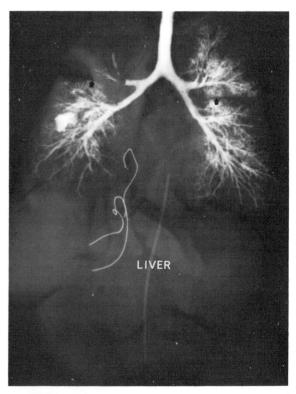

FIGURE 63–23. A postmortem tracheobronchogram from a newborn who died with the asplenia syndrome. The bronchial pattern is symmetric with the angulation, suggesting bilateral right lungs. The black arrows outline the minor fissure in each lung. The liver is midline and symmetric. (From Rowe, R. D.: The Neonate with Congenital Heart Disease. 2nd ed. Philadelphia, W. B. Saunders Company, 1981.)

counterclockwise loop in the frontal plane typical of an endocardial cushion defect. The configuration of the QRS complex depends on the position of the heart in the chest and the presence or absence of a ventricular septum. The P-wave axis is usually inferior and anterior with a normal P-R interval.

If a single ventricle is present, only one ventricular chamber and one A-V valve is present on the M-mode echocardiogram. On two-dimensional study, the complexity of the cardiovascular arrangement can usually be appreciated and most of the abnormalities sorted out.

At cardiac catheterization the catheter can be passed into all the heart chambers, but the total anomalous pulmonary venous return causes similar saturations in each chamber, and the large atrial and ventricular defects result in equal pressures in both atria and both ventricles, making chamber localization difficult. Angiocardiography in the ventricle(s), systemic veins, pulmonary veins, and ductus arteriosus is often necessary for outlining of the structures.

Differential Diagnosis. Infants with asplenia must be differentiated from those with large ventricular septal defect and pulmonary stenosis or atresia (TOF). The characteristic picture of abdominal heterotaxy with bilateral epiarterial bronchi on chest radiographs should alert one to the probability of the asplenia syndrome. Finding the inferior vena cava and abdominal aorta on the same side of the spine seems to be pathognomonic. The finding of Howell-Jolly and Heinz bodies in red cell smears is presumptive evidence of asplenia, and the absence of spleen on ultrasound or radionuclide scan is confirmatory.

It is often more difficult to differentiate between asplenia and polysplenia. In general, the heart disease is more complex with asplenia; the lungs are trilobed, the bronchi epiarterial, the P-wave axis normal, and the inferior vena cava present on the same side as the abdominal aorta. In the polysplenia syndrome, the lungs are bilobed, the bronchi hyparterial (bronchus beneath the pulmonary artery), the inferior vena cava absent, and the P-wave axis superior. Severe pulmonary stenosis is frequent in infants with asplenia and less common in polysplenia.

Treatment. Temporary infusion of prostaglandin E$_1$ helps those who depend on the ductus arteriosus for pulmonary blood flow (Freed et al., 1981), but the increased pulmonary blood flow may unmask latent pulmonary venous obstruction from the total anomalous pulmonary venous return (Freedom et al., 1978). Palliation in the form of systemic-to-pulmonary artery shunts (Blalock-Taussig, Waterston) has been somewhat successful, except in those with severe obstruction of pulmonary venous return.

The Fontan operation that directly connects the systemic venous return to the pulmonary arteries, leaving the single ventricle to pump the pulmonary venous blood to the body, has been attempted in some centers for asplenia and polysplenia. The largest series, from the Mayo Clinic, had a 43 per cent (21 of 49 patients) mortality rate overall but had a mortality rate of only 27 per cent (6 of 22 patients) in 1985 to 1986 (Humes et al., 1988). The risks for children with asplenia were higher than for those with polysplenia.

Since children without spleens have a high risk of sepsis and, at least in our experience, a higher rate of mortality from sepsis than from their heart disease, we believe that pneumococcal vaccine and prophylactic antibiotics should be administered to all asplenic patients who survive beyond the neonatal period (Waldman et al., 1977).

Prognosis. In the 1970s, the prognosis for the symptomatic newborn was grim. In the NERICP, more than two-thirds of the infants were dead by 1 year of age; other reports have not been much more positive. Survivors have been reported into adulthood; however, these children almost invariably have just the right amount of pulmonary stenosis to restrict pulmonary blood flow and prevent heart failure but not enough to cause severe hypoxemia. Better results in the era of less risky palliative operation and Fontan repair are expected.

POLYSPLENIA

Anatomy. In polysplenia there is "bilateral leftsidedness." Multiple splenules are usually present, with the mass of splenic tissue approximating that in the normal spleen. The lungs are usually bilobed, with bilateral hyparterial bronchi (bronchus beneath the pulmonary artery) present in about two-thirds of the cases. The liver is often midline, and, in most infants, the stomach is on the right side (Van Mierop et al., 1972). The heart disease may be as complex as that in the infants with asplenia but often is limited to abnormalities of pulmonary venous and systemic venous return. Absence of the renal to hepatic portion of the inferior vena cava is very common, with the hepatic veins draining directly into the right atrium and the lower inferior vena cava into the right or left superior vena cava via an azygos or hemiazygos connection. The superior vena cava is frequently bilateral, and the pulmonary veins often enter separately into both atria, with the right and left veins draining into the ipsilateral atrium. Large atrial septal defects are common, and a common atrium is not unusual. Other cardiac anomalies less frequently seen include pulmonary stenosis, double outlet right ventricle, and endocardial cushion defects. Infants with transposition of the great arteries and single ventricle are uncommon (Van Mierop et al., 1972).

Incidence. (See discussion of asplenia.)

Hemodynamics. The prenatal and postnatal hemodynamics depend on the lesions present. If only abnormalities of pulmonary venous and systemic venous return are present, the children are rarely symptomatic as newborns. If an endocardial cushion type of ventricular septal defect without pulmonary stenosis is present, congestive failure may occur as the pulmonary vascular resistance drops. Less commonly, the pulmonary stenosis is severe, and cyanosis from a right-to-left shunt predominates.

Clinical Manifestations. The clinical findings depend on the associated lesions present. Cyanosis may be present if there is pulmonary stenosis or atresia; congestive failure predominates if there is an endocardial cushion defect without pulmonary obstruction.

The most distinctive feature of the electrocardiogram is

the superior P-wave axis, usually known as a "coronary sinus rhythm," with a negative P wave in leads II, III, and AVF (Freedom and Ellison, 1973). If an endocardial cushion defect is present, the QRS axis is often superior (0 to -90 degrees) with a counterclockwise loop in the frontal plane.

The chest radiograph is also often distinctive, with a transverse midline liver, right-sided stomach, and absence of the inferior vena cava shadow above the diaphragm in the lateral projection. If the technique is optimal, the bilateral hyparterial bronchi can often be seen.

Two-dimensional echocardiography is usually helpful in defining the status of the venous return, A-V valves, and ventricular chambers.

Diagnosis. (See discussion of asplenia.)

Treatment and Prognosis. The precise defect determines the treatment. Those with atrial anomalies alone rarely require treatment in the neonatal period. In infants with more complex anatomy, congestive failure may be prominent and pulmonary artery banding may be necessary to reduce pulmonary blood flow. In the rare child with severe pulmonary stenosis and cyanosis, a palliative shunt to increase pulmonary flow may be beneficial.

The prognosis of these infants depends on the lesions present but is overall somewhat better than that associated with asplenia, since the heart disease is rarely as complex (Humes et al., 1988).

■ ACYANOTIC CONGENITAL HEART DISEASE

COARCTATION OF THE AORTA

Anatomy. The sine qua non of this anomaly is the presence of a constriction in the aorta distal to the left subclavian artery, usually at the site of insertion of the ductus arteriosus. There may be, in addition, tubular hypoplasia of the aortic arch and intracardiac anomalies. Coarctation of the aorta formerly was classified as infantile, or preductal, usually with tubular hypoplasia, or adult, or postductal, without tubular hypoplasia. This seems to be an oversimplification, because the preductal type can be seen in older children and a discrete juxtaductal or post-ductal obstruction can appear in some infants. We prefer the anatomic-physiologic classification suggested in 1972 by Rudolph and co-workers of aortic isthmus narrowing, including complete interruption, and discrete juxtaductal aortic obstruction. Infants with the aortic isthmus narrowing usually have intracardiac defects such as ventricular septal defect, double outlet right ventricle, or tricuspid atresia, and it seems likely that the tubular hypoplasia is due to decreased flow through the aortic arch in utero. The cause of the discrete juxtaductal coarctation is probably different, because the arch is otherwise normal and there are rarely other cardiac anomalies.

One theory is that muscular tissue from the ductus arteriosus extends into the aorta, and when the ductus closes after birth, the aorta is constricted by this ductal muscle (Ho and Anderson, 1979). Although many still adhere to this theory, histologically the obstruction appears to be on the posterior wall of the aorta, the side opposite

to ductal insertion. More recently, it has been suggested that some abnormality of fetal flow or direct injury before birth causes a proliferation of smooth muscle cells and fibrous tissue on the posterior wall of the aorta, resulting in the formation of a shelf of tissue (Rudolph et al., 1972; Talner and Berman, 1975). While the ductus is open in utero or after birth, this shelf is nonobstructive, but when the ductus arteriosus closes, obstruction results.

Incidence. There were 158 cases of infants with coarctation as their primary lesion in the NERICP, representing an incidence of one per 7000 live births. Only 35 (17 per cent) of these had juxtaductal coarctation alone; another 35 had coarctation with a ductus arteriosus. There were 73 with a ventricular septal defect with or without a ductus arteriosus, with the remaining 15 having more complex anomalies associated with coarctation. An additional 51 infants had coarctation as a secondary lesion, that is, associated with more complex congenital disease (e.g., single ventricle, transposition of the great arteries, hypoplastic left heart syndrome). Coarctation is the most common congenital heart disease presenting in the 2nd week of life.

Hemodynamics. Since there is normally little flow across the aortic isthmus in utero, the tubular hypoplasia of the arch does not affect fetal growth and development. In the presence of a posterior shelf, there is also no significant hemodynamic difficulty, because the flow is small and the large ductus arteriosus allows ample room for it to bypass the narrowing (Fig. 63–24).

After birth, the constriction in the aorta increases left ventricular afterload. In the presence of a ventricular septal defect, this increased systemic resistance leads to a large left-to-right shunt. As the pulmonary vascular resistance falls, the left-to-right shunt increases, resulting in a volume as well as a pressure overload of the left ventricle. In addition to congestive heart failure, there is failure of the

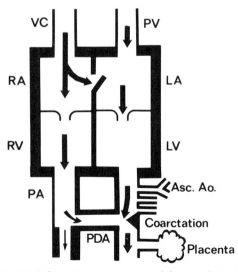

FIGURE 63–24. Schematic representation of the circulation in a fetus with coarctation of the aorta. The intracardiac blood flow is relatively normal. In utero, the constriction in the aorta is of no physiologic significance, since the open ductus arteriosus allows blood to go around the obstruction. After birth, when the ductus closes, the narrowing is exhibited. The abbreviations are the same as those used in Figure 63–2.

blood to pass from ascending to descending aorta if the coarctation is severe. The results are tissue hypoxia, lactic acidosis, and eventual death after the ductus arteriosus closes.

Those infants with a juxtaductal coarctation but no associated anomalies have a slightly different hemodynamic picture. In these newborns, closure of the ductus arteriosus leads to an acute increase in afterload to the left ventricle, because blood must be pumped through the narrowed segment. Since no obstruction was present in utero, no collateral vessels have developed. Owing in part to a reduced number of sympathetic receptors, the neonatal myocardium is not able to respond to increased work as well as the left ventricle of an older child or adult can. Consequently, congestive heart failure, with elevation of left ventricular end-diastolic, left atrial, and pulmonary venous pressures follows. Occasionally, the acute left atrial dilatation causes the septum primum to become incompetent, resulting in an atrial left-to-right shunt. If the coarctation is not too severe, congestive failure may be mild, and there may be time for compensatory mechanisms (e.g., left ventricular hypertrophy or collateral vessels that bypass the obstruction) to develop.

Clinical Features. The newborn with coarctation of the aorta presents with the usual signs and symptoms of congestive heart failure: dyspnea, tachypnea, tachycardia, hepatomegaly, poor feeding, and increased perspiration. A careful examination of the peripheral pulses demonstrates that pulses and blood pressure (by Doppler or flush method) in the legs are diminished compared with those in the arms. Blood pressure in both arms must be measured, because it may be diminished in the left arm if the coarctation involves the origin of the left subclavian artery and it may be decreased in the right arm in the rare situation in which the right subclavian arises anomalously below the coarctation as the last vessel of the aortic arch rather than as the first branch of the innominate. Occasionally, the pulses in the legs "wax and wane" as the ductus arteriosus opens and closes. In the newborn with an isolated juxtaductal coarctation, there may be no murmur or, occasionally, a short systolic ejection murmur in the axilla or back. In newborns with tubular hypoplasia and a ventricular septal defect, there is usually a harsh pansystolic murmur at the left lower sternal border, but its absence does not rule out a ventricular defect.

In the absence of complex intracardiac anomalies, there is right axis deviation and right ventricular hypertrophy on the electrocardiogram reflecting normal intrauterine blood flow. On the chest radiograph, the heart is enlarged with the pulmonary vascularity congested, and if a left-to-right shunt is present from a stretched foramen ovale, the heart is actively engorged. Poststenotic dilatation in the descending aorta and rib notching, usually present in older children with coarctation, are not seen in newborns.

The two-dimensional echocardiogram using a subxiphoid or suprasternal view usually demonstrates the site of obstruction and allows one to estimate the size of the aortic arch. However, some care must be taken, since the isthmus normally is small compared with the ascending and descending aorta in newborns. Because of the excellent images obtained, some centers no longer consider catheterization and angiography necessary for this group of patients (Glasow et al., 1988).

Cardiac catheterization and angiocardiography can define the site of obstruction and the size of the aortic arch and document the presence of associated cardiac anomalies, if any. In the newborn with isolated juxtaductal coarctation, there is usually no intracardiac shunting, although a left-to-right shunt at the atrial level may be found. A difference in systolic pressure between the left ventricle or ascending aorta and descending aorta is found. Angiocardiography in the left ventricle, after insertion of a venous catheter through the foramen ovale, demonstrates the site of obstruction (Fig. 63–25). In those with more complex disease, the catheterization findings depend on the anomalies present. There is often a left-to-right shunt at the ventricular level, so the pulmonary artery is opacified on a left ventricular injection, making it difficult to visualize the aortic arch. A retrograde study from the umbilical or femoral artery may be necessary to see the coarctation, but we have occasionally been able to show the aortic isthmus from an angiocardiogram done through a #23 indwelling cannula in the radial or brachial artery or from an angiogram in the descending aorta, usually through the ductus arteriosus, with balloon occlusion of the descending aorta where flow beyond the catheter is blocked by the inflated balloon catheter.

Diagnosis. The diagnosis of coarctation of the aorta is obvious if there is a marked discrepancy in blood pressure between the arms and legs. As already mentioned, however, in some newborns the pulses "wax and wane," presumably as the ductus arteriosus closes. Therefore, one must check the pulses and blood pressure more than once if there is any possibility of coarctation.

Coarctation of the aorta must be differentiated from other causes of congestive heart failure in the 1st or 2nd

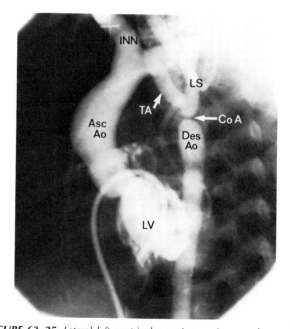

FIGURE 63–25. *Lateral left ventricular angiogram in a newborn with coarctation of the aorta without a ventricular septal defect. There is a discrete narrowing in the aorta just distal to the origin of the left subclavian artery. The transverse aortic arch between the innominate artery and the left subclavian is moderately hypoplastic. Asc Ao, ascending aorta; Co A, coarctation of the aorta; Des Ao, descending aorta; INN, innominate artery; LS, left subclavian artery; LV, left ventricle; TA, transverse aortic arch.*

week of life (see Differential Diagnosis). The hypoplastic left heart syndrome usually causes a symmetric decrease in pulses with equal blood pressures in the arms and legs and severe right ventricular hypertrophy on the electrocardiogram. Aortic stenosis also causes a symmetric decrease in pulses but is usually associated with left ventricular hypertrophy and ST–T changes on the electrocardiogram. Echocardiography or catheterization may be necessary to differentiate these lesions if no difference in pulses or blood pressure is apparent.

Treatment. The medical treatment of a newborn with congestive failure from coarctation of the aorta includes digitalis and diuretics and, if acidosis or low output is present, prostaglandin E_1 to dilate the ductus arteriosus (Freed et al., 1981). Newborns who present later in the 1st month with a juxtaductal coarctation and no other associated anomalies can occasionally be managed with anticongestives only. In this group, we have postponed surgery until later in the 1st year of life if heart failure can be controlled and an adequate weight gain sustained. Most newborns who present with coarctation of the aorta, however, have tubular hypoplasia and associated cardiac anomalies. In these infants, heart failure can rarely be controlled and relief is eventually mandatory. Some specialists have advocated balloon dilation of the narrowed segment (Morrow et al., 1988), but the role of this procedure in the newborn has not yet been determined. The most widely used surgical approach has been resection of the abnormal segment of aorta and end-to-end anastomosis of the noninvolved area. Long-term follow-up has demonstrated a relatively high incidence of residual obstruction at the anastomotic site that is due to either incomplete initial relief or, more likely, inadequate growth of the aorta at the anastomotic site through childhood. The subclavian patch plasty has gained favor (Waldhausen et al., 1964) because it avoids a circumferential suture line. With a left thoracotomy, the left subclavian artery is divided, opened lengthwise, turned down, and applied as a patch across the area of obstruction. The initial results of this operation are gratifying, although it is still unclear whether or not this approach is better than the conventional end-to-end anastomosis (Trinquet et al., 1988).

Some controversy remains about how to deal with the associated anomalies. If the intracardiac anatomy is complex (single ventricle, transposition with a ventricular defect) and associated with pulmonary hypertension and a large left-to-right shunt, we place a band around the pulmonary artery to increase pulmonary resistance and reduce pulmonary blood flow at the time of coarctation repair. If the intracardiac anatomy is more straightforward (e.g., a ventricular septal defect or atrioventricular canal), we repair the coarctation using the left thoracotomy and do not band the pulmonary artery. If congestive heart failure cannot be controlled in the postoperative period or if the child cannot be weaned from the respirator, our surgeons repair the intracardiac defect from a midline approach using deep-hypothermic circulatory arrest. Many surgeons, however, would choose to band these latter infants as well at the time of coarctation repair and postpone definitive repair until later in infancy.

Prognosis. In the NERICP extending from 1969 to 1974, only 74 per cent of infants with simple juxtaductal

coarctation of the aorta survived to their first birthday. For those with more complex anomalies, the prognosis was even poorer, with less than 50 per cent of infants surviving to 1 year. Surgery in the 1st week was especially hazardous, with 15 of 17 (88 per cent) newborns dying. Late mortality, usually due to the associated cardiac anomaly, was not uncommon.

More recently, there has been a significant improvement that is due to better preoperative care with prostaglandins, improved surgery, and better perioperative and postoperative management. We have recently reviewed 100 consecutive newborns who underwent repair between 1972 and 1984—29 with simple coarctation, 32 with an additional ventricular septal defect, and 39 with complex heart disease. The early mortality rate was 11.4 per cent for those with subclavian flap plasty, and of those patients, 75 per cent did not need reoperation after 5 years. The overall actuarial survival rate at 4 years was 86 per cent for those with coarctation, 80 per cent for those with coarctation and ventricular septal defect, and 43 per cent for those with complex heart disease (Ziemer et al., 1986).

INTERRUPTED AORTIC ARCH

Anatomy. Infants with an interrupted aortic arch have a discontinuity between the ascending and descending aorta. Celoria and Patton classified children with an interrupted aortic arch according to the site of the discontinuity: Type A, distal to the left subclavian artery (42 per cent of cases); Type B, distal to the left common carotid artery (53 per cent of cases); and Type C, distal to the innominate artery (4 per cent of cases) (Van Praagh et al., 1971). Almost any cardiac anomaly can be associated with interrupted aortic arch, but a patent ductus arteriosus and a ventricular septal defect are almost invariably present, and aortic stenosis, double outlet right ventricle, truncus arteriosus, and single ventricle are not uncommon.

The embryologic defect in interrupted aortic arch is not known, but Van Praagh and co-workers suggest that a leftward shift of the crista supraventricularis in the developing heart obstructs the subaortic region, reducing antegrade flow through the aortic valve and diverting flow away from the ascending aorta (arches 3 and 4) and toward the pulmonary artery (arch 6). This results in inappropriate involution of a portion of the transverse arch. More than two-thirds of the newborns with interrupted aortic arch have been found to have DiGeorge syndrome (Van Mierop and Kutsche, 1986).

Incidence. In the NERICP, there were 21 infants with interrupted aortic arch, an incidence of one per 50,000 live births; these infants represent about 1 per cent of critically ill infants with congenital heart disease.

Hemodynamics. In the normal fetus, the left ventricle supplies the ascending aorta and the right ventricle supplies the descending aorta through the ductus arteriosus, with only 10 per cent of combined ventricular output passing through the arch of the aorta from ascending to descending aorta (Rudolph, 1974). In the fetus with an interrupted aortic arch, no blood passes through the aortic isthmus, but this results in no major observable hemodynamic abnormalities (Fig. 63–26). After birth, however, the descending aorta continues to depend on the ductus

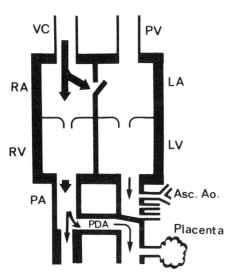

FIGURE 63–26. *Schematic diagram of the circulation in a fetus with an interrupted aortic arch. The intracardiac flow is normal. Blood from the right atrium passes through the right ventricle, pulmonary artery, and ductus arteriosus to the descending aorta and placenta. Flow to the ascending aorta is derived from blood passing through the foramen ovale and left heart chambers. No blood crosses from ascending to descending aorta. After birth, when the ductus arteriosus constricts, blood supply to the lower half of the body is compromised. The abbreviations are the same as those used in Figure 63–2.*

arteriosus to provide systemic output. When the ductus begins to close, flow to the descending aorta diminishes, and tissue hypoxia, acidosis, and death follow. Rarely, the ductus arteriosus remains open. In these infants, congestive heart failure occurs as the pulmonary vascular resistance falls over the first weeks of life and pulmonary blood flow increases.

Clinical Manifestations. The clinical presentations of the various types of interruption are similar. As the pulmonary vascular resistance falls, the newborns develop the signs and symptoms of congestive heart failure: respiratory distress, tachypnea, tachycardia, hepatomegaly, poor feeding, and increased perspiration. As the ductus arteriosus closes, the pulses and perfusion in the lower body diminish and mottling appears. Although differential cyanosis should be observable, because the upper body receives fully saturated blood from the left ventricle and the lower body receives desaturated venous blood from the pulmonary artery, it is rarely clinically apparent because a large left-to-right shunt through a ventricular septal defect tends to increase the pulmonary artery oxygen saturation and pulmonary venous desaturation from pulmonary edema lowers the aortic saturation, making the differences minimal and not clinically visible, even to the experienced observer. The presence of strong pulses in the left carotid but not in the left subclavian artery or in the right carotid but not left carotid artery can often localize the site of the interruption. Heart murmurs are rarely impressive in these infants, but a systolic murmur can sometimes be heard along the left sternal border, presumably from the ventricular septal defect. The second sound is usually loud and single.

Since intrauterine flows are normal, the electrocardiogram is rarely helpful at birth; there is usually right axis deviation and right ventricular hypertrophy that is normal

for age. No specific anomalies are present on the chest radiograph other than generalized cardiac enlargement and increased pulmonary vascular markings often associated with pulmonary venous congestion.

On two-dimensional echocardiography, the site of the interruption can usually be seen on a high parasternal or suprasternal notch view, whereas apical two-chamber or subcostal views usually define the intracardiac anatomy.

At cardiac catheterization, the systolic pressures in both ventricles, ascending aorta, and main pulmonary artery are equal because of the large ventricular septal defect. Frequently, there is a gradient between the main pulmonary artery and descending aorta reflecting the closing ductus arteriosus. Although anatomically there is often evidence of subaortic narrowing secondary to the leftward shift of the crista supraventricularis, we have rarely measured a gradient between the left ventricle and the ascending aorta at catheterization, probably because of reduced antegrade flow.

Angiocardiography in the left and right ventricle usually outlines the site of the interruption, but occasionally the catheter must be passed from the left ventricle to the ascending aorta to view optimally the site of interruption and to determine the distance between ascending and descending aorta (Fig. 63–27).

Diagnosis. The diagnosis of an interrupted aortic arch is difficult but should be suspected in any newborn with early congestive heart failure. The finding of differential blood pressures between the arms and legs suggests either coarctation of the aorta or interruption: differences in the pulse between the right and left carotid arteries make the latter condition more probable. The distinction between a Type A interruption (distal to the left subclavian) and coarctation is angiocardiographic. Other acyanotic heart

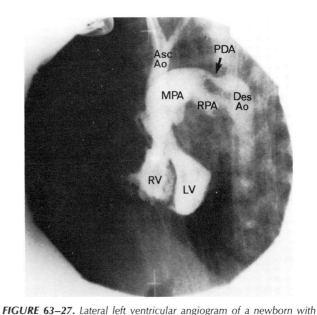

FIGURE 63–27. *Lateral left ventricular angiogram of a newborn with an interrupted aortic arch. There is no connection between the ascending and descending aorta; blood flow to the descending aorta is derived from the pulmonary artery through a closing ductus arteriosus. A ventricular septal defect connecting the right and left ventricle is present. Asc Ao, ascending aorta; Des Ao, descending aorta; LV, left ventricle; MPA, main pulmonary artery; PDA, patent ductus arteriosus; RPA, right pulmonary artery; RV, right ventricle.*

diseases in the newborn in which congestive heart failure occurs (e.g., aortic stenosis and hypoplastic left heart syndrome) can usually be excluded by the differential pulses in interrupted aortic arch or by the electrocardiographic finding of left ventricular hypertrophy and strain in aortic stenosis and the echocardiographic demonstration of a small ascending aorta in the hypoplastic left heart syndrome.

Treatment. Although the initial treatment of newborns with an interrupted arch is medical (digoxin, diuretics, and prostaglandin E_1 to dilate the ductus arteriosus), the prognosis is grim without surgical intervention. We prefer total correction of infants with an interrupted aortic arch and a ventricular septal defect (Collins-Nakai et al., 1976).

From a left thoracotomy, a Dacron conduit is attached to the descending aorta. The left thoracotomy is closed, and from a midline sternotomy, the proximal part of the conduit is attached to the ascending aorta, the patent ductus arteriosus is ligated, and the ventricular septal defect is closed using deep-hypothermic circulatory arrest. Occasionally, the ascending aorta and descending aorta can be brought together without a conduit from a midline approach. Recently, the surgical results for this abnormality have dramatically improved, with a probability of dying within 2 weeks of surgery (by a multivariate analysis of our recent data) dropping to 7 per cent (Sell et al., 1988). For infants with an interrupted aortic arch associated with more complex intracardiac anatomy, repair of the aortic arch, and pulmonary artery banding are probably the procedures of choice.

Prognosis. In the NERICP, the prognosis for this group was poor (Collins-Nakai et al., 1976). Of nine patients who were treated medically, eight died at a median age of 4 days. Of the 21 treated surgically, one-third had a ventricular septal defect, one-third had a ventricular defect and left ventricular outflow obstruction, and one-third had complex intracardiac anomalies. The overall mortality was 76 per cent. Our more recent data from the late 1970s and early 1980s had an actuarial survival rate of 1, 5, and 10 years of 52, 48, and 47 per cent, respectively (Sell et al., 1988). Improvements in early management in the late 1980s quoted earlier should lead to better survival in the decade ahead.

AORTIC STENOSIS

Anatomy. Although left ventricular outflow obstruction in childhood may occur below or above the valve, for all practical purposes only valvular aortic stenosis causes severe symptoms in the neonatal period. The valve is usually unicommissural and unicuspid (Moller et al., 1966), and the tissue is thickened, nodular, and severely deformed. The myocardium is always very hypertrophied, but the left ventricular cavity varies in size. It may be dilated, normal, or hypoplastic; when small, the defect gradually becomes a part of the hypoplastic left heart syndrome. In many infants, the left ventricular endocardium is thickened and covered with a gray layer of fibrous and elastic tissue that may involve the papillary muscles, resulting in mitral regurgitation. This "endocardial fibroelastosis" is probably secondary to myocardial hypoxia

from the very thick myocardium, which, in the presence of high intracavitary pressures, cannot be adequately perfused in the endocardial layers.

Associated lesions such as coarctation of the aorta and ventricular or atrial septal defects are occasionally seen.

Incidence. In the Baltimore-Washington Infant Study, aortic stenosis occurred in 0.8 of 10,000 live births, slightly higher than the 0.4 per 10,000 in the NERICP; overall, it occurred in about 1 in 16,000 live births and represented 2 per cent of infants seen with critical heart disease.

Hemodynamics. In utero, the presence of left ventricular outflow obstruction imposes a pressure load on the left ventricle. If the stenosis occurs early in gestation and is severe, the afterload reduces flow through the ventricle, and left ventricular hypoplasia and hypoplastic left heart syndrome may result (Rudolph, 1974). If the stenosis is less severe, the left ventricular size is normal, but the myocardium is very hypertrophied and fibroelastosis from inadequate endocardial perfusion may be present.

After birth, the left ventricular output normally must increase by about 50 per cent with the switch from a parallel to an in series circulation. In the presence of severe aortic obstruction, the marginally compensated left ventricle may be unable to handle increased volume load. If the foramen ovale is closed, the left atrial pressure rapidly increases, leading to pulmonary edema. Occasionally, left atrial dilatation makes the septum primum incompetent, allowing the left atrium to decompress through the foramen ovale. This left-to-right shunt at the atrial level may exacerbate the congestive heart failure.

Clinical Manifestations. The infant with critical aortic stenosis is usually normal at birth. A systolic murmur is invariably audible along the left sternal border with radiation to the right upper sternal border but may be only grade 2 or 3/6. The symptoms of congestive heart failure—respiratory distress, poor feeding, and tachypnea—may be delayed by hours to weeks; however, once symptoms occur, they may progress very rapidly, leading to a low output state with cool, mottled extremities, very diminished pulses, and a murmur that is barely audible.

The murmur is rarely associated with a thrill, even when output is adequate, but a systolic ejection click at the apex may be present. In stark contrast with its radiographically visible enlargement, the heart is rarely hyperactive on palpation.

The most frequent electrocardiographic pattern is left ventricular hypertrophy with inverted T waves over the left precordium, suggesting left ventricular ischemia (Fig. 63–28). Occasionally, right ventricular hypertrophy may be seen, but in our experience (Keane et al., 1975), this is associated with at least some hypoplasia of the left ventricle. Even in those with right ventricular predominance, inverted T waves over the left precordium are common.

In infants with congestive heart failure, the heart is invariably enlarged on chest radiographs and may be massive. The pulmonary vessels are indistinct owing to pulmonary venous congestion and may also be actively engorged if there is a large left-to-right shunt at the atrial level from a stretched foramen ovale.

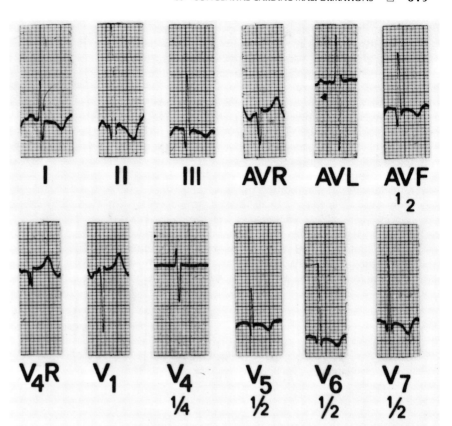

FIGURE 63–28. *Electrocardiogram in a newborn with aortic stenosis. There is left ventricular hypertrophy for age. The inverted T waves in the left precordium suggest left ventricular strain (ischemia).*

Using long-axis view of the left ventricular outflow tract, two-dimensional echocardiography shows severe immobility of the aortic valve with little or no systolic opening, left ventricular hypertrophy, left atrial dilatation, and post-stenotic dilatation in the ascending aorta. Evaluation of the ascending aorta with Doppler technique shows increased velocity of blood flow, allowing estimation of the gradient.

At cardiac catheterization, the left ventricle can usually be approached through the foramen ovale, but occasionally a retrograde study across the aortic valve or even a transatrial septal puncture may be necessary. There is usually a pressure gradient of greater than 40 mm Hg between the left ventricle and ascending aorta, with the left ventricular systolic pressure exceeding 120 mm Hg, but occasionally in children with severe congestive heart failure the left ventricle cannot generate such a high pressure, and the gradient may be less. The left ventricular end-diastolic pressure is invariably elevated and has been observed to be as high as 35 mm Hg. If the foramen ovale is incompetent, a left-to-right shunt at the atrial level may be present, with the pulmonary flow–to–systemic flow ratio occasionally exceeding 3:1. A left ventricular angiocardiogram in the left anterior oblique projection outlines the domed and thickened aortic valve.

Diagnosis. Aortic stenosis must be differentiated from other causes of heart failure in the 1st month of life. With aortic atresia and the hypoplastic left heart syndrome, there is congestive failure but no left ventricular hypertrophy on the electrocardiogram. In coarctation of the aorta with or without a ventricular septal defect, the pulses are weak or absent in the legs but are usually palpable in the arms and carotids, and left ventricular strain on the electrocardiogram is usually not present. The murmur of aortic stenosis is loudest at the right or left upper sternal borders, whereas in infants with coarctation the murmur is louder at the lower left sternal border or into the axilla. Finally, aortic stenosis is associated with an ejection click that is rarely present in the newborn with coarctation of the aorta.

With acyanotic lesions causing congestive heart failure such as ventricular septal defects, atrioventricular canal defects, and patent ductus arteriosus, there is usually a very hyperactive precordium associated with the large left-to-right shunts. In tricuspid atresia, truncus arteriosus, and single ventricle, there is usually cyanosis with crying.

Treatment. These infants are usually very sick when first seen, and the usual medical management with digoxin, diuretics, and correction of acidosis must be accomplished without delay. Because a progressive downhill course is almost inevitable once an infant becomes symptomatic, prompt catheterization and surgery are indicated. Aortic valvotomy, under inflow occlusion or cardiopulmonary bypass, has been the procedure of choice. The operative risk remains high, in part owing to hypoplasia of the ventricle and aortic annulus or coexisting fibroelastosis, and repeat surgery is not infrequently necessary because of inadequate relief or restenosis (Keane et al., 1975). Recently, balloon dilation of the aortic valve has been attempted in this group of critically ill newborns with results equal to or better than the surgical approach (Zeevi et al., 1988 b and c).

Prognosis. In the NERICP, the overall survival rate to the first birthday was only 22 of 45 infants, or 49 per cent (Fyler et al., 1980), with a 68 per cent mortality rate among infants undergoing surgery prior to 2 months of age. Of 18 infants surviving surgery who were followed by Keane and co-workers, residual abnormalities were present in most, and six required repeat operation to relieve residual stenosis or regurgitation. In 1981, Edmunds and co-workers reported a 50 per cent mortality rate among 14 newborns undergoing aortic valvotomy. They correlated the angiocardigraphically determined left ventricular size with operative risk and found that seven of eight newborns with a normally sized ventricle survived valvotomy, with six remaining alive 1½ to 6½ years after operation. Of six patients with a small left ventricle (end-diastolic volume of less than 30 ml/m²) all succumbed. The Toronto group has also recently reported fairly dismal results, with a long-term survival rate among 40 newborns with critical aortic stenosis of only 32 per cent (Pelech et al., 1987).

HYPOPLASTIC LEFT HEART SYNDROME: AORTIC OR MITRAL ATRESIA OR SEVERE STENOSIS WITH A HYPOPLASTIC LEFT VENTRICLE

Anatomy. On gross pathologic examination, the hearts of children with "hypoplastic left heart syndrome" (Noonan and Nadas, 1958) are all similar, with severe hypoplasia of the left ventricle and ascending aorta and a dilated right ventricle and pulmonary artery. The aortic valve may be atretic with a complete absence of any recognizable valve tissue or may be fused and domed with an eccentric pinhole orifice. The mitral valve is atretic in one-fourth of the cases and hypoplastic in the rest. The left ventricle may be slitlike if both mitral and aortic valves are atretic but is somewhat more developed when there is some flow through the mitral valve. The ascending aorta is hypoplastic between the coronaries and the innominate artery, and a coarctation of the aorta may be present. Ventricular septal defects are uncommon.

Incidence. In the NERICP, there were 177 cases of infants with hypoplastic left heart syndrome reported between 1969 and 1974, representing an incidence of one per 6000 live births. The syndrome was the fifth most common form of all congenital heart diseases, the second most common heart disease presenting in the 1st week of life (after transposition), and the third most common appearing in the 2nd week of life (following coarctation of the aorta and ventricular septal defect).

Hemodynamics. In a fetus with a hypoplastic left heart, the right ventricle must support the entire circulation (Fig. 63–29). Almost all the systemic venous return that enters the right atrium passes into the right ventricle and is ejected into the pulmonary artery. A small portion of blood may pass through the foramen ovale, but with mitral or aortic atresia this is minimal. Since the pulmonary resistance is high, virtually all the blood entering the pulmonary artery is diverted through the ductus arteriosus into the aorta rather than passing into the lungs. Most goes to the descending aorta and placenta, but some goes

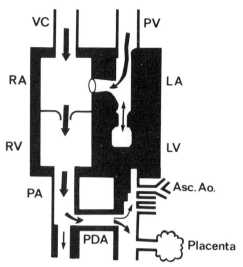

FIGURE 63–29. *Schematic diagram of the circulation in a fetus with hypoplastic left heart syndrome. There is aortic atresia and hypoplasia of the left ventricle, left atrium, and mitral valve. The systemic venous return from the vena cava passes through the right heart chambers into the ductus arteriosus and then to the descending aorta and placenta as well as the ascending aorta. The pulmonary venous return goes through a foramen ovale into the right atrium. After birth, the foramen may be obstructive as pulmonary flow increases. When the ductus arteriosus constricts, flow to the systemic circulation is reduced, and low output shock and death follow. The abbreviations are the same as those used in Figure 63–2.*

retrograde into the aortic arch and ascending aorta to the subclavian, carotid, and coronary arteries. The ascending aorta is small because the coronary arteries are the only continuation after the takeoff of the innominate artery.

After birth, the pulmonary vascular resistance falls and the systemic resistance increases so that an increasing proportion of blood from the single pulmonary trunk goes to the lungs rather than through the ductus arteriosus. The increased pulmonary blood flow leads to an increase in pulmonary venous return that cannot freely exit from the left atrium because of hypoplasia of the left atrium and foramen ovale, and it results in pulmonary venous hypertension and pulmonary edema. As the ductus arteriosus begins to close at 12 to 48 hours of age, the perfusion to the systemic circulation is reduced, resulting in systemic and coronary ischemia. Understandably, newborns with this disease are the sickest patients seen by the pediatric cardiologist, with the median age of death 4½ days in untreated infants (Watson and Rowe, 1962).

Clinical Features. The infants are usually normal at birth, but tachypnea and dyspnea soon develop as the pulmonary blood flow increases. Cyanosis is rarely prominent, despite the total mixing of the systemic and pulmonary circulations, because the pulmonary blood flow is so increased. Congestive heart failure with tachypnea, hepatomegaly, and poor feeding are usually present by 24 to 48 hours of age. Finally, as the ductus arteriosus begins to close, the signs of low output—mottling, grayness of the skin, and markedly diminished pulses—follow. One-third are in vascular collapse by the time they reach the physician, with blood pressures of 40 mm Hg or less, and they are hypothermic, hypoglycemic, and ashen in color. Auscultation is rarely helpful because prominent murmurs are unusual and the second heart sound is single.

The electrocardiogram reflects the intrauterine circulation, showing right axis deviation and right ventricular predominance that may be normal for age. Occasionally, diminished left-sided forces due to left ventricular hypoplasia can be appreciated. Right atrial hypertrophy is seen in about two-thirds of the infants. Coronary ischemia frequently results in ST–T wave changes. A marked sinus tachycardia is usually present.

The heart is markedly enlarged on chest radiographs, with both increased pulmonary blood flow and pulmonary venous congestion prominent.

On the two-dimensional echocardiogram using the subxiphoid and precordial views, the markedly enlarged right-sided chambers and hypoplastic left-sided chambers can be seen.

Cardiac catheterization may be performed to confirm the clinical and echocardiographic findings and to rule out correctable heart disease if the echocardiogram is equivocal. The pulmonary venous and left atrial pressures are elevated. The right ventricular and pulmonary artery pressures are increased and often exceed the systolic pressure in the aorta, reflecting the gradient across the closing ductus arteriosus. There is a large increase in oxygen saturation between the vena cava and the right atrium that is due to the torrential flow of pulmonary venous return from the left to the right atrium.

An angiocardiogram in the right ventricle, pulmonary artery, or aorta is usually diagnostic (Fig. 63–30). The ascending aorta is opacified retrograde from the ductus arteriosus and is extremely hypoplastic with little, if any, flow of unopacified blood through the aortic valve. In the presence of mitral stenosis rather than atresia, a left atrial injection demonstrates the size of the left ventricle.

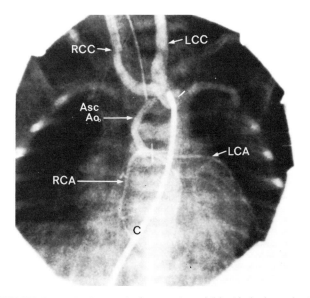

FIGURE 63–30. Angiogram in the aorta in a child with the hypoplastic left heart syndrome with aortic atresia. There is no antegrade flow through the aortic valve. Blood flow to the hypoplastic ascending aorta is retrograde from the ductus arteriosus. Asc Ao, ascending aorta; C, catheter; LCA, left coronary artery; LCC, left common carotid artery; RCA, right coronary artery; RCC, right common carotid artery.

Diagnosis. Infants with the hypoplastic left heart syndrome must be differentiated from those with other causes of respiratory distress in the 1st month of life.

In the early stages, the tachypnea may suggest lung disease, but the appearance of congestive heart failure with tachycardia, hepatomegaly, and cardiac enlargement on radiographs should allow the two to be differentiated. Nonstructural heart diseases, myocarditis, transient myocardial ischemia, and intrauterine supraventricular tachycardia must be ruled out as must other causes of vascular collapse such as sepsis.

After the onset of congestive heart failure, hypoplastic left heart must be differentiated from the two other common structural causes of failure early in the 1st week of life: aortic stenosis and the coarctation syndrome. There is usually left ventricular hypertrophy on the electrocardiogram in the former, and a difference in pulses and blood pressure between the upper and lower extremities is normally present in the latter.

The differentiation of low output shock, secondary to hypoplastic left heart syndrome, from the other causes of shock in the newborn is usually straightforward if the index of suspicion of heart disease is high.

Treatment. Since the hypoplastic left heart syndrome has been uniformly fatal, treatment has usually been terminated at the time of definitive diagnosis. Recently, some centers have suggested palliative operations in an attempt to improve the poor prognosis. In infants for whom palliative procedures are being considered, congestive failure should be treated with digoxin and diuretics. Prostaglandin E_1 infusion often dilates the ductus arteriosus (Freed et al., 1981) and improves perfusion. Bicarbonate should be given to treat the metabolic acidosis, but the quantity of sodium given must be carefully monitored so as not to create a hyperosmolar state.

The most common surgical approach turns the defect into a single ventricle that can later be repaired by a modified Fontan approach, but this must be done in two stages because high pulmonary resistance precludes an early Fontan operation.

In the first stage, which is performed in the newborn period, the ascending aorta is augmented, usually using pulmonary homograft; the main pulmonary artery is transsected, with the proximal end connected to the augmented aorta and the distal end patched closed; the atrial septum is removed to relieve any pulmonary venous obstruction; and a systemic to pulmonary artery connection, frequently a Blalock-Taussig shunt, is created to supply pulmonary blood flow.

Blood then passes from systemic and pulmonary veins into the right atrium and right ventricle and out the pulmonary valve to the reconstructed ascending aorta with pulmonary flow from the shunt (Pigott et al., 1988).

A Fontan procedure, partitioning the right atrium so that systemic venous blood passes to the pulmonary artery and pulmonary venous blood passes into right ventricle and aorta, closing the shunt, can be done when the infant is older than 6 months of age, when pulmonary vascular resistance has reached its nadir. These operations are difficult, with limited success thus far, prompting at least one center to consider orthotopic heart transplantation for this group of newborns (Bailey et al., 1988).

Prognosis. All 86 infants with aortic atresia in the NERICP were dead by the first anniversary of their birth. Of those with mitral atresia and hypoplasia of the left ventricle, only 10 of 60 (17 per cent) survived to their first birthday. With palliation, the results are somewhat better.

Of 104 newborns undergoing a Norwood first-stage repair between 1985 and 1987, there were 30 early and 11 late deaths (Pigott et al., 1988), a mortality rate of 40 per cent. There are little data so far on the second stage of repair, but it appears that about two-thirds have survived this operation for an overall survival of this two-stage palliative approach of 25 to 33 per cent.

Early results of the orthotopic transplantation have demonstrated 21 survivors out of 25 newborns operated on with no late deaths, with 4 to 40 months follow-up and no major complications thus far (Boucek et al., 1990).

Which of these approaches (or others that may come along) is superior will become more obvious in the years to come, but therapy for these newborns remains a major challenge.

VENTRICULAR SEPTAL DEFECTS

Anatomy. Ventricular septal defects may be isolated, part of a more complex cardiac anomaly such as TOF, or associated with other congenital cardiac defects such as coarctation of the aorta with a ventricular defect. In this section, only the isolated defect will be considered; the more complicated types are discussed further on in the chapter. Ventricular defects have been classified according to their location in the ventricular septum. The most common site is the membranous portion of the septum that lies between the crista supraventricularis and the papillary muscle of the conus when the heart is viewed from the right ventricular side. Less common sites are the area above crista (subpulmonary), the muscular portion of the septum below the tricuspid valve (atrioventricular canal), and the anterior trabecular portion of the ventricular septum near the apex of the right ventricle. The size of ventricular septal defects varies: They can be as small as a pinhole or large enough to make the ventricular septum almost completely absent. In about 10 per cent of infants, multiple defects are present.

Incidence. Ventricular septal defects are the most common congenital cardiac anomaly. Rowe and co-workers found 20 newborns with ventricular septal defects among 13,653 live births in New Zealand between 1960 and 1963. In the NERICP, there were 374 cases of infants with *large* ventricular defects among slightly more than 1,000,000 live births in the six New England states between 1969 and 1974, representing an incidence of one per 3000 live births. If results from echocardiograph are included, the incidence was 0.869 per 1000 live births in the Baltimore-Washington Infant Study (Ferencz et al., 1985).

Hemodynamics. Since the right and left sides of the heart are arranged in parallel before birth, the presence of a large communication at the ventricular level in addition to the normal ductus connection at the great vessel level does not significantly alter the fetal circulation. After birth, the hemodynamics depend on the size of the defect and the pulmonary and systemic vascular resistances. If the defect is large (>1 cm^2/m^2 body size or equal to at least half the size of the aortic valve), it offers no resistance to flow. The systolic pressures in both ventricles and both great vessels are approximately equal, and the degree of intracardiac shunting is determined by the systemic and pulmonary vascular resistances. For the first few hours of life, the resistances are about equal, and little shunting (left-to-right or right-to-left) occurs. Over the following hours, days, and weeks, the pulmonary vascular resistance gradually falls, increasing the proportion of blood ejected by the left ventricle that goes through the ventricular septal defect into the pulmonary artery. When the pulmonary blood flow is about three times greater than the systemic flow, the left ventricle can no longer accommodate the volume load, and signs and symptoms of congestive heart failure develop. In full-term infants with an isolated ventricular defect, this usually occurs late in the 1st or during the 2nd month of life, but failure is occasionally seen earlier, sometimes in the 1st week, presumably owing to a more rapid fall in the pulmonary vascular resistance. The left-to-right shunting at the ventricular level results in increased flow in the pulmonary artery, pulmonary vein, left atrium, and left ventricle, with the latter chamber ejecting blood directly into the pulmonary artery. The right atrium and right ventricle are not volume overloaded, but in the presence of a large defect the right ventricle must generate pressures equal to those of the left ventricle, so there is usually right ventricular hypertrophy without significant dilation.

If the ventricular defect is small, it does offer resistance to flow, and the pressures in the two ventricles may differ. These infants are a heterogeneous group, with the hemodynamics depending on the size of the hole rather than the pulmonary vascular resistance. If the defect is very small, the right ventricular and pulmonary artery pressures may be normal and the pulmonary blood flow less than twice the systemic flow. These infants are rarely symptomatic, and a murmur is usually the sole indication of heart disease. If the defect is larger, the right heart pressures may be close to systemic pressures, with flow ratios exceeding 3:1. These infants may have congestive heart failure.

Clinical Features. Newborns with a small ventricular septal defect have a grade 2 or 3/6 high-pitched, pansystolic murmur along the left sternal border and are asymptomatic.

Even if the defect is large, the elevated pulmonary resistance prevents significant shunting in the first few days and weeks of life, so heart failure is unusual. Later, as the left-to-right shunt increases, signs and symptoms of congestive failure—tachypnea, tiring with feeding, poor weight gain, diaphoresis, and hepatomegaly—develop.

On physical examination, the cardiac impulse is usually hyperactive and the apex is displaced laterally. A systolic thrill and grade 4/6 pansystolic murmur can be appreciated along the left sternal border. If the left-to-right shunt is large, a mid-diastolic rumble is audible at the apex from the increased flow across a structurally normal mitral valve. If the pulmonary artery pressure is increased, the pulmonary component of the second heart sound is single or narrowly split and accentuated.

Although the electrocardiogram is usually an accurate tool for assessing the hemodynamics in older children with a ventricular septal defect, it is less valuable in the newborn because the normal pattern of right ventricular predominance masks the typical changes. A normal progression from right to left ventricular predominance over the 1st month is usual for a small ventricular septal defect, and an increase in both right and left ventricular forces over the 1st month of life is typical of a large ventricular defect with pulmonary hypertension.

The chest film is a better tool than the electrocardiogram in the evaluation of a newborn with a ventricular defect. If the heart is normal in size and the pulmonary vascular markings are normal, the left-to-right shunt is small. With large shunts, the cardiac silhouette is enlarged, and the pulmonary vascular markings are increased and, if there is an elevated pulmonary venous pressure, indistinct (Fig. 63–31). The two-dimensional echocardiogram can usually allow visualization of defects that are larger than 2 mm and rule out associated cardiac anomalies (Bierman et al., 1980) (Fig. 63–32). Doppler assessment of the flow through the defect gives an estimate of the interventricular gradient and may be helpful to estimate the size. Color Doppler can frequently pick up very small defects that cannot be imaged otherwise.

Cardiac catheterization is unnecessary in asymptomatic newborns. In symptomatic infants, we defer catheterization until surgery is contemplated if the ventricular septal defect has been localized and more complicated disease ruled out on two-dimensional echocardiogram. The purposes of the catheterization are to measure the magnitude of the left-to-right shunt and pulmonary artery pressure and resistance, to locate the position and number of the ventricular defect(s), and to exclude other anomalies. There is a large increase in saturation between the superior vena cava and pulmonary artery that is usually located between the right atrium and ventricle but occasionally seen between the vena cava and right atrium if an atrial septal defect or stretched foramen ovale is present. Angio-

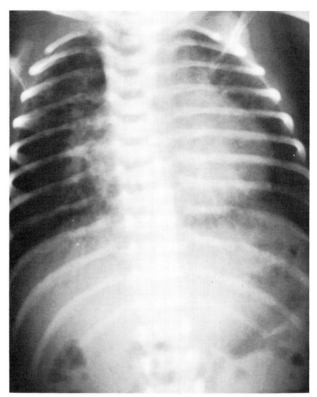

FIGURE 63–31. Plain anteroposterior chest radiograph in a newborn with a large ventricular septal defect. The heart is enlarged, and the pulmonary blood flow is increased.

cardiography in the left ventricle in the left anterior oblique position with cranial angulation (axial oblique) outlines most of the membranous ventricular septum, and the four-chamber, or hepatoclavicular, view outlines the posterior septum (Fig. 63–33). An aortogram is necessary to exclude a coexisting patent ductus arteriosus if the pulmonary artery pressure is elevated.

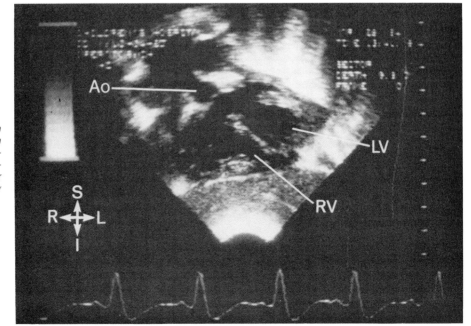

FIGURE 63–32. Perimembranous VSD in subxiphoid long-axis view. (Reprinted from Sanders, S. P.: Echocardiography and related techniques in the diagnosis of congenital heart defects: Part II, atrioventricular valves and ventricles. Echocardiography 1:333, 1984.)

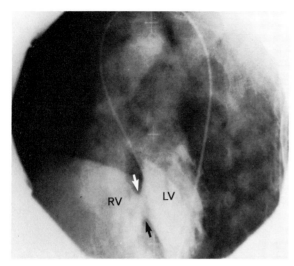

FIGURE 63–33. Left ventricular angiogram in the hepatoclavicular "four-chamber" projection using 40 degrees of left anterior obliquity and 40 degrees of cranial angulation. A large midmuscular ventricular septal defect is outlined by the arrows. LV, left ventricle; RV, right ventricle.

Diagnosis. As emphasized by Rowe and co-workers, a baby who has congestive heart failure and a systolic murmur in the first 2 weeks of life is not likely to have an isolated ventricular defect. If cyanosis is absent, coarctation (with or without a ventricular defect), critical aortic stenosis, or the hypoplastic left heart syndrome is more likely. They can usually be differentiated by the absence of femoral pulses in coarctation, the presence of left ventricular hypertrophy with strain on the electrocardiogram in aortic stenosis, and the appearance of a shock-like picture in the hypoplastic left heart syndrome. If cyanosis is present, truncus arteriosus, tricuspid atresia, or TOF must be considered. In the asymptomatic newborn with a murmur, mild aortic stenosis, valvular or peripheral pulmonary stenosis, and TOF can be confused, especially if the lesions are mild.

Treatment. One must treat newborns with a ventricular septal defect with the knowledge that many, if not most, of small defects will close spontaneously and that up to 20 per cent of large defects will also get much smaller or close (Fyler et al., 1980; Mesko et al., 1973).

Newborns with a small or moderate size ventricular septal defect often require no treatment. For those with mild heart failure, digoxin and diuretics and the usual anticongestive measures often suffice. Afterload reduction with hydralazine is conceptually attractive but has not yet had a controlled trial to demonstrate efficacy or safety. Occasionally, a child with a large defect responds poorly to anticongestive measures with continued severe heart failure and poor weight gain in spite of maximal medical management. For these infants, reparative surgery is necessary.

Prognosis. The prognosis for the newborn with a small ventricular septal defect is excellent. In one study of 50 children, it was predicted from actuarial analysis that 75 per cent of the defects would close by 10 years of age (Alpert et al., 1979). Many of the large defects that present during the first weeks of life will also become significantly smaller, and some of these will close. Even for the large defect that requires surgical closure, the results have dramatically improved in the past few years, so that correction can be accomplished with risks of 5 per cent or less (Rein et al., 1977).

ATRIOVENTRICULAR CANAL DEFECTS

Anatomy. The atrioventricular canal portion of the heart is formed from the endocardial cushions, a mass of embryonic mesenchymal tissue that forms the structures in the middle portion of the heart: the lower portion of the atrial septum, the upper portion of the ventricular septum, and the septal portions of the mitral and tricuspid valves. Any one or all of the components may be abnormal in an endocardial cushion defect, with the spectrum of abnormalities ranging from an isolated cleft in the mitral or tricuspid valve to a complete atrioventricular canal with a huge deficiency of the atrial and ventricular septum and a common atrioventricular valve (Piccoli et al., 1979). A variety of classifications have been proposed, but the tremendous spectrum of variations makes sharp distinctions difficult, and we prefer a description of the anomalies: atrial septal defect of the ostium primum type, ventricular septal defect of the A-V canal type, clefts of the mitral or tricuspid valve, single atrioventricular valve, and complete atrioventricular canal. Atrioventricular canal defects are the most common type of heart disease present in Down syndrome. In Fyler's 1980 series, 45 per cent of infants with atrioventricular canal defects had trisomy 21. Other cardiac anomalies are often present in association with atrioventricular canal defects. Heterotaxy syndromes, single ventricle, double outlet right ventricle, transposition, and pulmonary stenosis are the most common.

Incidence. There were 119 infants with atrioventricular canal defects in the NERICP, an incidence of one per 9000 live births. Infants with atrioventricular canal defects represented about 5 per cent of all infants with heart disease.

Hemodynamics. The hemodynamics of atrioventricular canal defects may be complex. In 1974, Rudolph noted that shunting in these infants may be dependent or obligatory. Dependent shunting through either an atrial or ventricular septal defect is a function of the pulmonary and systemic vascular resistance. In the newborn period, when the pulmonary vascular resistance is high, little left-to-right shunt may be present. As the pulmonary resistance drops over the first days and weeks of life, the pulmonary blood flow will increase, eventually leading to congestive heart failure as the left ventricle becomes overloaded. Obligatory shunting occurs from a high pressure chamber to a low pressure chamber, usually from ventricle to atrium, and is independent of resistance. In atrioventricular canal defects, obligatory shunting is usually from left ventricle through the mitral portion of the A-V valve into the left atrium and across the atrial defect into the right atrium or, less frequently, directly into the right atrium. This left-to-right shunt due to A-V valve regurgitation is independent of the status of the pulmonary vasculature and may occur even with the high pulmonary vascular resistance seen in the newborn period.

The degree of intracardiac shunting at any given time is the result of a complex interplay between the pulmonary and systemic resistances affecting the dependent shunting and the obligatory shunting. In the first weeks of life, however, when the pulmonary vascular resistance tends to be high, the newborns who present with congestive failure tend to have obligatory shunts due to A-V valve regurgitation.

Clinical Manifestations. When there is only an ostium primum atrial defect present, the children rarely, if ever, are seen in the neonatal period. Infants with an isolated ventricular defect present similarly to the previously described newborns with membranous or muscular ventricular defects.

The age at presentation of infants with a complete A-V canal is related to the presence of A-V valve regurgitation; if it is severe, the infants may present in the first 1 or 2 weeks of life with the usual manifestations of heart failure, tachycardia, tachypnea, feeding difficulties, and sweating. If the atrioventricular valves are competent, infants present later in the 1st month or even in the 2nd month of life. The precordium is usually hyperactive on palpation, with the maximal impulse displaced laterally and inferiorly. A thrill at the lower left sternal border is often present. If there is significant atrial shunting, the first heart sound is accentuated. In the usual case with pulmonary hypertension, the pulmonary component of the second heart sound is loud. Heart murmurs may be quite variable, but usually there is a loud pansystolic murmur at the lower left sternal border and a flow rumble across the mitral valve best heard at the apex. In the presence of mitral regurgitation, a pansystolic murmur at the apex is audible, but it may be hard to distinguish from the murmur of the ventricular septal defect.

The electrocardiographic features in infants with atrioventricular canal defects are very characteristic. Because of posterior displacement of the atrioventricular node, His bundle, and distal left bundle as well as hypoplasia of the anterior portion of the left fascicle and an early origin of the left bundle, there is a characteristic superior QRS axis (0 to −150 degrees) that on vectorcardiogram is inscribed counterclockwise in the frontal plane (Feldt and Titus, 1976). These children also have a prolonged P–R interval, biatrial hypertrophy, and biventricular hypertrophy (Fig. 63–34).

The heart is almost invariably enlarged on the chest radiograph, and the pulmonary blood flow is increased and often congested. The size of the cardiac silhouette is often out of proportion with the increased pulmonary blood flow, presumably owing to the A-V valve regurgitation.

On two-dimensional echocardiogram, the characteristic features of complete A-V canal are visible on subxiphoid four-chamber views, and these features include the posterior inflow ventricular defect and the common atrioventricular valve. Color flow Doppler studies are useful for the identification and quantification of A-V valve regurgitation (Fig. 63–35).

At cardiac catheterization, there is a great step-up in saturation between the vena cava and the right atrium that is due to the left-to-right shunt at the atrial level; an

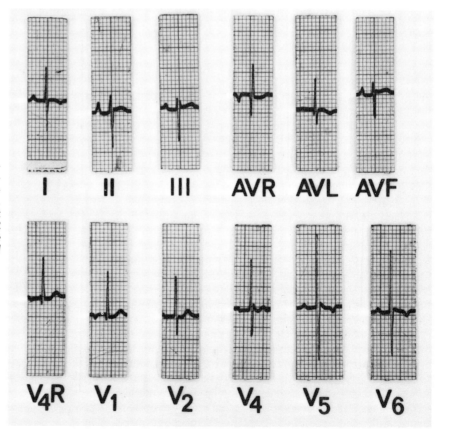

FIGURE 63–34. Electrocardiogram of a 1-week-old newborn with a complete atrioventricular canal. The QRS axis is −90 degrees with a predominant negative deflection in leads II, III, and AVF. The tall peaked P wave in lead II reflects right atrial hypertrophy, and the upright T waves in V₄R and V₁ suggest right ventricular hypertrophy. There is also first degree heart block with a P-R interval of 0.17 seconds.

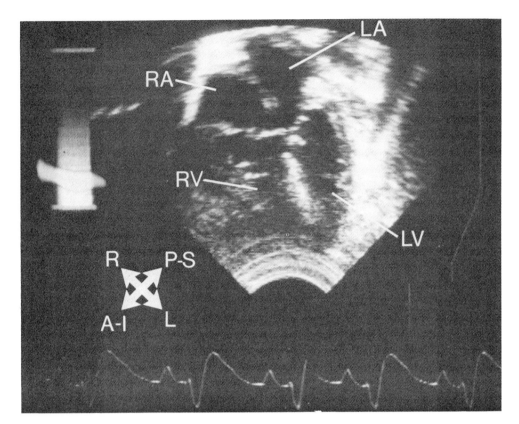

FIGURE 63–35. Apical four-chamber view in complete atrioventricular canal. Notice defect in the lower portion of the atrial septum, AV canal portion of the ventricular septum, and common AV valve bridging the defect. LA, left atrium; LV, left ventricle; RA, right atrium; RV, right ventricle. (Reprinted from Sanders, S. P.: Echocardiography and related techniques in the diagnosis of congenital heart defects: Part II, atrioventricular valves and ventricles. Echocardiography 1:333, 1984.)

additional step-up at the ventricular level is often present. The right and left atrial pressures are equal, as are the right and left ventricular pressures. In the absence of pulmonary stenosis, the systolic pressures in the pulmonary artery and aorta are equal, but the diastolic pressure in the pulmonary artery may be lower because of increased compliance of the pulmonary bed. In the past, we have used the right and left anterior oblique projections for our left ventricular angiocardiogram. In the early 1980s, we switched to the hepatoclavicular, or four-chambered, view because this allows optimal visualization of the atrioventricular valve(s), ventricular septum, and degree of regurgitation (Soto et al., 1981) (Fig. 63–36).

Diagnosis. Atrioventricular canal defects should be considered in all children who show congestive heart failure, a left-to-right shunt, and a superior axis on the electrocardiogram. Infants with tricuspid atresia without significant pulmonary stenosis may also demonstrate a large heart with increased pulmonary blood flow on the radiograph and a superior axis on the electrocardiogram, but they are desaturated and almost invariably have pure left ventricular hypertrophy on the electrocardiogram, as opposed to the right or biventricular hypertrophy seen in infants with atrioventricular canal defects. Echocardiography can resolve any remaining questions.

Treatment. When congestive failure is present, the usual medical management consisting of digoxin, diuretics, and high-calorie formula should be started. In some infants, this will suffice for many months, but frequently surgery is required because of persistent congestive heart failure and failure to thrive. Banding of the pulmonary

artery to increase pulmonary resistance and thus decrease pulmonary flow has been the procedure of choice. In the past the risks have been considerable in some series (30 to 40 per cent) (Epstein et al., 1979) probably due to the fact that the band is excellent palliation for dependent

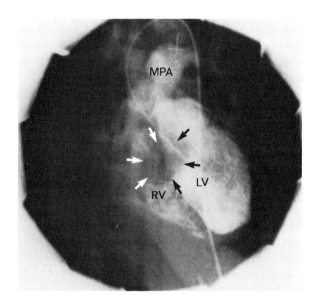

FIGURE 63–36. A left ventricular angiogram in the hepatoclavicular "four-chamber" projection in a newborn with a complete atrioventricular canal. The ventricular defect allows dye to enter the right ventricle. During atrial systole, unopacified blood is pumped into the ventricles, outlining the common atrioventricular valve (arrows) straddling the ventricular septum. LV = left ventricle; MPA = main pulmonary artery; RV = right ventricle.

shunting but has no benefit and, in fact, may be detrimental if there is obligatory shunting. Recently surgical risks in this group have been reduced to approximately 5 per cent (Silverman et al., 1983). Some have attempted to repair infants with A-V canal in a primary operation by dividing the atrioventricular valve, closing the atrial and ventricular portions of the defect, and suspending the reconstructed mitral and tricuspid valves on the patch. Although, this remains a significant undertaking, especially in the newborn, the risks (current mortality rate at Children's Hospital in Boston from 1987 to 1988 of 4 per 72 infants, or 6 per cent) seem better than those associated with banding.

Prognosis. In 1980, Fyler and co-workers reported that in the Regional Infant Cardiac Program (1969 to 1974), the 1-year survival rate for all patients with atrioventricular canal was only 44 per cent. If the infants with Down syndrome are excluded, the survival rates are only slightly better, 50 per cent. The high mortality is probably partly due to the high incidence of severe extracardiac anomalies present in this group of newborns. Recent advances in surgical techniques have undoubtedly increased the survival rates.

ARTERIOVENOUS FISTULAS

Anatomy. Arteriovenous fistulas are a rare cause of congestive heart failure in the newborn. There are two types of fistulous connections: a direct communication between an artery and vein bypassing the capillary bed and, less commonly in the newborn, an angioma with multiple arterial and venous supply. Although A-V fistulas causing heart failure have been described in the subclavian, internal mammary, and vertebral arteries and hemangiomas may be found in the skin, pelvis, and coronary arteries, most of the newborns with heart failure have either a cerebral A-V fistula or a hemangioma of the liver (Quero Jimenez et al., 1977).

Incidence. In the NERICP, there were 11 arteriovenous fistulas, representing an incidence of one per 100,000 live births. There were eight cerebral A-V fistulas and three systemic fistulas—one in the arm, one in the neck, and one in the liver (Fyler et al., 1980).

Hemodynamics. Atrioventricular fistulas are present in utero but do not seem to cause significant hemodynamic embarrassment. At birth, the babies are well developed without evidence of heart failure, but profound heart failure may develop within a few hours. This dramatic change is a result of the shift from the parallel to the in series circulation after birth. In utero, the systemic venous return including the A-V fistula is divided into two streams. Part of the venous return goes through the right heart chambers into the pulmonary artery and the rest goes through the foramen ovale to the left-sided heart chambers. After birth, the entire systemic return including return from the fistula must pass through the right heart as well as the pulmonary arteries and then to the left heart and aorta. In addition, the removal of the low resistance placenta circuit after birth increases the systemic resistance and forces more blood through the A-V fistula. These

changes occurring with the transitional circulation suddenly impart a large volume overload to the right and left sides of the heart. The neonatal heart is unable to tolerate the increased venous return, and heart failure and circulatory collapse result.

Clinical Manifestations. Congestive heart failure with tachypnea, dyspnea, and feeding difficulties are usually present within the first few days of life. Cyanosis is occasionally seen secondary to pulmonary venous desaturation and right-to-left shunting at the atrial or ductal levels (Cumming, 1980). The peripheral pulses are generally diminished but may be increased in the arteries feeding the fistula. Infants with a cerebral A-V fistula may have dilated veins in the neck. Cardiac enlargement with a hyperdynamic cardiac impulse is present on palpation, and a soft systolic ejection murmur over the semilunar valves or a diastolic flow murmur across the atrioventricular valves may be audible on auscultation. Occasionally, a continuous bruit may be heard over the fistula.

Right axis deviation, right ventricular hypertrophy, and ST–T wave changes are usually present on the electrocardiogram.

On the chest radiograph, there is generalized cardiac enlargement with increased pulmonary blood flow and pulmonary venous congestion. In infants with a cerebral A-V fistula, the superior mediastinum is often widened because of dilatation of the ascending aorta, carotid arteries, jugular vein, and superior vena cava. All cardiac chambers are enlarged on M-mode echocardiogram, and the two-dimensional study demonstrates the enlarged vessels in the superior mediastinum of an infant with a cerebral A-V fistula or in the liver of an infant with a hepatic hemangioma.

At catheterization, the oximetry data demonstrate a high saturation in the vessels returning from the fistula. The pulmonary artery pressure may be elevated, often above systemic levels. Because of the large aortic run-off, the pulse pressure is usually widened. A very high systemic venous saturation in the superior vena cava with a widened pulse pressure and normal pulmonary venous return to the left atrium is diagnostic of a cerebral A-V fistula. Rather than wasting an angiocardiogram in the left ventricle to confirm the diagnosis, one should immediately perform cerebral angiography in the hope of finding a surgically responsive lesion (Holden et al., 1972) (Fig. 63–37).

Diagnosis. The presence of vascular collapse and congestive heart failure in the 1st week of life suggests myocarditis or a left-sided obstructive lesion such as hypoplastic left heart, coarctation of the aorta, or aortic stenosis. If there is a bruit over the head with normal or brisk pulses in the head vessels and dilated veins in the neck, a fistula is likely. Occasionally, the clinical diagnosis remains unclear, and echocardiography or catheterization is necessary.

Treatment. For the newborn with circulatory collapse, the usual treatment of congestive heart failure, including correction of acidosis and administration of digoxin and diuretics followed rapidly by diagnostic study, is mandatory. For newborns with cerebral A-V fistulas, there has

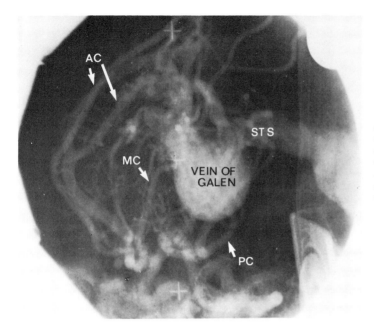

FIGURE 63–37. A lateral view of the head in a newborn with a cerebral A-V fistula. The dye was injected in the aortic arch. Large branches of the anterior, middle, and cerebral arteries drain into a dilated vein of Galen and then into the straight sinus. Both the number and the size of the arteries are abnormal. AC = anterior cerebral arteries; MC = middle cerebral arteries; PC = posterior cerebral arteries; STS = straight sinus.

been limited success with clipping the afferent vessels (Holden et al., 1972), but most infants die from congestive heart failure or neurologic complications or as a result of surgery. The treatment of infants with hepatic hemangioendothelioma is also a challenge. There have been some successes with hepatic arterial ligation, hepatic lobectomy, radiation, coil embolization and steroids, but no one method appears superior in all cases and individualization is necessary.

Prognosis. Johnston and associates (1987) reviewed the 13 patients of cerebral A-V fistula that they cared for and reviewed the literature, which included an additional 232 patients, 80 of whom were newborns. For the 70 patients in whom details were available, the mortality rate was 91 per cent (64 of 70 patients), which was equally bad whether these patients were treated medically or surgically. It remains to be seen whether or not there will be any major impact from earlier diagnosis and referral, more efficient evaluation with echocardiography or computerized tomography, and improved neurosurgical or interventional catheterization techniques.

■ DIFFERENTIAL DIAGNOSIS OF HEART DISEASE IN THE NEWBORN

The principal characteristics of common congenital and acquired diseases of the heart have been reviewed in preceding discussions and are also considered in the next chapter. In this section, the distinctive features of each condition are used to arrive at the correct diagnosis. Since most of the readers of this book are pediatricians or neonatologists rather than pediatric cardiologists, the differential diagnosis is based on the tools available to the noncardiologist in a hospital setting (i.e., history, physical examination, chest radiograph, electrocardiogram, and arterial blood gases).

Differential diagnosis is difficult in some respects. One problem is the considerable overlap in the clinical manifestations of congenital and acquired heart disease in the

newborn. Also, common diseases occasionally present with uncommon manifestations, and features of uncommon diseases may mimic the typical characteristics of their more common counterparts. Nevertheless, it is still worthwhile to attempt some distinctions without specialized tests, because the management of the newborn with, for example, a small ventricular septal defect differs so greatly from that of the infant with transposition. It must be remembered, however, that several studies have confirmed that even experienced pediatric cardiologists diagnose correctly in only 60 to 70 per cent of cases in which neither echocardiography nor cardiac catheterization is used.

As mentioned in Chapter 62, infants with heart disease present with heart murmurs, dysrhythmias, cyanosis, or congestive heart failure. In the absence of one or more of the latter manifestations of heart disease, heart murmurs do not indicate medical emergencies, although a persistent murmur probably warrants further studies, including chest radiography, electrocardiography, and elective referral to a pediatric cardiologist.

It is easy for one to auscultate a significant dysrhythmia using a stethoscope. Symptomatic dysrhythmias are usually tachyarrhythmias (supraventricular tachycardia) or bradyarrhythmias (heart block) and are reviewed in Chapter 65.

The diagnostic dilemmas in neonatal heart disease involve the infant with profound cyanosis or congestive failure. Neonates with profound cyanosis rarely have significant heart failure, and infants with congestive heart failure are rarely profoundly cyanotic, although they may have some arterial hypoxemia. Each group is reviewed separately.

CYANOSIS

"Profound cyanosis" by definition involves a PaO$_2$ of less than 50 mm Hg in both room air and 100 per cent O$_2$. A schema for the differential diagnosis of cyanotic newborns, based on findings obtained from chest radio-

TABLE 63–3. Cyanotic Congenital Heart Disease (Pao₂ <50 mm Hg, Fio₂ 0.21, 1.0)

DISEASE	RADIOGRAPH		ELECTROCARDIOGRAM		MURMURS
	Pulmonary Blood Flow	Heart Size	Ventricular Predominance	QRS Axis	
Transposition with IVS	Normal or increased				
TAPVR	Congested				
Ebstein anomaly	Decreased	Massive	RVH		
Tricuspid atresia	Decreased	Normal	LVH	0 to −90	
Pulmonary atresia, IVS	Decreased	Increased	LVH	30 to +90	Regurgitant
Pulmonary stenosis, IVS	Decreased	Increased	RVH	30 to +90	Ejection
Tetralogy of Fallot, VSD, and pulmonary stenosis	Decreased	Normal	RVH	>90	Ejection
Tetralogy of Fallot with pulmonary atresia	Decreased	Normal	RVH	>90	None or continuous

Abbreviations: IVS = intact ventricular septum, LVH = left ventricular hypertrophy, RVH = right ventricular hypertrophy, TAPVR = total anomalous pulmonary venous return, VSD = ventricular septal defect.

graphs, electrocardiograms, and physical examination, is presented in Table 63–3. Newborns with heart disease may be profoundly cyanotic because of either right-to-left intracardiac shunting or transposition of the great arteries with poor mixing between the systemic and pulmonary circuits. In the former case, the pulmonary blood flow is markedly reduced because of shunting away from the lungs; in the latter situation, pulmonary blood flow is normal or increased. Thus, a newborn who is profoundly cyanotic but who shows normal or increased pulmonary blood flow on radiographs almost certainly has *transposition of the great arteries with an intact ventricular septum*. Another virtually pathognomonic pattern of the chest radiograph in a profoundly cyanotic neonate is pulmonary venous congestion that suggests *total anomalous pulmonary venous return with obstruction*. The remainder of newborns with severe cyanosis have decreased pulmonary vascular markings on chest radiographs. If the heart is massively enlarged on the radiograph and the degree of right ventricular hypertrophy on the electrocardiogram is normal, the newborn probably has *Ebstein disease* with severe tricuspid regurgitation. Left ventricular hypertrophy on the electrocardiogram in the newborn with cyanosis and diminished pulmonary blood flow on the radiograph suggest a hypoplastic right ventricle. If the QRS is superior (−0 to −90 degrees) in the standard limb leads, *tricuspid atresia* is probably present. If the QRS axis is inferior (+30 to 90 degrees), *pulmonary stenosis with an intact ventricular septum (IVS)* is the most likely diagnosis if the child has an ejection murmur at the left upper sternal border. *Pulmonary atresia with an intact ventricular septum* is the most probable diagnosis if there is no murmur or only a regurgitant murmur of tricuspid incompetence along the left lower sternal border.

If the cyanotic infant with decreased pulmonary blood flow has right ventricular predominance on the electrocardiogram and cardiac enlargement on the radiograph, pulmonary stenosis without right ventricular hypoplasia is usually present. If cardiac size is normal, TOF *(ventricular septal defect and pulmonary stenosis)* is the most likely diagnosis if there is an ejection murmur. *Ventricular septal defect with pulmonary atresia* is the most likely diagnosis if there are no murmurs or continuous murmurs from aortopulmonary collaterals.

This schema does not differentiate the rare and more complex forms of cyanotic heart disease, such as single ventricle, L or D transposition, or atrioventricular canal defects with pulmonary stenosis or atresia. One must employ either echocardiography or angiography in order to distinguish these conditions.

CONGESTIVE HEART FAILURE

Myocardial dysfunction, pressure overload, and obligatory volume overload lesions are usually observed during the 1st week of life; dependent volume overload lesions are not usually seen until the 2nd to 4th weeks, when the pulmonary vascular resistance has dropped enough to allow significant left-to-right shunting. The most common causes of congestive heart failure during the 1st week of life are listed in Table 63–4.

Newborns with *transient myocardial ischemia* almost invariably have a history of prenatal or perinatal distress. They often have low Apgar scores and very early onset of respiratory distress. The newborn with in utero *dysrhythmias*, usually supraventricular tachycardia or complete heart block, may have heart failure before or immediately after birth; these infants are distinguished by a

TABLE 63–4. Causes of Congestive Heart Failure in the First Week of Life

DISEASE	HISTORY	PULSES	EKG	PRECORDIUM
Transient myocardial ischemia	+			
Dysrhythmias	±			
Arteriovenous fistula	—	Increased		
Coarctation of the aorta (interrupted aortic arch)	—	Asymmetric		
Aortic stenosis	—	Decreased	LVH	
Hypoplastic left heart syndrome	—	Decreased	RVH	Hyperactive
Myocarditis	—	Decreased	RVH	Decreased

very rapid or slow pulse. Newborns with cerebral or, less commonly, hepatic *arteriovenous fistulas* usually have a wide pulse pressure and bounding pulses, especially in the arteries feeding the fistula, in contrast with the diminished pulses expected in a newborn with severe heart failure and low cardiac output. In the infant with *coarctation of the aorta or interrupted aortic arch,* the pulses are usually asymmetric; that is, they may be normal or increased in the right arm proximal to the obstruction and diminished in the legs. The pulse in the left arm is variable, since the left subclavian artery may be proximal or distal to the obstruction. Newborns with aortic stenosis, hypoplastic left heart syndrome, and myocarditis have diminished pulses throughout. Those with *aortic stenosis* and a normal-sized left ventricle usually have left ventricular hypertrophy with strain on the electrocardiogram, whereas those with the hypoplastic left heart syndrome or myocarditis have the normal right ventricular predominance for age. One can usually distinguish these latter two lesions on the basis of precordial features. In the infant with *hypoplastic left heart syndrome,* there is a hyperactive precordium, which reflects increased pulmonary blood flow; in the newborn with *myocarditis,* the precordium is quiet. If doubt remains, the M-mode echocardiogram demonstrates a dilated, minimally contractile left ventricle in myocarditis and hypoplasia of the ascending aorta in the hypoplastic left heart syndrome.

The differential diagnosis of the infant with congestive heart failure between the 2nd and 4th weeks of life is complex, since in addition to the previously discussed lesions that occasionally are first seen late, there are many cases of dependent left-to-right intracardiac shunting that appear as the pulmonary resistance falls over the 1st month. One helpful way of distinguishing these conditions is to separate those patients with left-to-right or no shunting (who are acyanotic) from those with intracardiac right-to-left shunting who have some degree of arterial hypoxemia. If the newborns in the former group are placed in 100 per cent oxygen for 10 minutes, the PaO_2 increases considerably, usually above 150 to 200 mm Hg. In those infants with right-to-left intracardiac shunting, the PaO_2 may increase little with the increase in dissolved oxygen in the pulmonary veins, but the mixture of pulmonary venous with systemic venous blood prevents the PaO_2 from exceeding 150 mm Hg.

Acyanotic newborns (Table 63–5) may have cardiac failure with pressure overload (coarctation of the aorta, aortic stenosis), myocardial dysfunction (myocarditis, endocardial fibroelastosis), or volume overload (patent ductus arteriosus, aortopulmonary window ventricular septal defect, atrioventricular canal defects, arteriovenous fistula). Occasionally, a lesion causes both a volume and pressure overload, as is seen in coarctation of the aorta with a ventricular septal defect.

Children with isolated pressure overload or cardiomyopathies show cardiac enlargement with pulmonary venous congestion on radiographs but do not usually have increased pulmonary blood flow. Those with isolated *coarctation of the aorta* have differential pulses and blood pressure between the arms and legs. Newborns with *aortic stenosis* show a systolic ejection murmur at the right upper sternal border, a systolic click at the apex, and left ventricular hypertrophy with strain on the electrocardiogram.

TABLE 63–5. Causes of Congestive Heart Failure During the 2nd Through 4th Weeks of Life

Acyanotic (PaO$_2$ > 150 mm Hg in 100 per cent O$_2$)
　Coarctation of the aorta
　Aortic stenosis
　Myocarditis
　Endocardial fibroelastosis
　Patent ductus arteriosus
　Aortopulmonary window
　Arteriovenous fistula
　Ventricular septal defect
　Atrioventricular canal defects

Cyanotic (PaO$_2$ < 150 mm Hg in 100 per cent O$_2$)
　Hypoplastic left heart syndrome
　Total anomalous pulmonary venous return
　Truncus arteriosus
　Transposition and a ventricular septal defect
　Tricuspid atresia and a ventricular septal defect
　Single ventricle

Often one may need to initiate anticongestive measures in order to improve cardiac output enough for the murmur to be audible. Newborns with cardiomyopathies have symmetric pulses and no murmurs or, rarely, a murmur of mitral regurgitation. Those infants with *myocarditis* usually have diminished QRS voltages with ST–T wave changes, whereas those with *endocardial fibroelastosis* have increased QRS voltages, especially across the left precordium.

Left-to-right shunting is the most common cause of heart failure late in the 1st month of life. Characteristically, there is increased pulmonary blood flow with cardiomegaly on the chest radiograph (see Fig. 63–5C). The shunting is usually at the great vessel or ventricular level, because the relative ventricular compliances prevent a large shunt at the atrial level in this age range. Great vessel shunts are characterized by left ventricular volume overload, with enlargement of the left atrium and left ventricle and bounding pulses due to run-off from the aorta in diastole. Differentiation between *patent ductus arteriosus* and *aortopulmonary window* is accomplished with echocardiography or angiography, although even in full-term newborns, the incidence of patent ductus arteriosus is more than 16 times greater than that of aortopulmonary window. Infants with arteriovenous fistulas usually have a bruit over the head or liver.

Newborns with ventricular level shunts show cardiomegaly and increased blood flow on radiographs, with normal or symmetrically diminished pulses. Those infants with a ventricular septal defect usually have a rightward QRS axis (+90 to +180 degrees), whereas those with an endocardial cushion defect have a superior counterclockwise loop in the frontal plane, with a QRS axis of −30 to −120 degrees.

The differential diagnosis of the remaining lesions, those that present with arterial hypoxemia (PO$_2$ < 150 in 100 per cent oxygen) and congestive heart failure later in the 1st month of life (Table 63–5), is especially difficult because the signs and symptoms are remarkably similar and exact diagnosis is usually impossible without echocardiography and, frequently, angiocardiography.

Both *hypoplastic left heart syndrome* and *total anomalous pulmonary venous return* are associated with pulmonary venous obstruction on the chest radiograph and right ventricular predominance on the electrocardiogram. Infants with hypoplastic left heart syndrome often are grayish and have diminished pulses throughout as the ductus arteriosus constricts and consequently obstructs systemic blood flow. One may use either M-mode or two-dimensional echocardiography in determining the diagnosis.

One can usually discriminate newborns with *truncus arteriosus* on the basis of the mild cyanosis, bounding pulses, and increased pulmonary blood flow visible on chest radiographs. Infants who present with a clinical picture similar to that of a large ventricular septal defect (with gradually increasing congestive heart failure, a hyperactive precordium, and cardiomegaly) and who, on the hyperoxia test demonstrate that they are cyanotic, usually have (1) *transposition of the great arteries with a ventricular septal defect* if the electrocardiogram shows right ventricular hypertrophy, (2) *tricuspid atresia* if the electrocardiogram reveals left ventricular hypertrophy with a superior QRS axis (0 to −90 degrees), or (3) a *single ventricle* of the left ventricular type if there is left ventricular hypertrophy and an inferior QRS axis (+90 to +180 degrees).

■ REFERENCES

Alboliras, E. T., Julsrud, P. R., Danielson, G. K., et al.: Definitive operation for pulmonary atresia with intact ventricular septum. Results in twenty patients. J. Thorac. Cardiovasc. Surg. *93*:454, 1987.

Alpert, B. S., Cook, D. H., Varghese, P. J., and Rowe, R. D.: Spontaneous closure of small ventricular septal defects: Ten year follow up. Pediatrics *63*:204, 1979.

Anderson, C., Edmonds, L., and Erickson, J.: Patent ductus arteriosus and ventricular septal defect: Trends in reported frequency. Am. J. Epidemiol. *107*:281, 1978.

Bailey, L. L., Assaad, A. N., Trim, R. F., et al.: Orthotopic transplantation during early infancy as therapy for incurable heart disease. Ann. Surg. *208*:279, 1988.

Bierman, F. Z., Fellows, K., and Williams, R. G.: Prospective identification of ventricular septal defects in infancy using subxiphoid two-dimensional echocardiography. Circulation *62*:807, 1980.

Boucek, M. M., Kanakriyeh, M. S., Mathis, C. M., et al.: Cardiac transplantation in infancy: Donors and recipients. J. Pediatr. *116*:171, 1990.

Calder, A. L., Co, E. E., Sage, M. D.: Coronary arterial abnormalities in pulmonary atresia with intact ventricular septum. Am. J. Cardiol. *59*:436, 1987.

Calder, L., Van Praagh, R., Van Praagh, S., et al.: Truncus arteriosus communis. Clinical, angiocardiographic and pathologic findings in 100 patients. Am. Heart J. *92*:23, 1976.

Castaneda, A. R., Norwood, W. I., Jonas, R. A., et al.: Transposition of the great arteries and an intact ventricular septum: Anatomic repair in the neonate. Ann. Thorac. Surg. *35*:438, 1984.

Celoria, G. C., and Patton, R. B.: Congenital absence of the aortic arch. Am. Heart J. *58*:4-7, 1959.

Chin, A. J., Sanders, S. P., Sherman, F., et al.: Accuracy of subcostal two-dimensional echocardiography in prospective diagnosis of total anomalous pulmonary venous connection. Am. Heart J. *113*:1153, 1987.

Coceani, F., and Olley, P. M.: The response of the ductus arteriosus to prostaglandins. J. Physiol. Pharmacol. *51*:220, 1973.

Collins-Nakai, R. L., Dick, M., Parisi-Buckley, L., Fyler, D. C., and Castaneda, A. R.: Interrupted aortic arch in infancy. J. Pediatr. *88*:959, 1976.

Cumming, G. R.: Circulation in neonates with intracranial arteriovenous fistula and cardiac failure. Am. J. Cardiol. *45*:1019, 1980.

Delisle, G., Ando, M., Calder, A. L., et al.: Total anomalous pulmonary venous connection: Report of 93 autopsied cases with emphasis on diagnostic and surgical considerations. Am. Heart J. *91*:99, 1976.

Dick, M., Fyler, D. C., and Nadas, A. S.: Tricuspid atresia: Clinical course in 101 patients. Am. J. Cardiol. *36*:327, 1975.

Ebert, P. A., Turley, K., Stanger, P., et al.: Surgical treatment of truncus arteriosus in the first six months of life. Ann. Surg. *200*:451, 1984.

Ebstein, W.: Über einen sehr seltenen Fall von Insufficienz der Valvula Tricuspidalis, bedingt durch eine angeborene hochgradige Missbildung derselben. Arch. Anat. Physiol. Wissensch. Med. 238, 1866.

Edmunds, L. H., Wagner, H. R., and Heymann, M. A.: Aortic valvulotomy in neonates. Circulation *61*:421, 1981.

Edwards, J. E.: Persistent truncus arteriosus. Am. Heart J. *92*:1, 1976.

Edwards, J. E., and Burchell, H. B.: Congenital tricuspid atresia. A classification. Med. Clin. North Am. *33*:1177, 1949.

Epstein, M. L., Moller, J. H., Amplatz, K., and Nicoloff, D. M.: Pulmonary artery banding in infants with complete atrioventricular canal. J. Thorac. Cardiovasc. Surg. *78*:28, 1979.

Feldt, R. H., and Titus, J. L.: The conduction system in persistent common atrio-ventricular canal. In Feldt, R. H. (Ed.): Atrio-Ventricular Canal Defects. Philadelphia. W. B. Saunders Co., 1976, p. 36.

Ferencz, C., Rubin, J. D., McCarter, R. J., et al.: Congenital heart disease: Prevalence of live birth. The Baltimore-Washington Infant Study. Am. J. Epidemiol. *121*:31, 1985.

Ferencz, C., Rubin, J. D., McCarter, R. J., et al.: Cardiac and noncardiac malformations: Observations in a population-based study. Teratology *35*:367, 1987.

Ferrer, P. L.: Arrhythmias in the neonate. In Roberts, N. K., and Gelband, H. (Eds.): Cardiac Arrhythmias in the Neonate, Infant, and Child. New York, Appleton-Century-Crofts, 1977.

Fontan, F., and Baudet, E.: Surgical repair of tricuspid atresia. Thorax *26*:240, 1971.

Freed, M. D., Heymann, M. A., Lewis, A. B., Roehl, S. L., and Kensey, R. C.: Prostaglandin E₁ in infants with ductus arteriosus dependent congenital heart disease. Circulation *64*:899, 1981.

Freed, M. D., Rosenthal, A., Bernhard, W. F., Litwin, S. B., and Nadas, A. S.: Critical pulmonary stenosis with a diminutive right ventricle in neonates. Circulation *48*:875, 1973.

Freedom, R. M., and Ellison, R. C.: Coronary sinus rhythm in the polysplenia syndrome. Chest *63*:952, 1973.

Freedom, R. M., Olley, P. M., Coceani, F., and Rowe, R. D.: The prostaglandin challenge test to unmask obstructed total anomalous pulmonary venous connections in asplenia syndrome. Br. Heart J. *40*:91, 1978.

Fyler, D. C., Buckley, L. P., Hellenbrand, W., et al.: Report of the New England Regional Infant Cardiac Program. Pediatrics *65*(suppl.):375, 1980.

Garson, A., Gillette, P. C., and McNamara, D. G.: Propranolol: preferred palliation for tetralogy of Fallot. Am. J. Cardiol. *47*:1098, 1981.

Gathman, G. E., and Nadas, A. S.: Total anomalous pulmonary venous connection. Clinical and physiologic observations of 75 pediatric patients. Circulation *42*:143, 1970.

Glasow, P. F., Huhta, J. C., Yoon, G. Y., et al.: Surgery without angiography for neonates with aortic arch obstruction. Int. J. Cardiol. *18*:417, 1988.

Hamilton, W. J., and Mossman, H. W.: Hamilton, Boyd, and Mossman's Human Embryology: Prenatal development of form and function. 4th ed. Baltimore, Williams & Wilkins Co., 1972.

Ho, S. Y., and Anderson, R. H.: Coarctation, tubular hypoplasia and the ductus arteriosus. Histologic study of 35 specimens. Br. Heart J. *41*:268, 1979.

Holden, A. M., Fyler, D. C., Shillito, J., Jr., and Nadas, A. S.: Congestive heart failure from intracranial arterio-venous fistula in infancy. Pediatrics *49*:30, 1972.

Humes, R. A., Feldt, R. H., Porter, C. J., et al.: The modified Fontan operation for asplenia and polysplenia syndromes. J. Thorac. Cardiovasc. Surg. *96*:212, 1988.

Ilbawi, M. N., Grieco, J., DeLeon, S. Y., et al.: Modified Blalock-Taussig shunt in newborn infants. J. Thorac. Cardiovasc. Surg. *88*:770, 1984.

Jatene, A. D., Fontes, V. F., Paulista, P. P., et al.: Anatomic correction of transposition of the great arteries. J. Thorac. Cardiovasc. Surg. *72*:364, 1976.

Johnston, I. H., Whittle, I. R., Besser, M., and Morgan, M. K.: Vein of Galen malformation: Diagnosis and management. Neurosurgery *20*:747, 1987.

Keane, J. F., Bernhard, W. F., and Nadas, A. S.: Aortic stenosis surgery in infants. Circulation *52*:1138, 1975.

Keith, J. D., Rowe, R. D., and Vlad, P.: Heart Disease in Infancy and Childhood. New York, The Macmillan Co., 1958.

Kirklin, J. W., Blackstone, E. H., Shimazaki, Y., et al.: Survival, functional status and reoperations after repair of tetrology of Fallot with pulmonary atresia. J. Thorac. Cardiovasc. Surg. *96*:102, 1988.

Kirklin, J. W., et al.: Complete transposition of the great arteries: Treatment in the modern era. Pediatr. Clin. North Am. 37:171, 1990.

Kumar, A. E., Fyler, D. C., Miettinen, O. S., and Nadas, A. S.: Ebstein's anomaly: Clinical profile and natural history. Am. J. Cardiol. 28:84, 1971.

Langman, J.: Medical Embryology. 4th ed. Baltimore, Williams & Wilkins Co., 1981.

Lev, M., and Saphir, O.: Truncus arteriosus communis persistens. J. Pediatr. 20:74, 1942.

Liebman, J., Cullum, L., and Belloc, N. B.: Natural history of transposition of the great arteries. Anatomy and birth and death characteristics. Circulation 40:237, 1969.

Lightfoot, N. E., Coles, J. G., Dasmahapatra, H. K., et al.: Analysis of survival in patients with pulmonary atresia and intact ventricular septum treated surgically. Int. J. Cardiol. 24:159, 1989.

Lillehei, C. W., Varco, R. L., Cohen, M., et al.: The first open-heart corrections of tetralogy of Fallot. A 26–31 year follow-up of 106 patients. Ann. Surg. 204:490, 1986.

Long, W. A.: Fetal and Neonatal Cardiology. Philadelphia, W. B. Saunders Company, 1990.

Lucas, R. V., Jr., and Kraybill, K. A.: Anomalous venous connection, pulmonary and systemic. In Adams, F. H., Emmanouilides, G. C., Riemenschneider (Eds.): Heart Disease in Infants, Children and Adolescents, 4th ed. Baltimore, Williams & Wilkins, 1989.

Lundstrom, N. R.: Echocardiography in the diagnosis of Ebstein's anomaly of the tricuspid valve. Circulation 47:597, 1973.

Mair, D. D., Rice, M. J., Hagler, D. J., et al.: Outcome of the Fontan procedure in patients with tricuspid atresia. Circulation 72(II):88, 1985.

Mair, D. D., Seward, J. B., Driscoll, D. J., and Danielson, G. W.: Surgical repair of Ebstein's anomaly: Selection of patients and early and late operative results. Circulation 72(II):870, 1985.

Mesko, Z. G., Jones, J. E., and Nadas, A. S.: Diminution and closure of large ventricular septal defects after pulmonary artery banding. Circulation 43:847, 1973.

Moller, J. H., Nakib, A., Eliot, R. S., and Edwards, J. E.: Symptomatic congenital aortic stenosis in the first year of life. J. Pediatr. 69:728, 1966.

Moller, J. H., and Neal, W. A.: Fetal, Neonatal and Infant Heart Disease. New York, Appleton and Lange, 1990.

Morrow, W. R., Vick, G. W., III, Nihill, M. R., et al.: Balloon dilation of unoperated coarctation of the aorta: short and intermediate term results. J. Am. Coll. Cardiol. 11:133, 1988.

Mustard, W. T., Keith, J. D., Trusler, G. A., Fowler, R., and Kidd, L.: The surgical management of transposition of the great vessels. J. Thorac. Cardiovasc. Surg. 48:953, 1964.

Noonan, J. A., and Nadas, A. S.: The hypoplastic left heart syndrome. Pediatr. Clin. North Am. 5:1029, 1958.

Nora, J. J.: Etiologic aspects of congenital heart disease. In Moss, A. J., Adams, R. H., and Emmanouilides, G. C. (Eds.): Heart Disease in Infants, Children, and Adolescents. 2nd ed. Baltimore, Williams & Wilkins, 1977, p. 3.

Nora, J. J., Nora, A. H.: Maternal transmission of congenital heart diseases: New recurrence risk figures and vulnerability to teratogens. Am. J. Cardiol. 59:459, 1987.

Norwood, W. I., Hougen, T. J., and Castaneda, A. R.: Total anomalous pulmonary venous connection: Surgical considerations. In Engle, M. E. (Ed.): Pediatric Cardiovascular Disease. Cardiovascular Clinics, Philadelphia, F. A. Davis Co., 1980.

Olley, P. M., Coceani, F., and Bodach, E.: E type prostaglandins: a new emergency therapy for certain cyanotic congenital heart malformations. Circulation 53:728, 1976.

Pelech, A. N., Dyck, J. D., Trusler, G. A., et al.: Critical aortic stenosis. Survival and management. J. Thorac. Cardiovasc. Surg. 94:510, 1987.

Piccoli, G. P., Gerlis, L. M., Wilkinson, J. L., Lozadi, K., Macartney, F. J., and Anderson, R. H.: Morphology and classification of atrioventricular defects. Br. Heart J. 42:621, 1979a.

Piccoli, G. P., Wilkinson, J. L., Macartney, F. J., Gerlis, L. M., and Anderson, R. H.: Morphology and classification of complete atrioventricular defects. Br. Heart J. 42:633, 1979b.

Pigott, J. D., Murphy, J. D., Barber, G., Norwood, W. I.: Palliative reconstructive surgery for hypoplastic left heart syndrome. Ann. Thorac. Surg. 45:122, 1988.

Poirier, R. A., Berman, M. A., and Stansel, H. C., Jr.: Current status of the surgical treatment of truncus arteriosus. J. Thorac. Cardiovas. Surg. 69:169, 1975.

Pyeritz, R. E., Murphy, E. A.: Genetics and congenital heart disease: perspectives and prospects. J. Am. Coll. Cardiol. 13:1458, 1989.

Quaegebeur, J. M., Rohmer, J., Ottenkamp, J., et al.: The arterial switch operation: An eight year experience. J. Thorac. Cardiovasc. Surg. 92:361, 1986.

Quero Jimenez, M., Acerete Guillen, F., and Castro Guissoni, M. C.: Arterio-venous fistulas. In Moss, A. J., Adams, F. H., and Emmanouilides, G. C. (Eds.): Heart Disease in Infants, Children, and Adolescents. Baltimore, Williams & Wilkins, 1977, p. 470.

Radford, D. J., Graff, R. F., and Neilson, G. H.: Diagnosis and natural history of Ebstein's anomaly. Br. Heart J. 54:517, 1985.

Rashkind, W. J., and Miller, W. W.: Creation of an atrial septal defect without thoracotomy: A palliative approach to complete transposition of the great arteries. J.A.M.A. 196:991, 1966.

Rein, J. G., Freed, M. D., Norwood, W. I., and Castaneda, A. R.: Early and late results of closure of ventricular septal defects in infancy. Ann. Thorac. Surg. 24:19, 1977.

Rose, V., Izukawa, T., and Moes, C. A. F.: Syndromes of asplenia and polysplenia: A review of cardiac and non-cardiac malformations in 60 cases with special reference to diagnosis and prognosis. Br. Heart J. 37:840, 1975.

Rowe, R. D., Freedom, R. M., Mehrizi, A., and Bloom, K. R.: The Neonate with Congenital Heart Disease. 2nd ed. Philadelphia, W. B. Saunders Co., 1981.

Rudolph, A. M.: Congenital Diseases of the Heart. Chicago, Year Book Medical Publishers, 1974.

Rudolph, A. M., Heymann, M. A., and Spitznas, U.: Hemodynamic considerations in the development of narrowing of the aorta. Am. J. Cardiol. 30:514, 1972.

Sanders, S. P., Bierman, F. Z., and Williams, R. G.: Conotruncal malformations: diagnosis in infancy using two-dimensional echocardiography. Am. J. Cardiol. 50:1361, 1982.

Sell, J. E., Jonas, R. A., Mayer, J. E., et al.: The results of a surgical program for interrupted aortic arch. J. Thorac. Cardiovasc. Surg. 96:864, 1988.

Senning, A.: Surgical correction of transposition of the great vessels. Surgery 45:966, 1959.

Shimazaki, Y., Maehara, T., Blackstone, E. H., et al.: The structure of the pulmonary circulation in tetralogy of Fallot with pulmonary atresia. A quantitative cineangiographic study. J. Thorac. Cardiovasc. Surg. 95:1048, 1988.

Silverman, N., Levitsky, S., Fisher, E., et al.: Efficacy of pulmonary artery banding in infants with complete atrioventricular canal. Circulation 68(II):148, 1983.

Soto, B., Bargeron, L. M., Jr., Pacifico, A. D., et al.: Angiography of the atrio-ventricular canal defects. Am. J. Cardiol. 48:492, 1981.

Talner, N. S., and Berman, M. A.: Postnatal development of obstruction in coarctation of the aorta: Role of the ductus arteriosus. Pediatrics 56:562, 1975.

Trinquet, F., Vouhe, P. R., Vernant, F., et al.: Coarctation of the aorta in infants: Which operation? Ann. Thorac. Surg. 45:186, 1988.

Trusler, G. A., Williams, W. G., Duncan, K. F., et al.: Results with the Mustard operation in simple transposition of the great arteries 1963–1985. Ann. Surg. 206:251, 1987.

Van Mierop, L. H. S., and Kutsche, L.: Cardiovascular anomalies in DiGeorge syndrome and importance of neural crest as a possible pathogenic factor. Am. J. Cardiol. 58:133, 1986.

Van Mierop, L. H. S., Gessner, I. H., and Schiebler, G. L.: Asplenia and polysplenia syndrome. Birth Defects 8:36, 1972.

Van Mierop, L. H. S., Oppenheimer-Dekker, A., and Bruins, C.: Embryology and Teratology of the Heart and Great Arteries. Leiden, The Netherlands, Leiden University Press, 1978.

Van Praagh, R., Ando, M., Van Praagh, S., et al.: Pulmonary atresia: anatomic considerations. In Kidd, B. S. L., and Rowe, R. D. (Eds.): The Child with Congenital Heart Disease after Surgery. Mt. Kisco, N. Y., Futura Publishers, Inc., 1976, p. 103.

Van Praagh, R., Bernhard, W. F., Rosenthal, A., Parisi, L. F., and Fyler, D. C.: Interrupted aortic arch: surgical treatment. Am. J. Cardiol. 27:200, 1971.

Van Praagh, R., and Van Praagh, S.: The anatomy of common aorto-pulmonary trunk (truncus arteriosus communis) and its embryologic implications. A study of 57 necropsy cases. Am. J. Cardiol. 16:406, 1965.

Van Praagh, R., and Van Praagh, S.: Isolated ventricular inversion: Consideration of the morphogenesis, definition and diagnosis of non-transposed and transposed great arteries. Am. J. Cardiol. 17:395, 1966.

Waldhausen, J. A., Nahrwold, D. L., Lurie, P. R., and Shumaker, H. B., Jr.: Management of coarctation in infancy. J.A.M.A. 187:270, 1964.

Waldman, J. D., Rosenthal, A., Smith, A. L., Shurin, S., and Nadas, A. S.: Sepsis and congenital asplenia. J. Pediatr. *90*:555, 1977.

Walsh, E. P., Rockenmacher, S., Keane, J. F., et al.: Late results in patients with tetralogy of Fallot repaired during infancy. Circulation *77*:1062, 1988.

Watson, D. G., and Rowe, R. D.: Aortic-valve atresia. Report of 43 cases. J.A.M.A. *179*:14, 1962.

Watson, H.: Natural history of Ebstein's anomaly of the tricuspid valve in children and adolescents: an international cooperative study of 505 cases. Br. Heart J. *36*:417, 1974.

Wernovsky, G., Hougen, T. J., Walsh, E. P., et al.: Midterm results after the arterial switch operation for transposition of the great arteries with an intact ventricular septum: Clinical hemodynamic, echocardiographic and electrophysiologic data. Circulation *77*:1333, 1988.

Whittemore, R., Robbins, J. C., and Engle, M. A.: Pregnancy and its outcome with and without surgical treatment of congenital heart diseases. Am. J. Cardiol. *50*:641, 1982.

Yacoub, M., Bernhard, A., Lange, P., et al.: Clinical and hemodynamic results of two-stage anatomic correction of simple transposition of the great arteries. Circulation *62*(suppl):190, 1980.

Yee, E. S., Turley, K., Hsieh, W. R., and Ebert, P. A.: Infant total anomalous venous connection: Factors influencing timing of presentation and operative outcome. Circulation *76*(III):83, 1987.

Zeevi, B., Keane, J. F., Castaneda, A. R., et al.: Neonatal critical aortic stenosis: Surgery vs. balloon dilation. Circulation *78*(II):490, 1988a.

Zeevi, B., Keane, J. F., Fellows, K. E., and Lock, J. E.: Balloon dilation of critical pulmonary stenosis in the first week of life. J. Am. Coll. Cardiol. *11*:821, 1988b.

Zeevi, B., Perry, S. B., and Keane, J. F.: Interventional cardiac procedures in neonates and infants: State of the art. Clin. Perinatol. *15*:633, 1988c.

Ziemer, G., Jonas, R. A., Perry, S. B., et al.: Surgery for coarctation of the aorta in the neonate. Circulation *74*(I):25, 1986.

CARDIOMYOPATHIES 64

Michael D. Freed

There are several diseases of the newborn in which the myocardium is affected without primary abnormalities of the valves, great vessels, or septum. The heart may be affected by hypoxia and acidosis (transient myocardial ischemia), infection with virus, bacteria, or toxoplasmosis (myocarditis), infiltrative diseases (e.g., glycogen storage disease), tumor (rhabdomyoma, fibroma), or diseases of uncertain etiology (e.g., endocardial fibroelastosis, diabetic myopathy). Although none of the diseases are common, cumulatively they do account for a significant proportion of the heart disease in the newborn. Each is briefly reviewed in this chapter.

■ TRANSIENT MYOCARDIAL ISCHEMIA

Over the past few years, it has been recognized that a number of newborns suffer a form of myocardial ischemia that frequently is transient but that may be associated with significant cardiovascular symptoms and even death (Rowe et al., 1979). In some of these infants, the signs of respiratory distress and congestive heart failure or shock are predominant (Rowe and Hoffman, 1972); in others, myocardial dysfunction and tricuspid regurgitation are the presenting symptoms (Boucek et al., 1976; Bucciarelli et al., 1977).

Pathologic examination of the most severely affected newborns reveals dilated hearts and, frequently, anoxic petechial hemorrhages. On histologic examination, there is often smudging and edema of the myocardial fibers throughout the heart in those infants who die early in the course of their disease and areas of focal myocardial necrosis in those surviving for 3 or 4 days (Rowe et al., 1979).

Since the disease is frequently self-limited and many of these newborns can be saved with careful management, it is important to recognize these infants and institute prompt treatment.

Clinical Features. The infants are usually born at term by a delivery complicated by hypoxic stress that occurs before or during birth. Fetal scalp pH measurement is in the range of 6.9 to 7.1 in those in whom it is measured. The Apgar score is usually less than 3 at 1 minute. Respiratory distress and cyanosis are frequently present soon after birth, with the newborns developing the signs and symptoms of congestive heart failure (tachypnea, tachycardia, hepatomegaly, and a gallop rhythm) within a few hours. Some go on to develop hypotension and cardiovascular collapse and shock. About half the newborns have systolic heart murmurs. In most, the murmur is at the left lower sternal border and suggests tricuspid regurgitation, but in a few the murmur is loudest at the apex and sounds like mitral regurgitation.

The chest radiograph invariably shows cardiomegaly.

There is usually a diffuse haziness with pulmonary venous congestion in those with predominantly left-sided heart failure. In those with right-sided heart failure, the congestion may be absent with diminished pulmonary blood flow in those with cyanosis due to right-to-left atrial shunting.

The electrocardiogram shows right ventricular predominance that is normal for age and right atrial hypertrophy in the majority. Diffuse ST–T changes are usually present, with the most common pattern being ST depression in the midprecordium and persistent T-wave inversion over the left precordium.

On two-dimensional echocardiograms the cardiac structures are normal, but tricuspid regurgitation and decreased left ventricular contraction, especially of the left ventricular posterior wall, may be seen in those with left-sided heart failure.

A few newborns with transient myocardial ischemia have been catheterized. In some of these infants, there is persistent pulmonary hypertension with right-to-left shunting through the fetal pathways, the ductus arteriosus, and the foramen ovale. The ventricular end-diastolic pressures are usually elevated, reflecting ventricular dysfunction (Rowe et al., 1979). In another subgroup, tricuspid regurgitation predominates (Boucek et al., 1976; Bucciarelli et al., 1977). In these newborns the pulmonary artery pressure is only mildly increased but there is severe tricuspid regurgitation evident on angiocardiogram with right-to-left shunting at the atrial level. In both groups, arterial hypoxemia is almost invariably present but is rarely severe.

Diagnosis. Transient myocardial ischemia should be suspected in all newborns who experience a traumatic birth involving hypoxia and who have respiratory distress, cyanosis, or signs of congestive failure soon after birth. Since this picture may occasionally be seen in newborns with congenital heart disease, the performance of echocardiography is essential if congestive failure or cyanosis is prominent. Echocardiography is also helpful in distinguishing infants who have tricuspid regurgitation associated with transient ischemia from those who have tricuspid regurgitation caused by Ebstein disease of the tricuspid valve or critical pulmonary stenosis or pulmonary atresia with an intact ventricular septum.

Treatment. The treatment is symptomatic. Digitalis and diuretics should be given for congestive heart failure, and the metabolic abnormalities of hypoglycemia and acidosis should be corrected promptly. Those with severe respiratory distress may need intubation and assisted ventilation; those with cardiovascular collapse may benefit from inotropic support with isoproterenol or dopamine (Walther et al., 1985). Afterload reduction with nitroprusside should be reserved for the most severely affected.

Prognosis. In the infants without cardiogenic shock,

the prognosis is good. In the series of Bucciarelli and co-workers and of Boucek and colleagues involving only patients with severe tricuspid regurgitation, 16 of 18 newborns survived, usually with disappearance of the murmur within a couple of weeks and resolution of the electrocardiographic abnormalities within a few months. Five of the 16 survivors had cardiac catheterization 4½ months to 5 years later, with hemodynamics subsequently returning to normal.

In those who are first seen with severe acidosis and cardiogenic shock, the prognosis remains grim, with death likely occurring from heart failure, low output, or failure of a necessary organ system.

■ MYOCARDITIS

Myocarditis occurs in all age groups, but there is higher frequency in the 1st month than in any other period of life. It is a well-recognized entity with a clinical pattern sufficiently distinctive for one to make an antemortem diagnosis. Although often a fulminant disease, it is not invariably fatal, and early recognition and prompt treatment may alter the outcome.

Incidence. For the 50 years following Fiedler's original description of primary myocarditis, only a few isolated cases had been reported in the 1st month of life. Since 1950, there has been a striking increase in the number of reported cases particularly among newborn infants. Group B Coxsackie virus infections may be as common as 1 in 2000 live births (Kaplan et al., 1983). Recent nursery outbreaks have been reported (Drew, 1973; Hall and Miller, 1969). In the Regional Infant Cardiac Program reviewing critical heart disease in New England between 1969 and 1974, there were 13 infants with myocarditis, an incidence of 1 of every 80,000 live births (Fyler et al., 1980).

Etiology. Any infective agent can cause myocarditis, although the enteroviruses, particularly Coxsackie B and ECHO viruses, are the most common (Lerner et al., 1975). In 1961, Kibrick reported 54 cases in the neonatal period that were due to group B Coxsackie viruses. Of this group, 28 were infected during nursery outbreaks, with the mother as the original source of the infection in many instances. Among the 26 sporadic cases, there were a significant number in whom the infant's illness was associated with a febrile illness in the mother. There is some evidence that in a few patients the infection was acquired in utero (Kaplan et al., 1983), but the majority appear to have been acquired postnatally, probably from contact with a maternal source of the virus such as blood or respiratory tract secretions. Asymptomatic infants in the nursery or nursery personnel may also be a source of infection (Brightman et al., 1966).

Neonatal myocarditis may be caused by viruses other than Coxsackie B. Herpes simplex virus has been isolated from the heart of a newborn infant dying of disseminated disease (Wright and Miller, 1965). Myocarditis may be caused by the rubella virus, although this agent has never been isolated from the heart. It has been suggested that rubella myocarditis occurs in utero and may progress after

birth, leaving myocardial damage (Ainger et al., 1966; Harris and Nghiem, 1972).

Pathology. On gross examination, the heart is enlarged and dilated. The cardiac muscle feels flabby and is often pale or nutmeg-like in color. Microscopic examination reveals a multicellular infiltration of the myocardium (Fig. 64–1). Lymphocytes, large mononuclear cells, eosinophils, and polymorphonuclear leukocytes are present in varying numbers with either patchy or diffuse distribution. Necrosis and fragmentation of muscle fibers may be present (Burch et al., 1968). Although rare in patients with primary myocarditis, involvement of the endocardium and pericardium may occur. When the Coxsackie virus is the etiologic agent, involvement of other organs, particularly the central nervous system, is common. Involvement of multiple organs is even more common with rubella and herpes viruses.

Clinical Findings. Most serious Coxsackie virus infections occur in the first 10 days of life. The clinical course of young infants with myocarditis is variable. The initial symptoms may be mild and include lethargy, failure to feed, vomiting, or diarrhea. Jaundice may be present, and evidence of a mild upper respiratory tract infection is sometimes noted. In the milder forms of the disease, clinical manifestations may be limited to slight tachypnea, tachycardia, and poor heart sounds. Frequently, there are no premonitory symptoms whatsoever. The infant becomes seriously ill very suddenly. Respirations increase, become labored, and are often accompanied by a grunt. The infant appears restless and anxious. The skin is pale, mottled, and mildly cyanotic. The temperature may be slightly or greatly elevated or subnormal. the pulse rate is usually rapid, between 150 and 200, and weak. Occasionally, bradycardia is present. The percussion note over the chest may be normal or hyperresonant. Dullness is uncommon. The breath sounds are usually harsh, and rales may be heard at the bases. Although there is always some degree of cardiac enlargement, it is often difficult to detect clinically. The heart sounds are mushy, particularly the first sound, and a gallop rhythm may be present. The liver is almost invariably enlarged. Edema is an uncommon finding, and venous engorgement is almost never detected. There may be signs referable to central nervous system involvement, including lethargy, seizures, or coma with occasional focal signs suggesting meningoencephalitis.

Chest radiographs show generalized cardiac enlargement as well as haziness of the lung fields. At times, it is not possible to make the distinction between congestion and pneumonia (Fig. 64–2). Electrocardiograms often show abnormalities. Low-voltage QRS complexes and low, isoelectric, or inverted T waves are the most frequent findings. There may also be significant disturbances in conduction such as heart block, extrasystoles, and ventricular or atrial tachycardia (Fig. 64–3). The electrocardiographic abnormalities are frequently transient. Although usually not helpful in the acute stage, viral studies should be carried out. Elevations of aspartate transaminase, lactic dehydrogenase, and cardiac creatinine phosphokinase are variably present with levels dependent on the extent of tissue damage.

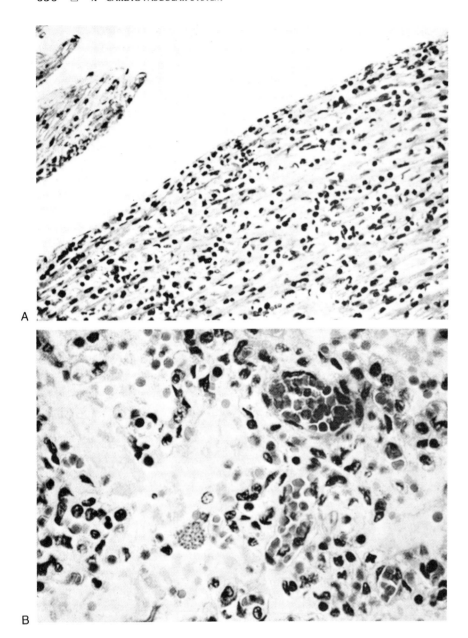

A

B

FIGURE 64–1. A, *Low-power microscopic view of section of the heart in a patient with myocarditis showing diffuse cellular infiltration in the myocardium.* B, *Higher-power microscopic view of section of myocardium showing cellular infiltration and toxoplasma.*

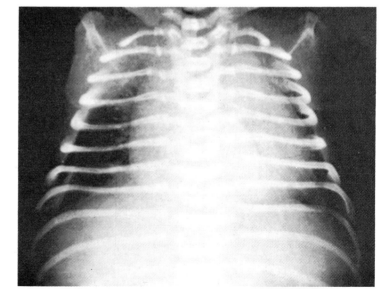

FIGURE 64–2. *Generalized cardiac enlargement caused by myocarditis.*

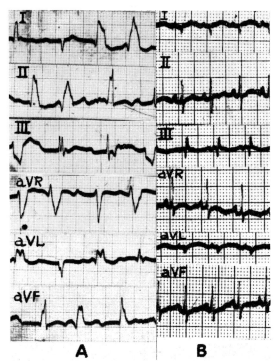

FIGURE 64–3. A, *Standard and unipolar limb leads showing conduction disturbances with variable atrioventricular block, bundle branch block, and multifocal ventricular complexes in a child with myocarditis.* B, *Standard and unipolar limb leads showing return to normal rhythm 24 hours later.*

The echocardiogram is helpful in ruling out associated structural heart disease and assessing myocardial function. In infants in whom neither congestive heart failure nor cardiac enlargement appears on the chest radiograph, the echocardiogram is usually normal. When cardiac enlargement does appear on the radiograph, the left atrium and left ventricle are usually dilated, with little change in left ventricular dimensions between systole and diastole, findings that reflect poor ventricular function.

Diagnosis. The diagnosis of myocarditis should be suspected in any newborn with congestive heart failure in whom structural heart disease has been excluded by two-dimensional echocardiogram. The suspicion should be heightened if there is a known respiratory infection in the mother or proved viral illness in other nursery infants. The diagnosis can be confirmed by the recovery of virus from the nasopharynx and the stool or by the development of neutralizing antibodies.

The acute form of myocarditis is commonly mistaken for overwhelming *sepsis* or a *severe lower respiratory tract infection*. This is especially true for the latter, since cyanosis and respiratory distress may initially suggest pneumonia. Myocarditis should be suspected if there are an inordinate tachycardia, poor heart sounds with or without gallop rhythm, a degree of dyspnea disproportionate with the pulmonary findings, and radiographic evidence of cardiac enlargement.

Myocarditis must also be differentiated from other cardiac conditions that may occur in the neonatal period, such as congenital heart disease with congestive failure precipitated by infection, the acute form of endocardial fibroelastosis, and paroxysmal tachycardia.

Congenital Heart Disease. The absence of heart murmurs does not rule out this possibility. Occasionally, infants with a large left-to-right shunt have an insignificant murmur in the neonatal period. Coarctation of the aorta, a not uncommon cause of heart failure in the newborn, must always be excluded by careful evaluation of the arm-leg pulses and blood pressure.

Endocardial Fibroelastosis. In this condition, there is usually left ventricular hypertrophy indicated in electrocardiographic tracings by high-voltage R waves in precordial leads taken over the left side of the heart. However, the left ventricular pattern may not be as striking in the first few days or weeks of life. In myocarditis, low-voltage complexes are characteristic and are the result of severe disturbances in myocardial function. Occasionally, infants with endocardial fibroelastosis in severe heart failure may have low voltage temporarily.

Paroxysmal Tachycardia. Congestive heart failure is frequently present, but in this condition the heart rate is usually much more rapid than in myocarditis. Almost invariably it is greater than 240 beats per minute if severe enough to cause heart failure.

Mild forms of myocarditis are particularly difficult to recognize. Signs of heart failure may not be prominent or may be absent entirely. The clinical manifestations may include pallor, slight increase in the respiratory rate, tachycardia, and poor heart sounds. Such findings in an infant who has signs of infection and who appears to have a disproportionate degree of cardiac embarrassment should suggest the possibility of myocarditis. Although electrocardiographic studies may aid in the diagnosis, there is no specific pattern, nor does a normal tracing rule out the disorder.

Treatment. Young infants with myocarditis may become critically ill with such rapidity that treatment should be instituted as soon as the diagnosis is suspected. Minimal handling is essential, since restlessness and agitation seem to worsen the cardiac involvement, a factor consistent with the more than 500-fold increase in the replication of Coxsackie virus in mice forced to exercise during experimental infection (Gatmanitan et al., 1970).

Oxygen therapy and digitalization should be started at once with the usual anticongestive measures. We usually prefer diuretics to digoxin in milder cases, since patients with myocarditis may be unusually sensitive to digitalis.

Since the efficiency of the heart muscle is weakened by the infection, recent efforts have been directed at reducing the work of the heart. It has been found that since cardiac work is a function of the volume of blood ejected during systole and the pressure that the heart must generate, reducing systemic resistance and arterial pressure allows a higher cardiac output to be maintained. Vasodilators such as nitroprusside (0.1 to 5 μg/kg/min) and hydralazine have been found to reduce the "afterload" of the heart and to improve peripheral perfusion in the most severely affected newborns. Inotropic support with isoproterenol or dopamine may improve cardiac contractility and increase cardiac output in those who are most critically ill. Immunosuppressive therapy in adults with myocarditis is contraindicated in the initial phase of the disease since it may increase viral replication, but it may be useful later in the disease; no data are yet available for infants or children. Gamma globulin has been tried with some success but a large trial has not yet proved its efficacy.

Although the etiologic agent in myocarditis is frequently viral, bacterial infections of the lung are common and antibiotics should be given. After the initial digitalization, the patient should be maintained on digitalis until the heart has returned to normal size and the pulse is within normal limits.

Prevention. The fact that viral and bacterial agents may cause neonatal myocarditis emphasizes the need for preventive measures in carrying out nursery routine. The Coxsackie virus may cause minor or inapparent illnesses in adults and yet lead to serious, often fatal disease in newborn infants. Reports of outbreaks in nurseries suggest the infectious nature of this disorder. For these reasons, stress must be placed on the absolute necessity for careful isolation of the mother and the newborn during the course of even mild respiratory infections.

Prognosis. The prognosis for infants with fulminating disease is poor. Patients are occasionally victims of "crib deaths" or arrive at the hospital moribund. Among the 54 cases reported by Kibrick, 12 patients survived. Undoubtedly, milder forms of the disease occur, and the recovery rate in this group is high, although more recent studies continue to show a high mortality rate, approximately 50 per cent (Rowe et al., 1981). In a study of children 13 years after each had suffered an attack of neonatal myocarditis, no clinical or laboratory abnormalities were found, although others have found ventricular dysfunction persisting long after the initial episode (Rozkovec et al., 1985). It is possible that, as the awareness of neonatal myocarditis as a clinical entity increases, earlier diagnosis and more vigorous supportive treatment will improve the overall mortality rate.

■ ENDOCARDIAL FIBROELASTOSIS

Endocardial fibroelastosis may occur as an isolated or primary condition or in association with a variety of congenital and acquired cardiac lesions. In the latter groups, the clinical entity is that of the underlying cardiac disease, and the fibroelastosis is a secondary finding on postmortem examination. The description that follows is limited mainly to infants with the primary or isolated form of endocardial fibroelastosis.

Etiology. Recently, the concept of primary endocardial fibroelastosis has been challenged by Lurie (1988) who argues that all endocardial fibroelastosis is secondary to a "reactive process set off in the endocardium by stress of the myocardium" during fetal life. The stress may be due to inflammatory myocarditis (Fruhling et al., 1962; Hastreiter and Miller, 1964; Hutchins and Vie, 1972), mitochondrial cardiomyopathy (Neustein et al., 1979), or other causes.

Incidence. The reports on incidence are confusing because of the inclusion of large numbers of cases with the secondary form of this disease. The 1956 study by Kelly and Anderson makes this distinction clear. In their series from the Babies Hospital, there were 17 instances among 237 necropsy patients with congenital heart disease, an incidence of 7 per cent. Family occurrences were noted in three of the 17 cases. There are several additional reports that record the disease among multiple births and siblings.

Primary endocardial fibroelastosis may be becoming rarer. Mitchell and co-workers found an incidence of 1 in every 5000 to 6000 births in a prospective national collaborative study during the early 1960s; in the New England Regional Infant Cardiac Program during the early 1970s, endocardial fibroelastosis occurred in only 14 of 1,000,000 live births, an incidence of 1 of 70,000 live births (Fyler et al., 1980). There does not appear to be any relation to birth weight, sex, or race.

Pathology. Gross enlargement of the heart is a constant finding. The weight is increased, and there are hypertrophy and dilatation of one or more chambers. This is especially true of the left ventricle, which is the most frequent site of endocardial thickening. Involvement of the left atrium is fairly common, but less than half have an additional lesion of the right ventricle and right atrium. Fibroelastosis confined to the right side of the heart is rare. On gross examination, the endocardium is diffusely thickened and smooth and has a porcelain-white appearance (Fig. 64–4). About half the cases show involvement of one or more valves, the mitral more commonly than the others. In contrast to the usual pattern of congenital abnormalities, there is a striking absence of other malformations.

Microscopic examination shows an increase in the fibrous and elastic tissue within the endocardium with some extension into the myocardium. When the valves are involved, the picture is similar to that of the endocardium. There is no evidence of inflammation in the heart. Pneumonia and signs of congestive heart failure are commonly associated autopsy findings.

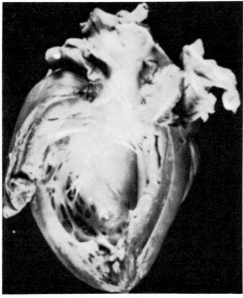

FIGURE 64–4. Endocardial fibroelastosis in an infant who died at the age of 9 days. The endocardium of both ventricles is thickened and porcelain-white in appearance.

Clinical Course. Many infants have symptoms early in the course of the disease. In a recent study, the median age of presentation was 8.8 months, but 40 per cent were seen in the first 3 months of life (Ino et al., 1988), and heart failure in utero has been reported (Harris and Nghien, 1972). In the acute form, the presentation can be fulminant, with a previously well infant becoming sick over a few hours and succumbing to the disease. The more typical case, however, exhibits the signs and symptoms of congestive heart failure, including tachypnea and retractions (71 per cent); gastrointestinal symptoms, including vomiting, diarrhea, or poor feeding (33 per cent); fever (17 per cent); poor weight gain (15 per cent); and neurologic symptoms, such as lethargy or hypotonia (10 per cent) (Ino et al., 1988). The heart rate is variable, with tachycardia that is occasionally due to a paroxysmal atrial rhythm (Hung and Walsh, 1962), although heart block, either partial or complete, has also been reported (Fig. 64–5) that may be present in utero (Anderson and Kelly, 1956).

On auscultation, the heart sounds may be normal or muffled and a third heart sound is frequently present. Heart murmurs may be present in more than 50 per cent of patients, usually a Grade I to Grade II pansystolic murmur at the apex from mitral regurgitation secondary to papillary muscle dysfunction. Diastolic murmurs are very uncommon. Chest roentgenographs invariably show cardiac enlargement that is usually significant, with increased pulmonary vascularity secondary to pulmonary venous congestion with left atrial enlargement being common (Fig. 64–6).

The electrocardiogram almost invariably reveals left ventricular hypertrophy with tall R waves over the left precordium, frequently associated with prominent Q waves and T-wave inversion (Ino et al., 1988; Lambert et al., 1953). Supraventricular or nodal tachycardia, complete heart block, or other arrhythmias may occasionally be seen.

On echocardiogram the left ventricular end-diastolic and end-systolic dimensions are usually increased with a reduced fractional shortening. The left atrial size is also increased, with normal to slightly increased left ventricular septal and free-wall thicknesses. The thickened endocardium may be visualized in some cases on two-dimensional study.

At cardiac catheterization the left ventricular end-diastolic pressure, as well as left atrial and pulmonary arterial wedge pressures, are increased. The pulmonary artery pressure is elevated commensurate with the pulmonary venous pressures, but it is uncommon to have peak

pulmonary artery pressures of greater than 40 mm Hg. The cardiac index is usually reduced, and left ventriculography reveals a global reduction in wall motion with decreased ejection fraction. The surface of the left ventricle may be unusually smooth (porcelainized), with the common finding of mitral valve regurgitation.

Diagnosis. Endocardial fibroelastosis should be suspected in the newborn if abnormalities of cardiac rhythm (e.g., heart block, atrial tachycardia) are present. In the most acute form, diagnosis is difficult. These infants often resemble patients with sepsis or pneumonia. The presence of tachycardia, cardiomegaly, and hepatomegaly should lead to the suspicion of heart failure due to primary heart disease. Differentiation from primary myocarditis may be particularly difficult. The findings in both conditions are remarkably similar. One distinguishing feature is the strikingly low voltage noted on the electrocardiogram in severe myocarditis, but this may occasionally occur in endocardial fibroelastosis. The left ventricular pattern commonly found in endocardial fibroelastosis may be slight or absent in the patient less than 1 week old with an acute case.

The chronic form of the disease may cause symptoms from birth, but the diagnosis is rarely suspected until the signs of heart failure are fairly well developed. At times, the wheezing or labored respirations are wrongly interpreted as signs of asthma, an enlarged thymus, or some other obstructive abnormality. The diagnosis should be suspected in any young infant with an enlarged heart, particularly when there is little or no cyanosis and no audible heart murmurs. Absence of the latter signs should exclude most other forms of congenital heart disease. The presence of palpable femoral pulsations eliminates coarctation of the aorta. Infants with anomalous origin of the left coronary artery may have a similar clinical and radiographic picture. The electrocardiogram in this condition is often distinctive, however, and shows a pattern of coronary insufficiency with inverted T waves in leads I and II plus a prominent Q wave in lead I.

Glycogen storage disease of the heart is a rare cause of cardiac enlargement in infancy. Here, the enlargement is usually globular, without specific chamber enlargement. The electrocardiographic pattern is more bizarre in glycogen storage disease, and a short P–R interval is often present. A specific diagnosis can be made by analysis of the glycogen content of skeletal muscle.

Treatment. Treatment is directed toward the control of heart failure. Oxygen therapy is indicated. Digitalization should be started immediately. If the patient is extremely

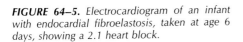

FIGURE 64–5. Electrocardiogram of an infant with endocardial fibroelastosis, taken at age 6 days, showing a 2.1 heart block.

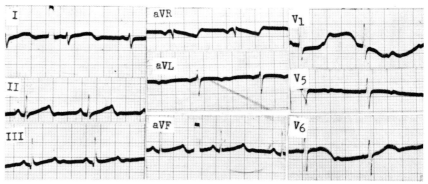

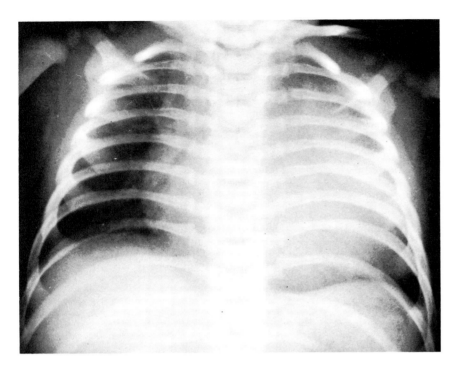

FIGURE 64–6. *Endocardial fibroelastosis in a 6-week-old infant. The heart is diffusely enlarged.*

ill, one of the more rapid-acting digitalis preparations should be used. The prolonged use of digitalis has been recommended as an important aspect of therapy.

Diuretics should be reserved for infants who have clinical evidence of edema or who fail to respond to oxygen and digitalis. More complete details on the dosage of anticongestive drugs are presented elsewhere.

In the critically ill infant, reducing the work of the heart by decreasing afterload with nitroprusside or hydralazine may be helpful.

Prognosis. A small number of patients fail to respond to all measures and die within 1 day to 2 weeks after onset of the illness. In a larger group, the response to anticongestive treatment is good, even dramatic at times. Of 19 patients with symptoms before 1 month of life, ten lived from 3 months to 3 years (Kelly and Anderson, 1956). In general, the earlier the onset, the worse the prognosis. Symptoms recur intermittently until death. The terminal illness is usually brief and is the result of heart failure often complicated by pneumonia. The prognosis in infants with the familial type of endocardial fibroelastosis is generally poor.

It is still not certain that endocardial fibroelastosis is an invariably fatal disease. Linde and Adams described 17 patients in whom a presumptive diagnosis of primary endocardial fibroelastosis was made. Of these, four have had completely normal findings over a period of 3 to 10 years. Reviewing 52 patients seen since 1970 at the Hospital for Sick Children in Toronto, Ino and colleagues found an actuarial survival rate of 93 per cent at 6 months, 83 per cent at 1 year and 77 per cent at 4 years. Poor outcome was associated with low LV ejection fraction and cardiac index at catheterization. Further observations will be necessary before the overall prognosis in this condition is known. In the meantime, early recognition and vigorous treatment make a favorable outcome possible in some patients.

■ HYPERTROPHIC CARDIOMYOPATHY OF THE INFANT OF THE DIABETIC MOTHER

Since the widespread availability of M-mode echocardiography, it has become evident that many large for gestational age infants born to diabetic mothers have an asymmetric hypertrophic cardiomyopathy involving primarily the ventricular septum (Gutgesell et al., 1976; Poland et al., 1975; Way et al., 1975). In 1980, Breitweser and co-workers found an excellent correlation between the degree of neonatal hypoglycemia and the thickness of the interventricular septum on echocardiogram in 18 infants of diabetic mothers and in one infant of a nondiabetic mother with nesidioblastosis (ductoinsular cell proliferation), and they have postulated that fetal hyperinsulinemia contributes directly to the observed septal hypertrophy. Microscopic examination has demonstrated hypertrophy of the fibers with areas of cellular disarray (Gutgesell et al., 1976). The exact mechanism of the cardiac hypertrophy and the reason that the hypertrophy primarily affects the ventricular septum remain a matter of conjecture, but the hypertrophy appears not to be related to maternal diabetic control (Sheehan et al., 1986).

This syndrome does not affect all infants of diabetic mothers. Only 3 of 23 asymptomatic infants had disproportionate thickening of the septum, compared with 10 of 26 symptomatic infants in one study (Gutgesell et al., 1980).

Clinical Features. The involved infants, who are usually puffy and plethoric, may present with the signs and symptoms of congestive heart failure: tachypnea, tachycardia, and hepatomegaly. They usually have respiratory distress and frequently cyanosis from birth. Systolic ejection murmurs are common and, at least according to one study, seem to be correlated with the degree of obstruction to left ventricular ejection by the septal hypertrophy (Way et al., 1979).

Cardiac enlargement on the chest radiograph is almost universal, and pulmonary venous congestion is seen in most symptomatic patients (Way et al., 1979). These abnormalities, however, do not correlate with the echocardiographic findings of wall or septal thickness (Gutgesell et al., 1980).

The electrocardiographic findings are quite variable. Among 24 symptomatic infants studied in 1980 by Gutgesell and co-workers, the electrocardiogram was normal in 12, showed right ventricular hypertrophy in seven, and demonstrated biventricular hypertrophy in five. Although all five newborns who had significant left ventricular outflow obstruction had an abnormal electrocardiogram, there was no consistent pattern between the electrocardiographic evidence of hypertrophy and the echocardiographic measurements of wall thickness.

On echocardiographic evaluation of symptomatic infants, the right ventricular anterior wall, the ventricular septum, and the left ventricular posterior wall are thickened, but the septal wall is disproportionately hypertrophied so that the septal-wall-to-left-ventricular-posterior-wall ratio is increased above normal in about one half of infants (Gutgesell, 1980). The internal dimensions of the right and left ventricle were normal, as was the percentage of dimensional change, a measure of cardiac function in this study. In five of the 24 infants, there was evidence of left ventricular outflow tract obstruction due to apposition of the anterior leaflet of the mitral valve to the hypertrophied interventricular septum during systole.

Only a few newborns have undergone cardiac catheterization. Three of five newborns catheterized within the first 2 weeks of life by Way and co-workers in 1979 had a gradient between the left ventricle and the aorta, ranging from 20 to 74 mm Hg. In one, the gradient increased from 20 to 80 mm Hg between catheterization performed at 1 day and 3 weeks of age. Left ventricular angiograms in these infants showed hypertrophy of the papillary muscles, interventricular septum, and left ventricular posterior wall with complete emptying and obliteration of the left ventricular cavity, as frequently seen in older children with the familial form of the disease.

Diagnosis. The echocardiogram is diagnostic and should be performed on all infants of diabetic mothers with signs or symptoms of respiratory distress or congestive heart failure. Other forms of heart disease must be excluded, since the incidence of congenital heart disease in infants of diabetic mothers is five times that of the normal population (Rowland et al., 1973).

Treatment. The treatment is symptomatic. Hypoglycemia, hypocalcemia, hypomagnesemia, and polycythemia should be corrected, and maintenance fluids should be provided intravenously if oral intake is not possible. Occasionally, increasing respiratory distress requires intubation and assisted ventilation. Unless severely depressed myocardial contractibility can be demonstrated on echocardiogram, digitalis and other inotropic agents are contraindicated, since they may lead to increased left ventricular outflow obstruction (Rowe et al., 1981).

Prognosis. In contrast to the outlook for older children and adults with the progressive familial form of hypertrophic cardiomyopathy with asymmetric hypertrophy, the prognosis in this group of newborns is excellent. Of 11 symptomatic infants reported by Way and colleagues in 1979, all were asymptomatic by 1 month of age, with the radiograph in all and the electrocardiogram in 10 returning to normal. Echocardiograms showed regression of septal thickness in all the patients, and repeat cardiac catheterizations in two of the 11 have shown normal hemodynamics with elimination of gradients of 30 and 74 mm Hg between the left ventricle and the aorta. The findings of Gutgesell and co-workers are similar.

■ GLYCOGEN STORAGE DISEASE OF THE HEART

Glycogen storage disease is a rare condition that may produce symptoms from birth. There are at least 22 types of which only three affect the heart. The most common is Pompe disease, usually classified as Type IIa. It is transmitted through a single recessive autosomal gene. The defect is due to the congenital absence of alpha 1, 4 glycosidase (lysosomal acid maltose) from intracellular lysosomes (Hers, 1963). This results in the accumulation of normal glycogen in lysosomal sacs of virtually all tissues, where it cannot be degraded by glycolytic enzymes.

Pathology. The heart is always enlarged, often to enormous proportions. The walls of both ventricles are thick, but the atria are normal. Microscopic examination shows infiltration of the muscle fibers with large vacuoles of glycogen. Varying amounts of glycogen deposition are also found in the skeletal muscles, liver, kidneys, and central nervous system (Fig. 64–7).

Clinical Features. Symptoms were noted from birth in about one-fourth of the 54 cases summarized by Ehlers and co-workers. Frequently, the infant appears normal at birth but goes on to have a history of poor feeding, lassitude, a feeble cry, protruding tongue, and failure to gain weight. Hypotonia may be striking, and the tongue may appear thick. Cardiac enlargement is the rule. A systolic heart murmur may be noted, but it is often soft and variable. The liver is not usually enlarged.

The usual parameters for glycogen metabolism are normal, including glucose tolerance and response to epinephrine and glucagon. These infants do not suffer from hypoglycemia. Radiologic examination shows gross generalized cardiomegaly, although the heart need not be enlarged at birth (Fig. 64–8). The electrocardiogram may show abnormalities at birth or after a period of some weeks: The presence of a short P–R interval, huge precordial voltages, and evidence of left ventricular hypertrophy is universal. T-wave inversion, ST–T elevation, and deep Q waves are frequently seen (Caddell and Whittemore, 1962) (Fig. 64–9).

On echocardiogram, Bloom and co-workers discovered thickening of the left ventricular free wall disproportionate to the thickness of the interventricular septum. Cardiac catheterization and angiography are rarely indicated.

Diagnosis. The diagnosis is rarely made in the neonatal period unless there is a family history of the disease. The early symptoms are ill defined and, with the exception of

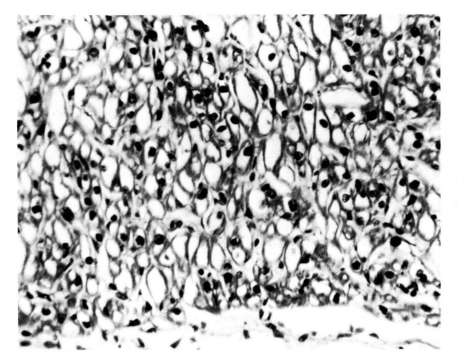

FIGURE 64–7. *Microscopic section of the myocardium of an infant with glycogen storage disease of the heart. Note the vacuolization among the myofibers. These vacuoles were filled with glycogen when appropriately stained.*

intermittent episodes of dyspnea, do not suggest a cardiac abnormality. The patient is more likely to be several weeks or months old before the cardiac enlargement is detected. The diagnosis should be suspected in any infant with an enlarged heart in the absence of structural heart disease, especially if the enlargement is great. Muscle weakness is an important additional clue. Macroglossia is often present and may be confused with cretinism or Down syndrome.

This condition must be distinguished from other causes of cardiac enlargement in early infancy. The absence of cyanosis and significant murmurs excludes many of the congenital defects. *Endocardial fibroelastosis* and *anomalous left coronary artery* are the two conditions that most frequently enter into the differential diagnosis. The left ventricular component in the radiograph is more striking in both the aforementioned conditions, whereas the heart in glycogen storage disease is larger and more globular.

All three entities may show a left ventricular pattern and striking T-wave changes in the electrocardiogram. In the anomalous left coronary artery, the electrocardiographic changes resemble more closely those seen with a posterior infarct. In endocardial fibroelastosis, the T-wave changes are restricted to the left side of the precordium, whereas they are often present in all leads in glycogen storage disease. A short P-R interval does not occur in endocardial fibroelastosis or with an anomalous coronary artery. Pompe disease should be differentiated from other storage diseases, other genetic metabolic diseases, and mitochondrial disorders (Kohlschutter and Hausdorf, 1986).

The diagnosis of glycogen storage disease can be confirmed by demonstration of increased glycogen in a biopsy of skeletal muscle. It can be more readily confirmed by examination of blood lymphocytes for glycogen content (Nihill et al., 1970). Although this may be unreliable,

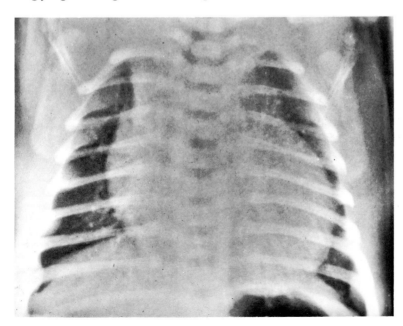

FIGURE 64–8. *X-ray film of the chest of a 12-hour-old infant with glycogen storage disease of the heart. There is considerable cardiac enlargement.*

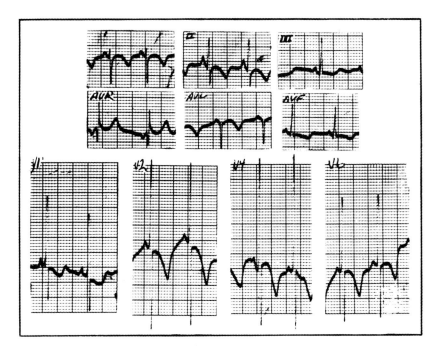

FIGURE 64–9. *Electrocardiogram of a 1-day-old infant with glycogen storage disease of the heart. Note the short P-R interval, increased voltage, and deeply inverted T waves in leads I, II, AVL, and V_2–V_6.*

prenatal diagnosis by amniocentesis or chorionic villus sampling is now available.

Prognosis. Death due to heart failure almost always occurs by 4 to 8 months of life, frequently from aspiration pneumonia. Among 54 cases proved at autopsy and reviewed by Keith and Sass-Kortsak, 10 patients died in the first 2 months of life.

Treatment. There is no satisfactory treatment for this condition. Anticongestive therapy and treatment of intercurrent infection may be instituted in an attempt to prolong life although digoxin may aggravate left ventricular outflow tract obstruction.

■ TUMORS OF THE HEART

Cardiac tumors are uncommon, but when present, the manifestations of heart disease may appear infrequently in the neonatal period. Several types of tumors have been described—rhabdomyomas are the most common (Bigelow et al., 1954; Nadas and Ellison, 1968; Williams et al., 1972) and are frequently associated with tuberous sclerosis. Most commonly, the tumors are multiple, but occasionally only one is found (Fig. 64–10). They are situated in the walls of the right or left ventricle or occasionally in the interventricular septum and, on occasion, project into the lumen and obstruct one of the valves or the outflow tract of the right and left ventricle (Shahar et al., 1972; Van der Hauert, 1971). Histologically, they consist of numerous nodular areas with vacuoles that contain glycogen. On electronmicroscopy the glycogen is seen in the cytoplasm and in the mitochondria. Fibromas, solitary tumors in the septal or parietal wall of the left ventricle, are usually not encapsulated with tissue mixing with the myocardial cells in the wall. They have been described in the neonatal period (Bigelow et al., 1954) and occasionally cause problems by compressing the anterior descending coronary artery, interfering with the conduction system, or obstructing right or left ventricular

outflow. Other tumors, including teratoma, lipoma, hemangioma, hamartoma, and sarcoma, are considerably less common, especially in the perinatal period.

The clinical picture is extremely variable. Many infants, especially those with multiple intramural rhabdomyomas, are asymptomatic and are identified on two-dimensional echocardiogram performed because minor obstructions lead to turbulence and murmurs. Occasionally, newborns present with arrhythmias, including atrial flutter or fibrillation, ventricular tachycardia, or complete heart block because of interference with the conduction system. Heart murmurs are usually not present unless the tumor projects into the cardiac cavity and obstructs blood flow. Changes in the cardiac examination depend on the location and severity of the intracavitary obstruction to flow. The electrocardiographic findings are variable, with right, left, and combined ventricular hypertrophy being reported, although occasionally the electrocardiogram is normal. Often there is evidence of abnormal repolarization with inverted T waves (Fig. 64–11). On chest x-ray studies, the heart is usually normal in the absence of significant

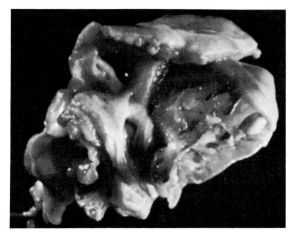

FIGURE 64–10. *Age 1 month. Multiple rhabdomyomas. Gross specimen of the opened heart shows numerous nodular masses within the walls of the ventricle that protrude into the chamber of the heart.*

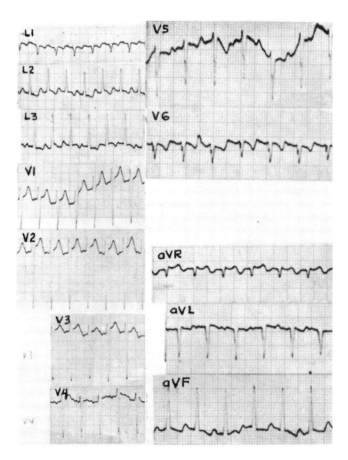

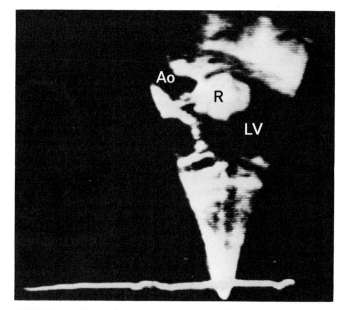

FIGURE 64–11. Age 7 weeks. Multiple rhabdomyomas of the heart. The electrocardiogram is abnormal. There is T-wave inversion in the limb leads and over the left side of the precordium. The S waves are abnormally deep over the right and left sides of the precordium. The over-all pattern is bizarre.

hemodynamic disruption, although in children with large fibromas the tumor may distort the cardiac contour. Two-dimensional echocardiogram with Doppler imaging is now the best tool to evaluate the size, location, number, and hemodynamic severity of the tumor or tumors (Fig. 64–12).

Most rhabdomyomas and fibromas need no therapy. The natural history has not been determined conclusively since these tumors are so uncommon. However, most of the intramural lesions do not progress and enlarge, and some may become relatively smaller with time. Successful surgical removal has been accomplished when the tumors are hemodynamically significant (Van der Hauwaert, 1971; Williams et al., 1972; Shaher et al., 1972; and Skillington et al., 1987). Occasional improvement in arrhythmias has been noted after surgical excision when an obvious area of abnormal tissue can be located electrophysiologically and anatomically (Garson et al., 1987). The finding of multiple rhabdomyomas in an asymptomatic or symptomatic child on echocardiogram raises the strong possibility of tuberous sclerosis, even if the other systemic findings are not yet present.

■ CARDIOMYOPATHY SECONDARY TO HUMAN IMMUNODEFICIENCY DISEASE

Myocardial dysfunction with dilated cardiomyopathy, myocarditis, pericardial effusion, infarction, and direct infectious or neoplastic involvement of the myocardium has been described in adults with acquired immunodeficiency disease (AIDS). To date, however, little information has been obtained on infants with congenital or perinatally acquired infection. Estimates of the Centers for Disease Control suggest that the number of cases of congenitally acquired HIV disease will soon dwarf that of other fatal congenital infections, making preventive efforts mandatory. As of this writing, since most data have been pre-

FIGURE 64–12. A subxiphoid view on two-dimensional echocardiogram of the left ventricle (LV) and aorta (Ao) in a 1-week-old child with tuberous sclerosis. Note the rhabdomyoma (R) that is arising just below the aortic valve and that projects into the lumen of the left ventricle, causing subaortic stenosis. Compare this with Figure 26–2, a normal view of the LV and Ao on two-dimensional echocardiogram. (Courtesy of Roberta G. Williams, M.D.)

sented only in abstract form, conclusions must be viewed as very preliminary.

Prospective data based on a very small number of patients with short-term follow-up have shown neonatal infection rates in the range of 20 to 50 per cent (Feinkind and Minkoff, 1988). The finding of an AIDS embryopathy and isolation of the virus from the thymus of newborns delivered in midpregnancy suggest that, at least in many infants, the infection is acquired prior to birth. It is possible, however, that in some children the infection is transmitted by body fluids (blood, amniotic fluid, and vaginal secretions) at birth.

To date, little information is available concerning the natural history of the cardiac disease associated with AIDS. In a group of eight children with symptomatic cardiac dysfunction reviewed by Stewart and associates (1989), all had hepatosplenomegaly, fever, pneumonia, tachycardia, tachypnea, and anemia. An S3 gallop was present in six of the eight children. The electrocardiograms showed flattened T waves in five, with left ventricular hypertrophy, right ventricular hypertrophy, or both, in seven. Echocardiography showed diminished left ventricular function in all eight children, with a dilated right ventricular myopathy in six, concentric left ventricular wall thickening in two, enlarged right ventricle in two, and pericardial fluid in three.

In a larger study of 31 patients with human immunodeficiency viral infection (Lipschultz et al., 1989), abnormalities of left ventricular function were seen in 93 per cent and were independent of the progression of HIV infection. Two patterns were noticed; 63 per cent of the patients had hyperdynamic left ventricular performance with enhanced contractility and reduced afterload, whereas 26 per cent of the patients had a dilated cardiomyopathy. Pericardial effusions without tamponade were seen in 26 per cent. Twenty-four–hour Holter monitors showed atrial ectopy in 40 per cent and ventricular ectopy in 30 per cent. High-grade ventricular ectopy, including couplets and ventricular tachycardia, was present in six patients, or 20 per cent.

For symptomatic patients, the usual medical therapy including digoxin and diuretics seems to improve cardiac function. The prognosis for this group of patients appears poor. Although in the study of Stewart none of the patients died from cardiac causes, in 4 of 10 patients who died in the study of Lipschultz, the mortality was attributable to probable cardiac causes (two patients with a dilated myopathy, one patient with depressed contractility, and one patient with sudden unexplained death). Postmortem examination of the heart frequently, but not invariably, showed focal myocarditis with mononuclear infiltration and myocardial fibroid necrosis. Pericardial effusions and inflammation of the conduction system were occasionally seen.

■ REFERENCES

Ainger, L. E., Lawyer, N. G., and Fitch, C. W., et al.: Neonatal rubella myocarditis. Br. Heart J. 28:691, 1966.

Anderson, D. H., and Kelly, J.: Endocardial fibroelastosis associated with congenital malformations of the heart. Pediatrics 18:513, 1956.

Bigelow, N. H., Klinger, S., and Wright, A. W.: Primary tumors of the heart in infancy and childhood. Cancer 7:549, 1954.

Bloom, K. R., Hug, G., Schubert, W. K., and Kaplan, S.: Pompe's disease and the heart. Circulation, 50(Suppl. III):56, 1974.

Boucek, R. J., Graham, T. P., Jr., Morgan, J. P., et al.: Spontaneous resolution of massive congenital tricuspid insufficiency. Circulation 54:795, 1976.

Breitweser, J. A., Meyer, R. A., Sperling, M. A., et al.: Cardiac septal hypertrophy in hyperinsulinemic infants. J. Pediatr. 96:535, 1980.

Brightman, V. J., Scott, T. F., Westphal, M., and Boggs, T. R.: An outbreak of Coxsackie B–5 virus infection in a newborn nursery. J. Pediatr. 69:179, 1966.

Bucciarelli, R. L., Nelson, R. M., Eagan, E. A., II, et al.: Transient tricuspid insufficiency of the newborn: A form of myocardial dysfunction in stressed newborns. Pediatrics 59:330, 1977.

Burch, G. E., Sun, S., Chu, K., et al.: Interstitial and coxsackievirus B myocarditis in infants and children. J.A.M.A. 203:1, 1968.

Caddell, J., and Whittemore, R.: Observations on generalized glycogenesis with emphasis on electrocardiographic changes. Pediatrics 29:743, 1962.

Di Sant'Agnese, P., Anderson, D. H., and Mason, H. H.: Glycogen storage disease of the heart. Pediatrics 6:607, 1950.

Drew, J. H.: ECHO II virus outbreak in a nursery associated with myocarditis. Aust. Pediatr. J. 9:90, 1973.

Ehlers, K. H., Hagstrom, J. W., Lukas, D. S., et al.: Glycogen-storage disease of the myocardium with obstruction to left ventricular outflow. Circulation 25:96, 1962.

Feinkind, L., and Minkoff, H. L.; HIV in pregnancy. Clin. Perinatol. 15:189, 1988.

Fiedler, A.: Ueber akute interstitielle Myocarditis. Zendtralbl. inn. Med. 21:212, 1900.

Fruhling, L., Korn, R., Lavillaureix, J., et al.: Chronic fibroelastic myoendocarditis of the newborn and the infant (fibroelastosis). Ann. Anat. Path. (Paris) 7:227, 1962.

Fyler, D. C., Buckley, L. P., Hellenbrand, W., et al.: Report of the New England Regional Infant Cardiac Program. Pediatrics 65(suppl.):375, 1980.

Garson, A., Jr., Smith, R. T., Jr., Moak, J. P., et al.: Incessant ventricular tachycardia in infants: myocardial hamartomas and surgical cure. J. Am. Coll. Cardiol. 10:619, 1987.

Gatmanitan, B. G., Chason, J. L., Lerner, A. M.: Augmentation of the virulence of murine coxsackie virus B3 myocardiopathy by exercise. J. Exp. Med. 131:1121, 1970.

Gutgesell, H. P., et al.: Transient hypertrophic subaortic stenosis in infants of diabetic mothers. J. Pediatr. 89:120, 1976.

Gutgesell, H. P., Speer, M. E., and Rosenberg, H. S.: Characterization of the cardiomyopathy in infants of diabetic mothers. Circulation 61:441, 1980.

Hall, C. B., and Miller, D. G.: The detection of silent Coxsackie B–5 virus perinatal infection. J. Pediatr. 75:124, 1969.

Harris, L. C., and Nghiem, Q. X.: Cardiomyopathies in infants and children. Prog. Cardiovasc. Dis. 15:255, 1972.

Hastreiter, A. R., and Miller, R. A.: Management of primary endomyocardial disease. Pediatr. Clin. North Am. 11:401, 1964.

Hers, H. G.: Alpha glucosidase deficiency in generalized glycogen storage disease (Pompe's disease). Biochem. J. 86:11, 1963.

Hung, W., and Walsh, B. J.: Congenital auricular fibrillation in a newborn infant with endocardial fibroelastosis. J. Pediatr. 61:65, 1962.

Hutchins, G. M., and Vie, S. A.: The progression of interstitial myocarditis to idiopathic endocardial fibroelastosis. Am. J. Pathol. 66:483, 1972.

Ino, T., Benson, L. M., Freedom, R. M., and Rowe, R. D.: Natural history and prognostic risk factors in endocardial fibroelastosis. Am. J. Cardiol. 62:431, 1988.

Kaplan, M. H., Klein, S. W., McPhee, J., et al. Group B Coxsackie virus infections in infants younger than three months: A serious childhood illness. Rev. Infect. Dis. 5:1019, 1983.

Keith, J. D., and Sass-Kortsak, A.: Glycogen storage disease of the heart. In Keith, J. D., Rowe, R. D., and Vlad, P.: Heart Disease in Infancy and Childhood. 3rd ed. New York, Macmillan Publishing Co., 1978.

Kelly, J., and Anderson, D. H.: Congenital endocardial fibroelastosis. II. A clinical and pathologic investigation of those cases without associated cardiac malformations, including report of two familial instances. Pediatrics 18:539, 1956.

Kibrick, S.: Viral infections of the fetus and newborn. In Pollard, M. (Ed.): Perspectives in Virology. Vol. II. Minneapolis, Burgess Publishing Co., 1961, pp. 140–157.

Kohlschutter, A., and Hausdorf, G.: Primary (genetic) cardiomyopathies in infancy. A survey of possible disorders and guidelines for diagnosis. Eur. J. Pediatr. 145:454, 1986.

Lambert, E. C., Shumway, C. N., and Terplan, K.: Clinical diagnosis of endocardial fibrosis. Analysis of literature with report of four new cases. Pediatrics 11:255, 1953.

Lerner, A. M., Wilson, F. M., and Reyes, M. P.: Enteroviruses and the heart: epidemiological and experimental studies. I. Mod. Concepts Cardiovasc. Dis. 44:7, 1975.

Linde, L. M., and Adams, F. H.: Prognosis in endocardial fibroelastosis. Am. J. Dis. Child. 105:329, 1963.

Lipshultz, S. E., Chanock, S., Sanders, S. P., et al.: Cardiovascular manifestations of human immunodeficiency virus infections in infants and children. Am. J. Cardiol. 63:1489, 1989.

Lurie, P. R.: Endocardial fibroelastosis is not a disease. Am. J. Cardiol. 62:468, 1988.

Mitchell, S. C., Forehlich, L. A., Banas, J. S., and Gilkerson, M. R.: An epidemiologic assessment of primary endocardial fibroelastosis. Am. J. Cardiol. 18:859, 1966.

Nadas, A. S., and Ellison, R. C.: Cardiac tumors in infancy. Am. J. Cardiol. 21:363, 1968.

Neustein, H. B., Lurie, P. R., Dahms, B., and Takahash, M.: An x-linked recessive cardiomyopathy with abnormal mitochondria. Pediatrics 64:24, 1979.

Nihill, M. R., Wilson, D. S., Hugh-Jones, K., et al.: Generalized glycogenosis type II (Pompe's disease). Arch. Dis. Child. 45:122, 1970.

Poland, R. L., Walther, L. T., and Chang, C.: Hypertrophic cardiomyopathy in infants of diabetic mothers. Pediatr. Res. 9:269, 1975.

Rozkovec, A., Cambridge, G., King, M., and Hallidie-Smith, K. A.: Natural history of left ventricular function in Coxsackie myocarditis. Pediatr. Cardiol. 6:151, 1985.

Rowe, R. D., Finley, J. P., Gilday, D. L., et al.: Myocardial ischaemia in the newborn. In Godman, M. J., and Marquis, R. M. (Eds.): Pediatric Cardiology. Vol. 2. Heart Disease in the Newborn. Edinburgh, Churchill-Livingstone, 1979.

Rowe, R. D., Freedom, R. M., Mehrizi, A., and Bloom, K. R.: The Neonate with Congenital Heart Disease. Philadelphia, W. B. Saunders Co., 1981.

Rowe, R. D., and Hoffman, T.: Transient myocardial ischemia of the newborn infant. A form of severe cardio-respiratory distress in full-term infants. J. Pediatr. 81:243, 1972.

Rowland, T. W., Hubbell, J. P., and Nadas, A. S.: Congenital heart disease in infants of diabetic mothers. J. Pediatr. 83:815, 1973.

Shaher, R. M., Mintzer, J., Farina, M., Alley, R., and Bishop. M.: Clinical presentation of rhabdomyoma of the heart in infancy and childhood. Am. J. Cardiol. 30:95. 1972.

Sheehan, P. Q., Rowland, T. W., Shah, B. L., et al.: Maternal diabetic control and hypertrophic cardiomyopathy in infants of diabetic mothers. Clin. Pediatr. 25:266 1986.

Skillington, P. D., Brawn, W. J., and Edis, B. D.: Surgical excision of primary cardiac tumors in infancy. Aust. N. Z. J. Surg. 57:599, 1987.

Stewart, J. M., Kaul, A. Fromisch, D. S., et. al.: Symptomatic cardiac dysfunction in children with human immunodeficiency virus infection. Am. Heart J. 117:140 1989.

Van der Hauwaert, L. G.: Cardiac tumors in infancy and childhood. Br. Heart J. 33:125, 1971.

Walther, F. J., Siassi, B., Ramadan, N. A., and Wu, P. Y.: Cardiac output in newborn infants with transient myocardial dysfunction. J. Pediatr. 107:781, 1985.

Way, G. L., Wolfe, R. R., Pettet, G., et al.: Echocardiographic assessments of ventricular dimensions and myocardial function in infants of diabetic mothers. Pediatr. Res. 9:273, 1975.

Way, G. L., Wolff, R. R., Eshaghpour, E., et al.: The natural history of hypertrophic cardiomyopathy of infants of diabetic mothers. J. Pediatr. 95:1020, 1979.

Williams, W. G., Trusler, G. A., Fowler, R. S., et al.: Left ventricular myocardial fibroma: Case report and review of cardiac tumors in children. J. Pediatr. Surg. 7:324, 1972.

Wright, H. T., and Miller, A.: Fatal infection in a newborn infant due to herpes simplex virus. J. Pediatr. 67:130, 1965.

CARDIAC DYSRHYTHMIAS 65

Michael D. Freed

Cardiac dysrhythmias are not uncommon in the newborn, accompanying the significant changes in circulatory hemodynamics and gas exchange that occur with the switch from the in utero to extrauterine circulations. In a recent review of more then 3000 apparently normal newborns (Southall et al., 1981), about 1 per cent revealed dysrhythmias on a routine 10-second electrocardiogram prior to discharge. The vast majority of these dysrhythmias were of little significance, but life-threatening arrhythmias may occur on rare occasions. Excellent reviews of this topic have recently been published (Ferrer, 1977; Gillette and Garson, 1981; Losekoot and Lubbers, 1979).

◼ SINUS ARRHYTHMIA, SINUS TACHYCARDIA, AND SINUS BRADYCARDIA

Sinus arrhythmia is a phasic variation of the sinus node discharge that may occur either in cycle with respiration or independent of it. It is quite common and, as far as can be determined, is of no clinical significance. On electrocardiogram, the P–P interval is irregular and the P wave, P–Q interval, and QRS complexes are normal.

Sinus tachycardia can be defined as a heart rate that exceeds the upper range of normal, usually 175 to 190 beats/min in a full-term infant and 195 beats/min a premature infant. The P–P interval is short, but the P wave, P–Q interval, and QRS complexes are normal. It is usually a manifestation of increased adrenergic activity that may be the result of crying, feeding, or blood letting, but it may also be secondary to congestive heart failure, shock, anemia, or fever. No treatment is necessary if the significant secondary causes of the tachycardia can be ruled out.

Sinus bradycardia is a heart rate that falls below what is generally accepted as normal (i.e., below 90 to 100 beats/min), with a normal P wave preceding each QRS. Occasionally, the sinus mechanism is so depressed that the junctional tissue depolarizes first, resulting in a junctional escape rhythm. Sinus bradycardia has been associated with defecation, hiccupping, yawning, and nasopharyngeal stimulation, probably as a result of parasympathetic stimulation, and is frequently seen with prolonged apnea. Also, it may be seen with severe systemic disease, particularly that associated with acidosis, hypoxemia, or increased intracranial pressure. Occasionally, otherwise normal infants have a sinus bradycardia of 80 to 90 beats/min in the absence of other findings, probably because of immaturity of the autonomic nervous system and increased vagal tone. Careful monitoring, possibly with a 24-hour Holter ECG recording, may be indicated to ensure that more severe dysrhythmias do not coexist. If they can be ruled out and if severe systemic disease can be excluded, no treatment is necessary.

◼ ECTOPIC BEATS: SUPRAVENTRICULAR AND VENTRICULAR

Although during routine predischarge screening in one series the incidence of ectopic beats was less than 1 per cent (Southall et al., 1981), continuous monitoring of healthy newborns shows that the incidence of ectopic beats is much greater, as high as 13 per cent according to one report (Ferrer et al., 1977).

Supraventricular ectopic beats are usually preceded by a P wave with an abnormal contour, have a normal-appearing QRS, and are followed by an incomplete compensatory pause before the next P wave. Ventricular ectopic beats usually have a wide abnormal QRS, a tall T wave in the opposite direction from the QRS, and a full compensatory pause.

These arrhythmias may be seen with metabolic abnormalities, hypoxia, or digoxin toxicity or following cardiac surgery, but they are also frequently seen in otherwise normal newborns.

Treatment includes correction of the predisposing factors when possible; in otherwise normal infants no treatment is necessary unless couplets or atrial or ventricular tachycardia is present, since the prognosis is excellent, with ectopy usually disappearing within the 1st month of life.

◼ PAROXYSMAL SUPRAVENTRICULAR TACHYCARDIA

Paroxysmal supraventricular tachycardia (SVT) is one of the most common serious dysrhythmias occurring in the fetus and newborn. Although precise incidence data are not available, the generally accepted frequency is approximately 1 of every 25,000 children. Although usually relatively benign in the older child, the dysrhythmias may be life-threatening in the fetus or newborn, who generally has a higher ventricular rate and is less able to rely on other mechanisms for support of a failing circulation.

On electrocardiogram there is a rapid regular rhythm, usually 230 to 320 beats/min, that originates in the atria or junctional region with either normal, abnormal, or inapparent P waves, a normal or slightly widened QRS,

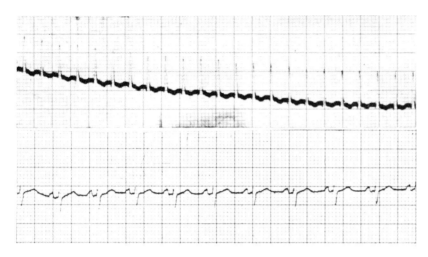

FIGURE 65–1. The upper tracing is lead III in a 7-day-old infant during a paroxysm of supraventricular tachycardia. The lower tracing (lead I) is in the same infant after the attack.

and ST segments that are normal or slightly depressed (Fig. 65–1). Several mechanisms play a part in the genesis of supraventricular tachycardias, but a rapid ectopic pacemaker or a circus type of re-entry secondary to different refractory periods of adjacent conducting bundles is the most common. Wolff-Parkinson-White syndrome, in which there is a direct muscular connection between the atrium and ventricle that allows re-entry, is recognizable on the electrocardiogram by a short P–Q interval and slow initial ventricular depolarization (delta wave) and is present in about 50 per cent of the cases (Fig. 65–2).

Clinical Manifestations. SVT may occur in the fetus (Newburger and Keane, 1979). It may not cause symptoms before birth, but occasionally the rapid rate may lead to in utero congestive heart failure with fetal edema or hydrops and fetal death. Rarely, the fetal SVT is intermittent, and we have observed infants with hydrops born with normal EKGs who subsequently demonstrate recurrent SVT.

The newborn with SVT presents with signs and symptoms of low cardiac output and congestive heart failure; fussiness, refusal to feed, vomiting, tachypnea, and hepatomegaly are common. At first, the infants have some duskiness or cyanosis of the skin, but later their skin turns ashen grey and their extremities become cool owing to extreme peripheral vasoconstriction. Cardiac examination usually reveals no problem other than tachycardia. Underlying heart disease may be difficult to detect, even if present, because of the rapid heart rate.

At first, the chest radiograph may be normal, but, by

the time symptoms occur, there is usually cardiac enlargement, often with pulmonary venous congestion. The echocardiogram is helpful in ruling out associated heart disease.

Diagnosis. SVT is diagnosed electrocardiographically. Occasionally, normal newborns with increased adrenergic activity may have heart rates exceeding 200 beats/min, but these infants do not have congestive failure and the rate slows down when they are quiet. Occasionally, however, it may be difficult to distinguish newborns with a tachycardia associated with severe congestive failure caused by myocarditis or congenital heart disease from those with SVT. Rates of 220 or more in the newborn are rarely, if ever, of sinus origin and thus require treatment. Rates of 220 or less in the newborn usually represent sinus rhythm. The presence of heart failure with a rate of 200 to 220 suggests underlying heart disease, since this rate alone is rarely rapid enough to cause significant congestive heart failure in the newborn. Another helpful electrocardiographic sign is that SVT is almost always very regular, with variation in heart rate of more than 1 to 2 beats/min being an unusual occurrence. Therefore, any variation in rate with crying or feeding is likely to signify a sinus mechanism. Rarely, a therapeutic trial of digoxin may be necessary to sort out the underlying mechanism.

Treatment. Supraventricular tachycardia in a newborn represents an emergency, and treatment should not be delayed. Vagal stimulation including gagging, carotid sinus massage, or ice compresses to the head should be tried but are rarely effective. For those infants who are not

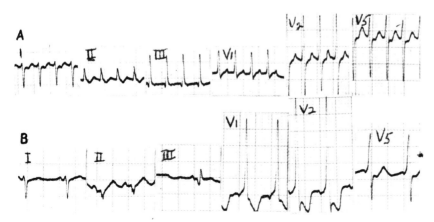

FIGURE 65–2. Electrocardiogram in a 4-day-old infant. A, Supraventricular tachycardia. B, Tracing after the tachycardia stopped shows a typical Wolff-Parkinson-White pattern with a short P-R interval and a wide QRS. The delta waves can be seen just before the upstroke of the R waves in the precordial leads.

critically ill, we continue to administer digoxin with half the total digitalizing dose of 0.04 mg/kg given stat and the rest in divided doses over the next 12 to 18 hours. If the newborn is sicker, three-fourths of the total digitalizing dose can be given immediately intravenously, with the remainder administered within 4 to 8 hours. Other regimens that can be used in an emergency include overdrive atrial pacing (Garson, 1981), DC cardioversion (0.25 to 1 joule/kg) synchronized to the peak of the QRS complex to avoid the vulnerable period of the T wave, propranolol (0.01 to 0.1 mg/kg IV), phenylephrine (0.01 to 0.1 mg/kg IV), or edrophonium (0.2 mg/kg IV). After conversion of SVT, we usually continue administering digoxin for about 1 year. If "breakthroughs" occur, we now use esophageal electrophysiologic drug testing to guide therapy.

Prognosis. The long-term prognosis is good. Recurrences occur in about 25 per cent of the infants, but these are usually easily controlled with drug therapy. Rarely, surgery or catheterization lab ablation is necessary to interrupt a bypass tract that is facilitating a re-entry tachycardia.

■ ATRIAL FLUTTER

Atrial flutter is a relatively rare dysrhythmia in the neonatal period. The atrial rate ranges between 360 and 480 beats/min, with the ventricular response one-half or, less commonly, one-third of that. The atrial activity is best seen as a saw-toothed pattern of the P waves in leads II and V_{4R} to V_2. Newborns with atrial flutter may have congestive heart failure from the tachycardia, but more commonly the 2:1 or 3:1 block reduces the ventricular rate so that the dysrhythmia is well tolerated (Fig. 65–3).

The treatment involves digitalization and, if this fails to revert the rhythm to sinus, cardioversion. The prognosis is not as favorable as with atrial tachycardia, since recurrences are more common, but most infants without associated structural heart disease usually do well. Ongoing treatment with digoxin is usually successful in preventing recurrences. If this approach is not successful, propranolol or quinidine can be added.

■ VENTRICULAR TACHYCARDIA

Ventricular tachycardia (3 or more premature complexes in a row) in the newborn is uncommon. When it does occur, it is usually in association with structural heart disease and is triggered by cardiac catheterization, surgery, anesthesia, metabolic abnormalities, or digitalis toxicity. The QRS complexes are wide and tall, and the T waves are directed opposite to the QRS complex. The rate is usually less than 200, but higher rates have been reported. The initial treatment should be lidocaine (1 mg/kg IV) or cardioversion. Other drugs that may occasionally be useful include phenytoin (diphenylhydantoin), procainamide, quinidine, and propranolol. In the idiopathic variety, echocardiography and angiocardiography should be performed to rule out the possibility that a resectable tumor is the source of the tachycardia. Treatment must be individualized, with the long-term prognosis depending primarily on the underlying cardiac problem.

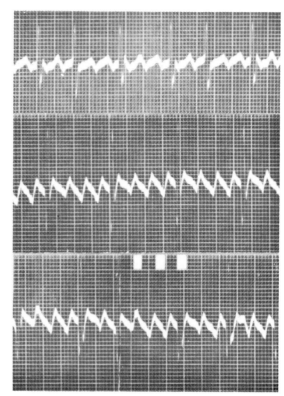

FIGURE 65–3. Standard limb leads during an attack of atrial flutter.

■ ATRIOVENTRICULAR BLOCK

First and Second Degree Heart Block. First degree heart block is a prolongation of the P–R interval beyond the normal limits, 0.14 second. It is of no hemodynamic significance by itself and requires no treatment. In second degree heart block, there is an intermittent failure of impulse transmission from atria to ventricles. It may be exhibited as a progressive prolongation of the P–R interval in successive cycles followed by an unconducted atrial impulse (Wenkebach or Mobitz type I) or failure of atrial impulse transmission with dropped ventricular beats and no progressive prolongation of the P–R interval (Mobitz type II). Both type I and type II may be manifestations of infection or digitalis toxicity. Neither type needs treatment, but both should be watched carefully, since either may lead to third degree or complete heart block.

Third Degree Heart Block. In complete heart block (CHB) there is complete failure of the atrial impulse to lead to a ventricular response; the atria and ventricles beat independently, with the latter having a slower rate. On the surface EKG, there is no fixed relationship between the P waves and the QRS complex (Fig. 65–4). CHB is a relatively common problem in the newborn, occurring in 1 of every 15,000 to 20,000 live births.

Histologically, there may be an absence of a connection between the atrial conduction tissue and the atrioventricular node, absence or degeneration of the connection between the A–V node tissue and the distal conducting tissue, or a lesion beyond the A–V node that interrupts the bundle of His (Lev, 1972). Intracardiac electrophysiologic studies obtained during cardiac catheterization on 24 older children with congenital complete heart block

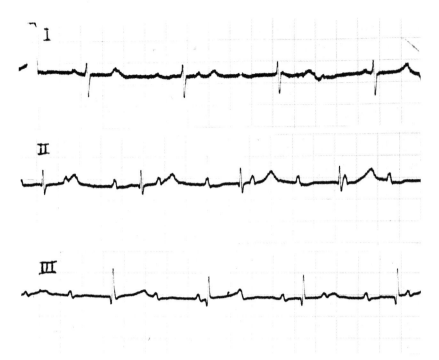

FIGURE 65–4. Age 4 days. Standard limb leads. Complete heart block is present. The ventricular rate is 90, the atrial rate 120.

demonstrated block above or in the A–V node in 79 per cent, within the bundle of His in 13 per cent, and more distal in the conducting system in 4 per cent. The site of block could not be determined in 4 per cent (Karpawich et al., 1981).

Approximately 40 per cent of infants with congenital complete heart block have associated structural heart disease (Michaelsson and Engle, 1972), with corrected transposition of the great arteries, single ventricle, and the heterotaxy syndrome the most common, although virtually any type of heart disease can occasionally be found.

Increasing evidence has accumulated suggesting an autoimmune component in the cause of congenital complete heart block in many if not all newborns without other structural heart disease. Taylor and colleagues (1988) have found autoantibodies to ribonucleoprotein antigens using immunofluorescence and western blots in all of 55 mothers with babies with complete heart block, in 10 of 29 women with connective tissue disease who did not have babies with heart block, and 4 of 445 normal pregnant women. Of 10 babies with complete heart block who were less than 3 months old, all had Ro (SSA) or La (SSB) antibodies, usually in lower titers than their mothers, suggesting deposition in the babies' tissues. Infants of mothers with lupus erythematosus seem especially vulnerable.

Clinical Manifestations. The block is often suspected or diagnosed in utero during the third trimester or during labor because of the persistent slow heart rate of the fetus, about 50 to 80 beats/min. More than half the babies are delivered by emergency cesarean section owing to the mistaken belief that the bradycardia represents fetal distress (Esscher and Michaelsson, 1979). The majority of newborns are symptom free; those newborns with associated structural congenital heart disease or ventricular rates of less than 50 beats/min are the most likely to have the symptoms of heart failure.

In the child without associated structural heart disease

or heart failure, the large stroke volume often results in soft systolic flow murmurs across the aortic or pulmonary valves, and the atrioventricular dissociation with variable flow across the A–V valves may produce a variable first heart sound and intermittent flow rumble across the mitral or tricuspid valves. On the radiograph, the heart may be slightly enlarged, but the pulmonary vascular markings are normal and pulmonary venous congestion is absent.

In the newborn with heart failure, the usual manifestations are usually present, with dyspnea, tachypnea, hepatomegaly, and feeding difficulties common. The findings on physical examination and radiographs usually depend on the associated cardiac lesions.

Treatment. Most newborns without structural heart disease are asymptomatic; for these, careful observation will suffice. For the rare child without associated anomalies in whom bradycardia causes heart failure unresponsive to diuretics, a pacemaker is necessary. Isoproterenol may be of temporary help. Although temporary pacing can usually be established by a transvenous catheter route, the possibility of cardiac perforation, emboli from the catheter, and the difficulties encountered with linear growth of the child make epicardial pacing desirable after a thoracotomy for placement of the wires. For newborns with symptoms due to CHB accompanying structural heart disease, treatment usually involves palliation or correction of the underlying cardiac anomaly with epicardial pacing.

Prognosis. The prognosis greatly depends on the presence and nature of associated structural heart disease. In a group of 118 newborns with complete heart block but without structural heart disease followed for a median interval of 9 years, there were 21 deaths (18 per cent), 15 of them occurring before 2 weeks of age and the remainder before 5 years of age. Thirteen required permanent pacemakers (Esscher and Michaelsson, 1979). In contrast, of 80 newborns with CHB diagnosed soon after birth who had associated heart disease, 34 (43 per cent) died, almost all in the 1st week of life (Michaelsson and Engle, 1972).

Most of the available data reflect management in the 1960s and early 1970s; with better corrective and palliative surgery as well as microcircuitry and miniaturization of pacemakers, results will likely improve in the next decade.

■ REFERENCES

Esscher, E., and Michaelsson, M.: Assessment and management of complete heart block. *In* Godman, M.J., and Marquis, R.M. (eds.): Pediatric Cardiology. Vol 2. Heart Disease in the Newborn. Edinburgh, Churchill-Livingstone, 1979.

Ferrer, P. L.: Arrhythmias in the neonate. *In* Roberts, N. K., and Gelband, H. (Eds.): Cardiac arrhythmias in the neonate, infant, and child. New York, Appleton-Century-Crofts, 1977.

Ferrer, P. L., Gelband, H., Garcia, O. I., et al.: Occurrence of arrhythmias in the newborn period. Clin. Res. 25:64A, 1977.

Garson, A., Jr.: Supraventricular tachycardia. *In* Gillette, P. C., and Garson, A., Jr. (Eds.): Pediatric Cardiac Dysrhythmias. New York, Grune & Stratton, 1981.

Gillette, P. C., and Garson, A.: Pediatric Cardiac Dysrhythmias. New York, Grune & Stratton, 1981.

Gillette, P. C., Garson, A., Jr., Crawford, F., et al.: Dysrhythmias. *In* Adams, F. H., Emmanouilides, G. C., and Riemenschneider, T. A. (Eds.): Moss' Heart Disease in Infants, Children, and Adolescents. Baltimore, Williams & Wilkins, 1989.

Karpawich, P. P., Gilette, P. C., Garson, A., et al.: Congenital complete atrio-ventricular predictors of need for pacemaker insertion. Am. J. Cardiol. 48:1098, 1981.

Lev, M.: Pathogenesis of congenital atrio-ventricular block. Prog. Cardiovasc. Dis. 15:145, 1972.

Losekoot, T. G., and Lubbers, W. J.: Arrhythmias in the neonate. *In* Godman, M. J., and Marquis, R. M. (Eds.): Pediatric Cardiology. Vol 2. Heart Disease in the Newborn. Edinburgh, Churchill-Livingstone, 1979.

McCue, C. M., Mantakas, M. E., Tingelstad, J. B., and Ruddy, S.: Congenital heart block in newborns of mothers with connective tissue disease. Circulation 56:82, 1977.

Michaelsson, M., and Engle, M. A.: Congenital complete heart block: an international study of the natural history. *In* Engle, M. A. (Ed.): Pediatric Cardiology, Cardiovascular Clinics. Philadelphia, F. A. Davis Co., 1972.

Newburger, J. W., and Keane, J. F.: Intrauterine supraventricular tachycardia. J. Pediatr. 95:780, 1979.

Southall, D. P., and Johnson, A. M., Shinebourne, E. A., Johnston, P. G., and Vulliamy, D. G.: Frequency and outcome of disorders of cardiac rhythm and conduction in a population of newborn infants. Pediatrics 68:58, 1981.

Taylor, P. V., Taylor K. F., Norman, A., Griffiths, S., and Scott, J. S.: Prevalence of maternal R$_o$(SSA) and L$_a$(SSB) autoantibodies in relation to complete heart block. Br. J. Rheumatol. 27:128, 1988.

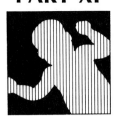

PART XI

THE GASTROINTESTINAL SYSTEM

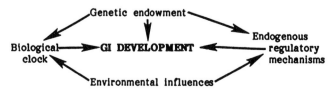

GENERAL **66** CONSIDERATIONS

William J. Byrne and Arthur E. D'Harlingue

■ HISTORICAL PERSPECTIVE

The human embryo . . . is a living theatre in which a weird transformation scene is being enacted, and in which countless strange and uncouth characters take part. Some of these characters are well-known to science, some are strangers.

—DRUMMOND, 1895

The study of gastrointestinal development dates back to the time of the ancient Greeks. Aristotle coined the term "meconium" because of its likeness to material obtained from the poppy (mekonion). He felt that this material was responsible for keeping the fetus asleep in the womb. Hippocrates hypothesized that the presence of meconium in the fetal intestine was proof that the fetus sucks in the womb. In 1874, Langendorff found pepsin in the fetal stomach and confirmed the findings of Elsasser that the gastric mucosa of the human fetus was capable of digesting albumin (Grand et al., 1976). At the turn of the century, Berry (1900) published a number of important observations about the morphologic development of the small intestine. He noted that villi were absent in the 1.7-cm (7-week-old) fetus, limited to the duodenum in the 2.6-cm (8- to 9-week-old) fetus, but present along the entire length of the small intestine in the 8-cm (12-week-old) fetus. In 1909, Ibrahim confirmed Langendorff's earlier observations about the presence of trypsin activity in the pancreas at 4 months' gestation. Further, he showed that enterokinase from the newborn duodenum was able to increase this activity. Later Ibrahim (1910) described the presence of sucrase in the small intestine by 14 weeks' gestation and lactase by 25 weeks' gestation. These early observations provided the foundation for subsequent studies upon which we base our current understanding of the ontogeny of the gastrointestinal tract.

■ CONCEPTUAL FRAMEWORK

From a conceptual point of view, the development of the gastrointestinal tract results from the interaction of four determinants (Fig. 66–1) (Lebenthal and Lee, 1983).

Genetic endowment plays the major role in the differentiation and maturation of tissue. The biological clock, the second determinant, refers to the genetically predetermined developmental sequence. Using the tools of molecular biology, Tilghman and Belayew (1982) observed the stage-specific regulation of gene expression for alphafetoprotein and albumin in the rat fetus. The biologic clock is species-specific and therefore creates problems when trying to extrapolate animal data to humans. For example, rat pups do not secrete hydrochloric acid in the stomach until the time of weaning (Ackerman, 1982; Ikizaki and Johnson, 1983). However, even in premature infants of 32 weeks' gestation, acid secretion is present in the human newborn 1 week after birth (Euler et al., 1979; Hyman et al., 1985).

The third determinant of gastrointestinal development, regulation by endogenous substances, is also known to be genetically mediated. These substances may in turn impact on gastrointestinal development. The best-known endogenous regulators are hormones, specifically T_3, glucocorticoids, and epidermal growth factor. The administration of glucocorticoids or thyroxine to suckling mice or rats before a critical stage in maturation results in an increase in the brush border activity of sucrase, alkaline phosphatase, and enteropeptidase. There is also increasing evidence that epidermal growth factor is important both prenatally and postnatally in gut development. Epidermal growth factor is a small polypeptide (molecular weight 6050 daltons) found in saliva, gastrointestinal secretions, colostrum, and breast milk. It is also present in human amniotic fluid by midgestation, but the cellular site

FIGURE 66–1. *Interaction of determinants in the ontogeny of the gastrointestinal tract. (From Lebenthal, E. M., and Lee, P. C.: Pediatr. Res. 17:20, 1983.)*

653

of origin is unknown (Barka et al., 1978). Epidermal growth factor stimulates epithelial cell proliferation and accelerates maturation (Conteas et al., 1986; Goodlad et al., 1985; Lebenthal and Leung, 1987), decreases gastric acid secretion by parietal cells (Elder et al., 1975), and inhibits gut prostaglandin synthesis (Konturek et al., 1981). These actions—mitogenesis, antisecretion, and cytoprotection—may be particularly important during the perinatal period of adaptation from intrauterine to extrauterine nutrition.

Finally, postnatal environmental influences may alter the timing of developmental stages by affecting endogenous regulatory mechanisms. For example, in suckling rats, sucrose infusion stimulates the production of sucrase and isomaltase but not lactase (Lebenthal et al., 1972). Lactose infusion has the same effect on lactase and decreases its rate of postnatal decline (Lebenthal et al., 1973). Malnutrition slows down the biological clock and delays development. Rats undernourished during the suckling period have decreased intestinal weights owing to decreased cell number and DNA content (Hatch et al., 1979a). Pancreatic enzyme content is also decreased with lipase being the most severely affected (Hatch et al., 1979b). In humans, severe malnutrition results in atrophy of the pancreas and intestinal mucosa (Martins Campos et al., 1979; Thompson and Trowell, 1951). These changes are correctable if the malnutrition is reversed.

■ EMBRYOLOGY

Highlights of the morphologic development of the gastrointestinal tract, pancreas, and liver are presented in Table 66–1. By the 4th week of gestation, the primitive gut is recognizable as a tubular structure. Rapid elongation during the 5th and 6th week results in a looping of the gut into the umbilical cord (Fig. 66–2A). At this same time the dorsal border of the cranial end of the gut elongates at a more rapid rate than the ventral border, producing a convexity that becomes the greater curvature of the stomach. The enlarging liver anlage displaces the stomach to the left, creating a "bridge" that eventually becomes the fundus. Late in the 6th week, the stomach undergoes a 90-degree clockwise rotation, positioning the dorsal surface (greater curvature) to the left side of the abdomen and the ventral surface (lesser curvature) to face the right (Fig. 66–2B). At about this same time, the small intestine rotates counterclockwise around the axis of the superior mesenteric artery. Thick bands fix the duodenum and splenic flexure of the colon, preventing their entrance into the cord. The small intestine continues to elongate. At 10 weeks' gestation, it reenters the abdominal cavity. The jejunum returns first, filling the left half and the ileum fills the right half (Fig. 66–2C and 66–2D). The colon enters last. The cecum becomes fixed in the right lower quadrant with the ascending and transverse colon slanting upward and across the abdomen to the splenic flexure. Later elongation of the colon results in the establishment of the hepatic flexure and transverse colon.

STOMACH

In the stomach, circular smooth muscle is present by the 9th week. Formation of the glandular pits is complete

TABLE 66–1. Development of the Human Gastrointestinal Tract

AGE (Weeks)	CROWN-RUMP LENGTH (mm)	STAGE OF DEVELOPMENT
2.5	1.5	Gut not distinct from the yolk sac
3.5	2.5	Fore and hindgut present
		Liver bud present
		Yolk sac broadly attached to the midgut
4	5	Esophagus short
		Stomach spindle-shaped
		Intestine present as a simple tube
		Liver cords, ducts, and gallbladder form
		Pancreatic buds appear as outpouching of the gut
	7.5	Esophagus clearly differentiated from the stomach
5	8	Intestine lengthens into a loop
6	12	Stomach rotates
		Intestinal loop undergoes torsion
		Parotid and submandibular buds appear
7	17	Stomach attains final position
		Circular muscle layer present
		Duodenum temporarily occluded
		Intestine herniates into the umbilical cord
	19	Villi begin to appear
8	23	Taste buds appear
		Gastric pits present in the fundus and body of the stomach
		Villi lined by a single layer of cells
10	40	Gastric pits in the pylorus and cardia of the stomach
		Intestine reenters the abdominal cavity
		Active transport of glucose present
		Dipeptidases present in the small intestine
12	56	Parietal cells detectable in the stomach
		Intestinal muscle layers present
		Active transport of amino acids present
		Colonic haustrations appear
		Pancreatic islets appear
		Bile secreted
	78	Circular folds appear in the small intestine
16		Meconium present in the gut
	120	Glucose transport in jejunum increasing
		Dipeptidase and disaccharidase activities increase
20	160	Peyer patches present in the intestine
		Muscularis mucosa present
24	203	Ascending colon recognizable
		Paneth cells appear
28	242	Esophageal glands appear
38	350	Maturity achieved

(Adapted from Grand, R. J., Watkins, J. B., and Torti, F. M.: Development of the human gastrointestinal tract. Gastroenterology 70:790, 1976. Reprinted with permission.)

by 12 weeks, and parietal cells are detectable. Chief cells and mucous neck cells are present by 14 weeks, and by 16 weeks mucus production in the stomach is present.

SMALL INTESTINE

Villi begin to form in the duodenum by 7 weeks' gestation. Differentiation progresses distally so that by 14 weeks the entire small intestinal mucosa is lined by villi. Circular folds appear at 12 weeks in the middle of the small intestine and are present throughout by 32 weeks. The Auerbach and Meissner plexuses appear by 9 and 13

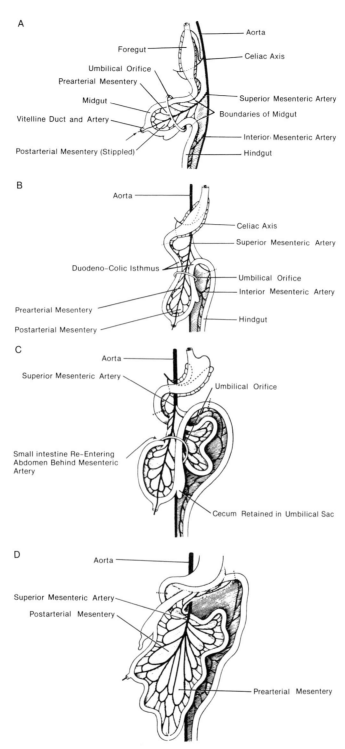

A

Aorta

Foregut

Celiac Axis

Umbilical Orifice

Prearterial Mesentery

Superior Mesenteric Artery

Midgut

Boundaries of Midgut

Vitelline Duct and Artery

Interior Mesenteric Artery

Postarterial Mesentery (Stippled)

Hindgut

B

Aorta

Celiac Axis

Superior Mesenteric Artery

Duodeno-Colic Isthmus

Umbilical Orifice

Interior Mesenteric Artery

Prearterial Mesentery

Postarterial Mesentery

Hindgut

C

Aorta

Superior Mesenteric Artery

Umbilical Orifice

Small intestine Re-Entering Abdomen Behind Mesenteric Artery

Cecum Retained in Umbilical Sac

D

Aorta

Superior Mesenteric Artery

Postarterial Mesentery

Prearterial Mesentery

FIGURE 66–2. Diagram showing normal rotation of alimentary tract. A, Fifth week of intrauterine life (lateral view). The foregut, midgut, and hindgut are shown with their individual blood supply supported by the common dorsal mesentery in the sagittal plane. The midgut loop has been extruded into the umbilical cord. B, Eighth week of intrauterine life (anteroposterior view). The first stage of rotation is being completed. Note the narrow duodenocolic isthmus from which the midgut loop depends and the right-sided position of the small intestine and left-sided position of the colon. Maintenance of this position within the abdomen after birth is termed "nonrotation." C, About the tenth week of intrauterine life, during the second stage of rotation (anteroposterior view). The bowel in the temporary umbilical hernia is in the process of reduction; the most proximal part of the prearterial segment entering the abdomen to the right of the superior mesenteric artery is held forward close to the cecum and ascending colon, permitting the bowel to pass under it. As the coils of small intestine collect within the abdomen, the hindgut is displaced to the left and upward. D, Eleventh week of intrauterine life at the end of the second stage of rotation. From its original sagittal position, the midgut has rotated 270 degrees in a counterclockwise direction about the origin of the superior mesenteric artery. The essentials of the permanent disposition of the viscera have been attained. (From Gardner, C. E., Jr., and Hart, D.: Arch. Surg. 29:942, 1934. Copyright 1934, American Medical Association.)

weeks, respectively. Peristalsis can be detected at this time. Lymphopoiesis is present at 15 weeks, and the Peyer patches are well developed by 20 weeks. Disaccharidases, peptidases, and the processes of glucose and amino acid transport are detectable by 15 weeks. Their functional capabilities increase with time. The regulatory peptides of the gut (gastrin, secretin, motilin, gastric inhibitory peptide, vasoactive intestinal peptide, enteroglucagon, and somatostatin) are detectable in the small intestine as early as 8 weeks, while neurotensin is not present until 12 weeks. Adult patterns of distribution are achieved by 24 weeks. Of the peptide hormones, only vasoactive intestinal peptide is localized to nerve fibers, and these are present in both enteric plexuses. Concentrations of the peptides increase steadily until term when they approach adult levels. Aynsley-Green (1985) has shown postnatal surges of these hormones following enteral feedings in preterm infants.

COLON

Critical to the development of the colon is the fusion of the rectum, which is derived separately as a subdivision of the cloaca, to the digestive tube by the 8th fetal week. There is a cranial-to-caudal migration of ganglion cells during the 5th to 12th weeks. Except for an area of hypoganglionosis 1 cm above the anal verge, a normal distribution of ganglion cells is present by 24 weeks. Taeniae appear and haustra begin forming by 12 weeks. Peristalsis in the colon has been detected as early as the 8th week (Pace, 1971).

PANCREAS

The dorsal and ventral pancreatic buds are detectable by the 4th week and fusion occurs by the 7th week. The head and body of the mature pancreas arise from the ventral primordium; the distal body and tail from the dorsal primordium. The pancreatic ducts join to form the duct of Wirsung, although the proximal portion of the duct from the dorsal bud may persist as the duct of Santorini. Acinar cells and the islets of Langerhans are present by the 12th week. Well-differentiated zymogen granules in the acinar cells can be seen by 20 weeks (Conklin, 1962; Liu and Potter, 1962).

LIVER

The hepatic anlage appears during the 4th week of gestation as a diverticulum arising from the duodenum. The cranial portion of this diverticulum differentiates into hepatic glandular tissue and bile ducts. The caudal portion forms the gallbladder and cystic duct. Hepatic lobes are identifiable by the 6th week. By the 10th week, the rapidly growing liver reaches its peak relative size, constituting 10 per cent of the fetal weight. During development, changes in the hepatic anlage occur. The liver initially contains more hematopoietic cells than functioning hepatocytes. These hepatocytes are small and contain little glycogen. As gestation progresses, hepatocytes increase in size, number, and glycogen content, while the number of hematopoietic cells decreases.

BILIARY SYSTEM

Well-developed bile canaliculi have been found as early as 6 weeks. Formation of intrahepatic bile ducts from cell plates derived from the hepatic duct is complete by the 3rd month of gestation (Koga, 1971). The cystic duct and gallbladder, initially solid epithelial cylinders, canalize by the 8th week (Grand et al., 1976).

■ SYMPTOMS OF GASTROINTESTINAL DISORDERS

VOMITING

Regurgitation of the first few feedings is not uncommon. However, the newborn who vomits should be observed and examined frequently. The nature of the material regurgitated furnishes useful clues to the location of obstruction. Pure mucus or a mixture of mucus and saliva alone denotes obstruction proximal to the stomach and suggests esophageal atresia. Unaltered or coagulated milk, unstained with bile, suggests gastroesophageal reflux or obstruction at the pylorus or in the duodenum proximal to the ampulla of Vater. Bile-stained vomitus suggests narrowing or obstruction of the intestinal lumen distal to the ampulla. The presence of bile in vomitus is suggestive, but not absolutely diagnostic, of organic obstruction. Fecal vomitus indicates obstruction low in the intestinal tract.

When blood is mixed with the vomitus, it may be difficult to ascertain its source. It should not be forgotten that such blood may be maternal in origin, ingested with the amniotic fluid after placental hemorrhage or ingested with the milk when the nipple is cracked and bleeding. With the Apt test fetal blood may be differentiated from maternal blood, since fetal red cells resist alkali denaturation.

In addition to gastrointestinal lesions, there are numerous other causes of vomiting. Intracranial lesions, chiefly subdural hemorrhage and hydrocephalus, commonly produce vomiting. Infections of almost any system may present with vomiting, and in some cases, the vomiting may continue until the infection is controlled. Metabolic disorders, such as galactosemia, hereditary fructose intolerance, tyrosinemia, and adrenal cortical hyperplasia, also often cause vomiting.

CONSTIPATION

The first meconium stool is passed by 69 per cent of healthy infants within 12 hours, by 94 per cent within 24 hours, and by 99.8 per cent within 48 hours (Sherry and Kramer, 1955). In 1973, Mangurten and Slade confirmed these findings and could discover "no relationship among birth weight, gestational age, Apgar score, or age at first feeding and age at first stool." Failure to pass stool within the first 24 hours should always be regarded with suspicion. In addition to obstruction and sepsis, delayed stooling may be the earliest sign of Hirschsprung disease.

After the first 2 days, during which pure meconium is passed, the newborn's stools consist of part meconium and part fecal matter for another day or two, after which they become entirely fecal. The number of stools passed by the healthy infant is extremely variable—for some, as few as one every 2nd or 3rd day; for others, as many as

10 every 24 hours. In general, the stools of the breast-fed infant are more frequent and more liquid than those of the formula-fed infant. However, it is not uncommon or abnormal for a breast-fed infant to have stools every 48 to 72 hours or even less frequently. This does not represent constipation unless the stools passed are hard and dry. At times, this may be the result of inadequate fluid intake. When intake is adequate and the consistency of stool is not abnormal, infrequent bowel movements may be considered normal.

In some newborns, especially premature infants, "functional" constipation may become a problem. Stools not only are passed at long intervals but also, when passed, are small, hard, and dry. Constipation in these tiny infants may produce anorexia, distention, and vomiting. Laxative medications in general should be avoided, but a glycerin suppository (usually only a fraction of one is necessary) is permissible and often effective. The exact cause of this type of constipation is not known, but weakness of the intestinal and abdominal musculature may play an important role. Infants of mothers with preeclampsia who may be hypermagnesemic are lethargic and flaccid, and their passing of meconium may be delayed.

DIARRHEA

Diarrhea is usually defined as the passage of an excessive number of liquid stools. This definition requires several qualifying statements. The breast-fed infant may pass as many as 10 stools in the course of 24 hours, yet appear well, and continue to thrive. Often the bowel movements follow a feeding. In this case, the term "diarrhea" should not be applied. Other infants, however, may have only two or three large liquid stools, yet look ill and become dehydrated and acidotic with great rapidity. Such a situation fulfills the definition of diarrhea.

Diarrhea in the newborn is usually due either to an intolerance to formula protein or to enteral infection. Rarely, it is caused by disaccharidase deficiency, and even more rarely, it may be the result of deficiency of monosaccharide absorption (Table 66–2).

GASTROINTESTINAL BLEEDING

The vomiting of blood or blood-stained gastric contents and the passage of bloody stools are not infrequent occurrences in the neonatal period. As mentioned earlier, the physician's first task is to determine whether this blood is maternal in origin or whether the infant is bleeding internally. As little as 3.0 ml of blood ingested by the infant may produce one or more bloody stools that appear 7 to 17 hours after ingestion.

Apt Test. Maternal blood may be distinguished from the infant's because of the high percentage of fetal hemoglobin (hemoglobin F), which is resistant to both alkali and acid in the newborn in contrast with its virtual absence in the adult. The Apt test for the differentiation of fetal blood from that of adult is performed by first mixing the specimen under study with an equal quantity of tap water. Either centrifuge the mixture or strain it through filter paper. If the supernatant or the filtrate is pink, hemoglobin may be present. To five parts of this supernatant or filtrate, add one part of 0.25 per cent sodium hydroxide. The pink color should deepen and persist for more than 2 minutes if hemoglobin F is present. If it turns yellow within 2 minutes, it is hemoglobin A.

Fetal blood indicates one of a variety of lesions, and its source may be difficult to determine. Bloody vomitus may be due to esophagitis. Although peptic ulcer of the stomach or duodenum occurs in the newborn, it may not be readily recognizable on radiographic contrast studies, and therefore, diagnosis rests on endoscopic evaluation after other causes of bleeding have been excluded. These include deficiencies in the clotting mechanism and pulmonary hemorrhage. Rarely, the newborn bleeds from peptic ulcers in unusual locations, such as in a Meckel diverticulum. Duplications of the bowel may also bleed and, more uncommonly, intussusception or hemangiomas in the bowel may occur.

ANOREXIA

Some newborns eat poorly at first. The reason in any particular case usually becomes obvious with careful observation and follow-up. On occasion, there seems to be a complete lack of the sensation of hunger. Neurologic disorders may present in this fashion. Choanal atresia may also present with poor feeding because of the inability of the newborn to breathe while feeding.

■ REFERENCES

Ackerman, S. H.: Ontogeny of gastric acid secretion in the rat: Evidence for multiple response systems. Science *217*:75–80, 1982.

Aynsley-Green, A.: Metabolic and endocrine interrelations in the human fetus and neonate. Am. J. Clin. Nutr. *41*:399–417, 1985.

Barka, T., Van der Noen, H., Gresik, E. W., et al.: Immunoreactive epidermal growth factor in human amniotic fluid. Mt. Sinai J. Med. *45*:679–684, 1978.

Berry, J. M.: On the development of the villi of the human intestine. Anat. Anz. *17*:242–249, 1900.

Bryant, M. G., Buchan, A. M. J., Gregor, M., et al.: Development of intestinal regulatory peptides in the human fetus. Gastroenterology *83*:47–54, 1982.

Conklin, J. L.: Cytogenesis of the human fetal pancreas. Am. J. Anat. *11*:181–203, 1962.

Conteas, C. N., De Morrow, J. M., and Majunder A. P. N.: Effect of epidermal growth factor on growth and maturation of fetal and neonatal rat intestine in organ culture. Experientia *42*:950–952, 1986.

Drummond, H.: The Ascent of Man, 5th ed. New York, James Pott and Co., 1895.

TABLE 66–2. Conditions Associated with Diarrhea from the Time of Birth

Absorptive disorders (symptoms brought on by feeding)
    Formula protein intolerance
    Glucose-galactose malabsorption
    Sucrase-isomaltase deficiency
    Lactase deficiency
    Enterokinase deficiency
    Cystic fibrosis
Secretory disorders
    Congenital chloridorrhea
    Tumors:
        Ganglioneuroma
        Neuroblastoma
Other
    Neonatal necrotizing enterocolitis
    Hirschsprung disease
    Intractable diarrhea of infancy
    Familial enteropathy

Elder, J. B., Ganguli, P. C., and Gillespie, J. E.: Effect of urogastrone on gastric secretion and plasma gastrin levels in normal subjects. Gut 15:887–893, 1975.

Euler, A. R., Byrne, W. J., Meis, P. J., et al.: Basal and pentagastrin stimulated acid secretion in newborn human infants. Pediatr. Res. 13:36–39, 1979.

Goodlad, R. A., Wilson, T. J. G., Lenton, W., et al.: Urogastrone-epidermal growth factor is trophic to the intestinal epithelium of parenterally fed rats. Experientia 41:1161–1163, 1985.

Grand, R. J., Watkins, J. B., and Torte, F. M.: Development of the human gastrointestinal tract. Gastroenterology 70:790–810, 1976.

Hatch, T. F., Lebenthal, E., Branski, D., et al.: The effects of early postnatal malnutrition on intestinal growth, disaccharidases and enterokinase. J. Pediatr. Gastroenterol. Nutr. 109:1874–1878, 1979a.

Hatch, T. F., Lebenthal, E., Krasner, J., et al.: Effect of postnatal malnutrition on pancreatic zymogen enzymes in the rat. Am. J. Clin. Nutr. 32:1224–1230, 1979b.

Hyman, P. E., Clarke, M. D., Everett, S. L., et al.: Gastric acid secretory function in preterm infants. J. Pediatr. 106:467–471, 1985.

Ibrahim, J.: Trypsinogen und enterokinase beim menschlichen neugeborenen und embryo. Biochem. Zeitschr. 23:24–32, 1909.

Ibrahim, J.: Die doppelzuckerfermente (lactase, maltase, invertin) beim menschlichen neugeborenen und embryo. Hoppe Seylers Z. Physiol. Chem. 66:19–52, 1910.

Ikizaki, M., and Johnson, L. R.: Development of sensitivity to different secretogogues in the rat stomach. Am. J. Physiol 244:G165, 1983.

Koga, A.: Morphogenesis of intrahepatic bile ducts of the human fetus: Light and electron microscopic study. Z. Anat. Entevichl-Geschrift 135:156–184, 1971.

Konturek, S. J., Radecki, T., and Brzozoeski, T.: Gastric cytoprotection by epidermal growth factor: The role of endogenous prostaglandins and DNA synthesis. Gastroenterology 81:438–443, 1981.

Lebenthal, E., and Lee, P. C.: Review article. Interactions of determinants in the ontogeny of the gastrointestinal tract: A unified concept. Pediatr. Res. 17:19–24, 1983.

Lebenthal, E., and Leung, Y. K.: Epidermal growth factor (EGF) and the ontogeny of the gut. J. Pediatr. Gastroenterol. Nutr. 6:1–6, 1987.

Lebenthal, E., Sunshine, P., and Kretchmer, N.: Effect of carbohydrate and corticosteroids on activity of alpha-glucosidases in intestine of the infant rat. J. Clin. Invest. 51:1244–1249, 1972.

Lebenthal, E., Sunshine, P., and Kretchmer, N.: Effect of prolonged nursing on the activity of intestinal lactase in rats. Gastroenterology 64:1136–1140, 1973.

Liu, H. M., and Potter, E. L.: Development of the human pancreas. Arch. Pathol. 74:439–452, 1962.

Mangurten, H. H., and Slade, C. I.: First stool in the preterm, low birth-weight infant. J. Pediatr. 82:1033–1038, 1973.

Martins Campos, J. V., Fagundes Neto, V., Patricio, F. R. S., et al.: Jejunal mucosa in marasmic children. Clinical, pathological and prestructural evaluation of the effect of protein energy malnutrition and environmental contamination. Am. J. Clin. Nutr. 32:1575–1580, 1979.

Pace, J. L.: Age of appearance of haustra of human colon. J. Anat. 109:75–80, 1971.

Sherry, S. N., and Kramer, I.: The time of passage of the first stool and the first urine by the newborn infant. J. Pediatr. 46:158–162, 1955.

Thompson, M. D., and Trowell, H. C.: Pancreatic enzyme activity in duodenal contents of children with a type of kwashiorkor. Lancet 1:1031–1033, 1951.

Tilghman, S. M., and Belayew, A.: Transcriptional control of the murine albumin-fetoprotein locus during development. Proc. Natl. Acad. Sci. U.S.A. 79:5254–5257, 1982.

FETAL, TRANSITIONAL, AND NEONATAL PHYSIOLOGY

67

William J. Byrne

By the 28th week of gestation, the morphologic development of the gastrointestinal tract is nearly complete. Yet, from the clinical experience of the past decade with very-low-birth-weight infants, it is obvious that the "organ" of nutrition often does not function in a manner sufficient to allow nutritional support by enteral means. Further, since the gastrointestinal tract is a major interface between the host and the environment, functional immaturity compromises the newborn's ability to protect himself from microorganisms and foreign proteins. The period between 28 and 38 weeks' gestation is critical for the maturation of essential biochemical and physiologic processes that are not only necessary for digestion and absorption but also for the propulsion of luminal contents down the gut (Balesteri, 1988; Henning, 1985).

■ PROTEIN DIGESTION AND ABSORPTION

Protein digestion begins in the stomach and requires hydrochloric acid and pepsin (Table 67–1). Discrepancies exist regarding the pattern of gastric acid production during the first several weeks of life. Euler and co-workers (1979) showed that, during the first 3 days of life, term infants secrete acid in the basal state and in response to penta-

gastrin. Harris and Frasier (1986) found that after 2 days of age, gastric acid secretion declined rapidly and was maintained at a low level for 3 weeks. Agunod and colleagues (1969) demonstrated that, following histamine stimulation, hydrochloric acid, pepsin, and intrinsic factor were present in the stomach of 12-hour-old term newborns. This response increased during the first 3 months of life, and by that age, intrinsic factor and acid secretion on a weight basis were similar to adult levels. Pepsin secretion, however, was only about 50 per cent of adult values. Hyman and associates (1985) studied gastric acid secretion in premature infants and found that initial concentrations of hydrochloric acid were less than for term infants (Fig. 67–1). However, after 4 weeks, regardless of gestational age, basal acid output and acid output in response to pentagastrin reached levels seen in older infants. A plateau was then observed. In addition, the presence of hydrochloric acid is critical for limiting the microbial colonization of the proximal gut. Pepsin is present by 16 weeks of gestation, suggesting that both the preterm and term newborn are capable of initiating limited protein digestion in the stomach. Yahav and co-workers (1987) found that pepsinogen secretion in preterm infants is significantly lower than in term infants (1/20 of that in term infants at 1 to 6 months of age); nonetheless, they demonstrated a pepsinogen secretory response to feeding in preterm infants at 3 to 4 weeks of age.

Most protein hydrolysis occurs in the proximal small intestine and depends on enterokinase, pancreatic proteases, and brush border and cytosolic peptidases (see Table 67–1). Duodenal enterokinase activates the pancreatic proteolytic enzyme trypsinogen, converting it to trypsin. Trypsin then converts the bulk of trypsinogen and the other zymogens (chymotrypsinogen, proelastase, and procarboxypeptidase) into their active proteolytic components. Antonowicz and Lebenthal (1977) measured small bowel enterokinase levels from human fetuses at between 21 and 40 weeks' gestation. Between 26 and 30 weeks' gestation, levels are only one-third of those found at term. By 32 weeks they are similar to levels found at term; however, term infants have levels only 10 per cent of those found in adults. The relative deficiency of enterokinase activity, however, is not rate-limiting in terms of protein digestion. Trypsin activity is present in the small bowel in response to pancreozymin and secretin (Fig. 67–2) (Zoppi et al., 1972) in both premature and term newborns (Lebenthal and Lee, 1980a). Protein in the diet stimulates trypsin production in both preterm and term

TABLE 67–1. Appearance of the Components of Digestion

COMPONENT	FIRST DETECTABLE (Weeks of Gestation)	34 WEEKS (Per cent of Term Infants)	TERM NEWBORN (Per cent of Adults)
Protein			
HCl	at birth	at birth	30
Pepsin	16		10
Trypsin	20	100	10–60
Chymotrypsin	20		10–60
Carboxypeptidase B	20		
Enterokinase	24	100	10
Peptidases (brush border and cytosolic)	15	100	100
Fat			
Bile salts	22	30	50
Pancreatic lipase	34	50	5–10
Lingual lipase	30	50	100
Carbohydrate			
Alpha amylase			
Salivary	16		10
Pancreatic	22	20	2
Sucrase-isomaltase	10	70	100
Lactase	10	30	100
Glucoamylase	10	100	50–100

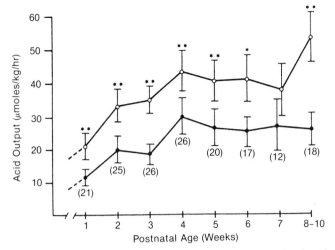

*FIGURE 67–1. Basal acid output (●) and pentagastrin-stimulated acid output (○) in preterm infants. Number of subjects studied at each age is given in parentheses. *P <0.05. **P <0.01. (From Hyman, P. E., Clarke, D. D., and Everett S. L.: Gastric acid secretory function in preterm infants. J. Pediatr. 106:468, 1985.)*

infants, and while levels are lower than those in older children, they are sufficient to permit the efficient digestion of protein. In addition to the trypsin response, Lebenthal and Lee (1980a) documented the presence of chymotrypsin and carboxypeptidase B in the small bowel.

The final phase of protein digestion involves the hydrolysis of small peptides by brush border and cytosolic peptidases. By 22 weeks' gestation, all peptidases except aminopeptidase A are present in adult levels (Auricchio et al., 1981). The absorption of amino acids and peptides involves an active transport process, which appears to be well developed by 28 weeks' gestation (Leven et al., 1968; Rubino and Guadalini, 1977). One interesting adaptation in the newborn may be a special mechanism for taurine absorption. Taurine, a sulfur-containing amino acid, is present in high concentrations in human milk and, because of limited endogenous production, is considered essential. In rat pups, a sodium-dependent transport mechanism for taurine exists in the jejunum until the pups are weaned and then disappears (Moyer et al., 1985).

In addition to the digestion of peptides and amino acids, the absorption of large macromolecules has been documented. This process appears to be more marked in term than in premature infants and subsequently decreases with postnatal age (Eastham et al., 1978, Rotherberg, 1969; Walker, 1978). In animal models, this enhanced permeability has been attributed to the increased lipid-to-protein ratio in the intestinal microvillous membrane in older infants (Pang et al., 1983). Macromolecules may stimulate development of the intestinal mucosal barrier and contribute to the protection of the infant (Tomasi et al., 1980). On the other hand, this process of immunologic stimulation may predispose to allergic and inflammatory processes. Despite the immaturity of these systems, however, protein absorption and peptide hydrolysis are essentially normal in both preterm and term infants.

■ FAT DIGESTION AND ABSORPTION

Fat is the main energy source for the newborn, providing 40 to 50 per cent of total calories. Fats provide fatty

acids for brain development, are an integral part of all cell membranes, and are the vehicle for absorption of fat-soluble vitamins. The absorption of fat takes place in two phases. The *luminal phase* involves the emulsification and hydrolysis of triglycerides to free fatty acids and a beta-monoglyceride. Bile acids aggregate to form micelles, into which free fatty acids and monoglycerides enter to form mixed micelles. The *mucosal phase* involves the passage of these mixed micelles though an "unstirred" water layer at the mucosal cell surface. The monoglycerides and free fatty acids are released and diffuse into the cell. In the cell, cytosol reesterification of the free fatty acids and monoglycerides to triglycerides takes place. The triglycerides are assimilated into chylomicrons before release from the mucosal cell and into the blood via the lymphatic vessels. While the mucosal phase is well developed in the newborn, the luminal phase is poorly developed. Estimations of lipid absorption for the premature infant vary from 38 to 88 per cent, and for the term infant from 71 to 95

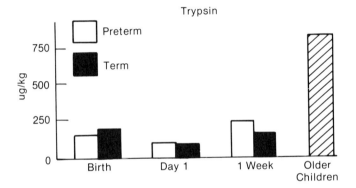

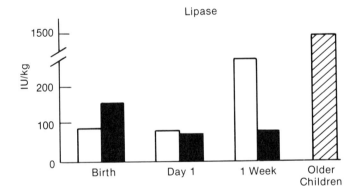

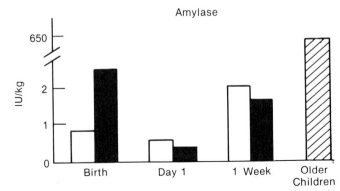

FIGURE 67–2. Pancreatic enzyme activity in preterm (32- to 34-week gestational age) and full-term infants fed a balanced formula. (Data are drawn from Zoppi et al., 1972, and represent mean values).

per cent (Barltrop and Oppe, 1973; Foman et al., 1970; Katz and Hamilton, 1974). Not until 4 to 5 months of age do fat digestion and absorption achieve adult levels of efficiency.

Fat digestion in the luminal phase is dependent upon the composition of the diet, a critical intraluminal bile acid concentration, and the presence of intraluminal lipase. Medium-chain triglycerides (MCTs) that are digested and absorbed more readily than long-chain triglycerides (LCTs) do not require bile salts for emulsification or solubilization (Roy et al., 1975). In addition, they are not reesterified, and therefore do not form chylomicrons but instead move directly across the mucosal cell and are delivered to the body by the splanchnic capillary system and the portal vein. Vegetable fats, in general, are absorbed more efficiently than animal fats. Some controversy exists with respect to the effect of formulas containing MCT or LCT on gastric lipolysis and fat absorption in preterm infants. Hamosh and co-workers (1989) recently reported no significant difference in fat absorption with MCT formulas versus LCT formulas in 6-week-old, healthy preterm infants. However, Jensen and colleagues (1986) reported slightly better fat absorption with MCT (95 per cent) versus LCT (90 per cent).

In premature infants between 32 and 36 weeks' gestation, bile salt synthesis and bile salt pool size are low, as compared with term infants and adults (Watkins et al., 1973) (Fig. 67–3). This reduced bile salt pool size contributes to decreased intraluminal bile salt concentration in newborns, frequently to concentrations less than 2 micromoles per liter, the critical micellar level essential for effective solubilization of fat into micelles. The result is fat malabsorption (Fig. 67–4). In addition, pancreatic lipase

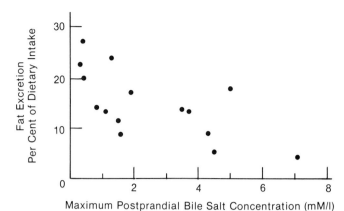

FIGURE 67–4. *Relationship between maximum postprandial bile salt concentration and fat excretion during the first 2 months of life in 15 infants with birth weights under 1300 g. (From Katz, L., and Hamilton, J. R.: Fat absorption in infants of birth weight less than 1,300 gm. J. Pediatr 85:609, 1974.)*

activity in the newborn is only 5 to 10 per cent of that in older children and adults (see Fig. 67–2).

Therefore, to explain the newborn's ability to absorb fat as a principal energy source, alternative mechanisms for digestion must be present. Lingual lipase is produced in the lingual serous glands located below the circumvallate papillae in the posterior third of the tongue. Its presence has been detected as early as 26 weeks of gestation, and by 34 weeks, levels similar to those found in term infants are present. This is not surprising, since nutritive sucking is the stimulus for secretion. Lingual lipase is active in the stomach, where it hydrolyzes triglycerides, diglycerides, and monoglycerides into free fatty acids and glycerol. The pH optimum of 3.5 to 5.5 is markedly different from that of pancreatic lipase and is ideally suited to the stomach. Bile salt concentrations below the critical micellar concentration also facilitate lingual lipase activity in the duodenum. Another lipase, referred to as "bile-salt–stimulated lipase," is present in breast milk after 26 weeks' gestation (Hamosh, 1982). As its name implies, it requires low concentrations of primary and secondary bile acids for activity, and it hydrolyzes both long-chain triglycerides and fatty acid esters. The pH optimum for this lipase is 7.5 to 9.0, but the enzyme is stable for 1 hour at a pH of 3.5, allowing its survival during passage through the stomach. The lack of bile-salt–stimulated lipase may explain the greater amount of fat malabsorption noted in formula-fed versus breast-fed infants.

Another lipase, gastric lipase, is secreted by the gastric glands in the stomach in response to feeding and provides for some intragastric lipolysis of fat (De Nigris et al., 1985; Salzmann-Mann et al., 1982). The combined action of intragastric lipolysis by lingual and gastric lipases and intestinal lipolysis by the bile-salt–stimulated lipase of human milk, thus, effectively substitutes for pancreatic lipase and compensates for the low levels of bile salts found in the newborn.

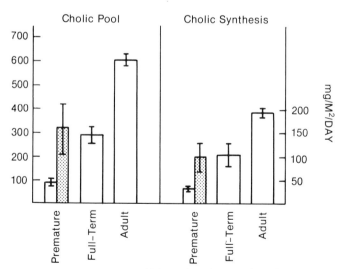

FIGURE 67–3. *Comparison of bile acid pool size and synthesis rate in premature infants, full-term infants, and adults, corrected for body surface area. Shaded bars refer to premature infants whose mothers had received prenatal treatment with dexamethasone or phenobarbital. (Data are mean +/− SE. Values for premature infants are from Watkins, J. B., Szczepanik, P., Gould, J. B., et al.: Bile salt metabolism in the premature infant. Preliminary observations of pool size and synthesis rate following prenatal administration of dexamethasone and phenobarbital. Gastroenterology 69(3):706, 1975; those for term infants are from Watkins, J. B., Ingall, D., Szczepanik, P., et al.: Bile-salt metabolism in the newborn: Measurement of pool size and synthesis by stable isotope technique. N. Engl. J. Med. 288:431, 1973; and those for adults are from Vlahcevic et al., 1971. Figure courtesy of Dr. John B. Watkins, Children's Hospital, Philadelphia.)*

■ CARBOHYDRATE DIGESTION AND ABSORPTION

Carbohydrate contributes 35 to 55 per cent of the calories in the newborn diet. Sucrase and maltase first appear at 10 weeks' gestation (Antonowicz and Lebenthal, 1977). By the 28th week, levels of sucrase and maltase reach 70 per cent of those found at term. Lactase is a late-developing enzyme with activity beginning at 28 to 32 weeks, at about 30 per cent of the level found at term (Fig. 67–5). The optimal amounts of disaccharide that can be hydrolyzed by the small bowel at various gestational ages have been estimated (Auricchio et al., 1965), although these are very rough calculations based on length of bowel, weight, and amount of enzyme as determined at necropsy. At 32 weeks, the gut has the capacity to hydrolyze 70 g of maltose, 35 g of sucrose, and 6 g of lactose per day; at term the values are 107 g of maltose, 72 g of sucrose, and 60 g of lactose. Despite an apparent lactase deficiency, healthy preterm infants are able to tolerate lactose-containing formulas while exhibiting normal growth and no diarrhea (MacLean and Fink, 1980; Mayne et al., 1986). This can be explained on the basis of conversion of malabsorbed lactose to volatile organic acids by colonic bacteria and their subsequent absorption. This salvage mechanism minimizes energy losses. However, preterm infants fed a high-lactose formula, such as breast milk, normally have a measurable amount of disaccharide present in their stools.

Glucose polymers are by-products of the partial hydrolysis of starch. Pancreatic amylase, which is the most efficient enzyme for starch and glucose polymer hydrolysis, is essentially absent in the newborn (see Fig. 67–2). However, the principal mechanism for glucose polymer digestion in newborns is the small intestinal brush border glycosidase, glucoamylase, which is present at 50 to 100 per cent of the adult activity level (Lebenthal and Lee, 1980b). Glucoamylase has maximal activity against polymers with a chain length of 5 to 9 units (Kerzner et al., 1981). Salivary amylase is present early in gestation and increases gradually with advancing gestational age. While the potential contributions of its activity to glucose polymer hydrolysis are significant, it falls far short of what pancreatic amylase achieves in later life (Murray et al., 1986). In contrast, breast-milk amylase activity is substantial in the newborn, but breast-fed infants seldom receive glucose polymers. The colonic flora that are important for lactose absorption in the premature infant (MacLean and Fink, 1980) also contribute to glucose polymer assimilation (Shulman et al., 1983). The ability of premature and term infants to utilize glucose polymers is the basis for their use as an alternative or supplemental carbohydrate source. The mechanism for the acute transport of monosaccharide develops between 10 and 20 weeks of gestation but may still be less efficient in the newborn than in the adult.

■ ELECTROLYTE, VITAMIN, MINERAL, AND METAL ABSORPTION

Electrolytes. Animal studies suggest that newborns may have unique fluid and electrolyte fluxes. Rat pups initially show a net secretion of water in the small intestine, which is reversible by the addition of glucose (Younoszai et al., 1978). Compared with 7-week-old rats, intraluminal osmotic loads in 2-week-old pups cause a greater increase in water, sodium, and chloride secretion by the small intestine, and other data show similar findings in humans.

Vitamin Absorption. Limited data are available regarding vitamin absorption in the newborn. The capacity to absorb folate is lower than that found in adults, and in addition, the reduced secretion of intrinsic factor by the stomachs of term and preterm infants may affect the absorption of vitamin B_{12}. Intrinsic factor is secreted by 3 months of age in term infants in amounts similar to those in adults. Stores at birth last almost 12 months.

Calcium is absorbed primarily in the duodenum by an active transport process (Koo and Tsang, 1988; Tsang and Nichols, 1988). Early studies suggested that the amount of calcium absorbed was dependent on gestational age and postnatal age and independent of the source, i.e., cow's milk versus human milk (Shaw, 1976); however, more recent data in the preterm infant show that up to 90 per cent of calcium in breast milk may be absorbed (Chappell et al., 1986; Ehrenkranz et al., 1985).

Phosphorus is absorbed principally in the jejunum by simple diffusion and an active transport process that is vitamin-D dependent. In preterm infants fed human milk with low phosphorus content, phosphorus absorption approaches 90 per cent of intake (Senterre et al., 1983). The process does not appear to be affected by vitamin-D

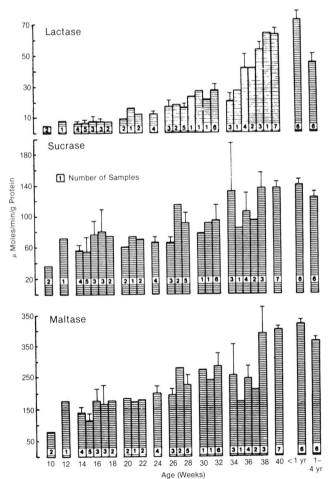

FIGURE 67–5. *Developmental patterns of jejunal disaccharidase activities in human fetuses. (From Antonowicz, I., and Lebenthal, E.: Developmental pattern of small intestinal enterokinase and disaccharidase activities in the human fetus. Gastroenterology 72:1301, 1977.)*

intake. The percentage of phosphorus absorbed in infants decreases as phosphorus intake increases. Excessive amounts of either calcium or phosphorus decrease the absorption of the other because of the precipitation of insoluble calcium phosphate (see Chapter 75).

Magnesium absorption occurs throughout the entire gastrointestinal tract at a similar rate and does not appear to vary with either gestational age or postnatal age (Tantibhedhyakul and Hashim, 1978). Magnesium absorption is 43 to 73 per cent when intake is normal (Greer and Tsang, 1985). Isolated deficiencies of magnesium absorption have also been described.

Copper is absorbed in the duodenum. Ehrenkranz and co-workers (1986) demonstrated that 53 per cent of copper was absorbed in formula-fed preterm infants. This increased to 72 per cent when preterm infants were fed human milk.

Zinc is absorbed in the duodenum and proximal jejunum. In newborns, absorption rates vary from 32 per cent with cow's milk to 52 per cent with human milk. Voyer and colleagues (1982) showed that in preterm infants of 30 to 32 weeks' gestation, zinc absorption could be enhanced by the addition of medium-chain triglycerides to formula or breast milk, suggesting that the process is linked to fat absorption. Higashi and associates (1988) studied zinc balance in premature infants given the minimum dietary zinc requirement and showed that zinc balance changes from negative to positive at about 36 weeks. They suggest that oral zinc supplementation in preterm infants of less than 36 weeks' gestation may lead to an increase in fecal extraction and that intravenous supplementation seems necessary to obtain a zinc retention rate similar to the fetal rate.

Iron for the newborn is provided as iron salts of nonheme iron. Absorption of the small amount of iron in breast milk approaches 50 per cent, even in the preterm infant. Because iron absorption is only 4 per cent from both fortified and nonfortified formulas, iron supplementation is necessary (Rios et al., 1975).

■ MOTILITY OF THE DIGESTIVE SYSTEM

The major limitations to enteral alimentation do not appear to be digestion or absorption but the propulsion of chyme along the gastrointestinal tract. Careful studies have documented swallowing in the human fetus as early as 17 weeks of gestation. The mechanism initiating swallowing is unknown, as is the exact role swallowing plays in the regulation of amniotic fluid volume. Increased amniotic fluid (hydramnios) is often seen in pregnancies in which fetal swallowing is impaired, such as when esophageal atresia or upper intestinal atresia are present. Exposure to factors in amniotic fluid appears to be important for gastrointestinal development. For example, mucosal maturation in the stomach is delayed by experimental ligation in rabbits and returns to normal if exposure to amniotic fluid or epidermal growth factor occurs.

In both premature and term infants younger than 12 hours of age, peristalsis in the body of the esophagus is poorly coordinated in response to swallowing. Simultaneous nonperistaltic contractions are often present along the entire length of the esophagus. Lower esophageal sphincter pressure is frequently decreased. Gastric emptying in the premature and young newborn is slow, compared with emptying in older children. Cavell (1979) showed that the emptying pattern for breast milk in healthy preterm infants was more rapid than for formula and was biphasic in nature. The emptying pattern for infant formula, however, was linear. As in adults, meal composition also affects gastric emptying, with delay occurring as caloric density increases. Emptying is also delayed more with glucose or lactose than with glucose polymers, and with long-chain triglycerides than with medium-chain triglycerides (Siegel et al., 1985). This last finding, however, has not been documented in preterm infants of fewer than 32 weeks' gestation.

McLain (1963) in one of the earliest studies of small bowel motility in human newborns suggested that motility increases with advancing gestational age. Until 30 weeks, contrast material did not progress through the small intestine of the fetus; however, at 32 weeks, contrast material passed through the small bowel to the colon in 9 hours, compared with a transit time of 4.5 to 7 hours in term infants. Worniak and co-workers (1983) studied jejunal motility in premature infants and identified three patterns similar to those described in newborn puppies and lambs (Table 67–2). Migrating motor complexes, first seen around 33 weeks of gestation, are an interdigestive phenomenon that functions to "sweep" gut contents over long segments of intestine between meals. This phenomenon may be a developmental mechanism related to prevention of bacterial overgrowth, similar to adult peristaltic motion. This pattern is inhibited by eating, which initiates postprandial mixing-type contractions. In the term infant, the time between migrating motor complexes is 44 minutes, or about half the time observed in older children. The propagation rate, however, is 3.1 cm/minute in term infants, compared with 8.2 cm/minute for older children, and the duration time is 10.9 minutes in infants, compared with 7.2 minutes for older children. Eating does not abolish the migrating motor complex in newborns, as it does in older children; in fact, Berseth (1989) has suggested that early feeding may be important in hastening the maturation of motility in the preterm infant.

Meconium is the thick black material that collects in the

TABLE 67–2. The Development of Small Intestinal Motility in the Human Newborn

GESTATIONAL AGE (Weeks)	PATTERN
26–30	*Disorganized random contractions* without periodicity or rhythmicity: No propagation along the intestine.
30–33	*Fetal complex:* Regular contractions every 5 minutes, lasting 30 to 90 seconds; 90 per cent are propagated.
33–36	*MMC-like patterns:* 11 cycles/minute; activity always aborally propagated but at variable intervals over variable lengths of time (2 to 16 minutes).
36–40	Clear-cut migrating motor complexes with clearly defined fasting activity.

distal portion of the small intestine and colon of the fetus and consists of intestinal secretions, bile, desquamated cellular debris, and amniotic fluid. Ninety-four per cent of newborns pass a meconium stool within 24 hours after birth. In premature infants, rectal sphincteric reflexes may be absent or impaired, and fecal passage is therefore delayed. Other bases for the failure of meconium passage have also been suggested, i.e., the absence of colonic bulk movement or of giant migrating complexes, but no data have been reported to clarify what causes failure to stool.

■ DEVELOPMENT OF HEPATIC FUNCTION

Bile secretion begins by the 12th week of gestation, with both qualitative and quantitative differences in bile acid composition between the fetus and newborn (Balesteri et al., 1983). In the fetus, taurine-conjugated chenodeoxycholic acid predominates rather than cholic acid. Bile flow and the biliary excretion of other compounds are bile-acid–dependent. Abnormal bile acids (Street et al., 1985), a reduced bile salt pool (Watkins et al., 1973), decreased uptake and excretion of bile acids by hepatocytes (Suchy et al., 1985), and an inefficient ileal active-transport mechanism for enterohepatic circulation (Moyer et al., 1985) all contribute to reduced bile flow in the newborn. Gallbladder contractility is also an important factor affecting bile flow. In newborn guinea pigs, Cox and co-workers (1987) demonstrated an association between functional immaturity of the biliary tree and reduction of bile flow, although a clear cause-effect relationship was not established. By 4 weeks of age, biliary motility was similar to that of adult guinea pigs. No similar studies in human newborns have been reported.

Hepatic metabolic function is known to be immature in the newborn. For example, UDP-glucouronyl transferase activity is decreased—the rate-limiting step in bilirubin extraction (Kawade and Oriski, 1983). Postnatal development of this enzyme occurs regardless of gestational age at birth. *Drug metabolism* in newborn infants is also inefficient. This may be related to low levels of activity of the hepatic cytochrome P450 mono-oxygenase system (Soyka and Redmond, 1981) (see Chapters 31 and 74).

■ ACKNOWLEDGEMENT

The editors appreciate the editorial review of Dr. Colin Rudolph.

■ REFERENCES

Agunod, M., Yamaguchi, N., Lopez, R., et al.: Correlative study of hydrochloric acid, pepsin and intrinsic factor secretion in newborns and infants. Am. J. Digest. Dis. *14*:400–414, 1969.

Antonowicz, I., and Lebenthal, E.: Developmental pattern of small intestinal enterokinase and disaccharidase activities in the human fetus. Gastroenterology *723*:1299, 1977.

Auricchio, S., Rubino, A., and Murset, C.: Intestinal glucosidase activities in the human embryo, fetus and newborn. Pediatrics *35*:944, 1965.

Auricchio, S., Stellato, A., and De Vizio, B.: Development of brush border peptidases in human and rat small intestine during fetal and neonatal development. Pediatr. Res. *15*:991, 1981.

Balesteri, W. F., Heubi, J. E., and Suchy, F. J.: Immaturity of the enterohepatic circulation in early life: Factors predisposing to "physiologic" maldigestion and cholestasis. J. Pediatr. Gastroenterol. Nutr. *2*:346, 1983.

Balesteri, W. F.: Anatomic and biochemical ontogeny of the gastrointestinal tract and liver. *In* Tsang, R. C., and Nichols, B. L. (Eds.): Nutrition During Infancy. Philadelphia, Hanley and Belfus, 1988, pp. 35–57.

Barltrop, D., and Oppe, T. E.: Absorption of fat and calcium by low birth weight infants from milk containing butter fat and olive oil. Arch. Dis. Child. *48*:496, 1973.

Berseth, C. L.: Gestational evolution of small intestine motility in preterm infants. J. Pediatr. *115*:646, 1989.

Cavell, B.: Gastric emptying in preterm infants. Acta Pediatr. Scand. *68*:725, 1979.

Chappell, J. E., Clandinin, M. T., and Kearney-Volpe, C.: Fatty acid balance studies in premature infants fed human milk or formula. Effect of calcium supplementation. J. Pediatr. *108*:439, 1986.

Cox, K. L., Cheung, A. T., Losche, C. L., et al.: Biliary motility: Postnatal changes in guinea pigs. Pediatr. Res. *21*:170, 1987.

De Nigris, S. J., Hamhosh, M., Kasbekar, D. K., et al.: Human gastric lipase: Secretion from dispersed gastric glands. Biochim. Biophys. Acta *836*:67, 1985.

Eastham, E. J., Lichanco, T., Grady, M. I., et al.: Antigenicity of infant formulas: Role of immature intestine on protein permeability. J. Pediatr. *93*:561, 1978.

Ehrenkranz, R. A., Ackerman, B. A., Nelli, C. M., et al.: Absorption of calcium in premature infants as measured with a stable isotope ^{46}Ca extrinsic tag. Pediatr. Res. *19*:178, 1985.

Ehrenkranz, R. A., Nelli, C. M., and Geltner, P. A.: Determination of copper absorption in premature infants with ^{65}Cu as an extrinsic stable isotope tracer. Pediatr. Res. *20*:209, 1986.

Euler, A. R., Byrne, W. J., Meis, P. J., et al.: Basal and pentagastrin stimulated acid secretion in human newborn infants. Pediatr. Res. *13*:36, 1979.

Foman, S. J., Ziegler, E. E., and Thomas, L. M.: Excretion of fat by normal full-term infants fed various milks and formulas. Am. J. Clin. Nutr. *23*:1299, 1970.

Greer, F. R., and Tsang, R. C.: Calcium, phosphorus, magnesium and vitamin D requirements for the preterm infant. *In* Tsang, R. C. (Ed.): Vitamin and Mineral Requirements in Preterm Infants. New York, Marcel Dekker, 1985, pp. 99–136.

Hamosh, M.: Lingual and breast milk lipases. Adv. Pediatr. *29*:33, 1982.

Hamosh, M., Bitman, J., Liao, T. H., et al.: Gastric lipolysis and fat absorption in preterm infants: Effect of medium-chain triglyceride or long-chain triglyceride-containing formulas. Pediatrics *83*:86, 1989.

Harris, J. T., and Frasier, A. J.: The acidity of the gastric contents of premature babies during the first 14 days of life. Biol. Neonat. *12*:186, 1986.

Henning, S. S.: Ontogeny of enzymes in the small intestine. Ann. Rev. Physiol. *47*:231, 1985.

Higashi, A., Ideda, T., Irube, K., et al.: Zinc balance in premature infants given the minimum dietary zinc requirement. J. Pediatr. *112*:262, 1988.

Hyman, P. E., Clarke, D. D., Everett, S. L., et al.: Gastric acid secretory function in preterm infants. J. Pediatr. *106*:467, 1985.

Jarvenpaa, A. L.: Feeding the low birth weight infant. Fat absorption as a function of diet and duodenal bile acids. Pediatrics *72*:684, 1983.

Jensen, C., Buist, N. R. M., and Wilson, T.: Absorption of individual fatty acids from long chain or medium chain triglycerides in very small infants. Am. J. Clin. Nutr. *43*:745, 1986.

Johnson, L. R.: Functional development of the stomach. Ann. Rev. Physiol. *47*:199, 1985.

Katz, L., and Hamilton, J. R.: Fat absorption in infants of birth weight less than 1300 gm. J. Pediatr. *85*:608, 1974.

Kawade, N., and Oriski, S.: The prenatal and postnatal development of UDP-glucouronyltransferase activity towards bilirubin and the effect of premature birth on activity in human liver. Biochem. J. *196*:257, 1983.

Kerzner, B., Sloan, H. R., Haase, G. L., et al.: The jejunal absorption of glucose oligomers in the absence of pancreatic enzymes. Pediatr. Res. *15*:250, 1981.

Koo, W. W. K., and Tsang, R. C.: Calcium, magnesium and phosphorus in nutrition during infancy. *In* Tsang, R. C., and Nichols, B. S. (Eds.): Nutrition During Infancy. Philadelphia, Hanley and Belfus, 1988, pp. 175–189.

Lebenthal, E., and Lee, P. C.: Development of functional response in human exocrine pancreas. Pediatrics *66*:556, 1980a.

Lebenthal, E., and Lee, P. C.: Glucoamylase and disaccharidase activities in normal subjects and in patients with mucosal injury of the small intestine. J. Pediatr. *97*:389, 1980b.

Lee, P. C.: Alternative pathways in starch digestion—their importance in premature and young infants. *In* Lifshitz, R. (Ed.): Carbohydrate Intolerance in Infancy. New York, Marcel Dekker, 1982, pp. 223–233.

Leven, R. H., Doldovsky, O., and Hoskova, J.: Electrical activity across human small intestine associated with the absorption processes. Gut 9:206, 1968.

MacLean, W. C., and Fink, B. B.: Lactose malabsorption by premature infants: Magnitude and clinical significance. J. Pediatr. 97:383, 1980.

Mayne, A. J., Brown, G. A., Sule, D., et al.: Postnatal development of disaccharidase activities in jejunal fluid of preterm neonates. Gut 27:1357, 1986.

McLain, C. R.: Amniography studies of the gastrointestinal motility of the human fetus. Am. J. Obstet. 86:1079, 1963.

Moyer, M. S., Goodrich, A. L., and Suchy, F. J.: Ontogenesis of intestinal taurine transport: Evidence for a carrier system in developing rat jejunum. Gastroenterology 90:1558, 1985.

Murray, R. D., Kerzner, B., Sloan, H. R., et al.: The contribution of salivary amylase to glucose polymer hydrolysis in premature infants. Pediatr. Res. 20:186, 1986.

Pang, K. Y., Bresson, J. L., and Walker, W. A.: Development of the gastrointestinal mucosal barrier. Evidence for structural differences in microvillous membranes from newborn and adult rabbits. Biochim. Biophys. Acta 717:201, 1983.

Rios, E., Hunter, R. E., and Cook, J.: The absorption of iron as supplements in infant cereal and infant formulas. Pediatrics 55:686, 1975.

Rotherberg, R. M.: Immunoglobulin and specific antibody synthesis during the first weeks of life of premature infants. J. Pediatr. 75:391, 1969.

Roy, C. C., Ste.-Marie, M., Chartrand, L., et al.: Correction of the malabsorption of the preterm infant with a medium chain triglyceride formula. Pediatrics 86:446, 1975.

Rubino, A., and Guadalini, S.: Dipeptide transport in the mucosa of developing rabbits. *In* Elliot, D., and O'Connor, M. (Eds.): Peptide Transport and Hydrolysis. CIBA Foundation Symposium 50. Amsterdam, Elsevier, 1977, pp. 61–71.

Salzmann-Mann, C., Hamosh, M., and Sevasubramanian, K. N.: Congenital esophageal atresia: Lipase activity is present in the esophageal pouch and in the stomach. Dig. Dis. Sci. 27:124, 1982.

Senterre, J., Putet, G., Salle, B., et al.: Effects of vitamin D and phosphorus supplementation on calcium retention in preterm infants fed banked human milk. J. Pediatr. 103:305, 1983.

Shaw, J. C. L.: Evidence of the defective skeletal mineralization in low birth weight infants: The absorption of calcium and fat. Pediatrics 57:16, 1976.

Shulman, R. J., Wong, W. W., Irving, C. S., et al.: Utilization of dietary cereal by young infants. J. Pediatr. 103:223, 1983.

Siegel, M., Krantz, B., and Lebenthal, E.: Effect of fat and carbohydrate composition on the gastric emptying of isocaloric feedings in premature infants. Gastroenterology 89:785, 1985.

Southgate, D. A. T., Widdowson, E. M., Smits, B. J., et al.: Absorption and excretion of calcium and fat by young infants. Lancet 1:487, 1969.

Soyka, L. F., and Redmond, G. P.: Drug Metabolism in the Immature Human. New York, Raven Press, 1981.

Street, J. M., Balesteri, W. F., and Stechell, K. D. R.: Bile acid metabolism in the perinatal period—excretion of conventional and atypical bile acids in meconium. Gastroenterology 90:1773, 1985.

Suchy, F. J., Couchine, S. M., and Blitzer, B. L.: Taurocholate transport by basolateral plasma membrane vesicles isolated from developing rat liver. Am. J. Physiol. 248:G648, 1985.

Tomasi, T. B., Larson, L., Challacombe, S., et al.: Mucosal immunity: The origin and migration of cells in the secretory system. Allergy Clin. Immunol. 65:12, 1980.

Tomomasa, R., Hyman, P. E., Itoh, K., et al.: Gastroduodenal motility in neonates: Response to human milk compared with cow's milk formula. Pediatrics 80:434, 1987.

Tsang, R. C., and Nichols, B. F. (Eds.): Nutrition During Infancy. Philadelphia, Hanley and Belfus, 1988.

Voyer, M., Davakis, M., Antener, I., et al.: Zinc balances in preterm infants. Biol. Neonate 42:87, 1982.

Walker, W. A.: Antigen handling by the gut. Arch. Dis. Child. 53:527, 1978.

Watkins, J. B.: Lipid digestion and absorption. Pediatrics 75(Suppl):151, 1985.

Watkins, J. B., Ingall, D., Szczepanik, P., et al.: Bile-salt metabolism in the newborn: Measurement of pool size and synthesis by stable isotope technique. N. Engl. J. Med. 288:431, 1973.

Worniak, E. R., Fenton, T. R., and Milla, P. J.: The development of fasting small intestine motility in human neonates. *In* Roman, C. (Ed.): Gastrointestinal Motility. London, Lancaster Press, 1983, pp. 265–270.

Yahav, J., Carrion, V., Lee, P. D., et al.: Meal-stimulated pepsinogen secretion in premature infants. J. Pediatr. 110:949, 1987.

Younoszai, M. K., Sapario, R. S., Laughlin, M., et al.: Maturation of jejunum and ileum in rats. Water and electrolyte transport during in vivo perfusion of hypertonic solutions. J. Clin. Invest. 62:271, 1978.

Zoppi, G., Andreotti, G., Pajno-Ferrara, F., et al.: Exocrine pancreas function in premature and full-term neonates. Pediatr. Res. 6:880, 1972.

DISORDERS OF 68
THE TEETH, MOUTH, AND NECK

William J. Byrne

■ TEETH

Infants may be born with one or more erupted teeth. These are usually lower incisors, which are called "natal teeth," to differentiate them from neonatal teeth, which erupt during the 1st month. Since the roots are poorly formed, these teeth are almost always loose, present a danger of aspiration, and therefore should be extracted.

■ MOUTH

Tiny cystic lesions may be visible in the mouths of up to 80 per cent of newborns. Those located on the hard palate on either side of the raphe are referred to as *Epstein pearls,* while those seen on the mandibular and maxillary alveolar ridges are called *Bohn* nodules. Ranula is a retention cyst of the sublingual salivary gland that presents as a pea-sized mass on the anterior floor of the mouth and is filled with a yellow fluid. Most disappear within 1 month, but larger ones or those interfering with feeding need to be removed surgically.

Tumors of the mouth are rare in the newborn; however, when they are present, careful evaluation with computed tomography is necessary to define the anatomy and exclude a connection with the central nervous system. *Epignathus* defines any type of growth arising from the upper jaw or palate and projecting from the mouth (Fig. 68–1). These tumors may be polyps, dermoids, or teratomas. Although most are benign, their size and location often result in respiratory or feeding difficulty. The definitive treatment is surgical removal.

Congenital epulis is a misnamed tumor arising from the upper or lower jaw that projects into the mouth and makes sucking impossible. These tumors arise from tissue overlying bone. Langley and Davson (1950) found 23 cases in the literature and reported on three of their own. The tumors were covered with squamous epithelium and contained vascular connective tissue, large polyhedral round cells, and spindle-shaped cells. They are considered benign since at the time of excision there has been no evidence of local invasion, and following excision, there has been no recurrence or metastasis (see Chapter 23).

Salivary gland lesions are also rare in the newborn. Tumors or infection (sialadenitis) may arise anywhere salivary gland tissue is present, including the floor of the mouth and the parotid regions. Hemangioma, usually present at birth, is the most common tumor, followed by lymphangioma (Welch and Trump, 1979). Both of these benign lesions are usually confined to the intracapsular portion of the gland. A surface sentinel lesion may provide a clue to the diagnosis. Treatment consists of histologic diagnosis via open biopsy and then careful observation. Juxtaparotid lymphangioma with histologic invasion of the gland should be locally excised. Suppurative parotitis may present during the 1st month of life in otherwise healthy infants. One or both of the parotid glands may be involved. The gland becomes swollen and the overlying skin erythematous. Pus can be expressed from the Stensen duct by putting gentle pressure on the gland. The infant may become septic; extension to the submaxillary gland is not uncommon. The offending organism is usually *Staphylococcus aureus* or *Escherichia coli,* but broad-spectrum antibiotic coverage is necessary until the organism has been identified and sensitivities established.

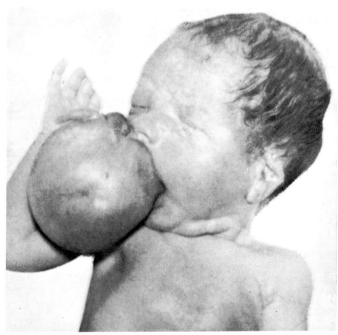

FIGURE 68–1. *Infant with epignathus: The orange-sized mass attached to the maxilla protrudes grotesquely from the mouth. (From Wynn, S.K., Waxman, S., Ritchie, G., and Askofsky, M.: Am. J. Dis. Child. 91:495, 1956. Copyright 1956, American Medical Association.)*

■ TONGUE

Aglossia congenita, or congenital absence of the tongue, has been described. Taste sensation is present and these children can learn to speak.

Ankyloglossia inferior (tongue-tie) is common in newborns. The frenulum of the newborn is normally short, but this does not interfere with sucking and swallowing, and with time it can be expected to lengthen; therefore, the frenulum should not be cut.

Ankyloglossia superior, attachment of the tongue to the roof of the mouth, is a rare anomaly that must be recognized at birth since respiratory obstruction may occur. Other lesions, including micrognathia, macroglossia, and cleft palate, are frequently associated with it (Spivack and Bennett, 1968).

True macroglossia, or enlargement of the tongue, results in continuous protrusion of this structure from the mouth making feeding difficult and respiration noisy. Minor degrees of enlargement may be present in otherwise normal newborns and do not constitute true macroglossia. Macroglossia is seen in Down syndrome and is associated with omphalocele and hyperglycemia (Beckwith syndrome). Lymphangioma and idiopathic muscular hypertrophy, however, are much more common causes. Characteristically, the gross appearance of a lymphangioma is that of a raised firm mass in the tongue with a warty-looking surface. Koop and Moschakis (1961) reported early hygromas in their three cases. Definitive diagnosis requires a biopsy. The treatment for a lymphangioma is surgical removal, if possible, or reduction of the tumor bulk with reshaping of the tongue. Infants with idiopathic muscular hypertrophy should be treated conservatively since reduction of the relative size of the tongue along with growth of the mandible may make the lesion less obvious.

Thyroid tissue may persist as a solid or cystic mass in the posterior midline of the tongue or under it. Since it represents a failure of migration, no other thyroid may exist. A thyroid scan should be performed in the evaluation of midline lingual tumors.

■ NASOPHARYNX

Nasopharyngeal tumors are rare and are either polyps, dermoids, or teratomas. Often these lesions are on a stalk and project into the mouth. Those not projecting externally may be palpated as a moveable, sausage-shaped mass in the pharynx. These lesions should be removed urgently since acute respiratory distress may occur if the nasopharynx is obstructed.

■ NECK

Cystic hygroma is the most common lateral neck mass in the newborn (Fig. 68–2). Derived from lymphatic tissue, these multilobular, multicystic masses may rapidly enlarge resulting in respiratory compromise. They are superficial and readily transilluminate. Excision is the treatment of choice.

Branchial cleft anomalies including skin tags, pits, sinuses, fistulas, and cysts present as preauricular and lateral neck lesions. Most are remnants of the second branchial

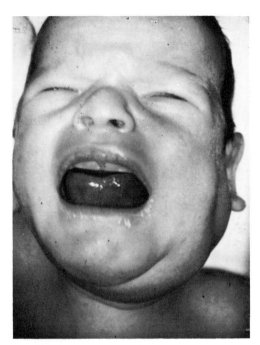

FIGURE 68–2. *Hygroma of the neck and tongue.*

cleft and pouch, and 10 to 15 per cent are bilateral (Bill and Vadheim, 1955). Sinuses and fistulas may be discovered during the newborn period, but cysts require time to fill and are usually not diagnosed until childhood. Ultrasound (Badami and Athey, 1981) and/or CT scan (Som et al., 1985) of the neck may be useful in the differential diagnosis of neck masses as well as in defining their anatomic relationships. Surgical removal is the treatment of choice.

Sternomastoid "tumor" can be seen and palpated within the body of the sternocleidomastoid muscle as a hard, smooth oval mass. The pathologic abnormality consists of endomysial fibrosis and the deposition of collagen and fibroblasts around individual muscle fibers that undergo atrophy. The etiology is unknown, but the incidence is 7 times higher following breech delivery, suggesting that the fetal position may play a role (Ling and Low, 1973). Torticollis is not always present. More often in the newborn there is rotation of the head to the side opposite the tumor. Cranial and facial asymmetry may also occur. In most infants the lesion resolves within 6 to 12 months. Surgical splitting of the muscle is indicated if severe hemihypoplasia develops (Jones, 1979).

Midline neck masses in newborns include cystic hygromas, hemangiomas, teratomas, goiter, ectopic thyroid tissue, and ectopic thymic tissue (Fig. 68–3). Goiter may be visible at birth as an enlargement of the lateral lobes and thyroid isthmus and may be hypo-, hyper-, or euthyroid. The second most common location for ectopic thyroid tissue is the anterior midline of the neck, just at or below the hyoid bone (Meyerowitz and Buchholz, 1969). This tissue may be easily mistaken for a thyroglossal duct cyst. However, as a differential point, thyroglossal duct cysts rarely present in the newborn. CT scan may be helpful with the differential diagnosis (Reede et al., 1985; Som et al., 1985). Prior to removal, it must be determined if this is the infant's only functioning thyroid tissue.

Thymic tissue arises high in the embryo as two lateral

A

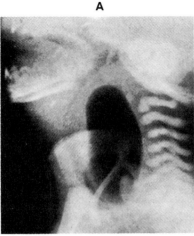

FIGURE 68–3. A, Lateral radiograph of the neck shows an air-containing cyst displacing the air passages and esophagus forward. B, Lateral view of the the neck with patient quiet, demonstrating straight, unobstructed tracheal air column. C, Lateral view of the neck with patient crying demonstrates mass lesion between the manubrium and the trachea, displacing the lower cervical trachea backward and moderately narrowing this portion of the trachea. (From Thompson, R.E., and Love, W.G.: Persistent cervical thymoma apparent with crying. Am. J. Dis. Child. 124:761, 1972. Copyright 1972, American Medical Association.)

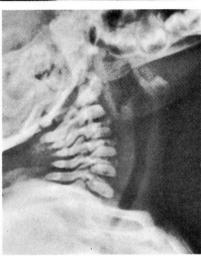

B

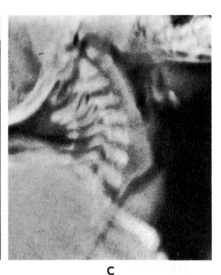

C

buds. They migrate caudad and join in the anterior mediastinum. Abnormal migration results in ectopic location and/or cyst formation, which may present as a lateral or midline neck mass (Thompson and Love, 1972), and requires surgical removal.

■ REFERENCES

Badami, J. P. and Athey, P. A.: Sonography in the diagnosis of branchial cysts. Am. J. Radiol. 137:1245–1248, 1981.

Beckwith, J. B.: Macroglossia, omphalocele, adrenal cytomegaly, gigantism and hyperplastic visceromegaly. Birth Defects 5: 188–198, 1969.

Bill, A. H., and Vadheim, J. L.: Cysts, sinuses and fistulas of the neck arising from the first and second branchial clefts. Ann. Surg. 142:904–912, 1955.

Jones, P. C.: Torticollis. In Ravitch, M. M. (Ed.): Pediatric Surgery. Chicago, Year Book Medical Publishers, 1979, pp. 386–390.

Koop, C. E., and Moschakis, E. A.: Capillary lymphangioma of the tongue complicated by glossitis. Pediatrics 27:800–805, 1961.

Langley, F. A., and Davson, J.: Epulis in the newborn. Arch. Dis. Child. 25:89–94, 1950

Ling, C. M., and Low, Y. S.: Sternomastoid tumor and muscular torticollis. J. Bone Joint Surg. 55:236–241, 1973.

Meyerowitz, B. R., and Buchholz, R. B.: Midline cervical ectopic thyroid tissue. Surgery 65:358–363, 1969.

Reede, D. L., Bereron, R. T., and Som, P. M.: CT of thyroglossal duct cyst. Radiology 157:121–125, 1985.

Som, P. M., Sacker, M., and Lanzieri, C.F.: Parenchymal cysts of the lower neck. Radiology 157:399–406, 1985.

Spivack, J., and Bennett, J. E.: Glossopalatine ankylosis. Plast. Reconstr. Surg. 42:129–134, 1968.

Thompson, R. E. and Love, W. G.: Persistent cervical thymoma apparent with crying. Am. J. Dis. Child. 124:761–766, 1972.

Welch, K. J., and Trump, D. S.: The oropharynx and jaws. In Ravitch, M. M. (Ed.): Pediatric Surgery. Chicago, Year Book Medical Publishers, 1979, p. 308.

DISORDERS OF THE ESOPHAGUS 69

William J. Byrne

■ ESOPHAGEAL ATRESIA WITH TRACHEO-ESOPHAGEAL FISTULA

Definition. Esophageal atresia and tracheo-esophageal fistula may occur as separate congenital defects, but more frequently they are seen together as a compound defect (Fig. 69–1). Esophageal atresia with distal tracheo-esophageal fistula is by far the most common form, accounting for 85 per cent of the cases.

Epidemiology. The incidence figures for esophageal atresia with tracheo-esophageal fistula vary from one per 3000 to one per 4000 live births (Meyers, 1974; Raffensperger, 1990). Most series show a slight male predominance and an increased incidence in premature infants (Reckham, 1981). The role genetic factors play is unclear; however, sibling involvement has been described and documented in both members of identical twins (Hausmann et al., 1957; Woolley et al., 1961). Vertical transmission of the lesion has also been reported by Engel (1970) and Ericksen (1981) and their colleagues.

Etiology. The anomaly occurs before the eighth week of gestation, but the exact mechanism is unknown. The foregut divides into a ventral and a dorsal tube by the folding-in of its lateral walls, giving rise to the trachea and esophagus, respectively. Problems with this division or the later compression of these primitive tubes by an extrinsic structure, such as an anomalous blood vessel, may result in one of the manifestations of this lesion. Associated anomalies occur in as many as 40 per cent of infants with tracheo-esophageal atresias. These are usually gastrointestinal (anal atresia, pyloric stenosis, duodenal obstruction, and malrotation) or cardiovascular (Greenwood and Rosenthal, 1976). Cardiovascular lesions, such as ventricular septal defect and patent ductus arteriosus, are seen when gastrointestinal anomalies are absent, whereas tetralogy of Fallot and atrial septal defect are usually seen in conjunction with gastrointestinal anomalies. One cluster seen more frequently in infants of diabetic mothers has been named the VATER association (Vertebral anomalies, Anal anomalies, Tracheo-esophageal fistula with Esophageal atresia, and Radial limb dysplasia and renal anomalies) by Quan and Smith (1973). An extension of this is the VACTERAL association, which includes Cardiac and Limb anomalies.

Diagnosis. Polyhydramnios is present in approximately one-third of the mothers bearing infants with esophageal atresia since the fetus is unable to swallow amniotic fluid. Within hours after birth, these infants are noted to accumulate large amounts of oral secretions, which require frequent suctioning and may precipitate coughing and respiratory distress. Attempts at feeding are followed by immediate vomiting, and if the infant has a distal tracheo-esophageal connection, abdominal distention may ensue as the intestine fills with air. A flat or gasless abdomen would suggest esophageal atresia without tracheo-esophageal fistula (see Fig. 69–1B). The most critical scenario occurs in those infants with a tracheo-esophageal fistula proximal to the esophageal atresia (see Fig. 69–1D, 69–1E and 69–1G). They develop life-threatening respiratory failure from aspiration almost immediately after birth.

Infants with the H-type tracheo-esophageal fistula (see Fig. 69–1F) do not have the severe regurgitation, mucus accumulation, and severe respiratory distress seen with the other types. Depending on the size of the fistula, they usually present with a history (over months to years in duration) of mild respiratory distress related to feeding or recurrent pneumonias.

If a diagnosis of esophageal atresia is suspected, a soft 5 or 8 French feeding tube can be passed into the esophagus until it meets an obstruction. On occasion, the tube coils in a blind pouch, creating the false impression that the esophagus is patent. A plain film confirms the position of the tube and frequently demonstrates the air-filled upper esophageal pouch. A film of the abdomen for presence of gas determines the presence or absence of a distal tracheo-esophageal fistula. Final proof of the diagnosis (usually not necessary) can be obtained by the instillation of 0.5 ml of contrast material into the proximal esophagus (Fig. 69–2). The pouch is not only clearly delineated by the study but may reveal a proximal fistula.

Treatment. The treatment of esophageal atresia begins with the insertion of a sump suction catheter into the proximal esophageal pouch for the continuous evacuation of secretions. The infant should also be placed in the upright position to help avoid the reflux of gastric secretions through the fistula and into the lungs. Hydration is maintained by intravenous fluids and surgical repair is undertaken when the infant's general condition permits.

The operation of choice for esophageal atresia with tracheo-esophageal fistula is division of the fistula with primary anastomosis between the proximal and distal esophageal segments. This is accomplished by an extrapleural or transpleural approach with an end-to-end or end-to-side anastomosis. Usually, a gastrostomy is also placed.

Postoperative care consists of respiratory support, antibiotics, and intravenous nutritional support. Small amounts of oral feedings may be started 7 to 10 days

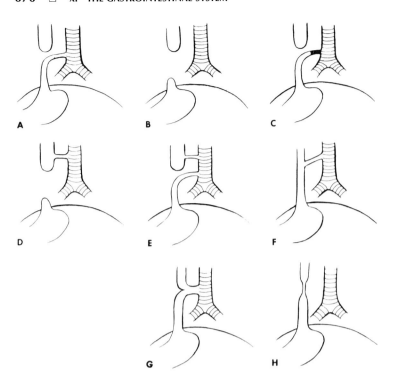

FIGURE 69–1. Types of tracheosophageal fistulas: A is overwhelmingly the most common, accounting for over 85 per cent of esophageal malformations. B is next most common and can be distinguished from A by the absence of air in the intestinal tract on roentgenogram. All the other types have been noted sporadically. (From Avery, M.E., et al.: The Lung and Its Disorders in the Newborn Infant. 4th ed. Philadelphia, W. B. Saunders Company, 1981.)

postoperatively after confirmation by radiographic contrast study that there are no esophageal anastomotic leaks. Enteral feedings via a gastrostomy or a transpyloric tube may be started on the 3rd or 4th postoperative day. These are initially given by continuous infusion. Bolus feedings may be introduced once full enteral alimentation is achieved.

Prognosis. The overall survival rate in term infants without respiratory complications preoperatively approaches 95 per cent (Holder and Ashcraft, 1970). Among premature infants or those with moderate to severe respiratory disease, survival is 85 per cent, while infants with multiple anomalies or those with severe respiratory disease

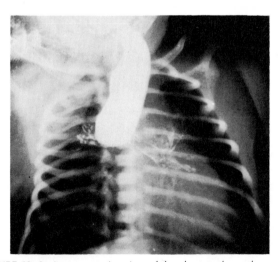

FIGURE 69–2. Anteroposterior view of the chest made on the second day of life, after an iodized oil (Lipiodol) swallow. A large dilated upper esophageal pouch ending blindly in the midchest can be seen. There is no air in the abdomen, a fact suggesting either that there is no fistula or that, if one is present, it is an upper one. Some dye has seeped into the lungs and an outline of a broad fistula tract coursing to the left of the lower end of the pouch is visible.

have a 75 per cent survival rate. Leakage from the anastomotic site may be relatively insignificant or life-threatening with mediastinitis, sepsis, and thoracic empyema, a stormy postoperative course, and a possible unsuccessful outcome. Minor leaks, if self-contained, will form small pseudodiverticula which usually resolve spontaneously or may occasionally form an esophagocutaneous fistula. If the lung remains inflated, these will close spontaneously.

Virtually all infants with esophageal atresia have residual problems with strictures and abnormal esophageal motility and swallowing. Esophageal stricture at the anastamotic site should be suspected if feeding diffculty develops, particularly after the 3rd week. Tension on the anastomosis predisposes to this problem. Repeated dilation may be necessary.

Recurrent stricture formation associated with chronic cough and persistent pneumonias has been attributed to gastroesophageal reflux. Gastroesophageal reflux has been reported in up to 70 per cent of patients following tracheo-esophageal fistula repair (Roberts et al., 1980). Mechanisms include lower esophageal sphincter incompetence and abnormal motility in the body of the esophagus (Whitington et al., 1977). Medical therapy may be successful initially, but most patients require antireflux surgery.

■ TRACHEO-ESOPHAGEAL FISTULA WITHOUT ESOPHAGEAL ATRESIA

Tracheo-esophageal fistula without esophageal atresia is rare. Only 5 per cent of tracheo-esophageal fistulas occur in the absence of esophageal atresia. Most are located superior to the second thoracic vertebra and can be repaired via a neck incision. A few also occur at the carina. Symptoms, which may begin in the newborn period, include coughing and cyanosis with feeding and recurrent episodes of pneumonia. The differential diag-

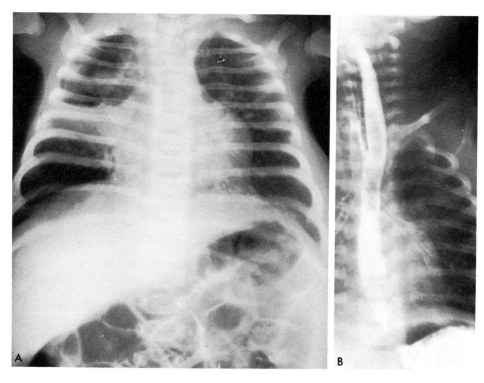

FIGURE 69–3. A, Anteroposterior view of chest of an infant 6 months old. There is atelectasis of the right middle lobe, hyperinflation of the right lower lobe, and some patchy opacification eleswhere. B, Spot film taken after barium swallow outlines the esophagus and a fistula of large caliber coursing from it upward toward the trachea. A faint bronchogram is visible. There is no atresia or stenosis of the esophagus. A tracheosophageal fistula without esophageal atresia was found at autopsy. (Courtesy of Dr. Thomas D. Michael of Baltimore.)

nosis includes gastroesophageal reflux with aspiration or pharyngeal incoordination during swallowing. If the diagnosis of tracheo-esophageal fistula is suspected, oral feedings should be withheld and replaced by gavage feedings until resolution of symptoms. A thick barium upper gastrointestinal series should be done to demonstrate the lesion (Figs. 69–3 and 69–4). If this is unsuccessful, simultaneous endoscopic examination of the trachea and esophagus may be done; the injection of a small amount of methylene blue into the trachea and its subsequent appearance in the esophagus may be diagnostic. The treatment is surgical ligation of the fistula.

■ LARYNGO-TRACHEO-ESOPHAGEAL CLEFT

Laryngo-tracheo-esophageal cleft is a communication of the larynx and trachea with the esophagus. Burroughs and Leape (1974) reviewed the literature and found 33 cases. The defect varies in length with the shortest being the length of the arytenoid cartilages between which the cleft lies, and the longest extending the entire length of the trachea (Fig. 69–5). It is due to a failure of the rostral advance and fusion of the lateral ridges of the laryngotracheal groove between the 5th and 7th weeks of gestation. One-fifth of the clefts are associated with esophageal atresia with tracheo-esophageal fistula. Clinical presentation occurs early in the newborn period and is similar to that for esophageal atresia with tracheo-esophageal fistula, except that stridor may also be present. A carefully done esophageal dye study should establish the diagnosis. However, tracheal spillover may be interpreted as a high H-type fistula or incoordination of the swallowing mechanism. Patients with this finding should have a carefully done bronchoscopic examination with immediate surgical repair. Temporary tracheostomy is necessary since breakdown of the closure is common, but with successful repair, normal survival is possible.

■ ESOPHAGEAL STENOSIS

The lumen of the esophagus may be narrowed due to congenital stenosis, webs, external pressure, or acquired strictures.

CONGENITAL STENOSIS

There are two forms of congenital stenosis. In one, the stenosis is associated with abnormal tissue in the esopha-

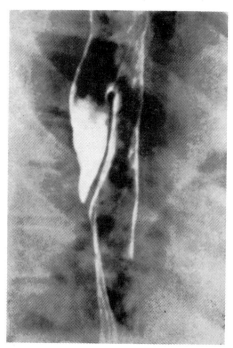

FIGURE 69–4. Roentgenogram after barium swallow, showing diverticulum before operation. The fistula is not demonstrated. (Robb, D.: Aust. N.Z. J. Surg. 22:120, 1952.)

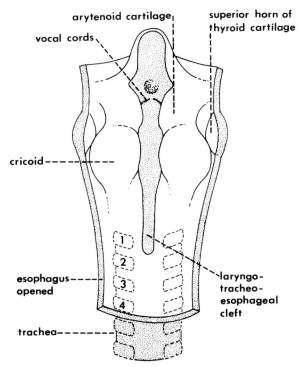

FIGURE 69–5. Illustration of the anatomy of a laryngo-tracheo-esophageal cleft. (From Burrough, N., and Leape, L.L.: Laryngotracheoesophageal cleft: Report of a case successfully treated and review of the literature. Pediatrics 53:517, 1974. Reproduced by permission of Pediatrics.)

geal wall, such as repiratory tissue including cartilage and ciliated epithelium (Ohkawa et al., 1975). The lesion is usually seen in the distal third of the esophagus. Most of these infants do well until solids are introduced into the diet. Vomiting and discomfort are then noted during or shortly after feeding. The diagnosis is made from a radiographic contrast study. The treatment, surgical resection of the short affected segment with primary anastomosis, has generally been successful.

The second type of stenosis is in fact a variant of esophageal atresia with the segments juxtaposed but separated by either a full thickness of esophageal wall or a thin diaphragm of mucous membrane. The diaphragm or web does not completely occlude the lumen. As with the first type, vomiting, particularly after taking solid foods, is the presenting complaint. The diagnosis can be made on a barium study of the esophagus. A thin membrane may respond to dilation, but in some cases surgical resection may be necessary.

■ ESOPHAGEAL DUPLICATIONS

Esophageal duplications make up 10 to 15 per cent of all gastrointestinal duplications. They occur when vacuoles formed during obliteration of the esophageal lumen coalesce during recanalization. The cysts are usually small and take on a spherical configuration, but they may also be tubular extending along the entire length of the esophagus. Sixty per cent are located in the distal esophagus. Dysphagia or vomiting is the usual presenting manifestation, unless the cyst is large, in which case respiratory symptoms may occur. These lesions seldom present in the neonatal period.

■ HIATUS HERNIA

Definition and Incidence. "Hiatus hernia," "congenitally short esophagus," and "partial thoracic stomach" are terms used interchangeably. In Great Britain the lesion is far more commonly reported than in the United States. This may be accounted for by the different techniques applied during upper gastrointestinal series. For purposes of this discussion, hiatus hernia refers to a defect in which at least 15 to 20 per cent of the stomach is in the chest (Fig. 69–6).

Etiology. In the newborn hiatus hernia is due to either abnormal development of the diaphragm or a failure of the esophagus to elongate and the stomach to migrate rapidly in the caudal direction. The result is a short esophagus with the stomach completely or partially trapped above the diaphragm. Botha (1958) carefully studied the anatomy of the diaphragmatic hiatus in newborns. Encircling fibers of two limbs of the right diaphragmatic crus surround the esophagus and overlap to produce a constricted oblique tunnel. This muscular ring is firmly attached to the lower esophagus and cardia by a strong phrenoesophageal membrane. Failure of this complex anatomy to form allows the stomach to pass freely into the chest.

Diagnosis. The primary symptom is vomiting, which may begin with the first feeding or weeks later. Volume and frequency of the vomiting depend on the size of the defect. Aspiration is a potential complication. The diagnosis may be made on an upper gastrointestinal series (see Fig. 69–6).

Treatment and Prognosis. Large defects require surgical closure of the diaphragmatic defect and the performance of a Nissan fundoplication (Johnson, 1986).

■ GASTROESOPHAGEAL REFLUX

Definition. Gastroesophageal reflux is the return of gastric contents into the esophagus. Vomiting is the return of gastric contents into the mouth. Therefore, reflux may occur without vomiting. Approximately 80 per cent of infants under 3 months of age vomit at least once daily (Oski, 1980). How many of these infants have "pathologic" reflux is unknown. Carre (1959) estimated the number to be one in 1000. Experience in this country would suggest a higher number, even if those infants with predisposing conditions, such as severe neurologic damage or bronchopulmonary dysplasia, or following tracheoesophageal fistula repair are excluded. Gastroesophageal reflux is also seen in newborns with apnea (Herbst et al., 1979). The significance of this observation in terms of cause and effect is controversial.

Etiology. Four factors together or alone are major determinants in the etiology of gastroesophageal reflux: (1) hiatus hernia, (2) decreased lower esophageal sphincter pressure, (3) inappropriate relaxation of the lower esophageal sphincter, and (4) abnormal motility in the

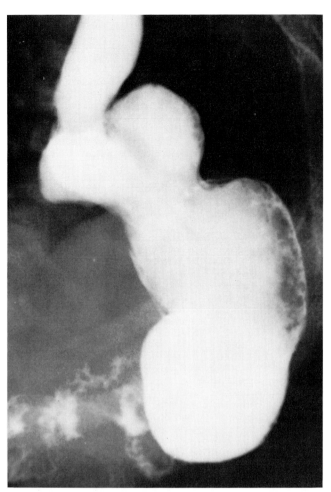

FIGURE 69–6. *Upper gastrointestinal series from a 1-month-old showing a large hiatus hernia and gastroesophageal reflux. The infant presented with massive vomiting following feeding. (Courtesy of Dr. Hoosang Taybi, Children's Hospital, Oakland, Calif.)*

stomach or proximal small bowel, which delays gastric emptying (Hillemeier et al., 1983; Werlin et al., 1980). This classification excludes anatomic partial obstruction by lesions such as an antral diaphragm, a duodenal web, or an annular pancreas. In addition to the four major factors listed earlier, a number of other minor functional factors contribute to reflux in the infant. Newborns eat frequently and not infrequently are overfed. The stomach therefore is often full. If an infant cries or strains, the increase in intra-abdominal pressure may result in reflux. Finally, position is important in preventing reflux. Vandenplas and Sacre-Smits (1985) demonstrated in normal newborns that reflux occurred least often in the prone position.

Diagnosis. In the young infant vomiting is the most common symptom. Complications that may ensue include aspiration pneumonia and failure to thrive. In most infants there is no association between apnea and reflux except during awake apneic episodes (Spitzer et al., 1984). An upper gastrointestinal series is the first study that should be done. This excludes anatomic lesions including malrotation. If there are no complications related to the vomiting, no further testing is necessary. Further studies to document the severity of reflux and its possible etiology include prolonged intraesophageal pH monitoring, esoph-

ageal manometry, technetium-labeled gastric emptying study, and upper endoscopy (Herbst, 1981).

Treatment. Except when there is a large hiatus hernia or gross aspiration on an upper gastrointestinal series, medical therapy for reflux should always be tried first. Carre (1959) estimated that 95 per cent of infants would respond and that vomiting would cease by 18 months in 60 per cent, with the greatest improvement occurring between the ages of 8 and 10 months. Medical treatment includes prone positioning with the head of the crib elevated 10 to 20 degrees, feedings every 3 hours with sufficient volume to provide adequate calories for growth, and frequent effective burping during and after the feeding. The efficacy of thickening feedings with rice cereal is controversial, but it does seem to decrease vomiting (Orenstein et al., 1987). Two pharmacologic agents are available, metoclopramide and bethanechol. Both raise lower esophageal sphincter pressure if it is low and facilitate gastric and esophageal motility. However, controlled studies demonstrating the efficacy of these agents for the treatment of reflux in the newborn are lacking. Further, these agents are not approved for use in infants and should be used only when reflux is carefully documented with pH monitoring. Antacids or H_2 blocking agents are indicated only if esophagitis is documented endoscopically or on esophageal biopsy.

Prognosis. Ninety-five per cent of infants respond to medical measures and do not require surgery. This figure does not include infants with severe CNS lesions or lung disease, one-half to two-thirds of whom need surgery. The antireflux procedure of choice is the Nissan fundoplication. A gastrostomy is constructed at the same time for feeding purposes and to allow venting should the gas bloat syndrome occur.

■ ACHALASIA

Achalasia is an idiopathic primary motility disorder of the esophagus characterized by: (1) an increased lower esophageal sphincter pressure, (2) failure of the lower esophageal sphincter to relax, and (3) a loss of effective peristalsis in the body of the esophagus. Fewer than 20 infants with this disorder have been described (Asch et al., 1974). Presenting symptoms include vomiting and recurrent aspiration pneumonia. The diagnosis can be made from an upper gastrointestinal series, which shows a symmetric beaklike narrowing at the gastroesophageal junction, with moderate to advanced dilation above this stenotic point. Esophageal manometry is necessary to confirm the diagnosis. In infants, the treatment of choice is the Heller myotomy. The major complication following surgery is reflux, and an antireflux procedure at the time of the myotomy has been proposed (Lemmer et al., 1985).

■ CRICOPHARYNGEAL DYSFUNCTION

Some newborns aspirate at times despite what appears to be a normal sucking and swallowing mechanism. If the problem is persistent, evaluation with a cineradiographic swallowing study is indicated. Diagnostic considerations include cricopharyngeal achalasia, familial dysautonomia, or myasthenia gravis. Blank and Silbiger (1972) described a newborn with cricopharyngeal achalasia. On barium swallow, a transverse submucosal bar was seen that was indistinguishable from the cricopharyngeus muscle. Treatment consisted of repeated bougienage. Linde and Westover (1962) called attention to the fact that infants with familial dysautonomia have pharyngeal incoordination beginning at birth that leads to chronic aspiration. In addition, poor esophageal peristalsis delays esophageal emptying.

■ DIFFUSE ESOPHAGEAL SPASM

The author has seen one newborn with this problem, and Fontan and co-workers (1984) described another. This esophageal motility disorder is characterized by tertiary esophageal peristaltic waves of increased amplitude and duration. It presents with symptoms of extreme agitation and vomiting during feeding. The diagnosis can be made from a barium study of the esophagus or esophageal manometry. Glycopyrrolate provided successful therapy in Fontan's patient. More extensive experience from adult series report success with nitroglycerin or calcium channel blocking agents.

■ RUPTURE OF THE ESOPHAGUS

Esophageal perforation has been found in premature infants secondary to malpositioned endotracheal tubes as well as stiff nasogastric tubes (Krasna et al., 1987). Five newborns have been described with spontaneous rupture of the esophagus. In one instance, the rupture occurred just proximal to a stenosing web, but in the other four, the ruptures were unexplained. Hematemesis followed by the development of a hydropneumothorax was the presenting manifestation. An esophagram can confirm the diagnosis and emergent surgical repair is necessary.

■ FAMILIAL DYSAUTONOMIA

Linde and Westover (1962) have called attention to the esophageal abnormalities one may expect in familial dysautonomia. Severe swallowing difficulties and recurrent pneumonitis, probably from aspiration, characterize many of these infants from birth. These observers noted, in addition to pharyngeal incoordination, weak peristaltic action that delayed esophageal emptying in the supine position. In the erect position, gravity facilitated passage of food into the stomach. They found it necessary to feed each swallow to one of their infants in the supine position, so that milk could reach the hypopharynx, then to sit him up so that it could traverse the esophagus.

■ ACKNOWLEDGMENT

We are grateful to Dr. Scott Adsick for his review of this chapter.

■ REFERENCES

Asch, M. J., Liebman, W., Lachman, R. S., et al.: Esophageal achalasia: Diagnosis and cardiomyotomy in a newborn infant. J. Pediatr. Surg. 9:911–912, 1974.

Blank, R. H., and Silbiger, M.: Cricopharyngeal achalasia as a cause of respiratory distress in infancy. J. Pediatr. 81:95–98, 1972.

Botha, G. S. M.: The gastro-esophageal region in infants: Observations in anatomy, with special reference to the closing mechanism and partial thoracic stomach. Arch. Dis. Child. 33:78–83, 1958.

Burroughs, N., and Leape, L. L.: Laryngotracheoesophageal cleft: Report of a case successfully treated and review of the literature. Pediatrics 53:516–522, 1974.

Carre, I. J.: The natural history of the partial thoracic stomach ("hiatal hernia") in children. Arch. Dis. Child. 34:344–353, 1959.

Engel, P., Vos, L., and Kuller, P. J.: Esophageal atresia with tracheoesophageal fistula in mother and child. J. Pediatr. Surg. 5:564–569, 1970.

Ericksen, C., Hauge, M., and Madsen, C. M.: Two generation transmission of oesophageal atresia with tracheo-oesophageal fistula. Acta. Pediatr. Scand. 70:253–258, 1981.

Fontan, J. P., Heldt, G. P., Heyman, M. B., et al.: Esophageal spasm associated with apnea and bradycardia in an infant. Pediatrics 73:52–55, 1984.

Greenwood, R. D., and Rosenthal, A.: Cardiovascular malformations associated with tracheoesophageal fistula and esophageal atresia. Pediatrics 57:87–93, 1976.

Grunwald, P.: Asphyxia, trauma and shock at birth. Arch. Pediatr. 67:103–121, 1950.

Hausmann, P. F., Close, A. S., and Williams, L. P.: Occurrence of tracheoesophageal fistula in three consecutive siblings. Surgery 41:542–547, 1957.

Herbst, J. J.: Gastroesophageal reflux. J. Pediatr. 98:859–870, 1981.

Herbst, J. J., Minton, S. D., and Book, L. S.: Gastroesophageal reflux causing respiratory distress and apnea in newborn infants. J. Pediatr. 95:763–768, 1979

Hillemeier, A. C., Grill, B. B., McCallum, R., et al.: Esophageal and gastric motor abnormalities in gastroesophageal reflux during infancy. Gastroenterology 84:741–746, 1983.

Hohf, R. P., Kimball, E. R., and Ballenger, J. J.: Rupture of the esophagus in the neonate. J.A.M.A. 181:939–945, 1962.

Holder, T. M., and Ashcraft, K. W.: Esophageal atresia and tracheoesophageal fistula (collective review). Ann. Thorac. Surg. 9:445, 1970.

Johnson, D. G.: The Nissan fundoplication. In Ashcraft, K. W., and Holder, T. M. (Eds.): Pediatric Esophageal Surgery. Orlando, Fla., Grune & Stratton, 1986, pp. 193–208.

Krasna, I. H., Rosenfeld, D., Benjamin, B. G., et al.: Esophageal perforation in the neonate: An emerging problem in the nursery. J. Pediatr. Surg. 22:784–790, 1987.

Lemmer, J. H., Coran, A. G., Wesley J. R., et al.: Achalasia in children: Treatment by anterior esophageal myotomy (modified Heller operation). J. Pediatr. Surg. 20:333–338, 1985.

Linde, L. M., and Westover, J. L.: Esophageal and gastric abnormalities in dysautonomia. Pediatrics 29:303–308, 1962.

Merriam, J. C., Jr., and Benirschke, K.: Esophageal erosions in the newborn. Lab. Invest. 8:39–47, 1959.

Meyers, N. A.: Oesophageal atresia: The epitome of modern surgery. Ann. R. Coll. Surg. Engl. 54:312–318, 1974.

Ohkawa, H., Takahashi, H., Hoshino, Y., et al.: Lower esophageal stenosis in association with tracheobronchial remnants. J. Pediatr. Surg. 10:453–458, 1975.

Orenstein, S. R., Magill, H. L. and Brooks, P.: Thickening of infant feedings for therapy of gastroesophageal reflux. J. Pediatr. 110:181–186, 1987.

Oski, F. A.: Iron-fortified formulas and gastrointestinal symptoms in infants: A controlled study. Pediatrics 66:168–170, 1980.

Quan, L., and Smith, D. W.: The VATER association: Vertebral defects, anal atresia, T-E fistula with esophageal atresia, radial and renal dysplasia. A spectrum of associated defects. J. Pediatr. 104:7–12, 1973.

Raffensperger, J. G.: Esophageal atresia and tracheoesophageal stenosis. In Raffensperger, J. G. (Ed.): Swenson's Pediatric Surgery. 5th ed. Norwalk, Conn., Appleton and Lange, 1990, pp. 697–717.

Randolph, J. G., Lilly, J. R., and Anderson, K. D.: Surgical treatment of gastroesophageal reflux in infants. Ann. Surg. 180:479–486, 1974.

Reckham, P. P.: Infants with esophageal atresia weighing under 3 pounds. J. Pediatr. Surg. 16:595–601, 1981.

Roberts, C. C., Herbst, J. J., Jolley, S. G., et al.: Evaluation of tests for gastroesophageal reflux in patients operated on for tracheoesophageal fistula. Pediatr. Res. *14*:509–514, 1980.

Spitzer, A. R., Boyle, J. T., Tuchman, D. N., et al.: Awake apnea associated with gastroesophageal reflux: A specific clinical syndrome. J. Pediatr. *104*:200–205, 1984.

Vandenplas, T., and Sacre-Smits, L.: Seventeen-hour continuous esophageal pH monitoring in the newborn: Evaluation of the influence of position in asymptomatic and symptomatic babies. J. Pediatr. Gastroenterol. Nutr. *4*:356–361, 1985.

Walsh, J. K., Farrell, M. K., Keenan, W. J., et al.: Gastroesophageal reflux in infants: Relation to apnea. J. Pediatr. *99*:197–201, 1981.

Werlin, S. L., Dodds, W. J., Hogan, W. J., et al.: Mechanisms of gastroesophageal reflux in children. J. Pediatr. *97*:244–249, 1980.

Whitington, P. F., Shermeta, D. W., Eto, D. S. Y., et al.: Role of lower esophageal sphincter incompetence in recurrent pneumonia after repair of esophageal atresia. J. Pediatr. *91*:550–554, 1977.

Woolley, M. M., Chinnock, R. F., and Paul, R. H.: Premature twins with esophageal atresia and tracheoesophageal fistula. Acta. Paediatr. *50*:423–428, 1961.

DISORDERS OF THE 70 STOMACH

William J. Byrne

■ HYPOPLASIA OF THE STOMACH

Hypoplasia of the stomach (congenital microgastria) is an exceedingly rare lesion in which fetal rotation of the stomach does not occur, and there is no differentiation into a fundus, body, antrum, and pyloric canal. The gastroesophageal junction is incompetent, and the esophagus takes over the storage function of the stomach. Malrotation, tracheo-esophageal fistula, and other anomalies may be present. Vomiting from birth is the principal clinical presentation. Survival is possible (Blank and Chisholm, 1973).

■ GASTRIC DUPLICATION

More than a hundred cases of gastric duplication have been reported in the English literature (Wieczorek et al., 1984), making up approximately 4 per cent of all enteric duplications. Thirty-six per cent are diagnosed before 3 months of age. Gastric duplications are spherical or hollow-tubular structures that: (1) are lined by a mucosal layer comprised of gastric, small bowel, or colonic epithelium, (2) contain a smooth muscle coat contiguous with the muscle of the stomach, and (3) are contiguous with the stomach wall. Most do not communicate with the gastric lumen and are usually located along the greater curvature. Embryologically, the lesion arises during the 4th week of gestation when, normally, the embryonic notochordal plates and endoderm separate. A band between them may cause a traction diverticulum leading to gut cyst formation (McLetchie et al., 1954). This would explain in part the associated anomalies that occur in 50 per cent of the patients, the most frequent being esophageal duplication and vertebral abnormalities. Sixty-one per cent present with vomiting, and 65 per cent have a palpable abdominal mass. The treatment is complete surgical excision of the cyst.

■ PYLORIC ATRESIA

Pyloric atresia accounts for less than 1 per cent of all atresias. The etiology may be vascular compromise, similar to the origin of small bowel or colonic atresias. As with other high atresias, history of polyhydramnios plus vomiting from birth are the usual presenting symptoms. A gasless abdomen on a plain film and the failure of contrast material to leave the stomach on an upper gastrointestinal series are suggestive and warrant urgent operative intervention. Simple excision of the diaphragm may be adequate, but some patients may require gastroduodenostomy or gastrojejunostomy.

■ ANTRAL WEB OR DIAPHRAGM

Antral webs or diaphragms are usually incomplete or contain an orifice and therefore produce only a partial gastric outlet obstruction. Forty-four cases in patients under 16 years of age were reported in a literature review by Bell and co-workers (1977). Sixty per cent were diagnosed before 3 months of age. The lesion is best explained by excessive local endodermal proliferation. Nonbilious vomiting is the most common presenting symptom. A careful upper gastrointestinal series (Fig. 70–1) may demonstrate the web, but upper gastrointestinal endoscopy may be necessary for diagnosis in some cases. Surgical intervention usually consists of excision of the web and pyloroplasty.

■ PYLORIC STENOSIS

Definition and Epidemiology. Hypertrophy of the pyloric muscle in early infancy results in partial gastric outlet obstruction. The incidence is 1 to 3 per 1000 live births with males being affected four times as often as females and firstborns accounting for half of the cases. Whites are at greater risk than blacks (Laron and Horne,

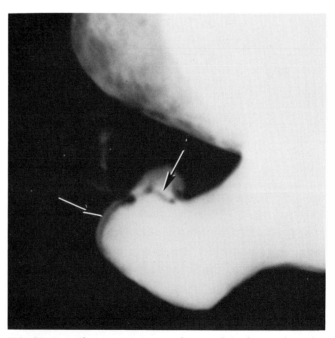

FIGURE 70–1. The arrows point to a thin antral diaphragm, the orifice of which can be seen. This infant began vomiting at 2 weeks of age. The film was taken at 2 months of age. (Courtesy of Dr. Paul Nancarrow, Children's Hospital, Oakland, Calif.)

676

1957). Premature infants are affected with the same frequency as term infants.

Etiology. The exact cause of pyloric stenosis is unknown. Hypergastrinemia has been found in some infants, but animal studies have been unable to reproduce pyloric hypertrophy with gastrin infusion. Hereditary factors have also been implicated since there is a 7 per cent incidence in siblings of affected patients.

Diagnosis. Vomiting is the primary presenting symptom. It may begin at any time from birth to the 12th week, but most often begins between the 3rd and 5th weeks. In premature infants, the onset follows the same pattern postnatally, bearing no relation to the postconceptual age. At first, the vomiting is infrequent and may be small in volume. With time, the frequency and volume of the emesis increase, and projectile vomiting develops. In five per cent of the patients, the vomitus may be brownish or contain some bright red blood. Weight loss, dehydration, and metabolic alkalosis usually ensue as a consequence of the vomiting. Gastric peristaltic waves may be seen passing obliquely from the left upper quadrant across the midline, a pattern that can sometimes be accentuated by feeding the infant an ounce of glucose water. Jaundice may occasionally occur with an elevation of indirect bilirubin that recedes 5 to 10 days after pyloromyotomy. In most instances of pyloric stenosis, a definite tumor, or "olive," can be felt either in the epigastric area or just to the right of the midline in the right upper quadrant. When the clinical presentation is atypical, the lesion can be demonstrated on an upper gastrointestinal series. The most significant radiographic sign is curvature, elongation, and narrowing of the pyloric channel, the "string sign" (Fig. 70–2). More recently, ultrasound has been used to make the diagnosis (Fig. 70–3) (Khamapirad and Athey, 1983).

Treatment. The stomach should be decompressed and dehydration and metabolic alkalosis corrected with intravenous fluids prior to surgery. Pyloromyotomy (Fredet-Ramstedt operation) involves splitting the hypertrophied pyloric muscle. Feedings may be started 8 to 12 hours after surgery and quickly advanced so that by 24 hours the infant is on formula or breast milk. Some vomiting may occur in the postoperative period and persist for up to 1 week.

Prognosis. Overall, the mortality from this operation is less than 0.5 per cent (Scharli et al., 1969). Perforation of the stomach at the time of surgery is seen in less than 2 per cent, and these are recognized and closed at the time of surgery. Incomplete pyloromyotomy is rare.

■ MOTILITY DISORDERS

Disruption of normal motility in the stomach and proximal small bowel delays gastric emptying. The result is vomiting, which clinically may be indistinguishable from that seen with pyloric stenosis, antral diaphragm, or malrotation. While delayed gastric emptying can be documented on a technetium meal gastric emptying scan, the pathophysiologic etiologies for this finding remain elusive.

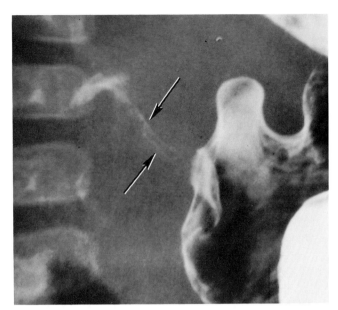

FIGURE 70–2. Upper gastrointestinal series illustrating the "string sign" (arrows) diagnostic for pyloric stenosis. This 2-month-old infant began vomiting at 3 weeks of age. (Courtesy of Dr. Paul Nancarrow, Children's Hospital, Oakland, Calif.)

DELAYED GASTRIC EMPTYING

Problems with gastric emptying are not uncommon in the newborn, especially in premature infants recovering from respiratory distress syndrome. The onset of vomiting is usually early, sooner than that seen with pyloric stenosis. In general, the vomiting is not forceful, but the frequency and quantity may result in significant caloric loss and failure to thrive. Abnormal patterns of myoelectrical activity in the fundus (tachygastria) have been described in

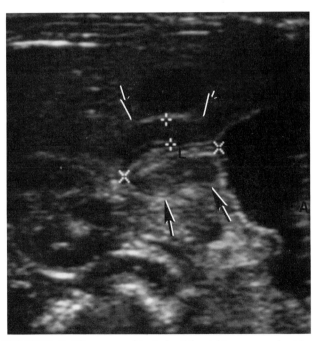

FIGURE 70–3. Ultrasonographic study of the right upper quadrant in a 1-month-old infant with a 1-week history of vomiting. The length (+) of the pylorus is 18.4 mm (normal up to 16 mm) and wall thickness (×) is 4.5 mm (normal is up to 4.0 mm). The arrows outline the muscular wall and point to the lumen (L). A is the antral lumen. (Courtesy of Dr. Ronald M. Cohen, Children's Hospital, Oakland, Calif.)

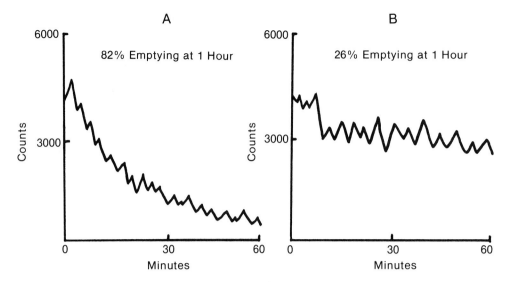

FIGURE 70–4. *Gastrointestinal scintigraphy in a normal infant (A) and in an infant with chronic vomiting, but without anatomic obstruction (B). The time activity curves are constructed by scanning over the stomach for one hour following the ingestion of 90 cc of formula containing 100 microcuries of technetium-99 sulfur colloid.*

older children and adults (Cucchiara et al., 1986). In addition, using perfused catheter systems, abnormal patterns of muscular contraction in the fundus, antrum, and duodenum of adults have all been shown to delay gastric emptying (Malagelada and Stanghellini, 1985). Although there are no data for newborns, several factors are known to affect the physiology of emptying. The prone or right lateral position favors emptying, rather than the supine or left lateral position (Yu, 1975). Isocaloric starch meals empty more rapidly than glucose or lactose, and medium-chain triglycerides empty more rapidly than long-chain triglycerides (Siegel et al., 1985). In piglets, hypoxemia results in decreased blood flow to the gut and delays emptying (Szabo et al., 1985a). Contrary to what might be expected, one study found nutritive and nonnutritive sucking have no effect on gastric emptying (Szabo et al., 1985b). Widstrom and co-workers (1988) found that sucking on a pacifier during tube feedings delayed gastric emptying.

Once anatomic lesions have been excluded by contrast radiography and delayed emptying documented using scintigraphy (Fig. 70–4), medical therapy can be initiated. This includes small frequent feedings, i.e., every 3 hours, right lateral or prone positioning, and the use of metoclopramide, which increases emptying in infants (Hyman et al., 1985). Continuation of this regimen for several months with concurrent growth should make surgical intervention unnecessary.

PYLOROSPASM

Infantile pylorospasm is a radiologic diagnosis and must be differentiated from pyloric stenosis. Radiographically, infants with pylorospasm show a narrow distal antrum, but unlike pyloric stenosis, the caliber of the channel changes. Peristalsis is present in the affected area, and there are no features of muscular hypertrophy, as seen with pyloric stenosis. During the examination, an initial delay in the passage of barium may be followed by a sudden emptying of the stomach. The etiology of pylorospasm is unknown. Conservative medical management similar to that outlined for delayed emptying is all that is necessary. Atropine, 1 drop of a 1:1000 solution, 15 minutes before each meal, may be more successful than

metoclopramide. Pylorospasm usually resolves within 1 to 2 weeks with a disappearance of the vomiting.

■ PEPTIC ULCER DISEASE

Definition and Epidemiology. Ulceration of the gastric or duodenal mucosa is rare in the newborn. Peptic ulcers may be classified as primary if they occur in otherwise healthy individuals or secondary if they are seen in association with underlying systemic disorders. In the newborn most ulcers are secondary and are found in the duodenum (Bell et al., 1981).

Etiology. The etiology of peptic ulcer disease is unknown but is probably multifactorial even in patients with secondary ulcers (Byrne, 1985). Genetic factors, emotional factors, dietary and environmental factors, the amount of hydrochloric acid, and local tissue resistance factors contribute in the older child and adolescent. In the newborn a breakdown of local tissue resistance plays the major role. Normally, a complex barrier protects the mucosal cell, which involves gastric mucus, the secretion of bicarbonate by the mucosal cell, the "alkaline tide," mucosal blood flow, and prostaglandins. Drugs, such as indomethacin which block prostaglandin synthesis, or acidosis and shock, which affect blood flow and bicarbonate production, may lead to a disruption of this barrier and the back-diffusion of hydrochloric acid. The result is mucosal cell destruction, inflammation, and the potential for ulceration.

Diagnosis. In the newborn hematemesis, hematochezia, and perforation of the stomach or duodenum are presenting clinical manifestations. At times, the loss of blood may be considerable, causing a rapid drop in the hematocrit and the development of shock. At other times the bleeding is gradual and recognized only by the vomiting of "coffee grounds" or a Hemoccult-positive stool. A plain radiograph may detect the presence of free air in the abdomen indicating perforation. In general, however, radiographic studies in the newborn are not useful in demonstrating ulceration or gastritis. Upper gastrointestinal fiberoptic endoscopy can be done in the smallest of infants. For suspected peptic ulcer disease, endoscopy is the procedure of choice.

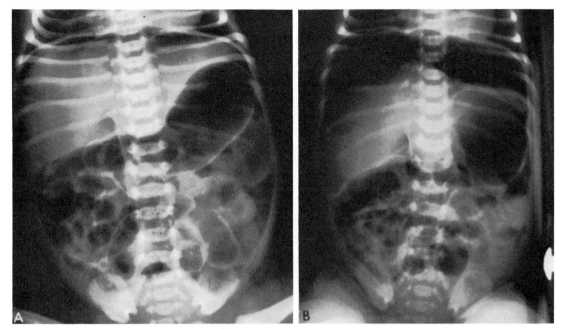

FIGURE 70–5. A, *Anteroposterior view of abdomen taken in the erect position at 72 hours of age. There is air in the stomach and intestines, and one gets the distinct impression that some of the air is outside the lumen of the bowel. A layer of air is clearly visible above the liver and below the diaphragm. B, Ten hours later. By now, there is a huge accumulation of air between the diaphragm and the liver.*

Treatment. Blood loss into the gastrointestinal tract requires prompt and adequate replacement. A nasogastric tube should be passed and the stomach lavaged with room-temperature saline (Andrus and Ponsky, 1987). This is stopped once the material aspirated is only pink-tinged. Antacid therapy 1 ml/kg every 2 hours is then begun. If there is no further bleeding after 24 hours, feedings may be started. The antacids should be continued at the same dose and given 1 hour after each feeding, for 6 to 8 weeks.

■ GASTRIC PERFORATION

Spontaneous perforation of the stomach in the new-born occurs most often during the first 5 days of life (Fig. 70–5) (Bell, 1985). Perinatal stress leading to localized ischemia appears to be the causative mechanism in 80 per cent of the cases. However, in 20 per cent of the cases, no etiology can be identified. Potential causes include rapid overdistention, trauma from passage of a nasogastric tube, and spontaneous rupture of weak points in the gastric wall along the greater curvature where muscle is deficient. Shaw and co-workers (1965) showed that the stomach of a normal infant, when sufficiently distended with air to raise intragastric pressure to a critical level, would rupture.

Sixty-five per cent of the affected infants are of low birth weight. Ordinarily, pregnancy, labor, and delivery are uncomplicated. The infants initially seem well. On the 2nd to 5th day, refusal of food is followed by vomiting, abdominal distention, and respiratory distress. Plain films of the abdomen show free air and fluid. Immediate decompression, fluid resuscitation, and broad-spectrum antibiotic administration should be followed by immediate surgical intervention to close the tear. Early recognition and treatment result in an overall survival rate of 90 per cent (Bell, 1985). The surgeon should always search for possible multiple sites of rupture and rule out distal obstruction.

■ ACKNOWLEDGMENT

The editors are grateful to Dr. Scott Adsick for his review of this chapter.

■ REFERENCES

Andrus, C. H., and Ponsky, J. L.: The effects of irrigant temperature in upper gastrointestinal hemorrhage: A requiem for iced saline lavage. Am. J. Gastroenterol. *82*:1062–1063, 1987.

Bell, J. J.: Perforation of the gastrointestinal tract and peritonitis in the neonate. Surg. Gynecol. Obstet. *160*:20–26, 1985.

Bell, M. J., Keating, J. P., Ternberg, J. L., et al.: Perforated stress ulcers in infants. J. Pediatr. Surg. *16*:998–1002, 1981.

Bell, M. J., Ternberg, J. L., McAlister, W., et al.: Antral diaphragm—a cause of gastric outlet obstruction in infants and children. J. Pediatr. *90*:196–202, 1977.

Blank, E., and Chisholm, A. J.: Congenital microgastria: A case report with 26 year follow-up. Pediatrics *51*:1037–1045, 1973.

Byrne, W. J.: Diagnosis and treatment of peptic ulcer disease in children. Pediatr. Rev. *7*:182–190, 1985.

Cucchiara, S., Janssens, J., and Vantrappen, G.: Gastric electrical dysrhythmias (tachygastria and tachyarrhythmia) in a girl with chronic intractable vomiting. J. Pediatr. *108*:264–267, 1986.

Hyman, P. E., Abrams, C., and Dubois, A.: Effect of metoclopramide and bethanechol on gastric emptying in infants. Pediatr. Res. *19*:1029–1032, 1985.

Khamapirad, T., and Athey, P. A.: Ultrasound diagnosis of hypertrophic pyloric stenosis. J. Pediatr. *102*:23–26, 1983.

Laron, Z., and Horne, L. M.: The incidence of infantile pyloric stenosis. Am. J. Dis. Child. *94*:151–154, 1957.

McLetchie, N. G. B., Purves, J. K., and Saunders, R. L.: The genesis of gastric and certain intestinal diverticula and enterogenous cysts. Surg. Gynecol. Obstet. *99*:135–141, 1954.

Malagelada, J. R., and Stanghellini, V.: Manometric evaluation of functional upper gut symptoms. Gastroenterology *88*:1223–1231, 1985.

Scharli, A., Sieber, W. K., and Kiesewetter, W. B.: Hypertrophic pyloric stenosis at the Children's Hospital of Pittsburgh from 1912 to 1967. J. Pediatr. Surg. *4*:108–114, 1969.

Shaw, A., Blanc, W. A., Santulli, T. V., et al.: Spontaneous rupture of the stomach: A clinical and experimental study. Surgery 58:561–571, 1965.

Siegel, M., Krantz, B., and Lebenthal, E.: Effect of fat and carbohydrate composition on the gastric emptying of isocaloric feedings in premature infants. Gastroenterology 89:785–790, 1985.

Szabo, J. S., Stonestreet, B. S., and Oh, W.: Effects of hypoxemia on gastrointestinal blood flow and gastric emptying in the newborn piglet. Pediatric. Res. 19:466, 469, 1985a.

Szabo, J. S., Hillemeier, A. C., and Oh, W.: Effect of nonnutritive and nutritive suck on gastric emptying in premature infants. J. Pediatr. Gastroenterol. Nutr. 4:348–351, 1985b.

Widstrom, A. M., Marchini, G., and Uvnas-Moberg, K.: Nonnutritive sucking in tube-fed preterm infants: Effects on gastric motility and gastric contents of somatostatin. J. Pediatr. Gastro. Nutr. 7:517–523, 1988.

Wieczorek, R. L., Seidman, I., Ranson, J. H. C., et al.: Congenital duplication of the stomach: Case report and review of the English literature. Am. J. Gastroenterology 79:597–602, 1984.

Yu, V. Y. H.: Effect of body position on gastric emptying in the neonate. Arch. Dis. Child. 50:500–504, 1975.

DISORDERS OF THE INTESTINES AND PANCREAS

William J. Byrne

■ MECHANICAL OBSTRUCTION

CONGENITAL LESIONS

Complete or partial obstruction of the small bowel or colon is not unusual in the newborn. A variety of lesions, intrinsic or extrinsic, may be responsible (Table 71–1). Success or failure in terms of morbidity and mortality depends not so much on pinpointing the exact location of the lesion as it does on correctly diagnosing obstruction as a cause of the clinical symptoms and then instituting prompt operative intervention.

Vomiting, particularly of bile-stained material, with abdominal distention and/or the failure to pass meconium are highly suggestive symptoms. If the obstruction is high or complete, symptoms start soon after birth. Vomiting of bile suggests that the lesion is distal to the ampulla of Vater, whereas sporadic vomiting may be seen in patients with partial obstruction such as occurs with malrotation, duplications, or annular pancreas. Abdominal distention may be present soon after birth, reaching a peak at 24 to 48 hours with visible peristaltic waves. Failure to pass meconium within 24 hours after birth suggests a colonic lesion. Infants with high obstruction or even those with obstruction as low as the ileum pass meconium, so this finding by itself does not exclude obstruction. Prenatal diagnosis of gastrointestinal obstruction has been successful and is becoming more common (Langer et al., 1989).

Palpation of the abdomen may reveal a solid or cystic mass. Occasionally, hard masses are palpable throughout the abdomen, a finding consistent with meconium ileus.

The initial radiographic studies obtained should be plain films in the supine and left lateral position. Normally, air fills the stomach immediately after birth, the small bowel within 12 hours, and the colon within 24 hours. When obstruction exists, the air pattern will stop abruptly at one point, leaving the remainder of the bowel airless. Obstruction at the pylorus produces one large bubble outlining a dilated stomach, whereas duodenal obstructions produce a "double-bubble" picture (Fig. 71–1). Distal obstructions show a series of dilated, air- and fluid-filled loops of intestine. Obstruction due to meconium ileus is an exception in that air-fluid levels usually are not seen. In an incomplete obstruction gas may be seen distal to dilated loops of bowel.

If the diagnosis is in doubt or a meconium plug is suspected, a contrast enema can be done. The finding of a microcolon is suggestive of small bowel atresia or

meconium ileus. An upper gastrointestinal series is done only if the plain film and enema are nondiagnostic.

INTRINSIC OBSTRUCTION

Atresias

Definition and Etiology. Atresia, complete obstruction of the lumen of the bowel should be distinguished from stenosis, which is a narrowing of the lumen. Atresias account for a third of all intestinal obstructions in the newborn, occurring in one of every 1500 live births. Sites of occurrence, in order of frequency, are jejunoileal, duodenal, and colonic. Failure of the gut to recanalize during the 8th to 10th weeks of gestation seems to be the most likely etiology for duodenal atresia. In the jejunum, ileum, and colon, vascular compromise early in gestation may be responsible for bowel atresias (Louw, 1966). Other potential causes in utero include incarceration of the physiologic umbilical hernia, localized volvulus, intussusception, focal peritonitis, and peritoneal band formation.

Duodenal Atresia. Thirty per cent of all atresias occur in the duodenum and the majority are distal to the ampulla. There is a high incidence (70 per cent) of associated anomalies including, in order of frequency, Down syndrome, annular pancreas, cardiovascular malformations, malrotation, esophageal atresia, small bowel lesions, and anorectal lesions (Young and Wilkinson, 1968). Anatomically, duodenal atresia may occur in sev-

TABLE 71–1. Causes of Intestinal Obstruction in the Newborn

MECHANICAL		FUNCTIONAL
Congenital	**Acquired**	
Intrinsic	Necrotizing enterocoli-	Hirschsprung
Atresias	tis	disease
Stenoses	Intussusception	Meconium
Meconium ileus	Peritoneal adhesions	plug
Anorectal malformations		syndrome
Enteric duplications		Ileus
		Peritonitis
Extrinsic		Intestinal
Volvulus		pseudo-
Peritoneal bands		obstruction
Annular pancreas		syndrome
Cysts and tumors		
Incarcerated hernias		

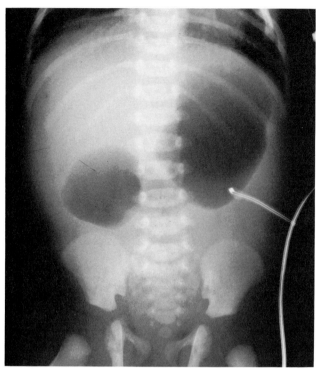

FIGURE 71–1. *Abdominal film from a 12-hour-old infant with vomiting. A "double-bubble" sign is present. At laparotomy duodenal atresia was found. (Courtesy of Dr. Ronald M. Cohen, Children's Hospital, Oakland, Calif.)*

eral forms (Fig. 71–2). Bile-stained vomiting on the 1st day of life and a history of polyhydramnios are common presenting symptoms. Abdominal distention is usually absent. Dehydration with a metabolic alkalosis rapidly ensues. The diagnosis may be made on plain abdominal films with the appearance of the "double-bubble" sign (see Fig. 71–1). Medical therapy consists of the passage of a nasogastric tube and correction of dehydration and electrolyte abnormalities. Urgent surgical intervention is necessary. Because of the high incidence of multiple atresias (15 per cent), inspection of the entire bowel is carried out before constructing a duodenojejunostomy or, more recently, a duodenoduodenostomy (Weber et al., 1986). Mortality following surgery is less than 10 per cent (Mooney et al., 1987). Most deaths that now occur are due to related major anomalies.

Jejunoileal Atresia. Fifty-five per cent of intestinal atresias occur in the jejunum or ileum. Of these 31 per cent occur in the proximal jejunum, 20 per cent in the distal jejunum, 13 per cent in the proximal ileum, and 36 percent in the distal ileum (De Lorimier et al., 1969). Associated extraintestinal anomalies are infrequent (7 per cent), and unlike in duodenal atresia, Down syndrome is uncommon (1 per cent). A useful classification is shown in Figure 71–3 (Martin and Zerella, 1976). Signs and symptoms of jejunoileal atresia include maternal polyhydramnios, bilious vomiting, abdominal distention, which may not become obvious until the 2nd or 3rd day of life, failure to pass meconium, and jaundice. On a plain film, dilated loops of bowel with no gas in the rectum are seen (Fig. 71–4). Contrast enema using Gastrografin or barium may not reach the obstruction, but the appearance of a

microcolon in the normal anatomic position makes other lesions, such as malrotation, colonic atresia, and aganglionosis unlikely. Meconium ileus can also be excluded. The type of surgical operation depends on the lesion, but the procedure of choice is primary closure with end-to-end anastomosis. Survival rate now, with the availability of postoperative intravenous nutritional support, exceeds 90 per cent.

Colonic Atresia. Less than 10 per cent of atresias occur in the colon, and stenosis is even less common. Seventy-five per cent of the atresias are found proximal to the splenic flexure, usually in the ascending colon (Sturum and Ternberg, 1966), with a significant amount of colon missing in most infants and associated anomalies of the gastrointestinal wall occurring in one-third of the infants. Clinical symptoms of colonic atresia include abdominal distention and vomiting beginning on the 2nd or 3rd day of life, and failure to pass meconium. On plain radiographs, dilated loops of bowel will be present, but a contrast enema is essential for definitive diagnosis. One surgical approach involves primary anastomosis, whereas another involves initial colostomy or ileostomy with subsequent anastomosis. Survival with the second approach is greater than 90 per cent (Boles et al., 1976).

Stenosis. Duodenal stenosis may be secondary to an intrinsic defect (see Fig. 71–3) or the result of compression by extrinsic lesions. These include annular pancreas, peritoneal bands, aberrant superior mesenteric artery, or a preduodenal portal vein. Depending on the degree of obstruction, vomiting may begin at any time after birth. Since most lesions involve the second or third portion of the duodenum, the vomiting is bilious. Plain films are

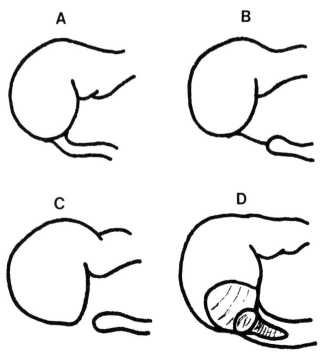

FIGURE 71–2. *Forms of intrinsic duodenal obstruction: A, Duodenal atresia with continuity of the bowel wall. B, Duodenal atresia with a fibrous cord joining segments. C, Complete atresia with two separate segments. D, Wind sock deformity.*

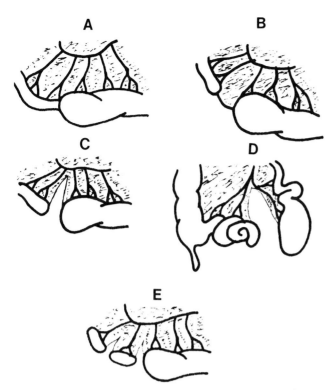

FIGURE 71–3. *Classification of intestinal atresias: A, Mucosal atresia with intact bowel wall and mesentery. B, Blind ends joined by a fibrous cord. C, Blind ends separated by a mesenteric defect. D, Blind ends with the "apple-peel" atresia. E, Multiple atresias.*

usually not diagnostic, but on upper gastrointestinal series the area of stenosis can be delineated; differentiation of the cause may not be possible before surgery.

Meconium Ileus

Definition and Etiology. Meconium ileus refers to an intraluminal intestinal obstruction produced by thick inspissated meconium. Ninety per cent of patients with meconium ileus have cystic fibrosis (CF). Indeed 10 to 15 per cent of CF patients present with meconium ileus. Recently, DNA markers for the cystic fibrosis gene have been identified and localized on chromosome 7 (Rommens et al., 1989). Mornet and co-workers (1988) showed different haplotypic variants for CF chromosomes in families with meconium ileus as compared with families with no meconium ileus. To explain this finding they suggested there were different mutations at the same locus: one for CF and one for meconium ileus. However, Kerem and colleagues (1989) were unable to verify this observation.

Severe pancreatic involvement is not a consistent finding in cystic fibrosis patients presenting with meconium ileus (Waters et al., 1990). In utero, some cystic fibrosis fetuses produce exceptionally viscid secretions from the mucous glands of the small intestine. The meconium formed is dry and contains higher than usual concentrations of protein, including albumin (Schwachmann and Antonowicz, 1981). The abnormal meconium adheres firmly to the mucosal surface of the distal small bowel, creating an intraluminal obstruction. Histologically, the goblet cells and mucous glands are prominent and distended with an eosinophilic material that merges with the intraluminal meconium for a cast of the crypts and villi. Proximal to the obstruction there may be intestinal muscular hypertrophy.

Diagnosis. Prenatal diagnosis of cystic fibrosis is now a possibility (Lemna et al., 1990). A family history of cystic fibrosis should alert one to the possibility of meconium ileus. In the simple form where obstruction occurs in the middle and distal ileum without perforation and peritonitis, signs of obstruction appear within the first 48 hours in an otherwise healthy infant. Abdominal distention is noticed between 12 and 24 hours, followed by vomiting. No meconium is passed. Physical examinations may reveal hard palpable masses throughout the abdomen that are freely movable in any direction. Meconium ileus complicated by volvulus, atresias, meconium peritonitis, or pseudocyst formation is found in one-third of the patients. Newborns with these complications present earlier than those with simple meconium ileus, usually within the first 24 hours of life. They appear sicker, with severe vomiting, signs of neonatal sepsis, and more marked distention causing respiratory distress.

Radiographic examination in the erect position shows dilated loops of bowel. Fluid levels are inconspicuous owing to the viscous nature of the meconium, which produces a coarse granular, or ground-glass, appearance. The abdominal film in addition to the distended gas-filled loops may show intra-abdominal calcification indicative of meconium peritonitis (Fig. 71–5). A cross-table lateral film with the baby in the prone position helps determine if air is in the rectum. Air-fluid levels suggest jejunal or ileal

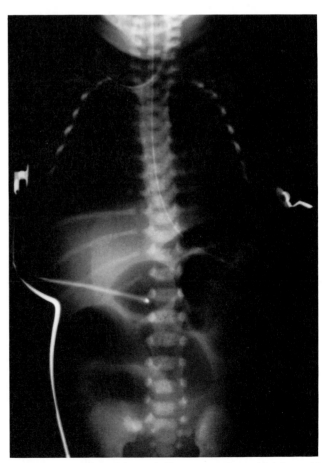

FIGURE 71–4. *Plain abdominal film in a 24-hour-old infant with vomiting and abdominal distention. Multiple dilated bowel loops are present. No gas is seen in the rectum. At surgery proximal ileal atresia was found. (Courtesy of Dr. Ronald M. Cohen, Children's Hospital, Oakland, Calif.)*

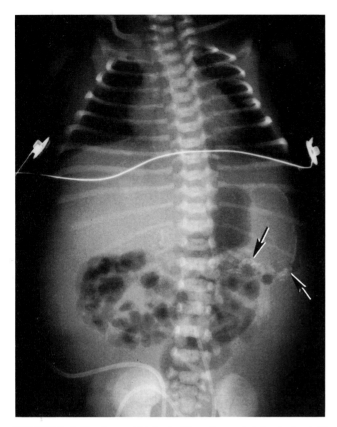

FIGURE 71–5. *Ten-hour-old infant with ascites and abdominal calcification (arrows) secondary to meconium peritonitis. No gas is present in the rectum. The infant had ileal atresia and a subsequent sweat chloride was positive. (Courtesy of Dr. Ronald M. Cohen, Children's Hospital, Oakland, Calif.)*

atresia. A single grossly distended loop of bowel suggests postnatal volvulus. Perforations after birth result in free intraperitoneal air.

All newborns with meconium ileus should be evaluated for cystic fibrosis. Boat and co-workers (1989) have reviewed the clinical, physiologic, and genetic aspects of cystic fibrosis. The identification and cloning of the primary cystic fibrosis gene and the ability to identify mutations causing cystic fibrosis have advanced our ability to provide accurate diagnosis as well as counseling (Kerem et al., 1989; Lemna et al., 1990; Rommens et al., 1989).

Treatment. In simple meconium ileus about 60 per cent of the infants have their obstructions successfully relieved by a hyperosmolar enema (Noblett, 1969). Before the hyperosmolar enema is given, other complications, such as perforation, volvulus, or atresia, must be excluded. The hypertonic enema draws water into the intestinal tract dislodging and breaking up the meconium. Because of rapid fluid shifts, great care must be taken to maintain fluid and electrolyte balance. Failure to pass meconium within several hours after the enema is an indication for surgical intervention, not another enema. If the enema is successful, meconium passage continues for 24 to 48 hours. Acetylcysteine, 5 ml every 6 hours for 5 days, is given via a nasogastric tube. Broad-spectrum antibiotics are also advisable.

Surgical intervention in simple meconium ileus may consist of enterotomy with irrigation and immediate closure, resection of the ileum with irrigation and primary anastomosis, or in the past, resection of the ileum and construction of a Mikulicz-type ileostomy or a Bishop-Koop ileostomy. More recently, the need for an ileostomy has been questioned (Nguyen et al., 1986). Complicated meconium ileus always requires surgical intervention. The operative procedure depends on the pathologic findings.

Prognosis. Operative mortality is well under 20 per cent for simple meconium ileus. The severity of pulmonary involvement affects eventual outcome.

Anorectal Malformations

Definition and Epidemiology. Anorectal anomalies occur in one out of every 5000 births and are slightly more common in males (deVries and Cox, 1985). Associated anomalies occur in over half of these infants and are more frequent in cases where the rectal pouch lies above the puborectalis sling. Vertebral malformations are the most common, followed by genitourinary malformations (28 per cent) and gastrointestinal malformations (13 per cent) (Kiesewetter and Chang, 1977).

Etiology. The proctoderm comprises the anus and a canal that extends cephalad a short distance to meet the blind end of the hindgut, which has simultaneously moved caudad. Around the 7th to 8th weeks of gestation these should make contact, separated only by an anal membrane. At the same time, the lower urinary tract develops alongside the lower intestinal tract, separated by the urorectal membrane. Anal malformations arise locally from maldevelopment within the proctoderm. Atresias, stenosis, and fistulas arise from imperfect resolution of the anorectal membrane with or without concomitant failure of the urorectal membrane to separate completely the rectal and genitourinary anlagen.

Diagnosis and Treatment. Inspection of the perianal area will reveal abnormal anatomy. Table 71–2 lists the various types and relative frequencies of anorectal anomalies.

Anal Stenosis. Anal stenosis accounts for about 8 per cent of anorectal anomalies. The lesion represents a narrowing of a normally formed anorectum at its lowermost extremity. The onset of symptoms varies depending upon the size of the opening. Defecation is difficult and the stools may be ribbon-like. Treatment consists of dilation but in some cases it may be necessary to excise the fibrous tissue and mobilize the rectum, suturing it to the lower part of the anal canal. The prognosis is good, since the anorectal region is basically normal.

Imperforate Anal Membrane. An imperforate anal membrane accounts for 6 per cent of all anorectal anomalies. The newborn fails to pass meconium. On inspection of the perineum, a greenish bulging membrane of epithelium is seen overlying the anal orifice. Excision of the membrane relieves the problem, and sphincter function is usually normal.

Anal Agenesis. Anal agenesis without fistulas accounts for 7 per cent of the lesions and is seen almost exclusively in males. Normal bowel descends through the levator sling, but because of abnormal anal development, only an anteriorly placed dimple is present externally. These infants fail to pass meconium. Anoplasty is the procedure of choice.

Anal agenesis with "fistula" formation occurs in 29 per cent of patients. The fistulas are, in fact, ectopic openings of the anus. In males, the fistula is almost always

TABLE 71–2. Anatomic Classification of Anorectal Malformations

	LESION	FREQUENCY (PER CENT)			SURVIVAL (PER CENT)
		Overall	Male	Female	
Low (below the levator)	Anal stenosis	8			100
	Imperforate anal membrane	6			95
	Anal agenesis	36			84
	No fistula	7	7	0	
	Fistula	29	8	21	
	Anovulvar		1	14	
	Anoperineal		8	7	
High (above the levator)	Rectal agenesis	47			72
	No fistula	13	11	2	
	Fistula	31	21	10	
	Rectourethral		24		
	Rectovesical		1		
	Rectovaginal			8	
	Rectocloacal			3	
	Rectal atresia	3	1	2	57
Overall					80

(Data from Kiesewetter, W. B., and Chang, J. H. T.: Imperforate anus: A five to thirty year follow-up perspective. Prog. Pediatr. Surg. *10*:81–90, 1977.)

to the perineum but rarely to the urethra. In females, it may be either to the vulva (63 per cent) or to the perineum (37 per cent). Any opening or the presence of a spot of meconium in the vulva, or along the perineal raphe in a male, should suggest this lesion. There are a number of anoplasty techniques to move the anus to its normal anatomic location.

Rectal Agenesis. These lesions make up 47 per cent of anorectal anomalies. In the female, these high supralevator lesions occur both with and without fistula. Meconium is either not passed at all or is passed through the fistula, which is not visible on the perineum. The fistula opens either into the vagina or into the urogenital sinus, which is a common passageway for the urethra and vagina. Males may also have rectal agenesis with or without fistula formation. Fistulas in the male are rectourethral or rectovesical and can be detected by examining the urine for meconium in an infant who fails to pass meconium rectally. Patients with high anomalies are treated initially with diverting colostomy, followed by a pull-through procedure between 1 and 2 years of age.

Rectal Atresias. These are rare lesions that present as a bowel obstruction with the failure to pass meconium. The obstructing membrane lies just above the levator sling. This lesion is managed surgically in a manner similar to rectal agenesis.

Prognosis. Early survival figures given in Table 71–2 are dependent primarily on the absence of associated anomalies. From the same series, with a follow-up period of 5 to 30 years, continence was achieved in 75 per cent (Kiesewetter and Chang, 1977). In another 14 per cent, soiling occasionally occurred, but the patient had a socially acceptable degree of continence. Ditesheim and Templeton (1987) reported continence rates of 65 to 70 per cent in their 25-year follow-up of patients operated on for high imperforate anus. In this series quality of life correlated closely with the establishment of continence. Iwai and co-workers (1988), using electromyography and anal manometry, stated that problems with continence following repair of high imperforate anus were due to external anal sphincter dysfunction. Posterior sagittal anorectoplasty promises to revolutionize the surgical approach and outcome for imperforate anus (Pena, 1985).

Enteric Duplications. Duplications of the gastrointestinal tract are relatively rare. Sixty-five per cent are located in the small bowel with over half of these occurring in the ileum (Favara et al., 1971). Thirty per cent are associated with other anomalies, the most common being intestinal atresias. Spherical duplications are more common than tubular ones. Duplications are generally located on the mesenteric side of the lumen, are lined by intestinal mucosa, and share a common wall and mesenteric blood supply with the adjacent intestine, but usually do not communicate with the gut lumen. At least half of the patients are diagnosed in the neonatal period (Grosfeld et al., 1970). Presenting symptoms include vomiting and signs of obstruction with the presence of a palpable mass. Plain films of the abdomen may show displacement of adjacent viscera by a mass. Upper gastrointestinal series and barium enema demonstrate a filling defect or, rarely, may show a communication between the cyst and normal bowel. Treatment is surgical excision with primary anastomosis.

EXTRINSIC OBSTRUCTION

Malrotation with Volvulus
Definition, Epidemiology, and Etiology. Anomalies of intestinal rotation occur in one per 6000 live births. Malrotation of the gut occurs between the 8th and 10th weeks of gestation when the elongating intestine returns to the abdominal cavity. If the mesenteric attachments do not develop properly, the midgut lies free, attached to the posterior abdominal wall at only two points, the duodenum and the proximal colon. It may therefore twist in either direction, but when volvulus occurs it is usually in the clockwise direction. The twisting may make several complete turns, resulting in obstruction of the duodenojejunal junction. Compromise of the circulation of the twisted bowel leads to the rapid development of gangrene.

Diagnosis. Of symptomatic cases, 80 per cent present with evidence of high intestinal obstruction during the 1st month of life. Bilious vomiting, once it begins, occurs after each meal. Since the obstruction is often incomplete, all gradations of distention are seen. Interruption of blood flow leads to peritonitis, sepsis, and shock. Plain film of the abdomen may show dilated stomach and duodenum with little air in the distal bowel. An upper gastrointestinal series should be done initially. If the diagnosis is unclear, a barium enema is indicated (Fig. 71–6).

Treatment. Immediate operation is imperative to prevent irreversible ischemic damage to the gut. The volvulus is reduced by counterclockwise rotation, and the Ladd bands are divided. Nonviable bowel can be resected, but in the absence of perforation, many pediatric surgeons take a conservative approach and wait to resect bowel at a second procedure 24 to 36 hours after the initial operation. During this interval the infant is treated with volume expanders and broad-spectrum antibiotics.

Prognosis. Operative mortality is less than 15 per cent and depends on the infant's clinical condition at the time of surgery. Morbidity depends on the amount of bowel resected and the need for long-term parenteral nutrition.

Annular Pancreas. Annular pancreas is an uncommon lesion that arises from a persistence of the dorsal pancreatic bud, which develops into its own lobe and grows around the left side of the duodenum to join the bilobate ventral pancreatic bud. In 10 to 20 per cent of cases, there are associated anomalies including duodenal atresia, malrotation, duodenal diaphragm, and Down syndrome (Kiernan et al., 1980) Most cases, however, are not diagnosed until adulthood. Symptoms in the newborn are those of partial obstruction, i.e., vomiting and abdominal distention. Treatment is surgical. The procedure of choice is duodenoduodenostomy or duodenojejunostomy. No attempt should be made at operative dissection or division of the pancreatic annulus.

ACQUIRED LESIONS

NECROTIZING ENTEROCOLITIS

Definition. Necrotizing enterocolitis (NEC) is the most common acquired gastrointestinal emergency in the new-

born. The ileum is usually affected, followed, in order of frequency, by the ascending colon, cecum, transverse colon, and rectosigmoid.

Epidemiology. In the United States, between 2000 and 4000 infants each year develop NEC with the majority of cases occurring in infants weighing less than 1500 g (Wilson et al., 1983). Nonetheless, 10 per cent of patients are term infants. The incidence varies among hospitals, but averages from 1 to 5 per cent of admissions to the neonatal intensive care unit. Even within the same hospital, the incidence varies during different periods, owing to epidemics or clustering of cases superimposed on less frequent, endemic cases (Moomjian et al., 1978).

Etiology. The etiology of NEC remains unknown, but it is no doubt multifactorial (Walsh et al., 1988). Hypoxia, acidosis, and hypotension lead to selective circulatory ischemia of the gut wall, which is an essential component of this disorder. The mechanism for this ischemia is unknown since factors controlling mesenteric blood flow in the newborn are poorly understood. Mesenteric thromboemboli from umbilical arterial catheters or direct interference by the catheter with mesenteric blood flow has been proposed to contribute to the ischemia, but pathologic studies have found neither of these to be present in the majority of cases (Kliegman et al., 1982). The "dive reflex," which is the shunting of blood away from the intestine in hypoxic newborn animals, has been postulated as a mechanism for the intestinal ischemia in human newborns. However, when patients with NEC are compared to age-matched controls, no risk factors for this reflex are consistently identified (Wilson et al., 1983). A patent ductus arteriosus with a large left-to-right shunt producing relative bowel ischemia has been identified as an associated factor (Palder et al., 1988). Clinical trials with the prophylactic use of indomethacin in premature infants have not produced consistent results (Clyman and Campbell, 1987). Cassady and co-workers (1989) con-

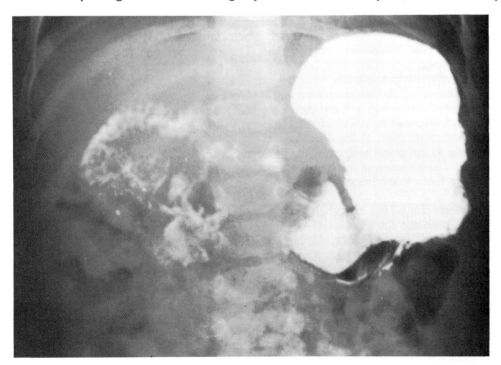

FIGURE 71–6. *Unequivocal malrotation, proved by the presence of the cecum and appendix in the left lower quadrant; the lower end of the midgut mesentery is therefore improperly located. There is also barium in the stomach, but the duodenum and ligament of Treitz are not shown.*

ducted a randomized controlled trial of very early prophylactic surgical ligation of the ductus arteriosus in infants weighing less than 1000 g. They showed a reduction in the incidence of NEC in the operated group but no difference in the frequency of death, bronchopulmonary dysplasia, retinopathy of prematurity, or intraventricular hemorrhage compared with the control group.

Neonatal polycythemia occurs more frequently among infants with NEC and thus appears to be a risk factor (Black et al., 1985). How hyperviscosity affects intestinal blood flow is unknown.

Certain colonic bacteria play an important role in the pathogenesis of NEC. During periods of intestinal ischemia, these bacteria appear to be able to penetrate the mucosal barrier resulting in sepsis. Support for the above comes from studies in germ-free animals, which when subjected to intestinal ischemia, survived longer than animals with enteric organisms (Yales et al., 1974). Epidemiologic observations also support a role for microorganisms or their toxins in the development of NEC. Epidemics of NEC have been reported with *Escherichia coli, Klebsiella, Enterobacter, Pseudomonas,* salmonella, *Clostridium difficile, C. perfringens,* coronavirus, rotavirus, and enteroviruses (Kliegman and Fanaroff, 1984).

Enteral alimentation has traditionally been considered a risk factor for NEC. However, in a composite review of six studies involving 537 infants with NEC, Kliegman and Fanaroff (1984) found that 6.8 per cent of the patients had never been fed. Formula hyperosmolarity and the absence of immunoprotective factors in proprietary preparations were felt to play contributing roles. Today hypertonic formulas are rarely used in the nursery, and care should be taken when administering hypertonic medications (Muty and Obladen, 1985). Because the newborn has a limited ability to mount local immune responses, breast milk has been advocated as a means of providing immunoprotection. Unfortunately, NEC has occurred in infants fed exclusively human milk regardless of whether it was refrigerated, frozen, or pasteurized (Moriartey et al., 1979). A possible protective effect of oral IgA-IgG was reported but requires confirmation (Eibl et al., 1988). Volume of feeding and the rate of volume increments do not appear to be important variables in the pathogenesis of NEC. Recent data suggest that early dilute enteral feedings in premature infants do not predispose to the development of NEC (La Gamma et al., 1985; Ostertag et al., 1986).

Additional factors that may predispose to NEC include enteral and parenteral preparations of vitamin E (Johnson et al., 1985), indomethacin (Nagaraj et al., 1981), and xanthines (Grosfeld et al., 1983). Functional immaturity of the gut, beyond the decreased motility previously mentioned, may play a role. The bile salt pool of the premature infant is smaller than that of the term infant, and bile salts neutralize endotoxin. Animal studies have shown that in newborn rats, the enteric administration of bile salts protects against enterocolitis (Diaz et al., 1980). Bauer and co-workers (1984) demonstrated that the antenatal administration of glucocorticoids to mothers, which has been shown to increase bile salt pool size and hasten gut maturation, decreased the incidence of NEC among preterm infants entered in the U.S. Collaborative Trial of Prenatal Glucocorticoids.

Diagnosis. NEC may present with a wide spectrum of manifestations ranging from a benign gastrointestinal disturbance characterized by mild feeding intolerance, delayed gastric emptying, abdominal distention, diarrhea, and occult or frank blood in the stool to a more fulminant process in which the above are followed rapidly by perforation, sepsis, and shock. Some infants have nonspecific findings such as apnea, bradycardia, and temperature instability that precede the gastrointestinal manifestations. On physical examination the abdomen may be distended and firm with visible loops of bowel and decreased bowel sounds. Marked erythema of the abdominal wall usually represents peritonitis, although rarely it may initially be a local cellulitis in response to underlying inflamed bowel.

Two or more clinical findings suggestive for NEC warrant radiographic evaluation. The radiographic hallmark of NEC is pneumatosis intestinalis (Fig. 71–7) (Mata and Rosenpart, 1980). Air may also be seen in the biliary tree (Fig. 71–8). Free air in the abdomen, usually seen under the diaphragm, is indicative of advanced disease with intestinal perforation. Some infants will not show these specific radiographic findings. A large distended immobile intestinal loop on repeated x-rays suggests a gangrenous loop of bowel. A gasless abdomen may indicate perforation and peritonitis.

Treatment. The use of staging criteria is helpful in guiding therapy (Table 71–3). Broad-spectrum antibiotic coverage should be started immediately. Shock should be treated with sufficient volumes of colloid or crystalloid fluid and pressors to maintain blood pressure and urine output. Enteral feedings should be stopped, and the

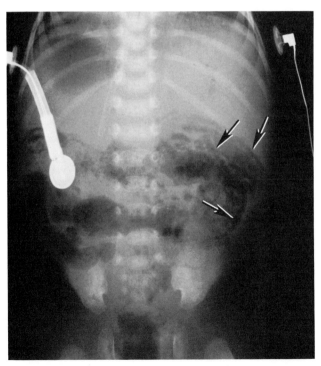

FIGURE 71–7. *Premature infant, 21 days old, who was doing nicely on enteral feedings when she developed abdominal distention, vomiting, and tachycardia. Abdominal plain film shows air in the bowel wall—pneumatosis intestinalis* (arrows). *(Courtesy of Dr. Ronald M. Cohen, Children's Hospital, Oakland, Calif.)*

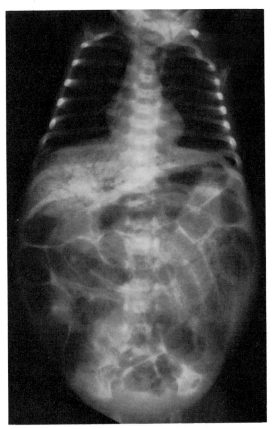

FIGURE 71–8. This film of the chest and abdomen, obtained because of abdominal distention and bloody stools 5 days after birth, shows extensive gaseous distention of the intestines. The distention clearly involves the small bowel and probably involves the colon as well. Fine linear lucencies projected over the left side of the abdomen represent either intramural gas (pneumatosis intestinalis) or gas in the smaller tributaries of the mesenteric veins. The most striking finding is in the liver; the branching lucent shadows are cast by gas widely distributed in the intrahepatic branches of the portal vein. The radiologic findings strongly support the clinical impression of necrotizing enterocolitis. Patient weighed 1650 grams at birth with a gestational age of 28 weeks.

stomach decompressed with a nasogastric tube. Abdominal roentgenograms should be done every 6 hours during the acute period to monitor for perforation. Many infants develop apnea and acidosis and require intubation and ventilation. Disseminated intravascular coagulation (DIC) should be managed with fresh frozen plasma and platelet transfusions. Care must be taken when administering plasma or blood products. Although a rare occurrence, life-threatening hemolysis after transfusion has been reported in infants with NEC (Seges et al., 1981). The hemolysis was attributed to the interaction of anti-T antibody from the transfusion product with exposed T-antigen on the infant's red cells. The T-antigen exposure was caused by the action of bacterial neuraminidase. Enteral aminoglycosides are not indicated since they do not alter the course of the disease. The exception to this statement occurs during epidemics of NEC associated with a specific organism. Under these circumstances, appropriate antimicrobial prophylaxis may be beneficial.

Once the patient has stabilized, total parenteral nutrition should be started to prevent nutritional deterioration. Infants should not be fed for at least 5 days after their gastrointestinal function, abdominal examination, and ab-dominal roentgenogram are normal (usually 10 to 14 days from onset). Antibiotics are continued for 10 to 14 days.

Intestinal perforation is an absolute indication for surgery. Ideally, however, surgery should be performed before the peritoneum is soiled with fecal matter. Findings suggestive of ischemic bowel and impending perforation include: shock unresponsive to volume replacement and pressors, persistent thrombocytopenia, neutropenia, metabolic acidosis, the persistence of a dilated loop of bowel on serial radiographs, a right lower quadrant mass, and abdominal wall erythema. The surgical procedure of choice has been limited resection with diverting ostomy and subsequent closure at a later time; however, primary anastomosis is coming into favor in selected instances (Harberg et al., 1983). On occasion, the entire bowel may appear gangrenous. Under these circumstances, repeat laparotomy in 12 to 48 hours may better delineate viable from nonviable bowel and prevent the need for massive resection.

Prognosis. Mortality is still between 20 and 40 per cent. A significant number of survivors develop strictures (either single or multiple) that usually produce symptoms 2 to 8 weeks after the acute episode (Schwartz et al., 1982). Infants without the chronic sequelae of short bowel syndrome and parenteral nutrition cholestasis have the same long-term prognosis as their peer group of low-birth-weight infants (Abbasi et al., 1984; Stevenson et al., 1980).

SHORT BOWEL SYNDROME

Definition and Etiology. Although a congenital short bowel syndrome has been described (Dorney et al., 1986), short bowel syndrome per se is usually the consequence of surgical resection for an abdominal catastrophe. Traditionally, it has been accepted that if the infant's intestine is to adapt sufficiently for long-term survival, a minimum of 38 cm of jejunoileum without the ileocecal valve or a minimum of 15 cm of jejunoileum with the ileocecal valve must remain (Wilmore, 1972). Dorney and co-workers (1985) extended these observations to minimums of 25 cm without the ileocecal valve and 11 cm with the ileocecal valve.

After small intestinal resection, the residual bowel dilates, and both crypt depth and villus height increase as the result of mucosal hyperplasia. This results in increased absorption area per unit length of intestine. With linear growth of the infant, the intestine also elongates, further increasing the absorptive area. Adaptive changes occur more readily in the ileum than in the jejunum, which does not appear to acquire the specialized transport functions of the ileum. The mechanism or mechanisms responsible for adaptation are complex and poorly understood. Pancreatic and biliary secretions play a role, as do certain hormones such as enteroglucagon and, to a lesser degree, gastrin (Sagor and Bloom, 1983). However, critical to the adaptive process is early enteral alimentation with a balanced formula of peptides, some long-chain fats, and carbohydrates.

Treatment. Management of short bowel syndrome depends on an appreciation of its pathophysiology. In the

TABLE 71–3. Modified Bell's Staging Criteria for Necrotizing Enterocolitis

STAGE	SYSTEMIC SIGNS	INTESTINAL SIGNS	RADIOLOGIC SIGNS	TREATMENT
I. Suspected				
A	Temperature instability, apnea, bradycardia	Elevated pregavage residuals, mild abdominal distention, occult blood in stool	Normal or mild ileus	NPO, antibiotics × 3 days
B	Same as IA	Same as IA, plus gross blood in stool	Same as IA	Same as IA
II. Definite				
A: Mildly ill	Same as IA	Same as above, plus absent bowel sounds, abdominal tenderness	Ileus, pneumatosis intestinalis	NPO, antibiotics × 7 to 10 days
B: Moderately ill	Same as I, plus mild metabolic acidosis, mild thrombocytopenia	Same as above, plus absent bowel sounds, definite abdominal tenderness, abdominal cellulitis, right lower quadrant mass	Same as IIA, plus portal vein gas, with or without ascites	NPO, antibiotics × 14 days
III. Advanced				
A: Severely Ill, bowel intact	Same as IIB, plus hypotension, bradycardia, respiratory acidosis, metabolic acidosis, disseminated intravascular coagulation, neutropenia	Same as above, plus signs of generalized peritonitis, marked tenderness, and distention of abdomen	Same as IIB, plus definite ascites	NPO, antibiotics × 14 days, fluid resuscitation, inotropic support, ventilator therapy, paracentesis
B: Severely Ill: bowel perforated	Same as IIIA	Same as IIIA	Same as IIB, plus pneumoperitoneum	Same as IIIA, plus surgery

(From Walsh, M. C., Kliegman, R. M., and Fanaroff, A. A.: Necrotizing enterocolitis: A practitioner's perspective. Pediatr. Rev. 9:225, 1988. Reproduced by permission of Pediatrics.)

immediate postoperative period, nutritional requirements can be met with total parenteral nutrition. Gastric hypersecretion may be a problem in some infants, and can be controlled with H_2 blockers. As soon as possible, enteral alimentation with a semielemental formula (Pregestimil) should be started by continuous infusion. Advancement of the enteral alimentation and the gradual decrease of the parenteral nutrition depend upon stool output and fluid and electrolyte balance. The goal is to discontinue the parenteral nutrition in order to stop ongoing liver damage and reduce the risk of gallstone formation. Along with continuous gastrostomy, or nasogastric tube feedings, oral stimulation, with small feedings and a pacifier, is critical to maintain normal oral motor development. This will be important later when oral feeding is attempted. Considerations in the transition from parenteral to enteral nutrition should focus on stool losses secondary to malabsorption. Supplemental sodium, potassium bicarbonate, magnesium, or calcium may be necessary, particularly in infants with an ileostomy or jejunostomy. Careful monitoring is essential. Except for vitamin B_{12}, which is absorbed in the distal ileum, water-soluble vitamin absorption is not a major problem, and the daily administration of a multivitamin preparation is all that is usually necessary. Vitamin B_{12} is given every 6 months by intramuscular injection. Fat-soluble vitamin levels should be monitored every 3 months once full enteral alimentation is achieved. Supplementation is provided as necessary. Additional iron is usually also required, and this can be given enterally.

Severe diarrhea is best controlled by manipulating feedings. Cholestyramine, which binds malabsorbed bile acids, may reduce stool frequency by interfering with the bile acids' secretory effect on the colon, but antimotility drugs should be avoided in infants. A number of surgical

alternatives have been proposed for the management of short bowel syndrome. These include antiperistaltic segments, intestinal tapering and lengthening, and recirculating loops (Thompson and Rikkers, 1987). Only very limited success has been achieved.

Prognosis. With aggressive support, survival rates for infants with short bowel syndrome approach 70 to 80 per cent. Morbidity and mortality are related primarily to parenteral nutrition. In a long-term follow-up study, Ralston and co-workers (1984) reported normal cognitive and motor development in most of these patients.

INTUSSUSCEPTION

Intussusception is the invagination of one loop of bowel into a loop distal to it. Although intussusception is a relatively common cause of intestinal obstruction in infants 6 to 18 months old, it is extremely rare in the 1st month of life. Talwalker (1962) reviewed the case histories of 24 newborns with intussusception (Table 71–4). Eight arose in the jejunum, which resulted in an unusually high proportion of jejunal to ileocecal intussusceptions. Vomiting and blood in the stools were almost always present. Unlike in the older infants, pain and a palpable mass were rare. Plain films show dilated loops above the obstruction with an almost gasless abdomen distally. Barium enema shows the column ending in a meniscus with a coiled-spring pattern extending proximally. The passage of blood or blood-stained mucus, with signs of obstruction clinically and on plain films, warrants the performance of a proctoscopic examination and barium enema. In older infants, a barium enema is not only diagnostic but in 81 per cent of the patients is also therapeutic (Gierup et al., 1972).

TABLE 71–4. Intussusception in the Newborn

| TYPE | METHODS OF TREATMENT | | | |
	Number	Reduction	Resection	None
Ileocecal	12	6	3	3
Jejunal	8	2	6	–
Ileal	3	2	1	–
Colonic	1	–	1	–

Adapted from Talwalker, V. C.: Intussusception in the newborn. Arch. Dis. Child. 37:203–208, 1962.

Hydrostatic reduction in the newborn has been successful in only 40 per cent, and surgical reduction is therefore usually necessary.

PERITONEAL ADHESIONS

Obstruction may follow the development of adhesions between one hollow viscus and another as a result of healed peritonitis. The initial inflammation may have taken place weeks to months before. Causes include bacterial infection, chemical irritation, such as that occurring with bile peritonitis, or mechanical irritation from a previous laparotomy.

MESENTERIC THROMBOSIS

Thrombosis of the mesenteric veins has been a well-recognized entity in adults since the 1940s. Pathologists have called our attention to mesenteric arterial thrombosis, most often involving the superior mesenteric artery, for almost as long. In the newborn we encounter both: the venous form almost always secondary to abdominal inflammatory disease—perhaps with dehydration, shock, and increased blood viscosity playing a role—and the arterial form to emboli, either septic or nonseptic—perhaps arising in the contracting ductus arteriosus. In the past decade, this syndrome has been associated with umbilical artery catheterization, sepsis, and shock. Infants of poorly controlled diabetic mothers are susceptible to thromboses in many organs, one of which is the mesentery (Oppenheimer and Avery, 1968).

Prevention and Treatment. Mesenteric thrombosis is probably rare now because of vigorous initial stabilization of blood pressure and attention to hydration. Better control of diabetes in pregnancy has been associated with fewer complications, including venous thromboses.

Once the lesion is suspected, correction of hemoconcentration is mandatory, and consultation with a pediatric surgeon is appropriate to discuss the necessity for and timing of surgical exploration.

■ FUNCTIONAL OBSTRUCTION

HIRSCHSPRUNG DISEASE

Definition and Epidemiology. Hirschsprung disease is a lower intestinal obstruction due to agenesis of ganglion cells in the Auerbach and Meissner plexuses. The lesion originates in the rectum and extends proximally over a variable distance. In 80 to 90 per cent of the patients, involvement does not extend more proximally than the sigmoid colon. With involvement limited to the rectosig-

moid, males predominate 4:1. Both sexes are equally affected in long-segment disease. Aganglionic megacolon occurs in one in 5000 live births and accounts for 5 per cent of neonatal intestinal obstructions. It is uncommon in low-birth-weight infants and not infrequently associated with Down syndrome (up to 15 per cent) and other chromosomal disorders.

Diagnosis. Delay in the passage of meconium beyond 24 hours occurs in 95 per cent of newborns with this disease. Other clinical findings include evidence of lower intestinal obstruction (abdominal distention and vomiting), obstipation, and failure to thrive. The development of enterocolitis may lead to diarrhea, dehydration, and shock. In some patients, the disease resembles the meconium plug syndrome, initially responding to an enema with the passage of meconium. However, within a few days the symptoms of constipation recur.

A barium enema may not be diagnostic in the newborn. Only rarely does one see the characteristic narrowed rectosigmoid segment distal to a dilated sigmoid segment. The typical caliber differential does not become apparent until 3 or 4 weeks of age. However, the persistence of barium in the rectum and sigmoid for more than 24 hours after the examination is highly suggestive of Hirschsprung disease.

The definitive diagnosis may be made on rectal suction biopsy (Campbell and Noblett, 1969). If ganglion cells are not present in three specimens of sufficient depth after serial sectioning, a full-thickness biopsy can be done prior to diverting colostomy.

Treatment. Definitive treatment for Hirschsprung disease is operative. Most pediatric surgeons defer definitive repair until 8 to 12 months of age, temporizing by performing a colostomy. A number of definitive procedures are available, including the Swenson pull-through, the Duhamel operation, and the Soave endorectal pull-through (Joseph and Sim, 1988; Vane and Grosfeld, 1986). All have their proponents, and the choice depends on the experience of the surgeon.

Prognosis. Mortality for enterocolitis is 20 per cent. Prompt diagnosis and therapy should improve this figure. Operative mortality is less than 5 per cent, and a good surgical outcome in terms of continence can be expected in 80 per cent.

MECONIUM PLUG SYNDROME

Meconium plug syndrome was initially described as an intestinal obstruction in the newborn that is relieved by the passage of an inspissated gray plug of meconium from the distal colon (Ellis and Clatworthy, 1966). It was initially thought that the meconium itself was abnormal. However, this syndrome is now considered to be a form of colonic dysmotility without an abnormality of intramural ganglion cells.

These infants pass no meconium for the first 24 to 48 hours of life and eventually develop symptoms of distal intestinal obstruction. Contrast enema may be both diagnostic and therapeutic. Because half of these patients eventually are diagnosed with Hirschsprung disease, careful follow-up is necessary.

ILEUS

Ileus is defined as a derangement impairing the proper distal propulsion of intestinal contents that is not due to a mechanical cause. The etiology may be infectious, metabolic, chemical, neurologic, or idiopathic (Table 71–5). Abdominal distention is always present, and bowel sounds may be decreased or absent.

PERITONITIS

Causes of peritonitis may not be clinically obvious in the newborn. Two entities, isolated perforation of the bowel and acute appendicitis, are discussed here.

Perforation. Perforation of the gastrointestinal tract may be spontaneous or associated with a history of asphyxia, prematurity, diagnostic procedures, or the use of positive pressure in the treatment of respiratory disorders. Perforation has also been reported in newborns given indomethacin for the treatment of patent ductus arteriosus (Aschner et al., 1988; Nagaraj et al., 1981) and in premature infants whose mothers underwent chronic tocolysis with indomethacin (Vanhaesebrouck et al., 1988). Tucker and co-workers (1975) described 53 cases of gastrointestinal perforation, 72 per cent of which presented during the 1st week of life, and 25 per cent of which occurred in the small intestine or colon. Sudden clinical deterioration with the presence of free air in the abdomen warrants exploration to repair the perforation. Mortality in Tucker's series was 50 per cent.

Acute Appendicitis. More than 100 cases have been reported in newborns (Parsons et al., 1970). It is difficult

TABLE 71–5. Nonmechanical Causes of Ileus in Infancy

Infections
    Generalized sepsis
    Peritonitis
Metabolic
    Hypokalemia
    Hypo- or hypermagnesemia
    Hypocalcemia
    Hypophosphatemia
    Azotemia
Endocrine
    Hypothyroidism
    Hypoparathyroidism
Pharmacologic
    Narcotics
    Barbiturates
    Ganglionic block agents
    Tricyclic antidepressants
    Phenothiazines
Neurologic
    Severe anoxic brain damage
    Spinal cord injury or transection
    Myotonic dystrophy
    Familial dysautonomia
Miscellaneous
    Chronic idiopathic intestinal pseudo-obstruction
    Megacystitis–microcolon–intestinal hypoperistalsis syndrome
    Congestive heart failure

to diagnose and may be confused with necrotizing enterocolitis. An association with Hirschsprung disease has been noted. The high mortality of 80 per cent has been attributed to: (1) a delay in diagnosis until perforation occurs, (2) a small omentum, which does not seal off the process, and (3) impaired defense mechanisms (Shaul, 1981).

CHRONIC IDIOPATHIC INTESTINAL PSEUDO-OBSTRUCTION SYNDROME

The chronic idiopathic intestinal pseudo-obstruction syndrome lumps together a group of motility disorders of both muscular and neurogenic origin. Patients may become symptomatic at any time, including during the neonatal period (Anuras et al., 1986; Byrne et al., 1977). Symptoms include abdominal distention and vomiting. With onset in the newborn period, there is unlikely to be a "resolution" of the obstruction, as is seen in older patients. Pharmacologic agents such as metoclopramide, cisapride, bethanechol chloride, prostaglandins, cholecystokinin, pentagastrin, ceruletide, and acetylcholine have been tried without success (Golladay and Byrne, 1981). Surgical intervention is usually not successful and should be avoided. Treatment consists of long-term parenteral nutritional support.

A variant of pseudo-obstruction is the megacystis–microcolon–intestinal hypoperistalsis syndrome, as described by Berdon and associates (1981) and recently reviewed by Vintzileos and co-workers (1986). Rarely seen in males, this disorder presents in the newborn period with signs of a bowel obstruction. In addition, bilateral flank masses (hydronephrotic kidneys) and a single large midline abdominal mass (megacystis) suggest an obstructive uropathy. Ultrasound, voiding cystourethrogram, and barium enema are diagnostic. Surgical exploration usually reveals a massively dilated bladder and a short, malfixed small intestine with a microcolon. Adequate peristalsis never returns, so that long-term parenteral nutrition is necessary.

■ DISORDERS OF THE PANCREAS
EXOCRINE PANCREATIC INSUFFICIENCY

Cystic Fibrosis. The usual presentation of this disorder in the newborn period is meconium ileus. However, this diagnosis should be considered in the young infant with failure to thrive and hypoalbuminemia, even in the absence of respiratory disease. Incidence figures for whites vary from one in 600 to one in 2500 and for American blacks, one in 17,000. Cystic fibrosis is an autosomal recessive disorder. (See the discussion of genetic diagnosis with meconium ileus earlier in this chapter.) In addition to being concerned about failure to thrive and hypoalbuminemia, parents may complain that the infant is constipated or passes large, very malodorous stools. The diagnosis can be made on a sweat test. Nutritional therapy is directed at providing adequate calories for growth and improving protein digestion and absorption. Predigested formulas with a significant percentage of their fat as medium-chain triglycerides often accomplish this goal. If the infant is fed regular formula or breast milk, enzyme supplementation is necessary. Even with more elemental formulas, enzymes may increase absorption by 50 per cent. Half of a capsule with feedings is usually sufficient. Fat-soluble vitamin supplementation is not usually necessary in these infants but vitamin levels should be followed at 4- to 6-month intervals.

Shwachman Syndrome. Shwachman syndrome is characterized by pancreatic insufficiency and bone marrow dysfunction (Aggett et al., 1980). The defect appears to be with enzyme secretion and acinar function, not bicarbonate secretion and duct function (Hill et al., 1982). Microscopically, there is an absence of acinar tissue with preservation of the islets and ducts. The hematologic defect is primarily a severe neutropenia, although mild anemia and thrombocytopenia may be present. The etiology of Shwachman syndrome is genetic, but the mode of inheritance is unknown. Clinically, the infants present with neutropenia and failure to thrive. Pancreatic enzyme replacement improves nutrition, but mortality during childhood remains high (30 per cent) because of recurrent infections and the development of leukemia (Woods et al., 1981).

Pancreatic Agenesis. Several forms of insulin-requiring diabetes have been described in the newborn period. One form of pancreatic agenesis also includes exocrine pancreatic insufficiency (Howard et al., 1980). In addition to diabetes, the clinical presentation includes edema, hypoproteinemia, and failure to thrive. Steatorrhea can be documented. Therapy includes enzyme replacement and insulin. Survival is possible.

Isolated Enzyme Defects. Isolated deficiencies of trypsinogen (Townes et al., 1967) and lipase have been reported. Trypsinogen deficiency presents with hypoproteinemia, edema, and failure to thrive. With lipase deficiency, steatorrhea and poor growth are the presenting manifestations.

■ ACKNOWLEDGMENT

We are grateful to Dr. Scott Adsick for his review and contributions to this chapter.

■ REFERENCES

Abbasi, S., Pereira, G. R., and Johnson, L.: Long-term assessment of growth, nutritional status, and gastrointestinal function in survivors of necrotizing enterocolitis. J. Pediatr. *104*:550–554, 1984.

Aggett, P. J., Cavanaugh, N. P. C., and Matthew, D. J.: Shwachman's syndrome. Arch. Dis. Child. *55*:331–347, 1980.

Anuras S., Metros, F. A., Soper, R. T., et al.: Chronic intestinal pseudoobstruction in young children. Gastroenterology *91*:62–70, 1986.

Aschner, J. L., Deluga, K. S., Metlay, L. A., et al.: Spontaneous focal gastrointestinal perforation in very low birth weight infants. J. Pediatr. *113*:364–367, 1988.

Bauer, C. R., Morrison, J. C., Poole, W. K., et al.: A decreased incidence of necrotizing enterocolitis after prenatal glucocorticoid therapy. Pediatrics *73*:682–688, 1984.

Berdon, W. E., Baker, D. N., Blank, W. A., et al.: Megacystis-microcolon-intestinal hypoperistalsis syndrome: A new cause of intestinal obstruction in the newborn. Report of radiologic findings in five newborn girls. AJR *137*:749–755, 1981.

Black, V. D., Rumack, C. M., Lubchenco, L. O., et al.: Gastrointestinal injury in polycythemic term infants. Pediatrics *76*:225–231, 1985.

Boat, T. F., Welsh, M. J., Beaudet, A. L., et al.: Cystic fibrosis. *In* Scriver, C. R., Beaudet, A. L., Sly, W. S., et al. (Eds.): The Metabolic Basis of Inherited Disease. 6th ed. New York, McGraw-Hill, 1989, pp. 2649–2680.

Boles, E. T., Vassy, L. E., and Ralston, M.: Atresia of the colon. J. Pediatr. Surg. *11*:69, 1976.

Byrne, W. J., Cipil, L., Euler, A. R., et al.: Chronic idiopathic intestinal pseudo-obstruction syndrome in children—clinical characteristics and prognosis. J. Pediatr. *90*:585–589, 1977.

Campbell, P. E., and Noblett, H. R.: Experience with rectal suction biopsy in the diagnosis of Hirschsprung's disease. J. Pediatr. Surg. *4*:410–415, 1969.

Cassady, G., Crovse, D. T., and Phillips, J. B.: A randomized, controlled trial of very early prophylactic ligation of the ductus arterosus in babies who weighed 1000 gm or less at birth. N. Engl. J. Med. *320*:1511–1516, 1989.

Clyman, R. I., and Campbell, D.: Indomethacin therapy for patent ductus arteriosus: When is prophylaxis not prophylactic? J. Pediatr. *111*:718, 1987.

De Lorimier, A. A., Fonkalsrud, E. W., and Hays, D. W.: Congenital atresia and stenosis of the jejunum and ileum. Surgery *65*:819–827, 1969.

deVries, P. A., and Cox, K. L.: Surgery of anorectal anomalies. Surg. Clin. N. Am. *65*:1139–1169, 1985.

Diaz, J., Samson, H., and Kessler, D.: Experimental necrotizing enterocolitis: The possible role of bile salts in its etiology and treatment. Pediatr. Res. *14*:595, 1980.

Ditesheim, J. A., and Templeton, J. M.: Short-term versus long-term quality of life in children following repair of high imperforate anus. J. Pediatr. Surg. *22*:581–587, 1987.

Dorney, S., Ament, M. E., Berquist, W. E., et al.: Improved survival in very short small bowel of infancy with the use of long-term parenteral nutrition. J. Pediatr. *107*:521–525, 1985.

Dorney, S. F., Byrne, W. J., and Ament, M. E.: Case of congenital short small intestine: Survival with the use of long-term parenteral feeding. Pediatrics *77*:386–389, 1986.

Eibl, M. M., Wolf, H. M., Furnkranz, H., et al.: Prevention of necrotizing enterocolitis in low-birth-weight infants by IgA-IgG feeding. N. Engl. J. Med. *319*:1–7, 1988.

Ellis, D. G., and Clatworthy, H. W.: The meconium plug syndrome revisited. J. Pediatr. Surg. *1*:54–61, 1966.

Favara, B. E., Franciosi, R. A., and Akers, D. R.: Enteric duplications: 37 cases, a vascular theory of pathogenesis. Am. J. Dis. Child. *122*:501–506, 1971.

Gierup, J., Jorulf, H., and Levaditis, A.: Management of intussusception in infants and children: A survey based on 288 consecutive cases. Pediatrics *50*:535–540, 1972.

Golladay, E. S., and Byrne, W. J.: Intestinal pseudo-obstruction. Surg. Gynec. Obset. *153*:257–273, 1981.

Grosfeld, J. L., Dalsing, M. C., Hull, M., et al.: Neonatal apnea xanthines and necrotizing enterocolitis. J. Pediatr. Surg. *18*:80–84, 1983.

Grosfeld, J. L., O'Neill, J. A., and Clatworthy, H. W.: Enteric duplications in infancy and childhood: An 18 year review. Annals Surg. *172*:83–90, 1970.

Gross, R. E.: The Surgery of Infancy and Childhood. Philadelphia, W. B. Saunders Company, 1953.

Harberg, F. J., McGill, C. W., Saleen, M. M., et al.: Resection with primary anastomosis in necrotizing enterocolitis. J. Pediatr. Surg. *18*:743, 1983.

Hill, R. E., Durie, P. R., and Gaskin, K. J.: Steatorrhea and pancreatic insufficiency in Shwachman's syndrome. Gastroenterology *83*:22–27, 1982.

Howard, C. P., Go, V. L. W., Infante, A. J., et al.: Long-term survival in a case of functional pancreatic agenesis. J. Pediatr. *97*:786–789, 1980.

Iwai, N., Yanagihara, J., and Takahasi, T.: Voluntary anal continence after surgery for anorectal malformations. J. Pediatr. Surg. *23*:393–397, 1988.

Johnson, L., Bowen, F. W., Affasi, S., et al.: Relationship of prolonged pharmacologic serum levels of vitamin E to incidence of sepsis and necrotizing enterocolitis in infants of birth weight 1,500 grams or less. Pediatrics *75*:619–638, 1985.

Joseph, V. T., and Sim, C. K.: Problems and pitfalls in the management of Hirschsprung's disease. J. Pediatr. Surg. *23*:398–402, 1988.

Kerem, E., Corey, M., and Levison, H.: Clinical and genetic comparisons of patients with cystic fibrosis, with or without meconium ileus. J. Pediatr. *114*:767–773, 1989.

Kerem, B. S., Rommens, J. M., Buchanan, J. A., et al.: Identification of the cystic fibrosis gene: genetic analysis. Science 245:1073, 1989.

Kiernan, P. D., Remine, S. G., Kiernan, P. C., et al.: Annular pancreas. Arch. Surg. 115:46–50, 1980.

Kiesewetter, W. B., and Chang, J. H. T.: Imperforate anus: A five to thirty year follow-up perspective. Prog. Pediatr. Surg. 10:81–90, 1977.

Kliegman, R. M., and Fanaroff, A. A.: Necrotizing enterocolitis. N. Engl. J. Med. 310:1093–1103, 1984.

Kliegman, R. M., Hack, M., Jones, P., et al.: Epidemiologic study of necrotizing enterocolitis among low-birth-weight infants. J. Pediatr. 100:440–444, 1982.

La Gamma, E. F., Ostertag, S. G., and Birenbaum, H.: Failure of delayed oral feedings to prevent necrotizing entercolitis. Am. J. Dis. Child. 139:385–389, 1985.

Langer, J. C., Adzick, N. S., Filly, R. A., et al.: Gastrointestinal tract obstruction in the fetus. Arch. Surg. 124:1183–1187, 1989.

Lemna, W. K., Feldman, G. L., Bat-Sheva Kerem, et al.: Mutation analysis for heterozygote detection and the prenatal diagnosis of cystic fibrosis. N. Engl. J. Med. 322:291–296, 1990.

Louw, J. H.: Jejunoileal atresia and stenosis. J. Pediatr. Surg. 1:8–15, 1966.

Martin, L. W., and Zerella, J. T.: Jejunoileal atresia: A proposed classification. J. Pediatr. Surg. 11:399–406, 1976.

Mata, A. G., and Rosenpart, R. M.: Interobserver variability in the radiographic diagnosis of necrotizing enterocolitis. Pediatrics 66:68–71, 1980.

Mooney, D., Lewis, J. E., and Weber, T. R.: Newborn duodenal atresia: An improving outlook. Am. J. Surg. 153:347–349, 1987.

Moomjian, A. S., Peckham, G. J., and Fox, W. W.: Necrotizing enterocolitis—Endemic versus epidemic form. Pediatr. Res. 12:530, 1978.

Moriartey, R. R., Finer, N. N., and Cox S. F.: Necrotizing enterocolitis and human milk. J. Pediatr. 94:295–296, 1979.

Mornet, E., Serre, J. L., and Farrell, M.: Genetic differences between cystic fibrosis with and without meconium ileus. Lancet 1:376–378, 1988.

Muty, A. E., and Obladen, M. W.: Hyperosmolar oral medications and necrotizing enterocolitis. Pediatrics 75:371, 1985.

Nagaraj, H. S., Sandhu, A. M., Cook, L. N., et al.: Gastrointestinal perforation following indomethacin therapy in very low birth weight infants. J. Pediatr. Surg. 16:1003–1007, 1981.

Nguyen, L. T., Youssef, S., Guttman, I. M., et al.: Meconium ileus: Is a stoma necessary? J. Pediatr. Surg. 21:766, 1986.

Noblett, H. R.: Treatment of uncomplicated meconium ileus by Gastrografin enema: a preliminary report. J. Pediatr. Surg. 4:190–195, 1969.

Oppenheimer, E. N., and Avery, M. E.: Clinical-pathologic conference. J. Pediatr. 73:143, 1968.

Ostertag, S. G., La Gamma, E. F., Reisin, C. E., et al.: Early enteral feeding does not affect the incidence of necrotizing enterocolitis. Pediatrics 77:275–280, 1986.

Palder, S. B., Schwartz, M. Z., Tyson, K. R., et al.: Association of closure of patent ductus arteriosus and development of necrotizing enterocolitis. J. Pediatr. Surg. 23:422–423, 1988.

Park, R. W., and Grand, R. J.: Gastrointestinal manifestations of cystic fibrosis: A review. Gastroenterology 81:1143–1161, 1981.

Parsons, J. M., Miscall, B. G., and McSherry, C. K.: Appendicitis in the newborn infant. Surgery 67:841–843, 1970.

Pena, A.: Surgical treatment of high imperforate anus. World J. Surg. 9:236–245, 1985.

Ralston, C. W., Ament, M. E., Berquist, W., et al.: Somatic growth and developmental functioning in children receiving prolonged home total parenteral nutrition. J. Pediatr. 105:842–847, 1984.

Rommens, J. M., Zengerling, S., and Burns, J.: Identification and regional localization of DNA markers on chromosome 7 for cloning of the cystic fibrosis gene. Am. J. Hum. Genet. 43:645–663, 1989.

Rothschild, H. B., Storch, A., and Meyers, B.: Mesenteric occlusion in a newborn infant. J. Pediatr. 43:569–571, 1953.

Sagor, G. R., and Bloom, S. R.: Evidence for a humoral mechanism after small intestinal resection. Gastroenterology 84:902–906, 1983.

Schwachmann, H., and Antonowicz, I.: Studies on meconium. In Lebenthal E. (Ed.): Textbook of Gastroenterology and Nutrition in Infancy. New York, Raven Press, 1981.

Schwartz, M. Z., Hayden, C. K., Richardson, C. J., et al.: A prospective evaluation of intestinal stenosis following necrotizing enterocolitis. J. Pediatr. Surg. 17:764–770, 1982.

Seges, R. A., Kenny, A., Bird, G. W., et al.: Pediatric surgical patients with severe anaerobic infection: report of 16 T-antigen positive cases and possible hazard of blood transfusion. J. Pediatr. Surg. 16:905–910, 1981.

Shaul, W. L.: Clues to the early diagnosis of neonatal appendicitis. J. Pediatr. 98:473–476, 1981.

Stevenson, D. K., Kerner, J. A., and Malachowki, N.: Late morbidity among survivors of necrotizing enterocolitis: A case control study. J. Pediatr. 96:447–451, 1980.

Sturum, H. S., and Ternberg, J. L.: Congenital atresia of the colon. Surgery 59:458–465, 1966.

Talwalker, V. C.: Intussusception in the newborn. Arch. Dis. Child. 37:203–208, 1962.

Thompson, J. S., and Rikkers, L. F.: Surgical alternatives for the short bowel syndrome. Am. J. Gastroenterol. 82:97–106, 1987.

Townes, P. L., Bryson, M., and Miller, C.: Further observations on trypsinogen deficiency disease: Report of a second case. J. Pediatr. 71:220–224, 1967.

Tucker, A. S., Soine, L., and Izant, R. E.: Gastrointestinal perforations in infancy. Am. J. Roentgenol. 123:755–790, 1975.

Vane, D. W., and Grosfeld, J. L.: Hirschsprung's disease. Experience with the Duhamel operation in 195 cases. Ped. Surg. Int. 1:95–99, 1986.

Vanhaesebrouck, P., Thiery, M., Leroy, J. G., et al.: Oligohydramnios, renal insufficiency and ileal perforation in preterm infants after interuterine exposure to indomethacin. J. Pediatr. 113:738–743, 1988.

Vintzileos, A. M., Eisenfeld, L. I., Herson, V. C., et al.: Megacystismicrocolon-intestinal hypoperistalsis syndrome. Am. J. Perinatol. 3:297–302, 1986.

Walsh, M. C., Kliegman, R. M., and Fanaroff, A. A.: Necrotizing enterocolitis: A practitioner's perspective. Pediatr. Rev. 9:219–223, 1988.

Waters, D. L., Dorney, S. F., Gaskin, K. J., et al.: Pancreatic function in infants identified as having cystic fibrosis in a neonatal screening program. N. Engl. J. Med. 322:303, 1990.

Weber, T. R., Lewis, J. E., Mooney, D., et al.: Duodenal atresia: A comparison of techniques of repair. J. Pediatr. Surg. 21:1133–1136, 1986.

Wilmore, D. W.: Factors correlating with successful outcome following extensive intestinal resection in newborn infants. J. Pediatr. 80:88–93, 1972.

Wilson, R., del Portillo, M., Schmidt, E., et al.: Risk factors for necrotizing enterocolitis in infants weighing more than 2,000 grams at birth: A case-control study. Pediatrics 71:19–22, 1983.

Woods, W. G., Roloff, J. S., Lukens, J. N., et al.: The occurrence of leukemia in patients with the Shwachman syndrome. J. Pediatr. 99:425–428, 1981.

Yales, C. E., Balish, E., and Wu, J. P.: The bacterial etiology of pneumatosis cystoides intestinalis. Arch. Surg. 198:89–94, 1974.

Young, D. G., and Wilkinson, A. W.: Abnormalities associated with neonatal duodenal obstruction. Surgery 63:832–840, 1968.

Zachary, R. B.: Meconium and faecal plugs in the newborn. Arch. Dis. Child. 32:22–27, 1957.

DISORDERS OF THE UMBILICAL CORD, ABDOMINAL WALL, URACHUS, AND OMPHALOMESENTERIC DUCT

William J. Byrne

The umbilical region is a very busy locale during embryonic life. Originally the widely open communication between the yolk sac and primitive gut, it becomes a narrow aperture through which course the umbilical arteries and vein, omphalomesenteric (vitelline) duct, and urachus. In the interim, the entire midgut passes through it into a large physiologic umbilical hernia, remains there several weeks, and returns to take its position in the abdominal cavity. Alterations in this orderly process sometimes lead to serious congenital anomalies.

■ UMBILICAL CORD LESIONS

Single Umbilical Artery. Normally, the umbilical cord consists of two arteries and a vein. After birth the umbilical arteries contract, blood flow ceases, their internal and medial layers undergo aseptic necrosis, and the stump separates. Granulation tissue develops that is covered by epithelium. Single umbilical artery occurs in 1 per cent of single births and 7 per cent of twin births. Associated anomalies occur in about one-third of these, with gastrointestinal obstructive lesions and urogenital lesions being the most common. Careful physical examination and a high index of suspicion detect these early.

Granuloma of the Umbilicus. Delay in separation of the umbilical stump 5 to 8 days after birth or infection may result in the production of granulation tissue that must be differentiated from everted gastric or intestinal mucosa. A granuloma is solid whereas everted mucosa permits the entrance of a fine probe. Treatment for both is desiccation with silver nitrate.

Delay in Separation of the Cord. If the umbilical cord fails to separate after more than 14 days, then investigation for a possible defect in neutrophil function and chemotaxis should be undertaken.

Umbilical Infection. Serous, purulent, or sanguineous drainage from the umbilicus for a number of days after the cord has separated is an early clinical presentation of omphalitis. Infection may remain restricted to the cord or may spread to involve the surrounding skin. Parenteral antibiotics including antistaphylococcal coverage are indicated if the discharge is frankly purulent or there is evidence of spread.

Septic Umbilical Arteritis. In this relatively uncommon disorder, bacteria may invade or spread along the lumen, the inner necrosing coats, or the mantle of loose connective tissue of the umbilical artery. If both the iliac and abdominal ends of the artery are sealed, the infection forms an abscess, whereas if the artery remains patent externally, the umbilicus drains purulent material. If the mantle zone is involved, spread may lead to peritonitis. Infection may also track along the course of the artery to point as an abscess in the scrotum or thigh. If the iliac end of the umbilical artery is patent, the patient becomes septic.

■ ABDOMINAL WALL DEFECTS

OMPHALOCELE

Definition and Epidemiology. Omphalocele refers to a congenital defect in the formation of the umbilical and supraumbilical portions of the abdominal wall that is larger than 4 cm in diameter (Table 72–1 and Figs. 72–1 and 72–2). The defect occurs in from one in 6000 to one in 10,000 live births. Most have no fixation of the midgut, and rotation is incomplete.

Etiology. The midgut normally returns from the umbilical cord into the abdomen by the 10th week of gestation. The developing somatic layers of the cephalic, caudal, and lateral folds join to close the defect in the abdominal wall. For unknown reasons, this closure may

TABLE 72–1. Characteristics of Gastroschisis and Omphalocele

DEFECT	GASTROSCHISIS	OMPHALOCELE
Covering sac	Absent	Present, but may be torn
Fascial defect	Small	Small or large
Cord attachment	Onto the abdominal wall	Onto the sac
Herniated bowel	Edematous	Normal
Prematurity (%)	50–60	10–20
Associated anomalies (%)	10–15	45–55
Gastrointestinal	18	37
Cardiac	2	20
Trisomy syndromes	–	30
Necrotizing enterocolitis (%)	18	Only if sac is ruptured
Malabsorption	Common	Only if sac is ruptured

not take place. Two types of omphalocele are now recognized (Margulies, 1945). In the first type, the failure of closure begins early, about the 3rd week of gestation, and the defect is large. Three subtypes make up this first type. An epigastric omphalocele occurs with abnormal development of the cephalic fold that is associated with a lower thoracic wall malformation, cleft sternum, diaphragmatic defect, pericardial defect, and cardiac anomaly (Cantrell pentalogy). The classic omphalocele occurs from an interruption in lateral fold development. The defect lies between the epigastric and hypogastric regions. The umbilicus arises from an anterior position on the omphalocele, and the muscular abdominal wall is normal. Caudal fold abnormalities result in a hypogastric omphalocele. Associated defects include bladder exstrophy and imperforate anus (Fig. 72–3). The second type of omphalocele is more often referred to as an umbilical hernia. By definition, this is no bigger than 4 cm in diameter and contains only loops of small bowel in the sac (Fig. 72–4). It arises between the 8th and 10th weeks owing to a failure of closure of the umbilical ring (see next section).

Diagnosis. The diagnosis may be made prenatally with ultrasound. Ultrasound can distinguish omphalocele from gastroschisis. Since the association of cardiac anomalies and chromosomal disorders is high, fetal echocardiogra-phy and amniocentesis should also be performed. Vaginal delivery does not adversely affect outcome, and therefore, the need for cesarean section should be based on obstetric indications alone (Bond et al., 1988; Langer et al., 1988).

If not discovered prenatally, the diagnosis is obvious at birth. If the sac ruptures, the bowel loops may be edematous and matted together and can mimic gastroschisis.

Treatment. When the omphalocele is first seen, the sac should be kept moist by wrapping it with gauze sponges soaked in normal saline. A plastic covering is then wrapped around the defect to limit water and heat loss. These should not apply any pressure. A nasogastric tube is passed to decrease the accumulation of air in the bowel. The infant is started on 1.5 times maintenance intravenous fluids and broad-spectrum antibiotics.

Operative repair should be done as soon as possible. Small defects can be closed with a single-stage repair. For larger defects, attempts at primary repair may lead to respiratory failure and compression of the vena cava. In these infants staged repair using a prosthetic material to cover the defect, with gradual reduction into the abdominal cavity over 7 to 10 days, is usually successful (Schuster, 1979). Postoperatively, protracted ileus usually necessitates prolonged parenteral nutrition. Attention must also be directed to the diagnosis and management of associated anomalies.

Prognosis. Mortality with associated heart disease is 80 per cent. Without heart disease, 70 per cent survive.

UMBILICAL HERNIA

Umbilical hernia differs from omphalocele in that skin and subcutaneous tissue cover the original defect while separation of the rectus muscle persists. These lesions are found in 30 per cent of black infants and 4 per cent of white infants under 6 weeks old. The condition is more common in infants under 1500 g, 75 per cent of whom have small hernias. The hernia aperture, located at the umbilicus, varies in size from less than 1 cm to up to 4 cm in diameter. The sac may contain a loop of bowel that

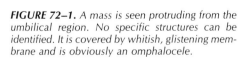

FIGURE 72–1. A mass is seen protruding from the umbilical region. No specific structures can be identified. It is covered by whitish, glistening membrane and is obviously an omphalocele.

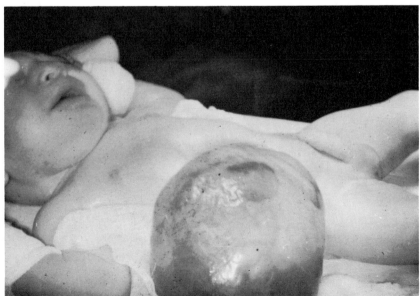

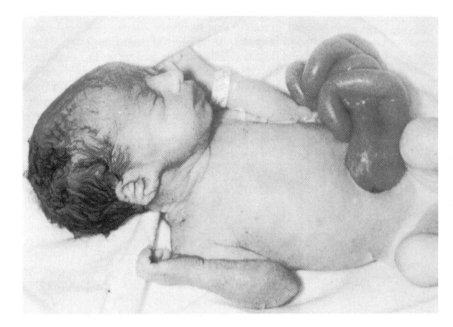

FIGURE 72–2. Omphalocele in which the containing amniotic-peritoneal membrane must have been torn away during delivery. Loops of bowel lie free upon the abdominal wall. (Courtesy of Dr. Arnold Tramer of Baltimore.)

may easily be pushed back into the abdomen. Small umbilical hernias, smaller than 2 cm in diameter, will close on their own (Fig. 72–5). Taping does not accelerate the healing process, and ordinarily, at least 2 years should be allowed for spontaneous closure before surgery is considered. Larger hernias, however, may require surgical intervention (Fig. 72–6) (Lassaletta et al., 1975).

GASTROSCHISIS

Definition and Epidemiology. Gastroschisis is the herniation of abdominal contents through an abdominal wall defect, usually occurring on the right side of a normally positioned umbilical cord (see Table 72–1). The lesion occurs with about one-third the frequency of omphalocele, and associated anomalies are less frequent and usually gastrointestinal in origin, including malrotation and atresias. Infants with gastroschisis tend to have intrauterine growth retardation.

Etiology. These lesions are not felt to represent a ruptured omphalocele but rather to be of vascular etiology. Intrauterine interruption of the omphalomesenteric artery

has been proposed, an explanation that nicely accounts for many of the clinically observed differences between this lesion and omphalocele (Hoyme et al., 1981).

Diagnosis and Treatment. As with an omphalocele, gastroschisis may be correctly diagnosed by prenatal ultrasound (Bond et al., 1988). The severity of the lesion in addition to bowel dilation and mural thickening can be assessed. The latter are associated with advanced intestinal dysmorphia and a poorer prognosis. The infants may benefit from early delivery. As with omphalocele, the need for cesarean section should be restricted to obstetric indications only (Langer et al., 1987).

If not diagnosed prenatally, the lesion is obvious at birth. Preoperatively, the bowel contents should be kept moist by wrapping them in gauze sponges soaked in normal saline. The defect should then be covered with a

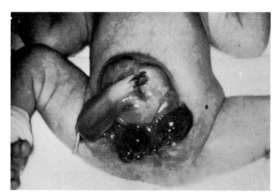

FIGURE 72–3. A combination of omphalocele and ectopia vesicae. The bright structure below the omphalocele is an everted, exstrophic bladder.

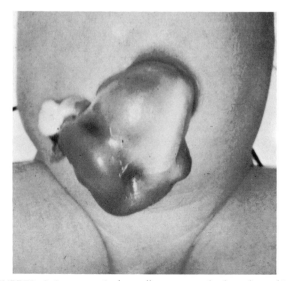

FIGURE 72–4. A comparatively small mass protrudes from the umbilical region and a loop of bowel can be readily recognized running around its lower margin. The mass is completely covered by shiny transparent membrane—clearly an umbilical cord hernia.

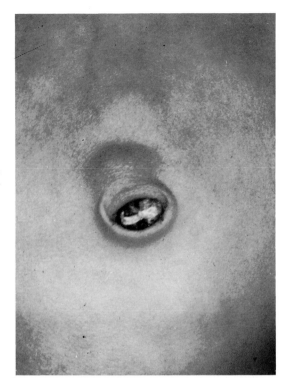

FIGURE 72–5. Two definite bulges are seen cephalad to the umbilicus, one above the other. Two distinct apertures could be felt in the midline. This represents a minor defect of the abdominal wall.

plastic insulating material to prevent heat and water loss. A nasogastric tube is passed for decompression, and 1.5 times maintenance intravenous fluids given. Broad-spectrum antibiotics should also be started. Primary closure is often possible, but larger defects may require staged repair. Postoperatively, prolonged ileus may require long-term parenteral nutrition. These infants are at increased risk for necrotizing enterocolitis. Prolonged obstruction and malabsorption are frequent complications in the postoperative period.

Prognosis. Reported mortality figures vary from 10 to 30 per cent.

PRUNE BELLY SYNDROME

Prune belly syndrome refers to a triad of anomalies consisting of a deficiency of abdominal musculature, cryptorchidism, and urinary tract abnormalities. The most frequent urinary tract anomalies occurring individually or in combination are megaloureter, cystic renal dysplasia, urethral obstruction, and megacystis (Lattimer, 1958). Associated gastrointestinal (malrotation) and cardiac anomalies occur in 30 and 20 per cent, respectively. Only rarely is the syndrome found in females. The exact etiology is unknown. One theory proposes a failure in the development of the abdominal wall between the 6th and 8th weeks of gestation. A second theory holds that there is a primary urethral obstruction with early bladder distention giving rise to abdominal distention and other secondary anomalies (Moerman et al., 1984). At birth the defect is obvious. The abdomen is shapeless and the skin hangs in wrinkled folds. There may be an open patent urachus, which by itself signals a poor prognosis. Of immediate concern is the evaluation and relief of urinary tract obstruction. Overall, mortality is 50 per cent (Rogers and Ostrow, 1973).

INGUINAL HERNIA

The incidence of demonstrable inguinal hernia is higher in low-birth-weight and very-low-birth-weight infants than in normal term newborns. Comparable figures are as follows: 500 to 1000 g, 42 per cent; 1000 to 1500 g, 10 per cent; and 1500 to 2000 g, 3 per cent (Peevy et al., 1986). Sex and race do not appear to be significant factors. Among infants under 32 weeks' gestational age, intrauterine growth retardation increases the risk. By 32 weeks in the male, the testes have entered the scrotum and contracture of the inguinal canal around the spermatic cord has begun. In the female a similar contracture of the inguinal canal also occurs by 32 weeks. With preterm delivery and the accompanying increase in intra-abdominal pressure, testicular descent and inguinal canal closure do not take place, thus explaining the increased incidence of inguinal hernia. Because there is a high frequency of incarceration in these hernias, it is imperative that bilateral elective surgical repair is accomplished, preferably prior to discharge.

DIAPHRAGMATIC HERNIA

Definition and Epidemiology. Diaphragmatic hernias may be of two types: through a posterolateral defect (foramen of Bochdalek) or through a retrosternal defect (foramen of Morgagni). Ninety-eight per cent are of the posterolateral variety, and 90 per cent of these involve the left leaf of the diaphragm. The incidence of diaphragmatic hernia is one in 4000 live births.

Etiology. These lesions arise due to a failure of fusion of the diaphragmatic leaflets during the 8th to 10th weeks of gestation (Bloss et al., 1981).

Diagnosis and Treatment. Bochdalek hernias are usually large. Ultrasound can identify many of the hernias in

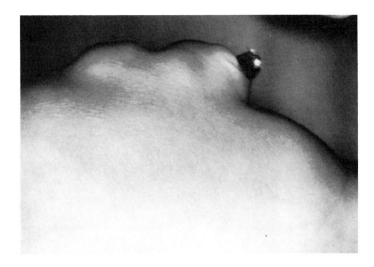

FIGURE 72–6. Large triangular herniation of and above the umbilicus. The bulge contained easily reducible bowel. A large aperture could be felt just above the umbilicus and a second, smaller one several centimeters above it. Between them the rectus muscles were diastatic. This is a large defect of the abdominal wall demanding surgical closure.

the fetus, and thus, delivery can be planned at a center equipped to treat the infant (Adsick et al., 1989). At birth the infant may appear normal, but as gas fills the bowel, severe respiratory distress occurs. Breath sounds are absent on the affected side. Right-sided posterolateral and retrosternal hernias are usually much smaller, so the onset of respiratory distress may be delayed. Chest films show gas-filled bowel loops in the chest (Fig. 72–7).

Once the diagnosis is made, the infant should be intubated and ventilated and a nasogastric tube passed to decompress the stomach. If the patient can be stabilized, then surgical repair should proceed. However, Langer and co-workers (1988) have suggested that delaying surgery to allow stabilization may lead to improved outcome. Some physicians feel that critically ill infants, whose respiratory and metabolic statuses are difficult to stabilize, may benefit from the pre- or postoperative use of extracorporeal membrane oxygenation (ECMO).

Prognosis. Mortality is still high (30 to 50 per cent) even with improved techniques of respiratory support. This in large part is thought to be due to pulmonary hypoplasia, which results from compression of the developing lung buds (Harrison et al., 1978). In addition, pathologic studies have shown thickening of the pulmonary artery musculature, which contributes to the development of pulmonary hypertension and further complicates ventilation.

URACHAL LESIONS

The urachus is that remnant of the allantois that extends from the bladder portion of the cloaca to the umbilicus. The urachus may remain completely patent throughout its length or fail to obliterate (Ney and Friedenberg, 1968) (Fig. 72–8). All varieties of this defect are rare.

Completely Patent Urachus. This lesion presents with the passage of urine from the umbilicus. Injection of radiopaque contrast into the orifice outlines the urachal tract and fills the bladder. Treatment consists of surgical excision of the umbilicus along with the entire urachus and a small portion of the bladder. Results are usually good.

Blind External Type. When only the distal end of the urachus fails to obliterate, a draining sinus results. Drainage of urine begins sometime after the cord separates. Treatment consists of surgical excision of the sinus tract.

Blind Internal Type. Failure of obliteration of the proximal end of the urachus results in a bladder diverticulum. It produces no symptoms and may be coincidentally discovered on cystogram. Nothing needs to be done surgically.

Urachal Cyst. Incomplete obliteration of the midportion of the urachus leads to the development of a urachal cyst. Cysts may present at birth, or may grow slowly and

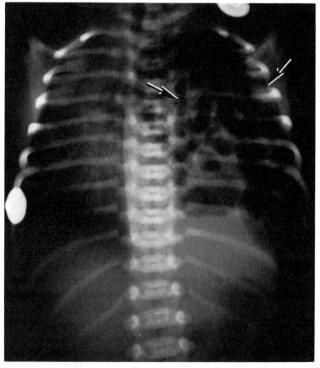

FIGURE 72–7. Plain film of the abdomen and chest of a 2-hour-old infant who developed severe respiratory distress. Loops of bowel are present in the chest with a shifting of the mediastinum to the right (arrows). (Courtesy of Dr. Ronald M. Cohen, Children's Hospital, Oakland, Calif.)

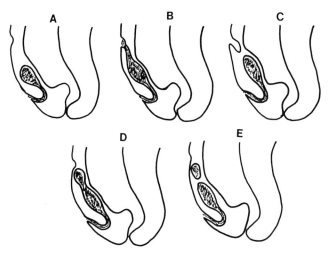

FIGURE 72–8. Urachal anomalies: A, Normal anatomy, B, completely patent urachus, C, blind external tract–urachal sinus, D, blind internal tract–bladder diverticulum, and E, urachal cyst.

become obvious at anytime during infancy or childhood. The cysts frequently become infected. Plain films may show the lesion just beneath the abdominal wall. Surgical excision should be performed.

■ MALFORMATIONS OF THE OMPHALOMESENTERIC DUCT

In the developing embryo the omphalomesenteric (vitelline) duct connects the yolk sac to the primitive midgut through the umbilical cord. In the normal course of ontogeny, the duct becomes obliterated and disappears. Under certain circumstances, all or portions of the duct may persist (Fig. 72–9).

Patent Omphalomesenteric Duct. Over 200 cases of patent omphalomesenteric duct (enteroumbilical fistula) have been reported. It presents with the passage of meconium and fecal matter through the umbilicus. This may begin at birth or occur within 1 to 2 weeks. The most significant danger with this lesion is evagination of the small bowel through the umbilical orifice. Mortality increases five-fold when this occurs. Once this lesion is diagnosed, it should be corrected by surgical excision of the umbilicus and the duct.

Omphalomesenteric Sinus. Failure of distal closure of the duct leads to the formation of a sinus. Persistent watery discharge from the umbilical cord is the initial presentation. Examination of the umbilicus reveals a red nodule projecting from the base. Gentle massage results in the extrusion of mucus, which differentiates this from an umbilical granuloma. Injection of radiopaque contrast outlines the sinus tract. Treatment consists of surgical excision.

Omphalomesenteric Duct Cyst. When the middle portion of the omphalomesenteric duct persists and eventually fills with secretions, a cyst forms. This may be detected as an enlarging umbilical mass. Treatment consists of surgical excision.

MECKEL DIVERTICULUM

When the proximal, or intestinal, end of the omphalomesenteric duct fails to become obliterated completely, an outpouching of the ileum persists. The diverticulum may be as short as 2 cm or as long as 90 cm. It is usually tent-shaped, but it may be tubular. It may arise from any point of the small intestine as close as 3 cm proximal to the cecum or as far as 100 cm distant from it. The junction usually lies at some point in the ileum, rarely in the jejunum, and exceptionally in the duodenum. It must arise from the antimesenteric side of the bowel, a fact that distinguishes Meckel diverticulum from duplications. Its distal end usually lies free in the peritoneal cavity, but some are attached to the umbilicus by a fibrous cord, and a small minority remain patent to the umbilicus (omphalomesenteric fistula) (Fig. 72–10). Its structure simulates that of small bowel, with well-defined mucosa, submucosa, muscularis, and serosa. Unfortunately, in about one-fifth of the cases, it is the site of ectopic pancreatic or gastric tissue. Aberrant pancreatic tissue is usually present as a small mass in the wall, while gastric mucosa replaces or overlies the usual intestinal mucosa at some point or points. A pancreatic mass may act as a leader to produce intussusception. Gastric mucosa may cause peptic ulceration and bleeding; the latter is the sign almost always the presenting one if Meckel diverticulum becomes symptomatic. The fibrous cord, if present, may produce intestinal obstruction. Rarely, inflammation of the diverticulum may lead to peritonitis.

Incidence. A Meckel diverticulum can be discovered in 1.5 to 2 per cent of all persons. Only a small proportion of these ever become symptomatic, and when they do, this usually happens beyond the age of 4 months. The youngest infant to become symptomatic in our experience presented with intestinal obstruction from a volvulus around the diverticulum at 10 days of age (Meguid et al., 1974). Only exceptionally do they cause illness in the neonatal period. Males outnumber females by 3 to 5:1.

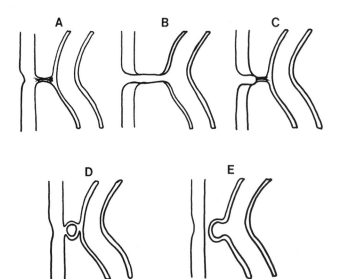

FIGURE 72–9. Omphalomesenteric (vitelline) duct anomalies: A, Normal anatomy, B, patent omphalomesenteric duct, C, blind external tract–umbilical sinus, D, omphalomesenteric duct cyst, and E, blind internal tract–Meckel diverticulum.

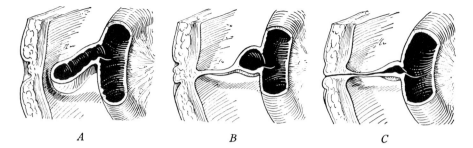

FIGURE 72–10. Meckel diverticulum of the ileum: A, Ordinary blind sac. B, Diverticulum continued to umbilicus as a cord. C, Diverticulum with fistulous opening of umbilicus. (From Arey, L.B.: Developmental Anatomy. Revised 7th ed. 1974.)

Diagnosis. Hemorrhage from the bowel is the definitive sign of Meckel diverticulum. A few cases in older children and adults may produce the signs and symptoms of diverticulitis, but this condition has never been described in young infants. Hemorrhage is often sudden and catastrophic, causing a precipitous fall in the hematocrit level and a shocklike state within a few hours. The first few stools passed may be composed almost entirely of unchanged blood; later, they become burgundy-colored, then tarry. In other instances, bleeding is constant and occult. About 25 per cent of individuals with Meckel diverticulum present with intussusception.

Meckel diverticulum must be differentiated from the other disorders that produce gross bleeding from the bowel. These are peptic ulcer, duplication, and intestinal polyp for the most part. Intussusception, intestinal hemangioma, and a few other even rarer entities may be responsible for an occasional case. Blood dyscrasias usually cause bleeding into the skin and from other sites simultaneously. Fissure in ano, proctitis, and ulcerative colitis ordinarily do not lead to gross hemorrhage, blood loss being confined to the passage of bloody mucus or of stools containing a surface accumulation of blood. Polyps, too, are seldom responsible for massive hemorrhage, so that bleeding peptic ulcer and duplication are the only conditions left that are difficult to distinguish from bleeding Meckel diverticulum. The most useful differential point is that hematemesis usually coexists with rectal bleeding in the case of peptic ulcer, whereas hematemesis is extremely rare in Meckel diverticulum. The mass of duplication is sometimes palpable.

We no longer advocate barium studies, since they rarely demonstrate the lesion and may interfere with a technetium scan.

Scans after intravenous injection of ^{99m}technetium pertechnetate are often, but not always, diagnostic of Meckel diverticulum, since the technetium is concentrated in gastric mucosa. Pentagastrin or cimetidine is useful in enhancing the image of gastric mucosa on subsequent technetium scans (Fig. 72–11).

Treatment. Blood replacement therapy is the prime indication in massive hemorrhage regardless of its cause. If bleeding ceases and the diagnosis has not been ascertained, it is permissible to keep the infant under observation and do nothing more. In the newborn a peptic ulcer, once healed, is not likely to cause further trouble. A second episode of bleeding at some future date strongly suggests some other diagnostic possibility, and Meckel diverticulum takes first place in this list. Laparotomy is therefore indicated after a recurrent bout of hemorrhage. If a diverticulum is discovered, it must be excised. After its resection, no additional trouble is to be anticipated.

■ ACKNOWLEDGMENTS

We are grateful for the editorial review and contributions of Dr. Scott Adsick.

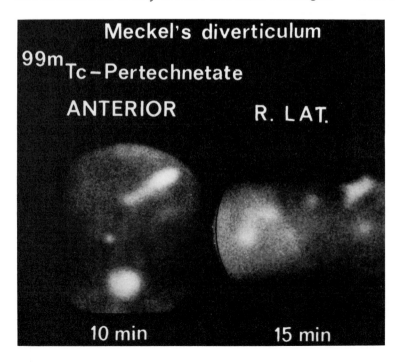

FIGURE 72–11. Anterior gamma camera view of the abdomen of a 2-year-old infant. Note the small well-defined area of increased uptake located in the right lower quadrant. The stomach and bladder are also visualized. On the lateral view, some radioactivity is evident on the diaper as well. (Courtesy of Dr. S. Treves, Children's Hospital, Boston, Mass.)

■ REFERENCES

Abrahamson, J.: Repair of inguinal hernias in infants and children. Clin. Pediatr. *12*:617–623, 1973.

Adsick, N.S., Vacanti, J. P., Lillehei, C. W., et al.: Fetal diaphragmatic hernia: Ultrasound diagnosis and clinical outcome in 38 cases. J. Pediatr. Surg. 24: 654–657, 1989.

Bloss, R. S., Aranda, J. V., and Beardmore, H. E.: Congenital diaphragmatic hernia: Pathophysiology and pharmacologic support. Surgery *89*:518–524, 1981.

Bond, S., Harrison, M. R., and Golbus, M. S.: Severity of intestinal damage in gastroschisis: Correlation with prenatal sonographic findings. J. Pediatr. Surg. *23*:520–535, 1988.

Greenwood, R. D.: Cardiovascular malformation associated with omphalocele. J. Pediatr. *85*:818–824, 1974.

Harrison, M. R., Bjordal, R. I., Langmark, F., et al.: Congenital diaphragmatic hernia: The hidden mortality. J. Pediatr. Surg. *13*:227–230, 1978.

Hoyme, H. E., Higginbottom, M. C., and Jones, K. L.: The vascular pathogenesis of gastroschisis: Intrauterine interruption of the omphalomesenteric artery. J. Pediatr. *98*:228–231, 1981.

Langer, J. C., Filler, R. M., Bohn, D. J., et al.: Timing of surgery for congenital diaphragmatic hernia: Is emergency operation necessary? J. Pediatr. Surg. *23*:731–734, 1988.

Langer, J. C., Harrison, M. R., Adzich, N. S., et al.: Perinatal managament of the fetus with an abdominal wall defect. Fetal Ther. *2*:216–221, 1987.

Lassaletta, L., Fonkalsrud, E. W., Tovar, J.A., et al.: Management of umbilical hernias in infancy and childhood. J. Pediatr. *10*:405–410, 1975.

Lattimer, J. K.: Congenital deficiency of the abdominal musculature and associated genitourinary anomalies: A report of 22 cases. J. Urol. *79*:343–348, 1958.

Margulies, L.: Omphalocele. Am. J. Obstet. Gynecol. *49*:695–710, 1945.

Meguid, M., Canty, T., and Eraklis, A. J.: Complications of Meckel's diverticulum in infants. Surg. Gynecol. Obstet. *139*:541–546, 1974.

Moerman, P., Fryns, J., Goddeeris, P., et al.: Pathogenesis of the prune-belly syndrome: A functional urethral obstruction caused by prostatic hypoplasia. Pediatrics *73*:470–475, 1984.

Ney, C., and Friedenberg, R. M.: Radiographic findings in anomalies of the urachus. J. Urol. *99*:288–294, 1968.

Peevy, K. J., Speed, F. A., and Hoff, C. J.: Epidemiology of inguinal hernia in preterm neonates. Pediatrics 77:246–247, 1986.

Rogers, L. W., and Ostrow, P. T.: The prune belly syndrome. J. Pediatr. *83*:786–793, 1973.

Schuster, S.: Omphalocele, hernia of the umbilical cord and gastroschisis. *In* Ravitch, M. M. (Ed.): Pediatric Surgery. Chicago, Year Book Medical Publishers, 1979, pp. 778–900.

ASCITES AND PERITONITIS

William J. Byrne

■ ASCITES

Accumulation of fluid in the abdomen of the fetus may be so massive as to necessitate cesarean section and may produce respiratory distress after birth (Fig. 73–1). Immediate aspiration just below the umbilicus may be both diagnostic (Table 73–1) and therapeutic. Radiographic studies are useful in less acutely ill infants (Griscom et al., 1977). Ascites may be chylous, urinary, biliary, or pancreatic. It may be secondary to neonatal hydrops or congestive heart failure or caused by the rupture of a large ovarian cyst in the fetus during delivery.

Chylous Ascites. In the newborn chylous ascites is usually due to a congenital failure of the lymphatic channels to communicate (Cochran et al., 1985). Since it may also be seen with malrotation and incomplete volvulus, infants should be evaluated for malrotation. The lesion is slightly more common in males. In most cases, pathologic findings are limited to the abdomen. In the newborn, the initial paracentesis may yield clear fluid. Following the feeding of formula containing long-chain fats, abdominal distention becomes more marked and repeat paracentesis yields a milky fluid high in triglyceride content. An abdominal film and, if necessary, an upper gastrointestinal series should be done to exclude malrotation. Treatment consists of repeated paracentesis to relieve distention. The use of

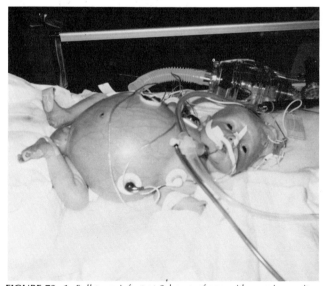

FIGURE 73–1. Full-term infant at 2 hours of age with massive ascites, which subsequently proved to be chylous. The distention was controlled with repeated paracentesis and an elemental diet. By 6 months of age paracentesis was no longer necessary. At 13 months of age the infant remains on an elemental diet growing and developing normally.

TABLE 73–1. Laboratory Studies Useful in the Evaluation of Ascites

ROUTINE	SPECIAL
Red cell count	Triglycerides
White cell count with differential	Amylase
Specific gravity	Bilirubin
Total protein	
Culture	

a formula whose fat source is primarily medium-chain triglycerides decreases the formation of chyle. If despite the specialized formula, chyle formation persists, intravenous alimentation may be necessary. Most patients undergo spontaneous remission, and the outlook for total recovery is good.

Urinary Ascites. This finding is due to an obstructive uropathy. The male-to-female ratio is 5:1. Posterior urethral valves are the most common cause (Mann et al., 1974). Other responsible lesions include ureteroceles, urethral atresia, bladder neck obstruction, neurogenic bladder, and bladder hematoma. Perforation of the bladder has also been found. The infants present with abdominal distention. Paracentesis yields urine. Evaluation should include an abdominal ultrasound, intravenous pyelogram, and voiding cystourethrogram to delineate the cause. Surgical decompression of the urinary tract or definitive correction of the lesions should be performed with urgency.

Biliary Ascites. Biliary ascites is caused by spontaneous perforation of the biliary tree. In 68 per cent, the perforation is in the main biliary tree. The remainder are located at the junction of the cystic and common ducts or in an accessory bile duct. Two clinical forms are apparent. In the acute form, the infant presents with signs of an acute abdomen: distention, vomiting, absent bowel sounds, and unstable vital signs. Clinical jaundice may not be present. In the more chronic form, which occurs in about 80 per cent of reported cases, clinical jaundice appears early, followed by gradual abdominal distention. Paracentesis reveals fluid with a bilirubin content above 4 g/dl. Technetium liver scan is confirmatory (So et al., 1983). Laparotomy with a biliary drainage procedure is essential for survival. Survival following surgery is 80 per cent.

Pancreatic Ascites. This extremely rare lesion may be the presenting manifestation of pancreatitis secondary to a pancreatic duct anomaly. Except for abdominal distention, the infants are asymptomatic. Urine and serum amylase levels may be normal. The diagnosis depends on finding a markedly elevated amylase and lipase in the paracentesis fluid. Most infants require a surgical drainage procedure.

Ruptured Ovarian Cyst. Ahmed (1971) reported this complication in a review of newborns with ovarian cysts. The presenting symptoms at birth included ascites or hemoperitoneum.

■ PERITONITIS

Peritonitis in the newborn can be classified as either bacterial or chemical (Fonkalsrud et al., 1966). Bacterial peritonitis occurs as the result of perforation of a hollow viscus, contiguous spread of an inflammatory process (acute appendicitis or gangrenous bowel), or septicemia.

Chemical peritonitis may be due to meconium or bile. Bile peritonitis results in the development of ascites, as previously discussed. Meconium peritonitis may result from intrauterine perforation or perforation shortly after birth. Ninety per cent of these are secondary to bowel obstruction with almost half due to meconium ileus (Santulli, 1980). At autopsy or surgery, the tear may be obvious or may have healed over. In addition to meconium ileus and bowel atresia, which are the most common causes, meconium peritonitis has been reported with intussusception, volvulus, incarcerated internal hernia, imperforate anus, and meconium plugs. To explain bowel rupture without obstructions, various hypotheses have been proposed. The bowel wall may have been congenitally weak from a localized defect or may have been weakened as the result of a vascular accident. Perforation can take place anytime after the 5th month, once the fetus has begun to swallow.

■ REFERENCES

Ahmed, S.: Neonatal and childhood ovarian cysts. J. Pediatr. Surg. 6:702–708, 1971.

Cochran, W. J., Klish, W. J., Brown, M. R., et al.: Chylous ascites in infants and children: A case report and literature review. J. Pediatr. Gastroenterol. Nutr. 4:668–673, 1985.

Fonkalsrud, E. W., Ellis, D. G., and Clatworthy, H. W.: Neonatal peritonitis. J. Pediatr. Surg. 1:227–233, 1966.

Griscom, N. T., Colodny, A. H., and Rosenberg, H. K.: Diagnostic aspects of neonatal ascites: Report of 27 cases. Am. J. Roentgenol. 128:961–967, 1977.

Kalwinsky, D., Frittelli, G., and Oski, F. A.: Pancreatitis presenting as unexplained ascites. Am. J. Dis. Child. 128:734–736, 1974.

Mann, C. M., Leape, L. L., and Holder, T. M.: Neonatal urinary ascites: A report of 2 cases of unusual etiology and a review of the literature. J. Urol. 111:124–130, 1974.

Prevot, J., Rickham, P. P., and Hecker, W. C.: Acute biliary peritonitis. Prog. Pediatr. Surg. 1:196–201, 1971.

Santulli, T. V.: Meconium ileus. In Holder, T. M., and Ashcraft, K. W. (Eds.): Pediatric Surgery. Philadelphia, W. B. Saunders Company, 1980, pp. 367–372.

So, S. K. S., Lindahl, J. A., Sharp, H. L., et al.: Bile ascites during infancy: Diagnosis using Tc-99m sequential scintiphotography. Pediatrics 71:402–405, 1983.

DISORDERS OF THE LIVER 74

William J. Byrne

Bilirubin metabolism in the newborn and causes of conjugated and unconjugated hyperbilirubinemia are discussed in Part XIII.

■ HEPATITIS

Infectious Causes. A number of infectious agents, both viral and bacterial, may cause neonatal hepatitis. Every effort should be made to make a specific diagnosis.

Women who have acute hepatitis B in the first or second trimester rarely transmit the infection to their infants. However, in mothers who are infected during the third trimester or at the time of delivery, the risk of transmission is 60 per cent. Mothers who are asymptomatic but carriers of hepatitis B surface antigen (HBsAg) put their infants at risk. This risk of transmission reaches 90 per cent if the mothers are also positive for the early antigen (HBeAg) (Stevens et al., 1979). Most infants are probably infected at the time of delivery. Fulminant infections are uncommon, and most infants remain clinically asymptomatic. Liver function tests become abnormal during the 6th to 8th weeks, and the abnormalities persist for a year. Chronic active hepatitis may develop in some. Fifty per cent of the infants who are infected with hepatitis B virus in the newborn period become chronic HBsAg carriers and therefore face the risk of developing primary liver cancer. These infants need careful follow-up for clearance of the antigenemia. Prevention of hepatitis B in the newborn depends on maternal screening for HBsAg. Infants born to positive mothers should receive both hepatitis B hyperimmune globulin (0.5 ml/kg IM) and hepatitis B vaccine (0.5 ml IM) within 12 hours of birth. Booster vaccinations should be given at 1 and 6 months of age. The infant should be tested at 1 year of age for antibody to HBsAg to document response to the vaccine.

Hepatitis A is transmitted only if the mother has clinical disease during the perinatal period. Little is known about the vertical transmission of hepatitis non-A–non-B viruses. Only recently has a serologic marker for one of this group, hepatitis C virus, become available. Vertical transmission of this has yet to be documented. Rubella, cytomegalovirus, herpes simplex, coxsackievirus, Epstein-Barr, and adenovirus may all present with cholestatic hepatitis. Serologic studies, liver biopsy, and viral isolation establish the diagnosis. The majority of patients recover without sequelae.

Hepatitis due to syphilis is now being seen more frequently. Newborns present with hepatosplenomegaly and jaundice during the 1st month of life. Serum transaminase levels may reach 500 IU. Liver biopsy shows a picture consistent with giant cell hepatitis. Even after

penicillin therapy, liver dysfunction may persist for up to 2 months (Long et al., 1984).

Bacterial hepatitis may produce cholestasis by two mechanisms. The first is associated with generalized sepsis with bacterial invasion of the liver and markedly elevated transaminase levels, hepatomegaly, and liver necrosis. Treatment and prognosis are the same as for neonatal sepsis. The second mechanism is a "toxic cholestasis." No direct invasion or destruction of the hepatocytes occurs. Therefore, transaminases are usually normal or only slightly elevated. This form is usually seen with severe urinary tract infections caused by *Escherichia coli* or *Proteus* or with pneumonia and generalized sepsis from pneumococcus. The mechanism is thought to be due to a toxin that inhibits hepatic excretory function. Successful treatment of the infection results in resolution of the cholestasis.

■ INHERITED AND METABOLIC LIVER DISORDERS

Alpha₁-antitrypsin Deficiency. This disorder is due to the accumulation of alpha₁-antitrypsin in the hepatocyte with subsequent hepatocellular necrosis (Morse, 1978; Talamo, 1975). Alpha₁-antitrypsin is an alpha₁-globulin and is a major serum protease inhibitor. It is inherited as an autosomal recessive trait. Although there are several phenotypes, only the homozygous Pi (protease inhibitor) ZZ and, rarely, the MZ types have been associated with liver disease in infancy. The ZZ phenotype occurs in one in 2000 live births, but only 10 per cent develop cholestasis in the neonatal period. The absence of the alpha₁-globulin fraction on a serum electrophoresis is highly suggestive of the disorder. Definitive diagnosis depends on finding a reduced serum alpha₁-antitrypsin level, Pi typing, and a liver biopsy that shows periodic acid–Schiff (PAS)–positive cytoplasmic granules with variable degrees of hepatic necrosis and fibrosis. There is no specific treatment. The course is quite variable, but some infants have progressive liver disease and require transplantation.

Cystic Fibrosis. Cholestasis in early infancy can be an initial presentation of cystic fibrosis (Park and Grand, 1981). Half of the infants presenting in this fashion also have meconium ileus. Liver disease eventually occurs in up to 50 per cent of cystic fibrosis patients. Five per cent develop cirrhosis, but only 2 per cent have clinical findings. Liver biopsy in the infants shows evidence of excessive biliary mucus with mild periportal inflammation and fibrosis. Bile duct plugging may also be present. Focal biliary cirrhosis, characterized by inspissated granular eosinophilic material in ductules and bile duct proliferation, develops later and may progress to multilobular biliary cirrhosis.

Galactosemia. Galactosemia is an autosomal recessive disorder of carbohydrate metabolism that results from deficient galactose-1-phosphate uridyltransferase activity. Accumulation of galactose-1-phosphate results in cholestasis, hepatomegaly, hypoglycemia, cataracts, vomiting, and failure to thrive. The diagnosis is made by demonstrating low levels of erythrocyte galactose-1-phosphate uridyltransferase activity. Treatment consists of removing all sources of galactose (lactose) from the diet.

Hereditary Fructose Intolerance. This congenital deficiency of fructose-1-phosphatase results in the accumulation of fructose and fructose-1-phosphate in body tissues. Introduction of fructose into the diet results in vomiting, hepatomegaly, and jaundice. The treatment is eliminating fructose and sucrose from the diet (Odievre et al., 1978).

Tyrosinemia. This is a rare autosomal recessive disorder characterized by decreased activity of p-hydroxyphenylpyruvic acid oxidase, methionine-activating enzyme, and cystathionine synthetase. Both acute and chronic forms have been described. The acute form presents with vomiting, failure to thrive, liver failure, and renal tubular dysfunction, usually within the first 3 to 6 weeks of life (Carson et al., 1976). Plasma and urine aminograms reveal elevated levels of tyrosine and its metabolites. Dietary restriction of tyrosine and phenylalanine may slow the progress of the liver disease, but without a liver transplant, most infants die during the 1st year of life.

Lipid Storage Diseases. Niemann-Pick disease, Gaucher disease, Wolman disease, and cholesterol ester storage disease are rare genetic disorders of lipid metabolism. They present with hepatosplenomegaly and varying degrees of liver dysfunction, including cholestasis.

Familial Recurrent Cholestasis. Familial recurrent cholestasis (Byler disease) is an autosomal recessive disorder characterized by episodic cholestasis. The initial presentation is within the first 6 months of life. The cholestatic episodes may last weeks to months. Cirrhosis eventually develops. Death from liver failure occurs between 2 and 15 years of age.

Recurrent Cholestasis with Lymphedema. Recurrent cholestasis with lymphedema (Aagenaes syndrome) is a rare genetic disorder characterized by cholestasis and lymphedema of the lower extremities. Cirrhosis develops in some patients.

Cerebrohepatorenal Syndrome. Cerebrohepatorenal (Zellweger) syndrome is one of a group of disorders of peroxisomal dysfunction. Inherited as an autosomal recessive trait, it presents in the neonatal period with cholestasis, hepatomegaly, profound hypotonia, and dysmorphic features (Moser et al., 1984). The diagnosis is made by demonstrating abnormal very-long-chain fatty acid levels in the serum.

■ TOTAL-PARENTERAL-NUTRITION–ASSOCIATED CHOLESTASIS

Definition and Epidemiology. Fifty per cent of infants with birth weights less than 1000 g develop cholestasis after 2 weeks of parenteral nutrition (Merritt, 1986). In newborns with birth weights between 1000 and 2000 g, the incidence is 15 per cent. The incidence increases with the duration of parenteral nutrition. After 13 weeks of total parenteral nutrition, up to 90 per cent of low-birth-weight infants develop cholestasis.

Etiology. No precise etiology has been found, but a number of factors appear to be important. These include immaturity of biliary excretion, lack of oral feedings, toxicity of certain amino acid components of the parenteral nutrition solution, and inadequate intake of certain nutrients such as taurine. Lipid infusion does not appear to play a role. The final common pathway may be the accumulation in the serum and bile of toxic bile acids, such as glycolithocholate.

Diagnosis. Serum bile salt concentrations rise before clinical jaundice becomes obvious. After 2 weeks or more on total parenteral nutrition, there is a gradual rise in the conjugated bilirubin with a modest rise in the serum transaminases and alkaline phosphatase (Fig. 74–1). Physical findings are limited to jaundice and hepatomegaly. In some infants the gallbladder becomes hydropic and is palpable. The diagnosis is made by excluding other causes of cholestasis. Histologic changes on liver biopsy are nonspecific and therefore not diagnostic.

Treatment. Treatment consists of the introduction of enteral alimentation and the discontinuation of intravenous nutrition. If total parenteral nutrition must be contin-

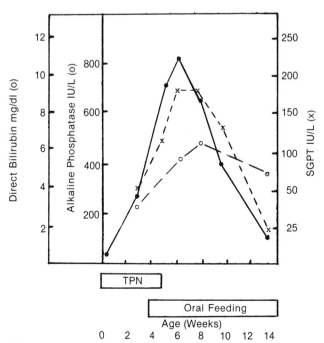

FIGURE 74–1. Typical pattern of liver function tests in a premature infant on total parenteral nutrition.

ued, sufficient protein (at least 8 per cent of the total calories) should be provided to prevent hepatic steatosis.

Prognosis. After discontinuation of the parenteral nutrition, liver function abnormalities usually resolve after 4 to 12 weeks. Gallbladder hydrops also resolves with the institution of feedings. Some infants develop gallstones that necessitate cholecystectomy. A small number of infants may develop progressive cirrhosis despite discontinuation of the parenteral nutrition (Table 74–1). Deaths have been reported from liver failure and from hepatic carcinoma. Liver transplantation may be required.

■ DRUG-INDUCED CHOLESTASIS

As part of the evaluation of cholestasis in the newborn, each drug the infant is receiving should be carefully considered as a potential cause or contributing factor. The following is a partial list: erythromycin estolate, ampicillin, oxacillin, diazepam, phenothiazines, and thiazide diuretics. Stricker and Spoelstra (1985) provide a more comprehensive review.

■ HYPERAMMONEMIA

Hyperammonemia in the first few days of life is due to either a urea cycle disorder or transient hyperammonemia of the newborn. Later in the neonatal period, fulminant hepatic failure may result in hyperammonemia.

Urea Cycle Disorders. Congenital urea cycle enzymopathies present during the first few days of life with vomiting, lethargy, seizures, and coma (Batshaw and Brusilow, 1980). Of the major enzyme deficiencies, ornithine transcarbamylase deficiency is the most common. Serum ammonia levels rise rapidly following the provision of enteral or parenteral protein and exceed 500 micromol/l. The diagnosis can be made on plasma and urine aminograms with confirmation provided by enzyme analysis of a liver biopsy specimen. Once a provisional diagnosis of a urea cycle enzymopathy has been made, therapeutic measures should be started at once. Protein intake is restricted. Intravenous arginine at a dose of 4 micromol/kg/day (8 ml/kg/day of 10 per cent arginine

TABLE 74–1. Hepatic Histologic Changes Observed in Pediatric Patients Receiving Total Parenteral Nutrition (TPN)

HISTOLOGIC LESION	DURATION OF TPN (DAYS)			
	0–10	10–30	30–60	>60
Steatosis	+ +	+	+	
Extramedullary erythropoiesis	+ +	+ +	+	
Periportal inflammation	+	+	+ +	+ + +
Cholestasis		+ +	+ + +	+ + +
Fibrosis		+	+	+ + +
Ductular proliferation		+	+	+ + +
Cirrhosis			+	+→+ + +

+, Mild or inconsistent finding; + +, consistent finding or generally more than mild when present; + + +, frequently seen and moderate to severe when present.

(From Merritt, R. J.: Cholestasis associated with total parenteral nutrition. J. Pediatr. Gastroenterol. Nutr. 5:10, 1986. Reprinted with permission.)

hydrochloride) should be started. Peritoneal dialysis should also begin. Sufficient nonprotein calories to prevent gluconeogenesis should be provided. Survival rate is 50 per cent, and the incidence of neurologic sequelae is high (see Chapter 18).

Transient Hyperammonemia of the Newborn. A syndrome of transient hyperammonemia of the newborn has been described by Ballard and co-workers (1978). It presents in the first few days of life with lethargy and coma. Urea cycle defects must be excluded. Aggressive treatment as outlined above, including peritoneal or hemodialysis to reduce the ammonia to nontoxic levels, is usually rewarded with permanent resolution of the hyperammonemia within 1 to 2 weeks. Feedings are tolerated, and there are no known long-term neurologic sequelae.

■ FULMINANT HEPATIC FAILURE

Fulminant hepatic failure results from massive hepatocellular injury (Russell et al., 1987). In addition to encephalopathy, coagulopathy due to impaired hepatic clotting factor synthesis (I, II, V, VII, IX, and X), hypoglycemia, and infection may complicate the course. Early perinatal causes include herpesvirus, adenovirus, and echovirus. In addition to the above, late perinatal causes are Epstein-Barr virus, tyrosinemia, fructose intolerance, and galactosemia. Treatment is supportive and includes placement of a central venous catheter and an arterial line. Blood sugar is maintained with hypertonic dextrose along with 2.5 g/kg/day of amino acids, which prevents tissue catabolism and maintains nitrogen balance. Special hepatic formulations of amino acids are of no proven benefit in acute hepatic failure. Vitamin K, 1 mg/day, may be given parenterally. The prothrombin time is monitored daily. If it falls below 20 per cent of control, then fresh frozen plasma should be administered to correct the prothrombin time and prevent bleeding. A nasogastric tube should be passed and placed to gravity drainage. Lactulose is administered via the tube, 5 ml every 6 hours, to induce a catharsis and perhaps reduce the colonic production of ammonia and other toxins. Antacids, 1 ml/kg, every 3 hours via the tube may reduce the risk of stress-related gastrointestinal bleeding. With vigorous support, recovery without permanent hepatic damage, depending on the etiology, is possible.

■ LIVER TRANSPLANTATION

Recent advances in techniques for liver transplantation have made successful treatment of liver failure possible in many infants (Esquivel et al., 1987; Starzl et al., 1989a and 1989b).

■ REFERENCES

Ballard, R. A., Vinocur, B., Reynolds, S. W., et al.: Transient hyperammonemia of the preterm infant. N. Engl. J. Med. *299:*920–925, 1978.

Batshaw, M. L., and Brusilow, S. W.: Treatment of hyperammonemic coma caused by inborn errors of urea synthesis. J. Pediatr. *97:*893–900, 1980.

Carson, N. A. J., Biggart, J. D., Bittles, A. H., et al.: Hereditary tyrosinaemia. Clinical, enzymatic and pathological study of an infant with the acute form of the disease. Arch. Dis. Child. *51:*106–110, 1976.

Esquivel, C. O., Shunzaburo, I., Gordon, R. D., et al.: Indications for pediatric liver transplantation. J. Pediatr. *111*:1039–1045, 1987.

Gordon, E. R., Shaffer, E. A., and Sass-Kortsak, J.: Bilirubin secretion and conjugation in the Crigler-Najjar syndrome type II. Gastroenterology *70*:761–764, 1976.

Long, W. A., Ulshen, M. H., and Lawson, E. E.: Clinical manifestations of congenital syphilitic hepatitis: Implications for pathogenesis. J. Pediatr. Gastroenterol. Nutr. *3*:351–355, 1984.

Maisels, M. J.: Jaundice in the newborn. Pediatr. Rev. *3*:305–319, 1982.

Merritt, R. J.: Cholestasis associated with total parenteral nutrition. J. Pediatr. Gastroenterol. Nutr. *5*:9–22, 1986.

Morse, J. O.: Alpha-1-antitrypsin deficiency. N. Engl. J. Med. *299*:1045–1048; 1099–1105, 1978.

Moser, A. E., Singh, I., Brown, F. R., et al.: The cerebrohepatorenal (Zellweger) syndrome. N. Engl. J. Med. *310*:1141–1146, 1984.

Odievre, M., Gentil, C., Gautier, M., et al.: Hereditary fructose intolerance in childhood: Diagnosis, management and course in 55 patients. Am. J. Dis. Child. *132*:605–610, 1978.

Park, R. W., and Grand, R. J.: Gastrointestinal manifestations of cystic fibrosis: A review. Gastroenterology *81*:1143–1161, 1981.

Russell, G. J., Fitzgerald, J. F., and Clark, J. H.: Fulminant hepatic failure. J. Pediatr. *111*:313–319, 1987.

Starzl, T. E., Demetris, A. J., and Thiel, D. V. Liver transplantation. Part I. N. Engl. J. Med. *321*:1014, 1989a.

Starzl, T. E., Demetris, A. J., and Thiel, D. V.: Liver transplantation. Part II. N. Engl. J. Med. *321*:1092, 1989b.

Stevens, C. E., Neurath, R. A., Beasley, R. P., et al.: HBeAg and anti-HBe detection by radioimmunoassay: Correlation with vertical transmission of hepatitis B virus in Taiwan. J. Med. Virol. *3*:237–241, 1979.

Stricker, B. H., and Spoelstra, P.: Drug-Induced Hepatic Injury. New York, Elsevier, 1985.

Talamo, R. C.: Basic and clinical aspects of alpha-1-antitrypsin deficiency. Pediatrics *56*:91–99, 1975.

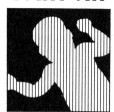
NUTRITION IN THE 75 NEWBORN

Arthur E. D'Harlingue and William J. Byrne

Advances in cardiopulmonary and nutritional care have greatly improved the outcome of sick premature and term newborns. Important advances in nutritional management include the development of various enteral feeding techniques, formulas adapted to the special needs of the premature infant, elemental formulas, and the provision of total parenteral nutrition (TPN). Current practice generally results in adequate postnatal growth. However, many very-low-birth-weight (VLBW) infants fail to establish growth comparable with the third trimester intrauterine growth rate. Also, much remains to be learned about the composition and quality of postnatal growth in both premature and sick term newborns.

■ NUTRITIONAL REQUIREMENTS OF THE NEWBORN

FETAL GROWTH AND NUTRITION

A knowledge of fetal growth and body composition during the third trimester is useful in understanding the nutritional needs of the newborn. Fetal growth in the third trimester is characterized by rapid weight gain (10 to 15 g/kg/day) with a quadrupling of fetal mass. This growth is fueled by a constant flux of transplacental glucose, amino acids, minerals, and vitamins. Inadequate delivery of nutrients and oxygen results in intrauterine growth retardation, and in some cases, fetal demise. In contrast, excessive glucose delivery in a diabetic pregnancy predisposes the fetus to hyperinsulinemia and macrosomia.

During the third trimester, fetal protein increases 2 g/kg/day. Due to increasing adipose tissue, the fetal composition increases from 1 per cent fat at 28 weeks' gestation to 15 per cent at term. In contrast to the accumulation of protein and fat, only a limited amount of carbohydrate is stored as hepatic glycogen. Calcium, phosphorus, and magnesium accumulate rapidly. At term, calcium content is 28 g with 98 per cent in bone. Similarly, phosphorus content at term is 16 g with 80 per cent in bone, while magnesium content is 0.8 g with 60 per cent

in bone. Iron content of the fetus, which averages 75 mg/kg, increases proportionately with weight during the third trimester. Most of the fetal iron is incorporated into hemoglobin, whereas other tissue stores are limited. Hence, any factor that results in rapid postnatal expansion of the red blood cell mass (e.g., recovery from perinatal hemorrhage, or prematurity with rapid postnatal growth) may result in iron deficiency unless iron intake is increased. Some trace minerals are stored in large amounts during the third trimester. Hepatic copper concentration accumulates to levels higher than that at any other time in life. Zinc accumulates at 250 mcg/kg/day during the third trimester. Most water-soluble vitamins are generally not stored in tissues and must be provided postnatally. However, fetal hepatic folate content does increase toward term. Even stores of fat-soluble vitamins are limited. Hepatic retinol increases during the third trimester, but both term and premature infants frequently have a hepatic retinol concentration considered to be deficient in adults (< 20 mcg/gram). Vitamin E stores in the fetus increase in parallel with fetal fat content. Hence, prematurely delivered infants are at greater risk for vitamin E deficiency. When the rapid growth of the third trimester is interrupted by premature delivery, the infant is particularly at risk for the development of both macro-nutrient and micronutrient deficiencies.

POSTNATAL GROWTH AND NUTRITION

WATER

There are large shifts in water balance during the postnatal period, such that the fluid needs of sick term and premature infants must be closely monitored. The full-term infant normally loses about 10 per cent of body weight postnatally partially due to a contraction of the extracellular fluid space. Preterm infants younger than 32 weeks' gestation may experience a postnatal weight loss of up to 20 per cent of birthweight with the nadir occurring at about 2 weeks of age. (Shaffer et al., 1987). A number

TABLE 75–1. Water Requirements (ml/kg/day) of Newborns

BIRTHWEIGHT	AGE (DAYS)		
	1 to 2	**3 to 7**	**7 to 30**
<750	100 to 250	150 to 300	120 to 180
750 to 1000	80 to 150	100 to 150	120 to 180
1000 to 1500	60 to 100	80 to 150	120 to 180
1500 to 2500	60 to 80	100 to 150	120 to 180
Term	60 to 80	100 to 150	120 to 180

of other factors affect water requirements of the newborn (see Fluid and Electrolyte Management/Acid Base, Chapter 28). One of the most important factors for the extremely premature infant (< 1000 g) is transepidermal water loss, which can exceed 200 ml/kg/day. The caloric density of parenteral and enteral nutrition also affects water requirements. In order to provide 120 kcal/kg/day, an infant must be given 180 ml/kg/day of 20 kcal/oz formula or 150 ml/kg/day of 24 kcal/oz formula. The water intake of an infant receiving peripheral TPN is necessarily much higher than that with central TPN so that the same amount of calories are provided. Suggested ranges for water intake for infants are summarized in Table 75–1.

ENERGY REQUIREMENTS

Whereas the term healthy infant can regulate its energy intake from its sense of hunger, sick premature and term infants must have their energy needs considered and appropriate calories provided. The caloric needs of the newborn are divided into expenditure, excretion, and storage (Table 75–2). Energy expenditures are divided between the resting metabolic rate, activity, thermoregulation, and tissue synthesis. Activity is not a major factor in most newborns, but it may be very important in infants with a large energy cost due to excessive work of breathing (e.g., bronchopulmonary dysplasia). The energy used for thermoregulation can be minimized by maintaining the infant in a thermoneutral environment. Although only a small allowance must be made for fat and carbohydrate malabsorption in infants receiving enteral nutrition, this is a major source of energy loss in infants with short bowel syndrome. Once the energy needs of maintenance metabolism, thermoregulation, and activity are met, the remaining energy can be used for tissue synthesis and storage of energy. These two latter factors contribute to the cost of growth, which is approximately 4 to 6 kcal for each gram

TABLE 75–2. Energy Requirements in Enterally Fed Premature Infants

	kcal/kg/day
Total intake	100–165
Expenditure	
resting metabolic rate	45–60
activity	4–10
thermoregulation	5–10
synthesis	10–35
Excretion	7–30
Storage	20–70

(Data from Reichman, B. L., Cheesex, P., Putet, G., et al.: Partition of energy metabolism and energy cost in the very low-birth-weight infant. Pediatrics 69:446–451, 1982; and Schulze, K. F., Stefanski, M., Masterson, J., et al.: Energy expenditure, energy balance, and composition of weight gain in low birth weight infants fed diets of different protein and energy content. J. Pediatr. 110:753–759, 1987.)

of weight gain. Some of the variation in energy requirements is due to differences in the composition of growth. The synthesis of fatty tissue has a higher cost than that of muscle or lean body mass, which is composed primarily of protein and water.

Healthy enterally fed term infants generally require 100 to 120 kcal/kg/day for appropriate postnatal growth in the first few months of life. However, by 4 months of age, caloric requirements decrease to 70 to 95 kcal/kg/day in term infants (Butte et al., 1984). Optimal growth of premature infants (comparable to the intrauterine rate) is achievable with a caloric intake of approximately 115 to 130 kcal/kg/day (AAP, Committee on Nutrition, 1985; European Society of Paediatric Gastroenterology and Nutrition, 1987 Kashyap et al., 1986). The caloric intake of sick newborns may need to be higher in order to achieve appropriate growth, varying with different clinical conditions. Infants with intrauterine growth retardation may require up to 150 kcal/kg/day to support rapid postnatal "catch up" growth. Severe congenital heart disease puts an infant at risk for growth failure and malnutrition due to malabsorption and elevated metabolic rate (Sondheimer and Hamilton, 1978). Infants with severe bronchopulmonary dysplasia have an increased caloric requirement, as demonstrated by high rates of oxygen consumption and associated growth failure (Kurzner et al., 1988). Such infants should be fed formulas with a high caloric density in order to avoid fluid overload. Infants with short gut syndrome lose large amounts of energy because of malabsorption and may require 150 kcal/kg/day or more to achieve appropriate growth. Owing to minimal fecal energy losses during TPN, parenteral caloric requirements are usually less than with enteral nutrition. During the total parenteral nutrition of premature infants, positive nitrogen balance and protein sparing are possible with 60 nonprotein kcal/kg/day and 2.5 grams/kg/day of amino acids (Anderson et al., 1979), whereas growth requires 70 to 100 kcal/kg/day (Zlotkin et al. 1981). After surgery, full-term newborns appear to have similar parenteral protein and energy requirements (Zlotkin, 1984).

PROTEIN REQUIREMENTS

Adequate protein intake of good quality is essential to the growth and development of the newborn (Raiha et al., 1985). Generally, 8 to 12 per cent of nutritional calories should be provided as protein. The protein needs of term infants have been determined from the intake of breast-fed infants, and it is reasonable to assume that the plasma and amino acid profile of the infant fed breast milk represents the "gold standard" that should be achieved in feeding all infants. Human milk contains relatively low amounts of protein (1 to 2 g/dl in the 1st month and 0.9 g/dl in mature milk). However, it also contains nonprotein nitrogen, which may be available for amino acid metabolism. The protein intake of breast-fed term infants is about 2 g/kg/day in the 1st month, declining to about 1 g/kg/day by 6 months of age. During the third trimester, the fetus accretes 320 to 480 mg/kg/day of nitrogen or about 2 to 3 g/kg/day of protein (Ziegler et al., 1981). It is assumed that the premature infant should ideally continue to accrete nitrogen postnatally at this rate. The amount of enteral protein required to achieve this rate of nitrogen retention has been estimated by the factorial method to be 3.5 to 4.0 g/kg/day (Ziegler et al., 1981).

A number of studies of infant feeding have evaluated weight gain and nitrogen retention in premature infants. By increasing the protein content of formula, the rate of weight gain and nitrogen retention in premature infants can also be increased (AAPCON, 1977; Babson and Bramhall, 1969, Davidson, 1967). Some of this weight gain has been attributed to the higher ash and electrolyte content of high-protein formulas. Protein intakes of 2.25 to 5.0 g/kg/day appear to be without major adverse effects, whereas intakes of 6–9 g/kg/day are associated with lethargy, hyperpyrexia, acidosis, increased BUN, and elevated amino acids in premature infants (AAPCON, 1977). Excessive protein intake and an abnormal plasma aminogram may put the infant at risk for neurologic injury. Protein intakes of more than 6 g/kg/day resulted in lower developmental quotient and increased strabismus as compared with intakes of 3–3.6 g/kg/day (Goldman, 1974). Elevated plasma tyrosine in infants receiving a high-protein formula was associated with a lower IQ (Menkes et al., 1972). Both the absolute amount and ratio of protein and energy are important for optimal weight gain and nitrogen retention in the premature infant. Kashyap and colleagues (1986) demonstrated better nitrogen retention and growth with the administration of 3.6 g/kg/day of protein as compared with that of 2.24 g/kg/day (both groups received 115 kcal/kg/day). Increasing the caloric intake to 149 kcal/kg/day with 3.6 g/kg/day of protein did not improve growth but did increase the deposition of fat (Schulze et al., 1987).

The quality of ingested protein is important to amino acid and protein metabolism. Should any essential amino acid be limited in supply, then protein synthesis could be impaired. The premature infant may have a nutritional requirement for several amino acids (cysteine, tyrosine, histidine, taurine) that are nonessential in older infants. Human fetuses and premature infants have been shown to have low levels of hepatic cystathionase, which is important in the conversion of methionine to cysteine. Taurine is important in the conjugation of bile acids and in retinal and CNS function (Gaull, 1989). Unless taurine is supplied to the infant, plasma taurine levels decline. Human milk is high in taurine (40 mg/l). Taurine is now added to most infant formulas and recommended in parenteral amino acid preparations.

CARBOHYDRATE REQUIREMENTS

Carbohydrate provides a major portion of an infant's energy needs. In utero, the newborn is provided with a continuous supply of transplacental glucose. At birth, this glucose flux is interrupted and the infant is dependent on gluconeogenesis until enteral or parenteral nutrition is provided. The term and particularly the premature newborn has very limited glycogen stores, which may have been depleted by intrauterine growth retardation, perinatal stress, or tocolytic therapy with beta-mimetic drugs. The endogenous glucose production rate is approximately 4 mg/kg/min. Hence, parenteral glucose administration to sick newborns should approximate this rate, and this may be achieved by infusing 10 per cent dextrose at 60 ml/kg/

day or comparable amounts of intravenous glucose. Lactose is the major carbohydrate source from human milk and bovine formulas. Intestinal mucosal lactase activity rises slowly in the third trimester but remains low at term. Lactose malabsorption is common in newborns, but bacterial fermentation and colonic salvage of unabsorbed carbohydrate occurs. Other carbohydrates, such as glucose polymers or sucrose, have been added to infant formulas, and these appear to be easily hydrolyzed and absorbed.

FAT AND ESSENTIAL FATTY ACIDS REQUIREMENTS

Infants should receive between 10 and 50 per cent of their energy from fat. Pancreatic lipase levels are low in the newborn. However, lingual lipase and human milk lipases (bile salt–activated lipase and a lipoprotein lipase) are effective in hydrolyzing triglycerides. A critical level of intraluminal bile acids is important for micelle formation, activation of bile salt–dependent lipase, and absorption of triglycerides. Hence, the diminished capacity for bile acid secretion and reduced pool size in newborns predisposes the infant to fat malabsorption. Generally, unsaturated fatty acids are absorbed better than saturated fat. Long-chain fatty acids require micelle formation for efficient absorption. Medium-chain triglycerides are absorbed without the need for micelle formation.

Aside from its important role as an energy source, fat must be provided to prevent essential fatty acid deficiency. Linoleic acid (C18:2ω6) is the only fatty acid proven to be essential in the human. Linoleic is further metabolized to arachidonic acid (C20:4ω6), which is important in platelet function and further metabolism to prostaglandins. There are data suggesting that linolenic acid (C18:3ω3) and longer chain ω–3 fatty acids may also be essential in the human (Anderson et al., 1979; Holman et al., 1982). Essential fatty acid deficiency in the newborn is associated with a scaly dermatitis, alopecia, platelet dysfunction, thrombocytopenia, infections, and failure to thrive. Because of a low adipose composition (as little as 1 per cent in VLBW infants), essential fatty acid deficiency develops rapidly in premature infants on a fat-free diet. Biochemical evidence for essential fatty acid deficiency includes increased 5,8,11-eicosatrienoic acid (C20:3ω9) and a triene/tetraene ratio of > 0.4. Approximately 2 to 4 per cent of caloric intake as linoleic acid is needed to prevent essential fatty acid deficiency. This is provided by 0.5 to 1.0 g/kg/day of intravenous lipids.

MACROMINERALS

Newborns generally require between 1 to 3 mEq/kg/day of both sodium and potassium. Premature infants are prone to hyponatremia due to increased renal excretion of sodium and may occasionally require up to 6 to 8 mEq/kg/day of sodium (Kumar and Sacks, 1978). However, excess sodium administration may be associated with water retention, generalized edema, and continuing serum hyponatruria. Sodium and potassium requirements are increased with the administration of diuretics or excessive gastrointestinal losses. Inadequate chloride intake (Grossman et al., 1980) or chloride depletion in association with diuretics predisposes the infant to metabolic alkalosis and growth failure. (See also Chapter 28.)

Adequate intake of calcium and phosphorus is important for bone mineralization. Nutritional deficiencies of these macrominerals are seldom a problem in term infants, who consume either human milk or standard infant formulas. Hypocalcemic tetany with hyperphosphatemia has been reported in some term infants fed bovine formulas, and this may have been due to inadequate renal excretion of phosphorus. The premature infant has a much higher nutritional requirement for calcium and phosphorus as compared with the term infant. During the third trimester, calcium and phosphorus accrete at 100 to 150 mg/kg/day and 75 to 100 mg/kg/day, respectively. Achieving such high levels of retention, especially in the VLBW infant, is often not possible because of the low solubility of calcium and phosphorus salt in TPN solutions. Osteopenia and rickets of prematurity are preventable common problems due to a combination of phosphorus depletion and inadequate calcium intake. Vitamin D deficiency is rarely responsible.

Iron deficiency anemia remains another common preventable problem in infancy. Term infants fed human milk probably require no iron supplementation until they are 6 months of age. Formula-fed infants should receive iron supplemented formula (12 mg/l) from birth. The iron stores of a rapidly growing premature infant become readily depleted unless supplementation is provided. Infants who are being regularly transfused for anemia of prematurity often have a normal or elevated serum iron levels and probably do not require supplementation. Otherwise, enterally fed premature infants should be supplemented with ferrous sulfate (2 mg/kg/day of elemental iron) starting at 2 weeks to 2 months of age (see also Chapter 86).

TRACE MINERALS

Zinc deficiency is associated with growth failure, diarrhea, and a rash that tends to be localized to the perineal and perioral areas and distal extremities. It may occur as a result of the autosomal recessive disorder acrodermatitis enteropathica, which is thought to be a defect in intestinal absorption of zinc that can be cured with oral zinc therapy for life. Zinc deficiency also occurs during TPN if zinc is not provided in the TPN solution (Sivasubramanian and Henkin, 1978) (see Chapter 76).

Copper deficiency is exhibited by neutropenia, bony changes (flaring and cupping of long bones), failure to thrive, and microcytic anemia (Sutton et al., 1985). Most enterally fed premature infants are in negative copper balance during the first postnatal weeks, but hepatic stores may protect against deficiency. The AAPCON recommends a copper intake of 90 micrograms/100 kcal for premature infants. Those at greatest risk for the development of copper deficiency are premature infants on TPN particularly those who also experienced intrauterine growth retardation (see also Chapter 76).

Selenium, cobalt, molybdenum, and chromium are required in trace amounts, but there are little data available. Infants fed enterally with human milk or infant formula do not develop clinical deficiencies of these trace minerals. Selenium deficiency may develop in patients on

very prolonged TPN (Lockitch et al., 1989; Vinton et al., 1987). Symptoms of selenium deficiency include cardiomyopathy, muscle pain, red blood cell fragility, macrocytosis, and pseudoalbinism. Fluoride supplementation should be provided to infants who reside in areas where the water supply has a fluoride content of < 0.3 ppm (AAPCON, 1986).

VITAMINS

The vitamin requirements of the newborn are not well defined. A recommended daily allowance has been set for most vitamins (Table 75–3), but such guidelines are more applicable for term newborns and older infants than for premature infants (see also Chapter 76).

ENTERAL NUTRITION

The preferred route to feed the newborn is enteral. Besides its simplicity, enteral nutrition has trophic effects on gastrointestinal growth and function. However, enteral nutrition is often precluded by cardiopulmonary or gastrointestinal disease in the premature or sick newborn. Although partial or total parenteral nutrition are often required in caring for these infants, the ultimate goal should be to establish full enteral feedings.

FEEDING HEALTHY TERM INFANTS

The timing and choice of the first feeding for the healthy term newborn is decided more by custom and tradition than clear scientific data. The first feeding should be delayed until it is clear that the newborn has made a stable transition to extrauterine life. There should be no respiratory distress or neurologic depression. For the newborn who is clearly doing well, feedings may commence within an hour of birth. Because of concerns of possible

TABLE 75–3. Recommended Daily Dietary Allowances for Infants

NUTRIENTS	0–0.5 YEAR	0.5–1 YEAR
Calories (kcal/kg)	115 (95–145)	105 (80–135)
Protein (g/kg)	2.2	1.6
Vitamin A (μg RE)*	375	375
Vitamin D (μg)	7.5	10
Vitamin E (mg α-TE)†	3	4
Vitamin C (mg)	30	35
Vitamin K (μg)	5	10
Thiamin (mg)	.3	.4
Riboflavin (mg)	.4	.5
Niacin (mg)	5	6
B_6 (mg)	.3	.6
Folate (μg)	25	35
B_{12} (μg)	.3	.5
Calcium (mg)	400	600
Phosphorus (mg)	300	500
Magnesium (mg)	40	60
Iron (mg)	6	10
Zinc (mg)	5	5
Iodine (μg)	40	50
Selenium (μg)	10	15

*RE, retinol equivalents
†alpha-tocopherol equivalents
(Adapted from National Research Council, Subcommittee on the Tenth Edition of the RDAs: Recommended Dietary Allowances, 10th Edition. Washington, D.C., National Academy Press, 1989).

aspiration, the first feeding has often been sterile water. Sterile water has no nutritional value, does not buffer gastric secretions, and does not support blood glucose. Therefore, this practice should be seriously reevaluated and probably abandoned.

Breast-fed infants should be fed on demand, usually resulting in 8 to 12 feedings per day. Frequent feedings establish the mother's milk flow, prevent dehydration, and reduce breast-feeding associated jaundice (De Carvalho et al., 1982). Breast-feeding brings the infant and mother into close physical contact. This appears to promote mothering behaviour and facilitates the bonding process (Fig. 75–1). Although breast-feeding is the preferred mode of nutrition for the term infant, bottle-feeding of formula certainly does not preclude the development of a healthy relationship between the infant and the mother. Bottle-fed infants may be similarly fed on demand, although the frequency of the feedings may be less than that of the breast-fed infant. Bottle-fed infants take only ½ to 1 ounce per feeding in the 1st day, but this increases to 2 to 3 ounces by several days of age. A number of proprietary formulas are currently available (Table 75–4). Routinely, a standard 20 kcal/oz bovine milk formula should be used. The newborn generally requires no other nutritional source than human milk or standard infant formula for the first 3 to 6 months of life.

HUMAN MILK

With relatively few exceptions, human milk is the preferred feeding for the newborn. The composition of human milk (Table 75–4) is affected by several factors, such as the time of day, fore or hindmilk, and premature versus term delivery (Jenness 1979). Human milk from a mother who has delivered a term infant has a protein content of about 2 g/dl in the 1st week. Thereafter, the protein content steadily declines to about 0.9 g/dl in mature milk at several months. For mothers delivering prematurely, human milk contains 2 to 3 g/dl of protein in the 1st week, and declines to 1.8 g/dl at 1 month (Gross et al., 1980). Human milk protein is two-thirds whey and one-third casein. The remaining nitrogen in human milk is nonprotein nitrogen, which may be available for incorporation into protein by amination of keto acids. In contrast, cow's milk protein is about 80 per cent casein and 20 per cent whey. Cow's milk is lower in cysteine and taurine and higher in tyrosine, phenylalanine, valine, and methionine than human milk. Human milk contains between 60 and 75 kcal/100 ml. Most of this variation is due to the wide range of fat in human milk (3 to 5 g/100 ml). The lactose content is less variable (6.8 to 7.2 g/100 ml).

Much of an infant's passive immunity at birth is derived from transplacental IgG. However, human milk, particu-

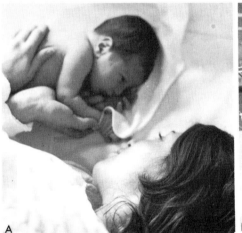

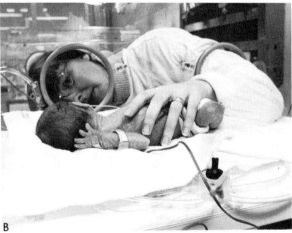

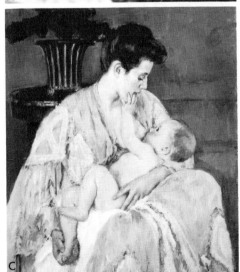

FIGURE 75–1. *Mothers in the "en face" position. En face is defined as occurring when the mother's face is rotated such that her eyes and those of the infant meet full in the same vertical plane of rotation. A, A mother and her full-term infant. B, A mother and her premature infant. C, Mother and Child, by Mary Cassatt. (A and B, Klaus, M., and Kennell, J.: In The Care of the High-risk Neonate. Philadelphia, W. B. Saunders Company, 1973. C, Courtesy of the Art Institute of Chicago, Chicago, Illinois.)*

TABLE 75–4. Comparison of Human Milk and Infant Formulas (Per 100 ml)

	HUMAN MILK*	ENFAMIL	SIMILAC	SMA	SOY-BASED FORMULA†	EPF-24	SSC-24	PREGESTIMIL
kcal	68	68	68	68	68	81	81	68
mOsm/kg/H$_2$O	300	300	290	300	200–296	300	300	300
protein (g)	0.9	1.5	1.5	1.5	1.8 to 2.1	2.4	2.2	1.9
source	human	bovine	bovine	bovine	soy	bovine	bovine	casein
whey:casein (%)	60:40	60:40	18:82	60:40	—	60:40	60:40	hydrolysate
carbohydrate (g)	6.8–7.2	6.9	7.2	7.2	6.8–6.9	8.9	8.6	7.0
source	lactose	lactose	lactose	lactose	corn syrup solids and/or sucrose	lactose, glucose polymers (40:60)	lactose, glucose polymers (50:50)	corn syrup solids, glucose, starch
fat (g)	3–5	3.8	3.6	3.6	3.6 to 3.7	4.1 40% MCT	4.4 50% MCT	3.8 60% MCT
sodium (mEq)	0.8	0.8	1.0	0.7	0.9 to 1.4	1.4	1.7	1.4
potassium (mEq)	1.4	1.8	2.1	1.4	1.9 to 2.4	2.1	2.9	1.9
calcium (mg)	30	46	51	44	63 to 70	134	144	63
phosphorus (mg)	15	31	39	33	44 to 50	68	72	42
vitamin A, IU	190	210	203	200	200 to 211	970	552	254
vitamin D, IU	2	42	41	40	40 to 42	220	122	51
vitamin E, IU	.18	2	2	1	1 to 2	3.7	3.2	2.5

*Term mature human milk.
†Range for Prosobee, Isomil, Nursoy.
MCT, medium-chain triglycerides.

larly colostrum, is very high in secretory IgA. The mother and infant together form an enteromammary cycle (Kleinman, 1979). Antigens present in the maternal gut are processed by intestinal macrophages and lymphocytes, resulting in T-lymphocyte activation. The T lymphocytes migrate to mammary tissue where these cells secrete specific antibodies to these antigens into human milk. Although little of this IgA is absorbed by the infant, it is available in the gut lumen to bind to antigens and infectious agents. This may be the primary mechanism by which human milk protects against bacterial and viral gastroenteritis. There are a number of other antiinfective properties of human milk (Welsh and May, 1979). Lysozyme acts with vitamin C and IgA to lyse *Escherichia coli*. Lactoferrin binds to enteric iron, making it unavailable for bacterial metabolism. *Lactobacillus bifidus* growth factor is active against gram-negative enteric organisms, which may then allow the proliferation of *Lactobacillus* in breast-fed infants. Intact maternal macrophages and lymphocytes are excreted in breast milk, but their role in the infant's GI tract is unknown. The exclusively breast-fed infant has a predominantly gram-positive flora, whereas the formula-fed infant has more gram-negative organisms. However, the colonization patterns in breast-fed infants in an intensive care nursery do not show a significant difference from those of bottle-fed infants. Despite feeding with human milk, infants in an intensive care nursery still develop abnormal colonization patterns with a predominance of gram-negative coliforms or *Staphylococcus epidermidis*.

A number of hormones and other proteins are secreted into human milk (Koldovsky and Thornburg, 1987). Epidermal growth factor, lactoferrin, thyroid hormone, gastrin, and prolactin are important for gastrointestinal development and mucosal growth. These proteins or other trophic factors (e.g., nonprotein nitrogen) may explain the better intestinal growth seen in neonatal animals fed their own mother's milk rather than an artificial formula.

All breast-feeding mothers should be aware of the potential passage of medications, alcohol, and illicit drugs into their milk. Detailed reviews of this subject are available (American Academy of Pediatrics, Committee on Drugs,

1989; Briggs et al., 1990; Lawrence, 1989). Although most drugs given to lactating women are passed into breast milk to some extent, documentation of adverse effects in infants are limited; even so, when prescribing drugs for lactating women, the potential risk to the infant must be considered. Most antibiotics do not pose any risk to the breast-fed infant, but some caution should be taken for mothers receiving metronidazole, clindamycin, or chloramphenicol. Antineoplastic agents could have adverse effects on multiple organ systems in the infant, thus precluding breast-feeding. Radionucleotides for diagnostic studies are also excreted in human milk. Breast-feeding may resume when the radioactivity of the milk is eliminated. Maternal use of cocaine causes hypertension and seizures in breast-fed infants (Chaney et al., 1988; Chasnoff et al., 1987). Maternal opiates are generally excreted into human milk in small amounts, and this may be a concern only in the narcotic-addicted mother. Table 75–5 lists some of the drugs for which breast-feeding may be precluded or for which special precautions are indicated.

Hepatitis B virus is excreted into human milk. If the mother is known to be HBsAg positive, the infant should be appropriately treated with hepatitis B immune globulin and hepatitis B vaccine. The current recommendations of the World Health Organization and the American Academy of Pediatrics do not preclude breast-feeding for the HBsAg-positive mother, but this is controversial. Both herpes simplex and human immunodeficiency virus are excreted into human milk, and neonatal disease acquired by this route has been documented. Cytomegalovirus is excreted into human milk. It is inactivated by pasteurization or freezing ($-20°$ C [$-68°$ F]).

STANDARD INFANT FORMULAS

When breast-feeding is not possible, standard 20 kcal/oz bovine or soy infant formulas offer a safe and nutritionally complete alternative, which is preferable to cow's milk (see Table 75–4). Although an infant will generally grow well without major nutritional problems on infant formulas, there are a number of aspects that make them

TABLE 75–5. Maternal Drugs and Breast Milk

MATERNAL DRUGS	EFFECTS ON INFANT OR PRECAUTIONS
Contraindicated Drugs	
Radioactive agents	Resume breast-feeding when radioactivity has been eliminated from milk
Anticancer drugs	Gastrointestinal system, bone marrow, immune system
Chloramphenicol	Gray baby syndrome
Cimetidine	Central nervous system stimulation, decreased gastric acidity
Cocaine	Hypertension, seizures
Ergotamine	Vomiting, diarrhea, seizures
Heroin	Sedation, withdrawal, HIV risk
Metronidazole	Hematologic, central nervous system, mutagenic
Drugs Used With Precautions	
Alcohol	Safe in moderation
Anticholinergics (atropine)	Tachycardia
Beta blockers	Bradycardia
Clindamycin	Colitis
Diazepam	Sedation, slow clearance
Methadone	Associated heroin use, HIV risk
Phenobarbital	Sedation
Propylthiouracil	Inhibits thyroid function
Sulfisoxazole	Displacement of bilirubin from albumin
Theophylline	Irritability
Warfarin	Monitor prothrombin time
Probably Safe Drugs	
Aminoglycosides	Alters gastrointestinal flora, poor gastrointestinal absorption
Cephalosporins	Alters gastrointestinal flora, some displace bilirubin from albumin
Furosemide	Poor gastrointestinal absorption
Heparin	Does not enter breast milk
Hydralazine	Watch for changes in blood pressure or perfusion
Magnesium sulfate	Little effect upon milk mg^{++} level
Methyldopa	Watch for changes in blood pressure or perfusion
Penicillins	Alters gastrointestinal flora

inferior to human milk. Formulas lack the many immunologic, anti-infective, hormonal, and trophic factors present in human milk. Improper mixing of formula, resulting in hypocaloric or hypercaloric concentrations, can cause hyponatremia or hypernatremia and growth disturbances. Formula feeding of infants is generally safe from bacterial or toxin contamination in developed nations, but this is not true in the third world. Infant mortality due to infection, chronic diarrhea, and malnutrition clearly rise with increased use of infant formula in underdeveloped areas.

Whereas human milk contains mostly whey protein, the protein in bovine formulas is predominantly casein (e.g., 82 per cent in Similac) unless additional whey is added to the formula (e.g., 60:40 whey:casein ratio in PM 60:40, Enfamil, and SMA). In premature infants, the administration of casein-predominant formulas are associated with metabolic acidosis. However, generally either whey-predominant or casein-predominant formulas are well tolerated in term infants. Some plasma amino acids are relatively more elevated in whey-predominant (threonine) or casein-predominant (phenylalanine, tyrosine) formulas as compared with human milk (Jarvenpaa et al., 1982). Janas and associates (1985) showed that the addition of whey to cow's milk formulas does not result

in a plasma aminogram similar to that of human milk. Bovine infant formulas contain higher levels of protein than mature human milk, resulting in higher levels of BUN and certain amino acids. Although it is unclear whether this higher protein content in bovine formulas is either necessary or harmful, it may provide a margin of safety should bovine protein be less efficacious than human milk protein for infant metabolism and growth.

Standard bovine formulas contain lactose as the major carbohydrate. Although term infants often have some intestinal lactose malabsorption, the colon does absorb some of this malabsorbed carbohydrate after bacterial fermentation. In addition, lactose may improve calcium absorption. Fat in infant formulas is not as well absorbed as in human milk, despite the generally high content of polyunsaturated fatty acids in formula. Vitamin and mineral supplementation of standard formulas are sufficient to prevent deficiency in healthy term infants. Formula-fed term infants should receive an iron-containing formula from birth in order to prevent iron deficiency anemia.

There are limited indications for the use of soy formulas in the newborn, including galactosemia, secondary lactose intolerance, and congenital lactase deficiency (rare). Although soy formulas have been used in infants who have developed or who are at risk for bovine protein sensitivity, there is no clear basis for this practice. Infants sensitive to bovine milk protein may also develop soy protein sensitivity (Powell, 1978). A more rational practice for infants with protein intolerance is to encourage breast-feeding or to use a formula containing only hydrolyzed protein.

FEEDING PREMATURE INFANTS

There has been considerable controversy regarding the timing of initial enteral feedings for premature infants. For the larger healthy premature (birth weight > 1500 g) without lung disease, feedings may be started in the 1st day at a volume of 3 to 5 ml/kg every 3 hours. The feedings may be advanced by 3 to 5 ml/kg/day until 120 kcal/kg/day is achieved. For the VLBW infant or the premature infant requiring ventilation for lung disease, the correct time to start feedings is less clear. It has been a common practice to delay feedings in such infants due to the increased risk of necrotizing enterocolitis in those infants. However, prospective randomized studies of early hypocaloric feedings versus delayed feedings in sick VLBW infants showed no difference in the incidence of necrotizing enterocolitis between groups. Early feedings are associated with earlier full enteral nutrition, fewer days of parenteral nutrition, a lower incidence of cholestasis, and improved calcium metabolism (Dunn et al., 1988; LaGamma et al., 1985; Ostertag et al., 1986; Slagle and Gross, 1988). Some of these beneficial effects may be due to the induction of gastrointestinal mucosal enzymes and improved bowel motility. Despite these encouraging results with early enteral nutrition in sick premature infants, it is prudent to delay feedings in any infant with shock, hypotension, or signs of ileus until such symptoms resolve.

The choice of feeding for the premature infant is limited to several options, each with specific advantages or disadvantages. If maternal milk is available, this should be given unless there are specific contraindications. Banked pooled human milk, which is donated by women delivering term infants, has been fed to premature infants for many years. This mature milk differs in composition from human milk produced by women delivering prematurely, the latter containing higher levels of protein and sodium. In addition, lactating women who donate to milk banks must be carefully screened for infectious viruses (e.g., HIV, hepatitis B) and instructed in the expression and storage of milk (Asquith 1987). Human milk can be refrigerated and used for up to 24 hours, or it can be frozen for future use. Freezing will kill maternal white blood cells in human milk, but levels of immunoglobulins, C3, lactoferrin, and lysozyme are unchanged. Levels of these factors are appreciably reduced by pasteurization at 62.5° C (144.5° F).

Although human milk is ideal for the term infant, there are some nutritional deficiencies in its use for the VLBW infant. The protein content of mature human milk (0.9 g/100 ml) does not fulfill the needs of the rapidly growing premature. The milk of women who deliver prematurely does have a higher protein content during the 1st month (2 to 3 g/100 ml) decreasing to lower values thereafter. Gross (1983) evaluated growth parameters in a population of premature infants fed human milk from mothers who delivered prematurely, pooled banked human milk, and a formula for premature infants. He found that premature infants fed human milk from mothers who delivered prematurely or the formula for premature infants had weight gain and head growth that was comparable with the intrauterine rate and exceeded that of infants fed mature banked human milk. These differences were attributed to the higher protein content of the human milk from mothers who delivered prematurely and the formula for premature infants. Whereas mature banked human milk does not meet the needs of the VLBW weight infant, supplementation of banked milk with human or bovine milk protein can result in growth and nitrogen retention similar to the intrauterine rate (Putet et al., 1987; Ronnholm et al., 1986; Schanler et al., 1985).

The mineral content of human milk also may not be suitable for the premature infant. Mature human milk is low in sodium, which predisposes the premature infant to hyponatremia. The higher sodium content of human milk from mothers who delivered prematurely (1 to 2 mEq/100 ml) and formulas for premature infants is more appropriate for VLBW infants, who have higher nutritional requirements for sodium. The calcium and phosphorus content of premature and term human milk are similar, and both are inadequate for the VLBW infant (Atkinson et al., 1983). Intrauterine rates of calcium and phosphorus accretion can be met by supplementation of human milk with calcium and phosphorus salts. Use of unsupplemented human milk in the premature infant, especially in infants weighing less than 1000 g, may result in osteopenia and rickets of prematurity.

For the larger premature infant (> 1500 g), supplementation of premature human milk may not be necessary. However, the VLBW infant receiving human milk alone is at risk for the development of osteopenia, hypoalbuminemia, and poor weight gain and head growth. In order to increase the caloric density of human milk and to supplement protein and mineral levels, a powdered supplement has been developed for use in the premature infant (Modanlou et al., 1986). Alternatively, human milk can be mixed with formulas for premature infants in a 1:1 ratio. Addition of calories alone (e.g., medium-chain triglyceride, glucose polymers) to human milk without additional protein is not advisable. Such a practice may result in an excessively high non-nitrogen calorie to protein ratio and may lead to fat deposition and inadequate nitrogen retention.

The composition of formulas for premature infants (see Table 75–4) is based on our current understanding of the gastrointestinal development of the fetus and newborn (Lebenthal et al., 1983). The higher protein content as compared with standard formulas or term human milk is necessary to achieve nitrogen accretion at the intrauterine rate. The 60:40 whey-to-casein ratio in formulas for premature infants is preferred over a predominance of casein because the casein-predominant formula is associated with metabolic acidosis and low plasma tyrosine and phenylalanine in premature infants (Raiha, 1976; Rassin et al., 1977). Since intestinal lactase activity is low in the premature infant, only approximately half of the carbohydrate is provided as lactose. The remaining carbohydrate is glucose polymers, which can be hydrolyzed by intestinal glucoamylase and sucrase-isomaltase. Premature infants do not absorb 10 to 25 per cent of ingested fat owing to reduced bile salt concentration, decreased bile pool size, and decreased pancreatic lipase secretion. Since medium-chain triglyceride does not require micelle formation for absorption, approximately half of the fat in premature formulas is provided as medium-chain triglyceride. After delivery via the portal venous system, hydrolyzed medium-chain triglyceride is rapidly oxidized by the liver, which may be disadvantageous to overall energy metabolism (Bach and Babayan, 1982). Earlier studies showed improved fat absorption with medium-chain triglyceride (Roy et al., 1975). More recent studies have demonstrated no difference in fat or energy absorption (Hamosh et al., 1989, Whyte et al., 1986) or nitrogen and mineral retention (Huston et al., 1983; Whyte et al., 1986) between formulas with and without medium-chain triglyceride. Further studies are needed in premature infants regarding the efficacy and metabolic fate of medium-chain triglyceride in order to determine whether or not its continued use is warranted.

Higher levels of calcium and phosphorus are provided in premature formulas (see Table 75–4). Studies of formulas for premature infants have demonstrated calcium and phosphorus retention and bone mineralization comparable with the intrauterine rate (Chan et al., 1986; Greer et al., 1982). However, when these formulas are fed by continuous nasogastric infusion, there is significant binding of calcium and phosphorus to the tubing (Bhatia and Fomon, 1983). Sodium, zinc, and copper are provided at higher levels than those in standard formulas to meet the increased requirements of the premature.

Premature infants may be switched to unsupplemented human milk or standard term infant bovine formulas with iron when they have achieved a weight of 2000 g. Soy formulas are not recommended for routine use in premature infants (AAPCON, 1983). Phosphorus absorption and serum phosphorus levels are lower with soy formulas as compared with bovine formulas in the premature infant (Shenai et al., 1981). This may be due to binding of calcium by plant phytates in the gut lumen with subsequent malabsorption. Prolonged use of soy formulas may put the premature at risk for osteopenia or rickets of prematurity.

SPECIALIZED FORMULAS

The term elemental is used to describe formulas composed of pre-hydrolyzed protein and that are adapted to improve carbohydrate and fat absorption. Protein is provided as a hydrolysate in order to improve absorption and minimize immunogenicity. Carbohydrate is provided as glucose polymers and other simple sugars but not as lactose. The majority of fat is provided as medium-chain triglyceride, which does not require micelle formation for absorption. Elemental formulas are indicated for newborns after surgery for necrotizing enterocolitis, abdominal wall anomalies, or intestinal atresias. Infants with short bowel syndrome have malabsorption related to decreased intestinal length and mucosal mass for the hydrolysis and absorption of nutrients. These infants particularly benefit from the administration of elemental formulas. Infants with ileostomies should be fed an elemental formula in order to reduce water and electrolyte loss. Elemental formula should also be considered for infants with pancreatic insufficiency due to cystic fibrosis or for infants with malabsorption secondary to gastroenteritis. Infants with protein sensitivity should benefit from elemental formulas because it prevents further sensitization and gastrointestinal mucosal injury. Supplementation with calcium and phosphorus may be indicated for premature infants on such formulas for optimal bone mineralization.

Infants with chronic lung disease have increased caloric needs because of elevated metabolic rates and associated growth failure (Kurzner et al., 1988). Providing adequate caloric intake to these infants is complicated by fluid retention and lung edema. The needs of infants with chronic lung disease, for example, can be met by increasing the caloric density of enteral feedings without increasing water intake. For small infants with chronic lung disease (< 3 kg), 24 calorie/oz formulas should be used in order to limit water intake. For the older infant with chronic lung disease, Merritt (1988) has described the addition of Polycose, corn oil, and protein to standard 24 calorie/oz formula, yielding a caloric density of 30 to 34 calories/oz. Addition of calories alone (as glucose polymers or fat) without added protein should be done cautiously because inadequate protein intake may impair growth.

ENTERAL FEEDING TECHNIQUES

Although nipple feedings, whether by breast or bottle, is the simplest and most desirable way to feed infants, this modality is often not possible in the premature or sick newborn. Although the ability to suck may be present as early as 24 weeks' gestation, most premature infants do not have an effective and coordinated sucking and swallowing ability until the age of 34 postconceptional weeks. In the VLBW infant or in infants with central nervous system disorders, cardiopulmonary disease, or major gastrointestinal anomalies, nipple feeding may be impossible or inadequate to maintain good nutrition. In such instances, tube feeding is necessary until full nipple feedings are established.

BOLUS NASOGASTRIC FEEDINGS

Bolus nasogastric feeding has remained the most common method of feeding for small premature infants in the modern era of newborn intensive care (Churella et al., 1985). A 5 or 8 French feeding tube is passed through the nose or mouth to the stomach. Feedings are started at a volume of 3–5 ml/kg/feeding and are gradually increased until adequate enteral calories are provided. Gastric residuals are checked prior to each feeding and a volume of ≥ 20 per cent of the previous feeding suggests inadequate gastric emptying or feeding intolerance. This technique is well tolerated by most premature and term infants and requires little equipment. Bolus nasogastric feeding relies on adequate gastric emptying, which can be decreased in premature or neurologically depressed infants. Although gastric emptying is decreased with increasing caloric density and glucose concentration, the actual delivery of nutrients to the small intestine is similar when either 20- or 24-calorie/oz. formula is used. Gastroesophageal reflux can be a problem with bolus nasogastric feedings, which may lead to aspiration or inadequate caloric intake. Bolus gavage feedings have been associated with apnea, cyanosis, and decreased pH and PaO_2 (Krauss et al., 1978). Some of these effects may be due to gastric distention, increased intra-abdominal pressure, and elevation of the diaphragm. Changes in pulmonary mechanics include decreased functional residual capacity, decreased lung and chest wall dynamic compliance, and increased minute ventilation and diaphragmatic work (Heldt, 1988). For the premature infant recovering from lung disease, these changes may compromise the infant and may lead to apnea, respiratory distress, or oxygen desaturation. Repeated passage of a nasogastric tube may result in traumatic injury or perforation into the esophagus or stomach. Whether continuous feeding has any advantage over bolus feeding in reducing these problems is not well studied.

CONTINUOUS NASOGASTRIC FEEDINGS

This technique involves the continuous slow drip of formula to the stomach via a nasogastric tube and a constant infusion pump. Although there are reports regarding the use of continuous nasogastric feedings in infants and premature infants (Valman et al., 1972; Vanderhoof et al., 1982), prospective controlled studies are limited. Better nitrogen, fat, and mineral absorption has been demonstrated with continuous nasogastric feeding than with bolus nasogastric feeding in infants with diarrhea and malnutrition and in infants with short bowel syndrome (Parker et al., 1981). Limited data in premature infants weighing less than 1250 g suggest that weight gain may be better with continuous NG than bolus gavage (Krishman and Satish, 1981; Toce et al., 1987). Continuous nasogastric feedings are useful in VLBW infants, in whom bolus gavage feeds increase intra-abdominal pressure and impair lung function. Infants with poor gastric emptying and gastroesophageal reflux and those who are at risk for aspiration also benefit from continuous nasogastric feedings. Continuous indwelling nasogastric tubes become colonized, which may predispose the infant to bacterial overgrowth in the gastrointestinal tract. With continuous nasogastric feedings, large amounts of calcium and phosphorus bind to the tubing and are not delivered to the infant. Gastrointestinal hormonal regulation is influenced by the type of feeding. Aynsley-Green (1983) showed that there are surges in the blood levels of insulin and other gastrointestinal hormones in response to bolus feedings. These levels then return to baseline between feedings. With continuous nasogastric feedings, these hormones remain at steady state baseline levels without such surges, and it is possible that this factor is disadvantageous to the infant's nutrition.

TRANSPYLORIC FEEDINGS

Transpyloric feedings are indicated in infants with poor gastric emptying, severe gastroesophageal reflux, or infants at risk for aspiration. The efficacy of this method of feeding in premature infants has been documented (Cheek and Staub, 1973; Rhea and Kilby, 1970). Transpyloric feedings require passage of a soft tube (Silastic or polyurethane) into the distal duodenum or proximal jejunum. Although stiffer tubes of polyethylene or polyvinyl chloride have been used, the risk of perforation is greater. Confirmation of tube placement through x-ray examination is necessary. Although some controlled prospective studies demonstrated better weight gain with transpyloric feedings as compared with nasogastric feedings (Van Caillie and Powell, 1975; Wells and Zachman, 1975), this has not been found by others (Pereira et al., 1981; Roy et al., 1977). Since hyperosmolar feedings given directly into the intestine may not be well tolerated, especially in premature infants, iso-osmolar feedings are recommended. Complications related to transpyloric feedings include intestinal perforation, necrotizing enterocolitis, intussusception, and malabsorption (Boros and Reynolds, 1975, Chen and Wong, 1975, Roy et al., 1977). Since a transpyloric tube bypasses the stomach and often the sphincter of Oddi, the digestive effects of lingual lipase and pancreatobiliary secretions may be decreased. Malabsorption can result from migration of the tube into more distal jejunum.

GASTROSTOMY FEEDINGS

Although used in the past as a routine method to feed premature infants (Berg et al., 1964; Vengusamy et al., 1969), this modality is now reserved for special situations in sick premature and term newborns. Any infant who is anticipated to require tube feedings for more than 3 to 6 months is a candidate for gastrostomy. Such infants include infants with central nervous system disorders and infants with severe bronchopulmonary dysplasia who require very prolonged ventilatory support. Infants should be evaluated for gastroesophageal reflux before the tube is placed, since surgical Stamm gastrostomy predisposes the infant to reflux and, therefore, may worsen preexisting reflux (Mollitt et al., 1985). There are several different types of gastrostomy tubes. The "button" gastrostomy tube has enjoyed recent popularity, because of its ease of use, physical appearance, and relative freedom from complications. Feedings through the gastrostomy tube may be started within 48 to 72 hours of placement and may follow the same guidelines for nasogastric feedings.

PARENTERAL NUTRITION

When enteral feedings are not possible, the use of parenteral nutrition (PN) is essential to the care of the sick newborn. The goals of PN are severalfold: (1) to promote nitrogen retention and protein-sparing, (2) to provide energy for metabolic processes, and (3) to establish growth and maturation during the critical postnatal period. The premature newborn has limited glycogen and fat stores, which become rapidly depleted with starvation. The premature infant who weighs less than 1500 g and who has respiratory disease or other contraindications to enteral feedings should be started on intravenous glucose during the first hours of life. Electrolyte and calcium supplementation should begin by 12 to 24 hours after birth, and amino acids should be started by 3 days of age. Larger premature and sick term newborns may be maintained on only glucose and electrolyte solutions, if it is anticipated that full enteral feedings will be tolerated by 5 to 7 days of age. Since VLBW prematures develop biochemical evidence of essential fatty acid insufficiency within 3 days of fat-free nutrition, low doses (0.5 to 1 g/kg/day) of intravenous lipid should be started within 1 week and preferably within 3 days of starting PN. The infant with necrotizing enterocolitis or gastrointestinal anomalies, once stable from a metabolic and cardiopulmonary standpoint, should be started on PN. Parenteral nutrition in concert with slowly progressive enteral feedings has become a standard method of nourishing premature infants. This method allows enteral feedings to be advanced slowly, while stimulating intestinal enzyme induction, growth, and maturation. The balance of nutrition is provided by PN until full feedings are established. Whether using total PN or PN with enteral feedings, the goal is to reverse postnatal weight loss and to establish quality growth at a rate comparable with in utero growth for the premature and normal postnatal growth for the term infant.

PROTEIN AND ENERGY

The recommended intakes of energy and macro- and micronutrients during total PN are summarized in Table 75–6. The American Academy of Pediatrics Committee on Nutrition (1983) recommends that premature infants receive 2–3 g/kg/day of amino acids. Positive nitrogen balance has been demonstrated in premature infants who receive 2.5 g/kg/day of amino acids and 60 kcal/kg/day (Anderson et al., 1979). However, sick premature and term newborns generally require more than 70 kcal/kg/day and 2.5 to 3.5 g/kg/day of amino acids to support growth and nitrogen retention as compared with the intrauterine rate (Zlotkin et al., 1981). Since protein-calorie malnutrition has been seen in some infants despite provision of the recommended amounts of protein and energy, close monitoring is essential (Shulman et al., 1986). More than 3 g/kg/day of amino acids may be needed in certain cases.

Crystalline amino acid solutions should be used, which provide adequate amounts of both essential and nonessential amino acids. Besides the essential amino acids listed in Table 75–7, the premature infant may also require histidine, tyrosine, cysteine, and taurine. Supplementation of PN with cysteine and taurine has been advocated, but

TABLE 75–6. Maintenance Requirements and Example Solutions for Total Parenteral Nutrition

COMPONENT	MAINTENANCE (AMOUNT PER KG/DAY)	PERIPHERAL TPN* (PER 100 ML)	CENTRAL TPN† (PER 100 ML)
fluid (ml)	100 to 150		
calories (kcal)	80 to 110	40 to 50	60 to 80
protein (g)	2.5 to 3.0	1.5 to 2	2 to 3
glucose (g)	10 to 20	10 to 12.5	15 to 20
fat (g)	1 to 3	separately as 10 or 20% emulsion	
sodium (mEq)	2 to 4	2	3
potassium (mEq)	2 to 4	2	2
acetate (mEq)	1 to 2	1	1
Ca gluconate (mg)	300 to 600	400	600
phosphorus (mg)	30 to 60	30	45
magnesium (mEq)	.4	.3	.4
zinc (mcg)‡	100,300§	70, 200	100, 300
copper (mcg)‡	20	13	20
manganese (mcg)‡	1 to 5	3.3	5
chromium (mcg)‡	.14 to .2	.11	.17
MVI-Pediatric (vial/day)	<1 kg 30% 1 to 2 kg 65% > 3 kg 100%	same	same

*Assumes intake of 150 ml/kg/day.
†Assumes intake of 100 ml/kg/day.
‡Recommendation of AMA (Nutrition Advisory Group) except for lower range for Mn.
§Zinc: 100, 300 mcg/kg/day, term and prematures, respectively.

the efficacy of these practices is still unproved (Cooke et al., 1984; Gaull, 1989; Geggel et al., 1985, Malloy et al., 1984). Table 75–7 lists some of the available amino acid solutions for use in the newborn. Amino acid solutions designed primarily for use in adults have been widely used in newborns. New pediatric solutions, which are formulated to achieve aminograms similar to those of the postprandial breast-fed infant are now available (Heird et al., 1987, 1988). In two groups of newborns who underwent surgery and were placed on total PN, Helms and co-workers (1987) demonstrated better nitrogen balance

and weight gain in the group that received a pediatric solution with added cysteine as compared with the group that received a standard adult amino acid solution. There are little data otherwise available to judge whether or not these amino acid solutions marketed for pediatric use offer any distinct advantage over the standard adult preparations. Because the solubility of calcium and phosphorus salts improves with increasing acidity, a low pH is preferred for amino acid solutions used in neonatal PN. Complications of PN related to amino acids include azotemia, hyperammonemia, hyperchloremic metabolic acidosis, an

TABLE 75–7. Composition of Amino Acid Solutions (Each Individual Amino Acid Expressed as mg/g of Total Mixture)

AMINO ACIDS	TROPHAMINE 10% (KENDALL MC GAW)	AMINOSYN-PF 10% (ABBOTT)	AMINOSYN 10% (ABBOTT)	FREAMINE III 10% (KENDALL MC GAW)
Essential				
Isoleucine	82	76	72	69
Leucine	114	120	94	91
Lysine	82	68	72	73
Methionine	34	18	40	53
Phenylalanine	48	43	44	56
Threonine	42	51	52	40
Tryptophan	20	18	16	15
Valine	78	67	80	66
Nonessential				
Alanine	54	70	128	71
Arginine	112	123	98	95
Aspartic acid	32	53	—	—
Glutamic	50	82	—	—
Proline	68	81	86	112
Serine	38	50	42	59
Glycine	36	39	128	140
Histidine*	48	31	30	28
Tyrosine*	24*	4	4	—
Taurine*	2	7	—	—
Cysteine*	<2**	—	—	<2
pH	5–6	5.4	5.3	6.5

*Possibly essential in the premature.
†Includes 7 mg tyrosine and 17 mg as N-acetyl-L-tyrosine.
‡Cysteine HCl may be added at 40 mg/g of amino acids.

(Adapted from AHFS Drug Information, American Society of Hospital Pharmacists, 1989.)

abnormal aminogram, and an increased risk of infection. The amino acids, in particular tryptophan, are postulated to play a primary role in PN-related liver disease (Merritt 1984, 1986).

CARBOHYDRATE

Carbohydrate as glucose is essential in PN to maintain glucose homeostasis and to provide energy. The concentration of glucose usually starts at D5 per cent in the infant weighing more than 1000 g and D10 per cent in larger infants. The concentration of glucose may be advanced in increments of 2.5 per cent on a daily basis, usual maximum concentration of D12.5 per cent in peripheral and D25 per cent in central lines. Glucose tolerance should be monitored by blood micromethods and urine dipstick for glucose. The blood glucose should be maintained between 40 and 150 mg/dl by adjusting the rate of glucose infusion. Predisposing factors for glucose intolerance and hyperglycemia include prematurity (particularly infants weighing < 1000 g), sepsis, respiratory disease, and intravenous lipid infusion. Complications of hyperglycemia include osmotic diuresis and dehydration. If persistent hyperglycemia limits adequate energy intake to establish weight gain, then insulin may be given by continuous intravenous infusion (Binder et al., 1989; Ostertag et al., 1986; Vaucher et al., 1982) or by subcutaneous injection (Pildes, 1986). Usually no more than 20 grams/kg/day of glucose is needed, provided intravenous lipids are also given. Excessive carbohydrate infusion may contribute to PN cholestasis, and it also complicates respiratory disease by causing excessive CO_2 production and O_2 consumption (Sauer et al., 1986).

FAT

The development of safe intravenous lipid solutions was an important advance in the science of total PN. In contrast to the frequent and severe allergic and hematologic complications that were seen with an earlier cottonseed oil preparation, current soybean and combined soybean/safflower products can generally be administered with few complications. Intravenous fat products are triglyceride emulsions stabilized by the addition of egg phospholipid, resulting in artificial chylomicrons, whose metabolism is similar to naturally occurring chylomicrons. The chylomicrons of infused lipids are hydrolyzed by

lipoprotein lipase and hepatic lipase releasing free fatty acids, which are then available for oxidation in tissues or synthesis of stored triglyceride in fat. Circulating free fatty acids are bound to albumin. They may be cleared by the liver and oxidized or incorporated into lipoproteins. Although concurrent heparin and lipid infusion increases plasma lipolytic activity and free fatty acid levels, the metabolism of triglyceride and free fatty acid is limited in premature infants and in infants who are small for gestational age (Andrew et al., 1976; Spear et al., 1988). The composition and osmolality of available products are summarized in Table 75–8. Both 10 and 20 per cent lipid emulsions are available. The 20 per cent emulsions are particularly useful for fluid-restricted infants. Currently marketed products are high in linoleic acid, which is an essential nutrient. Without a source of linoleic acid, the premature infant develops biochemical evidence of essential fatty acid deficiency (triene/tetraene ratio >0.4, presence of 5,8,11-eicosatrienoic acid) in several days (Friedman et al., 1976). A minimum of 2 to 4 per cent of an infant's calories should be provided as linoleic acid in order to prevent or reverse clinical and biochemical evidence of essential fatty acid deficiency, and this is achieved with about 0.5 to 1.0 g/kg/day of intravenous lipids (Cooke et al., 1987, Farrell et al., 1988). There are limited data suggesting that linolenic acid may also be essential in the human (Anderson and Connor, 1989, Holman 1982). For this reason consideration should be given to using only preparations containing both linoleic and linolenic acid (Byrne, 1982).

Intravenous lipid solutions may be given through a peripheral or central venous line via a Y or T connector, distal to the filter. It may also be admixed directly with the amino acid/glucose solution. Although an admixture of lipids and amino acid/glucose solutions is widely used in adults, experience in pediatric patients, particularly in the newborn, is limited. The usual starting dose for intravenous lipid administration in the newborn is 0.5 to 1.0 g/kg/day, advancing by 0.5 g/kg/day increments to a maximum of 3 g/kg/day. Since bolus administration is associated with hypertriglyceridemia, intravenous lipid should be administered by continuous infusion at a rate of ≤ 0.15 g/kg/hr over 18 to 24 hours (Gustafson et al., 1974; Kao et al., 1984).

Intravenous lipid infusion can have adverse effects on several organ systems (Stahl et al., 1986). Vileisis and associates (1982) demonstrated a glycemic response with lipid infusion, which generally is mild and does not limit

TABLE 75–8. Composition of Intravenous Fat Emulsions

	INTRALIPID (KABIVITRUM)	LIPOSYN II (ABBOTT)	SOYACAL (ALPHA THERAPEUTIC)
Source	Soybean	Soybean/safflower	Soybean
Egg phospholipid	1.2%	1.2%	1.2%
Glycerin	2.25%	2.5%	2.21%
Fatty acids			
Linoleic	50%	65.8%	49 to 60%
Oleic	26%	17.7%	21 to 26%
Palmitic	10%	8.8%	9 to 13%
Linolenic	9%	4.2%	6 to 9%
Stearic	3.5%	3.4%	3 to 5%
Calories (kcal/ml)			
10%	1.1	1.1	1.1
20%	2.0	2.0	2.0

(Adapted from AHFS Drug Information, American Society of Hospital Pharmacists, 1989.)

fat or glucose intake. The infusion of IV lipid is associated with a rise in total cholesterol, triglycerides, phospholipids, and free fatty acids, often resulting in hyperlipidemia. Low-density lipoproteins also rise and lipoprotein X appears. Preliminary data show that there is a greater rise in triglycerides, total cholesterol, phospholipids, low-density lipoproteins, and lipoprotein X with the use of 10 per cent intravenous lipid than with 20 per cent intravenous lipid, and that this is due to the higher phospholipid/triglyceride ratio in the 10 per cent preparations (Haumont et al., 1988, Tashiro et al., 1989). Despite these abnormalities, the metabolism of high-density lipoproteins improves during PN with intravenous lipid (Forte et al., 1988). Whether the occurrence of hyperlipidemia early in life increases the risk for atherosclerosis later in life is unknown. In order to prevent hyperlipidemia and its complications, intravenous lipid administration should be closely monitored. Since serum turbidity and nephelometry have been shown to be poor predictors of hyperlipidemia (D'Harlingue et al., 1983; Schreiner et al., 1979), triglycerides and cholesterol should be measured. It is recommended to maintain the plasma triglyceride levels less than 150 mg/dl and total cholesterol less than 200 mg/dl. Free fatty acids compete with bilirubin for binding to albumin. A molar ratio of free fatty acids to bilirubin of greater than 6:1 causes displacement of bilirubin from albumin and may increase the risk for kernicterus in jaundiced newborns. Intravenous lipid should be discontinued when the serum bilirubin approaches a level at which exchange transfusion would be considered. Infants with only mild jaundice tolerate 2 g/kg/day of lipid without a significant increase in the unbound bilirubin (Spear et al., 1988).

Lipid infusion with marked hypertriglyceridemia may result in the fat overload syndrome characterized by thrombocytopenia and disseminated intravascular coagulation (Heyman et al., 1981). Although thrombocytopenia is uncommon with intravenous lipid administration (Cohen et al., 1977; Kerner et al., 1983), it has been reported (Lipson et al., 1974; Goulet et al., 1986), but most cases of neonatal thrombocytopenia are due to causes other than intravenous lipid administration (Castle et al., 1986). Since essential fatty acid deficiency causes platelet dysfunction (Friedman et al., 1977), parenteral fat should not be withheld in infants with thrombocytopenia unless there is marked hypertriglyceridemia or coagulation abnormalities. If thrombocytopenia persists and other causes are not identified, a trial period off intravenous lipid administration may then be warranted.

At autopsy, Friedman and colleagues (1978) and others reported the deposition of fat globules in the pulmonary vasculature of newborns who had received intravenous lipid. Subsequent reports suggested that such findings were postmortem artifacts (Hertel et al., (1982), but this theory remains controversial (Shulman et al., 1987). Lipid infusion can cause a block in the pulmonary diffusion of oxygen and a decrease in PaO_2 (Pereira et al., 1980). These factors may not be clinically significant with slow continuous infusion over 24 hours (Brans et al., 1986). Teague and co-workers (1987) demonstrated in lambs that lipid infusion results in a dose-related increase in pulmonary artery pressure and lung lymph flow due to an increase in thromboxane B_2. This mechanism may be responsible for the finding of an increased rate of pulmo-

nary morbidity with the early use of intravenous lipid in premature infants with respiratory distress syndrome (Hammerman and Aramburo, 1988). Although some studies suggest that lipids in vitro impair neutrophil function, neutrophils from newborns treated with intravenous lipid have normal function (Usmani et al., 1988).

Lipid infusion is associated with *Malassezia furfur* infection. Symptoms generally resolve after removing the central venous catheter and discontinuing the administration of lipids (Azimi et al., 1988).

Carnitine is important to fat metabolism as a cofactor for transport of long chain fatty acids into mitochondria for oxidation. Carnitine is synthesized in the liver and kidney from the essential amino acids lysine and methionine. The newborn has low plasma and tissue levels and poorly developed biosynthetic capabilities, resulting in a low plasma level (Borum, 1983). Infants receiving prolonged total PN develop evidence of carnitine deficiency. Although supplementation with carnitine during lipid infusion has been recommended, it is not clear whether it is truly required or beneficial (Schmidt-Sommerfeld et al., 1983; Orzali et al., 1984.). Intravenous carnitine supplementation remains experimental at this time.

CALCIUM, PHOSPHORUS, AND MAGNESIUM

It is recommended that calcium gluconate rather than calcium chloride be used in neonatal PN. Phosphorus may be given as sodium or potassium phosphate; magnesium may be given as its sulfate salt. The amount of calcium and phosphorus provided in parenteral solutions is limited primarily by their solubility, which is affected by amino acid concentration and pH. Up to 400 mg of calcium gluconate and 1 mmole of phosphorus (31 mg) per 100 ml will generally stay in solution in the presence of 2 per cent amino acids, but reference should be made to solubility curves specific to the amino acid source (Fitzgerald and McKay, 1986; Poole et al., 1983). Since a number of other factors also affect the calcium phosphorus solubility product, all total PN solutions should be visually inspected for precipitate prior to administration.

Table 75–6 lists the recommended intravenous intake of calcium, phosphorus, and magnesium. Calcium and phosphorus deficiency causes osteopenia, rickets, and fractures. Calcium deficiency results from inadequate intake or excessive losses in the urine. Hypercalciuria occurs with furosemide therapy, inadequate phosphorus intake, glucosuria, and high vitamin D intake. Excessive calcium intake may result in hypercalcemia with central nervous system and renal toxicity. Deficiency of phosphorus not only results in bone demineralization, but extreme hypophosphatemia leads to muscle paralysis and respiratory failure. Hyperphosphatemia due to excessive loading of phosphorus causes hypocalcemic tetany and secondary hypoparathyroidism. Magnesium is incorporated into bone and is a cofactor in many enzymatic reactions. Hypermagnesemia causes central nervous system depression; hypomagnesemia is associated with seizures.

ZINC, COPPER AND OTHER TRACE MINERALS

The recommendations of the AMA Nutrition Advisory Group (Shils et al., 1979) and the American Society for

TABLE 75–9. Recommended Doses of Parenteral Trace Minerals (mcg/kg/day)

	AMA(NAG)	ASCN
Zinc		
Premature	300	400
Term	100	250 <3 mo
		100 >3 mo
Copper	20	20
Manganese	2 to 10	1
Chromium	0.14 to 0.2	0.2
Selenium	—	2
Molybdenum	—	0.25
Iodide	—	1

AMA (NAG), American Medical Association Nutrition Advisory Group; ASCN, American Society for Clinical Nutrition.

(Data from Shils, M. E., Burke, A. W., Greene, H. L., et al.: Guidelines for essential trace element preparation for parenteral use: A statement by an expert panel, AMA Department of Foods and Nutrition. J.A.M.A. *241*:2051–2054; and Greene, H. L., Hambridge, K. M., Schanler, R. and Tsang, R. C.: Guidelines for the use of vitamins, trace elements, calcium, magnesium, and phosphorus in infants and children receiving total parenteral nutrition; Report of the Subcommittee on Pediatric Parenteral Nutrient Requirements from the Committee on Clinical Practice Issues of the American Society for Clinical Nutrition. Am. J. Clin. Nutr. *48*:1324:1342, 1988.)

Clinical Nutrition (Greene et al., 1988) for trace mineral supplementation are summarized in Table 75–9. Currently, zinc, copper, manganese, and chromium are supplied in most trace mineral solutions for PN. Also, there is inherent trace mineral contamination in the additives used for PN solutions. Owing to the very limited data available on supplementation of selenium, molybdenum, and iodine, it may be prudent to consider supplementation of these trace minerals only in patients requiring more than 2 months of total PN. In the presence of significant cholestatic jaundice, copper and manganese should be removed from the PN solution, because these elements are excreted by the liver and are potentially hepatotoxic. Selenium, chromium, and molybdenum are excreted by the kidneys and should be deleted in patients with renal failure. Aluminum is not an essential trace element, but it heavily contaminates PN solution primarily via the added calcium gluconate. Aluminum may contribute to metabolic bone disease and PN-associated osteopenia (Koo and Kaplan, 1988).

Prior to the routine supplementation of trace minerals, zinc and copper deficiency were a common complication during PN. If recommended doses of copper and zinc are provided, then symptomatic deficiency of these minerals is only likely to occur if there are excessive losses (see also Chapter 76).

VITAMIN SUPPLEMENTATION

The AMA Nutrition Advisory Group (1979) recommendations for vitamin supplementation in PN are summarized in Table 75–10. Currently, only one PN-specific multivitamin supplement for pediatric patients is marketed in the United States, MVI-Pediatric (Armour) (Table 75–10). This preparation has been studied in newborns and is generally safe and efficacious (Greene et al., 1987). The manufacturer recommends a dose of 30 per cent, 65 per cent, and 100 per cent of a vial (5 ml) for infants weighing less than 1 kg, 1 to 3 kg, and more than 3 kg, respectively. Greene and associates (1988) recommended a dose of 40 per cent of a vial/kg of MVI-Pediatric. However, owing to binding to intravenous tubing, delivery of vitamin A (retinol) in MVI-Pediatric is inadequate. Addition of MVI-Pediatric to intravenous lipids results in better delivery of retinol (Baeckert et al., 1988; Greene et al., 1987), but further investigation is needed. MVI-Pediatric contains vitamin K, so this vitamin does not need to be supplemented separately. Vitamin E levels were readily maintained within the range of 0.5 to 3.0 mg/dl for premature infants weighing less than 1 kg and those weighing more than 1 kg given 50 per cent and 65 per cent of a vial, respectively (Phillips et al., 1987). The amounts of some water-soluble vitamins in MVI-Pediatric may be excessive for premature infants (Greene et al., 1988), but toxicity has not been reported (see also Chapter 76).

PERIPHERAL VERSUS CENTRAL PARENTERAL NUTRITION

Table 75–6 lists maintenance requirements and recommended solutions for peripheral and central parenteral nutrition. The peripheral route is suitable for short-term PN (1 to 2 weeks) for infants who can tolerate up to 150

TABLE 75–10. Composition of MVI-Pediatric (Armour) and Recommended Intake of Parenteral Vitamins

VITAMIN	MVI-PEDIATRIC (VIAL)	AMA(NAG), ASCN (Dose/kg/day for Term Infants)	ASCN* (Dose/kg/day for Premature Infants)
A (mcg)	700	700	500
D (IU)	400	400	160
E, alpha tocopherol (mg)	7	7	2.8
K (mcg)	200	200	80
Ascorbic acid (mg)	80	80	25
Thiamin (mg)	1.2	1.2	0.35
Riboflavin (mg)	1.4	1.4	0.15
Pyridoxine (mg)	1	1	0.18
Niacin (mg)	17	17	6.8
Pantothenate (mg)	5	5	2
Biotin (mcg)	20	20	6
Folate (mcg)	140	140	56
B$_{12}$ (mcg)	1	1	0.3

*ASCN recommends a dose of 40 per cent of a vial of MVI-Pediatric/kg/day for premature infants pending the availability of a new formulation that meets the ASCN recommendations.

AMA(NAG), American Medical Association Nutrition Advisory Group; ASCN, American Society for Clinical Nutrition.

ml/kg/day of fluid. There are few complications of peripheral PN. Since hyperosmolality may cause phlebitis and intravenous infiltration may result in tissue injury, the osmolality of peripheral PN solutions should be less than or equal to 900 mOsm/l (AAPCON 1983). For the VLBW premature infant, repeated needle sticks for intravenous access can be very stressful and may compromise cardiopulmonary status. No more than 12.5 per cent glucose, 2 per cent amino acids, and 400 mg/dl calcium gluconate should be given by peripheral vein. Central total PN is preferred for the provision of long-term PN in critically ill newborns because it allows the delivery of hyperosmolar solutions into large veins. The catheter tip preferably should be placed in the superior vena cava, but the subclavian, innominate, or inferior vena cava are acceptable. If the catheter tip is in the right atrium, there is a risk for cardiac perforation and tamponade. Catheter material of low thrombogenicity is preferred (e.g., Silastic). Techniques that have been useful in the newborn include percutaneous Silastic catheters and the Broviac catheter. Glucose concentrations may be routinely increased to 20 per cent, and amino acids may be increased to 3 per cent in central lines. Higher concentrations should be used with caution because of the risk for central vein thrombosis.

COMPLICATIONS

Many of the complications of PN are catheter related (Table 75–11). In some cases of catheter-related bacterial sepsis (particularly with *Staphylococcus epidermidis*), the infection can be treated with antibiotics alone, without removal of the central line. Infections due to *Staphylococcus aureus, Candida,* and *Malassezia furfur* require removal of central catheters. The incidence of sepsis with surgically placed central venous catheters is 10 to 15 per cent. However, recent experience with percutaneous Silastic central catheters provides evidence of infection rates of only 1 per cent (Lefrak et al., 1984). Ziegler and associates (1980) found a 9 per cent and a 20 per cent incidence of combined vascular and infectious complications with peripheral and central PN, respectively. However, the incidence of complications per patient day was no different between the groups. Vascular perforation, thrombosis, and superior vena cava syndrome are infrequent but major complications of central PN. Umbilical artery catheters have been used to administer PN (Hall and Rhodes 1976), but central venous catheters are preferred over this method. A controversial route of administration is the use of umbilical vein catheters positioned in the inferior vena cava or right atrium. Provided an umbilical vein catheter is not used for blood sampling, it may be used for central PN for a short period of time with a low risk of infection (Ewing and Durand, 1989).

MONITORING

In monitoring PN, the goals are to prevent complications and to assess the efficacy of the therapy. Guidelines for monitoring are provided in Table 75–12. Despite the problems of water balance in sick newborns, change in body weight is the single most useful parameter to monitor to assess growth during the administration of PN. For premature infants, the goal is to achieve postnatal weight

TABLE 75–11. Complications of Parenteral Nutrition

COMPLICATIONS RELATED TO CATHETER INSERTION AND USE
Thrombosis
Superior vena cava syndrome
Perforation of central vessels
Infiltration with tissue injury
Pneumothorax
Hydrothorax and hemothorax
Hydro-pericardium and hemopericardium
Catheter sepsis

METABOLIC COMPLICATIONS
Electrolyte imbalance
Hypoglycemia and hyperglycemia
Abnormal plasma aminogram
Hyperammonemia
Azotemia
Hyperchloremic metabolic acidosis
Hyperlipidemia
Essential fatty acid deficiency
Osteopenia
Cholestatic liver disease
Trace mineral deficiencies
Vitamin deficiencies

HEMATOLOGIC COMPLICATIONS
Thrombocytopenia
Fat overload syndrome/DIC
Bilirubin displacement from albumin
Iron deficiency anemia

PULMONARY COMPLICATIONS
Oxygen diffusion block
Lipid deposition
Pulmonary artery hypertension
Malassezia furfur vasculitis

gain comparable with the intrauterine growth rate. Although more difficult to measure reliably, head circumference and length should be measured weekly. Triceps skinfold thickness and the midarm circumference/head circumference ratio have been used for nutritional assessment, but these measurements are difficult to perform reliably in the newborn. Measurement of rapid-turnover serum proteins (retinol-binding protein, prealbumin, and

TABLE 75–12. Monitoring of Neonatal Total Parenteral Nutrition

MEASUREMENT	BASELINE AND 1st WEEK	AFTER 1st WEEK
Weight	daily	daily
HC, length	weekly	weekly
Fluid (cc/kg/day)	daily	daily
Calories (kcal/kg/day)	daily	daily
Hemogram/Hct	2 to 3 times/week	weekly
Platelet count	weekly	weekly
Na, K, Cl, CO_2	daily	2 to 3 times week
Blood glucose*	3 or more/day	daily or more often
Urine glucose (dipstick)	3 or more/day	daily or more often
Calcium	daily	1 to 2 times week
Phosphorus	1 to 2 times/week	weekly
Magnesium	weekly	weekly
Total protein, albumin	weekly	weekly
BUN, creatinine	1 to 2 times/week	weekly
Direct bilirubin	weekly	weekly
SGOT or SGPT	weekly	weekly
Alkaline phosphatase	weekly	weekly
Triglyceride	weekly	weekly
Cholesterol	weekly	weekly
Ammonia	prn lethargy	prn lethargy
Zinc, copper	monthly	monthly

*Micromethods are suitable.

transferrin) may be more useful than serum albumin for nutritional assessment during the administration of PN.

■ REFERENCES

American Academy of Pediatrics,Committee on Drugs: Transfer of drugs and other chemicals into human milk. Pediatrics 84:924–936, 1989.

American Academy of Pediatrics, Committee on Nutrition (AAPCON): Nutritional needs of low-birth-weight infants. Pediatrics 60:519–530, 1977.

American Academy of Pediatrics, Committee on Nutrition (AAPCON): Soy-protein formulas: Recommendations for use in infant feeding. Pediatrics 72:359–363, 1983.

American Academy of Pediatrics, Committee on Nutrition (AAPCON): Commentary on parenteral nutrition. Pediatrics 71:547–552, 1983.

American Academy of Pediatrics, Committee on Nutrition (AAPCON): Nutritional needs of low-birth-weight infants. Pediatrics 75:976–986, 1985.

American Academy of Pediatrics, Committee on Nutrition (AAPCON): Fluoride supplementation. Pediatrics 77:758–761, 1986.

American Medical Association, Department of Foods and Nutrition: Multivitamin preparations for parenteral use: A statement by the Nutrition Advisory Group. J.P.E.N. 3:258–265, 1979.

Anderson G. J., and Connor W. E.: On the demonstration of ω–3 essential-fatty-acid deficiency in humans. Am. J. Clin. Nutr. 49:585–587, 1989.

Anderson, T. L., Muttart, C. R., Bieger, M. A., et al.: A controlled trial of glucose versus glucose and amino acids in premature infants. J. Pediatr. 94:947–951, 1979.

Andrew, G., Chan, G., and Schiff, D.: Lipid metabolism in the neonate. J. Pediatr. 88:273–278, 1976.

Asquith, M. T., Pedrotti, P. W., Stevenson, D. K., and Sunshine, P.: Clinical uses, collection, and banking of human milk. Clin. Perinatol. 14:173–185, 1987.

Atkinson, S. A., Radde, I. C., and Anderson, G. H.: Macromineral balances in premature infants fed their own mothers' milk or formula. J. Pediatr. 102:99–106, 1983.

Aynsley-Green, A.: Hormones and postnatal adaptation to enteral nutrition. J. Pediatr. Gastroenterol. Nutr. 2:418–427, 1983.

Azimi, P. H., Levernier, K., Lefrak, L. M., et al.: Malassezia furfur: A cause of occlusion of percutaneous central venous catheters in infants in the intensive care nursery. Pediatr. Infect. Dis. J. 7:100–103, 1988.

Babson, S. G., and Bramhall, J. L.: Diet and growth in the premature infant: The effect of different dietary intakes of ash-electrolyte and protein on weight gain and linear growth. J. Pediatr. 74:890–900, 1969.

Bach, A. C., and Babayan, V. K.: Medium-chain triglycerides: An update. Am. J. Clin. Nutr. 36:950–962, 1982.

Baeckert, P. A., Greene, H. L., Fritz, I., et al.: Vitamin concentrations in very low birth weight infants given vitamins intravenously in a lipid emulsion: Measurement of vitamins A, D, and E and riboflavin. J. Pediatr. 113:1057–1065, 1988.

Bell, E. F., Brown, E. J., Milner, R., et al.: Vitamin E absorption in small premature infants. Pediatrics 63:830–832, 1979.

Berg, R. B., Schuster, S. R., and Colodny, A. H.: The use of gastrostomy in feeding premature infants. Pediatrics 33:287–289, 1964.

Bhatia, J., and Fomon, S. J.: Formulas for premature infants: Fate of the calcium and phosphorus. Pediatrics 72:37–40, 1983.

Binder, N. D., and Raschko, P. K., Benda, G. I., and Reynolds, J. W.: Insulin infusion with parenteral nutrition in extremely low birth weight infants with hyperglycemia. J. Pediatr. 114:273–280, 1989.

Borum, P. R.: Carnitine. Am. Rev. Nutr. 3:233, 1983.

Boros, S. J., and Reynolds, J. W.: Duodenal perforation: A complication of neonatal nasojejunal feeding. J. Pediatr. 85:107–108, 1975.

Brans, Y. W., Dutton, E. B., Andrew, D. S., et al.: Fat emulsion tolerance in very low birth weight neonates: Effect on diffusion of oxygen in the lungs and on blood pH. Pediatr. 78:79–84, 1986.

Briggs, G. G., Freeman, R. K., and Yaffe, S. J.: Drugs in Pregnancy and Lactation. 3rd ed., Baltimore, MD, Williams & Wilkins, 1990.

Butte, N. F., Garza, C., Smith, O., and Nichols, B. L.: Human milk intake and growth in exclusively breast fed infants. J. Pediatr. 104:187–195, 1984.

Byrne, W. J.: Intralipid or Liposyn-comparable products? (Editorial.) J. Pediatr. Gastroenterol. Nutr. 1:7–8, 1982.

Castle, V., Andrew, M., Kelton, J., et al.: Frequency and mechanism of neonatal thrombocytopenia. J. Pediatr. 108:749–755, 1986.

Chan, G. M., Mileur, L., and Hansen, J. W.: Effects of increased calcium and phosphorous formulas and human milk on bone mineralization in preterm infants. J. Pediatr. Gastroenterol. Nutr. 5:444–449, 1986.

Chaney, N. E., Franke, J., and Wadlington, W. B.: Cocaine convulsions in a breast-feeding baby. J. Pediatr. 112:134–135, 1988.

Chasnoff, I. J., Lewis, D. E., and Squires, L.: Cocaine intoxication in a breast-fed infant. Pediatrics 80:836–838, 1987.

Cheek, J. A., and Staub, G. F.: Nasojejunal alimentation for premature and full-term newborn infants. J. Pediatr. 82:955–962, 1973.

Chen, J. W., and Wong, P. W.: Intestinal complications of nasojejunal feeding in low-birth-weight infants. J. Pediatr. 85:109–110, 1975.

Churella, H. R., Bachhuber, W. L., and MacLean, W. C. Jr: Survey: Methods of feeding low-birth-weight infants. Pediatrics 76:243–249, 1985.

Cohen, I. T., Dahms, B., and Hays, D. M.: Peripheral total parenteral nutrition employing a lipid emulsion (Intralipid): Complications encountered in pediatric patients. J. Pediatr. Surg. 12:837–845, 1977.

Cooke, R. J., Whitington, P. F., and Kelts, D.: Effect of taurine supplementation on hepatic function during short-term parenteral nutrition in the premature infant. J. Pediatr. Gastroenterol. Nutr. 3:234–238, 1984.

Cooke, R. J., Yeh, Y., Gibson, D., et al.: Soybean oil emulsion administration during parenteral nutrition in the preterm infant: Effect on essential fatty acid, lipid, and glucose metabolism. J. Pediatr. 111:767–773, 1987.

D'Harlingue, A., Hopper, O., Stevenson, D. K., et al.: Limited value of nephelometry in monitoring the administration of intravenous fat in neonates. J.P.E.N. 7:55–58, 1983.

Davidson, M., Levine, S. Z., Bauer, C. H., and Dann, M.: Feeding studies in low-birth-weight infants: I. Relationships of dietary protein, fat, and electrolyte to rates of weight gain, clinical courses, and serum chemical concentrations. J. Pediatr. 70:695–713, 1967.

De Carvalho, M., Klaus, M. H., and Merkatz, R. B.: Frequency of breast-feeding and serum bilirubin concentration. Am. J. Dis. Child. 136:737–738, 1982.

Dunn, L., Hulman, S., Weiner, J., and Kliegman, R.: Beneficial effects of early hypocaloric enteral feeding on neonatal gastrointestinal function: Preliminary report of a randomized trial. J. Pediatr. 112:622–629, 1988.

European Society of Paediatric Gastroenterology and Nutrition, Committee on Nutrition of the Preterm Infant: Acta Paediatr. Scand. (Suppl). 336:1–14, 1987.

Ewing, C. K., and Durand, D. J.: Use of umbilical venous catheters: A study of 100 patients. Pediatr. Res. 25:214A, 1989.

Farrell, P. M., Gutcher, G. R., Palta, M., and DeMets, D.: Essential fatty acid deficiency in premature infants. Am. J. Clin. Nutr. 48:220–229, 1988.

Fitzgerald, K. A., and MacKay, M. W.: Calcium and phosphate solubility in neonatal parenteral nutrient solutions containing Trophamine. Am. J. Hosp. Pharm. 43:88–93, 1986.

Forte, T. M., Genzel-Boroviczeny, O., Austin, M. A., et al.: Effect of total parenteral nutrition with intravenous fat on lipids and high density lipoprotein heterogeneity in neonates. JPEN, 13:490, 1989.

Friedman, Z., Danon, A., Stahlman, M. T., and Oates, J. A.: Rapid onset of essential fatty acid deficiency in the newborn. Pediatrics 58:640–649, 1976.

Friedman, Z., Lamberth, E. L., Stahlman, M. T., and Oates, J. A.: Platelet dysfunction in the neonate with essential fatty acid deficiency. J. Pediatr. 90:439–443, 1977.

Friedman, Z., Marks, K. H., Maisels, M. J., et al.: Effect of parenteral fat emulsion on the pulmonary and reticuloendothelial systems in the newborn infant. Pediatrics 61:694–698, 1978.

Gaull, G. E.: Taurine in pediatric nutrition: Review and update. Pediatrics 83:433–442, 1989.

Geggel, H. S., Ament, M. E., Heckenlively, J. R., et al.: Nutritional requirement for taurine in patients receiving long-term parenteral nutrition. N. Engl. J. Med. 312:142–146, 1985.

Goldman, H. L., Goldman, J. S., Kaufman, I., Liebman, O. B.: Late effects of early dietary protein intake on low-birth-weight infants. J. Pediatr. 85:764–769, 1974.

Goulet, O., Girot, R., Maier-Redelsperger, M., et al.: Hematologic disorders following prolonged use of intravenous fat emulsions in children. J.P.E.N. 10:284–288, 1986.

Greene, H. L., Moore, M. C., Phillips, B., et al.: Evaluation of a pediatric multiple vitamin preparation for total parenteral nutrition. II. Blood levels of vitamins A, D and E. Pediatrics 77:539–547, 1986.

Greene, H. L., Phillips, B. L., Franck, L., et al.: Persistently low blood retinol levels during and after parenteral feeding of very low birth weight infants: Examination of losses into intravenous administration sets and a method of prevention by addition of a lipid emulsion. Pediatrics 79:894–900, 1987.

Greene, H. L., Hambidge, K. M., Schanler, R., and Tsang, R. C.: Guidelines for the use of vitamins, trace elements, calcium, magnesium, and phosphorus in infants and children receiving total parenteral nutrition: Report of the Subcommittee on Pediatric Parenteral Nutrient Requirements from the Committee on Clinical Practice Issues of the American Society for Clinical Nutrition. Am. J. Clin. Nutr. 48:1324–1342, 1988.

Greer, F. R., Steichen, J. J., and Tsang, R. C.: Effects of increased calcium, phosphorus, and vitamin D intake on bone mineralization in very-low-birth-weight infants fed formulas with Polycose and medium-chain triglycerides. J. Pediatr. 100:951–955, 1982.

Greer, F. R., and Tsang, R. C.: Calcium, phosphorus, magnesium, and vitamin D requirements for the preterm infant. In Tsang, R. C. (Ed.), Vitamin and Mineral Requirements in Preterm Infants. New York, Marcel Dekker, Inc., 1985.

Gross, S. J., David, R. J., Bauman, L., and Tomarelli, R. M.: Nutritional composition of milk produced by mothers delivering preterm. J. Pediatr. 96:641–644, 1980.

Gross, S. J.: Growth and biochemical response of preterm infants fed human milk or modified infant formula. N. Engl. J. Med. 308:237–241, 1983.

Grossman, H., Duggan, E., McCamman, S., et al.: The dietary chloride deficiency syndrome. Pediatrics 66:366–374, 1980.

Gustafson, A., Kjellmer, I., Olegard, R., and Victorin, L.: Nutrition in low-birth-weight infants. Acta. Paediat. Scand. 63:177–182, 1974.

Hall, R. T., and Rhodes, P. G.: Total parenteral alimentation via indwelling umbilical catheters in the newborn period. Arch. Dis. Child. 51:929–934, 1976.

Hammerman, C., and Aramburo, M. J.: Decreased lipid intake reduces morbidity in sick premature neonates. J. Pediatr. 113:1083–1088, 1988.

Hamosh, M., Bitman, J., Liao, T. H., et al.: Gastric lipolysis and fat absorption in preterm infants: Effect of medium-chain triglyceride or long-chain triglyceride-containing formulas. Pediatrics 83:86–92, 1989.

Haumont, D., Deckelbaum, R. J., Richelle, M., et al.: Phospholipid content of lipid emulsions determines plasma lipids and lipoproteins in low birth weight infants. Pediatr. Res. 23:304A, 1988.

Heird, W. C., Dell, R. B., Helms, R. A., et al.: Amino acid mixture designed to maintain normal plasma amino acid patterns in infants and children requiring parenteral nutrition. Pediatrics 80:401–408, 1987.

Heird, W. C., Hay, W., Helms, R. A., et al.: Pediatric parenteral amino acid mixture in low birth weight infants. Pediatrics 81:41–50, 1988.

Heldt, G. P.: The effect of gavage feeding on the mechanics of the lung, chest wall, and diaphragm of preterm infants. Pediatr. Res. 24:55–58, 1988.

Helms, R. A., Christensen M. L., Mauer E. C., and Storm M. C.: Comparison of a pediatric versus standard amino acid formulation in preterm neonates requiring parenteral nutrition. J. Pediatr. 110:466–470, 1987.

Hertel J., Tygstrup, I., and Andersen, G. E.: Intravascular fat accumulation after Intralipid infusion in the very low-birth-weight infants. J. Pediatr. 100:975–976, 1982.

Heyman, M. B., Storch, S., and Ament, M. E.: The fat overload syndrome. Am. J. Dis. Child. 135:628–630, 1981.

Higashi, A., Ikeda, T., and Matsuda, I.: Zinc balance in premature infants given the minimal dietary zinc requirement. J. Pediatr. 112:262–266, 1988.

Hittner, H. M., Godio, L. B., Rudolph, A. J., et al.: Retrolental fibroplasia: Efficacy of vitamin E in a double-blind clinical study of preterm infants. N. Engl. J. Med. 305:1365–1371, 1981.

Holman, R. T., Johnson, S. B., and Hatch, T. F.: A case of human linolenic acid deficiency involving neurologic abnormalities. Am. J. Clin. Nutr. 35:617–623, 1982.

Huston, R. H., Reynolds, J. W., Jensen, C., and Buist, N. R. M.: Nutrient and mineral retention and vitamin E absorption in low-birth-weight infants: Effect of medium-chain triglycerides. Pediatrics 72:44–48, 1983.

Janas, L. M., Picciano, M. F., and Hatch, T. F.: Indices of protein metabolism in term infants fed human milk, whey-predominant formula or cow's milk formula. Pediatrics 75:775–784, 1985.

Jarvenpaa, A. L., Rassin, D. K., Raiha, N. C. R., and Gaull, G. E.: Milk

protein quantity and quality in the term infant. II. Effects on acidic and neutral amino acids. Pediatrics 70:221–230, 1982.

Jenness R.: The composition of human milk. Semin. Perinatol. 3:225–239, 1979.

Johnson, L., Bowen, F. W., Abbasi, A., et al.: Relationship of prolonged pharmacologic serum levels of vitamin E to incidence of sepsis and necrotizing enterocolitis in infants with birth weight 1500 grams or less. Pediatrics 75:619–638, 1985.

Kao, L. C., Cheng, M. H., and Warburton, D.: Triglycerides, free fatty acids, free fatty acids/albumin molar ratio, and cholesterol levels in serum of neonates receiving long-term lipid infusions: Controlled trial of continuous and intermittent regimens. J. Pediatr. 104:429–435, 1984.

Kashyap, S., Forsyth, M., Zucker, C., et al.: Effects of varying protein and energy intakes on growth and metabolic response in low birth weight infants. J. Pediatr. 108:955–963, 1986.

Kashyap, S., Schulze, K. F., Forsyth, M., et al.: Growth, nutrient retention, and metabolic response in low birth weight infants fed varying intakes of protein and energy. J. Pediatr. 113:713, 1988.

Kerner, B., Sloan, H. R., Lubin, A. H., et al.: The use of intralipid 10% and 20% in very low birthweight premature infants. Acta Chir. Scand. (Suppl.) 517:135–148, 1983.

Kleinman, R. E., and Walker, W. A.: The enteromammary immune system. Dig. Dis. Sci. 24:876–882, 1979.

Koldovsky, O., and Thornburg, W.: Hormones in milk. J. Pediatr. Gastroenterol. Nutr. 6:172–196, 1987.

Koo, W. W. K., and Kaplan, L. A.: Aluminum and bone disorders: With specific reference to aluminum contamination in infant nutrients. J. Am. Coll. Nutr. 7:199–214, 1988.

Krauss, A. N., Brown, J., Waldman, S., et al.: Pulmonary function following feeding in low-birth-weight infants. Am. J. Dis. Child. 132:139–142, 1978.

Krishnan, V., and Satish, M.: Continuous vs. intermittent nasogastric feeding in very low birth weight infants. Pediatr. Res. 15:537, 1981.

Kumar, S. P., and Sacks, L. M.: Hyponatremia in very low birth weight infants and human milk feedings. J. Pediatr. 93:1026–1027, 1978.

Kurzner, S. I., Garg, M., Bautista, D. B., et al.: Growth failure in infants with bronchopulmonary dysplasia: Nutrition and elevated resting metabolic expenditure. Pediatrics 81:379–384, 1988.

LaGamma, E. F., Ostertag, S. G., and Birenbaum, H.: Failure of delayed oral feeding to prevent necrotizing enterocolitis: Results of study in very-low-birth-weight neonates. Am. J. Dis. Child. 139:385–389, 1985.

Lawrence, R. A.: Drugs in breast milk. In Breast Feeding: A Guide for the Medical Profession. St. Louis, MO, C.V. Mosby, 1989, pp. 256–284.

Lebenthal, E., Lee, P. C., and Heitlinger, L. A.: Impact of development of the gastrointestinal tract on infant feeding. J. Pediatr. 102:1–9, 1983.

Lefrak, L. A., Lund, C. H., D'Harlingue, A., et al.: Catheter life, infection rate and complications associated with the use of percutaneously inserted Silastic venous catheters in neonates. Clin. Res. 32:126A, 1984.

Lipson, A. H., Pritchard, J., and Thomas, G.: Thrombocytopenia after Intralipid infusion in a neonate. Lancet 2:1462–1463, 1974.

Lockitch, G., Jacobson, B., Quigley, G., et al.: Selenium deficiency in low birth weight neonates: An unrecognized problem. J. Pediatr. 114:865–870, 1989.

Malloy, M. H., Rassin, D. K., and Richardson, C. J.: Total parenteral nutrition in sick preterm infants: Effects of cysteine supplementation with nitrogen intakes of 240 and 400 mg/kg/day. J. Pediatr. Gastroenterol. Nutr. 3:239–244, 1984.

Martone, W. J., Williams, W. W., Mortensen, M. L., et al.: Illness with fatalities in premature infants: Association with an intravenous vitamin E preparation, E-Ferol. Pediatrics 78:591–600, 1986.

Menkes, J. H., Welcher, D. W., Levi, H. S., et al.: Relationship of elevated blood tyrosine to the ultimate intellectual performance of premature infants. Pediatrics 49:218–224, 1972.

Merritt, R. J., Sinatra, F. R., Henton, D., and Neustein, H.: Cholestatic effect of intraperitoneal administration of tryptophan to suckling rat pups. Pediatr. Res. 18:904–907, 1984.

Merritt, R. J.: Cholestasis associated with total parenteral nutrition. J. Pediatr. Gastroenterol. Nutr. 5:9–22, 1986.

Merritt, R. J., and Hack, S.: Infant feeding and enteral nutrition. Nutr. Clin. Pract. 3:47–64, 1988.

Modanlou, H. D., Lim, M. O., Hansen, J. W., and Sickles, V.: Growth, biochemical status, and mineral metabolism in very-low-birth-weight infants receiving fortified preterm human milk. J. Pediatr. Gastroenterol. Nutr. 5:762–767, 1986.

Mollitt, D. L., Golladay, E. S., and Seibert, J. J.: Symptomatic gastroesophageal reflux following gastrostomy in neurologically impaired patients. Pediatrics 75:1124–1126, 1985.

Moore, M. C., Greene, H. L., Phillips, B., et al.: Evaluation of a pediatric multiple vitamin preparation for total parenteral nutrition in infants and children. I. Blood levels of water-soluble vitamins. Pediatrics 77:530–538, 1986.

Orzali, A., Maetzke, G., Donzelli, F., and Rubaltelli, F.F.: Effect of carnitine on lipid metabolism in the neonate. II. Carnitine addition to lipid infusion during prolonged total parenteral nutrition. J. Pediatr. 104:436–440, 1984.

Ostertag, S. G., LaGamma, E. F., Reisen, C. E., and Ferrentino, F. L.: Early enteral feeding does not affect the incidence of necrotizing enterocolitis. Pediatrics 77:275–280, 1986.

Ostertag, S. G., Jovnaovic, L., Lewis, B., and Auld, P. A. M.: Insulin pump therapy in the very low birth weight infant. Pediatrics 78:625–630, 1986.

Parker, P., Stroop, S., and Greene, H.: A controlled comparison of continuous versus intermittent feeding in the treatment of infants with intestinal disease. J. Pediatr. 99:360–364, 1981.

Pereira, G. R., Fox, W. W., Stanley, C. A., et al.: Decreased oxygenation and hyperlipemia during intravenous fat infusions in premature infants. Pediatrics 66:26–30, 1980.

Pereira, G. R., and Lemons, J. A.: Controlled study of transpyloric and intermittent gavage feeding in the small preterm infant. Pediatrics 67:68–72, 1981.

Phelps, D. L., Rosenbaum, A. L., Isenberg, S. J., et al.: Tocopherol efficacy and safety for preventing retinopathy of prematurity: A randomized, controlled, double-masked trial. Pediatrics 79:489–500, 1987.

Phillips, B., Franck, L. S., and Greene H. L.: Vitamin E levels in premature infants during and after intravenous multivatimin supplementation. Pediatrics 80:680–683, 1987.

Pildes, R. S.: Neonatal hyperglycemia. J. Pediatr. 109:905–907, 1986.

Poole, R. L., Rupp, C. A., and Kerner, J. A.: Calcium and phosphorus in neonatal parenteral nutrition solutions. J.P.E.N. 7:358–360, 1983.

Powell, G. K.: Milk- and soy-induced enterocolitis of infancy: Clinical features and standardization of challenge. J. Pediatr. 93:553–560, 1978.

Putet, G., Rigo, J., Salle, B., and Senterre, J.: Supplementation of pooled human milk with casein hydrolysate: Energy and nitrogen balance and weight gain composition in very low birth weight infants. Pediatr. Res. 21:458–461, 1987.

Raiha, N. C. R., Heinonen, K., Rassin, D. K., and Gaull, G. E.: Milk protein quantity and quality in low-birthweight infants: I. Metabolic responses and effects on growth. Pediatrics 57:659–674, 1976.

Raiha, N. C. R.: Nutritional proteins in milk and the protein requirement of normal infants. Pediatrics 75(Suppl.):136–141, 1985.

Rassin, D. K., and Gaull, G. E., Raiha, N. C. R., and Heinonen, K.: Milk protein quantity and quality in low-birth-weight infants: IV. Effects on tyrosine and phenylalanine in plasma and urine. J. Pediatr. 90:356–360, 1977.

Reichman, B. L., Chassex, P., Putet, G., et al.: Partition of energy metabolism and energy cost of growth in the very low-birth-weight infant. Pediatrics 69:446–451, 1982.

Rhea, J. W., and Kilby, J. O.: A nasojejunal tube for infant feeding. Pediatrics 46:36–40, 1970.

Ronnholm, K. A. R., Perheentupa, J., and Siimes, M. A.: Supplementation with human milk protein improves growth of small premature infants fed human milk. Pediatrics 77:649–653, 1986.

Roy, C. C., Ste-Marie, M., Chartrand, L., et al.: Correction of the malabsorption of the preterm infant with a medium-chain triglyceride formula. J. Pediatr. 86:446–450, 1975.

Roy, R. N., Pollnitz, R. P., Hamilton, J. R., and Chance, G. W.: Impaired assimilation of nasojejunal feeds in healthy low-birth-weight newborn infants. J. Pediatr. 90:431–434, 1977.

Sauer, P. J. J., Van Aerde, J. E. E., Pencharz, P. B., et al.: Glucose oxidation rates in newborn infants measured with indirect calorimetry and [U-13C] glucose. Clin. Sci. 70:587–593, 1986.

Schanler, R. J., Garza, C., and Nichols, B. L.: Fortified mothers' milk of very low birth weight infants: Results of growth and nutrient balance studies. J. Pediatr. 107:437–445, 1985.

Schmidt-Sommerfeld, E., Penn, D., and Wolf, H.: Carnitine deficiency in premature infants receiving total parenteral nutrition: Effect of L-carnitine supplementation. J. Pediatr. 102:931–935, 1983.

Schreiner, R. L., Glick, M. R., Nordschow, C. D., and Gresham, E. L.: An evaluation of methods to monitor infants receiving intravenous lipids. J. Pediatr. 94:197–200, 1979.

Schulze, K. F., Stefanski, M., Masterson, J., et al.: Energy expenditure, energy balance, and composition of weight gain in low birth weight infants fed diets of different protein and energy content. J. Pediatr. 110:753–759, 1987.

Shaffer, S. G., Bradt, S. K., Meade, V. M., and Hall, R. T.: Extracellular fluid volume change in very low birth weight infants during the first 2 postnatal months. J. Pediatr. 111:124–128, 1987.

Shenai, J. P., Jhaveri, B. M., Reynolds, J. W., et al.: Nutritional balance studies in very low-birth-weight infants: Role of soy formula. Pediatrics 67:631–637, 1981.

Shenai, M. P., Kennedy, K. A., Chytil, F., and Stahlman, M. T.: Clinical trial of vitamin A supplementation in infants susceptible to bronchopulmonary dysplasia. J. Pediatr. 111:269–277, 1987.

Shils, M. E., Burke, A. W., Greene, H. L., et al.: Guidelines for essential trace element preparations for parenteral use: A statement by an expert panel, AMA Department of Foods and Nutrition. J.A.M.A. 241:2051–2054, 1979.

Shulman R. J., DeStefano-Laine L., Petitt R., et al.: Protein deficiency in premature infants receiving parenteral nutrition. Am. J. Clin. Nutr. 44:610–613, 1986.

Shulman, R. J., Langston, C., and Schanler, R. R.: Pulmonary vascular lipid deposition after administration of intravenous fat to infants. Pediatrics 79:99–102, 1987.

Sivasubramanian, K. N., and Henkin, R. I.: Behavioral and dermatologic changes and low serum zinc and copper concentration in two premature infants after parenteral alimentation. J. Pediatr. 93:847–851, 1978.

Slagle, T. A., and Gross, S. J.: Effect of early low-volume enteral substrate on subsequent feeding tolerance in very low birth weight infants. J. Pediatr. 113:526–531, 1988.

Sokol, R. J., Guggenheim, M. A., Heubi, J. E., et al.: Frequency and clinical progression of the vitamin E deficiency neurologic disorder in children with prolonged neonatal cholestasis. Am. J. Dis. Child. 139:121–1215, 1985.

Sondheimer, J. M., and Hamilton, J. R.: Intestinal function in infants with severe congenital heart disease. J. Pediatr. 92:572–578, 1978.

Spear, M. L., Stahl, G. E., Hamosh, M., et al.: Effect of heparin dose and infusion rate on lipid clearance and bilirubin binding in premature infants receiving intravenous fat emulsions. J. Pediatr. 112:94–98, 1988.

Stahl, G. E., Spear, M. L., and Hamosh, M.: Intravenous administration of lipid emulsions to premature infants. Clin. Perinatol. 13:133–162, 1986.

Sutton, A. M., Harvie, A., Cockburn, F., et al.: Copper deficiency in the preterm infant of very low birthweight: Four cases and a reference range for plasma copper. Arch. Dis. Child. 60:644–651, 1985.

Tashiro, T., Sanada, M., Mashina, Y., et al.: Lipoprotein metabolism during TPN with Intralipid 10% vs. 20%. J.P.E.N. 13(Suppl.):7S, 1989.

Teague, W. G. Jr, Raj, J. U., Braun, D., et al.: Lung vascular effects of lipid infusion in awake lambs. Pediatr. Res. 22:714–719, 1987.

Toce, S. S., Keenan, W. J., and Homan, S. M.: Enteral feeding in very-low-birth-weight infants. Am. J. Dis. Child 141:439–444, 1987.

Usmani, S. S., Harper, R. G., and Usmani S. F.: Effect of a lipid emulsion (Intralipid) on polymorphonuclear leukocyte functions in the neonate. J. Pediatr. 113:132–136, 1988.

Valman, H. B., Heath, C. D., and Brown, R. J.: Continuous ingastric milk feeds in infants of low birth weight. Br. Med. J. 3:547–550, 1972.

Van Caille, M., and Powell, G. K.: Nasoduodenal versus nasogastric feeding in the very low birthweight infant. Pediatrics 56:1065–1072, 1975.

Vanderhoof, J. A., Hofschire, P. J., Baluff, M. A., et al.: Continuous enteral feedings: An important adjunct to the management of complex congenital heart disease. Am. J. Dis. Child. 136:825–827, 1982.

Vaucher, Y. E., Walson, P. D., and Morrow, G.: Continuous insulin infusion in hyperglycemic, very low birth weight infants. J. Pediatr. Gastroenterol. Nutr. 1:211–217, 1982.

Vengusamy, S., Pildes, R. S., Raffensperger, J. F., et al.: A controlled study of feeding gastrostomy in low birth weight infants. Pediatrics 43:815–820, 1969.

Vileisis, R. A., Cowett, R. M., and Oh, W.: Glycemic response to lipid infusion in the premature neonate. J. Pediatr. 100:108–112, 1982.

Vinton, N. E., Dahlstrom, K. A., Strobel, C. T., and Ament, M. E.:

Macrocytosis and pseudoalbinism: Manifestations of selenium deficiency. J. Pediatr. *111*:711–717, 1987.

Wells, D. H., and Zachman, R. D.: Nasojejunal feedings in low-birthweight infants. J. Pediatr. *87*:276–279, 1975.

Welsh, J. K., and May, J. T.: Anti-infective properties of breast milk. J. Pediatr. *94*:1–9, 1979.

Whyte, R. K., Campbell, D., Stanhope, R., et al.: Energy balance in low birth weight infants fed formula of high or low medium-chain triglyceride content. J. Pediatr. *108*:964–971, 1986.

Ziegler, E. E., Biga, R. L., and Fomon, S. J. Nutritional requirements for the premature infant. *In* Suskind R.M. (Ed): Textbook of Pediatric Nutrition. New York, Raven Press, 1981, p. 29.

Ziegler, M., Jakobowski, D., Hoelzer, D., et al.: Route of pediatric parenteral nutrition: Proposed criteria revision. J. Pediatr. Surg. *15*:472–476, 1980.

Zlotkin, S. H., Bryan, M. H., and Anderson, G. H.: Intravenous nitrogen and energy intakes required to duplicate in utero nitrogen accretion in prematurely born human infants. J. Pediatr. *99*:115–120, 1981.

Zlotkin, S. H.: Intravenous nitrogen intake requirements in full-term newborns undergoing surgery. Pediatrics *73*:493–496, 1984.

VITAMINS AND TRACE MINERAL DISORDERS 76

Arthur E. D'Harlingue

■ VITAMINS

Clinically recognizable vitamin deficiency in newborns and young infants is rare in the United States and other developed nations in the absence of systemic illness or prematurity. Fetal stores of vitamins are generally sufficient at birth to prevent deficiency symptoms in the immediate postnatal period despite maternal deficiency states. However, the premature infant has lower total tissue stores of water and fat-soluble vitamins than the term infant. In critically ill newborns and premature infants, inadequate nutritional intake may deplete the limited neonatal stores of vitamins, resulting in deficiency. Subclinical deficiencies of vitamins (without overt symptoms) may adversely affect the course of neonatal lung disease, bone mineralization, gastrointestinal development, and retinal differentiation and function. Pharmacologic doses of vitamins are being studied in the prevention or treatment of retinopathy of prematurity, bronchopulmonary dysplasia, and intraventricular hemorrhage. Although some studies have demonstrated beneficial effects from pharmacologic doses of vitamins, results have been inconsistent and complications have been reported. In the attempt to optimally nourish the sick newborn, we must be careful to avoid toxicity and adverse effects due to vitamin therapy. This section of the chapter reviews vitamin requirements, deficiency, and toxicity in infants, with special emphasis on problems seen in the intensive care nursery.

VITAMIN A

Metabolism and Function. Vitamin A refers to several biologically active compounds of which retinol is the most important. Carotenes are a group of provitamins that can be metabolized to retinol. Oxidation of retinol to retinaldehyde is important for the biologic action of vitamin A in the retina. Further oxidation leads to retinoic acid, which can support all the biologic effects of vitamin A except for reproduction and vision. Retinol, which is the most active form of vitamin A, has wide effects in a variety of tissues. It is important in the growth and differentiation of epithelial tissues, including those of the lung, intestine, chondrocytes, retina, and cornea. The mechanism of action of retinol is only well understood in the retina, where retinaldehyde in ultimately incorporated into the visual pigment rhodopsin. Outside the retina the mechanism of vitamin A effects are less clear. After binding to a cellular retinol-binding protein, retinol and retinoic acid can effect changes in nucleic acid metabolism and glycoprotein synthesis (Goodman, 1984).

Retinol is transported across the placenta with retinol-binding protein, resulting in increasing total fetal liver stores of retinyl ester with advancing gestational age. The fetal lung is also high in retinyl esters, which may play a role in perinatal lung development (Zachman et al., 1984). Generally, there is a poor correlation between maternal and cord sera retinol levels. Supplementation of vitamin A to the mother appears to have little effect on cord blood levels unless the mother is vitamin A deficient. With enteral feeding of the infant, dietary carotenes and retinyl esters are converted to free retinol in the intestine by pancreatic and intestinal hydrolases. The free retinol is absorbed by the intestinal mucosal cell, re-esterified, and then released into the lymphatics incorporated into chylomicrons. After clearance from the circulation, retinol is stored primarily in the liver as retinol palmitate. The liver then regulates delivery of retinol to the tissues and serves as a reservoir for body needs. Prior to release into the circulation retinol is bound to retinol-binding protein. Retinol-binding protein is rapidly turned over in the plasma and its synthesis is affected by protein-calorie intake and zinc sufficiency. Retinol-binding protein and retinol are further bound in the plasma to transthyretin, and this complex is then carried to target tissues. Within the cells of target tissues, the free retinol is again bound by a cellular retinol-binding protein. The sites of action are within the nucleus or on glycoprotein synthesis.

Hepatic stores of retinol are the best indicator of retinol sufficiency. A liver retinol level of 20 mcg/g of protein is believed to be adequate in adults. Hepatic retinol levels in newborn, term, and premature infants are comparable, but are often below 20 mcg/g of protein (Iyengar and Apte, 1972). However, clinical signs of vitamin A deficiency in the newborn period are rare. The premature infant is at a disadvantage as compared with the term infant, because the term infant has greater total retinol stores. Since hepatic tissue is rarely available, blood levels of retinol have been used to assess vitamin A status. However, low blood levels of retinol do not necessarily reflect low hepatic stores unless the plasma retinol level is less than 5 mcg/dl. Plasma retinol levels of less than 10 mcg/dl are generally accepted to reflect vitamin A deficiency. Premature infants have mean plasma retinol levels of 15 to 19 mcg/dl as compared with 22 to 24 mcg/dl in term infants. Similarly, plasma retinol-binding protein levels are lower in premature infants as compared with those of term infants (Zachman, 1989).

Deficiency. Vitamin A deficiency remains a major problem in underdeveloped countries and is frequently seen in association with protein-calorie malnutrition. Ocular symptoms include night blindness, conjunctival xerosis, and progressive corneal changes leading to scarring and blindness. Vitamin A deficiency impairs differentiation of epithelial tissues, which becomes manifest in the respiratory tract as squamous metaplasia. Abnormalities of the electroretinogram of vitamin A–deficient animals have been described. Other symptoms include disturbances of growth and reproduction, respiratory infections, and increased intracranial pressure.

Classic symptoms of vitamin A deficiency are rarely seen in the intensive care nursery, but biochemical evidence (low plasma retinol levels) are commonly found in premature infants, particularly those with bronchopulmonary dysplasia. Infants receiving only parenteral nutrition for prolonged periods of time have low plasma retinol levels despite supplementation with pediatric parenteral multivitamin preparation containing retinol (Greene et al., 1986). Free retinol in multivitamin preparations binds to intravenous tubing, impairing its delivery to the patient. The problem of retinol delivery may be resolved by reformulating pediatric intravenous multivitamins with retinol palmitate, which does not bind to intravenous tubing (Gutcher et al., 1984). Alternatively, Baeckert and associates (1988) have shown that the addition of pediatric intravenous multivitamins to lipid emulsion results in adequate delivery of retinol to the patient. Infants with fat malabsorption are at risk for the development of fat-soluble vitamin deficiency. Hence, infants with biliary atresia, cystic fibrosis, or severe short bowel syndrome should be monitored for deficiencies of vitamin A and other fat-soluble vitamins.

Vitamin A deficiency may contribute to the development of bronchopulmonary dysplasia. The histologic changes in the respiratory epithelium of the airway in bronchopulmonary dysplasia are similar to those seen in vitamin A deficiency. The further observation of low retinol levels in infants with bronchopulmonary dysplasia (Hustead et al., 1984, Shenai et al., 1985) subsequently led to prospective trials of the therapeutic use of retinol to prevent the disorder. Shenai and colleagues (1987) conducted a randomized prospective study comparing the effects of supplemental intramuscular retinyl palmitate to those of a placebo in 40 premature infants of 700 to 1300 g who required oxygen and mechanical ventilation. Shenai and colleagues found that the retinol-supplemented group had higher plasma retinol and retinol-binding protein levels, a lower incidence of bronchopulmonary dysplasia (9 of 20 treatment versus 17 of 20 controls), and a reduced need for mechanical ventilation and oxygen as compared with the placebo group. Similar results were found by Papagaroufalis (1988). Despite these encouraging results, relatively little is known of the pharmacokinetics and toxicity of retinol in premature infants. The administration of parenteral or enteral vitamin A beyond standard recommended doses should be performed with great caution. Pharmacologic doses of retinol for the prevention of bronchopulmonary dysplasia should be considered experimental.

Toxicity. Toxicity can result from a massive acute ingestion or chronic excessive intake of vitamin A (Bendich and Langseth, 1989). Acute toxicity can result in infants with a single dose of 100,000 IU of vitamin A. Chronic toxicity has occurred in infants from the feeding of chicken liver or excessive vitamin supplementation. Symptoms include increased intracranial pressure, headache, alopecia, bone lesions, hepatic injury, and hypercalcemia. Patients with renal failure may develop toxicity while receiving standard doses of parenteral multivitamins due to impaired metabolism of vitamin A (Gleghorn et al., 1986). High doses of maternal vitamin A has been shown to be teratogenic in animal studies, but evidence for teratogenesis caused by vitamin A in humans is limited (Bendich and Langseth, 1989). Maternal use of isotretinoin (13-*cis*-retinoic acid) has been associated with congenital anomalies (microtia and anotia, cleft palate, central nervous system malformations, hydrocephalus, congenital heart disease, thymic abnormalities) in the newborn (Lammer et al., 1985).

Requirements. Although vitamin A activity may be provided from several sources, the preferred source for the infant is retinol. Vitamin A potency is as follows: 1 retinol equivalent = 1 mcg of retinol = 6 mcg of carotene = 3.3 IU. The recommended dietary allowance (RDA) for vitamin A is 375 mcg of retinol or retinol equivalents during the 1st year of life (National Research Council, 1989). Mature human milk contains about 670 ± 200 mcg retinol equivalents/l. The AAPCON (1977) recommends that infant formulas contain a minimum of 75 mcg of retinol equivalents/100 kcal. With infant formulas or breast-feeding, further supplementation of vitamin A is not indicated unless there are unusual requirements (e.g., fat malabsorption). Greene and co-workers (1986) measured serum retinol in premature and term infants who were given 455 and 700 mcg/day of retinol, respectively during total parenteral nutrition. The premature infants continued to have low retinol levels, whereas most term infants were generally within the reference range. As described above, retinol adheres to intravenous tubing, resulting in inadequate delivery of the vitamin during the administration of total parenteral nutrition. Baeckert and colleagues (1988) demonstrated better delivery of parenteral retinol when the pediatric multivitamins are admixed with the intravenous fat emulsion. With this technique, they found that 280 mcg/kg/day of retinol increased serum retinol in very-low-birth-weight (VLBW) infants from 11.0 ± 0.76 to 19.2 ± 0.97 mcg/dl. Until the current pediatric intravenous multivitamins are reformulated to contain retinol palmitate, it will continue to be difficult to achieve normal serum retinol values in premature infants receiving total parenteral nutrition.

VITAMIN D

Metabolism and Function. Vitamin D is essential for normal calcium homeostasis and bone mineralization (Reichel et al., 1989). Vitamin D is not an essential nutrient in the diet provided there is sufficient exposure to sunlight. In the epidermis, 7-dehydrocholesterol is converted to D_3 by the action of ultraviolet light of 290–320 nm. When sunlight exposure is limited, then dietary sources of vitamin D are essential. Vitamins D_2 (ergocalciferol) and D_3 (cholecalciferol) are derived from plant and animal sources, respectively. Both are equally potent sources of vitamin D, and 1 mcg of vitamin D is equivalent to 40 IU. Approximately 80 per cent of ingested vitamin D is absorbed in infants. Since it is fat soluble, vitamin D absorption is decreased in the presence of fat malabsorption. Transport of vitamin D in the blood occurs along with vitamin D–binding protein. In the liver, vitamin D is hydroxylated to 25-hydroxy D (25-OHD). This step appears to be relatively unregulated, and 25-OHD levels appear to be determined primarily by dietary intake and tissue stores. In the kidney, 25-OHD is converted to 1,25-dihydroxy D (1,25-OHD) by 1-α-hydroxylase. This step is highly regulated in such a way that levels of 1,25-OHD are determined primarily by calcium requirements. Synthesis of 1,25-OHD is increased with hypocalcemia and hypophosphatemia through the increased secretion and effects of parathyroid hormone. There is also feedback inhibition of 1-α-hydroxylase by its product, 1,25-OHD. 1,25-OHD has far-ranging effects on many tissues (Reichel et al., 1989), but its primary effects on mineral metabolism are the result of its actions on bone, intestine, parathyroid gland, and kidney. In the intestine, 1,25-OHD causes increased absorption of calcium and phosphorus. In the kidney 1,25-OHD acts to decrease its own synthesis from 25-OHD. In the parathyroid gland, 1,25-OHD decreases parathyroid hormone synthesis. 1,25-OHD acts to promote mobilization of calcium from bone. It is also essential for bone mineralization and remodeling.

During pregnancy, blood levels of 25-OHD have been reported to be lower than normal. However, a recent study of pregnant women showed that total 25-OHD and 1,25-OHD levels were similar to and higher than those of the adult reference range, respectively (Hoogenboezem et al., 1989). 1,25-OHD appears to be transported across the placenta to the fetus. At birth, levels of 25-OHD and 1,25-OHD in newborns are lower than maternal levels (Hoogenboezem et al., 1989). Maternal blood levels show a positive correlation with cord blood levels. Newborn levels of 1,25-OHD rise in the first 24 hours of life, coincident with the decline of serum calcium. Levels of vitamin D, vitamin D metabolites, and antirachitic activity measured by bioassay are very low in human milk (Specker et al., 1985; Weisman et al., 1982).

Deficiency. Vitamin D deficiency occurs when there is insufficient dietary intake or inadequate exposure to sunlight. Hence, due to the low levels of vitamin D in human milk, exclusively breast-fed infants are particularly at risk for the development of rickets (Bachrach et al., 1979, Edidin et al., 1980). This risk is greater during winter months in northern latitudes as a result of decreased exposure to sunlight. Maternal vitamin D deficiency predisposes the newborn to infantile rickets, and cases of congenital rickets have been reported. Rickets is prevalent among infants maintained on a macrobiotic diet, which is high in fiber and excludes dairy products (Dagnelie et al., 1990). Syndromes associated with fat malabsorption also predispose infants to vitamin D deficiency. Deficiency of vitamin D results in a wide spectrum of laboratory findings and clinical symptoms. Mild vitamin D deficiency may become manifest only in a low blood level of 25-OHD. Severe or prolonged deficiency may result in tetany, severe growth failure, and rachitic bone disease. Clinical signs of rickets include craniotabes, swelling at the costochondral junction, softening of cranial bones, flaring of the epiphyses at the wrists, bowed legs, and fractures.

Radiologic findings of rickets include rarefaction and irregular fraying of the zone of provisional calcification of the radius and ulna and splaying of the metaphyses. The histologic findings of vitamin D deficiency rickets are shown in Figure 76–1. Laboratory findings usually include a low or normal serum calcium level, hypophosphatemia, and an elevated alkaline phosphatase level. Blood levels of 25-OHD are usually less than 8–15 ng/ml in rickets (Arnaud et al., 1976; Garabedian et al., 1983). In contrast, the blood level of 1,25-OHD may be low, normal, or high (Markestad et al., 1984). It is important to recognize those patients who are at high risk for vitamin D deficiency in order to appropriately monitor for symptoms and to provide adequate vitamin D supplementation. Rickets has been treated with 2000 to 5000 IU/day of vitamin D. However, as little as 400 IU/day may be sufficient for healing rickets in infants.

Osteopenia of Prematurity. Osteopenia of prematurity, also known previously as rickets of prematurity, occurs primarily in infants whose birth weight is less than 1000 g. Clinical findings include fractures (especially of the humerus, femur, and ribs), bone demineralization on x-ray study, and decreased bone mineral content by bone densitometry. The serum calcium level is usually normal. Hypophosphatemia and an elevated alkaline phosphatase level are often present. Multiple factors have been found to contribute to this disorder. Osteopenia of prematurity has been treated with large doses of vitamin D in the past in the belief that vitamin D deficiency was a major etiologic factor. However, most premature infants with osteopenia have normal 25-OHD levels. It appears that inadequate intake and retention of calcium and phosphorus are the primary cause of this disorder (Greer and Tsang, 1985; Steichen et al., 1980, 1981). Other factors contributing to osteopenia include calcium-wasting from diuretics and aluminum loading. Osteopenia can be treated and prevented by sufficient enteral mineral intake to retain calcium and phosphorus at the intrauterine rate. This can be achieved by routine calcium and phosphorus supplementation of human milk or by feeding specialized premature infant formulas (Greer et al., 1982). Vitamin D should be provided at the recommended dose of 400 IU/day. High doses of vitamin D (2000 to 5000 IU/day) are not recommended in the treatment of osteopenia of prematurity. Such high doses may actually worsen osteopenia by increasing bone resorption.

Toxicity. Toxicity can occur with massive single doses or chronic high doses of vitamin D (Chesney, 1990). Symptoms of vitamin D toxicity include poor weight gain, increased deep tendon reflexes, irritability, and diarrhea. Hypercalcemia (up to 18 mg/dl), caused by increased calcium absorption and bone resorption, results in hypercalciuria, nephrocalcinosis, azotemia, polyuria, and hypokalemia. Blood levels of 25-OHD are elevated, but levels of 1,25-OHD are low or normal. An epidemic of hypercalcemia in children occurred in the United Kingdom after World War II. This epidemic was probably due to excessive vitamin D supplementation of cows' milk, cereals, and other foods resulting in some children receiving up to 4000 IU/day of vitamin D (AAPCON, 1963). The upper limit of a safe dose of vitamin D in infants, which does

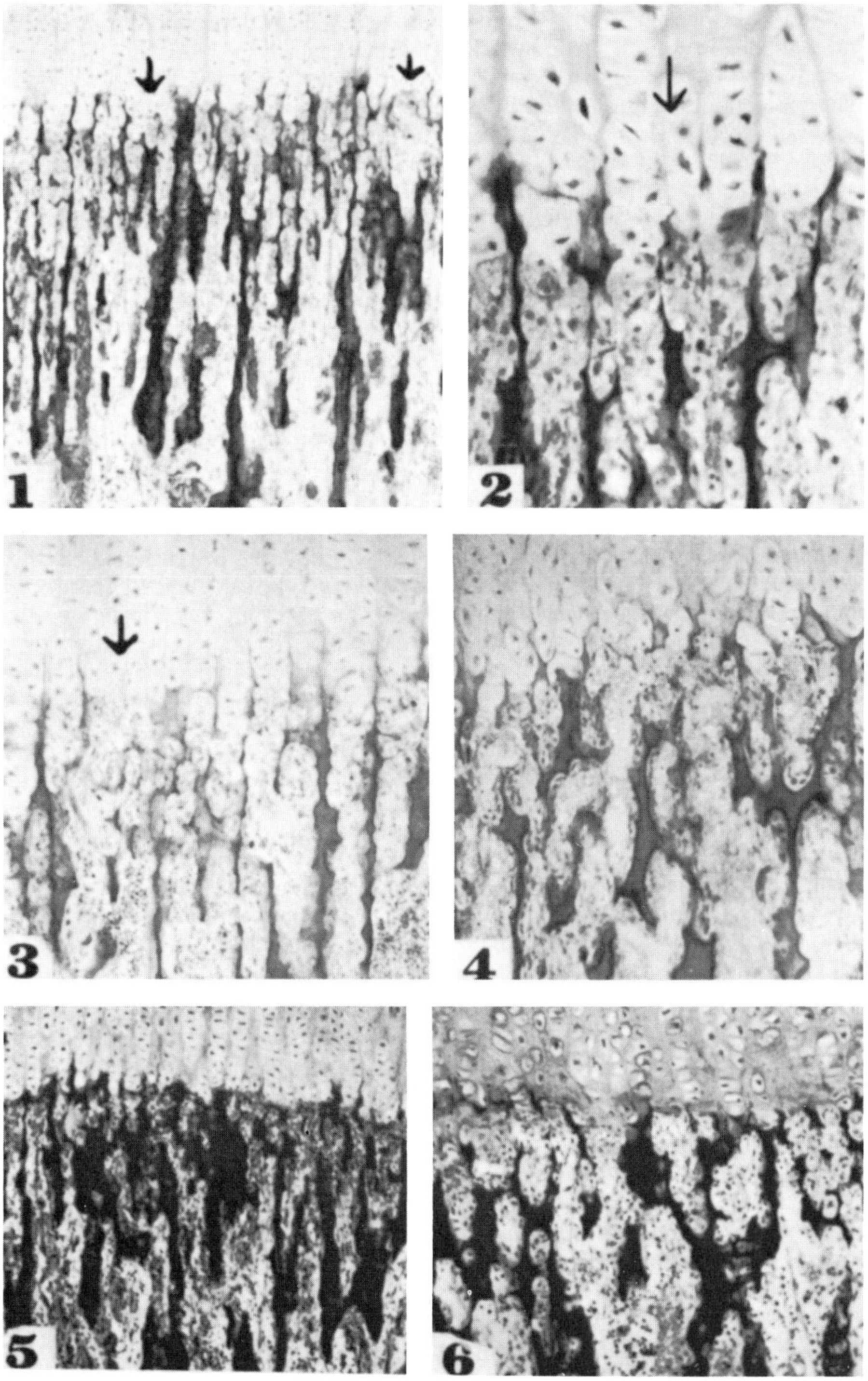

FIGURE 76–1. 1, Rickets, acute, slight. Arrows indicate several areas in cartilaginous matrix between hypertrophic cells where disposition of inorganic materials is lacking (as indicated by failure to stain with hematoxylin). 2, Rickets, acute, slight. Higher power to show area in matrix between several rows of hypertrophic cells where deposition of inorganic materials is faulty. 3, Rickets, acute, slight. Focus of defective calcification in cartilage. 4, Rickets, acute, moderate. Large focus of defective calcification in cartilage. 5, Rickets, acute, severe. Except for a few areas, there is virtual cessation of lime salt deposition in provisional zone of calcification. 6, Rickets, acute, severe. Sudden and complete cessation of deposition of inorganic materials in areas of hypertrophic cells. The suddenness is evidenced by the adequacy (dark staining materials) beneath. (From Follis, R. H., Park, E. A., and Jackson, D.: Bull. Johns Hopkins Hosp. 91:480, 1952.)

not cause toxicity, is not known with certainty. Doses of 1800 to 6300 IU/day have been reported to cause inhibition of linear growth in infants (Jeans and Stearns 1938). However, Fomon and co-workers (1966) found no difference in growth or serum calcium with doses of 300 to 2170 IU/day of vitamin D. Currently, vitamin D toxicity can occur with excessive supplementation (prescribed by physicians or administered by parents). Greer and associates (1984) reported an infant in which massive maternal vitamin D supplementation (100,000 IU/day resulted in a vitamin D concentration of 6700 to 7660 IU/liter in human milk. No toxicity was seen in the infant over 25 days of exclusive breast-feeding. However, it is possible that

chronic pharmacologic doses of maternal vitamin D could result in toxicity over a prolonged period of time in the breast-fed infant. Infants with vitamin D toxicity should have vitamin D excluded from the diet until symptoms subside and 25-hydroxy D levels return to normal. If hypercalcemia is severe and high output renal failure is present, then intravenous isotonic saline (150 to 200 ml/kg/day) and furosemide should be administered.

Williams syndrome is characterized by supravalvular aortic stenosis, mental retardation, elfin facies, and transient hypercalcemia. This disorder was once believed to be due to excessive vitamin D intake during pregnancy. The disorder appears to be much more complex. Many children with this syndrome do not have hypercalcemia, and 25-OHD and 1,25-OHD levels are usually normal. Williams syndrome may be associated in some cases with increased sensitivity to or abnormal synthesis and degradation of 1,25-OHD (Chesney, 1990; Garabedian et al., 1985).

Requirements. The recommended daily allowance of vitamin D for infants had previously been 400 IU/day. The new recommended daily allowance (1989) is 300 IU and 400 IU/day for 0 to 6 months and 6 to 12 months, respectively. The AAPCON (1977) recommends that standard infant formulas be supplemented at a minimum of 40 IU/100 kcal and a maximum of 100 IU/100 kcal.. Most standard infant formulas contain 400 to 420 IU/liter, and human milk is low in vitamin D. When assessed by antirachitic bioassay, human milk usually contains less than 20 to 40 IU of vitamin D per liter. Human milk contains about 315 ng/l (range 187 to 531) of total vitamin D_2 and D_3, 100 to 800 ng/l of 25-OHD, and 1–3 ng/l of 1,25-OHD (Hoogenboezem et al., 1989, Specker et al., 1985; Weisman et al., 1982). Levels of vitamin D in human milk correlate somewhat with maternal dietary intake (Specker et al., 1985). Maternal serum 25-OHD correlates with levels of 25-OHD in human milk (Hoogenboezem et al., 1989). Maternal supplemention of vitamin D (2500 IU/day) during lactation increased the vitamin D activity of human milk from less than 20 IU/l to 140 IU/l (Specker et al., 1988). There is considerable controversy regarding whether or not term healthy breast-fed infants require vitamin D supplementation. Most breast-fed term infants are free of clinical symptoms of rickets and appear to grow well without vitamin D supplementation. Roberts and colleagues (1981) found no difference in bone mineral content, serum calcium, phosphorus, or alkaline phosphatase between vitamin D–supplemented (400 IU/day) and unsupplemented term breast-fed infants. Levels of 25-OHD were lower in the unsupplemented group. However, Greer (1982) found lower bone mineral content and serum 25-OHD at 12 weeks of age in unsupplemented breast-fed infants as compared with a vitamin D–supplemented group (400 IU/day). Although differences in 25-OHD persisted at 6 months (but not 12 months), bone mineral content was similar between groups at 6 and 12 months of age. The 1985 AAPCON Pediatric Nutrition Handbook appears to recommend routine vitamin D supplementation in term breast-fed infants, but a definitive statement is not made to that effect. Based on available data, vitamin D supplementation at 400 IU/day should be strongly considered for all breast-fed infants. If maternal nutrition is marginal or if the infant receives limited sunlight exposure (e.g., in extremely northern latitudes), then vitamin D supplementation is clearly indicated.

Premature infants, whether fed human milk or formula, have low levels of 25-OHD unless vitamin D supplementation is provided (Senterre, 1982). Premature infant formulas in the United States contain between 480 to 2200 IU/L. The AAPCON (1985) recommends that premature infants be given 400 IU/day of vitamin D. Several studies support a recommended dose of vitamin D (beyond that in formula or human milk) in the range of 200 to 500 IU/day (Cooke et al., 1990; Huston 1983, Markestad 1984). It appears that with an intake 400 IU/day

of vitamin D, plasma levels of 25-OHD may be primarily determined by postconceptional age (Cooke et al., 1990). However, Hillman and co-workers (1985a) found that about half of a group of premature infants developed low levels of 25-OHD despite receiving a supplement of 400 IU/day of vitamin D. When premature infants were given a vitamin D supplement of 800 IU/day, this resulted in significantly higher 25-OHD levels than with 400 IU/day (Hillman et al., (1985b). Senterre and Sable (1982) found that higher doses of vitamin D (1200 to 2000 IU/day) resulted in improved calcium and phosphorus absorption. It is unclear whether or not such higher doses of vitamin D are more beneficial to the premature infant than the usual recommended dose of 400 IU.. The differences between studies may be a reflection of populations of premature infants with differing maternal and fetal vitamin D status at birth.

Parenteral vitamin D requirements are not well defined at this time. Greene and colleagues (1986) gave premature and term infants 260 IU and 400 IU/day of vitamin D intravenously, respectively. 25-OHD levels were within the reference range for both the premature and term groups of infants. However, the parenteral vitamin D requirement may actually be much lower. Koo (1987) provided 25 IU of vitamin D per 100 ml of fluid during total parenteral nutrition, resulting in a mean maximum dose of 31 IU/kg/day of vitamin D. Blood levels of 25-OHD increased to the normal range, which was maintained for up to 6 months. Baeckert (1988) found that 25-OHD levels were maintained in a normal range when premature infants were given 160 IU/kg/day of vitamin D (40 per cent vial/kg/day MVI-Pediatric mixed in with the IV fat). This dose of parenteral vitamin D is recommended by the American Society for Clinical Nutrition (Greene et al., 1988).

VITAMIN E

Metabolism and Function. Vitamin E, a fat-soluble vitamin, was discovered in 1922 as the nutritional factor necessary for successful reproduction in rats maintained on a diet using rancid lard as the fat source. Vitamin E now has a wide variety of indications for use in pediatric and adult medicine (Bell and Filer, 1981, Bieri et al., 1983). Vitamin E includes several isomers, the most potent of which is d-α-tocopherol. Other isomers include γ- and β- tocopherol, which have only 10 and 33 per cent of the activity of d-α-tocopherol. Vitamin E primarily functions as a biologic antioxidant by interrupting the sequence of lipid peroxidation of polyunsaturated fatty acids. In this process, vitamin E is itself oxidized to a quinone. Due to its lipid solubility, vitamin E is readily incorporated into the lipid bilayers of cells, which are rich in polyunsaturated fatty acids. In the red blood cell, vitamin E prevents lipid peroxidation of the red blood cell membrane and hemolysis. Vitamin E interacts with several other nutrients. Vitamin E requirements are increased when the diet is high in polyunsaturated fatty acids. Dietary iron interacts with vitamin E by two possible mechanisms. In the intestine, iron may interact with vitamin E, resulting in its oxidation prior to absorption. Perhaps more importantly, iron can increase the oxidation of polyunsaturated fatty acids, thus increasing the dietary vitamin E requirement.

There is also interaction between vitamin E and selenium, which is also an important antioxidant in the red blood cell. Provision of either vitamin E alone or with selenium results in a relative protection against deficiency of the other.

Although maternal plasma levels of d-α-tocopherol rise during pregnancy, cord levels are only one-fourth of maternal levels, suggesting a limited transfer of d-α-tocopherol across the placenta. Vitamin E is stored in lung, liver, muscle, and adipose, hence the third trimester of pregnancy is an important period for deposition of vitamin E in fetal tissues. Premature infants are particularly at risk for the development of vitamin E deficiency unless provided an exogenous source of vitamin E postnatally. Intestinal absorption of vitamin E is improved in the presence of bile salts, pancreatic enzymes, and fats. Infants with clinically significant fat malabsorption (e.g., cystic fibrosis, biliary atresia) are at risk for vitamin E deficiency. Absorption of vitamin E is decreased in premature infants of less than 32 weeks' gestation as compared with older infants (Melhorn and Gross 1971). After absorption, vitamin E is carried with lipoproteins into the lymphatics and bloodstream.

A number of techniques have been used to assess vitamin E sufficiency. Because most of the functional vitamin E activity in the body is accounted for by d-α-tocopherol, this isomer should be specifically measured. Older colorometric techniques measure total tocopherol, including the α, β, and γ isomers. Currently, high pressure liquid chromatography is the preferred method to measure d-α-tocopherol. Tissue measurements of d-α-tocopherol provide a more accurate reflection of vitamin E sufficiency. Because tissue is usually not available for d-α-tocopherol determinations, plasma levels are measured to assess vitamin E status. In adults, a d-α-tocopherol level of less than 0.5 mg/dl suggests vitamin E insufficiency. Populations of premature infants generally have a mean d-α-tocopherol below 0.5 mg/dl at birth (Gross and Gabriel, 1985, Zipursky et al., 1987). Although the tocopherol and lipid ratio has been useful in adults to assess vitamin E status, in infants plasma d-α-tocopherol levels appear to be the best predictor of vitamin E deficiency (Gutcher and Farrell, 1985).

Deficiency. Vitamin E deficiency in premature infants was reported by Oski and Barness (1967) and Ritchie and associates (1968) to cause hemolytic anemia, reticulocytosis, thrombocytosis, and edema. Subsequently, iron supplementation and the use of formulas high in polyunsaturated fatty acids were shown to increase vitamin E requirements and to result in anemia (Gross and Gabriel, 1985; Williams, 1975). Currently, such clinically evident symptoms attributable to vitamin E deficiency are unusual in premature infants. This may be due to better maternal nutrition, the judicious use of iron supplementation in premature infants, and to the attention now paid to the ratio of vitamin E to polyunsaturated fatty acids in infant formulas. However, biochemical evidence of vitamin E deficiency (plasma d-α-tocopherol < 0.5 mg/dl) is still common in premature infants. The Committee on Nutrition of the American Academy of Pediatrics (1977) recommended that premature infant formulas have a vitamin E to polyunsaturated fatty acid (mg of d-α-tocopherol to

grams of linoleic acid) ratio of greater than or equal to 1, and that a supplemental dose of 5–25 IU of vitamin E be given daily. Although routine provision of 25 IU of d-α-tocopherol to premature infants increases vitamin E levels to the normal adult range, it appears to have no effect on hemoglobin concentration, reticulocyte count, or red blood cell morphology (Zipursky et al., 1987). When studies of the routine use of vitamin E for the prevention of anemia and hyperbilirubinemia in premature infants were reviewed, mixed results were found (Bell and Filer, 1981).

Disorders of fat malabsorption often lead to deficiencies of fat-soluble vitamins. Vitamin E deficiency occurs by this mechanism in cystic fibrosis, abetalipoproteinemia, short gut syndrome, biliary atresia, and other cholestatic disorders (Muller et al., 1983; Sokol et al., 1985a). When vitamin E deficiency is longstanding, it results in a neurologic syndrome characterized by ataxia, absent deep tendon reflexes, ophthalmoplegia, and peripheral neuropathy. These neurologic symptoms can be prevented or ameliorated by the administration of vitamin E (Sokol et al., 1985b). Children with disorders of fat malabsorption should be monitored for vitamin E deficiency by measurement of d-α-tocopherol. Oral doses of 50–200 IU/kg/day of d-α-tocopherol may be needed to prevent or treat vitamin E deficiency in such cases. Some children require parenteral administration of vitamin E, at a dose much lower than oral therapy, in order to achieve adequate plasma levels. Treatment must be monitored by plasma levels in order to correct deficiency and prevent toxicity.

Pharmacologic Vitamin E Therapy. Because of its antioxidant properties, there have been multiple studies using pharmacologic doses of vitamin E to prevent neonatal diseases associated with oxygen-induced injury. Owens and Owens (1949) first demonstrated that large doses of vitamin E could prevent retinopathy of prematurity. Hittner and colleagues (1981) randomized 100 premature infants with respiratory distress to either placebo or 100 mg/kg/day of oral d-α-tocopherol. The overall incidence of retinopathy of prematurity was the same in both groups, but vitamin E did significantly reduce the incidence of severe (grade III and IV) retinopathy of prematurity. Other randomized studies have yielded inconsistent results regarding the effectiveness of vitamin E to prevent retinopathy of prematurity (Finer et al., 1982; Johnson et al., 1974; Puklin et al., 1982; Schaffer et al., 1985). Based on such findings, the Committee on Fetus and Newborn of the American Academy of Pediatrics (1985) recommended that the pharmacologic doses of vitamin E used to prevent retinopathy of prematurity should be considered experimental and not be given routinely. A large randomized study by Phelps and associates (1987) subsequently found no difference between the effects of placebo and vitamin E on the incidence or severity of retinopathy of prematurity. It would appear from the results cited earlier and in view of its potential toxic effects (see later) that pharmacologic doses of vitamin E are not indicated in the prevention of retinopathy of prematurity.

Pharmacologic doses of vitamin E have also been studied for the amelioration of bronchopulmonary dysplasia. After initial promising results were reported by Ehrenkranz and co-workers (1978), a more extensive study found no benefit from vitamin E in the prevention of bronchopulmonary dysplasia (Ehrenkranz et al., 1979). When all studies of vitamin E given for bronchopulmonary dysplasia were reviewed by Bell (1986), he concluded that vitamin E is not efficacious in the prevention of bronchopulmonary dysplasia. Vitamin E has also been proposed as a potential therapy to prevent subependymal hemorrhage and intraventricular hemorrhage in very-low-birth-weight infants. However, conflicting data have been reported. Some studies have shown a decrease in the incidence of subependymal hemorrhage and intraventricular hemorrhage with pharmacologic doses of vitamin E (Chiswick et al., 1983; Speer et al., 1984). In contrast, Phelps and associates (1987) found an increase in the incidence of severe intraventricular hemorrhage (grade III and IV) in infants weighing less than 1 kg when vitamin E was given as prophylaxis for retinopathy of prematurity. At this time, pharmacologic doses of vitamin E cannot be recommended for either the prevention of bronchopulmonary dysplasia or intraventricular hemorrhage.

Adverse Effects and Toxicity. As part of the monitoring of prospective studies of vitamin E for the prevention of retinopathy of prematurity, several potential adverse effects of high dose vitamin E have been identified. High doses of vitamin E predispose the infant to bacterial sepsis and necrotizing enterocolitis (Finer et al., 1984; Johnson et al., 1985). The association of pharmacologic doses of vitamin E with necrotizing enterocolitis may be partially explained by the use of hyperosmolar oral solutions of d-α-tocopherol or by effects on white blood cell function in the presence of high blood α-tocopherol levels. The administration of vitamin E through intramuscular injection has been reported to cause calcifications at the site of the injection (Barak et al., 1986).

A new syndrome, possibly due to vitamin E toxicity, was reported in a group of premature infants, who were treated with an intravenous preparation (E-Ferol) of d-α-tocopherol acetate (Lorch et al. 1985; Martone et al., 1986). Symptoms included ascites, hepatomegaly, azotemia, and thrombocytopenia. The affected infants were given a mean intravenous dose of d-α-tocopherol acetate of 37 IU/kg/day. Some of these infants had high serum and tissue levels of α-tocopherol. It remains unclear whether this syndrome was due to toxicity from vitamin E or polysorbate 80 (an emulsifier in E-Ferol) (Alade et al., 1986).

Requirements The Committee on Nutrition of the American Academy of Pediatrics (AAPCON) (1977) recommends that premature infant formulas have more than or equal to 0.7 IU vitamin E/100 kcal or a vitamin E to polyunsaturated fatty acid (mg of d-α-tocopherol to grams of linoleic acid) ratio of more than or equal to 1. Premature infants may also benefit from a supplemental dose of 5 to 25 IU/day of vitamin E. However, AAPCON was unable to recommend a specific dose of supplemental vitamin E in 1985. Formulas for term infants should have more than or equal to 0.3 IU vitamin E/100 kcal or a vitamin E to polyunsaturated fatty acid ratio of more than or equal to 0.7. The RDA of vitamin E for infants 0 to 6 months and 6 to 12 months of age is 3 and 4 mg of α-tocopherol equivalents, respectively (National Research Council, 1989). Healthy term infants who are fed human milk or standard infant formulas require no further supplementation of vitamin E. Premature infants may benefit from maintaining serum d-α-tocopherol levels in a range that is associated with vitamin E sufficiency (> 0.5 mg/dl), but below potentially toxic levels (> 3 mg/dl). The American Academy of Pediatrics Committee on the Fetus and Newborn (Poland, 1986) has suggested a target range of 1 to 2 mg/dl for d-α-tocopherol levels in premature infants.

Vitamin E requirements during total parenteral nutrition are less well defined. Gutcher and Farrell (1985) showed that 2 mg/kg/day of d-α-tocopherol acetate increased mean serum d-α-tocopherol levels from $0.37 \pm .09$ to $1.56 \pm .20$ mg/dl in 4 days. Phillips and co-workers (1987) found that 65 per cent of a vial of MVI-Pediatric (Armour, 7 mg d-α-tocopherol acetate/vial) per day for premature infants weighing 1 to 1.5 kg resulted in mean serum d-α-tocopherol levels between 1.44 to 1.87 mg/dl over 2 days to 4 weeks of parenteral nutrition. For infants weighing less than 1 kg and who were receiving 65 per cent of a vial of MVI-Pediatric (4.5 mg α-tocopherol), d-α-tocopherol levels were slightly higher (1.92 to 2.45 mg/dl), and 31 per cent of these infants had a level higher than 3.5 mg/dl. When only 30 per cent of a vial (0.21 mg α-tocopherol) was given to infants weighing less than 1 kg, 9 of 16 (56 per cent) had a d-α-tocopherol level of less than 1 mg/dl and 2 (18 per cent) had a level below 0.5 mg/dl. When very-low-birth-weight infants were given a dose of 2.8 mg/kg/day of d-α-tocopherol acetate (40 per cent of a vial of MVI-Pediatric/kg/day mixed in the daily dose of Intralipid), mean serum d-α-tocopherol levels were between 1.56 and 2.57 mg/dl (Baekert et al., 1988). The last-mentioned dose of α-tocopherol has been recommended by Greene (1988) for premature infants. However, in order to maintain serum d-α-tocopherol levels in the target range of 1 to 2 mg/dl (Poland, 1986) for the infant weighing less than 1000 g, as much as 3.5 mg/day of α-tocopherol may be needed (Amorde-Spalding et al., 1990).

VITAMIN K

Vitamin K is important in the carboxylation of coagulation factors and is therefore necessary for the synthesis of prothrombin and other factors. Normal intestinal bacteria synthesize the vitamin. Since the newborn infant's intestinal tract is not colonized at birth, vitamin K deficiency may occur at several days of life and result in hemorrhagic disease of the newborn. The American Academy of Pediatrics recommends a dose of 0.5 to 1.0 mg of vitamin K_1 oxide (phytonadione), administered intramuscularly, at birth. A similar dose is recommended by the Canadian and European Pediatric Societies (von Kries and Gobel, 1988; Fetus and Newborn Committee, CPS, 1988). Oral administration of vitamin K (2 mg) to healthy newborns is an alternative that remains controversial. Vitamin K_1 and vitamin K_3 are absorbed well from the gastrointestinal tract (McNinch et al., 1985; O'Connor and Addiego, 1986), and the oral route has been used successfully in some parts of Europe (McNinch, 1988). The levels achieved with oral vitamin K are much lower and widely variable (Ogata et al., 1988; Shinzawa, 1989; Matsuda,

1989). Oral vitamin K₁ should be used only in healthy term infants who do not have history of maternal drug exposure and should be given within the first 6 hours of life and before milk is given. Conditions associated with vitamin K deficiency include fat malabsorption (e.g., with cystic fibrosis, short bowel syndrome), the use of broad-spectrum antibiotics, and fetal exposure to phenytoin or other drugs that impair vitamin K metabolism (e.g., phenobarbital, rifampin, isoniazid, and coumadin).

ASCORBIC ACID

Metabolism and Function. Ascorbic acid, or vitamin C, is a water-soluble vitamin that has widespread functions in metabolism (Levine, 1986; Moran and Greene 1979). Deficiency of ascorbic acid leads to the clinical syndrome of scurvy. Ascorbic acid functions as a coenzyme in a variety of reactions that mostly involve hydroxylation steps. It is important in the synthesis of procollagen, acting as a cofactor for the hydroxylation of proline and lysine. Ascorbic acid also participates in the synthesis of carnitine and dopamine and in the amination of peptide hormones. Tyrosine metabolism is also affected by ascorbate, which increases the conversion of 4-hydroxyphenylpyruvic acid to homogentisic acid. The recycling of tetrahydrofolate is also improved by ascorbate. Ascorbic acid is one of a number of naturally occurring antioxidants and may be important in reducing oxygen toxicity in newborns who require oxygen therapy.

Cord blood levels of ascorbate are twice maternal levels. Vitamin C deficiency is extremely rare in infants fed fresh human milk, which contains 7 to 10 mg/100 kcal in healthy populations. Pasteurization of human milk significantly decreases the concentration of ascorbate. Term infants have plasma ascorbate levels of 1.4 ± 0.4 mg/dl at birth, and premature infants have similar levels during the 1st day of life (Heinonem et al., 1986). Plasma levels of more than 0.6 mg ascorbate/dl usually reflect vitamin C sufficiency. Levels less than 0.2 mg/dl are found in scurvy. Tissue stores are limited, and clinical deficiency results after 1 to 2 months without vitamin C intake. Iron absorption in the intestine is improved in the presence of ascorbic acid. Vitamin C is excreted in the urine.

Deficiency. Clinical deficiency resulting in scurvy is extremely rare in infants. It results from an inadequate intake of vitamin C from unsupplemented cow's milk, evaporated milk, or pasteurized pooled human milk. It does not seem to occur in the breast-fed infant. Symptoms include irritability, tender extremities (due to subperiosteal hemorrhage), swelling of the costochondral junction, and gingival bleeding (Grewar, 1965). Radiologic findings include generalized osteoporosis, thickening of the zone of provisional calcification, spur formation, and subperiosteal hemorrhage. These findings may be difficult to distinguish from copper deficiency or congenital syphilis. Untreated scurvy results in death. Ingalls (1938) reported the occurrence of scurvy in three premature infants fed pasteurized pooled human milk. Heinonem and co-workers (1986) reported low vitamin C levels in a group of premature infants who were not given supplemental vitamin C and were fed a combination of pooled pasteurized human milk and unpasteurized preterm maternal milk. Infantile scurvy has also been reported in infants whose mothers received megadoses of vitamin C during pregnancy (Moran and Greene, 1979).

When premature infants are given a high protein intake (> 5 g/kg/day), particularly with casein-predominant formulas, they develop transient hypertyrosinemia (Avery et al., 1967). This finding appears to be due to a low activity of 4-hydroxyphenylpyruvate dioxygenase in premature infants, which is increased with ascorbic acid supplementation. Transient hypertyrosinemia may result in neurologic injury (Menkes et al., 1972), but this was not found in other studies (AAPCON, 1985). Doses of 60 to 100 mg/day of vitamin C seem to be inconsistent in preventing hypertyrosinemia (AAPCON, 1985; Avery et al., 1967). Transient hypertyrosinemia no longer seems to be a clinically significant problem, because enteral protein intakes of premature infants now generally are kept below 4 g/kg/day.

Toxicity. Vitamin C toxicity has been described in adults receiving pharmacologic doses (Olson and Hodges, 1987). High doses of vitamin C can cause hemolytic anemia in patients with glucose–6-phosphate dehydrogenase deficiency. There is some evidence that even moderate supplementation of vitamin C may lead to adverse effects. Ballin and associates (1988) reported the occurrence of hemolytic anemia in a premature infant given 30 mg ascorbic acid per day in a standard multivitamin. Evidence was presented that ascorbic acid can act as an oxidant in neonatal erythrocytes. Pharmacologic doses of vitamin C should not be given to infants.

Requirements and Treatment. The recommended daily allowance for ascorbic acid is 30 mg in the first 6 months and 35 mg at age 6 to 12 months. Infants may actually require as little as 10 mg/day to prevent scurvy. The AAPCON (1977) recommends that formulas contain a minimum of 8 mg ascorbic acid/100 kcal. Human milk contains comparable amounts of vitamin C. For premature infants, the AAPCON (1985) recommends the usual dose of 35 mg of vitamin C in standard infant multivitamin preparations, depending on the amount of vitamin already in the infant feeding. Currently, clinical deficiency is not seen with standard premature formulas. Parenteral vitamin C requirements are not well defined. Moore and co-workers (1986) provided 52 and 80 mg of ascorbic acid to premature and term infants, respectively, in a pediatric parenteral multivitamin preparation. Ascorbic acid levels were above the reference range in the premature infants, suggesting that this dose may be excessive. The term infants had normal ascorbic acid levels. Greene and associates (1988) recommended a parenteral ascorbic acid dose of 32 mg/kg/day using current intravenous multivitamin formulations (40 per cent of a vial MVI-Pediatric/kg/day).

Grewar (1965) suggested that infantile scurvy be treated with 100 to 1000 mg/day of ascorbic acid. Because pharmacologic doses of vitamin C carry a potential for toxicity and antioxidant effects, a lower initial dose of 100 mg/day ascorbic acid, followed by 50 mg/day thereafter, seems to be more appropriate (Moran and Greene 1979).

THIAMINE

Metabolism and Function. Thiamine, or vitamin B₁, is important in carbohydrate metabolism. It acts as a coenzyme in the oxidative decarboxylation of pyruvate, α-keto acids, and branched-chain amino acids. Thiamine is also a coenzyme in the pentose shunt. Deficiency of thiamine causes beriberi. In the adult, withdrawal of thiamine from the diet produces symptoms within a week. Thiamine may be actively transported across the placenta. Cord blood levels of thiamine are higher than maternal levels (Baker et al., 1975). This fact may explain the rarity of congenital beriberi except in circumstances of extreme maternal deprivation. Thiamine is absorbed in the intestine, and excess of the vitamin is excreted by the kidneys. Human milk is relatively low in thiamine (210 ± 35 mcg/l). Thiamine sufficiency can be evaluated by measurement of erythrocyte transketolase activity.

Deficiency. Deficiency of thiamine affects infants in two age groups. A congenital form develops within the first few days of life, and an infantile form is seen after several months of age. Although beriberi is common in Asian countries, where polished rice is the main dietary staple, it is very rare in the United States. The congenital type occurs only in infants born to mothers who are thiamine deficient. The infantile form has been seen at 2 to 7 months of age in breast-fed infants whose mothers are thiamine deficient. The infant with thiamine deficiency presents with "wet beriberi," which is characterized primarily by congestive heart failure. Other symptoms include anorexia, lethargy, vomiting, aphonic cry, bulging fontanelle, seizures, coma, and death (Moran and Greene, 1979; Van Gelder and Darby, 1944). Thiamine deficiency in breast-fed infants has also been reported to cause central nervous system depression, progressing to coma and death (Fehily, 1944). In contrast to the infant, adults with thiamine deficiency present with "dry beriberi," which is characterized by peripheral neuropathy, paresthesias, and weakness. Other presentations of thiamine deficiency in adults include Wernicke encephalopathy and Korsakoff syndrome. Treatment of thiamine deficiency in infants includes supportive measures and the administration of thiamine 10 mg every 6 to 8 hours. The mother of an infant with congenital beriberi or the infantile form associated with breast-feeding may also require thiamine therapy.

RIBOFLAVIN

Metabolism and Function. Riboflavin in incorporated into the flavin nucleotides flavin mononucleotide and flavin adenine dinucleotide. These coenzymes are essential for the activity of glutathione reductase, xanthine oxidase and other flavoproteins. Cord blood values of riboflavin are greater than maternal levels, which is consistent with active placental transport of the vitamin (Dancis et al., 1985). Riboflavin is known to be light sensitive, resulting in degradation of the vitamin in human milk and total parenteral nutrition solutions exposed to light.

Deficiency. Symptoms of riboflavin deficiency include angular stomatitis, glossitis, cheilosis, seborrheic dermatitis, and corneal vascularization (Moran and Greene, 1979). Riboflavin status can be assessed by the measurement of red blood cell glutathione reductase activity. Clinically significant deficiency is extremely rare in term infants due to the adequate vitamin levels in human milk and infant formulas. Also, both fresh cow's milk and evaporated milk are high in riboflavin. A group of premature infants, who were fed pooled milk or their own mothers' human milk, were shown to have biochemical (but not clinical) evidence of riboflavin deficiency. Supplementation of premature infants with 0.3 mg/day of riboflavin had only a modest effect on their riboflavin status (Ronnholm, 1986). Premature infants were generally riboflavin sufficient when fed a formula containing 1.8 mg/l of riboflavin (Lucas and Bates 1984). Various studies have yielded conflicting results regarding degradation of riboflavin by phototherapy (Lucas and Bates, 1984; Meloni et al., 1982; Rudolph et al., 1985).

Toxicity. Toxicity from riboflavin does not appear to occur. Photo-oxidation of amino acids in the presence of riboflavin in total parenteral nutrition solutions could result, in theory, in the formation of toxic products (Bhatia et al., 1980). Similarly, phototherapy may lead to the formation of reactive photoproducts of riboflavin, which can react with cellular DNA (Ennever and Speck, 1983).

Requirements. The recommended daily allowance of riboflavin is 0.4 and 0.5 mg/day for infants of 0 to 6 and 6 to 12 months of age, respectively. Human milk contains an average of 0.049 mg/100 kcal (range 0.036 to 0.072 mg/100 kcal) of riboflavin (Schanler, 1988). AAPCON (1977) recommends that infant formula contain a minimum of 0.06 mg/100 kcal. Infant formulas for premature infants contain 0.16 to 0.62 mg/100 kcal of riboflavin. Further routine supplementation for both premature and term infants fed either human milk or infant formulas does not appear to be required. Premature infants who are fed human milk alone may benefit from 0.6 mg of riboflavin which is the standard dose in infant multivitamins. Additional riboflavin supplementation during phototherapy is not advisable based on available data. There are little data regarding riboflavin requirements during the administration of total parenteral nutrition. Moore and co-workers (1986) gave 0.9 and 1.4 mg riboflavin per day to premature and term infants, respectively, as part of a pediatric parenteral multivitamin supplement. By measurement of red blood cell glutathione reductase, neither group was deficient, but this test does not exclude excessively high levels. Baeckert and colleagues (1988) gave 0.68 mg/kg/day of parenteral riboflavin to premature infants and found plasma riboflavin levels to be excessively high.

VITAMIN B₆

Metabolism and Function. Vitamin B_6, which is widely distributed in nature, comprises the following active compounds: pyridoxine, pyridoxal, and pyridoxamine. These forms are converted in the body to pyridoxal–5'-phosphate, which is the major form of vitamin B_6 in the blood. Pyridoxal–5'-phosphate acts as a coenzyme in broad variety of reactions in amino acid, glycogen, and heme metabolism. Heller and associates (1973) noted that biochemical evidence of vitamin B_6 deficiency was common during pregnancy. Reflective of these increased vitamin B_6 requirements in pregnancy, the recommended daily allowance for pregnant women is 2.2 mg/day, rather than the 1.6 mg/day for adult women. The fetus seems to be relatively protected against vitamin B_6 deficiency. Vitamin B_6 is transported across the placenta in large amounts during the third trimester. Vitamin B_6 levels of cord blood, which is high in pyridoxal–5'-phosphate, pyridoxamine phosphate, and pyridoxic acid, are several times greater than maternal levels. Premature infants have been shown to have low cord levels of pyridoxal–5'-phosphate (Reinken and Mangold, 1973), which is consistent with the active placental transport of vitamin B_6 during the third trimester. Levels of vitamin B_6 in human milk increase with maternal dietary intake. Absorption of vitamin B_6 occurs in the upper intestine.

Deficiency. True pyridoxine deficiency is extremely rare. It does not occur at birth but is a result of inadequate vitamin B_6 intake over the first months of life. Symptoms include irritability, seizures, microcytic anemia, and growth failure (May, 1954; Snyderman et al., 1950). In the early 1950s a modification in the preparation of an infant formula resulted in inactivation of vitamin B_6. This vitamin B_6–deficient formula resulted in an epidemic of seizures, which occurred at 6 weeks to 4 months of age (May, 1954). The use of unfortified goat milk has also been associated with vitamin B_6 deficiency (Johnson, 1982). Current standard infant formulas contain a minimum of 0.035 mg/100 kcal of pyridoxine (AAPCON, 1985). Although human milk often contains less pyridoxine than is recommended for infant formulas and does not always provide the recommended daily allowance (0.3 mg/day), clinical symptoms of deficiency generally are not seen. Both malabsorption and inhibition by drugs such as isoniazid and penicillamine have caused vitamin B_6 deficiency in older children.

In animals, pyridoxine deficiency leads to impaired growth, anemia, changes in skin and hair, and seizures. These manifestations may be due to decreased production of gamma-aminobutyric acid, a central nervous system inhibitory neurotransmitter. The active form the vitamin appears to cocatalyze the conversion of glutamic acid to gamma-aminobutyric acid with the apoenzyme glutamic acid decarboxylase. Deficiency of gamma-aminobutyric acid predisposes the brain to hyperirritability and seizures.

The diagnosis of pyridoxine deficiency depends on identification of compatible symptoms and reversal of these symptoms by vitamin therapy. When possible, vitamin B_6 deficiency should be verified by measurement of blood levels or by use of the tryptophan loading test (Driskell, 1984)

Pyridoxine Dependency. Seizures associated with neonatal pyridoxine dependency occur when an apoenzyme requires an unusually high tissue level of pyridoxine for functional activity. In such cases, the blood or tissue levels of active vitamin B_6 are normal but higher levels are required to prevent clinical symptoms. Pyridoxine dependency usually is exhibited by irritability and seizures in the first days of life. Seizures may even occur in utero, and may be treatable with administration of vitamin B_6 to the mother (Bejsovec et al., 1967). In most cases, seizures have been brief and tonic-clonic in nature. An interesting feature is the inability of anticonvulsants to control this seizure disorder in contrast to the rapid control achieved

by a single dose of 50 mg of pyridoxine. This feature has been considered diagnostically useful. During continuous electroencephalographic recording, a single dose of 50 mg of intravenous pyridoxine is given as both a therapeutic and diagnostic trial. Control of seizures, as indicated by electroencephalography, within minutes after injection of the vitamin suggests that the patient has pyridoxine dependency. Although control of seizures may be rapid, it may require up to 24 hours before the electroencephalogram fully returns to normal. Other syndromes associated with pyridoxine dependency include pyridoxine responsive microcytic anemia, xanthenurenic aciduria, cystathioninuria, and homcystinuria (Moran 1979).

The early onset and high continuing vitamin requirements of pyridoxine dependency should distinguish it from simple pyridoxine deficiency. Quantitative measurements of plasma vitamin B_6 should be normal in pyridoxine dependency but low in pyridoxine deficiency. The tryptophan loading test, although normal in dependency states, results in an increase in xanthenurenic acid in true deficiency states. This is a result of the importance of vitamin B_6 as a coenzyme in the further breakdown of tryptophan and has been used to confirm the differentiation of these clinical entities.

Toxicity. Massive doses of pyridoxine have been reported to cause ataxia and sensory neuropathy in adults. Cases of toxicity have not been reported in infants.

Requirements and Treatment. The recommended daily allowance for pyridoxine is 0.3 mg/day for infants. Infant formulas should contain a minimum of .035 mg/ 100 kcal. Levels of pyridoxine in human milk (mean .205 ± .03 mg/l) vary with maternal supplementation. As little as 0.1 mg/day of puridoxine may be adequate for the newborn, and this amount is provided by standard infant formulas and human milk. During the administration of total parenteral nutrition, the provision of 0.65 and 1.0 mg/day of pyridoxine to premature and term infants, respectively, appeared to be sufficient (Moore et al., 1986). Treatment of pyridoxine deficiency would simply require replenishment of the body pool, and this could be accomplished by the administration of 50 to 100 mg per day of pyridoxine for several days, followed by provision of a diet adequate in vitamin B_6. Syndromes of pyridoxine dependency vary in the vitamin B_6 requirement. In general, 25 to 100 mg/day of pyridoxine is necessary to prevent irritability and seizures.

FOLATE

Metabolism and Function. Folate is a coenzyme in reactions involving single carbon transfer in protein and nucleic acid metabolism. Fetal plasma and red blood cell folate levels are much higher than maternal levels during the last trimester (Ek, 1980). Human milk contains a factor that facilitates the absorption of folate. Folate requirements in formula-fed infants may actually be higher than those fed human milk because of the absence of this factor in artificial formulas (Ek, 1982).

Deficiency. Folate deficiency is associated with growth retardation, megaloblastic anemia, and an increased frequency of gastroenteritis and infection. Premature infants are particularly at risk for the development of folate deficiency due to limited tissue stores. Premature infants develop megaloblastic anemia when fed a diet low in folate (Strelling et al., 1966). Megaloblastic anemia and intestinal lesions have been reported in infants fed unsupplemented goat's milk, which is deficient in folate (Davidson and Townley, 1977).

Toxicity. Folate toxicity does not appear to occur in infants.

Requirements. The new recommended daily allowance for folate is 25 and 35 mcg/day for infants 0 to 6 and 6 to 12 months, respectively, which is a decrease from the earlier recommendation of 50 mcg/day. Human milk contains 50 to 60 mcg/l of folate, which should readily provide the recommended daily allowance for folate in term infants. AAPCON (1977) recommended that infant formulas be supplemented with a minimum of 4 mcg folate per 100 kcal, although most formulas are supplemented at a higher level. The folate requirements of premature infants may be much higher due to lower tissue stores secondary to premature delivery and due to rapid postnatal growth. AAPCON (1985) suggested that folate supplementation (50 mcg/day) for premature infants be added separately to liquid pediatric multivitamins once full enteral feedings are established. However, this recommendation was not definitive and it was suggested that formula intake and vitamin content of the formula be considered. Ek (1985) studied two groups of premature infants (one supplemented with additional 50 mcg of folate, and the other had no supplement) who were fed a cow's milk formula containing 21 mcg/l of folate. He showed that the group given an additional 50 mcg of folate had higher plasma and red blood cell folate levels (similar to term breast-fed infants) at 2 to 6 months of age. Despite these differences in folate levels, there was no difference in hemoglobin or mean corpuscular volume between the groups. Ek (1985) calculated the folate requirement of the premature infant to be about 15 mcg/kg/day. Formulas for premature infants are high in folate. For infants who are fed a special formula that contains at least 35 mcg folate/100 kcal, an intake of at least 107 ml/day of 20-kcal/oz formula would provide the RDA for folate. Based on available data, it appears that premature infants do not require further folate supplementation beyond the amounts in formulas for premature infants. Human milk should meet the needs of the premature infant without difficulty. There is little information regarding folate requirements during the administration of total parenteral nutrition. Moore and colleagues (1986) found that the provision of 91 mcg/day of folate to premature infants and 140 mcg/day of folate to term infants results in normal or high red blood cell folate levels without signs of toxicity.

VITAMIN B₁₂

Metabolism and Function. Vitamin B_{12} is particularly important in DNA synthesis, red blood cell development, and biochemical reactions involving transfer of methyl groups. Vitamin B_{12} includes a number of compounds that can be converted to the active coenzymes methylcobalamin and 5′-deoxyadenosylcobalamin. Cord blood levels of vitamin B_{12} are twice maternal levels. Vitamin B_{12} is absorbed in the terminal ileum after it is bound to intrinsic factor, which is excreted by the stomach. Vitamin B_{12} is transported in the blood bound to transcobalamin II.

Deficiency. Vitamin B_{12} deficiency in the 1st year of life is very rare. Vitamin B_{12} deficiency does not become clinically evident until liver stores are depleted. Hence, intake and absorption of vitamin B_{12} can be inadequate for many months before clinical signs of deficiency become apparent. Symptoms in infants include megaloblastic anemia, immune suppression, pallor, failure to thrive, glossitis, developmental delay, involuntary motor movements, and coma (Higginbottom et al., 1978; Sadowitz et al., 1986). Vitamin B_{12} deficiency rarely occurs in breast-fed infants. However, it has been reported in breast-fed infants whose mothers are strict vegetarians and also B_{12} deficient. Although urinary excretion of methylmalonic acid (an index of vitamin B_{12} insufficiency) in healthy infants fed human milk is higher than those fed vitamin B_{12}–supplemented formula, the clinical significance of this finding is unknown (Specker et al. 1990). Vitamin B_{12} deficiency occurs after ileal resection for necrotizing enterocolitis and other neonatal gastrointestinal surgical disorders (Collins et al., 1984). A congenital defect in B_{12} absorption has been reported in children, but this does not appear in the first year of life. Clinical signs of vitamin B_{12} deficiency also occur in congenital defects of transcobalamin II, defects in vitamin B_{12} absorption, lack of intrinsic factor, and with adherence to a vegetarian diet.

Toxicity. Vitamin B_{12} toxicity does not appear to occur.

Requirements. The new recommended daily allowance for vitamin B_{12} is 0.3 mcg/day at age 0 to 6 months and 0.5 mcg/day at 6 to 12 months. Human milk contains 0.5 ± 0.2 mcg/l of vitamin B_{12}. Breast-fed infants whose mothers are at risk of becoming or who are indeed vitamin B_{12} deficient should receive supplemental vitamin B_{12}. AAPCON (1977) recommends that infant formulas be supplemented at a minimum of 0.15 mcg/100 kcal. Formulas for premature infants in the United States are supplemented at 0.3 to 0.55 mcg/100 kcal. Moore and co-workers (1986) reported blood vitamin B_{12} levels during parenteral nutrition with a pediatric intravenous multivitamin. Premature and term infants received 0.65 mcg/day and 1 mcg/day of vitamin B_{12}, respectively. In these infants, the blood vitamin B_{12} levels increased over several weeks to greater than 2 SD above the mean of a healthy reference population. No apparent toxicity was noted from these high blood levels. Greene and associates (1988) has recommended lowering the parenteral vitamin B_{12} intake of premature infants to 0.3 mcg/kg/day. After ileal resection, it is difficult to predict which infants will develop vitamin B_{12} deficiency. For infants who underwent more than 15 cm of distal ileal resection, it may be necessary to provide lifelong parenteral supplementation of vitamin B_{12} (Collins et al., 1984). An intramuscular dose of 50 to 100 mcg monthly for such infants should be sufficient.

NIACIN

Metabolism and Function. Niacin includes nicotinic acid and nicotinamide as forms of this vitamin. Nicotinamide is incorporated into nicotinamide-adenine dinucleotide and nicotinamide-adenine dinucleotide phosphate, which are important to a variety of oxidation and reduction reactions in carbohydrate, fat, and protein metabolism. About 1.5% of dietary tryptophan can be converted into niacin. Hence, dietary requirements are often expressed in niacin equivalents (NE)—1 mg of niacin equals 1 NE, and 60 mg tryptophan equals 1 NE. Pharmacologic doses of niacin have been used in the treatment of hyperlipidemias.

Deficiency. Deficiency of niacin leads to an illness called pellagra, which may actually be due to a deficiency of several vitamins beside niacin. This condition is characterized initially by a dermatitis, which begins in sunlight-exposed areas, and is followed by worsening skin, mucosal, and psychic symptoms (Moran and Greene, 1979). Deficiency of niacin is generally not seen in newborns.

Toxicity. Toxicity has only been seen with pharmacologic doses in adults, and the condition includes gastrointestinal, hepatic, and dermatologic symptoms (Moran 1979).

Requirements. The recommended daily allowance for niacin is 5 and 6 NE at 0 to 6 and 6 to 12 months, respectively. AAPCON (1977) recommends that infant formulas contain a minimum of 0.25 mg niacin/100 kcal. Human milk contains about this much niacin, and further niacin equivalents are contributed by tryptophan. Premature infants do not require further supplementation beyond the niacin present in human milk or premature infant formulas. Parenteral niacin requirements are not well studied. Moore and Greene (1986) gave 11 and 17 mg niacin/day to premature and term infants, respectively. Niacin levels were in an appropriate range for both groups. Greene and co-workers (1988) recommend a parenteral dose of 6.8 mg/kg/day of niacin, which is provided by a dose of 40 per cent of a vial/kg/day of MVI-Pediatric.

PANTOTHENIC ACID

Metabolism and Function. Pantothenic acid is incorporated into coenzyme A, which is important in a number of acylation reactions of carbohydrate, protein, and lipid metabolism. Neonatal levels of pantothenic acid are higher than maternal levels.

Deficiency. Deficiency of this vitamin was believed to be the cause of "burning feet syndrome," which occurred among prisoners of war in the Far East. Neonatal and infant deficiency of this vitamin does not appear to occur (Moran and Greene, 1979).

Toxicity. Toxicity from pantothenic acid does not appear to occur.

Requirements. The estimated safe and adequate daily dietary intake of pantothenic acid is 2 and 3 mg, respectively, for infants 0 to 6 and 6 to 12 months of age. Human milk contains approximately 0.3 mg/100 kcal. AAPCON (1977) recommends that infant formulas contain a minimum of 0.3 mg/100 kcal. During the administration of total parenteral nutrition, Moore and associates (1986) found that the administration of 5 mg pantothenic acid daily for term infants resulted in normal blood levels of the vitamin. Premature infants had excessively high levels when given 3.2 mg/day. Greene and co-workers (1988) recommend a dose of 2 mg pantothenic acid/kg/day for premature infants (40 per cent vial MVI-Pediatric/kg/day).

SUMMARY OF RECOMMENDATIONS FOR VITAMIN SUPPLEMENTATION

1. Term breast-fed infants: Strong consideration should be given to provide a supplement of 400 IU of vitamin D daily. Infants of vitamin D–deficient mothers or infants with limited sunlight exposure should definitely receive supplemental vitamin D on a daily basis.

2. Formula-fed term infants: Routine vitamin supplementation is not indicated, provided the formula meets AAPCON (1977) standards.

3. Premature infants fed human milk: These infants should receive the standard dose of infant multivitamins (e.g., 1 ml of Poly-Vi-Sol daily). This provides 400 IU vitamin D and further supplements vitamins (A, E, water soluble vitamins) that may be marginal in the sick premature infant. Consideration should be given to providing an additional 25 IU of vitamin E daily. Further folate supplementation (50 mcg daily) is probably not needed.

4. Premature infants fed specialized premature formulas: A vitamin D supplement of 400 IU daily should be provided. This is easily achieved by provision of the standard infant oral multivitamin (e.g., 1 ml Poly-Vi-Sol). Consideration should be given to providing an additional 25 IU of vitamin E daily. Further folate supplementation (50 mcg daily) is probably not needed.

5. Infants receiving total parenteral nutrition should be given MVI-Pediatric daily as follows: those weighing less than 1 kg, 30–50 per cent vial/day; those weighing 1 to 3 kg, 65 per cent vial/day, those weighing more than 3 kg, 100 per cent vial/day; or alternatively follow the recommendation of Greene (1988) of 40 per cent vial/kg/day.

■ TRACE MINERALS

Micromineral nutrient deficiencies rarely occur in enterally fed premature and term infants unless they are fed an inappropriate diet. The premature infant requires a higher intake of some trace minerals due to rapid postnatal growth, thus predisposing the premature to the development of nutrient deficiencies. With the widespread use of total parenteral nutrition in sick newborns, trace mineral requirements were initially provided in the past by fresh frozen plasma transfusions. It quickly became clear that this approach did not consistently meet the micromineral requirements of the parenterally fed infant. Zinc and copper are now routinely supplemented during the administration of total parenteral nutrition, and standard doses are fairly well established. However, studies of other trace minerals during the administration of total parenteral in newborns are limited and recommended doses are tentative (see Table 75–9). Toxicity from trace minerals due to inadvertent or injudicious administration can occur. Inherent contamination of parenteral infusates (e.g., with aluminum) can have toxic effects on the infant.

ZINC

Metabolism and Function. Zinc is essential to the function of a number of enzymes as a cofactor or as part of a metalloenzyme. Such enzymes include alkaline phosphatase, carbonic anhydrase, and superoxide dismutase. Zinc is particularly important in the metabolism of amino acids, RNA, and DNA (Gordon, 1981).

In the fetus, zinc accumulates during the third trimester at a rate of approximately 250 mcg/kg/day. Much of this zinc is incorporated into liver, muscle, and other fat-free tissues. Zinc, which has been ingested or released by the sloughing of intestinal cells, is absorbed in the proximal small bowel. Zinc absorption from human milk appears to be facilitated by a low molecular weight ligand that may be citrate. Human milk contains 0.47 ± 0.12 (mean ± SD) mg/l of zinc in the 1st month of lactation, declining to 0.29 ± 0.07 mg/l at 12 months (Casey et al., 1989). The zinc content of human milk of women who delivered prematurely appears to be similar (Atkinson et al., 1989; Zimmerman et al., 1982). Absorption rates vary widely (14 to 41 per cent) depending largely on the type of diet consumed (Sandstrom et al., 1983) and interactions of other nutrients. Absorption rates for zinc are better with human milk than with cow's milk formulas. Iron and copper may interfere with zinc absorption. Phytates in the diet can form an insoluble complex with zinc and calcium, preventing zinc absorption. Zinc absorption is regulated in the intestinal cell by metallothionein, which binds absorbed zinc. Zinc is transported in the blood bound to albumin and alpha–2-macroglobulin. Normal zinc concentrations in the adult are between 76 to 222 mcg/dL (Gordon et al., 1981). Both term and premature newborns generally start with serum zinc levels in this range, but then zinc levels often decline postnatally (Vileisis et al., 1981).

Deficiency. The classic picture of zinc deficiency is encompassed in the presentation of acrodermatitis enteropathica. Acrodermatitis enteropathica is an autosomal recessive disorder, which usually presents at the time of weaning from breast-feeding. The skin manifestations of acrodermatitis enteropathica dominate the clinical picture, which is true of zinc deficiency in general. Initially, the infant develops a perioral, perinasal, and perineal rash, which can be bullous, pustular, or erythematous. The rash then spreads to the limbs, with involvement of the extensor surfaces (elbows and knees), hands, and feet. Severe involvement leads to alopecia and loss of nails. Other symptoms include growth failure, pale bulky stools, impaired immune response, hypogeusesthesia, and malabsorption of carbohydrate and fat. Measurement of serum zinc levels should be obtained to confirm zinc deficiency. Human milk has been used in the treatment of acrodermatitis enteropathica. The benefits of human milk in acrodermatitis enteropathica are due to the efficient absorption of zinc from human milk. By chance observation it was found that the administration of diiodohydroxyquinoline improved the symptoms of acrodermatitis enteropathica. The mechanism of this effect is probably related to the zinc-binding properties of diiodohydroxyquinoline, which may have improved zinc absorption. With the recognition of the role of zinc deficiency in acrodermatitis enteropathica, specific therapy with zinc is clearly the treatment of choice (Neldner and Hambidge, 1975). Infants with acrodermatitis enteropathica should receive zinc sulfate at a dose of 1–2 mg/kg/day of elemental zinc.

There have been case reports of zinc deficiency occurring in both term and premature infants fed human milk (Aggett et al., 1980, Atkinson et al., 1989, Zimmerman et al., 1982). The breast milk from the mothers of these infants was found to be very low in zinc (0.05 to 0.130 mg/l in the 1st month and < 0.05 mg/l after 2 months) as compared with normal human milk. Zinc secretion from the mammary gland appears to be impaired in these women, and the condition does not improve with maternal zinc supplementation. Treatment of the infant with supplemental zinc (1 to 2 mg/kg/day of elemental zinc) should allow for continued breast-feeding. Kumar and Anday (1984) reported on a group of three premature infants who developed edema, hypoproteinemia, and hypozincemia. These infants were fed a combination of formula and human milk. Symptoms subsided with zinc supplementation. It is unclear whether these symptoms were due to zinc deficiency or to protein-calorie malnutrition.

Premature and term infants have been reported to develop symptoms of zinc deficiency during prolonged parenteral nutrition with inadequate amounts of zinc (Latimer et al., 1980; Srouji et al., 1978). Infants who have required gastrointestinal surgical procedures may be particularly at risk for the development of zinc deficiency. Such infants can lose large amounts of zinc in gastrointestinal secretions from nasogastric drainage, ileostomy fluid, and watery stools due to malabsorption. With the provision of a minimum of 300 mcg/kg/day of elemental zinc in the total parenteral nutrition infusate to premature infants, clinical zinc deficiency is now unusual. Term newborns recovering from gastrointestinal surgical procedures may require similar amounts of zinc supplementation during the administration of total parenteral nutrition.

Toxicity. Zinc is relatively nontoxic, and reported cases of toxicity are rare (Fosmire, 1990). Excessive oral doses of zinc are excreted largely in the stool. With intravenous administration, large amounts of zinc are excreted in the urine. Acute oral ingestions of large doses of zinc are associated with vomiting and diarrhea. An inadvertent acute intravenous dose of 1.5 grams of zinc resulted in death in an adult. Chronic zinc therapy has been reported to cause copper deficiency in older patients. High levels of zinc supplementation have been associated with a suppressed immune response, an increase in low density lipoproteins, and a decrease in high-density lipoproteins. All of these potential effects of zinc supplementation have not been adequately evaluated in term or premature infants. The safe upper limit of zinc supplementation in premature infants has not been defined. However, Higashi and associates (1988) found no effect upon copper retention in a group of premature infants who were receiving zinc-supplemented human milk (8.4 mg/l zinc). Until more information is available it would be prudent to avoid doses of zinc beyond the amounts usually recommended for premature infants unless there is evidence of zinc deficiency.

Requirements. Mature human milk contains about 0.5 mg of zinc/100 kcal, and AAPCON (1977) recommends that infant formulas contain a minimum of 0.5 mg/100 kcal. Most standard cow's milk and soy formulas for the term infant contain about 0.75 to 0.8 mg/100 kcal of zinc. In view of the better absorption of zinc from human milk, it appears to be prudent to provide this higher level of zinc in formula. The feeding of a cow's milk formula containing 1.8 mg/l of zinc resulted in significantly lower incremental growth (weight and length) in term male infants as compared with a formula containing 5.8 mg/l of zinc (Walravens and Hambidge, 1976). A more recent study, however, found no difference in growth between a group of term infants fed human milk and a group fed formula containing 1.0 or 3.2 mg/l of zinc (Matsuda et al., 1984). Although exclusively breast-fed term infants receive less than the recommended daily allowance (5 mg/day), clinical deficiency is rare.

The intrauterine accretion rate of zinc in the third trimester is about 250 mcg/kg/day. Despite zinc supplementation, premature infants tend to remain in negative zinc balance in the first two months of life due to large fecal losses. Urinary losses of zinc in the premature infant are also high (30 to 40 mcg/kg/day) in the first 2 months of life. Dauncey and colleagues (1977) reported that premature infants who were fed pooled pasteurized human milk remained in negative zinc balance until 60 days postnatal age. Higashi and co-workers (1988) studied two groups of premature infants who were fed either zinc-supplemented (8.4 ± 0.8 mg/L) or unsupplemented (2.2 ± 1.1 mg/l) human milk. Both groups of infants remained in negative zinc balance until 36 weeks postconceptional age. However, Mendelson and associates (1983) found that premature infants of a mean gestational age of about 29 weeks were in positive zinc balance at 1 to 4 weeks of age when they were fed their own mothers milk. The better zinc retention found in this study may reflect the higher zinc content of early premature milk as compared with mature pooled human milk. Tyrala (1986) was able to achieve intrauterine retention rates of zinc in 31 to 37 week postconceptional age premature infants who were fed a whey-predominant formula that contained 50 per cent of the fat as medium-chain triglycerdes and a total of 12.5 mg/l zinc. Despite some differences between studies, it is clear that the premature infant should benefit from zinc supplementation. Premature infant formulas (24 kcal/oz) contain between 8 to 12.7 mg/l of zinc, which should be sufficient to meet the needs of tissue growth and to prevent clinical signs of deficiency except in circumstances of unusual fecal losses. Premature infants may require higher levels of zinc than is available in mature pooled human milk.

Parenteral zinc requirements are much lower than oral requirements due to lower fecal losses in infants who are not being fed enterally. Term newborns may require only 150 to 175 mcg/kg/day of zinc in the 1st month of life (Greene et al., 1988; Zlotkin and Buchanan, 1983). The parenteral zinc requirements of older infants are between 30 and 100 mcg/kg/day unless there are increased gastrointestinal fluid losses (Greene et al., 1988; Shulman, 1989). Parenteral zinc requirements are much higher in the premature infant than in the term newborn. Zlotkin and Buchanan (1983) found that a parenteral zinc intake of more than 438 mcg/kg/day is necessary to achieve zinc retention rates comparable to those in utero in premature infants. Lockitch and co-workers (1983) and Friel and associates (1984) have reported that the administration of 400 and 350 mcg/kg/day of zinc, respectively, during total parenteral nutrition is sufficient to maintain stable serum zinc levels (mean > 113 mcg/dl) in premature infants older than 2 to 4 weeks of age. Parenteral zinc requirements can also vary with the amino acid preparation used. Urinary losses of zinc appear to be higher with some amino acid formulations (Greene et al., 1988; Zlotkin and Buchanan, 1983). The American Society for Clinical Nutrition recommends that premature infants be given 400 mcg/kg/day of zinc during the administration of total parenteral nutrition (Greene et al., 1988). The AMA Nutrition Advisory Group recommended 300 mcg/kg/day of zinc (Shils et al., 1979).

COPPER

Metabolism and Function. Copper is incorporated into a number of metalloenzymes. Cytosolic superoxidase dismutase scavenges superoxide ions, thus protecting against oxygen toxicity. Ceruloplasmin, which binds much of the copper in blood, has ferroxidase activity. Ceruloplasmin oxidizes ferrous iron released from tissues to ferric iron, which is then transported to bone marrow and other sites. Other copper-containing enzymes participate in collagen, dopamine, and melanin synthesis. The fetus accumulates large amounts of copper in the third trimester (approximately 50 mcg/kg/day). Most of this copper is stored in the fetal liver. Fetal liver copper concentration increases up to 200 mcg/g of dry weight, which is 10 to 20-fold greater than adult levels. The fetal liver stores the copper bound to metallothionein, which probably protects the fetal liver from copper toxicity. These high fetal hepatic stores of copper then act as a reservoir for postnatal needs. Little is known regarding changes in hepatic copper and metallothionein concentration. It is unknown whether it is advantageous or harmful to the liver of the premature infant to continue to accumulate hepatic copper at the intrauterine rate.

Absorption of copper by stable isotope methods appears to be more efficient with human milk (72 per cent) than with cow's milk formula (53 per cent) in premature infants (Ehrenkranz et al., 1986). Net absorption rates as a proportion of intake are much lower. Premature infants are often in negative copper balance during the first weeks of life (Dauncey et al., 1977; Tyrala, 1986). Tyrala found net absorption (per cent of intake) to be 12 to 14 per cent in formula-fed premature infants. Mendelson and colleagues (1983) reported greatly improved copper absorption in premature infants fed their own mothers' milk as compared with infant formula (52 to 76 per cent versus − 15 to + 15 per cent). Copper absorption in the intestine is reduced by excessive intakes of ascorbic acid, iron, and zinc. Copper is transported in the blood bound to ceruloplasmin, albumin, low molecular proteins, and amino acids. Copper is excreted primarily in the biliary tract, which explains the accumulation of copper in cholestatic disorders. Urinary excretion of copper is low (2 to 6 mcg/kg/day) in both enterally and parenterally fed infants (Mendelson et al., 1983; Zlotkin and Buchanan, 1983).

Serum copper levels are the most readily available method to assess copper status. Because serum copper levels do not always reflect hepatic stores, there are limitations in the use of this method. Serum copper levels are much lower in term (32 ± 21 mcg/dl) and premature infants (26 ± 17 mcg/dl) at birth as compared with those of adults (101 ± 20 mcg/dl) (Hillman 1981a). Similarly, ceruloplasmin levels are low in both term and premature infants. There is a postnatal maturational change in ceruloplasmin and copper levels, which appears to be somewhat independent of copper intake. Both copper and ceruloplasmin levels slowly rise to adult values over several months with a strong positive correlation to postceptional age in premature infants (Hillman et al., 1981a, 1981b; Salmenpera et at., 1986; Sutton et al., 1985). Hence, it is difficult to assess copper status in the first few months of life by measurement of serum copper alone. Comparison of results must be made with norms for the infant's gestational age.

Deficiency. Because of the large stores of copper available in liver at birth, copper deficiency appears in newborns at 2 to 3 months of age or older. Clinical findings include neutropenia, normocytic hypochromic anemia, pallor, and distended veins. Radiologic findings may include osteopenia, fraying, cupping, and splaying of the metaphyses of long bones on x-ray study, along with fractures. Because of similarities to the bony findings of osteopenia of prematurity, radiologic diagnosis alone is not sufficient. Serum copper levels and ceruloplasmin levels, which are generally low, must be compared with the appropriate norms for gestational age. Because premature infants have low serum copper levels in the first 2 months of life, the diagnosis should be made only in the setting of compatible clinical findings (hematologic and bone) and a positive response to copper supplementation.

Premature infants particularly are at risk for developing copper deficiency due to reduced hepatic stores from premature delivery. Sutton and associates (1985) reported on four premature infants who developed copper deficiency while being fed human milk or infant formulas relatively low in copper (39 mcg/100 ml). The enteral copper intake of these infants ranged between 25 and 64 mcg/kg/day, which is below the recommendation by the AAPCON (1977) of 90 mcg/100 kcal for premature infants. Term infants, who have been fed cow's milk, were reported to have copper deficiency, which appeared at age 6 months of age (Levy et al., 1985). Cow's milk is a poor source of copper because it contains only 10 mcg/100 ml. Copper deficiency occurs in infants given parenteral nutrition without supplemental copper over several months (Karpel and Peden, 1972) Menkes kinky hair syndrome is a complex autosomal recessive disorder that shares some common characteristics (bony changes) with nutritional copper deficiency. Serum and hepatic concentrations of copper are usually low, and intestinal absorption of copper is defective (Danks et al., 1972).

Treatment of copper deficiency may only require provision of recommended amounts of copper in enteral or parenteral nutrition. Supplemental oral copper sulfate (1 per cent solution) may be given at a dose of 200 to 800 mcg/kg/day of elemental copper until the serum copper is corrected to normal levels.

Toxicity. When copper accumulates to high levels in the liver, it can cause hepatotoxicity and cirrhosis. Wilson disease is an autosomal recessive disorder that presents later in childhood. It is associated with high hepatic copper concentration and low or normal ceruloplasmin levels. Clinical findings may include hepatitis, hemolytic anemia, coagulopathy, cataracts, renal tubular dysfunction, and neurologic and skeletal abnormalities. Copper toxicity can also occur when biliary excretion of copper is impaired, as in cholestatic disorders (e.g. biliary atresia). In theory, copper toxicity could occur with continued administration of parenteral copper in total parenteral nutrition associated cholestatic jaundice. Although it is recommended to delete copper from total parenteral nutrition solutions in the setting of total parenteral nutrition–associated cholestasis, copper toxicity has not been proved to occur with continued administration. Another example of copper excess is East Indian childhood cirrhosis, which presents in infancy. The pathogenesis of cirrhosis in East Indian children is not completely understood, but it appears to be the result of excessive copper intake resulting in hapatotoxicity. Infants affected by this disorder have often been fed copper-contaminated animal milk, which has been stored and prepared in copper-containing household containers (Tanner et al., 1983).

Requirements. Copper deficiency does not appear to occur in breast-fed term infants. Hence, human milk provides a good first estimate of copper requirements. In the 1st month of lactation, human milk (term and premature) contains 0.4 to 0.7 mg/l of copper, declining to 0.1 to 0.2 mg/l in term mature milk (Casey et al., 1989; Mendelson et al., 1983; Salmenpera et al., 1986). The intrauterine accretion rate of copper in the third trimester in calculated to be 50 mcg/kg/day. Premature infants fed their own mothers' milk are in positive copper balance, with copper retention above the in utero rate (Mendelson et al., 1983). However, studies in premature infants fed pooled pasteurized human milk and infant formula have shown that the infants were in negative copper balance in the 1st month of life (Dauncey et al., 1977; Tyrala, 1986). Tyrala (1986) was able to achieve the in utero copper retention rate in some premature infants by using a formula containing 1.2 mg of copper/liter. The copper requirements for tissue growth (retention of 20 mcg/kg/day) are much lower than the in utero retention rate. Because of the concern for hepatotoxicity with excessive copper and the fact that serum copper and ceruloplasmin are little affected by copper administration in the 1st month of life, it may be prudent to provide only the amount of copper required to maintain tissue growth. The current recommendations of the AAPCON (1977, 1985) readily meet these needs. Infant formulas for term and premature infants should contain 60 and 90 mcg of copper/100 kcal, respectively.

The primary goal of copper supplementation of infants

during the administration of total parenteral nutrition should be to prevent deficiency symptoms without toxicity. Hence, attempts to achieve in utero retention rates of copper are not prudent, as discussed earlier. Manser and associates (1980) found that serum copper rose in a group of premature infants during the administration of total parenteral nutrition without supplemental copper. This factor may have been the result of trace copper contamination in the total parenteral nutrition infusate or a rise in serum ceruloplasmin from multiple blood transfusions. Zlotkin and Buchanan (1983) found that the in utero copper retention rate is met by provision of at least 63 mcg/kg/day, whereas only 16 mcg/kg/day is required for positive copper balance and replacement of ongoing losses. Provision of 20 mcg/kg/day of copper to premature infants during the administration of total parenteral nutrition maintains a steady slow rise in serum copper over the 1st month (Friel et al., 1984). Lockitch and colleagues (1983) found no difference in serum copper and ceruloplasmin levels between doses of 20 and 40 mcg/kg/day in premature infants during the administration of total parenteral nutrition. The AMA Nutrition Advisory Group (Shils et al., 1979) and the American Society of Clinical Nutrition (Greene et al., 1988) recommend a parenteral copper dose of 20 mcg/kg/day.

SELENIUM

Metabolism and Function. The only known function of selenium is its incorporation into glutathione peroxidase, which protects against oxidative injury and lipid membrane peroxidation by acting on hydrogen peroxide. Selenium is easily absorbed (80 per cent), and serum levels are determined by dietary intake. Dietary intake is largely determined by the selenium content of the soil. Excretion of selenium is primarily from the kidneys. Levels of selenium in human milk are generally higher than those in infant formulas.

Deficiency. In endemic areas (e.g., certain parts of China), selenium deficiency causes cardiomyopathy and death in children and pregnant women (Keshan disease). Plasma glutathione peroxidase and selenium levels decline during the administration of total parenteral nutrition without selenium in premature infants and adults (Cohen et al., 1979; Huston et al., 1982; Van Ris et al., 1989). Clinical symptoms of selenium deficiency have been reported in pediatric and adult patients after prolonged total parenteral nutrition without selenium supplementation (Johnson et al., 1981; Kelly et al., 1988). Symptoms include muscle weakness and pain and cardiomyopathy. Vinton and co-workers (1987) described four pediatric patients with low serum selenium levels (38 ± 11 ng/ml) on total parenteral nutrition with selenium supplementation. A variety of symptoms including macrocytosis, skin and hair depigmentation, muscle weakness, and elevated transaminases were ascribed to selenium deficiency. Symptoms subsided with selenium supplementation (2 mcg/kg/day).

Toxicity. Acute ingestion of 5 mg/kg of selenium has been reported to cause death. Chronic excessive ingestion causes alopecia, nausea, and roughening of the nails.

Toxicity has been reported in animals in areas containing high levels of selenium.

Requirements and Treatment. Selenium requirements in infants are estimated to be 1 mcg/kg/day, which is an approximation based on the adult requirement (70 mcg/day). Although an recommended daily allowance of 10 mcg/day (0 to 6 months) and 15 mcg/kay (6 to 12 months) during infancy has been established, a safe range of selenium intake for premature infants is unknown. Human milk contains higher amounts of selenium in the first month, declining to 5 to 18 ng/ml in different populations. Infant formulas contain lower amounts of selenium (5.8 to 9.2 ng/ml) than human milk (Smith et al., 1982). Enterally fed infants receive adequate amounts of selenium from human milk or infant formulas, and no further supplementation is indicated. During total parenteral nutrition, most infants require no selenium supplementation over 1 to 2 months. Infants who require very prolonged total parenteral nutrition (> 2 months) should receive 1 to 2 mcg/kg/day of selenium. Because there is very little information on parenteral selenium in infants, serum selenium levels should be monitored during supplementation, if available. Since selenium is excreted by the kidneys, the parenteral dose of selenium should be reduced in renal failure.

OTHER TRACE MINERALS

Manganese is incorporated into mitochondrial superoxide dismutase and pyruvate carboxylase. Spontaneous human deficiency has not been reported. Neurologic toxicity occurs in work-related exposures among miners. Human milk levels of manganese are about 6 mcg/l early in lactation, declining to 4 mcg/l at 2 months (Vuori, 1979). Various infant formulas contain much higher amounts of manganese, up to 200 times the concentration found in human milk (Table 76–1). Despite a much higher manganese intake with formula, infants do not show signs of manganese toxicity. The fractional absorption of manganese from human milk (8 per cent) is higher than from cow's milk or infant formulas (0.7 to 7 per cent) (Davidsson et al., 1989). The recommended dose of manganese during total parenteral nutrition is 1 mcg/kg/day (Greene et al., 1988), but higher doses of 1 to 10 mcg/kg/day are used without apparent toxicity. Serum manganese levels are elevated in patients with cholestasis during total parenteral nutrition (Hambidge, 1989). Manganese should be reduced or removed from the total parenteral nutrition infusate in patients with cholestatic jaundice.

Iodine is essential for normal synthesis of thyroxine. Iodine accumulation in the fetus is estimated to be 1 mcg/kg/day. Human milk contains a mean of 178 mcg/l with a range of 29 to 470 mcg/l (Gushurst et al., 1984). Levels in human milk are affected by maternal dietary intake. AAPCON (1977) recommends that infant formula contain a minimum of 5 mcg/100 kcal. Infant formulas generally contain higher amounts of iodide that the minimum requirements (Table 76–1). Iodide deficiency is unlikely to occur in infants fed human milk or formula except in areas of endemic goiter. During total parenteral nutrition, it has been recommended to give 1 mcg/kg/day of iodide. Such supplementation is likely to be unnecessary except in

TABLE 76–1. Trace Mineral Composition of Human Milk and Infant Formulas: Comparison with
Postnatal Oral Requirements in the Premature Infant

TRACE MINERAL	MATURE HUMAN MILK*	PRETERM HUMAN MILK†	COWS' MILK FORMULA‡	FORMULA FOR PREMATURE INFANTS§	POSTNATAL REQUIREMENTS (mcg/kg/day)‖
Zinc (mg/l)	0.5 to 1.0	2 to 5	5.0 to 5.2	8 to 12.7	1250¶
Copper (mg/l)	0.1 to 0.3	0.6 to 0.7	0.47 to 0.63	0.7 to 2.03	100 to 120¶
Selenium (mcg/l)	5 to 18		5.1 to 7.9	13.4**	3
Manganese (mcg/l)	2 to 8		34 to 150	100 to 206	20¶
Iodide (mcg/l)	0.03 to 0.47		60 to 100	50 to 83	4¶

*Mature human milk after the 1st month.
†Premature milk during the 1st month.
‡Range of Enfamil 20 (Mead-Johnson), Similac 20 (Ross), and SMA 20 (Wyeth).
§Range of Enfamil Premature Formula 24 (Mead-Johnson), Similac Special Care 24 (Ross), and SMA Premie 24 (Wyeth).
‖Data from Hambidge, K. M.: Trace element requirements in premature infants. In Lebenthal, E. (Ed.): Textbook of Gastroenterology and Nutrition. New York, Raven Press, 1989, pp. 393–401.
¶Requirements may be lower with human milk.
**Value for Enfamil Premature Formula alone.

patients requiring prolonged total parenteral nutrition over several months. Cutaneous absorption of iodide from topical providone-iodine solutions represents a significant source of iodide in the newborn (Pyati et al., 1977). Neonatal thyroid suppression has been reported after the application of topical povidone-iodine (l'Allemand 1983).

Chromium deficiency or toxicity has not been reported in infants. Human milk contains 0.3 mcg of chromium per liter. Chromium deficiency has been reported to occur in adults during prolonged administration of total parenteral nutrition. Symptoms include glucose intolerance and peripheral neuropathy (Freund et al., 1979; Jeejeebhoy et al., 1977). The recommended dose of chromium during TPN is 0.14 to 0.2 mcg/kg/day (see Table 75–9).

Molybdenum is incorporated into xanthine oxidase and sulfite oxidase. A single case of deficiency has been reported in an adult during prolonged parenteral nutrition with symptoms of scotomas and progression to coma (Abumrad, 1984). Greene and colleagues (1988) recommends that molybdenum supplementation be provided only after prolonged TPN at a dose of 0.25 mcg/kg/day.

ALUMINUM TOXICITY

Aluminum has no known physiologic function in the human. However, because of its ubiquitous nature, aluminum is present in significant amounts in both enteral and parenteral nutrition. Hence, the potentially toxic effects of this trace mineral on sick infants must be considered. Aluminum is poorly absorbed by the intestine (< 2 per cent of intake). However, with large doses of aluminum (e.g., antacid therapy), up to 10 per cent absorption can occur. In the plasma, aluminum is highly protein bound. Aluminum is excreted almost exclusively by the kidneys. In the healthy infant exposed to small amounts of aluminum, any absorbed aluminum is readily excreted. When large amounts of aluminum are ingested or given by total parenteral nutrition, then aluminum loading occurs with deposition of aluminum in bone, liver, and brain.

In adults, aluminum toxicity has occurred in patients with renal failure with the use of dialysates high in aluminum. This resulted in fracturing dialysis osteodystrophy and dialysis encephalopathy (Ward et al., 1978). Subsequently, pediatric patients with renal failure, who were not on dialysis, were described with a similar encephalopathy

and bone disease. These patients were receiving high oral doses of aluminum-containing phosphate binders (Andreoli et al., 1984; Foley et al., 1981). Sedman and colleagues (1985) showed that premature infants who required IV therapy had high levels of plasma, urinary, and bone aluminum as compared with normal infants. Many components used for intravenous therapy and total parenteral nutrition are heavily contaminated with aluminum (AAPCON, 1986). However, calcium gluconate would appear to be the most important source of aluminum contamination in total parenteral nutrition, contributing about 88 per cent of the aluminum load (Koo and Kaplan, 1988a). Infants receiving parenteral nutrition are only able to excrete about 40 per cent of administered aluminum (Koo et al., 1986). Such infants are particularly at risk for deposition of aluminum into tissues and resulting toxicity. This risk is compounded by any component of renal failure. Despite the high tissue levels found in premature infants, it is unclear how much injury aluminum actually causes. Deposition of aluminum in rapidly growing bone may contribute to the osteopenia of prematurity (Koo and Kaplan, 1988a). In view of the encephalopathy seen in the past in patients with renal failure, studies are needed regarding the effects of aluminum loading on the neonatal brain.

Because the intestine is an effective barrier to the absorption of aluminum, the enterally fed infant is at much lower risk for aluminum toxicity, unless there is renal failure (Freundlich et al., 1985). Human milk is very low in aluminum (< 50 mcg/l). However, infant formulas are much higher in aluminum content, particularly soy formulas (Koo et al., 1988b). Some municipal water supplies are heavily contaminated with aluminum (> 1000 mcg/l).

The diagnosis of aluminum toxicity depends on the presence of osteopenia or encephalopathy with evidence of aluminum loading. Blood and urinary aluminum levels are usually elevated. Bone biopsy may show aluminum staining. The treatment of aluminum toxicity involves limiting the intake of both oral and intravenous aluminum. For patients who require total parenteral nutrition, every effort must be made to establish enteral feedings. Part or all of the calcium gluconate given intravenously could be replaced by a lower dose of calcium chloride (which is low in aluminum), but this requires close monitoring of the chloride level and acid-base status. Intravenous deferoxamine has been used to treat aluminum toxicity in older patients.

FLUORIDES

Fluoride prevents dental decay by its incorporation into teeth during infancy and childhood.

Fluoride supplementation is recommended in all breast-fed infants: no agreement has been reached as to when to start supplementation with 0.25 mg daily, but it is usually started after 2 weeks and before 6 months of age. Formula-fed infants require fluoride supplementation if the concentration in drinking water is less than 0.3 parts/million. Overdosage with fluoride can discolor teeth with white spots, a condition known as fluorosis.

SUMMARY OF TRACE MINERAL RECOMMENDATIONS

1. Term infants fed human milk or infant formula do not routinely require any further trace mineral supplementation.

2. Premature infants fed their own mothers' milk may have better zinc and copper balance than those fed pooled pasteurized human milk. However, premature infants weighing less than 1500 to 2000 g may benefit from zinc and copper supplementation to human milk. Supplemental zinc and copper can be provided by the addition of a powdered supplement (Enfamil Human Milk Fortifier, Mead-Johnson) to human milk.

3. Formula-fed premature infants weighing less than 1500–2000 g should be fed a premature infant formula high in zinc and copper.

4. Recommended doses of trace minerals during parenteral nutrition are summarized in Table 75–9.

■ REFERENCES

Abumrad, N. N.: Molybdenum—Is it an essential trace metal? Bull. N. Y. Acad. Med. 60:163–171, 1984.
Alade, S. L., Brown, R. E., and Paquet A., Jr: Polysorbate 80 and E-Ferol toxicity. Pediatrics 77:593–597, 1986.
Aggett, P. J., Atherton, D. J., More, J., et al.: Symptomatic zinc deficiency in a breast-fed, preterm infant. Arch. Dis. Child. 55:547–550, 1980.
American Academy of Pediatrics, Committee on Fetus and Newborn: Vitamin E and the prevention of retinopathy of prematurity. Pediatrics 76:315–316, 1985.
American Academy of Pediatrics, Committee on Nutrition (AAPCON): The prophylactic requirements and the toxicity of vitamin D. Pediatrics 31:512–525, 1963.
American Academy of Pediatrics, Committee on Nutrition (AAPCON): Nutritional needs of low-birth-weight infants. Pediatrics 60:519–530, 1977.
American Academy of Pediatrics, Committee on Nutrition (AAPCON): Nutritional needs of low-birth-weight infants. Pediatrics 75:976–986, 1985.
American Academy of Pediatrics, Committee on Nutrition (AAPCON): Vitamin and mineral supplement needs of normal children in the United States. In Forbes, G. B. (Ed.): Pediatric Nutrition Handbook. Elk Grove Village, IL, American Academy of Pediatrics, 1985, pp. 37–48.
American Academy of Pediatrics, Committee on Nutrition (AAPCON): Aluminum toxicity in infants and children. Pediatrics 78:1150–1154, 1986.
Amorde-Spalding, K. L., D'Harlingue, A. E., Phillips, B. L., et al.: Fifty percent of a vial of MVI-Pediatric maintains acceptable alpha-tocopherol levels in ≤ 1000 gram infants. Pediatr. Res. 27:279A, 1990.
Andreoli, S. P., Bergstein, J. M., and Sherrard, D. J.: Aluminum intoxication from aluminum-containing phosphate binders in children with azotemia not undergoing dialysis. N. Engl. J. Med. 310:1079–1084, 1984.
Arnaud, S. B., Stickler, G. B., and Haworth, J. C.: Serum 25-hydroxyvitamin D in infantile rickets. Pediatrics 57:221–225, 1976.
Atkinson, A. S., Whelan, D., Whyte, R. K., and Lonnerdal, B.: Abnormal zinc content in human milk. Am. J. Dis. Child. 143:608–611, 1989.
Avery, M. A., Clow, C. L., Menkes, J. H., et al.: Transient tyrosinemia of the newborn: Dietary and clinical aspects. Pediatrics 39:378–384, 1967.
Bachrach, S. J., Fisher, J., and Parks, J. S.: An outbreak of vitamin D deficiency rickets in a susceptible population. Pediatrics 64:871–877, 1979.
Baeckert, P. A., Green, H. L., Fritz, I., et al.: Vitamin concentrations in very low birth weight infants given vitamins intravenously in a lipid emulsion: Measurement of vitamins A, D, and E and riboflavin. J. Pediatr. 113:1057–1065, 1988.
Baker, H., Frank, O., Thomson, A. D., et al.: Vitamin profiles of 174 mothers and newborns at parturition. Am. J. Clin. Nutr. 28:56–65, 1975.
Ballin, A., Brown, E. J., Koren, G., and Zipursky A.: Vitamin C–induced erythrocyte damage in premature infants. J. Pediatr. 113:114–120, 1988.
Barak, M., Herschkowitz, S., and Montag, J.: Soft tissue calcification: A complication of vitamin E injection. Pediatrics 77:382–385, 1986.
Bejsovec, M., Kulenda, Z., and Ponca, E.: Familial intrauterine convulsions in pyridoxine dependency. Arch. Dis. Child. 42:201–207, 1967.
Bell, E. F., and Filer, L. J.: The role of vitamin E in the nutrition of premature infants. Am. J. Clin. Nutr. 34:414–422, 1981.
Bell, E. F.: Prevention of bronchopulmonary dysplasia: Vitamin E and other antioxidants. In Farrell, P. M., and Taussig, L. M. (Eds.): Bronchopulmonary Dysplasia and Related Chronic Respiratory Disorders. Report of the Ninetieth Ross Conference on Pediatric Research, 1986; pp. 77–82.
Bendich, A., and Langseth, L.: Safety of vitamin A. Am. J. Clin. Nutr. 49:358–371, 1989.
Bhatia, J., Mims, L. C., and Roesel, R. A.: The effect of phototherapy on amino acid solutions containing multivitamins. J. Pediatr. 96:284–285, 1980.
Biere, J. G., Corash, L., and Hubbard, V. S.: Medical uses of vitamin E. N. Engl. J. Med. 308:1063–1071, 1983.
Casey, C. E., Neville, M. C., and Hambidge, K. M.: Studies in human lactation: Secretion of zinc, copper, and manganese in human milk. Am. J. Clin. Nutr. 49:773–785, 1989.
Chesney, R. W.: Requirements and upper limits of vitamin D intake in the term neonate, infant, and older child. J. Pediatr. 116:159–166, 1990.
Chiswick, M. L.: Johnson, M., Woodhall, C., et al.: Protective effect of vitamin E (dl-alpha-tocopherol) against intraventricular hemorrhage in premature babies. Br. Med. J. 287:81–84, 1983.
Cohen, H. J., Brown, M. R., Hamilton, D., et al.: Glutathione peroxidase and selenium deficiency in patients receiving home parenteral nutrition: Time course for development of deficiency and repletion of enzyme activity in plasma and blood cells. Am. J. Clin. Nutr. 49:132–139, 1989.
Collins, J. E., Rolles, C. J., Sutton, H., and Ackery, D.: Vitamin B₁₂ absorption after necrotizing enterocolitis. Arch. Dis. Child. 59:731–734, 1984.
Cooke, R., Hollis, B., Conner, C., et al.: Vitamin and mineral metabolism in the very low birth weight infant receiving 400 IU of vitamin D. J. Pediatr. 116:423–428, 1990.
Dagnelie, P. C., Vergote, F. J., van Staveren, W. A., et al.: High prevalence of rickets in infants on macrobiotic diets. Am. J. Clin. Nutr. 51:202–208, 1990.
Dancis, J. Lehanka, J. and Mortimer, L.: Transfer of riboflavin by the perfused human placenta. Pediatr. Res. 19:1143–1146, 1985.
Danks, D. M., Campbell, P., Stevens, B., et al.: Menkes' kinky hair syndrome: An inherited defect in copper absorption with widespread effects. Pediatrics 50:188–201, 1972.
Dauncey, M. J., Shaw, J. C. L., and Urman, J.: The absorption and retention of magnesium, zinc, and copper by low birth weight infants fed pasteurized human breast milk. Pediatr. Res. 11:991–997, 1977.
Davidson, G. P., and Townley, R. R. W.: Structural and functional abnormalities of the small intestine due to nutritional folic acid deficiency in infancy. J. Pediatr. 90:590–594, 1977.
Davidsson, L., Cederblad, A., Lonnerdal, B., and Sandstrom, B.: Manganese absorption from human milk, cow's milk, and infant formulas in humans. Am. J. Dis. Child. 143:823–827, 1989.

Driskell, J. A.: Vitamin B$_6$. *In* Machlin, L. J., (Ed.): Handbook of Vitamins. New York, Marcel Dekker, 1984, pp. 379–401.

Edidin, D., Levitsky, L. L., Schey, W., Resurgence of nutritional rickets associated with breast-feeding and special dietary practices. Pediatrics 65:232–235, 1980.

Ehrenkranz, R. A., Bonta, B. W., Ablow, R. C., and Warshaw, J. B.: Amelioration of bronchopulmonary dysplasia after vitamin E administration: A preliminary report. N. Engl. J. Med. 299:564–569, 1978.

Ehrenkranz, R. A., Ablow, R. C., and Warshaw, J. B.: Prevention of bronchopulmonary dysplasia with vitamin E administration during the acute stages of respiratory distress syndrome. J. Pediatr. 95:873–878, 1979.

Ehrenkranz, R. A., Nelli, C. M., Gettner, P. A., et al.: Determination of copper (Cu) absorption in premature infants with ^{65}Cu as an extrinsic stable isotopic tracer. Pediatr. Res. 20:409A, 1986.

Ek, J.: Plasma and red cell folate values in newborn infants and their mothers in relation to gestational age. J. Pediatr. 96:288–292, 1980.

Ek, J.: Folic acid and vitamin B$_{12}$ requirements in premature infants. *In* Tsang, R. C. (Ed.), Vitamin and Mineral Requirements in Preterm Infants. New York, Marcel Dekker, 1985, pp. 23–38.

Ek, J., and Magnus, E.: Plasma and red cell folate values and folate requirements in formula-fed term infants. J. Pediatr. 100:738–744, 1982.

Ennever, J. F., and Speck, W. T.: Photochemical reactions of riboflavin: Covalent binding to DNA and to poly (dA), poly (dT). Pediatr. Res. 17:234–236, 1983.

Fehily, L.: Human milk intoxication due to B$_1$ avitaminosis. Br. Med. J. 2:590, 1944.

Fetus and Newborn Committee, Canadian Pediatric Society: The use of vitamin K in the perinatal period. Can. Med. Assoc. J. 139:127, 1988.

Finer, N. N., Schindler, R. F., Grant, G., et al: Effect of intramuscular vitamin E on the frequency and severity of retrolental fibroplasia: A controlled trial. Lancet 1:1087–1091, 1982.

Finer, N. N., Peters, K. L., Hayek, A., and Merkel, C. L.: Vitamin E and necrotizing enterocolitis. Pediatrics 73:387–393, 1984.

Foley, C. M., Polinsky, M. S., Gruskin, A. B., et al: Encephalopathy in infants and children with chronic renal disease. Arch. Neurol. 38:656–658, 1981.

Fomon, S. J., Younoszai, M. K., and Thomas, L. N.: Influence of vitamin D on linear growth of normal full-term infants. J. Nutr. 88:345–350, 1966.

Fosmire, G. J.: Zinc toxicity. Am. J. Clin. Nutr. 51:225–227, 1990.

Freund, H., Atamian, S., and Fischer, J. E.: Chromium deficiency during total parenteral nutrition. J. A. M. A. 241:496–498, 1979.

Freundlich, M., Zilleruelo, G., Abitbol, C. C., et al.: Infant formula as a cause of aluminum toxicity in neonatal uraemia. Lancet 2:527–529, 1985.

Friel, J. K., Gibson, R. S., Peliowski, A., and Watts, J.: Serum zinc, copper, and selenium concentrations in preterm infants receiving enteral nutrition or parenteral nutrition supplemented with zinc and copper. J. Pediatr. 104:763–768, 1984.

Garabedian, M., Vainsel, M., Mallet, E., et al.: Circulating vitamin D metabolite concentrations in children with nutritional rickets. J. Pediatr. 103:381–386, 1983.

Garabedian, M., Jacqz, E., Guillozo, H., et al.: Elevated plasma 1,25-dihydroxyvitamin D concentration in infants with hypercalcemia and an elfin facies. N. Engl. J. Med. 312:948–952, 1985.

Gleghorn, E. E., Eisenber, L. K., Hack, S., et al.: Observations of vitamin A toxicity in three patients with renal failure receiving parenteral alimentation. Am. J. Clin. Nutr. 44:107–112, 1986.

Goodman, D. S.: Vitamin A and retinoids in health and disease. N. Engl. J. Med. 310:1023–1031, 1984.

Gordon, E. F., Gordon, R. C., Passal, D. B.: Zinc metabolism: Basic, clinical, and behavioural aspects. J. Pediatr. 99:341–349, 1981.

Greene, H. L., Hambidge, K. M., Schanler, R., and Tsang, R. C.: Guidelines for the use of vitamins, trace elements, calcium, magnesium, and phosphorus in infants and children receiving total parenteral nutrition: Report of the Subcommittee on Pediatric Parenteral Nutrient Requirements from the Committee on Clinical Practice Issues of The American Society for Clinical Nutrition. Am. J. Clin. Nutr. 48:1324–1342, 1988.

Greene, H. L., Moore, C., Phillips, B., et al.: Evaluation of a pediatric multiple vitamin preparation for total parenteral nutrition. II. Blood levels of vitamins A, D, and E. Pediatrics 77:539–547, 1986.

Greer, F. R., Hollis, B. W., and Napoli, J. L.: High concentrations of vitamin D$_2$ in human milk associated with pharmacologic doses of vitamin D$_2$. J Pediatr 105:61–64, 1984.

Greer, F. R., Searcy, J. E., Levin, R. S., et al.: Bone mineral content and serum 25-hydroxyvitamin D concentrations in breast-fed infants with and without supplemental vitamin D: One year follow-up. J. Pediatr. 100:919–922, 1982.

Greer, F. R., Steichen, J. J., and Tsang, R. C.: Effects of increased calcium, phosphorus, and vitamin D intake on bone mineralization in very low-birth-weight infants fed formulas with Polycose and medium-chain triglycerides. J. Pediatr. 100:951–955, 1982.

Greer, F. R., and Tsang, R. C.: Calcium, phosphorus, magnesium, and vitamin D requirements for the preterm infant. *In* Tsang, R. C. (Ed.): Vitamin and Mineral Requirements in Preterm Infant. New York, Marcel Dekker Inc., 1985, pp. 99–136.

Grewar, D.: Infantile scurvy. Clinical Pediatrics 4:82–89, 1965.

Gross, S. J., and Gabriel E.: Vitamin E status in preterm infants fed human milk or infant formula. J. Pediatr. 106:635–639, 1985.

Gushurst, C. A., Mueller, J. A., Green, J. A., and Sedor F.: Breast milk iodide: Reassessment in the 1980s. Pediatrics 73:354–357, 1984.

Gutcher, G. R., and Farrell P. M.: Early intravenous correction of vitamin E deficiency in premature infants. J. Pediatr. Gastroenterol. Nutr. 4:604–609, 1985.

Gutcher, G. R., Lax, A. A., and Farrell, P. M.: Vitamin A losses to plastic intravenous infusion devices and an improved method of delivery. Am. J. Clin. Nutr. 40:8–13, 1984.

Hambidge, K. M.: Trace element requirements in premature infants. *In:* Lebenthal, E. (Ed.): Textbook of Gastroenterology and Nutrition. New York, Raven Press, Ltd., 1989a, pp. 393–401.

Hambidge, K. M., Sokol, R. J., Fidanza, A. J., and Goodall, M. A.: Plasma manganese concentrations in infants and children receiving parenteral nutrition. J. Parenter. Enter. Nutr. 13:168–171, 1989b.

Heinonem, K., Monomen, I., Mononen, T., et al.: Plasma vitamin C levels are low in premature infants fed human milk. Am. J. Clin. Nutr. 43:923–924, 1986.

Heller, S., Salkeld, R. M., and Korner, W. F.: Vitamin B$_6$ status in pregnancy. Am. J. Clin. Nutr. 26:1339, 1973.

Higashi, A., Ikeda, T., Iribe, K., and Matsuda, I.: Zinc balance in premature infants given the minimal dietary zinc requirement. J. Pediatr. 112:262–266, 1988.

Higginbottom, M. C., Sweetman, L., and Nyhan, W. L.: A syndrome of methylmalonic aciduria, homocystinuria, megaloblastic anemia, and neurologic abnormalities in a vitamin B$_{12}$–deficient breast-fed infant of a strict vegetarian. N. Engl. J. Med. 299:317–323, 1978.

Hillman, L. S.: Serial serum copper concentrations in premature and SGA infants during the first 3 months of life. J. Pediatr. 98:305–308, 1981a.

Hillman, L. S., Hoff, N., Salmons, S., et al.: Mineral homeostasis in very premature infants: Serial evaluation of serum 25-hydroxyvitamin D, serum minerals, and bone mineralization. J. Pediatr. 106:970–980, 1985a.

Hillman, L. S., Hollis, B., Salmons, S., et al.: Absorption, dosage, and effect on mineral homeostasis of 25-hydroxycholecalciferol in premature infants: Comparison with 400 and 800 IU vitamin D$_2$ supplementation. J. Pediatr. 106:981–989, 1985b.

Hillman, L. S., Martin, L., and Fiore, B.: Effect of oral copper supplementation on serum copper and ceruloplasmin concentrations in premature infants. J. Pediatr. 98:311–313, 1981b.

Hittner, H. M., Godio, L. B., Rudolph, A. J., et al.: Retrolental fibroplasia: Efficacy of vitamin E in a double-blind clinical study of preterm infants. N. Engl. J. Med. 305:1365–1371, 1981.

Hoogenboezem, T., Degenhart, H. J., De Muinck Keizer-Schrama, S. M. P. F., et al.: Vitamin D metabolism in breast-fed infants and their mothers. Pediatr. Res. 25:623–628, 1989.

Hustead, V. A., Gutcher, G. R., Anderson, S. A., and Zachman, R. D.: Relationship of vitamin A (retinol) status to lung disease in the preterm infant. J. Pediatr. 105:610–615, 1984.

Huston, R. K., Benda, G. I., Carlson, C. V., et al.: Selenium and vitamin E sufficiency in premature infants requiring total parenteral nutrition. J. Parenter. Enter. Nutr. 6:507–510, 1982.

Huston, R. K., Reynolds, J. W., Jensen, C., and Buist, N. R. M.: Nutrient and mineral retention and vitamin D absorption in low-birth-weight infants: Effect of medium-chain triglycerides. Pediatrics 72:44–48, 1983.

Ingalls, T. H.: Ascorbic acid requirements in early infancy. N. Engl. J. Med. 218:872–875, 1938.

Iyengar, L., and Apte, S. V.: Nutrient stores in human foetal livers. Br. J. Nutr. 27:313–317, 1972.

Jeans, P. C., and Stearns, G.: The effect of vitamin D on linear growth in infancy. II. The effects of intakes above 1800 USP units daily. J. Pediatr. 13:730–740, 1938.

Jeejeebhoy, K. N., Chu, R. C., Marliss, E. B., et al.: Chromium deficiency, glucose intolerance, and neuropathy reversed by chromium supplementation in a patient receiving long-term total parenteral nutrition. Am. J. Clin. Nutr. 30:531–538, 1977.

Johnson G. M.: Powdered goat's milk. Clin. Pediatr. 21:494–495, 1982.

Johnson, L., Bowen, F. W. Jr, Abbasi, S., et al.: Relationship of prolonged pharmacologic serum levels of vitamin E to incidence of sepsis and necrotizing enterocolitis in infants with birth weights 1,500 grams or less. Pediatrics 75:619–638, 1985.

Johnson, L., Schaffer, D. B., and Boggs, T. R., Jr: The premature infant, vitamin E deficiency, and retrolental fibroplasia. Am. J. Clin. Nutr. 27:1158–1173, 1974.

Johnson, R. A., Baker, S. S., Fallon, J. T., et al.: An occidental case of cardiomyopathy and selenium deficiency. N. Engl. J. Med. 304:1210–1212, 1981.

Karpel, J. T., and Peden, V. H.: Copper deficiency in long-term parenteral nutrition. J. Pediatr. 80:32–36, 1972.

Kelly, D. A., Coe, A. W., Shenkin, S., et al.: Symptomatic selenium deficiency in a child on home parenteral nutrition. J. Pediatr. Gastroenterol. Nutr. 7:783–786, 1988.

Koo, W. W. K., and Kaplan, L. A.: Aluminum and bone disorders: With specific reference to aluminum contamination of infant nutrients. J. Am. Coll. Nutr. 7:199–214, 1988a.

Koo, W. W. K., Kaplan, L. A., Bendon, R., et al.: Response to aluminum in parenteral nutrition during infancy. J. Pediatr. 109:877–883, 1986.

Koo, W. W. K., Kaplan, L. A., and Krug-Wispe, S. K.: Aluminum contamination of infant formulas. J. Parenteral Enteral Nutr. 12:170–173, 1988b.

Koo, W. W. K., Tsang, R. C., Steichen, J. J., et al.: Vitamin D requirement in infants receiving parenteral nutrition. J. Parenteral Enteral Nutr. 11:172–176, 1987.

Kumar, S. P., and Anday, E. K.: Edema, hypoproteinemia, and zinc deficiency in low-birth-weight infants. Pediatrics 73:327–329, 1984.

L'Allemand, D., Gruters, A., Heidemann, P., and Schurnbrand, P. I.: Iodine-induced alterations of thyroid function in newborn infants after prenatal and perinatal exposure to povidone iodine. J. Pediatr. 102:935–938, 1983.

Lammer, E. J., Chen, D. T., Hoar, R. M., et al.: Retinoic acid embryopathy. N. Engl. J. Med. 313:837–841, 1985.

Latimer, J. S., McClain, C. J., and Sharp, H. L.: Clinical zinc deficiency during zinc-supplemented parenteral nutrition. J. Pediatr. 97:434–437, 1980.

Levine, M.: New concepts in the biology and biochemistry of ascorbic acid. N. Engl. J. Med. 314:892–902, 1986.

Levy, Y., Zeharia, A., Grunebaum, M., et al.: Copper deficiency in infants fed cow milk. J. Pediatr. 106:786–788, 1985.

Lockitch, G., Godolphin, W., Pendray, M. R., et al.: Serum zinc, copper, retinol-binding protein, prealbumin, and ceruloplasmin concentrations in infants receiving intravenous zinc and copper supplementation. J. Pediatr. 102:304–308, 1983.

Lorch, V., Murphy, M. D., Hoersten, L. R., et al: Unusual syndrome among premature infants: Association with a new intravenous vitamin E product. Pediatrics 75:598–602, 1985.

Lucas, A., and Bates, C.: Transient riboflavin depletion in preterm infants. Arch. Dis. Child. 59:837–841, 1984.

McNinch, A. W.: Vitamin K prophylaxe in England. In Sutor, A. H., Göbel, U. (Hrsg.): Gegenwärtiger Stand der Vitamin-K-Prophylaxe in Deutschland, 1988.

McNinch, A. W., Upton, C., Samuels, M., et al.: Plasma concentrations after oral or intramuscular vitamin K_1 in neonates. Arch. Dis. Child. 60:814, 1985.

Manser, J. I., Crawford, C. S., Tyrala, E. E., et al.: Serum copper concentrations in sick and well preterm infants. J. Pediatr. 97:795–799, 1980.

Markestad, T., Halvorsen, S., Halvorsen, S., et al.: Plasma concentrations of vitamin D metabolites before and during treatment of vitamin D deficiency rickets in children. Acta Paediatr. Scand. 73:225–231, 1984.

Martone, W. J., Williams, W. W., Mortensen, M. L., et al: Illness with fatalities in premature infants: Association with an intravenous vitamin E preparation, E-Ferol. Pediatrics 78:591–600, 1986.

Matsuda, I., Higashi, A., Uehara, I., and Kuroki, Y.: Effects on zinc and copper content of formulas on growth and on the concentration of zinc and copper in serum and hair. J. Pediatr. Gastroenterol. Nutr. 3:421–425, 1984.

Matsuda, I., Nishiyama, S., Motohara, K., et al.: Late neonatal vitamin K deficiency associated with subclinical liver dysfunction in human milk–fed infants. J. Pediatr. 114:602, 1989.

May, C. D.: Vitamin B_6 in human nutrition: A critique and an object lesson. Pediatrics 14:269, 1954.

Melhorn, D. K., and Gross, S.: Vitamin E–dependent anemia in the premature infant. II. Relationships between gestational age and absorption of vitamin E. Eur. J. Pediatr. 79:581–588, 1971.

Meloni, T., Corti, R., Naitana, A. F., and Arese, P.: Lack of effect of phototherapy on red cell riboflavin status and on glucose–6-phosphate dehydrogenase activity in normal and G–6-PD–deficient subjects with neonatal jaundice. J. Pediatr. 100:972–974, 1982.

Mendelson, R. A., Bryan, M. H., and Anderson, G. H.: Trace mineral balances in preterm infants fed their own mother's milk. J. Pediatr. Gastroenterol. Nutr. 2:256–261, 1983.

Menkes, J. H., Welcher, D. W., Levi, H. S., et al.: Relationship of elevated blood tyrosine to the ultimate intellectual performance of premature infants. Pediatrics 49:218–224, 1972.

Moore, M. C., Greene, H. L., Phillips, B., et al.: Evaluation of a pediatric multiple vitamin preparation for total parenteral nutrition in infants and children. I. Blood levels of water-soluble vitamins. Pediatrics 77:530–538, 1986.

Moran J. R., and Greene H. L.: The B vitamins and vitamin C in human nutrition. Am. J. Dis. Child. 133:192–199, 308–314, 1979.

Muller, R. P., Lloyd, J. K., and Wolff, O. H.: Vitamin E and neurological function. Lancet 1:225–227, 1983.

National Research Council, Subcommittee on the Tenth Edition of the RDAs: Recommended Dietary Allowances, 10th Edition. Washington, D. C., National Academy Press, 1989.

Neldner, K. H., and Hambidge, M.: Zinc therapy of acrodermatitis enteropathica. N. Engl. J. Med. 292:879–882, 1975.

O'Connor, M. D. and Addiego, J. E.: Use of oral vitamin K_2 to prevent hemorrhagic disease of the newborn infant. J. Pediatr. 108:616, 1986.

Ogata, T., Motohara, K., Endo, F., et al.: Vitamin K effect in low birth weight infants. Pediatrics 81:423, 1988.

Olson, J. A., and Hodges, R. E.: Recommended dietary intakes (RDI) of vitamin E in humans. Am. J. Clin. Nutr. 45:693–703, 1987.

Oski, F. A., and Barness, L. A.: Vitamin E deficiency: A previously unrecognized cause of hemolytic anemia in the premature infant. J. Pediatr. 70:211–220, 1967.

Owens, W. C., and Owens, E. U.: Retrolental fibroplasia in premature infants. II. Studies on the prophylaxis of the disease: The use of alpha-tocopheryl acetate. Am. J. Ophthalmol. 32:1631–1637, 1949.

Papagaroufalis, C., Cairis, M., Pantazatou, E., et al.: A trial of vitamin A supplementation for the prevention of bronchopulmonary dysplasia in very-low-birth-weight infants. Pediatr. Res. 23:518A, 1988.

Pediatric Nutrition Handbook. Evanston, IL, American Academy of Pediatrics, 1985, p. 171.

Phelps, D. L., Rosenbaum, A. L., Isenberg, S. J., et al.: Tocopherol efficacy and safety for preventing retinopathy of prematurity: A randomized, controlled, double-masked trial. Pediatrics 79:489–500, 1987.

Phillips, B., Franck, L. S., and Greene, H. L.: Vitamin E levels in premature infants during and after intravenous multivitamin supplementation. Pediatrics 80:680–683, 1987.

Poland R.: Vitamin E: What should we do? (Letter.) Pediatrics 77:787–788, 1986.

Puklin, J. E., Simon, R. M., and Ehrenkranz, R. A.: Influence on retrolental fibroplasia of intramuscular vitamin E administration during respiratory distress syndrome. Ophthalmology 89:96–103, 1982.

Pyati, S. P., Ramamurthy, R. S., Krauss, M. T., and Pildes, R. S.: Absorption of iodine in the neonate following topical use of povidone iodine. J. Pediatr. 91:825–828, 1977.

Reichel, H., Kieffler, P., and Norman, A. W.: The role of the vitamin D endocrine system in health and disease. N. Engl. J. Med. 320:980–991, 1989.

Reinken, L., and Mangold, B.: Pyridoxal phosphate values in premature infants. Int. J. Vitam. Nutr. Res. 43:472–478, 1973.

Ritchie, J. H., Fish, M. B., McMasters, V., and Grossman, M.: Edema and hemolytic anemia in premature infants: A vitamin E deficiency syndrome. N. Engl. J. Med. 279:1185–1190, 1968.

Roberts, C. C., Chan, G. M., Folland, D., et al.: Adequate bone mineralization in breast-fed infants. J. Pediatr. 99:192–196, 1981.

Ronnholm, K. A. R.: Need for riboflavin supplementation in small prematures fed with human milk. Am. J. Clin. Nutr. 43:1–6, 1986.

Rudolph, N., Parekh, A. J., Hittelman, J., et al.: Postnatal decline in pyridoxal phosphate and riboflavin. Am. J. Dis. Child. 139:812–815, 1985.

Sadowitz, P. D., Livingston, A., and Cavanaugh, R. M.: Developmental regression as an early manifestation of vitamin B_{12} deficiency. Clin. Pediatr. 25:369–371, 1986.

Salmenpera, L., Perheentupa, J., Pakarinem, P., and Siimes M. A.: Cu nutrition in infants during prolonged exclusive breast-feeding: Low intake but rising serum concentration of Cu and ceruloplasmin. Am. J. Clin. Nutr. 43:251–257, 1986.

Sandstrom, B., Cederblad, A., and Lonnerdal, B.: Zinc absorption from human milk, cow's milk, and infant formulas. Am. J. Dis. Child. 137:726–729, 1983.

Schaffer, D. B., Johnson, L., Quinn, G. E., et al.: Vitamin E and retinopathy of prematurity: Follow-up at one year. Ophthalmology 92:1005–1011, 1985.

Schanler, R. J.: Water-soluble vitamins: C, B_1, B_2, B_6, niacin, biotin, and pantothenic acid. In Tsang, R. C. (Ed.): Nutrition During Infancy. Philadelphia, 1988, Hanley & Belfus, Inc., pp. 236–252.

Sedman, A. B., Klein, G. L., Merritt, R. J., et al.: Evidence of aluminum loading in infants receiving intravenous therapy. N. Engl. J. Med. 312:1337–1343, 1985.

Senterre, J., and Salle, B.: Calcium and phosphorus economy of the preterm infant and its interaction with vitamin D and its metabolites. Acta Paediatr. Scand. Suppl. 296:85–92, 1982.

Shenai, J. P., Chytil, F., and Stahlman, M. T.: Vitamin status of neonates with bronchopulmonary dysplasia. Pediatr. Res. 19:185–188, 1985.

Shenai, J. P., Kennedy, K. A., Chytil, F., and Stahlman, M. T.: Clinical trial of vitamin A supplementation in infants susceptible to broncho-pulmonary dysplasia. J. Pediatr. 111:269–277, 1987.

Shils, M. E., Burke, A. W., Greene, H. L., et al.: Guidelines for essential trace element preparations for parenteral use: A statement by an expert panel, AMA Department of Foods and Nutrition. J. A. M. A. 241:2051–2054, 1979.

Shinzawa, T., Mura, T., Tsunei, M., et al.: Vitamin K absorption capacity and its association with vitamin K deficiency. Am. J. Dis. Child. 143:686, 1989.

Shulman, R. J.: Zinc and copper balance studies in infants receiving total parenteral nutrition. Am. J. Clin. Nutr. 49:879–883, 1989.

Smith, A. M., Picciano, M. F., and Milner, J. A.: Selenium intakes and status of human milk and formula fed infants. Am. J. Clin. Nutr. 35:521–526, 1982.

Snyderman, S. W., Carretero, R., and Holt, E., Jr: Pyridoxine deficiency in the human being. Fed. Proc. 9:371, 1950.

Sokol, R. J., Guggenheim, M. A., Heubi, J. E., et al.: Frequency and clinical progression of the vitamin E deficiency neurologic disorder in children with prolonged neonatal cholestasis. Am. J. Dis. Child. 139:1211–1215, 1985a.

Sokol, R. J., Guggenheim, M. A., Iannaccone, S., et al.: Improved neurologic function after long-term correction of vitamin E deficiency in children with chronic cholestasis. N. Engl. J. Med. 313:1580–1586, 1985b.

Specker, B. L., Tsang, R. C., and Hollis, B. W.: Effect of race and diet on human-milk vitamin D and 25-hydroxyvitamin D. Am. J. Dis. Child. 139:1134–1137, 1985.

Specker, B. L., Greer, F., and Tsang, R. C.: Vitamin D. In Tsang, R. C., and Nichols, B. L. (Eds.): Nutrition During Infancy. Philadelphia, Hanley & Belfus, Inc., 1988, pp. 264–276.

Specker, B. L., Brazerol, W., Ho, M. L., and Norman, E. J.: Urinary methylmalonic acid excretion in infants fed formula or human milk. Am. J. Clin. Nutr. 51:209–211, 1990.

Speer, M. E., Blifeld, C., Rudolph, A. J., et al.: Intraventricular hemorrhage and vitamin E in the very low-birth-weight infant: Evidence for efficacy of early intramuscular vitamin E administration. Pediatrics 74:1107–1112, 1984.

Srouji, M. N., Balistreri, W. F., Caleb, M. H., et al.: Zinc deficiency during parenteral nutrition: Skin manifestations and immune incompetence in a premature infant. J. Pediatr. Surg. 13:570–575, 1978.

Steichen, J. J., Gratton, T. L., and Tsang, R. C.: Osteopenia of prematurity: The cause and possible treatment. J. Pediatr. 96:528–534, 1980.

Steichen, J. J., Tsang, R. C., Greer, F. R., et al.: Elevated serum 1,25 dihydroxyvitamin D concentrations in rickets of very low-birth-weight infants. J. Pediatr. 99:293–298, 1981.

Strelling, M. K., Blackledge, G. D., Goodall, H. B., and Walker, C. H. M.: Megaloblastic anemia and whole-blood folate levels in premature infants. Lancet 1:898–900, 1966.

Sutton, A. M., Harvie, A., Cockburn, F., et al.: Copper deficiency in the preterm infant of very low birthweight. Arch. Dis. Child. 60:644–651, 1985.

Tanner, M. S., Kantarjian, A. H., Bhave, S. A., and Pandit, A. N.: Early introduction of copper-contaminated animal milk feeds as a possible cause of Indian childhood cirrhosis. Lancet ii:992–995, 1983.

Tyrala, E. E.: Zinc and copper balances in preterm infants. Pediatrics 77:513–517, 1986.

Van Gelder, D. W., and Darby F. U.: Congenital and infantile beriberi. J. Pediatr. 25:226–235, 1944.

van Rij, A. M., Thomson, C. D., McKenzie, J. M., and Robinson, M. F.: Selenium deficiency in total parenteral nutrition. Am. J. Clin. Nutr. 32:2076–2085, 1979.

Venkataraman, P. S., Tsang, R. C., Buckley, D. D., et al.: Elevation of serum 1,25-dihydroxyvitamin D in response to physiologic doses of vitamin D_3 in vitamin D–deficient infants. J. Pediatr. 103:416–419, 1983.

Vileisis, R. A., Deddish, R. B., Fitzsimons, E., and Hunt, C. E.: Serial serum zinc levels in preterm infants during parenteral and enteral feedings. Am. J. Clin. Nutr. 34:2653–2657, 1981.

Vinton, N. E., Dahlstrom, K. A., Strobel, C. T., and Ament, M. E.: Macrocytosis and pseudoalbinism: Manifestations of selenium deficiency. J. Pediatr. 111:711–717, 1987.

von Kries, R., and Gobel, U.: Vitamin K prophylaxis in Europe. What is done, what should be done? Pediatr. Eur. 2:22, 1988.

Vuori, E.: A longitudinal study of manganese in human milk. Acta Paediatr. Scand. 68:571–573, 1979.

Walravens, P. A., and Hambidge, K. M.: Growth of infants fed a zinc supplemented formula. Am. J. Clin. Nutr. 29:1114–1121, 1976.

Ward, M. K., Feest, T. G., Ellis, H. A., et al: Osteomalacic dialysis osteodystrophy: Evidence for a water-borne aetiological agent, probably aluminum. Lancet 1:841–845, 1978.

Weisman, Y., Bawnik, J. C., Eisenberg, Z., and Spirer Z.: Vitamin D metabolites in human milk. J. Pediatr. 100:745–748, 1982.

Williams, M. L., Shott, R. J., O'Neal, P. L., and Oski F. A.: Role of dietary iron and fat on vitamin E deficiency anemia of infancy. N. Engl. J. Med. 292:887–890, 1975.

Zachman, R. D.: Retinol (vitamin A) and the neonate: Special problems of the human premature infant. Am. J. Clin. Nutr. 50:413–424, 1989.

Zachman, R. D., Kakkad, B., and Chytil, F.: Perinatal rat lung retinol (vitamin A) and retinyl palmitate. Pediatr. Res. 18:1297–1299, 1984.

Zimmerman, A. W., Hambidge, M., Lepow, M. L., et al.: Acrodermatitis in breast-fed premature infants: Evidence for a defect of mammary zinc secretion. Pediatrics 69:176–183, 1982.

Zipursky, A., Brown, E. J., Watts, J., et al.: Oral vitamin E supplementation for the prevention of anemia in premature infants: A controlled trial. Pediatrics 79:61–68, 1987.

Zlotkin, S. H., and Buchanan, B. E.: Meeting zinc and copper intake requirements in the parenterally fed preterm and full-term infant. J. Pediatr. 103:441–446, 1983.

PART XIII

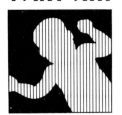

DISORDERS OF BILIRUBIN METABOLISM

GENERAL CONSIDERATIONS 77

Frank A. Oski

Jaundice is the visible manifestation of chemical hyperbilirubinemia. Most adults are visibly jaundiced when serum bilirubin concentrations exceed 2.0 mg/dl, whereas neonatal icterus is rarely perceptible until the serum bilirubin concentration exceeds 7.0 mg/dl.

Chemical hyperbilirubinemia, a serum bilirubin of 2.0 mg/dl or more, is virtually universal in newborns during the 1st week of life. Although some degree of jaundice may be considered a normal physical finding in both term and preterm infants, the findings from the National Collaborative Perinatal Project indicate that only 6.2 per cent of white infants and 4.5 per cent of black infants weighing more than 2500 g at birth will have bilirubin values in excess of 12.9 mg/dl (221 μmol/l). In contrast, 10 to 20 per cent of infants weighing less than 2500 g at birth will have bilirubin values that exceed 15 mg/dl during the 1st week of life.

■ BILIRUBIN FORMATION AND EXCRETION

Bilirubin is derived from the catabolism of heme proteins. Heme-containing proteins include hemoglobin, myoglobin, and heme-containing enzymes such as the cytochromes, catalase, and tryptophan pyrrolase. Virtually all cells of the body are a potential source of bilirubin, although, under usual circumstances, this pigment is primarily due to the destruction of hemoglobin contained within erythrocytes. The catabolism of 1 g of hemoglobin results in the production of 34 mg of bilirubin.

Bilirubin IXα, the naturally occurring isomer in humans, is ultimately derived from the enzymatic opening of the protoporphyrin IX ring of heme at the alpha carbon bridge (Fig. 77–1) with the initial formation of carbon monoxide and biliverdin. This oxidation is catalyzed by the enzyme microsomal heme oxygenase. Biliverdin, the initial tetrapyrrolic product of the ring-opening reaction, is then rapidly reduced to bilirubin by the enzyme, biliverdin reductase.

One molecule of carbon monoxide is produced for every molecule of bilirubin produced. This pathway represents the only known source of both bilirubin and carbon monoxide in humans. The measurement of either carbon monoxide production rates or carboxyhemoglobin levels has proved useful in documenting the magnitude of heme catabolism and in providing insights into the mechanism of hyperbilirubinemia in both infants and adults.

The destruction of circulating erythrocytes accounts for approximately 75 per cent of the daily bilirubin production in the normal newborn infant (Fig. 77–2). In the normal adult, the death of senescent red cells is the source of 85 to 90 per cent of the bilirubin produced each day. About 25 per cent of the daily bilirubin production in the newborn comes from sources other than the circulating red blood cell. These alternate sources include a nonerythrocytic component resulting from the catabolism of heme proteins and free heme, primarily in the liver, and an erythropoietic component that results from the destruction of red cell precursors in the bone marrow or soon after their release into circulation. This destruction of nonsenescent red blood cells is termed "ineffective erythropoiesis."

The normal newborn produces 8.5 ± 2.3 mg bilirubin per kilogram per day, which is more than double the bilirubin production of 3.6 mg per kilogram per day observed in the adult. This difference is a result of the fact that the newborn has a larger red cell mass per kilogram of body weight, red cells with a life span that is only two-thirds that of red cells produced by normal adults, and a larger production of bilirubin from nonerythrocytic sources. This increase in bilirubin production is reflected in the higher carbon monoxide production rates observed in normal term infants. Endogenous carbon monoxide production averages 14 to 15 μl/kg/hr in term infants as compared with an average value of 6.1 μl/kg/hr in normal adults. Carbon monoxide production rates in preterm infants display wide variability but average about 20 per cent more than those observed in term infants.

Bilirubin produced in the peripheral regions of the body and the reticuloendothelial system is transported, tightly bound to albumin, to the liver. Binding to albumin is

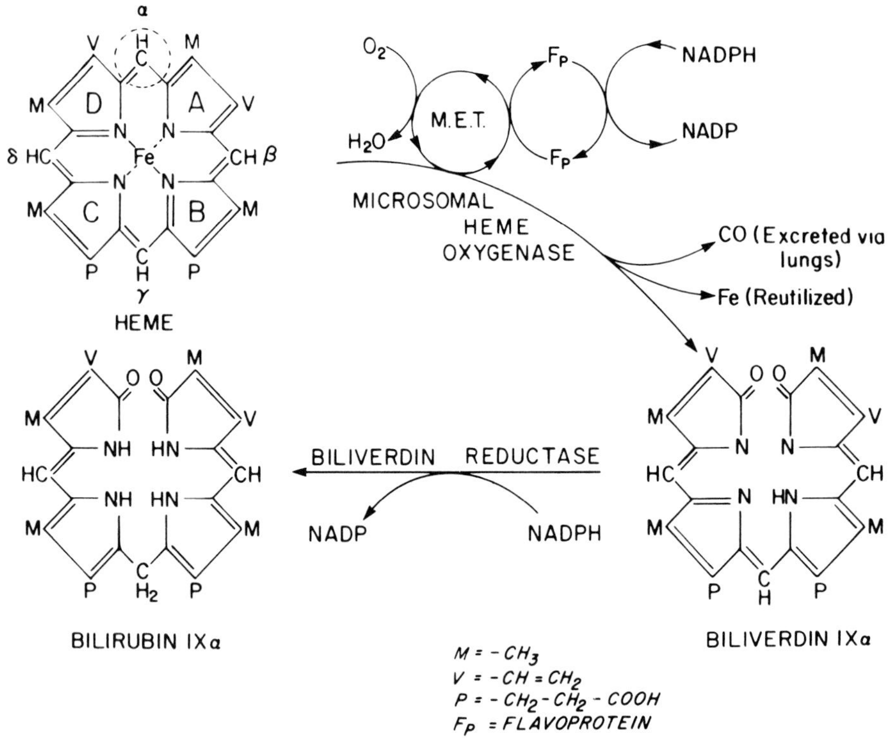

FIGURE 77–1. *Catabolism of heme to bilirubin IXα by microsomal heme oxygenase and biliverdin reductase. M.E.T. = microsomal electron transport system. (From Berlin, N. I., and Berk, P. D.: Quantitative aspects of bilirubin metabolism for hematologists. Blood 57:983, 1981.)*

essential for transport because the solubility of unbound bilirubin at pH 7.4 is extremely low, averaging 0.4 μg/dl. Uptake of the bilirubin from this bilirubin-albumin complex occurs on the surface of the liver parenchymal cells. Bilirubin, but not albumin, is transferred across the cell membrane into the hepatocyte, where it is bound to soluble intracellular proteins. The uptake from the circulation into the liver cell displays the kinetic properties of carrier-mediated transport and may be facilitated by a distinct bilirubin-binding protein located on the membrane surface of the hepatocyte.

Bilirubin within the hepatocyte is bound primarily to ligandin (Y protein, glutathione S-transferase B) but also to other glutathione S-transferases and to Z protein. This binding within the cell prevents backflow of bilirubin into the circulation. Phenobarbital increases the concentration of ligandin, thus providing more intracellular binding sites for bilirubin.

The bound intracellular bilirubin is next transported to the smooth endoplasmic reticulum for conjugation. The unconjugated (or indirect-reacting) bilirubin, which is poorly soluble in aqueous solutions at a pH of 7.4, is converted to its water-soluble conjugate, direct-reacting bilirubin, prior to excretion. In adults, the major product of conjugation is bilirubin diglucuronide. In newborns during the first 48 hours of life, only monoglucuronides are formed. After 48 hours of life, bilirubin diglucuronide is the major excretory product. It appears that two separate enzymes participate in the conjugation process. The first is bilirubin uridine diphosphate glucuronyl transferase (UDPG-T), an enzyme associated with the smooth endoplasmic reticulum and inducible by phenobarbital. UDPG-T catalyzes the formation of bilirubin monoglucuronide. This monoglucuronide may be excreted, stored, or converted to the diglucuronide. The formation of the bilirubin

diglucuronide appears to be catalyzed by a transferase enzyme located in the plasma membrane of the hepatocyte. This complex series of steps is diagrammatically illustrated in Figure 77–3.

After conjugation, bilirubin is excreted into the bile. This is an active, energy-dependent process because the conjugated bilirubin is excreted against a large concentration gradient. Conjugated bilirubin is not reabsorbed once it enters the intestinal tract. In the normal adult, most of the conjugated bilirubin is reduced to stercobilin by bacteria, and only a very small fraction is hydrolyzed to unconjugated bilirubin and reabsorbed via the enterohepatic circulation. In the sterile intestine of the newborn, the reduction of bilirubin to stercobilin does not occur. In addition, the newborn gut is rich in β-glucuronidase, an enzyme that hydrolyzes the ester linkage of bilirubin glucuronide yielding unconjugated bilirubin. This unconjugated bilirubin is now capable of being reabsorbed and returned to the circulation, where it must again be transported to the liver for conjugation and excretion. This enterohepatic phase of bilirubin metabolism appears to play a major role in the hyperbilirubinemia of some newborns.

■ FETAL BILIRUBIN METABOLISM

Bilirubin formed from heme catabolism during fetal life must also be eliminated. Disposal in utero appears to occur by two mechanisms. Bilirubin that enters the placental circulation is cleared across the placenta into the maternal circulation. The concentration of bilirubin in the venous blood returning from the placenta has been found to be lower than the concentration in the umbilical arteries that transport blood to the placenta. Only unconjugated bilirubin is cleared via the placental circulation. Conjugated

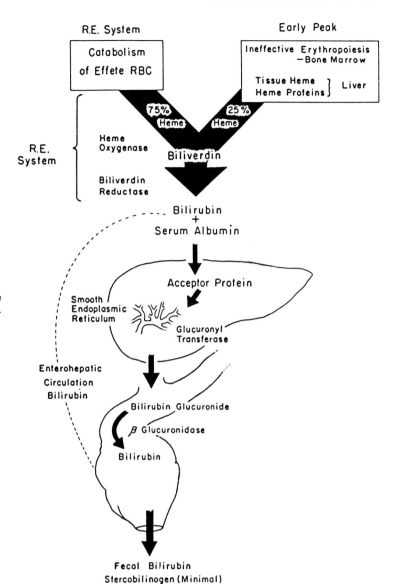

FIGURE 77–2. Bilirubin metabolism in the newborn. (From Maisels, M. J.: Jaundice in the newborn. Pediatr. Res. 3:306, 1982. Reproduced by permission of Pediatrics.)

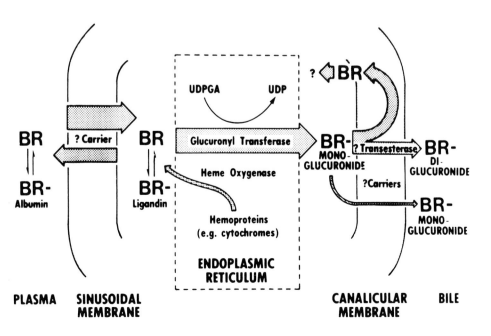

FIGURE 77–3. Bilirubin transport and conjugation in the hepatocyte. Bilirubin (BR) that has been transferred across the sinusoidal membrane is converted to bilirubin monoglucuronide by glucuronyl transferase located in the endoplasmic reticulum. The monoglucuronide is then either excreted into the bile or converted to bilirubin diglucuronide by a glucuronyl transferase believed to be located in the canalicular membrane. (From Schmid, R.: Bilirubin metabolism: state of the art. Gastroenterology 74:1307, 1978.)

bilirubin, when formed in utero, remains in the fetus and may accumulate in fetal plasma and other tissues. Infants with severe hemolytic disease may be born with increased concentrations of conjugated bilirubin in their blood.

The second route for bilirubin clearance in the fetus is by way of the fetal liver. This excretory pathway is limited in the fetus as a consequence of reduced hepatic blood flow, low levels of hepatocyte ligandin, and limited UDP glucuronyl transferase activity. Conjugated bilirubin that is excreted into the fetal gut is largely hydrolyzed and reabsorbed into the fetal circulation.

Bilirubin can be found in normal amniotic fluid at about the 12th week of gestation. It usually disappears from the amniotic fluid by the 36th to 37th weeks of pregnancy. Increased levels of bilirubin are found in the amniotic fluid of infants with severe hemolytic disease and in association with fetal intestinal obstruction.

The mechanism by which bilirubin gets into the amniotic fluid is still a matter of speculation. It has been suggested that bilirubin reaches the amniotic fluid from tracheobronchial secretions, fetal urine, meconium, diffusion across the umbilical vessels, diffusion from the skin, or direct transfer from the maternal circulation. In rabbits, there is a close relationship between the concentration of unconjugated bilirubin in the plasma and that found in tracheal fluid.

In the chapters to follow, the various causes of neonatal hyperbilirubinemia will be discussed. Jaundice is usually the result of one or more of the following mechanisms:

1. Overproduction of bilirubin.
2. Defective uptake and transport of bilirubin within the hepatocyte.
3. Impaired conjugation within the hepatic microsomes.
4. Defects in bilirubin excretion.
5. Increased reabsorption of bilirubin from the intestinal tract.

■ REFERENCES

Berlin, N. I., and Berk, P. D.: Quantitative aspects of bilirubin metabolism for hematologists. Blood 57:983, 1981.

Bernstein, L. H., Ezzer, J. B., Gartner, L., and Arias, I. M.: Hepatic intracellular distribution of tritium-labelled unconjugated and conjugated bilirubin in normal and Gunn rats. J. Clin. Invest. 45:1194, 1966.

Hardy, J. B., Drage, J. S., and Jackson, E. C.: The first year of life. The Collaborative Perinatal Project of the National Institutes of Neurological and Communicative Disorders and Stroke. Baltimore, The Johns Hopkins University Press, 1979, p. 104.

Maisels, M. J.: Neonatal jaundice. (Preface). Clin. Perinatol. 17(2):1, 1990.

Odell, G. B.: Neonatal Hyperbilirubinemia. New York, Grune & Stratton, 1980.

Paumgartner, G., and Reichen, J.: Kinetics of hepatic uptake of unconjugated bilirubin. Clin. Sci. Mol. Med. 51:169, 1976.

Schenker, S., Dawlser, N., and Schmid, R.: Bilirubin metabolism in the fetus. J. Clin. Invest. 43:32, 1964.

Schmid, R.: Bilirubin metabolism: State of the art. Gastroenterology 74:1307, 1978.

Stevenson, D. K., Ostrander, C. R., Cohen, R. S., and Johnson, J. D.: Relationship of heme catabolism to jaundice. Bilirubin production in infancy. Perinatol. Neonatol. 5:35, 1981.

Stevenson, D. K.: Estimation of bilirubin production. In Hyperbilirubinemia in the Newborn, Report of the Eighty-fifth Ross Conference on Pediatric Research. Columbus, Ohio, Ross Laboratories, 1983, pp. 64–74.

Tenhunen, R., and Marver, H. S.: The enzymatic conversion of heme to bilirubin by microsomal heme oxygenase. Proc. Natl. Acad. Sci. U.S.A. 61:748, 1968.

Wolkoff, A. W., Goresky, C. A., Sellin, J., Gatmaitan, Z., and Arias, I. M.: Role of ligandin in transfer of bilirubin from plasma into liver. Am. J. Physiol. 236:638, 1979.

PHYSIOLOGIC JAUNDICE 78

Frank A. Oski

An understanding of bilirubin production and catabolism, as described in the preceding chapter, provides a basis for an understanding of what has long been called "physiologic" jaundice of the newborn. The normal newborn has one or more defects in bilirubin metabolism and transport that regularly result in the occurrence of increased concentrations of serum unconjugated bilirubin during the 1st week of life.

The general limits of hyperbilirubinemia vary as a function of the gestational age and the race of the infant. In Tables 78–1 and 78–2, the results of the National Collaborative Perinatal Project are presented. In this project, serum bilirubin concentrations were obtained on more than 35,000 infants. Bilirubin concentration was measured at 48 hours of age and then repeated daily if the initial value exceeded 10 mg/dl. Sampling was continued until the serum bilirubin concentration decreased to less than 10 mg/dl. Although this project included all infants, both well ones and those with known hemolytic disease, in 97 per cent the maximum serum bilirubin concentration did not exceed 12.9 mg/dl before the use of phototherapy.

It is now recognized that infant feeding practices influence the maximum bilirubin values attained in healthy term infants. The data of Maisels and Gifford (1986) indicate that the 97th percentile for bilirubin is 12.4 mg/dl in the bottle-fed infant and 14.8 mg/dl in the breast-fed infant. Schneider (1986) from his analysis of pooled published studies concluded that only 4 per cent of bottle-fed infants achieve a bilirubin concentration greater than 12 mg/dl while 12.9 per cent of breast-fed infants have values that exceed that figure. Only 0.3 per cent of bottle-fed infants have a bilirubin concentration that reaches or exceeds 15.0 mg/dl while 2 per cent of breast-fed infants reach or exceed a bilirubin concentration of 15.0 mg/dl.

Studies of serum bilirubin values in seemingly normal term and preterm infants have provided guidelines for what is and is not physiologic jaundice. Maisels (1981) has proposed five criteria that can be used to exclude the diagnosis of physiologic jaundice (Table 78–3). It must be remembered, however, that the absence of these criteria does not guarantee that the jaundice is physiologic and that the infant has no underlying pathologic process.

This pattern of hyperbilirubinemia, physiologic jaundice, results from an interaction of several developmental abnormalities and has been classified by Gartner and co-workers (1977) into two functionally distinct periods. The first period, designated as Phase I, includes the first 5 days of life in the term infant and is characterized by a relatively rapid rise in serum unconjugated bilirubin concentrations from an average cord blood value of 1.5 mg/dl to a peak value of 6 to 7 mg/dl on the 3rd day of life. In the preterm infant, the peak value averages 10 to 12 mg/dl and does not occur until the 5th to 7th days of life. In the term infant, after the 3rd day of life, the bilirubin begins to decline quickly until the 5th day of life, at which point Phase II begins. Phase II is characterized by a relatively stable serum unconjugated bilirubin concentration of about 2 mg/dl that persists until the end of the 2nd week of life. After this time, the serum bilirubin concentration declines again to values observed in normal adults. Normal adults' serum bilirubin concentrations are usually less than 1.0 mg/dl. Phase II may persist in the preterm infant for a month or more, depending on the gestational age of the infant at birth.

Studies in newborn rhesus monkeys by Gartner and associates (1977) have disclosed a similar pattern, although the overall course of the disease is shorter. This animal model has provided insight into the biochemical basis for human neonatal physiologic jaundice. Phase I hyperbilirubinemia is caused by excessive bilirubin production coupled with deficient hepatic conjugation. The impaired hepatic conjugation appears to be primarily a

TABLE 78–1. Highest Total Serum Bilirubin by Birth Weight in White Newborns

mg/dl	UNDER 2500 g			OVER 2500 g			TOTAL		
	Live Births	Per cent	Cumulative Per cent	Live Births	Per cent	Cumulative Per cent	Live Births	Per cent	Cumulative Per cent
0–7	488	42.73	100.00	11908	73.73	100.00	12396	71.69	100.00
8–12	336	29.42	57.27	3243	20.08	26.27	3579	20.70	28.31
13–15	128	11.21	27.85	531	3.29	6.19	659	3.81	7.62
16–19	114	9.98	16.64	315	1.95	2.90	429	2.48	3.81
20+	76	6.65	6.65	153	0.95	0.95	229	1.32	1.32
Subtotal	1142	100.00		16150	100.00		17292	100.00	
Unknown	177	13.42		1012	5.90		1189	6.43	
TOTAL	1319	100.00		17162	100.00		18481	100.00	

(From Hardy, J. B., et al.: The Collaborative Perinatal Project of the National Institutes of Neurological and Communicative Disorders and Stroke. Baltimore, The Johns Hopkins University Press, 1979.)

TABLE 78–2. Highest Total Serum Bilirubin by Birth Weight in Black Newborns

mg/dl	UNDER 2500 gm			OVER 2500 gm			TOTAL		
	Live Births	Per cent	Cumulative Per cent	Live Births	Per cent	Cumulative Per cent	Live Births	Per cent	Cumulative Per cent
0–7	1137	50.29	100.00	11734	74.48	100.00	12871	71.45	100.00
8–12	719	31.80	49.71	3309	21.00	25.52	4028	22.36	28.55
13–15	225	9.95	17.91	412	2.62	4.51	637	3.54	6.19
16–19	113	5.00	7.96	202	1.28	1.90	315	1.75	2.66
20+	67	2.96	2.96	97	0.62	0.62	164	0.91	0.91
Subtotal	2261	100.00		15754	100.00		18015	100.00	
Unknown	356	13.60		1133	6.71		1489	7.63	
TOTAL	2617	100.00		16887	100.00		19504	100.00	

(From Hardy, J. B., et al.: The Collaborative Perinatal Project of the National Institutes of Neurological and Communicative Disorders and Stroke. Baltimore, The Johns Hopkins University Press, 1979.)

result of deficient glucuronyl transferase activity. The excessive bilirubin load presented to the liver is due to the accelerated destruction of red cells and the increased enterohepatic circulation of bilirubin. The exaggerated physiologic jaundice of the premature infant is the result of a delay in maturation of glucuronyl transferase activity coupled with an even greater rate of red cell destruction than is observed in the normal term infant.

Phase II physiologic jaundice is less well understood. Evidence derived from the study of rhesus monkeys suggests that this phase of hyperbilirubinemia results from the simultaneous occurrence of delayed hepatic uptake of bilirubin and a continued increased bilirubin load that is largely due to excessive enteric bilirubin absorption. This delay in maturation of hepatic bilirubin uptake may be a result of inadequate production of ligandin, the hepatic cytoplasmic bilirubin-binding protein that was discussed in Chapter 77.

Both term and premature newborns are in an ever-changing situation with respect to the various steps in bilirubin metabolism. Slight perturbations in any of the developmental processes may result in excessive hyperbilirubinemia. Some of these possibilities are listed in Table 78–4. It should be emphasized that although unconjugated hyperbilirubinemia may be a manifestation of either a pathologic process or an exaggerated developmental process, the presence of conjugated hyperbilirubinemia is always an indication of the presence of a pathologic process.

■ FACTORS INFLUENCING SERUM BILIRUBIN LEVELS

It is now recognized that genetic and ethnic factors, perinatal events, maternal diseases, drugs administered to

TABLE 78–3. Criteria That Rule Out the Diagnosis of Physiologic Jaundice

1. Clinical jaundice in the first 24 hours of life.
2. Total serum bilirubin concentration increasing by more than 5 mg/dl (85 μmol/l) per day.
3. Total serum bilirubin concentration exceeding 12.9 mg/dl (221 μmol/l) in a full-term infant or 15 mg/dl (257 μmol/l) in a premature infant.
4. Direct serum bilirubin concentration exceeding 1.5 to 2 mg/dl (26–34 μmol/l).
5. Clinical jaundice persisting for more than 1 week in a full-term infant or 2 weeks in a premature infant.

(From Maisels, M. J.: In Avery, G. B. (Ed.): Neonatology. 2nd ed. Philadelphia, J. B. Lippincott, 1981, p. 484.)

the mother, and infant feeding practices may all influence the degree and course of neonatal hyperbilirubinemia.

Serum bilirubin values appear to be significantly higher in apparently normal Chinese, Japanese, Korean, and American Indian infants. In certain areas of Greece, there is a very high incidence of hyperbilirubinemia of unexplained origin. It has not as yet been established whether this exaggerated hyperbilirubinemia is a consequence of increased bilirubin production or a maturational delay in bilirubin conjugation and excretion.

Perinatal events that have been reported to be associated with an increased incidence of hyperbilirubinemia include delayed cord clamping, delivery by vacuum extraction, the use of forceps, breech delivery, the use of oxytocin, and the administration of epidural (bupivacaine) analgesia to the mother. Delayed cord clamping is believed to result in higher peak bilirubin concentrations as a result of the fact that the infant has a larger red cell mass and thus a greater capacity to produce bilirubin. Vacuum extraction, the use of forceps, and breech delivery may all produce bruising in an infant, and the resorption of red cells from such entrapped hemorrhages will result in hyperbilirubinemia. Although not all surveys have demonstrated an association between the use of oxytocin and hyperbilirubinemia, Buchan (1959) has found that infants delivered following oxytocin induction had evidence of hemolysis. In addition, the oxytocin group had decreased erythrocyte deformability that was ascribed to osmotic swelling of the red cells produced by the action of oxytocin on the red cell membrane resulting in increased water uptake. The mechanism by which bupivacaine produces hyperbilirubinemia is presently unknown, but this agent is soluble in the membrane of the erythrocyte and may produce changes in red cell deformability that could result in accelerated destruction of the cell.

Infants of diabetic mothers are more likely to develop hyperbilirubinemia. This may be a consequence of hypoxia, plethora in the infant, or delay in the maturation of hepatic uptake of bilirubin. It has been observed that hyperbilirubinemia occurs only in macrosomic infants of diabetic mothers.

The introduction of early feeding, now a common practice, as opposed to a 48-hour fast after birth (a practice that was common in the 1950s), results in a lower peak serum bilirubin concentration. The feeding may stimulate gut motility and reduce the enterohepatic circulation of bilirubin. Delay in passage of the first stool is known to be associated with increased peak serum bilirubin concentrations.

TABLE 78–4. Possible Factors Involved in Producing "Physiologic Jaundice"

FACTOR	CLINICAL CORRELATE
1. Increased bilirubin load to liver cell. Newborns have increased blood volume, erythrocytes with a reduced life span, increased ineffective erythropoiesis, and increased bilirubin reabsorption from gut.	Bilirubin levels tend to be higher in infants with polycythemia or delayed cord clamping. Infants with reduced bowel motility tend to have higher bilirubin levels.
2. Defective uptake of bilirubin from the plasma. Decreased Y protein.	Caloric deprivation may reduce formation of hepatic binding proteins. Decreased caloric intake results in higher bilirubin levels.
3. Defective bilirubin conjugation. Decreased UDP glucuronyl transferase activity.	UDP glucuronyl transferase activity decreased with inadequate caloric intake. Enzyme may be inhibited by factors in some mothers' breast milk. Hypothyroidism reduces enzyme activity.
4. Defective bilirubin excretion.	Congenital infections.
5. Inadequate hepatic perfusion.	May occur with hypoxia or in patients with congenital heart disease. Both situations associated with increased incidence of hyperbilirubinemia.
6. Increased enterohepatic circulation of bilirubin.	Increased bilirubin values in babies with delayed passage of meconium or with intestinal obstruction.

BREAST-FEEDING AND HYPERBILIRUBINEMIA

Surveys have indicated that somewhere between one in 50 and one in 200 breast-fed infants will develop protracted hyperbilirubinemia. The recurrence rate in future siblings may approximate 70 per cent.

This form of neonatal jaundice was initially ascribed to the inhibition of hepatic glucuronyl transferase activity by an abnormal hormonal component in the human milk. More recent studies have not confirmed this hypothesis.

The typical late-onset breast-milk jaundice usually occurs after the 3rd day of life. Bilirubin concentration, rather than falling as is the usual course in the normal term infant, continues to rise and may achieve peak concentrations of 20 to 25 mg/dl by the end of the 2nd week of life. These infants do well with good appetites, good weight gain, and no evidence of hemolytic disease or other recognized causes of jaundice. If nursing continues, serum bilirubin concentrations gradually decline to normal over a period of 1 to 4 months. An interruption in nursing will produce a fall in serum bilirubin concentration in 24 to 72 hours. Failure of bilirubin concentration to decline significantly within 3 days of cessation of breast-feeding eliminates human milk as the cause of the jaundice. Resumption of breast-feeding is associated with either a cessation of the previously observed decline in serum bilirubin concentration or a rise of only 2 to 3 mg/dl. Kernicterus

TABLE 78–5. Guidelines for Use of Phototherapy in Newborn Period

BIRTH WEIGHT (g)	INDICATION FOR PHOTOTHERAPY
<1500	Start phototherapy during first 24 hours of life regardless of serum bilirubin concentration.
1500–1999	Without hemolysis start phototherapy at 10 mg/dl. With hemolysis start phototherapy at 8 mg/dl.
2000–2499	Without hemolysis start phototherapy at 12 mg/dl. With hemolysis start phototherapy at 10 mg/dl.
>2500	Without hemolysis in healthy infant withhold use of phototherapy. With hemolysis or in presence of factors that contraindicate use of exchange transfusion start phototherapy at 15 mg/dl.

Phototherapy to be continued until serum bilirubin concentration has stabilized or fallen.

(From Gartner, L. M.: Disorders of bilirubin metabolism. *In* Nathan, D. G., and Oski, F. A. (Eds.): Hematology of Infancy and Childhood. 3rd ed. Philadelphia, W. B. Saunders Company, 1987, p. 92.)

has never been reported with breast-milk jaundice, but long-term prospective studies have never been conducted. The mechanism for the association of breast-feeding with jaundice is still unsettled. It has been proposed that the milk of such mothers may contain large quantities of unsaturated fatty acids that may inhibit hepatic bilirubin conjugation. Perhaps more than one mechanism is responsible.

Temporary cessation of breast-feeding in a jaundiced infant should be performed only when bilirubin values have approached levels of approximately 20 mg/dl or when such interruption is crucial in establishing the etiology of the protracted jaundice.

Gourley and Arend (1986) found significantly more beta-glucuronidase activity in breast milk compared with formula, suggesting that increased production and absorption of unconjugated bilirubin in the gut contribute to breast-milk jaundice.

■ DIAGNOSIS AND MANAGEMENT

The diagnosis of physiologic jaundice remains largely a diagnosis of exclusion (see Table 78–3). The steps in the differential diagnosis of jaundice are described in Chapter 83. In brief, any infant in whom the serum bilirubin concentration exceeds the usual limits of normal for weight, gestational age, and feeding source should be studied. Initial evaluation consists of a review of the maternal and perinatal history, a repeat physical examination, and laboratory studies that consist of a hemoglobin or hematocrit, a reticulocyte count, a white cell count with differential, an examination of a peripheral blood film, blood typing of mother and infant, and the performance of direct and indirect Coombs test on the infant's erythrocytes and serum. It has been estimated that these simple procedures will provide clues to the correct diagnosis in one-half of all infants studied.

Blood tests as well as liver function studies will be normal in infants with physiologic jaundice.

Treatment is obviously directed to the prevention of bilirubin encephalopathy. Guidelines for the use of phototherapy are described in Table 78–5. Nomograms designed to reduce the need for phototherapy have been prepared by Cockington (1979) and may provide helpful guidance.

HEME OXYGENASE INHIBITORS

Several metalloporphyrins are capable of inhibiting heme oxygenase, thereby blocking the enzymatic process for the formation of bilirubin from heme. Initial studies have been done with tin protoporphyrin (Kappas et al., 1988), but concerns about photosensitization have been raised (McDonagh, 1988). Other metalloporphyrins, including zinc, manganese, and chromium, are currently being evaluated (Ekstrand et al., 1990) to identify compounds for use in infants with hemolytic jaundice who have high heme oxygenase inhibition activity and low photosensitization.

PHOTOTHERAPY

Cremer and co-workers reported in 1958 that the exposure of premature infants to sunlight or blue fluorescent light produced a decline in serum bilirubin concentration. Since that initial report, visible light has been used extensively for the prevention and treatment of hyperbilirubinemia. Brown and McDonagh (1980) have reviewed the efficacy, toxicity, and current concepts of the mechanism of action of phototherapy.

In a number of well-controlled studies, the effectiveness of phototherapy as a method of preventing or treating moderate degrees of hyperbilirubinemia has been documented. Prophylactic phototherapy in infants at 24 hours of age can reduce serum bilirubin levels by 30 to 50 per cent during the 1st week of life. Continuous phototherapy in preterm infants will result in bilirubin levels in excess of 12 mg/dl in only 8 per cent of the group; in a control group not receiving phototherapy, the incidence will be 44 per cent.

Data from the collaborative study on phototherapy sponsored by the National Institute of Child Health and Human Development indicate that when phototherapy is used prophylactically in preterm infants between 24 and 120 hours of age, the decrement in bilirubin is greatest in the first 24 hours of exposure. The decreases in serum bilirubin concentration attributable to phototherapy averaged 2.4 and 1.6 mg/dl/day for infants with birth weights below 1500 g and between 1500 and 1999 g, respectively. The use of phototherapy reduced the rate of exchange transfusion for infants weighing less than 2000 g from 24.4 per cent in the control group to 4.1 per cent in the treated group.

Phototherapy is thought to reduce serum bilirubin by two possible mechanisms. It was initially believed that light resulted in the photo-oxidation of bilirubin. Bilirubin absorbs light maximally in the blue wavelengths between 420 and 480 nm. Light reaching the bilirubin raises the pigment to a higher energy state. This energy is then transferred to oxygen with the production of singlet oxygen molecules. The singlet oxygen reacts with the bilirubin to produce a variety of oxidation products. The products of photo-oxidation include biliverdin, dipyrroles, and monopyrroles. Many of these products are colorless and, in the van den Bergh test, nonreactive, and they are presumably excreted by the liver and kidneys without requiring conjugation. Animal studies have suggested that these photo-oxidation products are nontoxic. Unfortunately, there is very little evidence to support the hypothesis that the photo-oxidation of bilirubin plays a major role in the lowering of serum bilirubin concentration by phototherapy.

Phototherapy reduces serum bilirubin primarily by facilitating biliary excretion of unconjugated bilirubin. The work of McDonagh and associates (1980) suggests that the major effect of phototherapy is the rapid conversion of unconjugated bilirubin to two configurational isomers termed "photobilirubin." A small percentage of bilirubin is also converted to the structural isomer "lumirubin."

The first step in the process occurs when light shines on the skin. Part of this light is absorbed by the tissues, and bilirubin IXα is instantly isomerized into photobilirubin, a more polar compound. Next, the photobilirubin moves from the tissues to the blood by a passive, diffusion-controlled reaction. In the blood, the photobilirubin is bound to albumin and transported to the liver, where the photobilirubin is removed from the circulation. Finally, the photobilirubin is secreted by the hepatocyte into the biliary canaliculus and excreted with normal bile into the duodenum. The excretion of photobilirubin is independent of the bilirubin concentration and does not require hepatic conjugation. Upon entry into the bile, the photobilirubin may be reisomerized to the original bilirubin IXα.

Various oxidation products of bilirubin are also formed when it is exposed to light in the presence of oxygen. These photodegradation products are excreted in the urine. Photoisomerization rather than photodegradation is believed to be the primary major mechanism by which phototherapy serves to reduce the concentration of bilirubin in the plasma. It is preferable to use either daylight lamps, which allow easy clinical monitoring with minimal side effects, or special blue lamps, which provide maximal therapeutic effect (Tan, 1989). Green lamps are less effective and have side effects for infants and staff.

The efficiency of phototherapy depends on the irradiance at the level of the infant's skin. (Irradiance is expressed as microwatts per square centimeter per nanometer.) It has been reported that most standard phototherapy units, fitted with eight 20-w daylight fluorescent lamps, will provide an irradiance of 5 to 6 μw/cm^2/nm at a distance of 42 to 45 cm below the lamp, inside the incubator. For most infants with nonhemolytic hyperbilirubinemia, this should produce an average fall in bilirubin of about 2.4 mg/dl in 24 hours. Raising the irradiance to 8.6 μw/cm^2/nm may produce a decrease in bilirubin of 3.5 mg/dl in 24 hours, but an increase above 8.6 μw/cm^2/nm confers no additional benefit and may, in fact, increase the incidence of undesirable side effects. A minimum irradiance of 4 μw/cm^2/nm appears to be necessary for effective phototherapy.

In 1981, Wu published the following recommendations regarding the indications and technique of phototherapy:

1. Individual centers should establish limits for serum bilirubin concentration that are acceptable for infants of various gestational ages and with various clinical conditions.

2. Phototherapy should be initiated in the presence of values 2.5 to 3 mg below this acceptable limit.

3. The light source should generally not be farther than 45 to 50 cm above the infant to provide an irradiance of 5 to 6 μw/cm^2/nm.

4. The irradiance should not be less than 4 μw/cm^2/nm at the effective spectral bandpass of 400 to 500 nm (maximum bilirubin reduction can be achieved with irradiances between 8 and 9 μw/cm^2/nm with a combination of 4 daylight and 4 blue 20-w lamps).

5. The phototherapy unit must have a thermoplastic cover (0.25 inch thick).

6. Infants, naked except for eye patches, can best be treated inside a servo-controlled incubator. Lights may be briefly discontinued and patches removed during feeding or visiting time of parents or relatives.

7. There should be a space of about 2 inches between the thermoplastic incubator hood and the cover of the lamp. This minimizes overheating of the incubator by allowing free flow of air between the two sections of thermoplastic.

8. The hospital line voltage should be no less than 100 v (preferably between 115 and 120 v).

9. Infants receiving phototherapy should be given extra fluid (10 to 15 ml per kilogram of body weight) to compensate for increased insensible water loss. When possible, caloric intake should be at least 60 calories per kilogram of body weight every 24 hours (preferably more), since oral caloric intake improves efficiency of phototherapy.

10. In infants weighing 1500 g with nonhemolytic jaundice, a rebound of 1 to 2 mg of bilirubin should be anticipated when phototherapy is discontinued after serum bilirubin concentration has decreased to <10 mg/dl and after the infant is 72 to 144 hours of age. For larger infants, overt rebound may not be present.

Phototherapy may produce a transient rash, transient loose green stools, lethargy, and abdominal distention. Phototherapy may result in the "bronze baby" syndrome, which occurs almost exclusively in infants with an increased concentration of direct-reacting bilirubin in their sera, usually as a result of associated liver disease.

Other metabolic effects of phototherapy include a mild reduction in the platelet count, a reduction in the serum calcium concentration, and an increase in water loss via the skin and respiratory tract. In view of this increased insensible water loss and the increase in stool water content, infants receiving phototherapy require an increase in fluid intake of approximately 15 to 25 ml/kg/24 hours.

During phototherapy, the infant's eyes should be shielded. If the eye shields remain in place and are opaque, damage to vision will not occur. It has been suggested that the phototherapy be intermittently discontinued and the eye shields removed so that the infant and mother may enjoy visual contact. Recently, a new technique utilizing a fiberoptic light source embedded in a blanket has been introduced that makes eye patches unnecessary and allows the infant to be held while receiving phototherapy (Gale et al., 1990).

■ REFERENCES

Balistreri, W. F., Heubi, J. E., and Suchy, F. J.: Immaturity of the enterohepatic circulation in early life: Factors predisposing to "physiologic" maldigestion and cholestasis. J. Pediatr. Gastro. Nutr. 2:346, 1983.

Brown, A. K., and McDonagh, A. F.: Phototherapy for neonatal hyperbilirubinemia: efficacy, mechanism and toxicity. Adv. Pediatr. 27:341, 1980.

Brown, A. K., and Wu, P. Y. K.: Efficacy of phototherapy in prevention of hyperbilirubinemia. Pediatr. Res. 13:277, 1979.

Brown, W. R., and Boon, W. H.: Ethnic group differences in plasma bilirubin levels of full-term healthy Singapore newborns. Pediatrics 36:745, 1965.

Buchan, P. C.: Pathogenesis of neonatal hyperbilirubinemia after induction of labor with oxytocin. Br. Med. J. 2:1255, 1959.

Chalmers, I., Campbell, H., and Turnbull, A. C.: Use of oxytocin and incidence of neonatal jaundice. Br. Med. J. 2:116, 1975.

Cockington, R. A.: A guide to phototherapy in the management of neonatal hyperbilirubinemia. J. Pediatr. 95:281, 1979.

Cohen, A. N., and Ostrow, J. D.: New concepts in phototherapy: photoisomerization of bilirubin IX alpha and potential toxic effects of light. Pediatrics 65:740, 1980.

Cremer, R. J., Perryman, P. W., and Richards, D. H.: Influence of light on the hyperbilirubinemia of infants. Lancet 1:1094, 1958.

Dahm, B. B., Krauss, A. N., Gartner, L. M., et al.: Breast feeding and serum bilirubin values during the first 4 days of life. J. Pediatr. 83:1049, 1973.

Davis, D. R., Yeary, R. A., and Lee, K.: The failure of phototherapy to reduce plasma bilirubin levels in the bile-ligated rat. J. Pediatr. 99:956, 1981.

De Carvalho, M., Robertson, S., and Klaus, M.: Fecal bilirubin excretion and serum bilirubin concentrations in breast-fed and bottle-fed infants. J. Pediatr. 107:786, 1985.

Ekstrand, B. D., Vreman, H. J., and Stevenson, D. K.: Selection of heme oxygenase inhibitors based on potency and photoreactivity. Clin. Res. 38:194A, 1990.

Gale, R., Dranitzki, A., Dollberg, S., et al.: A randomized controlled application of the Wallaby phototherapy system compared to standard phototherapy. Clin. Res. 38:194A, 1990.

Gartner, L. M., and Auerbach, K. G.: Breast milk and breastfeeding jaundice. Adv. Pediatr. 34:249, 1987.

Gartner, L. M., Lee, K. S., and Auerbach, K. G.: Development of bilirubin transport and metabolism in the newborn rhesus monkey. J. Pediatr. 90:513, 1977.

Gourley, G. R., and Arend, R. A.: Beta-glucuronidase and hyperbilirubinemia in breast-fed and formula-fed babies. Lancet 1:644, 1986.

Hardy, J. B., Drage, J. S., and Jackson, E. C.: The first year of life. The Collaborative Perinatal Project of the National Institutes of Neurological and Communicative Disorders and Stroke. Baltimore, The Johns Hopkins University Press, 1979, p. 104.

Kaplan, E., Herz, F., Scheye, E., and Robinson, L. D., Jr.: Phototherapy in ABO hemolytic disease of the newborn infant. J. Pediatr. 79:911, 1971.

Kappas, A., Drummond, G. S., Manola, T., et al.: Sn-protoporphyrin use in the management of hyperbilirubinemia in term newborns with direct Coombs-positive ABO incompatibility. Pediatrics 81:485, 1988.

Kopelman, A. E., Brown, R. S., and Odell, G. B.: The bronze baby syndrome: A complication of phototherapy. J. Pediatr. 81:466, 1972.

Kramer, L. I.: Advancement of dermal icterus in the jaundiced newborn. Am. J. Dis. Child. 118:454, 1969.

Lucey, J., Ferreiro, M., and Hewitt, J.: Prevention of hyperbilirubinemia of prematurity by phototherapy. Pediatrics 41:1047, 1968.

McDonagh, A. F.: Purple versus yellow: Preventing neonatal jaundice with tin-porphyrins. J. Pediatr. 113:777, 1988.

McDonagh, A. F.: Phototherapy: A new twist to bilirubin. J. Pediatr. 99:909, 1981.

McDonagh, A. F., Palma, L. A., and Lightner, D. A.: Blue light and bilirubin excretion. Science 208:145, 1980.

Maisels, M. J.: Neonatal jaundice. Clin. Perinatol. 17(2):1, 1990.

Maisels, M. J., and Gifford, K.: Bilirubin levels in the newborn and breast-feeding. Pediatrics 78:837, 1986.

Romagnoli, G., Polidore, L., Cataldi, G., et al.: Phototherapy-induced hypocalcemia. J. Pediatr. 94:815, 1979.

Saigal, S., Lunyk, O., Bennet, K. J., et al.: Serum bilirubin levels in breast- and formula-fed infants in the first 5 days of life. Can. Med. Assoc. J. 127:985, 1982.

Schneider, A. P., II: Breast milk jaundice in the newborn. A real entity. JAMA 255:3270, 1986.

Shennon, A. T.: The effect of phototherapy on the hyperbilirubinemia of Rh incompatibility. Pediatrics 54:417, 1974.

Tan, J. L.: Efficacy of fluorescent daylight. Blue and green lamps in the management of nonhemolytic hyperbilirubinemia. J. Pediatr. 114:132, 1989.

Winfield, C. R., and MacFaul, R.: Clinical study of prolonged jaundice in breast- and bottle-fed babies. Arch. Dis. Child. 53:506, 1978.

Wu, P. Y. K.: Phototherapy update. Factors affecting efficiency of phototherapy. Perinatol. Neonatol. 5:49, 1981.

UNCONJUGATED 79 HYPERBILIRUBINEMIA

Frank A. Oski

A variety of pathologic conditions may result in severe or prolonged jaundice in which the predominant or exclusive pigment that accumulates in the serum is unconjugated (indirect) bilirubin. The conditions in which unconjugated hyperbilirubinemia is primarily responsible for the jaundice are listed in Table 79–1. The most common cause of hyperbilirubinemia is hemolytic disease. The red cell disorders resulting in excessive bilirubin production are discussed in Chapter 86.

The role of swallowed blood and entrapped hemorrhage in the genesis of hyperbilirubinemia has been discussed in Chapter 78.

Intestinal obstruction is frequently associated with hyperbilirubinemia. Jaundice in such circumstances is believed to be the consequence of enhanced enterohepatic circulation of bilirubin and the impairment of hepatic bilirubin conjugation that results from inadequate caloric intake. When the passage of meconium is delayed, the bilirubin that has been excreted into the gut during fetal life may be reabsorbed. Bilirubin cleared from the circulation in the early neonatal period is also reabsorbed and results in presentation of an increased bilirubin load to the liver for repeated conjugation. Martin and Siebenthal (1955) were the first to describe the association of jaundice with hypertrophic pyloric stenosis. It has been estimated to occur with a frequency ranging from 2.6 to 17 per cent. No satisfactory explanation for this particular association

TABLE 79–1. Pathologic Causes of Unconjugated Hyperbilirubinemia

1. Hemolytic disorders:
   Isoimmunization
   Inherited defects of red cell metabolism
   Acquired hemolytic disorders secondary to infections, drugs, and microangiopathies
2. Extravasation of blood; petechiae, hematomas, pulmonary, cerebral, or retroperitoneal hemorrhages; cephalhematomas
3. Swallowed blood
4. Increased enterohepatic circulation of bilirubin:
   Intestinal obstruction
   Pyloric stenosis
   Meconium ileus
   Paralytic ileus, drug-induced ileus
   Hirschsprung disease
5. Hypothyroidism
6. Hypopituitarism
7. Familial nonhemolytic jaundice:
   Types 1 and 2
   Gilbert disease
8. Lucey-Driscoll syndrome
9. Mixed disturbances in which both unconjugated and conjugated hyperbilirubinemia may be present:
   Galactosemia
   Tyrosinosis
   Hypermethioninemia
   Cystic fibrosis

has yet been demonstrated, although liver biopsies obtained at operation in some infants with prolonged undernutrition have been found to have profoundly decreased glucuronyl transferase activity.

The association of congenital hypothyroidism with hyperbilirubinemia was first documented by Akerrén in 1954. Subsequent studies have found that approximately 10 per cent of all newborns with hypothyroidism will have protracted hyperbilirubinemia. When hyperbilirubinemia occurs in association with a gestation of 42 weeks, a birth weight of more than 4.0 kg, a large posterior fontanel, respiratory distress, hypothermia, peripheral cyanosis, hypoactivity, lethargy, lag in stooling beyond 20 hours of life, abdominal distention, or edema, a diagnosis of hypothyroidism should be strongly considered. It is unclear whether the protracted jaundice is a consequence of delayed maturation of hepatic conjugating capacity, but a similar picture of protracted jaundice, often in association with refractory hypoglycemia, is seen in infants with congenital hypopituitarism. The presence of a cleft palate or a small penis in association with hypoglycemia and jaundice should alert the physician to the possible presence of hypopituitarism.

The inherited disorders of bilirubin metabolism (the nonhemolytic unconjugated hyperbilirubinemias) can be conveniently, but perhaps simplistically, divided into three major types according to the degree of bilirubin–UDPG-T activity and their response to enzyme-inducing agents such as phenobarbital. The principal features of these three forms of the disorder are described in Table 79–2.

The Type I disorder was first described by Crigler and Najjar (1952) and often is referred to by this eponym. These authors described seven patients in whom the diagnosis was certain and eight others in whom the diagnosis seemed highly probable in retrospect. All fifteen patients could be traced to two common ancestors of a consanguineous marriage. This extremely rare disorder in the past often produced kernicterus, but now patients who are treated with phototherapy and agents that reduce the enterohepatic circulation of bilirubin may lead normal lives.

The Type II disorder is more frequently encountered but is difficult to recognize during the first week of life. The inheritance of the Type II disorder differs from that of Type I in that it is autosomal dominant. A conjugating defect can generally be demonstrated in one of the parents. Siblings or parents may have bilirubin concentrations in the 2.0 to 4.0 mg/dl range. The administration of phenobarbital will control the hyperbilirubinemia during the neonatal period and may be used in later life if the hyperbilirubinemia proves to be cosmetically unacceptable to the patient.

TABLE 79–2. Congenital Nonhemolytic Unconjugated Hyperbilirubinemia: Clinical Syndromes

CHARACTERISTICS	MARKED (CRIGLER-NAJJAR SYNDROME) (ARIAS TYPE I)	MODERATE (ARIAS TYPE II)	MILD (GILBERT DISEASE)
Steady-state serum bilirubin:	>20 mg/dl	<20 mg/dl	<5 mg/dl
Range of bilirubin values	14–50 mg/dl	5.3–37.6 mg/dl	0.8–10 mg/dl
Bilirubin in bile:			
Total	<10 mg/dl (increased with photo-therapy)	50–100 mg/dl	Normal
Conjugated	Absent	Present (only monoglucuronide)	Present (50% monoglucuronide)
Bilirubin–UDPG-T activity in vitro	None detected	None detected	20–30% of normal
Bilirubin clearance	Extremely decreased	Markedly decreased	20–30% of normal
Hepatic bilirubin uptake	Normal	Normal	Reduced
Glucuronide formation with other substrates	Decreased	Decreased	Decreased?
Response to phenobarbital:			
Plasma bilirubin	Unchanged	Decreased but remains above normal range	Within normal range
Bilirubin–UDPG-T activity	None detected	None detected	Within normal range
Glucuronidation of other substrates	Increased from previous subnormal levels	Increased from previous subnormal levels	Increased
Smooth endoplasmic reticulum	Hypertrophy	Hypertrophy	Hypertrophy
Bilirubin encephalopathy	Usually present	Uncommon. May occur only in the neonatal period	Not present
Genetics	Autosomal recessive. Parents often related, both demonstrate impairment of glucuronidation but have normal bilirubin levels.	Heterogeneity of defect distinctly possible. Autosomal dominant? Double heterozygotes? No parental consanguinity. Abnormal glucuronidation or Gilbert defect in one of the parents.	Autosomal dominant (heterozygotes). Usually one of the parents demonstrates similar abnormality

(From Valaes, T.: Bilirubin metabolism: Review and discussion of inborn errors. Clin. Perinatol. 3:177, 1976.)

Gilbert disease is probably the most common cause of mild, chronic, or intermittent unconjugated hyperbilirubinemia that occurs in the absence of a hemolytic disorder or intrinsic liver disease. The diagnosis is rarely made in infancy, the mean age of recognition being approximately 18 years, although about half the patients with confirmed Gilbert disease will have a history of significant neonatal hyperbilirubinemia. It is estimated that 2 to 6 per cent of the population have Gilbert disease. In view of the fact that caloric deprivation results in hyperbilirubinemia in the child or adult with this disease, it seems highly probable that many infants with unexplained hyperbilirubinemia are actually demonstrating the earliest manifestations of this disease. Unfortunately, no follow-up studies have been performed on infants with unexplained hyperbilirubinemia to determine whether they do, in fact, have Gilbert disease. The hyperbilirubinemia of this disease is also corrected with phenobarbital therapy.

The Lucey-Driscoll syndrome was originally described in 24 infants born of eight mothers. Four of the infants in the original report developed kernicterus as a result of their intense hyperbilirubinemia. The sera from the mothers of these infants contained a substance that markedly inhibited the conjugation, in vitro, of aglycones such as O-aminophenol. This inhibitory material was also detected in the sera of the infants and was postulated to have been transplacentally acquired. The substance eventually disappears from the circulation of both the mother and the infant and is believed to be a gestational hormone. This syndrome should be considered in those circumstances in which siblings experience intense, transient hyperbilirubinemia of unexplained cause.

■ REFERENCES

Akerrén, Y.: Prolonged jaundice in the newborn associated with congenital myxedema, a syndrome of practical importance. Acta Paediatr. 43:411, 1954.

Arias, I. M.: Inheritable and congenital hyperbilirubinemia. N. Engl. J. Med. 285:1416, 1971.

Bleicher, M. A., Reiner, M. A., Rapaport, S. A., and Track, N. S.: Extraordinary hyperbilirubinemia in a neonate with idiopathic hypertrophic pyloric stenosis. J. Pediatr. Surg. 14:527, 1979.

Copland, K. C., Franks, R. C., and Ramamurthy, R.: Neonatal hyperbilirubinemia and hypoglycemia in congenital hypopituitarism. Clin. Pediatr. 20:523, 1981.

Crigler, J. F., Jr., and Najjar, V. A.: Congenital familial nonhemolytic jaundice with kernicterus. Pediatrics 10:169, 1952.

Eden, A. N., and Weinstein, V.: Neonatal jaundice and cretinism. N.Y. State J. Med. 64:2914, 1964.

Lucey, J. F., Arias, I., and McKay, R.: Transient familial neonatal hyperbilirubinemia. Am. J. Dis. Child. 100:787, 1960.

McGillivray, M. H., Crawford, J. D., and Robey, J. S.: Congenital hypothyroidism and prolonged neonatal hyperbilirubinemia. Pediatrics 40:283, 1967.

Martin, J. W., and Siebenthal, B. J.: Jaundice due to hypertrophic pyloric stenosis. J. Pediatr. 47:95, 1955.

Porto, S. O.: Jaundice in congenital malrotation of the intestine. Am. J. Dis. Child. 117:684, 1969.

Powell, L. W., Hemingway, E., Billing, B. H., and Sherlock, S.: Idiopathic unconjugated hyperbilirubinemia (Gilbert's syndrome): a study of 42 families. N. Engl. J. Med. 227:1108, 1967.

Schärli, A., Sieber, W. K., and Kiesewetter, W. B.: Hypertrophic pyloric stenosis at the Children's Hospital of Pittsburgh from 1912 to 1967. J. Pediatr. Surg. 4:108, 1969.

Talamo, R. C., and Hendren, W. H.: Prolonged obstructive jaundice: report of a case with meconium ileus and jejunal atresia. Am. J. Dis. Child. 115:74, 1968.

Valaes, T.: Bilirubin metabolism. Review and discussion of inborn errors. Clin. Perinatol. 3:177, 1976.

Woolley, M. M., Felsher, B. F., Asch, M. J., et al.: Jaundice, hypertrophic pyloric stenosis, and glucuronyl transferase. J. Pediatr. Surg. 9:359, 1974.

KERNICTERUS 80

Frank A. Oski

In 1904, Schmorl coined the term "kernicterus" to describe the characteristic yellow staining of the nuclear centers of the brain that was commonly observed in jaundiced infants who died from severe erythroblastosis fetalis. In kernicterus, the basal ganglia, globus pallidus, putamen, and caudate nuclei are most intensely affected, but cerebellar and bulbar nuclei as well as white and gray matter of the cerebral hemispheres may also be involved. If the affected infant survives the neonatal period and subsequently dies, the yellow staining may no longer be present, but the basal ganglia will display microscopic evidence of cell injury, neuronal loss, and glial replacement (Hansen, 1986).

■ THE CLASSIC DISEASE

The classic form of the disease, which was generally observed in term infants with hemolytic disease, is virtually unknown today. In these infants, the earliest physical findings are a blunted Moro reflex with incomplete flexion of the extremities and opisthotonic posturing (Fig. 80–1). The suck becomes weak, and nursing is difficult. As the disease progresses, the Moro reflex disappears, and vomiting and a high-pitched cry are observed. Hyperpyrexia

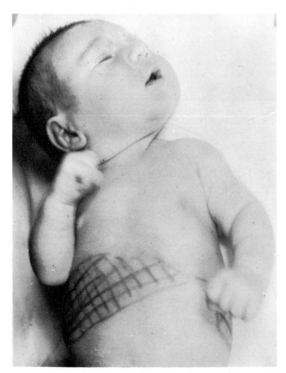

FIGURE 80–1. Infant with severe hemolytic disease of the newborn in whom kernicterus has developed. Note the enlarged liver and spleen. The posture is typical of athetosis, the head turned sharply to one side, one arm rigidly extended, the other just as rigidly flexed. Movements were characteristically writhing.

and seizures are frequently present. Muscle rigidity, paralysis of upward gaze, periodic oculogyric crises, and irregular respirations are often present in the terminal phases of the disease, and infants may die with oozing of bloody froth from the nose and pharynx as a result of pulmonary hemorrhage. Approximately 50 per cent of infants demonstrating these symptoms will die. Surviving infants display the postkernicteric syndrome consisting of high-frequency nerve deafness, choreoathetoid cerebral palsy, dental enamel dysplasia, and, less commonly, mental retardation. In such surviving infants, lessening of spasticity usually occurs at about the end of the first week of life and may incorrectly suggest that the infant has recovered from his neurologic insult. The late sequelae generally reappear by about 6 weeks of age, with neurologic evidence of spasticity progressing to choreoathetosis. Even infants with no apparent neurologic abnormalities during the newborn period may reveal subtle motor, cognitive, and behavioral disorders during subsequent follow-up.

Zuelzer and Kaplan (1954) diagnosed kernicterus in four of 38 ABO-incompatible infants with deep jaundice. Two died promptly, the third died at 6 months, and the fourth was grossly retarded at 8 months. One more of the group, undiagnosed in the neonatal period, demonstrated ataxia, athetosis, and mental retardation later in life. Crosse and her collaborators (1950) followed 16 survivors from a group of 60 kernicteric premature infants. At the age of 1 year, the 13 who could be examined were all retarded. Hearing was impaired in seven, speech delayed in all. Three were already rigid, six were having "stiffening spells," and four had oculogyric crises. Retrospective studies done in schools for cerebral spastics have been revealing. Asher and Schonell (1950) found 55 athetotics among 368 children in a school for "cerebral spastics." Nineteen of these had had hemolytic disease of the newborn, and 12 more had had severe jaundice in the neonatal period for other reasons. Among the 313 non-athetoid infants with spasticity, only seven gave such a history. The association of athetosis with deafness makes the retrospective diagnosis of neonatal kernicterus likely, although this combination is also frequent among children who survived fetal rubella.

Mental retardation without motor defect may follow untreated or incompletely treated hyperbilirubinemia of the newborn, according to Day (1956). He found highly significant differences between the I.Q.'s of untreated newborns with hemolytic disease of the newborn, who recovered without motor defect, and those of their "normal" siblings.

■ KERNICTERUS TODAY

In recent years, improved and aggressive therapy directed at controlling hyperbilirubinemia with phototherapy and exchange transfusions has virtually eliminated clear-cut clinical signs of kernicterus in infants. Unfortunately, kernicterus is still being observed at autopsy. At present, the population at greatest risk for the development of kernicterus appears to be sick, small premature infants. In these infants, kernicterus has been found even when bilirubin levels have remained in a range formerly regarded as "safe."

It has been postulated that kernicterus develops in such infants as a consequence of potentiating factors that act by affecting serum albumin binding of bilirubin or by enhancing the tissue uptake of bilirubin. Potentiating factors that have been proposed include birth weight of less than 1500 g, hypothermia, asphyxia, acidosis, hypoalbuminemia, sepsis, meningitis, and a variety of pharmacologic agents. Critical analysis of low-birth-weight infants who died and who were found at autopsy to have kernicterus has failed to reveal any relationship between these potentiating factors and the presence or absence of kernicterus. It may not be possible with presently available criteria to distinguish those infants who are at risk for kernicterus from other premature infants who appear to be as critically ill.

Despite this problem, it has been claimed that the incidence of kernicterus can be reduced by the use of phototherapy and exchange transfusion based on the use of critical bilirubin concentrations adjusted according to birth weight or gestational age and clinical status. Roth and Polin (1988) recently reviewed controversial topics in kernicterus and concluded that there is "still no clear standard of practice with regard to management. However, enough is known to allow the inquisitive pediatrician to analyze and treat each patient on an individual basis and to avoid the performance of both unnecessary and risky procedures."

Pathogenesis. Although there is a substantial body of evidence to implicate bilirubin in the pathogenesis of kernicterus, its precise role and the relevant modifying factors have not been thoroughly defined.

The direct association between severe unconjugated hyperbilirubinemia and neurologic damage was first convincingly demonstrated in 1952 by Hsia and co-workers and by Mollison and Cutbush (1954). Table 80–1 illustrates the data from which such conclusions were drawn. It should be noted that not all infants developed kernicterus, even when bilirubin concentrations reached values of 30 to 40 mg/dl.

It has been repeatedly demonstrated that exchange transfusions in term infants with hemolytic disease, designed to prevent the serum bilirubin level from exceeding 20 mg/dl, virtually eliminate the risk of kernicterus. Other studies have provided evidence that the risk of kernicterus is extremely low in infants weighing more than 1500 g with nonhemolytic hyperbilirubinemia if serum bilirubin concentrations are kept below 24 mg/dl.

Free bilirubin is presumed to have access to the brain because of its lipophilic characteristics, while albumin-bound bilirubin is believed to be restricted to the cerebral circulation by the blood-brain barrier. Although the free bilirubin theory does explain much of what we currently know about the toxicity of bilirubin, not all observations are consistent with this hypothesis. The most predominant of the alternative hypotheses regarding the genesis of brain injury with hyperbilirubinemia is that albumin-bound bilirubin enters the brain because of increased permeability of the brain-blood barrier. This alternative hypothesis has been convincingly demonstrated to hold true in animals in the work of Levine (1988).

The mechanism by which bilirubin produces neuronal injury once it gains entry into the cell is still a matter of speculation. It has been postulated that bilirubin may interfere with oxidative phosphorylation, cell respiration, protein synthesis, and glucose metabolism. Attempts to demonstrate mitochondrial poisoning in vivo through the perfusion of bilirubin into animals have been largely unsuccessful. In many animal models of kernicterus, asphyxiation in conjunction with bilirubin infusion is necessary to produce the characteristic lesion.

The fact that kernicterus may be observed both in the Gunn rat and in patients with the Crigler-Najjar syndrome, in which the cause of the hyperbilirubinemia is an absence of hepatic glucuronyl transferase activity, is persuasive evidence that unconjugated bilirubin, when present in high concentrations, can be neurotoxic. Even in the Gunn rat strain differences exist so that hyperbilirubinemia does not uniformly result in kernicterus. This implies the existence of a factor, or factors, other than glucuronyl transferase deficiency that influence the toxicity of bilirubin.

TABLE 80–1. Relation Between Maximum Bilirubin Concentration in the Plasma and Kernicterus in Hemolytic Disease of the Newborn

MAXIMUM BILIRUBIN CONCENTRATION (mg/dl)	TOTAL NUMBER OF CASES	NUMBER WITH KERNICTERUS
30–40	11	8
25–29	12	4
19–24	13	1
10–18	24	0

From the data of Mollison, P. L., and Cutbush, M.: Haemolytic disease of the newborn. *In* Gairdner, D. (Ed.): Recent Advances in Pediatrics. New York, Blakiston, 1954.

■ REFERENCES

Arnold, D. P., Witebsky, E., Selkirk, G. H., and Alford, K. M.: Clinical and serological experience in treating hemolytic disease of the newborn. J. Pediatr. 46:520, 1955.

Asher, P., and Schonell, F. E.: Survey of 400 cases of cerebral palsy in childhood. Arch. Dis. Child. 25:360, 1950.

Crosse, V. M., Meyer, T. C., and Gerrard, J. W.: Kernicterus and prematurity. Arch. Dis. Child. 25:360, 1950.

Day, R.: Kernicterus: further observations on the toxicity of heme pigments. Pediatrics 17:925, 1956.

Gartner, L. M.: Disorders of bilirubin metabolism. In Nathan, D. G., and Oski, F. A. (Eds.): Hematology of Infancy and Childhood. 2nd ed. Philadelphia, W. B. Saunders Company, 1981, pp. 86–118.

Gartner, L. M., Snyder, R. N., Chabon, R. S., and Bernstein, J.: Kernicterus: high incidence in premature infants with low serum bilirubin concentrations. Pediatrics 45:906, 1970.

Hansen, T. W. R., and Bratlid, D.: Bilirubin and brain toxicity (review article). Acta Paediatr. Scand. 75:513, 1986.

Harris, R. C., Lucey, J. F., and Maclean, J. R.: Kernicterus in premature infants associated with low concentrations of bilirubin in the plasma. Pediatrics 21:875, 1958.

Hsia, D. Y.-Y., Allen, F. H., Gellis, S. S., and Diamond, L. K.: Erythroblastosis fetalis. VIII. Studies of serum bilirubin in relation to kernicterus. N. Engl. J. Med. 247:668, 1952.

Johnson, L., Garcia, M. L., Figueroa, E., and Sarmiento, F.: Kernicterus in rats lacking glucuronyl transferase. A.M.A. J. Dis. Child. *101*:322, 1961.

Levine, R. L.: Neonatal jaundice. Acta Paediatr. Scand. *77*:177, 1988.

Meyer, T. C.: A study of serum bilirubin levels in relation to kernicterus and prematurity. Arch. Dis. Child. *31*:75, 1956.

Mollison, P. L., and Cutbush, M.: Haemolytic disease of the newborn. *In* Gairdner, D. (Ed.): Recent Advances in Pediatrics. New York, Blakiston, 1954.

Mollison, P. L., and Walker, W.: Controlled trials of the treatment of hemolytic disease of the newborn. Lancet *1*:429, 1952.

Pearlman, M. A., Gartner, L. M., Lee, K.-S., Morecki, R., and Horoupian, D. S.: Absence of kernicterus in low birth weight infants from 1971 through 1976: comparison with findings in 1966 and 1967. Pediatrics *62*:460, 1978.

Perlman, M., and Frank, J. W.: Bilirubin beyond the blood-brain barrier. Pediatrics *81*:304, 1988.

Roth, P., and Polin, R. A.: Controversial topics in kernicterus. Clin. Perinatol. *15*(4):965, 1988.

Schmorl, G.: Zur Kenntnis des Ikterus neonatorum, insbesondere der Dabei auftretenden Gehirnveranderungen. Verhand d. Deutsch Path. Ges. *6*:109, 1903.

Stern, L., and Denton, R. L.: Kernicterus in small premature infants. Pediatrics *35*:483, 1965.

Turkel, S. B., Guttenberg, M. E., Moynes, D. R., and Hodgman, J. E.: Lack of identifiable risk factors for kernicterus. Pediatrics *66*:502, 1980.

Wishingrad, L., Cornblath, M., Takakuwa, P., et al.: Studies of non-hemolytic hyperbilirubinemia in premature infants. Prospective randomized selection for exchange transfusion with observations on the levels of serum bilirubin with and without exchange transfusion and neurologic evaluations one year after birth. Pediatrics *36*:162, 1965.

Zuelzer, W. W., and Kaplan, E.: ABO heterospecific pregnancy and hemolytic disease: a study of normal and pathological variants. IV. Pathological variants. A.M.A. J. Dis. Child. *88*:319, 1954.

OBSTRUCTIVE JAUNDICE DUE TO BILIARY ATRESIA AND NEONATAL HEPATITIS

81

Frank A. Oski

In the last two decades we have witnessed a major reorientation in our thinking with respect to the entity termed *congenital atresia of the bile ducts.* In the past, clinicians attempted to distinguish hepatitis from atresia by a variety of diagnostic procedures and deferred operative intervention for several months in the hope that patients with hepatitis would get better, while assuming that little or nothing could be done for infants with anatomic abnormalities.

There is now a growing consensus that neonatal hepatitis and biliary atresia may be opposite ends of a single spectrum of disease and that the pathologic process observed is dynamic. The pathologic picture observed depends on the time and nature of intrauterine insult and the age at which the infant is examined.

Loose and ambiguous use of the term *biliary atresia* has led to confusion concerning the approach to therapy. Only surgical exploration, an operative cholangiogram if a gallbladder is present, a careful dissection of the porta hepatis, and microscopic examination of liver tissue can enable one to classify the patient's disease as intrahepatic or extrahepatic biliary obstruction with or without atresia.

With this information, one can make the following diagnostic classification:

1. Complete intrahepatic biliary atresia
   a. Normal extrahepatic biliary system
   b. Hypoplastic extrahepatic biliary system
   c. Complete extrahepatic biliary atresia
2. Complete extrahepatic biliary atresia
   a. Normal number of intrahepatic ducts
   b. Decreased number of intrahepatic ducts
3. Hypoplasia of the extrahepatic biliary trees
   a. Normal number of intrahepatic ducts
   b. Decreased number of intrahepatic ducts

Such classification is essential now that it has become apparent (owing to the pioneering work of Kasai and co-workers [1968] and the later success of Lilly [1975]) that infants with functioning intrahepatic ducts may benefit from surgical procedures that employ a variety of anastomotic techniques that result in adequate biliary drainage. Intrahepatic ducts may disappear over a period of several months in the presence of complete extrahepatic obstruction; thus, early surgical intervention is necessary in order

to be beneficial. Liver transplantation is emerging as a potential treatment for these infants (Starzl et al., 1989) (see Chapter 74).

Pathology. Almost every conceivable pattern of absence or atresia of one or more of the components of the biliary outflow tract has been encountered. All the extrahepatic ducts or, rarely, all the intrahepatic ducts may be absent. The hepatic, cystic, or common duct may be atretic. The gallbladder may be absent or hypoplastic, or it may have no connection with the liver or the duodenum. Stenosis rather than complete atresia may be found.

The liver shows all gradations of damage ranging from biliary stasis to advanced biliary cirrhosis, depending on the length of time the particular infant survives. (This is discussed in greater detail in the section entitled Liver Biopsy.) The spleen enlarges as portal hypertension advances. The bones may become rachitic or osteoporotic because of defective absorption of both vitamin D and calcium. In advanced cases, foci of destruction of skeletal muscle may be discovered after careful search. Weinberg and co-workers (1958) correlate this lesion with prolonged deprivation of vitamin E.

Etiology. There is little evidence that congenital biliary atresia is familial or hereditary. One must presume that it results from some noxious process that adversely affects the development of the bile duct system during gestation. Congenital rubella and cytomegalovirus infections have been associated with biliary atresia, as has prenatal infection by *Listeria monocytogenes.* The final pattern evolves from two distinct portions of the liver anlage: the larger cranial part forming parenchyma as well as hepatic and common ducts and the small caudal part eventuating in gallbladder and cystic duct. These two portions must accomplish juncture secondarily. Congenital defects of many kinds are the end results of imperfections in this complex evolution.

Diagnosis. The prime sign of congenital biliary atresia is persistent jaundice. Many times, the icterus appears to be a continuation of physiologic icterus of the newborn, and one begins to suspect serious trouble only when the color fails to fade at the expected time. In other cases, jaundice is not noted until 1, 2, or even 3 or more weeks have passed, after which it persists and deepens. A history dating the onset of jaundice after 6 weeks of age is good evidence (after 4 weeks, fair evidence) that the disorder is something other than atresia. Surprisingly enough, jaundice often appears variable in intensity, alternately deepening and lightening. Because one would expect complete atresia to give rise to jaundice that steadily increases in intensity, such variability tends to be misleading. The second diagnostic sign is absence of bile in the stools. In some cases, infants pass the typical clay-colored stools from the 4th or 5th day on. In other instances, confusion arises because stools fail to become absolutely white for several weeks or months or because some are clay-colored while others contain a tinge of brown or green. The usual phenomenon is that heavily jaundiced intestinal epithelial cells may be sloughed off and incorporated in the bulk of the stool. These two factors, variability in intensity of jaundice and delay and variability in absoluteness of acholia in stools, cause uncertainty regarding the congenital origin and completeness of the obstruction. One can only warn that not too much weight be assigned to these "red herrings." Within these limitations, jaundice and acholic stools constitute the pathognomonic signs. Jaundice steadily increases to its maximum degree, ultimately imparting to the infant a deep yellow color, due to bilirubin, that is mixed with a greenish discoloration, due to biliverdin. The liver soon becomes large and extremely firm. In the first few months, the baby does not appear or act as though he is ill. Venous dilatation appears over the surface of the protuberant abdomen, greatest over its upper half, and ascites develops. The spleen enlarges.

Fat-soluble vitamins are poorly absorbed in the absence of bile salts from the intestine, but deficiencies in vitamins A, D, and K do not become manifest until after the neonatal period. Vitamin E deficiency may be demonstrated by laboratory tests, and the absorption of an orally administered dose of Aquasol E has been proposed as a simple test for distinguishing hepatitis from biliary atresia.

Blood is normal in the neonatal period. Hemoglobin content and red and white blood cell counts fall within the usual range, and there is no excess of nucleated erythrocytes or reticulocytes. The urine contains bile in large quantities but no urobilinogen. By 4 to 6 weeks of age, most patients are anemic with elevations in their reticulocyte counts.

Serum bilirubin becomes elevated by the end of the 1st week and gradually rises to a maximum, where it remains throughout life, with minor fluctuations. Much of the bilirubin is of the direct type.

Liver function tests may indicate liver damage but not until considerably later in life, after cirrhotic alterations have begun to develop.

Blood cholesterol level tends to rise gradually pari passu with increasing liver damage. This never happens as early as the neonatal period.

Several transaminating enzymes have been measured in the sera of infants with persistent jaundice. Values for serum aspartate aminotransferase (AST) in normal adults range from 8 to 40 units (in normal newborns, from 13 to 120 units) per milliliter of serum per minute. From 5 to 35 units of alanine aminotransferase (ALT) are present in

adult serum, and in newborn serum there are 12 to 90 units (Kove et al., 1958). In bile duct atresia, the activities of these enzymes may increase to levels ranging from 500 to 700 units, whereas in hepatitis this figure may rise to as high as more than 1000 units. Unfortunately, there is a good deal of overlapping in these two conditions. The ratio of serum gamma-glutamyl transpeptidase to AST is elevated in infants with obstructive cholangiopathy. Platt and co-workers (1981) have proposed that the measurement of this ratio may be a sensitive means of distinguishing infants with extrahepatic biliary atresia from those with neonatal hepatitis. This distinction may be evident as early as 5 to 14 days of life. The ratio may also be elevated in neonates with alpha$_1$-antitrypsin deficiency who demonstrate bile duct proliferation.

A promising diagnostic aid is the measurement of serum alpha-fetoprotein. Zeltzer and co-workers (1974) found this to be elevated in 10 of 11 patients with neonatal hepatitis and in only 1 of 6 infants with biliary atresia.

Thaler and Gellis (1968) made a strong case for the rose bengal ^{131}I excretion test as the most reliable, although still not perfect, diagnostic test of biliary atresia. Excretion of less than 10 per cent of the dye in the stool was found in all their patients with extrahepatic obstructions, whereas in their patients with hepatitis, the average was 32 per cent. Nevertheless, 20 per cent of those infants in the latter group were obstructed also, with less than 10 per cent of the dye excreted. Most centers now employ rose bengal ^{131}I scintigraphy or other radionuclide biliary excretion tests in the initial evaluation of infants with obstructive jaundice.

In an infant with persistent jaundice and apparent biliary obstruction, efforts should be made by 6 to 8 weeks of age to determine the precise etiology. In addition to conventional measurements of liver enzymes, diagnostic procedures should include one or more of the following in an attempt to determine whether obstruction is present: rose bengal ^{131}I excretion, duodenal intubation and analysis for bile acids, and laparoscopy with biopsy and cholangiogram. If the tests are equivocal or indicate the presence of obstruction, surgery should be performed in an attempt to establish a precise diagnosis and possibly correct or ameliorate the problem. Surgery should be performed by a surgeon who is familiar with the problem and capable of performing an anastomosis if indicated. At the time of exploratory laparotomy, a cholangiogram as well as a liver biopsy should be obtained.

Liver Biopsy. There has been some alteration in the thinking of neonatal pathologists about the pictures that characterize biliary atresia versus those of the other causes of persistent neonatal jaundice with a high percentage of direct-reacting bilirubin. Brough and Bernstein (1969) believe, as did several others before them, that bile duct and ductular proliferation is the most reliable sign of biliary atresia. The second most accurate sign consists of hypertrophic changes in hepatic artery branches. Bile plugs in dilated ducts, fibrosis (largely portal), inflammatory changes, and giant-cell transformation are seen, but in fewer than half of the cases. These findings contrast with those of neonatal hepatitis, in which hepatocellular damage and inflammation, mostly portal infiltration with mononuclear cells, are the outstanding signs. Giant-cell trans-

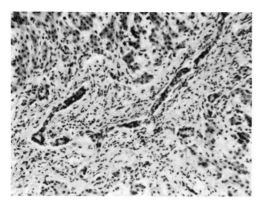
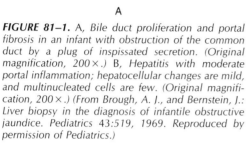

A

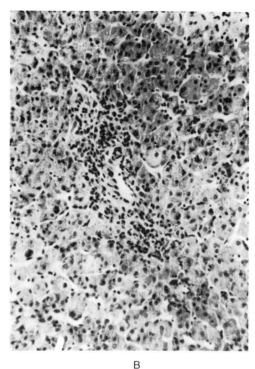

B

FIGURE 81–1. *A, Bile duct proliferation and portal fibrosis in an infant with obstruction of the common duct by a plug of inspissated secretion. (Original magnification, 200×.) B, Hepatitis with moderate portal inflammation; hepatocellular changes are mild, and multinucleated cells are few. (Original magnification, 200×.) (From Brough, A. J., and Bernstein, J.: Liver biopsy in the diagnosis of infantile obstructive jaundice. Pediatrics 43:519, 1969. Reproduced by permission of Pediatrics.)*

formation is far from universal in them, and duct proliferation is only rarely seen (Fig. 81–1).

Kasai (1980) reported the long-term follow-up results in his series of 189 proven cases of biliary atresia studied between 1953 and 1979. In one-third of the cases, the common bile duct or the common hepatic duct was involved; the atresia was therefore of the "correctable type." In general, the operative results have markedly improved in the last 10 years, with jaundice disappearing in 61 per cent of the patients who have been operated on since 1971. There was a close correlation between the postoperative bile flow and the age of the patient at operation: The younger the patient, the better the result. When the operation was performed before 60 days of age, 90 per cent of the infants achieved satisfactory bile drainage. In contrast, when the operation was performed after 120 days of life, no patient displayed active postoperative bile flow. The results of the Kasai experience are depicted in Tables 81–1, 81–2, and 81–3.

Late referral for surgery remains one of the major reasons for failure of surgery to improve the prognosis of

infants with extrahepatic biliary atresia. Mielli-Vergani and co-workers (1989) reported that the jaundice cleared in 12 of 14 infants operated on by 8 weeks of age but in only 13 of 36 operated on later. In their study all 25 children in whom surgery was successful were alive and well, while 13 of 25 with unsuccessful surgery died at a median age of 1 year.

If anastomosis proves impossible, one is left with the tasks of keeping the infant comfortable, as well-nourished as possible, and free of vitamin deficiencies and hoping to refer the patient for liver transplantation. Fat-soluble vitamins should be given in the water-miscible form. Drisdol with vitamin A is superior to oily preparations. Vitamin K_1 may be indicated later in the course. It is possible that added tocopherol may avert some muscle damage due to vitamin E deficiency. The distressing itching that is a feature in some infants may prove unresponsive to all forms of sedative and antihistaminic therapy. Treatment with cholestyramine is worthy of trial, although Lottsfeldt and co-workers (1963) believe that this anion-exchange resin will be ineffective in cases of complete biliary obstruction.

TABLE 81–1. Anatomic Distribution of the Atretic Areas in 189 Patients with Biliary Atresia Studied Between 1953 and 1979

	NUMBER (AND PER CENT) OF PATIENTS		
LEVEL OF ATRESIA	Total	Operated On	Whose Jaundice Disappeared
Common bile duct	29	29	15 (52)
Common hepatic duct	34	34	6 (18)
Total extrahepatic biliary system	126	124*	38 (31)
Total	189	187	59 (32)

*Nine underwent surgical exploration only.

(From Kling, S.: Neonatal jaundice: The surgical viewpoint. CMA Journal *123*:1218, 1980. Originally published in Canadian Medical Association Journal, December 20, 1980, Vol. 123.)

TABLE 81–2. Correlation Between Postoperative Bile Flow and Age of Patients at the Time of Surgical Correction of Biliary Atresia Between 1971 and 1979

	NUMBER (AND PER CENT) OF PATIENTS			
AGE (DAYS) AT TIME OF OPERATION	Total	Good Flow	Poor Flow	No Flow
≤60	13	12 (92)	1	0
61–70	21	13 (62)	7	1
71–90	16	8 (50)	7	1
≥91	7	2 (29)	2	3
Total	57	35 (61)	17	5

(From Kling, S.: Neonatal jaundice: The surgical viewpoint. CMA Journal *123*:1218, 1980. Originally published in Canadian Medical Association Journal, December 20, 1980, Vol. 123.)

TABLE 81–3. Outcome for 187 Patients with Biliary Atresia Treated Surgically Between 1953 and 1979

OUTCOME	NUMBER OF PATIENTS
Death	129
In hospital	44
After discharge	
Within 1 year	36
After 1 year	49
Survival	58
With jaundice	4
Without jaundice	54

(From Kling, S.: Neonatal jaundice: The surgical viewpoint. CMA Journal *123*:1218, 1980. Originally published in Canadian Medical Association Journal, December 20, 1980, Vol. 123.)

Prognosis. Death will supervene in all cases of biliary atresia that cannot be surgically corrected or receive a liver transplant. An occasional infant on whom this diagnosis has been made may suddenly and spontaneously be relieved of jaundice after many months. This does not mean that atresia is reversible but indicates that the diagnosis has been incorrect. Errors of this sort have been made even after careful exploration in reputable clinics. One must therefore qualify the grave prognosis when communicating it to the parents by pointing out that this slim possibility exists. Most deaths will be caused by either hepatic failure or the bleeding of portal hypertension and will occur between 6 months and 2 years of age. A few children live years longer. Kernicterus does not complicate biliary atresia because much of the accumulated bilirubin is of the direct kind, and dangerous levels of indirect hyperbilirubinemia are not reached.

■ ATRESIA OF THE INTRAHEPATIC BILE DUCTS

This extraordinary variant of the biliary atresia group has been studied most carefully and described most completely by Ahrens and colleagues (1951). Its clinical course differs in some particulars from that of atresia of extrahepatic ducts.

Incidence. Only 10 cases had been reported until 1951, when 264 cases of extrahepatic atresia appeared in the literature. Among 110 cases of neonatal obstructive jaundice, Danks and Bodian (1963) found seven of intrahepatic atresia versus 58 of the extrahepatic variety and 45 of neonatal hepatitis. It is therefore extremely infrequent.

Pathology. The absence of bile ducts of any size within the liver substance is characteristic. Bile capillaries are present within each lobule, and these often are dilated and contain plugs of inspissated bile. Extrahepatic ducts are usually absent also, but in three of the 10 early reported cases the extrahepatic duct system seemed perfectly normal. No remnants of compressed, chronically inflamed, or fibrosed ducts are found, and there is no apparent pericholangiolitis. Fibrosis is minimal, and cirrhosis develops extremely slowly and seldom reaches the degree it does when atresia is extrahepatic. Ahrens and co-workers (1951) believe that this slow development of cirrhosis stems from the absence of intrahepatic ducts, a condition in which there cannot, of course, be liver injury

by distention, backflow of bile, and periductal inflammation.

Diagnosis. The chief difference between intrahepatic and extrahepatic atresia regarding clinical course is that the former disease progresses more slowly than the latter. Jaundice appears at the same time and is equally persistent, but the liver enlarges much more slowly in intrahepatic atresia and does not become so hard and nodular. The nutritional state remains fairly good, and the life span is long. Infants with intrahepatic atresia show a great tendency to develop cutaneous xanthomatosis. This sign is not seen before 18 months of age, usually later, and it may be more apparent in this group because of the increased life expectancy of the infants. Xanthomas appear and disappear with fluctuations in the serum lipid content.

Laboratory Investigations. The blood, stool, and urine findings are exactly the same as those in extrahepatic atresia. Blood lipid content gradually increases over the course of months or years of biliary obstruction of any type.

Treatment. No specific treatment is available. Cholestyramine is more likely to produce lowering of the bilirubin level and subsidence of itching in this form of jaundice than in the extrahepatic obstructive variety.

Prognosis. As has been indicated, the life span of patients with this variety of biliary atresia appears to be considerably longer than that of those in the extrahepatic group. Patients living 10 years or more have been observed. The ultimate prognosis is grave without liver transplantation.

■ CHOLEDOCHAL CYST

Cystic dilatation of the common duct results from congenital defect of the duct wall, a mucosal valve, or abnormal course of the duct through the duodenal wall. The dilatation is confined to the common duct itself and does not involve the hepatic or cystic ducts or the gallbladder. It may reach the size of an orange or grow even larger.

Incidence. Over 200 cases have been reported in all age groups, but it is extremely rare for choledochal cyst to become symptomatic and to be diagnosed within the neonatal period. In Brough and Bernstein's experience (1969) with 39 proven cases of obstructive lesions causing persistent neonatal jaundice, 36 were extrahepatic atresias, one was an obstructive bile plug, and two were choledochal cysts.

Diagnosis. In older persons, a triad consisting of jaundice, abdominal pain, and an upper abdominal tumor strongly suggests the diagnosis. In the neonatal period, the mass is not necessarily large enough to palpate, but it may be huge, filling the entire abdomen. This was true in the last example we saw. Pain is not prominent or easy to localize. When a cystic mass is felt within the abdomen in the presence of jaundice, the possibility must be considered seriously. Wide fluctuations in the depth of the jaundice are highly suggestive. In the final analysis, differential diagnosis can be made only by cholecystography or by direct observation after laparotomy.

Laboratory Investigations. Since jaundice results from blockage by the expanding cyst of entry of bile into the duodenum, the findings will be those of obstructive jaundice. Stools become acholic, the urine contains bile but no urobilin, and the serum bilirubin level rises, with a large percentage of the total bilirubin being direct. Biopsy of the liver will reveal a picture indistinguishable from that of extrahepatic atresia.

Treatment. After the cyst has been visualized by cholecystography or by exploratory laparotomy, its walls should be anastomosed to that of the duodenum.

Prognosis. Cholecystoduodenostomy should result in cure. Again, if operative intervention is delayed, irreversible liver damage may occur.

▪ PSEUDOCHOLEDOCHAL CYST

Whereas choledochal cyst results from a congenital defect of the common duct, pseudocholedochal cyst is an iatrogenic disorder that follows injury to the common duct at operation.

▪ NEONATAL HEPATITIS

Between one-third and one-half of infants with persistent obstructive jaundice do not have primary biliary atresia. Although, as previously indicated, biliary atresia and neonatal hepatitis may be different behaviors of the same disease process, in many instances an entity defined as neonatal hepatitis can be recognized as distinct in its pathologic picture and clinical course. The distinctive pathologic picture is the presence of a cholestatic inflammatory process. Giant-cell transformation occurs, but significant bile duct proliferation is absent. Biopsy specimens may demonstrate disorganized lobular architecture, fibrosis, round cell infiltration, and extramedullary hematopoiesis.

Incidence. This disorder cannot be considered rare, since it is observed in two or three patients every year in most large children's hospitals. Milder forms of this entity are much more common and may occur in great numbers during certain viral epidemics such as rubella.

Etiology. Neonatal hepatitis has multiple etiologies. Viral agents recognized to produce the disease include rubella, cytomegalovirus, herpes simplex, Epstein-Barr virus, coxsackievirus, and the hepatitis B virus. Hepatitis may also be observed in infants born with congenital infections due to toxoplasmosis and syphilis. In addition, a clinical picture indistinguishable from that observed with infectious agents may be seen in some infants with severe hemolytic disease or galactosemia. In many instances, an etiologic agent is not determined. Familial cases do occur, and in such patients the disease appears to carry a much worse prognosis (see Chapters 36 and 82).

Pathology. The microscopic pictures of the livers of these children have been compared with those of children suffering from congenital extrahepatic duct atresias. In most but not all patients, the distinction can be made by the histologic pattern.

Diagnosis. Jaundice is the primary sign of neonatal hepatitis. It has been observed at birth, but usually it becomes apparent days or weeks after birth. Onset more than 4 weeks after birth probably, after 6 weeks surely, makes this diagnosis more likely than that of biliary atresia. Abdominal distention and hepatic enlargement appear with or soon after the jaundice. Later, with advancing cirrhosis, the liver may shrink in size and become hard. At this stage, splenomegaly becomes prominent, and ascites may develop. Fever is usually absent. These infants, in contrast to those with biliary atresia, may appear ill, eat poorly, and vomit. Stools become acholic within the first few weeks, but this sign may be intermittent. Striking intermittence may strongly, but not absolutely, indicate the absence of congenital atresia. The urine darkens at the same time that color disappears from the stool.

Fletcher and co-workers (1964) reported an extraordinary case of an infant with neonatal hepatitis who was born with massive ascites. He was greatly improved by exchange transfusion and, thanks to excellent supportive care, made a complete recovery after 7 weeks of being very ill.

In many instances, the clinical differentiation of hepatitis from biliary atresia is not possible with absolute certainty.

Laboratory Investigations. The differentiation between obstructive jaundice on the basis of hepatocellular disease due to neonatal hepatitis and that due to obstruction of the extrahepatic biliary tree is very difficult in many instances. This is because hepatitis often produces prolonged and essentially complete obstruction of the passage of bile from the liver into the gastrointestinal tract. Certain diagnostic procedures, however, may aid in making a distinction.

A gradually rising serum bilirubin level suggests atresia, whereas an irregularly declining serum bilirubin suggests hepatitis.

The presence of a serum that is positive for alphafetoprotein suggests the diagnosis of neonatal hepatitis.

The rose bengal radioactive test may also aid in diagnosis. Patients with obstructive jaundice who have patent bile ducts excrete 5 to 20 per cent of the injected dye in their stools, whereas those with biliary atresia excrete 8 per cent or less (in 72 hours). Newer radiopharmaceuticals such as technetium 99m derivatives of iminodiacetic acid are even better for visualization of the biliary tree.

The fat-soluble vitamin E is poorly absorbed when bile salts do not reach the small intestine. Measurement of vitamin E absorption as described by Lubin and co-workers (1971) or by Melhorn and associates (1972) is a simple procedure that correlates well with the results of rose bengal testing and the pathologic picture found at laparotomy.

Administration of phenobarbital or cholestyramine increases the rose bengal excretion and lowers the serum bilirubin and bile salts in many patients with intrahepatic obstruction.

Recovery of a viral agent or serologic demonstration of an infection with rubella, hepatitis B virus, cytomegalovirus, or toxoplasmosis strongly suggests the presence of neonatal hepatitis, although some of these agents may be observed in the presence of a pathologic picture of biliary atresia.

Many infants will ultimately require surgical exploration, cholangiography, and liver biopsy so that the etiology of the persistent jaundice may be determined. Before such procedures are performed, other diseases that may produce liver diseases must also be excluded. These include alpha$_1$-antitrypsin deficiency, galactosemia, tyrosinemia, and cystic fibrosis.

It is now the consensus that operative diagnosis should not be postponed beyond 2 months of age so that those patients with correctable forms of biliary atresia can be cured.

Prognosis. The prognosis for infants presenting with evidence of hepatitis is largely a function of the etiology of the disease. In general, the majority of infants with viral and bacterial causes of hepatitis recover without residual evidence of chronic liver disease of cirrhosis. Rapid resolution of hepatic dysfunction will occur in newborns with galactosemia if diagnosis is promptly established and galactose-containing feeds are removed from the diet. In contrast, hepatitis as a result of cystic fibrosis, alpha$_1$-antitrypsin deficiency, cystic fibrosis, or tyrosinemia often progresses to chronic liver disease. The prognosis for infants with idiopathic forms of neonatal giant cell hepatitis is extremely variable. Approximately 20 to 40 per cent of such patients die within the 1st year of life, another 20 to 40 per cent develop chronic liver disease, and the remainder recover entirely.

Prevention. Hepatitis B immune globulin is given to infants of infected mothers at birth, followed by hepatitis B vaccine within the first week. Repeat doses of immune globulin are given at 1 and 6 months.

■ REFERENCES

Ahrens, E. H., Harris, R. C., and MacMahon, H. E.: Atresia of the intrahepatic bile ducts. Pediatrics 8:628, 1951.

Alagille, D., Estrada, A., Hadchouel, M., et al.: Syndromic paucity of interlobular bile ducts (Alagille syndrome or arteriohepatic dysplasia): Review of 80 cases. J. Pediatr. 110:195, 1987.

Becroft, D. M. O.: Biliary atresia associated with prenatal infection by Listeria monocytogenes. Arch. Dis. Child. 47:656, 1972.

Brough, A. J., and Bernstein, J.: Liver biopsy in the diagnosis of infantile obstructive jaundice. Pediatrics 43:519, 1969.

Danks, D., and Bodian, M.: A genetic study of neonatal obstructive jaundice. Arch. Dis. Child. 38:378, 1963.

Danks, D., Campbell, P. E., Clarke, A. M., Jones, P. G., and Solomon, J. R.: Extrahepatic biliary atresia. The frequency of potentially operable cases. Am. J. Dis. Child. 128:684, 1974.

Dickinson, E. H., and Spencer, F. C.: Choledochal cyst: Report of a case with unusual features. J. Pediatr. 41:462, 1952.

Fletcher, C. B., Eakin, E. L., and Rothman, P. E.: Fetal ascites—liver giant-cell transformation. Am. J. Dis. Child. 108:554, 1964.

Gellis, S. S.: Biliary atresia. Pediatrics 55:8, 1975.

Gellis, S. S., Craig, J. M., and Hsia, D. Y.-Y.: Prolonged obstructive jaundice in infancy. IV. Neonatal hepatitis. J. Dis. Child. 88:285, 1954.

Henriksen, N. T.: Cholestatic jaundice in infancy. The importance of

familial and genetic factors in aetiology and prognosis. Arch. Dis. Child. 56:622, 1981.

Hsia, D. Y.-Y., Boggs, J. D., Driscoll, S. G., and Gellis, S. S.: Prolonged obstructive jaundice in infancy. V. The genetic component in neonatal hepatitis. J. Dis. Child. 95:485, 1958.

Hsia, D. Y.-Y., Patterson, P., Allen, F. H., Jr., et al.: Prolonged obstructive jaundice in infancy. Pediatrics 10:243, 1952.

Kasai, M., Kimura, S., Asakura, Y., et al.: Surgical treatment of biliary atresia. J. Pediatr. Surg. 3:665, 1968.

Kasai, M., Watanabe, I., and Ohi, R.: Follow-up studies of long-term survivors after hepatic portoenterostomy for "noncorrectable" biliary atresia. J. Pediatr. Surg. 10:173, 1975.

Kasai, M.: Long term follow-up after surgery for biliary atresia. In Long-term Follow-up in Congenital Anomalies. Paper and discussion presented at a Pediatric Surgical Symposium, Sept. 14 and 15, 1980, Children's Hospital of Pittsburgh; Kiesewetter, W. B., Coordinator and Editor. Cited by Kling, S.: Neonatal jaundice: The surgical viewpoint. CMA Journal 123:1218, 1980.

Kattamis, C. A., Demetrios, D., and Matsaniotis, M.: Australia antigen and neonatal hepatitis syndrome. Pediatrics 54:175, 1974.

Kohler, P. F., Dubois, R. S., Merrill, D. A., and Bowes, W. A.: Prevention of chronic neonatal hepatitis B virus infection with antibody to the hepatitis B surface antigen. N. Engl. J. Med. 291:1378, 1974.

Kove, S., Goldstein, S., and Wróbleski, F.: Serum transaminase activity in neonatal period: valuable aid in differential diagnosis of jaundice in the newborn infant. J.A.M.A. 168:860, 1958.

Landing, B. H.: Considerations of the pathogenesis of neonatal hepatitis, biliary atresia and choledochal cyst—the concept of infantile obstructive cholangiopathy. In Bill, A. H., and Kasai, M. (Eds.): Progress in Pediatric Surgery, vol. 2. Baltimore, University Park Press, 1974, pp. 113–139.

Lawson, E. E., and Boggs, J. D.: Long-term follow-up of neonatal hepatitis: Safety and value of surgical exploration. Pediatrics 53:650, 1974.

Lilly, J. R.: The Japanese operation for biliary atresia: Remedy or mischief? Pediatrics 55:12, 1975.

Lottsfeldt, F. I., Krivit, W., Aust, J. B., and Carey, J. B., Jr.: Cholestyramine therapy in intrahepatic biliary cirrhosis. N. Engl. J. Med. 269:186, 1963.

Lubin, B. H., Baehner, R. L., Schwartz, E., et al.: Red cell peroxide hemolysis test in differential diagnosis of obstructive jaundice in the newborn period. Pediatrics 48:562, 1971.

Melhorn, D. K., Gross, S., and Izant, R. J., Jr.: The red cell hydrogen peroxide hemolysis test and vitamin E absorption in the differential diagnosis of jaundice in infancy. J. Pediatr. 81:1082, 1972.

Mielli-Vergani, G., Portman, B., Howard, E. R., et al.: Late referral for biliary atresia—missed opportunity for effective surgery. Lancet 1:421, 1989.

Mowat, A. P., Psacharopoulos, H. T., and Williams, R.: Extrahepatic biliary atresia versus neonatal hepatitis. Review of 137 prospectively investigated infants. Arch. Dis. Child. 51:763, 1976.

Platt, M. S., Potter, J. L., Boeckman, C. R., and Jaberg, C.: Elevated SGTP/SGOT ratio. An early indicator of infantile obstructive cholangiopathy. Am. J. Dis. Child. 135:834, 1981.

Scott, R. B., Wilkens, W., and Kessler, A.: Viral hepatitis in early infancy. Pediatrics 13:442, 1954.

Spivak, W., Sarkar, S., Winter, D., et al.: Diagnostic utility of hepatobiliary scintigraphy with TC-99 DISIDA in neonatal cholestasis. J. Pediatr. 110:855, 1987.

Starzl, T. E., Demetris, A. J., and Thiel, D. V.: Liver transplantation (1st part). N. Engl. J. Med. 321:1014, 1989. (2nd part, N. Engl. J. Med. 321:1092, 1989.)

Stevens, C. E., Beasley, R. P., Tseu, J., and Lee, W. C.: Vertical transmission of hepatitis B antigen in Taiwan. N. Engl. J. Med. 292:771, 1975.

Thaler, M. M., and Gellis, S. S.: Studies in neonatal hepatitis. Am. J. Dis. Child. 116:257, 262, 271, 280, 1968.

Weinberg, T., Gordon, H. H., Oppenheimer, E. H., and Nitowsky, H. M.: Myopathy in association with tocopherol deficiency in cases of congenital biliary atresia and cystic fibrosis of the pancreas. Am. J. Pathol. 34:565, 1958.

Zeltzer, P. M., Neerhout, R. C., Fonkalsrud, E. W., and Stiehm, E. R.: Differentiation between neonatal hepatitis and biliary atresia by measuring serum-alpha-protein. Lancet 1:373, 1974.

OTHER CONJUGATED HYPERBILIRUBINEMIAS **82**

Frank A. Oski

Although the clinician commonly associates the accumulation of conjugated bilirubin in the serum of the newborn with the possible presence of either neonatal hepatitis or biliary atresia, it must be appreciated that a large number of heterogeneous disorders are associated with laboratory evidence of conjugated hyperbilirubinemia (Table 82–1).

■ METABOLIC DEFECTS

Conjugated bilirubin may be retained as a result of an isolated specific defect in hepatic bilirubin transport, as occurs in the Dubin-Johnson and Rotor syndromes, or as a result of a more generalized disturbance in hepatic biliary secretion. This more generalized defect is termed *cholestasis*. Obstruction of a mechanical nature may produce cholestasis, but not all cases of cholestasis result from obstructive jaundice.

Dubin-Johnson syndrome and Rotor syndrome are rarely diagnosed in the neonatal period, although both may initially manifest themselves during this period by the elevation in conjugated ("direct"-reacting) bilirubin. The Dubin-Johnson syndrome is caused by a deficiency in the canalicular secretion of conjugated bilirubin and other anions. Bile salt secretion occurs normally and affected patients are not pruritic. The most characteristic laboratory feature of this disease is the markedly increased urinary excretion of the Type I isomer of coproporphyrin. This metabolic error is inherited as an autosomal recessive trait. Liver biopsy is normal except for the presence of brownish-black granules that have many of the characteristics of melanin. Jaundice in patients with the Dubin-Johnson syndrome becomes more intense during the last trimester of pregnancy and when estrogen-containing oral contraceptives have been used prior to pregnancy.

Rotor syndrome is also inherited as an autosomal recessive trait and is characterized by the presence of life-long mild conjugated hyperbilirubinemia. No pigment accumulates in the liver of affected patients, in contrast to the biopsy findings in patients with the Dubin-Johnson syndrome. The defect in this disorder is believed to be the result of a disturbance in the hepatic storage of anions.

Other rare metabolic defects may produce injury to the hepatocytes and often, but not always, result in the retention of conjugated bilirubin. Alpha$_1$-antitrypsin deficiency may be the most common of the inherited metabolic defects associated with liver disease in the newborn period. Presentation in the neonatal period may mimic that of neonatal hepatitis with jaundice, abnormal liver function tests, and bilirubinuria. The homozygous form of the severe deficiency, designated as the PiZZ genotype by

TABLE 82–1. Disorders of the Newborn Associated with Conjugated (Direct-Reacting) Hyperbilirubinemia

I. *Obstruction to biliary flow:*
   1. Extrahepatic biliary atresia
   2. Paucity of intrahepatic ductules (intrahepatic biliary atresia)
   3. Choledochal cyst (bile duct stenosis)
   4. Bile-plug syndrome (inspissated bile syndrome)
   5. Cystic fibrosis
   6. Choledocholithiasis
   7. Tumors
   8. Hepatic hemangioendotheliomas
   9. Lymphadenopathy

II. *Hepatic cell injury:*
   1. Infection:
      Bacterial:
         Syphilis
         Listeriosis
         Tuberculosis
      Viral:
         Rubella
         Cytomegalovirus
         Herpes
         Coxsackie B
         Hepatitis B (?)
         Hepatitis A (?)
      Parasitic:
         Toxoplasmosis
      Idiopathic:
         Neonatal hepatitis (giant cell hepatitis)
   2. Toxic:
      Bacterial sepsis (*E. coli, Proteus, Pneumococcus*)
      Intravenous alimentation
      Drugs
   3. Metabolic errors:
      Galactosemia
      Fructosemia
      Tyrosinemia
      Alpha$_1$-antitrypsin deficiency
      Cystic fibrosis
      Infantile Gaucher disease
      Glycogenosis Type IV
      Wolman disease
      Idiopathic neonatal hemochromatosis
      Niemann-Pick disease
      Cerebro-hepato-renal syndrome (Zellweger disease)
      Byler disease
      Trihydroxycoprostanic acidemia
      Indian childhood cirrhosis (?)
      Rotor syndrome
      Dubin-Johnson syndrome

III. *Chronic bilirubin overload:*
   1. Erythroblastosis fetalis
   2. Glucose-6-phosphate dehydrogenase deficiency and other erythrocyte enzyme deficiencies
   3. Spherocytosis, elliptocytosis, pyknocytosis
   4. Congenital erythropoietic porphyria

(From Gartner, L. M.: Disorders of bilirubin metabolism. *In* Nathan, D. G., and Oski, F. A. (Eds.): Hematology of Infancy and Childhood. 2nd ed. Philadelphia, W. B. Saunders Company, 1981, p. 108.)

protein electrophoresis, is the only mutant form of the disease associated with liver disease in childhood. This same genotype is associated with emphysema in adults. It is estimated that between 10 and 20 per cent of individuals with the PiZZ genotype will present with conjugated hyperbilirubinemia or cirrhosis or both during infancy or early childhood. When the disease is symptomatic in the neonatal period, it usually leads to fatal cirrhosis. The finding of little or no alpha$_1$-globulin on routine protein electrophoresis suggests that the disease is present. The diagnosis can be made by demonstration that serum is deficient in trypsin-inhibitory activity and that the patient possesses a PiZZ type on electrophoresis. Liver biopsy in affected patients will demonstrate hepatocytes containing amorphous clumps of pink-staining material in the cytoplasm of the cell. These granules are PAS-positive and resistant to diastase digestion. Unfortunately, no effective therapy is presently available to halt the progress of the disease.

Galactosemia, tyrosinemia, fructosemia, Niemann-Pick disease, Gaucher disease, glycogenosis Type IV, and cystic fibrosis are other metabolic disorders in which conjugated hyperbilirubinemia may be observed in the newborn period. In general, other features of the disease dominate the clinical picture, and the patients rarely present as a simple problem in the differential diagnosis of conjugated hyperbilirubinemia.

Gatzimos and Jowitt (1955) first called attention to the association between jaundice and cystic fibrosis. Many of these infants may have a history of delayed passage of the first meconium stool. These infants can be demonstrated to have thick tenacious bile plugging their biliary tree. Needle biopsy of the liver may demonstrate the characteristic eosinophilic plugs in the portal bile ducts, which may be accompanied by hyperplasia. The jaundice usually resolves spontaneously. One can establish a diagnosis of cystic fibrosis in the newborn period by demonstrating the increased concentration of sweat chloride.

■ SEPSIS

Both generalized sepsis and severe urinary tract infections, particularly with *Escherichia coli*, during the first month of life may be accompanied by an increase in the serum concentration of conjugated bilirubin. Bacterial products are believed to produce a toxic injury to the hepatocellular excretory system. Liver biopsy of infected and jaundiced newborns reveals cholestasis, focal liver cell necrosis, and other nonspecific changes. Direct infection of the liver is not evident. Despite the marked increases in the concentration of bilirubin that may accompany infection, the serum values for alkaline phosphatase and the transaminases are either normal or only slightly elevated. Treatment of the infection produces a decline in the bilirubin concentrations without evidence of residual liver damage.

■ "TOXIC" HEPATITIS

Although bacterial infections may produce a toxic hepatitis, this term is more commonly applied to circumstances in which exposure to exogenous substances produces cholestasis with variable degrees of hepatocellular injury, inflammation, or fibrosis.

The most common cause of toxic hepatitis or cholestatic jaundice observed in neonatal intensive care nurseries at the present time is the prolonged use of total parenteral nutrition.

Cholestatic jaundice induced by parenteral nutrition is seen with greatest frequency in the most immature infants. It is estimated that at least 10 per cent of infants with a gestational age of less than 32 weeks will develop this complication if they receive parenteral nutrition for periods of 3 to 4 weeks. In contrast, only about 1 per cent of infants with gestational ages of more than 36 weeks will develop cholestatic jaundice under similar circumstances.

Bacterial infections appear to contribute to the development of cholestasis.

Liver biopsies in infants who develop cholestatic jaundice in association with parenteral nutrition demonstrate both hepatocellular damage and cholestasis. Giant-cell transformation may also be observed. The etiology of the cholestasis is unclear but may relate to the fact that amino acids inhibit bile flow. Evidence of hepatic dysfunction, but not clinical jaundice, can be demonstrated within 1 week of the initiation of total parenteral nutrition. This effect appears to be independent of the newborn's underlying condition and unrelated to the concomitant use of intravenous lipid. The initial effect of the amino acid infusion appears to be on the canalicular membrane and is reflected by increases in the serum concentrations of gamma glutamyl transpeptidase and 5'-nucleotidase.

Discontinuation of the parenteral nutrition usually produces a disappearance of the hepatic abnormalities, although evidence of hepatocellular damage and fibrosis may persist over several weeks. Newborns receiving total parenteral nutrition should be monitored, at least weekly, with conjugated bilirubin values and serum bile acids.

■ THE BILE-PLUG SYNDROME

It had been suspected for many years that obstructive jaundice could be caused by plugs in the extrahepatic bile ducts. Bernstein and co-workers (1977) proved this theory by demonstrating such plugs in two infants, one of whom became jaundiced as early as 6 days, and the other as late as 7 weeks of age. The second baby was saved after demonstration by cholangiogram of obstruction in the distal end of the common duct and following the removal of an impacted mass of dark, granular, bile-colored material.

■ REFERENCES

Bernstein, J., Braylan, R., and Brough, A. J.: Bile-plug syndrome. A correctable cause of obstructive jaundice in infants. Pediatrics 43:273, 1969.

Bernstein, J., Chang, C.-H., Brough, A. J., et al.: Conjugated hyperbilirubinemia in infants associated with parenteral alimentation. J. Pediatr. 90:361, 1977.

Black, D. D., Suttle, A., Whitington, P. F., et al.: The effect of short-term total parenteral nutrition on hepatic function in the human neonate: A prospective randomized study demonstrating alteration of hepatic canalicular function. J. Pediatr. 99:445, 1981.

Colon, A. R., and Sandberg, D. H.: Presently recognized forms of inherited jaundice in infancy. A summary and review. Clin. Pediatr. 12:326, 1973.

Escobedo, M. B., and Barton, L. L.: The frequency of jaundice in neonatal bacterial infections. Clin. Pediatr. *13*:656, 1974.

Gatzimos, C. D., and Jowitt, R. H.: Jaundice in mucoviscidosis (fibrocystic disease of the pancreas). J. Dis. Child. *80*:182, 1955.

Heathcote, J., Deodhar, K. P., Scheuer, P. J., et al.: Intrahepatic cholestasis in childhood. N. Engl. J. Med. *295*:801, 1975.

Mowat, A. P.: Liver Disorders in Childhood. London, Butterworth and Co., 1979.

Odievre, M., Martin, J. P., et al.: Alpha-1-antitrypsin deficiency in liver disease in children: phenotypes, manifestations, and prognosis. Pediatrics *57*:226, 1976.

Pereira, G. R., Sherman, M. S., DiGiacomo, J., et al.: Hyperalimentation-induced cholestasis. Increased incidence and severity in premature infants. Am. J. Dis. Child. *135*:842, 1981.

Taylor, W. F., and Qaqundah, B. Y.: Neonatal jaundice associated with cystic fibrosis. Am. J. Dis. Child. *123*:161, 1972.

Touloukian, R. J., and Downing, S. E.: Cholestasis associated with long-term parenteral hyperalimentation. Arch. Surg. *106*:58, 1973.

DIFFERENTIAL DIAGNOSIS OF JAUNDICE

83

Frank A. Oski

A thoughtful attempt should be made to establish the etiology of jaundice in all infants who meet one of the following criteria:

1. Clinical jaundice in the first 24 hours of life.
2. Total bilirubin concentration increasing at a rate in excess of 5 mg/dl/day.
3. Term infants in whom the total serum bilirubin concentration exceeds 12.9 mg/dl if bottle-fed, or 15.0 mg/dl if breast-fed.
4. Preterm infants in whom the total serum bilirubin concentration exceeds 15.0 mg/dl.
5. All infants in whom the conjugated bilirubin (direct) concentration exceeds 2.0 mg/dl or more than 15 per cent of the total bilirubin value.
6. The persistence of clinical jaundice beyond the 1st week of life in a term infant or the persistence of clinical jaundice beyond the 2nd week of life in a preterm infant.

The initial diagnostic procedures should be directed at determining whether the jaundice is a result of increased production of bilirubin, impaired bilirubin conjugation, impaired bilirubin excretion, increased reabsorption of bilirubin from the intestinal tract, or a combination of these factors.

Guidelines for the collection and interpretation of historical data, the pertinent physical findings, and laboratory tests are listed in Table 83–1. Maisels and Gifford (1975) have reported that the measurement of direct and total bilirubin and hemoglobin or hematocrit, performed with the determination of the blood type of mother and infant, direct Coombs test on the infant's erythrocytes, the measurement of the infant's reticulocyte count, and examination of the peripheral smear, will define or suggest the cause of jaundice in approximately 50 per cent of all infants with hyperbilirubinemia.

Jaundice that appears within the first 24 hours of life is usually due to increased production of bilirubin as a result of a hemolytic process. In general, the more severe hemolytic anemias will be manifested by early jaundice rather than by late appearance of pallor. Rh incompatibility and ABO incompatibility are the most common causes of hemolytic disease associated with jaundice during the 1st day of life. Other congenital defects of red cell metabolism may also be associated with jaundice during this period and must be considered in the differential diagnosis of an infant with unexplained hemolytic anemia. In some instances, jaundice associated with severe infection may

appear during the first day. Some features that are useful in distinguishing ABO, Rh, and infectious origins of jaundice are described in Table 83–2.

Physical examination supplies a few valuable differentiating points. If the newborn is jaundiced but neither sick nor pale, is not covered with petechiae and ecchymoses, and has little or no enlargement of the spleen or liver, ABO or mild Rh hemolytic disease is most likely the correct diagnosis. If the newborn looks very sick, he may have either severe hemolytic disease or nonbacterial infection. Skin hemorrhages and a large liver and spleen strongly suggest the latter.

Further diagnostic studies may have to be postponed and transfusion started at this point if the infant is in shock or is obviously very anemic. The first blood withdrawn will then be subjected to a number of tests. The mother's and father's blood may also have to be investigated.

One should act according to the following guidelines:

1. Evaluate the infant's hemoglobin, serum bilirubin and its partition, red blood cell count, number of spherocytes, nucleated red blood cell number, reticulocyte percentage, white cell count and differential platelet count, direct and indirect Coombs test results, and the infant's and parents' isoimmunologic and Rh grouping.
2. If Rh is negative and if direct Coombs test result is strongly positive, search for rare antigens (e.g., Kell, Duffy).
3. If Rh is positive and if direct Coombs test result is strongly positive, search for circulating Rh antibodies.
4. If Rh is negative and if direct Coombs test result is negative or weakly positive, and if infant belongs to group A or B and mother to group O, perform an indirect Coombs test and search for circulating anti-A or anti-B antibodies. Presence and number of spherocytes should be noted.
5. If no blood group incompatibility exists and if this observation is confirmed by negativity of both Coombs test results, perform blood culture, urine culture for viruses, and serologic studies. These latter tests should be performed on the mother's serum as well. The infant's IgM concentration and the presence or absence of IgMs against specific diseases will be extremely helpful.

One may interpret these results using the data in Table 83–2. The qualifications are pointed out in footnotes.

Jaundice beginning during the 2nd or 3rd day is probably physiologic. If, however, the infant appears ill, if

TABLE 83–1. Data Collection in the Diagnosis of Neonatal Jaundice

INFORMATION	SIGNIFICANCE
Family History	
Parent or sibling with history of jaundice or anemia	Suggests hereditary hemolytic anemia such as hereditary spherocytosis
Previous sibling with neonatal jaundice	Suggests hemolytic disease due to ABO or Rh isoimmunization
History of liver disease in siblings or disorders such as cystic fibrosis, galactosemia, tyrosinemia, hypermethioninemia, Crigler-Najjar syndrome, or alpha₁-antitrypsin deficiency	All associated with neonatal hyperbilirubinemia
Maternal History	
Unexplained illness during pregnancy	Consider congenital infections such as rubella, cytomegalovirus, toxoplasmosis, herpes, syphilis, hepatitis A or B, Epstein-Barr virus
Diabetes mellitus	Increased incidence of jaundice among infants of diabetic mothers
Drug ingestion during pregnancy	Ingestion of sulfonamides, nitrofurantoins, antimalarials may initiate hemolysis in G6PD deficient infant
History of Labor and Delivery	
Vacuum extraction	Increased incidence of cephalhematoma and jaundice
Oxytocin-induced labor	Increased incidence of hyperbilirubinemia
Delayed cord clamping	Increased incidence of hyperbilirubinemia among polycythemic infants
Apgar score	Increased incidence of jaundice in asphyxiated infants
Infant's History	
Delayed passage of meconium or infrequent stools	Increased enterohepatic circulation of bilirubin. Consider intestinal atresia, annular pancreas, Hirschsprung disease, meconium plug, drug-induced ileus (hexamethonium)
Caloric intake	Inadequate caloric intake results in delay in bilirubin conjugation
Vomiting	Suspect sepsis, galactosemia, or pyloric stenosis; all associated with hyperbilirubinemia.
Infant's Physical Exam	
Small for gestational age	Infants frequently polycythemic and jaundiced
Head size	Microcephaly seen with intrauterine infections associated with jaundice
Cephalhematoma	Entrapped hemorrhage associated with hyperbilirubinemia
Plethora	Polycythemia
Pallor	Suspect hemolytic anemia
Petechiae	Suspect congenital infection, overwhelming sepsis, or severe hemolytic disease as cause of jaundice
Appearance of umbilical stump	Omphalitis and sepsis may produce jaundice
Hepatosplenomegaly	Suspect hemolytic anemia or congenital infection
Optic fundi	Chorioretinitis suggests congenital infection as cause of jaundice
Umbilical hernia	Consider hypothyroidism
Congenital anomalies	Jaundice occurs with increased frequency among infants with trisomic conditions

Laboratory Data

INFORMATION	SIGNIFICANCE
Maternal	
Blood group and indirect Coombs test	Necessary for evaluation of possible ABO or Rh incompatibility
Serology	Rule out congenital syphilis
Infant	
Hemoglobin	Anemia suggests hemolytic disease or large entrapped hemorrhage. Hemoglobin above 22 g/dl associated with increased incidence of jaundice
Reticulocyte count	Elevation suggests hemolytic disease
Red cell morphology	Spherocytes suggest ABO incompatibility or hereditary spherocytosis. Red cell fragmentation seen in disseminated intravascular coagulation
Platelet count	Thrombocytopenia suggests infection
White cell count	Total white cell count less than 5000/mm³ or band/neutrophil ratio >0.2 suggests infection
Sedimentation rate	Values in excess of 5 during the first 48 hours indicate infection or ABO incompatibility
Direct bilirubin	Elevation suggests infection or severe Rh incompatibility
Immunoglobulin M	Elevation indicates infection
Blood group and direct and indirect Coombs test	Required to rule out hemolytic disease as a result of isoimmunization
Carboxyhemoglobin level	Elevated in infants with hemolytic disease or entrapped hemorrhage
Urinalysis	Presence of reducing substance suggests diagnosis of galactosemia

the liver or spleen is enlarged, if urobilin or bile appears in excess in the urine, or if conjugated bilirubin is found in the blood, other explanations should be sought.

Jaundice first appearing at 4 days or later is usually not due to hemolytic disease of the newborn. Intranatally or postnatally acquired virus infection (cytomegalic disease, generalized herpes simplex) must be thought of as well as the bacterial infections. Neonatal hepatitis cannot be ignored, since its onset may take place at any time from birth to 4 months.

Icterus that persists beyond the usual duration of physiologic jaundice may be hemolytic, functional, or obstructive. If hemolytic, it may be the result of persistent sepsis, pyelonephritis, hereditary erythrocyte malformation, or very rarely, congenital hemoglobin disorders or erythrocyte enzyme defects. The morphology of the red cells, their osmotic fragility, as well as electrophoretic studies, enzyme studies, and repeated blood cultures should differentiate this group.

If bilirubinemia is pronounced and if the serum bilirubin

TABLE 83–2. Laboratory Tests in Jaundice That Begins Within the First 24 Hours

DISEASE PROCESS	BLOOD SMEAR			INFANT'S ERYTHROCYTES			INFANT'S BILIRUBIN		ANTIBODIES			Special Tests for Infection
	Spherocytes	Erythroblasts	Reduced Platelets	Group O	Rh-Positive	Direct Coombs	Direct	Indirect	Indirect Coombs	A or B	Rh	
ABO hemolytic disease	+	+	Rarely and later	Never*	0 or +	Weak	No > 2.0 mg %	+	+	+	0	0
Rh hemolytic disease	0	+	Rarely and later	±	+†	+ and strong	Rarely > 2.0 mg %	+	+	0	+	0
Infection	0	+	+ often	±	0	0	+	+	0	0	0	+†‡

*The infant's blood group is usually A.
†In hR (little c, d, or e) sensitization and those caused by other rare antigens, the Rh will be negative.
‡In toxoplasmosis, Sabin's dye test becomes positive early, whereas complement fixation becomes positive later. At this stage, dye tests should be positive in the mother and infant, complement fixation only in the mother. If cytomegalic inclusion disease is the cause, the urinary sediment should show inclusion bodies and should yield the virus upon culture. Specific IgM tests are highly desirable.

is almost entirely of the indirect type when there is no evidence of increased hemolysis (reticulocytosis, normoblastosis, and erythroblastosis in the blood; increased urobilin in the stool or urine), one should think first of events that can predispose the patient to hepatic recirculation of bilirubin absorbed from the intestine and, if this is not the cause, should next consider hypothyroidism. If the latter diagnosis is also incorrect, one can then justifiably think seriously of congenital familial nonhemolytic jaundice.

Persistent obstructive jaundice is a sign that causes much diagnostic perplexity. Its characteristics include a high proportion of direct-reacting bilirubin in the serum (usually 35 per cent or more of the total), diminished or absent bilirubin and urobilin in stools, and increased bile in the urine. Diagnostic possibilities include (1) anatomic

obstructions (atresia of bile ducts, bile duct plug, choledochus or pseudocholedochus cyst, or rarely, cystic fibrosis, hypertrophic pyloric stenosis, intestinal atresia, or malrotation of the intestine); (2) neonatal hepatitis (following erythroblastosis fetalis or congenital or acquired hemolytic anemia or appearing independent of any known underlying disease); and (3) neonatal cirrhosis of the liver. Clinically, there are few features that allow one to differentiate among these possibilities. A fairly reliable one is that infants with bile duct atresia do not appear ill during the neonatal period. They eat well and gain fairly well at first. Likewise, those infants who have obstructive jaundice that follows hemolytic disease do not initially appear ill. Infants with hepatitis and especially those with cirrhosis look and act sick, eat poorly, and may have fever and may vomit often. Infants with hemolytic disease of the

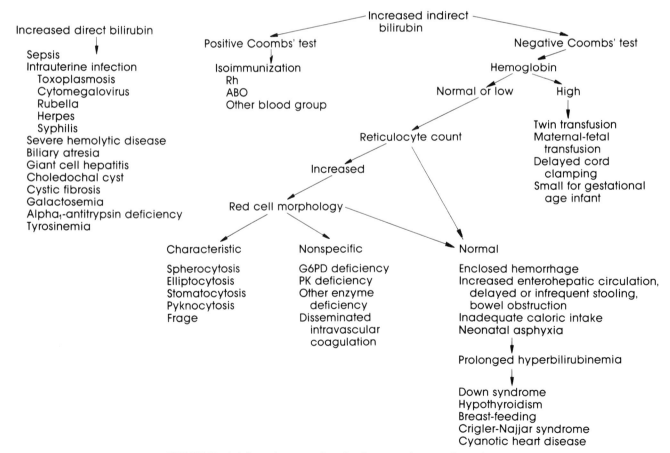

FIGURE 83–1. Schematic approach to the diagnosis of neonatal jaundice.

newborn usually have gone through a stage of nonobstructive jaundice within the 1st week of life, and the obstructive condition either has followed the first stage directly or has appeared a few days or weeks after subsidence of the nonobstructive episode. The knowledge that hemolytic disease had been manifest earlier makes the diagnosis of inspissated bile syndrome secondary to this disorder simple. If one does not have this knowledge, retrospective tests as described previously will still be diagnostic.

Liver function tests are of little differentiating value. The rose bengal excretion test may be of greater use, since the dye is well excreted in a large number of patients in the hepatitis group, but poorly in infants with atresia. Serum transaminase activities have some differential diagnostic value.

An approach to all the potential clinical possibilities discussed in the previous chapters is illustrated in Figure 83–1. It is designed to serve as a reminder of some of the less common clinical entities that often lead to diagnostic confusion.

■ REFERENCES

Adler, S. M., and Denton, R. L.: The erythrocyte sedimentation rate. J. Pediatr. *86*:942, 1975.

Alden, E. R., Lynch, S. R., Wennberg, R. P.: Carboxyhemoglobin determination in evaluating neonatal jaundice. Am. J. Dis. Child. *127*:214, 1974.

Freeman, L. M., and Weissmann, H. S. (Eds.): Nuclear Medicine Annual. New York, Raven Press, 1981.

Gartner, L. M.: Disorders of bilirubin metabolism. *In* Nathan, D. G., and Oski, F. A. (Eds.). Hematology of Infancy and Childhood. 2nd ed. Philadelphia, W. B. Saunders Company, 1981, pp. 86–118.

Maisels, M. J., and Gifford, K.: Neonatal jaundice and breast-feeding. Pediatr. Res. *9*:308, 1975.

Thaler, M. M.: Algorithmic diagnosis of conjugated and unconjugated hyperbilirubinemia. J.A.M.A. *237*:58, 1977.

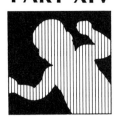
HEMOSTATIC 84 DISORDERS IN THE NEWBORN

Bertil E. Glader and Michael D. Amylon

■ PHYSIOLOGY OF NORMAL NEONATAL HEMOSTASIS

Normal hemostasis is a complicated process involving vascular integrity, platelets, and coagulation proteins (Fig. 84–1). The majority of neonatal bleeding disorders are due to deficiencies of coagulation proteins or thrombocytopenia. Hemorrhage caused by vascular problems (anatomic or physiologic) may be responsible for some of the serious bleeding episodes (pulmonary and CNS) seen in premature infants. Unfortunately, the pathophysiology of vascular-related bleeding is poorly understood.

Platelets. Platelets are activated following exposure to subendothelial collagen of the severed blood vessel. In the presence of collagen, platelets release several hemostatic factors including serotonin, adenosine diphosphate (ADP), and platelet membrane lipid (platelet factor 3). Serotonin enhances vasoconstriction. Platelet factor 3 is utilized in the clotting scheme (see subsequently). Released ADP causes platelets to aggregate reversibly into clumps, thus forming the primary, or loose, hemostatic plug. The platelet count in term and healthy premature infants is the same as that in older children. Previously, it was thought that premature infants had significantly lower platelet counts than normal term infants. In part, this was due to the fact that many laboratories included all premature infants in establishing their normal values. A platelet count of less than 100,000/μl is definitely abnormal.

Coagulation factors. In addition to platelets, coagulation factors are necessary for the production of a firm definitive hemostatic plug (Table 84–1). As seen in Figure 84–1, there are two different pathways for initiating the coagulation cascade. The "intrinsic pathway" is stimulated when factor XII reacts with subendothelial collagen. Following this, sequential interaction with other factors (XI, IX, VIII,

and platelet factor 3) results in the activation of factor X. The "extrinsic" pathway is stimulated when injured tissues release a tissue thromboplastin that reacts with factor VII to activate factor X. Thus, the intrinsic and extrinsic pathways activate factor X via different reactions, but beyond this step the clotting pathways are identical. Activated factor X, factor V, and platelet factor 3 together convert prothrombin (factor II) into thrombin. Thrombin is a proteolytic enzyme that converts fibrinogen (factor I) into a loose fibrin clot. Factor XIII (fibrin stabilizing factor) then converts the friable clot into tight fibrin polymers. The definitive hemostatic plug consists of irreversible platelet aggregates and tight fibrin polymers. Irreversible platelet clumps are formed when thrombin reacts with reversible platelet aggregates.

At the time of birth, levels of fibrinogen and factor VIII are the same as normal child or adult values while the activities of factors V and XIII are mildly decreased (Table 84–2). In contrast, the activities of factors II, VII, IX, X, XI, and XIII are significantly decreased, and this is more severe in premature infants than in term infants. Presumably, these low factor levels are a consequence of hepatic immaturity and decreased factor synthesis. However, some coagulation factors (II, VII, IX, X) are also dependent upon vitamin K for complete activation, and since newborns are vitamin K–deficient, this can add further to the normally reduced values seen during the newborn period (discussed later in the section on hemorrhagic disease of the newborn). In both term and premature newborns, all of the coagulation proteins increase to near-normal levels by 6 months of age.

In tandem with the coagulation process, there are physiologic controls that limit thrombus formation. Some of these controls function by regulating the generation of fibrin. Antithrombin III interacts with endogenous heparin to neutralize the varied actions of thrombin, including the conversion of fibrinogen to fibrin. Protein C is activated by thrombin in the presence of thrombomodulin (a recep-

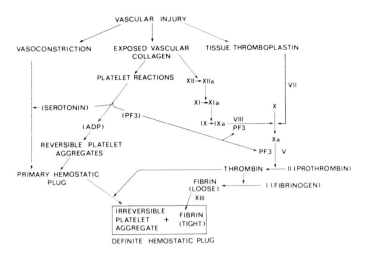

FIGURE 84–1. *Physiology of normal hemostasis.*

tor on endothelial cells). Activated protein C, in the presence of protein S (another cofactor), inhibits the activity of factors V and VIII, and thereby retards fibrin formation. As for coagulation proteins, the levels of anti-thrombin III, protein C, and protein S all are transiently reduced in newborns. Part of protein C and protein S deficiency may be related to the fact that these are vitamin K–dependent proteins. The "balanced" decrease in co-agulation and inhibitor proteins may explain why bleeding is seldom a problem in healthy newborns.

An alternative means of limiting the extent of thrombus formation is the lysis of fibrin after it has formed. This fibrinolytic activity is mediated by plasminogen following its activation to plasmin (Fig. 84–2). There are many physiologic activators of plasminogen, some of which also activate the coagulation cascade. The proteolytic activity of plasmin breaks down fibrin deposited at sites of vessel injury. In addition, plasmin degrades factors V, VIII, and fibrinogen. Together these highly regulated reactions limit the extent of fibrin formation and thereby maintain normal vascular patency. In pathologic states, such as dissemi-nated intravascular coagulation (DIC), persistent activation of clotting and fibrinolysis can deplete factors V, VIII, and fibrinogen and thereby lead to bleeding. Moreover, in-creased levels of the fibrin split products (FSPs) can enhance the hemorrhagic tendency by directly inhibiting the normal conversion of fibrinogen to fibrin.

TABLE 84–1. Blood Clotting Factors

NUMBER	SYNONYMS
I	Fibrinogen
II	Prothrombin
III	Thromboplastin
IV	Calcium
V	Proaccelerin (labile factor)
VI	Activated factor V (term not used)
VII	Proconvertin (stable factor)
VIII	Antihemophiliac factor (AHF)
IX	Plasma thromboplastin component (PTC) Christmas factor
X	Stuart-Power factor
XI	Plasma thromboplastin antecedent (PTA)
XII	Hageman factor, contact factor
XIII	Fibrin stabilizing factor

General Approach to the Bleeding Infant

Medical History and Physical Examination. Evalua-tion of any bleeding infant requires historical information regarding outcome of previous pregnancies, family bleed-ing problems, maternal illnesses (especially infections), drug administration (maternal and neonatal), and docu-mentation that vitamin K was given at birth. Simple observations on physical examination (localized versus diffuse bleeding; healthy or sick infant) have tremendous importance for classifying hemorrhagic disorders. Normal infants frequently have petechiae over presenting parts secondary to venous congestion and the trauma of deliv-ery. These petechiae are seen shortly after birth but gradually disappear and are not associated with bleeding. Infants with isolated platelet disorders generally appear healthy except for progressive petechiae, ecchymoses, and/or mucosal bleeding. Hemorrhages due to vitamin K deficiency or inherited coagulation defects characteristi-cally occur in apparently healthy children with large ec-chymoses or localized bleeding (large cephalohematomas, umbilical cord bleeding, or gastrointestinal hemorrhage). Bleeding due to DIC or liver injury generally is seen in sick infants with diffuse bleeding from several sites.

Laboratory Evaluation of Bleeding Infant. The etiol-ogy of hemorrhage frequently can be identified by simple diagnostic tests. A review of the common and esoteric methods used in studying neonatal hemostasis recently has been published (Corrigan, 1989). A differential diag-nosis based on the platelet count, prothrombin time (PT), and partial thromboplastin time (PTT) is presented in Table 84–3.

1. Platelet Count. In emergency situations or when quantitative platelet counts cannot be obtained, a reliable estimate of the platelet count can be made by examining the peripheral blood smear. The average number of platelets per high-power field is determined after observing several fields under the microscope. This number multi-plied by 15,000 is a valid estimate of the platelet count. For example, if one observes 50 platelets after examining 20 high-power fields, there is an average of 2.5 platelets per field, and the approximate platelet count is 37,500 (2.5 multiplied by 15,000). The peripheral blood smear

TABLE 84–2. Coagulation Profile of Newborn Infants

	NORMAL ADULT	TERM INFANT	PRETERM INFANT
Platelet count	150K–400K	150K–400K	150K–350K
Bleeding time	2–10 minutes	2–10 minutes	2–10 minutes
Prothrombin time	10.8–13.9 seconds	10.2–15.8 seconds	10.6–16.2 seconds
Activated PTT	26.6–40.3 seconds	31.3–54.5 seconds	27.5–79.4 seconds
Clotting Factors		**Term and Preterm Infants**	
Normal	All factors	Fibrinogen, VIII, vWF	
Slightly decreased	–	V, XIII	
Moderately decreased	–	II, VII, IX, X, XI, XII, and antithrombin III, protein C and S	

Data based on normal values published by Andrew, M., et al.: Blood 70:1651, 1987 and 72:1651, 1988, and normal values of the Stanford University Hospital and Children's Hospital at Stanford, Palo Alto, Calif.

also should include an evaluation of platelet size. Thrombocytopenia associated with normal-sized platelets generally reflects a bone marrow production defect, whereas the presence of large platelets indicates rapid production and destruction of circulating platelets.

The platelet count in term and healthy premature newborns is the same as that in older children.

2. Prothrombin Time and Partial Thromboplastin Time.
These two tests should be used as the initial coagulation screening procedures in any bleeding infant:

Prothrombin Time (PT). This test measures the extrinsic activation of factor X by factor VII as well as the remainder of the coagulation scheme (factors V, II, and fibrinogen).

Partial Thromboplastin Time (PTT). This test measures the intrinsic pathway (activation of factor X by factors XII, XI, IX, and VIII) as well as the final coagulation reactions (V, II, and fibrinogen). Most laboratories use an activated partial thromboplastin time (APTT). This test is similar to the PTT except that material is added to hasten the activation of factor XII and thereby speed up the overall reaction.

Two important variables must be considered when collecting venous blood for neonatal coagulation studies. First, the ratio of blood to anticoagulant (3.8 per cent sodium citrate) should be 19:1 (Koepke et al., 1975). The usual ratio (9:1) may give spurious results in newborns with hematocrits over 60 per cent. Second, *blood should not be drawn from heparinized catheters, since even minute amounts of this anticoagulant can prolong the PTT.*

As discussed previously, newborns have decreased levels of certain clotting factors, and, consequently, the PT and PTT in healthy term infants are slightly prolonged as compared with those of older children (see Table 84–2). These physiologic factor deficiencies are exaggerated in premature infants, and thus, the PT and PTT in prematures may be even more prolonged. It is important to emphasize that the differences in clotting parameters between older children and infants are physiologically normal because of impaired hepatic factor synthesis. Any questionable abnormality must be compared to these "normal" neonatal values. Furthermore, each individual hospital must establish its own normal values, since slight modifications in blood collection or assay methods exist between different laboratories.

3. Fibrinogen Determination.
One measures this factor when attempting to differentiate DIC or liver disease from other clotting abnormalities. Reduced fibrinogen synthesis occurs in liver disease. Increased degradation of fibrinogen is seen in DIC.

4. Fibrin Split Products (FSPs).
These degradation products of fibrin and fibrinogen are increased in patients with DIC. Increased levels occasionally are seen in liver disease and are possibly due to decreased clearance of FSPs. Since DIC frequently coexists with liver disease, it is often difficult to distinguish these two entities. Fibrin split products are not increased in normal infants when blood samples are properly collected.

5. Bleeding Time.
This test is a practical way to assess platelet interaction with vascular endothelium. It should not be performed in patients with thrombocytopenia. In older children and adults, it is a valuable procedure for identifying patients with von Willebrand disease or functional platelet disorders. This test is of questionable utility in the newborn period and is rarely used. No reliable techniques for the bleeding time have been described for newborns.

6. Apt Test.
This simple test distinguishes gastrointestinal blood loss due to neonatal hemorrhage from that caused by swallowed maternal blood.

a. Mix 1 volume of stool or vomitus with 5 volumes of water.

b. Centrifuge mixture and separate clear pink supernatant (hemolysate).

c. Add 1 ml of 1 per cent NaOH to 4 ml hemolysate. Mix and observe color change after 2 minutes. Hemoglobin A changes from pink to a yellow-brown color (this indicates maternal blood). Hemoglobin F resists denaturation and remains pink (this indicates fetal blood).

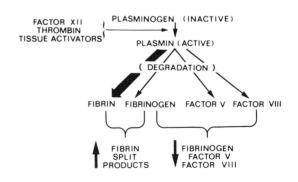

FIGURE 84–2. *Physiology of fibrinolysis.*

TABLE 84–3. Differential Diagnosis of Bleeding in the Neonate

CLINICAL EVALUATION	LABORATORY STUDIES			LIKELY DIAGNOSIS
	Platelets	PT	PTT	
"Sick"	↓	↑	↑	DIC
	↓	N	N	Platelet consumption (infection, necrotizing enterocolitis, renal vein thrombosis)
	N	↑	↑	Liver disease
	N	N	N	Compromised vascular integrity (associated with hypoxia, prematurity, acidosis, hyperosmolality)
"Healthy"	↓	N	N	Immune thrombocytopenia
				Occult infection or thrombosis
				Bone marrow hypoplasia (rare)
	N	↑	↑	Hemorrhagic disease of newborn (vitamin K deficiency)
	N	N	↑	Hereditary clotting factor deficiencies
	N	N	N	Bleeding due to local factors (trauma, anatomic abnormalities)

N, normal; ↑, increased; ↓ decreased.

Approximately 30 per cent of all episodes of gastrointestinal bleeding are due to swallowed maternal blood (Sherman and Clatworthy, 1967). In those cases in which there is true fetal blood loss, less than 25 per cent of infants have detectable platelet or coagulation abnormalities. Underlying abnormalities of the gastrointestinal tract are responsible for some of these bleeding episodes, although in many cases there is no *discernible cause* of hemorrhage.

■ BLOOD COMPONENTS USED IN THERAPY OF BLEEDING INFANTS

Platelet Transfusions. A unit of platelets is defined as that number of platelets obtained from one unit of blood. Platelets are suspended in plasma, approximately 1 unit of platelets in 15 ml of plasma. In order to prevent neonatal red blood cell injury, donor platelets should be type-specific (A, B, O), since the donor plasma may contain antibodies that react with recipient RBCs. Platelets do not contain the Rh antigen, but virtually all platelet concentrates contain some RBCs. Rh-negative infants, therefore, are given platelets from Rh-negative donors. If emergency conditions require that Rh-negative girls be given platelets from an Rh-positive donor, the use of anti-Rh immune globulin (RhoGAM) should be considered in order to protect against red blood cell isoimmunization. In cases of neonatal isoimmune thrombocytopenia, maternal platelets are obtained, washed free of antibody, and resuspended in AB-negative plasma. As a rule of thumb, the administration of 1 unit of fresh platelets to a *newborn* should elevate the platelet count to over 100,000/μl. Subsequently, the platelet count should decline slowly over 4 to 6 days. Failure to sustain a platelet increase indicates platelet incompatibility due to sensitization or increased platelet destruction (sepsis, DIC, antiplatelet antibody).

Fresh Frozen Plasma. Plasma that is frozen and stored immediately after separation contains adequate concentrations of all clotting factors. Fresh frozen plasma (10 ml/kg) given every 12 hours provides adequate hemostasis for most causes of bleeding due to lack of factors. Plasma also can be used to treat bleeding newborns known to have factor VIII deficiency (classic hemophilia) or factor

IX deficiency (Christmas disease). Whenever possible, infants with hemophilia should be treated with specific concentrates that have been purified of any viral contamination. Currently, several different processes are employed to inactivate human immunodeficiency virus (HIV), such as heat inactivation, monoclonal antibody purification, and detergent removal of the virus.

■ HEMORRHAGIC DISEASE OF THE NEWBORN

The American Academy of Pediatrics has defined hemorrhagic disease of the newborn (HDN) as any bleeding problem due to vitamin K deficiency and decreased activity of factors II, VII, IX, and X. The physiology and pathophysiology of vitamin K deficiency have recently been reviewed (Hathaway, 1987; Lane and Hathaway, 1985). The vitamin K–dependent clotting proteins are synthesized in the liver, but they are biologically inert until activated by vitamin K. The specific function of vitamin K is that of a cofactor in the carboxylation of glutamic acid residues, a reaction that provides the calcium-binding site required for coagulant activation. The precursors of these coagulation factors are referred to as PIVKA (proteins induced by vitamin K absence). In vitamin K deficiency PIVKA levels are elevated in plasma despite little or no measurable coagulant activity. Three different patterns of hemorrhage due to vitamin K deficiency are recognized: classic, early, and late hemorrhagic disease of the newborn.

CLASSIC HEMORRHAGIC DISEASE OF THE NEWBORN

As discussed previously, neonatal coagulant factor synthesis is modestly decreased because of hepatic immaturity. However, because there also is a relative deficiency of vitamin K, coagulant activity of these factors is further reduced. Vitamin K normally is obtained from the diet and from intestinal bacterial synthesis. Newborns, however, get variable amounts of dietary vitamin K during the first few days of life, and the intestine is not colonized with bacteria at birth. Therefore, as the limited amounts of maternally derived vitamin stores are depleted during the 1st day of life, vitamin K deficiency actually becomes worse, clotting studies become more abnormal, and significant bleeding problems can occur between 1 and 7 days of age. This has been referred to as classic hemorrhagic disease of the newborn.

Many years ago, the important observation was made that HDN could be prevented by early feeding with cow's milk. This beneficial effect was due to the significantly higher vitamin K content of cow's milk compared with that of breast milk (Dam et al., 1942). Subsequently, classic HDN has virtually disappeared as a clinical problem because vitamin K routinely is given to most infants at birth. Prior to this practice, the incidence of significant hemorrhage (i.e., classic HDN) was estimated to be one in 200 to 400 newborns. Today, bleeding due to HDN is unusual. It is seen under conditions in which vitamin K mistakenly was not given, or in some areas in which there are parents who elect not to have their infant administered this vitamin. In classic HDN, hemorrhage due to vitamin K deficiency characteristically occurs in otherwise healthy infants after 24 hours of age. Bleeding may be localized to one area (e.g., cephalohematoma or gastrointestinal bleeding), or there may be diffuse ecchymoses. The following laboratory test results suggest vitamin K deficiency: normal platelet count, prolonged PTT, and prolonged PT. Bleeding infants who have these results should be given vitamin K (1 mg intravenously). Within 4 hours the PT and PTT begin to normalize, and clinical bleeding ceases in those cases due to vitamin K deficiency. If clinical bleeding and coagulation tests do not improve after giving vitamin K, other diagnoses, such as liver disease or isolated factor deficiencies, must be considered. Life-threatening hemorrhages due to vitamin K deficiency are unusual, but if they occur, fresh frozen plasma (10 ml/kg) should be given in addition to vitamin K.

In most nurseries, prophylactic vitamin K (0.5 to 1.0 mg) is given intramuscularly following delivery. The minimal dose of vitamin K that prevents the fall in PT and bleeding is 0.025 mg; higher concentrations have no additional beneficial effect (Aballi and DeLamerens, 1962). Nevertheless, we continue to give doses that greatly exceed the minimum requirement. Previously, it was thought that premature infants did not respond to vitamin K. Aballi and co-workers (1957), however, have demonstrated that healthy prematures do respond, although sick prematures may manifest a less than optimal change in clotting studies. It is the authors' policy to administer vitamin K (0.5 mg) one to two times each week to ill prematures and infants receiving broad-spectrum antibiotics or total parenteral alimentation. Vitamin K given to mothers during labor has proved effective in preventing neonatal bleeding, although one is never quite certain how much actually crosses the placenta. For this reason, it makes more sense to administer vitamin K at the time of birth; the response following vitamin administration is rapid, and bleeding rarely occurs in the first 24 hours of life.

EARLY HEMORRHAGIC DISEASE OF THE NEWBORN

Occasionally, bleeding due to vitamin K deficiency occurs in newborns less than 24 hours old, and these cases are referred to as "early hemorrhagic disease of the newborn." Early HDN is seen in children born to epileptic mothers (under treatment with phenytoin or phenobarbital) or, less commonly, mothers with tuberculosis (under treatment with isoniazid or rifampin) (Mountain et al., 1970). These maternal drugs can interfere with the neonatal oxidation of vitamin K, thereby causing abnormal clotting studies, low clotting factor levels, and bleeding at birth. Bleeding in early HDN may vary from moderate skin and umbilical hemorrhage to fatal intrathoracic, intraabdominal, or intracranial hemorrhage. The precise risk of early HDNs developing in an infant of an epileptic mother receiving anticonvulsant therapy is unknown. Moreover, the most appropriate management of pregnancy to avoid early HDN in these cases also is not known. A reasonable and safe approach may be to give the mother oral vitamin K (20 mg/day) for 2 weeks prior to delivery (Deblay et al., 1982). Following birth, intramuscular vitamin K should be given as usual to the newborn. It should also be noted that infants born to mothers receiving coumarin compounds (vitamin K antagonists) may bleed because these drugs cross the placenta and interfere with neonatal vitamin K metabolism and coagulation factor synthesis. Heparin does not cross the placenta and therefore should be substituted for coumarin several days before delivery in those maternal conditions requiring anticoagulation therapy (Hirsh et al., 1970). Heparin also should be used instead of coumarin compounds in the first trimester of pregnancy, since coumarin has been associated with teratogenicity (Fillmore and McDevitt, 1970).

LATE HEMORRHAGIC DISEASE OF THE NEWBORN

In recent years, it has become apparent that hemorrhage due to vitamin K deficiency can occur beyond the immediate newborn period (1 to 12 months of age). Late HDN most commonly presents with CNS bleeding and widespread deep ecchymoses. Less commonly, the presenting manifestations relate to the gastrointestinal tract or superficial skin bleeding. Late HDN is seen primarily in clinical states associated with impaired vitamin K absorption. Moreover, the hemorrhagic manifestations may be the initial sign of an underlying problem, such as cystic fibrosis, biliary atresia, alpha$_1$-antitrypsin deficiency, hepatitis, abetalipoproteinemia, celiac disease, and chronic diarrhea with malabsorption. It is now recognized that prolonged diarrhea (over 1 week duration) in otherwise healthy breast-fed infants is a particularly worrisome problem, and the American Academy of Pediatrics has recommended that these infants receive at least one intramuscular injection of vitamin K (0.5–1.0 mg) during this illness. In some cases of late HDN, no cause is found, and these are considered to be idiopathic (Lane and Hathaway, 1985). Of interest, many of these idiopathic cases occur in breast-fed infants who have not received vitamin K at birth. The majority of idiopathic cases occur within 1 to 3 months of age, while other secondary cases occur any time during the 1st year of life. In any infant with late HDN one must look diligently for an underlying primary disease responsible for the vitamin K deficiency.

■ HEREDITARY CLOTTING FACTOR DEFICIENCIES

The vast majority of genetic coagulation disorders are due to factor VIII deficiency (hemophilia A, or classic hemophilia) or factor IX deficiency (hemophilia B, or Christmas disease). Other hereditary coagulation factor deficiencies associated with bleeding are extremely rare. The laboratory tests in hemophilia A and B reveal that the PTT is prolonged with the PT and platelet count usually normal. Neither bleeding nor abnormal coagulation studies respond to vitamin K.

FACTOR VIII DEFICIENCY

Hemophilia A is defined as deficiency of factor VIII coagulant activity. Factor VIII circulates in the plasma as a complex of two separate peptides: the factor VIII coagulant protein and von Willebrand factor (vWF). The function of factor VIII coagulant is to facilitate the generation of fibrin. The function of vWF is two-fold: to transport factor VIII coagulant and to facilitate platelet adhesion to vascular endothelium. Being two distinct polypeptides, the factor VIII protein complex is a product of two separate genes, one sex-linked and the other autosomal. The X chromosome contains the gene that regulates factor VIII coagulant production, while the autosomal gene on chromosome 12 regulates synthesis of vWF. Classic hemophilia is a sex-linked disorder characterized by diminished levels of factor VIII coagulant activity with normal amounts of the carrier protein (vWF) (Ratnoff, 1972). In contrast, von Willebrand disease is an autosomal disorder characterized by decreased levels of factor VIII carrier protein (vWF) with a correspondingly reduced level of factor VIII coagulant activity (Table 84–4).

The spectrum of problems in older hemophiliac children varies from mild soft tissue hemorrhages and frequent joint bleeds to life-threatening central nervous system hemorrhages. In newborns, however, severe bleeding due to factor VIII deficiency is unusual. Most commonly, it presents as cephalohematoma, gastrointestinal hemorrhage, or bleeding from the umbilical stump or following circumcision. It has been observed that up to 40 per cent of hemophiliacs may bleed following circumcision, but in most cases, the bleeding was not life-threatening (Baehner and Strauss, 1966). One reason for this may be that tissue injury liberates thromboplastin and thereby activates factor VII and the extrinisic pathway (which bypasses factor VIII). In rare cases, intracranial hemorrhage may be the initial presentation of newborns with hemophilia (Bray and

Luban, 1987; Yoffe and Buchanan, 1988). Despite this, vaginal delivery seems to be safe in the vast majority of pregnancies in which a fetus with hemophilia is at risk. In most centers, the appropriate indications for ceserean section are no different than in otherwise normal pregnancies. Beyond the neonatal period, de novo cases of hemophilia first may present following parental "jostling," intramuscular administration of immunizations, or injuries sustained after the baby becomes mobile.

As a sex-linked disorder, hemophilia affects only male children. In a newborn in whom the diagnosis of hemophilia is suspected, a specific factor assay should be done to confirm the type of factor deficiency (hemophilia A or B) and its magnitude. In infants with classic hemophilia, there is no problem assessing this, since factor VIII levels in the newborn are the same as in older children. The normal level of coagulation factor activity is considered to be 100 per cent (50 to 150 per cent range). Children with severe hemophilia have less than 1 per cent factor VIII activity, and clinically, this disorder is characterized by spontaneous hemorrhages. In contrast, children with moderate hemophilia have 1 to 5 per cent factor VIII activity, and bleeding usually occurs with trauma. The presence of 5 to 25 per cent normal coagulation factor activity is seen in mild hemophilia, which is characterized by hemorrhage only in the presence of severe trauma. Whenever a newborn is suspected of having hemophilia, it is critical to consult with a hematologist regarding the general care of the child and to discuss the treatment of specific bleeding episodes.

An important aspect of the routine care of infants with hemophilia includes preparing parents for what to anticipate. The soft tissue and joint hemorrhages characteristic of hemophilia in older children usually begin after a few months of age when infants begin to crawl. The signs of hemorrhage in young babies may be quite subtle, manifested only by irritability or limb disuse. Routine immunizations should be given subcutaneously (not intramuscularly) followed by an ice pack to the injection site. No factor replacement therapy is necessary if they are given in this manner. Also, infants with hemophilia should be immunized with recombinant hepatitis B vaccine. This is advisable despite the fact that all current hemophilia products are screened for hepatitis B.

Specific bleeding episodes are treated with factor concentrates. In small soft tissue and extremity bleeds, usually only one infusion is needed; however, sufficient factor VIII must be given to raise the plasma concentration to at least 40 per cent of normal. As a rule, one factor VIII unit administered per kilogram of body weight elevates the plasma concentration 2 per cent. Thus, to achieve a level that is 40 per cent of normal requires 20 factor VIII units/kg, or 60 factor VIII units for a 3-kg infant. In severe life-threatening hemorrhages, sufficient factor VIII must be administered to raise the level to 100 per cent. Moreover, in many of these life-threatening bleeds, and in surgery patients, it is necessary to maintain these elevated factor levels for a period of time. The in vivo half-life of factor VIII is approximately 12 hours, and thus, infusions need to be repeated twice daily. An initial dose of 50 units of factor VIII activity per kilogram of body weight followed by 25 units per kilogram every 12 hours should keep the factor VIII level at 50 to 100 per cent of normal and

TABLE 84–4. Factor VIII Complex Analysis

	FACTOR VIII	vWF	FACTOR VIII : vWF
Normal	1.0 (0.5–1.5)	1.0 (0.5–1.5)	1.0
Hemophilia A	0 (0–0.25)	1.0 (0.5–1.5)	0–0.25
Hemophilia A carrier	0.5 (0.25–0.75)	1.0 (0.5–1.5)	0.5
von Willebrand disease	0 (0.1–0.5)	0 (0.1–0.5)	1.0

The relative factor VIII coagulant activity, vWF concentration, and factor VIII : vWF ratio are depicted in normal individuals and individuals with hemophilia A, female hemophilia A carriers, and those with von Willebrand disease.

thereby control bleeding. As mentioned previously, all currently available concentrates for treating patients with hemophilia are prepared in such a way as to render them free of HIV and safe to use. However, a recombinant DNA factor VIII product has been developed and currently is undergoing limited clinical trials. It is anticipated that this new preparation soon will be the standard product for hemophilia A treatment.

The carrier state for hemophilia A can be detected in a majority of families where there is an affected individual. Measurement of factor VIII coagulant activity and vWF can identify 90 per cent of hemophilia A carriers (see Table 84–4). If there is a family member with hemophilia who is available for study, molecular biology techniques (i.e., restriction-fragment length polymorphisms, or RFLPs) can identify an even higher fraction of hemophilia carriers. Prenatal diagnosis also is possible in pregnant women known to be carriers of hemophilia A. The first step in prenatal diagnosis is amniocentesis to establish the sex of the fetus. This can be accomplished at 13 to 16 weeks of gestation, and using fibroblast DNA obtained at amniocentesis, RFLP analysis can be used to establish whether or not the fetus has hemophilia. Earlier in pregnancy (9 to 12 weeks of gestation), it also is possible to establish the diagnosis of hemophilia from DNA obtained by chorionic villus sampling. Both this procedure and amniocentesis have approximately a 0.5 per cent associated morbidity. If amniocentesis establishes that the fetus is a male, but DNA studies do not clearly establish the diagnosis of hemophilia, it is possible to obtain fetal blood samples using cordocentesis. Immunologic and/or functional coagulation studies on fetal blood can ascertain whether or not factor VIII coagulant is present.

VON WILLEBRAND DISEASE (vWD)

This common autosomal dominant disorder is due to decreased levels of von Willebrand factor, which results in proportionately lower levels of factor VIII coagulant activity (see Table 84–4). The bleeding manifestations in vWD are a consequence of the reduced vWF necessary for platelet adhesion to an area of endothelial injury. Newborns hardly ever are symptomatic, and very rarely is this a serious neonatal problem. A more common issue is the question of whether this disorder can be diagnosed in an infant born to a family where one parent is known to have vWD. In fact, it is extremely difficult to diagnose vWD in the newborn period (Weinger et al., 1980). In part, this is because the stress of delivery may cause a transient increase in vWF concentration. Definitive testing for vWD should be deferred until the infant is at least 1 month old (Corrigan, 1989). As discussed earlier, the definitive diagnosis of von Willebrand disease can usually be made by measuring levels of factor VIII carrier protein (vWF) and coagulant VIIIc). In vWD, the vWF and VIIIc are both depressed to the same degree (usually 15 to 40 per cent of normal activity).

FACTOR IX DEFICIENCY

Factor IX deficiency (Christmas disease, or hemophilia B) is less common than factor VIII deficiency, accounting for 15 per cent of all cases of hemophilia. This disorder is also sex-linked, and the clinical manifestations are indistinguishable from those of factor VIII deficiency. Measurement of factor IX activity in the newborn period can be diagnostic, although the exact factor level in moderate cases may not be established until after 2 months of age. The level of factor IX activity may be higher at a later date because of the decreased factor synthesis at birth. Carrier detection and prenatal diagnosis of factor IX deficiency are possible, but the level of diagnostic precision has not yet reached that seen for factor VIII deficiency.

In the case of a bleeding infant thought to have Christmas disease, it is essential that a hematologist be notified, since appropriate therapy for this specific type of hemophilia is undergoing marked changes. Fresh frozen plasma (10 ml/kg) can be given for most minor bleeds. Alternatively, virally purified factor IX concentrates also can be administered (1 unit of factor IX increases plasma IX activity by 1 per cent). For minor bleeding episodes, 20 to 30 factor IX units per kilogram of body weight should be given. With more severe bleeding, factor IX activity should be increased to 40 to 50 per cent of normal and repeated every 24 hours. With currently available products, this can be dangerous because "activated procoagulants" are present in the factor IX concentrates. The new monoclonal antibody purified factor IX preparations are expected to be free of contaminating activated coagulants and other infectious agents.

FACTOR XI DEFICIENCY

Factor XI deficiency (hemophilia C) is an extremely rare autosomal recessive disorder that occurs primarily in Jewish families. Bleeding rarely is a serious problem. It is difficult to diagnose in newborns, since factor XI levels remain low for the first several months of life. Factor therapy rarely is required. In a patient with factor XI deficiency who is bleeding, fresh frozen plasma (10 ml/kg) can be given.

FACTOR XIII DEFICIENCY

Factor XIII (fibrin stabilizing factor) deficiency, characterized by delayed bleeding from the umbilical stump, is a genetic disease that should be recognized by neonatologists. Hereditary deficiency of this factor results in an inability to cross-link fibrin, and thus, a very friable clot is produced. Initial hemostasis is apparently adequate, but after 24 to 48 hours, the clot begins to ooze. The screening coagulation tests (platelet count, PT, and PTT) are all normal. Diagnosis requires both a high index of suspicion and definitive laboratory tests. Normal fibrin clots are not dissolved by reagents such as 5M urea or monochloroacetic acid, whereas the friable clot produced in factor XIII–deficient plasma is rapidly broken down by these agents. Fibrin stabilizing factor is present in plasma, and therefore, plasma should be administered if there is significant bleeding.

MISCELLANEOUS FACTOR DEFICIENCIES

Hereditary deficiencies of virtually all clotting factors have been described. Most of these are extremely rare. Moreover, significant neonatal bleeding associated with these deficiencies is even more infrequent. Diagnosis of individual factor deficiencies is suggested by unexplained abnormalities in coagulation tests, but specific factor assays are required for confirmation. When in doubt, fresh frozen plasma should be given for serious hemorrhage in any bleeding newborn with an undiagnosed factor deficiency.

■ INTRAVASCULAR COAGULATION SYNDROMES

The intravascular coagulation syndromes are a consequence of altered endothelial cell function in response to local or systemic pathology. Physiologic and/or structural changes in endothelial cell function lead to activation of coagulation and fibrinolysis. The clinical effects of this occur for several reasons. One of the most important is that platelets and certain factors (II, V, VIII, and fibrinogen) are consumed when fibrin is formed. In addition, the stimulation of fibrinolysis generates fibrin split products (FSPs), which inhibit the normal conversion of fibrinogen to fibrin.

DISSEMINATED INTRAVASCULAR COAGULATION

Years ago, the term "secondary hemorrhagic disease" was applied to sick infants with severe bleeding not related to vitamin K deficiency. It is now apparent that this syndrome includes many infants with disseminated intravascular coagulation (DIC). DIC is associated with a variety of conditions in the newborn period: shock, sepsis, acidosis, hypoxia, hypothermia, abruptio placentae, and retention of a dead twin fetus. Unlike bleeding due to vitamin K deficiency or inherited factor deficiencies, *DIC occurs in sick infants*, most commonly in prematures (Table 84–5). The severity of DIC generally is related to the magnitude and duration of the activating stimulus. For example, in cases where there is self-limited coagulant activation, such as transient hypothermia or abruptio placentae, coagulation abnormalities are less severe. In contrast, in those conditions associated with more prolonged problems, such as sepsis, the coagulation abnor-

TABLE 84–5. Disseminated Intravascular Coagulation

Clinical Diagnosis
Sick infant
Usually diffuse petechiae/bleeding
Rarely diffuse thrombosis (skin necrosis)

Laboratory Diagnosis
Decreased platelets
Prolonged PT and PTT
Decreased factors V, VIII, and fibrinogen
Increased fibrin split products
Microangiopathic RBC changes

Therapy
1. Vigorous treatment of underlying condition (correction of hypoxia, acidosis, and hypovolemia; antibiotics)
2. Plasma and platelet infusions
3. If serious bleeding continues:
   (a) consider exchange transfusion
   (b) continue plasma and platelet infusions as required
4. If clinical presentation is mainly thrombotic:
   (a) administer heparin intravenously
   (b) after heparinization, give plasma and platelets

malities are more persistent. Some infants with DIC have no clinical manifestations despite marked laboratory abnormalities. In most DIC cases, however, there is diffuse bleeding characterized by petechiae, oozing from venipuncture sites, and gastrointestinal hemorrhage. In a small number of infants, the clinical picture also is associated with thrombosis (gangrenous necrosis of the skin or purpura fulminans). The diagnosis of DIC is characterized by several distinct laboratory abnormalities. Invariably, there is thrombocytopenia due to increased platelet utilization. The PT and PTT are prolonged due to factor depletion. Fibrinogen, factor V, and factor VIII levels are usually decreased. Fibrin split products are increased because of enhanced fibrinolysis. Microangiopathic erythrocyte changes (RBC fragments) are seen on the peripheral blood smear. These red cell fragments are a consequence of RBC interactions with fibrin on endothelial cells.

The treatment of children with DIC is two-fold: to correct the underlying pathophysiology responsible for coagulant activation and to limit hemorrhage. There is universal agreement that the most important aspect of managing infants with DIC is to remove the conditions activating coagulation. Thus, therapy must be directed at correcting the underlying infection, hypoxia, acidosis, and/or hypotension. In treating the bleeding problems, the most basic consideration is to replace platelets and plasma (every 12 hours), although sometimes cryoprecipitate is used as a source of fibrinogen. Occasionally, this replacement therapy is all that is necessary in newborns who are not very ill and who have minimally abnormal clotting studies. If severe bleeding persists after plasma and platelet replacement, it is not unreasonable to consider an exchange transfusion using red blood cells reconstituted with fresh frozen plasma (hematocrit of 50 to 60) and also giving platelets. This procedure provides clotting factors and platelets, but it also may remove fibrin split products and some of the toxic factors causing DIC. In addition, adult red blood cells deliver oxygen more readily than do neonatal red blood cells, and at least in principle, this may reduce tissue damage from hypoxia. Gross and Melhorn (1971) have reported the beneficial effects of exchange transfusion in several infants with DIC. In some of these newborns, exchange transfusion corrected bleeding and coagulation problems before the associated conditions (sepsis, respiratory distress) were under control. However, it should be noted that there are few published data to support the concept that specific coagulopathy therapy alters survival (Gross et al., 1982).

In some less common cases, infants with DIC may have bleeding and gangrenous necrosis of the skin (purpura fulminans). Rarely, DIC produces kidney necrosis caused by the thrombosis of large renal vessels. In each of these cases, there appears to be a relative impairment of the fibrinolytic activation that normally occurs in DIC. In part, this may be due to a protein C or protein S deficiency, which is greater than that normally occurring in newborns. A logical therapeutic approach to children with DIC and thrombotic problems is to anticoagulate with heparin (15 mg/kg/hr intravenously for a total duration of 2 to 3 days). Once heparin is started, platelet and plasma transfusions can safely be given despite the thrombotic problems. From a theoretical perspective, it seems important to give platelets and plasma after the heparin; otherwise, one may only provide substrate for further thrombus formation. Some physicians have employed heparin in cases of DIC in which there is bleeding without significant thrombosis. This approach is based on the assumption that heparin, by inhibiting coagulation, allows coagulation factors to regenerate and thereby decreases bleeding. There are several reports that heparin corrects the laboratory abnormalities in DIC. However, the studies of Corrigan and Jordan (1970) clearly demonstrate that heparin has no effect on the overall mortality from DIC.

LOCALIZED INTRAVASCULAR COAGULATION

Several disorders are associated with platelet deposition and fibrin formation in a focal area of specific pathology. Occasionally, this localized coagulation has more widespread effects with the systemic depletion of platelets and/or coagulation factors. This type of localized intravascular coagulation is seen in renal vein thrombosis, portal vein thrombosis, necrotizing enterocolitis, hemolytic uremic syndrome, and large hemangiomas (see section on thrombocytopenia). These disorders are recognized by their underlying pathology and the associated coagulation abnormalities. Just as for DIC, treatment of these conditions is aimed at rectifying the underlying disorder. Any bleeding problems are treated with platelet transfusions, if there is significant thrombocytopenia, and with fresh frozen plasma, if there are factor deficiencies.

BLEEDING ASSOCIATED WITH LIVER DISEASE

Since the liver produces virtually all coagulation factors, it is not surprising that bleeding is a complication of serious liver disease. Neonatal bleeding due to liver injury generally occurs *in sick infants* following hypoxia or hypotension. The characteristics of this type of bleeding are very similar to those of DIC (which frequently is associated with liver disease). The PT and PTT are both prolonged, and there is no significant change following vitamin K administration. The platelet count usually is normal, but it may be decreased, depending upon whether there is associated DIC. Fibrin split products may be increased owing to decreased hepatic clearance, even in the absence of DIC. A presumptive diagnosis of bleeding due to liver disease is made on the basis of clinical findings, hepatic chemistry alterations, and coagulation abnormalities, as previously described. A more precise diagnosis is arrived at by measuring coagulation factors (II, VII, IX, and X), which remain depressed even following vitamin K administration. Of interest, although factor VIII probably is made in the liver, levels of this coagulant often remain normal even in severe liver disease. Therapy for bleeding due to liver disease requires fresh frozen plasma to replace coagulation factors (10 ml fresh frozen plasma/kg every 12 hours). Factor concentrates (which contain factors II, VII, IX, and X) used to treat hemophilia B should not be used in children with liver disease because of their thrombotic potential. Platelets are given only if there is associated thrombocytopenia.

■ PLATELET DISORDERS

Platelet-related bleeding usually is due to thrombocytopenia, although hereditary and acquired platelet dysfunction are seen rarely. Bleeding due to platelet disturbances generally is petechial and superficial (skin and mucosa) in contrast to the large ecchymoses and muscle hemorrhages seen in coagulation disturbances. The physiologic causes of thrombocytopenia are impaired platelet production, accelerated platelet destruction, and combinations of both disordered production and destruction. The vast majority of neonatal thrombocytopenic disorders are due to immune-mediated thrombocytopenia, infections, and DIC.

NEONATAL ALLOIMMUNE THROMBOCYTOPENIA

Neonatal alloimmune thrombocytopenia (NAIT) is analogous to erythroblastosis due to ABO and Rh incompatibility. The infant's platelets express an antigen that is lacking on maternal platelets. During pregnancy, fetal platelets enter the maternal circulation and stimulate antibody production against the unique fetal platelet antigens (Harrington et al., 1953). Maternal platelets are not affected by the antibody, which crosses the placenta and destroys fetal platelets. In almost all cases, the antibody is directed against the PL^{A1} antigen (mother is PL^{A1}-negative, father and infant are PL^{A1}-positive) (Shulman et al., 1964). There is fetal-maternal PL^{A1} incompatibility in approximately 1 in 50 pregnancies since the antigen is present in 98 per cent of individuals and lacking in 2 per cent. However, the incidence of NAIT is much less than the frequency of fetal-maternal incompatibility, occurring in 1 in 2000 to 3000 babies. The reason for this is that sensitization has been found to be limited to the 10 per cent of mothers who have HLA-B8 and DR3; the frequency of this combination is approximately 1 in 500 pregnancies (Reznikoff-Etievant et al., 1983). The associated immune responsiveness of this particular HLA and DR type only applies to the PL^{A1} antigen.

There are two major issues regarding this disorder: (1) the recognition and treatment of first affected newborns, and (2) the management of subsequent pregnancies of PL^{A1}-negative sensitized women.

Diagnosis and Treatment of NAIT. The clinical spectrum of infants with alloimmune thrombocytopenia is quite variable. In mild cases there may be only a low platelet count in an otherwise healthy infant, or there may be increasing petechiae and mucosal bleeding during the first 48 hours of life (Deaver et al., 1986; Pearson et al., 1964). In other cases, accounting for 25 per cent of affected infants, there is central nervous system bleeding, which may cause death or severe neurologic impairment. In large part, this CNS bleeding is a consequence of birth trauma. However, it now is recognized that antenatal CNS bleeding also may occur, and this may be associated with porencephalic cyst formation (Herman et al., 1986). It is this antenatal and perinatal CNS bleeding that is the major reason for concern in managing subsequent pregnancies.

In babies with NAIT, the platelet count is decreased, often to less than 10,000/μl. Coagulation studies are normal. The mother has a normal platelet count, and her platelet morphology is normal. In the absence of sepsis, this constellation of findings is presumptive evidence for the diagnosis of NAIT. If the infant's blood is tested for the presence of antiplatelet antibody, it generally is positive against random platelets, but nonreactive against the mother's platelets. Moreover, the mother's serum contains antibodies that also react against random platelets. When tested against a panel of platelets of known antigenicity, the specific antigen involved (almost always PL^{A1}) can often be identified and will be one that is lacking on the mother's platelets but present in the father and the newborn.

In cases where there is clinical bleeding, or when the platelet count is very low (less than 30,000/μl), the affected newborn should be infused with compatible antigen-negative platelets. In the usual clinical setting of a firstborn infant for whom NAIT is unsuspected, bleeding usually is treated with random donor platelets from the blood bank. Transfusion of random donor platelets, however, is of little value in the large majority of NAIT cases, in particular those where the antibody is directed against the PL^{A1} antigen, since 97 per cent of donors are PL^{A1}-positive. A more useful approach is to transfuse with PL^{A1}-negative platelets, which should increase the neonatal platelet count in the majority of cases. Alternatively, and always a safer product, maternal platelets can be used for transfusion. These have the advantage of also being effective in that minority of cases not caused by the PL^{A1} antigen. The failure to see an increased platelet count following a transfusion with random donor platelets, but an increase in the platelet count after giving maternal platelets, is virtually diagnostic of NAIT. Intravenous immunoglobulin (500 mg/kg/day for 2 days) has been used successfully in cases where antigen-negative platelets are not readily available. Steroids and exchange transfusions have little or no clinical role in the management of NAIT. Clinically, significant bleeding usually does not occur in the first few days of life. The platelet count in the infant may remain low, however, until the maternally derived antibody is cleared, which usually takes 4 to 8 weeks.

Management of the Pregnancy at Risk for NAIT. Alloimmune thrombocytopenia differs from Rh disease in that 50 per cent of cases occur in the first pregnancy (Shulman et al., 1964). Furthermore, once this entity has occurred, there is a 70 to 85 per cent probability of recurrence in subsequent pregnancies. For this reason, once a case of NAIT is identified, all subsequent pregnancies must be considered to be at high risk. There is at present no satisfactory assay to predict whether or not an infant will be thrombocytopenic. Maternal antibody titers have been followed, but have not been of prognostic value. In high-risk pregnancies (where a previous case of alloimmune thrombocytopenia has occurred), it is the standard of care to deliver these infants by cesarean section. Prior to delivery, maternal platelets can be obtained and transfused to the newborn immediately after birth.

Since there now is a high level of concern for antenatal CNS hemorrhage, it also is becoming common practice to consider intrauterine therapy. This is accomplished by monitoring fetal platelet counts by cordocentesis. More-

over, just as intrauterine red blood cell transfusions are utilized for severe Rh incompatibility, platelet transfusions now are being administered to fetuses with alloimmune thrombocytopenia (Daffos et al., 1988; Kaplan et al., 1988). In centers where this is done, platelets are given during the last trimester, since this is the period when almost all fatal CNS hemorrhages occur (Herman et al., 1986). In many hospitals it may be difficult to obtain appropriate platelets for these fetuses. Moreover, many medical centers do not have the ability to do fetal blood sampling and intrauterine fetal transfusions. For this reason, there is a growing interest in using noninvasive therapies such as the maternal administration of intravenous immunoglobulin (IVIG). Bussel and co-workers (1988) observed that weekly IVIG administered to pregnant mothers prevented serious fetal bleeding in families where there previously had been an infant severely affected with NAIT, including three with CNS hemorrhage. The exact time to begin maternal IVIG therapy is not known, although Bussel and co-workers recommend beginning when the fetal platelet count is low.

IMMUNE THROMBOCYTOPENIA SECONDARY TO MATERNAL IDIOPATHIC THROMBOCYTOPENIA

In contrast to alloimmune thrombocytopenia, immune thrombocytopenia secondary to maternal idiopathic thrompocytopenia (ITP) involves a transplacental antibody directed against a public antigen on maternal platelets, but the infant's platelets are affected as well as the mother's. The likelihood that thrombocytopenia will develop in a baby is determined in part by the state of the maternal disease. If the mother has a history of childhood ITP, but now has a normal platelet count, there is virtually no risk that the infant will be thrombocytopenic. On the other hand, if the mother continues to have evidence of active disease and a low platelet count, the risk to the infant is much higher. Also, if the mother has undergone splenectomy for chronic ITP, she may have a normal platelet count but still have significant antiplatelet antibody titers, and thus, the infant may be at risk. The measurement of maternal antiplatelet antibody titers unfortunately has not been particularly useful in predicting the likelihood of a given fetus being affected. In pregnant women with ITP, it has been demonstrated that the administration of steroids during the last few days of pregnancy decreases the risk of significant neonatal thrombocytopenia, although this does not affect the maternal platelet count (Karpatkin et al., 1981). Moreover, maternally administered IVIG reportedly has been useful in preventing fetal thrombocytopenia (Newland et al., 1984). It should be noted that pregnancy is generally well tolerated in women with ITP, even with platelet counts of 30,000 to 50,000/μl. There are few data indicating that maternal ITP gets worse with pregnancy. There are no reported deaths of pregnant mothers with ITP in the last 20 years.

The major risk to an infant born to a mother with ITP is CNS hemorrhage due to the trauma of delivery. In contrast to NAIT, however, severe bleeding in this secondary ITP is much less common. Cesarean section generally is recommended in all cases where the mother has active ITP. Some authors also advocate cesarean delivery if the mother has been splenectomized or has a platelet count of less than 100,000/μl at the time of delivery (McMillan, 1981). The previously used technique of fetal scalp sampling to determine the platelet count, and thereby provide guidelines for the obstetrician, generally is being replaced by fetal cordocentesis.

Bleeding is rarely severe and usually confined to the first few days of life. Any infant with significant bleeding or very low platelet count (less than 20,000/μl) should be given IVIG (500 mg/kg/day for 2 days). In contrast to the management of alloimmune thrombocytopenia, platelet transfusion is seldom indicated in these infants. Since the maternal antibody is generally directed against a public antigen that will be present on random donor platelets, transfused platelets do not produce a sustained rise in the platelet count because they also are rapidly removed from the circulation. Nevertheless, in the case of life-threatening hemorrhage, random donor platelets may have transient activity and should be given.

IMMUNE THROMBOCYTOPENIA DUE TO OTHER CAUSES OF MATERNAL ANTIBODY

In addition to maternal ITP, any disease that causes the production of antiplatelet antibodies in a pregnant woman can lead to thrombocytopenia in the newborn. Women with lupus or who are taking certain drugs may develop antiplatelet antibodies that can affect the fetus. For example, some drugs (quinine, quinidine, sulfonamides, digitoxin) given to mothers can cause both maternal and neonatal thrombocytopenia on an immune basis (Mauer et al., 1957). An antibody to the drug is produced by the mother. This antibody reacts with the drug, and the drug-antibody complex then attaches to the platelets ("innocent bystanders"), resulting in the removal of coated platelets from the circulation. The newborn is affected to the extent that drug and antibody cross the placenta into the fetal circulation. These children are clinically indistinguishable from other newborns with thrombocytopenia due to maternal disease. Significant bleeding is rare.

THROMBOCYTOPENIA ASSOCIATED WITH INFECTION

Thrombocytopenia frequently is seen in bacterial sepsis, cytomegolovirus (CMV) infection, toxoplasmosis, syphilis, rubella, disseminated herpes, and human immunodeficiency virus infection. These infants may be relatively asymptomatic or severely ill. Rarely is thrombocytopenia the only abnormality, and in most cases it is not the major problem. Occasionally, however, significant bleeding may occur. Hepatosplenomegaly is a common clinical finding not seen in the other neonatal thrombocytopenias.

The mechanism of thrombocytopenia is multifactorial:

1. Many infections are associated with DIC, a common cause of decreased platelets.
2. Megakaryocyte platelet production may be inhibited directly by causative agents or their metabolites.
3. Reticuloendothelial hyperplasia associated with infection may lead to platelet sequestration.
4. Infectious agents may react with circulating platelets

(similar to platelet plus antibody), which thereby leads to their sequestration and removal.

In the absence of DIC, thrombocytopenia rarely is severe enough to cause serious bleeding. The major therapeutic effort must be directed to the underlying infection. There is no documented role for IVIG administration, but steroids are of no value. If serious bleeding does occur, platelet transfusions are indicated.

THROMBOCYTOPENIA ASSOCIATED WITH GIANT HEMANGIOMAS

Hemangiomas commonly appear in the neonatal period, grow during the first few months of life, and then begin to recede in size. Occasionally, large superficial hemangiomas are associated with thrombocytopenia and bleeding (Kasabach and Merritt, 1940). Studies with [51]chromium-labeled platelets have demonstrated that thrombocytopenia is due to sequestration and destruction of platelets within the vascular tumor (Kontras et al., 1963). In addition, decreased levels of factors V, VIII, and fibrinogen are present in many patients, thus suggesting that localized intravascular coagulation also occurs in these lesions.

Hemorrhage most commonly occurs after several weeks of age when the tumors are largest. One rare exception is an angioma of the placenta (chorioangioma), which can cause neonatal thrombocytopenia. Bleeding hemangiomas characteristically darken in color, enlarge, and become firm to palpation. Petechiae may appear around the periphery of the hemangioma as well as at distant sites. Systemic bleeding secondary to thrombocytopenia or depletion of clotting factors or both may occur. In some cases, however, the most worrisome clinical problems are not due to blood loss but rather are secondary to compression of vital structures (i.e., airway obstruction) as bleeding occurs into the hemangioma.

THROMBOCYTOPENIA DUE TO BONE MARROW HYPOPLASIA

Thrombocytopenia due to decreased platelet production is usually associated with other congenital abnormalities or evidence of systemic disease. The diagnosis of a production defect is suggested by a decreased quantity of normal-sized platelets on peripheral blood smear. Examination of the bone marrow is mandatory in cases of suspected marrow failure in order to rule out aplasia, leukemia, and other neoplasms. Bleeding episodes are treated with platelet transfusions.

Thrombocytopenia and Bilateral Absence of Radii. Several cases of these two isolated congenital abnormalities have been reported (Hall et al., 1969). These infants frequently manifest a leukemoid reaction (markedly elevated leukocyte count with many immature forms) in the peripheral blood. Bleeding should be treated with platelet transfusions. Beyond the neonatal period, the platelet count usually increases over the next several years.

Fanconi Hypoplastic Anemia. This syndrome usually

becomes apparent later in childhood, at which time there is pancytopenia (anemia, neutropenia, thrombocytopenia). In rare instances, thrombocytopenia during infancy may be the initial manifestation of this disorder. Invariably, most patients have one or more congenital abnormalities, such as short stature, renal deformities, skeletal defects, hyperpigmentation, and microphthalmia. Patients with Fanconi hypoplastic anemia manifest increased chromosomal breakage in the presence of certain alkylating agents. This DNA abnormality can be used advantageously in diagnosing this autosomal recessive disorder prenatally (chorionic villus DNA) or immediately after birth (peripheral blood lymphocytes) (Auerbach and Alter, 1989).

Congenital Leukemia. Bleeding due to thrombocytopenia may be the presenting sign of congenital leukemia (see Chapter 85).

Thrombocytopenia Secondary to Maternal Drug Ingestion. Although the maternal ingestion of thiazides was previously considered to be a relatively common cause of neonatal thrombocytopenia, the general consensus now is that this is an extremely rare cause, if it exists at all (Merenstein et al., 1970). It is difficult to document maternal drug ingestion as a cause of neonatal megakaryocyte failure when maternal platelets are not affected. In this category of thrombocytopenia the physician must rely upon a diagnosis of exclusion, since it is much more important not to overlook other, more subtle, causes of decreased platelet production.

HEREDITARY THROMBOCYTOPENIAS

Wiskott-Aldrich Syndrome. Thrombocytopenia, eczema, and frequent infections due to immunologic defects characterize this disorder. In rare instances, bleeding in the neonatal period may be the initial manifestation. Thrombocytopenia is due to an intrinsic platelet defect leading to decreased platelet survival. Unlike the large platelets seen in other thrombocytopenias characterized by a decreased life span, those in the Wiskott-Aldrich syndrome are much smaller than normal (microplatelets). This is a sex-linked disorder affecting male children. The prognosis is poor, and children die of severe infections during the first years of life. Bone marrow transplantation has been successful in curing some of these infants.

Miscellaneous Hereditary Thrombocytopenias. This group includes several poorly understood thrombocytopenias caused by either decreased platelet life span or decreased platelet production. Family members frequently manifest thrombocytopenia. Serious neonatal bleeding problems are unusual.

Hemorrhage Due to Platelet Dysfunction. Platelet function can be assessed in vivo by the bleeding time or in vitro by observing platelet aggregation in response to known stimulants (ADP, thrombin, collagen). Neonatal platelet aggregation reportedly is abnormal, but this must not be of major significance, since the bleeding time of infants and older children is the same. In rare instances, hereditary disorders of platelet function (Glanzmann thrombasthenia) may present with bleeding in the newborn period. A more important fact, however, is that newborns frequently acquire platelet dysfunction secondary to drug exposure.

Aspirin is known to cause abnormal platelet function. (Acetylation of platelet membrane by aspirin inhibits release of platelet ADP and thereby prevents platelet aggregation.) In some individuals, this results in bleeding. Several studies have demonstrated that aspirin taken by mothers within 2 or 3 days of delivery produces both maternal and neonatal platelet dysfunction (Bleyer and Breckenridge, 1970; Corby and Schulman, 1971). Furthermore, some infants with aspirin-induced platelet dysfunction have had suspicious hemorrhages (large cephalohematomas). Other drugs also have been implicated in neonatal platelet abnormalities. Corby and Schulman observed decreased platelet aggregation in newborns born to mothers given Demerol (meperidine) and Phenergan (promethazine) prior to delivery. No effect on maternal platelet function was noted.

■ HEMOSTATIC ABNORMALITIES ASSOCIATED WITH SERIOUS LOCAL HEMORRHAGE

We have become relatively sophisticated in our understanding of normal hemostasis, and many major bleeding problems are currently being studied at the molecular level. The pathophysiology of the most serious neonatal bleeding problems, however, remains to be defined. Major pulmonary and central nervous system hemorrhages are discussed elsewhere. The point to be emphasized here is that fatal bleeding episodes in newborn infants are not necessarily due to coagulation or platelet abnormalities. Massive pulmonary hemorrhage is occasionally associated with laboratory evidence of DIC or liver injury, but usually no hemostatic abnormality is detected. Similarly, coagulation abnormalities (liver injury, DIC) often are seen with the respiratory distress syndrome (RDS), and children with RDS frequently have intraventricular hemorrhages. Clotting defects, however, are seen in only a small number of these infants with CNS hemorrhages. In most cases of intraventricular hemorrhage, local vascular factors must be important, since there often is no bleeding outside the CNS.

■ REFERENCES

General and Neonatal Hemostasis

Andrew, M., Paes, B., Milner, R., et al.: Development of the human coagulation system in the full-term infant. Blood 70:165, 1987.

Andrew, M., Paes, B., Milner, R., et al.: Development of the human coagulation system in the healthy premature infant. Blood 72:1651, 1988.

Corrigan, J. J.: Neonatal disorders. In Alter, B. P. (Ed.): Methods in Hematology. Perinatal Hematology. Edinburgh, Churchill Livingstone, 1989, pp. 165–193.

Craig, W. S.: On real and apparent external bleeding in the newborn. Arch. Dis. Child. 36:575, 1961.

Fogel, B. J., Arias, D., and Kung, F.: Platelet counts in healthy premature infants. J. Pediatr. 73:108, 1968.

Koepke, J. A., Rodgers, J. L., and Ollivier, M. J.: Preinstrumental variables in coagulation testing. Am. J. Clin. Pathol. *64*:591, 1975.

Oski, F. A., and Naiman, J. L.: Hematologic Problems in the Newborn. 3rd ed. Philadelphia, W. B. Saunders Company, 1982.

Sell, E. J., and Corrigan, J. J., Jr.: Platelet counts, fibrinogen concentrations, and factor V and factor VIII levels in healthy infants according to gestational age. J. Pediatr. *82*:1028, 1973.

Sherman, N. J., and Clatworthy, H. W., Jr.: Gastro-intestinal bleeding in neonates: a study of 94 cases. Surgery *62*:614, 1967.

Hemorrhagic Disease of the Newborn

Aballi, A. J., and DeLamerens, S.: Coagulation changes in neonatal period and early infancy. Pediatr. Clin. North Am. *9*:785, 1962.

Aballi, A. J., Lopez Banus, V., DeLamerens, S., and Rozengvaig, S.: Coagulation studies in the newborn period. I. Alterations of thromboplastin generation and effects of vitamin K on full-term and premature infants. Am. J. Dis. Child. *94*:594, 1957.

Committee on Nutrition, American Academy of Pediatrics: Vitamin K compounds and the water-soluble analogues: Use in therapy and prophylaxis in pediatrics. Pediatrics *28*:501, 1961.

Dam, H., Glavind, J., Larsen, H., and Plum, P.: Investigations into the cause of physiological hypoprothrombinemia in newborn children. IV. The vitamin K content of woman's milk and cow's milk. Acta Med. Scand. *112*:210, 1942.

Deblay, M. F., Vert, P., Andre, M., et al.: Transplacental vitamin K prevents haemorrhage disease of the infant of epileptic mother (letter). Lancet *1*:1247, 1982.

Fillmore, S. J., and McDevitt, E.: Effects of coumarin compounds on the fetus. Ann. Intern. Med. *73*:731, 1970.

Gellis, S. S., and Lyon, R. A.: The influence of diet of the newborn infant on the prothrombin index. J. Pediatr. *19*:495, 1941.

Hathaway, W. E.: New insights on vitamin K. Hematology/Oncology Clin. North Am. *1*:367, 1987.

Hilgartner, M. W., Solomon, G. E., and Kutt, H.: Diphenylhydantoin induced coagulation abnormalities. Pediatr. Res. *5*:408, 1971.

Hirsh, J., Cade, J. F., and O'Sullivan, E. F.: Clinical experience with anticoagulant therapy during pregnancy. Br. Med. J. *1*:270, 1970.

Lane, P. A., and Hathaway, W. E.: Vitamin K in infancy. J. Pediatr. *106*:351, 1985.

Lucey, J. F., and Dolan, R. G.: Hyperbilirubinemia of newborn infants associated with the parenteral administration of a vitamin K analogue to the mothers. Pediatrics *23*:553, 1959.

Mountain, K. R., Hirsh, J., and Gallus, A. S.: Neonatal coagulation defect due to anticonvulsant drug treatment in pregnancy. Lancet *1*:265, 1970.

Townsend, C. W.: The hemorrhagic disease of the newborn. Arch. Pediatr. *11*:559, 1894.

Hereditary Clotting Factor Deficiencies

Abildgaard, C. F.: Current concepts in the management of hemophilia. Semin. Hematol. *12*:223, 1975.

Baehner, R. L., and Strauss, H. S.: Hemophilia in the first year of life. N. Engl. J. Med. *275*:524, 1966.

Bray, G. L., and Luban, N. L. C.: Hemophilia presenting with intracranial hemorrhage. Am. J. Dis. Child. *141*:1215, 1987.

Britten, A. F. H.: Congenital deficiency of factor XIII (fibrin-stabilizing factor). Am. J. Med. *43*:751, 1967.

Cade, J. F., Hirsh, J., and Martin, M.: Placental barrier to coagulation factors: its relevance to the coagulation defect at birth and to haemorrhage in the newborn. Br. Med. J. *1*:281, 1969.

Ratnoff, O. D.: The molecular basis of hereditary clotting disorders. In Spaet, T. (Ed.): Progress in Hemostasis and Thrombosis, vol. 1. New York, Grune & Stratton, 1972, pp. 39–74.

Weinger, R. S., Cecalupo, A. J., Olson, J. D., and Frankel, L.: Neonatal von Willebrand's disease: Diagnostic difficulty at birth. Am. J. Dis. Child. *134*:793, 1980.

White, G. C., and Shoemaker, C. B.: Factor VIII gene and hemophilia A. Blood *73*:1, 1989.

Yoffe, G., and Buchanan, G. R.: Intracranial hemorrhage in newborn and young infants with hemophilia. J. Pediatr. *113*:333, 1988.

Intravascular Coagulation Syndromes

Abildgaard, C. F.: Recognition and treatment of intravascular coagulation. J. Pediatr. *74*:163, 1969.

Chessells, J. M., and Wigglesworth, J. S.: Secondary haemorrhagic disease of the newborn. Arch. Dis. Child. *45*:539, 1970.

Chessells, J. M., and Wigglesworth, J. S.: Coagulation studies in preterm infants with respiratory distress and intracranial haemorrhage. Arch. Dis. Child. *47*:564, 1972.

Corrigan, J. J., and Jordan, C. M.: Heparin therapy in septicemia with disseminated intravascular coagulation. N. Engl. J. Med. *283*:778, 1970.

Gross, S. J., Filston, H. C., and Anderson, J. C.: Controlled study of treatment for disseminated intravascular coagulation in the neonate. J. Pediatr. *100*:445, 1982.

Gross, S., and Melhorn, D. K.: Exchange transfusion with citrated whole blood for disseminated intravascular coagulation. J. Pediatr. *78*:415, 1971.

Platelet Disorders

Anthony, B., and Krivit, W.: Neonatal thrombocytopenic purpura. Pediatrics *30*:776, 1962.

Auerbach, A. D., and Alter, B. P.: Prenatal and postnatal diagnosis of aplastic anemia. In Alter, B. P. (Ed.): Methods in Hematology. Perinatal Hematology. Edinburgh, Churchill Livingstone, 1989, pp. 225–251.

Bleyer, W. A., and Breckenridge, R. T.: Studies in the detection of adverse drug reactions in the newborn. II. The effects of prenatal aspirin on newborn hemostasis. J.A.M.A. *213*:2049, 1970.

Bussel, J. B., Berkowitz, R. L., McFarland, J. G., et al.: Antenatal treatment of neonatal alloimmune thrombocytopenia. N. Engl. J. Med. *21*:1374, 1988.

Corby, D. G., and Schulman, I.: The effects of antenatal drug administration on aggregation of platelets of newborn infants. J. Pediatr. *79*:307, 1971.

Corrigan, J. J.: Thrombocytopenia: a laboratory sign of septicemia in infants and children. J. Pediatr. *85*:219, 1974.

Daffos, F., Forestier, F., Kaplan, C., and Cox, W.: Prenatal diagnosis and management of bleeding disorders with fetal blood sampling. Am. J. Obstet. Gynecol. *158*:940, 1988.

Daffos, F., Forestier, F., Muller, J. Y., et al.: Prenatal treatment of alloimmune thrombocytopenia. Lancet *2*:632, 1984.

Deaver, J. E., Leppert, P. C., and Zaroulis, C. G.: Neonatal alloimmune thrombocytopenic purpura. Am. J. Perinatol. *3*:127, 1986.

DeVries, L. A., Connell, J., Bydder, G. M., et al.: Recurrent intracranial haemorrhages in utero in an infant with alloimmune thrombocytopenia. Case report. Br. J. Obstet. Gynaecol. *95*:299, 1988.

Duncan, W., and Halnan, K. E.: Giant hemangioma with thrombocytopenia. Clin. Radiol. *15*:224, 1964.

Editorial: Management of alloimmune neonatal thrombocytopenia. Lancet *1*:137, 1989.

Fost, N. C., and Esterly, N. B.: Successful treatment of juvenile hemangiomas with prednisone. J. Pediatr. *72*:351, 1968.

Goodhue, P. A., and Evans, T. S.: Idiopathic thrombocytopenic purpura in pregnancy. Obstet. Gynecol. Surg. *18*:671, 1963.

Hall, J. G., Levin, J., Kuhn, J. P., et al.: Thrombocytopenia with absent radius. Medicine *48*:411, 1969.

Harrington, W. J., Sprague, C. C., Minnich, V., et al.: Immunologic mechanisms in idiopathic and neonatal thrombocytopenic purpura. Ann. Intern. Med. *38*:433, 1953.

Herman, J. H., Jumbelic, M. I., Ancona, R. J., and Kickler, T. S.: In utero cerebral hemorrhage in alloimmune thrombocytopenia. Am. J. Pediatr. Hematol. Oncol. *8*:312, 1986.

Kaplan, C., Daffos, F., Forestier, F., et al.: Management of alloimmune thrombocytopenia: Antenatal diagnosis and in utero transfusion of maternal platelets. Blood *72*:340, 1988.

Karpatkin, M., Porges, R. F., and Karpatkin, S.: Platelet counts in infants of women with autoimmune thrombocytopenia. N. Engl. J. Med. *305*:936, 1981.

Kasabach, H. H., and Merritt, K. K.: Capillary hemangioma with extensive purpura. Report of a case. Am. J. Dis. Child. *59*:1063, 1940.

Kontras, S. B., Green, O. C., King, L., and Duran, R. J.: Giant hemangioma with thrombocytopenia; case report with survival and sequestration studies of platelets labeled with chromium 51. Am. J. Dis. Child. *105*:188, 1963.

McIntosh, S., O'Brien, R. T., Schwartz, A. D., and Pearson, H. A.: Neonatal isoimmune purpura: response to platelet infusions. J. Pediatr. *82*:1020, 1973.

McMillan, R.: Chronic idiopathic thrombocytopenic purpura. New Engl. J. Med. *304*:1145, 1981.

Mauer, A. M., DeVaux, L. O., and Lahey, M. E.: Neonatal and maternal thrombocytopenic purpura due to quinine. Pediatrics 19:84, 1957.

Merenstein, G. B., O'Loughlin, E. P., and Plunket, D. C.: Effects of maternal thiazides on platelet counts of newborn infants. J. Pediatr. 76:766, 1970.

Newland, A. C., Boots, M. A., Patterson, K. G., et al.: Intravenous IgG for ITP in pregnancy (Letter). N. Engl. J. Med. 310:261, 1984.

Pearson, H. A., Shulman, N. R., Marder, V. J., and Cone, T. E., Jr.: Isoimmune neonatal thrombocytopenic purpura. Clinical and therapeutic considerations. Blood 23:154, 1964.

Reznikoff-Etievant, M. F., Muller, J. Y., Julien, F., and Patereau, C.: An immune response gene linked to MHC in man. Tissue Antigens 22:312, 1983.

Shulman, N. R., Marder, V. J., Hiller, M. C., and Collier, E. M.: Platelet and leukocyte isoantigens and their antibodies: Serologic, physiologic and clinical studies. Progr. Hematol. 4:222, 1964.

Skacel, P. O., and Contreras, M.: Neonatal alloimmune thrombocytopenia. Blood Rev. 3:174, 1989.

LEUKOCYTE 85 DISORDERS IN THE NEWBORN

Bertil E. Glader and Theodore Zwerdling

Leukocytes have a central role in host defense against infection. The pathophysiology of lymphocyte disorders is discussed in Chapter 34. This chapter is concerned with quantitative and qualitative disorders of blood neutrophils, congenital leukemia, and the transient myeloproliferative syndrome. Many infants with granulocyte abnormalities have clinical problems in the newborn period. In most cases, however, the diagnosis of specific neutrophil disorders occurs after repeated infectious episodes, generally a few weeks to months after birth.

■ NORMAL GRANULOCYTE PHYSIOLOGY

Several growth factors recently have been identified that promote differentiation of stem cells into the different types of myeloid cells. These factors have been referred to as "lymphokines," although the term "cytokine" is more appropriate, since many cell types besides lymphocytes are able to produce these factors. Some of these colony-stimulating factors, such as interleukin-3 (IL-3) and granulocyte-macrophage colony-stimulating factor (GM-CSF), are necessary for the differentiation of all types of myeloid cells (i.e., granulocytes, basophils, eosinophils, and monocytes) as well as for the differentiation of erythroid and megakaryocyte precursors. In contrast, other colony-stimulating factors have more specific regulatory roles, such as in the differentiation of granulocytes (G-CSF) or monocytes (M-CSF). The physiology and molecular biology of these growth factors are an area of intense scientific inquiry. The genes for certain of these growth factors have been cloned, and recombinant colony-stimulating factors soon may be available for clinical disorders.

Development of myeloid cells into circulating neutrophils takes 6 to 10 days (Fig. 85–1). Approximately one-third of bone marrow myeloid cells are in some phase of cell division (blasts, promyelocytes, myelocytes), while the remaining, more differentiated cells (metamyelocytes, bands, mature granulocytes) are maintained in a storage pool. In newborns it is particularly important that this neutrophil storage pool is easily depleted during bacterial infections, as this may relate to an increase in mortality from sepsis (Christensen and Rothstein, 1980). Myeloid cells continue to mature in this storage pool, although they can be released if needed in the periphery. After release from the bone marrow, neutrophils are equally distributed between circulating cells and granulocytes mar-

ginated on the vascular wall. The peripheral blood count measures only circulating cells. Granulocytes remain in the circulation for less than 24 hours before being mobilized into peripheral tissues. It is here that neutrophils begin their major function, phagocytosis of bacteria.

The term "phagocytosis" includes several independent but related processes: chemotaxis, opsonization, ingestion, and intracellular killing (Fig. 85–2). *Chemotaxis* is the directed movement of neutrophils to areas of injury or bacterial infection. This is a metabolically dependent response of granulocytes to chemoattractants in peripheral tissues. Factors known to stimulate leukocyte migration include soluble bacterial products, complement components, and antigen-antibody complexes. In vivo, chemotaxis is assessed by sequential observation of cell migration into an abraded area of skin pretreated with chemoattractants such as DPT or typhoid vaccine (Rebuck skin window). Under these conditions, granulocytes initially appear within 3 to 6 hours, but by 12 hours monocytes predominate. In vitro, chemotaxis is evaluated by measuring the rate at which granulocytes traverse a filter that separates cells and chemotactically active material (Boyden chamber). This method is useful in determining what substances have chemotactic activity, but it is of questionable validity when used to compare chemotactic function of different granulocytes. Leukocyte migration through filters is a measure of several cell properties in addition to chemotactic responsiveness.

Opsonization is the process whereby bacteria are made more "edible" for phagocytes. The granulocyte ingestion of bacteria normally is a very slow process unless the bacterial membrane surface is first modified by various serum proteins. There are three fundamental modes of opsonization:

1. Rarely, increased concentrations of specific antibody alone can prepare bacteria for ingestion.
2. More commonly, opsonization follows the reaction of small amounts of antibody with complement proteins.
3. Opsonization can also occur by bacterial complement fixation in the presence of properdin proteins. This properdin-dependent, or "alternate," pathway is important, since it does not require antibody.

Ingestion is an active metabolic process in which the neutrophil membrane surrounds opsonized bacteria and forms an internalized vacuole, or phagosome. This ingestion-related movement (as well as chemotaxis itself) prob-

COMPARTMENT	RELATIVE SIZE	TIME	FUNCTION
BONE MARROW	20-30	6-10d	1/3 PRODUCTION (BLASTS → MYELOCYTES) 2/3 STORAGE (METAMYELOCYTES → MATURE NEUTROPHILES)
VASCULAR	1	<1d	1/2 CIRCULATING (MEASURED BY WBC COUNT) 1/2 MARGINATED ON VASCULAR WALL
TISSUE	?	?	PHAGOCYTOSIS

FIGURE 85–1. Neutrophil life cycle.

ably depends on contractile proteins. It has been suggested that reversible polymerization and depolymerization of neutrophil "actin" is responsible for this active motion.

Intracellular killing is the last stage of phagocytosis. One of the essential reactions in this process is the generation of superoxide and hydrogen peroxide in the area of the phagosome. The specificity and intracellular location of the enzyme responsible for this reaction are not definitely known. An equally important process is the fusion of neutrophilic granules with the phagosome, following which digestive enzymes are thrust upon the enclosed bacteria. Neutrophils contain two types of granules. Primary granules are first noted in young myeloid cells (promyelocytes) and contain several hydrolytic enzymes, including myeloperoxidase. This enzyme potentiates the bactericidal effect of hydrogen peroxide. The secondary, or specific, granules develop in older cells (late myelocytes). These secondary lysosomal structures contain alkaline phosphatase in addition to other hydrolytic enzymes.

■ GRANULOCYTE PHYSIOLOGY AND NEONATAL INFECTION

In older infants and children, the total and differential leukocyte count can be used to diagnose infection and frequently can help distinguish between bacterial and viral processes. During the neonatal period, wide variations in the quantity and distribution of leukocytes limit the utility of these simple laboratory measurements. The total white blood cell (WBC) count shortly after birth ranges from 10,000 to 30,000 per μl, owing mainly to an increase in neutrophils, bands, and metamyelocytes (Table 85–1). Occasionally, younger myeloid forms are seen also, particularly in premature infants. During the first week of life, the WBC count decreases (6000 to 15,000 per μl), immature myeloid cells disappear, and neutrophils decrease to a level that equals the number of lymphocytes. Xanthou (1970) has noted that the absolute neutrophil count (4000 to 7000 per μl) actually is quite stable in healthy infants after 72 hours of age. Furthermore, she observed that newborns with suspected or proved infec-

tion (after 3 days of age) manifested significant qualitative or quantitative neutrophil changes or both. Either the absolute granulocyte count was elevated above 7000/μl or there was an increased number of circulating immature myeloid cells (Christensen et al., 1981; Manroe et al., 1979; Zipursky et al., 1976). Under these conditions, the absolute band count is not elevated, although the *ratio* of immature granulocytes to mature segmented cells is increased (Christensen et al., 1981). Neonatal infections are not always associated with neutrophilia; in fact, *neutropenia is much more common*. The reason for the neutropenia, as stated previously, is that the marrow storage pool of myeloid cells is easily depleted during bacterial infections. Moreover, this storage pool depletion may relate to the increased morbidity and mortality associated with neonatal sepsis.

Each stage of phagocytosis has been examined in neonatal granulocytes. The in vivo movement of neutrophils to an area of inflammation is normal, although there is a delay in the subsequent appearance of mononuclear cells. The clinical significance of this is not known. In vitro studies (Boyden chamber) suggest that chemotaxis is decreased in neonatal granulocytes. For the aforementioned reasons, however, it is not clear whether this reflects abnormal chemotaxis or merely some other physical property regulating neonatal neutrophil movement. Decreased opsonic activity of neonatal serum is one phagocytic abnormality on which there is general agreement. This may be due to decreased IgM, low complement levels (C3), or defects in the properdin pathway. Approximately 15 per cent of newborns are severely deficient in certain properdin proteins. Once bacteria are opsonized, neonatal granulocytes are capable of normal ingestion and intracellular killing.

■ GRANULOCYTE TRANSFUSIONS

Neutrophil transfusions have been used to treat gram-negative bacterial infections in neutropenic children and adults with hematologic malignancies. However, there now is somewhat less emphasis on utilizing granulocyte

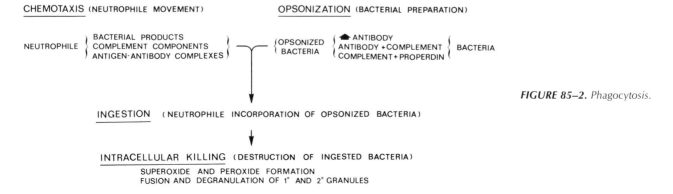

FIGURE 85–2. Phagocytosis.

TABLE 85–1. Leukocyte Values in Term and Premature Infants (10³ Cells/μl)

AGE (hrs)	TOTAL WBC	NEUTROPHILS	BANDS/METAS	LYMPHOCYTES	MONOCYTES	EOSINOPHILS
Term infants						
0	10.0–26.0	5.0–13.0	0.4–1.8	3.5–8.5	0.7–1.5	0.2–2.0
12	13.5–31.0	9.0–18.0	0.4–2.0	3.0–7.0	1.0–2.0	0.2–2.0
72	5.0–14.5	2.0–7.0	0.2–0.4	2.0–5.0	0.5–1.0	0.2–1.0
144	6.0–14.5	2.0–6.0	0.2–0.5	3.0–6.0	0.7–1.2	0.2–0.8
Premature infants						
0	5.0–19.0	2.0–9.0	0.2–2.4	2.5–6.0	0.3–1.0	0.1–0.7
12	5.0–21.0	3.0–11.0	0.2–2.4	1.5–5.0	0.3–1.3	0.1–1.1
72	5.0–14.0	3.0–7.0	0.2–0.6	1.5–4.0	0.3–1.2	0.2–1.1
144	5.5–17.5	2.0–7.0	0.2–0.5	2.5–7.5	0.5–1.5	0.3–1.2

(Data from Xanthou, M.: Leukocyte blood picture in healthy full-term and premature babies during neonatal period. Arch. Dis. Child. 45:242, 1970.)

transfusions. In part this is because of the availability of new and better broad-spectrum antibiotics. Currently, there are no clear-cut indications for granulocyte transfusions in patients with hematologic or oncologic disorders. Similarly, the role of granulocyte transfusions in septic newborns remains an area of controversy. Leukocyte chemotaxis and opsonization may be slightly impaired in newborns. However, the main reason for using leukocyte transfusions is that newborns may have a decreased marrow granulocyte storage pool and, thereby, a limited capacity to mobilize granulocytes in the face of infection. In the few studies that have been published, the transfusion of granulocytes appears to have a significant beneficial effect in reducing mortality from neonatal sepsis (Christensen et al., 1982; Cairo, 1989). Despite this, it currently is not possible to provide firm guidelines for the use of granulocyte transfusions in newborns with sepsis or presumed sepsis. Some of the questions that need to be answered include how leukocytes should be procured and how many infusions are necessary. Potential side effects of granulocyte transfusions given to newborns include volume overload, transmission of certain infectious agents, leukocyte aggregation, allosensitization to leukocyte antigens, and occasionally, granulocyte sequestration syndromes in the lungs and/or brain. Granulocyte donors should be antibody-negative for cytomegalovirus (CMV). In addition, before transfusing the granulocytes, the preparation should be radiated in order to prevent graft-versus-host disease.

■ NEUTROPENIC DISORDERS

Neutropenia is defined as an absolute granulocyte count less than 1500 cells per μl. This may occur as a transient phenomenon associated with infection (discussed previously) or as a chronic process. The general mechanisms of neutropenia are the same as those that produce anemia and thrombocytopenia: decreased production and increased destruction or utilization. Viral infections are the most common cause of transient neutropenia, presumably owing to suppression of normal myeloid production. This form of neutropenia is of little consequence. Bone marrow aplasia or neoplasia also can present with neutropenia, but in addition there almost always are other hematologic abnormalities and/or abnormal physical findings. In these cases, it is mandatory to examine the bone marrow to rule out leukemia or other marrow disorders. Also, a bone marrow examination is necessary for newborns with persistent neutropenia and frequent bacterial infections since

these children may have severe agranulocytosis (Kostmann syndrome). However, in the vast majority of newborns with isolated neutropenia, but who are otherwise healthy and without bacterial infections, bone marrow examination is not needed. A simple diagnostic approach to infants with persistent neutropenia is presented in Table 85–2.

The spectrum of clinical severity in neutropenic children is extremely variable. Most children have no clinical problems, some manifest frequent infections of moderate severity, and a few develop serious life-threatening infections. The difference between children with mild disease and those with severe disease is related to the capacity for neutrophils to be mobilized at sites of infection, and this probably is a function of the absolute neutrophil count. Severe infections are unusual with consistent mean granulocyte levels greater than 500 cells/μl. At lower neutrophil levels, however, the frequency and severity of infections increase dramatically. The degree of monocytosis may be important also, since these macrophages can partially compensate for the loss of neutrophil phagocytic function. In the absence of infection, no treatment for neutropenic children is indicated. Steroids have no role in the management of these disorders. If infection is present, however, vigorous antibiotic therapy with bactericidal drugs is indicated.

ALLOIMMUNE NEUTROPENIA

This disorder is the neutrophil equivalent of alloimmune thrombocytopenia and alloimmune anemia (ABO and Rh incompatibility). Fetal granulocytes possess an antigen not present on maternal neutrophils, and maternal sensitiza-

TABLE 85–2. Diagnostic Evaluation of Infants with Persistent Neutropenia

In association with other hematologic and/or physical examination abnormalities:
1. *Bone marrow examination* to rule out leukemia, neoplasm, or aplastic anemia.
In the absence of other hematologic abnormalities:
1. *Maternal neutrophil counts* to rule out maternal disease or drugs.
2. *Neutrophil counts on family members* to rule out hereditary neutropenia.
3. *Antineutrophil antibody determination* to rule out immune neutropenia.
4. *Repeat neutrophil counts on baby* (two times per week for 6 weeks) to rule out cyclic neutropenia.
5. *Bone marrow examination if associated with frequent bacterial infections* to rule out agranulocytosis (Kostmann syndrome).

tion results in antibody production against fetal granulocytes. Maternal neutrophils are not affected. The measurement of neutrophil antibodies is more difficult than the detection of antibodies in other alloimmune disorders. Consequently, these assays are done only in specialized laboratories. The clinical significance of antigranulocyte antibodies is not completely understood, since 20 to 25 per cent of all multiparous women have antineutrophil antibodies, yet neutropenia rarely is seen in these infants. The prognosis for infants with alloimmune neutropenia is very good. Fever and skin infections due to *Staphylococcus aureus* may occur. Severe pulmonary and urinary tract infections, as well as septicemia, are very unusual. The granulocytopenia resolves as soon as the infant clears maternal antibody (6 to 12 weeks). An increase in the neutrophil count after this period of time also helps differentiate this alloimmune disorder from other nonimmune causes of neutropenia.

NEUTROPENIA ASSOCIATED WITH MATERNAL DISEASE

Antibodies that cause maternal neutropenia may passively cross the placenta and secondarily injure fetal granulocytes. Rare cases of maternal idiopathic neutropenia have been associated with neonatal granulocytopenia. Similarly, maternal lupus erythematosus has been implicated as a cause of immune neonatal neutropenia. In association with maternal systemic disease, however, anemia and thrombocytopenia frequently are present and usually are more important than any coexistent neutropenia.

SEVERE CONGENITAL NEUTROPENIA

This profound neutropenia (also called Kostmann syndrome) is characterized by the neonatal onset of fulminant infections and early death. The bone marrow manifests marked myeloid hypoplasia, although rarely are there adequate early myeloid precursors. In all cases there is a marked depletion of mature neutrophils in the marrow and the absolute granulocyte count in the peripheral blood is usually less than 200 cells/μl. The hemoglobin and platelet count are normal. Some cases are familial where it appears as an autosomal recessive disorder. It is of interest that preliminary studies indicate that recombinant growth factor (GM-CSF) has been successful in treating children with this disorder (Bonilla et al., 1989).

A rare and unusual variant of this disorder is known as reticular dysgenesis. Infants with this syndrome have no circulating neutrophils or lymphocytes. Similarly, the bone marrow contains no myeloid or lymphoid elements. All children reported with reticular dysgenesis have died within the first weeks of life.

BENIGN CONGENITAL NEUTROPENIA

In these disorders neutropenia often is discovered accidentally when a blood count is done on an otherwise healthy child. The neutropenia first may be noticed in the neonatal period but rarely do these infants have serious infections. The fact that this is a benign disorder is established by the fact that neutropenia persists for months to years without any increased frequency of bacterial infections. In most cases the bone marrow contains adequate numbers of myeloid precursors, and the degree of granulocytopenia is not as low as in the severe syndromes. The platelet count and hemoglobin concentration are normal. Beyond the newborn period children with benign congenital neutropenia who become febrile require no special therapy; prophylactic antibiotics are not indicated.

CYCLIC NEUTROPENIA

This is another variant of neutropenia characterized by a fluctuating granulocyte count that cycles approximately every 21 days. At the nadir of the neutropenia, there often is an increased incidence of fevers and mild infections (stomatitis, gingivitis). This disorder is not recognized in the immediate neonatal period. It is only considered a diagnostic possibility in patients with persistent neutropenia with periodic infections.

NEUTROPENIA SECONDARY TO DRUGS

Many drugs have been implicated in the etiology of neutropenia. Phenothiazines, antithyroid medications, and certain antibiotics (chloramphenicol, sulfonamides) have gained the most notoriety. In addition, gentamicin, some penicillins, cephalosporins, phenytoin, and thiazides have all been shown to cause neutropenia. Thus, in any neutropenic newborn receiving medications the possibility of a toxic drug effect always should be considered.

■ DISORDERS OF LEUKOCYTE FUNCTION

Recurrent bacterial infections can occur in the presence of adequate numbers of circulating and bone marrow neutrophils. Most commonly, these infections are due to decreased serum opsonic activity caused by a lack of specific antibody (i.e., hypogammaglobulinemic states). Occasionally, abnormal granulocyte function itself is responsible. The diagnosis of neutrophil dysfunction syndromes rarely is made in the newborn period, although these infants frequently are infected. A few of these functional disorders are outlined below. A much more detailed review of all leukocyte dysfunction disorders has been published elsewhere (Curnutte and Boxer, 1987.)

CONGENITAL NEUTROPHIL MEMBRANE GLYCOPROTEIN DEFICIENCY

This clinical disorder is characterized by recurrent bacterial infections, periodontitis, leukocytosis, and in some newborns, delayed separation of the umbilical cord (Crowley et al., 1980; Anderson and Springer, 1987). The most unique abnormality seen in this disorder is that neutrophils fail to accumulate at sites of infection despite elevated granulocyte counts in the peripheral blood. The failure of neutrophils to migrate to sites of inflammation is not due to defective granulocyte chemotaxis or to deficiencies in the production of chemotactic factors. Rather, neutrophils from these patients are unable to adhere to surfaces, a process that is a necessary prerequisite for normal cell migration and for opsonization. There are no abnormalities in degranulation or in the oxidative metabolism of stimulated neutrophils. The molecular defect in this disorder is that neutrophils, monocytes, and lymphocytes have reduced or absent expression of several cell membrane glycoproteins. This neutrophil membrane glycoprotein disorder is inherited in an autosomal recessive fashion. As is the case for other qualitative neutrophil abnormalities, treatment of this disorder is largely supportive. Patients with recurrent infections sometimes are maintained on prophylactic antibiotics, such as trimethoprim-sulfamethoxazole. More serious infections need to be treated vigorously with appropriate antibiotics.

CHRONIC GRANULOMATOUS DISEASE

Chronic granulomatous disease (CGD) is a rare hereditary disorder characterized by recurrent granulomatous infections involving lymph nodes, skin, viscera, and bones. After the first few months of age hepatosplenomegaly is present. The peripheral blood neutrophil count and bone marrow are entirely normal. Chemotaxis is normal, ingestion is intact, and there are no opsonic defects. The fundamental abnormality in this condition is an inability of neutrophils to kill certain ingested bacteria. Pathologically, the persistence of viable intracellular bacteria stimulates granulomata formation in tissues to which neutrophils are transported. The molecular basis for decreased intracellular killing is not completely understood, although it is related to reduced hydrogen peroxide production in the phagosome. When CGD granulocytes ingest latex particles coated with an enzyme that generates peroxide, the intracellular killing defect is corrected. This finding partially explains the spectrum of clinical infections in children with CGD. Severe problems commonly are due to *Staphylococcus aureus*, although infections also occur with *Klebsiella, Escherichia coli, Serratia marcescens*, and *Candida albicans*. Each of these microorganisms contains catalase, an enzyme potentially capable of destroying whatever small amounts of peroxide are formed in the phagosome. Infections with organisms lacking catalase are not a clinical problem; presumably, the trivial amount of peroxide present in CGD neutrophils is bactericidal for these agents. CGD is diagnosed by observing granulocyte inability to kill catalase-positive organisms or by failure of nitroblue tetrazolium (NBT) reduction in circulating neutrophils. (NBT dye reduction correlates with intracellular peroxide formation.) The clinical course of children with CGD is quite variable. No specific therapy is available to correct the intracellular lesion. In view of the predominance of staphylococcal infections, patients commonly are maintained on prophylactic dicloxacillin. Chronic granulomatous disease is classically a sex-linked disorder affecting male children, although some cases may be autosomal recessive. In accord with the Lyon hypothesis, female carriers have both normal and abnormal neutrophils, and this is seen most clearly when the NBT slide test is performed. Clinically, female CGD carriers manifest no increased evidence of infection. Prenatal diagnosis of CGD can be made by doing an NBT test on fetal neutrophils obtained by cordocentesis (Newburger et al., 1979). Also, since the CGD gene has been cloned, prenatal diagnosis should be possible using amniotic fluid fibroblasts.

CHÉDIAK-HIGASHI SYNDROME

This autosomal recessive disorder is characterized by oculocutaneous albinism, photophobia, and recurrent infections. During the course of disease, hepatosplenomegaly also develops. Most patients ultimately die from infection, although death is occasionally due to a lymphoma-like illness. Thrombocytopenia is frequently present. Anemia is rare. The total white blood cell count can be normal, but neutropenia is common in severe cases. The pathognomonic laboratory finding is the presence of large granules in granulocytes and lymphocytes. Within neutrophils, these giant lysosomal structures contain peroxidase activity, and thus represent abnormal primary granules. It has been observed that these giant lysosomes fail to degranulate their contents into phagocytic vacuoles at a normal rate, and intracellular killing of certain bacteria also is abnormal. In spite of these interesting findings, however, increased susceptibility to infections is correlated best with the degree of neutropenia. The relationship of granule abnormalities to rare malignant transformation is unknown.

EOSINOPHILIA IN PREMATURE INFANTS

Eosinophilia (>500 eosinophils/μl) in older children is associated with allergy, drug reactions, parasitic infestations, immunodeficiency syndromes, collagen-vascular diseases, and adrenal insufficiency. Eosinophilia also frequently is observed in premature infants, although the significance of this finding is unknown. Usually, there are no obvious explanations for this eosinophilia. A recent report suggests eosinophilia in premature infants may reflect a normal growth process, the onset of positive nitrogen balance (Gibson et al., 1979).

■ MYELOPROLIFERATIVE DISORDERS IN THE NEWBORN

The newborn who presents with hepatosplenomegaly, nucleated red blood cells in the peripheral blood, and an elevated white blood cell count is a clinical challenge. Diagnostic possibilities include the following: congenital infection (e.g., toxoplasmosis, rubella, herpes, cytomegalovirus, syphilis), hematologic disease of the newborn, acute leukemia, and the transient myeloproliferative syndrome. The latter two conditions are discussed in this section.

NEONATAL LEUKEMIA

Leukemia during the neonatal period is extremely rare. Almost all congenital leukemias are either acute lymphoblastic leukemia (ALL) or acute nonlymphocytic leukemia (ANLL). In contrast to leukemia in older children where the incidence of ALL to ANLL is about 4 to 1, a reverse ratio is observed in neonatal leukemia, with ANLL being much more common. The most frequent subtypes of acute myelogenous leukemia in newborns are acute monocytic and myelomonocytic leukemia, which are associated with a high incidence of extramedullary leukemia especially involving the skin and central nervous system. The clinical presentation of ALL in infants differs from that seen in older children in that newborns present with higher white blood cell counts, more severe thrombocytopenia, more hepatosplenomegaly, and a higher incidence of CNS leukemia. In older children with ALL, the majority of lymphoblasts express the common acute lymphoblastic leukemia antigen (CALLA positive), whereas most lymphoblasts in neonatal ALL are CALLA-negative. In addition, many infants with ALL manifest a high incidence of chromosome translocations, again being much higher than that seen in older children with ALL (Pui et al., 1987). *Infants with ALL and ANLL have a much poorer prognosis* than older children with these same disorders (Reaman et al., 1985; Crist et al., 1986). Whenever a newborn is suspected of having congenital leukemia, it is imperative that a pediatric hematologist/oncologist be consulted.

TRANSIENT MYELOPROLIFERATIVE SYNDROME

This disorder has been described as a transient acute leukemia. It is characterized by ineffective regulation of granulopoiesis and occurs almost exclusively in children with Down syndrome (Weinstein, 1978). Rarely, this disorder is seen in phenotypically normal infants who are mosaics for trisomy 21. This syndrome becomes apparent shortly after birth and has many of the clinical and hematologic features of ANLL. Usually, these infants have hepatosplenomegaly, leukocytosis with white cell counts over 100,000/μl, and frequently thrombocytopenia. Bone marrow aspirate may reveal an increased number of blasts, often indistinguishable from acute leukemia. If only supportive care is given, the hematologic status returns to normal in a few weeks to months. Several children have died of cardiac or pulmonary disease years after the resolution of this myeloproliferative disorder, and in these cases, there was no evidence of leukemia at autopsy. However, a few rare cases have been described in which leukemia evolved after spontaneous regression of the original myeloproliferative syndrome.

In an infant with Down syndrome it can be difficult to distinguish acute leukemia from the transient myeloproliferative syndrome. Moreover there is an equal chance of a child with trisomy 21 having either a transient myeloproliferative syndrome or acute leukemia. The absence of cutaneous leukemia may favor a transient myeloproliferative syndrome, whereas cytogenetic studies that demonstrate chromosomal abnormalities in addition to the trisomy 21 suggest acute leukemia. Often, however, these two disorders are distinguished only after a period of weeks to months of patient observation with supportive care. Specific antileukemic chemotherapy is not indicated unless there is hematologic progression of disease. Again, it is critical that a hematologist/oncologist be involved in the management of these infants.

■ REFERENCES

Normal Granulocyte Physiology

Christensen, R., and Rothstein, G.: Exhaustion of mature marrow neutrophils in neonates with sepsis. J. Pediatr. *96*:316–318, 1980.

Stossel, T. P.: The phagocyte system: Structure and function. *In* Nathan, D. G., and Oski, F. A. (Eds.): Hematology of Infancy and Childhood. Philadelphia, W. B. Saunders Company, 1987, pp. 779–796.

Granulocyte Physiology and Neonatal Infection

Christensen, R. D., Bradley, P. B., and Rothstein, G.: The leukocyte shift in clinical and experimental sepsis. J. Pediatr. *98*:101, 1981.

Gregory, J., and Hey, E.: Blood neutrophil response to bacterial infection in the first month of life. Arch. Dis. Child. *47*:747, 1972.

Manroe, B. L., Weinberg, A. G., Rosenfeld, C. R., and Browne, R.: The neonatal blood count in health and disease. I. Reference values for neutrophilic cells. J. Pediatr. *95*:89, 1979.

Miller, M. E.: Chemotactic function in the human neonate: humoral and cellular aspects. Pediatr. Res. *5*:492, 1971.

Miller, M. E.: Phagocytosis in the newborn infant: humoral and cellular factors. J. Pediatr. *74*:255, 1969.

Xanthou, M.: Leukocyte blood picture in healthy full-term and premature babies during neonatal period. Arch. Dis. Child. *45*:242, 1970.

Xanthou, M., Tsomides, K., Nicolopoulos, D., and Matsaniotis, N.: Leukocyte blood picture in newborn babies during and after exchange transfusion. Pediatr. Res. *6*:59, 1972.

Zipursky A., Palko J., Milner, R., et al.: The hematology of bacterial infections in premature infants. Pediatrics *57*:839–853, 1976.

Granulocyte Transfusions

Cairo, M. S.: Neutrophil transfusions in the treatment of neonatal sepsis. Am. J. Pediatr. Hematol/Oncol. *11*:227–234, 1989.

Christensen, R. D., Rothstein, G., Anstatt, H. B., and Bybee, B.: Granulocyte transfusions in neonates with bacterial infection, neutropenia, and depletion of mature marrow neutrophils. Pediatrics *70*:1–6, 1982.

Neutropenic Disorders

Bonilla, M. E., Gillo, A. P., Ruggeiro, M., et al.: Effects of recombinant human granulocyte colony-stimulating factor on neutropenia in patients with congenital agranulocytosis. N. Engl. J. Med. *320*:1574–1580, 1989.

de Vaal, O. M., and Seynhaseve, V.: Reticular dysgenesia. Lancet *2*:1123, 1959.

Lalezari, P., Nussbaum, M., Gelman, S., and Spaet, T. H.: Neonatal neutropenia due to maternal isoimmunization. Blood *15*:236, 1960.

Laurenti, F., Ferro, R., Isacchi, G., et al.: Polymorphonuclear leukocyte transfusion for the treatment of sepsis in the newborn infant. J. Pediatr. *98*:118, 1981.

Shwachman, H., Diamond, L. K., Oski, F. A., and Khaw, K. T.: The syndrome of pancreatic insufficiency and bone marrow dysfunction. J. Pediatr. *65*:645, 1964.

Disorders of Leukocyte Function

Anderson, D. C., and Springer, T. A.: Leukocyte adhesion deficiency: An inherited defect in the Mac-1, LFA-1, and p150, 95 glycoproteins. Ann. Rev. Med. *38*:175–194, 1987.

Baehner, R. L., and Johnston, R. B., Jr.: Chronic granulomatous disease: correlation between pathogenesis and clinical findings. Pediatrics *48*:730, 1971.

Baehner, R. L., Nathan, D. G., and Karnovsky, M. L.: Correction of the metabolic deficiencies in the leukocytes of patients with chronic granulomatous disease. J. Clin. Invest. *49*:860, 1970.

Blume, R. S., and Wolff, S. M.: The Chédiak-Higashi syndrome: studies in four patients and a review of the literature. Medicine *51*:247, 1972.

Boxer, L. A., and Anderson, D. C.: Leukocyte abnormalities of the newborn. *In* Alter, B.P. (Ed.): Methods in Hematology, vol. 21. Perinatal Hematology. Edinburgh, Churchill Livingstone, 1989, pp. 194–224.

Crowley, C. A., Curnutte, J. T., Rosin, R. E., et al.: An inherited abnormality of neutrophil adhesion. Its genetic transmission and its association with a missing protein. N. Engl. J. Med. *302*:1163–1168, 1980.

Curnutte, J. T., and Boxer, L. A.: Disorders of granulopoiesis and granulocyte function. *In* Nathan, D. G., and Oski, F. A. (Eds.): Hematology of Infancy and Childhood. Philadelphia, W. B. Saunders Company, 1987, pp. 797–847.

Newburger, P. E., Cohen, H. J., Rothchild, S. B., et al.: Prenatal diagnosis of chronic granulomatous disease. N. Engl. J. Med. *300*:178–181, 1979.

Eosinophilia in Premature Infants

Gibson, E. L., Vaucher, Y., and Corrigan, J. J.: Eosinophilia in premature infants: relationship to weight gain. J. Pediatr. 95:99, 1979.

Myeloproliferative Disorders in the Newborn

Crist, W., Pullen, J., Boyett, J., et al.: Clinical and biologic features predict a poor prognosis in acute lymphoid leukemias in infants: A Pediatric Oncology Group study. Blood 67:135, 1986.

Pui, C. -H., Raimondi, S. C., Murphy, S. B., et al.: An analysis of leukemic cell chromosomal features in infants. Blood 69(5):1289–1293, 1987.

Reaman, G., Zeltzer, P., Bleyer, W. A., et al.: Acute lymphoblastic leukemia in infants less than one year of age: A cumulative experience of the Children's Cancer Study Group. J. Clin. Oncol. 3:1513, 1985.

Weinstein, H. J.: Congenital leukaemia and the neonatal myeloproliferative disorders associated with Down's syndrome. Clin. Haematol. 7:147–154, 1978.

ERYTHROCYTE DISORDERS IN INFANCY 86

Bertil E. Glader and J. Lawrence Naiman

■ NORMAL ERYTHROCYTE PHYSIOLOGY IN THE FETUS AND NEWBORN

FETAL ERYTHROPOIESIS

Fetal erythropoiesis occurs in three different sites: yolk sac, liver, and bone marrow. Yolk sac formation of red blood cells (RBCs) is maximal between the 2nd and 10th weeks of gestation. The liver is a major site of erythropoiesis between the 10th and 26th weeks of gestation. Myeloid, or bone marrow, production of red blood cells begins around the 18th week, and by the 30th week of fetal life bone marrow is the major erythropoietic organ. At birth, almost all RBCs are produced in the bone marrow, although a low level of hepatic erythropoiesis persists through the first few days of life. Sites of fetal erythropoiesis are occasionally reactivated in older patients with hematologic disorders such as myelofibrosis, aplastic anemia, and severe hemolytic anemia.

RBC production in extrauterine life is controlled in part by erythropoietin, a humoral erythropoietic stimulating factor (ESF) produced by the kidney. The role of erythropoietin in the developing fetus has not been completely defined. Current thoughts are that ESF does not influence yolk sac or hepatic erythropoiesis, but it may partially regulate myeloid RBC production (Finne and Halvorsen, 1972). ESF is detected in fetal blood and amniotic fluid during the last trimester of pregnancy. The concentration of this hormone increases directly with the period of gestation, and thus, erythropoietin levels in term newborns are significantly higher than in premature infants. This difference may reflect some degree of fetal hypoxia during late intrauterine life. Increased ESF titers also are seen in placental dysfunction, fetal anemia, and maternal hypoxia (Finne, 1966). Fetal RBC formation is not influenced by maternal erythropoietin, since transfusion-induced maternal polycythemia (decreased maternal ESF levels) has no effect on fetal erythropoiesis (Jacobson et al., 1959). Maternal nutritional status also is not a significant factor in the regulation of fetal erythropoiesis, because iron, folate, and vitamin B_{12} are trapped by the fetus irrespective of maternal stores. Most studies have demonstrated that women with severe iron deficiency bear children with normal total body hemoglobin content (Lanzkowsky, 1961).

Hemoglobin, hematocrit, and RBC count increase throughout fetal life (Table 86–1). Extremely large RBCs (mean corpuscular volume [MCV] of 180) with an in-

creased hemoglobin content (mean corpuscular hemoglobin [MCH] of 60) are produced early in fetal life. The size and hemoglobin content of these cells decrease throughout gestation, but the mean corpuscular hemoglobin concentration (MCHC) does not change significantly. Even at birth, the MCV and MCH are greater than those seen in older children and adults. Many nucleated RBCs and reticulocytes are present early in gestation, and the percentage of these cells also decreases as the fetus ages.

Hemoglobin production increases markedly during the last trimester of pregnancy. The actual hemoglobin concentration increases, but, more importantly, body weight, blood volume, and total body hemoglobin triple in size during this period. Fetal iron accumulation parallels the increase in total body hemoglobin content. The neonatal iron endowment at birth, therefore, is directly related to total body hemoglobin content and length of gestation. Term infants have more iron than premature infants.

RED BLOOD CELL PHYSIOLOGY AT BIRTH

In utero, fetal blood (umbilical vein) is approximately 50 per cent saturated with oxygen. This relative hypoxia may be responsible for the increased content of erythropoietin and signs of active erythropoiesis (nucleated RBCs, increased reticulocytes) seen in newborns at birth. When lungs become the source of oxygen, hemoglobin-O_2 saturation increases to 95 per cent and erythropoiesis decreases. Within 72 hours after birth, erythropoietin is undetectable, nucleated RBCs disappear, and reticulocytes decrease to less than 1 per cent.

The concentration of hemoglobin during the first few hours of life increases to values greater than those seen in cord blood. This is a relative increase due to a reduction in plasma volume (Gairdner et al., 1958) and an absolute increase due to placental blood transfusion (Usher et al., 1963). The umbilical vein remains patent long after umbilical arteries have constricted, and thus transfusion of placental blood occurs when newborns are held at a level below the placenta. The placenta contains approximately 100 ml of fetal blood (30 per cent of the infant's blood volume). Approximately 25 per cent of placental blood enters the newborn within 15 seconds of birth, and by 1 minute, 50 per cent is transfused. The time of cord clamping is thus a direct determinant of neonatal blood volume. The blood volume of term infants (mean of 85 ml/kg) varies considerably (50 to 100 ml/kg) because of

TABLE 86–1. Mean Red Blood Cell Values During Gestation

AGE (Weeks)	Hb (g/dl)	HEMATO-CRIT (%)	RBC (10⁶/mm³)	MEAN CORPUSCULAR VOLUME (fl)	MEAN CORPUSCULAR Hb (pg)	MEAN CORPUSCULAR Hb CONCEN-TRATION (g/dl)	NUCLEATED RBC (% of RBCs)	RETIC-ULOCYTES (%)	DIAMETER (μ)
12	8.0–10.0	33	1.5	180	60	34	5.0–8.0	40	10.5
16	10.0	35	2.0	140	45	33	2.0–4.0	10–25	9.5
20	11.0	37	2.5	135	44	33	1.0	10–20	9.0
24	14.0	40	3.5	123	38	31	1.0	5–10	8.8
28	14.5	45	4.0	120	40	31	0.5	5–10	8.7
34	15.0	47	4.4	118	38	32	0.2	3–10	8.5

(From Oski, F. A., and Naiman, J. L.: Hematologic Problems in the Newborn. 3rd ed. Philadelphia, W. B. Saunders Company, 1982.)

different degrees of placental transfusion (Usher et al., 1963). These differences are readily apparent when the effects of early versus delayed cord clamping are compared at 72 hours of age: 82.3 ml/kg (early clamping) versus 92.6 ml/kg (delayed clamping). These changes are largely due to differences in RBC mass (early clamping 31 ml/kg, delayed clamping 49 ml/kg). The blood volume of premature infants (89 to 105 ml/kg) is slightly greater than that of term infants, but in large part this is due to an increased plasma volume (Usher and Lind, 1965). The RBC mass of premature infants is the same as in term newborns.

FETAL AND NEONATAL HEMOGLOBIN FUNCTION

A variety of hemoglobins are present during fetal and neonatal life (see discussion under Hemoglobinopathies). Fetal hemoglobin (Hgb F) is the major hemoglobin in utero, whereas hemoglobin A is the normal hemoglobin of extrauterine life. Both are present in the same cell, but the relative proportion of each varies with gestational and postnatal age. One major difference between hemoglobins A and F is related to oxygen transport.

The transport of oxygen to peripheral tissues is regulated by several factors, including blood oxygen capacity, cardiac output, and hemoglobin-oxygen affinity. (1) Oxygen capacity is a direct function of hemoglobin concentration (1 g hemoglobin combines with 1.34 ml oxygen). (2) Compensatory changes in cardiac output can maintain normal O_2 delivery under conditions in which oxygen capacity is significantly reduced. (3) The oxygen affinity of hemoglobin also influences oxygen delivery to tissues. Hemoglobin A is 95 per cent saturated at arterial oxygen tensions (100 mm Hg), but this decreases to 70 to 75 per cent saturation at a venous Po_2 of 40 mm Hg. The difference in O_2 content at arterial and venous oxygen tensions reflects the amount of oxygen that can be released. Changes in hemoglobin affinity for oxygen can influence O_2 delivery (Fig. 86–1). At any given Po_2, more oxygen is bound to hemoglobin when oxygen affinity is increased. Stated in physiologic terms, increased hemoglobin-oxygen affinity reduces oxygen delivery, whereas decreased hemoglobin-oxygen affinity increases oxygen release to peripheral tissues.

The oxygen affinity of hemoglobin A in solution is greater than that for hemoglobin F. Paradoxically, however, whole blood from normal children (Hgb A) has a lower oxygen affinity than neonatal blood (Hgb F) (Allen et al., 1953). This difference is related to an intermediate of RBC metabolism known as 2,3-diphosphoglycerate

(2,3-DPG). This organic phosphate compound interacts with hemoglobin A to decrease its affinity for oxygen and thereby enhance O_2 release. Fetal hemoglobin does not interact with 2,3-DPG to any significant extent (Bauer et al., 1968); consequently, cells containing hemoglobin F have a higher oxygen affinity than those containing hemoglobin A.

The increased oxygen affinity of fetal RBCs is obviously advantageous for extracting oxygen from maternal blood within the placenta. A few months after birth, however, infant blood acquires the same oxygen affinity as that of older children (Fig. 86–2). The postnatal decrease in O_2 affinity is due to a reduction in hemoglobin F and an increase in hemoglobin A (which interacts with 2,3-DPG). It is an interesting fact that oxygen delivery (the difference in arterial and venous O_2 content) actually increases while oxygen capacity (hemoglobin concentration) decreases during the 1st week of life (Fig. 86–3). This enhanced delivery is largely a reflection of the decreased oxygen affinity of infant blood (Delivoria-Papadopoulos et al., 1971). The oxygen affinity of blood from premature infants is higher than that of term infants, and the normal postnatal changes (decrease in oxygen affinity, increase in

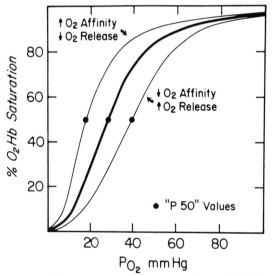

FIGURE 86–1. The oxygen dissociation curve of normal adult hemoglobin (dark line). The per cent oxygen saturation (ordinate) is plotted for arterial oxygen tensions between 0 and 100 mm Hg (abscissa). As the curve shifts to the right, more oxygen is released at any given Po_2. Conversely, as the curve shifts to the left, more oxygen is retained on hemoglobin at any given Po_2. The "P 50" refers to that Po_2 in which hemoglobin is 50 per cent saturated with oxygen. This term is useful in comparing the oxygen affinity of different hemoglobins. (Oski, F. A., and Delivoria-Papadopoulos, M.: The red cell, 2,3-diphosphoglycerate, and tissue oxygen release. J. Pediatr. 77:941, 1970.)

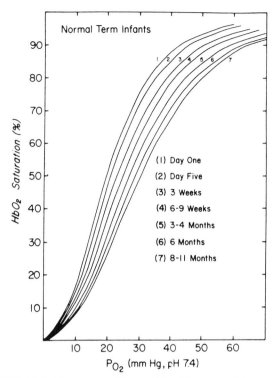

FIGURE 86–2. The oxygen affinity of blood from term infants at birth and at different postnatal ages. The gradual rightward shift of the oxygen saturation curve indicates increased oxygen release from hemoglobin as infants get older. This decreased oxygen affinity is due to a decrease in hemoglobin F and an increase in hemoglobin A. (Oski, F. A., and Delivoria-Papadopoulos, M.: The red cell, 2,3-diphosphoglycerate, and tissue oxygen release. J. Pediatr. 77:941, 1970.)

oxygen delivery) occur much more gradually in premature infants (Fig. 86–3).

■ GENERAL APPROACH TO ANEMIC INFANTS

Medical History and Physical Examination. The etiology of anemia frequently can be ascertained by medical history and physical examination. Particular importance is given to family history (anemia, cholelithiasis, unexplained jaundice, splenomegaly), maternal medical history (especially infections), and obstetric history (previous pregnancies, length of gestation, method and difficulty of delivery). The age at which anemia becomes manifest also is of diagnostic importance. Significant anemia at birth invariably is due to blood loss or alloimmune hemolysis. After 24 hours, internal hemorrhages and other causes of hemolysis become manifest. Anemia that appears several weeks after birth can be caused by a variety of conditions, including abnormalities in the synthesis of hemoglobin-beta chains, hypoplastic RBC disorders, and the physiologic anemia of infancy or prematurity.

Infants with anemia due to chronic blood loss may appear pale, without other evidence of clinical distress. Acute blood loss can produce hypovolemic shock and a clinical state similar to severe neonatal asphyxia. Newborns with hemolytic anemia frequently show a greater than expected degree of icterus. In addition, hemolysis

often is associated with hepatosplenomegaly, and in cases due to congenital infection, other stigmata may be present.

Laboratory Evaluation of Anemia. A simple classification of neonatal anemia based on physical examination and simple laboratory tests is presented in Table 86–2. References to more esoteric RBC tests (as well as methodologies for the study of neonatal coagulation and leukocyte abnormalities) recently have appeared in a monograph on perinatal hematology (Alter, 1989).

RBC Count, Hemoglobin, Hematocrit, and RBC Indices. Red blood cell values during the neonatal period are more variable than at any other time of life. The diagnosis of anemia must therefore be made in terms of "normal" values appropriate for an infant's gestational and postnatal age. The mean cord blood hemoglobin of healthy term infants ranges between 14 and 20 g/100 ml (Table 86–3). Shortly after birth, however, hemoglobin concentration increases. This increase is both relative (owing to a reduction of plasma volume) and absolute (owing to placental RBC transfusion). Failure of hemoglobin to increase during the first few hours of life may be the initial sign of hemorrhagic anemia. RBC values at the end of the 1st week are virtually identical with those seen at birth. Anemia during the 1st week of life is thus defined as any hemoglobin value less than 14 g/100 ml. A significant hemoglobin decrease during this time, although within the normal range, is suggestive of hemorrhage or hemolysis. For example, 14.5 g hemoglobin at 7 days of age is abnormal for a term infant whose hemoglobin was 18.5 g at birth. A slight hemoglobin reduction normally occurs in premature infants during the 1st week. Beyond the 1st week, however, the hemoglobin concentration decreases in both term and premature infants (see Physiologic Anemia of Infancy and Prematurity).

The electronic equipment currently used for blood counts also gives statistical information regarding erythrocyte size (mean corpuscular volume [MCV] and hemoglobin content (mean corpuscular hemoglobin [MCH]). The normal MCV ($\mu\mu$) in older children ranges from 75 to 90. Mean corpuscular volumes of less than 75 are considered microcytic, whereas those over 100 indicate macrocytosis. Normal infant RBCs are large (MCV 105 to 125), and not until 8 to 10 weeks of age does cell size approach that of older children. Neonatal microcytosis is defined as an MCV of less than 95 at birth. The RBC hemoglobin content of neonatal cells (MCH 35 to 38) is greater than that seen in older children (MCH 30 to 33). Neonatal hypochromia is defined as an MCH of less than 34. Hypochromia and microcytosis generally occur together, and invariably these abnormalities are due to hemoglobin production defects. Neonatal hypochromic microcytosis is seen with iron deficiency (chronic blood loss, late anemia of prematurity) and thalassemia disorders (alpha and gamma thalassemias).

The site at which blood is obtained is important, since peripheral stasis leads to higher hemoglobin concentrations in capillary blood compared with simultaneously obtained central venous samples. This difference can be minimized by warming an extremity to obtain "arterialized capillary blood" (Oh and Lind, 1966). In the face of acute hemorrhage, however, central venous samples must be obtained because of marked peripheral vasoconstriction.

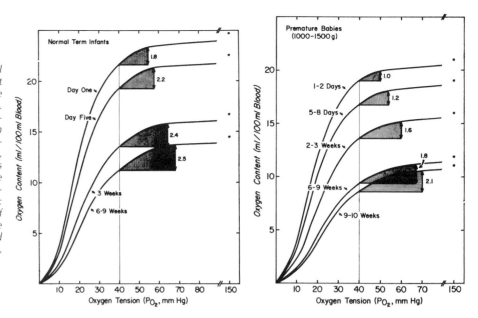

FIGURE 86–3. Oxygen delivery in normal term and premature infants. Oxygen content (a function of total hemoglobin) is on the ordinate. Oxygen tension is on the abscissa. Oxygen delivery is measured by the difference in oxygen content at arterial (100 mm Hg) and venous (40 mm Hg) oxygen tensions. For both term and premature infants, oxygen delivery (shaded areas) increases with age. This occurs in spite of a decrease in oxygen content. (Delivoria-Papadopoulos, M., Roncevic, N. P., and Oski, F. A.: Postnatal changes in oxygen transport of term, premature, and sick infants: The role of red cell 2,3-diphosphoglycerate and adult hemoglobin. Pediatr. Res. 5:235, 1971.)

Reticulocyte Count. The normal reticulocyte count of children and older infants is 1 to 2 per cent. The reticulocyte count in term infants ranges between 3 and 7 per cent at birth, but this decreases to 1 to 3 per cent by 4 days and to less than 1 per cent by 7 days of age (Table 86–3). In premature infants, reticulocyte values at birth are higher (6 to 10 per cent) and may remain elevated for a longer period of time. Nucleated red blood cells are seen in newborn infants, but they generally disappear by the 3rd day of life in term infants and in 7 to 10 days in premature infants. The persistence of reticulocytosis or nucleated RBCs suggests the possibility of hemorrhage or hemolysis. Hypoxia, in the absence of anemia, also can be associated with increased release of reticulocytes and nucleated RBCs.

Peripheral Blood Smear. Examination of the peripheral blood smear is an invaluable aid in the diagnosis of anemia. In particular, the smear is evaluated for alterations in the size and shape of RBCs as well as abnormalities in leukocytes and platelets. Erythrocytes of older children are approximately the size of a small lymphocyte nucleus, whereas those of newborns are slightly larger. Red blood cell hemoglobinization (e.g., hypochromia) is estimated by observing the area of central pallor, which is one-third the diameter of normal RBCs and over one-half the diameter of hypochromic cells. Spherocytes are detected by the complete absence of central pallor. The degree of reticulocytosis can be estimated, since these cells are larger and have a bluish coloration.

Serum Bilirubin. Bilirubin is a normal breakdown product of hemoglobin. In cases of hemolytic anemia (increased RBC destruction), bilirubin levels are increased to above normal neonatal levels. Hyperbilirubinemia is not seen with anemia caused by external hemorrhage, although resorption of blood from large enclosed hemorrhages can produce icterus.

Haptoglobin. This glycoprotein binds free hemoglobin, and the hemoglobin-haptoglobin complex is cleared from the circulation. Decreased serum haptoglobin is a sign of hemolysis in older children, but it is not a useful measurement in newborns, since haptoglobin is normally decreased at this time of life. Normal haptoglobin levels generally are present by 3 months of age.

Coombs Test. The vast majority of neonatal hemolytic anemias are due to isoimmunization. The Coombs test detects the presence of antibody on RBCs (direct Coombs) or in the plasma (indirect Coombs). The direct Coombs test also is known as the direct antiglobulin test (DAT). One must search diligently to rule out an isoimmune disorder before embarking on a more esoteric work-up of hemolysis.

Blood Transfusions in the Treatment of Anemia. A hemoglobin of 15 g/100 ml corresponds to an RBC mass of 30 ml/kg. This implies that a transfusion of 2 ml RBC/kg increases the hemoglobin concentration 1 g/100 ml. Packed RBCs (hematocrit approximately 67 per cent) contain 2 ml of RBC/3 ml packed RBC. Whole blood (hematocrit approximately 33 per cent) contains 2 ml RBC/6 ml whole blood. Thus, the transfusion of 3 ml packed RBC/kg or 6 ml whole blood/kg increases hemoglobin concentration 1 g/100 ml.

TABLE 86–2. Differential Approach to Anemia in Newborn Period

HEMOGLOBIN	RETICULOCYTES	BILIRUBIN	COOMBS TEST	CLINICAL CONSIDERATIONS
Decreased	Normal/decreased	Normal	Negative	Physiologic anemia of infancy and prematurity Hypoplastic anemia
Decreased	Normal/increased	Normal	Negative	Hemorrhagic anemia
Decreased	Normal increased	Increased	Positive	Immune-mediated hemolysis
Decreased	Normal/increased	Increased	Negative	Acquired or hereditary RBC defects Enclosed hemorrhage with resorption of blood Coombs-negative ABO incompatibility

TABLE 86–3. RBC Values in Term and Premature Infants During the 1st Week of Life

	Hgb (g/100 ml)	Hct (%)	RETICULOCYTES (%)	NUCLEATED RBCs (cells/1000 RBCs)
Term				
Cord blood	17.0	53.0	<7	<1.00
	(14–20)	(45–61)		
Day 1	18.4	58.0	<7	<0.40
Day 3	17.8	55.0	<3	<0.01
Day 7	17.0	54.0	<1	0
Premature (weighing less than 1500 g)				
Cord blood	16.0	49	<10	<3.00
	(13.0–18.5)			
Day 7	14.8	45	<3	<0.01

EXAMPLE. A 3.5-kg infant with a hemoglobin of 6.5 g/100 ml is to be transfused to a hemoglobin of 12.0 g/100 ml. The difference between the desired and present hemoglobin is 5.5 g/100 ml. The volume of packed RBCs to be administered is 58 ml (3.5 kg × 5.5 g/100 ml hemoglobin difference × 3 ml packed RBC/kg).

Packed RBCs are the product of choice when transfusion is necessary for simple anemia, as occurs in hemolysis. If anemia is accompanied by hypovolemia from acute blood loss, volume expansion must be achieved promptly, using either whole blood or packed red cells and a colloid such as 5 per cent serum albumin or plasma protein fraction (infused separately). Because of the reduced availability of whole blood owing to the demand for components, the usual choice is packed red cells and colloid. The previously common practice of reconstituting red cells with fresh frozen plasma to make "whole blood" is no longer acceptable because the increased donor exposure increases the risk of transmitting infectious disease. When packed red cells need to be diluted to facilitate nonurgent transfusion, isotonic saline is the preferred diluent. If exchange transfusion is needed for hemolysis with hyperbilirubinemia, the need for albumin to improve bilirubin binding and removal is ample reason to request whole blood. Although fresh blood less than 2 days old is ideal because of the reduced risk of hyperkalemia, this is not usually available. An acceptable substitute is packed cells less than 4 to 5 days old. These packed cells provide adequate oxygen delivery; hyperkalemia can be prevented by washing the cells once in saline, then reconstituting with fresh frozen plasma. Washing is not required for the usual small simple transfusions of packed red cells where the small volume of plasma negates any toxic effect of increased concentration of potassium in the plasma.

Blood currently available in most blood banks is anticoagulated with citrate-phosphate-dextrose (CPD) or CPD-adenine (CPDA-1), with shelf lives of 21 and 35 days respectively. Hematocrit usually ranges between 65 and 80 per cent for packed RBCs. Near-normal 2,3-DPG levels are maintained for up to 12 to 14 days, which is advantageous when transfusing infants with acute hypoxia or those receiving large volumes of blood. Newer additive preparations in which most of the plasma is replaced by a solution containing saline, adenine, glucose (and in some preparations, mannitol) support storage of red cells up to 42 days. (Although these are the predominant red cells available today, the longer shelf life is of no advantage for newborns in whom fresher cells are preferred.) Hematocrits range from 55 to 65 per cent, thus facilitating

flow during infusion. Limited experience suggests these preparations are well tolerated by newborns.

Preterm infants born weighing less than 1250 g are uniquely susceptible to potentially serious cytomegalovirus (CMV) infection from transfused blood, particularly if they lack immunity due to seronegativity of their mothers. This can be prevented by using blood products only from seronegative donors (Yeager et al., 1981). Since approximately 40 to 60 per cent of adults are seropositive, this limits the availability of seronegative donors. Reserving seronegative blood for the minority of infants who are seronegative can reduce the demand for such donors. Alternatively, since CMV resides mainly in leukocytes, removal of such cells could prevent transmission of the virus. Frozen thawed, deglycerolized red cells (Brady et al., 1984) and newer high-efficiency leukocyte depletion filters (Gilbert et al., 1989) have proved effective. Conventional saline-washed red cells are not effective, presumably because they contain greater numbers of residual leukocytes (Demmler et al., 1986). A potential disadvantage of using CMV-seronegative blood in CMV-positive infants receiving large amounts of blood is dilution of infant's antibody level, resulting in increased susceptibility to nursery-acquired CMV infection.

Graft-versus-host (GVH) reaction rarely follows transfusion and occurs mainly in certain newborns at risk. For this to occur, viable lymphocytes in cellular blood products must be able to engraft and react against foreign antigens on tissues of the recipient. Infants at risk include those with congenital or acquired defects of cellular immunity, fetuses receiving intrauterine transfusion of red cells or platelets, newborns receiving exchange transfusion following intrauterine transfusion (Naiman et al., 1969; Parkman et al., 1974), and infants receiving directed blood donations from first-degree relatives (whose genetic similarity may increase the likelihood of engraftment). Irradiation of red cells, whole blood, platelets and granulocytes with a minimum of 1500 r has proved effective in preventing GVH. Reports of GVH after red cell transfusion in very premature infants without known risk factors (Enoki et al., 1985; Sanders et al., 1989) has prompted some workers to recommend irradiation of blood given to all infants with this condition. Logistic difficulties in providing routine irradiation preclude general endorsement of such recommendations at present.

■ HEMORRHAGIC ANEMIA

Anemia frequently follows fetal blood loss, bleeding from obstetric complications, and internal hemorrhages associated with birth trauma (Table 86–4). The clinical presentation of anemia depends on the magnitude and acuteness of blood loss.

Infants with anemia subsequent to moderate hemorrhage or chronic blood loss are generally asymptomatic. The only physical findings are pallor of the skin and mucous membranes. Laboratory studies can range from a mild normochromic-normocytic anemia (hemoglobin 9 to 12 g/100 ml) to a more severe hypochromic-microcytic anemia (hemoglobin 5 to 7 g/100 ml). The only therapy required for asymptomatic children is iron (2 mg elemental iron/kg, t.i.d. for 3 months). RBC replacement is indicated only if there is evidence of clinical distress (tachycardia, tachypnea, irritability, feeding difficulties). In most cases, raising the hemoglobin to 10 to 12 g/100 ml removes all signs and symptoms associated with anemia. Since severely anemic infants are frequently in incipient heart failure, however, these children should be transfused very slowly (2 ml/kg/hr). If signs of congestive heart failure appear, a rapid-acting diuretic (furosemide, 1 mg/kg intravenously) should be given before proceeding with the transfusion. An alternative approach is to administer an exchange transfusion with packed RBCs for anemic whole blood to severely anemic infants. This increases the hemoglobin concentration without the danger of increasing blood volume and precipitating congestive heart failure.

A simple formula for the volume of RBC needed in a partial exchange transfusion to correct severe anemia has been described by Nieburg and Stockman (1977): Packed RBC volume needed (ml) = body weight (kg) × 75 ml/kg × desired Hgb change/[22 g/dl − Hgb$_w$], where 75 ml/kg approximates the average blood volume and 22 g/dl represents the Hgb concentration of packed red blood cells. The term Hgb$_w$ is a reflection of the hemoglobin removed during the exchange transfusion, and this is approximated by (initial Hgb + desired Hgb)/2. For each infusion and withdrawal, syringe volumes up to 5 per cent of the blood volume are well tolerated. For example, in the case of a 3-kg newborn with a hemoglobin of 3 g/dl that needs to be raised to a hemoglobin of 10 g/dl, approximately 100 ml of packed RBCs are needed for the procedure; syringe volumes of 15 ml can be used for each cycle of infusion and withdrawal of blood.

TABLE 86–4. Hemorrhagic Anemia in Newborns

Fetal hemorrhage
  Spontaneous fetomaternal hemorrhage
  Hemorrhage following amniocentesis
  Twin–twin transfusion
  Nuchal cord

Placental hemorrhage
  Placenta previa
  Abruptio placentae
  Multilobed placenta (vasa previa)
  Velamentous insertion of cord
  Placental incision during cesarean section

Umbilical cord bleeding
  Rupture of umbilical cord with precipitous delivery
  Rupture of short or entangled cord

Postpartum hemorrhage
  Bleeding from umbilicus
  Cephalhematomas, scalp hemorrhages
  Hepatic rupture, splenic rupture
  Retroperitoneal hemorrhages

TABLE 86–5. Comparative Clinical Findings in Neonatal Asphyxia and Acute Hemorrhage

	NEONATAL ASPHYXIA	ACUTE BLOOD LOSS
Heart rate	Decreased	Increased
Respiratory rate	Decreased	Increased
Intercostal retractions	Present	Absent
Skin color	Pallor with cyanosis	Pallor without cyanosis
Response to oxygen and assisted ventilation	Marked improvement	No significant change

Infants who rapidly lose large volumes of blood appear in acute distress (pallor, tachycardia, tachypnea, weak pulses, hypotension, and shock). This presentation is distinct from that seen in neonatal respiratory asphyxia (slow respirations with intercostal retractions, bradycardia, and pallor with cyanosis) (Table 86–5). The clinical response to assisted ventilation and oxygen is also different: Infants with respiratory problems demonstrate a marked improvement, whereas there is little change in anemic newborns. Cyanosis is not a feature of severe anemia because the hemoglobin concentration is too low (clinical cyanosis indicates at least 5 g/100 ml of deoxygenated hemoglobin). The hemoglobin concentration immediately after an acute hemorrhage may be normal, since the initial response to acute volume depletion is vasoconstriction. A decreased hemoglobin may not be seen until the plasma volume has re-expanded several hours later. In view of these hemodynamic considerations, it is apparent that the diagnosis of acute hemorrhagic anemia is based largely on physical findings and evidence of blood loss. It is important to recognize these clinical features because immediate therapy is required. Treatment is directed at rapid expansion of the vascular space (20 ml fluid/kg). This is most quickly accomplished by rapid infusion of either isotonic saline or 5 per cent albumin, followed by either type-specific, cross-matched whole blood, or packed red cells resuspended with saline depending on availability. Fresh frozen plasma, formerly used for reconstituting red cells, is no longer acceptable because of the increased donor exposure with resultant increased risk of transfusion-transmissible infection. In infants in whom anemia and hypoxia are severe, uncross-matched group O, Rh-negative red cells are an acceptable alternative. Infants with hypovolemic shock due to acute external blood loss usually show marked clinical improvement after this treatment. A poor response is seen in newborns with severe internal hemorrhage.

FETAL HEMORRHAGE

Fetomaternal Hemorrhage. Significant bleeding into the maternal circulation occurs in approximately 8 per cent of all pregnancies and thus represents one of the most common forms of fetal bleeding. Small amounts of fetal blood are lost in most cases, but in 1 per cent of pregnancies fetal blood loss may be as great as 40 ml (Cohen et al., 1964). Fetomaternal hemorrhage occasionally follows amniocentesis and placental injury (Zipursky et al., 1963), although anemia is seen only after unsuccessful amniocentesis or when there is evidence of a bloody tap (Woo Wang et al., 1967). For this reason, infants born to mothers who have had amniocentesis should be observed closely for signs of anemia. The effects of anemia due to fetomaternal hemorrhages are variable. Large acute hemorrhages can produce hypovolemic shock (Raye et al., 1970), whereas slower, more chronic blood loss results in hypochromic microcytic anemia due to iron deficiency (Pearson and Diamond, 1959). Some infants with severe chronic anemia (hemoglobin as low as 4 to 6 g/100 ml) may have minimal symptoms. An examination of the maternal blood smear for the presence of fetal cells (Kleihauer-Betke preparation) is necessary in any infant with suspected fetomaternal hemorrhage. This test is based on the principle that hemoglobin A is eluted from RBCs at an acid pH, whereas hemoglobin F is not affected by these conditions. Consequently, when alcohol-fixed and acid-treated RBCs are stained with eosin, those containing hemoglobin A are colorless, whereas those containing hemoglobin F (fetal RBCs) appear normally colored. Approximately 50 ml of fetal blood must be lost to produce significant neonatal anemia. This volume is greater than 1 per cent of the maternal blood volume, and therefore fetal cells within the maternal circulation may be detected readily. This test is not valid when there is coexistence of maternal hemoglobinopathies with increased hemoglobin F levels. In addition, fetomaternal ABO incompatibility may cause rapid removal of fetal RBCs and thus obscure any significant hemorrhage. For this reason, it is important to examine maternal blood as soon as anemia due to fetal hemorrhage is suspected. An unusual form of fetal blood loss is presumed to occur in infants born with a nuchal cord. In these cases, anemia is due to compression of the umbilical vein preventing placental blood from returning to the fetus (Shepherd et al., 1985).

Twin–Twin Transfusion. Transfusion of blood from one homozygous twin to another can result in anemia in the donor twin and polycythemia in the recipient. Significant hemorrhage is seen only in monochorionic monozygous twins (approximately 70 per cent of all monozygous twins). In approximately 15 per cent of these pregnancies, there is a twin–twin transfusion (Rausen et al., 1965). Bleeding occurs because of vascular anastomosis in monochorionic placentas. The anemic donor twin is usually smaller than the polycythemic recipient, with a greater than 20 per cent difference in birth weight. Polyhydramnios is frequently seen in the recipient twin and oligohydramnios is seen in the donor. Twin–twin transfusions should be suspected when the hemoglobin concentration of identical twins differs by more than 5 g/100 ml; however, such a difference in hemoglobin concentration does not prove there has been a twin–twin transfusion. Recent studies indicate that this major hemoglobin difference can exist in some dichorionic twins, in whom there are no vascular anastamoses and therefore no possibility for twin–twin transfusion (Danskin and Neilson, 1989).

PLACENTAL BLOOD LOSS

Placental bleeding during pregnancy is common, but in most cases hemorrhage is from the maternal aspect of the placenta. In placenta previa, however, the thin placenta overlying the cervical os frequently results in fetal blood loss. The vascular communications between multilobular placental lobes are also very fragile and are easily subjected to trauma during delivery. Vasa previa is the condition in which one of these connecting vessels overlies the cervical os and thus is prone to rupture during delivery. The perinatal death rate in vasa previa may be greater than 50 per cent. Abruptio placentae generally causes fetal anoxia and death, although some infants survive but can be severely anemic. Bleeding also follows inadvertent placental incision during cesarean sections (Montague and Krevans, 1966), and thus the placenta should be inspected for injury following all cesarean sections.

UMBILICAL CORD BLEEDING

The normal umbilical cord is resistant to minor trauma and does not bleed. The umbilical cord of dysmature infants, however, is weak and liable to rupture and hemorrhage (Raye et al., 1970). In cases of precipitous delivery, a rapid increase in cord tension can rupture the fetal aspect of the cord and cause serious acute blood loss. Short or entangled umbilical cords and abnormalities of umbilical blood vessels (velamentous insertions into the placenta) are also liable to rupture and hemorrhage. Bleeding from injured umbilical cords is rapid but generally ceases after a short period of time, owing to arterial constriction. The umbilical cord should always be inspected for abnormalities or signs of injury, particularly after unattended, precipitous deliveries.

CASE 86–1

A 2950-g white male infant was born by vaginal delivery to a gravida 1, para 0, white female at 38 weeks' gestation. Vaginal bleeding was excessive at the time of delivery, and inspection of the cord and placenta revealed a velamentous insertion of umbilical vessels into the placenta. The infant's Apgar score was 7, although he was pale and demonstrated moderate tachycardia and tachypnea. There were no intercostal retractions or cyanosis. Spleen and liver were not palpable. The hemoglobin concentration of blood from the umbilical vein was 13.4 g/100 ml. Bilirubin was 2.3 mg/dl. The infant was transfused with 30 ml of fresh frozen plasma followed by 30 ml of packed RBCs, following which his color improved and cardiac and respiratory status returned to normal. Eight hours after the blood transfusion, the infant's hemoglobin was 14.4 g/100 ml. The infant's subsequent clinical course was unremarkable, and no further transfusions were required.

Comment. Physical findings and a history of excessive bleeding at birth suggested some degree of blood loss. The nearly normal hemoglobin concentration at birth probably was due to immediate vasoconstriction associated with loss of blood volume. Transfusion with RBCs in colloid certainly improved the infant's clinical state, although the increase in hemoglobin was less than expected. This case clearly demonstrates the dramatic response to blood transfusion given to newborns with moderate but self-limited blood loss. Presumably this reflects that the infant was vasoconstricted and hypovolemic.

HEMORRHAGE AFTER DELIVERY

Hemorrhagic anemia due to internal bleeding is occasionally associated with birth trauma. Characteristically, internal hemorrhages are asymptomatic during the first 24 to 48 hours of life, with signs and symptoms of anemia developing after this time. Cephalhematomas can be sufficiently large to cause anemia and hyperbilirubinemia, owing to the resorption of blood (Leonard and Anthony, 1961). Scalp hemorrhages ("hemorrhagic caput") also can produce severe anemia (Pachman, 1962). These hemorrhages are frequently more extensive than cephalhematomas, since bleeding is not limited by periosteum. Adrenal and kidney hemorrhages occasionally follow difficult breech deliveries. Splenic rupture and hemorrhage occur most commonly in association with splenomegaly, as in erythroblastosis fetalis. Hepatic hemorrhages are generally subcapsular and may be asymptomatic. Rupture of the hepatic capsule results in hemoperitoneum and hypovolemic shock. Hepatic hemorrhages are suspected when a previously healthy infant goes into shock with clinical manifestations of an increasing right upper quadrant abdominal mass, shifting dullness on percussion, and evidence of free fluid on abdominal radiographs. In contrast to newborns with acute blood loss due to fetomaternal or umbilical vessel bleeding, infants with hepatic hemorrhage generally demonstrate a poor clinical response to blood replacement.

■ HEMOLYTIC ANEMIA

Red blood cells from children and adults normally circulate for 100 to 120 days. Erythrocyte survival in newborns is somewhat shorter: 70 to 90 days in term infants, 50 to 80 days in premature infants (Pearson, 1967). Hemolytic anemia is the clinical consequence of RBC abnormalities leading to shorter than normal erythrocyte survival (Table 86–6). The precise mechanism of cell destruction is not known, although membrane deformability is thought to be an important determinant (LaCelle, 1970). Erythrocytes are 7 to 8 μm wide, whereas the vascular diameter in some areas of the microcirculation may be less than 3 μm. Consequently, RBCs must deform their membranes and intracellular contents in order to pass through these narrow channels. This is no problem for normal RBCs. Abnormalities in RBC metabolism,

TABLE 86–6. Hemolytic Anemia During the Newborn Period

Immune
  Isoimmune: Rh and ABO incompatibility
  Maternal immune disease: autoimmune hemolytic anemia, systemic lupus erythematosus
  Drug induced: penicillin

Acquired RBC disorders
  Infection: CMV, toxoplasmosis, syphilis, bacterial sepsis
  Disseminated and localized intravascular coagulation, respiratory distress syndrome

Hereditary RBC disorders
  Membrane defects: hereditary spherocytosis, hereditary elliptocytosis
  Enzyme abnormalities: G6PD, pyruvate kinase
  Hemoglobinopathies: alpha-thalassemia syndromes, gamma/beta-thalassemia

hemoglobin, or cell shape, however, all lead to decreased RBC membrane deformability. The consequence of this decreased membrane flexibility is RBC sequestration and removal by reticuloendothelial cells of the spleen and liver.

In older infants and children, the usual response to increased RBC destruction is enhanced erythropoiesis, and there may be little or no anemia if the rate of production matches the accelerated rate of destruction. In these cases of well-compensated hemolysis, the major manifestations are due to increased erythrocyte destruction (hyperbilirubinemia) and augmented erythropoiesis (reticulocytosis). During the early neonatal period, however, increased oxygen-carrying capacity of blood (see Physiologic Anemia of Infancy) may obviate any compensatory erythropoietic activity in cases of mild hemolysis. Consequently, hyperbilirubinemia in excess of normal neonatal levels may be the only apparent manifestation of hemolysis. In most cases of significant hemolysis, however, some degree of reticulocytosis is usually present. The degree of hyperbilirubinemia and reticulocytosis obviously must be interpreted in terms of values appropriate for gestational and post-gestational age.

THERAPEUTIC CONSIDERATIONS FOR INFANTS WITH HEMOLYTIC DISEASE

As for older children and adults, the general therapeutic principles for newborns with hemolytic disease include maintenance of normal oxygen delivery (adequate levels of circulating hemoglobin) and rectification of causative hemolytic factors (treatment of infection, removal of hemolytic drugs). An additional important therapeutic consideration is prevention of kernicterus. This condition is a clinical consequence of increased unconjugated bilirubin levels, transport of "free" bilirubin (not bound to albumin) across the blood-brain barrier, and bilirubin-staining of the cerebellum and basal ganglia. The molecular explanation for bilirubin toxicity in neural tissue is not understood. Kernicterus generally does not occur at bilirubin levels less than 20 mg/dl, although numerous factors modify this (acidosis, low serum albumin, prematurity), and serious problems can occur at lower bilirubin concentrations. It should be noted, however, that hyperbilirubinemia is not a problem for erythroblastotic fetuses, since bilirubin is effectively cleared by the placenta and maternal liver. Since normal infant bilirubin levels may reach 12 to 15 mg/dl, the increased bilirubin load due to hemoglobin degradation (1 g hemoglobin = 34 mg bilirubin) may further aggravate the "physiologic" hyperbilirubinemia. Clinical features of kernicterus include lethargy, poor feeding, loss of Moro reflex, high-pitched crying, and spasms leading to opisthotonos. Once these clinical signs of kernicterus appear, over 75 per cent of affected infants die. Surviving infants have problems ranging from moderate hearing loss to spastic diplegia, choreoathetosis, and mental retardation. Thus, to prevent kernicterus, one should attempt to keep bilirubin levels reduced. This is accomplished by two different procedures: exchange transfusion and phototherapy.

Exchange transfusion is an effective means of reducing serum bilirubin concentration and removing potential sources of bilirubin (i.e., RBCs). The usual two-volume exchange transfusion effectively removes 85 per cent of circulating RBCs, although the resultant serum bilirubin decrease is less than expected from the removed blood volume. This discrepancy reflects that bilirubin is distributed in both extracellular fluid and intracellular compartments. During exchange transfusion, bilirubin rapidly equilibrates between blood and interstitial fluids, but there is a much slower bilirubin redistribution between tissues and extracellular fluid. Consequently, there commonly is a "rebound" increase in bilirubin within 30 to 60 minutes after an exchange transfusion. Exchange transfusion is much more effective for removing "potential bilirubin" than for lowering the actual serum bilirubin concentration, and, thus, it is important to consider early exchange transfusion for those neonatal conditions in which persistent RBC destruction is likely (i.e., hemolysis due to Rh incompatibility).

Phototherapy (see Part XIII). This therapy is based on the principle that light (450 to 460 nm) and oxygen convert bilirubin to water-soluble degradation products that are excreted in bile and urine. These photodegradation products are relatively nontoxic and do not cause or influence the development of kernicterus. Occasional mild complications of phototherapy include transient bronze skin discoloration, skin rashes, and frequent loose stools. The rate of light-induced bilirubin oxidation is relatively slow, and thus the value of this procedure is limited to conditions associated with mild hyperbilirubinemia. It has proved particularly effective in the hyperbilirubinemia of prematurity, in mild cases of ABO incompatibility, and as an adjuvant procedure following exchange transfusions. It should not be used as the initial treatment for marked hyperbilirubinemia or when significant RBC destruction is likely. Also, once phototherapy is instituted, it is necessary to monitor the serum bilirubin concentration closely, because photo-oxidation nullifies the use of "jaundice" as a clinical sign of hyperbilirubinemia.

Tin-protoporphyrin. The enzyme heme oxygenase catalyzes a critical reaction in the degradation of heme to bilirubin. It has been observed that tin (Sn)-protoporphyrin, a synthetic metalloporphyrin, inhibits heme oxygenase and decreases bilirubin levels in animals and humans (Kappas et al., 1988). The use of Sn-protoporphyrin remains experimental but, in the future, this may provide a chemical means of preventing hyperbilirubinemia in hemolytic states (see ABO Hemolysis).

IMMUNE HEMOLYSIS

The most common cause of neonatal hemolysis is transplacental passage of maternal antibodies that injure fetal erythrocytes. Maternal antibodies generally are directed against specific antigens on fetal RBCs, and thus hemolysis occurs only in the fetus. Previously this process was referred to as isoimmune hemolysis, but currently the preferred terminology is alloimmune hemolysis. Occasionally, autoimmune maternal antibodies produce hemolysis in both mother and newborn.

Rh Hemolytic Disease (Erythroblastosis Fetalis). The role of the Rh antibody in classic erythroblastosis fetalis was first elucidated in 1941 by Levine and Katzin. It is now recognized that the Rh antigen is a large protein molecule with several antigenic sites and that each of these antigens reflects a specific chemical or structural protein characteristic. There are several recognized Rh antigens (C, c, D, E, e), each of which is detected by specific antibodies. The most important of these is the D antigen, and RBCs possessing this antigen are Rh-positive. The symbol "d" (used to denote the absence of D, or Rh-negative) is not a specific antigen, since no anti-d serum has been identified. Proteins are produced under the direction of paired chromosomes, and thus red blood cell Rh proteins have two determinants of each antigen (CC, cc, or Cc; DD, dd, or Dd; and EE, ee, or Ee). Individuals with DD or dD are considered Rh-positive, whereas those with dd are Rh-negative. The frequency of the Rh-negative genotype varies in different racial groups. It is high in whites (15 per cent), lower in American blacks (5 per cent), and virtually nonexistent in Orientals. The frequency of Rh-incompatible matings in Caucasians is relatively high (85 per cent Rh-positive × 15 per cent Rh-negative = 12.5 per cent, or one of every eight matings).

The pathophysiology of alloimmune hemolysis due to Rh incompatibility includes the following: (1) an Rh-negative mother, (2) an Rh-positive fetus, (3) leakage of fetal RBCs into maternal circulation, (4) maternal sensitization to D antigen on fetal RBCs, (5) production and transplacental passage of maternal anti-D antibodies into fetal circulation, (6) attachment of maternal antibodies to Rh-positive fetal RBCs, and (7) destruction of antibody-coated fetal RBCs. Rh hemolytic disease is rare (1 per cent) during the first pregnancy involving an Rh-positive fetus, but the likelihood of having an affected infant increases with each subsequent pregnancy. The first pregnancy generally is characterized by maternal sensitization to fetal RBCs. Small volumes of fetal RBCs enter the maternal circulation throughout gestation, although the major fetomaternal bleeding responsible for sensitization occurs during delivery (Zipursky et al., 1963) (see discussion of prevention of Rh sensitization further on). When significant hemolysis occurs in the first pregnancy, this is usually ascribable to prior maternal exposure to Rh-positive RBCs resulting in primary immunization, as occurs after obstetric mishaps leading to fetomaternal transfusion (e.g., abortion, ruptured tubal pregnancy) or mismatched blood transfusion. Small booster fetomaternal transfusions during the current pregnancy provoke rises in antibody concentration to levels sufficient to cause hemolysis in the fetus.

The initial antibody response in the mother consists of the production of IgM anti-D, a saline agglutinin, followed by IgG anti-D, which is best demonstrated by the indirect antiglobulin (Coombs) reaction. Since only the IgG antibody crosses the placenta, quantification of this antibody provides the best serologic measure of clinically significant maternal sensitization.

In the fetus, absorption of this antibody by Rh-positive red cells results in a positive direct antiglobulin (Coombs) reaction. Depending on the amount of anti-D absorbed, varying degrees of fetal hemolysis occur, leading to anemia, hepatosplenomegaly (due to marked extramedullary hematopoiesis), and increased bilirubin formation. In utero, bilirubin is removed by transfer across the placenta into the maternal circulation, and therefore hyperbilirubinemia is not a problem until after delivery, when levels in the fetal blood may rise sharply. The main threat to the fetus is severe anemia leading to hydrops fetalis and intrauterine death. The spectrum of severity has been classified from mild through moderate to severe (Bowman, 1975), as illustrated in Table 86–7.

Mild Hemolytic Disease. Approximately 50 per cent of affected infants with a positive direct Coombs test have a minimal hemolysis associated with no anemia (cord blood hemoglobin greater than 14 g/dl) and minimal hyperbilirubinemia (cord blood bilirubin less than 4 mg/dl). Aside from early phototherapy, these newborns generally do not require specific therapy unless the postnatal bilirubin rise is greater than expected (Fig. 86–4). Infants who do not become sufficiently jaundiced to require exchange transfusion are at risk of developing severe anemia associated with a low reticulocyte count, around 3 to 6 weeks of age. It is therefore important to carefully monitor hemoglobin levels after discharge in the event simple transfusion (of Rh-negative packed red cells) is needed.

Moderate Hemolytic Disease. In approximately 25 per cent of affected infants there is significant hemolysis, associated with mild to moderate anemia (cord blood hemoglobin less than 14 g/dl) and increased cord blood bilirubin levels (greater than 4 mg/dl). The peripheral blood of moderately affected newborns may contain numerous nucleated RBCs, decreased numbers of platelets, and, occasionally, a leukemoid reaction with marked numbers of immature granulocytes. The etiology of thrombocytopenia is not understood, but it is unlikely that it is due to an immune reaction, since platelets lack the Rh antigen. Similarly, the cause of leukemoid reactions is not defined, although these rarely may be of such a magnitude as to be confused with congenital leukemia. Infants with leukemoid reactions also may exhibit marked hepatosplenomegaly, a consequence of several factors: extramedullary hematopoiesis, sequestration of antibody-coated RBCs, and reticuloendothelial hyperplasia. This group of newborns will develop kernicterus if not treated, and thus early exchange transfusion with type-specific Rh-negative fresh RBCs is mandatory. There is minimal morbidity and mortality from this procedure, and clearly it has been responsible for the favorable outcome of this group of infants with moderate isoimmune hemolysis. It is not uncommon for newborns treated with exchange transfu-

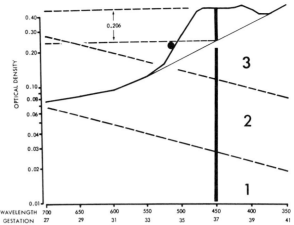

FIGURE 86–4. *This composite graph depicts how spectrophotometric estimation of amniotic fluid bilirubin levels can be utilized as an indicator of fetal jeopardy from hemolytic disease. (1) The optical density of amniotic fluid (ordinate) is measured from 700 to 350 nm (abscissa—top). This absorption curve is depicted as the heavy solid line. (2) The contribution of bilirubin to this absorption is then calculated by subtracting the optical density of the projected baseline (fine solid line) from the measured optical density at 450 nm. In this case, the calculated value is 0.206. (3) This calculated contribution of bilirubin is then plotted as a function of gestational age (abscissa—bottom). In this particular patient, the gestational age of 34.5 weeks and the bilirubin absorption of 0.206 determine the point indicated by the solid dot. (4) The dashed lines demarcate three zones (1, 2, and 3): Zone 1 indicates an Rh negative infant or very mild hemolytic disease. Zone 2 indicates mild to moderate hemolytic disease. Zone 3 represents severe hemolytic disease with impending fetal death. Since the bilirubin concentration of amniotic fluid decreases with gestational age, the absolute optical density that places a fetus in zone 3 decreases as the length of gestation increases. In the case depicted here, an absorption of 0.206 at 34.5 weeks' gestation indicated this fetus was in zone 3 and thus seriously at risk. (From Bowman, J. M., and Pollock, J. M.: Amniotic fluid spectrophotometry and early delivery in the management of erythroblastosis fetalis. Pediatrics 35:815, 1965. Reproduced with permission from Pediatrics.)*

sion to demonstrate a lower than normal hemoglobin at the nadir of their physiologic anemia. This may reflect the decreased p50 and enhanced oxygen delivery of adult RBCs used for the exchange process.

Severe Hemolytic Disease. A significant fraction of remaining affected infants (25 per cent) have more severe disease and are either stillborn or hydropic at birth. The pathophysiology of hydrops fetalis, originally attributed to high-output cardiac failure secondary to severe anemia, is not clear. Blood volume and intravascular pressure studies of Phibbs and colleagues (1974, 1976) do not support cardiac failure in the majority of cases. Two other consequences of anemia have been proposed by these workers as contributing to the edema of hydrops: (1) low colloid osmotic pressure due to hypoalbuminemia (possibly a consequence of hepatic dysfunction due to severe extramedullary hematopoiesis); and (2) a capillary leak syndrome secondary to tissue hypoxia. Therapy for these seriously affected fetuses is directed at prevention of severe anemia and death. In order to accomplish this, it is first necessary to identify the "severely" affected fetus and then to institute appropriate therapy.

As discussed previously, elevated maternal titers of IgG anti-D indicate maternal sensitization but do not accurately predict the severity of fetal hemolysis. A better correlation can be obtained by spectrophotometric estimation of bile pigment in amniotic fluid, as measured by the deviation

TABLE 86–7. Clinical and Laboratory Features of Immune Hemolysis Due to Rh Disease and ABO Incompatibility

	Rh DISEASE	ABO INCOMPATIBILITY
Clinical Features		
Frequency	Unusual	Common
Pallor	Marked	Minimal
Jaundice	Marked	Minimal to moderate
Hydrops	Common	Rare
Hepatosplenomegaly	Marked	Minimal
Laboratory Features		
Blood type		O
Mother	Rh(−)	A or B
Infant	Rh(+)	Minimal
Anemia	Marked	Frequently negative
Direct Coombs test	Positive	Usually positive
Indirect Coombs test	Positive	Variable
Hyperbilirubinemia	Marked	Spherocytes
RBC morphology	Nucleated RBCs	

in optical density at 450 nm (Fig. 86–4). (Chemical measurement is unreliable because the concentration of bilirubin in amniotic fluid of affected infants is usually under 1 mg/dl). Plotting the "delta O.D. 450 nm" against fetal age, Liley (1961) demonstrated a good correlation with the severity of fetal hemolysis during the third trimester, as illustrated in Figure 86–4. The trend of two or more values was subsequently shown to be a more reliable predictor of severity of fetal disease. Since amniocentesis may provoke fetomaternal hemorrhage with stimulation of maternal antibody production, it should be reserved for pregnancies in which the probability of severe fetal hemolysis is great, as suggested by an adverse outcome of previous pregnancy and/or an anti-D titer exceeding the so-called critical level for that laboratory (usually in the range of 1:16 or 1:32 by the indirect antiglobulin method). Fetuses with amniotic fluid delta O.D. values in zone 3 or rising toward zone 3 were shown to be at great risk of intrauterine death from severe anemia and hydrops fetalis. If they were younger than 32 weeks and their lungs were not sufficiently mature to enable them to survive outside the uterus, they were given repeated intrauterine intraperitoneal transfusions, a technique first developed by Liley (1963a and b). This procedure ameliorated the anemia sufficiently to save many otherwise doomed fetuses. If hydrops fetalis was already present, however, the success rate was much lower, owing to the fact that absorption of blood from the peritoneal cavity was too slow (due to ascites) to reverse the effects of severe anemia and hypoxia.

Some fetuses are so severely affected that they are hydropic by 20 to 22 weeks. The Liley amniocentesis curves, derived from studies after 27 weeks' gestation, often failed to predict severe disease when applied at this stage of gestation (Nicolaides et al., 1986). With the development of high-resolution ultrasound, major advances in fetal diagnosis and therapy became possible. Serial ultrasound not only facilitated detection of early signs of hydrops (ascites and edema), but also enabled direct percutaneous umbilical blood sampling (PUBS; cordocentesis) for determination of red cell antigen typing and measurement of fetal hematocrit or hemoglobin levels. Although cordocentesis in severe Rh hemolytic disease was first employed successfully through the fetoscope by Rodeck and associates in 1981, it was associated with a 2 to 5 per cent mortality rate due to fetal trauma from the large size of the instrument (16 gauge). Ultrasound permitted sampling through a 22-gauge spinal needle, reducing the fetal mortality to 1 to 2 per cent. Rodeck showed that fetal hydrops did not occur until the hemoglobin of the fetus fell below 4 g/dl (or hematocrit fell below about 15 per cent). In addition to providing more precise assessment of the severity of fetal hemolysis, cordocentesis enables direct intravascular transfusion to rapidly correct severe life-threatening anemia, with prompt reversal of established hydrops in 80 to 90 per cent of cases (Grannum et al., 1988; Rodeck et al., 1984). This technique is illustrated in Figure 86–5. Depending on the age of the fetus and the severity of the anemia, most workers transfuse 15 to 100 ml of packed red cells, aiming for a post-transfusion hematocrit of approximately 35 to 45 per cent. Of interest, with transfusion-induced reversal of hydrops the serum albumin rises, supporting the role of anemia in

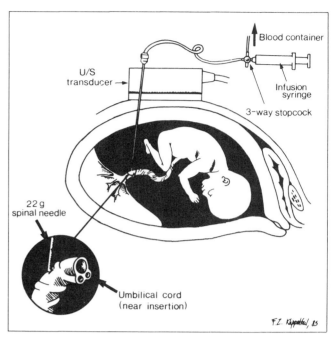

FIGURE 86–5. Diagrammatic view of in utero direct intravascular transfusion. (U/S, ultrasound.) (From Grannum, P. A., Copel, J. A., Plaxe, S. C., et al.: In utero exchange transfusion by direct intravascular injection in severe erythroblastosis fetalis. N. Engl. J. Med. 314:1431, 1986. Reprinted, by permission of the New England Journal of Medicine.)

the pathogenesis of low albumin levels. The Yale group, concerned about hypervolemia from simple transfusion, performed successful intrauterine intravascular exchange transfusions in a number of fetuses (Grannum et al., 1986). Others prefer simple transfusion because of its shorter duration, aiming for a post-transfusion hematocrit no greater than 45 per cent to avert circulatory overload.

Since hemoglobin concentration of normal fetuses rises gradually during the latter part of pregnancy, interpretation of hemoglobin results in affected fetuses requires comparison with normals for the state of gestation. Nicolaides and co-workers (1988), using data collected from over 200 fetuses from 17 to 40 weeks' gestation, established both a reference range for normal fetuses and the ranges observed in fetuses with varying degrees of hemolysis (Fig. 86–6). Expressing the degree of anemia as "hemoglobin deficit" (gram per deciliter below the normal mean hemoglobin value for age), they defined three zones of severity: I (mild): deficit less than 2 g/dl; II (moderate): deficit 2 to 7 g/dl; and III (severe, hydropic): deficit 7 to 10 g/dl. Their observation of hydrops in 32- to 34-week-old fetuses with hemoglobin concentrations as high as 6 g/dl is explainable by reference to the rising normal values with gestation.

The results of cordocentesis and intravascular transfusion are impressive and reflect the accumulated experience and skill of perinatal teams in a few tertiary referral centers. With the successful use of Rh immune globulin to prevent Rh sensitization, the dwindling numbers of severely affected fetuses who are suitable candidates for such treatment is a strong argument for referring patients to these centers.

Among infants born after intrauterine transfusions, hyperbilirubinemia (often with elevation of the conjugated fraction) is common and may require multiple exchange

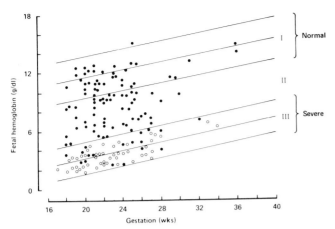

FIGURE 86–6. *Fetal hemoglobin concentration of 48 hydropic (open circles) and 106 nonhydropic (solid circles) fetuses from red cell isoimmunized pregnancies at time of first fetal blood sampling. Values are plotted on the reference range of fetal hemoglobin for gestation. The individual 95 per cent confidence intervals of the normal hemoglobin for gestation define zone I and the individual 95 per cent confidence intervals of the hemoglobin for gestation define zone III. Zone II indicates moderate anemia. (From Nicolaides, J. H., Soothill, P. W., Clewell, W. H., et al.: Fetal hemoglobin measurement in the assessment of red cell isoimmunization. Lancet 1:1073, 1988.)*

transfusions. This reflects the severity of hemolysis and its effects on the fetal liver. Anemia may be minimal or absent, along with a negative finding on the direct antiglobulin test, if recently transfused Rh-negative red cells predominate. Such infants may not require exchange transfusion.

As seen in Figure 86–7, neonatal exchange transfusion, amniocentesis, selective-early induction of delivery, and intrauterine fetal blood transfusions all have reduced the neonatal death rate from Rh incompatibility. Without question, however, the major factor responsible for the reduced death rate has been the development of Rh immune globulin to prevent maternal sensitization. Approaches toward this goal initially were based on two separate observations: (1) The bulk of fetomaternal RBC transfer (and presumably sensitization) occurs during delivery. (2) The frequency of Rh immune hemolytic disease is much lower in ABO-incompatible pregnancies (maternal RBC type O, fetal RBC type A or B). The beneficial effect of ABO incompatibility presumably is mediated by maternal alloantibodies that cause the destruction of fetal RBCs before sensitization occurs. On the basis of these observations, attempts were made to prevent maternal Rh sensitization by injection of potent anti-D serum. The success of these experiments and the later availability of a concentrated Rh immune globulin preparation led to its routine use for prevention of sensitization in all unsensitized Rh-negative pregnant women (Freda et al., 1975). Initially, it was given to the mother as a single intramuscular dose of 300 mcg within 72 hours of delivery of an Rh-positive infant. The few failures were attributed to either fetomaternal bleeding greater than 30 ml or bleeding occurring antenatally. The former should be detected by routine testing of mothers for large fetomaternal bleeding at delivery, and the dose of Rh immune globulin should be increased proportionally. The majority of the latter are preventable by routine administration of the immune globulin at 28 weeks' gestation, and also after

any event associated with an increased risk of fetomaternal hemorrhage during pregnancy (e.g., abortion, genetic amniocentesis, chorionic villus biopsy).

ABO Incompatibility. Hemolysis associated with ABO incompatibility is similar to Rh hemolytic disease in that maternal antibodies enter the fetal circulation and react with A or B antigens on the erythrocyte surface (Table 86–7). In type A and B individuals, naturally occurring anti-B and anti-A isoantibodies largely are IgM molecules that do not cross the placenta. In contrast, the isoantibodies present in type O individuals are predominantly IgG molecules (Abelson and Rawson, 1961). For this significant reason, ABO incompatibility is largely limited to type O mothers with type A or B fetus. The presence of IgG anti-A or anti-B antibodies in type O mothers also explains why hemolysis due to ABO incompatibility frequently occurs during the first pregnancy without prior "sensitization." A set-up for ABO incompatibility is present in approximately 12 per cent of pregnancies, although red blood cell–antibody reactions (i.e., positive direct Coombs test) are found in only 3 per cent of births, and less than 1 per cent of live births are associated with significant hemolysis (Kaplan et al., 1976; Zipursky et al., 1963).

The relative mildness of neonatal ABO hemolytic disease contrasts sharply with the findings in Rh incompatibility. In large part, this is because A and B antigens are present in many tissues besides RBCs; consequently, only a small fraction of anti-A or anti-B antibody that crosses the placenta actually binds to erythrocytes, the remainder being absorbed by other tissues.

Although hemolytic disease due to ABO incompatibility is clinically milder than that due to Rh disease, severe hemolysis occasionally occurs, and hydrops fetalis has been reported. In such cases it is essential to exclude other antibodies and other causes of hemolysis. In most cases, infants are minimally pale and jaundiced (Table 86–7). Hepatosplenomegaly is uncommon. Laboratory features

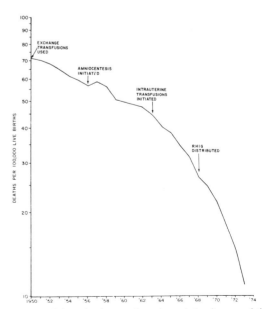

FIGURE 86–7. *Infant death rates from hemolytic disease of the newborn, United States, 1950 to 1973. (From Centers for Disease Control: Rh Hemolytic Disease Surveillance Annual Report, June 1975, with kind permission.)*

include minimal to moderate hyperbilirubinemia and, occasionally, some degree of anemia. The direct Coombs test frequently is negative, although the indirect Coombs test (neonatal serum plus type-specific adult RBCs) more commonly is positive. This paradox is related to the fact that adult RBCs, compared with neonatal erythrocytes, have more type-specific antigen on their surface (Voak and Williams, 1971). Heat-elution is the most sensitive test for anti-A or anti-B antibodies on infant red cells, but like the antiglobulin tests, it has poor predictive value for hemolysis. Recent studies of the subclass of the IgG anti-A and anti-B in maternal serum and on red cells of ABO-incompatible infants point to a possible explanation (Brouwers et al., 1988). The most common subclass is IgG2, which crosses the placenta but does not bind to Fc-receptors of phagocytic cells and therefore is incapable of causing cell lysis. This accounts for the frequent observation of positive indirect and direct Coombs tests with little or no hemolysis. On the other hand, IgG3 antibodies and to a lesser extent IgG1 antibodies, although present in lower concentrations on fetal red cells, do bind to Fc-receptors and have strong lytic activity. This seems to account for cases of hemolysis associated with a negative or only weakly positive direct antiglobulin test. The lytic activity of maternal serum, as measured in an antibody-dependent cell-mediated cytotoxicity assay (ADCC), was found by Brouwers and co-workers (1988) to be a sensitive predictor of hemolysis in the infant, particularly when used with determinations of the density of A and B antigens on cord red blood cells. The ADCC test, although not widely available, may be of value in predicting fetal involvement in the unusual group O mothers with a history of a previous severely affected infant. The peripheral blood smear is characterized by marked spherocytosis, which is thought to be due to the reduced RBC surface area that results as antibody and membrane are removed by splenic macrophages. Autoimmune hemolytic anemia in older children is associated with antibodies directed against the Rh locus, and these cases also are characterized by spherocytosis. For unknown reasons, however, spherocytes are not a prominent feature of neonatal hemolysis due to Rh incompatibility.

Hemolytic disease in ABO incompatibility is usually mild, presenting mainly with hyperbilirubinemia that is controllable by phototherapy; guidelines have been reviewed by Osborn and associates (1984). If hyperbilirubinemia is severe and not controlled by phototherapy, exchange transfusion will be necessary, using group O, Rh-compatible red cells. Recent studies have shown that tin-protoporphyrin, an inhibitor of heme catabolism to bilirubin, may help prevent hyperbilirubinemia in ABO-incompatible infants (Kappas et al., 1988).

Minor Blood Group Incompatibility. With the sharp decline in cases of hemolytic disease due to Rh incompatibility the *proportion* of cases due to other RBC antigens, both Rhesus (c, E) and non-Rhesus (Kell, Duffy, Kidd), has risen greatly from the previous estimates of 1 to 3 per cent. The pathophysiology of these disorders is similar to that of Rh and ABO incompatibility. The infrequency of minor group incompatibility is primarily a reflection of the lower antigenicity of these RBC antigens. Diagnosis of minor group incompatibility is suggested by

Coombs-positive hemolytic anemia in the absence of ABO or Rh incompatibility and a negative maternal direct Coombs test. Definitive diagnosis requires identification of the specific antibody in neonatal serum or an eluate from neonatal RBCs. This is readily accomplished by testing serum against a variety of known RBC antigens. Maternal serum should contain elevated titers of the antibody in question. With some antibodies such as Kell, antibody titer and amniocentesis findings may underestimate the severity of fetal hemolysis. Therefore, frequent ultrasound monitoring may be necessary, with fetal blood sampling in worrisome cases. Fetal blood sampling is also useful in determining whether or not a fetus of a heterozygous father has inherited the offending RBC antigen.

Immune Hemolytic Anemia Due to Maternal Disease. Maternal autoimmune hemolytic anemia (AIHA) during pregnancy may be associated with passive transfer of IgG antibody to the fetus. The degree of hemolysis in the fetus depends largely on amount and the specificity of transferred antibody. AIHA also occurs with connective tissue disorders such as lupus erythematosus and rheumatoid arthritis. In these cases, maternal antibody may not be specific for RBCs, and immune neutropenia or thrombocytopenia or both also occur (Seip, 1960). The diagnosis of neonatal hemolysis is suggested by the presence of Coombs-positive neonatal hemolytic disease, lack of set-up for Rh or ABO incompatibility, and Coombs-positive hemolysis in the mother. Treatment with prednisone (2 mg/kg/day) may reduce both maternal hemolysis and neonatal morbidity. As in other cases of neonatal hemolysis, attempts are made to prevent hyperbilirubinemia and kernicterus.

Drug-Induced Immune Hemolysis. The classic example of drug-induced immune hemolysis is seen with penicillin and appears when an antibody is directed to a complex of penicillin bound to the RBC membrane. No hemolysis occurs in the absence of penicillin, even though antibody persists in the circulation. This type of drug-mediated immune hemolysis has been reported in newborn infants. In a mother who had a penicillin antibody but who was not on penicillin, neonatal hemolysis occurred when the infant was given penicillin (Clayton et al., 1969). The Coombs test in these cases may be positive only when the test is done in the presence of penicillin. Hemolysis ceases once the drug is withdrawn.

NONIMMUNE ACQUIRED HEMOLYTIC DISEASE

Infection. Cytomegalic inclusion disease, toxoplasmosis, syphilis, and bacterial sepsis all can be associated with hemolytic anemia. In most of these conditions, some degree of thrombocytopenia also exists. Generally, there is hepatosplenomegaly. In cases of bacterial sepsis, both the direct and indirect bilirubin may be elevated. The mechanism of hemolysis is not clearly defined, but it may be related to RBC sequestration in the presence of marked reticuloendothelial hyperplasia associated with infection. Documentation of infection as the cause of hemolysis is made by the presence of other clinical and laboratory stigmata of neonatal infections. Hemolysis due to infections may be exhibited early in the neonatal period, or it can be delayed for several weeks.

Disseminated Intravascular Coagulation. This coagulation abnormality is discussed in detail elsewhere. The hemolytic component of this disorder is secondary to the deposition of fibrin within the vascular walls. When erythrocytes interact with fibrin, fragments of RBCs are broken off, producing fragile, deformed red blood cells, or schistocytes. These cells are relatively rigid and thus incapable of normal deformation within the microcirculation. The hemolytic-uremic syndrome represents a localized form of intravascular coagulation that is characterized by thrombocytopenia, renal disease, and hemolytic anemia. Hemolysis is characterized by RBC fragmentation, presumably for the aforementioned reasons.

HEREDITARY RBC DISORDERS

Membrane Defects. Several RBC membrane abnormalities are associated with hemolytic anemia, but aside from hereditary spherocytosis (HS) these disorders are relatively uncommon (Fig. 86–8).

HEREDITARY SPHEROCYTOSIS

This is an autosomal dominant disorder that becomes manifest by the presence of spherocytic RBCs. Spherocytes are characterized by a decreased membrane surface area to volume ratio. The volume (MCV) of HS red blood cells is relatively normal, and thus it is thought that spherocytes result from a decrease in membrane surface area. In fact, it has been established that HS erythrocytes lose membrane lipid during their life span. Spherocytes in vitro are susceptible to osmotic lysis (i.e., the release of hemoglobin when RBCs swell in hypotonic salt solutions). It is unlikely that this is an important hemolytic mechanism in vivo. More likely, the rigid membrane properties of spherocytes lead to splenic sequestration and hemolysis.

The clinical manifestations of HS include mild to moderate hemolysis with reticulocytosis, hyperbilirubinemia, and splenomegaly. This is usually a well-compensated process with little or no anemia. There is a neonatal history of hemolysis and hyperbilirubinemia in approximately 50 per cent of all cases (Stamey and Diamond, 1957). In over 70 per cent of patients, there is a family history of HS and either the mother or father also have the disorder. In the other 30 per cent of patients, HS is thought to be due to a new mutation. In a given family in which either the mother or father have HS, there is a 50 per cent chance that each of their children also will be affected.

The diagnosis of HS is suspected when there is laboratory evidence of hemolysis and presence of spherocytes on the peripheral blood smear. However, in contrast to HS in older children, spherocytes are seen less frequently in affected newborns. In addition, the osmotic fragility test, which is most useful for diagnosing HS in older children, has been considered to be less reliable in newborns because infant RBCs are normally more resistant to osmotic stress. Despite this, when the fresh and incubated osmotic fragility of RBCs from normal newborns and infants with HS are compared, erythrocytes from the

infants with HS clearly are osmotically more fragile (Schröter and Kahsnitz, 1983). A Coombs test and blood typing are essential in any case of spherocytosis, since the clinical and laboratory presentation of HS is similar to that seen in ABO incompatibility. Unfortunately, however, the result of the Coombs test in ABO incompatibility is occasionally negative, thus obscuring the correct diagnosis. Examination of family members for spherocytes may be useful in these cases. Alternatively, definitive diagnosis can be deferred until maternal antibody is cleared by the newborn (after 4 months). Persistence of spherocytes at this time indicates hereditary spherocytosis.

The important hemolytic role of the spleen in HS becomes manifest by the rapid decrease in bilirubin and reticulocytes following splenectomy. Spherocytes persist following surgery, but the survival of these cells is nearly normal once the spleen is removed. There is no question regarding the efficacy of splenectomy in reducing hemolysis in cases of HS. Nevertheless, surgery is usually deferred until the child is at least 5 years of age, since young splenectomized children have an increased susceptibility to overwhelming pneumococcal and H. influenzae sepsis (Diamond, 1969). The most important aspect of therapy in the neonatal period is prevention of kernicterus (by phototherapy, exchange transfusion). Packed RBCs should be given if there is significant anemia without hyperbilirubinemia.

HEREDITARY ELLIPTOCYTOSIS

The clinical course of hereditary elliptocytosis (HE) is extremely heterogenous. Most commonly, it is a morphologic abnormality without anemia; rarely, it is associated with a severe hemolytic process with marked dyserythropoiesis. During the newborn period, HE occasionally may cause hemolytic anemia and the peripheral smear may resemble that seen in patients with pyropoikilocytosis, with many budding erythrocytic forms (Austin and Desforges, 1969). In some infants, the characteristic elliptocytes may not appear until they are several months of age, at which time hemolysis may completely cease. In other infants, the rate of hemolysis continues with marked abnormalities in RBC morphology and an increased osmotic fragility of circulating RBCs. There is no easy test to distinguish those infants who will go on to have a mild course of nonhemolytic HE from those who will have significant hemolysis.

RBC ENZYME ABNORMALITIES

Hemolysis has been reported in association with several erythrocyte enzyme deficiencies, but only two of these are of major clinical significance: glucose-6-phosphate dehydrogenase (G6PD) deficiency and pyruvate kinase (PK) deficiency. An extensive review of all hereditary enzymopathies recently has been published in a monograph on congenital hemolytic disorders (Mentzer and Glader, 1989).

GLUCOSE-6-PHOSPHATE DEHYDROGENASE DEFICIENCY

This RBC enzyme deficiency affects millions of people throughout the world, with the highest frequency occurring

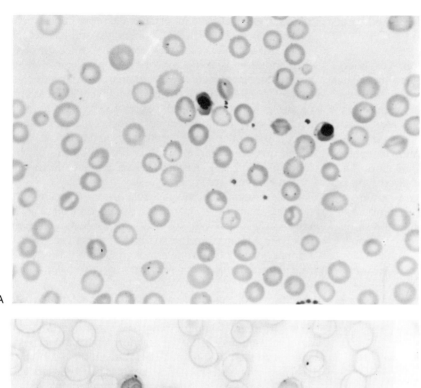

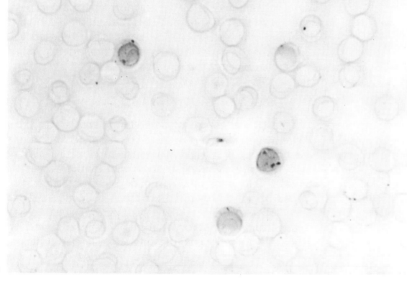

FIGURE 86–8. A, *Hypochromic-microcytic RBCs secondary to chronic fetal blood loss.* B, *Fetal RBCs in the maternal blood after a feto-maternal hemorrhage (acid-elution technique).*

in Mediterranean countries, Africa, and China. Approximately 10 per cent of blacks in the United States are G6PD deficient. Generally, this is a mild hemolytic disorder, although it can cause life-threatening anemia in certain individuals. Hemolysis occurs because enzyme-deficient RBCs are unable to defend against the external oxidant stresses associated with infection and the administration of certain drugs (Fig. 86–9). Generation of hydrogen peroxide near or within RBCs is the common denominator of all oxidants, and the intracellular accumulation of peroxide leads to an oxidative assault on the RBC membrane, enzymes, and hemoglobin. The oxidant attack on hemoglobin results in globin degradation (Heinz bodies), and this in turn produces membrane injury leading to decreased deformability and hemolysis. Normal RBCs contain reduced glutathione (GSH), a sulfhydryl-containing tripeptide that functions as an intracellular buffer that degrades peroxide and protects other cell proteins from oxidant injury. In G6PD-deficient RBCs, there is a limited capacity to sustain adequate levels of

GSH, and thus these cells are vulnerable to oxidant injury and hemolysis.

The severity of hemolysis in G6PD deficiency is related to the individual's racial origin and sex.

Race. The defect in G6PD-deficient black individuals is due to enzyme instability in old RBC, such that hemolysis is self-limited, affecting only the older erythrocytes. In contrast, in whites and Asians with G6PD deficiency, all RBCs are enzyme deficient and hemolysis often is severe. Rare cases of death due to erythrocyte G6PD deficiency have been reported in caucasians and asians. Favism is an idiopathic reaction resulting in massive and rapid hemolysis of G6PD-deficient RBCs after eating or inhaling pollen of the fava bean. The mechanism of this reaction is unknown. Favism is seen in caucasians and asians, but not in blacks with G6PD deficiency.

Sex. G6PD deficiency is a sex-linked disorder that causes hemolysis primarily in males. Females are variably

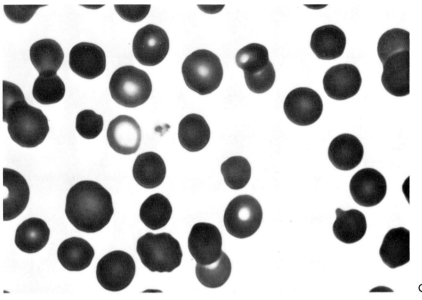

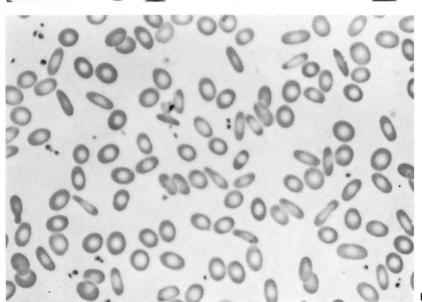

FIGURE 86–8 Continued. *C, Hereditary sphe-rocytosis. D, Hereditary elliptocytosis.*
Illustration continued on following page

affected, since they possess one normal X chromosome in addition to the X chromosome bearing the G6PD-deficient gene. In accord with the Lyon hypothesis, however, only one X chromosome is active in a given cell line, since the other chromosome is randomly inactivated early in embryonic life (Lyon, 1961). As a consequence of this factor, G6PD-deficient females are affected to the extent that they have lyophilized to the abnormal chromosome. A female with 50 per cent of normal G6PD activity has 50 per cent normal RBCs and 50 per cent G6PD-deficient cells. The deficient cells are as vulnerable to hemolysis as are deficient male RBCs.

The diagnosis of G6PD deficiency is suggested by Coombs-negative hemolytic anemia associated with drugs or infection. Cells that look as if a "bite" had been taken (due to splenic removal of Heinz bodies) occasionally are seen on the routine peripheral blood smear. Supravital stains of the peripheral blood (brilliant cresyl blue) may reveal Heinz bodies during hemolytic episodes. The specific diagnosis of G6PD deficiency can be made using a screening kit although it is the authors' policy to confirm

any enzyme abnormality with a specific quantitative test. Unfortunately, however, false negative results for G6PD deficiency are common with all tests, particularly during acute hemolytic episodes. In some cases it is necessary to wait until the hemolytic crisis is over and re-evaluate the patient when his or her RBC mass has been repopulated with cells of all ages (approximately 8 to 12 weeks).

Hemolysis due to G6PD deficiency is well documented in the newborn period. The usual causal factors (drugs and infection) can be responsible, although in many cases there is no obvious oxidant threat. It is generally agreed that term black infants with G6PD deficiency exhibit no increased incidence or severity of hemolysis and hyper-bilirubinemia (O'Flynn and Hsia, 1963). In premature black infants with G6PD deficiency, however, hyperbili-rubinemia has been reported, but significant hemolysis is rare (Eshaghpour et al., 1967). Severe hemolysis and hyperbilirubinemia are seen only in caucasians and asians with G6PD deficiency. In one study from Greece (Doxiadis and Valaes, 1964), approximately 30 per cent of all exchange transfusions for hyperbilirubinemia were done

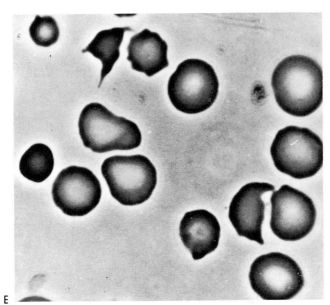

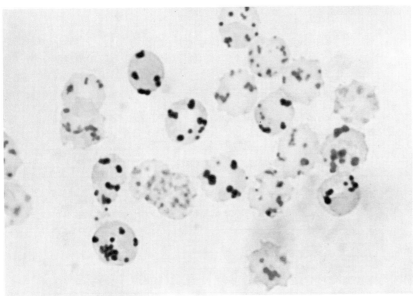

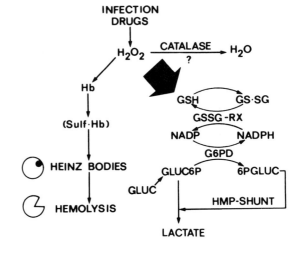

FIGURE 86–8 Continued. E, G6PD-deficient RBCs during acute hemolytic episode. F, Heinz bodies in patient with G6PD deficient hemolysis (stained with supravital dye).

FIGURE 86–9. G6PD hemolysis—pathophysiology.

in G6PD-deficient infants with no evidence of isoimmune hemolytic anemia.

Therapy for neonatal hemolysis due to G6PD deficiency is as follows: (1) Prevent kernicterus by managing hyperbilirubinemia with phototherapy or exchange transfusion or both. (2) Replace RBCs if there is significant anemia. Transfused cells will survive normally. (3) Attempt to remove all potential oxidants. Treat infections and avoid all possible offending drugs. In the absence of hemolysis, no specific therapy is required.

CASE 86-2 (MENTZER AND COLLIER, 1975)

A male infant weighing 2722 g was born at 38 weeks' gestation to a 30-year-old Chinese, gravida 3, para 1, aborta 1, mother. Apgar score at birth was 1. Despite intensive resuscitative measures, the infant died after 2 hours, never having established spontaneous respirations. Hemoglobin was 9.8 g/100 ml, and the WBC count was 7200. There was marked polychromatophilia (reticulocytosis), and numerous nucleated RBCs were seen in the peripheral smear. The infant's blood type was AB-positive, mother's blood type was B-positive, and the Coombs test (direct and indirect) was negative. Hemoglobin electrophoresis revealed 52 per cent hemoglobin F, 45 per cent hemoglobin A, and no evidence of Bart hemoglobin or hemoglobin H. Erythrocyte G6PD activity was decreased. The infant's mother also was G6PD-deficient (heterozygote). During her pregnancy, the mother had an upper respiratory infection 4 weeks prior to delivery. Ascorbic acid (250 to 500 mg/day) was administered for 2 weeks as therapy for this viral infection. On at least one occasion during the last month of pregnancy, she also ate fava beans.

Comment. Severe hemolysis and hyperbilirubinemia are not uncommon in G6PD-deficient whites and Asians. As a result of cases such as this, however, G6PD deficiency should also be considered in the differential diagnosis of hydrops fetalis. The reason for the disastrous course in this newborn is not known. Infection, ascorbic acid (an intracellular oxidant), or fava-bean exposure could have been responsible.

PYRUVATE KINASE DEFICIENCY

This autosomal recessive disorder occurs in all ethnic groups. Although its frequency is much less than that of G6PD deficiency, several hundred cases of hemolytic anemia due to this enzyme defect have been identified (Glader and Nathan, 1975; Tanaka and Paglia, 1971). Pyruvate kinase is one of two key enzymatic steps during which adenosine triphosphate (ATP) can be generated in RBCs. It is no surprise that impaired ATP production of PK-deficient cells leads to a short survival in the circulation.

Pyruvate kinase deficiency is characterized by a variable degree of anemia and hemolysis. Some children exhibit a moderate chronic hemolytic anemia (hemoglobin 8 to 10 g/100 ml, hyperbilirubinemia, reticulocytosis, and splenomegaly), whereas others may require frequent blood transfusions to maintain an adequate circulating hemoglobin. Most children with PK deficiency have neonatal jaundice, and many require exchange transfusion. Kernicterus has been reported in PK-deficient newborns.

The diagnosis of PK deficiency is considered in the presence of unexplained jaundice and a Coombs-negative hemolytic anemia not related to infection or drugs. The peripheral blood smear is nonspecific, although irregularly contracted and densely staining erythrocytes may be seen. Specific diagnosis requires a definitive enzyme assay for pyruvate kinase. Parents exhibit biochemical heterozygosity (decreased enzyme activity), but they are not anemic and there is no hemolysis.

Treatment of PK deficiency during the newborn period is symptomatic and directed at the prevention of kernicterus (phototherapy, exchange transfusion). In the presence of severe anemia, RBC transfusions should be given. Children who require frequent RBC transfusions may benefit from splenectomy, although this decision should be deferred for several years.

HEMOLYSIS DUE TO HEMOGLOBIN DISORDERS

In order to appreciate the unique hemoglobinopathies that occur in newborns, one must have an understanding of in utero hemoglobin production (Fig. 86-10). Hemoglobin is a tetrameric protein consisting of 4 hemes (iron-protoporphyrins), each of which is associated with a specific globin polypeptide chain. The heme groups in all known hemoglobins are identical, although there are major differences in the various globin chains (alpha, beta, gamma, delta, epsilon, and zeta). Most functional hemoglobins produced beyond early embryonic life consist of two alpha chains and two non-alpha globin chains.

Gower 1 (zeta 2, epsilon 2) is the earliest detectable embryonic hemoglobin. Currently, it is thought that zeta chains are the embryonic equivalent of alpha chains.

Gower 2 (alpha 2, epsilon 2) is another embryonic hemoglobin present in early fetal life.

Hemoglobin Portland (zeta 2, gamma 2) is the embryonic equivalent of fetal hemoglobin.

Fetal hemoglobin (alpha 2, gamma 2) accounts for 90 to 95 per cent of all hemoglobin production, and thus it is the major hemoglobin of fetal life. This maximal synthetic rate decreases after 35 weeks' gestation, and at birth fetal hemoglobin accounts for 50 to 60 per cent of hemoglobin production. This rate continues to decrease, and at 3 months of age only 5 per cent of synthesis is due to fetal hemoglobin (Fig. 86-11).

Hemoglobin A is the major extrauterine hemoglobin. At 20 weeks' gestation, Hgb A accounts for 5 to 10 per cent of hemoglobin synthesis, and this increases to 35 to 50 per cent of new hemoglobin production at birth.

The hemoglobin composition of cord blood is a reflec-

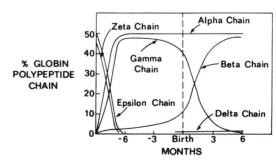

FIGURE 86-10. Fetal and neonatal hemoglobin production.

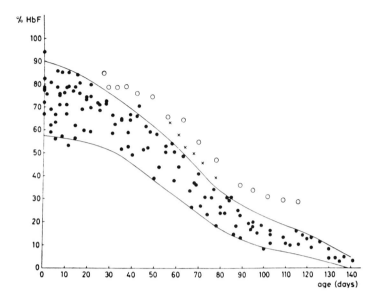

FIGURE 86–11. *Decreasing concentration of fetal hemoglobin after birth. (Garby, L., Sjölin, S., and Vuille, J. C.: Studies of erythro-kinetics in infancy. II. The relative rate of synthesis of haemoglobin F and haemoglobin A during the first months of life. Acta Paediatr. 51:245, 1962.)*

tion of past and present synthesis (Fig. 86–12). The concentration of hemoglobin F is 60 to 85 per cent, and the remaining 15 to 40 per cent is due to hemoglobin A. Trace amounts of other hemoglobins are also present in cord blood. Hemoglobin A_2 is a minor hemoglobin (less than 3 per cent of total hemoglobin in children and adults), and it may be present in small concentrations in cord blood. Bart hemoglobin is a tetramer of gamma chains (gamma 4) that is increased in alpha thalassemic disorders (see following discussion). Normal cord blood contains less than 1 per cent Bart hemoglobin.

Hemolysis is associated with quantitative and qualitative hemoglobin defects. Qualitative disorders are due to the production of abnormal globin chains (sickle cell disease). Quantitative disorders are due to decreased synthesis of normal globin chains (thalassemia syndromes). Hemoglobinopathies related to beta-chain abnormalities are usually not clinically apparent in the neonatal period. On the other hand, gamma-chain abnormalities may be clinically manifest in newborns and then disappear as infants get older and beta-chain synthesis increases. Alpha-chain disorders are seen in both infants and children.

THALASSEMIA SYNDROMES

This group of autosomal recessive disorders is a result of decreased synthesis of normal hemoglobin polypeptides. Decreased hemoglobin production leads to anemia characterized by small RBCs (microcytes) containing less hemoglobin per cell (hypochromia). An associated hemolytic component aggravates the magnitude of anemia. Hemolysis is a consequence of continued synthesis of the remaining globin chains (e.g., decreased beta-chain pro-

duction in beta thalassemia is associated with alpha-chain accumulation in developing RBCs). The excess of unbalanced globin chains interacts to form alpha globin chain aggregates, tetramers of beta globin chains (hemoglobin H) and tetramers of alpha globin chains (Bart's hemoglobin). These non-alpha globin chains are unstable and tend to precipitate and produce cell membrane injury.

Alpha Thalassemia. This form of thalassemia is seen worldwide with a particularly high incidence in Asia and Africa, although its manifestation is milder in blacks than in Asians. Defects in alpha-chain production are apparent at birth, since alpha chains constitute half the globin moiety of fetal hemoglobin. In the absence of alpha chains, gamma-chain tetramers (Bart hemoglobin) are formed. Severity of the alpha-chain defect is proportional to the cord blood content of Bart hemoglobin. The clinical and laboratory signs of alpha thalassemia are best understood if one accepts the theory that four genes (two from each parent) regulate the normal production of alpha polypeptide chains (Table 86–8).

Silent Carrier State. These individuals lack one of the four genetic loci regulating alpha-chain production. There are no clinical or hematologic abnormalities. Cord blood contains a slightly increased level of Bart hemoglobin (1 to 2 per cent).

Alpha Thalassemia Trait. Deficiency of two determinants of alpha-chain production results in a mild hypochromic microcytic anemia. There is no significant hemolysis or reticulocytosis. No therapy is required. In older children, the diagnosis is made by excluding iron deficiency, beta-thalassemia trait, and other causes of hypochromic microcytic anemia. In affected newborns, alpha-thalassemia trait is manifested by an MCV (less than 95) that is decreased compared with that of normal infants (100 to 120) (Schmaier et al., 1973). The content of Bart hemoglobin in cord blood is increased (5 to 6 per cent).

Hemoglobin H Disease. This disorder results from a deficiency of three determinants of alpha-chain production. One parent has alpha-thalassemia trait, whereas the other is a silent carrier. Anemia is more severe than in alpha-thalassemia trait, globin chain imbalance is greater,

	HEMOGLOBIN	GLOBIN POLYPEPTIDES	% IN CORD BLOOD
EMBRYONIC	GOWER -1	Zeta-2, Epsilon-2 ($\zeta_2\epsilon_2$)	0
	GOWER -2	Alpha-2, Epsilon-2 ($\alpha_2\epsilon_2$)	0
	PORTLAND	Zeta-2, Gamma-2 ($\zeta_2\gamma_2$)	0
FETAL	BARTS	Gamma-4 (γ_4)	<1%
	Hgb F	Alpha-2, Gamma-2 ($\alpha_2\gamma_2$)	60-85%
ADULT	Hgb A	Alpha-2, Beta-2 ($\alpha_2\beta_2$)	15-40%
	Hgb A_2	Alpha-2, Delta-2 ($\alpha_2\delta_2$)	<1%

FIGURE 86–12. *Hemoglobin composition of cord blood.*

TABLE 86–8. Alpha-Thalassemia Syndromes

		ANEMIA	HEMOLYSIS	α:β CHAIN SYNTHESIS	ABNORMAL HEMOGLOBINS	
					Cord Blood	Adult Blood
Normal	$\frac{\alpha/\alpha}{\alpha/\alpha}$	None	None	0.95–1.10	0–1% γ4	—
Silent carrier	$\frac{\alpha/—}{\alpha/\alpha}$	None	None	0.85–0.95	1–2% γ4	—
α-thalassemia trait	$\frac{—/—}{\alpha/\alpha}$	Mild Hypochromic Microcytic	None	0.72–0.82	5–6% γ4	—
Hemoglobin "H" disease	$\frac{—/—}{\alpha/—}$	Moderate Hypochromic Microcytic	Moderate	0.30–0.52	20–40% γ4 0–5% β4	20–40% β4
Homozygous α-thalassemia ("hydrops")	$\frac{—/—}{—/—}$	Severe Hypochromic Microcytic	Severe	0	70–80% γ4 15–20% β4 0–10% $\zeta_2\gamma_2$	

and hemolysis may be more intense. Bart hemoglobin accounts for 20 to 40 per cent of cord blood hemoglobin. Small amounts of hemoglobin H (β_4) also may be present. Both these tetrameric hemoglobins are readily detected on hemoglobin electrophoresis.

Homozygous Alpha Thalassemia (Hydrops). This disorder is caused by the absence of all four genetic loci for alpha-chain synthesis. Both parents have alpha-thalassemia trait. In the absence of alpha chains, cord blood contains Bart hemoglobin and hemoglobin H. In addition, small amounts of hemoglobin Portland, the embryonic form of fetal hemoglobin, can be present. (In the absence of alpha-chain production, zeta synthesis persists during fetal life.) Most affected infants are stillborn, although some may live for a few hours after birth. Death is due to severe anemia. The gamma- and beta-chain tetramers have a high oxygen affinity, which also contributes to the degree of asphyxia. These infants are hydropic at birth and thus are similar in appearance to newborns with severe erythroblastosis due to Rh incompatibility. Invariably, there is hepatosplenomegaly. The mother has a hypochromic microcytic anemia. There is no Rh or ABO incompatibility, and the Coombs test on cord blood is negative. This homozygous form of alpha thalassemia is seen only in asians. In at least two cases, homozygous alpha thalassemia has been diagnosed prenatally and the infants were delivered (at 28 and 32 weeks' gestation) when fetal distress became apparent (Beaudry et al., 1986; Bianchi et al., 1986). Following birth, both infants received red blood cell transfusions and the plan was to manage these newborns like children with beta thalassemia major or severe RBC aplasia. The ability to diagnose homozygous alpha thalassemia in utero raises several ethical questions. If prenatal diagnosis reveals that a child has homozygous alpha thalassemia, should interuterine RBC transfusions be employed? Moreover, if an infant with homozygous alpha thalassemia is born alive because of prenatal diagnosis and intrauterine red cell transfusions, should allogeneic bone marrow transplantation be considered? It is obvious that the answers to these questions are beyond the scope of this chapter.

Beta Thalassemia. This hemolytic anemia occurs throughout the world, but the incidence is particularly increased in countries surrounding the Mediterranean Sea. In the United States, it is the most common form of thalassemia seen in older caucasian children and adults.

This is not specifically a neonatal problem, because this disorder is due to decreased beta-chain production. Infants with beta thalassemia are not anemic at birth. Symptoms and signs first appear 2 or 3 months after birth, when the bulk of hemoglobin synthesis is due to beta-chain production. The heterozygous state (thalassemia minor) is characterized by a mild hypochromic microcytic anemia. This is a benign disorder that requires no specific therapy. Affected individuals have a normal life span. Conversely, homozygous beta thalassemia (thalassemia major, or Cooley anemia) is a severe hypochromic microcytic anemia associated with marked hemolysis (due to accumulation of alpha chains). Most children with this disorder have a lifelong RBC transfusion requirement. Death commonly occurs before 20 years of age, usually from complications of iron overload (iron from RBC transfusions and increased intestinal absorption). Most cases of thalassemia major are diagnosed after 3 months of age but before 1 year. A severe hemolytic anemia associated with marked hepatosplenomegaly occurs in late infancy. Hemoglobin analysis indicates that almost all hemoglobin is of the fetal type, with a small amount of hemoglobin A_2. There is virtually no hemoglobin A. It is of great importance that molecular biologic techniques now allow for prenatal diagnosis of beta thalassemia in most families at risk (Kazazian and Boehm, 1988). Rapid diagnosis is possible within a week of obtaining a chorionic villus sample (9 to 11 weeks' gestation) or cells from amniocentesis (15 to 17 weeks' gestation).

Hemoglobin E–Beta Thalassemia. Since the recent influx of Southeast Asians into the United States, a second type of thalassemia now commonly is recognized. This disorder, hemoglobin E–beta thalassemia, is the doubly heterozygous state for beta thalassemia trait and hemoglobin E. Hemoglobin E is a beta globin mutation commonly found in Southeast Asians (15 to 30 per cent of the population) where there is a single amino acid substitution on the beta chain (glutamine at the 26th position is replaced by lysine). In older children heterozygous hemoglobin E (Hgb AE) and homozygous hemoglobin E (Hgb EE) are mild, microcytic anemias similar to that seen in thalassemia trait (Hurst et al., 1983). In the patient who also has a beta thalassemia trait, however, the resultant hemoglobin E–beta thalassemia is a hemolytic anemia characterized by jaundice and splenomegaly. The degree of anemia is variable, ranging from a mild hemolytic process to a more severe disorder that requires frequent blood transfusions. It is the more severe disorder that often is indistinguishable from homozygous beta thalassemia. Hemoglobin E–beta thalassemia becomes a clinical problem in infants older than 4 months of age.

Gamma Thalassemia. The production of gamma polypeptides is regulated by four genes. The complete absence of gamma chains is incompatible with fetal life. Intermediate reduction of gamma-polypeptide synthesis may produce a mild to moderate neonatal anemia characterized by a reduced percentage of fetal hemoglobin (Stamatoyannopoulos, 1971). This type of anemia resolves when significant beta-chain synthesis begins.

CASE 86–3 (KAN ET AL., 1972)

A full-term 2300-g girl was noted to be jaundiced at 24 hours of age (bilirubin 13.7 mg). Hemoglobin was 10.4 g/100 ml, hematocrit 32 per cent, RBC count 3.8×10^6 μl, MCV 84 μ³, and MCH 27 pg. The reticulocyte count was 26 per cent, and there were 400 nucleated RBCs per 100 white cells. There was no Rh or ABO incompatibility, Coombs test was negative, iron and iron-binding capacity were normal, and there was no detectable RBC-enzyme deficiency. Hemoglobin F content was 52 per cent (normal 60 to 85 per cent), and no Bart's hemoglobin was detected. The infant was transfused with packed RBCs, and over the next few days nucleated RBCs disappeared, reticulocytes decreased, and the hematocrit remained stable. The infant's mother was hematologically normal, but her father had a hypochromic microcytic anemia that was diagnosed as beta-thalassemia trait. At several months of age, this infant was doing well, although she had a mild hypochromic microcytic anemia that clearly was due to beta-thalassemia trait.

Comment. We frequently see newborns with severe hemolytic anemia that spontaneously disappears by several months of age, thus suggesting that some unique feature of the fetal RBC is responsible for hemolysis. This case is such an example. The presence of a hypochromic microcytic anemia not related to iron deficiency (which occurs with chronic fetal blood loss) suggested one of the thalassemia disorders. Either alpha or gamma thalassemia could produce this degree of anemia. Alpha thalassemia was ruled out by the absence of Bart hemoglobin in cord blood. With special techniques to measure the synthesis of separate globin chains, it was found that this child produced decreased amounts of gamma chains (i.e., gamma-thalassemia trait). In addition, she exhibited a lower than anticipated rate of beta-chain synthesis (beta-thalassemia trait), and thus her defect is best described as beta-gamma thalassemia. Neonatal hemolytic anemia was presumably a result of increased alpha-chain accumulation in the absence of normal beta and gamma polypeptides. Hemolysis diminished as the infant got older and began to synthesize more beta chains. Her father had beta-thalassemia trait, and as the patient became older she also developed the classic laboratory evidence of heterozygous beta thalassemia.

SICKLE CELL ANEMIA

Sickle hemoglobin differs from hemoglobin A in that there is a single amino acid substitution whereby valine replaces glutamic acid as the sixth amino acid on the beta globin chain. This amino acid change itself is a reflection of a single base pair substitution in the DNA molecule at the beta-globin gene. The net result of these changes is the production of sickle hemoglobin. A unique property of hemoglobin S is that it gels at low oxygen tension and thereby distorts the cell membrane forming sickled cells. Approximately 10 per cent of all blacks in the United States are carriers of the sickle gene, and because this is an autosomal recessive disorder, one in 400 black infants has sickle cell anemia. Individuals heterozygous for this abnormality (sickle cell trait) are asymptomatic and are not anemic. Homozygotes have sickle cell anemia and suffer from all the known vaso-occlusive and infectious problems associated with this disease. During the immediate newborn period, children who are homozygous for sickle hemoglobin (i.e., destined to have sickle cell disease) have no anemia or vaso-occlusive problems because this is a beta chain abnormality. The first clinical problems due to sickle cell anemia usually appear after 4 months of age, the major problems being the hand-foot syndrome, splenic sequestration crises, and infection. The *hand-foot syndrome* is a unique bone crisis due to infarction of metacarpal and metatarsal bones, and often is the initial clinical manifestation of sickle cell anemia. This dactylitis is demonstrated by low grade fever and painful dorsal swelling of the hands and/or feet. There is no specific therapy other than fluids and analgesics. *Splenic sequestration crises* are a consequence of intrasplenic sickling, which leads to massive pooling of blood within the spleen. Immediate recognition of this disorder is critical because death due to vascular collapse is common. The cardinal manifestations are increasing severe anemia, splenomegaly, hypotension, and tachycardia. Parents of young children known to have sickle cell disease are taught how to palpate the spleen and recognize this problem. Treatment is directed at the restoration of intravascular volume with RBC transfusions. The spleen returns to normal size in a few days. However, since many children will have recurrent splenic sequestration crises, most hematologists currently recommend that splenectomy should be performed after the first episode. From the perspective of infection, it is not critical to retain the spleen because it is known that the large spleen in sickle cell patients is nonfunctional. *Infection* is another serious problem contributing to the morbidity and mortality of children with sickle cell disease. In large measure, the increased infections of young children with sickle cell disease are due to impaired splenic function. The particular infections that are most common are due to *Haemophilus influenzae* and *Streptococcus pneumoniae*. Fulminant pneumococcal sepsis is of special concern and, for this reason, once the diagnosis of sickle cell anemia is made in young infants, penicillin V prophylactic therapy should be instituted (125 mg b.i.d.). This recommendation is based on a report of a large study that examined the role of prophylactic daily penicillin given to newborns diagnosed with sickle cell anemia. In this study, there was an 8 per cent incidence of sepsis with a 25 per cent mortality rate in those infants not given penicillin (Gaston et al., 1986).

Because of the life-threatening problems that can occur in the 1st year of life, the current standard of practice is to diagnose sickle cell disease as early as possible, preferably in the newborn period. Once a child is identified as having sickle cell anemia, appropriate parental education and penicillin prophylaxis can be instituted. In many states hemoglobin identification currently is part of the overall newborn metabolic screening program. At a recent Sickle Cell Disease Consensus Conference held at the National Institutes of Health (1987), it was concluded that: (1) cord blood identification of sickle and other hemoglobinopathies can be readily accomplished using conventional hemoglobin electrophoresis in cellulose acetate at pH 8.6; (2) in those cord blood samples in which an abnormal hemoglobin is identified, a second confirming electrophoresis should be performed using citrate agar, pH 6.3; and (3) thin-layer isoelectric focusing can be used as an alternative to electrophoresis because this technique has the advantage of distinguishing abnormal hemoglobins using one test procedure. The metabisulfite "sickle prep" and sickle solubility tests are not used in newborns because of the low concentration of hemoglobin S and thereby many false negative results. Cord blood is the preferred sample for analysis although dried blood on filter paper can be used. An excellent review of the importance of neonatal screening for sickle cell anemia and the laboratory techniques utilized has been published in a supplement of *Pediatrics* (Newborn Screening, 1989).

Individuals heterozygous for the sickle gene and an additional hemoglobin abnormality may also have problems long after the newborn period (Fig. 86–13). Heterozygosity for the sickle gene and beta thalassemia (each parent must have one defect) produces sickle cell thalassemia. If one parent has hemoglobin C (another beta-chain variant) while the other carries the sickle gene, there is a 25 per cent chance that offspring will develop hemoglobin S-C disease. Both of these conditions (S-thalassemia and S-C disease) demonstrate many of the same problems seen in sickle cell anemia, although the overall course generally is milder.

Infants born to mothers with sickle cell disease present more of a neonatal problem than those destined to develop sickle cell anemia after several months of age. It is well established that maternal morbidity and mortality are increased in pregnant women with sickle cell disease, although recent studies suggest that good obstetric management can minimize these problems (Pritchard et al., 1973). Nevertheless, fetal wastage and prematurity remain

serious problems in these pregnancies. Approximately 35 per cent of all pregnancies end in early abortion, 17 per cent are associated with stillborns or neonatal deaths, and only 48 per cent result in surviving children. Furthermore, 40 per cent of all viable infants are born premature, and 15 per cent are small for gestational age. These statistics reflect the inordinate vulnerability of the placenta to sickling. The clinical problems of newborns born to mothers with sickle cell disease (SS, S-C, S-thalassemia) are directly related to their degree of prematurity. These infants have no hematologic disease, although they will be carriers of the S, C, or thalassemia gene as they begin to produce beta chains. In those cases in which the father also carries a gene for one of these hemoglobinopathies, the infant may develop hemolytic anemia at a later age.

■ HYPOPLASTIC ANEMIA

The two major causes of pure red cell aplasia in children are Diamond-Blackfan anemia (DBA) and transient erythroblastopenia of childhood (TEC).

Diamond-Blackfan Syndrome. This condition, also known as congenital hypoplastic anemia, is a consequence of impaired differentiation of developing erythroblasts. It is characterized by a lifelong anemia that usually presents in the first months of life, often at birth (Alter, 1980; Diamond and Blackfan, 1938). It is thought that this is a genetic disease because more than one family member may be affected. Often there is growth retardation or other congenital abnormalities. The diagnosis of DBA is suggested by anemia with reticulocytopenia presenting in the first 6 months of life. Moreover, red blood cells from patients with DBA have a variety of abnormal features (increased MCV, elevated fetal hemoglobin, increased activity of adenosine deaminase) and these persist throughout life independent of therapy, even when the patient is in clinical remission. The major therapeutic modalities for DBA are corticosteroids, RBC transfusions and, rarely, bone marrow transplantation. The outcome for the majority of patients with DBA who respond to steroids appears to be good. Iron overload in transfusion-dependent patients remains a serious problem, and several deaths due to hemosiderosis have occurred. There also is some concern that DBA may be a preleukemic syndrome because several cases of acute leukemia have occurred in older patients with DBA (Glader, 1987).

Transient Erythroblastopenia of Childhood. This condition is an RBC hypoplastic anemia which occurs in previously healthy children who develop pallor over a period of several weeks (Wranne, 1970). The cause of TEC is not known, although it is associated with a transient antibody-mediated suppression of normal erythropoiesis. It is not due to parvovirus infection, which is known to cause red cell aplasia in individuals with chronic hemolytic anemia. The degree of anemia is severe (3 to 6 g hgb/dl), and there is reticulocytopenia with a depletion of bone marrow erythroblasts. The platelet count often is increased while neutropenia is seen in some children (Rogers et al., 1989). This disorder occurs almost exclusively in young children (3 months to 4 years of age). Rarely, there have been cases of TEC in newborn infants, and these need to

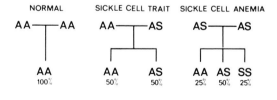

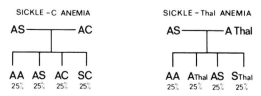

FIGURE 86–13. *Genetics of sickle cell variants.*

be distinguished from Diamond-Blackfan syndrome. In contrast to children with DBA, children with TEC have no increased incidence of congenital anomalies, and the abnormal RBC features seen in DBA are not present in TEC. The natural history of this disorder is one of spontaneous recovery over the period of a few weeks, and because most children are recognized at the nadir of their anemia, there occasionally is evidence of recovery at the time of diagnosis. A red blood cell transfusion may be indicated in children who are symptomatic from their anemia. Steroids have no role in the management of this disorder. There are no known long-term hematologic sequelae of TEC, and recurrences are very rare.

■ PHYSIOLOGIC ANEMIA OF INFANCY AND PREMATURITY

At birth, the mean hemoglobin of term infants (17.0 g/100 ml) is slightly greater than in premature infants (16.0 g/100 ml). The hemoglobin concentration in term infants subsequently decreases to a plateau at which it remains throughout the 1st year of life (Table 86–9). This is known as the *physiologic anemia of infancy*. A similar process occurs in premature infants except that hemoglobin falls more rapidly and reaches a lower concentration. This is known as the *anemia of prematurity*. After 1 year of age, there is little difference between the hemoglobin values of term and premature infants.

PHYSIOLOGIC ANEMIA OF INFANCY

The hemoglobin-oxygen saturation at birth increases from 50 per cent to 95 per cent, thus producing an increase in blood oxygen content and a cessation of erythropoiesis. Subsequently, the hemoglobin concentration begins to decrease because there is no replacement of aged RBCs as they are normally removed from the circulation. Iron from degraded RBCs is stored in tissue for future hemoglobin synthesis. The hemoglobin concentration continues to fall until a point is reached at which tissue oxygen needs are greater than oxygen delivery. This occurs sometime between 6 and 12 weeks of age, when hemoglobin has reached a level of 9.5 to 11.0 g/100 ml. Erythropoiesis resumes at this time, and iron previously stored in reticuloendothelial tissues is used for hemoglobin synthesis. These stores provide normal term infants with sufficient iron for hemoglobin synthesis until 20 weeks of age. It is unnecessary to administer iron during this period, since it does not prevent the physiologic

decrease in hemoglobin. Any iron that is given is added to stores for future use. It must be emphasized that this physiologic hemoglobin decrease does not represent "anemia" in the true sense of the term. Rather, it is a reflection of the excess oxygen delivery relative to tissue O_2 needs. There is no hematologic problem, and no therapy is required.

ANEMIA OF PREMATURITY

The magnitude of anemia in premature infants is directly related to birth weight, and in large measure it is an exaggeration of the physiologic anemia of infancy, although there are differences. One difference is that the hemoglobin nadir is reached at an earlier age (4 to 8 weeks), presumably owing to the decreased RBC survival of premature infants compared with that of term newborns (Pearson, 1967). A more significant difference is that the hemoglobin nadir in premature infants (6.5 to 9.0 g/100 ml) is lower than in term infants (9.5 to 11.0 g/100 ml), and this difference may be related to several different factors. In small part, this lower hemoglobin may be a reflection of the fact that *premature infants consume less oxygen* (ml O_2/kg/min) than do term newborns (Mestyan et al., 1964). The lower hemoglobin concentrations seen in premature infants thus may represent a balanced state of reduced oxygen-carrying capacity with decreased oxygen needs. Another partial explanation for the anemia of prematurity relates to *vitamin E deficiency*. Premature infants are endowed with significantly less vitamin E than term newborns, and this deficiency state persists for 2 to 3 months. Vitamin E is an antioxidant compound vital to the integrity of erythrocytes and, in its absence, RBCs are susceptible to lipid peroxidation and membrane injury. One clinical consequence of vitamin E deficiency is that hemolytic anemia can occur in small premature infants (weighing less than 1500 g) at 6 to 10 weeks of age (Oski and Barness, 1967; Ritchie et al., 1968). This hemolytic anemia, which is characterized by reduced vitamin E levels and increased RBC peroxide hemolysis (a measure of RBC vitamin E content), rapidly disappears following vitamin E administration. More pertinent, however, it also is now recognized that some degree of the anemia of prematurity may be due to vitamin E deficiency. This first was demonstrated by Oski and Barness (1967) who observed that premature infants given daily vitamin E (15 IU per day) had higher hemoglobin levels and lower reticulocyte levels than a control group not given the vitamin (Table 86–10). Currently it is standard practice in neonatal medicine to administer vitamin E to all premature

TABLE 86–9. Hemoglobin Changes During the 1st Year of Life

WEEK	TERM	PREMATURE (1.2–2.5 kg)	PREMATURE (<1.2 kg)
0	17.0 (14.0–20.0)	16.4 (13.5–19.0)	16.0 (13.0–18.0)
1	18.8	16.0	14.8
3	15.9	13.5	13.4
6	12.7	10.7	9.7
10	11.4	9.8	8.5
20	12.0	10.4	9.0
50	12.0	11.5	11.0
Lowest hemoglobin (mean)	10.3 (9.5–11.0)	9.0 (8.0–10.0)	7.1 (6.5–9.0)
Time of nadir	6–12 weeks	5–10 weeks	4–8 weeks

TABLE 86–10. Effect of Supplemental Vitamin E on Anemia of Prematurity*

	CONTROL	VITAMIN E (15 IU/DAY)
Birth weight	1176 ± 182 g	1278 ± 180 g
6–8 weeks of age		
Vitamin E (mg/100 ml)	0.22 ± 0.10	1.00 ± 0.25
H_2O_2 hemolysis (%)	66 ± 21	9 ± 9
Lowest Hgb (g/100 ml)	7.7 ± 1.5	9.2 ± 1.3
Highest reticulocytes (%)	6.7 ± 2.5	3.1 ± 0.7

*Premature infants were given prophylactic vitamin E (15 international units per day) and the vitamin E level, peroxide hemolysis, hemoglobin concentration, and reticulocyte count were measured after 6 to 8 weeks. These values were compared with a group of control infants not given vitamin E supplements. (Data from Oski, F. A., and Barness, L. A.: Vitamin E deficiency: A previously unrecognized cause of hemolytic anemia in the premature infant. J. Pediatr. 70:211, 1967.)

infants, but despite this practice the hemoglobin nadir in premature infants still is lower than that in term newborns.

The recent development of a sensitive radioimmune assay for measurement of erythropoietin has provided us with a better insight into the anemia of prematurity. Clearly, the most important reason for the lower hemoglobin concentration in premature infants is that the *erythropoietin response is blunted*. At birth, erythropoietin levels in premature infants are higher than in adults, but during the 2nd month of life, when the hemoglobin of the premature infant is much less than that of the normal adult, serum erythropoietin levels are the same as in adults (Brown et al., 1983). Moreover, premature infants have significantly lower erythropoietin levels compared with adults with the same hemoglobin concentration (Fig. 86–14) (Ross et al., 1989). It is not clear why the erythropoietin response in premature infants is blunted, although it may reflect neonatal immaturity, before the shift in erythropoietin production from the liver to the kidneys (Dallman, 1984). This possibility is intriguing since extrarenal production of erythropoietin (primarily hepatic) is much less responsive to hypoxia than is renal erythropoietin production.

RBC Transfusion Therapy in Premature Infants. Transfusions are usually given in the immediate neonatal period to replace blood drawn to monitor illness in sick newborns, and later on for symptoms attributable to so-called anemia of prematurity. In the first setting, most agree on the practice of giving small transfusions of packed RBCs whenever the volume of blood removed exceeds approximately 10 per cent of the estimated blood volume over a 48-hour period, aiming to maintain hemoglobin values of 12 g/100 ml or more or hematocrit values of 40 per cent or more. It is in the later period that controversy exists. Traditionally, RBCs have been recommended for symptoms presumed to reflect hypoxia (e.g., tachycardia, tachypnea, dyspnea, apneic spells, and poor feeding) (Oski and Naiman, 1982; Wardrop et al., 1978). However, studies to validate such practices have met with conflicting results. Studying the effect of transfusion on weight gain, Stockman and Clark (1984) showed a beneficial effect; this benefit could not be shown by Blank and co-workers (1984). With regard to apneic spells, beneficial effects of transfusions were reported by DeMaio and colleagues (1986), Joshi and associates (1987), and Ross and co-

workers (1989). No evidence of benefit was found by Blank and colleagues (1984) and Keyes and co-workers (1989). Presumably, differences in patient population and study design account for the differing conclusions. At present, therefore, no firm recommendation can be made about indications for transfusion in the late anemia of prematurity, and physicians must use their best judgment in individual cases. Since blood transfusions always carry some risk of transmitting disease in spite of all modern screening and precautions, one must administer them only when the perceived benefits exceed the risks. Decisions such as this may be moot if studies of recombinant human erythropoietin now in progress in prematures prove of value. In this regard, it should be noted that there are no abnormalities of erythroid progenitor cells in the anemia of prematurity and these red cell precursors demonstrate normal in vitro culture characteristics, including normal responsiveness to erythropoietin (Shannon et al., 1987).

Need for Iron Therapy. The hemoglobin concentration of premature and term infants is similar at birth, although the total body content of hemoglobin (and thereby iron) is significantly less in prematures, and iron depletion occurs earlier. Most premature infants are endowed with sufficient iron to maintain hemoglobin synthesis for 10 to 14 weeks. Iron administered to premature infants before this time does not influence the rate or level of the physiologic decrease in hemoglobin, but it is stored for later use (Schulman, 1959). After 2 months of age, however, iron supplements must be given in order to maintain hemoglo-

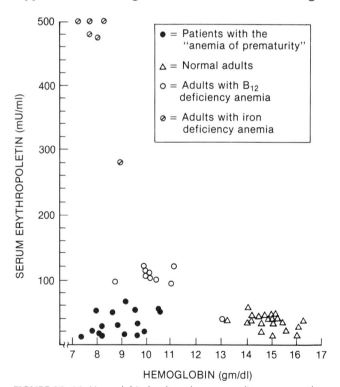

FIGURE 86–14. *Hemoglobin levels and corresponding serum erythropoietin levels are shown. Values from each of the study subjects, normal adults, adults with vitamin B_{12} deficiency anemia, and adults with iron deficiency anemia also are shown. (From Ross, M. P., Christensen, R. D., Rothstein, G., et al.: A randomized trial to develop criteria for administering erythrocyte transfusions to anemic preterm infants from 1 to 3 months of age. J. Perinatol. 9:246, 1989. Reprinted by permission of Appleton & Lange, Inc.)*

bin synthesis and to prevent iron deficiency (the late anemia of prematurity). Iron is given as ferrous sulfate (2 mg of elemental iron/kg/day for a period of 6 months). This iron requirement is satisfied by currently available iron-fortified formulas.

■ POLYCYTHEMIA

Polycythemia in older children is seen with arterial hypoxemia (cyanotic heart disease, pulmonary disorders), tumors (renal, hepatic, cerebellar), and abnormal hemoglobins (increased oxygen affinity). Polycythemia vera or primary erythrocytosis is rare. Neonatal polycythemia is usually due to either increased fetal erythropoiesis or fetal hypertransfusion. Specific conditions in each of these categories are listed in Table 86–11. In normal term infants, the most common cause is delayed cord clamping, resulting in increased placental transfusion. Although a number of conditions have been reported to cause increased fetal erythropoiesis and polycythemia, the most common are those associated with placental insufficiency and chronic intrauterine hypoxia, as manifested typically in small-for-gestational age infants. With acute intrapartum hypoxia, increased placental transfusion may account for the increased fetal RBC mass, according to animal studies by Oh and co-workers, 1975.

Blood viscosity increases at hematocrits greater than 60 per cent, and this in turn leads to a reduction of blood flow (Fig. 86–15). Oxygen transport, which is determined by hemoglobin (oxygen content) and blood flow, is maximal in the normal hematocrit range. At low hematocrits, oxygen transport is decreased because of limited oxygen capacity, whereas at higher hematocrits, decreased oxygen transport is due to reduced blood flow. These changes are further modified when the effects of normovolemia and hypervolemia are compared. Hypervolemia is advantageous, since this distends the vasculature, decreases peripheral resistance, and thereby increases blood flow and oxygen transport at any given hematocrit. These physiologic concepts are of therapeutic importance, since

TABLE 86–11. Etiology of Neonatal Polycythemia

ACTIVE (INCREASED INTRAUTERINE ERYTHROPOIESIS)	PASSIVE (SECONDARY TO ERYTHROCYTE TRANSFUSIONS)
Intrauterine hypoxia	Delayed cord clamping
Placental insufficiency	Intentional
Small-for-gestational-age infants	Unassisted delivery
Postmaturity	Maternofetal transfusion
Toxemia of pregnancy	Twin–twin transfusion
Drugs (propranolol)	
Severe maternal heart disease	
Maternal smoking	
Maternal diabetes	
Neonatal hyperthyroidism or hypothyroidism	
Congenital adrenal hyperplasia	
Chromosome abnormalities	
Trisomy 13	
Trisomy 18	
Trisomy 21 (Down syndrome)	
Hyperplastic visceromegaly (Beckwith syndrome)	
Decreased fetal erythrocyte deformability	

From Oski, F. A., and Naiman, J. L.: Hematologic Problems in the Newborn. 3rd ed. Philadelphia, W. B. Saunders Company, 1982.

most cases of polycythemia are associated with an increased blood volume (i.e., hypervolemia).

Most polycythemic infants are asymptomatic, particularly those diagnosed during routine neonatal screening. Symptoms, when present, are usually attributable to hyperviscosity and poor tissue perfusion or to associated metabolic abnormalities such as hypoglycemia and hypocalcemia. Common early symptoms include plethora, cyanosis (due to peripheral stasis), lethargy, hypotonia, poor suck and feeding, and tremulousness. Serious complications include cardiorespiratory distress (with or without congestive failure), seizures, peripheral gangrene, necrotizing enterocolitis, renal failure (occasionally due to renal vein thrombosis), and priapism. Hyperbilirubinemia is common, because the elevated RBC mass increases the production of bilirubin from catabolism of hemoglobin. This condition may lead to gallstones.

In the symptomatic infant, a venous hematocrit of 65 per cent or more (or a hemoglobin greater than 22 g/100 ml) points to the diagnosis of polycythemia. In screening apparently healthy newborns for polycythemia, however, diagnosis is complicated by the effects of a number of physiologic variables that influence "normal" values during the first 12 hours of life. These include: (1) *time of cord clamping*—immediate clamping (within 30 sec) minimizes placental transfusion; (2) *age at sampling*—values rise from birth to a peak at 2 hours, gradually falling to cord levels around 12 to 18 hours (Ramamurthy and Berlanga, 1987; Shohat et al., 1984); (3) *site of sampling*—values from blood extracted by the heelstick method exceed those from venous blood (the difference can be minimized by prewarming the heel); (4) *method of hematocrit determination*—spun values are higher than those obtained by Coulter counter, and show better correlation with blood viscosity (Villalta et al., 1988). With this in mind, screening can be standardized and simplified as follows: At birth, clamp the cord at about 30 to 45 seconds; at 4 to 6 hours of age obtain a blood sample from a warmed heelstick and perform a spun hematocrit—if this is greater than 70 per cent, repeat on a venous sample. A venous hematocrit of 65 per cent or more indicates polycythemia. Studies controlling most of these variables show that 1 to 5 per cent of newborns are polycythemic; the range largely reflects differences in altitude of the study population. Using a 65 per cent hematocrit as the criterion for diagnosis, it is not surprising that preterm infants under 34 weeks' gestation are not identified, because the range of normal rises with gestational age.

Once polycythemia is diagnosed, an attempt should be made to identify possible *causes*, as listed in Table 86–11). Polycythemia is particularly common in infants of diabetic mothers and in those with Down syndrome. However, no apparent cause is found in most cases. Studies to document the *effects* of polycythemia should include serum for bilirubin, glucose, calcium and renal function, along with other studies depending on the clinical findings.

In patients with any symptoms attributable to polycythemia, partial exchange transfusion (PET) is indicated to reduce red cell mass. Black and co-workers (1985) have observed necrotizing enterocolitis *following* PET with fresh frozen plasma (Black et al., 1985). This has not been a

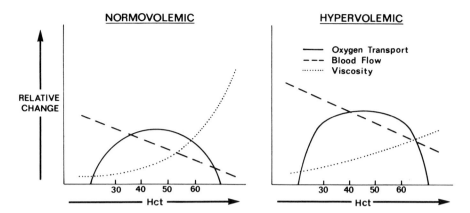

FIGURE 86–15. Effect of hematocrit on viscosity, blood flow, and oxygen transport.

problem with plasma protein fraction or 5 per cent albumin (Hein and Lathrop, 1987). For this reason, and also because these products are pasteurized and do not transmit infectious agents, they are the preferred diluents. Isotonic saline may also be used. As a further precaution against necrotizing enterocolitis, Hein advocates infusing the diluent through a peripheral vein while blood is slowly withdrawn from either a superficial vein or the umbilical vein. Practical difficulties often preclude use of small peripheral veins for withdrawing blood. If signs of congestive heart failure persist following hematocrit reduction, diuretics and digitalization are indicated. The general principles for the partial exchange have been outlined by Oski and Naiman:

EXAMPLE. Volume of blood exchanged for diluent =

$$\text{Blood volume} \times \frac{\text{Observed HcT} - \text{Desired Hct}}{\text{Observed Hct}}$$

Assume blood volume of 100 ml/kg. Desired Hct is 55 per cent, since viscosity is relatively normal at this level. Exchange should be done in syringe volumes of 3 ml blood/kg body weight.

EXAMPLE. A 3-kg dyspneic infant with an 80 per cent hematocrit requires a partial exchange.

Blood volume = 3 kg × 100 ml/kg = 300 ml

$$\frac{\text{Observed Hct} - \text{Desired Hct}}{\text{Observed Hct}} = \frac{80 - 55}{80} = 0.31$$

Therefore, volume of exchange = 300 ml × 0.31 = 93 ml.

In *asymptomatic* infants, management is less clear. Although such infants have an increased risk of late though mild neuropsychologic handicaps, prospective studies have failed to demonstrate major benefits from PET (Delaney-Black et al., 1989). We would reserve PET for those with venous hematocrits greater than 70 per cent. Since coexisting hypoglycemia is an important determinant of adverse neurologic outcome, careful monitoring and maintenance of adequate glucose levels and hydration is important.

CASE 86–6

A gravida 2, para 1, white female delivered a 2950-g male infant following a normal pregnancy, labor, and delivery. At birth, the child had an Apgar score of 6. Physical examination revealed a cyanotic infant with a grade III/VI systolic heart murmur. The liver edge was palpable 2 cm below the right costal margin, and the spleen tip was palpable. Chest radiograph revealed a markedly enlarged heart with increased pulmonary vascular markings. The hemoglobin was 26 g/100 ml, and the hematocrit was 79 per cent. There were no other hematologic abnormalities. The infant was partially exchanged with 5 per cent albumin and the post-exchange hematocrit was 62 per cent. Subsequently, the infant's color improved, the heart murmur disappeared, and there were no remaining signs of congestive heart failure.

Comment. The clinical findings in this infant were initially very suggestive of organic heart disease. All cardiac signs cleared rapidly once polycythemia was recognized and treated, thus indicating that the cardiac effects were secondary to polycythemia-induced hyperviscosity. This series of events is distinct from that seen in older children with cyanotic heart disease and polycythemia. The increased RBC mass in these infants represents a compensatory adjustment by which adequate oxygen transport is maintained in the presence of arterial hypoxemia. Consequently, phlebotomy of RBCs from these patients can produce an acute hypoxic insult. During the newborn period, however, infants with cyanotic heart disease are not polycythemic (Gatti et al., 1966), and it is extremely unlikely that neonatal polycythemia is due to underlying organic heart disease.

■ METHEMOGLOBINEMIA

Hemoglobin iron is normally in the reduced or ferrous (Fe^{++}) state. Methemoglobin is an oxidized derivative of hemoglobin in which iron is in the ferric (Fe^{+++}) state. In contrast to ferrohemoglobin, ferrihemoglobin (methemoglobin) does not complex with oxygen. Significant methemoglobinemia, therefore, reduces blood oxygen capacity and transport.

In vivo, small amounts of hemoglobin are continually being oxidized by endogenous agents including oxygen itself (auto-oxidation). Normally, however, less than 1 per cent of hemoglobin is methemoglobin, because RBCs can reduce the relatively low levels of ferrihemoglobin that are formed:

1. *NADH-methemoglobin reductase* (also known as cytochrome b_5 reductase) is the enzyme that catalyzes the reduction of methemoglobin under physiologic conditions.

Hereditary deficiency of this enzyme produces methemoglobinemia.

2. *NADPH-methemoglobin reductase* by itself is unable to reduce methemoglobin to any significant extent. Individuals lacking this enzyme do not have methemoglobinemia. In the presence of certain redox compounds (e.g., methylene blue), however, this enzyme rapidly reduces methemoglobin to ferrohemoglobin. Thus, this enzyme is important in the treatment of methemoglobinemia with methylene blue.

An increased methemoglobin concentration is caused by disruption of the delicate balance between oxidation and reduction of hemoglobin iron. Two forms of methemoglobinemia are seen: acquired or toxic methemoglobinemia (common) and congenital methemoglobinemia (rare).

Acquired methemoglobinemia occurs in normal individuals exposed to increased concentrations of chemicals that oxidize hemoglobin iron. During the first weeks of life, newborns are particularly susceptible to this form of methemoglobinemia for the following reasons: (1) Fetal hemoglobin is more readily oxidized to the ferric state than is hemoglobin A (Martin and Huisman, 1963). (2) Newborns are transiently deficient in NADH-methemoglobin reductase activity, a deficiency that persists for the first 3 or 4 months of life (Bartos and Desforges, 1966). One class of chemicals that readily oxidizes hemoglobin iron includes nitrite and nitrate compounds. Nitrite is the active agent. Nitrates are converted to nitrites by intestinal bacteria. Newborns fed with formula made from ''well water'' with an increased nitrate content occasionally develop methemoglobinemia (Comly, 1945). Also, the feeding of vegetable preparations with high levels of nitrate (cabbage, spinach, beets, and, occasionally, carrots) can produce methemoglobinemia in infants. Aniline derivatives constitute another class of chemicals that oxidizes hemoglobin, and methemoglobinemia has been caused in newborns by marking nursery diapers with aniline dyes. Drugs administered prior to delivery can also produce methemoglobinemia in mothers and newborn infants. Prilocaine, a local anesthetic used for obstetric purposes, is such an agent (Climie et al., 1967). It should be noted that most agents capable of oxidizing hemoglobin will, in fact, produce methemoglobin in normal individuals if the concentration of oxidant chemical is sufficiently high. Increased infant susceptibility to these chemicals during the first weeks of life is relative to fetal hemoglobin content and the degree of NADH-methemoglobin reductase deficiency.

Congenital methemoglobinemia can be due to inherited hemoglobin or enzyme abnormalities:

1. *Hemoglobin M disorders* are rare autosomal dominant defects brought about by amino acid substitutions in the normal globin chain. As a result of these substitutions, heme iron is more stable in the ferric than in the ferrous state. The normal methemoglobin reductive capacity cannot compensate for this instability of ferrous heme. Of the eight known M hemoglobins, three are due to alpha-chain variants, three are beta-globin variants, and two are gamma-globin chain mutations. As expected, only alpha- and gamma-chain variants are associated with neonatal methemoglobinemia and, of interest, methemoglobinemia

due to a gamma-chain variant disappears as beta-globin production increases. The two reported gamma-chain M hemoglobins are hemoglobin FM–Osaka (Hayashi et al., 1980), and hemoglobin FM–Fort Ripley (Priest et al., 1989). Heterozygotes have increased methemoglobin levels and some degree of cyanosis but otherwise are asymptomatic. No therapy is indicated (and none is possible). The homozygous state is obviously incompatible with life.

2. *NADH-methemoglobin reductase deficiency* is a rare autosomal recessive disorder in which the rate of ferrihemoglobin reduction is markedly reduced. Heterozygotes are asymptomatic and do not have methemoglobinemia unless challenged by toxic agents. Homozygote deficients generally have 15 to 40 per cent methemoglobin levels. These patients are cyanotic but otherwise asymptomatic.

The cardinal clinical manifestation of methemoglobinemia is cyanosis without evidence of cardiac or respiratory disease (normal physical examination, chest radiograph, EKG, and arterial Po_2). Cyanosis may be present at birth (suggesting hereditary methemoglobinemia) or may suddenly appear in an otherwise asymptomatic infant (suggesting toxic or acquired methemoglobinemia) (Table 86–12). Blood appears dark in color, but in contrast to deoxygenated blood, does not change in color to bright red when it is mixed with air. This is the basis of the following simple screening test for detection of methemoglobin (Harley and Celermajer, 1970):

A drop of blood is placed on filter paper and then allowed to dry while the filter paper is waved in air. Blood that is not saturated with oxygen turns red, whereas methemoglobin remains brown. This test detects levels of ferrihemoglobin greater than 10 per cent of total hemoglobin. Methemoglobin concentrations can be measured with spectrophotometric techniques in most laboratories (Evelyn and Malloy, 1938). Cyanosis is apparent at methemoglobin levels of 1.5 g/100 ml (10 per cent of total

TABLE 86–12. Approach to Infants with Cyanosis and Methemoglobinemia

Cyanosis associated with respiratory and cardiac findings
  Blood turns red when mixed with air
  Decreased arterial Po_2
  Consider pulmonary, cardiac, or CNS disease

Cyanosis with or without respiratory and cardiac findings
  Blood turns red when mixed with air
  Normal arterial Po_2
  Consider polycythemia syndromes (αOCBC)

Cyanosis without respiratory or cardiac findings
  Blood remains dark after mixing with air
  Arterial Po_2 normal
  Consider methemoglobinemia syndromes:
  1. Rapid clearing of methemoglobin following methylene blue
     a. Consider toxic methemoglobinemia (look for environmental oxidants)
     b. Consider NADH-methemoglobin reductase deficiency (perform enzyme assay)
  2. Reappearance of methemoglobinemia after initial response to methylene blue
     a. Consider NADH-methemoglobin reductase deficiency
  3. No change in methemoglobin following methylene blue
     a. Consider hemoglobin M disorders (perform hemoglobin electrophoresis)
     b. Consider associated G6PD deficiency (perform enzyme assay)

hemoglobin). Symptoms due to decreased oxygen transport are generally not apparent until 30 to 40 per cent of hemoglobin is oxidized to methemoglobin. Levels greater than 70 per cent are incompatible with life. Methemoglobinemia is not associated with anemia, hemolysis, or other hematologic abnormalities.

Newborns with greater than 15 to 20 per cent methemoglobin are treated with methylene blue (1 mg/kg as a 1 per cent solution in normal saline). The response to methylene blue is both therapeutic and diagnostic. A rapid decrease in methemoglobin occurs within 1 to 2 hours if the cause of methemoglobin is an acquired toxic agent or a deficiency of NADH-methemoglobin reductase. Failure to note improvement following the administration of methylene blue suggests one of the M hemoglobins, and this can be confirmed by hemoglobin electrophoresis. Decreased NADPH generation (i.e., G6PD deficiency) also produces a less than optimal response to methylene blue. (It should be pointed out that G6PD deficiency per se is not a cause of methemoglobinemia but rather a possible cause of poor response to methylene blue.) A reappearance of methemoglobinemia after an initial response to methylene blue suggests a deficiency of NADH-methemoglobin reductase, although the persistence of an occult oxidant must be kept in mind. The diagnosis of NADH-methemoglobin reductase deficiency requires an enzyme assay, which is done in specialized hematology laboratories. Most infants with hereditary methemoglobinemia are asymptomatic and require no therapy. In older children, therapy is occasionally given for cosmetic reasons to decrease cyanosis. This is readily accomplished with daily oral administration of ascorbic acid or methylene blue. Methylene blue produces blue urine, but this is harmless.

■ REFERENCES

Normal Erythrocyte Physiology in the Fetus and Newborn

Allen, D. W., Wyman, J., and Smith, G. A.: The oxygen equilibrium of fetal and adult hemoglobin. J. Biol. Chem. 203:81, 1953.
Bauer, C., Ludwig, I., and Ludwig, M.: Different effects of 2,3-diphosphoglycerate and adenosine triphosphate on oxygen affinity of adult and fetal hemoglobin. Life Sci. 7:1339, 1968.
Delivoria-Papadopoulos, M., Roncevic, N. P., and Oski, F. A.: Postnatal changes in oxygen transport of term, premature, and sick infants: The role of red cell 2,3-diphosphoglycerate and adult hemoglobin. Pediatr. Res. 5:235, 1971.
Finne, P. H.: Erythropoietin levels in cord blood as an indicator of intrauterine hypoxia. Acta Paediatr. Scand. 55:478, 1966.
Finne, P. H., and Halvorsen, S.: Regulation of erythropoiesis in the fetus and newborn. Arch. Dis. Child. 47:683, 1972.
Gairdner, D., Marks, J., Roscoe, J. D., and Brettell, R. O.: The fluid shift from the vascular compartment immediately after birth. Arch. Dis. Child. 33:489, 1958.
Jacobson, L. O., Marks, E. K., and Gaston, E. O.: Studies on erythropoiesis. XII. The effect of transfusion-induced polycythemia in the mother on the fetus. Blood 14:644, 1959.
Lanzkowsky, P.: The influence of maternal iron deficiency on the haemoglobin of the infant. Arch. Dis. Child. 36:205, 1961.
Oski, F. A., and Delivoria-Papadopoulos, M.: The red cell, 2,3-diphosphoglycerate, and tissue oxygen release. J. Pediatr. 77:941, 1970.
Usher, R., and Lind, J.: Blood volume of the newborn premature infant. Acta Paediatr. Scand. 54:419, 1965.
Usher, R., Shepard, M., and Lind, J.: The blood volume of the newborn infant and placental transfusion. Acta Paediatr. Scand. 52:497, 1963.

General Approach to Anemic Infants

Alter, B. E.: Methods in Haematology, Perinatal Haematology, Volume 21. Edinburgh, Churchill Livingstone, 1989.

Brady, M. T., Milam, J. D., Anderson, D. C., et al.: Use of deglycerolized red blood cells to prevent posttransfusion infection with cytomegalovirus in neonates. J. Infect. Dis. 150:334, 1984.
Demmler, G. J., Brady, M. T., Bijou, H., et al.: Posttransfusion cytomegalovirus infection in neonates; role of saline-washed red blood cells. J. Pediatr. 108:762, 1986.
Enoki, M., Goto, R., Goto, A., et al.: Graft-versus-host reaction in an extremely premature infant after repeated blood transfusions. Acta Neonatol Jpn. 21:696, 1985.
Gilbert, G. L., Hayes, K., Hudson, I. L., et al.: Prevention of transfusion-acquired cytomegalovirus infection in infants by blood filtration to remove leucocytes. Lancet 1:1228, 1989.
Naiman, J. L., Punnett, H. H., Lischner, H. W., et al.: Possible graft-versus-host reaction after intrauterine transfusion for Rh erythroblastosis fetalis. N. Engl. J. Med. 281:697, 1969.
Oh, W., and Lind, J.: Venous and capillary hematocrit in newborn infants and placental transfusion. Acta Paediatr. Scand. 55:38, 1966.
Parkman, R., Mosier, D., Umansky, I., et al.: Graft-versus-host disease after intrauterine and exchange transfusions for hemolytic disease of the newborn. N. Engl. J. Med. 209:359, 1974.
Sanders, M. R., Graeber, J. E., Vogelsang, G., et al.: Post-transfusion graft versus host disease in a premature infant without known risk factors. Pediatr. Res. 25:272A, 1989.
Schwartz, A. D.: Differential diagnosis of neonatal anemia. Paediatrician 3:107, 1974.
Yeager, A. S., Grumet, F. C., Hafleigh, E. B., et al.: Prevention of transfusion-acquired cytomegalovirus infections in newborn infants. J. Pediatr. 98:281, 1981.

Hemorrhagic Anemia

Becker, P. S., and Lux, S. E.: Hereditary spherocytosis and related disorders. Clin. Hematol. 14:15, 1985.
Cohen, F., Zuelzer, W. W., Gustafson, D. C., and Evans, M. M.: Mechanisms of isoimmunization. I. The transplacental passage of fetal erythrocytes in homo-specific pregnancies. Blood 23:621, 1964.
Danskin, F. H., and Neilson, J. P.: Twin-to-twin transfusion syndrome: What are appropriate diagnostic criteria? Am. J. Obstet. Gynecol. 161:365, 1989.
Leonard, S., and Anthony, B.: Giant cephalohematoma of newborn. Am. J. Dis. Child. 101:170, 1961.
Montague, A. C. W., and Krevans, J. R.: Transplacental hemorrhage in cesarean section. Am. J. Obstet. Gynecol. 95:1115, 1966.
Nieburg, P. I., and Stockman, J. A.: Rapid correction of anemia with partial exchange transfusion. Am. J. Dis. Child. 131:60, 1977.
Oski, F. A., and Naiman, J. L.: Hematologic Problems in the Newborn. 3rd. ed. Philadelphia, W. B. Saunders Company, 1982.
Pachman, D. J.: Massive hemorrhage in the scalp of the newborn infant. Hemorrhagic caput succedaneum. Pediatrics 29:907, 1962.
Pearson, H. A., and Diamond, L. K.: Fetomaternal transfusion. Am. J. Dis. Child. 97:267, 1959.
Philipsborn, H. F., Traisman, H. S., and Greer, D.: Rupture of the spleen: A complication of erythroblastosis fetalis. N. Engl. J. Med. 252:159, 1955.
Rausen, A. R., Seki, M., and Strauss, L.: Twin transfusion syndrome. A review of 19 cases studied at one institution. J. Pediatr. 66:613, 1965.
Raye, J. R., Gutberlet, R. L., and Stahlman, M.: Symptomatic posthemorrhagic anemia in the newborn. Pediatr. Clin. North Am. 17:401, 1970.
Shepherd, A. J., Richard, J., and Brown, J. P.: Nuchal cord as a cause of neonatal anemia. Am. J. Dis. Child. 139:71, 1985.
Woo Wang, M. Y. F., McCutcheon, E., and Desforges, J. F.: Fetomaternal hemorrhage from diagnostic transabdominal amniocentesis. Am. J. Obstet. Gynecol. 97:1123, 1967.
Zipursky, A., Pollock, J., Chown, B., and Israels, L. G.: Transplacental fetal maternal hemorrhage after placental injury during delivery or amniocentesis. Lancet 2:493, 1963.

Hemolytic Anemia

Abelson, N. M., and Rawson, A. J.: Studies of blood group antibodies. V. Fractionation of examples of anti-B, anti-A,B, anti-M, anti-P, anti-JKᵃ, anti-Leᵃ, anti-D, anti-CD, anti-K, anti-Fyᵃ, anti-S, and anti-Good. Transfusion 1:116, 1961.
Austin, R. F., and Desforges, J. F.: Hereditary elliptocytosis: An unusual presentation of hemolysis in the newborn associated with transient morphologic abnormalities. Pediatrics 44:196, 1969.

Bard, H.: The postnatal decline of hemoglobin F synthesis in normal full-term infants. J. Clin. Invest. 55:395, 1975.

Beaudry, M. A., Ferguson, D. J., Pearse, K., et al.: Survival of a hydropic infant with homozygous alpha-thalassemia-1. J. Pediatr. 108:713–716, 1986.

Bianchi, D. W., Beyer, E. C., Stark, A. R., et al.: Normal long-term survival with alpha-thalassemia. J. Pediatr. 108:716–718, 1986.

Boehm, C. D., Antonarakis, S. E., Phillips, J. A., et al.: Prenatal diagnosis using DNA polymorphisms. N. Engl. J. Med. 308:1054, 1983.

Bowman, J. M.: Rh erythroblastosis fetalis. Semin. Hematol. 12:110, 1975.

Brouwers, H. A. A., Overbeeke, M. A. M., van Ertbrugeen, I., et al.: What is the best predictor of the severity of ABO-haemolytic disease of the newborn? Lancet 2:641, 1988.

Clayton, E. M., Hyun, B. H., Palumbo, V. N., and Dean, V. M.: Penicillin induced positive Coombs' test in a newborn. Am. J. Clin. Pathol. 52:370, 1969.

Diamond, L. K.: Splenectomy in childhood and the hazard of overwhelming infection. Pediatrics 43:886, 1969.

Doxiadis, S. A., and Valaes, T.: The clinical picture of glucose-6-phosphate dehydrogenase deficiency in early infancy. Arch. Dis. Child. 39:545, 1964.

Eshaghpour, E., Oski, F. A., and Williams, M.: The relationship of erythrocyte glucose-6-phosphate dehydrogenase deficiency to hyperbilirubinemia in Negro premature infants. J. Pediatr. 70:595, 1967.

Forget, B. G., and Kan, Y. W.: Thalassemia and the genetics of hemoglobin. In Nathan, D. G., and Oski, F. A. (Eds.): Hematology of Infancy and Childhood. Philadelphia, W. B. Saunders Company, 1974, p. 450.

Freda, V. J., Gorman, J. G., Pollack, W., and Bowe, E.: Prevention of Rh hemolytic disease—10 years' clinical experience with Rh immune globulin. N. Engl. J. Med. 292:1014, 1975.

Gaston, M. H., Verter, J. I., Wood, G., et al.: Prophylaxis with oral penicillin in children with sickle cell anemia. N. Engl. J. Med. 314:1593, 1986.

Glader, B. E., and Nathan, D. G.: Haemolysis due to pyruvate kinase deficiency and other glycolytic enzymopathies. Clin. Haematol. 4:123, 1975.

Grannum, P. A., Copel, J. A., Plaxe, S. C., et al.: In utero exchange transfusion by direct intravascular injection in severe erythroblastosis fetalis. N. Engl. J. Med. 314:1431, 1986.

Grannum, P. A. T., Copel, J. A., Moya, F. R., et al.: The reversal of hydrops fetalis by intravascular transfusion in severe isoimmune fetal anemia. Am. J. Obstet. Gynecol. 158:914, 1988.

Hurst, D., Tittle, B., Kleman, K. M., et al.: Anemia and hemoglobinopathies in Southeast Asian refugee children. J. Pediatr. 102:692, 1983.

Kan, Y. W., Forget, B. G., and Nathan, D. G.: Gamma-beta thalassemia: A cause of hemolytic disease of the newborn. N. Engl. J. Med. 286:129, 1972.

Kaplan, E., Herz, F., and Scheye, E.: ABO hemolytic disease of the newborn, without hyperbilirubinemia. Am. J. Hematol. 1:279, 1976.

Kappas, A., Drummond, G. S., Manola, T., et al.: Sn-protoporphyrin use in the management of hyperbilirubinemia in term infants with direct Coombs-positive ABO incompatibility. Pediatrics 81:485, 1988.

Kazazian, H. H., and Boehm, C. D.: Molecular basis and prenatal diagnosis of beta-thalassemia. Blood 72:1107, 1988.

LaCelle, P. L.: Alteration of membrane deformability in hemolytic anemias. Semin. Hematol. 7:355, 1970.

Levine, P., Katzin, E. M., et al.: Isoimmunization in pregnancy, its possible bearing on the etiology of erythroblastosis fetalis. J.A.M.A. 116:825, 1941.

Liley, A. W.: Liquor amnii analysis in the management of pregnancy complicated by rhesus sensitization. Am. J. Obstet. Gynecol. 82:1359, 1961.

Liley, A. W.: Errors in the assessment of hemolytic disease from amniotic fluid. Am. J. Obstet. Gynecol. 86:485, 1963a.

Liley, A. W.: Intrauterine transfusion of foetus in hemolytic disease. Br. Med. J. 2:1107, 1963b.

Lyon, M. F.: Gene action in the X-chromosome of the mouse. Nature 190:372, 1961.

Mentzer, W., and Glader, B. E.: Disorders of erythrocyte metabolism. In Mentzer, W. C., and Wagner, G. M. (Eds.): The Hereditary Hemolytic Anemias. Edinburgh, Churchill Livingstone, 1989, pp. 267–318.

Mentzer, W. C., Jr., and Collier, E.: Hydrops fetalis associated with erythrocyte G-6-PD deficiency and maternal ingestion of fava beans and ascorbic acid. J. Pediatr. 86:565, 1975.

Newborn screening for sickle cell disease and other hemoglobinopathies. Pediatrics (Suppl.) 83(5):2, 1989.

Nicolaides, K. H., Rodeck, C. H., Mibashan, R. S., and Kemp, J. R.: Have Lily charts outlived their usefulness? Am. J. Obstet. Gynecol. 155:90, 1986.

Nicolaides, J. H., Soothill, P. W., Clewell, W. H., et al.: Fetal hemoglobin measurement in the assessment of red cell isoimmunization. Lancet 1:1073, 1988.

O'Flynn, M. E. D., and Hsia, D. Y.: Serum bilirubin levels and glucose-6-phosphate dehydrogenase deficiency in newborn American Negroes. J. Pediatr. 63:160, 1963.

Orkin, S. H., and Goff, S. C.: The duplicated human α-globin genes: Their relative expression as measured by RNA analysis. Cell 24:345, 1981.

Osborn, L. M., Lenarsky, C., Oakes, R. C., et al.: Phototherapy in full-term infants with hemolytic disease secondary to ABO incompatibility. Pediatrics 74:371, 1984.

Pearson, H. A.: Life-span of the fetal red blood cell. J. Pediatr. 70:166, 1967.

Phibbs, R. H., Johnson, P., and Tooley, R. H.: Cardiorespiratory status of erythroblastotic newborn infants. II. Blood volume, hematocrit, and serum albumin concentrations in relation to hydrops fetalis. Pediatrics 53:13, 1974.

Phibbs, R. H., Johnson, P., Kitterman, J. A., et al.: Cardiorespiratory status of erythroblastotic newborn infants. III. Intravascular pressure during the first hours of life. Pediatrics 58:484, 1976.

Pritchard, J. A., Scott, D. E., Whalley, P. J., et al.: The effects of maternal sickle cell hemoglobinopathies and sickle cell trait on reproductive performance. Am. J. Obstet. Gynecol. 117:662, 1973.

Rodeck, C. H., Holman, C. A., Karnicki, J., et al.: Direct intravascular fetal blood transfusion by fetoscopy in severe rhesus isoimmunization. Lancet 1:625, 1981.

Rodeck, C. H., Nicolaides, K. H., Warsof, S. L., et al.: The management of severe rhesus isoimmunization by fetoscopic intravascular transfusions. Am. J. Obstet. Gynecol. 150:769, 1984.

Schmaier, A. H., Maurer, H. M., Johnston, C. L., and Scott, R. B.: Alpha thalassemia screening in neonates by mean corpuscular volume and mean corpuscular hemoglobin determination. J. Pediatr. 83:794, 1973.

Schröter, W., and Kahsnitz, E.: Diagnosis of hereditary spherocytosis in newborn infants. J. Pediatr. 103:460, 1983.

Seip, M.: Systemic lupus erythematosus in pregnancy with hemolytic anemia, leucopenia and thrombocytopenia in the mother and her newborn infant. Arch. Dis. Child. 35:365, 1960.

Stamatoyannopoulos, G.: Gamma-thalassemia. Lancet 2:192, 1971.

Stamey, C. C., and Diamond, L. K.: Congenital hemolytic anemia in the newborn. Am. J. Dis. Child. 94:616, 1957.

Tanaka, K. R., and Paglia, D. E.: Pyruvate kinase deficiency. Semin. Hematol. 8:367, 1971.

Valaes, T., Karaklis, A., Stravrakakis, D., et al.: Incidence and mechanism of neonatal jaundice related to glucose-6-phosphate dehydrogenase deficiency. Pediatr. Res. 3:448, 1969.

Voak, D., and Williams, M. A.: An explanation of the failure of the direct antiglobulin test to detect erythrocyte sensitization in ABO hemolytic disease of the newborn and observations on pinocytosis of IgG anti-A antibodies by infant (cord) red cells. Br. J. Haematol. 20:9, 1971.

Zipursky, A., Pollock, J., Chown, B., and Israels, L. G.: Transplacental foetal hemorrhage after placental injury during delivery or amniocentesis. Lancet 2:493, 1963.

Hypoplastic Anemia

Alter, B. P.: Childhood red cell aplasia. Am. J. Pediatr. Hematol. Oncol. 2:121, 1980.

Diamond, L. K., and Blackfan, K. D.: Hypoplastic anemia. Am. J. Dis. Child. 56:464, 1938.

Glader, B. E.: Diagnosis and management of red cell aplasia in children. Hematol. Oncol. Clin. North Am. 1:431, 1987.

Rogers, Z. R., Bergstrom, S. K., Amylon, M. D., et. al.: Reduced neutrophil counts in children with transient erythroblastopenia of childhood. J. Pediatr. 15:746, 1989.

Wranne, L.: Transient erythroblastopenia in infancy and childhood. Scand. J. Haematol. 7:76, 1970.

Physiologic Anemia of Infancy and Prematurity

Blank, J. P., Sheagren, T. G., Vajaria, J., et al.: The role of RBC transfusion in the premature infant. Am. J. Dis. Child. 138:831, 1984.

Brown, M. S., Garcia, J. F., Phibbs, R. H., et al.: Decreased response of plasma immunoreactive erythropoietin to "available oxygen" in anemia of prematurity. J. Pediatr. *105*:793, 1984.

Brown, M. S., Roderic, R. H., Garcia, J. F., et al.: Postnatal changes in erythropoietin levels in untransfused premature infants. J. Pediatr. *103*:612, 1983.

Dallman, P. R.: Erythropoietin and the anemia of prematurity. J. Pediatr. *105*:756, 1984.

DeMaio, J. G., Harris, M. C., and Spitzer, A. R.: The response of apnea of prematurity to transfusion therapy. (Abstract.) Pediatr. Res. *20*:389A, 1986.

Joshi, A., Gerhardt, T., and Shandloff, P.: Blood transfusion effect on the respiratory pattern of preterm infants. Pediatrics *80*:79, 1987.

Mestyan, J., Fekete, M., Bata, G., and Jarai, I.: The basal metabolic rate of premature infants. Biol. Neonatol. *7*:11, 1964.

Oski, F. A., and Barness, L. A.: Vitamin E deficiency: A previously unrecognized cause of hemolytic anemia in the premature infant. J. Pediatr. *70*:211, 1967.

Oski, F. A., and Naiman, J. L.: Hematologic Problems in the Newborn. Philadelphia, W. B. Saunders Company, 1982.

Pearson, H. A.: Life-span of the fetal red blood cell. J. Pediatr. *70*:166, 1967.

Ritchie, J. H., Fish, M. B., McMasters, V., and Grossman, M.: Edema and hemolytic anemia in premature infants. N. Engl. J. Med. *279*:1185, 1968.

Ross, M. P., Christensen, R. D., Rothstein, G., et al.: A randomized trial to develop criteria for administering erythrocyte transfusions to anemic preterm infants 1 to 3 months of age. J. Perinatol. *9*:246, 1989.

Schulman, I.: The anemia of prematurity. J. Pediatr. *54*:663, 1959.

Shannon, K. M., Gordon, G. S., Torkildson, J. C., et al.: Circulating erythroid progenitors in the anemia of prematurity. N. Engl. J. Med. *317*:728, 1987.

Stockman, J. A., and Clark, D. A.: Weight gain: A response to transfusion in selected preterm infants. Am. J. Dis. Child. *138*:828, 1984.

Stockman, J. A. Anemia of prematurity: Current concepts in the issue of when to transfuse. Pediatr. Clin. North Am. *33*:111, 1986.

Wardrop, C. A. J., Holland, B. M., Veale, K. E. A., et al.: Nonphysiological anaemia of prematurity. Arch. Dis. Child. *53*:855, 1978.

Polycythemia

Black, V. D., Rumack, C. M., Lubchenko, L. O., et al.: Gastrointestinal injury in polycythemic term infants. Pediatrics *76*:225, 1985.

Delaney-Black, V., Camp, B. W., Lubchenko, L. O., et al.: Neonatal hyperviscosity association with lower achievement and IQ scores at school age. Pediatrics *83*:662, 1989.

Gatti, R. A., Muster, A. J., Cole, R. B., and Paul, M. H.: Neonatal polycythemia with transient cyanosis and cardiorespiratory abnormalities. J. Pediatr. *69*:1063, 1966.

Hathaway, W. E.: Neonatal hyperviscosity. Pediatrics *72*:567, 1983.

Hein, H. A., and Lathrop, S. S.: Partial exchange transfusion in term, polycythemic neonates: Absence of association with severe gastrointestinal injury. Pediatrics *80*:75, 1987.

Oh, W., Omori, K., Emmanouilides, G. C., and Phelps, D. L.: Placenta to lamb fetus transfusion in utero during acute hypoxia. Am. J. Obstet. Gynecol. *122*:316, 1975.

Ramamurthy, R. S., and Berlanga, M.: Postnatal alteration in hematocrit and viscosity in normal and polycythemic infants. J. Pediatr *110*:929, 1987.

Shohat, M., Merlob, P., and Reisner, S. H.: Neonatal polycythemia: I. Early diagnosis and incidence relating to time of sampling. Pediatrics *73*:7, 1984.

Methemoglobinemia

Bartos, H. R., and Desforges, J. F.: Erythrocyte DPNH dependent diaphorase levels in infants. Pediatrics *37*:991, 1966.

Climie, C. R., McLean, S., Starmer, G. A., and Thomas, J.: Methaemoglobinaemia in mother and foetus following continuous epidermal analgesia with prilocaine. Br. J. Anaesthesiol. *39*:155, 1967.

Comly, H. R.: Cyanosis in infants caused by nitrates in well water. J.A.M.A. *129*:112, 1945.

Evelyn, K. A., and Malloy, H. T.: Microdetermination of oxyhemoglobin, methemoglobin, and sulfhemoglobin in a single sample of blood. J. Biol. Chem. *126*:655, 1938.

Harley, J. D., and Celermajer, J. M.: Neonatal methaemoglobinaemia and the "red-brown" screening test. Lancet *2*:1223, 1970.

Hayashi, A., Fujita, T., Fujimura, M., et al.: A new abnormal fetal hemoglobin, Hb FM-Osaka. Hemoglobin *4*:447, 1980.

Martin, H., and Huisman, T. H. J.: Formation of ferrihaemoglobin of isolated human haemoglobin types by sodium nitrite. Nature *200*:898, 1963.

Priest, J. R., Watterson, J., Jones, R. T., et al.: Mutant fetal hemoglobin causing cyanosis in a newborn. Pediatrics *83*:734, 1989.

RHEUMATIC 87 DISORDERS

Mandel R. Sher

■ INFANTILE POLYARTERITIS NODOSA

Infantile polyarteritis nodosa (IPN) is an uncommon disease of early childhood and rarely occurs in newborns. The clinical presentation and pathologic findings of IPN differ from those of other forms of polyarteritis nodosa; however, IPN and the more recently described mucocutaneous lymph node syndrome (MLNS, or Kawasaki disease) are very similar. The clinical presentations of IPN and MLNS have common features, and the pathologic vasculitic lesions of both entities are indistinguishable (Fig. 87–1; Table 87–1). IPN is usually fatal, whereas MLNS is associated with a low mortality rate. Therefore, IPN and MLNS may represent different expressions of the same disease process.

IPN usually is associated with prolonged or intermittent fever, upper respiratory tract symptoms, and rash. The rash is typically erythematous and macular but can be urticarial or similar to erythema multiforme. Conjunctivitis, lymphadenopathy, hepatosplenomegaly, diarrhea, and peripheral edema are frequent clinical manifestations. Less frequent but significant clinical characteristics include nuchal rigidity, limb paresis, congestive heart failure, hypertension, and digital and extremity infarcts.

Leukocytosis and either pyuria or albuminuria are frequent findings. Cardiomegaly and pulmonic infiltrates can be seen on the chest roentgenogram. The ECG in 20 per cent of cases reveals evidence of left ventricular hypertrophy or myocardial ischemia. Cerebrospinal pleocytosis with increased protein occurs in 20 per cent of patients.

The course of IPN averages 27 days and usually terminates in sudden death from coronary thrombosis or rupture. The pathologic hallmark of IPN is the presence of coronary artery vasculitis, with thromboses and aneurysms seen in over 90 per cent of cases. Vasculitis and thrombosis of other medium-sized vessels are common. These include, in order of decreasing frequency, renal, periadrenal, intestinal, pancreatic, splenic, and iliac arteries. Myocardial and renal infarcts are frequently seen.

Pathology. The histologic appearance of IPN is primarily characterized by a segmental panarteritis of medium-sized vessels. Different stages of inflammation and repair can be seen in the same artery. The exudative phase is marked by intimal proliferation with destruction of the internal elastic lamina and media. Thrombi, when present, merge with the intima. Fibrinoid changes are not seen, because the rate of the disease process allows time for repair. However, aneurysms may develop during the reparative phase.

Diagnosis. Rarely has the diagnosis of IPN been made during life. Chamberlain and Perry (1971) as well as Glanz and colleagues (1976) diagnosed IPN in infants after documentation of coronary aneurysms by coronary angiography. The diagnosis of IPN should be suspected when the typical clinical characteristics are present. Documentation of coronary thromboses and aneurysms by two-dimensional echocardiography helps establish the diagnosis. Coronary angiography may be performed when a diagnosis cannot be confirmed by other means. Since this procedure has a significant risk in the presence of active coronary vasculitis, it should be performed only in the healing stages of disease. Differentiating IPN from MLNS may be difficult. Diagnostic criteria are established in MLNS (Table 87–2). Although the pathologies of MLNS and IPN are indistinguishable, very few cases of IPN fulfill the clinical criteria for a firm diagnosis of MLNS.

The diagnosis of IPN is even more difficult to make in the neonatal period. Of the 50 cases of documented IPN, five cases involved newborns presenting between 6 days and 5 weeks of age. Two of these five infants had the typical clinical course of IPN. Roberts and Fetterman (1963) reported a 5-week-old child with fever, upper respiratory infection, and macular rash who went on to develop congestive heart failure and arterial thrombosis of an arm and leg. Pathologic findings were typical of IPN.

Sanpawat and associates (1988) reported on a case of a newborn with fever, rash, rhinorrhea, alar nasi necrosis, bronchopneumonia, and hepatomegaly during the 1st week of life. The child developed skin nodules and ischemic necrosis of buccal mucosa, scrotum, and digits. Despite corticosteroid therapy, the child died at 24 days of age. Autopsy revealed necrotizing vasculitis with fibrinoid necrosis of small muscular arteries in multiple organs.

Wilmer (1945) reported two cases of newborns with IPN. The first child began to vomit on the 8th day and developed dyspnea on the 10th day. Purulent omphalitis was present, and the child died that day in shock. Necropsy revealed an umbilical arteritis and umbilical venous thrombosis in addition to vasculitis of many arteries. Wilmer's second patient presented with a rash and puffy eyelids during the 3rd week and went on to have fever, diarrhea, hematemesis, and petechiae. He developed thrombocytopenia and died after a right-sided convulsion. Necropsy revealed a large adrenal hemorrhage in addition to polyarteritis nodosa. In 1954, Liban and co-workers reported on a child who failed to thrive and had intermittent episodes of fever from birth. The child died at 9 months of age after developing progressive congestive heart failure. Necropsy revealed extensive vasculitic involvement of pulmonary and coronary arteries. Although

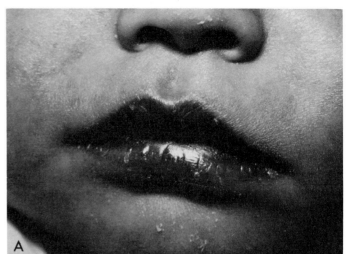

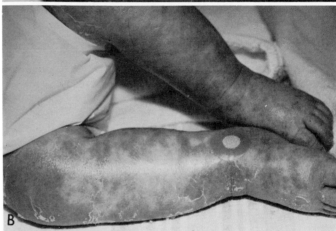

FIGURE 87–1. Eleven-week-old male infant with diagnosis of MLNS. *Erythematous macular rash, infected lips, and edema of extremities are also typical of IPN.*

Wilmer's cases are atypical, Liban's case could have been diagnosed today by echocardiography.

The pathogenesis of IPN is unknown. Studies by Rich and Gregory (1943) implicate a hypersensitivity mechanism in these forms of systemic vasculitis. This is supported by a report of increased serum concentrations of IgE in two patients with IPN.

Treatment. Treatment for this very rare condition remains controversial. Chamberlain and Perry (1971) as well as Glanz and co-workers (1976) treated their two patients with steroids and cytotoxic agents with satisfactory results. Older children and adults with polyarteritis nodosa respond well to this regimen. In contrast, steroids may be harmful to patients with the coronary aneurysms of MLNS, whereas treatment with high-dose intravenous gamma globulin and aspirin is efficacious (Newburger et al., 1986). Given the great similarities between IPN and MLNS, combined administration of corticosteroids and intravenous gamma globulin may be an appropriate therapy in IPN.

■ NEONATAL SYSTEMIC LUPUS ERYTHEMATOSUS (NSLE)

Neonatal systemic lupus erythematosus (NSLE) is a relatively uncommon syndrome. The clinical presentation

TABLE 87–1. Common Features of Infantile Polyarteritis Nodosa

SYMPTOM	FREQUENCY (Per Cent)
Fever	95
Upper respiratory symptoms	90
Rash	80
Conjunctivitis	50
Lymphadenopathy	40
Cardiomegaly	20
Digital desquamation	15
Hypertension	10
Extremity infarcts	10
Leukocytosis	95
Pyuria	45
Cerebrospinal fluid pleocytosis	20
ECG changes	20

TABLE 87–2. Diagnostic Criteria for Mucocutaneous Lymph Node Syndrome

1. Fever, persisting for more than 5 days
2. Bilateral conjunctival infection
3. Erythematous rash
4. Mucous membrane changes (at least one)
    a. Infected or fissured lips
    b. Infected pharynx
    c. Strawberry tongue
5. Extremity changes (at least one)
    a. Erythema of palms or soles
    b. Edema of the hands and feet
    c. Generalized or periungual desquamation
6. Cervical lymphadenopathy (at least one node 1.5 cm in diameter)

(From Report from MCLS Research Committee of the Ministry of Health and Welfare 1971–1972. Japanese Government, 1972, pp. 9–10.)

can vary from transient systemic phenomena to complete congenital heart block. Common to mothers and infants with NSLE are autoantibodies to antigens such as SS-A/Ro, SS-B/La, and U₁RNP. These antibodies are transferred across the placenta and appear to be critical to the syndrome's pathogenesis.

The incidence of NSLE is not known. The female-to-male ratio in NSLE is 2:1, whereas in adult SLE it is 9:1. A prospective study of 103 infants born to mothers with SLE or SLE-like disease revealed a 3 to 7 per cent incidence of NSLE (Lockshin et al., 1988). Forty per cent of mothers of infants with NSLE have clinical evidence of autoimmune disease at delivery, and an additional 25 to 40 per cent develop symptoms at a later date.

Transient symptoms of neonatal SLE typically include rash and, to a lesser extent, other systemic manifestations. The rash is usually erythematous and annular, exhibiting scaling telangiectasia or follicular plugging. The rash may be distributed over the face (particularly the periorbital area), trunk, and upper extremities. About 25 per cent of patients develop this rash after exposure to the sun or another source of ultraviolet light. The rash may be present at birth or may appear during the first several months of life; it commonly resolves by 6 months of age but may leave residual skin atrophy and telangiectasis. The skin lesions are similar to those seen in subacute cutaneous lupus syndrome, which occurs in older patients who tend to express anti-SS-A/Ro antibodies. The regression of NSLE skin lesions appears to correlate with decreasing levels of circulating anti-SS-A/Ro antibodies. SS-A/Ro antigen is present in fetal, neonatal, and adult skin and is expressed in photosensitive skin (Lee et al., 1985).

Hematologic abnormalities, including hemolytic anemia, leukopenia, and thrombocytopenia, occur in 10 to 20 per cent of patients. A review by Provost and co-workers of 32 NSLE infants with platelet count determinants revealed seven with thrombocytopenia (Provost et al., 1987a). The pathogenesis of the hematologic dysregulation is unknown and the role of antiplatelet antibodies remains unclear, although anti-SS-A/Ro antibodies may be involved. These antibodies have been observed in a small proportion of patients with idiopathic thrombocytopenic purpura. Less frequent transient manifestations of NSLE include hepatosplenomegaly and pericarditis (Nolan et al., 1979).

Congenital complete heart block (CCHB) represents the most severe expression of NSLE. The estimated incidence of CCHB in all infants is 1 in 20,000 births. As many as 80 per cent of these patients may be offspring of mothers with SLE or other autoimmune diseases; in this group, 84 per cent of mothers of infants with CCHB express anti-SS-A/Ro antibodies (Scott et al., 1983).

CCHB in these infants commonly presents antenatally or at birth with bradycardia. The diagnosis can be confused with bradycardia secondary to fetal distress, which may result in premature delivery of the infant. However, diagnosis of CCHB can be confirmed in utero using two-dimensional and M-mode fetal echocardiography (Truccone and Mariona, 1986). This method can detect associated congenital heart defects seen in over 25 per cent of cases. These defects include corrected transposition, patent ductus arteriosus, and partial anomalous venous return. Infants with CCHB can be asymptomatic or can present with congestive heart failure. A cardiomyopathy and associated congenital defects present in some of these infants may contribute to the development of heart failure. The mortality rate of CCHB in infants of mothers with SLE or connective tissue disease is 20 to 30 per cent. The frequency of congestive heart failure and the increased incidence of low birth weight and prematurity in infants of mothers with SLE contribute to this mortality rate. The development of heart block in NSLE is thought to result from inflammation of the fetal conduction system and myocardial tissue that causes malformations and scarring. Evidence supporting this theory includes the high concentration of anti-SS-A/Ro in heart tissue, the presence of this antibody in the normal fetal heart conduction tissue, and deposition of immunoglobulin in conductive systems of infants with CCHB (Deng et al., 1987; Litsey et al., 1985). Furthermore, transplacental passage of maternal antibodies is significantly increased after 20 weeks' gestation, correlating with the temporal development of CCHB.

Pathogenesis. The pathogenesis of NSLE syndrome is not fully known. NSLE appears to be associated with transplacental autoantibodies directed against fetal organs expressing the autoantigens. Although anti-SS-A/Ro is expressed in most mothers and infants with NSLE, anti-SS-B/La and anti-U₁RNP have also been associated with the development of NSLE. Since only a small number of infants with these autoantibodies express NSLE, other factors, i.e., genetic factors, must contribute to the development of the disease. Anti-SS-A/Ro expression is associated with HLA DR2 and DR3, and anti-SS-B/La with DR3. SLE mothers with NSLE infants tend to express DR3, whereas SLE mothers with normal infants express DR2 (Provost et al., 1987a).

Management. The cutaneous and hematologic manifestations of NSLE are usually benign and self-limited. A topical corticosteroid preparation such as hydrocortisone 1 per cent is effective for skin lesions but should be used cautiously to avoid skin atrophy. Avoidance of the sun is advised, and sunblocks are useful. Severe anemia and thrombocytopenia may benefit from oral corticosteroid therapy. Intravenous gamma globulin has been used successfully to treat two infants with NSLE thrombocytopenia and neutropenia (Hanada et al., 1987).

Asymptomatic infants with CCHB require only observation, whereas infants with both CCHB and congestive heart failure need meticulous medical management as well as cardiac pacing when indicated.

Maternal plasmapheresis in combination with corticosteroid therapy has been used without great success in attempts to reverse fetal complete heart block and myocarditis (Buyon et al., 1987; Herreman and Gaiezewski, 1985). Another approach is to identify risk factors that target those fetuses at greatest risk of NSLE and CCHB and to employ plasmapheresis at 20 weeks' gestation. Risk factors identified include maternal HLA DR3, high maternal titers of anti-SS-A/Ro or anti-SS-B/La, and the birth of a previous child with CCHB (Buyon et al., 1988).

Although cutaneous and hematologic manifestations are self-limited and cardiac defects are static, eight children with NSLE have developed rheumatic disorders in adolescence (Goldsmith, 1989).

■ INFANTILE (NEONATAL ONSET) MULTISYSTEM INFLAMMATORY DISEASE

Infantile or neonatal multisystem inflammatory disease is a recently described syndrome that appears in the neonatal period. Although this syndrome shares many features of systemic onset juvenile arthritis (SOJRA), it is distinctly different from the latter disease. Since Lorber first described this syndrome in 1973, 13 additional children (Table 87–3) have been reported with similar clinical characteristics (Lorber, 1973; Yarom et al., 1985).

Manifestations in the neonatal period include rash and, variably, hepatosplenomegaly, omphalocele, open fontanel, and macrocephaly. From 3 to 8 months of age, fever, lymphadenopathy, polyarticular arthritis, developmental delay, and neurologic abnormalities are observed. The rash, seen in all patients, occurs soon after birth. It has been described as urticaria or as a maculopapular, evanescent rash similar to that seen in SOJRA. The severe polyarticular arthritis leads to contractures, with bony involvement of joint spaces occurring more often than soft tissue swelling. Radiography also shows periosteal changes. Lymphadenopathy or hepatosplenomegaly is present in all cases. Uveitis, vitreous changes, and papilledema also can occur.

Central nervous system involvement is observed in all patients. Persistent, open fontanel and head enlargement are common. Cerebrospinal fluid pleocytosis may be exhibited as early as the 1st week of life. Other features of central nervous system involvement include developmental delay and mental retardation. Seizures and deafness may occur but are less frequent.

In addition, laboratory evaluation can reveal anemia, leukocytosis, an elevated sedimentation rate, and hypergammaglobulinemia.

Intermittent fever, evanescent rash, polyarthritis, orga-nomegaly, and the laboratory data are seen in both infantile (neonatal onset) multisystem inflammatory disease and SOJRA. However, SOJRA rarely occurs under 1 year of age, and central nervous system abnormalities and uveitis are uncommon in this form of juvenile arthritis. In addition, the arthritic manifestations of the two diseases are different: more bony and periosteal involvement and less synovial inflammation are observed in neonatal onset (infantile) multisystem inflammatory disease than in SOJRA. Synovial biopsies reveal mast cell accumulation and a paucity of synovial proliferation (Yarom et al., 1985).

The etiology of this disease is unknown. No infectious agent has been identified. The neonatal onset suggests in utero involvement with an ongoing inflammatory response to an infection or autoantigen. Other possibilities include an inherited metabolic disorder or a defect in an inflammatory inhibitor. No evidence has been found to support either hypothesis.

Management of this progressive disease is unsatisfactory. The arthritis is unresponsive to nonsteroidal anti-inflammatory drugs, gold, and penicillamine. Corticosteroids have some effect in slowing the progression of the arthritis and in reducing fever, rash, and organomegaly. Because the syndrome has only recently been characterized, overall prognosis is not known. However, three patients have died of myelomonocytic leukemia, bacterial meningitis, and necrotizing leukoencephalopathy (Prieur and Griscelli, 1982; Fajardo et al., 1982; Lampert et al., 1975).

■ REFERENCES

Ansell, B. M., Bywaters, E. G. L., and Elderkin, F. M.: Familial arthropathy with rash, uveitis and mental retardation. Proc. R. Soc. Med. *68*:584, 1975.

Beck, J. S., and Rowell, N. R.: Transplacental passage of antinuclear antibody. Lancet *1*:134, 1963.

Berlyne, G. M., Short, I. A., and Vickers, C. F. H.: Placental transmission of the LE factor. Lancet *2*:15, 1957.

Brustein, D., Rodriguez, J. M., Minkin, W., and Rabhan, N. B.: Familial lupus erythematosus. J.A.M.A. *238*:2294, 1977.

Buyon, J., Roubey, R., Swersky, S. H., et al.: Complete congenital heart block: Risk of occurrence and therapeutic approach to prevention. J. Rheumatol. *15*:1104, 1988.

Buyon, J. P., Swersky, S. H., Fox, H. E., et al.: Intrauterine therapy for presumptive fetal myocarditis with acquired heart block due to systemic lupus erythematosus. Arthritis Rheum. *30*:44, 1987.

Chamberlain, J. L., and Perry, L. W.: Infantile periarteritis nodosa with coronary and brachial aneurysms—a case diagnosed during life. J. Pediatr. *78*:1039, 1971.

Chameides, L., Truex, R. C., Vetter, V., et al.: Association of maternal systemic lupus erythematosus with congenital complete heart block. N. Engl. J. Med. *297*:1204, 1977.

Deng, J. S., Blair, L. W., Shen-Schwartz, S., et al.: Localization of SS-A/Ro antigen in the cardiac conduction system. Arthritis Rheum. *30*:1232, 1987.

Esscher, E., and Scott, J. S.: Congenital heart block and maternal systemic lupus erythematosus. Br. Med. J. *1*:1235, 1979.

Fajardo, J. E., Geller, T. J., Koenig, H. M., and Klrin, M. L.: Chronic meningitis, polyarthritis, lymphadenitis, and pulmonary hemosiderosis. J. Pediatr. *101*:738, 1982.

Fox, R. J., McCuistion, C. H., and Schoch, E. P.: Systemic lupus erythematosus. Arch. Dermatol. *115*:340, 1979.

Fraga, A., Mintz, G., Drozas, J., et al.: Sterility rates, fetal wastage and maternal morbidity in systemic lupus erythematosus. J. Rheumatol. *1*:293, 1974.

Glanz, S., Bittner, S. J., Berman, M. A., et al.: Regression of coronary artery aneurysms in infantile polyarteritis nodosa. N. Engl. J. Med. *294*:939, 1976.

TABLE 87–3. Clinical and Laboratory Data in 13 Children with Infantile Multisystem Inflammatory Disease

	n	PER CENT
Clinical data		
Age at onset	Birth to early infancy	
Sex (M/F)	6/7	
Arthritis	13/13	100
Evanescent rash	13/13	100
Adenopathy	13/13	100
Developmental delay	13/13	100
Fever	12/13	92
Persistent open fontanel	11/13	85
Head enlargement or hydrocephalus	9/13	69
Splenomegaly	9/13	69
Abnormal ossification	8/13	62
Papilledema	7/13	54
Uveitis	6/13	46
Convulsions	6/13	46
Hepatomegaly	5/13	38
Feeding problems	4/13	30
Deafness	3/13	23
Laboratory data		
Cerebrospinal fluid pleocytosis	10/10	100
Anemia	9/9	100
Leukocytosis	13/13	100
Elevated ESR	11/11	100
IgG elevation	8/10	80

(From Yarom A., Rennebohm, R. M., and Levinson, J. E.: Infantile multisystem disease; A specific syndrome? J. Pediatr. *106*:390, 1985.)

Goldsmith, D. P.: Neonatal rheumatic disorders. Rheum. Dis. Clin. North Am. *15*:207, 1989.

Hanada, T., Saito, K., Nagasawa, T., et al.: Intravenous gammaglobulin therapy for thromboneutropenic neonates of mothers with systemic lupus erythematosus. Eur. J. Haematol. *38*:400, 1987.

Harley, J. B., Kaine, J. L., Fox, O. F., et al.: Ro(SS-A) antibody and antigen in a patient with congenital complete heart block. Arthritis Rheum. *28*:1321, 1985.

Hassink, S. G., and Goldsmith, D. P.: Neonatal onset multisystem inflammatory disease. Arthritis Rheum. *26*:668, 1983.

Herreman, G., and Gaiezewski, N.: Maternal connective tissue disease and congenital heartblock. (Letter.) N. Engl. J. Med. *312*:1329, 1985.

Hess, E. V., and Spencer-Green, G.: Congenital heart block and connective tissue disease. Ann. Intern. Med. *91*:645, 1976.

Hogg, G. R.: Congenital acute lupus erythematosus associated with subendocardial fibroelastosis. Report of a case. Am. J. Clin. Pathol. *28*:648, 1957.

Hull, D., Binns, B. A. O., and Joyce, D.: Congenital heart block and widespread fibrosis due to maternal lupus erythematosus. Arch. Dis. Child. *41*:688, 1966.

Jackson, R., and Gulliver, M.: Neonatal lupus erythematosus progressing into systemic lupus erythematosus. Br. J. Dermatol. *101*:81, 1979.

Kasinath, B. S., and Katz, A. I.: Delayed maternal lupus after delivery of offspring with complete heart block. Arch. Intern. Med. *142*:2317, 1982.

Kato, H., Koike, S., and Yokoyama, T.: Kawasaki disease: Effect of treatment on coronary artery involvement. Pediatrics *63*:175, 1979.

Kawasaki, T., Kosaki, F., Okawa, S., et al.: A new infantile acute febrile mucocutaneous lymph node syndrome (MLNS) prevailing in Japan. Pediatrics *54*:271, 1974.

Kephart, D. C., Hood, A. F., and Provost, T.: Neonatal lupus erythematosus: New serologic findings. J. Invest. Dermatol. *77*:331, 1981.

Krous, H. F., Clausen, C. R., and Ray, C. G.: Elevated immunoglobulin E in infantile polyarteritis nodosa. J. Pediatr. *84*:841, 1974.

Lampert, F., Belohradsky, B. H., Forster, C., et al.: Infantile chronic relapsing inflammation of the brain, skin, and joints. Lancet *1*:1250, 1975.

Landing, B. H., and Larson, E. J.: Are infantile periarteritis nodosa with coronary artery involvement and fatal mucocutaneous lymph node syndrome the same? Comparison of 20 patients from North America with patients from Hawaii and Japan. Pediatrics *59*:651, 1977.

Lee, L. A., Bias, W. B., Arnett, F. C., et al.: Immunogenetics of the neonatal lupus syndrome. Ann. Intern. Med. *99*:592–596, 1983.

Lee, L. A., Harmon, C. E., Huff, J. C., et al.: The demonstration of SS-A/Ro antigen in human fetal tissues and in neonatal and adult skin. J. Invest. Dermatol. *85*:143, 1985.

Lee, L. A., Harmon, C. E., Huff, J. C., et al.: SS-A(Ro) antigen expression in human fetal, neonatal, and adult tissues. Arthritis Rheum. *27*:S20, 1984.

Liban, E., Shamir, Z., and Schorr, S.: Periarteritis nodosa in a nine month old infant. Am. J. Dis. Child. *88*:210, 1954.

Litsey, S. E., Noonan, J. A., O'Connor, W. N., et al.: Maternal connective tissue disease and congenital heart block. N. Engl. J. Med. *312*:98, 1985.

Lockshin, M. D., Bonfa, E., Elkon, K., et al.: Neonatal lupus risk to newborns of mothers with systemic lupus erythematosus. Arthritis Rheum. *31*:697, 1988.

Lorber, J.: Syndrome for diagnosis: Dwarfing, persistently open fontanelle, recurrent meningitis, recurrent subdural effusions with temporary alternate-sided hemiplegia, high-tone deafness, visual defect with pseudopapilloedema, slowing intellectual development, recurrent acute polyarthritis, erythema marginatum, splenomegaly, and iron-resistant hypochromic anemia. Proc. R. Soc. Med. *6*:1070, 1973.

McCue, C. M., Mantakas, M. E., Tingelstad, J. B., and Ruddy, S.: Congenital heart block in newborns of mothers with connective tissue disease. Circulation *56*:82, 1977.

McCune, A. B., Weston, W. L., and Lee, L. A.: Maternal and fetal outcome in neonatal lupus erythematosus. Ann. Intern. Med. *106*:518, 1987.

Mund, A., Simson, J., and Rothfield, N.: Effect of pregnancy on course of systemic lupus erythematosus. J.A.M.A. *183*:917, 1963.

Nathan, D. J., and Snapper, I.: Simultaneous placental transfer of factors responsible for LE cell formation and thrombocytopenia. Am. J. Med. *25*:647, 1958.

Newburger, J. W., Takahashi, M., Burns, J. C., et al.: The treatment of Kawasaki syndrome with intravenous gammaglobulin. N. Engl. J. Med. *315*:341, 1986.

Nice, C. M., Jr.: Congenital disseminated lupus erythematosus. Am. J. Roentgenol. Radium Ther. Nucl. Med. *88*:585, 1962.

Nolan, R. J., Shulman, S. T., and Victorica, B. E.: Congenital complete heart block associated with maternal mixed connective tissue disease. J. Pediatr. *95*:420, 1979.

Prieur, A., and Griscelli, C.: Arthropathy with rash, chronic meningitis, eye lesions, and mental retardation. J. Pediatr. *99*:79, 1982.

Provost, T. T., Watson, R., Gaither, K. K., and Harley, J. B.: The neonatal lupus erythematosus syndrome. J. Rheumatol. *14*:199, 1987a.

Provost, T. T., Watson, R., Gammon, W. R., et al.: The neonatal lupus syndrome associated with U_1RNP (mRNP) antibodies. N. Engl. J. Med. *316*:18, 1987b.

Ramsey-Goldman, R., Hom, D., Deng, J. S., et al.: Anti SS-A antibodies and fetal outcome in maternal systemic lupus erythematosus. Arthritis Rheum. *29*:1269, 1986.

Rich, A. R.: The role of hypersensitivity in periarteritis nodosa as indicated by 7 cases developing during serum sickness and sulfonamide therapy. Bull. Johns Hopkins Hosp. *71*:123, 1942.

Rich, A. R., and Gregory, J. E.: Experimental demonstration that periarteritis nodosa is a manifestation of hypersensitivity. Bull. Johns Hopkins Hosp. *72*:65, 1943.

Roberts, F. B., and Fetterman, G. H.: Polyarteritis nodosa in infancy. J. Pediatr. *63*:519, 1963.

Sanpawat, S., Chittinand, S., Pongprasit, P., and Viratchai, C.: Polyarteritis nodosa: Report in a newborn infant. J. Med. Assoc. Thai. *71*:297, 1988.

Schaller, J. G.: Lupus phenomena in the newborn. Proceedings of the first conference on childhood rheumatic diseases. Arthritis Rheum. (Suppl. 2) *20*:312, 1977.

Scott, J. S., Maddison, P. J., Taylor, P. V., et al.: Connective tissue disease, antibodies to ribonucleoprotein, and congenital heart block. N. Engl. J. Med. *309*:209, 1983.

Seip, M.: Systemic lupus erythematosus in pregnancy with hemolytic anaemia, leucopenia and thrombocytopenia in the mother and her newborn infant. Arch. Dis. Child. *35*:364, 1960.

Tanaka, N., Sekimoto, K., and Naoe, S.: Kawasaki disease. Relationship with infantile polyarteritis nodosa. Arch. Pathol. Lab. Med. *100*:81, 1976.

Taylor, P. V., Scott, J. S., Gerlis, I. M., et al.: Maternal antibodies against fetal cardiac antigens in congenital complete heart block. N. Engl. J. Med. *315*:667, 1986.

Truccone, N. J., and Mariona, F. G.: Prenatal diagnosis and outcome of congenital complete heart block: The role of fetal echocardiography. Fetal Therapy *1*:210, 1986.

Ty, A., and Fine, B.: Membranous nephritis in infantile systemic lupus erythematosus associated with chromosomal abnormalities. Clin. Nephrol. *12*:137, 1979.

Vonderheid, E. C., Koblenzer, P. J., Ming, P. M. L., and Burgoon, C. F.: Neonatal lupus erythematosus. Arch. Dermatol. *112*:698, 1976.

Watson, R. M., Kang, J. E., May, M., et al.: Thrombocytopenia in the neonatal lupus syndrome. Arch. Dermatol. *124*:560, 1988.

Watson, R. M., Lane, A. T., Barnett, N. K., et al.: Neonatal lupus erythematosus: A clinical, serologic, and immunogenetic study with review of the literature. Medicine (Baltimore) *63*:362, 1984.

Wilmer, H. A.: Two cases of periarteritis nodosa occurring in the first month of life. Bull. Johns Hopkins Hosp. *77*:275, 1945.

Yarom, A., Rennebohm, R. M., and Levinson, J. E.: Infantile multisystem disease: A specific syndrome? J. Pediatr. *106*:390, 1985.

HYDROPS FETALIS **88**

Roberta A. Ballard

Hydrops describes the infant who has generalized edema due to accumulation of excess fluid. The condition varies from mild, generalized edema to massive edema, with ascites and pleural and pericardial effusions and with peripheral edema so severe that the extremities are fixed in extension. Severely hydropic fetuses die in utero if they cannot be delivered under controlled circumstances, and even if delivered alive, they may die in the neonatal period from either the severity of their underlying disease or from severe cardiorespiratory failure caused by the hydrops.

■ HYDROPS FETALIS

Hydrops fetalis is the term used to describe hydrops that occurs as a result of end-stage, severe erythroblastosis fetalis (alloimmune hemolytic anemia). In the past, the great majority of cases were due to maternofetal incompatibility for the D-antigen in the Rh system. However, advances in the use of anti-D immune globulin to prevent maternal sensitization have markedly decreased the incidence of hydrops due to Rh disease (Phibbs and Naiman, 1989). Alloimmune disease does occur occasionally from incompatibility of other important blood group antigens and can be severe enough to cause hydrops (Baker et al., 1988; Beal, 1979). (See Hematology Section, Chapter 86 for further discussion of alloimmune hydrops.)

NONIMMUNE FETAL HYDROPS

Potter (1943) first distinguished between hydrops secondary to erythroblastosis fetalis and nonimmune hydrops in describing a group of infants with generalized body edema who did not have hepatosplenomegaly or abnormal erythropoiesis. With the decrease in incidence of alloimmune hydrops, it was estimated that by 1970 approximately 20 per cent of the cases of hydrops in western countries would be of the nonimmune type. With the nearly universal use of anti-D globulin and refinement of the schedule and doses for administration, the occurrence of immune hydrops has decreased still further. The increasing use of ultrasound in pregnancy has permitted early diagnosis (and, therefore, cataloguing) of more infants with nonimmune hydrops. Current estimates of incidence vary from 1 in 14,000 (Hutchinson et al., 1982)

to 1.7 per 1,000 (Tomic and McGillivray, 1985). In the group of patients undergoing prenatal ultrasound scans, half of the cases of hydrops reported by these authors were either due to cardiac lesions or to chromosomal abnormalities.

PATHOPHYSIOLOGY

Diamond and co-workers (1932) suggested three possible mechanisms that might be operative in infants with hydrops. These mechanisms included anemia, low colloid osmotic pressure with hypoproteinemia, and congestive heart failure with hypervolemia. Others (Barnes et al., 1977; Phibbs and Naiman, 1989) have reviewed these potential mechanisms, and they remain among central hypotheses addressed by investigators in this area.

Anemia. Infants with alloimmune hydrops (and several of the nonimmune hydrops conditions as well) have significant anemia. It has been proposed that anemia leads to congestive heart failure with increased hydrostatic pressure in the capillaries, causing vascular damage that results in edema. However, it has not been possible to reproduce hydrops in animal models with simple anemia, and, in addition, there is significant overlap in the hematocrit values of infants who do and who do not have hydrops, suggesting that anemia alone is not a satisfying explanation. However, in the most severely anemic fetuses it is probable that decreased oxygen transport causes tissue hypoxia, which in turn causes increased capillary permeability to both water and protein. It is probable that the changes in capillary permeability contribute to the development of hydrops. It is possible to produce some of the changes of hydrops using an animal model of capillary injury secondary to toxic shock (Gruenwald and Mayberger, 1950).

Low Colloid Osmotic Pressure with Hypoproteinemia. Infants who have erythroblastosis and hydrops seem to demonstrate a correlation between serum albumin concentration and the degree of hydrops (Phibbs et al., 1974). However, initial therapy after birth tends to raise the serum albumin toward normal very rapidly, and with diuresis, these infants appear to have normal albumin concentrations. This suggests that their hypoalbuminemia may have been the result of dilution rather than the cause of the hydrops. In addition, infants with congenital nephrotic syndrome usually do not develop hydrops.

Congestive Heart Failure with Hypervolemia. An animal model has been used to mimic this clinical picture by the induction of supraventricular tachycardia. The fetuses develop hydrops and have elevated venous pressure and elevated atrial natriuretic peptide levels, which is the same response seen in humans with congestive heart failure. However, most infants with hydrops due to erythroblastosis do not appear to be hypervolemic, but conversely, may have a low circulating blood volume and require transfusion after their asphyxia has been corrected (Phibbs et al., 1974).

GENERAL PRINCIPLES

In relation to the pathophysiology of fluid flux across an endothelial barrier, the factors that govern the transfer of fluid into the interstitium include (a) the surface area, (b) the permeability of the barrier to water and protein, (c) the hydrostatic pressure gradient between the vascular and interstitial space, and (d) the protein osmotic pressure difference between vascular and interstitial space. These general factors must be considered in the fetus in the context of the fact that, in utero, 40 per cent of fetal cardiac output goes through the placenta, allowing rapid transfer of water from the fetus to the mother. Because of this situation, it is unlikely that either low plasma colloid osmotic pressure or elevated capillary hydrostatic pressure could contribute to fluid retention in the fetus. On the other hand, increased capillary permeability, allowing water and protein to leak from the fetal circulation, would lead to higher colloid osmotic pressures in the tissues, including the interstitial spaces of the fetoplacental villi. Therefore, factors leading to increased capillary permeability, whether from severe anemia and hypoxia or from congestive heart failure, are more likely to contribute to hydrops.

DECREASED LYMPH FLOW

A fourth factor that might contribute to hydrops is decreased lymph flow (Brace, 1989; Gest et al., 1988). It is known that hydropic fetuses do not absorb the red blood cells from an intrauterine transfusion successfully. Since normal absorption is through the mesenteric and diaphragmatic lymphatics, it is clear that there is some type of lymphatic malfunction. In further investigating this relationship, Gest and colleagues (1988) were able to demonstrate that elevated central venous pressure was associated with reduced thoracic duct lymph flow and fetal hydrops in fetal lambs with tachycardia produced by electrical pacing.

Thus, the cause of hydrops appears to be multifactorial, with mechanisms that produce capillary leakage and impaired lymphatic drainage contributing to its development.

ETIOLOGY

Alloimmune hydrops is discussed in Chapter 86 and is most commonly associated with anti-D Rh-isoimmuniza-

tion. Nonimmune hydrops has been described in association with a wide range of conditions (Table 88–1). The majority of the conditions that have been associated with nonimmune hydrops would be expected to cause edema either through anemia with hypoxia and consequent capillary leak or through cardiovascular anomalies with heart failure. The latter may also result in tissue hypoxia with increased vascular permeability as well as decreased lymphatic flow. Other conditions associated with hydrops, such as arteriovenous malformations and pulmonary masses, may also act to increase the occurrence of capillary leak and may be associated with lymphatic abnormalities as well. The causal mechanism of hydrops in association with many other conditions is not clear.

ANTENATAL MANAGEMENT OF NONIMMUNE HYDROPS

The diagnosis of hydrops is now frequently made antenatally, as a result of evaluation of polyhydramnios, a pregnancy that is considered high risk for other reasons, or simply as part of a routine ultrasound screening. The goals of antenatal evaluation (Phibbs, 1989) are as follows:

1. *Identify conditions in which therapy is futile*, so that the mother is not subjected to unnecessary additional testing or unnecessary cesarean section for fetal distress.

2. *Identify those fetuses whose conditions can be corrected by intrauterine therapy*, for example, anemia, fetomaternal hemorrhage, or supraventricular tachycardia that can be corrected by treating the mother.

3. *Identify those conditions that can be corrected by appropriate care at the time of delivery*, such as elimination of a chorioangioma of the placenta or immediate neonatal surgical treatment. Obviously, these interventions need to be balanced against the degree of prematurity and the likelihood of the infant's surviving the problems of prematurity plus the treatment of the underlying cause of hydrops.

Carlton and associates (1989) have recently outlined a multidisciplinary approach to the evaluation and management of the mother, fetus, and newborn infant. Table 88–2 provides recommendations for the investigation of fetal hydrops. It is important in evaluating these mothers that one person coordinate the fetal assessment and serve as the consultant with the family. The suggested steps in evaluation are as follows:

1. A complete review of the mother's health history, as well as family and pregnancy history, should be performed, including documentation of ethnic origin, possibility of consanguinity, and history of similarly affected infants within the family. Maternal disorders such as diabetes, systemic lupus erythematosus, myotonic dystrophy, or any type of liver disease should also be noted.

2. Maternal blood studies should be obtained, including blood group typing, assessment for thalassemia, possible G6PD deficiency, or possible viral infection, and maternofetal hemorrhage should be ruled out.

3. Progressive ultrasound scans should be obtained during pregnancy, with attention to fluid accumulation, development of the fetus' cardiac structure and rhythm, assessment of limb shape (because of possible dwarfing), and fetal movement.

TABLE 88–1. Conditions Associated With Hydrops Fetalis

Hemolytic Anemias
  Alloimmune, Rh, Kell, c
  Alpha-chain hemoglobinopathies (homozygous alpha-thalassemia)
  Red blood cell enzyme deficiencies (glucose phosphate isomerase
    deficiency)
Other Anemias
  Fetomaternal hemorrhage
  Twin–twin transfusion
Cardiac Conditions
  Premature closure of foramen ovale
  Tricuspid insufficiency
  Hypoplastic left ventricle
  Subaortic stenosis with fibroelastosis
  Cardiomyopathy, myocardial fibroelastosis
  Myocarditis
  Right atrial hemangioma
  Intracardiac hamartoma or fibroma
  Tuberous sclerosis with cardiac rhabdomyoma
Cardiac Arrhythmias
  Supraventricular tachycardia
  Atrial flutter
  Congenital heart block
Vascular Malformations
  Hemangioma of liver
  Any large arteriovenous malformation
  Angiosteohypertrophy (Klippel-Treanaunay syndrome)
Vascular Accidents
  Thrombosis of umbilical vein or inferior vena cava
  Recipient in twin–twin transfusion
Infections
  Cytomegalovirus, congenital hepatitis, human parvovirus,
    other viruses
  Toxoplasmosis, Chagas disease
  Syphilis
  Leptospirosis
Lymphatic Abnormalities
  Lymphangiectasia
  Cystic hygroma
  Noonan syndrome
  Multiple pterygium syndrome
Nervous System Lesions
  Absent corpus callosum
  Encephalocele
  Cerebral arteriovenous malformation
  Intracranial hemorrhage (massive)
  Holoprosencephaly
  Fetal akinesia sequence

Pulmonary Conditions
  Cystic adenomatoid malformation of lung
  Mediastinal teratoma
  Diaphragmatic hernia
  Lung sequestration syndrome
  Lymphangiectasia
Renal Conditions
  Congenital nephrosis
  Renal vein thrombosis
Invasive and Storage Processes
  Tuberous sclerosis
  Neuroblastoma
  Gaucher disease
  Mucopolysaccharidosis
  Mucolipidosis
Chromosome Abnormalities
  Trisomy 13, trisomy 18, trisomy 21
  Turner syndrome
  XX/XY
Bone Diseases
  Osteogenesis imperfecta
  Achondroplasia
  Asphyxiating thoracic dystrophy
Gastrointestinal Conditions
  Bowel obstruction with perforation and meconium peritonitis
  Small-bowel volvulus
  Other intestinal obstruction
  Prune belly syndrome
Tumors
  Choriocarcinoma
  Sacrococcygeal teratoma
Maternal or Placental Conditions
  Maternal diabetes
  Maternal therapy with indomethacin
  Multiple gestation with parasitic fetus
  Chorioangioma of placenta, chorionic vessels, or umbilical vessels
  Toxemia
  Systemic lupus erythematosus
Miscellaneous
  Neu-Laxova syndrome
  Myotonic dystrophy
Idiopathic

TABLE 88–2. Investigation of Fetal Hydrops

Maternal
  Complete blood cell count and indices
  Hemoglobin electrophoresis
  Kleihauer-Betke stain of peripheral blood
  VDRL and TORCH titers
  Anti-Ro, systemic lupus erythematosus preparation, sedimentation
    rate
  Oral glucose tolerance test

Fetal
  Continued ultrasound cardiac assessment
  Limb length, fetal movement

Amniocentesis
  Karyotype
  Alpha-fetoprotein
  Viral cultures
  Establish culture for appropriate metabolic or DNA testing

Fetal Blood Sampling
  Karyotype
  Hemoglobin analysis
  IgM; specific cultures
  Albumin and total protein

(From McGillivray, B. C., and Hall, J. C.: Nonimmune Hydrops. Pediatr. Rev. 9(6):197, 1987. Reproduced by permission of Pediatrics.)

4. In addition, assessment of the fetus (via either amniocentesis or umbilical cord sampling) should include karyotyping, viral titers, metabolic testing, and determination of hemoglobin and protein levels.

5. It may be necessary to tap a fetal fluid cavity, such as the peritoneal or pleural cavity, for diagnosis or therapy.

6. Because of the possibility of fetal demise, preparations should be made for maximal evaluation at the time of delivery, including pathologic studies and radiographs.

7. Consideration should be given to possible therapeutic measures from nonspecific therapy, such as amniocentesis to remove excess fluid, increase maternal comfort, and decrease risk of premature labor, to specific therapy, such as treatment of fetal cardiac arrhythmia. In addition, plans should be made for delivery of the infant with a resuscitation team present, including special team members.

NEONATAL EVALUATION

Table 88–3 presents the diagnostic evaluation recommended for newborn infants with nonimmune hydrops of unknown cause (Carlton et al., 1989).

TABLE 88–3. Diagnostic Evaluation of Newborn Babies with Nonimmune Hydrops

SYSTEM	TYPE OF EVALUATION
Cardiovascular	Echocardiogram, electrocardiogram
Pulmonary	Chest radiograph, pleural fluid examination
Hematologic	Complete blood cell count, differential platelet count, blood type and Coombs test, blood smear for morphology
Gastrointestinal	Abdominal radiograph, abdominal ultrasound, liver function tests, peritoneal fluid examination, total protein, albumin
Renal	Urinalysis, BUN, creatinine
Genetic	Chromosomal analysis, skeletal radiographs, genetic consultation
Congenital infections	Viral cultures or serology (including TORCH agents and parvovirus)
Pathologic	Complete autopsy, placental examination

(Adapted from Carlton, D., et al., Clin. Perinatol. 16:844, 1989.)

CLINICAL COURSE AND OUTCOME

In spite of major advances in the ability to diagnose hydrops in utero by ultrasound techniques, the overall prognosis of patients with nonimmune hydrops remains poor. In cases in which the diagnosis is made antenatally, reported survival has ranged from 20 to 33 per cent (Holtzgreve et al., 1985; Tomic et al., 1985). Of those infants with hydrops who are born live, approximately 40 to 50 per cent survive; these figures are misleading, however, because many of the underlying conditions are lethal. Obviously, the degree of prematurity has a major impact on the overall mortality rate. As a group, the idiopathic cases currently seem to have the best prognosis.

Survival of the infant requires the presence of a resuscitation team at delivery and vigorous resuscitation (see Chapter 22). Survivors require initial mechanical ventilation because of respiratory failure due to either the underlying condition or hydrops itself. Carlton and co-workers (1989) reported on a group of 36 infants with nonimmune hydrops and noted that 90 per cent of those who died within 24 hours had pleural effusions compared with only 50 per cent of those who survived. They also noted that more than one-third of the infants in their study required thoracentesis in the delivery room to aid in lung expansion. All of the infants who lived more than 24 hours were mechanically ventilated and received supplemental oxygen. They required ventilation for an average of 11 days (range 2 to 48 days). Most of these infants lose a minimum of 15 per cent of their birth weight, and some lose as much as 30 per cent. Ordinarily, diuresis begins on the 2nd or 3rd day after birth and continues for a period of 2 to 4 days. Once the edema has resolved, the infants have normal levels of circulating protein and eventually appear to recover from their apparent capillary leak syndrome. If the hydrops is treated successfully, or if it is of the idiopathic variety, the long-term outcome is good in the absence of serious birth asphyxia.

■ ACKNOWLEDGMENT

The editors greatly appreciate the assistance of Roderic H. Phibbs, Professor of Pediatrics, University of California, San Francisco in the preparation of this chapter.

■ REFERENCES

Anand, A., Gray, E. S., Brown, T., et al.: Human parvovirus infection in pregnancy and hydrops fetalis. N. Engl. J. Med. 316:183, 1987.

Baker, J. W., Harrison, K. L., and Harvey, P. J.: Anti-C haemolytic disease requiring intrauterine and exchange transfusion. Med. J. Aust. 2:296, 1988.

Barnes, S. E., Bryan, E. M., Harris, D. A., et al.: Oedema in the newborn. Mol. Aspects Med. 1:187, 1977.

Bawle, E. V., and Black, V.: Nonimmune hydrops fetalis in Noonan's syndrome. Am. J. Dis. Child. 140:758, 1986.

Beal, R. W.: Non-rhesus (D) blood group isoimmunization in obstetrics. Clin. Obstet. Gynecol. 6:493, 1979.

Bierman, F. Z., Baxi, L., Jaffe, I., et al.: Fetal hydrops and congenital complete heart block: Response to maternal steroid therapy. J. Pediatr. 112:646, 1988.

Brace, R. A.: Effects of outflow pressure on fetal lymph flow. Am. J. Obstet. Gynecol. 160:494, 1989.

Carlton, D. P., McGillivray, B. C., and Schreiber, M. D.: Nonimmune hydrops fetalis: A multidisciplinary approach. Clin. Perinatol. 16 (4):839, 1989.

Diamond, L. K., Blackfan, K. D., and Baty, J. M.: Erythroblastosis fetalis and its association with universal edema of the fetus, icterus gravis neonatorum and anemia of the newborn. J. Pediatr. 1:269, 1932.

Etches, P. C., and Lemons, J. A.: Nonimmune hydrops fetalis: Report of 22 cases including three siblings. Pediatrics 64:326, 1979.

Gest, A. L., Martin, C. G., Moise, A. A., and Hansen, T. H.: Atrial pacing in fetal sheep causes reversal of blood flow. Pediatr. Res. 23:408A, 1988.

Gruenwald, P., and Mayberger, H. W.: Hydrops of the fetus: A manifestation of shock. Am. J. Med. Sci. 220:12, 1950.

Hutchinson, A. A., Drew, J. H., Yu, V. Y. H., et al.: Nonimmunologic hydrops fetalis: A review of 61 cases. Obstet. Gynecol. 59:347, 1982.

McGillivray, B. C., and Hall, J. G.: Nonimmune hydrops. Pediatr. Rev. 9(6):197, 1987.

Newburger, J. W., and Keane, J. F.: Intrauterine supraventricular tachycardia. J. Pediatr. 95:780, 1979.

Phibbs, R. H.: Hydrops fetalis and other causes of neonatal edema and ascites. In Polin, R. A., and Fox, W. W. (Eds.): Fetal and Neonatal Physiology. Philadelphia: W. B. Saunders Company, 1991 (in press).

Phibbs, R. H., Johnson, P., Kitterman, J. A., et al.: Cardiorespiratory status of erythroblastotic infants. I. Relationship of gestational age, severity of hemolytic disease and birth asphyxia to idiopathic respiratory distress syndrome and survival. Pediatrics 49:5, 1972.

Phibbs, R. H., Johnson, P., and Tooley, W. H.: Cardiorespiratory status of erythroblastotic newborn infants. II. Blood volume, hematocrit and serum albumin concentrations in relation to hydrops fetalis. Pediatrics 53:13, 1974.

Phibbs, R. H., and Naiman, J. L.: Hemolytic disease of the newborn. In Mentzer, W. C., and Wagner, G. H. (Eds.): Congenital Hemolytic Anemias. New Edinburgh, Churchill-Livingstone, 1989, pp. 319–390.

Potter, E. L.: Universal edema of the fetus unassociated with erythroblastosis. Am. J. Obstet. Gynecol. 46:30, 1943.

Ravindranath, U., Paglia, D. E., Warrier, I., et al.: Glucose phosphate isomerase deficiency as a cause of hydrops fetalis. N. Engl. J. Med. 316:258, 1987.

Tomic, S., and McGillivray, B. C.: A protocol for fetal hydrops: Summer Research Study. Vancouver, B. C., University of British Columbia, 1985.

PART XVI

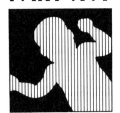

RENAL AND GENITOURINARY SYSTEMS

DISORDERS OF THE **89** KIDNEYS AND GENITOURINARY SYSTEM— INTRODUCTION, EMBRYOLOGY, AND MORPHOLOGY

Sudhir K. Anand

During fetal life, the body's homeostatic functions are primarily carried out by the placenta. Although the fetal kidneys elaborate urine beginning at the 12th week of gestation, their control of fetal fluid and electrolyte homeostasis is minimal. Babies born with bilateral renal agenesis have normal plasma composition at birth and develop signs of progressive renal failure only during the following few days. Appropriate development and maturation of kidneys during the intrauterine period are essential for normal adaptation to postnatal life. At birth, the kidneys assume the main responsibility of maintaining fluid and electrolyte homeostasis and excreting most nitrogenous waste products.

Renal function at birth is adequate for the usual needs of the newborn infant (but less so in the premature infant) and within reasonable limits can adapt to various stresses imposed by disease or injudicious management. When present in the neonatal period, nephrologic problems are usually a developmental defect of the urinary system, with or without an anatomic obstruction. With the increased use of ultrasound evaluation of the fetus during the last decade, congenital urinary disorders are often found prepartum. Such early recognition has assisted both in an early corrective surgery in the postnatal period and an

occasional use of corrective and/or first-step surgery in the fetus.

Also, during the past two decades, along with the development and provision of intensive care to newborns, acquired renal disorders, especially acute renal failure, have been recognized with increased frequency. In recent years, new technologic innovations (e.g., hemofiltration) have been developed for the evaluation and management of newborns with renal, fluid, and electrolyte disorders.

This section discusses anatomic development and maturation of function of various components of the genitourinary tract, clinical evaluation of renal function, various congenital disorders of the genitourinary tract, and disorders acquired during the neonatal period.

■ EMBRYOLOGY AND MORPHOLOGY OF THE GENITOURINARY TRACT

The human kidney develops from the nephrogenic ridge in three distinct but overlapping stages. The earliest structure, the pronephros, consists of a set of tubules in the 3-week-old embryo. The tubules join distally to form a duct that is the anlage of the mesonephric, or wolffian, duct. The pronephros degenerates, and more caudally, differentiation of the mesonephros occurs. The mesonephric duct eventually matures into the vas deferens, seminal vesicle, and epididymis in the male and into the vestigial Gartner duct in the female. One of the most significant events in the development of the urinary tract is the formation of a ureteric bud from the caudal portion of the mesonephric duct during the 5th week of gestation. The ureteric bud migrates cephalad and makes contact with the metanephric blastema, then induces the mass of metanephric cells to differentiate into the definitive kidney or metanephros (Fig. 89–1). The induction process is bidirectional, requiring both ureteric bud and metanephric cells to interact for normal development; just as failure of development of ureteric bud would lead to agenesis of kidney, without metanephric cells, complete maturation of the ureteric bud would not occur.

The ureteric bud at its growing end, or ampulla, goes through a series of dichotomous branchings and, in turn, forms the ureter, renal pelvis, calyces, and collecting tubules. The development of the renal pelvis and major

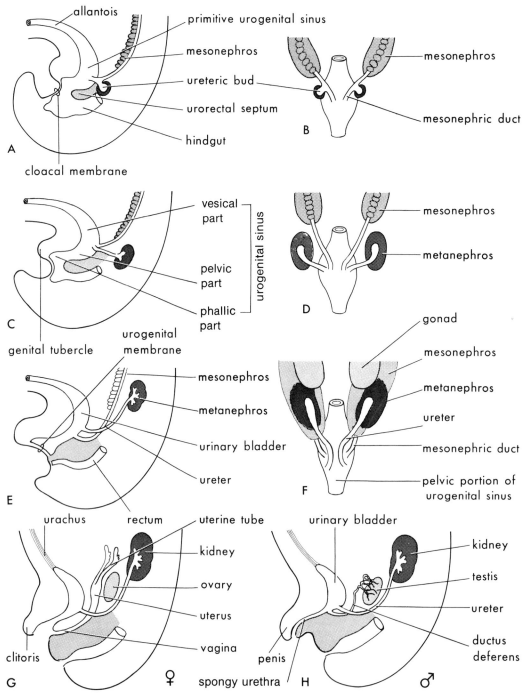

FIGURE 89–1. Embryology of the urogenital system from 5 to 12 weeks of gestation. Diagrams showing (1) division of the cloaca into the urogenital sinus and the rectum; (2) absorption of the mesonephric ducts; (3) development of the urinary bladder, urethra, and urachus; (4) changes in the location of the ureters; and (5) development of kidneys and gonads. A, C, E, G and H are lateral views; and B, D and F are dorsal views. Stage A is reached at 5 weeks, and stages G and H are reached by about 12 weeks. (Reproduced by permission from Moore, K. L. (Ed.): The Developing Human. Philadelphia, W. B. Saunders Company, 1988.)

and minor calyces is complete by 12 to 14 weeks' gestation. However, ampullary branching continues until nephrogenesis is complete.

The nephrons (exclusive of the collecting ducts) are formed from the metanephric blastema. The nephrons first develop as a rounded mass of cells on either side of the advancing ampulla. The spheroidal mass of cells then develops a central cavity, forming the renal vesicle. Thereafter, the renal vesicle grows, and the differential proliferation of epithelial cells results in elongation into an S-shaped vesicle. The S-shaped vesicle has three segments: The lower segment at the free end of the vesicle develops into the visceral and parietal epithelial layers of Bowman capsule; the middle segment develops into the proximal tubule and loop of Henle; and the upper segment develops into the distal tubule. Bernstein and his associates (1981) have shown that metanephric cells in culture produce glomeruli and tubules; these glomeruli, however, contain only epithelial cells and basement membrane but no mesangium or endothelial cells. A vessel from the interstitium grows into the primitive Bowman capsule and forms the endothelial layer of capillaries and mesangium of the glomeruli.

Nephrogenesis starts at 7 to 8 weeks and continues to 34 to 36 weeks, by which time all new nephrons have been formed. Subsequent to this, the nephrons gradually mature and grow in size, accompanied by a parallel increase in renal size and function. The development of nephrons proceeds in a centrifugal fashion, with juxtamedullary nephrons developing first and the superficial cortical nephrons developing later. At birth, the juxtamedullary nephrons are more mature than are superficial nephrons, both morphologically and functionally. In the small premature infant, nephrogenesis continues after birth.

The developing kidney is initially formed in the pelvis but later migrates cephalad to the renal fossa. As this ascent occurs, the renal collecting system (renal pelvis and ureter) rotates from an anterior position to its final medial location.

At 7 weeks' gestation, the urorectal septum divides the cloaca into the urogenital sinus anteriorly and the rectum posteriorly. Progressive absorption of the distal mesonephric duct by the urogenital sinus eventually results in separate opening sites for the mesonephric (ejaculatory)

duct and the ureteral orifice. The bladder forms from the urogenital sinus (see Fig. 89–1).

The gonads begin differentiation into testes or ovaries during the 7th week of gestation. A normal testis secretes müllerian inhibiting factor and prevents formation of the proximal vagina, uterus, and fallopian tubes from the paramesonephric, or müllerian duct. The external genitalia also develop under hormonal influence at between 7 and 14 weeks' gestation.

Defects in the development of the genitourinary system have a direct expression in congenital anomalies observed in some newborn infants. The reader is referred to the following references for further study of genitourinary embryology: Kissane, 1983, McCrory, 1972, 1987; Moore, 1988; Potter, 1972; Resnick et al., 1976.

■ RENAL ANATOMY AND MORPHOLOGY

At birth, both kidneys together weigh about 25 g compared with about 300 g in the adult. The kidneys measure about 4.5 cm in length in the newborn versus about 11.5 cm in the adult. The surface of the kidney appears lobulated; the lobulations persist for several months before becoming smooth as in the adult. Each kidney contains about 1 million nephrons, which is the full complement of nephrons in the adult kidney. However, glomerular and tubular size at birth is much smaller than in an older child or an adult. Fetterman and his associates (1965) have shown that in the newborn, the average glomerular diameter is about two-fifths that of adults (110 μm versus 280 μm) and the average proximal tubular length is about one-tenth (2 mm versus 20 mm) that of adults. Moreover, there is a greater heterogeneity among nephrons in newborn infants. The deeper (juxtamedullary) nephrons are larger and more mature than are the outer (superficial cortical) nephrons. These morphologic differences in the neonatal kidney find their functional correlates in significant differences between renal function of newborn infants and that of older children and adults.

The glomerular capillary consists of a fenestrated endothelial cell layer, the basement membrane, and the epithelial cell layer. The foot processes of epithelial cells are embedded in the outer aspect of the basement membrane. The epithelial cells in the newborn are more cuboidal and have a prominent nucleus, giving a hyper-

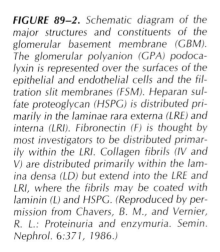

FIGURE 89–2. Schematic diagram of the major structures and constituents of the glomerular basement membrane (GBM). The glomerular polyanion (GPA) podocalyxin is represented over the surfaces of the epithelial and endothelial cells and the filtration slit membranes (FSM). Heparan sulfate proteoglycan (HSPG) is distributed primarily in the laminae rara externa (LRE) and interna (LRI). Fibronectin (F) is thought by most investigators to be distributed primarily within the LRI. Collagen fibrils (IV and V) are distributed primarily within the lamina densa (LD) but extend into the LRE and LRI, where the fibrils may be coated with laminin (L) and HSPG. (Reproduced by permission from Chavers, B. M., and Vernier, R. L.: Proteinuria and enzymuria. Semin. Nephrol. 6:371, 1986.)

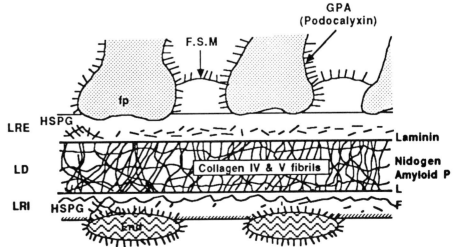

cellular appearance to the newborn glomeruli. The glomerular basement membrane is arranged in three layers: lamina rara interna, lamina densa, and lamina rara externa (Fig. 89–2). The glomerular basement membrane is a complex structure made of types IV and V collagen, Goodpasture antigen (in NC1 component of Type IV collagen), heparan sulfate proteoglycan, and large glycoproteins including laminin, fibronectin, and entactin (Chavers and Vernier, 1986; Kashtan and Fish, 1989; Michaels et al., 1984).

The magnitude of filtration of water and small molecular substances across the glomerular capillary is several times higher than in most other capillaries in the body and occurs as ultrafiltration whereby very little plasma protein enters the proximal tubule. The barrier to plasma proteins is both size and charge selective (Brenner et al., 1978). Neutral molecules of less than 15,000 daltons are freely permeable across the capillary, whereas the capillary is fairly impermeable to neutral particles larger than 80,000 daltons. Neutral particles with intermediate molecular weights have variable penetrance. The glomerular capillaries are negatively charged at the level of all three layers, and they impede filtration of negatively charged particles in plasma. Plasma albumin, which has a molecular weight of 68,000 and is highly anionic, does not normally filter across the glomerular capillary in contrast to equal-sized neutral or cationic proteins.

In some clinical disorders, the glomerular capillary negative charge is reduced and this phenomenon very likely contributes to the proteinuria observed in such disorders (Vernier et al., 1983). In others, proteinuria occurs secondary to alterations in the size-selective barrier (Dean et al., 1985).

The thickness of the glomerular basement membrane in the newborn is 100 nm compared with 300 nm in an older child and adult (Bloom et al., 1959). The chemical composition of neonatal glomerular basement membrane appears to be similar to that of adult glomerular basement membrane; however, neonatal glomerular basement membrane lacks Goodpasture antigen that is normally present in the glomerular basement membrane of older children and adults (Anand et al., 1978). As the glomeruli mature, the surface area of glomerular basement membrane increases, contributing to an increased glomerular filtration rate. Larsson and Maunsbach (1980) and Spitzer (1982) have proposed that, despite its thinness, permeability of the neonatal glomerular basement membrane is lower than that later in life and may contribute to the reduced glomerular filtration rate. More recently, Savin and associates (1985) have demonstrated that permeability of the glomerular basement membrane of the neonatal rat is greater than that in more mature rats. What role, if any, the thinness of the glomerular basement membrane

and the lack of Goodpasture antigen in newborn infants play in the observed differences in glomerular filtration rate and various glomerular diseases of the newborn versus those in children and adults is largely unknown at present.

■ REFERENCES

Anand, S. K., Landing, B. H., Heuser, E., et al.: Changes in glomerular basement membrane antigen(s) with age. J. Pediatr. 92:952, 1978.

Bernstein, J., Cheng, F., and Roska, J.: Glomerular differentiation in metanephric culture. Lab. Invest. 45:183, 1981.

Bloom, P. M., Hartmann, J. F., and Vernier, R. L.: An electron microscopic evaluation of the width of normal glomerular basement membrane in man in various ages. Anat. Record 133:251, 1959.

Brenner, B. M., Hostetter, T. H., and Humes, H. D.: Molecular basis of proteinuria of glomerular origin. N. Engl. J. Med. 198:826, 1978.

Chavers, B. M., and Vernier, R. L.: Proteinuria and enzymuria. Semin. Nephrol. 6:371, 1986.

Dean, W. M., Bridges, C. R., Brenner, B. M., et al.: Heteroporous model of glomerular size selectivity: Applications to normal and nephrotic humans. Am. J. Physiol. 249:374, 1985.

Fetterman, G. H., Shuplock, N. A., Phillipp, F. S., et al.: The growth and maturation of human glomeruli and proximal convolutions from term to adulthood. Studies by microdissection. Pediatrics 35:601, 1965.

Kashtan, C., and Fish, A. J.: Basement membrane and cellular components of the nephron. In Massary, S. G., and Glassock, R. J. (Ed.): Textbook of Nephrology. Baltimore, Williams & Wilkins, 1989, p. 28.

Kissane, J. M.: Development of the kidney. In Heptinstall, R. H. (Ed.): Pathology of the Kidney. Boston, Little, Brown and Company, 1983, p. 61.

Larsson, L., and Maunsbach, A. B.: The ultrastructural development of the glomerular filtration barrier in the rat kidney: A morphometric analysis. J. Ultrastr. Res. 72:392, 1980.

McCrory, W. W.: Developmental Nephrology. Cambridge, Harvard University Press, 1972, Chapter 1.

McCrory, W. W.: Renal structure and development. In Holliday, M. A., Barratt, T. M., and Vernier, R. L. (Eds.): Pediatric Nephrology. Baltimore, Williams & Wilkins, 1987, p. 31.

Michaels, A. F., Falk, R. J., Platt, J. L., et al.: Antigens of the human glomerulus. Adv. Nephrol. 13:203, 1984.

Moore, K. L. (Ed.): The Developing Human: Clinically Oriented Embryology. Philadelphia, W. B. Saunders Company, 1988.

Potter, E. L.: Normal and Abnormal Development of the Kidney. Chicago, Year Book Publications, 1972, Chapter 1.

Resnick, J. S., Brown, D. M., and Vernier, R. L.: Normal development and experimental models of cystic renal disease. In Gardner, K. D. (Ed.): Cystic Diseases of the Kidney. New York, John Wiley, 1976, p. 221.

Savin, V. J., Beason-Griffin, C., and Richardson, W. P.: Ultrafiltration coefficient of isolated glomeruli of rats aged 4 days to maturation. Kidney Int. 28:926, 1985.

Spitzer, A.: Factors underlying the increase in glomerular filtration rate during postnatal development. In Spitzer, A. (Ed.): The Kidney During Development. Morphology and Function. New York, Masson Publishing, 1982, p. 127.

Vernier, R. L., Klein, D. J., Sisson, S. P., et al.: Heparan sulfate rich anionic sites in the human glomerular basement membrane. Decreased concentration in congenital nephrotic syndrome. N. Engl. J. Med. 309:1001, 1983.

MATURATION OF **90**
RENAL FUNCTION

Sudhir K. Anand

Although the contribution of the fetal kidney to excretory function throughout gestation is minimal, fetal urine production does play an important role in maintenance of amniotic fluid volume. Our understanding of maturation of fetal renal function, especially in early gestation, is still limited. In the past two decades, with chronically implanted catheters in fetal vessels and the urinary bladder, a number of physiologic studies have been carried out in sheep to study the maturation of renal function in the latter half of gestation. Development and maturation of renal function during fetal and neonatal period proceed at different rates in various animal species; therefore, one must use caution in applying these results to humans.

The maturation of renal function occurs in parallel with the morphologic maturation of the fetus. There is gradual increase in renal blood flow, glomerular filtration rate, and ability to conserve sodium and fluid. Several hormonal systems including aldosterone, renin-angiotensin, arginine vasopressin, atrial natriuretic peptide, prostaglandins, and kallikrein and their receptors also mature and interact with the growing kidney. The role and regulatory mechanisms of these hormones in the fetus and in newborns are still only partially understood. Also, one should differentiate between effects observed during administration of large pharmacologic doses of these hormones and their physiologic functions in the fetus and newborn. The reader is referred to several recent reviews of maturation of renal function for detailed discussions: Arant, 1981; Robillard, 1987, 1988 a,b; Spitzer, 1985; Yared 1984.

■ RENAL BLOOD FLOW (RBF)

In sheep and other animals, during fetal life only 2 to 3 per cent of cardiac output goes to the kidney compared with about 6 per cent during the 1st week of life, 15 to 18 per cent by the end of the 1st month and 20 to 25 per cent in the adult (Paton et al., 1973; Robillard et al., 1988a; Rudolph and Heymann, 1970). The low renal blood flow in fetal and newborn animals is associated with a higher renal vascular resistance and a lower perfusion pressure compared with adult animals (Aperia et al., 1977a; Gruskin et al., 1970). During the first 24 hours after birth in sheep, renal blood flow does not significantly increase, nor is there much decrease in renal vascular resistance even though the glomerular filtration rate (GFR) during this time increases almost three-fold (Nakamura et al., 1987). Subsequently, the renal blood flow gradually increases, primarily due to a decrease in renal vascular resistance (Gruskin et al., 1970; Robillard et al., 1981a) (Fig. 90–1). An increase in blood pressure after birth also

appears to play a limited role in the increase in RBF (Robillard et al., 1981a).

Renal plasma flow and renal blood flow in newborns have been estimated by clearance of para-amino hippurate (PAH) (Calcagno and Rubin, 1963). PAH extraction rate by the kidney in older children and adults is over 90 per cent. However, in newborns, the extraction rate is only 60 per cent, which causes PAH clearance to be an underestimation of the true effective renal plasma flow. When corrected for body surface area, the PAH clearance and renal plasma flow are still low at birth, double in the first 2 weeks, and reach mature levels by 12 to 24 months of age (Calcagno and Rubin, 1963; Guignard et al., 1975).

During fetal life, outer cortical glomeruli are relatively underperfused compared with inner cortical (juxtamedullary) glomeruli. Following birth, renal perfusion to superficial cortical nephrons rises compared with deeper glomeruli (Aperia et al., 1977a; Robillard et al., 1981a). These changes in intrarenal blood flow distribution parallel the changes in glomerular morphologic and functional maturation (Spitzer and Brandis, 1974).

Various hormones that regulate fetal and neonatal renal blood flow and its intrarenal distribution include catecholamines, the renin-angiotensin system, prostaglandins, and kallikreins. The levels of circulating catecholamines and plasma renin activity and angiotensin II levels are elevated in newborn infants and fetal and neonatal animals when compared with adults (Eliot et al., 1980; Kotchen et al., 1972, Sulyok et al., 1979a). However, the exact role these elevated hormone levels play in the observed increased renal vascular resistance is still unclear. The response to exogenous hormones in various experiments is often different among fetal, neonatal, and adult animals, and there are also differences between various species (Robillard et al., 1988a). Inhibition of angiotensin II synthesis using captopril does not produce renal hemodynamic changes in immature fetal lambs (<120 days gestation) but decreases resistance in near-term fetuses (>130 days) and newborn lambs (Robillard et al., 1982). Also, infusion of angiotensin II antagonist in puppies does not modify renal blood flow (Jose, 1975).

Renal blood flow is affected by changes in tissue oxygenation and blood pressure. Hypoxemia, both in the fetal and newborn lamb, results in a marked increase in epinephrine and norepinephrine levels, a limited increase in plasma renin activity, an increase in renal vascular resistance, and a decrease in renal blood flow (Robillard et al., 1981b; Sidi et al., 1983; Weismann and Clark, 1981; Weismann and Robillard, 1988). The effects of hypoxemia on renal blood flow appear to be significantly more pronounced in the fetal lamb than in the newborn

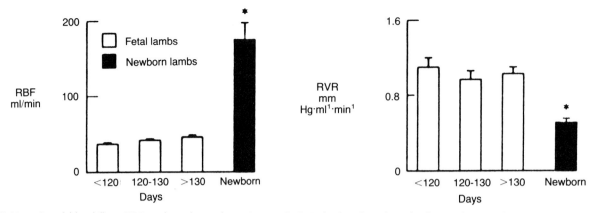

FIGURE 90–1. *Renal blood flow (RBF) and renal vascular resistance (RVR) in fetal and newborn lambs (newborn lambs were studied between 3 and 19 days postnatally). Values expressed as means ± SEM. Newborn values were significantly different from fetal values (P<0.05). (Reproduced by permission from Robillard, J. E.: Development of function in fetal kidney. In Holliday, M. A., Barratt, M. A., and Vernier, R. L. (Eds.): Pediatric Nephrology. Baltimore, Williams & Wilkins, 1987, p. 902.)*

lamb (Weismann and Robillard, 1988). Renal blood flow measured as PAH clearance is reduced in infants with respiratory distress syndrome (Guignard et al., 1976).

Autoregulation of renal blood flow allows the kidney to maintain relatively constant glomerular perfusion despite wide changes in mean arterial blood pressure. However, in adults, mean blood pressure below 80 mm Hg limits the ability of the kidney to autoregulate glomerular perfusion, resulting in decreased glomerular filtration (Brenner et al., 1986a; Navar, 1978). The kidney's ability to autoregulate is based on the interaction of various vasoactive hormones, on glomerular afferent and efferent arterioles, and the innate ability of arterioles to dilate or contract by myogenic reflex in response to alterations in perfusion pressure. The mean arterial blood pressure is relatively low in newborns (especially premature infants) (Adelman, 1988; Versmold et al., 1981; see Chapter 102). The minimal critical pressure above which the neonatal kidney can autoregulate renal blood flow is set at a lower level than in an adult animal (Chevalier, 1983; Jose, 1975). Whereas Jose and associates have suggested that autoregulation may be less than in the adult animal, Chevalier and associates have reported that young animals can effectively autoregulate renal blood flow.

■ GLOMERULAR FILTRATION RATE (GFR)

Glomerular filtration begins between the 9th and 12th week of gestation in humans. Fetal urine is a major constituent of amniotic fluid, and the urinary flow rate increases from 12 ml/hr at 32 weeks' gestation to 28 ml/hr at 40 weeks' gestation (Campbell et al., 1973) or about 7 ml/kg body weight/hr. In fetal sheep, the GFR increases three-fold during the last trimester (Robillard et al., 1975). Similar increases are described during the maturation of premature newborns from 28 to 40 weeks (see later).

The GFR is relatively low at birth, especially in the premature infant, even when corrected for surface area to adult values of 1.73 m². The GFR during the first 24 hours after birth in term infants is about 2 to 3.5 ml (15 to 25 ml/min/1.73 m²). The values of GFR nearly double between 3 and 7 days, and thereafter GFR continues to increase, so that by 1 to 2 years of age the GFR corrected to 1.73 m² is the same as in an older child or an adult

(Table 90–1). In premature infants, the GFR after birth is low (< 1 ml/min) and is directly related to the gestational age of the infant (Fig. 90–2) (Leake et al., 1976a). Also, the maturation of renal function in the premature infant is slower than that in term infants and GFR remains close to that of a fetus of corresponding conceptual age (Arant 1978; Leake et al., 1976a, 1977; Vanpee et al., 1988) (Table 90–1). There are marked variations in GFR among individual newborn infants within the same study and among different studies. The values for inulin clearance and creatinine clearance are generally concordant (Aperia et al., 1981a; Stonestreet et al., 1979) and have been used interchangeably in Table 90–1.

The glomerular filtration rate at the level of a single nephron (SNGFR) is dependent on glomerular perfusion rate, transcapillary hydraulic and oncotic pressure gradients, and the ultrafiltration coefficient of the capillary wall (Brenner and Humes, 1977; Brenner et al., 1986b). These authors have correlated SNGFR with other variables:

$$SNGFR = P_{UF} \times K_f$$

Where P_{UF} refers to net ultrafiltration pressure across glomerular capillary wall and K_f to ultrafiltration coefficient of capillary wall. The net ultrafiltration pressure is based on the balance of hydrostatic pressure in the glomerular capillary (P_{GC}) opposed by the plasma oncotic pressure (π_{GC}) and hydrostatic pressure in the proximal tubule (P_T) [$P_{UF} = P_{GC} - (\pi_{GC} + P_T)$]. The ultrafiltration coefficient depends on both the intrinsic hydraulic permeability of the capillary wall (k) and the surface area of the capillary wall (A) ($K_f = k \times A$).

The SNGFR equation does not include reference to renal plasma flow. However the plasma flow rate affects SNGFR by indirectly affecting the π_{GC} along the length of glomerular capillaries. The GFR of the whole kidney is based on cumulation of various SNGFR and, thus, is based on renal perfusion, the surface area of glomerular capillaries, and their permeability properties. In neonatal animals, values of most of these variables are decreased and account for the low GFR (Spitzer, 1982, 1985). The GFR increases from neonatal to adult values mostly because of increases in glomerular capillary surface area with limited contributions by the increase in glomerular capillary

TABLE 90–1. Changes in GFR with Age*

AGE	GFR ml/min	GFR ml/min/1.73m	SERUM CREATININE mg/dl
Premature			
<30 week	0.3 to 0.5	5 to 8 ml	<1.6
30 to 34 weeks	0.5 to 1.0	5 to 10 ml	<1.2
Full Term			
<24 hour	2 to 3.5	15 to 25	0.6 to 1.0
3 days to 3 weeks	4 to 8	30 to 50	0.5 to 0.6
1 to 2 months	10 to 12	60 to 70	0.4 to 0.5
3 to 4 months	18 to 20	70 to 80	0.3 to 0.4
6 months to 1 year	25 to 30	80 to 100	0.4 to 0.5
Adult	120 + 20	120 ± 20	0.6 to 1.4 (male)
			0.6 to 1.1 (female)

*Values based on data from several studies, including Aperia et al., 1981a; Arant, 1978; Fawer et al., 1979; Feldman and Guignard, 1982; Guignard et al., 1975; Leake and Trygstad, 1977; Oh et al., 1966; Schwartz et al., 1984; Stonestreet and Oh, 1978.

pressure (Ichikawa et al., 1979; Spitzer, 1982; Robillard, 1987). Changes in hydraulic permeability (as discussed in Chapter 89) contribute minimally to postnatal increase in GFR. The mean blood pressure in newborn animals is low, resulting in decreased glomerular capillary pressure (P_{GC}); however, net ultrafiltration pressure (P_{UF}) is maintained by coexisting decreased plasma oncotic pressure (π_{GC}) due to decreased plasma protein concentration (Spitzer, 1985).

The GFR in sheep increases three-fold during the first 24 hours following delivery (Nakamura et al., 1987). However, because there is no associated increase in renal plasma flow during this time, the increase in GFR probably occurs secondary to redistribution of intrarenal blood flow with increase in flow to superficial nephrons, which in turn increase renal GFR. The kidney is able to autoregulate GFR by autoregulation of glomerular perfusion (see earlier); however, this ability in the fetus and newborn may be limited (Robillard et al., 1981a; Yared and Yoshioka, 1989). Large intravenous fluid loads (Leake et al., 1976b) and placental transfusions (Oh et al., 1966) increase GFR in newborn infants, whereas hypoxemia reduces GFR (Robillard et al., 1981b; Guignard et al., 1976).

Inulin clearance has been the standard measure for GFR; however, the procedure is cumbersome and impractical for routine use because it requires urinary catheterization, inulin infusion, and timed collections of urine and blood. Techniques that obviate the need for urinary collection include plasma disappearance rates of [51]CrEDTA and ^{131}I sodium iodothalamate and constant infusion of inulin; however, these methods tend to overestimate GFR in the newborn. Serial measurements of serum creatinine are usually sufficient for clinical evaluation of glomerular filtration and, if necessary, may be accompanied by urine collection to measure creatinine clearance (see Chapter 91).

■ SODIUM REGULATION

Sodium plays a primary role in maintenance of extracellular fluid volume, serum osmolality, and overall fluid homeostasis. Urinary sodium excretion rate and fractional excretion of sodium (FENa) are both increased during fetal life but tend to decrease as gestation progresses. Gresham and associates (1972) reported daily urinary sodium excretion rate in fetal sheep (late in gestation) to

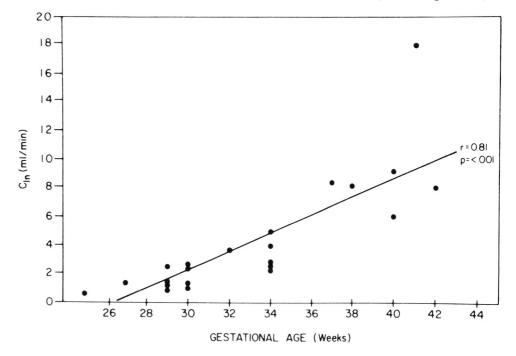

FIGURE 90–2. Correlation of glomerular filtration rate (GFR measured as inulin clearance) and gestational age in two- to three-day-old infants. (Reproduced by permission from Leake, R. D., Trygstad, C. W., and Oh, W.: Inulin clearance in the newborn infant: Relationship to gestational and postnatal age. Pediatr. Res. 10:759, 1976a.)

be 6 MEq/kg body weight. The FENa varies between 5 and 10 per cent (Robillard et al., 1977a). During the first hour after birth in the newborn lamb, FENa transiently increases to nearly 10 per cent before starting to decline to 1 per cent by 24 hours of age (Nakamura et al., 1987). Whether or not a similar transient increase in FENa occurs in newborn infants during the first few hours after birth is not known.

Most newborns during the first few days of life have an initial diuresis and weight loss associated with reduction in total body and extracellular fluid volume. Thereafter term infants are in a positive sodium balance; sodium retention is a normal component of physical growth. In term infants, the kidney efficiently conserves sodium. The daily urinary excretion of sodium is less than 0.5 mEq/kg body weight and FENa less than 0.5 per cent (Arant, 1978; Siegel and Oh, 1976). This capacity is essential because mature breast milk (after the 1st week) at a daily intake of 150 ml/kg body weight provides only 1 mEq/kg/day sodium intake. However, premature infants do not conserve sodium as efficiently as term infants, and normal very premature infants may have FENa of 5 per cent or higher (Siegel and Oh, 1976) (Fig. 90–3). Premature newborns often develop hyponatremia (in some infants there may be an initial episode of hypernatremia in the first days of life due to a great amount of insensible water loss through the skin) and are in a negative sodium balance for several days to a few weeks (Al-Dahan et al., 1983a, b; Engelke et al., 1978; Roy et al., 1976; Shaffer and Meade, 1989; Sulyok et al., 1979b). These infants require substantially larger daily sodium intake (usually 3 mEq/kg but occasionally as much as 12 mEq/kg for short periods in the least mature infants) than term newborns. The sodium absorption from the gut is also less efficient in premature infants than in term infants. Administration of large volumes of fluids to premature infants may also result in hyponatremia due to water retention (Rees et al., 1984a, b).

The data from growing animals suggest that the ability of the kidney to efficiently conserve sodium probably occurs secondary to enhanced sodium absorption in distal tubular sites and not in the proximal tubule (Aperia and Elinder, 1981b; Spitzer, 1985). The mechanism of enhanced sodium absorption in distal sites in the term newborn and a lack of the same in the premature newborn is not clearly understood. Spitzer (1985) and Sulyok and associates (1979b, c) have suggested that the elevated levels of aldosterone in term infants may be responsible for augmented sodium absorption at distal sites, whereas the premature newborn may have a diminished response to aldosterone.

Atrial natriuretic peptide(s) (ANP) is a peptide hormone secreted by the atria. The values of plasma ANP are increased both in fetal and newborn humans and animals when compared with the adult (Robillard and Weiner, 1988c; Robillard et al., 1988d; Shine et al., 1987; Tulassay et al., 1986), and increase further during volume expansion (Robillard and Weiner, 1988c; Ross et al., 1987). When ANP is exogenously administered, it causes increased natriuresis and diuresis (Atlas and Laragh, 1987; Ballerman and Brenner, 1987). The natriuresis is associated with both an increase in GFR and decreased tubular reabsorption of sodium in adult humans and animals and in 112- to 115-day-old sheep (Shine et al., 1987) but has limited action in 130-day-old fetal sheep (Hargrave et al., 1989; Robillard and Nakamura, 1988d) and young rats (Chevalier et al., 1988). The exact physiologic role of ANP in sodium homeostasis of the fetus and the newborn infant (including transient diuresis after birth) is still not clear (Shaffer and Meade, 1989).

Newborn infants and animals, when given large sodium loads, increase their urinary sodium excretion; however, this ability is reduced compared with adults (Aperia et al., 1977b, Goldsmith et al., 1979, Leake et al., 1976b). Excess fluid and sodium loads in newborns may lead to edema and heart failure, especially in infants with myocardial dysfunction. Patent ductus arteriosus with left-to-right shunt and bronchopulmonary dysplasia (Bell et al., 1980) are exacerbated by excess fluid and sodium loads in premature infants.

Hyponatremia and hypernatremia are seen in a variety of conditions, in both the term and premature infants. Their causes and management are discussed in Chapter 28.

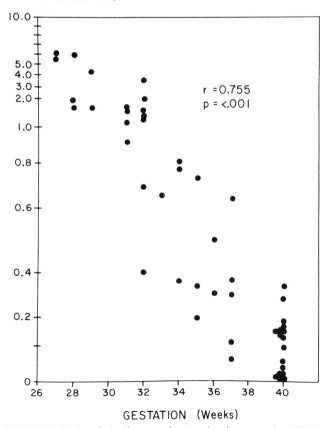

FRACTIONAL SODIUM EXCRETION (% FILTERED Na)

r =0.755
p = <.001

GESTATION (Weeks)

FIGURE 90–3. Correlation between fractional sodium excretion (FENa) and gestational age in human infants. (Reproduced by permission from Siegel, S. R., and Oh, W.: Renal functional maturation in human infants. Acta Paediatr. Scand. 65:481, 1976.)

■ **URINE DILUTING AND CONCENTRATING ABILITY**

The fetal urine in mammals is usually hypotonic to plasma, but the fetal kidney can concentrate or dilute urine depending on the state of maternal and, hence, fetal hydration (Ross et al., 1988; Smith and Robillard, 1989). The ability of the fetal kidney to maximally concentrate urine to adult values, however, is limited even during vasopressin infusions (Robillard, 1987; Smith and Robillard, 1989). The fetal pituitary gland produces arginine vasopressin (AVP), and both osmotic and volume regulation of AVP is intact in the fetus (Robillard et al., 1979; Weitzman et al., 1978).

The urine diluting capacity of newborn and premature infants is well developed, and these infants are capable of diluting urine to osmolality less than 40 mOsm/kg water, values well below those observed in older children and adults (Aperia et al., 1974). Despite the greater ability to excrete maximally dilute urine, the ability of newborn kidney to excrete a hypotonic fluid load is limited (Fisher et al., 1963), presumably due to low GFR.

In contrast, the urinary concentrating capacity in the newborn is limited. Following water deprivation, the newborn kidney is able to concentrate to 700 to 800 mOsm/kg water (Hansen and Smith, 1953; Edelmann et al., 1960). In the premature infant, maximal urinary osmolality may only reach 500 mOsm/kg water. The inability of the newborn kidney to concentrate urine to values of 1200 to 1400 mOsm/kg observed in older children and adults is due to several factors: anatomic immaturity with short renal medulla (Spitzer, 1985); limited solute (urea) excretion, resulting in a low renal medullary concentration gradient (Edelmann et al., 1960); and decreased sensitivity of collecting tubules to AVP due to decreased AVP receptors, decreased cyclic AMP production, and prostaglandin inhibition (Robillard, 1987). Asphyxia and acute renal failure also limit ability of the kidney to concentrate urine.

■ ACID-BASE REGULATION (also see Chapters 28 and 105)

The role of the kidneys in the regulation of acid-base balance of the fetus is limited; however, the fetal kidney is involved in regulation of acid-base balance (Kesby and Lumbers, 1986; Smith and Robillard, 1989). After birth, the kidney is capable of excreting hydrogen ion (nonvolatile acid) produced by metabolism of certain amino acids, phosphoesters, nucleic acid, and incomplete oxidation of organic acids. The newborn kidney, as the adult, first reclaims the filtered bicarbonate (primarily in the proximal tubule) and then generates bicarbonate by excreting net acid in form of titratable acid or ammonium ion. The renal threshold for bicarbonate, however, in the term infant is close to 20 to 22 mEq/l and in the preterm infant 18 to 20 mEq/l compared with 24 to 26 mEq/l in the older child and adult (Edelmann et al., 1967; Portale et al., 1987; Schwartz et al., 1979). The basis for this low threshold in the newborn is not known but may be related to greater heterogeneity of nephrons or expanded ECF volume (Edelmann et al., 1967; Robillard et al., 1977b; Moore 1972). However, in the newborn, the bicarbonate threshold may increase in a variety of conditions including volume depletion (diuretic use), chloride or potassium depletion, and chronic respiratory acidosis.

The normal newborn, in the first few days of life, may not be able to lower the urinary pH below 6.0 (Sulyok et al., 1972). However, by the 1st week of life, urinary pH below 6.0 occurs with systemic acidosis. Thereafter, urine pH varies between 5.0 and 8.0. During exogenous acid loading, ammonium excretion does not increase to adult levels. However, this incapacity is compensated for by an increase in excretion of titratable acid (Edelmann et al., 1967; Svenningsen, 1974). In the premature infant, these abilities are limited compared with term infants (Sulyok 1971; Sulyok et al., 1972).

■ POTASSIUM REGULATION

Potassium (K) is the predominant intracellular cation; only 2 per cent of total body potassium is located in the extracellular fluid compartment. The intracellular potassium concentration is about 150 mEq/l, and the extracellular potassium concentration is 3.5 to 5 mEq/l. The serum K concentration in the normal newborn is higher than in the older child and adult, and values as high as 6.0 mEq/l are not uncommon, especially in the premature infant (Day et al., 1976). The significance of the higher serum K values observed in the newborn is not known. It is generally believed that both term and premature infants are in a consistently positive potassium balance (Day et al., 1976; Guignard and John, 1986; Sulyok, 1971); however, Engle and Arant (1984) have reported that many critically ill newborns are in negative potassium balance. Also, in sick newborns, lack of potassium administration in intravenous fluid for the initial few days, use of diuretics, and maintenance of high urine flow rates may exaggerate the K losses. During the first 1 to 2 weeks of life, urinary K/Na ratio is usually less than one, both in term and premature infants (Vanpee et al., 1988); however, after that, urinary K/Na ratio exceeds one until age 6 months to 2 years when sodium supplemented foods are added to the diet in most societies. Potassium content of mature breast milk is 13 mEq/l versus 7 mEq/l for sodium, and this is the basis for urinary K/Na ratios greater than one. The higher urinary K/Na ratio after first 2 weeks of life may also reflect increased responsiveness of distal renal tubular sites to aldosterone.

■ REFERENCES

Adelman, R. D.: The hypertensive neonate. Clin. Perinatol. 15:567, 1988.

Al-Dahan, J., Haycock, G. B., Chantler, S., et al.: Sodium homeostasis in term and preterm neonates: I Renal aspects. Arch. Dis. Child. 58:335, 1983a.

Al-Dahan, J., Haycock, G. B., Chantler, S., et al.: Sodium homeostasis in term and preterm neonates: II Gastrointestinal aspects. Arch. Dis. Child. 58:343, 1983b.

Aperia, A., Broberger, O., Thodenius, K., et al.: Developmental study of the renal response to an oral salt load in preterm infants. Acta Pediatr. Scand. 63:517, 1974.

Aperia, A., Broberger, O., Herin, P., et al.: Renal hemodynamics in the perinatal period: A study in lambs. Acta Physiol. Scand. 99:261, 1977a.

Aperia, A., Borberger, O., Herrine, P., et al.: A comparative study of the response to an oral NaCl and NaHCO₃ found in newborn preterm and full term infants. Pediatr. Res. 11:1109, 1977b.

Aperia, A., Borberger, O., Herin, P., et al.: Sodium excretion in relation to sodium intake and aldosterone in newborn preterm and full term infants. Acta Pediatr. Scand. 68:813, 1979.

Aperia, A., Borberger, O., Elinder, G., et al.: Postnatal development of renal function in preterm and full term infants. Acta Pediatr. Scand. 70:183, 1981a.

Aperia, A., and Elinder, G.: Distal tubular sodium reabsorption in the developing rat kidney. Am. J. Physiol. 240:F487, 1981b.

Arant, B. S.: Developmental patterns of renal functional maturation compared in the human neonate. J. Pediatr. 92:705, 1978.

Arant, B. S.: Nonrenal factors influencing renal function during perinatal period. Clin. Perinatol. 8:225, 1981.

Atlas, S. A., and Laragh, J. H.: Physiological actions of natriuretic factor. In Murlow, P. J., and Shrier, R. (Eds.) Atrial Hormones and Other Natriuretic Factors. Baltimore, Williams & Wilkins, 1987, p. 53.

Ballermann, B. J., and Brenner, B. M.: Atrial natriuretic peptides and the kidney. Am. J. Kidney Dis. 10:7, 1987.

Bell, E. F., Warburton, D., Stonestreet, B. S., et al.: Effects of fluid administration on the development of symptomatic patent ductus arteriosus and congestive heart failure in premature infants. N. Engl. J. Med. 302:59, 1980.

Brenner, B. M., and Humes, H. D.: Mechanics of glomerular ultrafiltration. N. Engl. J. Med. 297:148, 1977.

Brenner, B. M., Zatz, R., and Ichikawa, I.: The renal circulations. In Brenner, B. M., and Rector, F. C. (Eds.) The Kidney. Philadelphia, W. B. Saunders Company, 1986a, p. 93.

Brenner, B. M., Dworkin, L. D., and Ichikawa, I.: Glomerular ultrafiltration. In Brenner, B. M., and Rector, F. C. (Eds.), The Kidney. Philadelphia, W. B. Saunders Company, 1986b, p. 124.

Calcagno, P. L., and Rubin, M. I.: Renal extraction of para amino hippurate in infants and children. J. Clin. Invest. 42:1632, 1963.

Campbell, S. W., Ladimiroff, J. W., and Dewhurst, C. J.: The antenatal measurement of fetal urine production. J. Obstet. Gynecol. 80:680, 1973.

Chevalier, R. L., and Kaiser, D. L.: Autoregulation of renal blood flow in the rat. Effects of growth and uninephrectomy. Am. J. Physiol. 244:F483, 1983.

Chevalier, R. L., Gomez, A., Carey, R. M., et al.: Renal effects of atrial natriuretic peptide infusion in young and adult rats. Pediatr. Res. 24:333, 1988.

Day, G. M., Radde, I. C., and Balfe, J. W.: Electrolyte abnormalities in very low birth weight infants. Pediatr. Res. 10:522, 1976.

Edelmann, C. M., and Barnett, H. L.: Role of the kidney in water metabolism in young infants. Physiologic and clinical considerations. J. Pediatr. 56:154, 1960.

Edelmann, C. M., Soriano, J. R., Boichis, H., et al.: Renal bicarbonate reabsorption and hydrogen ion excretion in normal infants. J. Clin. Invest. 46:1309, 1967.

Eliot, R. J., Lam, R., Leake, R. D., et al.: Plasma catecholamine concentration in infants at birth and during the first 48 hours of life. J. Pediatr. 96:311, 1980.

Engelke, S. C., Shah, B. L., Vasan, U., et al.: Sodium balance in very low birth weight infants. J. Pediatr. 93:837, 1978.

Engle, W. D., and Arant, B. S.: Urinary potassium excretion in the critically ill neonate. Pediatrics 74:259, 1984.

Fawer, C. L., Torrado, A., and Guignard, J. P.: Maturation of renal function in full term and preterm neonates. Helv. Pediatr. Acta 34:11, 1979.

Feldman, H., and Guignard, J. P.: Plasma creatinine in the first month of life. Arch. Dis. Child. 57:123, 1982.

Fisher, D. A., Pyle, H. R., Porter, J. C., et al.: Control of water balance in the newborn. Am. J. Dis. Child. 106:137, 1963.

Goldsmith, D. I., Drukker, A., Blaufox, M. D., et al.: Hemodynamic and excretory responses of the neonatal canine kidney to acute volume expansion. Am. J. Physiol. 237:F392, 1979.

Gresham, E. L., Rankin, J. H. G., Makowshi, E. L., et al.: An evaluation of fetal renal function in chronic sheep preparation. J. Clin. Invest. 51:149, 1972.

Gruskin, A. B., Edelmann, C. M., and Yaun, S.: Maturational changes in renal blood flow in piglets. Pediatr. Res. 4:7, 1970.

Guignard, J. P., and John, E. G.: Renal function in the tiny premature infant. Clin. Perinatol. 13:377, 1986.

Guignard, J. P., Torrado, A., Da Cunha, O., et al.: Glomerular filtration rate in the first three weeks of life. J. Pediatr. 87:268, 1975.

Guignard, J. P., Torrado, A., and Mazouni, S. M.: Renal function in respiratory distress syndrome. J. Pediatr. 88:845, 1976.

Hansen, J. D. L., and Smith, C. A.: Effects of withholding fluid in the immediate postnatal period. Pediatrics 12:99, 1953.

Hargrave, B. Y., Iwamoto, H. S., and Rudolph, A. M.: Renal and cardiovascular effects of atrial natriuretic peptide in fetal sheep. Pediatr. Res. 26:1, 1989.

Ichikawa, I., Maddox, D. A., and Brenner, B. M.: Maturational development of glomerular ultrafiltration in the rat. Am. J. Physiol. 36:F465, 1979.

Jose, P. A., Slotkoff, L. M., Montgomery, S., et al.: Autoregulation of renal blood flow in the puppy. Am. J. Physiol. 229:983, 1975.

Kesby, G. J., and Lumbers, E. R.: Factors affecting renal handling of sodium, hydrogen ions, and bicarbonate by the fetus. Am. J. Physiol. 251:F226, 1986.

Kotchen, T. A., Strickland, A. L., Rice, T. W., et al.: A study of the renin-angiotensin system in newborn infants. J. Pediatr. 80:938, 1972.

Leake, R. D., Trygstad, C. W., and Oh, W.: Inulin clearance in newborn infant: Relationship to gestational and postnatal age. Pediatr. Res. 10:759, 1976a.

Leake, R. D., Zakauddin, J., Trygstad, C. W., et al.: The effects of large volume intravenous fluid infusion on neonatal renal function. J. Pediatr. 89:968, 1976b.

Leake, R. D., and Trygstad, C. W.: Glomerular filtration rate during the period of adaptation to extrauterine life. Pediatr. Res. 11:959, 1977.

Moore, E. S., Fine, B. P., Satrasook, S. S., et al.: Renal reabsorption of bicarbonate in puppies. Effect of extracellular volume contraction on the renal threshold for bicarbonate. Pediatr. Res. 6:859, 1972.

Nakamura, K. T., Matherne, G. P., McWeeny, O. J., et al.: Renal hemodynamics and functional changes during the transition from fetal to newborn life in sheep. Pediatr. Res. 21:229, 1987.

Navar, L. E.: Renal autoregulation: Prospectives from whole kidney and single nephron studies. Am. J. Physiol. 234:F357, 1978.

Oh, W., Oh, M. A., and Lind, J.: Renal function and blood volume in newborn infants related to placental transfusion. Acta Pediatr. Scand. 56:197, 1966.

Paton, J. B., Fisher, D. E., Peterson, E., et al.: Cardiac output and organ blood flows in baboon fetus. Biol. Neonate 22:50, 1973.

Portale, A. A., Booth, B. E., and Morris, R. C.: Renal tubular acidosis. In Holliday, M. A., Barratt, T. M., and Vernier, R. L. (Eds.): Pediatric Nephrology. Baltimore, Williams & Wilkins 1987, p. 606.

Rees, L., Shaw, J. C. L., Brook, C. G. D., et al.: Hyponatremia in the first week of life in preterm infants. Part I. Arginine vasopressin secretion. Arch. Dis. Child. 59:414, 1984a.

Rees, L., Shaw, J. C. L., Brook, C. G. D., et al.: Hyponatremia in the first week of life in preterm infants. Part II. Sodium and water balance. Arch. Dis. Child. 59:423, 1984b.

Robillard, J. E.: Development of function in fetal kidney. In Holliday, M. A., Barratt, T. M., and Vernier, R. L. (Eds.): Pediatric Nephrology. Baltimore, Williams & Wilkins, 1987, p. 901.

Robillard, J. E., Kulvinskas, C., Sessions, C., et al.: Maturational changes in the fetal glomerular filtration rate. Am. J. Obstet. Gynecol. 122:601, 1975.

Robillard, J. E., Sessions, C., Kennedy, R. L., et al.: Interrelationship between glomerular filtration rate and renal transport of sodium and chloride during fetal life. Am. J. Obstet. Gynecol. 128:727, 1977a.

Robillard, J. E., Sessions, C., Burmeister, L., et al.: Influence of fetal extracellular volume contraction on renal absorption of bicarbonate in fetal lamb. Pediatr. Res. 11:649, 1977b.

Robillard, J. E., Weitzman, R. E., Fisher, D. A., et al.: The dynamics of vasopressin release and blood volume regulation during fetal hemorrhage in the lamb fetus. Pediatr. Res. 13:606, 1979.

Robillard, J. E., Weismann, D. N., and Herin, P.: Ontogeny of single glomerular perfusion rate in fetal and newborn lambs. Pediatr. Res. 15:248, 1981a.

Robillard, J. E., Weitzman, R. E., Burnmeister, L., et al.: Developmental aspects of renal response to hypoxemia in lamb fetus. Circ. Res. 48:128, 1981b.

Robillard, J. E., Gomez, R. A., Van Orden, D., et al.: Comparison of adrenal and renal response to angiotensin II in fetal lambs and adult sheep. Circ. Res. 50:140, 1982.

Robillard, J. E., Nakamura, K. T., Matherne, G. P., et al.: Renal hemodynamics and functional adjustments to postnatal life. Semin. Perinatol. 12:143, 1988a.

Robillard, J. E., and Nakamura, K. T.: Hormonal regulation of renal function during development. Biol. Neonate 53:201, 1988b.

Robillard, J. E., and Weiner, C.: Atrial natriuretic factor in the human fetus: Effect of volume expansion. J. Pediatr. 113:552, 1988c.

Robillard, J., Nakamura, K. T., Varille, V. A., et al.: Ontogeny of renal response to natriuretic peptide in sheep. Am. J. Physiol. 254:F634, 1988d.

Ross, M. G., Ervin, M. G., Lam, R. W., et al.: Plasma atrials natriuretic peptide response to volume expansion in the ovine fetus. Am. J. Obstet. Gynecol. 157:1292, 1987.

Ross, M. G., Sherman, D. J., Ervin, M. G., et al.: Maternal dehydration rehydration: Fetal plasma and urinary responses. Am. J. Physiol. 255:E674, 1988.

Roy, R. N., Chance, G. W., Radde, I. C., et al.: Late hyponatremia in very low birth weight infants (<1.3 kilograms). Pediatr. Res. *10*:526, 1976.

Rudolph, A. M., and Heymann, M. A.: Circulatory changes during growth in fetal lamb. Circ. Res. *26*:289, 1970.

Schwartz, G. J., Haycock, G. B., Chir, B.: Late metabolic acidosis. A reassessment of definition. J. Pediatr. *95*:102, 1979.

Schwartz, G. J., Feld, L. G., and Langford, D. J.: A simple estimate of glomerular filtration rate in full term infants during the first year of life. J. Pediatr. *104*:849, 1984.

Shaffer, S. G., and Meade, V. M.: Sodium balance and extracellular volume regulation in very low birth weight infants. J. Pediatr. *115*:285, 1989.

Shine, P., McDougall, J. G., Towstoless, M. K., et al.: Action of atrial natriuretic peptide in immature ovine kidney. Pediatr. Res. *22*:11, 1987.

Sidi, D., Kuipers, J. R. G., Teitel, D., et al.: Developmental changes in oxygenation and circulatory responses to hypoxemia in lambs. Am. J. Physiol. *245*:H674, 1983.

Siegel, S. R., and Oh, W.: Renal functional maturation in human infants. Acta Pediatr. Scand. *65*:481, 1976.

Smith, F. G., and Robillard, J. E.: Pathophysiology of fetal renal disease. Semin. Perinatol. *13*:305, 1989.

Spitzer, A., and Brandis, M.: Functional and morphologic maturation of the superficial nephrons. Relationship to total kidney function. J. Clin. Invest. *53*:279, 1974.

Spitzer, A.: Factors underlying the increase in glomerular filtration rate during postnatal development. *In* Spitzer, A. (Ed.): The Kidney During Development: Morphology and Function. New York, Masson Publishing, 1982, p. 127.

Spitzer, A.: The developing kidney and the process of growth. *In* Seldin, D. W., and Giebisch, G. (Eds.): The Kidney: Physiology and Pathophysiology. New York, Raven Press, 1985, p. 1979.

Stonestreet, B. S., Bell, E. F., and Oh, W.: Validity of endogenous creatinine clearance in low birth weight infants. Pediatr. Res. *13*:1012, 1979.

Stonestreet, B. S., and Oh, W.: Plasma creatinine levels in low birth-weight infants during the first three months of life. Pediatr. *61*:788, 1978.

Sulyok, E.: The relationship between electrolyte and acid-base balance in the premature infants during early postnatal life. Biol. Neonate *17*:227, 1971.

Sulyok, E., Heim, T., and Soltesz, G.: The influence of maturity on renal control of acidosis in newborn infants. Biol. Neonate *21*:418, 1972.

Sulyok, E., Nemeta, M., Tenyi, I., et al.: Relationship between maturity, electrolyte balance and the function of renin-angiotension-aldosterone system in newborn infants. Biol. Neonate *35*:60, 1979a.

Sulyok, E., Varger, F., Gyory, E., et al.: Postnatal development of sodium handling in premature infants. J. Pediatr. *95*:787, 1979b.

Sulyok, E., Nemeta, M., and Tenyi, I.: Postnatal development of renin angiotensin-aldosterone system (RAAS) in relation to electrolyte balance in premature infants. Pediatr. Res. *13*:817, 1979c.

Svenningsen, N. W.: Renal acid-base titration studies in infants with and without metabolic acidosis in the postnatal period. Pediatr. Res. *8*:659, 1974.

Tulassay, T., Rascher, W., Seyberth, H. W., et al.: Role of atrial natriuretic peptide in sodium homeostasis in premature infants. J. Pediatr. *109*:1023, 1986.

Vanpee, M., Herin, P., and Zeterstrom, R.: Postnatal development of renal function in very low birth weight infants. Acta Pediatr. Scand. *77*:191, 1988.

Versmold, H. T., Kitterman, J. A., Phibbs, R. H., et al.: Aortic blood pressure during the first 12 hours of life in infants with birth weight 610 to 4220 grams. Pediatrics *67*:607, 1981.

Weismann, D. N., and Clark, W. R.: Postnatal age related renal responses to hypoxiemia in lambs. Circ. Res. *49*:1332, 1981.

Weismann, D. N., and Robillard, J. E.: Renal hemodynamic responses to hypoxemia during development. Relationships to circulating vasoactive substances. Pediatr. Res. *23*:155, 1988.

Weitzman, R. E., Fisher, D. E., Robillard, J. E., et al.: Arginine vasopressin response to an osmotic stimulus in the fetal sheep. Pediatr. Res. *12*:35, 1978.

Yared, A., Kon, V., and Ichikawa, I.: Functional development of the kidney. *In* Tune, B. M., and Mendoza, S. A. (Eds.): Pediatric Nephrology. New York, Churchill-Livingstone, 1984, p. 61.

Yared, A., and Yoshioka, T.: Autoregulation of glomerular filtration in the young. Semin. Nephrol. *9*:94, 1989.

CLINICAL EVALUATION 91
OF RENAL DISEASE

Sudhir K. Anand

Renal disease in some newborns may be obvious on the basis of the history and physical examination. Renal disease should be suspected even though the presenting clinical features are nonspecific, e.g., fever, reduced appetite, limited weight gain, or weight loss. Renal disease should be anticipated in infants born with multiple congenital anomalies; after difficult labor and asphyxia; or in those who receive nephrotoxic medications. With increased use of antenatal ultrasonography, presence of renal structural problems is often known or suspected before birth.

■ HISTORY

Family History. Hereditary clinical disorders that primarily involve kidneys and that are present at birth include autosomal recessive (infantile) polycystic kidney disease, Finnish type congenital nephrotic syndrome, and nephrogenic diabetes insipidus. Autosomal dominant (adult) polycystic kidney disease usually presents in the fourth decade; however, cases have been reported in newborns and young infants (see Chapter 94). Vesicoureteral reflux is often present in siblings of patients with severe reflux. Renal dysplasia and agenesis have sometimes been reported to be familial (Kissane, 1976; Roodhooft et al., 1984). Several syndromes with multiple congenital anomalies that include kidneys are also hereditary, as discussed later.

Gestational History. A history of oligohydramnios suggests the presence of renal agenesis, severe dysplasia, or an obstructed urinary tract. The presence of polyhydramnios suggests esophageal atresia (occasionally with associated renal anomalies), swallowing disorders, CNS malformations, and rarely, the presence of nephrogenic diabetes insipidus.

Perinatal History. Delivery is sometimes difficult in newborns with large renal masses. Infants with Finnish type congenital nephrotic syndrome are born with a large placenta that weighs more than 25 per cent of birth weight. Newborns who develop distress due to asphyxia, hypoxia, hypotension, or hemorrhage may develop acute renal failure. Infants born to mothers who have received indomethacin before delivery often develop transient reduction in renal function (Heijdan et al., 1988), as do newborns given indomethacin for closure of patent ductus arteriosus (Halliday et al., 1979).

Time of First Voiding, Urinary Volume and Stream. Most infants void within 24 hours of birth. Sherry and

Kramer (1955) found that 17 per cent void in the delivery room, up to 92 per cent void by 24 hours and 99 per cent by 48 hours. Clark (1977) in a study of 500 newborns observed that 100 per cent of them voided during the first 24 hours. If the child has not voided by 48 hours, hypovolemia, urinary obstruction, bilateral renal agenesis or severe dysplasia, or renal tubular or cortical necrosis should be suspected.

The daily urinary volume is 15 to 60 ml/kg (0.5 to 2.5 ml/kg/hour) for the first 2 days, and after the first week urine volume measures 25 to 125 ml/kg/day (1 to 5 ml/kg/hour) (Goellner et al., 1981; Guignard, 1987). Newborns void two to six times during the first 2 days and five to 25 times per day thereafter. In patients with a posterior urethral valve or neurogenic bladder, the urinary stream is often weak or interrupted, or there may be dribbling of urine.

The history of edema, hematuria, or turbid urine is also helpful and is discussed later.

■ PHYSICAL EXAMINATION

Both kidneys, especially the left kidney, are normally palpable in most newborns.

Abdominal Mass. A palpable abdominal mass is present in approximately 0.5 per cent of all newborns (Museles et al., 1971; Perlman and Williams, 1976; Sherwood et al., 1956). Most abdominal masses in newborns are renal (65 per cent); the remaining 35 per cent are adrenal (10 per cent), female genitalia (10 per cent), and intestinal or hepatic (15 per cent) in origin. The etiology of various renal masses as defined by several studies is outlined in Table 91–1. More recent data from ultrasonography or

TABLE 91–1. Distribution of Renal Masses in 191 Newborn Infants*

LESION	NUMBER	PERCENTAGE
Hydronephrosis	74	39
Multicystic dysplasia	59	31
Polycystic kidneys	16	8
Ectopia	12	6
Tumor	10	5
Renal vein thrombosis	5	3
Horseshoe kidney	4	2
Other†	11	6

*Data from Sherwood et al. (1956), Griscom (1965), Emanuel and White (1968), Raffensperger and Abousleiman (1968), and Wedge et al. (1971).

†"Other" includes multilocular cysts, multiple cysts, solitary cysts, leiomyoma, cystic hamartoma, rupture of renal pelvis, abscess, agenesis, malrotation, and duplication.

renal scans show similar results (Clarke et al., 1989, Kirks et al., 1981, Wilson, 1982). The most common cause of a renal mass in the newborn is hydronephrosis, followed by multicystic (dysplastic) kidney (see Table 91–1). Most of the renal masses are unilateral (hydronephrosis, multicystic kidney) but some are bilateral (polycystic kidney disease).

The bladder is an extrapelvic organ in the newborn, and may be palpable in normal newborns before voiding. A distended bladder may be present in patients with posterior urethral valves or neurogenic bladder.

External genitalia in the male should be evaluated for penile size, prepuceal opening, and presence of hypospadias. The foreskin cannot be retracted in most normal newborns and no attempt should be made to forcibly retract it. Testes are descended bilaterally in most term infants but may be in the inguinal canal in premature infants. In the female newborn, the labia minora are hypertrophied due to maternal estrogen. Whitish mucus discharge is normally present over the hymenal opening. The urethral opening should be identified separately from the vaginal opening.

Examination of the lumbosacral area may demonstrate a dimple, spina bifida, or myelomeningocele, all of which are associated with increased urinary malformations.

Edema. The accumulation of interstitial edema is based upon the imbalance of Starling forces created by increased capillary hydrostatic pressure, decreased colloid osmotic pressure, decreased interstitial hydrostatic pressure, or decreased lymph removal. At birth, in the term infant, total body water content is about 75 per cent of body weight (35 per cent ICF, 40 per cent ECF) compared with about 65 per cent in a one-year-old (40 per cent ICF, 25 per cent ECF) and 60 per cent in the adult. In the premature infant (28 weeks' gestation), total body water content may be 85 per cent or more of body weight (30 per cent ICF, 55 per cent ECF) (Brans, 1986; Friis-Hansen, 1971; Shaffer et al., 1987). Edema on the dorsum of hands and feet (also called physiologic edema) is often observed during the first week of life in the normal premature infant and is unrelated to pathologic conditions. Occasionally, nonpathologic edema may also be seen in the term infant, especially after a cesarean section or in an infant born to a diabetic mother. This edema is thought to be due to excessive total body fluid (prior to physiologic diuresis), increased capillary permeability, and low colloid osmotic pressure. Physiologic edema requires no therapy and usually spontaneously resolves by the end of the 1st week.

Edema may be observed in a wide variety of renal and nonrenal disorders, for example, after severe shock and/or hypoxia (from any cause) with generalized capillary leak, acute renal failure, congenital nephrotic syndrome, congestive heart failure, cold stress, severe hypoproteinemia due to liver failure, protein-losing enteropathy, or congenital analbuminemia (Table 91–2). Localized edema may be observed as lymphedema of distal extremities in gonadal dysgenesis (Turner syndrome) or Milroy disease.

Ascites. Ascites may be seen in congenital nephrotic syndrome, congenital syphilis, and severe hepatobiliary disease. Newborns with obstructive urinary tract disorders

TABLE 91–2. Etiology of Edema in the Newborn

GENERALIZED EDEMA

Physiologic edema (especially in the premature infant and infant of a diabetic mother)

Severe shock, hypoxia, or sepsis due to generalized capillary leak

Renal disorders
  Acute renal failure
  Congenital nephrotic syndrome

Gastrointestinal—hepatic disorders
  Severe hepatobiliary disease
  Protein-losing enteropathy

Congestive heart failure
  Congenital heart defect
  Cardiac arrhythmia
  Multiple arteriovenous fistulas

Severe anemia
  Immune hemolytic
  Nonimmune anemia

Congenital infections
  Syphilis, cytomegalovirus, toxoplasmosis

Excessive fluid administration
  Fluid overload
  Inappropriate ADH syndrome

Miscellaneous
  Congenital analbuminemia
  Vitamin E deficiency

LOCALIZED EDEMA

Gonadal dysgenesis (Turner syndrome)
Milroy disease

(especially posterior urethral valves) occasionally develop urinary ascites. The urinary leakage is generally thought to have originated from a ruptured calyx or renal pelvis.

Generalized hydrops usually does not occur secondary to a renal disorder; however, it may be seen in an association with several congenital disorders including severe fetal anemia (immune or nonimmune), congenital heart disease or arrhythmia, or congenital infections.

Hypertension. Many neonatal renal disorders are associated with hypertension. Hypertension is discussed in Chapter 102.

■ DYSMORPHIC DISORDERS WITH RENAL MALFORMATIONS

A large number of clinical disorders with dysmorphic features have associated renal abnormalities that may manifest at birth or later in life. Some of the more common and important disorders associated with renal involvement are listed in Table 91–3. The reader is referred to reviews for a more comprehensive list of the disorders (Gilbert and Opitz, 1979; Gilli et al., 1987; Temple and Shapira, 1981).

■ URINALYSIS

Urinary findings in normal newborns are summarized in Table 91–4. The normal newborn urine is pale in color. Urates may be present in the first few voidings and may sometimes give the urine a pinkish tinge or stain the diaper a faint red.

Specific gravity of the newborn's urine is usually about 1005. The specific gravity can range from 1001 to 1020

TABLE 91–3. Renal Abnormalities in Various Dysmorphic, Chromosomal, or Hereditary (Single-gene Mutation) Disorders

DYSMORPHIC FEATURE OR SYNDROME	URINARY TRACT ABNORMALITY
Dysmorphic Disorders	
Potter syndrome	Bilateral renal agenesis or bilateral severe renal dysplasia
Small deformed ears or low-set ears	Ipsilateral renal agenesis or dysplasia
Anal atresia (high imperforate anus)	Unilateral renal agenesis or dysplasia; rectovaginal, rectovesical, or rectourethral fistula
VATER (or VACTERL) syndrome	Unilateral renal agenesis or dysplasia, renal ectopia, persistent urachus, penile deformities
Myelomeningocele	Neurogenic bladder, vesicoureteral reflux, hydronephrosis
Caudal regression syndrome	*Mild cases:* neurogenic bladder, renal dysplasia; *severe cases:* absent bladder, unilateral or bilateral renal agenesis, dysplasia
Prune belly syndrome	*Mild cases:* large atonic bladder with hydroureter and hydronephrosis; *severe cases:* dysplastic kidney, hydroureters, megacystis, patent urachus
Beckwith-Wiedemann syndrome	Enlarged kidneys, medullary dysplasia omphalocele
Hemihypertrophy	Enlarged kidneys, Wilms tumor, nephrocalcinosis
Aniridia	Wilms tumor (with or without chromosome 11 deletion)
Fetal alcohol syndrome	Hypoplastic kidney, unilateral agenesis, duplications
Chromosomal Disorders	
Trisomy 13	Cortical renal cysts, unilateral renal agenesis, duplication of ureters
Trisomy 18	Horseshoe kidney, duplication of ureters, cortical renal cysts
Turner syndrome	Horseshoe kidney, duplication of renal pelvis and ureters
Hereditary Disorders	
Autosomal Recessive	
Zellweger (cerebrohepatorenal) syndrome	Cortical renal cysts, dysplastic kidneys
Meckel syndrome	Cystic dysplastic kidneys, hydronephrosis
Smith-Lemli-Opitz syndrome	Hypospadias, focal renal dysplasia
Laurence-Moon-Biedel syndrome	Interstitial nephritis, peritubular fibrosis, renal failure
Asphyxiating thoracic dystrophy (Jeune syndrome)	Glomerular sclerosis, cystic dysplasia, renal failure
Autosomal Dominant	
Nail-patella syndrome	Proteinuria, nephrotic syndrome
Tuberous sclerosis	Polycystic kidneys or angiolipomas (usually manifest after neonatal period
Ehlers-Danlos syndrome	Various disorders including polycystic kidneys and renal tubular acidosis
Branchio-oto-renal or Branchio-oto-ureteral syndrome	Renal dysplasia, hypoplasia, duplication of ureters
X-linked	
Lowe syndrome	Renal tubular acidosis, Fanconi syndrome
Orofaciodigital syndrome, type I	Renal cortical cysts

with an osmolality of 40 to 800 mOsm/kg water. In the premature infant, maximal urinary osmolality may reach only 500 mOsm/kg water. The inability of the newborn to concentrate urine to values of 1200 to 1400 mOsm/kg water as found in older children is related in part to excretion of a small solute load (Edelmann et al., 1960). With increased solute load, the neonatal kidney by 4 weeks of age may be able to concentrate urine to 1000 mOsm/kg water. Urine specific gravity is increased in newborns with cardiac failure, dehydration, respiratory distress, and inappropriate antidiuretic hormone (ADH) secretion. In addition, urine specific gravity may be elevated by high-molecular-weight solutes such as radiographic contrast material, sugars, and protein.

Urine pH in the newborn varies between 4.5 and 8;

TABLE 91–4. Urinalysis in Normal Newborns

	PREMATURE	TERM INFANT	
	<34 weeks	First 3 days	2 to 3 weeks
Specific gravity	1002–1015	1001–1020	1001–1025
Osmolarity (mOsm/kg water)	40–500	40–800	40–900
pH	5.0–8.0	4.5–8.0	4.5–8.0
Glucose (by dipstick)	Negative to ++	Negative	Negative
Protein (by dipstick)	Negative to ++	Negative to +	Negative to trace
Blood dipstick or <2 RBC/HPF	Negative	Negative	Negative
Leukocytes dipstick or <5 WBC/HPF	Negative	Negative	Negative

however, during the first few days of life, in most newborns the urine pH is about 6.0. Urine pH should always be interpreted in relationship to plasma bicarbonate values. An alkaline urine in the face of metabolic acidosis may be seen in renal tubular acidosis (Edelmann et al., 1967) or urinary infection due to a urea-splitting organism.

The urine of healthy term newborns contains trace amounts of glucose. Premature infants, less than 34 weeks' gestation, may show glucosuria during the 1st week of life with plasma glucose values less than 150 mg/dl and occasionally even less than 100 mg/dl (Arant, 1978; Brodehl et al., 1972). This finding probably reflects heterogeneity of maturing nephrons. Sick or stressed newborns (especially premature) receiving treatment with glucose-containing intravenous fluids often show intermittent glucosuria (Stonestreet et al., 1980).

Proteinuria. Small amounts of protein are excreted in the urine of normal newborns. Arant (1978) in a study of 90 newborns of various gestational ages (28 weeks to 40 weeks) observed that during the first 48 hours, urinary protein excretion, measured with qualitative reagent strips, was negative in 24 per cent, trace in 55 per cent, 1+ in 18 per cent, and 2+ in 3 per cent. Quantitative protein excretion measured by sulfosalicylic acid varied with gestational age with peak mean of 2.5 mg/hr/m^2 (range 0 to 13.2) at 34 weeks. After the first 2 weeks of life in normal infants, protein excretion is minimal, and albumin is the most abundant of the plasma proteins in the urine (Karlsson et al., 1979). Other urinary proteins are secreted by the tubules.

Usually, only small amounts of protein pass through the glomerular basement membrane, and the majority of this filtered protein is reabsorbed in the proximal tubule. Administration of large amounts of plasma proteins or albumin to newborns can be associated with transient proteinuria, which may represent a saturation of the tubular reabsorptive mechanism.

Mild proteinuria may be seen with dehydration, cardiac failure, cyanotic heart disease, or after shock and asphyxia. Massive proteinuria usually indicates glomerular injury, and persistent massive proteinuria in the newborn suggests congenital nephrotic syndrome (see Chapter 104). Renal biopsy may be necessary to establish the diagnosis. Tubular injury without glomerular disease usually results in a modest increase in protein excretion.

Several other low-molecular-weight proteins and enzymes, e.g., β_2-microglobulin, lysozymes, proximal tubular epithelial cell antigen, adenosine deaminase–binding protein, N-acetyl-betaglucosaminidase, and alanine aminopeptidase, are excreted in the urine of newborns and older patients (Aperia and Borberger, 1979; Assadi et al., 1985; Chavers and Vernier, 1986; Schardijn and Statius van Eps, 1987; Tolkoff-Rubin, 1983). The urinary excretion of these proteins and enzymes may be increased in several renal tubular disorders including severe hypoxia, acute renal failure, aminoglycoside nephrotoxicity, pyelonephritis, interstitial nephritis, renal cystic disease, heavy-metal poisoning, and malignancy. Although measurements of these proteins may be useful in diagnosing early tubular dysfunction (Schardijn and Statius van Eps, 1987; Tack et al., 1988; Tolkoff-Rubin, 1983), they have not proved to be efficacious in the differential diagnosis of renal disorders (Chavers and Vernier, 1986).

Hematuria. The red cell excretion rate in the normal newborn is less than 100,000 red cells per 12 hours, and under usual circumstances no hematuria is detected either by dipstick or by examination of the urinary sediment (normally 0 to 2 RBC/HPF). Hemoglobinuria due to intravascular hemolysis and myoglobinuria due to rhabdomyolysis are also read as positive for blood on dipstick. When hematuria is detected its origin must be determined. Red blood cells can enter the urinary tract anywhere from the renal parenchyma to urethra. The presence of red cell casts indicates renal parenchymal disease. Various causes of hematuria in the newborn include perinatal asphyxia; acute renal failure due to tubular, cortical, or medullary necrosis; congenital urinary malformations; obstructive uropathy; infections; trauma; neoplasia; renal artery or vein thrombosis; disseminated intravascular coagulation; or blood dyscrasias (Table 91–5). Other sources of blood in the urine, such as the vagina or penile meatus, must be considered. Gross hematuria, however, is an uncommon disorder in the newborn (Emanuel and Aronson, 1974; and personal observations). The etiology of hematuria in 35 newborns reported by these authors was renal vein thrombosis (20 per cent), obstructive uropathy (20 per cent), infantile (autosomal recessive) polycystic kidney (17 per cent), and miscellaneous causes in the remaining patients.

Leukocyturia. Leukocyturia, or pyuria, is defined as more than 5 WBC/HPF on examination of a centrifuged

TABLE 91–5. Etiology of Hematuria in the Newborn

Hypoxic and vascular damage
    Perinatal asphyxia
    Acute tubular necrosis
    Renal medullary necrosis
    Renal cortical necrosis
    Renal artery thrombosis
    Renal vein thrombosis

Bleeding and clotting disorders
    Disseminated intravascular coagulation
    Thrombocytopenia
    Clotting factor deficiency

Trauma
    Traumatic delivery
    Suprapubic puncture

Congenital anomalies and obstructive disorders
    Hydronephrosis
    Polycystic kidney disease

Urinary tract infections

Miscellaneous
    Vaginal bleeding
    Severe diaper rash
    Meatitis

Nonhematuria red urines
    Hemoglobinuria   (positive dipstick and
    Myoglobinuria   negative smear)
    Urate stain
    Colored diaper syn-   (both negative
      drome   dipstick and smear)

urine sample. The most common cause of leukocyturia is urinary tract infection. However, leukocyturia can be associated with any type of inflammatory process within the genitourinary tract, such as glomerular disease, tubular disease, interstitial nephritis, fever, acidosis and dehydration, and following instrumentation. White blood cell casts are always an indication of renal parenchymal disease.

Casts. Casts are the only definitive evidence of upper urinary tract involvement found on examination of the urine. Casts are formed from precipitation of Tamm-Horsfall protein, which is secreted only in the ascending limb of the loop of Henle. Hyaline casts may be seen in the urine of normal newborns as well as in dehydrated infants and those with proteinuria. Red blood cell casts are most commonly seen in glomerular injury. White blood cell casts may be seen with infection, interstitial injury, or tubular damage. Epithelial cell casts, which may be difficult to distinguish from white blood cell casts, are seen with tubular or interstitial injury. Granular casts usually represent partially decomposed cellular casts. They can be seen in dehydration, interstitial injury, or tubular injury.

■ BLOOD EXAMINATION

Newborns with renal disorder may show abnormalities in a variety of blood chemical determinations, or these tests may be normal. The most common tests used to assess renal function are plasma creatinine (PCr) and urea nitrogen (BUN or SUN). Renal disorders may also be associated with hypo- or hypernatremia, hypo- or hyperkalemia, acidosis or alkalosis with alterations in pH and bicarbonate values, hypo- or hyperchloremia, hypo- or hyperphosphatemia, hypocalcemia, hypo- or hypermagnesemia, and hyperuricemia.

Plasma Creatinine. Plasma creatinine continues to be the most useful and simple laboratory measure to assess renal function in the newborn. The values of plasma creatinine at birth reflect those of maternal plasma creatinine and may be normal even in newborns with renal agenesis. Subsequent values of plasma creatinine are dependent on glomerular filtration rate (see Table 90–1) and muscle mass. In term infants mean plasma creatinine at birth (in cord blood) is about 0.8 mg/dl, rises to 0.9 mg/dl at day 1, and then gradually decreases to a value of 0.5 mg/dl by 1 week of age (Feldman and Guignard, 1982; Rudd et al., 1983; Schwartz et al., 1984). Thereafter, as the glomerular filtration rate (GFR) further increases, the plasma creatinine decreases to 0.4 mg/dl between 1 month and 1 year of age (Schwartz et al., 1984). After 1 year of age the GFR remains fairly stable; however, plasma creatinine gradually rises due to increasing muscle mass. In premature infants, serum creatinine values at birth are increased compared with term infants (Rudd et al., 1983; Stonestreet and Oh, 1978). Stonestreet and Oh (1978) reported that the mean plasma creatinine in newborns with gestation ages of 26 to 36 weeks was 1.3 mg/dl (range 0.8 to 1.8 mg/dl) during the first 10 days of life. After 1 month of age the mean creatinine in these premature infants fell to less than 0.6 mg/dl. Ketones and bilirubin may falsely increase plasma creatinine values as measured by Jaffe's reaction (in most clinical laboratories); a modified autoanalyzer technique may be used to measure true creatinine (Arant et al., 1972). Serial measurements of plasma creatinine generally provide a reasonable estimate of changes in renal function, and a sudden increase in plasma creatinine may signify a substantial decrease in the glomerular filtration rate.

Urea Nitrogen. Blood urea nitrogen (BUN) is another measure commonly used to assess renal function. However, values of BUN depend upon several factors including urinary flow rate, state of hydration, protein intake, and tissue catabolism. Therefore, BUN measurement is much less reliable in assessment of renal function in comparison to plasma creatinine. BUN values in term newborns vary between 5 and 20 mg/dl.

Uric Acid. During the first 3 to 4 days of life, serum uric acid values in newborns are elevated compared with those of older children and adults. The values average between 6 and 7 mg/dl. In premature infants and those that experience asphyxia or respiratory distress, the uric acid values are higher (Marks et al., 1968; Raivio, 1976). The uric acid values in the healthy term infants decrease to 3 to 5 mg/dl (same as in older children) by the end of the 1st week. The fractional excretion of uric acid, however, is inversely related to age, being 70 per cent in the premature (at 30 weeks' gestation), 40 per cent at term, and reaching adult values of 6 to 12 per cent by 1 year of age (Stapleton, 1983). The increased initial serum uric acid values in the newborn, despite the considerably increased fractional excretion of uric acid, are secondary to increased uric acid production (due to greater purine and nucleic acid turnover associated with rapid growth) and a reduced GFR. The ratio of daily uric acid to creatinine excretion in newborns exceeds 1, whereas in older children and adults the value is 0.5 or less (Marks

et al., 1968; Raivio, 1976). Acute urate nephropathy leading to acute renal failure is rare in the newborn, despite the high daily urinary uric acid excretion (Ahmadian and Lewy, 1977). This finding is probably due to the newborn's excretion of dilute urine with a pH greater than 6.0 in which uric acid precipitation is unlikely.

■ DIAGNOSTIC IMAGING OF THE GENITOURINARY SYSTEM

Ultrasonography, conventional voiding cystourethrography (VCUG), excretory urography, radionuclide renal imaging, radionuclide voiding cystourethrography, renal angiography, computed tomography (CT), and magnetic resonance imaging (MRI) are available for evaluation of the genitourinary tract in the newborn. It is often necessary to use more than one technique. Further details are included in recent reviews (Gordon, 1987; Lebowitz, 1985). Figure 91–1 outlines an algorithm for imaging evaluation of a newborn with a renal mass or other renal disorder.

Ultrasonography. Over the past decade, ultrasonography has emerged as the primary method for evaluation of newborns with genitourinary disorders because it is noninvasive, it can image the kidney and other abdominal or pelvic masses regardless of kidney function, and it can be performed on critically ill newborns who cannot be easily transported. Ultrasonography can confirm the presence or absence of kidneys, determine their size and position, identify the origins of a mass and indicate whether the mass is cystic or solid. In the evaluation of an infant with an abdominal mass, ultrasonography is useful in distinguishing hydronephrosis, cystic kidney, and renal tumors. In a newborn with renal failure, ultrasonography can assist in distinguishing renal agenesis or hypoplasia, obstructive urinary disorders, and intrinsic renal failure. Ultrasonography can demonstrate nephrocalcinosis, which may be seen in newborns or young infants receiving prolonged furosemide treatment and in infants with renal tubular acidosis or renal cortical necrosis. Newborns with multiple anomalies and specific syndromes should have screening with ultrasonography to identify the presence of associated renal abnormalities. Many pediatric nephrologists have switched from excretory urography to ultrasonography (in conjunction with conventional voiding cystourethrography) in the evaluation of newborns with urinary tract infection (UTI). Other pediatric nephrologists continue to prefer excretory urography in the evaluation of UTI because ultrasonography does not permit visualization of ureters (unless they are very dilated, hydroureters, duplicated ureters, or ectopically inserted ureters may be missed). If renal disease is suspected on the basis of an antenatal abdominal ultrasound of the mother, the study must be repeated after birth because, in some cases, the antenatal findings cannot be confirmed (Grupe, 1987).

The use of the Doppler technique can further enhance the usefulness of ultrasonography by identifying aortic or renal arterial clots or deformities and renal vein and/or inferior vena cava thrombosis.

Although ultrasonographic images have considerably improved over the past decade, inaccurate diagnoses may

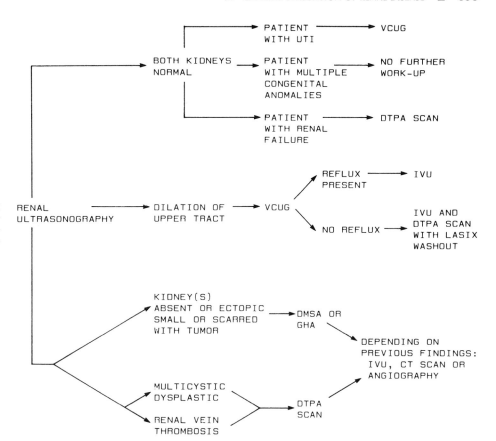

FIGURE 91–1. *Schema of diagnostic imaging in a newborn with known or suspected renal mass or some other renal disorder. (Please note that many cases do not need all the tests shown.)*

still be made (Clarke et al., 1989). Also, the image details are often limited and an excretory urogram or a radionuclide scan may still be necessary, either for further detail (especially ureters) and/or for functional evaluation of the urinary tract.

Voiding Cystourethrography. The VCUG is important in outlining the bladder and the urethra and in determining the presence and degree of vesicoureteral reflux. It is an essential part of the radiologic evaluation of newborns who have dilated upper tracts on ultrasound in order to determine whether the dilatation is due to an obstruction or high-grade reflux. Moreover, VCUG may allow visualization of the collecting system if reflux is present, even when the patient's GFR is reduced. Grade V (international classification I-V) reflux may be present in a newborn with a UTI even though the renal ultrasound or excretory urogram is normal. This finding is in contrast to observations in older children, in whom grade V reflux is usually associated with an anatomic abnormality of the upper tract. VCUG should also be performed in evaluation of newborns with urinary tract infection, urinary dribbling, outlet obstruction due to posterior or anterior urethral valves, neurogenic bladder, vesicovaginal or vesicorectal fistula, and patent urachus. A 15 per cent solution of diatrizoate, instilled at no more than 100 mm H_2O by gravity drip infusion under fluoroscopic control in the unanesthetized child using a straight catheter (not a Foley), provides proper and safe filling and yields the most useful information.

Excretory Urography. Excretory urography gives far more detailed views of the patient's upper urinary tract than either ultrasonography or radionuclide scanning.

Moreover, because intravenous urography (IVU) is based upon excretory function of the kidney, it gives a partial assessment of renal function by indicating a delay in excretion of the contrast agent. However, evaluation of the anatomy of the neonatal urinary tract may be difficult because newborns have a relatively low GFR and poor ability to concentrate urine. Larger doses of radiopaque material are usually required for satisfactory visualization. Because the radiopaque contrast agents commonly used are hyperosmolar, excessive doses must be avoided, particularly in ill infants. Excretory urograms done after the 1st week of life usually depict better images than those done during the first few days of life. The time sequence of normal infant IVU is prolonged, and delayed films are necessary for visualization in newborns with obstructive uropathy.

Radionuclide Imaging. Renal scans and renograms provide both anatomic and functional information about the kidneys and have the advantage of requiring considerable less irradiation than conventional IVU. These techniques can help determine the size, shape, and location of kidneys, detect renal obstruction, measure renal function and blood flow, and determine the relative contribution of each kidney to overall renal function.

The common radionuclide reagents used for renal scanning are ^{99m}Tc-labeled diethylenetriamine pentaacetic acid (DTPA), dimercaptosuccinic acid (DMSA), glucoheptonate (GHA), and ^{123}I-hippuran. A DTPA scan is studied in three phases: the uptake, transit, and excretory phases. The uptake phase enables assessment of differential renal function. Analysis of the excretory phase done in conjunction with furosemide-induced diuresis may help differentiate nonobstructed dilatation of calyces and/or renal pelvis from an obstructive hydronephrosis. The test occasionally may be falsely positive in the presence of renal failure or gross dilatation with obstructive hydronephrosis. DMSA and GHA are both taken up by proximal tubular cells and are more useful than DTPA in imaging of renal parenchyma. Both of them are helpful in detection of ectopic kidneys, presence of renal scars and other parenchymal lesions. GHA exposes the infant to less radiation, but DMSA provides a better quality image.

Radionuclide VCUG using ^{99m}Tc pertechnetate can be performed like a conventional VCUG with 1/20 irradiation, especially to the genitals. Although it is an excellent technique for detecting the presence or absence of reflux, the test fails to provide anatomic detail to grade adequately the severity of reflux. Moreover, in the male it does not adequately demonstrate the urethra or urethral valves. Both in the male and female this technique misses some bladder lesions, e.g., diverticulum, and consequently has limited use in the evaluation of newborns. It is more useful in older infants and children to determine resolution of reflux during follow-up.

Renal Angiography. Aortography and renal arteriography are primarily used in the evaluation of newborns with hypertension that may be secondary to persisting clots following umbilical artery catheterization. Inferior venacavography and renal venography are performed to confirm the diagnosis of renal vein thrombosis with or without extension into the inferior vena cava.

Computed Tomography and Magnetic Resonance Imaging. CT and MRI both offer high-resolution images. However, these procedures are expensive, time-consuming, and require sedation and immobilization. Moreover, they seldom add additional information to that already obtained with other procedures. Therefore, CT and MRI are usually reserved for difficult cases to answer specific questions raised by earlier investigations and in cases where damage may have occurred to multiple abdominal organs, as in trauma.

■ RENAL BIOPSY

Indications for performing renal biopsy in newborns are limited. However, in an occasional infant in whom a specific renal disorder (e.g., the Finnish type of congenital nephrotic syndrome versus nail-patella syndrome) is suspected, renal biopsy is valuable in establishing the diagnosis. The renal biopsy may be performed as a percutaneous biopsy or as a surgical (open) biopsy. If a biopsy is performed, it should be appropriately evaluated by light microscopy, immunofluorescence, and electron microscopy.

■ REFERENCES

Ahmadian, Y., and Lewy, P. R.: Possible urate nephropathy of the newborn infant as a cause of transient renal insufficiency. J. Pediatr. 91:96, 1977.

Aperia, A., and Borberger, U.: β₂-microglobulin, an indicator of renal tubular maturation and dysfunction in the newborn. Acta Pediatr. Scand. 68:699, 1979.

Arant, B. S., Edelmann, C. M., and Spitzer, A.: The congruence of creatinine and inulin clearances in children: Use of Technicon analyzer. J. Pediatr. 81:559, 1972.

Arant, B. S.: Developmental patterns of renal functional maturation compared in the human neonate. J. Pediatr. 92:705, 1978.

Assadi, F. K., John, E. G., Justice, P., et al.: β₂-microglobulin clearance in neonates: Index of tubular maturation. Kidney Int. 28:153, 1985.

Brans, Y. W.: Body fluid compartments in neonates weighing 1000 grams or less. Clin. Perinatal. 13:403, 1986.

Brodehl, J., Franken, A., and Gellissen, K.: Maximum tubular reabsorption of glucose in infants and children. Acta Pediatr. Scand. 61:413, 1972.

Chavers, B. M., and Vernier, R. L.: Proteinuria and enzymuria. Semin. Nephrol. 6:371, 1986.

Clark, D. A.: Times of first void and first stool in 500 newborns. Pediatrics 60:457, 1977.

Clarke, N. W., Gough, D. C. S., and Cohen, S. J.: Neonatal urological ultrasound: Diagnostic inaccuracies and pitfalls. Arch. Dis. Child. 64:578, 1989.

Edelmann, C. M., Barnett, H. C., and Troupkou, V.: Renal concentrating mechanisms in newborn infants. Effects of dietary protein and water content, role of urea and response to antidiuretic hormone. J. Clin. Invest. 399:1062, 1960.

Edelmann, C. M., Soriano, J. R., Boichis, H., et al.: Renal bicarbonate reabsorption and hydrogen ion excretion in normal infants. J. Clin. Invest. 46:1309, 1967.

Emanuel, B., and Aronson, N.: Neonatal hematuria. Am. J. Dis. Child. 128:204, 1974.

Emanuel, B., and White, H.: Intravenous pyelography in the differential diagnosis of renal masses in the newborn period. Clinic Pediatr. 7:529, 1968.

Feldman, H., and Guignard, J. P.: Plasma creatinine in the first month of life. Arch. Dis. Child. 57:123, 1982.

Friis-Hansen, B.: Body composition during growth. Pediatrics (suppl.) 47:264, 1971.

Gilbert, E., and Opitz, J.: Renal involvement in genetic hereditary malformation syndromes. In Hamburger, J., Crosuier, J., and Grunfeld, J. P.: (eds.): Nephrology. New York and Paris, Wiley-Flamarion, 1979, p. 909.

Gilli, G., Berry, A. C., and Chanther, C.: Syndromes with a renal component. In Holliday, M. A., Barratt, T. M., and Vernier, R. L. (Eds.): Pediatric Nephrology. Baltimore, Williams & Wilkins, 1987, p. 384.

Goellner, M. H., Ziegler, E. E., and Foman, S. J.: Urination during the first three years of life. Nephron 28:174, 1981.

Gordon, I.: Imaging the urinary tract. In Holliday, M. A., Barrat, T. M., and Vernier, R. L. (Eds.): Pediatric Nephrology. Baltimore, Williams & Wilkins, 1987, p. 300.

Griscom, N. T.: The roentgenography of neonatal abdominal masses. Am. J. Roengen. 93:447, 1965.

Grupe, W. E.: The dilemma of intrauterine diagnosis of congenital renal disease. Pediatr. Clin. North Am. 34:629, 1987.

Guignard, J. P.: Neonatal nephrology. In Holliday, M. A., Barratt, T. M., Vernier, R. L. (Eds.): Pediatric Nephrology. Baltimore, Williams & Wilkins, 1987, p. 921.

Halliday, H. L., Hirata, T., and Brady, J. P.: Indomethacin therapy for large patent ductus arteriosus in the very low birth weight infant: Results and complications. Pediatrics 64:154, 1979.

Heijden, A. J., Provoost, A. P., Nauta, A. J., et al.: Renal functional impairment in preterm neonates related to intrauterine indomethacin exposure. Pediatr. Res. 24:644, 1988.

Karlsson, F. A., Hardell, L. I., and Hellsing, K.: Prospective study of urinary proteins in early infancy. Acta Pediatr. Scand. 68:663, 1979.

Kirks, D. R., Merten, D. F., Grossman, H., et al.: Diagnostic imaging of pediatric abdominal masses: An overview. Radiol. Clin. North Am. 19:527, 1981.

Kissane, J. M.: The morphology of renal cystic disease. In Gardner, K. D. (Ed.): Cystic Diseases of the Kidney. New York, John Wiley and Sons, 1976, p. 31.

Lebowitz, R. L.: Pediatric uroradiology. Pediatr. Clin. North Am. 32:1353, 1985.

Marks, J. F., Kay, J., Baum, J., et al.: Uric acid levels in full term and low birth weight infants. J. Pediatr. 73:609, 1968.

Museles, M., Gaundry, C. L., and Bason, M. W.: Renal anomalies in the newborn found by deep palpation. Pediatrics 47:97, 1971.

Perlman, M., and Williams, J.: Detection of renal anomalies by abdominal palpation in newborn infants. Br. Med. J. 2:347, 1976.

Raivio, K. O.: Neonatal hyperuricemia. J. Pediatr. 88:625, 1976.

Raffensperger, J., and Abousleiman, A.: Abdominal masses in children under one year of age. Surgery 63:514, 1968.

Roodhooft, A. M., Birnholz, J. C., and Holmes, L. B.: Familial nature of congenital absence and severe dysgenesis of both kidneys. N. Engl. J. Med. *310*:341, 1984.

Rudd, P. T., Hughes, B. A., and Placzek, M. M.: Reference ranges for plasma creatinine during the first month of life. Arch. Dis. Child. *58*:212, 1983.

Schardijn, G. H. C., and Statius van Eps, L. W.: β_2-microglobulin: Its significance in the evaluation of renal function. Kidney Int. *32*:635, 1987.

Schwartz, G. J., Feld, L. G., and Lagford, D. L.: A simple estimate of glomerular filtration rate in full-term infants during the first year of life. J. Pediatr. *104*:849, 1984.

Shaffer, S. G., Bradt, S. K., Meade, V. M., et al.: Extracellular fluid volume changes in very low birth weight infants during first two postnatal months. J. Pediatr. *111*:124, 1987.

Sherry, S. N., and Kramer, I.: The time of passage of first stool and first urine by newborn infant. J. Pediatr. *46*:158, 1955.

Sherwood, D. W., Smith, R. C., Lemmon, R. H., et al.: Abnormalities of the genitourinary tract discovered by palpation of the abdomen of the newborn. Pediatrics *18*:782, 1956.

Stapleton, F. B.: Renal uric acid clearance in human neonates. J. Pediatr. *103*:290, 1983.

Stonestreet, B. S., and Oh, W.: Plasma creatinine levels in low birth weight infants during the first three months of life. Pediatriacs *61*:788, 1978.

Stonestreet, B. S., Rubin, L., Pollak, A., et al.: Renal functions of low birthweight infants with hyperglycemia and glucosuria produced by glucose infusions. Pediatrics *66*:561, 1980.

Tack, E. D., Perlman, J. M., and Robson, A. M.: Renal injury in sick newborn infants: A prospective evaluation using urinary β_2-microglobulin concentration. Pediatrics *81*:432, 1988.

Temple, J. K., and Shapira, E.: Genetic determinants of renal disease in neonates. Clin. Perinat. *8*:361, 1981.

Tolkoff-Rubin, N. E.: Monoclonal antibodies in the diagnosis of renal disease. Kidney Int. *29*:142, 1983.

Wedge, J. J., Grosfeld, J. L., and Smith, J. P.: Abdominal masses in the newborn: 63 cases. J. Urol. *106*:770, 1971.

Wilson, D. A.: Ultrasound screening for abdominal masses in the neonatal period. Am. J. Dis. Child. *136*:147, 1982.

PRENATAL DIAGNOSIS AND MANAGEMENT OF URINARY ABNORMALITIES 92

Sudhir K. Anand, Randal A. Aaberg, and Martin A. Koyle

Maternal ultrasonography has become widely used to evaluate the fetus. The prevalence of structural fetal abnormalities detected by maternal ultrasonography is approximately 1 per cent (Grisoni et al., 1986; Hill et al., 1985; Jassani et al., 1982); 20 per cent of these anomalies are genitourinary in origin (approximately 1 per 500 ultrasounds). This prevalence is less than the estimated prevalence of congenital urologic abnormalites in the general population (1 per cent), suggesting that ultrasonography does not detect all renal abnormalities, especially those not associated with renal enlargement or oligohydramnios.

The fetal bladder may be visualized by the 14th week of gestation, and most kidneys can be identified by the 18th week (Kramer, 1983). Jeanty and associates (1982) have described standards for normal fetal renal size and growth. Fetal sex may be ascertained by ultrasonography during second trimester if the penis, scrotum, or both labia majora can be unequivocally visualized (Birnholz, 1983; Stephens and Sherman, 1983). Amniotic fluid volume can be assessed by ultrasonography and oligohydraminios correctly identified.

The most common urologic abnormality detected by ultrasonography is hydronephrosis due to ureteropelvic junction (UPJ) obstruction (Table 92–1 and Figure 92–1). Other disorders include multicystic dysplastic kidneys, pelvic or pelvocalyceal dilatation, megaureter or megacal-ices, posterior urethral valves, reflux, duplex system, renal agenesis, prune belly syndrome, and polycystic kidney disease (Ahmed and Le Quesne, 1988; Colodny, 1987; Grisoni et al., 1986). The most difficult distinction to make antenatally is between UPJ obstruction and a multicystic dysplastic kidney. Oligohydramnios would suggest presence of bilateral renal agenesis, bilateral severe hydronephrosis due to posterior urethral valves or bilateral UPJ obstruction, bilateral multicystic kidneys, or severe autosomal recessive (infantile) polycystic kidneys. Also, severe oligohydramnios would suggest lung hypoplasia and nonviability of the fetus after birth.

Mild dilatation of the pelvocalyceal system may be visualized during the third trimester in the normal fetus without any anatomic urologic obstruction. This finding has been termed "physiologic hydronephrosis" (Colodny, 1987; Elder and Duckett, 1987) and may be due to high fetal urine production (see Chapter 90) or reflux of urine from the bladder to the kidney (Blane et al., 1983). Several authors in the past have reported these findings as unilateral or bilateral hydronephrosis that spontaneously resolved postnatally (Hellstrom et al., 1984; Hobbins et al., 1984).

■ POTENTIAL ERRORS IN DIAGNOSIS

The accuracy of prenatal diagnosis by ultrasonography has remarkably improved over the past decade. However,

TABLE 92–1. Urinary Abnormalities Detected By Fetal Ultrasound

	AHMED AND LE QUESNE (1988) N = 148	COLODNY (1987) N = 187	GRISONI ET AL. (1986) N = 31	TOTAL N N = 366
UPJ obstruction	40	63	16	119
Multicystic kidney	12	22	8	42
Nonobstructive pelvic or pelvocalyceal dilatation	28	–	–	28
Primary megaureter	–	23	–	23
Posterior urethral valves (bilateral hydro-nephrosis)	5	19	5	29
Duplication	13	19	–	32
Reflux	8	17	–	25
Prune belly syndrome	2	6	–	8
Miscellaneous*	16	17	2	35
Normal	24	1	–	25

*Miscellaneous includes renal agenesis, ureteroceles, ectopic ureters, ureterovesical junction obstruction, malrotated kidneys, and mesoblastic nephroma.

856

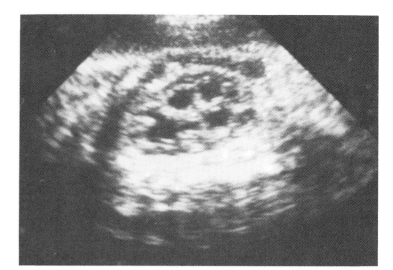

FIGURE 92–1. Prenatal ultrasound showing mild hydronephrosis. (From Colodny, A. H.: Antenatal diagnosis and management of urinary abnormalities. Pediatr. Clin. North Am. 34:1371, 1987.)

Grupe (1987) and Clarke and associates (1989) have pointed out that potential for error exists even in experienced hands, and Colodny (1987) has reported that an incorrect diagnosis is made in 30 per cent of the cases. The usual errors in prenatal diagnosis include normally lucent renal pyramids (Fig. 92–2), physiologic pelvocalyceal dilatation, and pelvocalyceal and ureteric dilation due to reflux being misinterpreted as obstructive hydronephrosis.

■ ANTENATAL MANAGEMENT

Intrauterine decompression of fetal urinary obstruction (Harrison et al., 1982) is a dramatic treatment. However, after careful evaluation of fetal benefits versus fetal and maternal risks, in the opinion of most fetal and neonatal urologists, intrauterine intervention is rarely indicated (Colodny, 1987; Elder and Duckett, 1988). The initial enthusiasm for fetal surgery overestimated the potential benefits and underestimated the possible fetal and maternal risks. In humans, urinary obstruction during the first trimester probably results in renal dysplasia; however, fetal detection and surgery at this stage are currently not practical (Elder and Duckett, 1987 and 1988).

Patients with unilateral obstruction or those with bilateral obstruction not accompanied by oligohydramnios have relatively good renal function and are managed expectantly. Because of the possible error in prenatal diagnosis and incidence of physiologic dilatation, these patients are reevaluated postpartum, and management decisions are made at that time. Early delivery is also an option.

Patients with bilateral obstruction and oligohydramnios require an evaluation of renal function by measurement of fetal urinary sodium and chloride concentration and osmolarity (Glick et al., 1985). If renal function is poor, intrauterine intervention should not be considered. In the presence of other fetal anomalies, termination of pregnancy is an option (Glick et al., 1985).

The rare patient with acceptable renal function, bilateral obstruction, and diminishing amniotic fluid may benefit from intrauterine intervention. Intrauterine decompression may be achieved by introducing a thin needle into the distended fetal bladder or kidney and placing a short indwelling catheter. It may also be possible to perform cutaneous ureterostomies or a vesicostomy. In rare instances, needle aspiration to decompress a large cystic mass may prevent dystocia (Manning et al., 1986). Elder

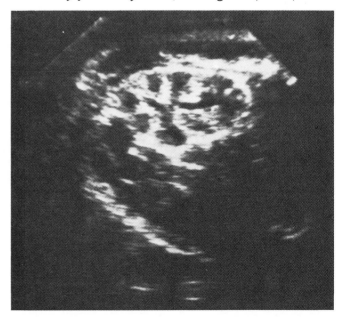

FIGURE 92–2. Prenatal ultrasound showing a normal fetal kidney. Note the normal lucent pyramids. They have been confused with cystic disease or hydronephosis. (From Colodny, A. H.: Antenatal diagnosis and management of urinary abnormalities. Pediatr. Clin. North Am. 34:1377, 1987.)

and associates (1987) in their review of intrauterine intervention in the management of obstructive urologic disorders found an overall complication rate of 45 per cent. The common complications were shunt failure or migration (20 per cent), onset of premature labor within 48 hours (10 per cent), chorioamnionitis (6 per cent) and urinary ascites (6 per cent). They did not find that intervention definitively improved renal function in any fetus.

■ REFERENCES

Ahmed, S., and Le Quesne, G. W.: A nine-year experience with urological anomalies detected by fetal ultrasound. Austral. Pediatr. J. 24:178, 1988.

Birnholz, J. C.: Determination of fetal sex. N. Engl. J. Med. 309:942, 1983.

Blane, C. E., Koff, S. A., Bowerman, R. A., et al.: Nonobstructive fetal hydronephrosis. Sonographic recognition and therapeutic implications. Radiology 147:95, 1983.

Clarke, N. W., Gough, D. C. S., Cohen, S. J.: Neonatal urological ultrasound: Diagnostic inaccuracies and pitfalls. Arch. Dis. Child. 64:578, 1989.

Colodny, A. H.: Antenatal diagnosis and management of urinary abnormalities. Pediatr. Clin. North Am. 34:1365, 1987.

Colodny, A. H.: The role of fetal ultrasounds. Problems in Urology 2:1, 1988.

Elder, J. S., and Duckett, J. W.: Perinatal urology. In Gillenwater, J. Y., Grayhack, J. T., Howards, S. S., and Duckett, J. W. (Eds.): Adult and Pediatric Urology. Chicago, Year Book Medical Publishers, 1987, p. 1528.

Elder, J. S., and Duckett, J. W.: Management of the fetus and neonate with hydronephrosis detected by prenatal ultrasonography. Pediatr. Ann. 17:19, 1988.

Elder, J. S., Duckett, J. W., and Snyder, H. M.: Intervention for fetal obstructive uropathy. Has it been effective? Lancet 2:1007, 1987.

Glick, P. L., Harrison, M. R., Golbus, M. S., et al.: Management of the fetus with congenital hydronephrosis II: Prognostic criteria and selection for treatment. J. Pediatr. Surg. 20:376, 1985.

Grisoni, E. R., Gauderer, M. W. L., Wolfson, R. N., et al.: Antenatal ultrasonography. The experience in a high risk perinatal center. J. Pediatr. Surg. 21:358, 1986.

Grupe, W.: The dilemma of intrauterine diagnosis of congenital renal disease. Pediatr. Clin. North Am. 34:629, 1987.

Harrison, M. R., Golbus, M. S., Filly, R. A., et al.: Fetal surgery for congenital hydronephrosis. N. Engl. J. Med. 306:591, 1982.

Hellstrom, W. J. G., Kogan, B. A., Jeffrey, R. B., et al.: The natural history of prenatal hydronephrosis with normal amounts of amniotic fluid. J. Urol. 132:947, 1984.

Hill, L. M., Breckle, R., and Gehrking, W. C.: Prenatal detection of congenital malformations by ultrasonography. Mayo Clinic experience. Am. J. Obstet. Gynecol. 151:44, 1985.

Hobbins, J. C., Romero, R., Grannum, P., et al.: Antenatal diagnosis of renal anomalies with ultrasound: I. Obstructive Uropathy. Am. J. Obstet. Gynecol. 148:868, 1984.

Jassani, M. N., Gauderer, M. W. L., Fanaroff, A. A., et al.: A perinatal approach to the diagnosis and management of gastrointestinal malformations. Obstet. Gynecol. 59:33, 1982.

Jeanty, P., Dramix-Wilmet, M., Elkhazen, N., et al.: Measurement of fetal kidney growth on ultrasound. Radiology 144:159, 1982.

Kramer, S. A.: Current status of fetal intervention for congenital hydronephrosis. J. Urol. 130:641, 1983.

Manning, F. A., Harrison, M. R., Rodeck, C., et al.: Catheter shunts for fetal hydronephrosis and hydrocephalus. Report of the International Fetal Surgery Registry. N. Engl. J. Med. 315:336, 1986.

Stephens, J. D., and Sherman, S.: Determination of fetal sex by ultrasound. N. Engl. J. Med. 309:984, 1983.

DEVELOPMENTAL ABNORMALITIES OF THE KIDNEYS

Randal A. Aaberg, Sudhir K. Anand, and Martin A. Koyle

Most authors estimate that significant genitourinary anomalies are present in approximately 1 per cent of live births (Steinhart et al., 1988). They are frequently associated with abnormalities of other organ systems. Many of these anomalies are of no clinical significance, while others pose significant threats.

UNILATERAL RENAL AGENESIS

Unilateral renal agenesis occurs when the ureteral bud fails to form or the metanephric blastema is absent on one side. The incidence of unilateral renal agenesis is about one in 500 live births (Longo and Thomson, 1952; Potter, 1972). The contralateral kidney is generally normal and shows compensatory hypertrophy. The disorder usually goes unrecognized and is compatible with normal life. However, we have seen several infants with unilateral agenesis and either ureteropelvic junction obstruction or ureterovesical reflux of the contralateral kidney. Moreover, an increased risk of renal insufficiency in adulthood has been reported in individuals born with a solitary kidney (Kiprov et al., 1982; Bhathena et al., 1985). Unilateral renal agenesis has been frequently associated with VAC-TERL complex and supralevator imperforate anus (Fleisher et al., 1985). Also, unilateral agenesis is often associated with cardiac (ventricular septal defect), nervous system (myelomeningocele), gastrointestinal (strictures, esophageal atresia, or tracheoesophageal fistula), and genital (absent vas deferens or vagina, bicornate uterus) anomalies (Kissane, 1983; Koff et al., 1987; Stephens, 1983). The ipsilateral adrenal gland is absent in 10 per cent of cases.

Ultrasonography is the best screening test (after palpation) for unilateral renal agenesis, but confirmation must be obtained by renal scan to rule out ectopia. If unilateral agenesis is incidentally found during prenatal or postnatal sonography, the contralateral kidney must be evaluated to be certain it is normal.

BILATERAL RENAL AGENESIS

Bilateral renal agenesis (Potter syndrome) occurs in one of every 3000 births and is incompatible with life. It is associated with oligohydramnios and pulmonary hypoplasia as well as the characteristic Potter facies: wide-set eyes, a prominent skinfold below the lower eyelid extending from medial canthus to the cheek, a parrot-beak nose,

pliable low-set ears, and receding chin (Fig. 93–1). These features presumably occur secondary to oligohydramnios and compression of the fetal face in restricted amniotic space. Mauer and associates (1974) have described an interesting case of monoamniotic twins, one of whom had bilateral renal agenesis. This twin did not have the usual Potter facies nor pulmonary hypoplasia. The other twin provided an adequate amount of fluid in their shared amniotic sac. Newborns with bilateral renal agenesis usually die within a few days because of pulmonary problems or renal failure. However, some newborns may survive 3 to 4 weeks despite no urinary output throughout this period.

The clinical diagnosis is usually confirmed by the absence of kidneys on renal ultrasonography and radionuclide scan. Patients with bilateral multicystic (dysplastic) kidneys and severe polycystic kidney disease may have oligohydramnios and features of Potter syndrome; however, both these disorders have large palpable kidneys in contrast to agenesis.

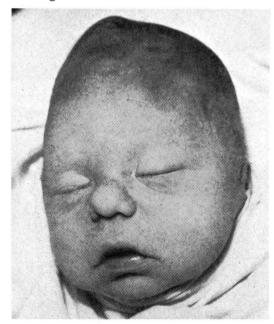

FIGURE 93–1. *Newborn with Potter facies. Note the prominent eyes, the fold sweeping in an arc from the inner canthus downward and outward, the depressed nasal bridge and retroussé nose, and the low-set ears. In this case, there was complete absence of the right kidney and hypoplasia of the left kidney. (Reprinted by permission of the Western Journal of Medicine. From Kirshbaum, J. D.: California Med. 71:148, 1949.)*

Renal agenesis is usually not considered to be a hereditary condition. However, Roodhooft and associates (1984) have described increased incidence of unilateral renal agenesis (4.5 per cent versus 0.3 per cent in controls) and other asymptomatic urinary abnormalities in parents and siblings of patients affected by bilateral agenesis.

RENAL ECTOPIA

Renal ectopia is caused by abnormal cephalad migration of the kidney to a thoracic, pelvic, or lumbar position. The left side is more commonly ectopic than the right. Because migration into the renal fossa is incomplete, rotational anomalies often coexist, thus altering the pyelocaliceal axis and producing an unusual radiographic appearance. Most ectopic kidneys are located in the pelvis (Fig. 93–2), function poorly, and are difficult to visualize radiographically. Vesicoureteral reflux is common. An ectopic kidney is usually asymptomatic but may be discovered as an abdominal mass. It is more prone to injury because of its poorly protected location. Frequently, the ectopic kidney is associated with a renal fusion abnormality (Stephens, 1983).

HORSESHOE KIDNEY

The horseshoe kidney is the most common type of renal fusion abnormality, occurring in one of every 400 persons with a male predominance (Perlmutter et al.,

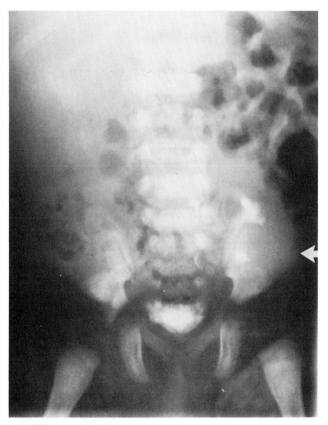

FIGURE 93–2. Ectopic left kidney. Excretory urogram of a 5-day-old infant born with two separate abdominal masses—one in left lower quadrant and the other in right flank. The former turned out to be an ectopic kidney, whereas the right mass was a nonfunctional multicystic kidney (arrow).

1986). It is thought to develop during the 5th to 6th week of embryogenesis. After the ureteric buds have encountered the metanephric blastema and induced early kidney formation, the lower poles touch and fuse in the midline, forming an isthmus. This fusion may interfere with complete rotation of the kidneys, and ureters may appear to arise anteriorly. Moreover, the fusion may arrest renal ascent at the level of the inferior mesenteric artery.

Two-thirds of horseshoe kidneys remain asymptomatic throughout life. If symptoms do develop, they are most commonly related to hydronephrosis, infection, or calculi formation. The most common abnormal finding in the horseshoe kidney is ureteropelvic junction obstruction with hydronephrosis (Whitehouse, 1975). Vesicoureteral reflux is common, and ureteral duplication is present in about 10 per cent of the patients. Hypospadias and undescended testes occur in 4 per cent of males, and bicornate uterus or septate vagina in 7 per cent of females (Boatman et al., 1972). Horseshoe kidney is often associated with orofaciodigital syndrome, Turner syndrome, trisomy 18, and spina bifida (Stephens, 1983). Wilms tumor or renal cell carcinoma may occur in a horseshoe kidney. However, in most patients, the presence of a horseshoe kidney does not adversely affect long-term survival (Glenn, 1959).

CROSSED FUSED ECTOPIA

Crossed fused ectopia is the second most common renal fusion abnormality (Fig. 93–3). The incidence is estimated to be one per 1000 live births, and it occurs twice as often in males as females. The left kidney crossing to the right side is more common. The right kidney usually lies superior with its lower pole fused to the upper pole of the ectopic left kidney. The left ureter crosses the midline to enter the bladder in a normal anatomic location. The disorder may be completely asymptomatic or may be diagnosed as an abdominal mass. Hydronephrosis may occur if there is obstruction of the ectopic ureter. Reflux is a common finding in the ectopic kidney, whereas most orthotopic (nonectopic) renal units are normal (Abeshouse and Bhisitkul, 1959).

RENAL HYPOPLASIA

Renal hypoplasia is defined as a congenital decrease in the amount of normal renal tissue. The number of renal lobules may be normal or reduced to five or less with a corresponding decrease in the number of calices. The nephrons appear normal or hypertrophied microscopically, with no histologic features of dysplasia. All small kidneys are not hypoplastic, and indeed many so-called hypoplastic kidneys are small dysplastic kidneys (Bernstein and Meyer, 1964). Hypoplasia is usually bilateral and the total mass of functioning renal tissue may be inadequate to sustain normal growth and development. Clinical recognition may be as early as several weeks of age or as late as the 2nd decade. Qazi and associates (1979) observed unilateral or bilateral hypoplasia in infants suffering from fetal alcohol syndrome. The two main recognized types of hypoplasia are oligomeganephronia and segmental hypoplasia.

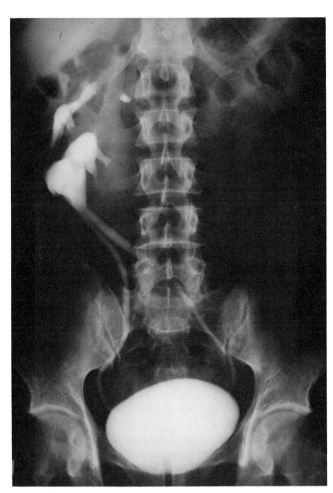

FIGURE 93–3. *Crossed fused ectopia: Excretory urogram in an infant who was found to have a right abdominal mass. The left kidney has crossed to the right and fused with the lower pole of right kidney. Notice the left ureter crossing the midline and inserting in normal location in the bladder.*

OLIGOMEGANEPHRONIA

Oligomeganephronia is a bilateral developmental abnormality characterized by a reduced number of nephrons and hypertrophy of those that remain (Fig. 93–4) (Fetterman and Habib, 1969; Royer et al., 1962; Scheinman and Abelson, 1970). The number of total nephrons is reduced to 100,000 or 200,000. One-third of infants are of low birth weight (<2500 g). Affected males outnumber females by 3 to 1. There is no clear familial tendency. Abnormalities in other organ systems are unusual. Pyelography and ultrasonography reveal small kidneys with normal calices. During the neonatal period and early infancy, the disorder may be asymptomatic or manifest as cyclic vomiting, dehydration, and fever. Tubular dysfunction is prominent, leading to polyuria, polydipsia, decreased concentrating ability, salt wasting, and acidosis. Mild to moderate proteinuria is often present. The onset of renal insufficiency occurs in the neonatal period or early infancy but may then remain stable for many years. Most infants and children with the disorder fail to grow adequately. Hypertension is unusual, even as renal failure progresses. End-stage renal disease usually develops between ages 5 and 15 years, and until then, these patients can be managed satisfactorily by the usual measures

required for treatment of chronic renal failure. Thereafter, they are good candidates for dialysis and transplantation.

SEGMENTAL HYPOPLASIA

Segmental hypoplasia (Ask-Upmark kidney) was originally thought to be a congenital developmental abnormality (Ask-Upmark, 1929; Royer et al., 1971); however, most authors now consider it to be an acquired condition secondary to reflux and scarring due to pyelonephritis (Arant et al., 1979). Most reported patients are older than 10 years. Only one premature infant has been reported with an Ask-Upmark kidney, which may be further support for the hypothesis that this is an acquired disease (Valderram and Berkman, 1979). Hypertension is the most prominent clinical feature and distinguishes segmental hypoplasia from other developmental renal abnormalities. The lesion is usually unilateral but can occasionally be bilateral. Partial or total nephrectomy for a unilateral lesion is associated with disappearance of hypertension and complete recovery.

RENAL DYSPLASIA

Renal dysplasia implies parenchymal maldevelopment and results from the abnormal differentiation of nephrogenic tissue in utero. Most dysplastic kidneys are grossly malformed and histologically are poorly organized with no differentiation between the cortex and medulla. Glomeruli and tubules appear primitive and are surrounded by abundant fibrous tissue. Dilated primitive ducts lined by tall columnar epithelium surrounded by fibromuscular collar, and nests of abnormal mesenchymal tissues, e.g., cartilage, smooth muscle cells, or hematopoietic tissue, are present (Bernstein, 1968; Kissane, 1976). Most dysplastic kidneys are cystic and, in early childhood, are the most common basis for renal cysts. The cystic dysplastic kidneys may be large, normal, or small. Although dysplasia usually affects the whole kidney, it may affect only a segment of it. Dysplastic kidneys or dysplastic segments usually have no or minimal function.

Dysplastic kidneys are associated with obstructive abnormalities of the ureter or lower urinary tract in about 90 per cent of patients; in others, it is a primary developmental abnormality (Bernstein, 1968 and 1971; Kissane, 1976). If high-grade urinary obstruction occurs early in gestation, it results in dysplasia; if obstruction occurs late, hydronephrosis develops (Beck, 1971; Glick et al., 1984; Rattner et al., 1963). Cystic dysplasia may be observed not only with anatomic obstruction, e.g., uteropelvic junction obstruction or posterior urethral valves, but also with intrauterine functional obstructions, e.g., prune belly syndrome. Other mechanisms that have been proposed to cause dysplasia include: (1) abnormal metanephric blastema, (2) abnormal induction of metanephric blastema by the ureteral bud, and (3) lateral ectopia of the ureteral bud causing induction of the metanephric blastema in an abnormal location (Elder and Duckett, 1987; Maisels and Simpson, 1983; Schwartz et al., 1981). In patients with duplicated ureters, when one is obstructed, cystic dysplasia occurs only in that segment of the kidney drained by the abnormal ureter (Bernstein, 1971).

In newborn and young infants with severe obstructive

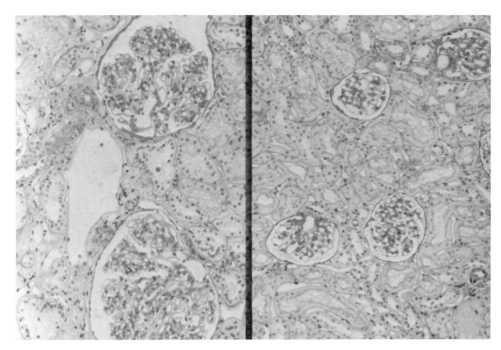

FIGURE 93–4. Oligomeganephronia: Notice the large glomeruli on the left from a young child with oligomeganephronia. For comparison, note normal glomeruli on the right. (Courtesy of Dr. Arthur Cohen.)

uropathy and significant dysplasia, relief of obstruction does not necessarily lead to the return of normal renal function (Anand et al., 1984). Most such infants achieve only temporary improvement in renal function following surgical correction of the obstructive lesion, and their renal function over the following months to years decreases.

Cystic dysplastic kidneys are also present in many newborns with multiple congenital anomalies or syndromes. Rarely, generalized renal dysplasia may be observed in the absence of obstruction or malformation of other organs, and the disease may be familial (Bernstein, 1971; Kissane, 1976; Roodhooft et al., 1984).

MULTICYSTIC KIDNEY

Multicystic kidney is a distinct type of dysplastic cystic kidney. A large renal mass contains numerous gross cysts (Figs. 93–5 and 93–6). Multicystic kidney is usually unilateral but on occasion may be bilateral. The ureter and/or the renal pelvis on the affected side are either occluded or atretic (Bernstein, 1971; Kissane, 1976). A unilateral

multicystic kidney usually manifests as an asymptomatic flank mass in a newborn. It is the second most common cause of an abdominal mass in a newborn after hydronephrosis (Griscom, 1965; Wilson, 1982). Increasingly, the disorder has been detected antenatally by ultrasound. The mass is occasionally associated with abdominal distention and hypertension. In unilateral disease, it is often assumed that the contralateral kidney is normal. However, Greene and associates (1971) and King (1988) have pointed out that significant disease may be present in the other kidney in 20 to 50 per cent of the patients. When

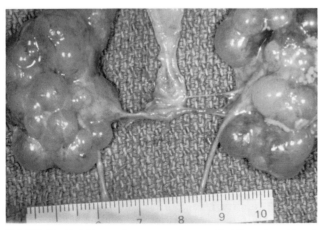

FIGURE 93–5. Kidneys from a newborn with bilateral multicystic kidneys. Both ureters were atretic. (Courtesy of Dr. Arthur Cohen.)

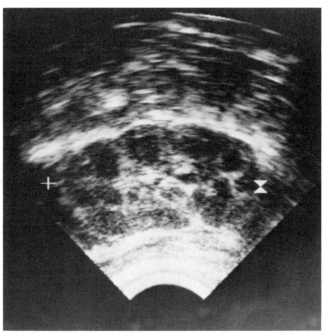

FIGURE 93–6. Multicystic kidney. Renal ultrasound of a 2-day-old newborn with right flank mass. The sonogram shows multiple lucent areas in the kidney. The kidney is outlined by the + and ⊻ marks. DTPA scan showed nonfunctioning right kidney and normal left kidney. VCUG showed no reflux.

both kidneys are multicystic, the clinical presentation mimics that of bilateral renal agenesis with Potter facies, anuria, and pulmonary hypoplasia.

The initial diagnostic evaluation of multicystic kidney usually consists of routine blood chemistries for evaluation of renal function and ultrasonography to differentiate the mass(es) from hydronephrosis and polycystic kidneys. Excretory urography usually reveals a nonfunctioning kidney. A voiding cystourethrogram is useful for evaluating reflux and associated bladder or urethral lesions.

The management of a multicystic kidney is controversial. Some authors recommend surgical removal between 6 months and 1 year of life because of potential for hypertension, infection, or the rare complication of neoplasia (King, 1988). Others including the authors advocate following these patients with serial abdominal ultrasonography (yearly or every 2 years) and monitoring the size of the kidneys. The kidney is removed if the diagnosis is in question, the mass changes in size, or hypertension, infection, or hemorrhage occur. Many parents have preferred elective nephrectomy rather than extensive follow-up and imaging studies.

■ REFERENCES

Abeshouse, B. S., and Bhisitkul, I.: Crossed renal ectopia with or without fusion. Urol. Int. 9:63, 1959.

Anand, S. K., Alon, U., and Chan, J. C. M.: Cystic diseases of the kidney in children. Adv. Pediatr. 31:371, 1984.

Arant, B. S., Sotello-Avilla, C., and Bernstein, J.: Segmental hypoplasia of the kidney. J. Pediatr. 95:931, 1979.

Ask-Upmark, E.: Über juvenile maligne Nephrosklerose und ihr Verhältnis zu Störungen in der Nierenentwicklung. Acta Pathol. Microbiol. Scand. 6:383, 1929.

Beck, A. D.: The effects of intrauterine obstruction upon the development of the fetal kidney. J. Urol. 106:939, 1971.

Bernstein, J.: Developmental abnormalities of the renal parenchyma: Renal hypoplasia and dysplasia. In Sommers, S. C. (Ed.): Pathology Annual. New York, Appleton-Century-Crofts, 1968.

Bernstein, J.: The morphogenesis of renal parenchymal maldevelopment. Pediatr. Clin. North Am. 18:395, 1971.

Bernstein, J., and Meyer, R.: Some speculations on the nature and significance of developmentally small kidneys (renal hypoplasia). Nephron 1:137, 1964.

Bhathena, D. B., Julian, B. A., McMorrow, R. G., et al.: Focal sclerosis of hypertrophied glomeruli in solitary functioning kidneys of humans. Am. J. Kidney Dis. 5:226, 1985.

Boatman, D. L., Kollin, C. P., and Flacks, R. H.: Congenital anomalies associated with horseshoe kidney. J. Urol. 107:205, 1972.

Elder, J. S., and Duckett, J. W.: Perinatal urology. In Gillenwater, J. Y., Grayhack, J. T., Howards, S. S., and Duckett, J. W. (Eds.): Adult and Pediatric Urology. Chicago, Year Book Medical Publishers, 1987, p. 1512.

Fetterman, G. H., and Habib, R.: Congenital bilateral oligomeganephronic renal hypoplasia with hypertrophy of nephrons (oligomeganephronia): Studies by microdissection. Am. J. Clin. Path. 52:199, 1969.

Fleisher, M. H., McLorie, G. A., Churchill, B. M., et al.: The yield of investigation of urinary tract in imperforate anus. J. Urol. 133:142, 1985.

Glenn, J. F.: Analysis of 51 patients with horseshoe kidney. N. Engl. J. Med. 261:684, 1959.

Glick, P. L., Harrison, M. R., Adzick, N. S., et al.: Correction of congenital hydronephrosis in utero. IV. In utero decompression prevents renal dysplasia. J. Pediatr. Surg. 19:649, 1984.

Greene, L. F., Feinzeig, W., and Dahlin, D. W.: Multicystic dysplasia with special references to the contralateral kidney. J. Urol. 105:482, 1971.

Griscom, N. T.: The roentgenography of neonatal abdominal masses. Am. J. Roentgen. 93:447, 1965.

King, L. R.: The management of multicystic kidney and uretero pelvic junction obstruction. In King, L. R. (Ed.): Urologic Surgery in Neonates and Young Infants. Philadelphia, W. B. Saunders Company, p. 140.

Kiprov, D. D., Colvin, R. B., and McCluskey, R. T.: Focal and segmental glomerulosclerosis and proteinuria associated with unilateral renal agenesis. Lab. Invest. 46:275, 1982.

Kissane, J. M.: The morphology of renal cystic disease. In Gardner, K. D. (Ed.): Cystic Diseases of the Kidney. New York, John Wiley and Sons, 1976, p. 31.

Kissane, J. M.: Congenital malformations. In Heptinstall, R. H. (Ed.): Pathology of the Kidney. Boston, Little, Brown & Co., 1983, p. 83.

Koff, S. A., Hayden, L. J., and Wise, H. A.: Anomalies of the kidney. In Gillenwater, J. Y., Grayhack, J. T., Howards, S. S., and Duckett, J. W. (Eds.): Adult and Pediatric Urology. Chicago, Year Book Medical Publishers, 1987.

Longo, V. J., and Thomson, G. J.: Congenital solitary kidney. J. Urol. 68:63, 1952.

Maisels, M., and Simpson, S. B.: Primitive ducts of renal dysplasia induced by culturing ureteral buds denuded of condensed renal mesenchyme. Science 21:509, 1983.

Mauer, S. M., Dobrin, R., and Vernier, R. L.: Unilateral and bilateral renal agenesis in monoamniotic twins. J. Pediatr. 84:236, 1974.

Perlmutter, A. D., Retik, A. B., and Bauer, S. B.: Anomalies of the upper urinary tract. In Walsh, P. C., Gittes, R. F., Perlmutter, A. D., and Stamey, T. A. (Eds.): Campbell's Urology. Philadelphia, W. B. Saunders Company, 1986.

Potter, E. L. (Ed.): Normal and Abnormal Development of the Kidney. Chicago, Year Book Medical Publishers, 1972.

Qazi, Q., Masakawa, A., Milman, D., et al.: Renal anomalies in fetal alcohol syndrome. Pediatrics 63:886, 1979.

Rattner, W. H., Meyer, R., and Bernstein, J.: Congenital abnormalities of the urinary system. IV. Valvular obstruction of the posterior urethra. J. Pediatr. 63:84, 1963.

Roodhooft, A. M., Birnholz, J. C., and Holmes, L. B.: Familial nature of congenital absence and severe dysgenesis of both kidneys. N. Engl. J. Med. 310:341, 1984.

Royer, P., Habib R., Broyer, M., et al.: Segmental hypoplasia of the kidney in children. Adv. Nephrol. 1:145, 1971.

Royer, P., Habib, R., Mathieu, H., et al.: L'Hypoplasie rénale bilatérale congénitale avec réduction du nombre et hypertrophie des nephrons chez l'enfant. Ann. Pediatr. (Paris) 38:133, 1962.

Scheinman, J. I., and Abelson, H. T.: Bilateral renal hypoplasia with oligonephronia. J. Pediatr. 76:369, 1970.

Schwartz, R. D., Stephens, F. D., Cussen, L. J.: The pathogenesis of renal dysplasia. II. The significance of lateral and medical ectopy of ureteral orifice. Invest. Urol. 19:97, 1981.

Steinhart, J. M., Kuhn, J. P., Eisenberg, B., et al.: Ultrasound screening of healthy infants for urinary tract abnormalities. Pediatrics 82:609, 1988.

Stephens, F. D.: Congenital Malformations of the Urinary Tract. New York, Praeger, 1983.

Valderram, E., and Berkman, J. I.: The Ask-Upmark kidney in a premature infant. Clin. Nephrol. 11:313, 1979.

Whitehouse, G. H.: Some urologic aspects of the horseshoe kidney anomaly: A review of 59 cases. Clin. Radiol. 26:107, 1975.

Wilson, D. A.: Ultrasound screening for abdominal masses in the neonatal period. Am. J. Dis. Child. 136:147, 1982.

CYSTIC DISEASES OF THE KIDNEYS

94

Sudhir K. Anand

Cystic diseases of the kidney are a heterogeneous group of disorders that may be hereditary, developmental, or acquired. The cysts in these disorders may be discovered as an incidental finding or they may cause severe derangements in renal function. Renal cysts may arise from any part of the nephron or collecting tubule and may be located in the cortex, medulla, or both. Renal cysts have been classified in a number of ways (Bernstein, 1973; Osthanondh and Potter, 1964; Resnick et al., 1976) and the classifications have often been confusing. Clinically, the most useful classifications are those that incorporate clinical, genetic, radiologic, functional, and morphologic features (Table 94–1).

Most renal cystic lesions in newborns result from dysplastic development of the kidneys secondary to intrauterine obstruction of the urinary tract (see Chapter 93). "Multicystic" dysplastic kidney is the most common type of cystic disorder in the newborn. The term "polycystic kidney" is restricted to a small group of hereditary renal disorders generally with diffuse bilateral involvement. Labeling every renal disorder with multiple cysts as "polycystic" is incorrect. Juvenile nephronophthisis and medullary cystic kidneys are important causes of renal failure in older children and young adults; however, the disorders are rarely seen before 5 years of age. Although simple renal cysts are the most common cystic disorder in adults, they are extremely uncommon in the newborn. Renal cysts are also present in several hereditary syndromes with multiorgan involvement (see Chapter 91).

Pathogenesis: The pathogenesis of polycystic kidney disease and nonobstructive renal cysts has been investigated in a number of experimental in vivo and in vitro models (Avner, 1988; Crocker et al., 1971; Gardner, 1988; Resnick et al., 1976). The in vivo studies have primarily focused on cyst induction by various chemicals in a number of animal species or on the development of cysts in inbred animal models. The in vitro studies have focused on development of cysts in cell cultures from murine metanephric tissue or cells from autosomal dominant polycystic kidneys. About 20 agents, including steroids, diphenylamine, and nordihydroguaiaretic acid, are known to cause cystic disease when given to neonatal or fetal animals (Resnick et al., 1976). None of these chemicals are known to cause renal cystic disease in humans.

Three separate hypotheses explain the pathogenesis of cysts (Gardner, 1988). The first postulates increased compliance of the tubular basement membrane. The second implicates epithelial cell hyperplasia and/or micropolyp formation leading to partial obstruction of tubular flow and dilatation of tubules from increased intraluminal pressure. The third hypothesis suggests unidirectional influx

TABLE 94–1. Classification of Cystic Diseases of Kidney

Polycystic Kidney Disease
  Autosomal recessive (infantile)*†
  Autosomal dominant (adult)*†
Cystic Dysplasia
  Cystic dysplasia with obstructive urinary tract*
  Multicystic kidney*
  Hereditary cystic dysplasia*†
Syndromes and Systemic Disorders with Multiple Renal Cysts
  Meckel syndrome*†
  Zellweger (cerebrohepatorenal) syndrome*†
  Ivemark syndrome*†
  Tuberous sclerosis†
  Trisomy 13 and 18*†
Renal Cortical Cysts
  Glomerulocystic disease
  Microcystic disease (congenital nephrotic syndrome)*†
Renal Medullary Cysts
  Juvenile nephronophthisis†
  Medullary cystic kidney†
  Renal retinal dysplasia†
  Medullary sponge kidney
Isolated Renal Cysts
  Simple cysts (solitary or multiple)
  Multilocular cysts
Acquired and Miscellaneous Cysts
  Acquired cysts during chronic dialysis
  Pyelocalyceal cysts
  Medullary necrosis cysts
  Tumor necrosis cysts
  Dysontogenic cysts
  Perinephric pseudo cysts

*May be seen in newborns.
†Inherited disorder.
(Adapted from Bernstein (1973) and Kissane (1983).)

instead of the normal efflux of solutes and water from the epithelium of the affected tubular segment (Gardner, 1988).

Polycystic kidney disease (PKD) has traditionally been divided into infantile and adult types (Bernstein, 1973), with infantile PKD being usually diagnosed during the neonatal period or early infancy and the adult variety during the 3rd or 4th decade. During the past two decades, it has become evident that the infantile variety of PKD may first become apparent in young adults and the adult variety may occasionally manifest in early infancy. Therefore, most authors now prefer the terms autosomal recessive (infantile) and autosomal dominant (adult) PKD, which are discussed in detail below.

■ AUTOSOMAL DOMINANT POLYCYSTIC KIDNEY DISEASE

Autosomal dominant (adult) polycystic kidney disease (ADPKD) is a common inherited disorder with a prevalence of about 1:500 to 1:1000 in the general population (Dalgaard, 1957; Grantham, 1988). Moreover, it is responsible for nearly 10 per cent of all patients developing end-stage renal disease both in Europe (Robinson and Hawkins, 1980) and the United States (Vollmer et al., 1983).

In ADPKD, only 1 to 2 per cent of tubules are affected by cystic lesions (Grantham, 1988). The renal cysts in ADPKD are usually globular in shape and may arise from any portion of the tubule. However, only 25 per cent of these cysts are connected to the tubules (Grantham et al., 1987). The pathogenesis of the remaining 75 per cent of cysts is not known but may be due to net transepithelial secretion.

ADPKD usually presents in the 3rd to 5th decade with symptoms and signs of flank and/or back pain, abdominal mass or enlargement, gross hematuria, hypertension, or nocturia (Dalgaard, 1957; Gabow and Shrier, 1989; Grantham, 1988; Zeier et al., 1988). Thereafter, the disease progresses to end-stage renal disease within months or years. Although ADPKD generally has bilateral diffuse involvement of the kidneys, on occasion the lesions can be asymmetrical with one kidney being considerably more affected than the other (Gardner, 1988; Porch et al., 1986). By ultrasound screening of families with ADPKD, the disorder has often been recognized in children under 10 years of age (Sedman et al., 1987), and there are several reports describing the disorder in newborns and young infants (Fig. 94–1) and occasionally also in fetuses (Bear et al., 1984; Chevalier et al., 1981; Cole et al., 1987; Fellows et al., 1976; Kaye and Lewy, 1974; Mehrizi et al., 1964; Proesmans et al., 1982; Sedman et al., 1987; Shokeir, 1978; Taitz et al., 1987; Zerres et al., 1985).

The clinical course in newborns with ADPKD has been variable. Some have been asymptomatic while others have been born with bilateral large cystic renal masses with the clinical course complicated by hypertension, early

renal failure, and death. Occasionally, infants have been stillborn or have died within a few days of birth.

Although the morbidity and mortality in ADPKD is primarily associated with the presence of renal cysts, the disorder affects many other organs—hepatic cysts, pancreatic cysts, and cerebral aneurysms. Hossack and coworkers (1988) have reported increased prevalence of mitral valve prolapse and incompetence of mitral, tricuspid, and aortic valves. Colonic diverticula may also be present (Scheff et al., 1980). These findings suggest that ADPKD is a systemic disorder with a defect in the synthesis of extracellular matrix (Carone et al., 1988; Gabow and Shrier, 1989; Grantham, 1988).

A positive family history for ADPKD is important diagnostic information for an infant with bilateral cystic renal masses. Ultrasonography demonstrates the presence of bilateral multiple cysts of variable sizes, and this test alone is adequate to confirm the diagnosis if family history is definitely positive. If a detailed family history is not available and ADPKD is suspected in a young child, both parents should be screened by ultrasonography for renal cysts. If the diagnosis is in doubt, CT scanning of the kidneys should be performed. Excretory urography may demonstrate cysts and calyceal displacement, although the technique is less sensitive and findings are often nonspecific. While the excretory urographic appearances of ADPKD and ARPKD are usually different, at times the two are hard to differentiate (Cole et al., 1987). On rare occasions, a liver biopsy is necessary to differentiate ADPKD from ARPKD. Bile duct hyperplasia and/or hepatic fibrosis are only seen in ARPKD, whereas in ADPKD a liver biopsy is usually normal (except for large hepatic cysts).

Reeders and associates (1985) reported that the gene for ADPKD is located on the short arm of chromosome 16 closely linked to the alpha-hemoglobin gene complexes. Subsequently, they have reported a technique for

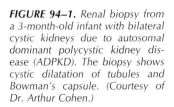

FIGURE 94–1. Renal biopsy from a 3-month-old infant with bilateral cystic kidneys due to autosomal dominant polycystic kidney disease (ADPKD). The biopsy shows cystic dilatation of tubules and Bowman's capsule. (Courtesy of Dr. Arthur Cohen.)

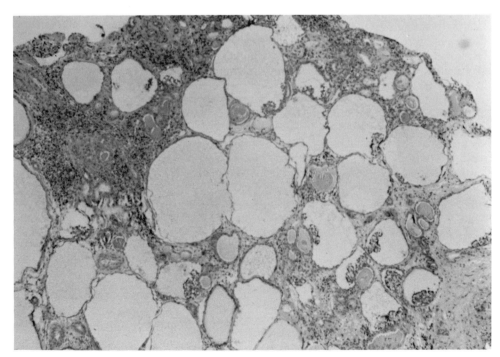

prenatal diagnosis of ADPKD with a DNA probe (Reeders et al., 1986). However, Kimberling and associates (1988) have failed to show alpha-hemoglobin gene linkage to ADPKD in a large family with ADPKD, suggesting that more than one abnormal gene may cause the disease.

■ AUTOSOMAL RECESSIVE POLYCYSTIC KIDNEY DISEASE

The incidence of ARPKD is about 1 in 40,000 births. The renal lesion manifests as cystic dilatation (ectasia) of the collecting tubules. Invariably, all patients also have hepatic involvement in the form of bile duct hyperplasia, dilatation (ectasia), and hepatic fibrosis (Bernstein, 1971; Gagnadoux et al., 1989; Lieberman et al., 1971). No other organ systems are affected in ARPKD in contrast to ADPKD which is a multisystem disorder.

The clinical presentation varies between patients depending upon the extent of kidney and hepatic involvement. At initial presentation, newborns and young infants have severe kidney and minimal hepatic involvement in contrast to older children and adults who primarily have hepatic damage (portal hypertension) and minimal renal involvement. Depending upon the age of presentation, clinical findings, and pathologic findings, Lieberman and associates (1971) have classified ARPKD into two subtypes: infantile polycystic kidney disease and congenital hepatic fibrosis. Blyth and Ockenden (1971) have divided ARPKD into four genetic subtypes: perinatal, neonatal, infantile, and juvenile. Juvenile ARPKD is synonymous with congenital hepatic fibrosis. Blyth and Ockenden suggest that a different mutant gene is involved in each of the four forms of ARPKD; however, most other authors (Anand et al., 1984; Gagnadoux et al., 1989; Resnick and Vernier, 1981) consider Blyth's classification as too rigid and believe that ARPKD and congenital hepatic fibrosis are a spectrum of the same inherited disorder with variations in clinical presentation among different patients and affected members of the same families.

Most newborns and young infants with ARPKD have a distended abdomen with massively enlarged kidneys (Blyth and Ockenden, 1971; Lieberman et al., 1971; Resnick and Vernier, 1981). Frequently, the liver is also enlarged. The bilateral renal enlargement is often diagnosed antenatally. Severely affected newborns have oligohydramnios and typical Potter facies. Labor is often difficult due to massive renal enlargement and cesarean section is sometimes necessary. Respiratory distress is common in affected newborns due to pulmonary hypoplasia, pneumothoraces, and/or upward compression of the diaphragm by massively enlarged kidneys. If patients survive beyond the neonatal period, the pulmonary problems usually resolve. Severely affected newborns have minimal urinary output, and they die because of renal failure or pulmonary problems.

The clinical course of infants with ARPKD who live beyond the neonatal period is often complicated by failure to thrive, hypertension, congestive heart failure, mild to moderate polyuria, and progressive renal failure. A few newborns and young infants with ARPKD have normal or near-normal renal function, and their growth may also be normal (Cole et al., 1987; Lieberman et al., 1971). As children grow, the kidney size remains enlarged but their size in proportion to the abdomen diminishes. The majority of children with ARPKD who have not developed end-stage renal disease by 5 years of age develop portal hypertension, esophageal varices, and splenic enlargement (Cole et al., 1987; Lieberman et al., 1971).

The diagnosis of ARPKD is confirmed by clinical findings, ultrasonography, and excretory urography; occasionally, CT scanning or renal biopsy may be necessary. Ultrasonography confirms the renal enlargement and demonstrates multiple small cysts. The excretory urogram is usually characteristic and helps differentiate ARPKD from other disorders causing bilateral renal enlargement. Typically, the urogram shows massive renal enlargement with alternating streaked radiodensities and radiolucencies (Fig. 94–2). The kidneys retain their reniform shape and have a smooth surface. Some patients have an irregularly mottled nephrogram instead of a streaked appearance. Marked delay in the excretion of contrast is usually present, and the urinary bladder may not be visualized for several hours. The contrast agent may be retained in the kidneys (in dilated collecting tubules) for several days.

Morphologically, the kidneys may be massively enlarged and show innumerable, tiny 1 to 5 mm cysts. The cysts are dilatations of collecting tubules and are arranged radially from the subcapsular cortex to medulla (Fig. 94–3). In severely affected newborns 90 per cent or more

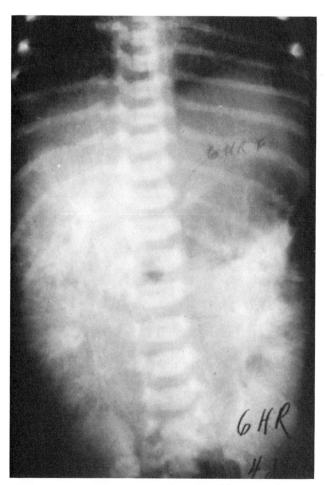

FIGURE 94–2. Excretory urogram of a 4-day-old infant with ARPKD, showing massive enlargement of both kidneys. The roentgenogram also shows radially oriented streaked densities in renal cortex. This roentgenogram was taken 6 hours after injection of contrast.

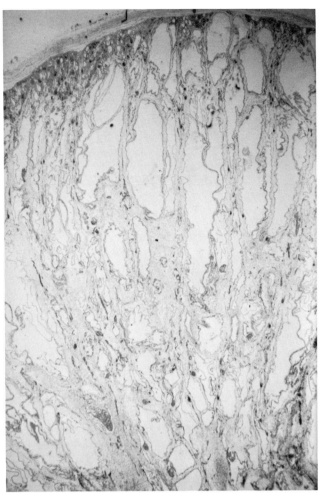

FIGURE 94–3. *Kidney biopsy from a newborn infant with ARPKD demonstrating radially arranged cystic dilatations of collecting tubules (From Anand, S. K., Alon, U., and Chan, J. C. M.: Cystic diseases of the kidney in children. Adv. Pediatr. 31:371, 1984; photograph courtesy of Dr. Arthur Cohen.)*

tubules may show cystic dilatation. In newborns the glomeruli, interstitium, and remaining parts of tubules appear normal, but later, atrophy and fibrosis may be present. Glomerular cysts are never found in ARPKD, unlike ADPKD (Kissane, 1983). In patients with clinical onset of ARPKD in later childhood, the cystic dilatation of tubules is limited both in number (10 per cent or less) and magnitude. The liver is usually enlarged. The portal areas show bile duct hyperplasia, dilatation, and tortuosness surrounded by periportal fibrosis. In newborns the biliary cysts are microscopic and fibrosis is minimal. Later, fibrosis becomes more evident, and the cysts may become macroscopic.

The treatment of ARPKD is primarily supportive until end-stage renal disease (ESRD) or severe portal hypertension develops. Systemic hypertension, if present, should be aggressively treated to prevent congestive heart failure and delay the development of ESRD. Children with ARPKD are good candidates for both chronic peritoneal or hemodialysis and renal transplantation.

■ REFERENCES

Anand, S. K., Alon, U., and Chan, J. C. M.: Cystic diseases of the kidney in children. Adv. Pediatr. *31*:371, 1984.

Avner, E. D.: Renal cystic disease: Insight from recent experimental investigation. Nephron *48*:89, 1988.

Bear, J. C., McManamon, P., Morgan, J., et al.: Age at clinical onset and at sonographic detection of adult polycystic kidney disease. Am. J. Med. Genet. *18*:45, 1984.

Bernstein, J.: Heritable cystic disorders of the kidney: The mythology of polycystic disease. Pediatr. Clin. North Am. *18*:435, 1971.

Bernstein, J.: The classification of renal cysts. Nephron *11*:91, 1973.

Blyth, H. M., and Ockenden, B. G.: Polycystic disease of kidneys and liver presenting in childhood. J. Med. Genet. *8*:257, 1971.

Carone, F. A., Makino, H., and Kanwar, Y. S.: Basement membrane antigens in renal polycystic disease. Am. J. Pathol. *130*:466, 1988.

Chevalier, R. L., Garland, T. A., and Buschi, A. J.: The neonate with adult-type autosomal dominant polycystic kidney disease. Int. J. Pediatr. Nephro. *2*:73, 1981.

Cole, B. J., Conley, S. B., and Stapleton, F. B.: Polycystic kidney disease in the first year of life. J. Pediatr. *111*:693, 1987.

Crocker, J. F. S., Brown, D. M., and Vernier, R. L.: Development defects of the kidney. Pediatr. Clin. North Am. *18*:355, 1971.

Dalgaard, O. Z.: Bilateral polycystic disease of the kidneys: A follow-up of 284 patients and their families. Acta Med. Scand. *328*(suppl.):3, 1957.

Fellows, R. A., Leonidas, J. C., and Beatty, E. C.: Radiologic features of "adult type" polycystic kidney disease in the neonate. Pediatr. Radiol. *4*:87, 1976.

Gabow, P. A., and Shrier, R. W.: Pathophysiology of adult polycystic kidney disease. Adv. Nephrol. *18*:19, 1989.

Gagnadoux, M., Habib, R., Levy, M., et al.: Cystic renal disease in children. Adv. Nephrol. *18*:33, 1989.

Gardner, K. D.: An overview of cystic renal disease. In Gardner, K. D. (Ed.): Cystic Disease of the Kidney. New York, John Wiley & Sons, 1976, p. 1.

Gardner, K. D.: Cystic kidneys. Kidney Int. *33*:610, 1988.

Grantham, J. J.: Polycystic kidney disease—an old problem in a new context. N. Engl. J. Med. *319*:944, 1988.

Grantham, J. J., Geiser, J. L., and Evan, A. P.: Cyst formation and growth in autosomal dominant polycystic kidney disease. Kidney Int. *31*:1145, 1987.

Hossack, K. F., Leddy, C. L., Johnson, A. M., et al.: Echocardiographic findings in autosomal dominant polycystic kidney disease. N. Engl. J. Med. *319*:907, 1988.

Kaye, C., and Lewy, P. R.: Congenital appearance of adult-type (autosomal dominant) polycystic kidney disease: Report of a case. J. Pediatr. *85*:807, 1974.

Kimberling, W. J., Fain, P. R., Kenyon, J. B., et al.: Linkage heterogeneity of autosomal dominant polycystic kidney disease. N. Engl. J. Med. *319*:913, 1988.

Kissane, J. M.: Congenital malformations. In Heptinstall, R. H. (Ed.): Pathology of the Kidney. Boston, Little, Brown & Co., 1983, p. 83.

Lieberman, E., Salinas-Madrigal, L., Gwinn, J. L., et al.: Infantile polycystic disease of the kidneys and liver: Clinical, pathological and radiological correlations and comparison with congenital hepatic fibrosis. Medicine *50*:277, 1971.

Mehrizi, A., Rosenstein, B. J., Pusch, A., et al.: Myocardial infarction and endocardial fibroelastosis in children with polycystic kidneys. Bull. Johns Hopkins Hosp. *115*:92, 1964.

Osthanondh, V., and Potter, E. L.: Pathogenesis of polycystic kidneys. Arch. Pathol. *77*:459, 1964.

Porch, P., Noe, H. N., and Stapleton, F. B.: Unilateral presentation of adult polycystic kidney disease in children. J. Urol. *135*:744, 1986.

Proesmans, W., Van Damme, B., Caesar, P., et al.: Autosomal dominant polycystic kidney disease in the neonatal period; associated with cerebroarteriovenous malformation. Pediatrics *70*:971, 1982.

Reeders, S. T., Breuning, M. H., Davies, K. E., et al.: A highly polymorphic DNA marker linked to adult polycystic kidney disease on chromosome 16. Nature *317*:542, 1985.

Reeders, S. T., Zerres, K., Gal, A., et al.: Prenatal diagnosis of autosomal dominant polycystic kidney disease with a DNA probe. Lancet *2*:6, 1986.

Resnick, J. S., Brown, D. M., and Vernier, R. L.: Normal developmental and experimental models of cystic renal disease. In Gardner, K. D. (Ed.): Cystic Disease of the Kidney. New York, John Wiley & Sons, 1976, p. 221.

Resnick, J. S., and Vernier, R. L.: Cystic disease of the kidney in the newborn infant. Clin. Perinatol. *8*:375, 1981.

Robinson, B. H. H., and Hawkins, J. B. (Eds.): Proceedings of the European Dialysis and Transplant Association, vol. *17*. London, Pitman Books Limited, 1980, p. 20.

Scheff, R. T., Zuckerman, G., Haster, H., et al.: Diverticular disease in patients with chronic renal failure due to polycystic kidney disease. Ann. Int. Med. 92:202, 1980.

Sedman, A., Bell, P., Manco-Johnson, M., et al.: Autosomal dominant polycystic kidney disease in childhood: A longitudinal study. Kidney Int. 31:1000, 1987.

Shokeir, M. H.: Expression of adult polycystic renal disease in the fetus and newborn. Clin. Genet. 14:61, 1978.

Taitz, L. S., Brown, C. B., Blanck, C. E., et al.: Screening for polycystic kidney disease: Importance of clinical presentation in the newborn. Arch. Dis. Child. 62:45, 1987.

Vollmer, W. M., Wahl, P. W., and Blagg, C. R. Survival with dialysis and transplantation in patients with end-stage renal disease. N. Engl. J. Med. 308:1553, 1983.

Zeier, M., Geberth, S., Ritz, E., et al.: Adult dominant polycystic kidney disease. Clinical problems. Nephron 49:177, 1988.

Zerres, K., Hansmann, M., Knopfle, G., et al.: Prenatal diagnosis of genetically determined early manifestation of autosomal dominant polycystic kidney disease. Hum. Genet. 71:368, 1985.

TUMORS OF THE KIDNEY 95

Randal A. Aaberg, Martin A. Koyle, and Sudhir K. Anand

■ CONGENITAL MESOBLASTIC LYMPHOMA

Congenital mesoblastic nephroma (CMN) is the most common renal neoplasm encountered in the newborn (Howell et al., 1982). A review of 3340 patients entered into the National Wilms Tumor Study from 1969 to 1984 revealed 24 renal malignancies in children under 30 days of age. Eighteen of these (75 per cent) were CMN and only four were considered true Wilms tumors (Hrabovsky et al., 1986). The mean age at diagnosis of CMN is 3.4 months. Males are affected 1.5 times more often than females.

Bolande and associates (1967) clearly distinguished CMN from Wilms tumor by its benign clinical behavior, preponderance of mesenchymal derivatives, and the lack of a malignant-appearing epithelial component. CMN has a tendency for local invasion unlike hamartomas, which have a more limited growth potential.

The most common clinical presentation is that of an asymptomatic, palpable mass noted during the newborn examination. The mass is solid and unilateral and can attain a large size (Fig. 95–1). The differential diagnosis should include multicystic dysplastic kidney or hydronephrosis, each of which will be sonolucent and can be distinguished from CMN by ultrasound alone. Hematuria (18 per cent), renin-mediated hypertension (4 per cent), hypercalcemia, and congestive heart failure secondary to arteriovenous shunting in the tumor may occur. Maternal polyhydramnios and premature birth have been noted frequently, but their etiology is unknown. The incidence of associated congenital anomalies is similar to that seen with Wilms tumor (14 per cent), although hemihypertrophy has been reported only once.

Nephrectomy is the treatment of choice for CMN, and the prognosis is excellent. Adjuvant chemotherapy or radiation is generally not necessary and is reserved for incompletely resected tumors or those in which intraoperative rupture has occurred.

■ WILMS TUMOR

Wilms tumor, or nephroblastoma, is named for the German surgeon Max Wilms, who identified seven new cases and published a monograph in 1899. A dramatic improvement in patient survival and increased understanding of this disease has occurred in the last two decades from collaborative efforts of the National Wilms Tumor Study group (Mesrobian, 1988).

Epidemiology. Wilms tumor is the most common malignancy of the genitourinary tract in children and accounts for approximately 8 per cent of all childhood malignancies. The risk of developing Wilms tumor is one in 10,000 live births, and approximately 500 new cases are reported annually. The peak incidence is 3.5 years of age with males and females being affected equally (Breslow and Beckwith, 1982).

Wilms tumor is associated with other genitourinary anomalies in 4.4 per cent of the patients, including hypospadias, cryptorchidism, ureteral duplication, ambiguous genitalia, and renal fusion abnormalities (Pendergrass, 1976). Hemihypertrophy occurs in 2.4 per cent of the children, and aniridia occurs in 1.1 per cent (Green, 1985).

Wilms tumor is also associated with heritable genetic abnormalities. Karyotype analysis of the Wilms tumor–aniridia complex demonstrates a deletion in the short arm of chromosome 11 (Riccardi et al., 1978). Furthermore, children with sporadic aniridia have a 1 in 3 chance of developing Wilms tumor, necessitating ultrasound screening in these patients (Pilling, 1975). Wilms tumor occurs bilaterally in 5 per cent of the children, most of whom display hereditary transmission (Matsunaga, 1981).

Pathology. Wilms tumor is usually a solitary encapsulated mass composed of nephrogenic, stromal, and epithelial components. Unfavorable prognostic factors include anaplastic histology, presence of hematogenous or lymph node metastases, large tumor volume, direct extension, vascular involvement, and operative spill of tumor.

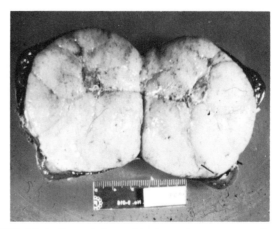

FIGURE 95–1. Congenital mesoblastic nephroma compressing and nearly totally replacing the kidney.

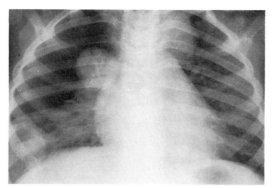

FIGURE 95–2. Pulmonary metastases of Wilms tumor.

Clinical Features. Wilms tumor presents as a palpable abdominal mass in 90 per cent of the patients. Classically, the mass is smooth and firm to palpation and does not cross the midline. Fever or pain may be present in 25 per cent of the patients. Gross hematuria occurs rarely, but microscopic hematuria has been detected in 50 per cent of the patients. Hypertension is present in up to 60 per cent of the patients and usually resolves after excision of the tumor. The initial laboratory evaluation of any child with a retroperitoneal mass includes a complete blood count, urinalysis, electrolytes, and renal and liver function tests. Urinary or plasma catecholamines are measured to rule out neuroblastoma. Bone marrow metastases are rare with Wilms tumor, and bone marrow biopsy is not necessary unless neuroblastoma is suspected.

Preoperative radiographic evaluation should document the presence of an intrarenal versus extrarenal mass, establish that the contralateral kidney is normal, determine the patency of the inferior vena cava, and document the presence or absence of pulmonary metastases (Fig. 95–2). Ultrasound is performed initially to determine the nature of the mass. Excretory urography is used much less frequently today. CT scanning is used if a Wilms tumor is suspected on ultrasound, to document the extent of the disease. MRI and, rarely, vena cavography may be necessary to evaluate vena cava extension.

Treatment. Surgical resection remains the cornerstone of therapy and staging in children with Wilms tumor (Table 95–1). Intraoperatively, it is important not only to stage the disease surgically but care must be taken to prevent spillage of tumor cells that would increase the tumor staging and make additional treatment necessary.

Bilateral Wilms tumors occur in 5 per cent of children, and one-third of these cases are not appreciated preoperatively. A renal parenchymal sparing approach is necessary, relying on chemotherapy and second-look surgical procedures for cure (Koyle and Ehrlich, 1988). Fortunately, bilateral Wilms tumor tends to be less malignant than unilateral lesions and is more often associated with favorable histology and thus better survival (Mesrobian, 1988).

A dramatic improvement in survival has occurred over the past two decades, due to successful multidisciplinary treatment with radiation and chemotherapy (Table 95–2).

■ NEUROBLASTOMA

Neuroblastoma is a malignant neoplasm originating from neural crest tissue. It is the most common solid tumor

TABLE 95–1. Current Staging of Wilms Tumor

Stage I
Tumor limited to kidney and completely resected.

Stage II
Tumor extending beyond kidney but completely resected. Regional extension of tumor, vessel infiltration, biopsy, or local spillage of tumor confined to the flank.

Stage III
Residual nonhematogenous tumor confined to the abdomen including lymph nodes, diffuse peritoneal contamination by tumor spillage, tumor extending beyond the surgical margins, or tumor not completely resectable because of local infiltration into vital structures.

Stage IV
Hematogenous metastases beyond the abdomen to lung, liver, bone, brain, or lymph nodes.

Stage V
Bilateral renal involvement at diagnosis.

of childhood and accounts for as many as 14 per cent of childhood malignancies and 50 per cent of neonatal malignancies. Most patients have metastatic disease at diagnosis. Although the prognosis for newborns is remarkably good, the overall prognosis for neuroblastoma remains poor in comparison to advances made in the treatment of Wilms tumor and other childhood malignancies.

Epidemiology. Neuroblastoma ranks just behind leukemia, lymphoma, and central nervous system tumors in prevalence but exceeds that of Wilms tumor and rhabdomyosarcoma. The peak age of presentation is at 1.5 years, with 25 to 33 per cent being diagnosed within the first year of life (Grosfeld and Bachner, 1980). Neuroblastoma "in situ" has been found at autopsy in infants under 3 months of age with a frequency of 40 times that of clinical neuroblastoma (Beckwith and Perrin, 1963). This suggests that only a small portion of these tumors become clinically evident.

Pathology. Neuroblastoma represents a spectrum of differentiation of the neuroblast including ganglioneuroma, which is a benign tumor composed of mature ganglion cells; ganglioneuroblastoma, which forms an intermediate group; and neuroblastoma, which is the most immature

TABLE 95–2. Survival of Patients With Wilms Tumor

	TWO-YEAR SURVIVAL (per cent)
Stage	
I	95
II	90
III	84
IV	54
Histologic Pattern	
Unfavorable	54
Favorable	90
Lymph Nodes	
Negative	82
Positive	54

(From D'Angio, G. J., Evans, A., Breslow, N. E., et al.: The treatment of Wilms tumor. Results of the second National Wilms Tumor Study. Cancer 47:2302, 1981.)

and malignant. Neuroblastoma is capable of differentiating into the more mature ganglioneuroma and ganglioneuroblastoma (Greenfield and Shelley, 1965). Spontaneous regression of these tumors has been noted many times, even in patients with metastatic disease (Schwartz et al., 1974).

Clinical Features. The majority of primary tumors are abdominal in origin; 40 per cent arise from the adrenal medulla, and 25 per cent arise from intra-abdominal sympathetic ganglia. Fifteen per cent arise from sympathetic ganglia in the chest (Rosen et al., 1984). Other primary sites account for 20 per cent of neuroblastomas and include sympathetic ganglia in the neck and pelvis. Bone marrow metastases are present in 70 per cent of the patients, and rosettes of neuroblastoma cells are pathognomonic (Fig. 95–3). Other common metastatic sites include the skull, diaphyses of the long bones, central nervous system, liver, and orbit (Grosfeld and Bachner, 1980). Local extension to the spinal canal may also occur (Punt et al., 1980).

A palpable, nontender, abdominal mass often crossing the midline in a sickly appearing child is present in half of the patients. With local extension of the tumor or involvement of secondary organs by metastases, the patient may lose weight or develop other nonspecific gastrointestinal complaints. Intractable diarrhea with secondary metabolic disturbances may be found in some patients because of increased levels of vasoactive intestinal polypeptide. Neuroblastoma has also been associated with an acute encephalopathy consisting of opsoclonus, truncal ataxia, and myoclonus. Horner syndrome may be present in an occasional patient.

Neuroblastoma in the newborn usually presents with hepatomegaly, unlike the presentation in older infants and children. Schneider and associates (1965) reviewed 56 cases of neonatal neuroblastoma recorded in the English literature since 1940. Of these, 52 per cent had metastases at the time of diagnosis; the liver was involved in 65 per cent, and subcutaneous nodules were seen in 32 per cent (Table 95–3). Metastases to lungs, bones, skull, and orbit are rare in the newborn, although rosettes of tumor cells are often found in bone marrow aspirates.

Punctate calcifications on an abdominal radiograph suggest neuroblastoma and are present in 50 per cent of the patients. The excretory urogram classically demonstrates a displaced kidney without distortion of the col-

lecting system. Ultrasound and computerized tomography are the most frequently used modalities for staging and follow-up. Magnetic resonance imaging, effective for visualizing the adrenal gland, may play a more prominent role in the future (Koyle, 1986).

Numerous studies have demonstrated the association between neuroblastoma and elevated urinary levels of norepinephrine and its precursors and metabolites. Elevated levels of homovanillic acid (HVA) or vanillylmandelic acid (VMA) are found in up to 95 per cent of patients.

Treatment. The most commonly used staging system is that reported by Evans and associates (1971) (Table 95–4). A unique group of patients are those with stage IV-S disease. They have disseminated disease to bone marrow, skin, or liver but no radiologic evidence of bony metastases. The 2-year survival in this category is 78 per cent for all age groups (95 per cent if less than 1 year old) versus 6 per cent for stage IV disease (28 per cent if less than 1 year old). Stage IV-S patients have normal serum ferritin levels, which can help distinguish them from patients with stage IV disease (Hann et al., 1981). Elevated serum ferritin levels have been associated with a worse prognosis in all stages of disease (Hann et al., 1985).

Surgery alone may be curative in stages I, II, and IV-S disease. Stage IV-S tumor may regress spontaneously

TABLE 95–3. Incidence of Metastases in the Newborn with Neuroblastoma

SITE	NUMBER	PERCENTAGE	ALL AGES (per cent)
Liver	20	64.6	24.3
Subcutaneous nodules	10	32.3	2.6
Marrow	3	9.7	
Lung	2	6.5	13.2
Spleen	2	6.5	2.0
Kidney	2	6.5	2.0
Pancreas	2	6.5	
Brain	2	6.5	15.8
Bone	1	3.2	47.4
Nodes	1	3.2	32.2
Pleura	1	3.2	
Myocardium	1	3.2	
Periadrenal	1	3.2	

(From Schneider, K. M., Becker, J. M., and Krasna, I. H.: Neonatal neuroblastoma. Pediatrics 36:359, 1965. Reproduced by permission from Pediatrics.)

TABLE 95–4. Staging of Neuroblastoma

Stage I
Tumor confined to the organ or structure of origin.

Stage II
Tumor extending beyond the site of origin, not crossing the midline.

Stage III
Tumor extending beyond the midline. Lymph nodes may be involved.

Stage IV
Distant metastases to skeleton, bone marrow, soft tissue, or other organs

Stage IV-S
Patients who would be stage I or II but who have distant disease confined to the liver, skin, or bone marrow.

(From Evans, A. E., D'Angio, G. J., and Randolph, J.: A proposed staging system for children with neuroblastoma. Cancer 27:374, 1971.)

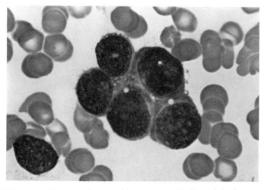

FIGURE 95–3. *Clump of neuroblastoma cells found in bone marrow aspiration.*

even without any treatment (Schwartz et al., 1974). Most patients, however, do not have Stage I or II tumors at initial diagnosis and are thus rarely curable. If unresectable disease is present, a biopsy from the most accessible site is obtained and chemotherapy is administered. If a significant response is demonstrated and no metastases are present, resection of all residual tumor may be an option (Smith et al., 1980). Even if the patient appears to have had a complete response to chemotherapy, surgery will often document residual microscopic tumor (Koop and Schnaufer, 1975).

The most effective chemotherapeutic agents are vincristine, doxorubicin, daunomycin, epipodophyllotoxin (VM-26), and cis-platinum, but despite inducing a high percentage of complete and partial responses, they have not affected long-term survival (Shafford et al., 1984). A recent approach to patients with recurrent disease is the use of supralethal chemotherapy and radiation, followed by bone marrow transplantation (August et al., 1984).

The most important prognostic factors in neuroblastoma are patient's age at diagnosis, tumor stage, and site of the primary lesion. Patients with supradiaphragmatic tumors located in the posterior mediastinum do better than patients with extensive intra-abdominal disease. Even with high-stage disease, newborns and infants fare better than older children with less disseminated disease. Two-year survival for infants diagnosed during the first year of life is 74 per cent. This decreases to 26 per cent during the 2nd year of life and to 12 per cent thereafter (Neifeld, 1988).

■ REFERENCES

August, C. S., Serota, F. T., Koch, P. A., et al.: Treatment of advanced neuroblastoma with supralethal chemotherapy, radiation, and allogeneic or autologous marrow reconstitution. J. Clin. Oncol. 2:609, 1984.

Beckwith, J. B., and Perrin, E. V.: In-situ neuroblastomas: A contribution to the natural history of neural crest tumors. Am. J. Pathol. 43:1089, 1963.

Bolande, R. P., Brough, A. J., and Izant, R. J., Jr.: Congenital mesoblastic nephroma of infancy: A report of eight cases and the relationship to Wilms tumor. Pediatrics 40:272, 1967.

Breslow, N. E., and Beckwith J. B.: Epidemiological features of Wilms tumor: Results of National Wilms Tumor Study. J. Natl. Cancer Inst. 68:429, 1982.

D'Angio, G. J., Evans, A., Breslow, N. E., et al.: The treatment of Wilms tumor. Results of the second National Wilms Tumor Study. Cancer 47:2302, 1981.

Evans, A. E., D'Angio, G. J., and Randolph, J.: A proposed staging system for children with neuroblastoma. Cancer 27:374, 1971.

Green, D. M.: The diagnosis and management of Wilms' tumor. Pediatr. Clin. North Am. 32:735, 1985.

Greenfield, L. J., and Shelley, W. M.: The spectrum of neurogenic tumors of the sympathetic nervous system: Maturation and adrenergic function. J. Nat. Cancer Inst. 35:215, 1965.

Grosfeld, J. L., and Baehner, R. L.: Neuroblastoma: An analysis of 160 cases. World J. Surg. 4:29, 1980.

Hann, H. L., Evans, A. E., Cohen, I. J., et al.: Biological differences between neuroblastoma stages IV-S and IV. Measurement of serum ferritin and E-rosette inhibition in 30 children. N. Engl. J. Med. 305:425, 1981.

Hann, H. L., Evans, A. E., Siegel, S. E., et al.: Prognostic importance of serum ferritin in patients with Stages II and IV neuroblastoma: The Children's Cancer Study Group experience. Cancer Res. 45:2843, 1985.

Howell, C. G., Othersen, H. B., Kiviat, N. B., et al.: Therapy and outcome in 51 children with mesoblastic nephroma: A report of the National Wilms' Tumor Study. J. Pediatr. Surg. 17:826, 1982.

Hrabovsky, E. E., Othersen, H. B., Jr., de Lorimier, A., et al.: Wilms' tumor in the neonate: A report from the National Wilms' Tumor Study. J. Pediatr. Surg. 21:385, 1986.

Koop, C. E., and Schnaufer, L.: The management of abdominal neuroblastoma. Cancer 35:905, 1975.

Koyle, M. A.: Neuroblastoma. In Rajfer, J. (Ed.): Urologic Endocrinology. Philadelphia, W. B. Saunders Company, 1986, pp. 106–111.

Koyle, M. A., and Ehrlich, R. M.: Wilms tumor in neonates and young infants: Current considerations and controversies. In King, L. R. (Ed.): Urologic Surgery in Neonates and Young Infants. Philadelphia, W. B. Saunders Company, 1988, p. 429.

Matsunaga, E.: Genetics of Wilms tumor. Hum. Genet. 57:231, 1981.

Mesrobian, H. -G.: J. Wilms' tumor: Past, present and future. J. Urol. 140:231, 1988.

Neifeld, J. P.: Neuroblastoma. In Broecker, B. H., and Klein, F. A. (Eds.): Pediatric Tumors of the Genitourinary Tract. New York, Alan R. Liss, 1988.

Pendergrass, T. W.: Congenital anomalies of children with Wilms tumor. Cancer 37:403, 1976.

Pilling, G. P.: Wilms' tumor in seven children with congenital aniridia. J. Pediatr. Surg. 10:87, 1975.

Punt, J., Pritchard, J., Pincott, J. R., et al.: Neuroblastoma: A review of 21 cases presenting with spinal cord compression. Cancer 45:3095, 1980.

Riccardi, V. M., Sujansky, E., Smith, A. C., et al.: Chromosomal imbalance in the aniridia—Wilms Tumor Association. interstitial deletion. Pediatrics 6:604, 1978.

Rosen, E. M., Cassady, J. R., Franz, C. N., et al.: Neuroblastoma: The Joint Center for Radiation Therapy/Dana-Farber Cancer Institute/Children's Hospital experience. J. Clin. Oncol. 2:719, 1984.

Schneider, K. M., Becker, J. M., and Krasna, I. H.: Neonatal neuroblastoma. Pediatrics 36:359, 1965.

Schwartz, A. D., Dadash-Zadeh, M., Lee, H., et al.: Spontaneous regression of disseminated neuroblastoma. J. Pediatr. 85:760, 1974.

Shafford, E. A., Rogers, D. W., and Pritchard, J.: Advanced neuroblastoma: Improved response rate using a multiagent regimen (OPEC) including sequential cisplatin and VM-26. J. Clin. Oncol. 2:742, 1984.

Smith, E. I., Krous, H. F., Tunnel, W. P., et al.: The impact of chemotherapy and radiation therapy on secondary operations for neuroblastoma. Am. Surg. 191:561, 1980.

Wilms, M.: Die Mischgeschwulste de Nieren. Leipzig, Arthur George, 1899, p. 1–90.

HYDRONEPHROSIS, MEGAURETER, AND OTHER ABNORMALITIES OF THE UPPER URINARY TRACT

96

Randal A. Aaberg, Sudhir K. Anand, and Martin A. Koyle

The upper urinary tract includes the kidneys, renal pelves, and ureters. In newborns and young infants, abnormalities of these structures often initially present with the recognition of a unilateral or bilateral abdominal mass(es). Various causes of unilateral and bilateral renal or pararenal masses are listed in Tables 96–1 and 96–2, respectively. Several of these disorders have been discussed in Chapters 93 to 95; the remaining are discussed here and in Chapter 101. One of the most common causes of abdominal mass in a newborn is hydronephrosis secondary to ureteropelvic junction obstruction. Hydronephrosis may also occur secondary to many other urinary lesions, as discussed later. Upper urinary tract disorders

TABLE 96–1. Etiology of a Unilateral Renal or Pararenal Mass

Hydronephrosis
    Ureteropelvic junction obstruction
    Ureterovesical junction obstruction
    Megaureter or megacalices (with or without reflux)

Cystic or Dysplastic Kidneys
    Multicystic kidney
    Other cystic disorders

Ectopic or Fused Kidneys
    Crossed fused renal ectopia
    Unilateral ectopic kidney
    Ectopic horseshoe kidney

Vascular Thrombosis
    Renal vein thrombosis
    Renal artery thrombosis

Renal Tumors
    Congenital mesoblastic nephroma
    Wilms tumor

Perirenal Masses
    Perirenal hematoma
    Perirenal abscess

Adrenal Mass
    Adrenal hematoma
    Neuroblastoma

may also present with urinary tract infection (UTI), renal failure, or electrolyte abnormalities, or they may be asymptomatic.

■ HYDRONEPHROSIS

Hydronephrosis denotes dilatation of the renal pelvis, usually associated with dilatation of the calyces. Hydroureteronephrosis can be subdivided into several categories on the basis of anatomic etiology (Table 96–3). Hydronephrosis confined to the kidney by an abnormality of the ureteropelvic junction is usually obstructive, although some patients with pelvocalyceal dilatation show no obstruction or dilatation of the ureter. Hydronephrosis accompanied by hydroureter is either a primary ureteral abnormality, such as obstruction, or an abnormality of the vesicoureteral junction leading to reflux. Lesions of the bladder, such as megacystis, or of the urinary outlet, such as urethral valves, can also result in hydronephrosis, as can extrinsic lesions, such as hydrometrocolpos or teratoma and other tumors. Identification and prompt diagnosis are of immense value, since the lesions are often treatable with at least some improvement. The infant

TABLE 96–2. Etiology of Bilateral Renal or Pararenal Masses

Bilateral Hydronephrosis
    Posterior urethral valve
    Bilateral uretropelvic junction obstruction
    Megacystis or megaureter (with or without reflux)

Cystic or Dysplastic Kidneys
    Autosomal recessive (infantile) polycystic kidneys
    Autosomal dominant (adult) polycystic kidneys
    Bilateral multicystic kidneys

Vascular Thrombosis
    Bilateral renal vein and/or inferior vena cava thrombosis
    Bilateral renal artery and/or aortic thrombosis

Tumors
    Bilateral congenital mesoblastic nephroma

TABLE 96–3. Hydroureteronephrosis in Newborns

AFFECTED NEWBORNS	CATEGORY	MALES	WITH FLANK OR SUPRAPUBIC MASS(ES)	WITH URINARY INFECTION OR SEPSIS	WITH IPSILATERAL OR CONTRALATERAL DYSPLASIA*	WITH OTHER URINARY STRUCTURAL ABNORMALITIES†	WITH EXTRAURINARY ANOMALIES
32	Ureteropelvic junction obstruction	18	26	2	7	9‡	6
27	Posterior urethral valves	27	12	2	0	2	6
20	Ectopic ureterocele	8	11	2	2	1§	3
18	Deficient abdominal musculature	18	4	3	6		6‖
11	Lower ureteral and ureterovesical obstruction	8	5	2	1	6	4
8	Infection without reflux or obstruction	6	1	8	1	3	5
7	Reflux without obstruction	4	2	2	2	2	3
7	Neurogenic hydronephrosis	2	1	0	0	0	0**
5	Bladder diverticulum or septation	4	3	0	1	2	2
4	Hydronephrosis of unknown cause	4	2	0	0	1	3
3	Obstruction of nonduplicated ectopic ureter	2	2	0	2	0	3
2	Simple ureterocele	1	2	0	1	0	0
2	Other urethral lesions	2	0	0	0	2	0
146							

*Probably an underestimate; does not include agenesis.
†Includes agenesis.
‡Does not include contralateral ureteropelvic obstruction.
§In addition to ipsilateral or bilateral duplication anomalies, which each of these children had.
‖In addition to undescended testicles and deficient musculature.
**Does not include myelomeningocele, which all these children had.
(From Lebowitz, R. L., and Griscom, N. T.: Neonatal hydronephrosis: 146 cases. Radiol. Clin. North Am. 15:49, 1977.)

kidney does not tolerate the destructive effects of obstruction well, especially when infection is added, as is frequently the case. Since urine is formed and excreted by the fetal kidney from the 12th week of gestation, the immature kidney has been exposed to abnormal drainage for months. It is not surprising, therefore, that considerable irreversible damage may be manifest at birth, and as discussed in Chapter 93, renal dysplasia may coexist with hydronephrosis. However, even significant renal insufficiency should not deter precise diagnosis and prompt therapy because of the remarkable capability of the immature kidney to hypertrophy after birth (Chevalier and Dahr, 1988).

CLINICAL PRESENTATION AND LABORATORY FINDINGS

Over half the infants present with one or more palpable abdominal masses, usually in the flank (see Table 96–3). In most series, hydronephrosis or hydroureteronephrosis is the most common reason for a neonatal abdominal mass, with multicystic dysplasia a close second (see Chapters 91 and 92). The mass, usually situated deep in the flank, is easily caught and rolled between the palpating hands and is firm, round, regular, and smooth. It is rarely tender and moves with respirations. Instances in which renal enlargement is extraordinarily advanced may manifest visible abdominal enlargement, with a fullness in one or both flanks. The larger ones transilluminate brightly. Although no other symptoms are evident in most, some infants may come to medical attention because of feeding problems, vomiting, failing to thrive, unexplained fevers, or urinary tract infection. In any newborn with sepsis, the possibility of a congenital urinary tract anomaly must be considered. More boys than girls are affected, except in instances of meningomyelocele and ectopic ureterocele.

Structural anomalies of the genitourinary tract other than hydronephrosis occur in approximately one-fourth of the patients, often on the contralateral side. Hydronephrosis sometimes exists with dysplasia of various types (see Chapter 93). Anomalies outside the urinary tract occur in approximately one-third of the patients and may be reason alone to suspect hydronephrosis (see Table 96–3). Such lesions include imperforate anus, congenital vertebral anomalies, malformed ears, facial skeletal anomalies, myelodysplasia, absent or deficient abdominal musculature, unexplained pneumothorax or pneumomediastinum, absence or dysplasia of the radius, hypoplasia of the bony pelvis, or severe hypospadias.

The urinalysis may be normal or may contain variable amounts of protein, white cells, and red blood cells. Blood urea nitrogen and serum creatinine may or may not be elevated, depending on the amount of functional renal tissue remaining.

Ultrasonography is the primary diagnostic tool utilized in making an initial distinction between hydronephrosis and multicystic kidney, polycystic kidney, a renal tumor, or other abdominal masses (Fig. 96–1). If hydronephrosis is suspected during an antenatal ultrasound, the diagnosis must be reconfirmed because up to 30 per cent of newborns with a prenatal diagnosis do not show hydronephrosis during the postnatal period (Clarke et al., 1979; Colodny, 1987).

Voiding cysturethrography (VCUG) is the next most useful test. If reflux is present, the ureter(s) and renal pelvis and calyces will be outlined on the affected side. If urethral obstruction (e.g., posterior urethral valves) is present, the anatomic site of obstruction will be visualized. Bladder dilatation, trabeculation, diverticuli, or ureteroceles may also be visualized. However, ureteroceles may sometimes be obscured by the density of the contrast material or collapsed by intravesicular pressure. Oblique

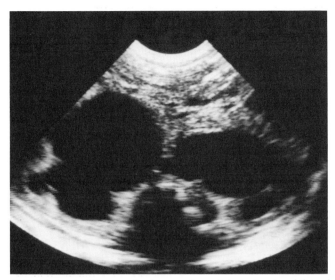

FIGURE 96–1. *Ultrasound of a newborn infant showing bilateral hydronephrosis.*

or lateral films during intravenous pyelography outline ureteroceles best.

Intravenous urography shows delayed excretion of contrast and in delayed films shows dilated pelvis and calyces. The calyces, when visualized, are full or have frankly globular cysts (Fig. 96–2). The ureter may not be visualized in ureteropelvic junction obstruction or may show dilatation and/or tortuousness in severe reflux, ureterovesical junction obstruction, and congenital megaureter. In those instances in which an umbilical artery catheter is present, an aortogram can be obtained as part of the intravenous pyelogram.

Radionuclide DTPA scan done in conjunction with furosemide-induced diuresis may help differentiate functional (nonobstructive) dilatation of calyces and/or renal pelvis from an obstructive hydronephrosis. Clearance of one-half ($T_{1/2}$) of the radioactivity in less than 10 minutes excludes obstruction, whereas a $T_{1/2}$ greater than 20 minutes confirms obstruction (Kass and Majd, 1985).

■ URETEROPELVIC JUNCTION OBSTRUCTION

Ureteropelvic junction (UPJ) obstruction is the most common cause of hydronephrosis in the newborn period. A palpable mass is present in 70 to 80 per cent of these infants. With increasing use of antenatal ultrasonography, the majority of patients are now discovered in utero (see Chapter 92). Other symptoms in the newborn may be urinary tract infection, urinary ascites, and hematuria. Males predominate and the disease is bilateral in 10 to 15 per cent of affected newborns. Anomalies in other parts of the genitourinary tract may occur with contralateral dysplasia, reflux, and agenesis.

Pathology. Most congenital UPJ obstructions are intrinsic in nature. Disoriented muscle fibers with excessive collagen deposition are seen microscopically in the area of the UPJ. Obstruction may result from failure of the ureter to recanalize during its embryologic development (Ruano-Gil et al., 1975). Other potentially obstructing intrinsic lesions at the UPJ include polyps, valves, persistent ureteral folds, and extrinsic fibrous bands. Although an accessory lower pole renal vessel crossing the ureter anteriorly is found in as many as 15 per cent of patients, it can rarely be incriminated as the cause of obstruction.

Diagnosis. The diagnostic work-up of a patient with UPJ obstruction and hydronephrosis is carried out as previously discussed. If an obstruction is not verifiable, the diagnosis may be confirmed noninvasively utilizing radionuclide scan or excretory urography with furosemide-induced diuresis. If the diagnosis is still equivocal, antegrade pyelography and pressure flow studies through a percutaneous catheter placed into the renal pelvis may be obtained. The antegrade pyelogram may help distinguish ureteropelvic obstruction from lower ureteral disease, and pressure flow studies may differentiate spurious from significant obstruction. With techniques currently available, it is rare that retrograde pyelography is required. In the evaluation of UPJ obstruction, a VCUG should also be performed because 10 per cent of such patients have coexisting ipsilateral reflux which may be high grade (Maizels et al., 1984).

Treatment and Prognosis. The treatment of UPJ obstruction requires operative correction of the anatomic defect. The timing of such surgery, neonatal versus delayed pyeloplasty is controversial (Elder and Duckett, 1987; Ransley and Manzoni, 1985). In the face of severe obstruction, obstruction of the only kidney, or other associated problems (e.g., infection or parental noncompliance), early surgery is clearly a logical choice. A dismembered pyeloplasty, in which the abnormal UPJ segment is excised and the ureter and renal pelvis are reanastomosed, is the most widely used and efficacious procedure. Using this technique, 95 per cent of the children (with no associated dysplasia) show improvement in renal function and radiologic appearance; however, residual dilatation of the renal pelvis often persists. With refinement of surgical and anesthetic techniques, earlier repair of UPJ obstruction has become possible, resulting in further improvement in renal function (King, 1988).

■ CONGENITAL MEGACALYCOSIS

Congenital megacalycosis is a disorder of the calices characterized by dilatation without obstruction. Since its description by Puigvert (1963), it has become recognized as a clinical and radiologic entity distinct from UPJ obstruction or hydronephrosis from other causes. Megacalices are covered by normal renal cortex. The medulla is underdeveloped, appearing as a thin crescent rather than as a full papilla. This results in flat calices that lack the normal cup shape, but they are not globular or convex as seen with obstruction or papillary necrosis.

Megacalycosis occurs predominantly in males and is usually asymptomatic. It may be detected during routine fetal ultrasonography and must be differentiated from congenital UPJ obstruction. It is usually detected during evaluation of a child with urinary tract infection (the two are not necessarily related). Some cases have been discovered in association with congenital malformations or hematuria. In adults, megacalices are usually discovered

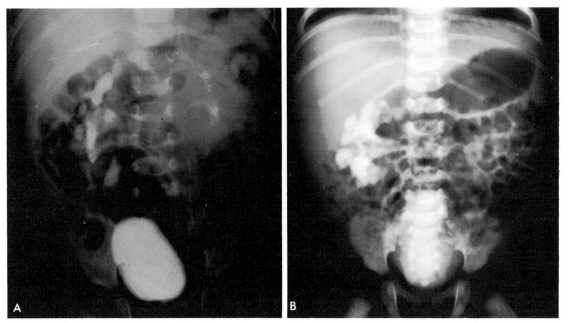

FIGURE 96–2. A, Intravenous pyelogram performed on the 5th day of life. The collecting system on the left appears to be perfectly normal. Calyces and pelvis of the right kidney are dilated, the calyces club-shaped. The right ureter cannot be seen. B, Later film shows that excretion from the right side is considerably slower than from the left. The enlargement and clubbing of calyces are more striking now, and the absence of right hydroureter strongly suggests obstruction of the ureteropelvic junction.

after the development of renal calculi. An associated megaureter is found in 10 to 20 per cent of patients (Gittes, 1984).

With intravenous pyelography, the calices appear dilated, but the infundibula, renal pelvis, and ureter are generally not enlarged. There is prompt excretion of contrast, and a renal scan shows normal function without obstruction. The number of calices may be increased (16 to 20) versus the normal 8 to 12, and the kidney may be enlarged. While the maximum concentrating ability of the kidney is often impaired, all other measures of renal function are normal.

It is important to recognize megacalycosis so that unnecessary surgery for nonexistent obstruction is avoided. Follow-up is important for infection during childhood and stone formation in adults (Gittes, 1984).

■ DUPLICATED URETERS

Duplication of the entire collecting system, including the renal pelvis may occur when two ureteral buds arise from the mesonephric duct. If a single ureteral bud forms and bifurcates early, a bifid renal pelvis with a single ureter results. Complete and partial duplications are frequently seen as normal variants in the urinary tract. Most are discovered as incidental findings without associated symptoms (Fig. 96–3). The reported incidence of various duplication anomalies ranges from 0.6 per cent in autopsy series to approximately 4 per cent in pyelogram reviews of patients with urinary symptoms. The most important aspects of ureteral duplication occur in the presence of a ureterocele or ectopic location or in association with obstruction or reflux (Kaplan and Packer, 1988).

Completely duplicated ureters are usually inserted in the normal location in the bladder; however, sometimes one or both may drain in abnormal or ectopic locations in the lower urinary tract. The ureter draining the upper

renal pole is usually the one that is ectopic, and it always enters distally in the lower urinary tract, crossing below the ureter from the lower renal pole. In the male, the upper pole ureter in a duplicated system might enter anywhere from the bladder trigone to the prostatic urethra, verumontanum, vas deferens, or seminal vesicle. Obstruction is characteristic of an ectopic ureter in the male and is visible as a nonfunctioning upper pole of the kidney on

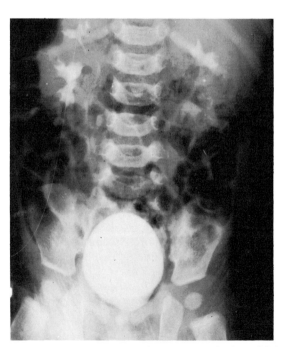

FIGURE 96–3. Excretory urogram demonstrating duplicated left collecting system with two ureters seen on that side. The right side was also duplicated but is not as clearly visible on the film. Despite this, the pelves are not enlarged, and all the calyces are delicate, sharply outlined, and concave. There is clearly no obstruction of urinary outflow at any point.

intravenous pyelography. In the female, the ectopic ureter may insert distal to the external urethral sphincter in the introitus causing urinary incontinence or infection (Stephens, 1983).

Ureteral duplications that are asymptomatic without obstruction, reflux, or ectopic insertion need no treatment. Surgical treatment is necessary for duplications associated with obstruction, ureterocele, or severe reflux (Caldamone, 1985).

▪ URETEROCELE

A ureterocele is a cystic dilatation of the terminal, intravesical ureter (Fig. 96–4). These can be insignificant in size or large enough to fill the bladder. Ureteroceles are classified as simple or ectopic. Simple ureteroceles are located within the bladder and are usually not associated with ureteral duplication. Ectopic ureteroceles are usually associated with the upper pole ureter in a duplicated system and may extend into the bladder neck, urethra, and introitus in the female (Fig. 96–5).

Children with ureteroceles usually present with urinary tract infections during the first few months of life. About 25 per cent of ureteroceles are discovered in newborns, and 90 per cent by 3 years of age (Caldamone, 1984; Gonzales and Deeter, 1988).

Ureteroceles are visualized best as filling defects in the bladder in lateral and oblique views during intravenous pyelography (IVP). In the presence of an ectopic ureterocele, IVP usually demonstrates an obstructed, dysplastic, or poorly functioning upper pole. Ultrasonography may demonstrate hydronephrosis of the upper pole as well as the ureterocele within the distended bladder. On a voiding

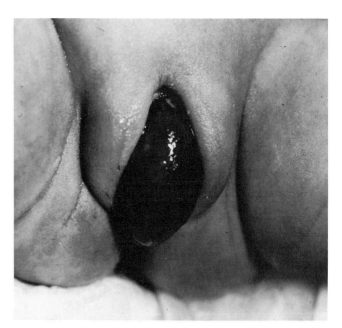

FIGURE 96–5. *Prolapsing ureterocele from the upper pole of a duplex system in a young girl who presented with fever and inability to void.*

cystourethrogram, ureteroceles usually appear as a characteristic filling defect, but careful observation is necessary because sometimes they are obscured by the density of contrast material. Vesicoureteral reflux is seen in 50 per cent of ipsilateral lower pole ureters in duplicated systems and in 15 per cent of contralateral ureters.

Surgical treatment is necessary for ureteroceles characterized by obstruction or infection or duplication anomalies (Caldamone, 1984). Early endoscopic surgery may be necessary for an obstructed, acutely septic patient (Tank, 1986). The usual therapy consists of excision of the obstructed pole (usually the upper pole) of the kidney together with its ureter to within a few centimeters of the bladder. The ureterocele is then left in situ, where it remains collapsed. With this approach, no additional surgery of the bladder is necessary, unless there is reflux of the other ipsilateral ureter. Salvage of the affected upper pole is rarely possible.

▪ MEGAURETER

Megaureter is a descriptive term applied to a ureter dilated out of proportion to the remainder of the urinary tract. When the dilatation is severe, the ureter appears tortuous. The dilatation of the ureter may be due to reflux or obstructions or idiopathic (nonrefluxing nonobstructed) (Table 96–4 and Fig. 96–6).

A refluxing megaureter may be due to primary vesicoureteral reflux or secondary reflux caused by high intravesical pressures from a neurogenic bladder or posterior urethral valve. An obstructed megaureter may be caused by extrinsic compression or an intrinsic aperistaltic segment located at the ureterovesical junction. Histologically, the aperistaltic segment contains fewer smooth muscle fibers and more connective tissue. The cause of nonrefluxing nonobstructed megaureter is unknown in most patients. In some it may be associated with diabetes insipidus or temporary ureteral atony secondary to severe urinary infection by endotoxins producing gram-negative bacteria

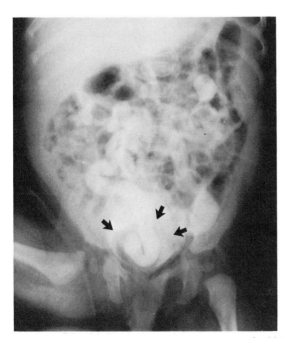

FIGURE 96–4. *Ureterocele: Excretory urogram in a 1-month-old infant who presented with fever and failure to thrive. Note the ureterocele (the nonfilling area marked by arrows) in the lower part of the bladder which also dips down in the region of urethra causing intermittent obstruction. In addition, bilateral hydronephrosis is present secondary to obstruction. The left side was not duplicated; however, the right side was duplicated and the ureterocele arose from the ureter draining a nonfunctional right upper pole.*

TABLE 96–4. International Classification of Megaureter

REFLUXING		OBSTRUCTED		NONREFLUXING NONOBSTRUCTED	
Primary	Secondary	Primary	Secondary	Primary	Secondary
Congenital (primary) reflux	High intravesical pressure from neurogenic bladder	Primary obstruction (adynamic distal segment)	Detrusor hypertrophy from neurogenic bladder	Idiopathic nonrefluxing nonobstructed	Diabetes insipidus
Megacystic mega-ureter syndrome	Posterior urethral valves	Ureterocele	Ureteral calculus		Infection
Ectopic ureter	Postoperative	Ectopic ureter	Extrinsic lesion	Residual dilatation following corrective surgery	
Prune-belly syndrome			Postoperative		

(Data from Smith et al.: Report of a working party to establish an international nomenclature for the large ureter. Birth Defects *13*(5):3, 1977.)

(Hanna, 1988; Pais and Retik, 1975). Most ureters that have been congenitally dilated or are dilated due to a prolonged obstruction may improve after relief of obstruction (or other corrective surgery); however, the majority have permanent residual dilatation.

Clinical presentation may include UTI (90 per cent), abdominal or flank pain (20 per cent), hematuria (10 per cent), or an abdominal mass (5 per cent) (Pfister and Hendren, 1978; McGowan et al., 1985). Some patients have also been diagnosed by prenatal ultrasonography (Hanna, 1988).

In primary obstructive megaureter the male-to-female ratio is approximately four to one, with the left ureter more commonly affected than the right. Bilateral obstructed megaureter may occur in 20 per cent of patients, and contralateral renal agenesis has been reported in 10 per cent of patients (King, 1985).

Megacystis megaureter is characterized by a large unob-

structed bladder and widely dilated, tortuous ureters. The bladder is thin-walled and shows no trabecuation or other evidence of obstruction and empties completely (in contrast to posterior urethral valves). Vesicoureteral reflux through gaping ureteral orifices is always present. The etiology of the disorder is unknown.

The treatment of a megaureter requires correction of all predisposing factors. Nonrefluxing nonobstructed ureters require no treatment, unless recurrent urinary tract infection develops, which would require low-dose antibiotic prophylaxis. There is controversy regarding management of refluxing megaureters because they are usually associated with grade 4 or 5 (International Reflux Grading Classification) (see Chapter 103). Although surgical correction of reflux has often been recommended, there is insufficient controlled data to substantiate its benefit. An obstructed megaureter requires surgical excision of the aperistaltic segment, ureteral tapering, and reimplantation. The indications for surgical intervention include demonstration of obstruction by furosemide-enhanced renogram, deterioration in renal function, increasing hydronephrosis, infection, pain, or formation of calculi (McGowan et al., 1985).

■ REFERENCES

Caldamone, A. A., Snyder, H. M., and Duckett, J. W.: Ureteroceles in children. Follow-up of management with upper tract approach. J. Urol. *131*:1130, 1984.

Caldamone, A. A.: Duplication anomalies of the upper tract in infants and children. Urol. Clin. North Am. *12*:75, 1985.

Chevalier, R. L., and El Dahr, S.: The case for early relief of obstruction in young infants. *In* King, L. R., (Ed.): Urologic Surgery in Neonates and Young Infants. Philadelphia, W. B. Saunders Company, 1988, p. 95.

Clarke, N. W., Gough, D. C. S., and Cohen, S. J.: Neonatal urological ultrasound. Diagnostic inaccuracies and pitfalls. Arch. Dis. Child. *64*:578, 1979.

Colodny, A. H.: Antenatal diagnosis and management of urinary abnormalities. Pediatr. Clin. North Am. *34*:1365, 1987.

Elder, J. S., and Duckett, J. W.: Perinatal urology. *In* Gillenwater, J. Y., Grayhack, J. T., Howard, S. S., and Duckett, J. W. (Eds.): Adult and Pediatric Urology. Chicago, Year Book Medical Publishers, 1987, p. 1554.

Gittes, R. F.: Congenital megacalices. *In* Stamey, T. A. (Ed.): Monographs in Urology. Princeton, N.J., Custom Publishing Services, 1984, p. 1.

Gonzales, E. T., and Deeter, R. M.: Management of ureteroceles in the newborn. *In* King, L. R. (Ed.): Urologic Surgery in Neonates and Young Infants. Philadelphia, W. B. Saunders Company, 1988, p. 204.

Hanna, M. K.: Megaureter. *In* King, L. R. (ed.): Urologic Surgery in Neonates and Young Infants. Philadelphia, W. B. Saunders Company, 1988, p. 160.

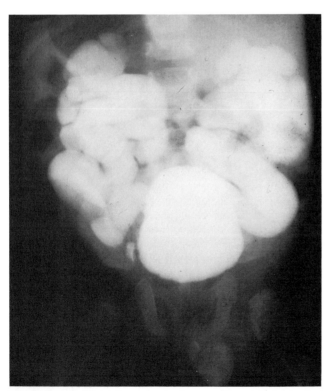

FIGURE 96–6. *Bilateral megaureter in a newborn infant who had bilateral grade 5 reflux (see Chapter 99). Note the dilated renal pelvis and clubbed calyces.*

Kaplan, G. W., and Packer, M. G.: Surgical management of ureteral duplications. Probl. Urol. *2*:69, 1988.

Kass, E. S., and Majd, M.: Evaluation and management of upper urinary tract obstruction in infancy and childhood. Urol. Clin. North Am. *12*:133, 1985.

King, L. R.: Ureter and ureterovesical junction. *In* Kelalis, P. P., King, L. R., and Belman, A. B. (Eds.): Clinical Pediatric Urology. Philadelphia, W. B. Saunders Company, 1985, p. 486.

King, L. R.: The case for repair of urologic obstructions in early infancy. Probl. Urol. *2*:18, 1988.

Lebowitz, R. L., and Griscom, N. T.: Neonatal hydronephrosis: 146 cases. Radiol. Clin. North Am. *15*:49, 1977.

McGowan, W., Snyder, H., and Duckett, J. W.: Current management of primary obstructive megaureter. J. Urol. *133*:115A, 1985.

Maizels, M., Smith, C. K., and Firlit, C. F.: Management of children with vesicoureteral reflux and ureteropelvic junction obstruction. J. Urol. *131*:722, 1984.

Pais, V. M., and Retik, A. B.: Reversible hydronephrosis in the neonate with urinary sepsis. N. Engl. J. Med. *292*:464, 1975.

Pfister, R. C., and Hendren, W. H.: Primary megaureter in children and adults. Clinical and pathological features of 150 ureters. Urology *12*:160, 1978.

Puigvert, A.: Megacalycosis: Diagnostico differential con la hidrocaliectasia. Med. Clin. *41*:294, 1963.

Ransley, P. G., and Manzoni, G. A.: Extended role of DTPA scan in assessing function and UPJ obstruction in neonate. Dialogues Pediatric Urol *8*:6, 1985.

Ruano-Gil, D., Coca-Payeras, A., and Tejedo-Mateu A.: Obstruction and normal recanalization of the ureter in the human embryo. Its relation to congenital ureteric obstruction. Eur. Urol. *1*:287, 1975.

Smith, E. D., Cussen, L. J., Glenn, J., et al.: Report of a working party to establish an international nomenclature for the large ureter. Birth Defects *13*(5):3, 1977.

Stephens, F. D.: Congenital Malformations of the Urinary Tract. New York, Praeger, 1983.

Tank, E. S.: Experience with endoscopic incision and open unroofing of ureteroceles. J. Urol. *136*:241, 1986.

DEVELOPMENTAL ABNORMALITIES OF THE LOWER URINARY TRACT

97

Randal A. Aaberg, Martin A. Koyle, and Sudhir K. Anand

■ PATENT URACHUS

The urachus is the obliterated remnant of the allantoic duct which connects the allantois to the urogenital sinus in the embryo. A patent urachus is due to the failure of the entire duct to obliterate. This is an extremely rare entity that results in drainage of urine through the umbilical area. A urachal sinus is more common—the bladder segment of the urachus does obliterate but the umbilical segment remains patent. Infection usually develops in the patent remnant, leading to an umbilical discharge. If only the bladder segment of the urachus fails to obliterate, a bladder diverticulum with the potential for urinary tract infection results. Finally, a urachal cyst develops when each end of the urachus obliterates, but the intervening area does not. This may cause a palpable intraumbilical mass which is often infected. The treatment of a urachal abnormality requires complete surgical excision. Persistent ductal tissue is at risk for the development of adenocarcinoma later in life.

■ EXSTROPHY OF BLADDER

Bladder exstrophy describes a condition in which the abdominal wall below the umbilicus is separated and replaced by an open bladder with everted bright red mucosa. The trigone and the ureteral orifices are exposed, and urine dribbles intermittently onto the mucosal surface. There is wide separation of the symphysis pubis.

In males, the penis is flattened, broad, and short. An opened fissure along the dorsal surface represents the epispadiac urethra (Fig. 97–1). The testes are usually undescended. In the female, the clitoris fails to fuse or is deeply fissured, and the labia are widely separated. The vagina may be absent, anteriorly dislocated, or replaced by a rectovaginal cloaca. Inguinal hernias are common (Fig. 97–2).

The incidence of classic bladder exstrophy is one in 30,000 births. It is twice as common in males as in females. Associated congenital anomalies, including those of the upper urinary tract, are unusual (Oesterling and Jeffs, 1987). Though rare, exstrophy is a striking abnormality, and it is important to reassure parents that the defect can be closed, genital function restored, and continence

achieved in the future. Multiple surgical procedures are generally necessary.

At birth, prompt evaluation and management by an experienced team is essential. The exposed mucosa is best covered with plastic (saran wrap) and the urine allowed to leak from underneath, keeping the mucosa warm and moist. Dressings invariably damage the mucosa, as may the umbilical clamp. The goals of management are to: (1) close the bladder, (2) reconstruct the external genitalia, (3) provide continence, and (4) correct vesicoureteral reflux. These goals are most successfully accomplished by staged surgical procedures.

Bladder closure is best performed within the first 48 hours postpartum. At this time, the anterior defect in the pelvic ring can usually be closed without iliac osteotomies. Successful initial closure is important to achieve sufficient bladder capacity in the future. A delay in closure necessitates iliac osteotomies to allow closure of the pelvic ring. If left exposed, the bladder mucosa may develop adenocarcinoma beyond the 3rd or 4th decades of life (Jordan and Gilbert, 1987).

Genital reconstruction in the male, by penile lengthening and tubularization of the urethra, is delayed until the 2nd year of life. This will lead to a greater bladder capacity and improved cosmetic results. In girls, the labia are approximated at a similar age. Finally, surgical therapy to correct incontinence and ureteral reflux is undertaken before school age, when continence becomes socially important. A bladder capacity of greater than 50 ml is required for bladder neck reconstruction without the need for bladder augmentation. With refinements in the use of artificial sphincters, bladder augmentation, and the acceptance of intermittent catheterization, previously "wet" exstrophy patients are now continent.

Newborns who undergo successful bladder closure have an excellent chance of healthy social adjustment, despite the need for subsequent reconstructive procedures. Mesrobian and co-workers (1988) reported complete or partial continence in 84 per cent of patients. Woodhouse and colleagues (1983) found 55 of 64 exstrophy patients to be normal and well-adjusted. Shapiro and associates (1984) reviewing 2500 exstrophy patients, identified 38 males who had fathered children, and 131 females who had given birth.

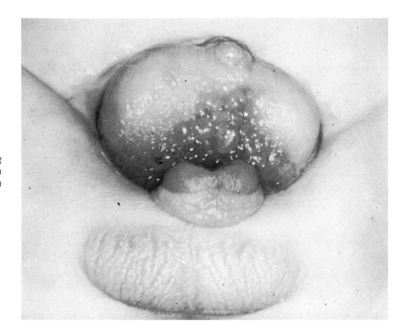

FIGURE 97–1. Exstrophy of bladder in a male. Bulging everted bladder lying below the umbilicus. Beneath this, a completely epispadiac penis is seen, and below that is a shallow, poorly developed scrotum devoid of testes.

■ CLOACAL EXSTROPHY

Cloacal exstrophy (vesicointestinal fissure) represents an extreme form of the exstrophy complex in which along with bladder exstrophy the urorectal septum fails to develop. This results in a large lower abdominal defect, an omphalocele, and an exposed midline strip of cecum representing the entire rudimentary hindgut, flanked by small hemibladders laterally and hemiphalluses caudally. Cloacal exstrophy is a more severe congenital anomaly than bladder exstrophy, and treatment is less successful. The incidence is approximately one in 250,000 live births or 8 infants per year in the United States. Most newborns with cloacal exstrophy should be raised as females because of the severe deformity and deficiency of the phallus. At birth the omphalocele is repaired, a terminal ileostomy or colostomy performed, and the bladder closed. A gonadectomy is done when sexual reassignment is indicated. Multiple surgeries, with varying degrees of success, are necessary to provide continence, resolve reflux, and reconstruct the vagina and external genitalia.

■ EPISPADIAS

Epispadias can exist in a wide spectrum ranging from its most severe form in association with exstrophy to its mildest form involving only the glans penis. Epispadias occurs in approximately one in 100,000 live births and is thus rarer alone than in combination with exstrophy. The male-to-female ratio is 3:1.

Anatomically, the glans penis is split dorsally and the urethra exposed anteriorly as a deep groove that may or may not extend proximally to the bladder neck. Incontinence occurs in 20 to 30 per cent of children with the most extensive defects. Continence may improve somewhat in males following puberty when the prostate enlarges. The goals of surgical correction are to provide a continent bladder neck, functional phallus in the male, and cosmetically acceptable appearance of the external genitalia. Surgery is best accomplished at approximately 2 years of age after toilet training and before beginning school.

■ PRUNE-BELLY SYNDROME

The prune-belly triad, or Eagle-Barrett syndrome, is characterized by a striking defect in which the abdominal wall is redundant, lax, and wrinkled due to the congenital absence of abdominal wall musculature (Fig. 97–3). The remainder of the triad includes undescended testes and urologic abnormalities (large hypotonic bladder, ureters, and collecting systems). The syndrome occurs in one of 30,000 live births, almost entirely males. Antenatally, oligohydramnios is common, but normal amounts of

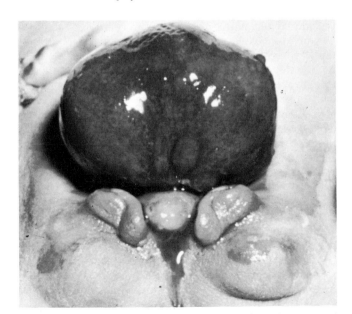

FIGURE 97–2. Exstrophy of a bladder in a female. Bulging everted bladder lies on the lower part of the abdomen. Below it, the three structures seen are a small, flattened clitoris in the midline and widely separated labia to either side. Below and lateral to these are the bulges of indirect inguinal hernias. (Courtesy of Dr. Martin A. Robbins of Baltimore.)

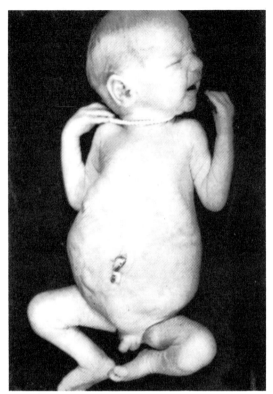

FIGURE 97–3. *Photograph at birth exhibits the characteristic appearance of the abdominal wall in an infant with prune belly syndrome. (From McGovern, J. M., and Marshall, V. F.: Surg. Gynecol. Obstet. 108:289, 1959. By permission of Surgery, Gynecology, and Obstetrics.)*

amniotic fluid may be detected. The etiology of this syndrome is unknown.

Abnormalities of the urinary tract are the major factors affecting prognosis. Megaureters are the most common abnormality, present in 80 per cent of the patients (see Chapter 96). Vesicoureteral reflux is present in 50 per cent of the patients. Histologically, the intrusion of fibrous tissue between sparse muscle layers is similar in the bladder and ureters. The prostatic urethra is also characteristically wide and elongated. Renal involvement ranges from agenesis or hypoplasia to normal function. Of patients affected, 20 per cent are stillborn or die in the neonatal period from renal failure or pulmonary hypoplasia associated with oligohydramnios. Another 30 per cent die of renal failure or urosepsis within the first 2 years of life. The remaining 50 per cent have various levels of renal function, often compatible with an extended life span (Greskovich and Muberg, 1988).

The newborn who has a lax abdominal wall and undescended testes must be assumed to have the prune-belly syndrome and undergo complete evaluation. A voiding cystourethrogram (VCUG), ultrasound, and a renal scan in combination with serum chemistries and urine culture provide an adequate assessment of the anatomy and function of the genitourinary tract.

In light of the broad clinical spectrum of patients with prune-belly syndrome, therapeutic options must be contemplated on a case-by-case basis. Most patients have only radiologic abnormalities but no obstruction and do not need any surgical intervention. Early surgical intervention, either by vesicostomy or ureterostomy, is reserved for infants with obstruction, decreasing renal function, or recurrent infection. Ureteral tapering and reduction cys-

toplasty are controversial aspects of treatment and are dependent on physician preference. Various abdominal wall plication techniques to improve cosmetic appearance are delayed until later childhood. Often an acceptable posture can be obtained with corsets alone.

The risk of malignancy in the undescended testes is the same in the prune-belly syndrome as in any other patient. While secondary sexual characteristics and libido are normal in these patients, there has never been reported fertility. Early orchidopexy (less than 6 months old) almost always allows the intra-abdominal testes to be brought into the scrotum without tension. Delayed surgery often necessitates a more extensive surgical technique to place the testes within the scrotum.

■ URETHRAL VALVES

Urethral valves have been described in both the anterior and posterior urethra. The disorder almost exclusively occurs in male patients. Anterior urethral valves are uncommon, but usually are obvious on VCUG by their association with a large ballooned proximal urethra. Posterior urethral valves (PUV) are the most common cause of bladder outlet obstruction in the male newborn. In 95 per cent of PUV patients, the obstruction is caused by enlarged and fused folds arising as a continuation of the caudal end of the verumontanum, extending distally to the external sphincter. These valves cause outflow obstruction only and allow easy retrograde catheterization.

In the past, half of the PUV patients presented during the neonatal period or during the first 6 months of life. Today, antenatal ultrasound allows diagnosis in many patients before clinical signs and symptoms are evident. Signs and symptoms include a palpable distended bladder, poor urinary stream, azotemia, and infection. A voiding cystourethrogram is diagnostic showing a dilated posterior urethra (Fig. 97–4), hypertrophy of the bladder neck, bladder trabeculation, and in 50 per cent of the patients, vesicoureteral reflux. Upper tract imaging is essential to evaluate the renal parenchyma and degree of hydroureteronephrosis. PUV is the second most common cause of hydronephrosis after ureteropelvic junction obstruction (see Table 96–3). Dysplastic kidneys are common along with significant dilatation of the upper urinary tract. Approximately one-third of PUV patients develop some degree of renal insufficiency (creatinine >2 mg/dl) (Hulbert and Duckett, 1988; Mininberg and Genvert, 1989). Patients who achieve a creatinine less than 1 mg/dl after treatment have the best prognosis for stable renal function.

Initial therapy is directed at the correction of any associated electrolyte abnormalities and infection. In the newborn, as a temporizing measure, a 5 French pediatric feeding tube is passed transurethrally to achieve urinary drainage. Once the overall medical condition is stabilized, the valves can be treated by endoscopic ablation. Premature or more seriously affected infants are initially treated with vesicostomy and delayed valve ablation. Great care must be taken not to damage and cause stricture of the delicate neonatal urethra. Spontaneous resolution of reflux occurs in at least 25 per cent of the patients once valve ablation has been performed. Children who continue to reflux are managed with prophylactic antibiotics and followed for breakthrough infections or

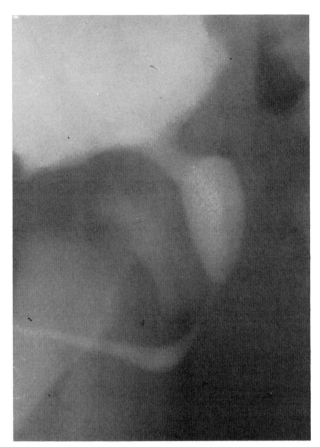

FIGURE 97–4. *Posterior urethral valve: Voiding cystourethrogram shows the greatly dilated posterior urethra, which then tapers to a fine point at the level of the external sphincter. Its caliber remains threadlike for several centimeters and then reverts to normal.*

poor renal growth. Early antireflux surgery is rarely required and may be difficult in the hypertrophied and trabeculated bladder. Some patients continue to have dilated upper urinary tracts after valve ablation without reflux. This phenomenon is termed the "valve bladder" (Mitchell, 1982) and is probably secondary to implantation of the ureters into the thick-walled, noncompliant, and hypertonic bladder. Bladder augmentation and ureteral reimplantation may be necessary in these patients (Glassberg, 1985).

■ MYELODYSPLASIA

Newborns with myelodysplasia (meningomyelocele) may have, or may develop, urologic abnormalities associated with their neurologic defect. Each child with spina bifida has a unique and evolving neurologic lesion, and thus, the neurovesical function can be expected to be similarly unique. On physical examination of the newborn,

one should include an assessment of renal size, bladder distention and emptying ability, abdominal muscle tone, anal sphincter tone, function of the sacral reflex arc (bulbocavernosus reflex), and function of the lower extremities. Serum chemistries and urinalysis are essential laboratory studies. Radiologic screening in the newborn is initially performed with ultrasonography. If the ultrasound is normal, further investigation is controversial. Some centers routinely perform urodynamic studies and a VCUG in all infants. In our institution, the renal ultrasound is repeated at 6-month intervals, and a urine culture and clinical evaluation are performed at 3-month intervals until 2 years of age. If abnormalities such as infection or upper tract damage are observed, a VCUG and urodynamic study are performed to guide diagnosis and treatment.

The urodynamic evaluation may be an important indicator of potential upper-tract deterioration. The most common abnormal findings are a hyper-reflexic detrusor muscle and detrusor sphincter dysfunction. Patients with intravesical leak pressures greater than 40 cm H_2O are at risk for reflux and progressive hydronephrosis. Clean intermittent catheterization is instituted in these infants as well as those with infections and hydronephrosis. Vesicostomy is reserved for those patients that do not respond to intermittent catheterization or for those who cannot comply. Anticholinergic medication is a helpful adjunct to intermittent catheterization. As the child grows, continence becomes an important factor, and bladder augmentation and/or the placement of an artificial urinary sphincter may be helpful in selected children (Kaplan, 1985).

■ REFERENCES

Glassberg, K. I.: Current issues regarding posterior urethral valves. Urologic Clinics North Am. *12*:175, 1985.

Greskovich, F. J., and Muberg, L. M.: The prune belly syndrome: A review of its etiology, defects, treatment, and prognosis. J. Urol. *140*:707, 1988.

Hulbert, W. C., and Duckett, J. W.: Current views on posterior urethral valves. Pediatr. Ann. *17*:31, 1988.

Jordan, G. H., and Gilbert, D. A.: Operative procedures for epispadias and exstrophy of the bladder. Semin. Urol. *5*:243, 1987.

Kaplan, W. E.: Management of myelomeningocele. Urol. Clin. North Am. *12*:93, 1985.

Mesrobian, H. G. J., Kelalis, P. P., and Kramer, S. A.: Long-term followup of 103 patients with bladder exstrophy. J. Urol. *139*:719, 1988.

Mininberg, D. T., and Genvert, H. P.: Posterior urethral valves: Role of temporary and permanent diversion. Urology *33*:205, 1989.

Mitchell, M. E.: Persistent ureteral dilatation following valve resection. Dial. Pediatr. Urol. *5*:8, 1982.

Oesterling, J. E., and Jeffs, R. D.: The importance of a successful initial bladder closure in the surgical management of classic bladder exstrophy: Analysis of 144 patients treated at the Johns Hopkins Hospital between 1975 and 1985. J. Urol. *137*:258, 1987.

Shapiro, E., Lepor, H., and Jeffs, R. D.: The inheritance of classical bladder exstrophy. J. Urol. *132*:308, 1984.

Woodhouse, C. R. J., Ransley, P. C., and Williams, D. I.: The exstrophy patient in adult life. Br. J. Urol. *55*:632, 1983.

ABNORMALITIES OF THE EXTERNAL GENITALIA

Martin A. Koyle and Sudhir K. Anand

▪ DISORDERS OF THE PENIS AND URETHRA

Most disorders of the penis and urethra are obvious on physical examination. Others are diagnosed following voiding or radiologic studies in infants who present with urinary symptoms.

HYPOSPADIAS

Phallic development is a hormone-dependent event that occurs between the 7th and 15th week of gestation. Hypospadias (from the Greek, *hypo*, below, and *spadon*, rent) is a congenital abnormality where there is incomplete formation of the anterior urethra. As a result, the urethral meatus may lie anywhere between the tip of the glans to as proximal a location as the perineum. The more proximal the location of the meatus, the more likely that there will be associated ventral curvature of the erect penis, due to the presence of chordee. Chordee is fibrotic tissue that replaces the normal Buck and dartos fascia.

Although there are many classifications of this deformity, Duckett (1987) has popularized the system of Barcat (1973) in which the location of the meatus, after the chordee has been released, defines the meatal location. Most (65 per cent) hypospadias are thus classified as being anterior, meaning that the urethra, after the release of chordee, lies in the glanular, coronal, or distal third of the shaft (anterior penile) of the penis. Fifteen per cent are midshaft hypospadias, and the remainder are considered posterior, where they lie in the posterior third of the shaft of the penis or proximal to such a location (Fig. 98–1).

The incidence of hypospadias is approximately one per 300 children (Sweet et al., 1974), and on occasion the disorder may be familial (Bauer et al., 1981), although the cause still remains unknown.

Especially in severe cases of hypospadias in which intersex is suspected, one must be observant for associated anomalies. When hypospadias is found in a situation of sexual ambiguity, mixed gonadal dysgenesis is the most common associated intersex state. Cryptorchidism and inguinal hernia are the most common abnormalities found in association with hypospadias. As the external genitalia are formed later in gestation than the upper urinary tract, the association between hypospadias and upper tract anomalies is infrequent.

The goal of hypospadias surgery is not only to recon-

struct a functional phallus, but to produce a cosmetically normal penis that is straight with a normal penile-scrotal junction, and with the meatus located at the tip of the glans. Preputial skin is the preferred tissue used in construction of a neourethra (urethroplasty). Thus, it is of paramount importance that neonatal circumcision not be performed on newborns with hypospadias. Today, most repairs can be done in one stage in an outpatient setting. The age of repair is progressively decreasing, with some surgeons performing such surgery as early as 3 to 6 months (Manley and Epstein, 1981).

Early complications associated with surgery include infection, skin loss, hemorrhage, and meatal stenosis. Later complications that may require secondary surgery include urethrocutaneous fistulas, residual chordee, stricture, diverticulum, the growth of hair in the urethra with subsequent stone formation and infection, and inflammation of the glans, including balanitis xerotica obliterans.

Occasionally, chordee or torsion anomalies of the penis can occur without hypospadias. Similar precautions regarding the foreskin should be exercised in such infants, as plastic repair of the phallus oftentimes with coincidental urethroplasty is necessary.

ABNORMALITIES OF PHALLIC NUMBER

Aphallia or duplication anomalies can occur and are obvious (Fig. 98–2). In patients without a penis, the scrotum is usually normally formed and located. Associated hydroceles, hernias, or cryptorchidism is common. The urethral meatus is usually just inside or anterior to the anus, often marked by a small skin tag. Various associated abnormalities are present, including imperforate anus, anal stricture, and rectovesical fistula. However, the infants are generally continent for urine. The lesion can be associated with renal dysplasia or agenesis or both. Endocrine and chromosomal abnormalities are not present. Other cosmetic deformities that may require reconstructive surgery include webbed penis and buried (concealed) penis.

URETHRAL ABNORMALITIES

Besides posterior urethral valves and hypospadias or epispadias, urethral abnormalities are unusual in newborns and young infants. Most diagnoses are made after symptomatic presentation that necessitate voiding studies and

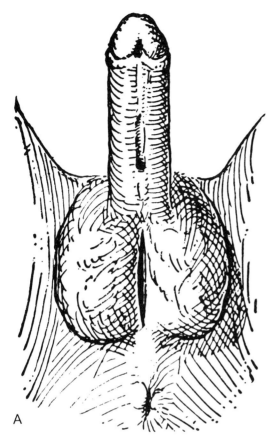

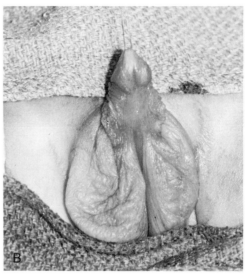

FIGURE 98–1. A, Hypospadias showing in one drawing a composite of all three locations. B, Posterior hypospadias with bifid scrotum.

A

B

FIGURE 98–2. Absence of external genitals, together with imperforate anus and facial characteristics suggestive of renal agenesis. (From Kirshbaum, J. D.: J. Pediatr. 37:102, 1950.)

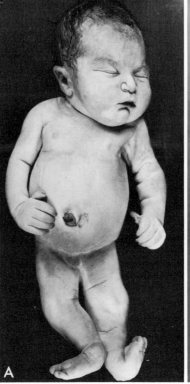

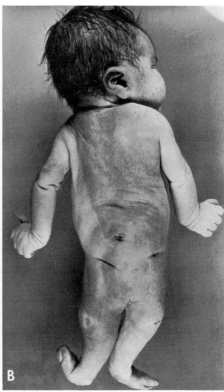

A

B

appropriate x-ray studies. These abnormalities include anterior urethral valves and diverticula, megalourethra, urethral duplications, congenital urethral stricture, urethral stenosis, and urethral prolapse (in girls).

MICROPENIS

Microphallus is defined as a normally formed phallus (that is, not a true hypospadias or a case of sexual ambiguity), with a length 2.5 standard deviations below the norm for that age. In the newborn, the stretched penis, when measured from the tip to the pubis, should be at least 2 cm. The etiology of this disorder is uncertain, but it is probably either due to insufficient androgen stimulation of the phallus itself, the inability of the phallus to respond to local androgens, or the failure of conversion of testosterone to the active dihydrotestosterone (5-alpha reductase deficiency). Lee and co-workers (1980) have shown that the majority of children who are diagnosed as having microphallus will be found to have a normal pituitary-testicular axis; that is, luteinizing hormone (LH) and follicle-stimulating hormone (FSH) will respond to exogenous gonadotropic-releasing hormone (Gn-RH), and testosterone will be secreted in a normal fashion in response to LH. In addition, the phallus itself may respond to exogenous testosterone. Thus, the defect appears to be primarily in the hypothalamus.

In the past, many of these children were raised as females; however, today the majority can be maintained as males with androgen stimulation beginning in the 1st year of life (Guthrie et al., 1973). It is preferable to administer androgens parenterally, rather than topically. Only in the rare child with obvious androgen insensitivity or in those who fail to respond to multiple courses of exogenous testosterone should gender conversion to female be considered.

■ INTERSEX

These problems are discussed in Chapter 108; therefore, only the surgical aspects are discussed here.

When evaluating the intersex patient, one must realize that the general appearance of the external genitalia is rarely of help in the differential diagnosis, except for the ability of the examiner to palpate gonads in the scrotum. Buccal smear, chromosome analysis, blood and urine steroids, and serum electrolytes are obtained. Cystovaginograms and pelvic ultrasonography are useful radiologic adjuncts in demonstrating the presence or absence of müllerian structures. Their presence excludes the male intersex states. Cystoscopy and vaginoscopy are often helpful in clarifying the anatomic appearance. In some circumstances, laparotomy with gonadal biopsy is necessary. After evaluation of all these studies, the team must reach an assignment of appropriate sex as early as possible. When coming to such a decision, one must take into account various factors, including gonadal potential, fertility, the potential success of corrective surgery, and the family's understanding and desires. Disorders of sexual differentiation can be broadly placed in one of the five following major classifications.

FEMALE PSEUDOHERMAPHRODITES

Female pseudohermaphrodites are 46,XX genetic females, who have been exposed to excessive androgen before the 12th week of gestation. Thus, internally they are female, but externally they demonstrate various degrees of masculinization. In the clinical examination of these newborns, it is important to verify the presence or absence of gonads because female pseudohermaphrodites never have palpable gonads. This group of disorders represents a true female with normal fertility potential, thus sex assignment should always be directed toward that goal.

Chromosome analysis is necessary, but definitive diagnosis relies on hormonal studies. Once diagnosed, treatment is instituted with exogenous hydrocortisone and, if necessary, mineralocorticoids. After stabilization, definitive surgical treatment can be appropriately implemented.

Exogenous maternal androgen administration also can lead to the development of female pseudohermaphrodites, but such occurrences are very uncommon (Wilkins, 1960).

MALE PSEUDOHERMAPHRODITES

Male pseudohermaphrotitism is a disorder in which the child is born with a Y chromosome but either has insufficient testosterone secretion due to a deficiency of 17α-hydroxylase, 17β-ketosteroid reductase, or other enzymes or fails to respond to the elaborated testosterone or to convert testosterone to dihydrotestosterone (5-alpha reductase deficiency). Most of these patients can be raised as males; however, if the phallus is very small, consideration should be given to raise them as females and appropriate plastic reconstruction performed.

TRUE HERMAPHRODITES

True hermaphrodites are born with both testicular and ovarian tissue internally, while externally, they present most often as males. However, they may present phenotypically anywhere within the spectrum of a feminine appearance to that of total masculinization. Over one-half of these patients are 46,XX karyotypes, but mosaics may be present as well. In this group, sex assignment is variable depending on appearance. Interestingly, instances of fertility both in children raised as males and as females have been documented. Gonadectomies and sexual reconstruction are planned after sex assignment has been made.

MIXED GONADAL DYSGENESIS

Mixed gonadal dysgenesis represents the second most common cause of intersexuality and occurs in patients with both a testes and a gonadal streak. The majority of these patients have been sex-assigned as females. XO/XY are the most common chromosome configurations identified in this group. It is the XO cell line that is responsible for the short stature often found in these patients, and they are always infertile. The gonads are prone to the development of gonadoblastoma, a potentially malignant tumor which may be associated with seminoma in later years.

PURE GONADAL DYSGENESIS

Phenotypically, patients with pure gonadal dysgenesis appear as normal females. They have bilateral streak gonads instead of ovaries. It is important in those who have a 46XY karyotype to realize that gonadoblastoma or dysgerminoma may develop in the streaks, and thus, gonadectomy is necessary in this subgroup.

■ DISORDERS OF THE TESTES AND SCROTUM

CRYPTORCHIDISM

Undescended testes, or cryptorchidism, is a common disorder of male children, with an incidence of approximately 1 per cent at age 1 year or older. The incidence of this problem at an earlier age is related primarily to the birth weight of the infant. In the full-term male with a birth weight over 2500 g, the incidence of cryptorchidism is approximately 3 per cent, while in the premature infant, it may approach as high as 30 per cent (Scorer and Farrington, 1971). In 10 per cent of the patients, this disorder is bilateral. In up to 4 per cent of the patients who present with unilateral or bilateral cryptorchidism, anorchidism is ultimately found.

The true defect responsible for testicular maldescent is unknown. About the 6th week of gestation, the primordial germ cells have made their way from the yolk sac to the genital ridges. During the 7th week of gestation, the gonads begin their differentiation. Mullerian inhibiting factor and testosterone are secreted by the 8th week of gestation. MIF, secreted by the Sertoli cells, is responsible for regression of the müllerian structures, whereas the testosterone secretion by the Leydig cells stimulates the development of the epididymis, vas deferens, and wolffian duct structures. By the time the external genitalia development is complete, that is, by the 15th week of gestation, the fetal testes still lie in an intra-abdominal position, proximal to the internal inguinal ring. Between the 12th week and 7th month of gestation, an outpouching of the peritoneum, called the processus vaginalis, reaches the scrotum. Between the 7th and 9th month, the testicles normally begin their descent into the scrotum. Thereafter, the processus vaginalis obliterates as the gubernaculum of the testes atrophies. Should the processus vaginalis not completely obliterate, a hernia or hydrocele develops.

Nonpalpable testes may be classified as cryptorchid, i.e., truly undescended, or retractile, i.e., a testis that has reached the scrotum but, for various reasons, spends periods of time outside the scrotum. In turn, the cryptorchid testes may be categorized as abdominal, canalicular, or ectopic. The practitioner must be able to differentiate the true cryptorchid testes from the much more common retractile testes. The latter is a benign condition that does not require surgical intervention. A true cryptorchid testis should have its position verified. Usually, those that have passed beyond the external ring and are ectopic reside in the superficial inguinal pouch and are palpable. The majority of nonpalpable testes are intracanalicular or intra-abdominal. When one finds bilateral nonpalpable testes, bilateral anorchia must be ruled out. The administration of human chorionic gonadotropin (HCG) (2000 units

intravenously three times per day) will not lead to a testosterone rise in the anorchid state, and usually in these patients, basal gonadotropin levels are extremely high. Many tests, including ultrasound, CT scanning, MRI, herniography, and testicular angiography have been utilized in an attempt to delineate the location of nonpalpable testes. None are satisfactory—the problems being that they are expensive and may require ionizing radiation and/or sedation or general anesthesia. More recently, laparoscopy has become popular as a helpful adjunct to locate the level of nonpalpable testes. The finding of blind-ending spermatic vessels is diagnostic of anorchia on that side. The surgeon should never, therefore, cease his exploration with the finding of a blind ending vas deferens alone. The termination of the spermatic vessels themselves must be identified. There is much theoretical and practical rationale for correcting the undescended testes, including cosmetic and psychological reasons. Undescended testes are more likely to develop malignancy and thus should be placed in a site where they can be easily palpated; in selected cases they should be removed. Ultrastructural changes have been described in the testes if orchidopexy is carried out after 2 years. It is unproved whether early orchidopexy at less than 1 year will improve fertility or ultimately reduce the incidence of malignancy. Moreover, all of these children have associated hernias and/or hydroceles and are more likely to have testes that may undergo torsion. The role of exogenous stimulation using HCG or Gn-RH analogues has not been substantiated in the treatment of true cryptorchidism (Koyle et al., 1988; Rajfer et al., 1986). There may be a place for the use of these substances, however, to identify the retractile testes in a child who presents with bilateral undescended testes.

SCROTAL SWELLINGS

The presence of acute scrotal swellings, particularly with an acute onset, often poses a diagnostic dilemma and may constitute a true emergency. Surgical exploration may be necessary, at times, to clarify the differential diagnosis.

ORCHITIS

Inflammation of the testes in the newborn infant is extremely rare. It may be part of generalized sepsis or occur secondary to associated epididymitis. It is treated with broad spectrum antibiotics.

TORSION OF THE SPERMATIC CORD AND TESTIS

Timely diagnosis is essential because torsion of the spermatic cord represents one of the few, true pediatric urological emergencies. Torsion can lead to irreversible damage of the testis within 6 hours of its occurrence.

Neonatal torsion, which is extravaginal torsion of the entire cord, usually presents as a painless swelling in a discolored hemiscrotum, as it most likely is a prenatal event. Testicular salvage is almost unheard of because this torsion probably occurs before birth during the process of testicular descent (usually beyond the seventh month of gestation). Regardless, it is the authors' preference to explore all such testes at birth. Also, despite controversy regarding this subject, we perform orchidectomy of the affected testes, with an orchidopexy on the contralateral side.

HERNIAS AND HYDROCELES

Both of these entities result from failure of obliteration of the processus vaginalis. Because of the risk of incarceration and strangulation, most hernias should be repaired soon after diagnosis. Controversy persists regarding the necessity of bilateral exploration in the event of clinical unilateral hernia. Suggestion of a strangulated hernia should lead to prompt admission, sedation, and placement of the child in a lateral decubitus position, with subsequent attempt at manual reduction. If successful, an elective hernia repair can follow a short time thereafter.

Virtually all hydroceles in infants are communicating. Even with the largest hydroceles, spontaneous closure of the processus is the rule in infants, rather than the exception. Thus, surgical repair should be reserved for the persistent hydrocele beyond the age of 1 year. After that age, the surgical repair of the congenital hydrocele should be performed through an inguinal incision so that high ligation of this sac, as with the hernia repair, can be accomplished.

TESTICULAR TUMORS

Although testicular tumors are rare causes of scrotal swelling in newborn boys, a high index of suspicion must be entertained. Ultrasonography is often useful in detailing the anatomy of these lesions. Most tumors of childhood occur around the 2nd birthday, with about 60 per cent being diagnosed before that date. Histologically, yolk sac tumors are the most common in this age group. They produce alpha-fetoprotein, and thus, this marker as well as the beta subunit of HCG should be measured prior to orchidectomy to follow such tumors. Radical inguinal orchidectomy remains the initial treatment of choice for all cases of yolk sac tumors. Further therapy, that is, retroperitoneal lymph node dissection versus radiation and chemotherapy, is controversial.

SCROTAL ABNORMALITIES

Bifid scrotum and transposition of the scrotum often are associated with intersex condition and severe hypospadias. These are dealt with at the time of definitive surgery of the associated defect.

■ FEMALE GENITAL ANOMALIES

HYDROCOLPOS AND HYDROMETROCOLPOS

Vaginal obstruction in the newborn is usually discovered by the presence of a lower abdominal mass, with associated urinary tract obstruction. Hydrocolpos is the distension of the vagina only, whereas hydrometrocolpos is the distension of both the vagina and uterus (Fig. 98–3). Vaginal obstruction in the newborn is most commonly due to imperforate hymen and less commonly to more proximal lesions, such as vaginal artresia or a high transverse vaginal septum. The secretions that accumulate in the distended organs are those from cervical glands that are secreted in response to maternal estrogens. An abdominal ultrasound usually reveals a large midline mass that displaces the bladder and the rectum, oftentimes with secondary obstruction. Usually, the imperforate hymen can be treated at birth, often without anesthetic. If vaginal atresia is responsible, an aggressive major surgical approach is indicated.

MAYER-ROKITANSKY-KÜSTER SYNDROME

Congenital vaginal agenesis, or the Mayer-Rokitansky-Küster syndrome, is due to a disorder of the vaginal plate or the uterovaginal canal. Although the disorder is present at birth, the diagnosis is rarely made in the newborn period. Typically, these patients are 46,XX females, who present with primary amenorrhea during adolescence. The patients have normal secondary sex characteristics. Indeed, a uterus, although it may be rudimentary, is present in most patients. At least one-third of such patients have associated upper urinary tract anomalies, so screening is warranted. The disorder may also occur as part of MURCS association (müllerian duct, renal, and cervical vertebral defects). The surgical treatment of vaginal agenesis is determined by the associated anatomy. If this syndrome

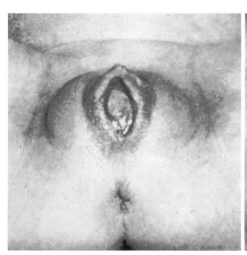
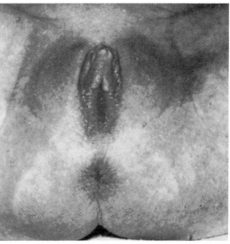

FIGURE 98–3. Hydrometrocolpos: A, *Appearance of external genitalia on admission. Note the bulge of the perineum, the widely spread labia, and the bulging hymen between. B, After spontaneous rupture of the hymen. The labia majora are still prominent from edema, but the perineal and hymeneal bulging has disappeared, and the labia minora have assumed a more normal approximation.*

is identified before puberty and a uterus is present, it is preferable to undertake vaginal reconstruction before the onset of menses.

OVARIAN CYSTS

Ovarian cysts in the newborn are uncommon. They usually present as an abdominal mass. They may be very large, often occupying the entire abdomen. Rupture or torsion may produce signs and symptoms of an acute abdomen. The cause of such cysts is unknown. Whenever possible, conservative surgical therapy that allows salvage of the ovary is indicated and should take place as soon as the diagnosis has been confirmed.

■ REFERENCES

Barcat, J.: Current concepts of treatment. *In* Horton, C. E. (Ed.): Plastic and Reconstructive Surgery of the Genital Area. Boston, Little, Brown & Co., 1973, p. 249.

Bauer, S. B., Retik, A. B., and Colodny, A. H.: Genetic aspects of hypospadias. Urol. Clin. North Am. *8*:559, 1981.

Donahoe, P. K.: The diagnosis and treatment of infants with intersex abnormalities. Pediatr. Clin. North Am. *34*:1333, 1987.

Duckett, J. W.: Hypospadias. *In* Gillenwater, J. Y., Grayhack, J. T.,

Howard, S. S., and Duckett, J. W. (Eds.): Adult and Pediatric Urology. Chicago, Year Book Medical Publishers, 1987, p. 1880.

Guthrie, R. D., Smith, D. W., and Graham, C. B.: Testosterone treatment for micropenis during childhood. J. Pediatr. *83*:247, 1973.

Koyle, M. A., Raffer, J., and Ehrlich, R. M.: The undescended testes. Pediatr. Ann. *17*:39, 1988.

Khuri, F. J., Hardy, B. E., and Churchill, B. M.: Urologic anomalies associated with hypospadias. Urol. Clin. North Am. *8*:565, 1981.

Lee, P. A., Mazur, T., Danish, R., et al.: Micropenis III—Primary hypogonadism, partial androgen insensitivity syndrome, and idiopathic disorders. Johns Hopkins Med. J. *146*:175, 1980.

Manley, C. B., and Epstein, E. S.: Early hypospadias repair. J. Urol. *125*:698, 1981.

Rajfer, J., Handlesman, D. J., Swerdloff, R. S., et al.: Hormonal therapy of cryptorchidism. N. Engl. J. Med. *314*:166, 1986.

Saenger, P., and Burk, R. D.: Probing the mysteries of maleness. J. Pediatr. *109*:831, 1986.

Scorer, C. G., and Farrington, G. H.: Congenital deformities of the testes and epididymus. New York, Appleton-Century-Crofts, 1971.

Snyder, H. M.: Management of ambiguous genitalia in the neonate. *In* King, L. R. (Ed.): Urologic Surgery in Neonates and Young Infants. Philadelphia, W. B. Saunders Company, 1988, p. 346.

Sweet, R. A., Schrott, H. G., Kurland, R., et al.: Study of the incidence of hypospadias in Rochester, Minnesota, 1940–70, and a case control comparison of possible etiologic factors. Mayo Clin. Proc. *49*:52, 1974.

Wilkins, L.: Masculinization of the female fetus due to the use of orally given progestins. J.A.M.A. *172*:1028, 1960.

NORMAL FORESKIN AND CIRCUMCISION 99

Sudhir K. Anand and Martin A. Koyle

The foreskin of newborn boys usually extends beyond the tip of glans penis and tapers down to a narrow point that, when spread, reveals an adequate preputial orifice. In most newborn boys the preputial opening is fairly tight and cannot be stretched to visualize the glans without tearing. Moreover, the inner layer of the foreskin is often adherent to the glans. Thus, in more than 95 per cent of newborn boys, the foreskin cannot be retracted. By six months of age the prepuce can be completely retracted in only 15 per cent of boys. By three years of age, 10 per cent still have unretractable foreskins (Gardner, 1949; Oster, 1968).

The epithelium covering the glans and inside of the prepuce gradually matures and separates. The shed epithelial cells produce a whitish cheesy material called "infant smegma" which naturally migrates to the tip of the foreskin, and is removed with routine cleaning (Duckett, 1988). No special care is required for the uncircumcised penis in infants and prepubertal boys except for external cleaning (Duckett, 1988; Osborn et al., 1981). During and after puberty, he should be taught to daily clean under the foreskin.

It is important that parents of uncircumcised boys be made aware that forcible attempts to retract the newborn foreskin should be avoided because it may lead to tearing, bleeding, secondary infection, scar formation, and later true phimosis.

■ CIRCUMCISION

Perhaps no topic in pediatric urology has stimulated more controversy than that of routine neonatal circumcision (Wallerstein, 1985). The American Academy of Pediatrics and the American College of Obstetricians and Gynecologists (1971, 1983) jointly have stated that there is no absolute medical indication for this procedure in the newborn. Despite these declarations circumcision continues to be widely practiced (70 to 85 per cent of newborn males) in the United States, primarily for religious, hygienic, and social reasons (Metcalf et al., 1983; Wiswell et al., 1987). With the advent of more lay groups and insurance companies advocating the abolishment of routine neonatal circumcision (Duckett, 1988), it appears that the number of newborns undergoing circumcision has declined (Wiswell et al., 1987).

Arguments supporting circumcision claim that this procedure may help to diminish the incidence of penile cancer, venereal diseases, balanoposthitis, balanitis, phimosis, and paraphimosis. Arguments against the procedure include that circumcision is a painful and unnatural procedure, that it is associated with medical complications

(discussed later), and that the disorders listed in the preceding sentence have many confounding factors involved with their pathogenesis.

Recently another provocative, but controversial, argument in support of circumcision has emerged. Wiswell and associates (1985, 1986, and 1989) and others (Ginsberg and McCracken, 1982) in retrospective analysis of urinary tract infections (UTI) in male infants reported a 10- to 20-fold higher incidence of UTI in uncircumcised versus circumcised infants. Wiswell's data show that incidence of UTI in uncircumcised and circumcised infant boys to be 4.1 per cent versus 0.21 per cent, respectively (among the 2502 male infants in the 1985 report), 1.12 per cent versus 0.11 per cent (among 217,116 male infants in the 1986 report), and 0.24 per cent versus 0.02 per cent (among 136,086 newborn boys in the 1989 report). Wiswell and associates (1988) also reported that circumcision reduced periurethral bacterial colonization, whereas the presence of foreskin is associated with increased colonization. They hypothesized that the latter finding may be pathogenetically related to the higher incidence of UTI. These studies have been criticized because they are retrospective, and they may also have methodologic flaws (American Academy of Pediatrics, 1989). Cunningham (1986) has suggested that the advice given to parents of uncircumcised infants by Wiswell and associates, to gently retract the foreskin and cleanse the exposed portion may have led to trauma of the prepuce and thereby opened a portal for entry of pathogenetic bacteria and contributed to increased UTI observed in the uncircumcised boys. Moreover, the opponents of circumcision have argued, that even if data for higher incidence of UTI in uncircumcised boys may be verified by prospective studies, the overall incidence of UTI is low, the disorder can be appropriately treated and this argument is not sufficient justification for routine circumcision. Lastly, Winberg and associates (1989) have proposed that

if increased incidence of UTI in uncircumcised newborns is confirmed, it will be the first instance of a potentially lethal disorder that would be preventable by removal of a normal body tissue. They further proposed that this would represent effects of one unphysiologic intervention counterbalancing effects of another unphysiologic state namely, colonization of newborns' gastrointestinal tract and genitalia in maternity and newborn units by E. coli strains of non-maternal origin against which the newborn has no passive immunity. As an alternative to circumcision, more natural colonization could be promoted by strict rooming-in of mother or baby or by active colonization of the baby with his mother's anaerobic gut flora.

The exact incidence of complications following circumcision is not known, but it is generally reported to be between 0.2 and 5.0 per cent (Ferguson et al., 1988; Kaplan, 1983; Wiswell and Geschke, 1989). Most complications are minor and include hemorrhage, local inflammation, or infection, urinary retention, and meatitis with secondary meatal stenosis. Meatitis is a superficial ulceration or redness of the meatal opening and is exclusively seen in the circumcised child. The disorder may be associated with some discharge, bleeding, crusting, and dysuria; however, it usually has no long-term consequences and is only rarely followed by meatal stenosis. The major complications following circumcision include removal of excessive foreskin leading to concealed penis, actual chordee, and even penile loss. Technical problems can also lead to the formation of skin bridges between glans and penile skin; unsuspected damage to the underlying urethra can lead to urethrocutaneous fistula (Kaplan, 1983; Duckett, 1988).

Infants undergoing circumcision without local anesthesia respond with pain and other transient physiologic and behavioral changes which usually last less than 24 hours (American Academy of Pediatrics, 1989; Anand and Hickey, 1987; Marshall et al., 1980). Dorsal penile nerve block may reduce pain and stress; however, experience with the procedure is limited, and it may cause local hematoma and skin necrosis (Kirya and Werthmann, 1978; Stang et al., 1988).

Costs of circumcision in the United States per year can be estimated conservatively by multiplying about 1 million circumcised males times $75 (physician's fee) times $150 (hospital fee) for a total of $225 million. This estimate ignores the added hospital days that accrue from the procedure.

In summary, as the American Academy of Pediatrics Task Force Report (1989) concluded, circumcision properly performed by experienced medical personnel is generally safe. The procedure has potential advantages and disadvantages, which should be explained to the parents. The emotional rhetoric both pro and con of circumcision can make counseling of parents difficult. When our advice has been sought, for routine circumcision, we have recommended against the procedure other than for religious reasons.

■ REFERENCES

American Academy of Pediatrics, Committee on Fetus and Newborn: Standards and Recommendations for Hospital Care of Newborn Infants, 5th ed. Evanston, Ill., American Academy of Pediatrics, 1971.

American Academy of Pediatrics, Committee on Fetus and Newborn: Guidelines for Perinatal Care, 1st ed. Evanston, Ill., American Academy of Pediatrics, 1983.

American Academy of Pediatrics: Report of the Task Force on Circumcision. Pediatrics 84:388, 1989.

Anand, K. J. S., and Hickey, P. R.: Pain and its effects in the human neonate and fetus. N. Engl. J. Med. 317:1321, 1987.

Cunningham, N.: Letter to the Editor. Pediatrics 77:267, 1986.

Duckett, J. W.: The neonatal circumcision debate. In King, L. R. (Ed.): Urologic Surgery in Neonates and Young Infants. Philadelphia, W. B. Saunders Company, 1988, p. 291.

Fergusson, D. M., Lawton, J. M., and Shannon, F. T.: Neonatal circumcision and penile problems: An 8 year longitudinal study. Pediatrics 81:537, 1988.

Gardner, D.: The fate of the foreskin. A study of circumcision. Br. Med. J. 2:1433, 1949.

Ginsberg, C. M., and McCracken, G. H.: Urinary tract infections in young infants. Pediatrics 89:409, 1982.

Kaplan, G. W.: Complications of circumcision. Urol. Clin. North Am. 10:543, 1983.

Kirya, C., Werthmann, M. W.: Neonatal circumcision and penile dorsal nerve block—a painless procedure. J. Pediatr. 92:998, 1978.

Marshall, R. E., Stratton, W. C., Moore, J. A., et al.: Circumcision: Effects upon newborn behavior. Infant Behav. Dev. 3:1, 1980.

Metcalf, T. J., Osborn, L. M., and Mariani, L. M.: Circumcision. A study of current practices. Clin. Pediatr. 22:575, 1983.

Osborn, L. M., Metcalf, T. J., and Mariani, E. M.: Hygienic care in uncircumcised infants. Pediatrics 67:365, 1981.

Oster, J.: Further fate of foreskin. Arch. Dis. Child. 43:200, 1968.

Stang, H. J., Cunnar, M. R., Snellman, L., et al.: Local anesthesia for neonatal circumcision: Effect on distress and cortisol response. J.A.M.A. 259:1507, 1988.

Wallerstein, E.: Circumcision: The uniquely American medical enigma. Urol. Clin. North Am. 12:1123, 1985.

Winberg, J., Bollgren, I., Gotheforsl, et al.: The foreskin: A mistake of nature? Lancet 1:598, 1989.

Wiswell, T. E., Smith, F. R., Bass, T. W., et al.: Decreased incidence of urinary tract infections in circumcised male infants. Pediatrics 75:901, 1985.

Wiswell, T. E., and Roscelli, J. D.: Corroborative evidence for the decreased incidence of urinary tract infection in circumcised male infants. Pediatrics 78:96, 1986.

Wiswell, T. E., Enzanaur, R. W., Holton, M. E., et al.: Declining frequency of circumcision: Implications for changes in the absolute incidence and male to female sex ratio of urinary tract infection in early infancy. Pediatrics 79:338, 1987.

Wiswell, T. E., Miller, G. M., Gelston, H. M., et al.: The effect of circumcision status on periurethral bacterial flora during the first year of life. J. Pediatr. 113:442, 1988.

Wiswell, T. E., and Geschke, D. W.: Risks from circumcision during the first month of life compared with those of uncircumcised boys. Pediatrics 83:1011, 1989.

ACUTE RENAL FAILURE*

Sudhir K. Anand

Acute renal failure (ARF) is defined as a sudden decrease in renal function resulting in progressive retention of nitrogenous waste products. Most newborns with ARF have associated reduced urine output, but in some, urine output may be normal. ARF may accompany a wide variety of medical disorders, especially in critically ill newborns. ARF has been classified into prerenal, intrinsic renal, and postrenal varieties, depending upon the site of lesion. This classification is useful because the diagnostic evaluation and treatment are quite different for these three types of ARF. Major causes of neonatal ARF are listed in Table 100–1.

The incidence of neonatal ARF depends upon the criteria used for defining ARF and the type of patients included in the study. Norman and Asadi (1979) observed that, of 314 newborns admitted to their neonatal intensive care units (most infants were transported from other hospitals), 72 had ARF; of these 72 per cent had prerenal and 28 per cent had intrinsic or obstructive ARF. Their criteria for defining ARF included BUN ≥20 mg/dl and urine output less than 1 ml/kg/hour. However, if the criteria for defining ARF are made more stringent, creatinine ≥1.8 mg/dl, BUN >25 mg/dl, and urine output ≤0.5 ml/kg/hour (<12 ml/kg/day), one would observe fewer newborns with ARF, but those identified would most likely have intrinsic ARF (Anand et al., 1978).

ARF should be anticipated in any newborn after difficult labor, hypoxia, hemorrhage, dehydration, or shock. ARF should be suspected if the newborn has anuria or a sustained decrease in urine output to <1 ml/kg/hour (after the first 48 hours), a BUN level >20 mg/dl, serum creatinine >1.0 mg/dl (1.5 mg/dl in the premature <34 weeks), and microscopic hematuria. Appropriate diagnostic evaluation and therapeutic intervention should be instituted to differentiate prerenal from intrinsic renal failure and, if possible, to prevent the development of intrinsic ARF.

■ PRERENAL ACUTE RENAL FAILURE

Prerenal ARF is the most common type of ARF in the newborn. Prerenal ARF results from hypoperfusion of an otherwise normal kidney, and the ARF is rapidly reversible early in the course of the disease if renal perfusion is improved. However, if hypoperfusion is prolonged, ischemic renal damage and intrinsic ARF will develop.

■ INTRINSIC ACUTE RENAL FAILURE

The term "intrinsic ARF" implies that renal failure is associated with damage to the kidneys. All disorders associated with prerenal disease may lead to intrinsic ARF if they produce prolonged renal ischemia. In most newborns with ARF, there is no preexisting renal disease. However, in a few patients with severe congenital anomalies, the renal impairment mimics that observed in acquired renal disorders (see Table 100–1).

Intrinsic acute renal failure usually occurs secondary to a major perinatal disorder, such as hyaline membrane disease, meconium aspiration, pneumonia, hemorrhage, dehydration, and sepsis or following surgery. Frequently, patients have more than one disorder (Anand et al., 1978; Chesney et al., 1975; Dauber et al., 1976; Norman and Asadi, 1979). Hypoxia, shock, and/or disseminated intravascular coagulation contribute to the development of acute renal failure in most of these conditions.

Renal artery or renal vein thrombosis are other important causes of acute renal failure in the newborn (Adelman, 1978, Anand et al., 1978; Arneil et al., 1973; Payne et al., 1989). (See Chapter 101.)

Indomethacin has emerged as an important cause of transient neonatal ARF when it has been used both postnatally for the closure of patent ductus arteriosus (Cifuentes et al., 1979; Halliday et al., 1979) and antenatally to prevent premature labor in the mother (Heijden et al., 1988). Aminoglycoside antibiotics are a frequent

---

TABLE 100–1. Etiology of Acute Renal Failure in Newborns

Prerenal Causes
1. Decreased plasma volume: hemorrhage, dehydration, or sepsis.
2. Other causes of renal hypoperfusion: hypoxia, shock respiratory distress syndrome, congestive heart failure, or hydrops fetalis.

Intrinsic Renal Causes
1. Prolonged ischemia: shock, hemorrhage, dehydration, sepsis, hypoxia, respiratory distress syndrome, meconium aspiration, complications of cardiac surgery, hydrops fetalis, or disseminated intravascular coagulation.
2. Vascular lesions: renal artery thrombosis or renal vein thrombosis.
3. Nephrotoxins: Indomethacin, aminoglycoside antibiotics, or radiologic contrast agents.
4. Pigments: myoglobinuria or hemoglobinuria.
5. Uric acid: hyperuricemia of the newborn.
6. Congential renal anomalies: bilateral agenesis, bilateral multicystic (dysplastic) kidneys, or infantile polycystic kidney disease.

Postrenal Causes
1. Bilateral obstruction: posterior urethral valves, trauma to urethra, imperforate prepuce, urethral diverticulum, neurogenic bladder, or bilateral ureteropelvic junction obstruction.
2. Obstruction of only functioning kidney: ureteropelvic junction obstruction.

---

*This chapter has been revised from a recent review by the author by permission of the publishers. Anand, S. K.: Acute renal failure in the newborn. Pediatr. Clin. North Am. 29:791, 1982.

cause of acute renal failure in adults. However, despite their widespread use in newborns, they have been reported to cause only a mild increase in serum creatinine but not ARF (Adelman et al., 1987; McCraken and Jones, 1970).

Large doses of contrast agents used in cardiac catheterization are occasionally associated with acute renal failure in newborns (Gruskin et al., 1970). However, nephrotoxicity resulting from use of contrast agents is relatively infrequent in newborns and children as compared with adults (Anderson and Shrier, 1980).

Rhabdomyolysis secondary to severe neonatal tissue trauma (e.g., due to difficult birth), hypoxia, intractable seizures, or sepsis may lead to myoglobinuria and ARF (Kojima et al., 1985). Severe acute hemolysis with hemoglobinuria may also lead to ARF. However, in newborns with hydrops fetalis who develop ARF, the renal failure probably results from heart failure and poor perfusion of the kidneys.

Infants born with agenesis, severe hypoplasia, or severe dysplasia of both kidneys, present with renal failure soon after birth. However, most newborns have characteristic clinical findings that suggest the underlying chronic nature of their illnesses.

Other causes of intrinsic acute renal failure in newborns are listed in Table 100–1. Renal parenchymal disorders (e.g., hemolytic uremic syndrome or rapidly progressive glomerulonephritis), which frequently cause acute renal failure in older infants and children, rarely cause ARF in newborns.

■ POSTRENAL ACUTE RENAL FAILURE

Postrenal ARF results from obstruction to the urinary flow after the urine has been formed by the kidneys. Therefore, the obstruction has to affect both kidneys unless the patient has only one functioning kidney. In the newborn, a variety of congenital urethral, bladder, or ureteral lesions can cause renal failure (see Table 100–1). The common disorders in this group include posterior urethral valves, a large ureterocele, and ureteropelvic junction obstruction. Because newborns with obstructive disorders may have associated renal dysplasia (Bernstein, 1971), kidney function may not return to normal even after the obstruction is relieved.

■ PATHOGENESIS OF ACUTE RENAL FAILURE

The pathogenesis of ARF in humans is controversial, and no single mechanism completely explains the sequence of events that lead to ARF (Epstein and Brown, 1988). Although intrinsic ARF secondary to renal hypoperfusion or nephrotoxins is often called acute tubular necrosis, in most humans, including newborns, the renal histology often shows minimal or no tubular necrosis (therefore, most authors prefer the term "ARF" rather than "acute tubular necrosis"). It is not understood why one finds a severe decrease or complete cessation of glomerular filtration even though renal blood perfusion often remains at 30 to 40 per cent of normal.

The four predominant hypotheses to explain the pathogenesis of ARF include: (1) tubular obstruction due to epithelial debris or cast formation (2) backleak of glomerular filtrate into the interstitium through the damaged epithelium, (3) renal vasoconstriction leading to hypoperfusion of the glomeruli and cortical and medullary tubules, and (4) decreased permeability of glomerular capillary due to altered filtration coefficient. In animals, depending upon the design of the experiment, one or more of these four mechanisms can be shown to contribute to the development of ARF and it is very likely that these mechanisms interact during development of ARF. Several renal hormonal and cellular-biochemical changes accompany ARF. Plasma and renal tissue renin and angiotensin II activity are often increased. The renal cellular energy production measured as high-energy phosphates (ATP and ADP) are decreased, and inorganic phosphates and AMP are increased. The decrease in cellular energy production probably leads to cell membrane damage and alterations in its functions leading to decreased sodium and potassium transport and cell swelling. Also, cell membrane damage leads to the entry of increased amounts of calcium into the cell. Further, cellular damage may occur from an increase in intracellular free radicals, e.g., superoxide, hydrogen peroxide. Sources of reviews on the pathogenesis of ARF are included in the reference list (Badr and Ichikawa, 1988; Brezis et al., 1986; Epstein and Brown, 1988; Gaudio and Siegel, 1987; Humes, 1986; Kon and Ichikawa, 1984; Myers and Moran, 1986).

The neonatal kidney may be especially vulnerable to the development of ARF because the renal blood flow is already proportionately less in newborns than in older children or adults (see Chapter 90). Hypoxemia, a common finding in newborn with respiratory distress syndrome further decreases renal blood flow and glomerular filtration rate both in newborns and animals (Torrado et al., 1974; Guignard et al., 1976; Weismann and Clark, 1981).

On pathological examination the kidneys of newborns dying with ARF may be normal or may show acute tubular necrosis, renal cortical and/or medullary necrosis, and renal artery or venous thrombosis, depending upon the etiology and severity of the ischemia (Anand et al., 1978; Bernstein and Meyer, 1961; Zuelzer et al., 1951).

■ CLINICAL AND LABORATORY FINDINGS

Clinical findings related specifically to acute renal failure include decreased urine output and edema if excessive fluids have been administered. With progression of renal failure, hyperkalemia with cardiac arrhythmia, hyperventilation due to acidosis, poor feeding, and vomiting due to uremia may be present. These findings are superimposed upon those of the primary condition.

Newborns with bilateral renal agenesis or severe dysplasia have features of Potter facies and usually have a history of oligohydramnios. Newborns with renal failure due to hydronephrosis, multicystic dysplastic kidneys, or infantile polycystic disease have large renal masses. Newborns with obstructive uropathy may have enlarged palpable bladder and occasionally urinary ascites.

Urine output <1 ml/kg/hour is the most important sign of acute renal failure. A small proportion of newborns may have normal or increased urine output, especially if acute renal failure is secondary to aminoglycoside antibiotics, nephrogenic diabetes insipidus, or partial urinary obstruction (Chevalier et al., 1984; Grylack et al., 1982). Most newborns with intrinsic acute renal failure have microscopic or gross hematuria (Anand et al., 1978; Norman and Asadi, 1979). The frequency of this finding appears to be higher than that observed in older children and adults with ARF. Mild proteinuria may accompany acute renal failure; however, severe proteinuria suggests congenital nephrotic syndrome as the primary disorder.

Newborns with acute renal failure whose fluid intake is not modified appropriately may develop edema, hyponatremia, congestive heart failure, or hypertension. Early in the course of acute renal failure, hypotension is a common finding; however, once the newborn's condition stabilizes, blood pressure is either normal or slightly increased. If the blood pressure is considerably increased, the possibility of renal cortical necrosis or renal artery thrombosis or embolism should be considered (Adelman, 1978; Anand et al., 1978).

The serum BUN and creatinine at birth reflect the values of the mother. Because during intrauterine life the excretory function of the body is performed predominantly by the placenta, renal function may be normal at birth even in infants with agenesis of the kidneys. With the onset of intrinsic renal failure, BUN rises daily by 5 to 20 mg/dl and serum creatinine by 0.5 to 1.0 mg/dl. Because most newborns with acute renal failure are quite sick, the usual symptoms of uremia, such as lethargy, nausea, and vomiting, are hard to discern. In those newborns whose condition stabilizes after recovery from the precipitating event, uremic symptoms sometimes become apparent.

Seizures are commonly observed in newborns with acute renal failure and may be due to hypoxia, intracranial hemorrhage, hypoglycemia, hypocalcemia, hypertension, uremia, or a combination of these factors.

■ DIFFERENTIAL DIAGNOSIS

The diagnostic work-up and treatment of acute renal failure must proceed simultaneously for successful management of the patient. After initial clinical evaluation, the following laboratory tests are advisable in all newborns suspected of having acute renal failure: complete blood count with red cell morphology and platelet count, prothrombin time, and partial thromboplastin time; serum sodium, potassium, bicarbonate, BUN, creatinine, uric acid, calcium, phosphorus, glucose, total protein, and albumin concentrations; blood pH, Po_2, and Pco_2; urinalysis and culture; and spot urinary sodium and creatinine concentration and osmolality. In addition, all infants should have an electrocardiogram and a chest roentgenogram.

The diagnosis of acute renal failure can be easily established by the above tests and the determination of urinary output over a timed interval. If the patient is not voiding frequently, it may be necessary to temporarily catheterize the bladder with a lubricated feeding tube (size 5 French in term infants) to obtain a urine specimen for analysis, to assess residual volume, to determine urinary flow rate, and to find out whether or not an outflow obstruction is present.

Tests that are helpful in differentiating prerenal from intrinsic renal failure include urinalysis, urine specific gravity or osmolality, urine to plasma creatinine ratio, urinary sodium concentration, fractional excretion of sodium (FENa) and renal failure index (RFI) (Table 100–2). It must be recognized that values for some of these tests in neonatal acute renal failure are different than those found in older children and adults with acute renal failure (Mathew et al., 1980; Miller et al., 1978). Moreover, these values are for full-term infants only and not the prematurely born. Normal premature infants may have FENa >5 per cent (Seigel and Oh, 1976), and no definite values for FENa in premature infants with ARF have been established.

Urinalysis in newborns with intrinsic acute renal failure often shows microscopic hematuria. Hematuria is rare in prerenal acute renal failure. The reliability of urinary osmolality and sodium concentration and urine to plasma creatinine ratio to differentiate intrinsic from prerenal ARF in the newborn is limited.

Mathew and associates (1980) in a prospective study of 42 newborns with oliguria, 22 with prerenal renal failure, 16 with intrinsic renal failure and 4 with probably early acute renal failure found that the most useful urinary indices to differentiate prerenal from intrinsic renal failure were FENa and the RFI (see Table 100–2). In prerenal disease the value of FENa was consistently <2.5 per cent (mean value, 0.9 per cent); in contrast, in intrinsic disease the values were >2.5 per cent (mean value, 4.2 per cent). The RFI in newborns with prerenal failure was consistently <3 (mean value, 1.3) versus >3 (mean value, 11.6) in intrinsic renal failure.

Although urinary indices are helpful in differentiating prerenal from intrinsic renal failure, a simple clinical method to distinguish between the two is a therapeutic trial of volume expansion (Norman and Asadi, 1979; Rahman et al., 1981). Once the possibility of congestive heart failure or urinary obstruction is excluded, 20 mg/kg of body weight of normal saline, 5 per cent albumin solution, or plasma (if appropriate) can be safely administered intravenously over 1 to 2 hours. If the oliguria persists at the end of this period, furosemide, 2 mg/kg of body weight, is administered. If no increase in urinary output is observed during the following hour, intrinsic renal failure should be suspected and fluid administration reduced. Some authors consider that furosemide may be

TABLE 100–2. Diagnostic Indices in Acute Renal Failure in the Term Infant

	PRERENAL	INTRINSIC
Urine osmolality (mOsm/kg of water)	>400	<400
Urinalysis	Normal	>5 RBC/HPF (often present)
Urine sodium (mEq/l)	31 ± 19	63 ± 35
U/P creatinine*	29 ± 16	10 ± 4
FENa per cent†	<2.5 (mean 0.9)	>2.5 (mean 4.2)
Renal failure index (RFI)‡	<3.0 (mean 1.3)	>3.0 (mean 11.6)

*U/P creatinine = Urinary to plasma creatinine ratio (both in mg/dl).

$$†FENa = \frac{UNa}{UCr} \times \frac{PCr}{PNa} \times 100$$

UNa = Urine sodium in mEq/l
UCr = Urine creatinine in mg/dl
PCr = Plasma creatinine in mg/dl
PNa = Plasma sodium in mEq/l

$$‡RFI = \frac{UNa}{UCr} \times PCr$$

(Data from Mathew and co-workers (1980) and the unpublished observations of the author.)

helpful in preventing imminent acute renal failure; however, its effectiveness has not been established. Once intrinsic renal failure has developed, repeated doses of furosemide are not beneficial and can cause toxicity, especially hearing loss.

The tests most helpful in differentiating intrinsic from postrenal renal failure in newborns are ultrasonography and voiding cystourethrography, respectively. Ultrasonography can identify the presence or absence of kidneys, enlarged kidneys, dilated pelvocalyceal system (i.e., hydronephrosis), or distended bladder. Voiding cystourethrography can identify posterior urethral valve or other lesions of the lower urinary tract that cause obstruction. Moreover, a large number of congenital renal anomalies that cause vesicoureteral reflux are identified by voiding cystourethrography. If the above tests are unable to identify a kidney, a diethylenetriamine pentaacedic acid (DTPA) and/or dimercaptosuccinic acid (DMSA) radionuclide scan may be helpful (see Chapter 91). Intravenous pyelography is occasionally helpful but is generally contraindicated because of the osmotic load of contrast agents. In selected patients who are suspected of having renal arterial or venous thrombosis, renal angiography through the umbilical or femoral vessels may establish the diagnosis, but in most other patients, angiography is contraindicated. The role of computed tomography of the abdomen and kidneys in newborns with acute renal failure is limited, and at present, this technique does not appear to offer any advantage over the other tests described above.

■ TREATMENT

Prompt recognition of prerenal ARF and its treatment with volume expanders may prevent the development of intrinsic renal failure. In newborns with obstructive uropathy, obstruction may be relieved by primary surgical repair, e.g., fulguration of posterior urethral valves, and if primary repair is not possible, a temporary drainage procedure may be employed (e.g., indwelling catheter, suprapubic drainage, or cutaneous ureterostomies) and definitive repair done later when the patient's condition stabilizes.

Currently, there is no treatment that enhances recovery of renal function in intrinsic renal failure. The therapeutic goal in these patients is to maintain normal body homeostasis as far as possible while awaiting spontaneous improvement.

Daily fluid intake is restricted to replacement of insensible water loss, urinary losses, and fluid losses from nonrenal sources, e.g., nasogastric drainage. From this value the amount of daily water produced by metabolism and tissue breakdown (about 10 to 20 ml/kg of body weight) is subtracted. Practically, for a full-term newborn, this means providing 30 ml of fluid per kilogram of body weight daily in addition to equal volume replacement of urinary and nonrenal losses. Premature infants have higher insensible fluid losses and, depending upon the gestation age and weight, may require 50 to 100 ml/kg daily for replacement of insensible losses.

Overhydration should be avoided in patients with acute renal failure because it can cause edema, congestive heart failure, hypertension, hyponatremia, encephalopathy, or seizures. To prevent its occurrence, fluid intake, fluid output, and body weight should be monitored at least every 12 hours. Newborns with acute renal failure should either maintain steady weight or lose about 1 to 2 per cent of body weight per day. Therefore, any infant with acute renal failure who gains weight is probably overhydrated.

Newborns with complete anuria require no electrolyte intake. Infants with urinary output should have daily measurement of urinary sodium losses, and the sodium losses should be replaced daily. Hyponatremia in acute renal failure is managed by fluid restriction and not by provision of extra sodium. Only if hyponatremia is symptomatic should hypertonic (3 per cent) sodium chloride or sodium bicarbonate (3 mEq/kg of body weight) be administered. (The dose is designed to raise serum sodium by 5 mEq/l using the formula: Dose of sodium in mEq = weight in kg × 5 × 0.6.)

Once acute renal failure is suspected, potassium intake from all sources should be restricted. By strict adherence to potassium restriction, severe hyperkalemia can be avoided in most cases in the early course of ARF. Serum potassium and electrocardiographic changes should be closely monitored. Electrocardiographic changes secondary to hyperkalemia include, in order of severity, tall peaked T waves, heart block with widening of QRS complex, arrhythmia, and cardiac arrest. Patients with mild hyperkalemia may be treated with ion exchange resins; sodium polystyrene sulfonate (Kayexalate) given by mouth or by retention enema (1 to 2 hours) is administered once every 4 to 6 hours. If the serum potassium has been rising slowly over several days and other indications for dialysis or hemofiltration exist (see later discussion), then dialysis or hemofiltration are more effective methods for treating hyperkalemia. If the newborn has severe hyperkalemia with venous serum potassium exceeding 7 mEq/l or if the electrocardiogram shows widening of the QRS complex and/or arrhythmias, treatment should begin immediately with intravenous calcium gluconate followed by sodium bicarbonate and glucose with insulin. The dose and duration of action of various drugs are summarized in Table 100–3. The doses described in Table 100–3 are based primarily on experience with treating older children and adults who have hyperkalemia but appear to be equally effective in newborns. Because the duration of action of these conservative measures is limited, arrangements should be made for peritoneal dialysis or hemofiltration (Lieberman et al., 1985; Ronco et al., 1986), if the infant is judged to be viable.

Hypertension in most newborns with acute renal failure is usually mild and the result of volume overload. Hypertension can be controlled in most cases by fluid restriction and administration of antihypertensive agents (see Chapter 102). Oral angiotensin-converting enzyme inhibitors (e.g., captopril and enalpril) should be used with caution because in newborns with renal artery thrombosis they may aggravate the renal failure (Adelman, 1988).

Mild metabolic acidosis is common in newborns and requires no treatment. If blood pH is <7.2 or serum bicarbonate concentration is <12 mEq/l, sodium bicarbonate may be administered, although caution is required to avoid hypertension, volume overload, hypertonicity, and intracerebral hemorrhage.

TABLE 100–3. Treatment of Hyperkalemia

DRUG	DOSE	ONSET OF ACTION	DURATION OF ACTION	REMARKS
Calcium gluconate 10 per cent solution	0.5–1.0 ml/kg	1–5 minutes	1/2–2 hours	Intravenously over 5–10 minutes while monitoring with electrocardiogram.
Sodium bicarbonate 3.75 per cent solution	2.0 mEq/kg	5–10 minutes	24 hours	Intravenously over 10–15 minutes.
Glucose 25 per cent solution	1–3 ml/kg/hour	1/2–1 hour	6–24 hours	Intravenously; do not exceed glucose 0.8 g/kg/hour.
Insulin	1 unit/5 g glucose			Always given with D_{25} glucose.
Sodium polystyrene sulfonate (Kayexalate) enema	1 g/kg dose in 4 ml/kg 10 per cent glucose	1–2 hours	4–6 hours	1 to 2 hours retention enema; may be repeated every 4–6 hours.
Peritoneal dialysis	–	2 + hours	As long as desired	Dialysis catheter may be inserted percutaneously or surgically.
Hemofiltration	–	2 + hours	As long as desired	Umbilical artery and vein may be used with minifilter.

In most newborns with acute renal failure hyperphosphatemia and hypocalcemia develop. In chronic cases, if serum phosphorus is more than 7.0 mg/dl, a formula containing low phosphorus, (e.g., breast milk, SMA, or PM 60:40) and phosphate binders, such as calcium carbonate mixed with formula, may be administered. If serum calcium concentration is <8.0 mg/dl, oral or intravenous calcium may be administered to prevent tetany. Hypocalcemia in acute renal failure tends to be refractory to treatment. Therefore, restoration of normal calcium values is often an unrealistic goal. Elemental calcium (50 to 100 mg/kg of body weight) is given daily in the form of calcium gluconate or calcium carbonate. Dihydrotachysterol (0.1 mg daily) or calciferol (1,25 $(OH)_2D_3$, 0.1 μg daily) may be administered to promote calcium absorption from the intestine. While these drugs are being used, the serum calcium level should be closely monitored to prevent hypercalcemia. Although administration of large doses of calcium and vitamin D analogues have the potential to cause soft tissue calcification, they are well tolerated by most newborns and young infants.

Adequate nutrition is important for newborns with acute renal failure because it prevents excessive tissue breakdown. If renal failure is of short duration (less than 3 or 4 days), most of the calories may be provided as carbohydrates. However, intake of fluid in most newborns with acute renal failure must be limited. Hence, the usual approach provides a limited amount of calories that are short of the daily requirements. In newborns in whom acute renal failure is expected to last beyond 3 or 4 days, all effort should be made to improve calorie intake. A limited amount of protein should also be provided to prevent or ameliorate negative nitrogen balance commonly present in patients with acute renal failure. If the newborn cannot take fluids orally, one should consider giving 25 or 50 per cent dextrose in water along with essential amino acids by an intravenous catheter placed in a large vein. The aim should be to provide 100 calories and 1 to 2 g of protein (amino acids) per kilogram of body weight, daily. For newborns who can tolerate oral fluids, low-protein formula (breast milk, PM 60:40, and SMA) should be administered along with high-caloric substances with low osmolality, e.g., polysaccharides (Polycose) and/or medium-chain triglycerides (MCT Oil), to provide sufficient calories. Although data for intensive nutrition of newborns with acute renal failure are limited, several pediatric nephrologists believe this approach prevents the severe malnutrition observed in many newborns with prolonged ARF.

Infection is an important cause of death in acute renal failure. Most newborns with acute renal failure are treated with antibiotics because of the primary condition. If possible, aminoglycoside antibiotics should be avoided, but if their use is considered imperative, doses should be modified. Proper serum levels of the antibiotic are the best guides for the dosage.

Many newborns with acute renal failure can be managed by the conservative techniques described above. However, if renal failure is prolonged beyond 7 or 10 days, or if complications arise, peritoneal dialysis should be performed. The usual indications for dialysis include volume overload, with potential for pulmonary edema or congestive heart failure, uncontrollable hyperkalemia or acidosis, and progressive uremia. Hemodialysis is technically quite difficult in the newborn and generally should be avoided. Dialysis should be performed while the newborn is stable, and one should not wait until the patient is moribund. The peritoneal catheter may be inserted percutaneously (Anand et al., 1975; Steel et al., 1987) or placed surgically (Tenckhoff catheter), especially if it is anticipated that peritoneal dialysis will be necessary for more than 2 or 3 days. Continuous arteriovenous hemofiltration through special blood filters utilizing the umbilical artery and vein as access sites is an efficient technique for removing extra fluid and sodium and may be used bedside in a regular neonatal intensive care as an alternative to peritoneal or hemodialysis. However, this technique is not efficient in removing urea or creatinine and cannot be used for a prolonged period due to clotting difficulties (Lieberman et al., 1985; Ronco et al., 1986).

CLINICAL COURSE

Oliguria in neonatal acute renal failure may last up to 3 weeks. Recovery is usually first indicated by an increase in urine output, which gradually increases over the next several days until it is normal or sometimes in the polyuric range. The BUN and serum creatinine may continue to rise during the first few days of diuresis before they start returning toward normal. During the diuresis, large quantities of sodium and potassium may be lost in the urine. Serum electrolytes should be closely monitored during this phase, and adequate replacement is needed to prevent hypokalemia and hyponatremia.

PROGNOSIS

The outcome in newborns with acute renal failure largely depends upon the primary condition, the extent of other organ damage, and the expertise in managing sick newborns. Chevalier and co-workers (1984) have demonstrated that newborns with nonoliguric renal failure have a better prognosis than those with oliguria. Patients with acute tubular necrosis usually have complete or nearly complete recovery. However, many newborns with renal cortical and/or medullary necrosis are left with renal functional impairment, chronic renal failure, and/or hypertension (Anand et al., 1978) (see Chapter 101).

■ REFERENCES

Adelman, R. D.: Neonatal hypertension. Pediatr. Clin North Am. 25:99, 1978.

Adelman, R. D.: The hypertensive neonate. Clin. Pernatol. 15:567, 1988.

Adelman, R. D., Wirth, R., and Rubio, T.: A controlled study of the nephrotoxicity of mezlocillin and amikacin in the neonate. Am. J. Dis. Child. 141:1175, 1987.

Anand, S. K.: Acute renal failure in the neonate. Pediatr. Clin. North Am. 29:791, 1982.

Anand, S. K., Northway, J. D., and Gresham, E.: Peritoneal dialysis catheter for newborn and small infants. J. Pediatr. 86:985, 1975.

Anand, S. K., Northway, J. D., and Crussi, F. G.: Acute renal failure in newborn infants. J. Pediatr. 92:985, 1978.

Anderson, R. J., and Shrier, R. W.: Clinical spectrum of oliguric and nonoliguric acute renal failure. In Brenner, B. M., and Stein, J. H. (Eds.): Acute renal failure. New York, Churchill Livingstone, 1980.

Arneil, G. C., MacDonald, A. M., Murphy, A. U., et al.: Renal vein thrombosis. Clin. Nephrol. 1:119, 1973.

Badr, K. F., and Ichikawa, I.: Prerenal failure: A deleterious shift from renal compensation to renal decompensation. N. Engl. J. Med. 319:623, 1988.

Bernstein, J.: The morphogenesis of renal parenchymal maldevelopment. Pediatr. Clin. North Am. 18:395, 1971.

Bernstein, J., and Meyer, R.: Congenital abnormalities of urinary system II. Renal cortical and medullary necrosis. J. Pediatr. 59:657, 1961.

Brezis, M., Rosen, S., and Epstein, F. H.: Acute renal failure. In Brenner, B. M., and Rector, F. C. (Eds.): The Kidney. Philadelphia, W. B. Saunders Company, 1986.

Chesney, R. W., Kaplan, B. S., Freedom, R. M., et al.: Acute renal failure: An important complication of cardiac surgery in infants. J. Pediatr. 87: 381, 1975.

Chevalier, R. L., Campbell, F., and Brenbridge, A. N.: Prognostic factors in neonatal acute renal failure. Pediatrics 74:265, 1984.

Cifuentes, R. F., Olley, P. M., Balfe, J. W., et al.: Indomethacin and renal function in premature infants with persistent patent ductus arteriousus. J. Pediatr. 95:583, 1979.

Dauber, I. M., Krauss, A. N., Symchych, P. S., et al.: Renal failure following perinatal anoxia. J. Pediatr. 88:851, 1976.

Epstein, F. H., and Brown, R. S.: Acute renal failure: A collection of paradoxes. Hosp. Prac. 23:171, 1988.

Gaudio, K., and Siegel, N. J.: Pathogenesis and treatment of acute renal failure. Pediatr. Clin. North Am. 34:771, 1987.

Gruskin, A. B., Oetliker, O. H., Wolfish, N. M., et al.: Effect of angiography on renal function and histology in infants and piglets. J. Pediatr. 76:41, 1970.

Grylack, L., Medani, C., Hultzen, C., et al.: Nonoliguric acute renal failure in the newborn. Am J. Dis. Child. 136:518, 1982.

Guignard, J. P., Torrado, A., Mazouni, S. M., et al.: Renal function in respiratory distress syndrome. J. Pediatr. 88:845, 1976.

Halliday, H. L, Hirata, T., and Brady J. P.: Indomethacin therapy for large patent ductus arteriosus in the very low birth weight infant: Results and complications. Pediatrics 64:154, 1979.

Heijden, A. J., Provoost, A. P., Nauta, A. J. et al.: Renal functional impairment in preterm neonates related to intrauterine indomethacin exposure. Pediatr. Res. 24:644, 1988.

Humes, H. D.: Role of calcium in the pathogenesis of acute renal failure. Am. J. Physiol. 250:F579, 1986.

Kojima, T., Kobayashi, T., Matsuzaki, S., et al.: Effects of perinatal asphyxia and myoglobinuria on development of acute neonatal renal failure. Arch. Dis. Child. 60:908, 1985.

Kon, V., and Ichikawa, I.: Research seminar: Physiology of acute renal failure. J. Pediatr. 105:351, 1984.

Lieberman, K., Nardi, L., and Bosch, J. P.: Treatment of acute renal failure in an infant using continuous arteriovenous hemofiltration. J. Pediatr. 106:646, 1985.

McCracken, G. H., and Jones, L. G.: Gentamicin in the neonatal period. Am J. Dis. Child. 120:524, 1970.

Mathew, O. P., Jones, A. S., James, E., et al.: Neonatal renal failure: Usefulness of diagnostic indices. Pediatrics 6557, 1980.

Miller, T. R., Anderson, R. J., Linas, S. L., et al.: Urinary diagnostic indices in acute renal failure. A prospective study. Ann. Intern. Med. 89:47, 1978.

Myers, B. D., and Moran, S. M.: Hemodynamically mediated acute renal failure. N. Engl. J. Med. 314:97, 1986.

Norman, M. E., and Asadi, F. K.: A prospective study of acute renal failure in the newborn infant. Pediatrics 63:475, 1979.

Payne, R. M., Martin, T. C., Bower, R. J.: Management and followup of arterial thrombosis in the neonatal period. J. Pediatr. 114:853, 1989.

Rahman, N., Boineau, F. G., and Lewy, J. E.: Renal failure in the perinatal period. Clin. Perinatol. 8:241, 1981.

Ronco, C., Brendolan, A., Bragantini, L., et al.: Treatment of acute renal failure in newborns by continuous arteriovenous hemofiltration. Kidney Int. 29:9008, 1986.

Siegel, S., and Oh, W.: Renal functional maturation in human infants. Acta Pediatr. Scand. 65:481, 1976.

Steel, B. T., Vigneux, A., Blatz, S., et al.: Acute peritoneal dialysis in infants weighing <1500 g. J. Pediatr. 110:126, 1987.

Torrado, A., Guignard, J. P., Predhom, L. S., et al.: Hypoxemia and renal function in newborns with respiratory distress syndrome. Helv. Pediatr. Acta 29:399, 1974.

Weismann, D. N., and Clark, W. R.: Postnatal age related renal responses to hypoxemia in lambs. Circ. Res. 49:1332, 1981.

Zuelzer, W. W., Charles, S., Kurnetz, R., et al.: Circulatory diseases of the kidneys in infancy and childhood. Am. J. Dis. Child. 81:1, 1951.

RENAL VASCULAR THROMBOSIS AND RENAL CORTICAL AND MEDULLARY NECROSIS

Sudhir K. Anand, Randal A. Aaberg, and Martin A. Koyle

Renal vascular occlusions in the newborn share the common pathogenic mechanism of altered parenchymal blood flow either through vasoconstriction or intravascular coagulation. In the past, renal venous thrombosis was more common. Renal arterial thrombosis, however, has become increasingly prevalent associated with the more frequent use of umbilical artery catheters.

The kidney in the newborn is particularly at risk for vascular thromboses. The vessels are small in caliber, the renal blood flow is relatively low, and the vascular resistance is comparatively high. Hypoxia and hypovolemia (hypotension) further decrease renal blood flow. There is a proportionately higher insensible water loss and fluid turnover, which places the infant at a greater risk for hypovolemia. The newborn is relatively more polycythemic. If an umbilical artery or venous catheter is used, it acts as a foreign body and can cause intimal damage (Chidi et al., 1983); both contribute to thrombus formation. Also, antithrombin III levels are low in the newborn, and the fibrinocytic system may be less mature (Corrigan, 1988). Therefore, small changes in any one or a combination of these factors provide ample opportunity for either arterial or venous thrombosis to occur.

The severity of renal parenchymal injury depends upon the extent of venous or arterial thrombosis. In limited disorders the thrombosis may be associated with focal zones of cortical or medullary necrosis or hemorrhagic infarction from which complete (or nearly complete) recovery of renal function may occur despite persistence of focal residual renal scarring. In more extensive thrombosis, complete renal infarction may occur with no or minimal recovery of renal function.

■ RENAL ARTERIAL THROMBOSIS

Thrombosis of the renal artery, until the advent of routine umbilical catheterization in critically ill newborns, was uncommon, and its incidence much less than renal venous thrombosis. During the past 20 years, however, concomitant with the use of umbilical artery catheters, the incidence of renal artery thrombosis has considerably increased and exceeds that of renal venous thrombosis. The disorder may be asymptomatic or lead to hypertension, renal failure, congestive heart failure, and death.

Incidence and Etiology. Zuelzer and co-workers in 1951 (in the preumbilical artery catheterization period) reported four cases of renal artery thrombosis among 2058 neonatal autopsies. The renal artery thrombosis in noncatheterized newborns was associated with hypovolemia, shock, coagulopathy, congestive heart failure, and embolism from ductus arteriosus (Adelman et al., 1978; Durante et al., 1976; Gross, 1945; Payne et al., 1989; Woodard et al., 1967).

Umbilical artery catheterization is frequently associated with thrombus formation in the aorta, renal, mesentric, and other arteries especially in critically ill infants who have medical problems similar to noncatheterized infants, as previously described (Caeton and Goetzman, 1985; Goetzman et al., 1975; Jackson et al., 1987; Neal et al., 1972; O'Neill et al., 1981; Schmidt and Zipurky, 1984; Stringel et al., 1985; Tyson et al., 1976; Wesstrom et al., 1979; Wiggers et al., 1970). The incidence of thrombosis in these studies is about 30 per cent (3 to 95 per cent), and a third to half of them have involvement of the renal artery. Also, the incidence of thrombus formation is probably related to the duration of catheterization (Jackson et al., 1987), the presence or absence of heparinization (Bosque and Weaver, 1986; Horgan et al., 1987; Rajani et al., 1979), the type of catheter used (Caeton and Goetzman, 1985; Jackson et al., 1987), and may be affected by the type of fluid infused. The level of the catheter tip placement (high or low) is controversial. Mokrohisky and associates (1978) reported increased complications with catheters placed low, whereas Adelman and co-workers (1978) have suggested that catheters placed in the thoracic aorta have more renal artery thrombosis. Most thrombi secondary to umbilical artery catheterization are asymptomatic; Goetzman and associates (1975) reported that in only 13 per cent of their patients the diagnosis was suspected prior to angiography. O'Neill and associates (1981) in their retrospective review of approximately 4000 cases of umbilical artery catheterization noted that only 1 per cent of the infants had severe symptomatic complications. Stringel and associates (1985) have reported an overall incidence of major complications to be 3 per cent.

Clinical Presentation and Laboratory Findings. The clinical findings caused by aortic and renal arterial thrombosis depend upon the severity of the thrombosis (Vailas et al., 1986). These findings are superimposed upon those of the primary disorder. Infants with minor thrombosis may be asymptomatic, or the only clinical manifestation may be systemic hypertension (Goetzman et al., 1975; Vailas et al., 1986). There is a controversy in the literature regarding the grading of the severity of thrombosis. Vailas and associates (1986) and others (Caplan et al., 1989) have used only clinical criteria to define minor, moderate, and major thrombosis. Minor thrombi are defined as thrombi with the presence of hypertension alone. Moderate thrombi are characterized by multiple signs including hypertension, congestive heart failure, decreased peripheral pulses, and gross or microscopic hematuria; however, urinary output remains normal, and the serum creatinine or BUN is either normal or minimally elevated. In cases with major thrombosis, these findings were exaggerated. Multiple organ failure, oliguria, and renal failure are present, and death invariably ensues in the neonatal period. Other authors (Krueger et al., 1985; Malin et al., 1985; Payne et al., 1989; and the present authors) would regard Vailas's classification as too rigid and have defined major aortic (or major branch) thrombosis by radiologic criteria (50 to 100 per cent occlusion); some of the patients with major thrombosis had oliguria and acute renal failure but still recovered. Patients with major thrombosis may develop complete renal infarction (Fig. 101–1). Depending upon what other major aortic branches are affected, bowel infarction due to mesenteric artery thrombosis, and gangrene of the skin, toes, or legs due to involvement of lower extremity arteries may occur. The kidney may be slightly enlarged due to renal artery thrombosis, but it is unusual to find a palpable renal mass in contrast to renal vein thrombosis (discussed later).

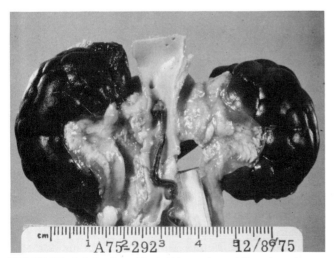

FIGURE 101–1. *Infarction of both kidneys due to bilateral renal artery thrombosis secondary to umbilical artery catheterization in a newborn. The thrombus in the aorta also occluded the mesenteric artery.*

Plain or Doppler ultrasonography can usually detect thrombi in the aorta and in the main renal arteries (Oppenheimer et al., 1982; Seibert et al., 1987). However, Vailas and associates (1986) have reported that in their series of 20 newborns with aortic thrombi (proven by aortography), ultrasonography failed to detect thrombi in four cases; three of these four had complete aortic obstruction on angiography. Radionuclide renography and scintigraphy using ^{99}Tc-DTPA may show reduced perfusion and renal function in the affected kidney(s). Aortography (usually via the umbilical artery catheter) remains the "gold standard" to document thrombus formation and should be performed in any case in which there is doubt about the diagnosis. Magnetic resonance imaging and computed tomography of the aorta and kidneys may also detect the thrombus but are usually not necessary.

Treatment. Aggressive medical support of the infant, including treatment of hypertension and renal failure is the most important part of the management. Meticulous attention should be paid to fluid and electrolyte balance, and if renal failure is severe, peritoneal dialysis or hemofiltration should be considered (see Chapter 100). Hypertension should be controlled with various antihypertensive medications (see Chapter 102). Captopril should be used with caution (if used at all) because it may worsen renal failure in infants with renal artery thrombosis (see Chapter 100).

There is considerable controversy regarding the use of heparin, thrombolytic treatment, or thrombectomy in the management of aortic and renal artery thrombosis (Schmidt and Andrew, 1988). The value of anticoagulation with heparin or thrombolytic treatment with urokinase or streptokinase has not been adequately established (Emani et al., 1987; Schmidt and Andrew, 1988) even though some reports support its use (Caplan et al., 1989; Flanigan et al., 1982). There is too little data to recommend the use of recently introduced tissue plasminogen activator (TPA). Some authors (Krueger et al., 1985; Payne et al., 1989) have recommended early surgical thrombectomy in cases with major aortic thrombosis and reported improved survival. Other authors (Malin et al., 1985) have reported equally good results in similar patients with aggressive medical treatment but without thrombectomy as anticoagulation. Schmidt and Andrew (1988) in their commentary on neonatal thrombotic disease concluded that the therapeutic efficacy of various currently used treatments is unproven and multicentered controlled clinical trials are needed to determine the risks and benefits of various treatment. In the interim they recommend appropriate supportive care.

Prognosis. Most patients with minor or moderate aortic or renal artery thrombi usually recover during the acute stage. However, mortality rates for major thrombosis with complete aortic occlusion are high (Caplan et al., 1989; Vailas et al., 1986). There is considerable long-term morbidity in newborns with moderate or major aortic or renal artery thrombosis who survive beyond the neonatal period. Hypertension often persists for weeks to months but usually becomes normal (without treatment) by 1 or 2 years of age (Adelman 1987; Caplan et al., 1989; Payne et al., 1989). Although most patients during the 1- to 6-

year follow-up have normal renal function, variable degrees of unilateral or bilateral renal atrophy (Figure 101–2) and renal insufficiency may develop in some survivors (Adelman, 1987; Payne et al., 1989).

■ RENAL VEIN THROMBOSIS

Renal vein thrombosis (RVT) may occur at any age, but the newborn is particularly prone to this accident. Over two-thirds of the patients with this disorder are under 1 month of age.

Incidence. The incidence of RVT in newborn nurseries is incompletely defined. Oppenheimer and Esterly (1965), in reviewing 4000 consecutive neonatal postmortem examinations, found 14 infants with renal vein thrombosis, five of whom were infants of diabetic mothers. The first diagnosis in vivo was made by Campbell and Matthews in 1942. Currently, renal venous thrombosis is recognized during life with increasing frequency. Nevertheless, most estimates of frequency are still based on postmortem examinations. Current estimates vary between 1.9 and 2.7 per cent of neonatal deaths (Arneil et al., 1973). Among surviving newborns the incidence is certainly much lower. In all series, more males than females are affected, and the ratio of may be as high as 2:1.

Etiology. Renal vein thrombosis is usually divided into primary and secondary forms, the latter resulting from extension of the thrombus from the vena cava. The primary form, in which thrombosis originates in the smaller intrarenal veins is the predominant form in the newborn. The most important predisposing factor is hypovolemia due to dehydration and other causes (Arneil et al., 1973; Clatworthy et al., 1953). In most instances, the thrombus probably starts in the small intrarenal veins due to venous stasis, subsequently spreading distally to involve the renal

cortex or medulla and simultaneously extending into larger veins (Arneil et al., 1973). In the secondary form, which is rare in the newborn and more common in adults, a thrombus in a main vein extends distally into the kidney.

Other factors contributing to venous stasis include hypotension, low renal plasma flow, polycythemia, anoxia, septicemia, cyanotic congenital heart disease, congenital renal anomalies, and severe pyelonephritis. Angiocardiography in infants with congenital heart lesions, possibly related to hyperosmolality, has also been implicated as a contributing factor. Thrombosis also has been reported in association with maternal diabetes mellitus or prediabetes (Avery et al., 1957; Oppenheimer and Esterly, 1965). This association, however, has not been as common in more recent years (Arneil et al., 1973). Injury from a severely traumatic or breech delivery has also been implicated. In many cases, however, no predisposing disorder has been discovered. There is clear evidence that the lesion can occasionally occur prenatally (Evans et al., 1981). In this situation, calcification of the kidney can be detected in utero or during the first weeks of life.

Clinical Presentation and Laboratory Findings. The characteristic presentation of renal vein thrombosis is the sudden enlargement of one kidney in association with a sudden deterioration of the infant's clinical status accompanied by gross hematuria, metabolic acidosis, tachypnea, and pallor. This usually occurs during the course of a complex illness or severe dehydration or several days after a traumatic delivery. A history of maternal diabetes, trauma, congenital cyanotic heart disease, recent arteriography, gastroenteritis, asphyxia, shock, or sepsis may be obtained. Renal vein thrombosis often affects both kidneys, but the involvement is usually asymmetric with one kidney more affected than the other. A unilaterally (or bilaterally) enlarged and firm kidney(s) is present in 60 per cent of the patients, and vomiting, abdominal distension, shock, and fever may appear along with enlargement. The blood pressure is usually normal or low, although hypertension can be present at levels generally not as severe as that seen with renal arterial thrombosis. Anuria or oliguria is present in 30 per cent of the cases, but edema is usually absent.

Gross hematuria is frequently present and may be the first sign. However, some cases have microscopic hematuria, and in other cases, hematuria may be absent entirely. The urine may also show increased protein and white cells. Azotemia is usual, and metabolic acidosis is present in half the infants. The serum sodium concentrations are variable, while the serum potassium level may be elevated.

Most infants have thrombocytopenia (90 per cent) and microangiopathic hemolytic anemia. Prothrombin time and partial thromboplastin time may be prolonged, and alterations in several coagulation factors may be present.

RVT must be differentiated from renal artery thrombosis and hemolytic uremic syndrome. Renal artery thrombosis generally occurs secondary to umbilical artery catheterization; the hypertension is usually more severe; and renal enlargement, if present, is lesser in magnitude. Hemolytic uremic syndrome is unusual in the newborn and does not cause renal enlargement; however, hematuria, anemia, thrombocytopenia, and renal insufficiency are similar to RVT.

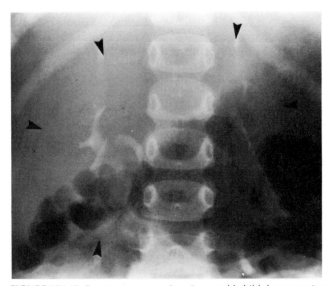

FIGURE 101–2. Excretory urogram in a 2-year-old child demonstrating marked atrophy of left kidney (the arrows outline upper, lateral, and lower borders of both kidneys). The patient as a newborn developed severe dehydration and fever, followed by left renal artery thrombosis, hypertension, and congestive heart failure. The hypertension initially required drug treatment, but by 1 year of age, blood pressure remained normal without medication.

Ultrasonography is the most useful initial diagnostic step and shows renal enlargement, loss of distinct corticomedullary junction and distorted echoes suggestive of areas of necrosis or hemorrhage within the parenchyma. Inferior vena cava thrombosis, if present, may be demonstrable by ultrasonography. A renal scan will demonstrate the degree of functional impairment. Excretory urography is not helpful in the presence of poor renal function, and the intravenous contrast medium may be harmful (Gilbert et al., 1970). If doubt persists, inferior vena cavagram and renal venogram may help establish the diagnosis.

Treatment. There is considerable controversy about the optimal treatment for RVT (Schmidt and Andrew, 1988) similar to that for renal artery thrombosis. All authors, however, agree that because most newborns with RVT are critically ill, the initial management should be supportive to correct hypovolemia, shock, hypoxia, acidosis, and hyperkalemia. If renal failure is severe, peritoneal dialysis or hemofiltration should be considered.

In the past, immediate nephrectomy or thrombectomy was considered the ideal treatment (Clatworthy et al., 1953). However, experience has clearly demonstrated that emergency surgery is rarely (if ever) indicated. Besides, the thrombosis usually begins in the small vessels of the kidney, making thrombectomy of little consequence to the kidney. Since the extent of kidney recovery is not predictable, emergency nephrectomy would also eliminate any chance of renal recuperation.

Belman and associates (1970) have demonstrated the effectiveness of medical treatment for unilateral renal vein thrombosis. Six of the seven infants they treated survived, and in only one of the survivors was the kidney found to be atrophic. Duncan and co-workers (1977), who used supportive therapy alone, avoiding the administration of anticoagulants, also reported encouraging results. Bilateral thrombosis is much more serious. Many have thrombosis of the vena cava as well. However, recent reports of recovery with conservative management and peritoneal dialysis are encouraging even in this serious state.

When there is evidence of continuing intravascular coagulation, such as worsening thrombocytopenia and decreasing fibrinogen and other clotting factors, or when there is bilateral disease with inferior vena cava thrombosis, heparin therapy along with infusion of fresh frozen plasma should be considered on an individual basis. The efficacy of heparin, however, has not been established (Schmidt and Andrew, 1988), and heparin may be associated with an increased risk of intraventricular hemorrhage in the premature (Lesko et al., 1986). A few infants have received urokinase or streptokinase (Gonzalez et al., 1982); however, no controlled studies have been done with their use or tissue plasminogen activator to recommend their routine use in the treatment of RVT.

Prognosis. Mortality rates as high as 60 per cent have been reported in the past. With improvements in management, the mortality rate has been reduced to less than 15 per cent (Schmidt and Zipurky, 1984; Schmidt and Andrew, 1988). The outcome during the acute stage to a large extent depends upon the severity of the underlying primary medical condition and not renal damage. Newborns with bilateral disease and inferior vena cava thrombosis generally do worse than infants with unilateral disease.

The affected kidney(s) may completely recover function; however, depending upon the severity of involvement, the kidney(s) may become completely fibrosed (shrunken) and nonfunctional or partially fibrosed with varying degrees of renal insufficiency (Keating and Althausen, 1985). Many patients show calyceal clubbing and renal calcification (Sutton et al., 1977). Some patients develop hypertension. Tubular dysfunction, including proteinuria, aminoaciduria, glycosuria, phosphaturia, metabolic acidosis with growth failure, and rickets also have been reported as late sequelae of renal venous thrombosis (Stark and Geiger, 1973).

■ RENAL CORTICAL AND MEDULLARY NECROSIS

It is appropriate to consider cortical and medullary necrosis together, because they are virtually indistinguishable clinically, often coexist, and are both the result of renal vascular compromise. Complete data concerning incidence or prevalence are not available. Davies and co-workers (1969) found 18 clinically unsuspected cases in 3516 autopsies. Nevertheless, it is probably misleading to give the impression that these conditions are rare.

Extensive renal cortical or medullary necrosis usually occurs in association with renal artery or venous thrombosis, but lesser degrees of cortical or medullary necrosis may occur without any demonstrable vascular thrombosis. The disorder commonly follows serious illness at birth, including profound perinatal asphyxia, hypovolemia due to dehydration or hemorrhage, shock, sepsis, severe anemia, pneumonia, hyperosmolality, congenital heart disease, obstructive uropathy with infection, and disseminated intravascular coagulation (Anand et al., 1977; Bernstein and Meyer, 1961; Chrispin, 1972; Davies et al., 1969; Gilbert et al., 1970). Cortical necrosis is the more common lesion associated with sepsis, while medullary necrosis is more commonly seen following hypovolemia or hyperosmolality.

Clinical Presentation and Laboratory Findings. Most newborns present with acute renal failure, and characteristically, there is complete anuria, or if urine is passed, it is scanty and nonconcentrated and contains protein and red blood cells. Occasionally, grossly bloody urine is present. The kidneys are often slightly enlarged. Severe hypertension may be present if there is coexisting renal artery thrombosis. The BUN and creatinine level are usually increased. When medullary necrosis occurs alone, the oliguria in a few days may be followed by polyuria and sodium wasting. In cortical necrosis, serum potassium may be elevated disproportionately to the degree of renal insufficiency. Thrombocytopenia and microangiopathic hemolytic anemia may be present as evidence of intravascular coagulation, as might other coagulation abnormalities.

Ultrasonography may reveal nephromegaly and internal echoes; however, similar findings may be observed in other disorders (Ogata et al., 1975). There is usually poor visualization of the kidneys by intravenous pyelography or nuclide scanning. When visualization is achieved, a prolonged nephrogram may be seen after some delay with dense opacification of the pyramids, which is characteristic of medullary necrosis (Fig. 101–3A). With cortical necrosis, the necrotic renal tissue calcifies in a few days, and both renal atrophy and calcifications may be visualized on a plain radiograph of the abdomen (Leonidas et al., 1971).

Treatment. Treatment consists of vigorous supportive care and careful management of fluid and electrolyte balance. If renal failure is severe or hyperkalemia is uncontrollable by the previously discussed measures, peritoneal dialysis or hemofiltration should be instituted.

Prognosis. The outcome depends on the degree to which the kidneys have been damaged. Severely affected infants commonly die within a few days. Most survivors have significant return of excretory function. Permanent impairment of concentrating ability may be present with medullary necrosis because of the extensive loss of juxtamedullary nephrons with their long loops of Henle. Growth of the kidney with either insult can be impaired, and variable degrees of focal scars or atrophy may be present.

Medullary necrosis, because of the location of the injury, will often demonstrate pyelocalyceal deformities, partial atrophy, irregular renal outlines, and clubbing of calyces on follow-up intravenous pyelography (Fig. 101–3B). Such deformities may be easily confused with chronic pyelonephritis, segmental renal hypoplasia, or dysplasia, unless previous knowledge of the infant's perinatal course is available (Anand et al., 1977; Mauer and Nosgrady, 1969). Within a few weeks, cortical necrosis will demonstrate a characteristic granular pattern of cortical calcification with occasional streaks radiating along the columns of Bertin into the medulla.

Reports of relatively longer survivals and recovery are increasing. Some of those who recover have late sequelae, including hypertension, tubular dysfunction (Groshong et al., 1971), and occasionally renal insufficiency (Anand et al., 1978), that eventually require dialysis and renal transplantation.

■ ADRENAL HEMORRHAGE

Small asymptomatic adrenal hemorrhage (hematoma) is a common finding at neonatal autopsies. However, adrenal hemorrhages large enough to cause a palpable abdominal mass are uncommon. Most adrenal hemorrhages follow a difficult vaginal delivery (Smith and Middleton, 1979) or are associated with hypoxia, shock, hemorrhagic disorders, and disseminated intravascular coagulation (Khuri et al., 1980). In 10 per cent of the patients adrenal hemorrhage is bilateral. The adrenal glands are relatively larger and hypervascular in the fetus and newborn than later in life, which perhaps makes them more vulnerable to hemorrhage.

Clinically, the disorder presents as an abdominal mass (85 per cent). Jaundice due to nonhemolytic indirect hyperbilirubinemia and mild anemia are also present in most patients. The diagnosis is confirmed by ultrasonography which can usually differentiate between adrenal hematoma and neuroblastoma. If there is any doubt about the nature of adrenal mass, vanilmandelic acid (VMA), homovanillic acid (HVA), should be collected to exclude neuroblastoma (see Chapter 95). The kidney is displaced

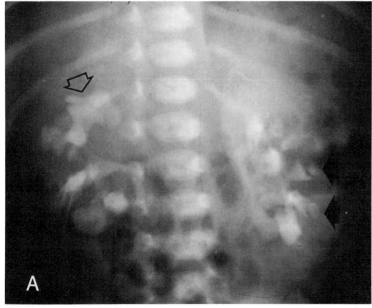
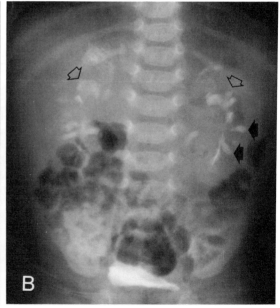

FIGURE 101–3. Medullary (papillary) necrosis. A, Excretory urogram in a 20-day-old infant exhibiting enlargement of both kidneys and dilated bizarre-appearing calices. Several calices in left kidney show intact fornices but have adjacent medullary cavities (solid arrows). Right lower and upper pole calices are replaced by large cavities suggestive of previously sloughed papillae (open arrow). B, Same patient age 2½ months. Excretory urogram shows bilateral bizarre-appearing calices and focal loss of renal cortex. Upper calices on both sides show large cavities (open arrows) whereas other calices appear fusiform (solid arrows). In left kidney fornices seen in earlier urogram are no longer discernible. Also note adrenal calcifications. (From Anand, S. K., Northway, J. D., and Smith, J. A.: Neonatal renal papillary and cortical necrosis. Am. J. Dis. Child. 131:773, 1977. Copyright 1977, American Medical Association.)

downward. A renal scan, an intravenous pyelogram, or magnetic resonance imaging may be occasionally necessary to differentiate adrenal hematoma from a renal mass or to detect a coexisting renal abnormality.

The disorder is usually self-limiting and requires no treatment. One initially needs to follow serial hemoglobin and bilirubin levels to detect worsening anemia or hyperbilirubinemia. The hematoma gradually regresses in size and is no longer palpable after a few weeks. As the hematoma resolves, calcification of the gland occurs and is usually detectable within 2 weeks of onset by ultrasonography or plain roentgenogram of the abdomen (Fig. 101–3B).

■ REFERENCES

Adelman, R. D.: Long-term follow-up of neonatal renovascular hypertension. Pediatr. Nephrol. *1*:36, 1987.

Adelman, R. D., Merten, D., Vogel, J., et al.: Non-surgical management of renovascular hypertension in the newborn. Pediatrics *62*:71, 1978.

Anand, S. K., Northway, J. D., and Crussi, F. G.: Acute renal failure in newborn infants. J. Pediatr. *92*:985, 1978.

Anand, S. K., Northway, J. D., and Smith, J. A.: Neonatal renal papillary and cortical necrosis. Am. J. Dis. Child. *131*:773, 1977.

Arneil, G. C., MacDonald, A. M., Murphy, A. V., et al.: Renal venous thrombosis. Clin. Nephrol. *1*:119, 1973.

Avery, M. E., Oppenheimer, E. M., and Gordon, H. J.: Renal vein thrombosis in newborn infants of diabetic mothers. N. Engl. J. Med. *256*:1134, 1957.

Belman, A. B., Susmano, D. F., Burden, J. J., et al.: Nonoperative treatment of unilateral thrombosis in the newborn. J.A.M.A. *211*:1165, 1970.

Bernstein, J., and Meyer, R.: Congenital abnormalities of the urinary system II. Renal cortical and medullary necrosis. J. Pediatr. *59*:657, 1961.

Bosque, E., and Weaver, L.: Continuous versus intermittent heparin infusion of umbilical artery catheters in the newborn infants. J. Pediatr. *108*:141, 1986.

Caeton, A. J., and Goetzman, B. W.: Risky business. Umbilical artery catheterization. Am. J. Dis. Child. *139*:120, 1985.

Campbell, M. F., and Matthews, W. F.: Renal thrombosis in infants: Report of two cases in male infants urologically examined and cured by nephrectomy at age 13 and 33 days of age. J. Pediatr. *20*:604, 1942.

Caplan, M. S., Cohn, R. A., Langman, C. B., et al.: Favorable outcome of neonatal aortic thrombosis and renovascular hypertension. J. Pediatr. *115*:291, 1989.

Chidi, C. C., King, D. R., and Boles, E. T.: An ultrastructural study of intimal injury induced by an indwelling umbilical artery catheter. J. Pediatr. Surg. *18*:109, 1983.

Chrispin, A. R.: Medullary necrosis in infancy. Br. Med. Bull. *28*:233, 1972.

Clatworthy, H. W., Jr., Dickens, D. R., and McClave, C. R.: Renal thrombosis complicating epidemic diarrhea in the newborn: Nephrectomy with recovery. N. Engl. J. Med. *248*:628, 1953.

Corrigan, J. J.: Neonatal thrombosis and the thrombolytic system. Am. J. Pediatr. Hematol. Oncol. *10*:83, 1988.

Davies, D. J., Kennedy, A., and Roberts, C.: Renal medullary necrosis in infancy and childhood. J. Pathol. *99*:125, 1969.

Duncan, R. E., Evans, A. T., and Martin, L. W.: Natural history and treatment of renal vein thrombosis in children. J. Pediatr. Surg. *12*:639, 1977.

Durante, E., Jones, D., and Spitzer, R.: Neonatal renal arterial embolism syndrome. J. Pediatr. *89*:978, 1976.

Emani, A., Saldanha, R., Knupp, C., et al.: Failure of systemic thrombolytic and heparin therapy in the treatment of neonatal aortic thrombosis. Pediatrics *79*:773, 1987.

Evans, D. J., Silverman, M., and Bowley, N. B.: Congenital hypertension due to unilateral renal vein thrombosis. Arch. Dis. Child. *56*:306, 1981.

Flanigan, D. P., Stolar, C. J. H., Pringle, K. L., et al.: Aortic thrombosis after umbilical artery catheterization. Arch. Surg. *17*:371, 1982.

Gilbert, E. F., Khoury, G. H., Hogan, G. R., et al.: Hemorrhagic renal necrosis in infancy: Relationship to radiopaque compounds. J. Pediatr. *76*:49, 1970.

Gonzalez, R., Schwartz, S., Sheldon, C. A., et al.: Bilateral renal vein thrombosis in infancy and childhood. Urol. Clin. North Am. *9*:279, 1982.

Goetzman, B. W., Stadalnik, R. C., Bogren, H. G., et al.: Thrombotic complications of umbilical artery catheter. A clinical and radiological study. Pediatrics *56*:374, 1975.

Groshong, T. D., Taylor, A. A., Nolph, K. D., et al.: Renal function following cortical necrosis in childhood. J. Pediatr. *78*:269, 1971.

Gross, R. E.,: Arterial embolism and thrombosis in infancy. Am J. Dis. Child. *70*:61, 1945.

Horgan, M. J., Bartoletti, A., Polansky, S., et al.: Effects of heparin infusates in umbilical arterial catheters on frequency of thrombotic complications. J. Pediatr. *111*:774, 1987.

Jackson, J. C., Truog, W. E., Watchko, J. F., et al.: Efficacy of thromboresistant umbilical artery catheter in reducing aortic thrombosis or related complications. J. Pediatr. *110*:102, 1987.

Keating, M. A., and Althausen, A. F.: The clinical spectrum of renal vein thrombosis. J. Urol. *133*:938, 1985.

Khuri, F. J., Alton, D. H., Hardy, B. E., et al.: Adrenal hemorrhage in neonates. Report of 5 cases and review of literature. J. Urol. *124*:684, 1980.

Krueger, T. C., Nebleh, W. W., O'Neill, J. A., et al.: Management of aortic thrombosis secondary to umbilical artery catheter in neonates. J. Pediatr. Surg. *20*::328, 1985.

Leonidas, J. C., Berdon, W. E., and Gribetz, D.,: Bilateral renal cortical necrosis in the newborn infant: Roentgenographic diagnosis. J. Pediatr. *79*:623, 1971.

Lesko, S. M., Mitchell, A. A., Epstein, M. F., et al.: Heparin use as a risk factor for intraventricular hemorrhage in low-birth-weight infants. N. Engl. J. Med. *314*:1156, 1986.

Malin, S. W., Baumgart, S., Rosenberg, H. K.., et al.: Nonsurgical management of obstructive aortic thrombosis complicated by renovascular hypertension in the neonate. J. Pediatr. *106*:603, 1985.

Mauer, S. M., and Nosgrady, M. B.: Renal papillary and cortical necrosis in a newborn infant: Report of a survivor with roentgenologic documentation. J. Pediatr. *74*:750, 1969.

Mokrohisky, S. T., Levine, R., Blumhagen, J. D., et al.: Low positioning of umbilical artery catheters increases associated complications in newborn infants. N. Engl. J. Med. *299*:561, 1978.

Neal, W. A., Reynolds, J. W., Jarvis, C. W., et al.: Umbilical artery catheterization: Demonstration of arterial thrombosis by aortography. Pediatrics *50*:6, 1972.

Ogata, E. S., Gooding, C. A., and Phibbs, R. H.: Angiographic and ultrasonographic appearance of renal cortical and medullary necrosis in the newborn. Pediatr. Radiol. *3*:226, 1975.

O'Neill, J. A., Neblett, W. W., and Born, M. L.: Management of major thromboembolic complications of umbilical artery catheters. J. Pediatr. Surg. *16*:972, 1981.

Oppenheimer, D. A., Carroll, B. A., and Garth, K. E.: Ultrasonic detection of complications following umbilical artery catheterization in the neonate. Radiology *145*:667, 1982.

Oppenheimer, E. H., and Esterly, J. R.: Thrombosis in the newborn; comparison between infants of diabetic and non-diabetic mothers. J. Pediatr. *67*:549, 1965.

Payne, R. M., Martin, T. C., and Bower, R. J.,: Management and follow-up of arterial thrombosis in the neonatal period. J. Pediatr. *114*:853, 1989.

Rajani, K., Goetzman, B. W., Wennberg, R. P., et al.: Effect of heparinization of fluids infused through an umbilical artery catheter on catheter potency and frequency of complications. Pediatrics *63*:552, 1979.

Schmidt, B., and Andrew, M.: Neonatal thrombotic disease: Prevention, diagnosis and treatment. J. Pediatr. *113*:407, 1988.

Schmidt, B., and Zipurky, A.: Thrombotic disease in newborn infants. Clin. Perinatal. *11*:461, 1984.

Seibert, J. J., Taylor, B. J., Williamson, S. L., et al.: Sonographic detection of neonatal umbilical artery thrombosis. AJR *148*:965, 1987.

Smith, J. A., and Middleton, R. G.: Neonatal adrenal hemorrhage. J. Urol. *122*:674, 1979.

Stark, H., and Geiger, R.: Renal tubular dysfunction following vascular accidents of the kidneys in the newborn. J. Pediatr. *83*:933, 1973.

Stringel, G., Mercer, S., Richler, M., et al.: Catheterization of the umbilical artery in neonates. Surgical implications. Can. J. Surg. *28*:143, 1985.

Sutton, T. J., Leblanc, A., Gauthier, N., et al.: Radiologic manifestations of neonatal renal vein thrombosis on follow-up examinations. Radiology *122*:435, 1977.

Tyson, J. E., deSa, D. J., and Moore, S.: Thromboatheromatous complications of umbilical arterial catheterization in the newborn period. Arch. Dis. Child. *51*:744, 1976.

Vailas, G. N., Brouillett, R. T., Scott, J. P., et al.: Neonatal aortic thrombosis: Recent experience. J. Pediatr. *109*:101, 1986.

Wesstrom, G., Finnstrom, O., and Stepport, G.: Umbilical artery catheterization in newborns I. Thrombosis in relation to catheter type and position. Acta Pediatr. Scand. *68*:575, 1979.

Wiggers, H. J., Bransilver, B. R., and Blanc, W. A.: Thrombosis due to catheterization in infants and children. J. Pediatr. *76*:1, 1970.

Woodard, J. R., Patterson, J. H., and Brinsfield, D.: Renal artery thrombosis in newborn infants. Am. J. Dis. Child. *114*:191, 1967.

Zuelzer, W. W., Kurnetz, R., and Newton, W. A., Jr.: Circulatory diseases of the kidneys in infancy and childhood. IV. Occlusion of the renal artery. Am. J. Dis. Child. *81*:21, 1951.

HYPERTENSION 102

Sudhir K. Anand

Until the early 1970s identification of hypertension in the newborn was infrequent (Adelman, 1978). Since then, hypertension has been recognized in the newborn, especially in neonatal intensive care units, with a much higher frequency. This may be the result of increased recognition due to closer blood pressure monitoring of the newborn with automated devices, increased renal artery (or peripheral branches) occlusion as a complication of indwelling umbilical artery catheterization, and perhaps survival of newborns who are at risk of development of hypertension, such as those with bronchopulmonary dysplasia (Abman et al., 1984; Adelman, 1988; Report of the Second Task Force, 1987).

■ MEASUREMENT OF BLOOD PRESSURE

Currently in the United States most blood pressure measurements in the newborn are performed by oscillometry or Doppler ultrasound techniques. With oscillometry (only Dynamap brand has been adequately tested so far), both systolic and diastolic blood pressure measurements closely resemble intra-arterial readings, whereas with Doppler ultrasound, correlation is good for systolic measurements and less so for diastolic measurements. In sick newborns with umbilical artery catheterization, direct intra-arterial blood pressure readings may be obtained with the help of a pressure transducer. Blood pressure values obtained from peripherally placed arterial catheters are not as reliable (Adelman, 1988). The palpation method (by palpating the brachial artery) is simple, but it only gives systolic pressure and values are 5 to 10 mm Hg lower than intra-arterial readings. Auscultatory and "flush" methods are difficult to implement in the newborn and have generally been replaced by oscillometry and ultrasound.

The blood pressure cuff width (inflatable bladder portion only) should cover approximately 75 per cent of the upper arm and nearly completely encircle the arm (or cuff width should be about half of arm circumference). Usually a 4 × 9-cm cuff works well in the newborn and a 2.5 × 5-cm cuff is used for the premature infant. The beginning of the Korotkoff I sound is used as the systolic blood pressure reading, and the beginning of the Korotkoff IV sound is used as the diastolic reading.

■ NORMAL BLOOD PRESSURE IN THE NEWBORN

Blood pressure in the newborn depends on the birth weight (maturity), postnatal age, and state of alertness. Several studies (deSwiet et al., 1980; Park and Lee, 1989; Report of the Task Force, 1987; Schachter et al., 1984; Uhari, 1980; Zinner et al., 1985) have described normal blood pressure values in term infants. Some of these studies describe blood pressure readings only at birth, whereas others describe serial blood pressure readings at 1- to 7-day intervals during the first month of life. Values in Table 102–1 are based on the data of Zinner and associates (1985). The systolic blood pressure during the first 36 hours in most studies averages approximately 70 mm Hg, and the diastolic value is 45 mm Hg. The systolic blood pressure during the first week after birth rises by 6 to 7 mm Hg (1 mm Hg/day) and thereafter increases about 2 mm Hg per week during the next 3 weeks. During the sleep state, blood pressure values are 5 to 10 mm Hg lower than during the awake state (deSwiet et al., 1980; Park and Lee, 1989; Zinner et al., 1985). In contrast, sucking, pain, crying, and other stresses (e.g., endotracheal suction) can raise the blood pressure as much as 10 to 20 mm Hg. The blood pressure in the lower extremities is almost the same (or minimally less) compared with that in the upper extremities (Park and Lee, 1989; Piazza et al., 1985).

Data on blood pressure values in the prematurely born infant, especially serial values with increasing postnatal age, are limited (Ingelfinger et al., 1983; Stork et al., 1984; Tan, 1988; Versmold et al., 1981). Figure 102–1 shows the systolic and diastolic blood pressure values in premature and term infants (from 610 to 4220 g) during the first 12 hours of life (Versmold et al., 1981). The systolic blood pressure in a 2.5-kg newborn is approximately 60 mm Hg (10 mm Hg less than that of a term infant), and in a 1.5-kg newborn it is approximately 50 mm Hg (20 mm Hg less than that of a term infant). Blood pressure values recently reported in premature infants in Singapore during the first 10 weeks of life are 5 to 10 mm Hg higher than in most other studies (Tan, 1988). Blood pressure in premature infants also rises with age (Stork et al., 1984; Tan, 1988). However, Tan (1988) did not find any difference in the blood pressure values

TABLE 102–1. Infant Blood Pressures*

AGE	NO.	SYSTOLIC	DIASTOLIC
1–2 d	127	69.7 ± 7.3	52.7 ± 7.5
3 d	382	71.4 ± 8.6	53.0 ± 7.3
4 d	155	75.7 ± 8.1	55.9 ± 7.7
5–7 d	90	76.1 ± 9.7	54.8 ± 10.7
8–14 d	566	77.5 ± 9.9	49.8 ± 9.0
15–21 d	77	79.3 ± 8.3	49.3 ± 8.2
1 mo	642	84.9 ± 10.2	46.2 ± 8.9
6 mo	525	92.2 ± 8.9	54.8 ± 8.6
12 mo	427	94.9 ± 7.9	55.6 ± 7.5
18 mo	335	96.1 ± 8.2	55.5 ± 8.0
24 mo	294	98.7 ± 7.5	57.9 ± 7.4

*Corrected for sleep/activity status to awake/quiet status. Values are mean ± SD in mm Hg.

(Reproduced by permission Zinner, S. H., Rosner, B., Oh, W., et al.: Significance of blood pressure in infancy: Familial aggregation and predictive effect on later blood pressure. Hypertension 7:411, 1985.)

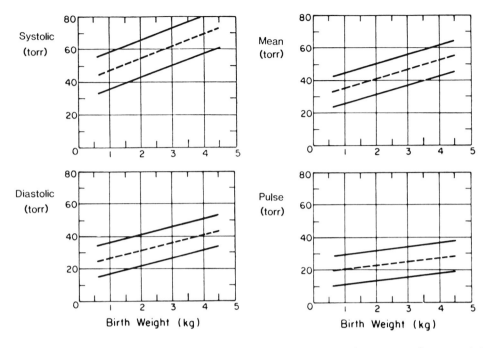

FIGURE 102–1. Systolic (top left), and diastolic (bottom left) aortic blood pressures; mean (top right) and pulse (bottom right) pressures during the first 12 hours of life in normal (term and premature) newborn infants grouped according to birth weight. Pressures were measured directly through umbilical artery catheter. Broken lines represent linear regressions, and solid lines represent 95 per cent confidence limits. (From Versmold, H. T., Kitterman, J. A., Phibbs, R. H., et al.: Aortic blood pressure during the first 12 hours of life in infants with birth weight 610 to 4220 g. Pediatrics 67:611, 1981. Reproduced by permission of Pediatrics.)

between the sleep or the awake state in the very premature infants, unlike findings observed in term infants.

DEFINITION AND INCIDENCE

The definition of hypertension in the newborn is controversial, just as it is in the older child. The report of the Second Task Force on Blood Pressure Control in Children (1987) defined hypertension as average systolic and/or diastolic blood pressure equal to greater than the 95th percentile for age and sex with measurements obtained on at least three occasions (Table 102–2). Similar definitions have been used by most neonatologists and other pediatricians to identify hypertension in the newborn. The task force further classified hypertension into two categories: (1) significant hypertension (blood pressure persistently between the 95th and 99th percentiles for age and sex) and (2) severe hypertension (blood pressure persistently at or above the 99th percentile for age and sex). Blood pressure values that qualify as significant or severe hypertension in newborns and in young infants are described in Table 102–3. Data for defining hypertension in the premature infant are limited; the numbers included in Table 102–3 are those culled from literature and based on my experience. As would be obvious from the previous definition of hypertension, 5 per cent of all newborns (>95th percentile) have hypertension, with 4 per cent

having significant and 1 per cent having severe hypertension. Ingelfinger (1982), however, recorded hypertension in only 20 of 10,000 deliveries, with an incidence of 0.2 per cent. Others (Adelman, 1988) report an incidence of 1 to 3 per cent.

Some studies have shown a significant degree of tracking (stability of percentile rank) of neonatal systolic blood pressure through infancy and early childhood (Zinner et al., 1985), whereas others have shown only a weak correlation between neonatal and later blood pressure (Uhari, 1980). Also, some authors have found familial aggregation of blood pressure, with the neonatal blood pressure percentiles correlating with those in mothers (Lee, 1976; Zinner et al., 1985).

ETIOLOGY

The two most common causes of neonatal hypertension are thrombosis of the renal artery or its branches (see Chapter 101) and coarctation of the aorta. There are many other neonatal disorders that may be associated

TABLE 102–2. Definitions of Hypertension

TERM	DEFINITION
High BP (hypertension)	Average systolic and/or average diastolic blood pressure ≥ 95th percentile for age and sex with measurements obtained on at least three occasions
Significant hypertension	Persistent blood pressure between the 95th and 99th percentiles for age and sex
Severe hypertension	Persistent blood pressure at or above the 99th percentile for age and sex

(Based on Report of the Second Task Force on Blood Pressure Control in Children—1987. Pediatrics 79:1, 1987.)

TABLE 102–3. Classification of Hypertension in Infants

AGE GROUP	SIGNIFICANT HYPERTENSION (mm Hg)	SEVERE HYPERTENSION (mm Hg)
PREMATURE*		
750–1000 g.	Systolic ≥ 60	Systolic ≥ 70
1500 g	Systolic ≥ 70	Systolic ≥ 80
2500 g	Systolic ≥ 80	Systolic ≥ 90
TERM NEWBORN†		
1 d	Systolic ≥ 90	Systolic ≥ 100
7 d	Systolic ≥ 96	Systolic ≥ 106
8–30 d	Systolic ≥ 104	Systolic ≥ 110
INFANT†		
< 2 yr	Systolic ≥ 112	Systolic ≥ 118
	Diastolic ≥ 74	Diastolic ≥ 82

*Premature and term newborns < 1 day old: data culled from literature.

†Data based on report of the Second Task Force on Blood Pressure Control in Children—1987. Pediatrics 79:1, 1987 (except values for 1 day old).

with neonatal hypertension (Table 102–4), but their frequency as a cause of neonatal hypertension is quite low. A variety of renal disorders, especially renal artery stenosis, polycystic kidney disease, and acute renal failure (Anand et al., 1978), are associated with hypertension. A common cause of the blood pressure reading being too high is the use of too small a cuff (e.g., a cuff appropriate for the premature infant being used on a term infant); this results in a factitiously increased blood pressure value.

Most reports on hypertension (usually symptomatic) in the newborn describe secondary causes and do not include essential hypertension as a cause of the disorder. However, a few authors (Adelman, 1988; Ogborn and Crocker, 1987; Sheftel et al., 1983) have reported significant hypertension in newborns and young infants for which no cause was found. In some of these infants blood pressure returned to normal spontaneously, whereas in others prolonged treatment was required. As mentioned earlier, 5 per cent of normal healthy-appearing infants have blood pressure readings above the 95th percentile (i.e., significant hypertension). Therefore, in asymptomatic newborns with blood pressure readings slightly higher than the 95th percentile, it would not be surprising to observe essential hypertension as the cause of the hypertension. Essential hypertension, however, must remain a diagnosis of exclusion.

■ CLINICAL PRESENTATION AND LABORATORY FINDINGS

In the past, most newborns with hypertension were reported to be symptomatic, presenting with congestive heart failure, seizures, acute renal failure, evidence of

TABLE 102–4. Causes of Neonatal Hypertension

VASCULAR
Coarctation of the thoracic aorta
Coarctation of the abdominal aorta
Hypoplasia of the aorta
Thrombosis of renal artery (and/or branches)
Stenosis of renal artery
RENAL
Polycystic kidney disease
Acute renal failure
Renal medullary or cortical necrosis
Obstructive uropathy with hydronephrosis
Horseshoe kidney
Crossed renal ectopia
Multicystic kidney
Renal hypoplasia
Renal tumors
ENDOCRINE
Neural crest tumors (neuroblastoma, ganglioneuroblastoma)
Adrenogenital syndrome (11-OH)
Cushing disease
Hyperthyroidism
DRUGS
Theophylline
Corticosteroids
Ocular phenylepinephrine
MISCELLANEOUS
Bronchopulmonary dysplasia
Increased intracranial pressure
Fluid overload
FACTITIOUS
Inappropriate cuff size
ESSENTIAL

peripheral arterial thrombosis, or failure to thrive. Now, many newborns with hypertension are asymptomatic or have nonspecific findings.

Each of the causes listed in Table 102–4 must be considered in the differential diagnosis, and appropriate laboratory studies should be performed based on the results of the initial clinical evaluation. Upper and lower extremity blood pressures must be measured to evaluate for coarctation of the aorta or aortic hypoplasia. Echocardiography, electrocardiography, and roentgenography of the chest should be performed to determine the presence of left ventricular hypertrophy and coarctation of the aorta.

In newborns with hypertension and indwelling umbilical artery catheter, in whom aortic or renal artery thrombosis is suspected, ultrasonography and Doppler flow study of the aorta and renal artery and radionuclide scintigraphy are usually adequate to confirm the diagnosis. If the diagnosis is in doubt and an umbilical artery catheter is in place, an aortogram and renal arteriogram can be safely completed through this route (see Chapter 101).

Urinalysis, tests of renal function, renal ultrasonography, radionuclide renal scan, and intravenous pyelography should also be performed to determine the presence of renal parenchymal disease and congenital abnormalities of the urinary tract. The routine measurement in every infant of urinary 17-hydroxysteroids, 17-ketosteroids, vanillylmandelic acid (VMA), catecholamines, and aldosterone, or plasma catecholamine and aldosterone without some other indication most often increases the expense and postpones definitive therapy with little diagnostic return. Measuring peripheral plasma renin activity (PRA) is helpful if the level is significantly elevated, but it may be deceiving if the level is normal. PRA levels in the newborn are significantly elevated compared with those of older children and adults. Kotchen and co-workers found that the mean PRA level for the newborn during the first 24 hours is 8.8 ng/ml/hr ± 2.8 S.E.M. By 3 to 6 days the PRA rises still higher to 11.6 ng/ml/hr. Three to 6 weeks later activity falls to 2.3 ng/ml/hr, but it is still higher than in the older child or adult. The peripheral PRA level is elevated in most, but not all, infants with renal vascular hypertension. However, levels may also be elevated in nonhypertensive infants with respiratory distress syndrome, renal failure, hypovolemia, and severe lung disease; an elevated PRA level in a hypertensive ill infant is not absolute evidence of renal artery disease.

The diagnosis of renal artery stenosis is best made by arteriography performed through the umbilical catheter or by percutaneous femoral puncture. Some authors recommend that renal vein samples for determination of PRA level be obtained at the same time that the arteriography is performed, while others advise this only in selected cases.

■ TREATMENT

The major reason for pursuing the clinical evaluation to completion and to a precise diagnosis is to provide sensible pharmacologic control and in select cases to provide the opportunity for surgical cure. Treatment must be individualized not only in terms of the type, amount, or combinations of antihypertensive agents but also in terms of the goal of the specific therapy. Information about the long-term effects of antihypertensive drugs begun in infancy or about the effects of these agents on growth and development in the immature infant is virtually non-existent. However, it is known that children with hypertension and normal renal function do not grow normally until the hypertension is brought under control. Therefore, patients with severe hypertension must be appropriately treated. Data are still inadequate to recommend drug treatment in asymptomatic newborns with blood pressures minimally above the 95th percentile and no cause for hypertension. In such patients, the author has usually withheld immediate drug treatment until a clear pattern of hypertension emerged or the patient developed clinical symptoms or echocardiographic evidence of left ventricular hypertrophy.

There is considerable controversy regarding the optimal management of neonatal hypertension due to renal artery thrombosis. As discussed in Chapter 101, most authors now recommend aggressive supportive therapy, including control of hypertension and management of fluid–electrolyte imbalance and renal failure if present. This treatment generally is sufficient and has comparable or better results than thrombectomy, nephrectomy, heparinization, or therapy with thrombolytic agents (e.g., streptokinase) (Adelman, 1988; see Chapter 101).

Mild hypertension if asymptomatic may be observed or may be treated with diuretics. In the majority of infants requiring further medication because of moderate or severe hypertension, a single antihypertensive agent can be used. Hydralazine and propranolol, either alone or in combination, are effective for most infants, provided sufficient medication is given. Methyldopa may be used as an alternative to either of these two drugs. Newborns seem to tolerate the higher dosages required to control hypertension from renal vascular disease (Table 102–5). Captopril, however, is usually effective at very low doses, and severe hypotension, renal failure, and cerebral ischemia with seizures may result with usual doses used in children and adults (Bifano et al., 1982; Mirkin and Newman, 1985; O'Dea et al., 1988; Perlman and Volpe,

1989; Tack and Perlman, 1988). Also, captopril is contraindicated in infants with bilateral renal artery stenosis or partial renal artery thrombosis because its use is frequently associated with acute renal failure. Experience with calcium channel blockers (e.g., nifedipine) to control hypertension in the newborn is limited, and some pediatric cardiologists do not recommend their use during the first month of life because of their potential myocardial depressant effects. Drugs such as guanethidine or reserpine are rarely indicated.

Hypertensive emergencies should be treated with parenteral medication. The drugs available include intravenous hydralazine, diazoxide, and nitroprusside. Many infants will respond promptly to hydralazine drips. Others would require diazoxide or nitroprusside (Adelman, 1988; Benitz et al., 1985). Gradually increasing doses of diazoxide or nitroprusside should be used to avoid the development of severe hypotension and cerebral ischemia. Often, these drugs will render the newborn more responsive to the oral drugs described previously.

Unilateral renal artery stenosis is often managed by unilateral nephrectomy because if it is diagnosed early enough, nephrectomy may be curative. Many authors believe that nephrectomy is better than attempts to reconstruct a renal artery, since most attempts at revascularization in the newborn result in thrombosis of the repaired vessels. However, as experience with vascular surgery in the newborn and young infant has improved, more successful attempts at vascular repair are being made. Balloon dilatation of the stenotic segment is still technically difficult in the newborn, but in the future it may become available as an alternate treatment. Bilateral stenotic disease is a more difficult problem. Infants with this disease are usually treated aggressively with medical treatment until they are large enough for surgical repair to be attempted on one side at a time.

■ PROGNOSIS

Until the early 1970s hypertension in the newborn was accompanied by 30 per cent mortality. During the past decade results with medical management have been encouraging (Adelman, 1978, 1988). This may reflect better medical management but perhaps also a different set of causes of hypertension, with renal artery thrombosis becoming predominant. In 1978, Adelman reported that in 17 newborns with renal arterial occlusion and hypertension all responded to pharmacologic treatment and none required nephrectomy. Three required less than 2 weeks of therapy, while in 13 others medication was discontinued 3 to 6 months later. More recently, Adelman (1987) has reported longer (5.75 years) follow-up in 12 newborns with hypertension. Blood pressure remained normal in all of these children on no medication, but several have residual renal abnormalities in the form of renal atrophy and abnormal function. Adelman's experience is not unique. Nevertheless, long-term follow-up of such infants is required, since the ultimate outcome of the survivors of neonatal hypertension is unclear and the possibility of reemergence of hypertension at a later age still remains, especially in children with renal atrophy.

TABLE 102–5. Medications Used in the Treatment of Neonatal Hypertension

MEDICATION	DAILY DOSAGE	COMMENTS
Furosemide	1–4 mg/kg IV, PO	May cause hyponatremia, hypokalemia, hypercalciuria
Chlorothiazide	20–50 mg/kg, PO	May cause hypokalemia, hyponatremia, hypochloremia
Hydralazine	1–9 mg/kg IV, PO	May cause tachycardia, paroxysmal atrial tachycardia
Methyldopa	5–50 mg/kg IV, PO	May cause somnolence
Propranolol	0.5–5.0 mg/kg, PO	May cause bronchospasm, bradycardia
Captopril	0.05–0.5 mg/kg/dose, PO	May cause oliguria, hyperkalemia
Diazoxide	2–5 mg/kg/dose IV	Effect highly variable; may cause hypotension and hyperglycemia
Nitroprusside	0.2–6.0 μg/kg/min IV	Monitor isothiocyanate levels

(From Adelman, R. D.: The hypertensive neonate. Clin. Perinatol. 15:567, 1988.)

■ REFERENCES

Abman, S. H., Warady, B. A., Lum, G. M., et al.: Systemic hypertension in infants with bronchopulmonary dysplasia. J. Pediatr. *104*:928, 1984.

Adelman, R. D.: Neonatal hypertension. Pediatr. Clin. North Am. *25*:99, 1978.

Adelman, R. D.: Long-term follow-up of neonatal renovascular hypertension. Pediatr. Nephrol. *1*:36, 1987.

Adelman, R. D.: The hypertensive neonate. Clin. Perinatol. *15*:567, 1988.

Anand, S. K., Northway, J. D., and Crussi, F. G.: Acute renal failure in newborn infants. J. Pediatr. *92*:985, 1978.

Benitz, W. E., Malachowski, N., Cohen, R. S., et al.: Use of sodium nitroprusside in neonates, efficacy and safety. J. Pediatr. *106*:102, 1985.

Bifano, E., Post, E. M., Springer, J., et al.: Treatment of neonatal hypertension with captopril. J. Pediatr. *100*:143, 1982.

deSwiet, M., Fayers, P., and Shinebourne, E. A.: Systolic blood pressure in a population of infants in the first year of life: The Brompton Study. Pediatrics *65*:1028, 1980.

Ingelfinger, J. R.: Hypertension in the first year of life. *In* Ingelfinger, J. R. (Ed.): Pediatric Hypertension. Philadelphia, W. B. Saunders Company, 1982.

Ingelfinger, J. R., Powers, L., and Epstein, M. F.: Blood pressure norms in low birth weight infants: Birth through four weeks. Pediatr. Res. *17*:319A, 1983.

Kotchen, T. A., Strickland, A. L., Rice, T. W., and Walters, D. R.: A study of the renin-angiotensin system in newborn infants. J. Pediatr. *80*:938, 1972.

Lee, Y. H., Rosner, B., and Gould, J. B.: Familial aggregation of blood pressure of newborn infants and their mothers. Pediatrics *58*:722, 1976.

Mirkin, B. L., and Newman, T. J.: Efficacy and safety of captopril in the treatment of severe childhood hypertension: Report of the International Collaborative Study Group. Pediatrics *75*:1091, 1985.

O'Dea, R. F., Mirkin, B. L., Alward, C. T., et al.: Treatment of neonatal hypertension with captopril. J. Pediatr. *113*:403, 1988.

Ogborn, M. R., and Crocker, J. F. S.: Investigation of pediatric hypertension: Use of a tailored protocol. Am. J. Dis. Child. *141*:1205, 1987.

Park, M. K., and Lee, D.: Normative arm and calf blood pressure values in the newborn. Pediatrics *83*:240, 1989.

Piazza, S. F., Chandra, M., Harper, R. G., et al.: Upper vs. lower limb blood pressure in full-term normal newborn. Am. J. Dis. Child. *139*:797, 1985.

Perlman, J. M., and Volpe, J. J.: Neurologic complications of captopril treatment of neonatal hypertension. Pediatrics *83*:47, 1989.

Report of the Second Task Force on Blood Pressure Control in Children—1987. Pediatrics *79*:1, 1987.

Schachter, J., Kuller, L. H., and Perfetti, C.: Blood pressure during the first five years of life: Relation to ethnic group (black or white) and to parental hypertension. Am. J. Epidemiol. *119*:541, 1984.

Sheftel, D. N., Hustead, V., and Friedman, A.: Hypertension screening in the follow-up of premature infants. Pediatrics *71*:763, 1983.

Stork, E. K., Carlo, W. A., Kleigman, R. M., et al.: Hypertension redefined for critically ill neonates. Pediatr. Res. *18*:321A, 1984.

Tack, E. D., and Perlman, J. M.: Renal failure in sick hypertensive premature infants receiving captopril therapy. J. Pediatr. *112*:805, 1988.

Tan, K. L.: Blood pressure in very low birth weight infants in the first 70 days of life. J. Pediatr. *112*:266, 1988.

Uhari, M.: Changes in blood pressure during the first year of life. Acta Pediatr. Scand. *69*:613, 1980.

Versmold, H. T., Kitterman, J. A., Phibbs, R. H., et al.: Aortic blood pressure during the first 12 hours of life in infants with birth weight 610 to 4220 grams. Pediatrics *67*:607, 1981.

Zinner, S. H., Rosner, B., Oh, W., et al.: Significance of blood pressure in infancy: Familial aggregation and predictive effect on later blood pressure. Hypertension *7*:411, 1985.

URINARY TRACT INFECTION AND VESICOURETERAL REFLUX

Sudhir K. Anand, Randal A. Aaberg, and Martin A. Koyle

Urinary tract infection (UTI) is a common problem in the newborn and sometimes is the source or result of neonatal sepsis. UTI is defined as significant bacteriuria irrespective of the site of infection in the urinary tract. UTI may be asymptomatic or may be associated with florid neonatal sepsis. In most newborns, UTI heals completely. However, in some infants, especially those with associated vesicoureteral reflux (VUR) and inadequate antibiotic treatment, UTI may lead to renal scarring and eventual hypertension and/or end-stage renal failure in later childhood. The reader is referred to recent comprehensive reviews for detailed discussions of this disorder (Govan and Lark, 1988; Winberg, 1986, 1987).

■ PREVALENCE

SCREENING BACTERIURIA

Asymptomatic bacteriuria is detected during surveys of healthy populations. We prefer to use the term *screening bacteriuria* because some of these patients may have low-grade symptomatology. The prevalence of screening bacteriuria in term newborns varies from less than 0.1 per cent (Edelmann et al., 1973; Randolph and Majors, 1970) to nearly 1 per cent (Abbott, 1972; Lincoln and Winberg, 1964; Littlewood et al., 1969; Wettergren et al., 1985). Bacteriuria rarely occurs during the first 4 to 5 days after birth and may have been responsible for the less than 0.1 per cent prevalence reported in some studies (Edelmann et al., 1973). Edelmann and associates (1973) reported the prevalence of bacteriuria in premature infants as approximately 3 per cent. In most series the prevalence of bacteriuria has been greater in newborn boys than newborn girls (Abbott, 1972; Lincoln and Winberg, 1964; Littlewood et al., 1969; Wettergren et al., 1985), whereas in others, the incidence has been greater (or equal) in girls compared with boys (Edelmann et al., 1973; McCarthy and Pryles, 1963; Randolph and Majors, 1970). Govan and Lark (1988), in their review of the literature, reported that 0.5 per cent of 1859 newborn girls and 1.4 per cent of 1883 boys had screening bacteriuria. Urine in most screening studies was collected by plastic bags usually after washing the genital region; therefore, these may be overestimates. Approximately 1 per cent of girls continue to have screening bacteriuria throughout childhood; however, screening bacteriuria is uncommon in boys after 1 year of age (Govan and Lark, 1988).

SYMPTOMATIC INFECTIONS

Most newborns and young infants present with symptoms of UTI and not asymptomatic bacteriuria. However, there are few studies that have prospectively studied the incidence or prevalence of UTI during the newborn period. Analysis by Winberg and associates (1974) suggests that overall the incidence of symptomatic UTI among 21,068 newborns is 0.25 per cent (males, 0.33 per cent and females, 0.16 per cent). Wiswell and Geschke (1989), based on retrospective studies, reported the incidence of symptomatic UTI in 136,086 newborn boys to be 0.08 per cent; the incidence, however, in uncircumcised boys was 12 times that in circumcised newborns, 0.24 per cent versus 0.02 per cent, respectively. Several authors (Bergstrom et al., 1972; Ginsberg and McCracken, 1982; Littlewood, 1972) have reported the incidence of UTI to be higher in newborn boys than in newborn girls; there has been only one report (Smellie et al., 1964) of a higher incidence of UTI in newborn girls than in newborn boys. Govan and Lark (1988), in their review of 305 newborns, reported UTI to be twice as common in newborn boys than in newborn girls (211 boys versus 94 girls). The higher incidence of UTI among male infants persists for the first 3 to 4 months of life, but thereafter the incidence and prevalence of UTI are considerably higher in females compared with males.

Maherzi and associates (1978), in a study of 1762 newborn infants admitted to a neonatal intensive care unit, reported the prevalence of UTI to be 1.9 per cent in 634 premature infants and 2.9 per cent in 1128 term or post-term infants. Seventy-nine per cent of these infants with UTI were symptomatic, and the remaining 21 per cent had no symptoms.

■ ETIOLOGY AND PATHOGENESIS

The pathogenesis of UTI involves interaction between various bacterial factors and protective host factors.

BACTERIAL ETIOLOGY

Escherichia coli accounts for 75 to 80 per cent of infections; the remainder are caused by other gram-negative enteric bacilli (*Klebsiella, Enterobacter,* and *Proteus*) and gram-positive cocci (enterococci, *Staphylococcus epidermidis,* and *S. aureus*). Of about 150 known *E. coli* groups (cell wall antigen), 8 to 10 of them cause about two thirds of all *E. coli* UTIs (Lindberg et al., 1975). Most organisms that cause UTI originate from the fecal flora.

Most patients with UTI have urine bacterial counts greater than 100,000 organisms per milliliter (i.e., significant bacteriuria). However, many adult women with symptomatic recurrent UTI have "clean catch" urine colony counts less than 1000/ml. Whether the same phenomenon applies to newborns and young infants is not known. Most authors reporting UTI in newborns and young infants have considered only 100,000 or more organisms per milliliter as significant, unless the urine sample was obtained by suprapubic puncture or catheterization.

ROUTE OF INFECTION

In older children and adult patients it is generally accepted that bacteria enter the urinary tract by the ascending route, and the increased prevalence of UTI in females is attributed to the short female urethra. In the newborn, it has generally been assumed (but not proven) that UTI results from a blood-borne infection. However, the work of Wiswell and associates (1986, 1988, 1989) suggests that UTI in newborn males may also be ascending and not blood borne. Bollgren and Winberg (1976) reported increased periurethral colonization among healthy newborn girls and boys (mostly uncircumcised) compared with girls and boys older than 5 years of age.

BACTERIAL ADHESION AND OTHER VIRULENCE FACTORS

The urinary pathogens that initiate colonization and induce UTI first must adhere to uroepithelium, otherwise the organisms will be swept away. Moreover, adhesion brings bacteria in direct contact with a rich source of nutrients that may be secreted by the host cell. The bacterial adhesion in *E. coli* is mediated by fimbriae, which are fine hairlike proteins emanating from the bacterial cell wall (Duguid et al., 1979). There are several types of *E. coli* fimbriae. The most important of these are P fimbriae and type 1 fimbriae. P fimbriae adhere to digalactoside (Gal-Gal) receptors, which form part of the blood group P antigen that is present on the uroepithelium and erythrocytes of most persons (Kallenius et al., 1980; O'Hanley et al., 1983). Winberg (1984, 1986) has reported that *E. coli* with P fimbriae was responsible for more than 90 per cent of cases of acute pyelonephritis in infants and children. However, in the presence of gross VUR, P-fimbriated *E. coli* is present in less than 50 per cent of cases (Lomberg et al., 1983, 1984). Harber and Asscher (1985) commented that although P fimbriae are associated with acute pyelonephritis, renal scar is more likely to be present in patients with VUR, most of whom have infection with

E. coli containing type 1 or other fimbriae but not type P fimbriae. There are many other bacterial virulence factors, including K and H antigens, hemolysin, serum resistance, colicins, and other proteins; however, their role in the pathogenesis of UTI is not well defined (Govan and Lark, 1988).

HOST FACTORS

Host factors that participate in the pathogenesis of UTI include age, sex, genetic structure, abnormal voiding urodynamics, VUR, and immune responses to infection. It is known that the uroepithelium of older girls and adult females who develop recurrent UTI binds *E. coli* more avidly than cells from nonsusceptible patients (Fowler and Stamey, 1977; Kallenius and Winberg, 1978). Women who develop frequent UTI show a higher density of receptors for P fimbriae (Svenson and Kallenius, 1983). It has been reported that women who are Lewis blood group nonsecretors or have a recessive phenotype are more likely to develop UTI (Sheinfeld et al., 1989). Whether similar host factors operate in newborns and infants is not known.

OBSTRUCTION

Obstruction is an uncommon finding in most newborns or young infants with UTI. Winberg and co-workers (1974) reported that obstruction was present in 10 per cent of males and 2 per cent of female children with UTI.

■ VESICOURETERAL REFLUX AND RENAL SCARRING (REFLUX NEPHROPATHY)

Retrograde passage of urine from the bladder to the ureter is called vesicoureteral reflux (VUR). The ureter enters the bladder obliquely, passes through the bladder wall, and then tunnels through the submucosa before it opens into the bladder lumen (Fig. 103–1). Under normal circumstances when the bladder is filled and during voiding, the submucosal segment is compressed, preventing reflux of urine into the ureter (Edelmann, 1988). VUR will occur when a ureter has a short submucosal segment. Reflux may occur in the presence of normal ureteral anatomy when bladder pressures exceed 40 cm H_2O, as seen in patients with posterior urethral valves or neurogenic bladder from myelodysplasia.

The magnitude of reflux is dependent on the length of the submucous tunnel, the diameter and location of the ureteral opening, and the voiding pressure within the bladder. The severity of VUR can be graded I to V (Fig. 103–2). Intrarenal reflux implies retrograde passage of urine from the renal pelvis into the collecting tubules (Fig. 103–3) and is observed in 5 to 10 per cent of newborns with VUR (Ransley and Risdon, 1978). Ransley and Risdon have also demonstrated that configuration of some renal papillae in infants is more concave than in later life and may make them more prone to develop intrarenal reflux.

The major long-term renal problem associated with UTI and VUR is renal scarring (reflux nephropathy). Renal scarring consists of calyceal clubbing or deformity with overlying corticomedullary scarring and atrophy.

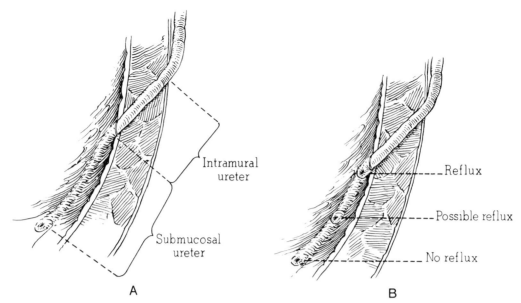

FIGURE 103–1. *A, Normal ureterovesical junction. Demonstration of length of intravesical submucosal ureteral segment. B, Refluxing ureterovesical junction. The same anatomic features as in the nonrefluxing orifice, except for inadequate length of intravesical submucosal ureter, are shown. Some orifices reflux intermittently with borderline submucosal tunnels. (From Glenn, J. [Ed.]: Urologic Surgery. 2nd ed. New York, Harper & Row, 1975.)*

VUR in most cases is considered to be a primary disorder owing to a congenital developmental defect of the ureterovesical junction. In recent years VUR has been recognized prenatally in some cases (Steele et al., 1989). VUR may also be a familial disorder and has been reported in 8 to 45 per cent of siblings of index cases (Jerkins and Noe, 1982; van den Abbeele et al., 1987). Although infection has been implicated in the etiology of secondary VUR (King et al., 1968), this question has not been resolved satisfactorily (Lerner et al., 1987). Most authors including ourselves consider that even though VUR and UTI often coexist, UTI does not cause VUR (Lerner et al., 1987). In animals in which VUR is induced by bladder

neck obstruction, UTI extends the duration of reflux following relief of obstruction (Roberts et al., 1988).

The prevalence of VUR in newborns and young infants with screening (asymptomatic) bacteriuria varies between 0 and 57 per cent (Abbott, 1972; Littlewood et al., 1969). Govan and Lark, in their review of the literature, reported VUR in 20 of 47 cases (43 per cent); of interest is that none of the patients had any renal scarring. However, in schoolage children with screening bacteriuria, whereas prevalence of VUR had decreased to 25 per cent, renal scarring and/or calyceal clubbing was recorded in 19 per cent of cases (Govan and Lark, 1988). A considerable number of these schoolage children had mild urinary

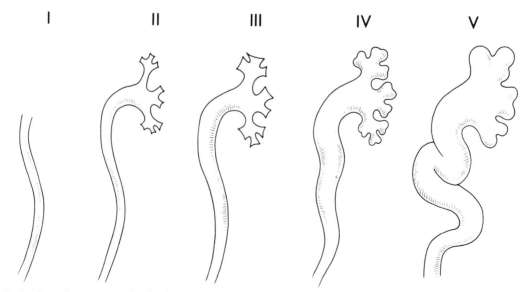

FIGURE 103–2. *Grading of vesicoureteral reflux by vesicoureterogram based on international classification. I, ureter only; II, ureter, pelvis and calyces but without dilatation; III, mild or moderate dilatation of ureter and mild or moderate dilatation of renal pelvis but no or slight blunting of fornices; IV, moderate dilatation and/or tortuosity of the ureter with moderate dilatation of renal pelvis and calyces and complete obliteration of the sharp angles of fornices but maintenance of papillary impressions in the majority of calyces; V, gross dilatation and tortuosity of ureters, renal pelves, and calyces; papillary impressions are no longer visible in the majority of calyces.*

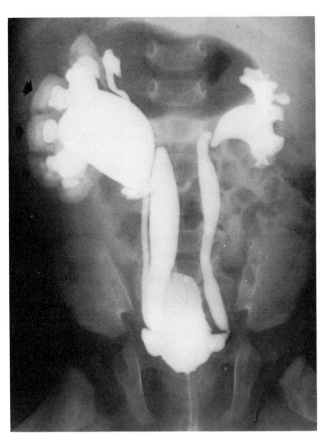

FIGURE 103–3. *Vesicoureterogram in a 2-month-old infant demonstrating grade III reflux on the left and grade IV reflux on the right. Note that the ureters on the right are duplicated. Also, note that most calyces on the right demonstrate reflux of dye into the renal cortex, i.e., intrarenal reflux or pyelotubular backflow (arrows).*

symptoms at the time of screening or had a history of previous symptomatic UTI. These observations suggest that continued asymptomatic bacteriuria beginning in infancy, previous symptomatic infections, VUR, or a combination of these factors may have led to the renal scarring observed on screening bacteriuria in schoolage children. Although the natural history of screening bacteriuria in the newborn is not clearly defined, the above observations offer a strong argument for treating any significant bacteriuria observed in the neonatal period or infancy.

The incidence of VUR in newborns with symptomatic UTI is approximately 41 per cent (70/170 cases), and none of the reported patients had renal scarring (Bergstrom et al., 1972; Govan and Lark, 1988). In infants beyond the neonatal period (1–12 months) with symptomatic UTI, the incidence of VUR is 37 per cent (184/497 cases) and approximately 10 per cent (range, 0 to 15 per cent) of these infants had renal scarring and/or calyceal clubbing (Bergstrom et al., 1972; Ginsburg and Mc-Cracken, 1982; Govan and Lark, 1988; Rolleston et al., 1970; Smellie et al., 1964). In schoolage children with symptomatic UTI, like in screening bacteriuria, the incidence of VUR is reduced to 20 to 30 per cent and renal scarring is increased up to 24 per cent.

A number of studies of UTI in infants and children have noted that although only 18 to 31 per cent of patients with refluxing ureters have associated renal scarring and calyceal clubbing, 75 to 91 per cent of patients with renal scarring have associated VUR (McKerrow et

al., 1984; Smellie et al., 1981). Moreover, the greater the severity of reflux, the greater has been the risk of reflux nephropathy (Govan and Lark, 1988; Rolleston et al., 1970; Smellie et al., 1975); patients with grade I to III reflux have no or minimal renal damage, whereas patients with grade IV to V reflux will have progressively more damage. The role of intrarenal reflux in renal scarring in humans is not clearly defined.

In a small number of infants and children with renal scarring and calyceal clubbing, no VUR is observed. The pathogenesis of renal scarring in these patients is not known. It may be secondary to reflux present at an earlier age that disappeared by the time of study (Govan and Lark, 1988). Alternatively, the renal scarring could be a consequence of pyelonephritis during infancy with a virulent organism even in the absence of any VUR (Winberg, 1986); the initial infection may have been recognized or remained unrecognized during infancy. It is known that renal scars may take several months to several years to be demonstrable radiographically.

The incidence of VUR in most patients with UTI or sterile reflux decreases with increasing age (Edwards et al., 1977; Heale, 1983; Report of the International Reflux Study Committee, 1981; Steele et al., 1989). This is considered a maturational change and probably occurs due to increased musculature in the bladder wall.

In animals, sterile VUR induced by partial bladder neck obstruction may lead to renal clubbing and scarring (Hodson et al., 1975; Roberts et al., 1982). However, in humans, most authors consider that VUR (primary) does not lead to scarring unless there is associated UTI (Govan and Lark, 1988; Lerner et al., 1987; Winberg, 1986). Prospective studies in children with persistent VUR have shown that emergence of new scars in the absence of infection is rare (Winberg, 1986).

In summary, patients most likely to develop renal clubbing and scarring are infants and young children (younger than age 3 years) with high-grade reflux and UTI. Also, early control of urinary tract infection may prevent development of renal scarring (Winberg, 1986).

■ CLINICAL PRESENTATION AND LABORATORY FINDINGS

The symptoms and signs of UTI in the newborn are varied and usually nonspecific. The clinical picture may resemble that of severe neonatal sepsis with temperature instability, cyanosis, and disseminated intravascular coagulation, or there may be an insidious onset with poor weight gain (or loss), low-grade fever, irritability, distended abdomen, diarrhea, vomiting, and jaundice. Patients with underlying urinary abnormalities may have additional manifestations, such as weak urinary stream or an abdominal mass. UTI is an uncommon finding in the evaluation of neonatal sepsis during the first 3 days of life (Visser and Hall, 1979; Winberg, 1987). After the first 3 days, however, UTI is present in a significant number of patients with suspected neonatal sepsis (Visser and Hall, 1979). Coexisting bacteremia is present in 10 to 40 per cent of patients (Visser and Hall, 1979; Wiswell and Geschke, 1989), and meningitis may coexist in 3 to 8 per cent of patients (Bergstrom et al., 1972; Wiswell and Geschke, 1989).

The diagnosis of UTI is established by finding a positive urine culture in a specimen obtained by bladder puncture or urinary catheterization. Most newborns with UTI have more than 100,000 organisms per milliliter of a single species; however, in some cases the colony count may be less and may vary between 1000 and 100,000 colonies per milliliter. A "bag urine" sample is valuable only if urine is sterile because the risk of contamination is high. Although studies of screening bacteriuria described earlier were performed with bag urine samples, the urine in these studies was usually collected under meticulous techniques rarely followed in most nurseries. Most patients with symptomatic UTI have leukocyturia; however, UTI may be present in the absence of leukocytes in urine. Moreover, leukocyturia may occur in other renal disorders in the absence of UTI. Also, tubular epithelial cells may sometimes be confused with leukocytes. Therefore, the diagnosis of UTI should never be made on the basis of leukocyturia alone.

Several methods, including sedimentation rate, C-reactive protein, urinary concentration, urinary lactic acid dehydrogenase isoenzymes, antibody-coated bacteria, and Fairleys technique, have been used with variable success to differentiate upper (renal) from lower (bladder) UTI in older children and adults. However, these methods have not been adequately evaluated in newborns or infants. Moreover, in newborns concern over upper or lower tract infection is not justified because UTI of either origin mandates complete evaluation for urinary anomalies and adequate treatment.

All newborns with UTI should have at least renal ultrasonography and contrast voiding cystourethrography (VCUG) performed. These two studies will detect most patients with structural renal anomalies and VUR. Renal ultrasound can be performed as soon as feasible after diagnosis. There is some controversy regarding the appropriate time for performing VCUG. Some pediatric nephrologists prefer to obtain VCUG 4 to 6 weeks after the onset of infection, to exclude the possibility of reflux secondary to UTI. This delay, however, entails antibiotic prophylaxis until completion of the study. Other nephrologists prefer to perform VCUG from the 7th to the 10th day of infection while the patient is in the hospital receiving antibiotic treatment. An excretory urogram is usually not necessary unless duplication or a ureterocele is suspected or adequate anatomic detail is not obtained by ultrasonography. Excretory urography is usually delayed until 2 weeks of age to obtain an adequate study (see Chapter 91).

■ TREATMENT

All newborns suspected of having UTI should have urine, blood, and cerebrospinal fluid samples taken for culture and sensitivity studies. The patient should be started on ampicillin and gentamicin (or cefotaxime), pending results of the studies; final antibiotic selection is based on the results of the studies. The treatment is continued for 10 to 14 days. Patients with obstruction require relief by appropriate corrective surgery or temporary diversion. In infants with VUR, low (prophylactic) doses of antibiotics are continued for at least 6 months to 1 year (up to age 6 weeks: amoxicillin, 20 mg/kg/day as a single dose, and after that, trimethoprim-sulfamethoxa-

zole, 2 mg/kg/day as a single dose). At the end of this period, a radionuclide VCUG is repeated to determine the disappearance of reflux. Development of renal scars can be best detected by DMSA scan (see Chapter 3). Most patients with VUR, including those with severe (grade IV–V) reflux, do not require surgical treatment because most grade I to III and 33 to 66 per cent of grade IV to V reflux in infants and young children disappears with increasing age (Govan and Lark, 1988; Steele, 1989). Moreover, the Birmingham Reflux Study group (1983) and preliminary results of the International Vesicoureteral Reflux Study group show no difference in the end result between prophylactic medical treatment designed to prevent infection and when surgical therapy was used. We recommend early surgery only for those patients who have poor medical compliance and break-through infections. Most urologists in the United States correct VUR by surgically reimplanting the ureter. A few urologists in Europe have used endoscopic injection with Teflon with equally good results (O'Donnell and Puri, 1984).

■ PROGNOSIS

Most newborns with UTI, if appropriately managed, recover completely and have normal renal growth and function. The frequency of renal scarring following UTI in newborns is not exactly known, irrespective of whether VUR was present or absent. About 25 per cent of newborns develop recurrence of infection during the following year. Therefore, repeat urine cultures should be done during follow-up in all infants, especially those with VUR, initially at 1- to 2-month intervals and later at 3- to 4-month intervals for at least 1 year or until disappearance of reflux. Infants with high-grade reflux and recurrent UTI are the ones most likely to develop renal scarring and calyceal clubbing and, eventually during later childhood or adolescence, hypertension, focal glomerulosclerosis, and end-stage renal disease (Chantler et al., 1980; Govan and Lark, 1988; Lerner et al., 1987). However, even in infants and children with severe reflux if infection is prevented, development of fresh scars is rare and renal function and growth remain normal (Smellie et al., 1975; Winberg, 1987).

■ REFERENCES

Abbott, G. D.: Neonatal bacteriuria: A prospective study in 1460 infants. Br. Med. J. 1:267, 1972.

Bergstrom, T., Larson, H., Lincoln, K., et al.: Studies of urinary tract infections in infancy and childhood: XII. Eighty consecutive patients with neonatal infection. J. Pediatr. 80:858, 1972.

Birmingham Reflux Study Group: Prospective trial of operative versus nonoperative treatment of severe vesicoureteral reflux: Two years' observation in 96 children. Br. Med. J. 287:171, 1983.

Bollgren, I., and Winberg, J.: The periurethral aerobic bacterial flora in healthy boys and girls. Acta Pediatr. Scand. 65:74, 1976.

Chantler, C., Carter, J. E., Bewick, M., et al.: 10-Year experience with regular hemodialysis and renal transplantation. Arch. Dis. Child. 55:435, 1980.

Duguid, J. P., Clegg, S., and Wilson, M. I.: The fimbrial and nonfimbrial hemagglutinins of E. coli. J. Med. Micro. 12:213, 1979.

Edelmann, C. M., Ogwo, J. E., Fine, B. P., et al.: The prevalence of bacteriuria in full-term and premature newborn infants. J. Pediatr. 82:125, 1973.

Edelmann, C. M.: Urinary tract infection and vesicoureteral reflux. Pediatr. Ann. 17:568, 1988.

Edwards, D., Normand, I. C. S., Prescod, N., et al.: Disappearance of vesicoureteral reflux during long-term prophylaxis of urinary tract infection in children. Br. Med. J. *2*:282, 1977.

Fowler, J. E., and Stamey, T. A.: Studies of introital colonization in women with recurrent urinary tract infection: VII. The role of bacterial adherence. J. Urol. *117*:472, 1977.

Ginsburg, C. M., and McCracken, G. H.: Urinary tract infection in young infants. Pediatrics *69*:409, 1982.

Govan, D. E., and Lark, D. L.: Urinary tract infection in neonates and infants. *In* King, L. R. (Ed.): Urologic Surgery in Neonates and Young Infants. Philadelphia, W. B. Saunders Company, 1988, p. 300.

Harber, M. J., and Asscher, A. W.: Virulence of urinary pathogens. Kidney Int. *28*:717, 1985.

Heale, W. F.: Prolonged follow-up of infants with reflux and reflux nephropathy. Eur. J. Pediatr. *140*:160, 1983.

Hodson, C. J., Maling, T. M. J., McManamon, B. J., et al.: The pathogenesis of reflux nephropathy: Chronic atrophic pyelonephritis. Br. J. Radiol. *48*(suppl. 13):1, 1975.

Jerkins, G. R., and Noe, H. N.: Familial vesicoureteral reflux: A prospective study. J. Urol. *128*:774, 1982.

Kallenius, G., Mollby, R., Swenson, S. B., et al.: The p^k antigen as receptor for the hemagglutinin of pyelonephritic *E. coli*. FEMS Microbiol. Lett. *7*:297, 1980.

Kallenius, G., and Winberg, J.: Bacterial adherence to periurethral epithelial cells in girls prone to urinary tract infections. Lancet *2*:540, 1978.

King, L. R., Surian, M. A., and Wendel, R. M.: Vesicoureteral reflux: A classification based on cause and results of treatment. J.A.M.A. *203*:169, 1968.

Lerner, G. R., Fleischmann, L. R., and Perlmutter, A. D.: Reflux nephropathy. Pediatr. Clin. North Am. *34*:747, 1987.

Lincoln, K., and Winberg, J.: Studies of urinary tract infections in infancy and childhood: II. Quantitative estimation of bacteriuria in unselected neonates with special reference to the occurrence of asymptomatic infections. Acta Pediatr. Scand. *53*:307, 1964.

Lindberg, U., Hanson, L. A., Jodal, U., et al.: Asymptomatic bacteriuria in school girls: II. Differences in *E. coli* causing asymptomatic and symptomatic bacteriuria. Acta Pediatr. Scand. *64*:432, 1975.

Littlewood, J. M.: Sixty-six infants with urinary tract infection in the first month of life. Arch. Dis. Child. *47*:218, 1972.

Littlewood, J. M., Kite, P., and Kite, B. A.: Incidence of neonatal urinary tract infection. Arch. Dis. Child. *44*:617, 1969.

Lomberg, H., Hanson, L. A., Jacobson, B., et al.: Correlation of P-blood group, vesicoureteral reflux, and bacterial attachment in patients with recurrent pyelonephritis. N. Engl. J. Med. *308*:1189, 1983.

Lomberg, H., Hellstrom, M., Jodal, U., et al.: Virulence-associated traits in *E. coli* causing first and recurrent episodes of urinary tract infection in children with or without vesicoureteral reflux. J. Infect. Dis. *150*:561, 1984.

Maherzi, M., Guignard, J. P., and Torrado, A.: Urinary tract infection in high-risk newborn infants. Pediatrics *62*:521, 1978.

McCarthy, J. M., and Pryles, C. V.: Clean voided and catheter neonatal urine specimens. Am. J. Dis. Child. *106*:85, 1963.

McKerrow, W., Davidson-Lamb, N., and Jones, P. F.: Urinary tract infection in children. Br. Med. J. *289*:299, 1984.

O'Donnell, B., and Puri, P.: Treatment of vesicoureteral reflux by endoscopic injection of Teflon. Br. Med. J. *289*:7, 1984.

O'Hanley, P., Lark, D., Normack, S., et al.: Mannose sensitive and Gal-Gal binding *E. coli* pili from recombinant strains: Chemical, functional and serologic properties. J. Exp. Med. *158*:1713, 1983.

Randolph, M. F., and Majors, F.: Office screening for bacteriuria in early infancy: Collection of a suitable urine specimen. J. Pediatr. *76*:934, 1970.

Ransley, P. G., and Risdon, R. A.: Reflux and renal scarring. Br. J. Radiol. *51*(suppl. 14):1, 1978.

Report of the International Reflux Study Committee: Medical versus surgical treatment of primary vesicoureteral reflux. Pediatrics *67*:392, 1981.

Roberts, J. A., Fischman, N. H., and Thomas, R.: Vesicoureteral reflux in the primate: IV. Does reflux harm the kidney? J. Urol. *128*:650, 1982.

Roberts, J. A., Kaack, M. B., and Morvant, A. B.: Vesicoureteral reflux in primate: IV. Infection as cause of prolonged high-grade reflux. Pediatrics *82*:91, 1988.

Rolleston, G. L., Shannon, F. T., and Utley, W. L. F.: Relationship of infantile vesicoureteral reflux to renal damage. Br. Med. J. *1*:460, 1970.

Sheinfeld, J., Schaeffer, A. J., Cordon-Cardo, C., et al.: Association of the Lewis blood-group phenotype with recurrent urinary tract infection in women. N. Engl. J. Med. *320*:773, 1989.

Smellie, J. M., Edwards, D., Hunter, N., et al.: Vesicoureteral reflux and renal scarring. Kidney Int. *8*:65, 1975.

Smellie, J. M., Hodson, C. J., Edward, D., et al.: Clinical and radiologic features of urinary tract infection in childhood. Br. Med. J. *2*:1222, 1964.

Smellie, J. M., Normand, I. C. S., and Katz, G.: Children with urinary infection: A comparison of those with and those without vesicoureteric reflux. Kidney Int. *20*:717, 1981.

Steele, B. T., Robitaille, P., and DeMaria, J.: Follow-up evaluation of prenatally recognized vesicoureteral reflux. J. Pediatr. *115*:95, 1989.

Svenson, S. B., and Kallenius, G.: Density and localization of P-fimbriae-specific receptors on mammalian cells: Fluorescence-activated cell analysis. Infection *11*:6, 1983.

van den Abbeele, A. D., Treves, S. T., Lebowitz, R. L., et al.: Vesico-ureteral reflux in asymptomatic siblings of patients with known reflux: Radionuclide cystography. Pediatrics *79*:147, 1987.

Visser, V. E., and Hall, R. T.: Urine culture in the evaluation of suspected neonatal sepsis. J. Pediatr. *94*:635, 1979.

Wettergren, B., Jodal, U., and Jonasson, G.: Epidemiology of bacteriuria during first year of life. Acta Pediatr. Scand. *74*:925, 1985.

Winberg, J.: P. fimbriae: Bacterial adhesion and pyelonephritis. Arch. Dis. Child. *59*:180, 1984.

Winberg, J.: Urinary tract infection in infants and children. *In* Walsh, P. C., Gittes, R. F., Perlmutter, A. D. (Eds.): Campbell's Urology. Philadelphia, W. B. Saunders Company, 1986, p. 831.

Winberg, J.: Clinical aspects of urinary tract infection. *In* Holliday, M. A., Burratt, M. A., Vernier, R. L. (Eds.): Pediatric Nephrology. Baltimore, Williams & Wilkins Company, 1987, p. 626.

Winberg, J., Andersen, H. J., Bergstrom, T., et al.: Epidemiology of symptomatic urinary tract infection in childhood. Acta Pediatr. Scand. *252*(suppl):1, 1974.

Wiswell, T. E., and Geschke, D. W.: Risks from circumcision during the first month of life compared with those of uncircumcised boys. Pediatrics *83*:1011, 1989.

Wiswell, T. E., Miller, G. M., Gelston, H. M., et al.: The effect of circumcision status on periurethral bacterial flora during the first year of life. J. Pediatr. *113*:442, 1988.

Wiswell, T. E., and Roscelli, J. D.: Corroborative evidence for the decreased incidence of urinary tract infection in circumcised male infants. Pediatrics *78*:96, 1986.

NEPHROTIC SYNDROME AND GLOMERULO-NEPHROPATHIES

104

Sudhir K. Anand

Nephrotic syndrome in the newborn is an infrequent disorder and is usually termed *congenital nephrotic syndrome* (CN). Like in the preschool or older child with nephrotic syndrome, CN is characterized by severe proteinuria, hypoalbuminemia, and generalized edema; however, the etiology, renal morphology, and clinical course of CN are very different from that seen in later childhood (Hallman et al., 1973; Mahan et al., 1984; Sibley et al., 1985). CN is a heterogeneous group of diseases that have in common only the fact that onset in all occurs during the first 3 months of life. Because the disorder is infrequent, no completely satisfactory classification has emerged; the classification listed in Table 104–1 is based on etiology, morphologic features, and clinical course.

■ FINNISH TYPE CONGENITAL NEPHROTIC SYNDROME

The majority of reported cases of CN are from Finland, and the disorder in most of these infants has been characterized by microscopic dilatation of tubules (Hallman and Hjelt, 1959; Hallman et al., 1973; Huttunen, 1976). Therefore, this type of CN has also been called Finnish type CN or microcystic disease. However, typical Finnish type CN has been reported from many other countries and in infants of other ethnic backgrounds; and, in fact, it is the most common cause of CN all over the world (Hoyer and Anderson, 1981; Mahan et al., 1984). The incidence of the disorder in Finland is approximately

TABLE 104–1. Classification of Congenital Nephrotic Syndrome

PRIMARY
Finnish type (i.e., microcystic disease)
Diffuse mesangial sclerosis
Mesangial proliferative glomerulonephritis
Focal segmental or diffuse glomerulosclerosis
Minimal change nephrotic syndrome
Interstitial nephritis
SECONDARY
Infections: congenital syphilis and toxoplasmosis, cytomegalovirus?
Nail-patella syndrome (i.e., onycho-osteodysplasia)
Vascular: renal vein thrombosis
Miscellaneous: nephroblastoma (Wilms tumor), gonadal dysgenesis, mercury poisoning

12 per 100,000 births, and it appears to be inherited in an autosomal recessive manner (Norio, 1966). Outside Finland, the disorder often appears to be sporadic. Males and females are equally affected. Prematurity with a large edematous placenta is common, as is a high incidence of toxemia during the pregnancy. The placenta may account for 40 per cent of the birth weight and be the most important early clue to the disease. Signs of fetal asphyxia are common, and many patients have a family history of high perinatal mortality.

Generalized edema is present in 50 per cent of the affected newborns during the 1st week of life and in all of them by 3 months of age. Ascites is usually present and may be extremely severe. Heavy proteinuria (more than 2 mg per milligram of creatinine in a spot urine test or more than 2 g/m²/day) is present in all cases. Microhematuria, glycosuria, and generalized aminoaciduria may be sometimes present. The serum albumin level is often less than 1 g/dl. Although hypercholesterolemia and hyperlipemia are also present, the serum lipid levels may not be as significantly elevated in the young infants as might be expected for the degree of hypoalbuminemia.

Renal function in the newborn period is normal. Hyponatremia and hypochloremia are often present (usually dilutional hyponatremia). Serum thyroxine levels are usually low, but thyroid stimulating hormone levels are normal. The decrease of thyroxine is attributed to urinary losses of thyroid binding proteins.

The characteristic renal lesion during the neonatal period is microcystic dilatation of the proximal tubules and Bowman capsule (Fig. 104–1). The dilated tubules have flattened epithelial cells and intact basement membranes. Small immature-appearing glomeruli (microglomeruli) within a dilated urinary space are common (Hoyer and Anderson, 1981; Sibley et al., 1985). The mature glomeruli usually show minimal abnormalities or mild mesangial hypercellularity. There are no immune deposits in the glomeruli or tubules early in the disease. Electron microscopy confirms the above finding and shows effacement (fusion) of epithelial foot processes. Although these morphologic changes are considered diagnostic of Finnish type CN, up to 25 per cent of cases do not show tubular dilatation but have a clinical course identical to those with microcystic changes (Hallman et al., 1973). Moreover, microcystic changes on occasion may be seen in newborns

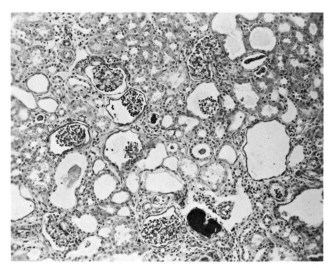

FIGURE 104–1. *Renal biopsy of a 7-week-old infant with congenital nephrotic syndrome. The biopsy shows several dilated tubules and small immature glomeruli within the dilated Bowman capsule. Although the morphologic picture is identical to Finnish type congenital nephrotic syndrome, the child recovered. (From Anand, S. K., Northway, J. D., and Vernier, R. L.: Congenital nephrotic syndrome: Report of a patient with cystic tubular changes who recovered. J. Pediatr. 95:265, 1979. Reproduced by permission of the publishers.)*

with CN owing to non–Finnish type etiology (Anand et al., 1979; Hoyer and Anderson, 1981). Several authors (Hoyer and Anderson, 1981; Rapola et al., 1984; Sibley et al., 1985) consider that microcystic dilatation probably is secondary to heavy proteinuria during gestation or the early newborn period and may be a nonspecific finding. This conclusion is strengthened by the disappearance of tubular dilatation on a second biopsy specimen following recovery in a newborn who initially presented with typical clinical and morphologic features of Finnish type CN (Anand et al., 1979). Vernier and co-workers (1983) have reported that heparan sulfate–rich anionic (negative) sites are decreased in the glomerular basement membrane of Finnish type CN and perhaps explain the severe proteinuria.

The diagnosis in any newborn with CN must be confirmed by percutaneous or surgical renal biopsy because of the universally poor prognosis of Finnish type CN and the possibility of finding some other type of renal lesion. Patients with Finnish type CN fail to respond to corticosteroids and cytotoxic drugs (Mahan et al., 1984; Mahan and Vernier, 1987). Moreover, infection is a major problem in these children, and it is in the child's best interest that corticosteroids or cytotoxic drugs not be tried.

Practically all patients fail to thrive and remain in poor general condition throughout the course of their disease. Growth is meager, bone age is severely retarded, and motor development is poor. Diarrhea, malnutrition, infections, and severe electrolyte disorders are the rule. In the experience of most physicians, death is inevitable before 4 years of age in the absence of dialysis and/or renal transplantation (Hallman et al., 1973; Hoyer et al., 1973; Mahan et al., 1984; Mahan and Vernier, 1987). Anand and associates (1979) and Sibley and co-workers (1985) have each described one patient with CN and microcystic changes who recovered. Until recently, more than half the children died during the 1st year of life and the cause of death usually was infection and not uremia (Hallman et

al., 1973; Huttunen, 1976). If children live beyond 1 year of age, slowly progressive uremia eventually ensues. Repeat renal biopsy specimens in these children show progressive focal and segmental glomerulosclerosis and interstitial fibrosis.

In recent years, several authors have recommended intensive nutritional support to maintain weight gain and improve the general condition and normal psychomotor development and have had variable rates of success with this regimen (Broyer et al., 1975; Mahan et al., 1984). This approach is maintained until children have grown to a size more favorable for successful dialysis and renal transplantation (Mahan et al., 1984).

Genetic counseling of the parents is very important, since there is one chance in four that subsequent children will be affected by the same lesion (Norio, 1966). Prenatal diagnosis as early as 15 weeks' gestation is possible by the detection of elevated levels of alpha-fetoprotein in both the amniotic fluid and the maternal plasma (Aula et al., 1978; Kjessler et al., 1975). Even though other fetal and obstetric problems can cause an elevated maternal plasma level of alpha-fetoprotein in the third trimester, the results to date have been quite accurate. Although this has led some investigators to recommend therapeutic abortion on the basis of the fact that the disease is universally fatal, recent improvements in survival with supportive therapy, infantile dialysis, and renal transplantation of the very young may warrant some modification of this recommendation.

■ FOCAL GLOMERULOSCLEROSIS AND OTHER MESANGIAL LESIONS

The kidney biopsy in some newborns and young patients with CN, instead of microcystic changes, shows diffuse mesangial sclerosis, mesangial proliferative glomerulonephritis, focal segmental or diffuse glomerulosclerosis (Beale et al., 1979; George et al., 1976; Habib and Bois, 1973; Moncrief et al., 1973; Sibley et al., 1985). Clinically these infants appear similar to infants with Finnish type CN. Familial involvement may be present in some of these cases. The disorder in most of these cases is slowly progressive, leading to end-stage renal disease by age 1 to 2 years; however, some of these patients go into remission and recover. Only supportive treatment is indicated.

■ MINIMAL CHANGE NEPHROTIC SYNDROME

The lesion of minimal change nephrotic syndrome is clinically and morphologically similar to the lipoid nephrosis more common in the older child. The renal histology by light microscopy appears entirely normal; immunofluorescence microscopy shows no evidence of antibody deposition, and only fusion of the epithelial cell foot processes is seen by electron microscopy. This disorder is extremely uncommon during the first 3 months of life, and when seen it occurs toward the end of the third month. Recovery from this disease, either spontaneously or following treatment with corticosteroids, is common. Although some infants progress to chronic renal insufficiency, their course is longer than those with the microcystic form of the disease. Clear definition by renal biopsy is essential in planning treatment.

■ INTERSTITIAL NEPHRITIS

One case, with onset at birth, has been described in which the primary renal abnormality was a chronic interstitial nephritis with widespread interstitial fibrosis (Grupe et al., 1966). There were collections of lymphocytes in the interstitium but no plasma cells and no polymorphonuclear leukocytes, with no indication of an infectious cause. The child had abnormal external genitalia and progressed to chronic renal failure and death at 9 months of age.

■ CONGENITAL SYPHILIS AND TOXOPLASMOSIS

Both congenital syphilis and congenital toxoplasmosis have been occasionally described to cause nephrotic syndrome in the newborn (Hill et al., 1972; Kaplan et al., 1972; McDonald et al., 1981; Shahin et al., 1974; Wickborn and Winberg, 1972). The frequency of renal lesions in these disorders is much less than that of neurologic, ophthalmic, or reticuloendothelial lesions. The newborns, like those with other types of CN, present with edema and proteinuria. Microscopic hematuria is frequently present. The kidney biopsy specimen shows variable thickening of the basement membrane and subepithelial immune deposits. Treponemal or *Toxoplasma* antigen may be demonstrable in the subepithelial immune deposits (Kaplan et al., 1972; Shahin et al., 1974). These disorders can be successfully treated by appropriate antimicrobial agents: penicillin for syphilis and a combination of pyrimethamine and sulfonamides for toxoplasmosis.

Cytomegalovirus infection has been occasionally described in association with CN; however, a causal relationship has not been established.

■ NAIL-PATELLA SYNDROME (HEREDITARY ONYCHO-OSTEODYSPLASIA)

Nail-patella syndrome is a rare disease that usually presents after 3 months of age, but it has been reported in the newborn (Simila et al., 1970). Renal disease is present in 30 to 40 per cent of patients with the syndrome. Inheritance is autosomal dominant. The clinical characteristics are malformed nails, absent or hypoplastic patella, abnormal radial head, and iliac horns. The radiographic demonstration of the iliac horns can be the presenting clue in the newborn. Proteinuria is the characteristic presentation of renal disease. The glomerular basement membrane is characteristically thickened on a renal biopsy (Hoyer et al., 1972); however, diagnosis can usually be made on a clinical basis. Approximately 25 per cent of those with the renal lesion will eventually suffer renal insufficiency.

■ RENAL VEIN THROMBOSIS

Renal vein thrombosis is frequently found in association with nephrotic syndrome in adults (Llach et al., 1980);

however, this finding is uncommon in childhood lipoid nephrosis or congenital nephrotic syndrome (Lewy and Jao, 1974). Renal vein thrombosis is now generally considered a consequence of the hypercoagulable state present in nephrotic syndrome and not a cause of nephrotic syndrome (Bernard, 1988).

■ MISCELLANEOUS DISORDERS WITH NEPHROTIC SYNDROME

Nephrotic syndrome has been reported in association with nephroblastoma and pseudohermaphroditism (Drash syndrome). Mercury intoxication, which may also be a cause, usually responds to withdrawal of the toxic agent.

■ OTHER GLOMERULONEPHROPATHIES

Immunologic renal disorders such as acute glomerulonephritis, IgA nephropathy, membranoproliferative glomerulonephritis, and chronic glomerulonephritis are extremely uncommon in the newborn period even though they are quite frequent in older children. The only immunologic renal disorders seen in the newborn are those related to congenital syphilis or congenital toxoplasmosis. There has been an occasional report of chronic glomerulonephritis in the newborn in the past (Collins, 1954), but now most cases with similar clinical findings in the newborn are attributable to other renal lesions described previously in the context of CN. The basis for the rarity of immunologic renal disease in the newborn is not known but may have to do with differences in immune maturation of the newborn versus that of the older child.

■ REFERENCES

Anand, S. K., Northway, J. D., and Vernier, R. L.: Congenital nephrotic syndrome: Report of a patient with cystic tubular changes who recovered. J. Pediatr. 95:265, 1979.

Aula, P., Rapola, J., Karjalanen, O., et al.: Prenatal diagnosis of congenital nephrosis in 23 high-risk families. Am. J. Dis. Child. 132:984, 1978.

Beale, M. G., Strayer, D. S., Kissane, J. M., et al.: Congenital glomerulosclerosis and nephrotic syndrome in two infants. Am. J. Dis. Child. 133:842, 1979.

Bernard, D. B.: Extrarenal complications of nephrotic syndrome. Kidney Int. 33:1184, 1988.

Broyer, M., Cathelineau, L., Loirat, C., et al.: Congenital nephrotic syndrome, Finnish type: A new therapeutic approach. Proceedings of the VII International Congress on Nephrology, 1975.

Collins, R. D.: Chronic glomerulonephritis in a newborn child. Am. J. Dis. Child. 87:478, 1954.

George, C. R. P., Hickman, R. O., and Stricker, G. E.: Infantile nephrotic syndrome. Clin. Nephrol. 5:20, 1976.

Grupe, W. E., Cuppage, F. E., and Heymann, W.: Congenital nephrotic syndrome and interstitial nephritis. Am. J. Dis. Child. 111:482, 1966.

Habib, R., and Bois, E.: Hétérogénéité des syndromes néphrotiques à debut précoce du nourrisson (syndrome néphrotique infantile). Helv. Paediatr. Acta 28:91, 1973.

Hallman, N., and Hjelt, L.: Congenital nephrosis syndrome. J. Pediatr. 55:152, 1959.

Hallman, N., Norio, R., and Rapola, J.: Congenital nephrotic syndrome. Nephron 11:101, 1973.

Hill, L. L., Singer, D. B., Falletta, J., and Stasney, R.: The nephrotic syndrome in congenital syphilis: An immunopathy. Pediatrics 49:260, 1972.

Hoyer, J. R., and Anderson, C. E.: Congenital nephrotic syndrome. Clin. Perinatol. 8:333, 1981.

Hoyer, J. R., Kjellstrand, C. M., Simmons, R. L., et al.: Successful renal transplantation in 3 children with congenital nephrotic syndrome. Lancet 1:1410, 1973.

Hoyer, J. R., Michael, A. F., and Vernier, R. L.: Renal disease in nail-patella syndrome: Clinical and morphologic studies. Kidney Int. 2:231, 1972.

Huttunen, N. P.: Congenital nephrotic syndrome of Finnish type: Study of 75 patients. Arch. Dis. Child. 51:344, 1976.

Kaplan, B. S., Wiglesworth, F. W., Marks, M. I., et al.: The glomerulopathy of congenital syphilis: An immune deposit disease. J. Pediatr. 81:1154, 1972.

Kjessler, B., Johansson, S. G. D., Sherman, M., et al.: Antenatal diagnosis of congenital nephrosis. Lancet 2:553, 1975.

Lewy, P. R., and Jao, W.: Nephrotic syndrome in association with renal vein thrombosis. J. Pediatr. 85:359, 1974.

Llach, F., Papper, S., and Massary, S. G.: The clinical spectrum of renal vein thrombosis: Acute and chronic. Am. J. Med. 69:819, 1980.

Mahan, J. D., Mauer, S. M., and Sibley, R. K.: Congenital nephrotic syndrome, evolution of medical management and results of renal transplantation. J. Pediatr. 105:549, 1984.

Mahan, J. R., and Vernier, R. L.: Congenital nephrotic syndrome. In Holliday, M. A., Barratt, T. M., and Vernier, R. L. (Eds.): Pediatric Nephrology. Baltimore, Williams & Wilkins Company, 1987, p. 457.

McDonald, R., Wiggelinkhuien, J., and Kaschula, R. O. C.: The nephrotic syndrome in very young infants. Am. J. Dis. Child. 122:507, 1981.

Moncrief, M. W., White, R. H. R., and Glasgow, E. F.: The familial nephrotic syndrome: II. A clinicopathological study. Clin. Nephrol. 4:220, 1973.

Norio, R.: Heredity in the congenital nephrotic syndrome. Ann. Paediatr. Fenn. 12(suppl. 27):1, 1966.

Rapola, J., Sariola, H., Ekblom, P., et al.: Pathology of fetal congenital nephrosis: Immunohistochemical and ultrastructural studies. Kidney Int. 25:701, 1984.

Shahin, B., Papadopoulou, Z. L., and Jenis, E. H.: Congenital nephrotic syndrome associated with congenital toxoplasmosis. J. Pediatr. 85:366, 1974.

Sibley, R. K., Mahan, J., and Mauer, S. M.: A clinicopathological study of forty-eight infants with nephrotic syndrome. Kidney Int. 27:544, 1985.

Simila, S., Vesa, L., and Wasz-Hockert, O.: Hereditary onycho-osteo-dysplasia (nail-patella syndrome) with nephrosis-like renal disease in a newborn boy. Pediatrics 46:61, 1970.

Vernier, R. L., Klein, D. J., Sisson, P., et al.: Heparan sulfate–rich anionic sites in the human glomerular basement membrane: Decreased concentration in congenital nephrotic syndrome. N. Engl. J. Med. 309:1001, 1983.

Wickborn, B., and Winberg, J.: Coincidence of congenital toxoplasmosis and acute nephritis with nephrotic syndrome. Acta Pediatr. Scand. 61:470, 1972.

Sudhir K. Anand

Renal tubular disorders are a heterogeneous group of disorders characterized by a defect in tubular reabsorptive or secretory function. The defect may be associated with dysfunction of a single tubular function (e.g., renal glycosuria) or of multiple tubular functions (e.g., Fanconi syndrome). The site of the disorder may be the proximal or the distal tubule. The glomerular filtration rate in most of these disorders is normal. Even if there is a mild decrease in the glomerular filtration rate the tubular dysfunction is still out of proportion to the degree of renal failure. A number of these disorders are listed in Table 105–1.

Renal tubular disorders may be primary or secondary to some other renal or systemic disease. Many of the primary renal disorders are hereditary conditions and have their onset during the newborn period, even though clinical detection usually occurs later in infancy or childhood. The presence of a positive family history should enable one to anticipate the disorder in subsequent births and make an early diagnosis. Moreover, telltale signs are sometimes present during the newborn period that should make possible early identification of the disorder and institution of appropriate therapy to prevent harmful consequences associated with a delay in diagnosis and treatment. Discussion of all of these disorders is beyond the scope of this chapter, and the reader is referred to other sections of this book and to the following references for further study: Chesney and Novello, 1989; Holliday et al., 1987; Scriver et al., 1989.

■ POLYURIA

The daily urine output in newborns after the first week of life varies between 50 and 150 ml/kg/day (2 to 6 ml/kg/hr). Urine output higher than 6 ml/kg/hr is usually considered polyuria. Various causes of polyuria in the newborn are listed in Table 105–2. The most common cause for polyuria is excessive oral or parenteral fluid administration. Polyuria is also commonly observed during recovery from edematous states and renal failure. Other causes of polyuria are uncommon but are important because they may be life-long disorders and, if treatment is started early, may have better long-term outcome. Congenital arginine vasopressin (AVP) deficiency may be an isolated defect or be associated with other central nervous system disorders. A variety of renal disorders may lead to polyuria, which may also be due to congenital renal anomalies, effects of drugs, or an isolated defect with end-organ resistance of action of AVP.

■ NEPHROGENIC DIABETES INSIPIDUS

Hereditary nephrogenic diabetes insipidus (H-NDI) is a congenital X-linked disorder characterized by severe poly-uria due to the inability of the kidneys to concentrate urine in response to AVP (Chesney and Novello, 1989; Kaplan, 1987; Reeves and Andreoli, 1989).

PATHOGENESIS

AVP increases water permeability in the collecting tubule and the distal tubule by first binding to hormone receptors located in the basolateral membrane of the tubular cells and then activating adenylate cyclase to produce cyclic adenosine monophosphate (AMP). Cyclic AMP, in turn, activates a protein kinase and other intermediate substances, which together increase water-specific channels in the luminal membrane and increase water reabsorption (Hays et al., 1987; Reeves and Andreoli, 1989). In patients with H-NDI there is end-organ refrac-

TABLE 105–1. Renal Tubular Disorders

SINGLE TUBULAR DYSFUNCTION
Water:
   Nephrogenic diabetes insipidus
   (hereditary X-linked)
Sodium:
   Pseudohypoaldosteronism
Potassium:
   Bartter syndrome
   Pseudohyperaldosteronism (Liddle syndrome)
   Renal tubular potassium secretion defect
   (Spitzer-Weinstein syndrome)
   Pseudohypoaldosteronism
H^+ ion:
   Renal tubular acidosis
     Type I: distal, classic
     Type II: proximal
     Type IV: hyperkalemic
Calcium and phosphorus:
   Familial hypophosphatemic rickets
   Vitamin D–dependent rickets
Magnesium:
   Hypomagnesemia
Carbohydrate:
   Renal glycosuria
   Pentosuria
Amino acids:
   Cystinuria
   Dibasic aminoaciduria
   Iminoglycinuria
   Hartnup disease
   Hyperdicarboxylic aminoaciduria
Uric acid:
   Hereditary renal hypouricemia

MULTIPLE TUBULAR DYSFUNCTION
Fanconi syndrome:
   Idiopathic
   Cystinosis
   Others

TABLE 105–2. Etiology of Polyuria in the Newborn

Excessive oral or parenteral fluid intake
Recovery from edematous states
Excessive urinary solute load: diabetes mellitus
Deficiency of arginine vasopressin
   Primary:
      Idiopathic sporadic or familial
   Secondary:
      Central nervous system disorders (e.g., trauma, tumors)
      Following recovery from meningitis
      Midline defects: holoprosencephaly
      Histiocytosis X
End-organ resistance to arginine vasopressin (nephrogenic diabetes
   insipidus)
   Primary:
      X-linked hereditary nephrogenic diabetes insipidus
   Secondary:
      During recovery from acute renal failure
      Following relief of urinary obstruction
      Acute pyelonephritis
      Polycystic kidney disease
      Dysplastic kidneys
      Hypoplastic kidneys
      Hypokalemia
      Hypercalcemia
      Renal papillary necrosis
      Sickle cell disease (only in older children)
      Drugs: diuretics, lithium

toriness to the action of AVP. The renal cellular defect in H-NDI may be either an impaired cyclic AMP production (type I H-NDI) or a reduced effect of normally produced cyclic AMP (type II H-NDI) (Bell et al., 1974; Ohzeki, 1985).

CLINICAL PRESENTATION

The disorder is clinically apparent in the first few days to weeks of life. Polyhydramnios may be present during gestation. Male newborns with H-NDI suck eagerly and appear always thirsty for milk or other fluids. However, they are irritable, often vomit, and have poor weight gain. Their diapers always seem wet, and constipation is common. These findings, however, are often ignored unless there was history of H-NDI in a previous family member. H-NDI may present as unexplained (dehydration) fever in newborns and young infants (Schrager et al., 1976). Episodes of hypernatremic dehydration are common, especially when fluid intake is temporarily limited owing to intercurrent upper respiratory tract infection or acute gastroenteritis. Failure to thrive and developmental delay are common during infancy, and older children with H-NDI often have mental retardation (Ruess and Rosenthal, 1963), which probably occurs because of repeated episodes of hypernatremic dehydration and its detrimental consequences on the brain (Finberg, 1969). Although the disorder is fully manifest in male infants only, variable degree of concentration defects may also be present in female infants.

DIAGNOSIS

In infants with H-NDI the urinary output while receiving free access to water often exceeds 10 ml/kg/hr (240 ml/kg/day). The urinary specific gravity usually varies between 1.001 to 1.002 and even during episodes of dehydration remains less than 1.010. The blood urea

nitrogen and serum creatinine values are normal except during episodes of dehydration. Serum AVP levels (if measured) are high normal or increased. The diagnosis of H-NDI is confirmed by failure of polyuria to respond to exogenously administered DDAVP (desmopressin) (intranasally), aqueous pitressin (intravenously or intramuscularly), or pitressin tannate in oil (intramuscularly). The response to intranasal DDAVP in the newborn and young infant may not be as reliable or reproducible as in the older child. The water deprivation test is usually not necessary, but if it is performed, close monitoring of urine output, weight loss, and serum sodium level must be done. The overnight water deprivation test should never be performed in infants and young children. These tests will exclude polyuria due to AVP deficiency states and excessive water intake. In other renal disorders associated with polyuria (e.g., cystic kidneys), the magnitude of polyuria is not as severe as in H-NDI and renal ultrasonography will detect the underlying anomalies.

TREATMENT

There is no specific therapy for H-NDI. Provision of substantial amounts of water during the day and night to meet the excessive urinary losses is the most important part of treatment. It is also important to reduce the solute intake by using milk or formulas with low protein and sodium content (e.g., breast milk, PM 60–40, SMA). Salt restriction must be used later in infancy and childhood. Thiazide diuretics (i.e., chlorothiazide, hydrochlorothiazide) may be used to reduce the urinary output by 25 to 40 per cent (Crawford and Kennedy, 1959; Early and Orloff, 1962). The paradoxic antidiuresis seen in H-NDI from diuretics results from their ability to interfere with tubular sodium absorption, which in turn reduces the renal ability to maximally dilute urine (during water diuresis). In addition, diuretics enhance proximal tubular sodium absorption, perhaps owing to a state of mild extracellular volume depletion. Hypokalemia should be prevented, which may aggravate further the renal concentrating defect. The potassium-sparing diuretic amiloride may be used instead of or in addition to thiazides (Alon and Chan, 1985). During states of dehydration and hypernatremia, fluid requirements in patients with H-NDI are higher than in other patients with hypernatremic dehydration (see Chapter 28); however, similar caution must be used in slowly lowering the serum sodium level (0.5 mEq/hr) to prevent brain damage.

PROGNOSIS

H-NDI is a life-long disease with good prognosis if dehydration and hypernatremia are prevented. However, mental retardation is often present in older children with H-NDI if the diagnosis is delayed (Ruess and Rosenthal, 1963). Children should be encouraged to urinate frequently to prevent development of large atonic bladders with hydroureter and hydronephrosis (ten Bensel and Peters, 1970). Genetic counseling should be provided to families. Recent reports suggest that the H-NDI gene is located on the long arm of the X-chromosome (Knoers et al., 1988), and prenatal diagnosis may be possible in the near future.

■ PSEUDOHYPOALDOSTERONISM

Pseudohypoaldosteronism is a renal tubular disorder characterized by urinary sodium wasting, hyponatremia, and hyperkalemia due to an inability of the distal tubule to respond to endogenous aldosterone or exogenously administered mineralocorticoids. See Chapter 107 for details.

■ BARTTER SYNDROME

Bartter syndrome is a renal tubular disorder characterized by renal potassium and chloride wasting, hypokalemia and hypochloremic metabolic alkalosis, increased plasma renin activity and angiotensin II and aldosterone levels, normal blood pressure and reduced sensitivity to angiotensin II, enhanced urinary prostaglandin excretion, and hyperplasia of the juxtaglomerular apparatus on renal biopsy (Dillon, 1987; Stein, 1985). In addition, several other abnormalities, including reduced tubular sodium reabsorption, defective renal acidification, magnesium deficiency, hypercalciuria, hypophosphatemia, renal failure, defective red blood cell sodium and potassium transport, and defective platelet aggregation have been reported occasionally (Dillon, 1987). Stein (1985) has proposed that Bartter syndrome may be a common expression of at least three well-defined defects in renal tubular function and has subdivided Bartter syndrome into type I, type II, and type III. A clinical picture similar to that of Bartter syndrome has been described in several infants who were accidentally fed a chloride-deficient formula (Roy and Arant, 1981). In older patients, diuretic or laxative abuse may also have similar clinical features.

CLINICAL PRESENTATION

The majority of patients first present during infancy with failure to thrive, periodic vomiting, and constipation. There may be a history of polyuria, polydipsia, and muscle weakness or hypotonia. Episodes of dehydration are common. Also, some patients have distinctive facial features with prominent forehead, drooping mouth, and protruding pinnae. Some infants may have developmental delay, but ultimate mental retardation is uncommon. Bartter syndrome may occasionally be present in siblings and is probably transmitted in an autosomal recessive fashion.

DIAGNOSIS

The diagnosis of Bartter syndrome is made when the following findings are present: hypokalemia, hypochloremic alkalosis, increased urinary potassium and chloride excretion, and hyperreninemia with normal blood pressure. Other disorders that may give rise to similar (but not identical) findings (e.g., diuretic abuse, hyperaldosteronism) must be excluded.

TREATMENT

Treatment is symptomatic. The goals of therapy are to maintain the serum potassium level consistently above 3.5 mEq/l. Potassium chloride supplements, 5 to 10 mEq/kg/day, are usually required in most patients. If this therapy fails (which it often does), indomethacin, triamterene, spironolactone, propranolol, enlapril, or ibuprofen may be tried with variable success. Potassium supplementation and indomethacin appear to be the most effective therapy.

PROGNOSIS

The long-term prognosis of Bartter syndrome is variable and to some extent depends on the severity of multiple defects present in the patient. Most children whose electrolyte balance is controlled to normal range have potential for normal stature and normal renal function. Some patients, especially those with glomerular or interstitial renal abnormalities and nephrocalcinosis, develop progressive renal failure.

■ RENAL TUBULAR ACIDOSIS

Renal tubular acidosis (RTA) is a clinical state characterized by hyperchloremic metabolic acidosis secondary to an impaired renal acidification (Chan, 1983; DuBose and Alpern, 1989; Kurtzman, 1987; Portale et al., 1987). The acidification defect may be an inability of the proximal tubule to reabsorb an adequate amount of filtered bicarbonate, called proximal RTA (i.e., type II); an inability of the distal tubule to generate enough hydrogen ion (H^+) gradient, called distal RTA (type I or classic); or a derangement of multiple distal tubular functions, called hyperkalemic RTA (type IV) due to associated hyperkalemia (types I and II RTA, in contrast, are frequently associated with hypokalemia). The term type III RTA is generally not used because the proposed type III RTA seems to be a variant of type I RTA. All three types of RTA may be primary (idiopathic) or secondary to a variety of medical disorders, as listed in Table 105–3.

NORMAL RENAL ACID-BASE REGULATION

The kidney regulates acid-base homeostasis by first reclaiming filtered bicarbonate and then generates bicarbonate by excreting net acid in the form of titratable acid and ammonium ion (NH_4^+). In older children and adults, approximately 2500 mEq/m^2 bicarbonate is filtered into the proximal tubule daily; in newborns the amount filtered is decreased owing to a reduced glomerular filtration rate and low plasma bicarbonate concentration (see also Chapter 90). In older children and adults nearly 85 per cent of the filtered bicarbonate is reabsorbed in the proximal tubule; in newborns only 65 to 70 per cent is reabsorbed in this segment (Chan, 1983). The remaining bicarbonate is reabsorbed in the loop of Henle and distal and collecting tubules. The renal threshold for bicarbonate in the term infant in usual states of hydration is close to 20 to 22 mEq/l and in the preterm infant, 18 to 20 mEq/l, compared with 24 to 26 mEq/l in the older child and adult (Edelmann et al., 1967; Portale et al., 1987; Schwartz et al., 1979) (see also Chapter 90).

The reabsorption of bicarbonate involves secretion of H^+ by the renal tubule. In the proximal tubule, the secretion of H^+ is primarily mediated by an electroneutral exchange of H^+ for sodium ion (Na^+) effected by a Na^+/H^+ antiporter (exchanger) located in the brush border

TABLE 105–3. Etiology of Renal Tubular Acidosis*

PROXIMAL RTA (TYPE II)
Isolated bicarbonate absorption defect
  Primary (idiopathic)†
    Sporadic or familial
  Carbonic anhydrase II deficiency
    Osteopetrosis†
Generalized defect (Fanconi syndrome)
  Primary (idiopathic)†
    Sporadic or familial
  Inborn errors of metabolism
    Cystinosis†
    Tyrosinemia†
    Wilson disease†
    Galactosemia†
    Lowe syndrome†
    Others
  Vitamin D deficiency or dependence†
  Toxins or drugs
    Heavy metal poisoning
    Outdated tetracycline

DISTAL RTA (TYPE I, CLASSIC)
Primary (idiopathic)
  Familial or sporadic†
Secondary (acquired)
  Genetic systemic diseases
    Hereditary elliptocytosis†
    Ehlers-Danlos syndrome
  Disorders with nephrocalcinosis
    Hypercalciuria†
    Hyperparathyroidism
    Vitamin D intoxication†
  Interstitial renal disease
    Obstructive uropathy (some patients)†
    Pyelonephritis
  Drugs and toxins
    Amphotericin B†
    Lithium

HYPERKALEMIC RTA (TYPE IV)
Aldosterone deficiency
  Adrenogenital syndrome†
  Primary hypoaldosteronism†
  Addison disease
Attenuated aldosterone response
  Pseudohypoaldosteronism†
  Obstructive uropathy (some patients)†
  Drugs
    Spironolactone
    Triamterene
    Amiloride
Hyporeninemic hypoaldosteronism
  Diabetes mellitus
  Obstructive uropathy (some patients)†
  Interstitial nephritis
  Lupus nephritis
  Uncertain pathophysiology

*This is an incomplete list of disorders. A more comprehensive list is found in the work of DuBose and Alpern (1989) and Portale and coworkers (1987).

†These disorders may be seen in the newborn period and early infancy.

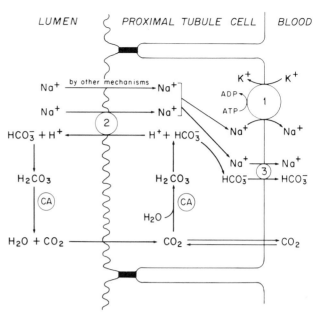

FIGURE 105–1. Proximal tubular cell secretion of H^+ into the lumen and reabsorption of HCO_3^- from the lumen. The energy for H^+ secretion is indirectly provided by ATP generated by Na/K ATPase (1) in the basolateral membrane. The secretion of H^+ ion into the lumen is mediated by Na^+/H^+ antiporter (2). The transfer of HCO_3 from cell to blood is mediated by Na^+/HCO_3^- Symporter (3). The luminal brush border of proximal tubule cells contains carbonic anhydrase (CA) that catalyzes the breakdown of carbonic acid to CO_2 (and the reverse inside the cell).

(DuBose and Alpern, 1989; Weinman et al., 1989). The bicarbonate generated inside the tubular cell during H^+ secretion is transported to blood with the help of a Na^+/HCO_3^- symporter (Figure 105–1) (DuBose and Alpern, 1989; Gluck, 1989). The energy for the H^+ secretion is indirectly provided by adenosine triphosphate (ATP) generated by sodium-potassium (Na^+/K^+)-ATPase located in the basolateral membrane of the tubular cell. The H^+ secreted in the proximal tubule combines with filtered bicarbonate to form carbonic acid, which dissociates into carbon dioxide and water. These reactions are catalyzed by carbonic anhydrase present in the brush border, whereby the proximal tubule can reabsorb large amounts of bicarbonate. Also, the proximal tubule is a "leaky" epithelium that prevents generation of a large electrical or H^+ concentration gradient. Thus, the proximal tubule is a high-capacity but low-gradient system and although large amounts of filtered bicarbonate are reabsorbed no net H^+ is excreted.

In the distal and collecting tubules, the secretion of H^+ is mediated by an electrogenic ATP-dependent proton pump (H^+-ATPase), located in the luminal membrane of selected cell types (Gluck, 1989). This electrogenic H^+ secretion (i.e., capability to transport a net positive charge in lumen) is not directly dependent on sodium absorption; however, the rate of H^+ secretion may be indirectly enhanced by the lumen's negative electrical potential difference generated by Na^+ reabsorption (Portale et al., 1987). Aldosterone also potentiates this H^+ secretion. The distal and collecting tubules have a "tight" epithelium that allows generations of steep H^+ concentration or electrical gradient. The urinary pH in the distal and collecting tubule may become as low as 4.4 (or 4.5), which is a 1000-fold higher H^+ concentration than in blood. The urinary excretion of free H^+ at pH 4.4, however, is less than one mEq/day, and the bulk of H^+ must be excreted in buffered form. The lowering of urinary pH to values less than 5.5 is essential in the distal tubule for adequate excretion of titratable acid and NH_4^+. There are several urinary buffer systems; the most important are the closed sodium hydrogen and dihydrogen phosphate (Na_2HPO_4/NaH_2PO_4) and the open ammonia and ammonium (NH_3/NH_4^+) systems (DuBose and Alpern, 1989). At low urine pH, H^+ is trapped with Na_2HPO_4 and excreted in urine as NaH_2PO_4. Urinary ammonia is produced from glutamine in all tubular segments but predominantly by the proximal tubule. In the loop of Henle, by a complex process, the ammonia effluxes into the medullary interstitium and later diffuses into the collecting tubule, where it is trapped as NH_4^+ (when luminar pH is low) and excreted in urine. Thus, the distal tubule is a low-capacity (for bicarbonate reabsorption) but high-gradient system, and it allows the body to excrete net acid to compensate for nonvolatile H^+ produced daily. Although distal and collecting tubules are generally thought of as sites where H^+ is actively secreted, data clearly show that specific distal and collecting tubular cells are also capable of directly secreting bicarbonate (in alkalotic states) into the urine (DuBose and Alpern, 1989; Gluck, 1989).

In adults the daily production and excretion of nonvolatile acid is approximately 1 mEq/kg/day, depending on the protein content of the diet. In newborns and infants, acid production and excretion has been estimated to be 2 to 3 mEq/kg/day (Chan, 1983). The higher H^+ excretion in the newborn has been partly explained on the basis of higher protein intake and accretion of calcium in bone that traps alkali but makes it necessary to excrete a corresponding amount of extra H^+ produced.

PATHOGENESIS

PROXIMAL RENAL TUBULAR ACIDOSIS

Proximal RTA results from reduced reabsorption of bicarbonate (Soriano et al., 1967), whereby, instead of reabsorbing the usual 85 per cent of filtered bicarbonate, the proximal tubule may reabsorb only 60 to 70 per cent (and in the newborn, even a lesser amount). Therefore, the distal tubular sites are presented with large amounts of bicarbonate that exceed their limited reabsorption capacity and as much as 15 to 20 per cent of filtered bicarbonate may be excreted (i.e., fractional excretion) in the urine. Due to urinary bicarbonate wasting, the serum bicarbonate value falls until the filtered bicarbonate level decreases to a point that most of it can be reabsorbed in the proximal tubule and the amount escaping to the distal tubule is sufficiently small that it can be completely reabsorbed. This new serum bicarbonate threshold level usually varies between 13 and 18 mEq/l. Because the distal tubular function is normal, when serum bicarbonate values fall below the threshold level, urine is appropriately acidified with pH less than 5.5 and titratable acid and ammonium excretion become normal (Soriano et al., 1967). Flooding of the distal tubule with sodium bicarbonate promotes sodium absorption in the distal tubule to prevent extracellular volume depletion and indirectly also increases potassium excretion. Depletion of extracellular volume also promotes chloride reabsorption (hyperchloremia) and aldosterone secretion, which may further enhance potassium losses.

Proximal RTA may occur as an isolated defect of acidification in the proximal tubule. The disorder is very uncommon, may be sporadic or familial, and is often transient. The isolated defect could be the result of a selective dysfunction of the Na^+/H^+ antiporter or carbonic anhydrase II located in the brush border or a defect in the Na^+/HCO_3^- symporter located in the basolateral membrane (DuBose and Alpern, 1989; Portale et al., 1987; Weinman et al., 1989).

More commonly, proximal RTA occurs as a generalized defect in proximal tubular function and patients have associated glycosuria, aminoaciduria, and phosphaturia (Fanconi syndrome). The cellular defect may be the result of an impairment of Na^+/K^+-ATPase or cellular phosphate depletion (DuBose and Alpern, 1989).

DISTAL RENAL TUBULAR ACIDOSIS

The pathogenesis of distal RTA is best explained by a reduced net rate of H^+ secretion by the distal and collecting tubules. The reduction of net H^+ secretion may result from (1) a reduced rate of H^+ secretion from distal tubular cell to lumen because of a defect in proton pump (H^+-ATPase), which makes it unable to secrete H^+ against a large plasma-to-lumen pH gradient; or (2) an increased tubular cell membrane permeability that allows passive back leak (from lumen to cell) of secreted H^+ or back leak of bicarbonate from cell to lumen (Portale et al., 1987). The reduction in net H^+ secretion decreases bicarbonate absorption in the distal sites; however, because most of bicarbonate has already been reabsorbed in more proximal sites, the fractional excretion of bicarbonate is less than 5 per cent. Moreover, because of reduced net H^+ secretion, the urinary pH cannot be reduced below 5.5 (usually >6) and urinary excretion of titratable acid and NH_4^+ is reduced despite severe metabolic acidosis (in contrast to proximal RTA). Hypokalemia, hypercalciuria, and hypocitraturia frequently accompany distal RTA, but proximal renal tubular functions are normal. Mild sodium wasting in untreated distal RTA is common. Contraction of the extracellular space stimulates secretion of renin and alodosterone, leading to potassium wasting. Hypercalciuria probably results from either a primary metabolic defect or from effects of persistent metabolic acidosis on bone (DuBose and Alpern, 1989; Portale et al., 1987). Nephrocalcinosis is common.

Distal RTA may be a primary inherited or a sporadic defect. It may also occur secondary to a number of disorders listed in Table 105–3.

HYPERKALEMIC RENAL TUBULAR ACIDOSIS

The acidification defect in this disorder may result from a defect in the generation of transepithelial potential difference in the collecting tubule, which impairs the ability to maximally secrete H^+ and also decreases K^+ secretion. The ability of the tubule to lower urine pH to values below 5.5, however, is maintained (DuBose and Alpern, 1989; Portale et al., 1987). The disorder is typically seen in patients with aldosterone deficiency or reduced tubular responsiveness to aldosterone. The excretion of NH_4^+ is also reduced, in part due to the associated hyperkalemia (Hulter et al., 1977).

CLINICAL PRESENTATION

In many patients with RTA (see Table 105–3) the disorder first manifests during the newborn period or early infancy. The usual findings are nonspecific and include failure to thrive, irritability, vomiting, constipation, polyuria, and polydipsia. Other clinical findings depend on the type of RTA and the primary disorder that led to the RTA. Patients with Fanconi syndrome may develop metabolic bone disease, patients with distal RTA may have nephrocalcinosis, and female infants with adrenogenital syndrome may show masculinization of the genitalia.

DIAGNOSIS

The diagnosis of RTA should be considered in any infant who presents with hyperchloremic metabolic acidosis (normal anion gap) and in whom other causes of metabolic acidosis (see Chapter 28) have been excluded. The urine pH should always be interpreted in relationship to plasma bicarbonate values. A persistently alkaline urine (or pH >6.0) irrespective of the severity of metabolic acidosis is strongly suggestive of distal RTA. A urine sample for the measurement of pH should be collected under a thin layer of mineral oil or taken up in a syringe to prevent loss of carbon dioxide and an increase of pH (Portale et al., 1987). The pH of urine is best measured with a pH meter.

Patients with proximal RTA frequently have an acid urine pH; however, when their serum bicarbonate level is raised above the threshold level by alkali therapy, the urine pH promptly becomes alkaline. Most patients with proximal RTA have multiple proximal renal tubular defects, and urine should be screened for aminoaciduria, phosphaturia, and glycosuria. Some patients have mixed type I and type II RTA and present both with decreased bicarbonate absorption in the proximal tubule and the inability to generate H^+ gradient in distal sites.

Diagnosis of type IV RTA is suggested when RTA is associated with hyperkalemia. Plasma renin and aldosterone levels should be measured to determine the cause of the type IV RTA (see Table 105–3).

In cases in which the diagnosis is in doubt, it may be necessary to measure urinary excretion of NH_4^+ and titratable acid following ammonium chloride loading (Edelmann et al., 1967). Other patients may occasionally require bicarbonate titration studies and measurement of fractional excretion of bicarbonate and urinary/blood PCO_2

gradient to differentiate between various types of acidosis (Table 105–4).

TREATMENT

The goals of therapy are to correct metabolic acidosis and maintain normal serum bicarbonate and potassium levels. Patients with severe metabolic acidosis and hypokalemia should be initially treated with intravenous therapy; otherwise, most patients can be managed by oral therapy. Patients may be given sodium bicarbonate or sodium citrate (Shohl solution). If potassium deficiency is present, potassium citrate should be added to the therapy. Most patients with distal RTA require 2 to 3 mEq/kg/day sodium bicarbonate (or citrate) in three to four divided doses. Patients with mixed distal and proximal RTA may require 5 to 10 mEq/kg/day of sodium bicarbonate. Patients with proximal RTA may require 5 to 20 mEq/kg/day of sodium bicarbonate to maintain normal serum bicarbonate and pH values. Some patients with proximal RTA who do not tolerate such high doses of bicarbonate therapy may benefit from thiazide diuretics (hydrochlorothiazide 1 mg/kg/day). The thiazide diuretics increase proximal tubular reabsorption of bicarbonate by inducing extracellular volume contraction. Patients with type IV RTA and aldosterone deficiency usually benefit from use of a mineralocorticoid (fluorohydrocortisone). Other patients with type IV RTA usually require 1 to 2 mEq/kg/day of sodium bicarbonate to correct acidosis.

PROGNOSIS

Most infants with isolated proximal RTA usually have a transient disorder lasting a few months to a couple of years. Although they initially require a large amount of bicarbonate therapy, their long-term prognosis is excellent. The prognosis in patients with Fanconi syndrome depends on the cause of the syndrome. Patients with primary distal RTA have a life-long disorder; however, with early recognition and adequate sustained therapy nephrocalcinosis may be prevented and normal growth achieved (McSherry and Morris, 1978). Patients with inadequate treatment

TABLE 105–4. Clinical and Laboratory Characteristics of Various Types of RTA

	TYPE I (DISTAL, CLASSIC)	TYPE II (PROXIMAL)	TYPE IV (HYPERKALEMIC)
During acidosis (low serum bicarbonate)			
Urine pH	> 6.0	< 5.5	< 5.5
Serum potassium	N or ↓	N or ↓	↑
Titratable acid and ammonium excretion	↓	N or ↓	↓
Urinary citrate	↓	↑	?
Aminoaciduria, glycosuria	—	±	—
Following therapy (normal bicarbonate)			
Fractional excretion of bicarbonate	3%–5%	> 15%	1%–15%
Serum potassium	N	N or ↓	N or ↑
Urinary-blood PCO_2 difference	< 20	> 20	< 20
Daily alkali treatment (mEq/kg/day)	1–4	5–20	1–4
Nephrocalcinosis	Common	Rare	Absent

N = normal.

(Data from Chan, J. C. M.: Renal tubular acidosis. J. Pediatr. *102:*32, 1983; DuBose, T. D., and Alpern, R. J.: Renal tubular acidosis. *In* Scriver, C. R., Beaudet, A. L., Sly, W. S., and Valle, D. [Eds.]: The Metabolic Basis of Inherited Disease. New York, McGraw-Hill Information Service Company, 1989, p. 2539; and Portale, A. A., Booth, B. E., and Morris, R. J.: Renal tubular acidosis. *In* Holliday, M. A., Barratt, T. M., and Vernier, R. L. [Eds.]: Pediatric Nephrology. Baltimore, Williams & Wilkins Company, 1987, p. 606.)

develop growth retardation, progressive nephrocalcinosis, and, ultimately, renal failure.

■ REFERENCES

Alon, U., and Chan, J. C.: Hydrochlorothiazide-amiloride in the treatment of congenital nephrogenic diabetes insipidus. Am. J. Nephrol. 5:9, 1985.

Bell, N. H., Clark, C. M., Avery, S., et al.: Demonstration of a defect in the formation of adenosine 3′,5′-monophosphate in vasopressin-resistant diabetes insipidus. Pediatr. Res. 8:223, 1974.

Chan, J. C. M.: Renal tubular acidosis. J. Pediatr. 102:32, 1983.

Chesney, R. W., and Novello, A. C.: Defects of renal tubular transport. In Massary, S. G., and Glassock, R. J. (Eds.): Textbook of Nephrology. Baltimore, Williams & Wilkins Company, 1989, p. 445.

Crawford, J. D., and Kennedy, G. C.: Chlorothiazide in diabetes insipidus. Nature 183:891, 1959.

Dillon, M. J.: Disorders of renal tubular handling of sodium and potassium. In Holliday, M. A., Barratt, T. M., and Vernier, R. L. (Eds.): Pediatric Nephrology. Baltimore, Williams & Wilkins Company, 1987, p. 598.

DuBose, T. D., and Alpern, R. J.: Renal tubular acidosis. In Scriver, C. R., Beaudet, A. L., Sly, W. S., and Valle, D. (Eds.): The Metabolic Basis of Inherited Disease. New York, McGraw-Hill Information Service Company, 1989, p. 2539.

Early, L. E., and Orloff, J.: The mechanism of antidiuresis associated with the administration of hydrochlorothiazide to patients with vasopressin-resistant diabetes insipidus. J. Clin. Invest. 41:1988, 1962.

Edelmann, C. M., Soriano, J. R., Boichis, H., et al.: Renal bicarbonate reabsorption and hydrogen ion excretion in normal infants. J. Clin. Invest. 46:1309, 1967.

Finberg, L.: Hypernatremic dehydration. Adv. Pediatr. 16:325, 1969.

Gluck, S. L.: Cellular and molecular aspects of renal H$^+$ transport. Hosp. Pract. 24(5):149, 1989.

Hays, R. M., Franki, N., Ding, G.: Effects of antidiuretic hormone on the collecting duct. Kidney Int. 31:530, 1987.

Holliday, M. A., Barratt, T. M., and Vernier, R. L. (Eds.): Pediatric Nephrology, section 8, Metabolic and Tubular Disease. Baltimore, Williams & Wilkins Company, 1987, p. 547.

Hulter, H. N., Ilnicki, L. P., Harbottle, J. A., et al.: Impaired renal H$^+$ secretion and NH$_3$ production in mineralocorticoid-deficient glucocorticoid-replete dogs. Am. J. Physiol. 232:F136, 1977.

Kaplan, S. A.: Nephrogenic diabetes insipidus. In Holliday, M. A., Barratt, T. M., Vernier, R. L. (Eds.): Pediatric Nephrology. Baltimore, Williams & Wilkins Company, 1987, p. 623.

Knoers, N. V., van der Heyden, H., van Vost, B. H., et al.: Nephrogenic diabetes insipidus: Close linkage with markers from the distal long arm of the human X chromosome. Hum. Genet. 80:31, 1988.

Kurtzman, N. A.: Renal tubular acidosis: A constellation of syndromes. Hosp. Pract. 22(11):173, 1987.

McSherry, E., and Morris, R. C.: Attainment and maintenance of normal structure with alkali therapy in infants and children with classic renal tubular acidosis. J. Clin. Invest. 61:509, 1978.

Ohzeki, T.: Urinary adenosine 3′,5′-monophosphate response to antidiuretic hormone in diabetes insipidus (DI): Comparison between congenital nephrogenic DI type 1 and 2 and vasopressin-sensitive DI. Acta Endocrinol. 108:485, 1985.

Portale, A. A., Booth, B. E., and Morris, R. J.: Renal tubular acidosis. In Holliday, M. A., Barratt, T. M., and Vernier, R. L. (Eds.): Pediatric Nephrology. Baltimore, Williams & Wilkins Company, 1987, p. 606.

Reeves, W. B., and Andreoli, T. E.: Nephrogenic diabetes insipidus. In Scriver, C. R., Beaudet, A. L., Sly, W. S., and Valle, D. (Eds.): The Metabolic Basis of Inherited Disease. New York, McGraw-Hill Information Service Company, 1989, p. 1985.

Roy, S., and Arant, B. S.: Hypokalemic metabolic alkalosis in normotensive infants with elevated plasma renin activity and hyperaldosteronism: Role of dietary chloride deficiency. Pediatrics 67:423, 1981.

Ruess, A. L., and Rosenthal, I. M.: Intelligence in nephrogenic diabetes insipidus. Am. J. Dis. Child 105:358, 1963.

Schrager, G. O., Josephson, B. H., Fine, B. F., et al.: Nephrogenic diabetes insipidus presenting as fever of unknown origin in the neonatal period. Clin. Pediatr. 15:1070, 1976.

Scriver, C. R., Beaudet, A. L., Sly, W. S., and Valle, D. (Eds.): The Metabolic Basis of Inherited Disease. New York, McGraw-Hill Information Service Company, 1989.

Schwartz, G. J., Haycock, G. B., and Chir, B.: Late metabolic acidosis: A reassessment of definition. J. Pediatr. 95:102, 1979.

Soriano, J. R., Boichis, H., Stark, H., et al.: Proximal renal tubular acidosis: A defect in bicarbonate absorption with normal urinary acidification. Pediatr. Res. 1:81, 1967.

Stein, J. H.: The pathogenetic spectrum of Bartter's syndrome. Kidney Int. 28:85, 1985.

ten Bensel, R. W., and Peters, E. R.: Progressive hydronephrosis, hydroureter and dilatation of the bladder in siblings with congenital nephrogenic diabetes insipidus. J. Pediatr. 77:439, 1970.

Weinman, E. J., Dubinsky, W. P., and Shenolikar, S.: Regulation of Na$^+$–H$^+$ exchanger. Hosp. Pract. 24(3):111, 1989.

PART XVII

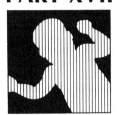

METABOLIC AND ENDOCRINE/EXOCRINE SYSTEMS

DISORDERS OF CALCIUM AND PHOSPHORUS METABOLISM

106

Constantine S. Anast*

■ GENERAL CONSIDERATIONS

The normal serum total calcium concentration varies only slightly with age and ranges between 8.8 and 10.6 mg/dl, with an average of 10 mg/dl. A normal serum calcium level of 10 mg/dl consists of approximately 5.5 mg/dl of diffusible calcium and 4.5 mg/dl of protein-bound calcium. Of the diffusible fraction, approximately 4.5 mg/dl is ionized, while the remainder is complexed to anions. The physiologically important fraction of extracellular calcium, which is the concentration that is closely controlled, is the ionized calcium. The serum inorganic phosphate concentration varies with age and sex and is highest during infancy, with a gradual decline to adulthood. Approximately 10 per cent of inorganic phosphate in serum is noncovalently bound to protein, while 90 per cent circulates as ions or complexes of HPO_4^{-2} and $H_2PO_4^{-1}$. The majority of total body calcium and phosphate is in the skeleton, in which hydroxyapatite, $Ca_5(OH)(PO_4)_3$, provides mechanical support as well as a reservoir of these important minerals. The principal hormones that control calcium and phosphate metabolism are parathyroid hormone, calcitonin, and vitamin D. The influence of these hormones on calcium and phosphorus metabolism is outlined in Figure 106–1.

Parathyroid hormone (PTH) is a single-chain polypeptide consisting of 84 amino acids with a molecular weight of 9500. The hormone is synthesized in the parathyroid gland as a larger molecule, proPTH, which is converted intracellularly into PTH by splitting off a hexapeptide at the aminoterminal end of the peptide chain. Following secretion, PTH is further cleaved into fragments. The aminoterminal portion (1–34) of the PTH molecule possesses full biologic activity, whereas the carboxyterminus is devoid of activity. Gel filtration studies indicate that most of the circulating immunoassayable PTH consists of a carboxyterminal fragment(s) and intact PTH. Immunocytologic studies indicate the presence of immunoreactive PTH-containing cells in the parathyroid gland of the fetus at 10 weeks' gestation (Leroyer-Alizon et al., 1981).

A fall in circulating ionized calcium level is the primary stimulus for secretion of PTH. The action of PTH at end organs is mediated through the adenylate cyclase–cyclic adenosine monophosphate (AMP) system. PTH promotes the resorption of calcium and phosphate from bone, increases the renal tubular absorption of calcium, and decreases the renal tubular reabsorption of phosphate. PTH stimulates the synthesis of 1,25-dihydroxyvitamin D in the kidney, which, in turn, increases the intestinal absorption of calcium and phosphate. The net effects of the action of PTH are an increase in circulating calcium and a decrease in circulating phosphate.

Calcitonin is produced by the parafollicular C cells of the thyroid gland. Immunocytologic studies indicate the presence of immunoreactive calcitonin in the C cells of the human fetal thyroid gland as early as 14 weeks' gestation (Leroyer-Alizon et al., 1980). The C-cell population and the concentration of immunoreactive calcitonin in the thyroid gland of newborns are much greater than in older subjects (Wolfe et al., 1975). Calcitonin is a single-chain polypeptide consisting of 32 amino acids with an aminoterminal seven-membered disulfide ring and a carboxyterminus of prolinamide. The primary stimulus for calcitonin secretion is a rise in the circulating calcium concentration. Calcitonin lowers the serum calcium and phosphate levels primarily by inhibiting bone resorption,

*Deceased.

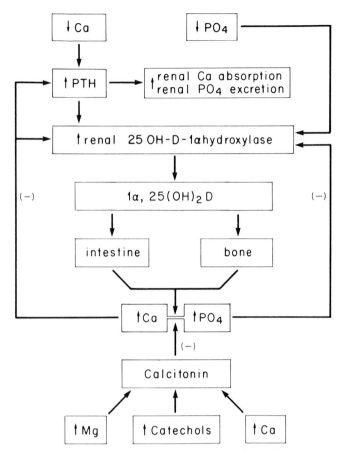

FIGURE 106–1. *Hormonal control of calcium and phosphorus metabolism.*

phate and acts on bone to enhance the resorption of calcium and phosphate.

■ PERINATAL CALCIUM METABOLISM

PARATHYROID HORMONE AND CALCITONIN

During pregnancy, the maternal total serum calcium concentration progressively declines, reaching a nadir at the middle of the third trimester and then increases slightly over the last 1 or 2 months of gestation (Pitkin and Gebhardt, 1977). Whether there is a significant change in maternal serum ionized calcium during pregnancy remains controversial. The maternal serum inorganic phosphate and magnesium levels exhibit patterns similar to that of total calcium during pregnancy. Although there is not complete agreement, most studies have demonstrated a gestational increase in maternal PTH levels. Several reports suggest that maternal levels of serum calcitonin increase during pregnancy. However, in one longitudinal study during pregnancy, 25 per cent of mothers exhibited relatively constant levels of calcitonin, 25 per cent had a progressive decline, and 50 per cent had a progressive increase to a maximum in the second trimester, followed by a decrement (Pitkin et al., 1979).

The total, ultrafilterable, ionized calcium and inorganic phosphate levels are higher in cord than in maternal plasma (Delivoria-Papadopoulis, 1967; Pitkin et al., 1979). This indicates that calcium and phosphate are transferred from mother to fetus against concentration gradients. There is no evidence that PTH and calcitonin cross the placenta. In normal newborns, the plasma calcium level decreases progressively after birth so that by the 2nd or 3rd day of life the level is lower than that found in older infants and children. The plasma calcium level usually returns to normal by 5 to 10 days of age in normal full-term infants. The serum PTH levels tend to be low in cord blood, whereas the calcitonin levels are normal or somewhat elevated (Anast and Dirksen, 1978; Hillman et al., 1977; Wieland et al., 1980). As the serum calcium level normally decreases during the first 48 hours of life, the serum PTH level increases to the normal range, and the serum calcitonin level increases sharply to peak at 13 to 24 hours of age. After 36 hours of age, there is a progressive decrease in the serum calcitonin level, but the level remains relatively high and above normal at the end of the 1st week of life (Hillman et al., 1977). The high serum calcitonin level in the neonatal period is consistent with the high C-cell population and calcitonin concentration in the thyroid gland of the newborn. It is possible that the elevated levels of calcitonin in the neonatal period contribute to the early fall in serum calcium level and that the serum PTH level increases as an appropriate physiologic response to the fall in the serum calcium level (Stevenson, 1983).

PERINATAL VITAMIN D METABOLISM

Maternal serum 25-OH-D varies with the season and vitamin D intake. The transport protein for vitamin D and its metabolites (DBP) increases in maternal serum during pregnancy (Bouillon and van Assche, 1982; Haddad et

although effects on urinary calcium and phosphate excretion as well as inhibition of intestinal mineral absorption have also been described.

Vitamin D, produced in the skin or absorbed by the gastrointestinal tract, is transported to the liver, where it is converted to 25-hydroxyvitamin D (25-OH-D). 25-OH-D is transported to the kidney, where it is converted to 1,25-dihydroxyvitamin D (1,25-$(OH)_2$-D) by renal tubular mitochondria. 1,25-$(OH)_2$-D is the most biologically active metabolite of vitamin D. The synthesis of 1,25-$(OH)_2$-D is increased by PTH and by phosphate depletion. Vitamin D, 25-OH-D, and 1,25-$(OH)_2$-D all circulate bound to an alpha-globulin (D-binding protein [DBP]). The normal circulating level of 25-OH-D is 10 to 50 ng/ml. The normal circulating concentration of 1,25-$(OH)_2$-D is approximately 1/1000 that of 25-OH-D and ranges from 30 to 75 pg/ml. Circulating 25-OH-D levels are increased by exposure to sunlight and by the ingestion of vitamin D and are decreased in vitamin D deficiency and in hepatocellular disorders. Circulating 1,25-$(OH)_2$-D levels are increased by hyperparathyroidism and in phosphate depletion and are reduced in hypoparathyroidism. Interestingly, circulating 1,25-$(OH)_2$-D levels may be either depressed or normal in vitamin D–deficient states (Chesney et al., 1981; Mawer, 1980). The normal levels are secondary to increased conversion of low substrate concentrations of 25-OH-D to 1,25-$(OH)_2$-D by increased circulating PTH levels and depressed circulating inorganic phosphate levels that occur in vitamin D deficiency. 1,25-$(OH)_2$-D acts on the intestine to increase the absorption of calcium and phosal., 1976). The calculated free concentration of 1,25-$(OH)_2$-D in maternal serum remains normal up to 35 weeks of gestation but increases significantly during the last 5 weeks of pregnancy. The human placenta can synthesize 1,25-$(OH)_2$-D, but the destination(s) of this placenta-produced vitamin D metabolite is uncertain (Tanaka et al., 1979; Weissman et al., 1979).

There is a close correlation between maternal and cord serum 25-OH-D levels consistent with a passive or facilitated transfer of this metabolite by the placenta (Bouillon and van Assche, 1982). Low levels may be found in infants born of mothers with low circulating levels of 25-OH-D resulting from poor dietary intake of vitamin D and lack of exposure to sunlight (Rosen et al., 1974). The serum 25-OH-D concentrations remain relatively stable during the 1st week of life in term infants, who will begin to correct low levels of this metabolite, if present. One study suggests that premature infants may have impaired ability to correct low levels or maintain normal serum levels of 25-OH-D (Hillman and Haddad, 1975).

Reports of the total cord serum levels of 1,25-$(OH)_2$-D at term vary. The reason for these divergent results is unknown. However, all studies agree that total cord serum levels of 1,25-$(OH)_2$-D at term are lower than the elevated maternal levels. The finding of higher levels of 1,25-$(OH)_2$-D in arterial than in venous cord blood suggests that the fetus might also synthesize this metabolite (Moore et al., 1985; Wieland et al., 1980).

■ NEONATAL CALCIUM METABOLISM

NEONATAL HYPOCALCEMIA

Neonatal hypocalcemia may be divided into the following clinical categories: (1) hypocalcemia occurring during the first 24 to 48 hours of life (early neonatal hypocalcemia), which is observed primarily in premature infants, sick infants, and in infants born after abnormal labor and pregnancy; (2) hypocalcemia found at the end of the 1st week of life (late neonatal hypocalcemia), which frequently appears in infants who have been fed cow's milk formulas that have an inherent high phosphorus load; (3) neonatal hypocalcemia associated with maternal hyperparathyroidism; (4) neonatal hypocalcemia associated with hypomagnesemia; and (5) other clinical entities, including primary hypoparathyroidism and renal abnormalities. These are summarized in Table 106–1. This classification is chosen for convenience, recognizing that in some cases the clinical separation may not be distinct.

Authors have variously defined neonatal hypocalcemia as a plasma calcium level less than 8 mg/dl, less than 7.5 mg/dl, or less than 7 mg/dl (Anast, 1975). The total circulating calcium concentration and the distribution between bound and ionized fractions are influenced by the protein concentration and pH of plasma. As indicated previously, 45 to 50 per cent of plasma calcium is bound to protein, but it is the ionized fraction that is biologically important. The determination of this ionized fraction is technically difficult, at present requiring large samples. Thus, most studies of neonatal calcium metabolism rely on measurements of total serum concentrations. Under basal conditions, the amount of total serum calcium is linearly correlated with levels of ionized calcium, and

TABLE 106–1. Causes of Neonatal Hypocalcemia

Early hypocalcemia (<48 hr of age)
  Prematurity
  Asphyxia/stress
  Infants of diabetic mothers
Late hypocalcemia (1st week of life)
  High phosphate load (of cow's milk)
  Relative maternal vitamin D deficiency
  Maternal hyperparathyroidism
  Hypomagnesemia
  Primary hypoparathyroidism
Miscellaneous disorders (may occur at any time)
  Therapy related
    Bicarbonate induced
    Transfusion of citrated blood
    Furosemide induced
    White light phototherapy
    Intravenous lipid administration
  Renal disease

various equations have been suggested that correct total serum calcium concentrations for pH and serum protein concentrations. However, these corrections are not valid in many of the pathophysiologic states in which they are employed. A precise definition of hypocalcemia in premature infants is particularly difficult and will probably be best defined by the level of ionized calcium. However, there is limited information regarding ionized calcium levels in premature infants, and a distinction between hypocalcemia and normocalcemia based on ionized calcium awaits further studies.

EARLY NEONATAL HYPOCALCEMIA

Early neonatal hypocalcemia is most frequently seen in premature infants as well as asphyxiated infants and infants of diabetic mothers. Premature infants demonstrate an exaggeration of the fall in serum calcium level seen in term infants, with a nadir occurring earlier (24 hours) and lower, with the decrease being inversely proportional to the gestation. The total serum calcium levels commonly fall below 7.0 mg/dl in premature infants. However, the fall in ionized calcium is not comparable to the fall in total calcium and the ratio of ionized to total calcium is higher in these infants (Scott et al., 1979). The reason for the maintenance of ionized calcium is uncertain but is probably related to the low serum protein concentration found in premature infants. This sparing effect of the ionized calcium may, in part, explain the frequent lack of signs of hypocalcemia in premature infants.

The pathogenesis of early neonatal hypocalcemia in premature infants is uncertain. The finding of elevated circulating levels of parathyroid hormone in several studies is consistent with an appropriate physiologic response of the parathyroid glands to hypocalcemia in premature infants (Anast and Dirksen, 1977, 1978; David et al., 1977, 1981; Hillman et al., 1977). Moreover, these studies indicate that factors other than parathyroid insufficiency act to lower the serum calcium in most premature infants.

The possibility that an abnormality in vitamin D metabolism plays a pathogenic role in the hypocalcemia of premature infants has been considered, but there is only limited information regarding this point. Studies have been performed on premature infants older than 31 weeks' gestation, and there is little or no information in infants of lower gestational age. There are studies that suggest impaired conversion of vitamin D to 25-OH-D by the liver. However, the presence of hypocalcemia in premature infants with normal circulating 25-OH-D and 1,25-(OH)$_2$-D levels suggests that impaired vitamin D metabolism is not the central factor in early hypocalcemia of prematurity (Glorieux et al., 1981).

Available evidence indicates that hypercalcitonemia may be an etiologic factor in the hypocalcemia of prematurity (Anast and Dirksen, 1977, 1978; David et al., 1977; Salle et al., 1977; Schedewie et al., 1978). An inverse correlation between gestational age and serum calcitonin levels as well as between serum calcitonin and serum calcium levels has been reported.

The finding of reduced phosphaturic and renal cyclic AMP responses to parathyroid extract in premature infants during the first few days of life suggests that refractoriness to PTH is a pathogenic factor (Linarelli et al., 1973). However, in contrast to the impaired renal response to parathyroid extract, a significant calcemic response to PTH administration in premature infants has been reported (Tsang et al., 1973). The role that refractoriness to PTH plays in the pathogenesis of neonatal hypocalcemia has not been clearly established.

Early neonatal hypocalcemia is frequently observed in asphyxiated infants. The etiology of this observation is probably complex. Levels of both circulating calcitonin and PTH have been reported to be elevated in these infants (Schedewie et al., 1978). Hyperphosphatemia resulting from increased tissue catabolism may induce a state of relative PTH resistance in these infants (Tsang et al., 1974). Furthermore, effective vitamin D hydroxylation is likely to be impaired in these infants, owing to effects of hyperphosphatemia and metabolic acidosis on renal 25-OH-D-1 hydroxylase activity. High levels of cortisol associated with neonatal distress may further antagonize the effects of vitamin D in intestinal absorption of calcium.

Early neonatal hypocalcemia is also frequent in infants of diabetic mothers. No consistent abnormality in vitamin D metabolism has been observed (Fleischman et al., 1978; Steichen et al., 1981), and the serum calcitonin level is not usually increased (Schedewie et al., 1979). A tendency to higher serum phosphorus concentration and to a delay in the neonatal increase in circulating PTH has been reported in infants of diabetic mothers (Schedewie et al., 1979; Tsang et al., 1975). Asphyxia and impaired placental function may also play a role promoting the hypocalcemia characteristic of infants of diabetic mothers.

LATE NEONATAL HYPOCALCEMIA

Late neonatal hypocalcemia most often occurs in fullterm infants. The incidence is higher in males than in females and varies according to feeding practice. The signs and symptoms of hypocalcemia usually occur at the end of the 1st week of life, most often in infants fed cow's milk formulas but occasionally in breast-fed infants. Human milk contains 150 mg/l of phosphorus as compared with 1000 mg/l in cow's milk and 500 mg/l in infant feedings prepared from cow's milk whey or isolated soy bean protein. Hyperphosphatemia is a prominent feature of late neonatal hypocalcemia. The ingestion of a relatively high phosphate load coupled with a low glomerular filtra-

tion rate in the neonatal period leads to an increase in serum phosphate levels and a reciprocal decrease in serum calcium levels. The usual physiologic response to hypocalcemia is an increase in PTH secretion, which would lead to an increase in both urinary excretion of phosphate and tubular resorption of calcium. However, low circulating PTH levels have been observed in infants with late neonatal hypocalcemia, reflecting a state of functional hypoparathyroidism (Fakhraee et al., 1980). An increase in the serum calcium level is frequently observed in these infants when they are placed on a milk formula with a low phosphate concentration and calcium supplements. After several days to weeks, the serum PTH level increases and the infants are able to tolerate higher phosphate loads. The pathogenesis of this "transient hypoparathyroidism" in infants with late neonatal hypocalcemia is unknown.

Some studies suggest that the incidence of late neonatal hypocalcemia is higher in infants of mothers who have low or marginal vitamin D intakes during pregnancy (Cockburn et al., 1980; Purvis et al., 1973). In addition, a high incidence of enamel hypoplasia of incisor teeth is reported in these infants, reflecting a defect in mineralization in the last trimester of pregnancy. However, it is not clear how the relative vitamin D deficiency would lead to impaired parathyroid secretion in the newborn. It is possible that impaired parathyroid secretion and relative maternal vitamin D deficiency are independent but additive factors in the pathogenesis of late neonatal hypocalcemia.

NEONATAL HYPOCALCEMIA ASSOCIATED WITH MATERNAL HYPERPARATHYROIDISM

Hypocalcemia is commonly observed in infants born of hyperparathyroid mothers (Anast, 1976; Hartenstein and Gardner, 1966). These infants frequently manifest symptoms of increased neuromuscular irritability during the first 3 weeks of life. The serum calcium levels range from 5.0 to 7.5 mg/dl, and the serum inorganic phosphate levels are usually 8.0 mg/dl or higher. The hypocalcemia and increased neuromuscular irritability appear to be more prominent in infants who receive cow's milk formulas with their inherent high phosphate loads. Indeed, there are reports of two infants born of hyperparathyroid mothers who exhibited symptoms of hypocalcemia for the first time at ages 5 months (Friderichsen, 1938) and 1 year (Bruce and Strong, 1955), respectively, shortly after addition of cow's milk to the infant's diet. In some instances the symptoms of hypocalcemia are severe in these infants, and they may be resistant to antitetany therapy. However, there is eventual improvement with calcium therapy, which in some cases must be continued for several weeks.

It is postulated that in maternal hyperparathyroidism, the increase in serum calcium and circulating maternal PTH facilitates calcium transport across the placenta to the fetus. As a result, fetal hypercalcemia develops and fetal parathyroid gland suppression may be even greater than in normal pregnancy. The reason for the hypomagnesemia observed in some infants born of hyperparathyroid mothers is uncertain but conceivably could be (1) secondary to maternal magnesium depletion, which could be a complication of hyperparathyroidism; (2) secondary to transient neonatal hypoparathyroidism; and (3) secondary to hyperphosphatemia, which may result from transient hypoparathyroidism or the high phosphate level of cow's milk formulas or both.

The mothers of affected infants are hypercalcemic and hypophosphatemic. They may also be asymptomatic, and hypocalcemic tetany occurring in the infant has led to the diagnosis of hyperparathyroidism in an asymptomatic mother.

NEONATAL HYPOCALCEMIA ASSOCIATED WITH HYPOMAGNESEMIA

Hypomagnesemia may impair parathyroid function by at least two mechanisms and thus produce hypocalcemia. Hypomagnesemia impairs PTH secretion (Anast et al., 1972, 1976; Rude et al., 1976), and also blunts the end-organ response to PTH (Rude et al., 1976). Newborns with depressed serum magnesium levels may be divided into two groups: (1) those with chronic congenital low serum magnesium levels or primary hypomagnesemia with secondary hypocalcemia and (2) those with transient low serum magnesium levels. Chronic congenital hypomagnesemia with secondary hypocalcemia is a relatively rare disease that is due to an isolated defect in the intestinal transport of magnesium. The serum magnesium level is frequently less than 0.8 mg/dl (normal, 1.6 to 2.8 mg/dl), and circulating levels of PTH are low despite the presence of hypocalcemia. The administration of magnesium to these patients leads to spontaneous parallel increases in serum PTH levels, serum calcium levels, and renal phosphate clearance.

Transient low serum magnesium levels in the newborn period occur in association with hypocalcemia; or less commonly, the plasma calcium level may be normal. The serum magnesium level in infants with transient hypomagnesemia is usually higher than in infants with chronic hypomagnesemia, frequently ranging from 0.8 to 1.4 mg/dl. In many infants with transient hypomagnesemia, the plasma magnesium level increases spontaneously as the plasma calcium level returns to normal following the administration of calcium supplements. However, in other cases the hypocalcemia responds poorly to calcium therapy, but when magnesium salts are given, the plasma calcium level as well as the plasma magnesium level rises.

CONGENITAL HYPOPARATHYROIDISM

On a rare occasion neonatal hypocalcemia is secondary to congenital hypoparathyroidism. The hypocalcemia is associated with hyperphosphatemia and low circulating PTH levels. The hypoparathyroidism in these infants is permanent. Congenital hypoparathyroidism may be due to the isolated absence of the parathyroid glands. Most cases are sporadic, but both X-linked recessive and autosomal recessive inheritance occur. Congenital absence of the parathyroid glands may be associated with congenital absence of the thymus and a variety of congenital aortic arch or conotruncal anomalies (DiGeorge syndrome). This syndrome occurs as a sporadic disorder in both males and females. Infants with congenital hypoparathyroidism require lifelong treatment with vitamin D preparations.

OTHER DISORDERS ASSOCIATED WITH HYPOCALCEMIA

Various common therapeutic interventions are associated with hypocalcemia. Bicarbonate therapy, as well as any form of alkalosis, decreases ionized levels of calcium and bone resorption of calcium. Citrated blood transfusions can form nonionized calcium complexes, thus decreasing ionized calcium levels. Furosemide therapy promotes calciuresis as well as nephrolithiasis. Continuous phototherapy with white light has been associated with hypocalcemia attributed to cortisol-related effects on bone metabolism. Lipid infusions may elevate serum free fatty acid levels, which form insoluble complexes with calcium. Most of these effects are transient, and cessation of therapy is associated with a return to normal of serum calcium levels. The major exception is furosemide therapy, which, when prolonged, leads to bone demineralization through continued calciuresis. The use of thiazide diuretics may obviate this effect.

CLINICAL FINDINGS

Signs and symptoms are variable and are not necessarily related to the degree of hypocalcemia. Although some infants are severely affected, others may be asymptomatic with equally depressed serum calcium levels.

The major manifestation of hypocalcemia is tetany, which is hyperexcitability of the central and peripheral nervous system. Increased neuromuscular irritability and convulsions are characteristic symptoms of neonatal tetany. Infants with tetany tend to be jittery and hyperactive, and they frequently exhibit muscle jerking and twitching. There may be a heightened response to sensory stimuli such as loud sounds or jarring of the bed. Laryngospasm with inspiratory stridor, at times severe enough to cause anoxia, is occasionally observed. Carpopedal spasm and ankle clonus may be present. Frank convulsions may occur at any time in the course of the disorder and may be focal or generalized. Vomiting occurs relatively frequently in neonatal tetany, and in a small number of cases there may be hematemesis or melena. At times, the gastrointestinal symptoms are severe enough to dominate the clinical picture and to suggest intestinal obstruction. It is possible that the vomiting results from spasms of the smooth muscles of the gastrointestinal tract that may be induced by hypocalcemia.

Other signs that have been described in neonatal tetany include apnea, tachycardia, tachypnea, and edema. It has not been established that the nonspecific manifestations of tetany are causally related to the concentration of calcium in the serum.

TREATMENT

There is no unanimity regarding indications for treatment of hypocalcemic infants who are completely asymptomatic. Decisions may be particularly difficult in premature infants with early neonatal hypocalcemia who are frequently asymptomatic. There are no known long-term consequences of transient neonatal early hypocalcemia in premature infants. Treatment of these infants may be associated with more morbidity than the condition itself.

Extravascular extravasation of calcium leads to skin necrosis, often requiring surgical intervention. Intravenous boluses of calcium salts are associated with bradyarrhythmias. Infusion of calcium into the umbilical vessels is particularly hazardous and to be avoided. Inadvertent intrahepatic injection of calcium through an umbilical venous catheter (due to failure to reach the inferior vena cava) can cause hepatic necrosis, and intra-aortic infusion has been shown to lead to vasospasm of the mesenteric arteries (and thus predipose to necrotizing enterocolitis). In making a decision regarding treatment of asymptomatic hypocalcemic infants, the serum protein concentration and pH should be taken into consideration. Values of total serum calcium less than 6.5 mg/dl and of serum ionized calcium less than 2.5 mg/dl are arbitrarily used as indications for treatment of asymptomatic hypocalcemia in premature infants with early neonatal hypocalcemia.

The treatment of neonatal hypocalcemia consists primarily of the administration of calcium salts. The commonly used compounds are calcium gluconate, calcium lactate, and calcium chloride. In evaluating these therapeutic agents, one should remember that the calcium content of calcium chloride is 30 per cent, as compared with 17 per cent in calcium lactate and 9 per cent in calcium gluconate.

For emergency treatment of acute tetany, a 10 per cent solution of calcium gluconate may be given intravenously at a rate not to exceed 1 ml/min. The calcium solution should be administered slowly to avoid reactions such as circulatory collapse or vomiting. Careful observation of the infant is essential, and the injection should be discontinued at the first sign of bradycardia or as soon as the desired clinical result is obtained. The intravenous dose of calcium gluconate necessary to stop convulsions usually is 1 to 3 ml. Toxic reactions may be avoided if the maximum intravenous dose of calcium gluconate administered at any one time does not exceed 2.0 ml/kg; doses above 3.0 ml/kg should be administered with caution. If necessary, intravenous calcium therapy may be repeated three or four times in 24 hours to help control acute symptoms. Because of its acidic properties, calcium chloride should not be given intravenously or by gavage into the stomach.

After acute symptoms have been controlled, calcium therapy should be continued as needed to maintain the serum calcium level above 7.0 mg/dl. In part, the level of serum calcium to be achieved will depend on the level of total serum protein. In hypoproteinemic infants, lower levels of total serum calcium are normally present. In premature and other infants in whom the oral intake is limited, 5.0 ml/kg of 10 per cent calcium gluconate may be infused with intravenous fluids over a 24-hour period. If oral feedings are tolerated, Neo-Calglucon (calcium glubionate), which contains approximately 24 mg of calcium per milliliter, may be given in a dose of 2 ml/kg/day divided into four to six doses. Intravenous or oral calcium supplements may be continued until the serum calcium level stabilizes.

In late neonatal tetany, dietary factors are of importance, and measures should be taken to reduce the phosphate load and to increase the calcium-phosphorus ratio of feedings to 4:1. This can be accomplished by the use of low phosphorus feedings such as human milk or Similac PM 60/40 in conjunction with calcium supplements. The serum calcium and phosphorus levels should be monitored weekly and the calcium supplements discontinued in a stepwise fashion after several weeks.

Although there are reports of the use of vitamin D metabolites in the treatment and prevention of early neonatal hypocalcemia in premature infants, this approach cannot be recommended at this time, especially in view of evidence that premature infants older than 31 weeks' gestation have the capacity to synthesize 25-OH-D and 1,25-$(OH)_2$-D. It is recommended that premature infants routinely receive 400 to 600 IU of vitamin D daily.

The administration of magnesium salts is indicated to infants with neonatal tetany who have depressed serum magnesium levels. Magnesium may be administered intramuscularly as a 50 per cent solution of magnesium sulfate (there are 4 mEq of magnesium in 1.0 ml of 50 per cent USP $MgSo_4 \cdot 7 H_2O$). The suggested intramuscular or intravenous dose of 50 per cent magnesium sulfate is 0.1 to 0.2 ml/kg. If given intravenously, the infusion should be introduced slowly and cautiously, with electrocardiographic monitoring to detect acute disturbances, which may include prolongation of atrioventricular conduction time and sinoatrial or atrioventricular block. The magnesium dose may be repeated every 12 to 24 hours, depending on clinical response and monitoring of serum magnesium levels. In many infants with transient hypomagnesemia, one to two injections of magnesium are sufficient. Serum magnesium levels should be carefully monitored to guard against hypermagnesemia. Infants with primary hypomagnesemia will have permanently low serum magnesium levels and require lifelong treatment with oral magnesium supplements.

NEONATAL HYPERCALCEMIA

Hypercalcemia may be defined as a total serum calcium concentration greater than 11.0 mg/dl and an ionized calcium concentration greater than 5.0 mg/dl. Neonatal hypercalcemia is found in association with a number of clinical entities and, if severe, presents as a medical emergency. The clinical findings in neonatal hypercalcemia include poor feeding, vomiting, hypotonia, lethargy, polyuria, hypertension, respiratory difficulties, and seizures. Hypercalcemia causes polyuria and polydipsia by interfering with the action of the antidiuretic hormone on renal collecting ducts, resulting in dehydration. The central nervous system manifestations result from a direct effect of calcium on nerve cells as well as from hypertensive encephalopathy and cerebral ischemia. The hypertension is probably secondary to a direct vasoconstriction effect of calcium as well as to increased activity of the renin-angiotensin system resulting from renal arteriolar constriction. Persistent hypercalcemia may result in calcification in the kidney, skin, subcutaneous tissue, falx cerebri, arteries, myocardium, lung, and gastric mucosa.

The first principle in the medical management of hypercalcemia is to increase the urinary excretion of calcium by maximizing glomerular filtration and the urinary excretion of sodium. In the normal kidney, sodium clearance and calcium clearance are very closely linked during water or osmotic diuresis. Infants with severe neonatal hypercalcemia are frequently dehydrated. Two thirds to full strength saline containing 30 mEq of potassium chloride per liter is infused intravenously at a rate to correct dehydration and maximize the glomerular filtration rate. After rehydration, furosemide in a dose of 1 mg/kg may be given intravenously at 6- to 8-hour intervals to inhibit tubular reabsorption of calcium as well as sodium and water. In situations in which severe hypercalcemia is associated with hypophosphatemia, oral or intravenous phosphorus may be given in a dose of 30 to 50 mg/kg/day of phosphorus as a phosphate salt. Unlike sodium, phosphate does not remove calcium from the body but causes a redistribution of calcium. The goal of phosphate therapy is to maintain serum inorganic phosphate levels in a range of 3 to 5 mg/dl. The oral route for phosphate therapy is preferable, since serious immediate reactions have been reported with intravenous phosphate treatment. Therapy usually results in a significant reduction in serum calcium concentration over a 24- to 48-hour period. In more severe and resistant cases, cortisone, 10 mg/kg up to 300 mg/day, or prednisone, 2 mg/kg up to 60 mg/day, can be added to the therapeutic regimen. The hypocalcemic effects of glucocorticoids result from decreased intestinal absorption of calcium as well as increased renal excretion. Although effective in several types of hypercalcemic states, glucocorticoids are relatively ineffective in the treatment of hypercalcemia associated with primary hyperparathyroidism. More definitive and specific therapy depends on the underlying cause of the hypercalcemia.

NEONATAL PRIMARY HYPERPARATHYROIDISM

Neonatal primary hyperparathyroidism is an uncommon but life-threatening disorder (Hillman et al., 1964; Marx et al., 1982; Pratt et al., 1947; Thompson et al., 1978). The infants usually appear normal at birth, but there are reported observations of a depressed sternum, elfin facies, thoracolumbar kyphosis, and one dysmature infant with a narrow thorax and short femurs. Symptoms of hypercalcemia usually develop during the early days of life. Repeated serum calcium levels usually range between 15 and 30 mg/dl, and the serum inorganic phosphate concentration is frequently less than 3.5 mg/dl. Anemia, splenomegaly, and hepatomegaly have been reported. Skeletal roentgenograms reveal demineralization, subperiosteal bone resorption, and pathologic fractures. Renal calcinosis is a common finding. In some cases, consanguinity in normocalcemic parents or hypercalcemia in siblings suggests autosomal recessive transmission. In others, the presence of hypercalcemia in one parent as well as in one or more siblings suggests an autosomal dominant transmission. Of great interest is the recent observation of an association between neonatal severe primary hyperparathyroidism and familial hypocalciuric hypercalcemia (FHH) (Marx et al., 1982). FHH is an autosomal dominant trait in which family members have modest and usually asymptomatic hypercalcemia. The reason for the occurrence of severe neonatal hyperparathyroidism in kindreds with FHH is unknown. It is apparent, however, that serum calcium determinations should be carried out on all family members of infants with neonatal primary hyperparathyroidism. Neonatal hyperparathyroidism may also occur as part of the syndrome of multiple endocrine adenomatosis.

Surgical intervention may be required for effective treatment.

NEONATAL HYPERPARATHYROIDISM ASSOCIATED WITH MATERNAL HYPOPARATHYROIDISM

Congenital hyperparathyroidism may occur in infants born to mothers with poorly treated idiopathic or surgical hypoparathyroidism (Anast, 1976; Bronsky et al., 1968; Landing and Kamoshita, 1970; Saan et al., 1976). In contrast to infants with neonatal primary hyperparathyroidism, these infants frequently have low birth weights, serum calcium levels that are frequently depressed or normal rather than elevated, and serum inorganic phosphate levels that are normal to somewhat elevated rather than depressed. The reason for these differences in biochemical findings between the two groups is unknown. In one hyperparathyroid infant born of a hypoparathyroid mother, there was radiographic evidence of rickets as well as hyperparathyroidism and the serum 25-OH-D level was low (Saan et al., 1976). The authors concluded that hyperparathyroidism in the infant induced a state of vitamin D deficiency, possibly by increasing the requirement for vitamin D, as has been reported in some adults with primary hyperparathyroidism. The mortality rate in infants born of poorly or untreated hypoparathyroid mothers is high, especially in infants with birth weights less than 2000 g. In the infants who survive, the osseous abnormalities regress spontaneously, and roentgenograms are normal by 4 to 7 months of age. Correction of hypocalcemia in hypoparathyroid women during pregnancy will prevent the development of hyperparathyroidism in the fetus.

IDIOPATHIC HYPERCALCEMIA

A large number of cases of hypercalcemia were observed in infants in Great Britain during and shortly after World War II (Harrison and Harrison, 1979). Findings consistent with hypervitaminosis D were found, including osteoporosis and dense bands of mineralization at the metaphyseal ends of long bones. These infants were receiving 3000 to 4000 units of vitamin D per day as part of a concerted effort to prevent nutritional deficiencies in infants subjected to the disruptions of wartime. With the reduction of vitamin D intake to 400 units per day, the incidence of "idiopathic hypercalcemia" decreased markedly.

Idiopathic hypercalcemia may be found in association with the Williams elfin facies syndrome (White et al., 1977; Williams et al., 1961). The phenotypic features of this syndrome include depressed nasal bone, receding mandible, prominent maxilla, hypertelorism, short turned-up nose, prominent upper lip, and low-set ears. Cardiovascular disturbances are common, including supravalvular aortic stenosis and peripheral pulmonic arterial stenosis. Many of the infants manifest a late psychomotor development. The hypercalcemia associated with normal or increased serum inorganic phosphate levels and the radiographic findings differentiate Williams syndrome from primary hyperparathyroidism. In some patients, the serum calcium level is normal, but the presence of nephrocalcinosis and other soft tissue calcification suggests the previous presence of hypercalcemia. In still other infants with phenotypic features of Williams syndrome there is neither present nor past evidence of hypercalcemia, as reflected in normal serum calcium levels and the absence of soft tissue calcification. One treats idiopathic hypercalcemia by feeding a low calcium, low vitamin D diet and by administering glucocorticoids.

NEONATAL HYPERCALCEMIA ASSOCIATED WITH SUBCUTANEOUS FAT NECROSIS

Infantile hypercalcemia occurs in association with subcutaneous fat necrosis (Sharlin and Koblenzer, 1970). In the afflicted infants, indurated subcutaneous masses with bluish-red discoloration of the overlying skin develop in the early weeks of life. The serum phosphate level and the alkaline phosphatase activity are normal. Radiographs of the long bones are usually normal, although periosteal elevation has been described in one case and findings similar to those in Williams syndrome were reported in another. Ectopic calcification may be present. The reason for the hypercalcemia in these infants is unknown but may be related to prostaglandin release (Veldhuis et al., 1979). It is known that prostaglandins have potent bone resorptive actions and can thus induce hypercalcemia. The hypercalcemia associated with subcutaneous fat necrosis may persist for several days or weeks and has primarily been treated with glucocorticoids and low calcium diet. If further studies confirm that prostaglandin production is a pathogenic factor in this disorder, inhibitors of prostaglandin synthetase such as aspirin or indomethacin may be effective therapeutic agents.

BLUE DIAPER SYNDROME

Blue diaper syndrome is a rare familial disease in which hypercalcemia and nephrocalcinosis are associated with a defect in the intestinal transport of tryptophan (Drummond et al., 1964). Bacterial degradation of the tryptophan in the intestine leads to excessive indole production, which is converted to indican in the liver. The oxidative conjugation of two molecules of indican following elimination from the body forms the water-insoluble dye indigotin (indigo blue), which results in blue discoloration of the diaper. The clinical course is characterized by failure to thrive, recurrent unexplained fever, infections, marked irritability, and constipation. The mechanism of the hypercalcemia is uncertain, although oral tryptophan loading in both humans and experimental animals produces an increase in the serum calcium level. Treatment consists of glucocorticoid administration and a low calcium, low vitamin D diet.

HYPERCALCEMIA ASSOCIATED WITH ADRENAL INSUFFICIENCY

Modest hypercalcemia may occur in acute adrenal failure. The pathogenesis is uncertain, but there is evidence that the total but not the ionized calcium concentration is increased in adrenal insufficiency. It has been suggested that three alterations combine to produce the hypercalcemia in adrenal failure (Walser et al., 1963): (1) an elevated plasma protein concentration due to hemoconcentration; (2) an increase in the affinity of plasma protein for calcium due to the hyponatremia and low ionic strength of plasma; and (3) an increase in calcium complexes, especially calcium citrate and calcium phosphate. The increased serum calcium concentration does not depend on increased intestinal absorption, since it occurs in the presence of a calcium-free diet. The serum calcium level returns to normal with glucocorticoid replacement.

HYPERCALCEMIA ASSOCIATED WITH PHOSPHATE DEPLETION

Hypercalcemia occurs in phosphate depletion, which, in the neonatal period, is seen most commonly in low-birth-weight infants who are fed human milk (Rowe et al., 1979; Sagy et al., 1980). The low phosphate concentration in human milk leads to hypophosphatemia, which, in turn, leads to an increase in circulating 1,25-$(OH)_2$-D with attendant increased intestinal absorption of calcium. In the presence of hypophosphatemia, only limited amounts of calcium can be deposited in bone and rickets with hypercalcemia and hypercalciuria results. The treatment of this condition is discussed in the following section.

OSTEOPENIA IN PREMATURE INFANTS

Osteopenia in the context of this discussion is defined as radiologic evidence of diminished bone density. Osteopenia is present in rickets, osteomalacia, and osteoporosis.

Rickets is defined as a disturbance in growing bone in which there is a lag in the mineralization of matrix so that uncalcified cartilage matrix and uncalcified bone matrix (osteoid) accumulate to an abnormal extent. Roentgenographic findings in rickets include osteopenia (decreased bone density) and characteristic findings at the cartilage-shaft junction of growing bones, including an increase in the width of the growth plate, cupping, and fraying. In rickets, the serum inorganic phosphate or calcium level or both are characteristically depressed and the serum alkaline phosphatase level is elevated.

Osteomalacia is rickets that occurs in the presence of little or no linear skeletal growth, such as might occur in some premature infants. Radiologically, osteomalacia is characterized by osteopenia but lacks the radiologic features of rickets at the cartilage-shaft junction.

Osteoporosis is defined as a state of reduced bone mass per unit volume with a normal ratio of mineral to matrix. Unlike rickets and osteomalacia, in which the primary abnormality is a defect in mineralization, the primary abnormality in osteoporosis is either a decrease in matrix formation or an increase in matrix and mineral resorption. Osteoporosis may not be distinguishable from osteomalacia radiographically, since both are characterized by an osteopenia without the characteristics of rickets at the cartilage-shaft junction. In contrast to patients with rickets and osteomalacia, patients with osteoporosis have normal serum concentrations of calcium, inorganic phosphate, and alkaline phosphatase. In some disorders, histologic examination reveals evidence of both osteoporosis and osteomalacia.

Osteopenia with or without radiologic evidence of rickets at the cartilage-shaft junction is commonly observed between 3 and 12 weeks of age in premature infants, especially those with birth weights less than 1500 g. There have been limited pathologic studies of osteopenic bones of premature infants, so that the relative contributions of osteoporosis and rickets or osteomalacia to the pathogenesis of the reduced bone density is uncertain. It is pertinent, however, that histopathologic studies in three preterm infants who died after prolonged intravenous feeding and artificial ventilation revealed pronounced osteoporosis in addition to osteomalacia (Oppenheimer and Snodgrass, 1980). It is possible, therefore, that osteoporosis, secondary to either reduced bone matrix formation or increased bone matrix destruction, is present to a degree in osteopenic bones of premature infants. Nevertheless, the remainder of this discussion will deal primarily with rickets and osteomalacia in the premature infant, since most studies and attention have been addressed to this defect in bone mineralization.

The clinical findings in premature infants with rickets include craniotabes, bony expansion at the wrists, costochondral beading, and fractured ribs (Geggel et al., 1978). Respiratory distress (tachypnea) may occur secondary to demineralization and softening of the thoracic cage (Glasgow and Thomas, 1977).

The biochemical findings of rickets in premature infants are similar to those found in older children and adults with rickets and osteomalacia and include a low to low-normal serum calcium level, low to low-normal serum inorganic phosphate level, elevated alkaline phosphatase activity, and elevated circulating PTH, which occurs secondary to the hypocalcemia. In premature infants there may not be a good correlation between serum alkaline phosphatase activity and the other biochemical or radiologic findings of rickets. Generalized aminoaciduria may be present and is secondary to elevated circulating PTH. The aforementioned biochemical abnormalities are found in infants with radiologic evidence of frank rickets and may be found in some infants with osteopenia in which there is no radiographic evidence of rickets (Hillman et al., 1979). The abnormal biochemical findings in the latter suggest a component of osteomalacia. Two factors have received primary consideration in the pathogenesis of a bone mineral defect in premature infants: (1) mineral deficiency and (2) relative vitamin D deficiency with possible impaired metabolism of vitamin D.

Until recently, the majority of premature infants in the United States were fed commercial formulas that contained from 440 to 550 mg/l calcium, from 330 to 460 mg/l phosphorus, and 400 IU/l vitamin D. Eighty per cent of bone mineralization in the fetus occurs during the last trimester, when fetal calcium and phosphorus requirements are 100 to 120 mg/kg/day and 60 to 75 mg/kg/day, respectively (Ziegler et al., 1976). Thus, mineral content of the standard commercial formulas coupled with a relatively low intestinal calcium absorption rate in premature infants does not allow for in utero accretion of calcium and phosphate. As a means of circumventing this problem, preterm milk formulas have been modified to contain approximately 1200 mg/l of calcium and 600 mg/l of phosphorus. Reported studies suggest that feeding these high mineral content formulas increases the retention of calcium and phosphorus to levels that approximate in utero accretion rates and increases bone mineral content

as evaluated by photon absorptiometry (Steichen et al., 1980). Moreover, rickets has been observed in low-birth-weight infants (800 to 1200 g) receiving standard formulas (Similac 20, Ross Laboratories, or ProSobee, Mead Johnson) and 400 to 800 IU of vitamin D per day. Rapid improvement was observed following the administration of high mineral content formulas (calcium, 1260 mg/l; phosphorus, 630 mg/l) and 800 to 1200 IU of vitamin D per day (Steichen et al., 1981).

Biochemical and radiologic evidence of rickets has been observed in very low-birth-weight infants (750 to 1160 g) in whom the serum 25-OH-D levels were extremely low (Hoff et al., 1979). Serum 1,25-(OH)$_2$-D levels were not measured. The infants had received either a low calcium, low phosphorus "human milk-like" (Similac PM 60/40) formula or a soy protein formula. The mean daily intake of vitamin D since birth had been 300 ± 181 IU. The administration of 4000 IU of vitamin D daily without a change in formula resulted in an increase in serum 25-OH-D to normal and healing of the rickets. The low circulating 25-OH-D levels in these infants suggests either reduced intestinal absorption of vitamin D or impaired conversion of vitamin D to 25-OH-D in the liver. Further work is needed to settle this issue more clearly. The available evidence indicates that the premature infant of postconceptual age greater than 31 weeks' gestation can hydroxylate 25-OH-D to 1,25-(OH)$_2$-D in the kidney (Glorieux et al., 1981). Whether or not premature infants of younger postconceptual age have this capacity is unknown.

For a variety of reasons, human milk has recently been prescribed as a food source for premature infants. Because human milk has a low phosphate content, feeding it to rapidly growing premature infants has resulted in rickets associated with phosphate depletion (Rowe et al., 1979; Sagy et al., 1980). Characteristically, these infants have hypophosphatemia, hypercalcemia, hypercalciuria, normal or depressed serum PTH levels, normal 25-OH-D levels, and elevated serum 1,25-(OH)$_2$-D levels. The hypophosphatemia is the stimulus for the production of 1,25-(OH)$_2$-D, which, in turn, increases the intestinal absorption of calcium. In the presence of hypophosphatemia, only limited amounts of calcium can be deposited in bone, and hypercalcemia and hypercalciuria result. The hypercalcemia inhibits PTH secretion. Rickets in this disorder does not respond to vitamin D therapy but responds promptly to an increase in the ingestion of inorganic phosphate. This can be accomplished either by supplementing human milk with 20 to 25 mg/kg/day of phosphorus as potassium phosphate or by switching from human milk to a proprietary formula with a higher phosphate content. The phosphate supplements may reduce serum calcium levels to subnormal values and require the addition of calcium supplements in a dose of 30 mg/kg/day of calcium. Human milk contains small quantities of 25-OH-D (0.3 μg/l) and 1,25-(OH)$_2$-D (5 ng/l) (Hollis et al., 1981). The total antirachitic activity is only 25 IU/l, and it is apparent that premature infants fed human milk should receive vitamin D supplements, probably at a dose of 400 to 600 IU daily.

Copper deficiency is an unusual cause of osteopenia in premature infants. In a case reported by Tanaka and co-workers in 1980, the osteopenia was associated with flaring and cupping of the metaphyses of the long bones and irregular thickening of the provisional zones of calcification. The serum copper and ceruloplasmin concentrations were decreased. The serum alkaline phosphate activity was increased, whereas the serum calcium, phosphate, and 25-OH-D levels were normal. The administration of copper sulfate resulted in marked improvement in the radiographic appearance of the bones. The copper deficiency was attributed to the low copper concentration of the milk formula fed to the infant.

■ NEONATAL MAGNESIUM METABOLISM

Magnesium is the second most common intracellular cation, and it is required for many enzymatic reactions, particularly those that also require adenosine triphosphate. About 50 per cent of total body magnesium is in bone, and most of the rest is intracellular. Normal serum magnesium levels range between 1.6 and 2.8 mg/dl. Roughly 35 per cent of total serum magnesium is bound to serum proteins. Fetal magnesium levels are higher than maternal levels because of active transport across the placenta. However, in experimental magnesium deficiency in rats, the fetus becomes relatively more deficient than the mother (Dancis et al., 1971). Following birth, there is a rise in serum magnesium levels, except in infants receiving cow's milk formulas with an inherent high phosphate load (Anast, 1964; David and Anast, 1974).

HYPOMAGNESEMIA

This condition is discussed in a preceding section entitled Neonatal Hypocalcemia Associated with Hypomagnesemia.

HYPERMAGNESEMIA

Magnesium sulfate continues to be used in the management of eclampsia. Magnesium given to the mother readily crosses the placenta and causes elevation of fetal magnesium levels and neurologic depression of the newborn. In 1967, Lipsitz and English studied 16 infants born to toxemic mothers who had received 16 to 60 g of magnesium by continuous intravenous infusion for 12 to 24 hours prior to delivery. The mothers' blood levels of magnesium ranged from 3.6 to 17 mg/dl, and the infants' levels were between 4.9 and 14.0 mg/dl. A majority of the infants were cyanotic, flaccid, and unresponsive. Others had less severe signs, including delayed passage of meconium. Nine infants required tracheal intubation and respiratory support. There was no absolute correlation between cord blood levels and depth of depression, but symptoms disappeared within 24 to 48 hours with the steady fall in magnesium levels. Infusion of calcium salts has been used to antagonize some of the adverse effects of excess magnesium (Lipsitz, 1971).

■ REFERENCES

Anast, C. S.: Serum magnesium levels in the newborn. Pediatrics 33:969, 1964.

Anast, C. S.: Tetany of the newborn. In Gardner, L. I. (Ed.): Endocrine and Genetic Diseases of Childhood and Adolescence. Philadelphia, W. B. Saunders Company, 1975, pp. 377–399.

Anast, C. S.: Parathyroid hormone during pregnancy and effect on offspring. In New, M. I., and Fiser, R. H. (Eds.): Diabetes and Other Endocrine Disorders During Pregnancy in the Newborn. New York, Alan R. Liss, 1976, pp. 235–248.

Anast, C., and Dirksen, H.: Neonatal hypocalcemia. In Norman, A. W., Schaefer, K., Coburn, J. W., et al. (Eds.): Vitamin D: Biochemical, Chemical and Clinical Aspects Related to Calcium Metabolism. New York, Walter de Gruyter and Company, 1977, p. 727.

Anast, C. S., and Dirksen, H.: Studies related to the pathogenesis of neonatal hypocalcemia. In Copp, D. H., and Talmadge, R. V. (Eds.): Endocrinology of Calcium Metabolism. Amsterdam, Excerpta Medica Foundation, 1978, vol 421, p. 12.

Anast, C. S., Mohs, J. M., Kaplan, S. L., and Burns, T. W.: Evidence for parathyroid failure in magnesium deficiency. Science 177:606, 1972.

Bouillon, R., and van Assche, F. A.: Perinatal vitamin D metabolism. Dev. Pharmacol. Ther. 4(suppl. 1):1–30, 1982.

Bronsky, D., Kiamko, R. T., Moncada, R., and Rosenthal, I. M.: Intrauterine hyperparathyroidism secondary to maternal hypoparathyroidism. Pediatrics 42:606, 1968.

Bruce, J., and Strong, J. A.: Maternal hyperparathyroidism and parathyroid deficiency in child, with account of effect of parathyroidectomy on renal function and attempt to transplant part of tumor. Q. J. Med. 24:307, 1955.

Chesney, R. W., Zimmerman, J., Hamstra, A., et al.: Vitamin D metabolite concentrations in vitamin D deficiency. Am. J. Dis. Child. 135:1025, 1981.

Cockburn, F., Belton, N. R., Purvis, R. J., et al.: Maternal vitamin D intake and mineral metabolism in mothers and their newborn infants. Br. Med. J. 288:11, 1980.

Dancis, J., Springer, D., and Cohlan, S. Q.: Fetal homeostasis in maternal malnutrition: II. Magnesium deprivation. Pediatr. Res. 5:131, 1971.

David, L., and Anast, C.: Calcium metabolism in newborn infants: The interrelationship of parathyroid function and calcium, magnesium, and phosphorus metabolism in normal, "sick," and hypocalcemic newborns. J. Clin. Invest. 54:287, 1974.

David, L., Salle, B., Chopard, P., and Grafmeyer, D.: Studies on circulating immunoreactive calcitonin in low birth weight infants during the first 48 hours of life. Helv. Paediat. Acta 32:39, 1977.

David, L., Salle, B. L., Putet, G., and Grafmeyer, D.: Serum immunoreactive calcitonin in low birth weight infants: Description of early changes; effect of intravenous calcium infusion; relationships with early changes in serum calcium, phosphorus, magnesium, parathyroid hormone, and gastrin levels. Pediatr. Res. 15:803, 1981.

Delivoria-Papadopoulis, M., Battaglia, F. C., Bruns, P. D., and Meschia, G.: Total, protein-bound, and ultrafilterable calcium in maternal and fetal plasma. Am. J. Physiol. 213:363, 1967.

DeLuca H. F.: The vitamin D story: A collaborative effort of basic science and clinical medicine. FASEB J. 2:224, 1988.

Drummond, K. N., Michael, A. F., Ulstrom, R. A., and Good, R. A.: The blue diaper syndrome: Familial hypercalcemia with nephrocalcinosis and indicanuria. Am. J. Med. 37:928, 1964.

Fakhraee, S., Bell, M., and Hillman, L. S.: Hypomagnesemia and parathyroid hormone (PTH) deficiency in classical late neonatal hypocalcemia (CLNH) and surgically related late neonatal hypocalcemia (SLNH). Pediatr. Res. 14:571, 1980.

Fleischman, A. R., Rosen, J. F., and Nathenson, G.: 25-Hydroxyvitamin D: Serum levels and oral administration of calcifediol in neonates. Arch. Intern. Med. 138:869, 1978.

Friderichsen, C.: Hypocalcemie bei einem Brustkind und Hypercalcemie bei der Mutter. Monatschr. Kinderheilkd. 75:146, 1938.

Geggel, R. L., Pereira, G. R., and Spackman, T. J.: Fractured ribs: Unusual presentation of rickets in premature infants. J. Pediatr. 93:680, 1978.

Glasgow, J. F. T., and Thomas, P. S.: Rachitic respiratory distress in small preterm infants. Arch. Dis. Child. 52:268, 1977.

Glorieux, F. H., Salle, B. L., Delvin, E. E., and David, L.: Vitamin D metabolism in preterm infants: Serum calcitriol values during the first five days of life. J. Pediatr. 90:64, 1981.

Haddad, J. G., Hillman, L., and Rojanasathit, S.: Human serum binding capacity and affinity for 25-hydroxyergocalciferol and 25-hydroxycholecalciferol. J. Clin. Endocrinol. Metab. 43:86, 1976.

Harrison, H. E., and Harrison, H. C.: Hypercalcemic states. In Harrison, H. E., and Harrison, H. C. (Eds.): Disorders of Calcium and Phosphate Metabolism in Childhood and Adolescence. Philadelphia, W. B. Saunders Company, 1979.

Hartenstein, H., and Gardner, L. I.: Tetany of the newborn associated with maternal parathyroid adenoma: Report of the seventh affected family. N. Engl. J. Med. *274*:266, 1966.

Hillman, D. A., Scriver, C. R., Pedvis, S., and Shragovitch, I.: Neonatal familial primary hyperparathyroidism. N. Engl. J. Med. *270*:483, 1964.

Hillman, L. S., and Haddad, J. G.: Perinatal vitamin D metabolism II: Serial concentrations in sera of term and premature infant. J. Pediatr. *86*:928, 1975.

Hillman, L., Hoff, N., Martin, L., and Haddad, J.: Osteopenia, hypocalcemia, and low 25-hydroxyvitamin D (25-OHD) serum concentrations with use of soy formula. Pediatr. Res. *13*:400, 1979.

Hillman, L., Rojanasathit, S., Slatopolsky, E., and Haddad, J.: Serial measurement of serum calcium, magnesium, parathyroid hormone, calcitonin, and 25-hydroxyvitamin D in premature and term infants during the first week of life. Pediatr. Res. *11*:739, 1977.

Hoff, N., Haddad, J., Teitelbaum, S., et al.: Serum concentrations of 25-hydroxyvitamin D in rickets of extremely premature infants. J. Pediatr. *94*:460, 1979.

Hollis, B. W., Roos, B. A., Draper, H. H., and Lambert, P. W.: Vitamin D and its metabolites in human and bovine milk. J. Nutr. *111*:1240, 1981.

Landing, B. H., and Kamoshita, S.: Congenital hyperparathyroidism secondary to maternal hypoparathyroidism. J. Pediatr. *77*:842, 1970.

Leroyer-Alizon, E., David, L., Anast, C. S., and Dubois, P. M.: Immunocytological evidence for parathyroid hormone in human parathyroid glands. J. Clin. Endocrinol. Metab. *52*:513, 1981.

Leroyer-Alizon, E., David, L., and Dubois, P. M.: Evidence for calcitonin in the thyroid gland of normal and anencephalic human fetuses: Immunocytological localization, radioimmunoassay, and gel filtration of thyroid extracts. J. Clin. Endocrinol. Metab. *50*:316, 1980.

Linarelli, L. G., Bobik, C., and Bobik, J.: Urinary cAMP and renal responsiveness to parathormone in premature hypocalcemic infants. Pediatr. Res. *7*:329, 1973.

Lipsitz, P. J.: The clinical and biochemical effects of excess magnesium in the newborn. Pediatrics *47*:501, 1971.

Lipsitz, P. J., and English, J. C.: Hypermagnesemia in the newborn infant. Pediatrics *40*:856, 1967.

Marx, S. J., Attie, M. F., Spiegel, A. M., et al.: An association between severe primary hyperparathyroidism and familial hypocalciuric hypercalcemia in three kindreds. N. Engl. J. Med. *306*:257, 1982.

Mawer, B. E.: Clinical implications of measurements of circulating vitamin D metabolites. Clin. Endocrinol. Metab. *9*:63, 1980.

Moore, E. S., Langman, C. B., Favis, M. J., and Coe, F. L.: Role of fetal 1-25 dihydroxy vitamin D production in intrauterine phosphorus and calcium homeostasis. Pediatr. Res. *19*:566, 1985.

Oppenheimer, S. J., and Snodgrass, G. J. A. I.: Neonatal rickets. Arch. Dis. Child. *55*:945, 1980.

Pitkin, R. M., and Gebhardt, M. P.: Serum calcium concentrations in human pregnancy. Am. J. Obstet. Gynecol. *127*:775, 1977.

Pitkin, R. M., Reynolds, W. A., Williams, G. A., and Hargis, G. K.: Calcium metabolism in pregnancy: A longitudinal study. Am. J. Obstet. Gynecol. *133*:781, 1979.

Pratt, E. L., Geren, B. B., and Neuhauser, E. B. D.: Hypercalcemia and idiopathic hyperplasia of the parathyroid glands in an infant. J. Pediatr. *30*:388, 1947.

Purvis, R., MacKay, G., Cockburn, F., et al.: Enamel hypoplasia of the teeth associated with neonatal tetany: A manifestation of maternal vitamin D deficiency. Lancet *2*:811, 1973.

Rosen, J. F., Roginsky, M., Nathenson, G., and Finberg, L.: 25-Hydroxyvitamin D: Plasma levels in mothers and their premature infants with neonatal hypocalcemia. Am. J. Dis. Child. *127*:220, 1974.

Rowe, J. C., Wood, D. H., Rowe, D. W., and Raisz, L. G.: Nutritional hypophosphatemic rickets in a premature infant fed breast milk. N. Engl. J. Med. *300*:293, 1979.

Rude, R. K., Oldham, S. B., and Singer, F. R.: Functional hypoparathyroidism and parathyroid hormone end-organ resistance in human magnesium deficiency. Clin. Endocrinol. *5*:209, 1976.

Saan, L., David, L., Thomas, A., et al.: Congenital hyperparathyroidism and vitamin D deficiency secondary to maternal hypoparathyroidism. Acta Paediatr. Scand. *65*:381, 1976.

Sagy, M., Birenbaum, E., Balin, A., et al.: Phosphate depletion syndrome in a premature infant fed human milk. J. Pediatr. *96*:683, 1980.

Salle, B. L., David, L., Chopard, J. P., et al.: Prevention of early neonatal hypocalcemia in low birth weight infants with continuous calcium infusion: Effect on serum calcium, phosphorus, magnesium, and circulating immunoreactive parathyroid hormone and calcitonin. Pediatr. Res. *11*:1180, 1977.

Schedewie, H., Fisher, D., Odell, W., et al.: Etiology of first day hypocalcemia (FDH) role of PTH and calcitonin? Pediatr. Res. *12*:512, 1978.

Schedewie, H. K., Odell, W. D., Fisher, D. A., et al.: Parathormone and perinatal calcium homeostasis. Pediatr. Res. *13*:1, 1979.

Scott, S. M., Ladenson, J. H., Aguanno, J. J., and Hillman, L. S.: Ionized calcium in the sick neonate. Pediatr. Res. *13*:505, 1979.

Sharlin, D. N., and Koblenzer, P.: Necrosis of subcutaneous fat with hypercalcemia: A puzzling and multifaceted disease. Clin. Pediatr. *9*:920, 1970.

Steichen, J. J., Gratton, T. L., and Tsang, R. C.: Osteopenia of prematurity: The cause and possible treatment. J. Pediatr. *96*:528, 1980.

Steichen, J. J., Tsang, R. C., Greer, F. R., et al.: Elevated serum 1,24-dihydroxyvitamin D concentrations in rickets of very low birth weight infants. J. Pediatr. *99*:293, 1981.

Steichen, J. J., Tsang, R. C., Ho, M., et al.: 1,25(OH)$_2$ vitamin D (1,25(OH)$_2$D) and incidence of hypocalcemia in infants of diabetic mothers (IDM) in relation to prospective randomized treatment during pregnancy. Pediatr. Res. *15*:683, 1981.

Stevenson, J. C.: Mineral needs of the fetus. Curr. Topics Exp. Endocrinol. *5*:177, 1983.

Tanaka, Y., Hatano, S., Nishi, Y., and Usui, T.: Nutritional copper deficiency in a Japanese infant on formula. J. Pediatr. *96*:255, 1980.

Thompson, N. W., Carpenter, L. C., Kessler, D. L., and Nishiyaa, R. H.: Hereditary neonatal hyperparathyroidism. Arch. Surg. *113*:100, 1978.

Tsang, R. C., Chen, I. W., Friedman, M. A., et al.: Parathyroid function in infants of diabetic mothers. J. Pediatr. *86*:399, 1975.

Tsang, R. C., Chen, I., Hayes, W., et al.: Neonatal hypocalcemia in infants with birth asphyxia. J. Pediatr. *64*:428, 1974.

Tsang, R. C., Light, I. J., Sutherland, J. M., and Kleinman, L. I.: Possible pathogenetic factors in neonatal hypocalcemia of prematurity. J. Pediatr. *82*:423, 1973.

Veldhuis, J. D., Kulin, H. E., Demers, C. M., and Lambert, P. W.: Infantile hypercalcemia with subcutaneous fat necrosis: Endocrine studies. J. Pediatr. *95*:460, 1979.

Walser, M., Robinson, B. H. B., and Duckett, J. W., Jr.: The hypercalcemia of adrenal insufficiency. J. Clin. Invest. *42*:456, 1963.

Weisman, Y., Harrell, A., Edelstein, S., et al.: 25-Dihydroxy vitamin D$_3$ and 24,25-dihydroxy vitamin D$_3$ in vitro synthesis by human decidua and placenta. Nature *281*:317, 1979.

White, R. A., Preus, M., Watters, G. V., and Fraser, F. C.: Familial occurrence of the Williams syndrome. J. Pediatr. *91*:614, 1977.

Wieland, P., Fischer, J., Trechsel, U., et al.: Perinatal parathyroid hormone, vitamin D metabolites, and calcitonin in man. Am. J. Physiol. *239*:E385, 1980.

Williams, J. C. P., Barratt-Boyes, B. G., and Lowe, J. B.: Supravalvular aortic stenosis. Circulation *24*:1311, 1961.

Wolfe, H., DeLellis, R., Voelkel, E., and Tashjian, A.: Distribution of calcitonin-containing cells in the normal neonatal human thyroid gland: A correlation of morphology with peptide content. J. Clin. Endocrinol. Metab. *41*:1076, 1975.

Ziegler, E. E., O'Donnell, A. M., Nelson, S. E., and Forman, S. J.: Body composition of the reference fetus. Growth *40*:329, 1976.

DISORDERS OF THE 107 ADRENAL GLAND*

Daniel H. Polk

■ GENERAL CONSIDERATIONS

The mammalian adrenal gland is a dual endocrine organ, consisting of a cortex and medulla within a common capsule. The two glands have distinct embryologic origins and different functions. In the 5th week of fetal life, the primitive adrenal cortex is formed from cells of the coelomic mesoderm. During the 7th week, the cortex is invaded by ectodermal neural crest cells that aggregate to form a central cell mass, the adrenal medulla.

Adrenal cortical cells produce a variety of steroid hormones, and the medulla produces the catecholamines norepinephrine and epinephrine. Adrenal catecholamines are important for successful neonatal adaptation. The consequences of catecholamine excess are discussed in the section on neuroblastoma. This chapter focuses on development and function of the adrenal cortex.

Adrenal steroid production can be detected by the 9th week of gestation, and by the 12th week the adrenal glands are as large as the kidneys. The primitive, or fetal, zone of the adrenal cortex accounts for most of its bulk. This zone involutes slowly during the 3rd trimester and more rapidly after birth. There is no intrinsic difference between male and female adrenal function in utero, and the adrenal does not contribute to normal genital differentiation. The primary role of the fetal adrenal appears to be production of inactive steroid precursors, such as dehydroepiandrosterone sulfate which the placenta can convert to estrogens.

During the second half of pregnancy, the permanent adrenal cortex emerges as a distinct anatomic structure and begins to synthesize the glucocorticoids and mineralocorticoids that are required for successful adaptation to extrauterine life (Fig. 107–1). Glucocorticoids, of which cortisol is the most important in humans, play a major role in carbohydrate metabolism. They promote gluconeogenesis and synthesis of liver glycogen and act to elevate blood glucose levels. Cortisol has enzyme-inducing capabilities that doubtless affect many organs and prepare the infant for postnatal life. This aspect of glucocorticoid action has been most completely delineated in the discussion of late fetal development (see Chapter 5).

Early evidence suggesting that human chorionic gonadotropin (hCG) is adrenocorticotropic in the fetus during the first half of pregnancy varies with recent reports failing to demonstrate such an effect (Walsh et al., 1979). In the second half of pregnancy, the growth and secretory activity of the adrenal depend on adrenocorticotropin hormone (ACTH).

The ACTH concentration is relatively high in fetal, neonatal, and maternal plasma (Simila et al., 1977; Winters et al., 1974). Winters and co-workers reported mean afternoon ACTH values of 43 ± 4 pg/ml in normal adults, 194 ± 29 pg/ml in maternal plasma during labor, 241 ± 33 pg/ml in cord blood prior to 34 weeks' gestation, 143 ± 7 pg/ml in cord blood at term, and 120 ± 8 pg/ml during the 1st week of life. Measurements of fetal and neonatal plasma ACTH levels reflect secretion of this hormone by the fetoplacental unit, since ACTH does not cross the placenta. There is evidence for placental as well as pituitary secretion of ACTH; proopiomelanocortin (POMC), the precursor peptide for ACTH, is demonstrable in placental extracts. Control of fetal ACTH production is uncharacterized. Large amounts of biologically active corticotropin-releasing hormone (CRH) are present in fetal and cord blood (Goland et al., 1988).

There is limited information regarding plasma cortisol concentrations during fetal life. In 1973, Beitins and co-workers reported a mean value of 2.1 ± 1.2 µg/dl in fetuses of 3 to 6 months gestation as compared with a mean value of 6.3 ± 2.9 µg/dl in the cord blood of infants born at term by cesarean section. Although the human fetal plasma cortisol concentration may increase between midpregnancy and term, there is not the abrupt increase in late pregnancy that has been observed in some nonprimate animals. Cortisol crosses the placenta, but approximately 80 per cent of maternal cortisol is converted to cortisone when it traverses the placenta (Campbell and Murphy, 1977). Cord arterial levels are higher than cord venous levels, indicating that a significant amount of circulating cord cortisol is of fetal origin. It has been estimated that near term, 50 to 75 per cent of fetal plasma cortisol is derived from the fetal adrenal, and 25 to 50 per cent originates from maternal cortisol that traverses the placenta (Beitins et al., 1973). The concentrations of corticosteroid-binding globulin (CBG), total cortisol, and unbound cortisol are lower in fetal than in maternal plasma (Ohrlander et al., 1976; Simmer et al., 1974).

Fetal plasma cortisol rises in association with a stress-induced increase in maternal plasma cortisol during labor (Ohrlander et al., 1976), and there is evidence to indicate that fetal plasma ACTH or cortisol is altered in response to fetal stress. Fetal plasma ACTH levels are elevated after labor and vaginal delivery when compared with elective cesarean section (Pohjavuori and Fyhrquist, 1983). Plasma levels of corticotropin-releasing factor (CRF) and arginine vasopressin (AVP), the primary hypothalamic peptides involved in stimulation of ACTH secretion, are also elevated at birth (Sasaki et al., 1984). The perinatal increase in ACTH is associated with fetal adrenal secretion of cortisol and pregnenolone (Arai and Yanaihara, 1977) as well as other POMC-derived peptides. In contrast to

---

*Revised from C. Anast, 5th edition.

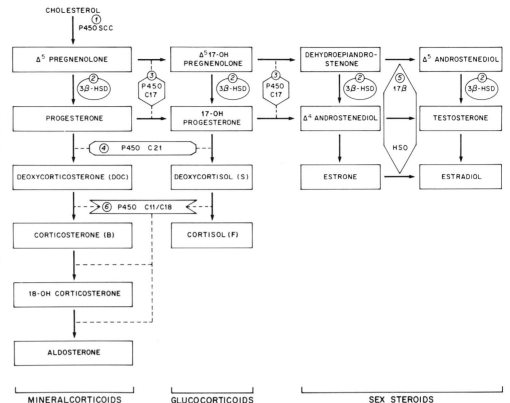

FIGURE 107–1. *Steroid biosynthetic pathways: 1, P450 SCC, formerly termed "20,22-desmolase," mediates side-chain cleavage and 20,22-hydroxylation of cholesterol. 2, 3β-hydroxysteroid dehydrogenase, a non-P450 enzyme. 3, P450 c17 mediates both 17-hydroxylation and 17,20-lyase activities. 4, P450 c21 mediates 21-hydroxylation. 5, 17β-hydroxysteroid oxido-reductase, a non-P450 enzyme. 6, P450 c11/c18 mediates three reactions: 11β-hydroxylation, 18-hydroxylation, and 18-methyl oxidation.*

reports in other species, there is no evidence to support the concept that the human fetal adrenal cortex plays a role in the initiation of labor.

The plasma cortisol concentration falls after birth, reaching a nadir at 24 to 36 hours of age, and then rapidly increases to levels that are equal to or greater than those later in infancy (Sperling, 1980). The response to exogenous ACTH is normal immediately after birth, but there is a smaller response in the initial days of life corresponding to the period of low plasma cortisol levels. After 5 days of life, there is a pronounced increase in serum cortisol in response to exogenous ACTH (Sperling, 1980). The age at which the circadian rhythm of ACTH and cortisol secretion becomes established is not known. The adult pattern of high morning and low nocturnal plasma 17-hydroxycorticosteroids does not appear to be present before 1 to 3 years of age (Franks, 1967).

ACTH contributes relatively little to the regulation of aldosterone synthesis. The main homeostatic mechanism involves release of renin from renal juxtaglomerular cells in response to diminished renal arteriolar pressure. Renin acts to increase angiotensin II, which in turn, increases aldosterone secretion, and also has a direct effect on vascular contractility. Increased intravascular pressure or volume acts to diminish renin production, thus closing the feedback loop. Low sodium and high potassium intakes also enhance aldosterone secretion, the latter by a mechanism that does not depend on the renin-angiotensin system.

The newborn is able to regulate aldosterone secretion in an appropriate manner. Kowarski and colleagues (1974) found that aldosterone levels in umbilical and newborn venous plasma were comparable to adult values. The levels rose to values above the adult range between 11 days and 1 year of age.

The fetus does not depend on endogenous glucocorticoid or mineralocorticoid production. Its needs can be met by transplacental passage of maternal hormones, and deficiencies, per se, are not evident at delivery. However, the catastrophic consequences of defective organogenesis or of enzymatic errors soon become apparent. Glucocorticoid deficiency can result in hypoglycemia within hours of birth, and mineralocorticoid deficiency manifests as salt loss and adrenal crisis within days or weeks after birth. The differential diagnosis of neonatal adrenal insufficiency is presented in the following sections and summarized in Table 107–1.

■ ADRENAL HEMORRHAGE

The large adrenal glands of the newborn are vulnerable to mechanical trauma during labor and delivery. Focal hemorrhage at the junction of the fetal zone and the

TABLE 107–1. Causes of Neonatal Adrenal Insufficiency

Adrenal hemorrhage
Transient adrenal insufficiency
Congenital adrenal hypoplasia
Primary: X-linked, autosomal recessive
Secondary: ACTH deficiency
Congenital adrenal hyperplasia
21-hydroxylase deficiency (P450 C21)
11β-hydroxylase deficiency (P450 C11/C18)
17-hydroxylase deficiency (P450 C17)
3β-hydroxysteroid dehydrogenase deficiency (3-HSD)
20,22-desmolase deficiency (P450 SCC)
Isolated aldosterone deficiency
18-hydroxylase deficiency (P450 C11/C18)
Pseudohypoaldosteronism
Congenital adrenal ACTH resistance
Neonatal adrenoleukodystrophy
Infantile glycerol kinase deficiency

permanent cortex is a common finding in infants dying of other causes (Boyd, 1967). Minor bleeding into the adrenal cortex may not produce symptoms but may be associated with adrenal calcifications noted incidentally later in life. In order to result in adrenal insufficiency, hemorrhage must involve both adrenals and at least 90 per cent of the adrenocortical tissue must be destroyed (Black and Williams, 1973). Massive adrenal hemorrhage is an uncommon but life-threatening event. Predisposing factors include large birth weight, prolonged or difficult labor, placental bleeding, and perinatal anoxia. Adrenal hemorrhage may occur in premature infants without obvious trauma. The adrenal may be a site of hemorrhage in infants with sepsis or with primary coagulopathies. In most published series, affected male infants outnumber females by three to one.

The affected infant may show signs of hypovolemic shock, but commonly presents with pallor, apnea, and hypothermia accompanied by a falling hematocrit and jaundice. A large flank mass may be palpated, more commonly on the right side. In only 5 to 10 per cent of cases the hemorrhage is bilateral. The condition must be differentiated from renal vein thrombosis. In both conditions, there may be azotemia, proteinuria, and hematuria, but in adrenal hemorrhage the hematuria is of a lesser degree. Intravenous pyelograms typically reveal no function on the affected side when a renal vein or artery has been thrombosed. Adrenal hemorrhage typically displaces the kidney downward and rotates it laterally, with flattening of the upper calyces.

Signs of adrenal insufficiency may be subtle and delayed. Even with extensive bilateral hemorrhage, functioning islands of zona gomerulosa cells are generally preserved. Hypoglycemia is a more common finding than is salt loss.

Immediate management is directed at blood and volume replacement. Indications for steroid replacement include bilateral hemorrhage, failure to respond to volume expansion, hypoglycemia, polyuria, hyponatremia, hyperkalemia, or anticipated general anesthesia.

Within 1 to 3 weeks after the hemorrhage, a thin zone of calcification appears at the periphery of the gland. As blood and necrotic adrenal tissue are resorbed, the area of calcification shrinks and assumes the shape and size of the original gland. Such calcification may persist for life. Adrenal function generally improves with resolution of the hemorrhage. ACTH stimulation with measurement of plasma or urinary corticoid responses is indicated after the acute phase of the illness; late adrenal insufficiency has been reported.

■ TRANSIENT ADRENAL INSUFFICIENCY

In 1946, Jaudon described a series of 14 infants with dehydration, salt loss, and failure to gain weight. All responded to steroid replacement, and in each case it was eventually possible to discontinue treatment without a recurrence of symptoms. Others have reported additional infants with an apparent delay in maturation of adrenal cortical function. Bongiovanni (1962) described a premature infant with marked hyponatremia and hyperkalemia and no detectable serum cortisol or urinary corticoids. The infant did well on cortisol replacement, and at age 6

months, following discontinuation of steroid treatment, he showed normal cortisol and aldosterone responses to ACTH. Kreines and DeVaux (1971) described a similar course in an infant born to a mother with Cushing's syndrome due to an adrenal adenoma.

Rarely, transient adrenal insufficiency is observed in a newborn whose mother received glucocorticoids during pregnancy. The type of glucocorticoid administered to the mother may be important in this regard. Substantial amounts of cortisol and prednisolone are converted to less active metabolites during their traversal across the placenta as well as in the fetal circulation by both the placenta and other fetal tissues. Thus, when the mother is treated with cortisol or prednisolone, the fetal plasma concentration of these active steroids is only a small fraction of that in the mother (Dorr et al., 1986). However, following administration of dexamethasone to the mother, the concentrations in fetal and maternal plasma are similar (Charnvises et al., 1985).

The combination of hyponatremia, hyperkalemia, and polyuria may occur in acutely ill infants under a variety of other circumstances that do not involve adrenal insufficiency. Infants recovering from hypovolemic shock and acute tubular necrosis demonstrate these features, as do infants treated with furosemide without replacement of sodium. In doubtful cases, one may collect serum and urine specimens during a therapeutic trial of desoxycorticosterone acetate. This agent, given intramuscularly in a dosage of 0.5 mg/kg/day, provides a potent mineralocorticoid effect and does not inhibit pituitary ACTH or interfere with serum cortisol or urinary corticoid estimation. If steroid measurements do not support a diagnosis of adrenal insufficiency and if serum sodium levels do not rise and serum potassium levels decline in response to desoxycorticosterone acetate, then the medication may safely be discontinued.

■ ADRENAL HYPOPLASIA

In the absence of pituitary gland function, the adrenal glands fail to develop normally. The adrenal glands of anencephalic infants weigh less than 0.5 g at birth, as opposed to normal combined weights greater than 6 g. Arrested development of the adrenals has been attributed to a lack of trophic stimulation of ACTH. Pituitary hypoplasia can also occur in infants without major central nervous system malformations. In these infants, severe hypoglycemia can result in death within the first 48 hours of life. Blizzard and Alberts (1956) described a male infant who had, in addition, microphallus and cryptorchidism. The association has been noted in several other cases and probably reflects a lack of trophic hormone stimulation of both adrenals and testes. Prompt glucocorticoid replacement is required.

Adrenal hypoplasia occurs in infants with anatomically and functionally intact pituitary glands (Pakravan et al., 1974; Roselli and Barbosa, 1965; Sperling et al., 1973). Isolated and familial forms, with either X-linked or autosomal recessive transmission, have been described. Early recognition, cortisol replacement, and prolonged survival have permitted studies of the mechanisms that underlie familial adrenal hypoplasia. The disease is manifested in infancy or early childhood by hyperpigmentation as a consequence of elevated ACTH levels and by hypoglycemia as a consequence of glucocorticoid deficiency. In contrast to congenital adrenal hyperplasia, familial adrenal hypoplasia has no associated excess of abnormal steroid metabolites. Mineralocorticoid production is generally unimpaired. A possible defect might involve the adrenal membrane receptor for ACTH (Migeon et al., 1968).

■ CONGENITAL ADRENAL HYPERPLASIA

Adrenal steroid biosynthesis requires a sequence of enzymatic reactions that are illustrated in Figure 107–1. Studies utilizing techniques of molecular biology have demonstrated that the synthesis of cortisol and aldosterone requires only five apoenzymes, some having more than one function. Four of these enzyme systems belong to the cytochrome P450 family of oxidases. The two mitochondrial P450 enzymes are involved in the side-chain cleavage of cholesterol (P450 SCC, formerly 20,22-desmolase) and the hydroxylation of cholesterol carbons C11 and C18 (P450 C11/C18). There are two microsomal P450 enzymes; one having 17-hydroxylase and 17,20-desmolase activities (P450 C17) and one with 21-hydroxylase activity (P450 C21). The fifth enzyme, microsomal in location, has 3β-hydroxysteroid dehydrogenase and Δ5–3 ketosteroid isomerase activities (3β-HSD). In recent years, complementary DNA probes have been cloned, permitting gene mapping and sequencing of these particular protein products (Miller, 1988). The disease states in this category have several features in common. Each condition is inherited in an autosomal recessive manner. Thus, multiple sibling involvement is common, and recurrence risk in subsequent pregnancies is 25 per cent. Each, with the exception of 18-hydroxysteroid dehydrogenase deficiency, involves hyperplasia of the adrenal cortex under the stimulus of elevated ACTH levels. In each case, the disorder may be managed quite well with appropriate steroid replacement.

Clinical manifestations of adrenal hyperplasia depend on the site and severity of the enzymatic block. With a block, precursors accumulate and are diverted into alternative metabolic pathways. Laboratory confirmation of a suspected defect involves measurement of these metabolites. The pathophysiology of all of these enzyme deficiencies is related to: (1) the specific enzyme involved and severity of the defect, (2) the amount and type of precursor overproduction, (3) the impact of precursors on differentiation of the external genitalia, (4) the severity of glucocorticoid deficiency, and (5) the severity of mineralocorticoid deficiency. The defects listed in Table 107–1 are discussed individually, as follows.

DEFICIENCY OF 21-HYDROXYLASE

The 21-hydroxylase deficiency is the most common form of congenital adrenal hyperplasia as well as the most common cause of ambiguous genitalia. The incidence of 21-hydroxylase deficiency is estimated to be one in 15,000 in Caucasians in the United States and Europe. However, the gene frequency varies in different ethnic groups, and an usually high incidence of the disorder (one in 490) has been reported in the Yupik Eskimos of Alaska (Hirschfeld and Fleishman, 1969). The gene that codes for 21-

hydroxylation is located on the short arm of chromosome 6 in proximity to the locus of the histocompatibility gene HLA-B and the loci for complement factors C4a and C4b (New et al., 1981). Knowledge of this genetic linkage has led to the use of human leukocyte antigen (HLA) typing in families with affected individuals for detection of heterozygotes as well as for the prenatal diagnosis of affected fetuses (Levine et al., 1980a; New et al., 1981; Pollack et al., 1981; Sherman et al., 1988).

Hydroxylation at the C21 position is required for synthesis of glucocorticoids and mineralocorticoids. There are two clinical syndromes of congenital adrenal hyperplasia due to a 21-hydroxylation defect: simple virilization and virilization with salt wasting. In both forms, defective cortisol synthesis leads to increased secretion of ACTH, which in turn, stimulates the adrenal to produce increased amounts of cortisol precursors, including androgens and androgen precursors. The plasma concentrations of 17-hydroxyprogesterone, androstenedione, and testosterone are elevated in affected patients, and the metabolites of these steroids result in increased urinary excretion of 17-ketosteroids and pregnanetriol. As a result of high levels of circulating fetal androgens, female newborns demonstrate varying degrees of virilization, ranging from mild to severe clitoral enlargement with complete labial fusion and a phallic urethra. Affected males are formed normally at birth. If untreated, both females and males show progressive virilization during infancy and early childhood with rapid linear growth and skeletal and somatic maturation. In addition to virilization, some infants show signs of salt wasting and aldosterone deficiency with failure to thrive, hyponatremia, hyperkalemia, and ultimately vascular collapse. Salt-losing crisis is uncommon before 6 days of age but occurs in about 50 per cent of affected infants between 6 and 14 days of age. Patients with virilization and salt wasting are aldosterone-deficient, as reflected by reduced circulating aldosterone levels and increased plasma renin activity. By contrast, patients with simple virilization have normal or elevated serum aldosterone levels and plasma renin activity in the baseline state that increase in response to sodium restriction. The reason for the increased circulating aldosterone in patients with simple virilization is uncertain.

The phenotype of 21-hydroxylase deficiency may encompass a variety of previously described abnormalities. Accumulated evidence suggests that classic congenital adrenal hyperplasia, "acquired or late onset" adrenal hyperplasia, and "cryptic" adrenal hyperplasia are all forms of 21-hydroxylase deficiency with a wide range of clinical abnormalities (Levine et al., 1980a; Lorenzen et al., 1980; New et al., 1981; Pollack et al., 1981).

Congenital adrenal hyperplasia should be suspected in all infants with ambiguous genitalia or a family history of either this condition or unexplained infant death and in all infants with vomiting, sluggish feeding, dehydration, or failure to thrive. The significant morbidity and mortality associated with this deficiency, especially in unrecognized males, has prompted screening by measurement of 17-OH progesterone in filter paper blood spots.

The evaluation of an infant with ambiguous genitalia is outlined in the next chapter. The steroidal biochemical findings in 21-hydroxylase deficiency include elevated urinary excretion of 17-ketosteroids and pregnanetriol and elevated plasma levels of 17-hydroxyprogesterone and Δ4 androstenedione. The most useful test is the determination of plasma 17-hydroxyprogesterone (17-OHP). The concentration of 17-OHP is normally elevated in umbilical cord blood with a mean value of 1700 ng/dl but rapidly decreases to 100 to 200 ng/dl after 24 hours of age (Grumbach and Conte, 1981). Although cord blood levels of 17-OHP may not be diagnostic of 21-hydroxylase deficiency, after 24 hours of age plasma 17-OHP and Δ4 androstenedione levels usually distinguish infants with 21-hydroxylase deficiency from normal infants. It is well to be aware, however, that sick unaffected infants may have elevated 17-OHP and Δ4 androstenedione levels that confuse the diagnosis of 21-hydroxylase deficiency. In affected patients, the plasma 17-OHP levels usually range from 3000 to 40,000 ng/dl, depending on the age and severity of 21-hydroxylase deficiency (Grumbach and Conte, 1981). Borderline normal levels of plasma 17-OHP are rarely reported in patients with mild 21-hydroxylase deficiency or in heterozygotes. In these instances, the effect of ACTH administration on the rise of plasma 17-OHP and the ratio of 17-OHP to cortisol will usually identify affected infants (Levine et al., 1981). It is important to note that cortisol levels may be normal in affected infants depending on the severity of the enzyme defect. In general, cortisol determinations are not useful in the diagnosis or management of this disease. In families with an affected member, HLA genotyping will distinguish between heterozygosity and a mild form of the disorder in a homozygous infant.

The urinary excretion of 17-ketosteroids and pregnanetriol have also been used in the diagnosis of 21-hydroxylase deficiency. It is necessary to be aware that during the first few days of life, the urinary 17-ketosteroids may be as high as 2 to 4 mg per 24 hours in normal infants, while urinary pregnanetriol may be normal in affected infants. After the early days of life, urinary 17-ketosteroid excretion values of greater than 2.5 mg per 24 hours and pregnanetriol values greater than 0.5 mg per 24 hours are diagnostic.

The combined use of HLA typing of amniotic fluid cells and the determination of 17-OHP and Δ4 androstenedione in amniotic fluid permits the definitive prenatal diagnosis of 21-hydroxylase deficiency. Amniotic fluid concentrations of 17-OHP and Δ4 androstenedione are elevated in affected fetuses between 14 and 20 weeks' gestation (Nagamani et al., 1978; Pang et al., 1980). HLA typing of amniotic fluid cells obtained from mothers who had a previously affected offspring permits identification of fetuses who are homozygous or heterozygous for 21-hydroxylase deficiency (Pollack et al., 1981). Various fetal treatment schemes have been employed to block the influence of unchecked ACTH stimulation on adrenal steroid production in affected fetuses (David and Forest, 1984). Maternal administration of dexamethasone will inhibit fetal ACTH overproduction until diagnostic procedures, such as chorionic villous sampling or amniocentesis, can be performed.

In the infant with severe salt loss, initial treatment requires volume expansion with isotonic saline in 5 or 10 per cent dextrose administered intravenously at a rate of 100 to 120 ml/kg/day with 25 per cent of this amount given in the first 2 hours. Fifty mg/m² of hydrocortisone

sodium succinate should be given as a bolus intravenously and another 50 to 100 mg/m² added to the infusion fluid over the first 24 hours. When hyponatremia and hyperkalemia are present, desoxycorticosterone acetate (DOCA) may be given intramuscularly in a dosage of 1 mg every 24 hours.

Chronic medical treatment of congenital adrenal hyperplasia requires the provision of sufficient cortisol to suppress adrenal androgen production and to protect against stress. The required dosage is generally in the range of 15 to 20 mg/m² of hydrocortisone per day, given in three divided oral doses. Cortisone acetate may be given intramuscularly every 3 days for long-term replacement. The dosage should be doubled or tripled during acute illnesses, and intramuscular cortisone acetate should be substituted in a dosage of 25 to 50 mg/m² per day during protracted vomiting or surgical stress. Inadequate dosage permits excessive production of androgens and excessively rapid growth and skeletal maturation. Overdosage produces slowing of growth and other features of the Cushing syndrome.

Infants with proven or suspected salt loss should also receive mineralocorticoid replacement and salt supplements (1 to 3 g/day orally). Fludrocortisone acetate (Florinef) in an oral dose of 0.025 to 0.1 mg/day is commonly used for mineralocorticoid replacement. During the first 2 years of life, some physicians prefer to implant one or two 125 mg DOCA pellets rather than prescribe Florinef. The pellets are absorbed slowly and last for 6 to 9 months. Suboptimal growth occurs with inadequate replacement, and excessive doses produce failure to thrive as well as hypertension.

Besides the evaluation of growth, skeletal maturation, and signs of virilization, adequacy of glucocorticoid therapy is assessed by monitoring urinary excretion of 17-ketosteroids and pregnanetriol and plasma levels of 17-OHP (Hughes and Winter, 1976). In this regard, plasma levels of 17-OHP have not been found more useful than urinary 17-ketosteroids (Grumbach and Conte, 1981). Indeed, there is uncertainty regarding the value of plasma 17-OHP measurements in assessing the quality of treatment (Frisch et al., 1981). Plasma levels of sodium and potassium and plasma renin activity are useful in evaluating the adequacy of mineralocorticoid therapy.

Surgical correction of mild to moderate clitoral enlargement is generally not required. Clitoral size tends to remain stable or even decrease as the child grows. When indicated, surgery may be performed at 4 to 12 months of age. The best age for correction of labial fusion is probably about 2 years. Some girls may require more complicated vaginoplasty at a later age. The prognosis for normal psychosexual development and reproductive function is excellent in boys and girls with 21-hydroxylase deficiency.

DEFICIENCY OF 11β-HYDROXYLASE

Hydroxylation at the C11 position is required for cortisol and aldosterone synthesis. As originally reported by Eberlein and Bongiovanni (1956), deficiency of 11β-hydroxylase results in virilization of the female infant together with a variable degree of hypertension. There is accumulation of the immediate precursors 11-deoxycortisol (compound S) and desoxycorticosterone (DOC) in the plasma and increased urinary excretion of their tetra-hydro metabolites. Whereas compound S is biologically inert, DOC has mineralocorticoid effects and contributes to the hypertensive state. Neither compound is recognized by the hypothalamic-pituitary regulatory system, and an increase in ACTH secretion occurs (Levine et al., 1980b). Hydrocortisone replacement suppresses ACTH production and thereby prevents further virilization and relieves hypertension. Transient hyponatremia and hyperkalemia may occur after the initiation of glucocorticoid therapy as a result of inhibition of ACTH-stimulated DOC secretion before the inhibited renin-angiotensin-aldosterone system has had time to recover (Holcombe et al., 1980). Monitoring of treatment requires determination of urinary 17-ketosteroid or tetrahydro-S excretion.

The 11β-hydroxylase gene is located on chromosome 8 and thus is not linked to the HLA loci. The frequency of 11β-hydroxylase deficiency is rare, comprising less than 3 per cent of the total cases of adrenal hyperplasia. In certain Middle Eastern populations, the two defects occur with equal frequency. The defect may be partial, and hypertension either may be absent or may not appear until late childhood or adulthood. Similarly, signs of virilization in the female may not appear until adolescence (Cathelineau et al., 1980).

DEFICIENCY OF 17-HYDROXYLASE

Hydroxylation at the C17 position is required for cortisol, androgen, and estrogen synthesis but is not involved in the synthesis of mineralocorticoids. Several different allelic gene defects for cytochrome P450 C17 have been associated with decreased activity of 17-hydroxylase. Biglieri and co-workers (1966) described four adult females with lack of secondary sexual development, hyperkalemic alkalosis, and hypertension who proved to have deficiency of this enzyme. They demonstrated excessive plasma levels of DOC and corticosterone and excessive excretion of their urinary metabolites. Aldosterone levels tended to be low, presumably owing to inhibition of the renin-angiotensin system. In affected XX females, both internal and external genitalia are normal. In males, impaired testosterone synthesis by the fetal testes results in either phenotypic female external genitalia or ambiguous genitalia, but the female müllerian duct derivatives are absent. Failure of pubertal development in females and defective virilization in males, as described by New and Suvannakul (1970), provide evidence that adrenal and gonadal 17-hydroxylase activities are under common genetic control. Cortisol replacement inhibits ACTH production and relieves hypertension. Exogenous androgens or estrogens are required at the age of puberty.

DEFICIENCY OF 3β-HYDROXYSTEROID DEHYDROGENASE

Conversion of pregnenolone to progesterone requires oxidation at the 3 position and isomerization of a double bond from the Δ5 to the Δ4 position. The defect results in defective synthesis of cortisol, aldosterone, and potent androgens and estrogens. Bongiovanni (1962) originally described several infants with defects in this crucial enzyme complex. These infants had severe salt and water loss

and, despite adequate steroid replacement, did not survive infancy. Urinary and plasma steroid metabolites are predominantly of the Δ5, β-hydroxy configuration and include pregnanetriol and dihydroepiandrosterone. However, during the first few weeks of life, the Δ5, 3β-hydroxysteroids may be elevated in normal premature and full-term infants. It is therefore necessary to interpret the levels of these steroids in early infancy in relation to normal values for age. As a result of accumulation of dihydroepiandrosterone, a weak androgen, and defective conversion to the more potent androgens, androstenedione and testosterone, both males and females have partial virilization. Males have hypospadias and may have a bifid scrotum with or without cryptorchidism. Females have slight to moderate clitoral enlargement, which may be associated with labial fusion. Affected males have developed gynecomastia at puberty. Mild forms of 3β-hydroxysteroid dehydrogenase deficiency may not become clinically evident until adolescence (Parks et al., 1971; Rosenfield et al., 1980). In infancy, urinary 17-ketosteroids and pregnanetriol are elevated. The latter finding differentiates the defect from the more common deficiency of 21-hydroxylase. Both glucocorticoid and mineralocorticoid replacement are required throughout life.

DEFICIENCY OF 20,22-DESMOLASE

Conversion of cholesterol to pregnenolone is an essential step in the synthesis of mineralocorticoids, glucocorticoids, androgens, and estrogens. In rare instances, infants with a homozygous defect in P450 SCC activity have been described. They cannot synthesize any glucocorticoid, mineralocorticoid, or sex steroid. Defects in this early set of reactions lead to severe salt and water loss and hypoglycemia. Female infants have normal genitalia at birth but are incapable of producing estrogens at the time of puberty. Male infants with this defect usually have feminized external genitalia with a blind vaginal pouch but no müllerian duct derivatives. Little or no C21 or C19 steroids are detectable in plasma or urine. The adrenal glands and gonads are enlarged and filled with cholesterol and other lipids, hence, the name "lipoid adrenal hyperplasia." Most patients have died in infancy, but in a few (who perhaps have had less severe defects), steroid treatment has permitted prolonged survival.

■ ISOLATED ALDOSTERONE DEFICIENCIES

DEFICIENCY OF 18-HYDROXYLASE

The final steps in aldosterone synthesis involve hydroxylation and dehydrogenation at C18. Deficiency at this level results in aldosterone deficiency and salt loss without any alteration in the synthesis of cortisol or the sex steroids. Several authors have postulated that the transient salt wasting of infancy described by Jaudon (1946) might be due to delayed maturation of these enzymes. Appropriate therapy consists of a mineralocorticoid and supplemental sodium chloride. Glucocorticoid replacement is not required.

■ PSEUDOHYPOALDOSTERONISM

Pseudohypoaldosteronism (end-organ unresponsiveness to aldosterone) is a salt-wasting disorder that results from renal tubular unresponsiveness to aldosterone (Proesmans et al., 1973). Characteristically, there is urinary sodium wasting, hyponatremia, hyperkalemia, vomiting, and dehydration in early infancy. Urinary 17-ketosteroids and plasma androgens are normal, whereas plasma aldosterone and renin concentrations are elevated. The infants do not respond to mineralocorticoid therapy, and treatment with supplemental sodium chloride is necessary.

■ CONGENITAL ADRENAL RESISTANCE TO ACTH

Infants affected by this entity present with recurrent hypoglycemia and skin hyperpigmentation. Serum electrolytes are normal, and there are no manifestations of mineralocorticoid deficiency. These findings suggest glucocorticoid deficiency and ACTH excess. Plasma concentrations of cortisol are low, while those of aldosterone and corticosterone are normal or elevated. Urinary 17-ketosteroids are low, while urinary aldosterone levels are elevated. Plasma ACTH levels are strikingly elevated, and there is no response in plasma 17-hydroxysteroids, cortisol, or aldosterone levels to pharmacologic doses of ACTH. Aldosterone levels do increase in response to sodium restriction. These findings suggest adrenal resistance to ACTH with preservation of a normal mineralocorticoid response to the renin-angiotensin system. Accordingly, the adrenal glands of affected patients are small, with atrophy of the zona fasciculata and sparing of the zona glomerulosa. Treatment consists of appropriate glucocorticoid replacement.

■ NEONATAL ADRENOLEUKODYSTROPHY

There seems to be a neonatal form of adrenoleukodystrophy, a chronic X-linked disease of childhood which is inherited as an autosomal recessive trait and may present in the weeks following birth. Jaffe and co-workers (1982) have described infants with craniofacial and central nervous system abnormalities that are associated with progressive adrenal insufficiency. They postulated that the progressive adrenal defects might be secondary to the primary disorder of fatty acid metabolism with effects on receptor binding of ACTH.

■ INFANTILE GLYCEROL KINASE DEFICIENCY

Infantile glycerol kinase deficiency is an X-linked disease that presents in male infants as an acute salt-wasting crisis with blood steroid determinations that suggest adrenal hypoplasia (Kohlschutter et al., 1987). They are distinguished from the latter by elevated blood glycerol and creatinine kinase levels. The diagnosis may be delayed until the onset of developmental and myopathic symptoms. The diagnosis is confirmed by demonstrating the mitochondrial enzyme defect in biopsy material. These patients may actually represent a deletion in the X-chromosome for three closely linked gene loci (glycerol kinase, adrenal hypoplasia, and progressive muscular dystrophy).

■ ADRENAL OVERACTIVITY

Glucocorticoid excess results in hyperphagia, obesity, and impairment of linear growth, together with hypertension, osteoporosis, and polycythemia. The Cushing syndrome is extremely rare in infancy except as a result of administration of glucocorticoids or ACTH. The cases that have been reported show a preponderance of adrenal tumors, both adenomas and carcinomas. There may be overproduction of androgens as well as glucocorticoids. There is no suppression of circulating corticoids with administration of dexamethasone. Surgical treatment involves extirpation with attendant glucocorticoid replacement to prevent acute adrenal insufficiency.

■ REFERENCES

Arai, K., and Yanaihara, T.: Steroid hormone changes in fetal blood during labor. Am. J. Obstet. Gynecol. *127*:879, 1977.

Beitins, I. Z., Bayard, F., Ances, I. G., et al.: The metabolic clearance rate, blood production, interconversion and transplacental passage of cortisol and cortisone in pregnancy near term. Pediatr. Res. 7:509, 1973.

Biglieri, E. G., Herron, M. A., and Brust, N.: 17-Hydroxylation deficiency in man. J. Clin. Invest. *45*:1946, 1966.

Black, J., and Williams, D. I.: Natural history of adrenal haemorrhage in the newborn. Arch. Dis. Child. *48*:183, 1973.

Blizzard, R. M., and Alberts, M.: Hypopituitarism, hypoadrenalism and hypogonadism in the newborn infant. J. Pediatr. *48*:782, 1956.

Bongiovanni, A. M.: Disorders of adrenal steroid biogenesis. *In* Stanbury, J. B., Wyngaarden, J. B., and Fredrickson, D. S. (Eds.): The Metabolic Basis of Inherited Disease. New York, McGraw-Hill, 1972, p. 857.

Bongiovanni, A. M.: Adrenogenital syndrome with deficiency of 3β-hydroxysteroid dehydrogenase. J. Clin. Invest. *41*:2086, 1962.

Boyd, J. F.: Disseminated fibrin thromboembolism among neonates dying within 48 hours of birth. Arch. Dis. Child. *42*:401, 1967.

Campbell, A. L., and Murphy, B. E. P.: The maternal-fetal cortisol gradient during pregnancy and delivery. J. Clin. Endocrinol. Metab. *45*:435, 1977.

Cathelineau, G., Brerault, J., Fiet, J., et al.: Adrenocortical 11β-hydroxylation defect in adult women with postmenarcheal onset of symptoms. J. Clin. Endocrinol. Metab. *51*:287, 1980.

Charnvises, S., de Fencl, M., Osthanondh, R., et al.: Adrenal steroids in maternal and cord blood after dexamethasone administration at midterm. J. Clin. Endocrinol. Metab. *61*:1220, 1985.

David, M., and Forest, M. G.: Prenatal treatment of congenital adrenal hyperplasia resulting from 21-hydroxylase deficiency. J. Pediatr. *105*:799, 1984.

Dorr, H. G., Versmold, H. T., Sippell, W. G., et al.: Antenatal betamethasone therapy: Effects on maternal, fetal and neonatal mineralocorticoids, glucocorticoids and progestins. J. Pediatr. *108*:990, 1986.

Eberlein, W. R., and Bongiovanni, A. M.: Plasma and urinary corticosteroids in hypertensive form of congenital adrenal hyperplasia. J. Biol. Chem. *223*:85, 1956.

Franks, R. D.: Diurnal variation of plasma 17-hydroxycorticosteroids in children. J. Clin. Endocrinol. Metab. *27*:75, 1967.

Frisch, H., Parth, K., Schober, E., et al.: Circadian patterns of plasma cortisol, 17-hydroxyprogesterone, and testosterone in congenital adrenal hyperplasia. Arch. Dis. Child. *56*:208, 1981.

Goland, R. S., Wardlow, S. L., Blum, M., et al.: Biologically active corticotropin-releasing hormone in maternal and fetal plasma during pregnancy. Am. J. Obstet. Gynecol. *159*:884, 1988.

Grumbach, M. M., and Conte, F. A.: Disorders of sex differentiation. *In* Williams, R. H. (Ed.): Textbook of Endocrinology. Philadelphia, W. B. Saunders Company, 1981, p. 423.

Hirschfeld, A. J., and Fleishman, J. K.: An unusually high incidence of salt-losing congenital adrenal hyperplasia in the Alaskan Eskimo. J. Pediatr. *75*:492, 1969.

Holcombe, J. A., Keenan, B., Nichols, B., et al.: Neonatal salt loss in the hypertensive form of congenital adrenal hyperplasia. Pediatrics 65:777, 1980.

Hughes, I. A., and Winter, J. S. D.: The application of a serum 17-OH-progesterone radioimmunoassay to the diagnosis and management of congenital adrenal hyperplasia. J. Pediatr. 88:766, 1976.

Jaffe, R., Cromline, P., Hashida, Y., et al.: Neonatal adrenoleukodystrophy. Clinical, pathological and biochemical delineation of a syndrome affecting both males and females. Am. J. Physiol. 198:100, 1982.

Jaudon, J. C.: Addisons's disease in an infant. J. Clin. Endocrinol. Metab. 6:558, 1946.

Kohlschutter, A., Willig, H. P., Schlamp, D., et al.: Infantile glycerol kinase deficiency—a condition requiring prompt identification. Eur. J. Pediatr. 146:575, 1987.

Kowarski, A., Katz, H., and Migeon, C. J.: Plasma aldosterone concentration in normal subjects from infancy to adulthood. J. Clin. Endocrinol. Metab. 38:498, 1974.

Kreines, K., and DeVaux, W. D.: Neonatal adrenal insufficiency associated with maternal Cushing's syndrome. Pediatrics 47:516, 1971.

Levine, L. S., Dupont, B., Lorenzen, F., et al.: Genetic and hormonal characterization of cryptic 21-hydroxylase deficiency. J. Clin. Endocrinol. Metab. 53:1193, 1981.

Levine, L. S., Dupont, B., Lorenzen, F., et al.: Cryptic 21-hydroxylase deficiency in families of patients with classical congenital adrenal hyperplasia. J. Clin. Endocrinol. Metab. 51:1316, 1980a.

Levine, L. S., Rauh, W., Gottediener, K., et al.: New studies of the 11β-hydroxylase and 18-hydroxylase enzymes in the hypertensive form of congenital adrenal hyperplasia. J. Clin. Endocrinol. Metab. 50:258, 1980b.

Lorenzen, F., Pang, S., New, M., et al.: Studies of the C-21 and C-19 steroids and HLA genotyping in siblings and parents of patients with congenital adrenal hyperplasia due to 21-hydroxylase deficiency. J. Clin. Endocrinol. Metab. 50:572, 1980.

Migeon, C. J., Kenny, F. M., and Kowarski, A.: The syndrome of congenital unresponsiveness to ACTH. Pediatr. Res. 2:501, 1968.

Miller, W. L.: Molecular biology of steroid hormone synthesis. Endocrinol. Rev. 9:295, 1988.

Nagamani, M., McDonough, P., Ellegood, J., et al.: Maternal and amniotic fluid 17α-hydroxyprogesterone levels during pregnancy. Diagnosis of congenital adrenal hyperplasia in utero. Am. J. Obstet. Gynecol. 130:791, 1978.

New, M. I., Dupont, B., Pang, S., et al.: An update of congenital adrenal hyperplasia. Recent Prog. Horm. Res. 37:105, 1981.

New, M. I., and Suvannakul, L.: Male pseudohermaphroditism due to 17α-hydroxylase deficiency. J. Clin. Invest. 49:1930, 1970.

Ohrlander, S., Genuser, G., and Encroth, P.: Plasma cortisol levels in the human fetus during parturition. Obstet. Gynecol. 48:381, 1976.

Pakravan, P., Kenny, F. M., Depp, R., et al.: Familial congenital absence of adrenal glands: Evaluation of glucocorticoid, mineralocorticoid, and estrogen metabolism in the perinatal period. J. Pediatr. 84:74, 1974.

Pang, S., Levine, L., Cederquist, M., et al.: Amniotic fluid concentrations of $\Delta 5$ and $\Delta 4$ steroids in fetuses with congenital adrenal hyperplasia due to 21-hydroxylase deficiency and in anencephalic fetuses. J. Clin. Endocrinol. Metab. 51:223, 1980.

Parks, G. A., New, M. I., Bermudez, J. A., et al.: A pubertal boy with the 3β-hydroxysteroid dehydrogenase defect. J. Clin. Invest. 33:269, 1971.

Pohjavuori, M., and Fyhrquist, F.: Vasopressin, ACTH and neonatal haemodynamics. Acta Pediatr. Scand. (Suppl.) 305:79, 1983.

Pollack, M. S., Levine, L. S., O'Neill, G. J., et al.: HLA linkage and B14, DR1, BfS haplotype association with the genes for late onset and cryptic 21-hydroxylase deficiency. Am. J. Hum. Genet. 33:540, 1981.

Proesmans, W., Geussens, H., Corbeel, L., et al.: Pseudohypoaldosteronism. Am. J. Dis. Child. 126:510, 1973.

Roselli, A., and Barbosa, L. T.: Congenital hypoplasia of the adrenal glands: Report of 2 cases in sisters, with necropsy. Pediatrics 35:70, 1965.

Rosenfield, R. L., Rich, B., Wolfsdorf, J., et al.: Pubertal presentation of congenital $\Delta 5$-3β-hydroxysteroid dehydrogenase deficiency. J. Clin. Endocrinol. Metab. 51:345, 1980.

Sasaki, A., Liotta, A. S., Luckey, M. M., et al.: Immunoreactive corticotropin-releasing factor is present in human maternal plasma during the third trimester of pregnancy. J. Clin. Endocrinol. Metab. 59:812, 1984.

Sherman, S. L., Aston, C. E., Morton, N. E., et al.: A segregation and linkage study of classical and nonclassical 21-hydroxylase deficiency. Am. J. Hum. Genet. 42(6):830, 1988.

Simila, S., Kauppila, A., Ulikorkala, O., et al.: Adrenocorticotrophic hormone during the first day of life. Eur. J. Pediatr. 124:173, 1977.

Simmer, H. H., Frankland, M. V., and Greipel, M.: Unbound unconjugated cortisol in umbilical cord and corresponding maternal plasma. Gynecol. Invest. 5:199, 1974.

Sperling, M. A.: Newborn adaptation: Adrenocortical hormones and ACTH. In Tulchinsky, D., and Ryan, K. J. (Eds.): Maternal-Fetal Endocrinology. Philadelphia, W. B. Saunders Company, 1980, p. 387.

Sperling, M. A., Wolfsen, A. R., and Fisher, D. A.: Congenital adrenal hypoplasia: An isolated defect of organogenesis. J. Pediatr. 82:44, 1973.

Winters, A. J., Oliver, S., Colston, C., et al.: Plasma ACTH levels in the human fetus and neonate as related to age and parturition. J. Clin. Endocrinol. Metab. 39:269, 1974.

Walsh, S. W., Normal, R. L., and Novy, M. J.: In utero regulation of Rhesus monkey fetal adrenals: Effects of dexamethasone, adrenocorticotropin, thyrotropin releasing hormone, prolactin, human chorionic gonadotropin and melanocyte stimulating hormone in fetal and maternal plasma steroids. Endocrinology 104:1805, 1979.

ABNORMALITIES OF SEXUAL DIFFERENTIATION* **108**

Daniel H. Polk

◾ GENERAL CONSIDERATIONS

Anatomic differentiation of the external genitalia is usually complete in the human infant by birth. This fortunate circumstance enables the obstetrician and proud parents to proclaim "It's a girl" or "It's a boy." Permanent gender assignment is made instantaneously. Occasionally, genital differentiation is incomplete or ambiguous. The physician's reactions to this medical emergency will have an immense impact on these children and their families. It is important to have a sound understanding of normal sexual development and to be able to initiate steps that will lead to appropriate gender assignment, diagnosis, and management.

Two principles emerge in the consideration of embryologic sexual differentiation. First, sexual organs at all three levels—gonads, internal duct structures, and external genitalia—develop from identical undifferentiated structures in the male and female fetus. Second, differentiation along female anatomic lines proceeds passively unless opposed by active male factors.

Male and female gonads develop from anlagen located on the urogenital ridge. Prior to 6 weeks of gestational age, testis and ovary are indistinguishable. In the fetus with a 46,XY chromosome constitution, definite testicular differentiation occurs rapidly over the ensuing weeks. By 12 weeks, both testicular testosterone concentration (Reyes et al., 1973) and the ability to convert pregnenolone to testosterone enzymatically (Siiteri and Wilson, 1974) are maximal. Peak concentrations of testosterone in the fetal circulation are reached at 16 weeks and are comparable to those of the adult male. Thereafter, the testosterone concentration falls, and after 24 weeks, the concentration is in the early pubertal range (Kaplan and Grumbach, 1978). In contrast, ovarian differentiation occurs later in gestation and is not a prerequisite for normal female genital development. In the fetus with a 46,XX chromosome complement, oocytes appear at about the 12th week. Primordial follicles, containing oocytes surrounded by a layer of granulosa cells, are recognizable by the 12th week. The circulating estrogens in the fetus are primarily of placental origin, with little contribution from the fetal ovary. The ovary has no apparent role in sex differentiation of the female genital tract.

The mechanism involved in the translation of genetic sex into a testis or ovary is poorly understood. Studies of the histocompatibility Y (H-Y) antigen provide some in-

sight into genes and testicular organogenesis (Ohno et al., 1979; Wachtel and Ohno, 1979). The H-Y antigen is a male-specific component that has been detected in the membranes of all cells from normal XY males except immature germ cells. The pericentromeric region of the Y chromosome contains a locus (or loci) that either codes for the plasma membrane H-Y antigen or regulates its expression. The H-Y antigen induces differentiation of the primitive gonad as a testis. The critical factor in testis organogenesis is not the presence or absence of a detectable Y chromosome but the expression of the H-Y antigen. The embryonic gonad has an inherent tendency to form an ovary in the absence of H-Y antigen or its specific receptor. Newer techniques have allowed Page and colleagues (1987a) to clone a part of the Y chromosome involved in testicular organogenesis. Further studies using this probe in normal and abnormal sexual development will result in a more comparable understanding of normal testicular development. Genes for normal ovarian differentiation are located on both the long and short arms of the human X chromosome. Accumulated evidence supports the view that two X chromosomes are required for differentiation of the indifferent gonad.

A schematic of fetal genital development is shown in Figure 108–1. At 7 weeks' gestation, the fetus has precursors of both male and female genital ducts. The müllerian ducts are anlagen of the fallopian tubes, uterus, and proximal vagina. Wolffian ducts are anlagen for the epididymis, vas deferens, seminal vesicles, and ejaculatory ducts of the male. The brilliant experiments of Josso (1972) have shown that the fetal testis produces a locally active macromolecular hormone that induces regression of the müllerian ducts. This action cannot be mimicked by androgens. However, high local concentrations of testosterone, produced by the fetal testis, are required for further development of the wolffian ducts. Genital duct development is nearly complete by 12 weeks of gestation.

Male and female external genitalia are identical during the 2nd month of pregnancy. Three structures are easily recognizable (see Fig. 108–1). These structures are the genital tubercle, the genital folds, and the genital swellings. Testosterone—and more specifically, its active intracellular metabolite dihydrotestosterone (DHT)—is required for male differentiation. Without testosterone, the genital tubercle remains small and forms the clitoris, the genital folds remain separate and form the labia minora, and the genital swellings form the labia majora. Under the influence of DHT, the genital tubercle enlarges and forms the penis, the genital folds fuse to form a phallic urethra, and

---

*Revised from C. Anast, 5th edition.

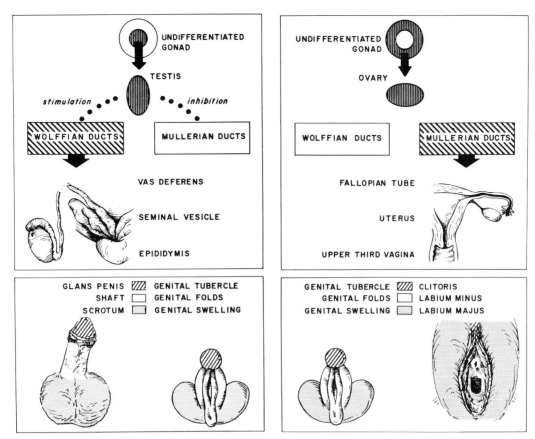

FIGURE 108–1. Outline of genital development. Note that gonadal development occurs from a common indifferent gonad, the internal genitalia develop from separate primordia present in both sexes, and the external genitalia develop in a continuous transformation of anlage common to both sexes. (From Fedeman, D.D.: Disorders of sexual development. N. Engl. J. Med. 277:351, 1967. Reprinted, by permission of the New England Journal of Medicine.)

the genital swellings fuse to form the scrotum. Fusion is complete by the 12th week of gestation, but phallic enlargement continues to term.

Most of the known errors of human sexual differentiation can be provisionally explained by genetic or biochemical alterations in the aforementioned sequence of events. Conte and Grumbach (1989) have written excellent detailed reviews of this area. This discussion follows the classification scheme shown in Table 108–1. The first category entails disorders of gonadal differentiation, usually in association with abnormal number or structure of the X or Y chromosomes. The second category involves virilization of the female fetus; the third, undervirilization of the male fetus. The last category involves anatomic defects that, in most cases, do not have a definite chromosomal or hormonal etiology.

■ DISORDERS OF GONADAL DIFFERENTIATION

KLINEFELTER SYNDROME

Klinefelter syndrome is one of the most common sex chromosome anomalies, occurring one in 1000 male births. The 47,XXY chromosome constitution arises during meiotic division in either parent or, less commonly, from mitotic nondisjunction in the zygote and is associated with advanced maternal age. Infants with 47,XXY karyotype as a group have lower birth weights than controls and have an increased incidence of major and minor congen-

ital anomalies, especially clinodactyly. Although the testes may be noticeably small during infancy, there are seldom any genital abnormalities, and the diagnosis is seldom made during early childhood. Presenting features in older children and adolescents include low verbal I.Q., behavioral disorders, poor gross motor control, eunuchoid habitus, gynecomastia, and variable virilization. Variants involving 46,XY/47,XXY individuals have been described. In addition 46,XX males occur with an incidence of one in 20,000 males. They share the endocrine manifestations of 47,XXY individuals but typically have normal stature. The biochemical basis for this defect is unknown but may involve Y chromosome translocations (Page et al., 1987b).

TURNER SYNDROME AND VARIANTS

Turner syndrome is defined as gonadal dysgenesis due to a missing or structurally defective X chromosome. The 45,X karyotype is associated with a high intrauterine mortality. Its frequency is one per 20 spontaneous abortuses but only one per 10,000 live newborn females. The incidence of 45,X karyotype is increased in the pregnancies of teenaged mothers. The condition should be suspected in female infants with webbing of the neck, edema of the extremities, or coarctation of the aorta. In the great majority of infants with gonadal dysgenesis, the external genitalia and internal duct structures are unequivocally female. Half the individuals with 45,X genotype also exhibit renal anomalies, some of which may not be suspected clinically (Shawker et al., 1987). More subtle

TABLE 108–1. Classification of Abnormalities of Sexual Differentiation

I. Disorders of gonadal differentiation
- A. Klinefelter syndrome: 47, XXY and variants
- B. Turner syndrome (gonadal dysgenesis): 45, X and variants
- C. Pure gonadal dysgenesis: 46, XX
- D. True hermaphroditism

II. Virilization of the female fetus: 46, XX
- A. Due to maternal ingestion of drugs
- B. Due to maternal overproduction of androgens
- C. Due to congenital adrenal hyperplasia
  1. P450 C21 deficiency
  2. 3 β-Hydroxysteroid dehydrogenase deficiency
  3. P450 C11/C18 deficiency

III. Undervirilization of the male fetus: 46, XY
- A. Anorchia, or vanishing testis syndrome
- B. Genetic defects in testosterone biosynthesis
  1. Defects common to cortisol and testosterone pathways
     a. 3β-Hydroxysteroid dehydrogenase deficiency
     b. P450 C17 deficiency
  2. Defects unique to androgen and estrogen synthesis
     a. 17, 20-Desmolase deficiency
     b. 17 β-Hydroxysteroid oxidoreductase deficiency
- C. End-organ insensitivity to testosterone
  1. 5 α-Reductase deficiency
  2. Testicular feminization
  3. Partial testicular feminization
- D. Testicular unresponsiveness to HCG and LH
- E. Maternal ingestion of progestins and estrogens

IV. Anatomic abnormalities
- A. As isolated findings
  1. Hypospadias
  2. Cryptorchidism
  3. Persistence of müllerian structures
- B. Associated with other birth defects

findings include low birth weight for gestational age, ptosis, hypertelorism, micrognathia, hypertension, low-set and/or deformed ears, cubitus valgus, and dysplasia of fingernails and toenails. In the newborn, pleural effusions and ascites that clear spontaneously are not uncommon, and pericardial effusion has been reported. In other affected girls, somatic abnormalities are minimal and the condition is suspected because of short stature, failure of breast development, and primary amenorrhea at the age of puberty. A lack of feedback inhibition of hypothalamic-pituitary axis by the dysgenic ovary is reflected in elevated serum FSH and LH levels in affected infants as early as 5 days of age (Conte et al., 1980).

Roughly 85 per cent of the girls with gonadal dysgenesis have a 45,X karyotype. The remainder have either mosaicism, or a structural abnormality of the X chromosome. Structural abnormalities include isochromosomes of either the short (XXpi) or long arm (XXqi), deletion of the short (XXp⁻) or long arm, or ring chromosomes. The diagnosis is thus confirmed by chromosome analysis and banding studies.

Suspicion and confirmation of gonadal dysgenesis in a newborn confers an unusual responsibility upon the physician. There is seldom any doubt about gender assignment, for these infants are females. However, their ovaries have in most instances regressed to vestigial streaks by the time of birth. The great majority of these girls will be short and infertile as adults. The parents should be told that their child will be shorter than average and probably infertile and will require hormone replacement at the age of puberty to foster a growth spurt, breast development, and menstrual cycles. However, it is well to be aware that

although streak gonads are the rule in 45,X gonadal dysgenesis, exceptions have been documented. Primary follicles have been observed in the ridges of some 45,X individuals in adolescence, and this correlates with the rare occurrence of menarche and a variable but attenuated period of regular menses. Moreover, conceptions have been documented in some women in whom extensive karyotypic studies revealed only 45,X cell line in multiple tissues (King et al., 1978; Kohn et al., 1980). Some fertile 45,X women may be unrecognized sex chromosome mosaics.

Mosaicism involving the Y chromosome is less common than classic Turner syndrome and produces a wider variety of phenotypes. Infants with 45,X/46,XY karyotypes commonly have ambiguous genitalia. Gender assignment should be in accordance with the expected potential for adult sexual function. Gonads in these individuals generally consist of bilateral dysgenic testis and a contralateral gonadal streak. Either or both gonads may have failed to produce müllerian-inhibiting substance, and there may be a uterus and unilateral or bilateral fallopian tubes. Depending on the extent and timing of intrauterine testosterone production, there may also be well-developed wolffian structures. Short stature and the somatic abnormalities of Turner syndrome are inconstant findings. Dysgenic gonads are predisposed to neoplasia and should be removed at an early age. Hormone replacement at the age of puberty must be concordant with the sex of rearing.

PURE GONADAL DYSGENESIS

"Pure gonadal dysgenesis" is a term applied to phenotypic females with bilateral streak gonads who lack the somatic stigmata of Turner syndrome and who are of normal or tall stature. Karyotype may be either 46,XX or 46,XY. The internal and external genitalia of the 46,XX individuals with gonadal dysgenesis are normal female. The 46,XX patients seldom show clitoral enlargement, may show ovarian function at puberty, and are not prone to gonadal neoplasms. Familial cases are not uncommon in 46,XX gonadal dysgenesis, and transmission is consistent with an autosomal recessive trait. Deafness is an associated finding in some families with 46,XX gonadal dysgenesis (Simpson, 1976). Inheritance consistent with an X-linked or male-limited dominant trait has been observed. Usually, the external and internal genital tract is completely female. However, clitoral enlargement occurs, and affected siblings may have ambiguous external genitalia and development of the genital ducts. Both H-Y antigen–positive and H-Y antigen–negative forms have been described, findings that further reflect the genetic heterogeneity of this syndrome.

TRUE HERMAPHRODITISM

True hermaphroditism is a rare condition that requires the presence of both ovarian and testicular tissue in the same individual. The tissue may be present in the same or opposite gonads. In almost half of the cases there is an ovotestis on one side and an ovary or testis on the other; in one-fifth there are bilateral ovotestes; and in one-third there is an ovary on one side and a testis on the other. The external genitalia are extremely variable, but roughly three-fourths of patients have phallic enlargement, generally with hypospadias, and many have been raised as males. Cryptorchidism is common, and an inguinal hernia that may contain a gonad or uterus is present in about half of the cases. A uterus is usually present and often asymmetric. Genital ducts develop in accordance with the function of the ipsilateral gonad. Most patients with an ovotestis have predominantly female development of the genital ducts. Chromosomal findings are varied and do not correlate with gonadal histology or external genital appearance. Approximately 70 per cent of true hermaphrodites are X chromatin-positive. Van Niekerk (1981) reported that of 148 patients, 89 were 46,XX, 18 were 46,XY, 21 were XX/XY chimeras, and the remainder were sex chromosome mosaics. All true hermaphrodites are H-Y antigen-positive. The presence of H-Y antigen in 46,XX true hermaphrodites supports the postulate that the structural gene for H-Y antigen is on an autosome and not the Y chromosome. Therefore, an autosomal mutation affecting the structural gene for H-Y antigen results in the differentiation of a testis or ovotestis in an XX individual (Fraccaro et al., 1979). However, until the sites of the putative regulatory genes that may affect the expression of H-Y are determined, the pathogenesis of true hermaphroditism in relationship to H-Y antigen remains uncertain.

At puberty, breast development is common; menses occurs in over half the patients; and a large number virilize. Although spermatogenesis is rare, ovulation is not uncommon, and pregnancy and childbirth have been observed in several patients with an XX karyotype (Kim et al., 1979).

True hermaphroditism should be considered in any infant or child with ambiguous genitalia in whom an alternative explanation cannot be established from chromosomal, hormonal, and radiologic contrast studies. Diagnosis requires laparotomy and biopsy of gonads. Management involves surgical removal of gonads, internal duct structures, and features of the external genitalia that are incongruous with gender assignment.

■ VIRILIZATION OF THE FEMALE FETUS

Virilization of the female fetus is the most common category of disorders producing ambiguity of the external genitalia. As previously stated, in the absence of androgens, external female genitalia will proceed to develop along female lines. Androgens, which may be derived from either maternal or fetal sources, can cause the external genitalia of otherwise normal 46,XX girls to virilize. In some cases, this process is so complete as to mimic the external genitalia of a cryptorchid male. Fusion of the genital folds or the genital swellings is a result of androgen exposure prior to the 12th gestational week. Clitoral enlargement can occur with androgen exposure at any time. Buccal smears are chromatin-positive, and karyotypes are 46,XX. Management of underlying pathological processes and surgical correction of anatomic abnormalities are followed by normal pubertal development and normal adult sexual and reproductive function.

VIRILIZATION BY MATERNAL INGESTION OF DRUGS

Virilization of the female fetus has been attributed to testosterone, the 19-nortestosterone progestins, progesterone, and even, paradoxically, diethylstilbestrol. In each case, a fairly small proportion of exposed infants had clinically evident virilization. There was seldom evidence of virilization in the mother (Jones, 1981). It is not known which of these compounds act directly on the external genitalia and which act indirectly through altering androgen synthesis by the mother or fetus. It seems reasonable to speculate that differences in maternal, placental, or fetal metabolism of the synthetic steroids determine which infants are affected.

The incidence of this condition has diminished as the use of synthetic estrogens and progestins for management of threatened abortion has waned. However, the condition is still seen in offspring of women who unknowingly continue to take birth control pills following conception. Severity of virilization is quite variable, ranging from mild clitoral enlargement to complete labial fusion with a phallic uretha. The infant does not show progressive virilization or accelerated growth and skeletal maturation after birth. Even in the presence of a positive history of maternal hormone ingestion, it is mandatory to obtain a buccal smear or a chromosome analysis and a determination of 17-ketosteroids or 17-hydroxyprogesterone to exclude other possible diagnoses.

VIRILIZATION BY MATERNAL OVERPRODUCTION OF ANDROGENS

Severe disorders of maternal androgen production generally preclude pregnancy. However, artificial induction of ovulation in a virilized woman or development of a virilizing neoplasm during pregnancy can set the stage for virilization of a female infant. In most cases, the mother has clinical signs of virilization, such as hirsutism, acne, clitoromegaly, and deepening of the voice. Virilization has been observed in a female infant born to a mother with a virilizing form of congenital adrenal hyperplasia (Kai et al., 1979). The clinical features of the offspring of virilized mothers are identical with those described previously for girls whose mothers received sex hormones. Diagnosis requires demonstration of elevated urinary 17-ketosteroids or plasma testosterone in the mother as well as exclusion of alternative diagnoses in the infant.

CONGENITAL ADRENAL HYPERPLASIA

The category of diseases encompassed by congenital adrenal hyperplasia is discussed more fully in Chapter 107. Inherited enzymatic blocks in the synthesis of cortisol lead to overproduction of androgens and virilization of the female fetus. Defects in P450 C21, 3β-hydroxysteroid dehydrogenase, or P450 C11/C18 can each produce this result. Buccal smear is chromatin-positive, and urinary excretion of 17-ketosteroids remains above 2.5 mg per 24 hours. In infants with a defect in 21-hydroxylase, the plasma 17-hydroxyprogesterone level is elevated. Treatment with cortisol suppresses adrenal androgen production and prevents further virilization and excessively rapid growth and skeletal maturation. In infants with salt-losing forms of congenital adrenal hyperplasia, cortisol and mineralocorticoid replacement are lifesaving.

■ UNDERVIRILIZATION OF THE MALE FETUS

Complete male genital differentiation requires the presence of testes, the ability of testes to produce testosterone, and the ability of the genital anlagen to recognize and respond to testosterone. Defects can occur at each of these levels and result in genitalia that are either ambiguous or unambiguously female. It is important to emphasize that the degree of virilization of 46,XX individuals can be remarkable, and that male sex assignment to infants born with bilateral cryptochordism may result in multiple surgical and medical interventions in what otherwise would have been a normal fertile female. The converse is also true, that is, that one should not hesitate to make an assignment of female gender to individuals with third-degree hypospadias and microphallus with bilateral anorchia despite the presence of a Y chromosome.

ANORCHIA

A spectrum of genital anomalies is observed in patients with a 46,XY karyotype resulting from cessation of testicular function during the critical stages of male sexual differentiation between 8 and 14 weeks' gestation. Deficiency of testicular function before 8 weeks' gestation results in female external and internal genitalia, whereas lack of testicular function beginning between 8 and 10 weeks' gestation results in ambiguous genitalia. Loss of testicular function after 14 weeks' gestation results in anorchia, or vanishing testes syndrome, in which there is normal male differentiation both internally and externally but no gonadal tissue. The diagnosis of anorchia is made in infants with apparent bilateral cryptorchidism, 46,XY karyotype, and elevated circulating gonadotropin levels, who fail to demonstrate a testosterone response to human chorionic gonadotropin administration (Lustig et al., 1987). As previously discussed, gender assignment in infants with this syndrome and ambiguous genitalia should be female, despite the presence of 46,XY karyotype.

GENETIC DEFECTS IN TESTOSTERONE BIOSYNTHESIS

In several varieties of congenital adrenal hyperplasia, the enzymatic defect is shared by adrenal and gonadal tissues. The result is undervirilization of the affected male due to impairment of fetal testosterone production. Specific defects include 3β-hydroxysteroid dehydrogenase and 17β-hydroxylase deficiencies, discussed in the previous chapter. In these conditions, the enzyme deficiency impairs synthesis of cortisol as well as testosterone.

Defects may also occur in metabolic pathways unique to the synthesis of sex steroids. The 17,20-desmolase enzyme converts 17α-hydroxypregnenolone to dihydroepiandrosterone and 17α-hydroxyprogesterone to androstenedione. Deficiency leads to severe hypospadias, with or without cryptorchidism, and an elevated urinary excretion of pregnenetriol and 11-ketopregnanetriol, suggesting elevated plasma levels of 17α-hydroxyprogesterone and 17α-hydroxypregnenolone. Occurrence in siblings and an "aunt" indicate X-linked recessive or male-limited autosomal-dominant inheritance. In 1976, Goebelsman and co-workers reported a 46,XY phenotypic female with normal external genitalia, no müllerian structures, atrophic wolffian derivatives, abdominal testes, and biochemical findings suggestive of a defect in 17,20-desmolase activity.

The next step in testosterone synthesis involves 17β-hydroxysteroid oxidoreductase, which converts dehydroepiandrosterone to 5-androstenediol, androstenedione to testosterone, and estrone to estradiol. Deficiency results in ambiguous genitalia and elevated plasma androstenedione and estrone levels in postpubertal patients (Conte and Grumbach, 1989). Puberty in the patients reported by Saez and colleagues (1972) was characterized by virilization and gynecomastia. The latter finding was attributed to elevated concentrations of the estrogen estrone.

END-ORGAN INSENSITIVITY TO TESTOSTERONE

DEFICIENCY OF 5α-REDUCTASE

The external genital anlagen of the fetus normally possess 5α-reductase activity and are able to convert testosterone to the active metabolite dihydrotestosterone. This compound is required for complete male genital development, and a defect at this level may explain an autosomal recessive condition known as "pseudovaginal perineoscrotal hypospadias." An interesting variant of this condition, known as the "penis at twelve" syndrome, involves marked virilization and phallic growth at puberty. This condition presumably results from an incomplete block in reductase activity which is overcome by increases in circulating testosterone which occur at puberty (Imperato-McGinley et al., 1984). Infants with 5α-reductase deficiency have 46,XY karyotype, normally differentiated testes, male internal ducts, and ambiguous external genitalia. Bilateral inguinal or labial masses, representing testes, may prompt evaluation, but usually these patients present during puberty.

TESTICULAR FEMINIZATION

Recognition of testosterone or dihydrotestosterone by target tissues requires the participation of a cytoplasmic receptor protein that binds the steroid, enters the nucleus, and interacts with nuclear chromatin. Genetic disorders in the rat and mouse involving receptor defects closely parallel the human condition of testicular feminization.

In the complete form of the disorder, 46,XY infants have unambiguously female external genitalia. Unless there are inguinal hernias containing testes, recognition may be delayed until puberty, when these girls show normal breast development but lack sexual hair and fail to menstruate. The vagina ends blindly, and the uterus and fallopian tubes are absent, reflecting the intrauterine production of and response to müllerian-inhibiting substance. The disorder is familial, with multiple sibling involvement and occurrence in maternal aunts suggesting

X-linked recessive or male-limited autosomal dominant inheritance. The gender assignment is unquestionably female. Gonads should be removed because of a recognized incidence of malignant degeneration. Estrogen replacement at puberty enhances breast development but does not induce menses because there is no uterus.

PARTIAL TESTICULAR FEMINIZATION

Partial testicular feminization implies a partial defect in the biological actions of testosterone with an attendant partial inhibition of male genital differentiation. Wilson and co-workers (1974) have suggested that many familial cases of microphallus, hypospadias, and gynecomastia with normal testosterone production at puberty fall in this category.

Studies of dihydrotestosterone binding by cultured fibroblasts from genital skin have shown two patterns in both the complete and partial forms of testicular feminization (Griffen and Wilson, 1980; Kaufman et al., 1979). In one, there are quantitatively reduced or absent (complete form) cytosol receptors for dihydrotestosterone and testosterone; in the other, cytosol binding and nuclear binding of dihydrotestosterone are normal. The latter presumably represents an as yet undefined postreceptor defect or subtle qualitative abnormality in the androgen receptor itself.

TESTICULAR UNRESPONSIVENESS TO HCG AND LH

Another form of male pseudohermaphroditism has been described in which there is Leydig cell hypoplasia or agenesis, apparently secondary to a deficiency or abnormality of the HCG-LH receptor on the plasma membrane of the fetal and postnatal Leydig cell (David et al, 1984). The external genitalia in these 46,XY patients were female except for slight posterior labial fusion and clitoromegaly in one patient. Separate vaginal and urethral openings were present, but uterus and fallopian tubes were absent. Plasma LH levels were elevated, and plasma FSH levels were normal. Plasma testosterone levels were low and did not increase in response to HCG. It is thought that the resistance of undifferentiated embryonic and fetal Leydig cells to HCG results in fetal testicular deficiency with female or predominantly female differentiation of the external genitalia.

MATERNAL INGESTION OF PROGESTINS AND ESTROGENS

Animal studies have suggested an antiandrogen effect of progestins on the male fetus. Maternal ingestion of progestins and estrogens has been implicated but not proved as a rare cause of male undervirilization in humans. Some studies have suggested an association between progestins and hypospadias (Aarskag, 1979); others have suggested that effects of maternal diethylstilbestrol ingestion during early pregnancy on male sexual differentiation are minimal (Leary et al., 1984). In vitro studies have demonstrated that progestins can inhibit 5α-reductase activity (Voight and Hsia, 1973), which as discussed earlier, converts testosterone to dihydrotestosterone, the active metabolite that is required for complete male development.

■ ISOLATED ANATOMIC ABNORMALITIES

A complete discussion of hypospadias and cryptorchidism is presented in Chapter 97. For purposes of this discussion, it is important to remember that virilization of otherwise functional 46,XX girls may at times be so remarkable as to result in the inappropriate assignment of male sex. Any child who presents with bilateral cryptorchidism and hypospadias should be carefully evaluated at the time of birth for the existence of a more serious underlying defect.

PERSISTENCE OF MÜLLERIAN DUCTS

A fully developed uterus and fallopian tubes may be discovered incidental to surgery in phenotypic males with normal 46,XY karyotypes. The theoretical explanation of this finding is a failure of production or recognition of müllerian-inhibiting substance. The condition may be transmitted as an autosomal recessive trait, although X-linked recessive inheritance and genetic heterogeneity have not been excluded (Summitt, 1979). Treatment consists of removal of organs that are discordant with the patient's gender.

■ ANATOMIC ABNORMALITIES IN ASSOCIATION WITH OTHER DEFECTS

Malformations of the external genitalia may be a part of a more complicated embryopathy. In females, genital abnormalities may be associated with imperforate anus, renal agenesis, congenital nephritis, and other congenital malformations of the lower intestine and genitourinary tract. Drash and co-workers (1970) have reported an association between degenerative renal disease, Wilms tumor, and ambiguity of the external genitalia in males. Rimoin and Schimke's monograph (1971) has an excellent discussion of associations between genital abnormalities and largely nonendocrine syndromes. In many instances, such infants have severe defects incompatible with life, but there is still the problem of assigning gender.

■ EVALUATION OF INFANTS WITH AMBIGUOUS GENITALIA

It is extremely important that the evaluation of a newborn with ambiguous genitalia be carried out immediately after birth. The flow chart in Figure 108–2 indicates studies that can be carried out to provide a provisional diagnosis and a firm gender assignment within the first 72 hours. The parents should be advised that their infant's genital development has not been completed by birth, that the baby is all girl or all boy and not a little of both, that tests will be done to determine the correct sex, and that announcement of the birth to friends and relatives should be delayed until the tests are returned.

Inspection of the external genitalia may reveal a phallic structure that is small for a male or large for a girl. There

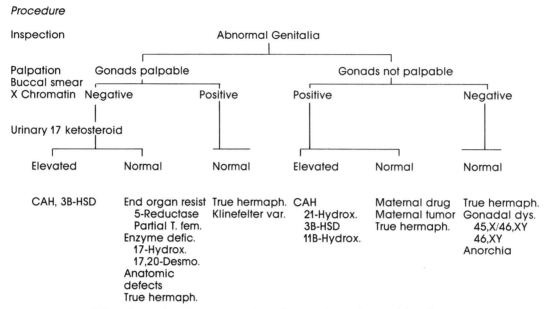

FIGURE 108–2. *Investigation of the infant with ambiguous genitalia. Palpation of gonads is useful in that it usually is associated with an X chromatin-negative buccal smear and a 46,XY karyotype. However, testicular nondescent can occur in virtually all of the enzymatic deficiency syndromes. Infants with 21-hydroxylase deficiency have elevated plasma levels of 17-hydroxyprogesterone. CAH = congenital adrenal hyperplasia; 3B-HSD = 3β-hydroxysteroid dehydrogenase.*

is likely to be chordee with hypospadias. The genitalia swellings may be fused or open. A urologic surgeon should be involved quite early in the examination of the infant. If the phallic structure shows little potential for penile function, a female gender assignment should be made regardless of further findings. However, the converse is not true; the degree of phallic enlargement should not preclude a female gender assignment. Palpation of the labial-scrotal structures for gonads is extremely important, for these gonads are usually testes.

The buccal smear for determination of sex chromatin should be done on the 1st day of life. Although the number of positive chromatin bodies may be diminished in comparison to adult values, there should be no overlap of results between 46,XX females and 46,XY males. The chromatin-positive infant should be considered to have virilizing congenital adrenal hyperplasia until proved otherwise. Lymphocyte karyotyping should be done on the same indications as the buccal smear, but analysis takes weeks rather than hours. Techniques utilizing actively dividing cells aspirated from bone marrow may shorten the time required for karyotyping.

Determination of 17-ketosteroid and pregnanetriol excretion can be accomplished in the first 72 hours. Infants with congenital adrenal hyperplasia due to a deficiency of 21-hydroxylase or 3β-hydroxysteroid dehydrogenase will show an increase rather than a decrease in 17-ketosteroid excretion during the first week, with levels remaining above 2.5 mg per 24 hours. A striking increase in plasma 17-hydroxyprogesterone is found in infants with defective 21-hydroxylation. Vomiting, dehydration, hyperkalemia, and hyponatremia are observed in salt-losing forms of 21-hydroxylase and 3β-hydroxysteroid dehydrogenase deficiencies.

Obtaining the history is extremely important. There should be a complete inquiry about all medications taken during pregnancy. Family history may reveal unexplained infant deaths among siblings of infants with salt-losing congenital adrenal hyperplasia. Infants with defects in testosterone synthesis or with partial testicular feminization commonly have hypogonadal maternal uncles, or maternal "aunts" with primary amenorrhea.

By 72 hours, a definite gender assignment will have been made in most cases. Chromatin-positive infants will almost always be female. Those who do not have congenital adrenal hyperplasia, virilization due to maternal drugs or tumor, or associated birth defects will probably require laparotomy and gonadal biopsy in later infancy. Chromatin-negative infants may have a male or female gender assignment, depending on phallic structure. They will require karyotyping to exclude 45,X/46,XY mosaicism, further serum and urinary steroid measurement to define rare abnormalities of adrenal or gonadal steroid synthesis, and contrast studies of the genitourinary tract to search for müllerian duct structures. Laparotomy and gonadal biopsy can safely be deferred to a later age.

The pioneering studies of Money and colleagues (1955) have shown that karyotype, gonads, internal ducts, and hormones have very little to do with behavior and psychosexual inclinations. These features are chiefly influenced by gender assignment and home environment. If the parents are secure about their boy or girl, the gender role is firmly established in early infancy and can rarely be reversed. The physician's role is to be sure that the physical and hormonal state of the growing child is not seriously at odds with the gender assignment. In the girl with congenital adrenal hyperplasia, this involves glucocorticoid replacement, consideration of clitorectomy and vaginoplasty if needed in infancy, and continued follow-up after maturity. In the male with hypospadias and deficient testosterone production, it means surgical repair of hypospadias and evaluation of the need for testosterone replacement at the age of puberty. The genetic male with a female gender assignment needs protection from confusing information about chromosomes and may require gonadectomy before puberty to prevent virilization.

■ PRENATAL DIAGNOSIS OF ABNORMALITIES OF SEXUAL DIFFERENTIATION

Amniocentesis, ultrasonography, and studies of maternal blood and urine provide tools for the prenatal diagnosis of abnormalities of sexual differentiation. Abnormalities of sex chromosome number and structure can be determined by karyotypic analysis of chromosomes from amniotic fluid obtained as early as 14 to 16 weeks' gestation and from chorionic villous biopsy specimens as early as 8 weeks' gestation. HLA typing of amniotic fluid cells may aid in the prenatal diagnosis of certain forms of congenital adrenal hypoplasia when HLA typing of previously affected family members is available. Moreover, elevated amniotic fluid levels of 17-hydroxyprogesterone and androstenedione are present in male and female fetuses with 21-hydroxylase deficiency (Pang et al., 1980). Similarly, a fetus affected with 11β-hydroxylase deficiency can be detected by measurement of 11-deoxycortisol in amniotic fluid or in maternal plasma and urine (Rosler et al., 1979; Schumert et al., 1980). Estriol concentrations in maternal plasma and urine reflect the functional integrity of the fetal adrenal and placenta; low levels are observed in disorders of fetal hypothalamic-pituitary-adrenal function (Davies, 1980). Fetal sexing is now possible with ultrasonography after 28 weeks' gestation (LeLann, 1979).

■ REFERENCES

Aarskog, D.: Maternal progestins as a possible cause of hypospadias. N. Engl. J. Med. 300::75, 1979.

Conte, F. A., and Grumbach, M. M.: Pathogenesis, classification, diagnosis and treatment of anomalies of sex. In DeGroot, L. J. (Ed.): Endocrinology. Philadelphia, W. B. Saunders Company, 1989, p. 810.

Conte, F. A., Grumbach, M. M., Kaplan, S. C., et al.: Correlation of luteinizing hormone–releasing factor, induced luteinizing hormone, and follicle-stimulating hormone release from infancy to 19 years with the changing pattern of gonadotropin secretion in agonadal patients: Relation to restraint of puberty. J. Clin. Endocrinol. Metab. 50:163, 1980.

David, R., Yoon, D. Y., Landin, L., et al.: A syndrome of gonadotropin resistance possibly due to a leutinizing hormone receptor defect. J. Clin. Endocrinol. Metab. 59:156, 1984.

Davies, J.: The fetal adrenal. In Tulchinksy, D., and Ryan, K. (Eds.): Maternal-Fetal Endocrinology. Philadelphia, W. B. Saunders Company, 1980.

Drash, A., Sherman, F., Hartmann, W. H., et al.: A syndrome of pseudohermaphroditism, Wilms' tumor, hypertension, and degenerative renal disease. J. Pediatr. 76:585, 1970.

Fraccaro, M., Tiepolo, L., Zuffardi, O., et al.: Familial XX true hermaphrodism and the H-Y antigen. Hum. Genet. 48:45, 1979.

Goebelsmann, U., Zachmann, M., Darajan, R., et al.: Male pseudohermaphrodism consistent with 17,20-desmolase deficiency. Gynecol. Invest. 7:138, 1976.

Griffen, J. E., and Wilson, J. D.: The syndrome of androgen resistance. N. Engl. J. Med. 302:198, 1980.

Imperato-McGinley, J., Peterson, R. E., and Gautier, T.: Primary and secondary 5α-reductase deficiency. In, Serio, M., Mota, M., Zanisc, M., et al.: (Eds.): Sexual Differentiation: Basic and Clinical Aspects. New York, Raven Press, 1984, p. 233.

Jones, H. W., Jr.: Nonadrenal female pseudohermaphroditism. In Josso, N. (Ed.): Pediatric and Adolescent Endocrinology, vol 8. Basel, Karger, 1981, p. 65.

Josso, N.: Permeability of membranes to the müllerian-inhibiting substance synthesized by the human fetal testis in vitro: A clue to its biochemical nature. J. Clin. Endocrinol. Metab. 34:265, 1972.

Kai, H., Nose, O., Iida, Y., et al.: Female pseudohermaphrodism caused by maternal congenital adrenal hyperplasia. J. Pediatr. 95:418, 1979.

Kaplan, N. M.: Male pseudohermaphrodism: Report of a case, with observations on pathogenesis. N. Engl. J. Med. 261:641, 1959.

Kaplan, S. L., and Grumbach, M. M.: Pituitary and placental gonadotropins and sex steroids in the human and sub-human primate fetus. Clin. Endocrinol. Metab. 7:487, 1978.

Kaufman, M., Pinsky, L., Baird, P. A., et al.: Complete androgen insensitivity with a normal amount of 5α-dihydrotestosterone–binding activity in labium majus skin fibroblasts. Am. J. Med. Genet. 4:401, 1979.

Kim, M. H., Gumpel, J. A., and Graff, P.: Pregnancy in a true hermaphrodite ("es"). Obstet. Gynecol. 53(3 Suppl.):4OS, 1979.

King, C. R., Magenis, E., and Bennett, S.: Pregnancy and the Turner syndrome. Obstet. Gynecol. 52:617, 1978.

Kohn, G., Yarkoni, S., and Cohen, M. M.: Two conceptions in a 45,X woman. Am. J. Med. Genet. 5:339, 1980.

Leary, F. J., Reseguie, L. J., Kurland, L. T., et al.: Males exposed in utero to diethylstilbestrol. J.A.M.A. 252:2984, 1984.

LeLann, D.: Diagnostic échographique antinatal du sexe masculin et féminin. Nouv. Presse Med. 8:2760, 1979.

Lustig, R. H., Conte, F. A., Kogan, B. A., et al.: Ontogeny of gonadotropin secretion in congenital anorchia: Sexual dimorphisim versus syndrome of gonadal dysgenesis and diagnostic considerations. J. Urol. 138:587, 1987.

Money, J., Hampson, J. G., and Hampson, J. L.: Hermaphroditism: Recommendations concerning assignment of sex, change of sex and psychologic management. Bull. Johns Hopkins Hosp. 96:253, 1955.

Ohno, S., Nagai, Y., Ciccarese, S., et al.: Testis-organizing H-Y antigen and the primary sex-determining mechanism of mammals. Recent Prog. Horm. Res. 35:449, 1979.

Page, D. C., Mosher, R., Simpson, E. M., et al.: The sex-determining region of the Y chromosome encodes a finger protein. Cell 51:1091, 1987a.

Page, D. C., Brown, L. G., and de la Chapelle, A.: Exchange of terminal portions of X and Y chromosomal short arms in human XX males. Nature 328:437, 1987b.

Pang, S., Levin, L. S., Cederquist, L. C., et al.: Amniotic fluid concentrations of Δ⁵ and Δ⁴ steroids in fetuses with congenital adrenal hyperplasia due to 21-hydroxylase deficiency and in anencephalic fetuses. J. Clin. Endocrinol. Metab. 51:223, 1980.

Reyes, F. I., Winter, J. S. D., and Faiman, C.: Studies on human sexual development. I. Fetal gonadal and adrenal sex steroids. J. Clin. Endocrinol. Metab. 37:74, 1973.

Rimoin, D. L., and Schimke, R. N.: Genetic Disorders of the Endocrine Glands. Saint Louis, C. V. Mosby, 1971.

Rosler, A., Leiberman, E., Rosenmann, A., et al.: Prenatal diagnosis of 11β-hydroxylase deficiency congenital adrenal hyperplasia. J. Clin. Endocrinol. Metab. 49:546, 1979.

Saez, J. M., Morera, A. M., dePeretti, E., et al.: Further in vivo studies in male pseudohermaphroditism with gynecomastia due to a testicular 17-ketosteroid reductase defect (compared to a case of testicular feminization). J. Clin. Endocrinol. Metab. 34:598, 1972.

Schumert, Z., Rosenmann, A., Landau, H., et al.: 11-Deoxycortisol in amniotic fluid: Prenatal diagnosis of congenital adrenal hyperplasia due to 11β-hydroxylase deficiency. Clin. Endocrinol. 12:257, 1980.

Shawker, T. H., Garra, B. S., Loriaux, D. L., et al.: Ultrasonography of Turner's syndrome. J. Ultrasound Med. 5:125, 1987.

Siiteri, P. K., and Wilson, J. D.: Testosterone formation and metabolism during male sexual differentiation in the human embryo. J. Clin. Endocrinol. Metab. 38:113, 1974.

Simpson, J. L.: Disorders of Sexual Differentiation: Etiology and Clinical Delineation. New York, Academic Press, 1976.

Summitt, R. L.: Genetic forms of hypogonadism in the male. In Steinberg, A. G., Bearn, A. G., Motulsky, A. G., et al. (eds.): Progress in Medical Genetics, Vol. 2. Philadelphia, W. B. Saunders Company, 1979.

van Niekerk, W. A.: True hermaphroditism. In Josso, N. (Ed.): Pediatric and Adolescent Endocrinology, vol.8. Basel, Karger, 1981, p. 80.

Voight, W., and Hsia, S. L.: Further studies on testosterone 5α-reductase of human skin: Structural features of steroid inhibitors. J. Biol. Chem. 248:4280, 1973.

Wachtel, S. S., and Ohno, S.: The immunogenetics of sexual development. In Steinberg, A. G., Bearn, A. G., Motulsky, A. G., et al. (Eds.): Progress in Medical Genetics, vol. 3. Philadelphia, W. B. Saunders Company, 1979.

Wilson, J. D., Harrod, M. J., Goldstein, J. L., et al.: Familial incomplete male pseudohermaphroditism, type I. Evidence for androgen resistance and variable clinical manifestations in a family with the Reifenstein syndrome. N. Engl. J. Med. 290:1097, 1974.

Daniel H. Polk and Delbert A. Fisher

■ EMBRYOGENESIS AND HISTOLOGIC DEVELOPMENT OF THE THYROID GLAND

The human thyroid gland is a derivative of the primitive buccopharyngeal cavity. It develops from contributions of two anlagen: (1) a midline thickening of the pharyngeal floor (median anlage) and (2) paired caudal extensions of the fourth pharyngobranchial pouch (lateral anlagen). All of these structures are discernible by day 16 or 17 of gestation; by the 24th day of gestation the median anlage has developed a thin flasklike diverticulum extending from the floor of the buccal cavity down to the fourth branchial arch. At 40 days of gestation, the median and lateral anlagen have fused, and by 50 days of gestation the buccal stalk has ruptured. During this period, the thyroid gland migrates caudally to its definitive location in the anterior neck, helped in part by its relationship with developing cardiac structures.

Developmental abnormalities of the thyroid gland usually represent defects in early morphogenesis resulting from aberrant thyroid tissue migration. The most common anomaly is the persistence of the thyroglossal duct. This is not usually associated with altered thyroid status in the newborn but may present in later life as an infected fistulous tract. Abnormalities of thyroid embryogenesis (thyroid dysgenesis) include agenesis or ectopic tissue in sublingual, cervical, mediastinal, or even intracardiac locations. Although ectopic thyroid tissue may manifest some function, these infants usually exhibit some degree of hypothyroidism. In addition, calcitonin deficiency is present in children with congenital hypothyroidism. However, hypoparathyroidism is not associated with thyroid dysgenesis, although the parathyroid glands may be ectopic in these children.

THYROID HORMONE SYNTHESIS

Circulating plasma iodide enters the thyroid follicular cells and is combined with tyrosine through a series of enzymatically mediated reactions to form the active thyroid hormones 3,5,3'triiodothyronine (T_3) and thyroxine (T_4). The steps in synthesis and release of thyroid hormones include: (1) active transport of inorganic iodide from plasma to thyroid cell; (2) synthesis of tyrosine-rich thyroglobulin which acts as the intermediate iodine acceptor; (3) organification of trapped iodide as iodotyrosines; (4) coupling of monoiodotyrosines (MIT) and diiodotyrosines (DIT) to form the iodothyronines, T_3 and T_4, with storage of iodotyrosines and iodothyronines in follicular colloid;

TABLE 109–1. Biochemical Steps to Thyroid Hormone Synthesis

STEP	INHIBITOR
Iodide transport	ClO_4^- and SCN^-
Thyroglobulin synthesis	protein synthesis inhibitors
Organification of iodide	PTU, MMI
MIT, DIT coupling	PTU, MMI
Thyroglobulin endocytosis and proteolysis	I^-, Li^-, colchicine, and cytochalasin B
Deiodination	dinitrotyrosine

MIT, monoiodotyrosine; DIT, diiodotyrosine.

(5) endocytosis and proteolysis of colloid thyroglobulin to release MIT, DIT, T_3, and T_4; and (6) deiodination of released iodotyrosines within the thyroid cell with reutilization of the iodine. These steps and their inhibitors are outlined in Table 109–1. Certain defects in these biochemical processes have been identified clinically leading in most cases to hypothyroidism. These are discussed in the section on congenital hypothyroidism.

FETAL-PLACENTAL-MATERNAL THYROID INTERACTION

The relative independence of the maternal and fetal hypothalamic-pituitary-thyroid hormone systems is suggested by several clinical observations. The placenta is impermeable to thyroid-stimulating hormone (TSH) and largely impermeable to the thyroid hormones. These data were recently reviewed by Roti (1988) and are summarized in Table 109–2. Direct evidence of placental transfer of thyroid hormones is provided by studies using various thyroid hormone analogues and tracers. Human studies have shown limited transfer from mother to fetus. Large doses of T_4 given to women produced only minor changes in cord serum concentrations of hormonal iodine. Supraphysiologic doses of T_3 chronically administered to pregnant women several weeks prior to delivery significantly

TABLE 109–2. Placental Permeability for Substances Affecting Thyroid Function

SUBSTANCE	PLACENTAL PERMEABILITY
I^-	+ + + +
TRH	+ + +
Thiourylenes	+ + +
IgG antibodies	+ + +
T_3	0
T_4	+
TSH	0

(Data from Roti, E.: Regulation of thyroid-stimulating hormone (TSH) secretion in the fetus and neonate. J. Endocrinol. Invest. *11*:145–150, 1988.)

increased maternal serum T_3 levels but only minimally lowered fetal T_4 values. Thus, it is clear that placental transfer of thyroid hormones is quite limited. This limitation is due, at least in part, to the presence in placental tissue of an inner (tyrosyl) ring iodothyronine deiodinase which converts T_4 to inactive reverse T_3 and converts T_3 to inactive diiodothyronine or T_2.

Maternal immunoglobulins of the IgG subclass are selectively transported across the placenta, particularly late in gestation. Hyper- or hypothyroidism has been reported in response to maternally derived TSH receptor-stimulating or TSH receptor-blocking antibodies. These syndromes are usually detected by either newborn screening or neonatal symptoms and signs (Matsurra et al., 1980; and Zakarija and McKenzie, 1983). Thyroid scanning in affected infants reveals the presence of a normally situated thyroid gland; the clinical abnormalities wane with degradation of the maternal antibody. The half-life in newborn blood for the maternally-derived IgG antibodies approximates 20 days.

The placenta is freely permeable to iodide, and the fetal thyroid is particularly sensitive to the inhibitory effects of iodine on thyroid function (Theodoropoulos et al., 1979). Relatively small amounts of maternal iodine exposure have been associated with transient neonatal hypothyroidism. The source may be radiopaque dyes used for radiographic procedures as well as maternal medications, including topically-applied iodine washes which may be absorbed across mucus membrane surfaces. This effect is more fully described in the section on neonatal hypothyroidism.

The thioureylene antithyroid drugs cross the placenta and may compromise fetal and neonatal thyroid function (Marchant et al., 1977). The placenta also is permeable to selected synthetic thyroid hormone analogues such as 3',5'-dimethyl, 5-isopropyl thyronine (DIMIT). However, there is no current rationale for use of these analogues due to their low biological activity. Finally, the placenta is permeable to the hypothalamic peptide thyrotropin-releasing hormone (TRH). This fact currently is being exploited clinically in attempts to modify pulmonary maturation in infants at risk for developing respiratory distress syndrome of prematurity. Both primate and human fetuses early in the third trimester respond to pharmacologic doses of exogenous TRH with an increase in serum TSH. However, little endogenous TRH is normally detected in adult humans due to the presence of TRH-degrading enzyme systems in the blood. Although the sera of pregnant women contain somewhat lower levels of these enzymes than nonpregnant sera, the nearly immeasurable levels of TRH in the maternal circulation have little effect on fetal thyroid function.

In addition to TRH, the placenta produces thyrotropin-like activity. The alpha subunit of TSH is identical to that of human chorionic gonadotropin (hCG), and the beta subunit of hCG has structural homology with the beta subunit of TSH; thus, hCG has some TSH-like bioactivity. However, the biological potency of hCG is only about 0.01 per cent that of TSH, and hCG normally has little influence on fetal thyroid system development or function. Because of the hyperthyroidism sometimes seen in patients with choriocarcinoma, a unique chorionic thyrotropin has been proposed, and a glycoprotein with thyro-

tropic activity has been isolated from human placenta. However, a structure has never been characterized, and it seems likely that this chorionic thyrotropin represents a variant form of hCG (Harada and Hershman, 1978).

In summary, placental permeability to maternal molecules might be a factor affecting fetal thyroid function as a result of maternal pathophysiologic states (acute iodide administration, autoimmune thyroid disease, or pharmacotherapy of thyrotoxicosis). However, the fetal pituitary-thyroid axis normally develops independently of the maternal thyroid axis influence. The placenta and selected fetal tissues may serve as sources of TRH or TSH, but the extent of this influence on fetal thyroid function is uncertain.

CONTROL OF THYROID HORMONE PRODUCTION

The pattern of perinatal thyroid hormone secretion in the human is shown in Figure 109–1. Maturation of thyroid system control can be considered in three phases—hypothalamic, pituitary, and thyroidal. Changes in these systems are complex and superimposed on the increasing production and increasing serum concentration of serum thyroid hormone–binding globulin (TBG) as well as the changing pattern of fetal tissue iodothyronine deiodination during gestation. Maturation of these latter systems is described in the next section.

Although the fetal thyroid gland is able to concentrate iodide and synthesize thyroglobulin at 70 to 80 days of gestation, little thyroid hormone synthesis occurs until about 18 weeks' gestation. At this time, thyroid follicular cell iodine uptake increases, and T_4 becomes measurable in the serum. Both total and free T_4 concentrations then increase steadily until the final weeks of pregnancy (Fisher, 1985). This pattern differs from the development of serum T_3 levels in the fetus. The fetal serum T_3 concentration is low (<15 $\mu g/dl$) until 30 weeks of gestation and then increases slowly in two distinct phases, a prenatal and a postnatal phase. Prenatally, serum T_3 increases slowly after 30 weeks of gestation to reach a level of approxi-

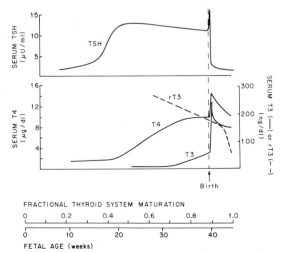

Maturation of Thyroid Hormone Secretion in the Human Fetus

FRACTIONAL THYROID SYSTEM MATURATION

FIGURE 109–1. Patterns of circulating levels of thyroid-stimulating hormone (TSH), rT_3, T_4, and T_3 in the fetus and newborn.

mately 50 μg/dl in term cord serum (Fisher and Klein, 1981). Postnatally, both T_3 and T_4 serum concentrations increase fourfold to sixfold within the first few hours of life, peaking at 24 to 36 hours after birth. These levels then gradually decline to adult values over the first 4 to 5 weeks of life. The prenatal increase in serum T_3 seems to be largely due to progressive maturation of hepatic type I (phenolic) outer ring iodothyronine deiodinase activity and increasing hepatic conversion of T_4 to T_3, although other tissue sources of deiodinase, such as brown fat and the kidney, may be involved.

Fetal serum TSH increases rapidly from a low level at 18 weeks' gestation to a peak value at 24 to 28 weeks' gestation then gradually declines until term. At the time of parturition, partly in response to cold stress, there is an acute release of TSH resulting in an elevated level by 30 minutes of life. The level of circulating TSH remains modestly elevated for 2 to 3 days after birth. The increases in thyroid hormone that occur immediately after birth are not totally dependent on TSH and may represent other influences in the thyroid gland at the time of parturition. The high postnatal T_3 levels in the days following birth are due to both TSH stimulation of thyroidal T_3 secretion and further rapid maturation of tissue outer ring mono-deiodinase activity.

Fetal thyroid gland function develops under the influence of a moderately elevated TSH level during the last half of gestation. The increase in serum T_4 that occurs during the last trimester is accompanied by a progressive decrease in serum TSH suggesting that changes in both thyroid follicular cell sensitivity to TSH and pituitary thyrotroph sensitivity to the negative feedback effect of thyroid hormones occur during this period. The pituitary gland contains a type II outer ring iodothyronine deiodinase which converts T_4 to active T_3, which in turn modulates TSH production. In most circumstances, it is circulating T_4 that is most important in TSH control. Thus, even when the circulating T_3 level is low (as in midgestation), there may be significant negative feedback control (by T_4) of pituitary TSH secretion.

The ontogeny of TRH secretion and function in the fetus remain somewhat obscure. TRH immunoactivity is detectable in the hypothalamus by midgestation, increasing markedly in the third trimester after the peak in serum TSH activity is noted. The premature infant (before 30 to 32 weeks) is characterized by low levels of T_4 and free T_4, a normal or low level of TSH, and a normal or prolonged TSH response to TRH indicating a state of physiologic TRH deficiency. The full-term human fetus responds to pharmacologic maternal doses of TRH with a somewhat prolonged increase in TSH suggesting a degree of relative hypothalamic (tertiary) hypothyroidism (Roti et al., 1981). Fetal sources of nonhypothalamic TRH (placenta and pancreas) probably contribute to the elevated circulating levels of fetal and cord blood TRH and presumably account for the high circulating TSH level characteristic of the midgestation fetus. However, the significance of ectopic TRH to the development of thyroid system control remains to be investigated.

In summary, the control of fetal thyroid hormone secretion can be characterized as a balance among increasing hypothalamic TRH secretion, increasing thyroid follicular cell sensitivity to TSH, and increasing pituitary sensi-

tivity to thyroid hormone inhibition of TSH release. The fetus progresses from a state of both primary (thyroidal) and tertiary (hypothalamic) hypothyroidism in midgestation through a state of mild tertiary hypothyroidism during the final weeks of pregnancy and to fully mature thyroid function in the perinatal period.

FETAL THYROID HORMONE METABOLISM

Although the thyroid gland is the sole source of T_4, most of the T_3 that circulates in the adult is derived from conversion of T_4 to T_3 via monodeiodination in peripheral tissues. Deiodination of the iodothyronines is the major route of metabolism, and monodeiodination may occur either at the outer (phenolic) ring or the inner (tyrosyl) ring of the iodothyronine molecule. Outer ring mono-deiodination of T_4 produces T_3, the active form of thyroid hormone with greatest affinity for the nuclear thyroid hormone receptor. Inner ring monodeiodination of T_4 produces reverse T_3 (rT_3), an inactive metabolite. In mature humans, between 70 to 90 per cent of circulating T_3 is derived from peripheral conversion of T_4, and 10 to 30 per cent from direct glandular secretion. Nearly all the circulating rT_3 derives from peripheral conversion with only 2 to 3 per cent coming directly from the thyroid gland. T_3 and rT_3 are progressively metabolized to diiodo, monoiodo, and noniodinated forms of thyronine, none of which possess biological activity.

Two types of outer-ring iodothyronine monodeiodinases (5'MDI) have been described. Type I 5'MDI, predominantly expressed in the liver and kidney, is an enzyme inhibited by propylthiouracil, and its activity is stimulated by thyroid hormone. Type II 5'MDI, predominantly located in the brain, pituitary, and brown adipose tissues, is insensitive to propylthiouracil, and its activity is inhibited by thyroid hormone (Refetoff and Larsen, 1989). Type I 5'MDI activity in the liver and perhaps the kidney and muscles probably accounts for most of the peripheral deiodination of T_4; type II 5'MDI acts primarily to increase local intracellular levels of T_3 in the brain and pituitary and is important to brown adipose tissue function during the immediate postnatal period. The outer ring iodothyronine deiodinase also deiodinates reverse T_3 to diiodothyronine.

Both type I and type II 5'MDI are present in third trimester fetuses (Polk et al., 1988b). Both deiodinase species are thyroid hormone responsive. However, hepatic type I 5'MDI activity becomes thyroid hormone responsive (e.g., activity decreases with hypothyroidism) only during the final weeks of gestation. Brain type II activity, in contrast, is responsive (increases with hypothyroidism) throughout the final trimester of gestation. Thus, type II deiodinase probably plays an important role to provide a source of intracellular T_3 to those tissues (such as the pituitary and in some species brown fat and the brain) dependent on T_3 during fetal life, while the ontogeny of the type I enzyme (to provide increased serum T_3 levels) increases only during the final weeks of gestation and during postnatal life.

An inner (tyrosyl) ring iodothyronine monodeiodinase (type III 5'MDI) has been characterized in most fetal tissues, including the placenta. This enzyme system catalyzes the conversion of T_4 to rT_3 and T_3 to diiodothyronine.

Fetal thyroid hormone metabolism is characterized by a predominance of type III enzyme activity, particularly in the liver, kidney, and placenta, and this accounts in part for the increased circulating levels of rT_3 observed in the fetus. Placental type III deiodinase contributes to amniotic fluid rT_3 levels and presumably also contributes to circulating fetal rT_3. However, the persistence of high circulating rT_3 levels for several weeks in the newborn indicates that type III 5'MDI activities expressed in nonplacental tissues are also important to the maintenance of high circulating rT_3 levels.

Both T_3 and T_4 in blood are associated with various plasma proteins including thyroxine-binding globulin (TBG), thyroxine-binding prealbumin (TBPA), and albumin. TBG serves as the primary transport protein for both T_3 and T_4; about 70 per cent of the total T_4 and 40 to 60 per cent of total T_3 are bound to TBG. The rest of the thyroid hormones are distributed almost equally between TBPA and albumin. The binding affinities of these proteins are such that adult free T_4 and T_3 concentrations are about 0.03 and 0.3 per cent, respectively, of the total hormone concentrations. TBG, TBPA, and albumin are produced by the liver, and production of these proteins increases progressively during the final half of gestation. Hepatic TBG production is stimulated by estrogen, and the increasing levels of estrogens during pregnancy account, at least in part, for the total plasma T_4 concentration which increases progressively from midgestation until 34 to 35 weeks' gestation.

THYROID SYSTEM EFFECTS AND ADAPTATION TO EXTRAUTERINE LIFE

In general, much of this fetal thyroid development is preparatory, providing for the relatively large amounts of thyroid hormones required for normal postnatal development. The production of active thyroid hormones is markedly increased in association with the events of parturition (see Fig. 109–1). During the first hours after birth, there are abrupt threefold to sixfold increases in circulating T_4 and T_3 levels, coincident with an increase in serum TSH concentrations. The initial increases in circulating thyroid hormone levels are due largely to increased hormone secretion from the thyroid gland. Substances other than TSH may also modulate the acute increases in circulating thyroid hormones at birth. A postnatal increase in serum catecholamine concentrations occurs at the time of parturition (Padbury et al., 1985), and the thyroid gland is adrenergically innervated. The cold-stimulated TSH surge is short-lived, and the decrease in TSH which follows during the 72 to 96 hours after birth is due to feedback inhibition by T_4 at either the hypothalamic or pituitary levels (or both). The serum TRH concentration is elevated in cord blood and falls in the days following birth. A clear increase in the serum TRH value coincident with the increase in TSH after parturition has not been reported, but the parallel increases in both TSH and prolactin levels in the early hours after birth support the view that the TSH surge is mediated by TRH (Roti, 1988). Thyroid hormone levels in the newborn gradually return to adult levels by about 1 month of age. The high level of circulating rT_3 characteristic of the fetus persists following

birth, gradually declining to the adult range by 4 to 6 weeks of age.

The metabolic significance of the neonatal thyroid hormone surge is not entirely clear. Physiologic processes known to be modulated by thyroid hormone in adults, such as thermogenesis and cardiovascular responses, clearly are important in the transition from intra- to extra-uterine life, and it is tempting to link these transitional events with changes in thyroid hormone metabolism. Several studies using animal models have attempted to establish such a link and support the view that the level of thyroid function during the final weeks of gestation is more important than the neonatal increases in T_3 and T_4 for successful neonatal transition (Polk et al., 1986a). The situation in the human newborn may be somewhat different. Newborns with congenital thyroid agenesis have few if any signs or symptoms of thyroid hormone deficiency, and their postnatal environmental adaptation usually is not impaired. The precise timing of maturation of thyroid hormone effects on thermogenesis and cardiovascular function in the human newborn has not been defined.

In humans thyroid hormone nuclear receptors have been reported in fetal lung, brain, heart, and liver at 13 to 19 weeks' gestation by Gonzales and Ballard (1981) and Bernal and Pekonen (1984). The only thyroid hormone actions that have been characterized in the fetus are the effects of hypothyroidism on serum TSH and bone maturation. Most effects of thyroid hormone on perinatal developmental processes occur postnatally (Fig. 109–2).

In summary, thyroid hormones affect important postnatal processes including growth, thermogenesis, and development. The largely successful transition of athyrotic infants to extrauterine life speaks to the limited importance of fetal thyroid hormones in all but the final weeks of gestation. An exception to this may be the fetal brain, a major site of type II iodothyronine monodeiodinase activity in the fetus. The presence of this enzyme system in the brain early in development as well as its demonstrated response to fetal hypothyroidism in the rat and sheep suggests that intracellular conversion of T_4 to T_3 in the brain is important in these species for normal development

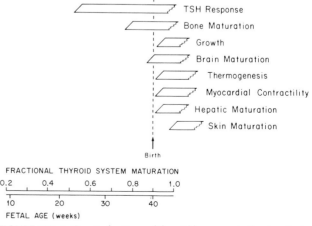

FIGURE 109–2. Onset of actions of thyroid hormone in the developing human. The left edge of the bar indicates the initiation of thyroid hormone responsiveness of the indicated parameter.

and differentiation of the central nervous system. The critical period for this effect is not known for the human fetus, but early treatment of congenital hypothyroidism in the newborn prevents mental retardation, suggesting that the period of thyroid dependency of the human brain extends into the postnatal period.

■ CONGENITAL HYPOTHYROIDISM

Congenital hypothyroidism has been recognized for centuries and its treatment known for decades, but only recently has the link between early treatment and the prevention of sequellae been proposed. With the emphasis now placed on early screening, many conditions that lead to the syndrome of congenital hypothyroidism have been recognized (Table 109–3). The importance of adequate neonatal screening in the management of newborn thyroid diseases cannot be overemphasized. Before the advent of screening, less than one-third of the infants found to ultimately have congenital hypothyroidism were diagnosed before 3 months of age, and only half were diagnosed by 6 months of age; most of these infants developed irreversible brain damage (Jacobsen and Brandt, 1981).

Newborn screening programs for congenital hypothyroidism are designed to detect elevated serum TSH levels in blood samples collected on filter paper. Some programs measure TSH directly, and others measure TSH in samples with low or low-normal T_4 concentrations. In most programs in the United States, an initial T_4 measurement is conducted, and TSH is measured in samples with the lowest 10 per cent of T_4 values. An elevated TSH level (>20 μU/ml) suggests primary hypothyroidism. Most screening programs are just that, and some infants with hypothyroidism are missed in the screening process. Thus, no infant who presents with signs or symptoms suggestive of thyroid dysfunction (Table 109–4) should be excluded from investigation on the basis of previous screening results. A determination of serum T_4 and TSH values is necessary in any infant with suspicious clinical or laboratory findings. With this as a background, we turn to a discussion of the major pathophysiologic states leading to

TABLE 109–3. Thyroid Disorders and Their Approximate Prevalences in the Neonatal Period

DISORDER	INCIDENCE
Thyroid Dysgenesis	1 : 4000
Agenesis	
Hypogenesis	
Ectopia	
Thyroid Dyshormonogenesis	1 : 30,000
TSH receptor defect	
Iodide trapping defect	
Organification defect	
Iodotyrosine deiodinase deficiency	
Defect in thyroglobulin	
Transient Hypothyroidism	1 : 40,000
Drug induced	
Maternal-antibody–induced	
Idiopathic	
Hypothalamic-Pituitary Hypothyroidism	1 : 100,000
Hypothalamic-pituitary anomaly	
Panhypopituitarism	
Isolated TSH deficiency	

TABLE 109–4. Clinical Signs and Symptoms of Congenital Hypothyroidism in Infancy

AGE	FREQUENCY (%)
0 to 7 Days	
Prolonged jaundice >3 days	73
Birth weight >4 kg	40
Poor feeding	40
Transient hypothermia	38
Large posterior fontanelle (>5 mm)	32
1 to 4 Weeks	
Failure to gain weight	45
Constipation	35
Hypoactivity	33
1 to 3 Months	
Failure to thrive	90
Umbilical hernia	49
Macroglossia	43
Myxedema	40
Hoarse cry	30

congenital thyroid dysfunction, as summarized in Table 109–3.

THYROID DYSGENESIS

The term thyroid dysgenesis describes infants with ectopic or hypoplastic thyroid glands (or both) as well as those with total thyroid agenesis. Thyroid dysgenesis is the etiologic factor in most infants with permanent congenital hypothyroidism detected in newborn screening programs. Some thyroid tissue probably is present in two-thirds of these infants, so that they represent a spectrum of severity of thyroid deficiency. A normal or near-normal circulating level of T_3 in the face of a low T_4 value suggests the presence of residual thyroid tissue, and this can be confirmed by a thyroid scan. A measurable level of serum thyroglobulin also indicates the presence of some thyroid tissue; athyrotic infants have no circulating thyroglobulin (Dammacco et al., 1985).

Thyroid dysgenesis occurs in 1:4000 live-born infants and is more prevalent in female than in male infants by a ratio of almost 2:1. Studies by Frasier and colleagues (1982) and Brown and co-workers (1981) suggest the disorder has been reported to be less common in black (1:32,000) than in white infants and may be more frequent (1:2000) in Hispanic infants. Although thyroid dysgenesis usually is sporadic, rare familial cases have been described, and the incidence is increased in infants with Down syndrome (Fort et al., 1984). Seasonal variations in incidence have been observed in Japan, Australia, and Canada. In isolated instances thyroid dysgenesis has occurred in association with maternal autoimmune thyroiditis. However, this may be coincidence; there usually is no correlation between thyroid dysgenesis and the presence of maternal autoimmune thyroiditis or circulating thyroid antimicrosomal or antithyroglobulin autoantibodies (Dussault et al., 1980). Immunoglobulins blocking TSH-stimulated thyroid cell growth in tissue culture have been reported in both maternal and newborn blood in about half of the cases of sporadic congenital hypothyroidism, but a role for such growth-blocking immunoglobulins in the pathogenesis of congenital hypothyroidism in vivo has not been established.

As already indicated, most newborns with thyroid dysgenesis are asymptomatic, and few infants have signs of hypothyroidism during the early weeks of life. Most affected infants have low serum T_4 and high TSH concentrations in cord blood or in filter-paper blood spots collected at 2 to 5 days of age. Ten to 20 per cent of hypothyroid infants have T_4 levels in the low-normal range with increased TSH values. These infants usually have ectopic functional thyroid tissue on scanning and significant levels of circulating thyroglobulin. Another 5 per cent have a delayed elevation of serum TSH and are missed in the screening process unless a second screening test is done (LaFranci et al., 1985). Again, thyroid function should be determined in any infant presenting with suspicious clinical signs or symptoms (see Table 109–4). Individuals with thyroid dysgenesis also show abnormalities of thyroidal C cells; calcitonin levels and responsiveness are reduced throughout infancy and childhood. Urinary calcium and hydroxyproline levels are increased, and there is a tendency toward osteopenia, but this seems of limited clinical significance (Kruse et al., 1987).

HYPOTHALAMIC-PITUITARY DEFECTS

Congenital hypothyroidism due to ineffective TSH stimulation of thyroid hormone secretion can result from a variety of abnormalities in TSH synthesis and metabolism. These include anomalous hypothalamic or pituitary development, isolated or familial deficiencies in TRH or TSH secretion, or TSH deficiency in association with other pituitary hormone deficiencies. Structurally abnormal forms of TSH, although theoretically possible, have not yet been described. Several TSH deficiency syndromes have been described: hypothalamic (tertiary) hypothyroidism with TRH deficiency or pituitary insensitivity (or both), isolated TSH deficiency, familial panhypopituitarism, congenital absence of the pituitary, and panhypopituitarism with absence of the sella turcica. The combined prevalence of these abnormalities associated with congenital hypothyroidism approximates one in 60,000 to 140,000 live births (Stanbury and Dumont, 1983).

INBORN DEFECTS OF THYROID HORMONE PRODUCTION

Infants with inborn defects in thyroid metabolism account for nearly 10 per cent of newborns with congenital nonendemic hypothyroidism (see Table 109–3). The defects in such patients include: (1) a decreased thyroid response to TSH; (2) decreased thyroid iodide trapping; (3) defective organification of trapped iodide; (4) decreased capacity for deiodinating iodotyrosines; and (5) abnormalities in thyroglobulin synthesis, storage, or release. These disorders usually are transmitted as autosomal recessive traits (Lever et al., 1983). Except for the familial incidence and tendency for affected individuals to develop goiter, the clinical manifestations of congenital hypothyroidism due to a biochemical defect are similar to those in infants with thyroid dysgenesis. Thyroid enlargement may be manifest at birth, but in many patients development of the goiter is delayed.

TRANSIENT CONGENITAL HYPOTHYROIDISM

Congenital hypothyroidism may present as a transient defect persisting for a variable period after birth. Usually, transient neonatal hypothyroidism is caused by maternal ingestion of goitrogenic substances that reach the fetus via placental transfer. One frequently ingested goitrogenic drug is iodide prescribed in expectorants for the treatment of asthma or as treatment for maternal thyrotoxicosis. The mothers of these infants often have taken large doses of iodide for many years without developing large goiters and have been euthyroid during pregnancy. The fetal thyroid gland is unusually sensitive to iodide-induced hypothyroidism because of immaturity of the mechanism(s) that decrease thyroid iodide uptake in response to high plasma iodide levels. Urine iodine concentrations in affected infants usually exceed 1 mg/l.

Other substances that have been associated with neonatal goiter include thioureylene (antithyroid) drugs, sulfonamides, and hematinic preparations containing cobalt. Neonatal goiters due to antithyroid drug administration are uncommon unless large doses of the drugs are given to the mother (more than 150 mg/day propylthiouracil or equivalent near term). Amniotic injection of radiographic contrast agents used during amniofetography also can lead to transient congenital hypothyroidism.

Maternal-to-fetal transfer of TSH-receptor–blocking antibodies also can lead to transient perinatal hypothyroidism (Drexhage and Bottazzo, 1985). This condition is rare but has been reported in the newborns of women with either euthyroid or hypothyroid autoimmune thyroid disease. In these infants, TSH-receptor autoantibodies are detectable in maternal and cord blood. These antibodies can be measured either as TSH-binding–inhibiting immunoglobulins (TBII) or TSH (cAMP) blocking antibodies (TBA). The duration of the hypothyroid state in these newborns is correlated with the initial titer of blocking antibody and the duration of its presence in newborn blood. Transient congenital hypothyroidism must be differentiated from transient hyperthyrotropinemia (see the section on thyroid function in preterm infants).

DIAGNOSIS AND MANAGEMENT

Infants with congenital hypothyroidism are born with little or no clinical evidence of thyroid hormone deficiency. Thus, detection based on signs and symptoms usually is delayed 6 to 12 weeks or longer. Even though the emphasis in diagnosis of congenital hypothyroidism now focuses on newborn screening, not all infants with congenital hypothyroidism will be detected by these systems. Early clinical diagnosis must be based on a high index of suspicion regarding nonspecific symptoms and signs. These are outlined in Table 109–4 along with their relative frequency. The diagnosis should be considered in any infant with prolonged jaundice, transient hypothermia, an enlarged (>1 cm) posterior fontanelle, failure to feed properly, or respiratory distress with feeding.

The classic signs evolve during the first weeks after birth. There is a rapid reduction in growth rate after birth and a progressive accumulation of myxedema in the subcutaneous tissues and in the tongue. The thickened tongue becomes protuberant, and the infant develops increasing difficulty in nursing and handling salivary secretions. The cry is hoarse because of myxedema of the vocal cords. There is marked muscular hypotonia, an umbilical hernia, constipation, bradycardia, and extremities that are cool to the touch and may exhibit pallor and circulatory mottling. The cardiac silhouette may be enlarged; the electrocardiogram shows low voltage and a prolonged conduction time. Some of the signs and symptoms are present by 6 to 12 weeks, especially lethargy, constipation, and the umbilical hernia. The cretinoid facies and growth retardation become progressively more obvious during the first several months of life.

As indicated earlier, infants can escape detection by screening because of a delayed elevation in serum TSH or due to errors in sample collection or laboratory routine; it is estimated that some 5 to 8 per cent of affected infants might be missed. Infants with TSH deficiency are not detected since most newborn screening programs report only those infants with elevated TSH levels. Congenital primary hypothyroidism is associated with a low serum T_4 and a high TSH concentration in individual cord blood or neonatal blood samples. A cord serum T_4 of 6.0 μg/dl or less with a TSH in excess of 80 μIU/ml suggests hypothyroidism. At 3 to 5 days of age, a serum T_4 less than 7 μg/dl with a serum TSH in excess of 20 μIU/ml suggests hypothyroidism. However, 10 to 20 per cent of infants with congenital hypothyroidism have T_4 values in the low-normal range (7 to 11 μg/dl). During the first 24 to 48 hours of life, serum TSH levels normally are elevated due to the neonatal TSH surge. Sampling infants during this time increases the number of false-positive results, but infants with congenital hypothyroidism are not usually missed.

The diagnosis of congenital hypothyroidism must be confirmed by measurement of serum T_4 and TSH concentrations in any infant with suspicious screening or neonatal sampling results. After 7 days of age a serum T_4 <6 μg/dl with a TSH >50 μIU/ml indicates primary hypothyroidism. A serum T_4 in the 6 to 11 μg/dl range with a TSH in the 20 to 50 μIU/ml range is suggestive, and repeat testing is necessary. Eight to 10 per cent of infants with congenital hypothyroidism will have screening TSH values <50 μIU/ml, and one in 12 to 24 hypothyroid infants (one in 50,000 to 100,000 newborns) will have a screening TSH level <20 μIU/ml with a delayed postnatal rise to hypothyroid levels.

Hypothalamic-pituitary hypothyroidism is more difficult to diagnose. The disorder is characterized by a low serum T_4 concentration with a normal TSH value. In contrast, a low T_4 and TSH pattern most commonly reflects prematurity or a low TBG concentration. Measurement of a low serum TBG concentration and/or a normal free T_4 level identifies the low TBG patients. An infant with a low free T_4 concentration should be carefully examined for evidence of hypothyroidism, and other tests of pituitary function should be conducted. A subnormal TSH response to TRH confirms a diagnosis of pituitary TSH deficiency. The TSH deficiency may be isolated or associated with other pituitary hormone deficiencies. If the peak level of TSH after TRH stimulation is normal and/or prolonged, hypothalamic TRH deficiency is likely.

The treatment of hypothyroidism relies on replacement with exogenous thyroid hormone. Sodium–L-thyroxine (Na T_4) is the drug of choice because of its uniform potency and reliable absorption. Appropriate doses of synthetic T_4 produce normal serum levels of T_3 via peripheral conversion. The best guide to adequacy of therapy is periodic measurement of circulating levels of T_4 and TSH; during the initial stages of treatment, a T_3 determination also may be of value. The history and physical examination are important in follow-up, but mild hypothyroidism or hyperthyroidism cannot always be excluded on clinical grounds. The usual starting dose of Na T_4 for hypothyroid infants is 10 to 15 μg/kg/day; we routinely begin treatment in term infants with a 50 μg T_4 tablet daily crushed and given orally in a small amount of liquid. Using Na T_4 for treatment, the goal of therapy is to maintain the serum T_4 in the upper normal range (10 to 16 μg/dl), which should result in normal serum T_3 levels (70 to 220 ng/dl).

Serum TSH levels may remain elevated in adequately treated patients. The thyroid hormone–pituitary feedback set-point seems to be altered in some infants with congenital hypothyroidism, and in such infants the serum TSH concentration remains elevated in the face of a normal or even elevated serum T_4 level (McCrossin et al., 1980).

Infants with presumably transient hypothyroidism due to maternal goitrogenic drugs need not be treated unless the low serum T_4 and elevated TSH levels persist beyond 2 weeks. Hyperthyroid mothers on antithyroid drugs may breast-feed their infants, since the concentration of drug in breast milk is very low. Infants with TSH-receptor–blocking antibody-induced hypothyroidism may require treatment for as long as 2 to 5 months.

Adequate dosage of thyroxine in the 1st year usually ranges between 25 and 50 μg daily. The growth rate should accelerate after initiation of therapy, and any growth deficit is commonly restored within a few months. Bone age is a sensitive index of thyroid deficiency, and delayed bone maturation suggests inadequate treatment even when other signs of hypothyroidism have ameliorated. Overtreatment can induce tachycardia, excessive nervousness, disturbed sleep patterns, and other findings suggesting thyrotoxicosis. Excessive thyroxine administered over a long period can produce premature synostosis of cranial sutures and undue advancement of bone age.

■ THYROID DYSFUNCTION SYNDROMES IN THE PREMATURE INFANT

Although the preterm infant is subject to the same pathophysiologic processes affecting the term infant, certain disorders of thyroid function are more common as a result of prematurity and are discussed in the following sections.

TRANSIENT HYPOTHYROXINEMIA

Serum T_4 concentrations increase progressively with gestational age (see Fig. 109–2). Most term infants have serum T_4 concentrations above 6.5 μg/dl; only 2 to 3 per cent have serum T_4 levels below this level. In contrast, some 50 per cent of premature infants delivered before 30 weeks' gestation have serum T_4 values below 6.5 μg/dl (Hadeed et al., 1981). These preterm infants with hypothyroxinemia also have relatively low levels of free T_4. These levels are not as low as those in newborns with congenital hypothyroidism; rather, they are similar to the levels in adults. These relatively low free T_4 levels in premature infants are associated with normal or even low serum TSH values and normal TSH and T_4 responses to TRH, indicating responsive pituitary and thyroid glands. The hypothyroxinemia is transient, correcting spontaneously (in 4 to 8 weeks) with progressive maturation. Because postnatal growth and development of these infants are normal, they do not require treatment, and treatment does not increase the growth rate (Chowdry et al., 1984). Thus, these infants appear to manifest a state of hypothalamic (or tertiary) hypothyroidism or immaturity which represents a normal stage of fetal thyroid system development. These infants are not detected in newborn screening programs unless low T_4 and TSH results are reported.

TRANSIENT PRIMARY HYPOTHYROIDISM

Transient hypothyroidism in the newborn, characterized by low serum T_4 and high TSH concentrations, is more common in Europe than in America; its prevalence varies geographically relative to iodine intake. In Belgium, it occurs in 20 per cent of premature infants, with the incidence increasing as gestational age decreases (Delange et al., 1985). Cord blood T_4 and TSH values in these infants are usually in the normal range for premature infants. However, premature infants require higher iodine intake levels than term infants to maintain a positive iodine balance in the extrauterine environment, so in iodine-deficient geographic areas, preterm infants may develop neonatal iodine deficiency. The primary hypothyroid state develops during the first weeks of extrauterine life and often is superimposed on the transient hypothyroxinemia characteristic of prematurity. Urinary iodine excretion and thyroid iodine content are low. The hypothyroidism is transient but may persist for 2 to 3 months so that treatment is recommended. Iodine treatment also corrects this transient primary hypothyroid state. The average time to recovery of function and discontinuation of treatment in Belgium was 50 days.

Premature infants also are particularly susceptible to transient, iodine-induced hypothyroidism (Delange et al., 1985). The mechanism by which the thyroid cell inhibits iodide transport in response to increased plasma iodide levels matures near term. Thus, either in utero or in the postnatal period, administration of iodine-containing drugs to the mother or amniotic injection of radiographic contrast agents for amniofetography has induced hypothyroidism. Premature infants are more susceptible, but term infants also can develop iodide-induced hypothyroidism. The dose of iodine required approximates 50 to 100 µg/kg/day. Urine iodine levels in iodine-induced hypothyroid infants usually exceed 1 mg/l. The hypothyroidism, with or without goiter, is characterized by low serum total T_4 and free T_4 concentrations and high levels of TSH and urinary iodide. Treatment of these infants is indicated.

TRANSIENT HYPERTHYROTROPINEMIA

Idiopathic hyperthyrotropinemia is a rare disorder. The serum TSH concentration is increased, often markedly,

but other thyroid function parameters are normal, and the infants are euthyroid. In Japan, Miyai and co-workers (1979) have reported an incidence of one in 15,000 to 20,000 newborns; the prevalence in Europe and America is not precisely known but is much lower. The serum TSH concentration may remain elevated for as long as 9 months before spontaneously normalizing. Affected infants do not require treatment, but prolonged follow-up is necessary to exclude the possibility of a permanent disorder, such as an ectopic thyroid gland, an inborn defect in thyroid hormonogenesis, or a thyroid hormone resistance syndrome. Transient hyperthyrotropinemia without hypothyroxinemia in the newborn also may occur in response to intrauterine antithyroid drug exposure, intrauterine iodine excess or deficiency, or a maternal TSH-receptor–blocking antibody and has been recorded as a TSH assay artifact. The mechanism of transient idiopathic hyperthyrotropinemia is not clear. Delayed maturation of thyroid responsiveness to TSH and/or of the iodothyronine feedback control of pituitary TSH secretion have been suggested.

LOW T_3 SYNDROME IN PREMATURES

In the preterm infant the changes in thyroid function parameters during neonatal adaptation are qualitatively similar to those in term infants but are quantitatively obtunded (Fisher and Klein, 1981). The neonatal TSH surge and the neonatal T_4 and T_3 peak responses decrease with decreasing gestational age, and the transient low T_3 state that follows probably is related to the state of relative undernutrition in the neonatal period. Premature infants have an increased susceptibility to neonatal morbidity including birth trauma, acidosis, hypoxia, hypoglycemia, hypocalcemia, and infection all superimposed on feeding disorders and relative malnutrition. All of these factors tend to inhibit peripheral T_4 to T_3 conversion and aggravate the extent of the low T_3 state characteristic of prematurity. Serum T_3 values may remain low in these infants for 1 to 2 months.

Features of the low T_3 syndrome in premature infants include a low serum T_3 concentration secondary to a decreased rate of conversion of T_4 to T_3, variable but usually elevated serum rT_3 levels, and normal or low total serum T_4 concentrations. Free T_4 levels usually are in the range of values for healthy premature infants of matched gestational age and weight. TSH values are low in these infants. Treatment is not warranted.

The wide application of neonatal screening programs for congenital hypothyroidism has resulted in the identification of other causes of low values of T_3 and T_4 in the newborn. Although physiologically these individuals are euthyroid, a discussion of these syndromes is warranted due to their impact on reported values of T_3 and T_4 in the perinatal period.

■ DISORDERS OF THYROID HORMONE CARRIER PROTEINS

The major determinants of the levels of circulating thyroid hormones are the concentrations of thyroid-hormone–binding proteins. As indicated earlier, thyroxine-binding globulin (TBG), thyroxine-binding prealbumin

(TBPA), and albumin all participate as thyroid hormone carrier proteins. Abnormalities of serum albumin concentration have been described; the major categories are dysalbuminemia and analbuminemia. However, albumin usually binds only about 10 per cent of the circulating T_4 and 30 to 50 per cent of T_3, and the concentrations of TBG and TBPA are normal or increased in these disorders. Consequently, the levels of thyroid hormones in these patients usually are in the normal range (Hollander et al., 1985). No confirmed primary disorder of TBPA resulting in abnormal thyroid hormone levels has been described to date. Thus, the plasma protein disorders associated with abnormal serum T_4 levels include only the variations in TBG and the recently described hyperthyroxinemic state "familial dysalbuminemic hyperthyroxinemia."

THYROXINE-BINDING GLOBULIN DEFICIENCY

The prevalence of TBG deficiency varies from one in 5000 to 12,000 newborns and is transmitted as an X-linked trait. Serum TBG levels are very low in affected males and approximately half normal in carrier females. In about half the families the TBG level by radioimmunoassay (RIA) is very low; in the other half the defect is partial; serum T_4 levels vary similarly. Affected subjects are euthyroid with normal serum TSH responses to exogenous TRH. Treatment is not indicated.

It is now clear that there are a variety of structural defects of the TBG molecule accounting for defective TBG-T_4 binding. Variants have been reported in Australian aborigines and American blacks as well as other families. These inherited defects seem not to be due to large fragment deletions, insertions, or rearrangements of DNA; consequently, polymorphism studies have not been helpful in detection or screening. A single amino acid substitution (asparagine for isoleucine) at position 96 of the TBG molecule accounts for the marked reduction of T_4-binding capacity of TBG-Gary (Takamatsu et al., 1987). Table 109–5 summarizes the reported properties of several variant TBG molecules investigated. Most patients with partial TBG deficiency demonstrated elevated levels of denatured TBG measured by RIA, and each manifested a defective molecule with reduced stability and decreased binding capacity. Patients with severe TBG deficiency

TABLE 109–5. Properties of Reported Abnormal Thyroxine-Binding Globulin (TBG) Molecules

	TBG CONCENTRATIONS		T_4 CONCEN-TRATION	TBG AFFINITY
	Normal	Denatured		
Normal TBG	100	100	100	100
TBG-S	88	100	84	100
TBG-A	74	100	58	54
TBG-Quebec	16	260	41	70
TBG-Montreal	14	390	38	<3
TBG-Gary	1	1000	24	<5

Values listed as percentage of values in normal subjects. Normal absolute values for the measured parameters are: TBG RIA 1.1 to 2.1 mg/dl; TBG-denatured <2 to 8 μg/dl; T_4 5 to 12 μg/dl; TBG affinity constant for T_4, 0.7 to 1.35 × 10^{-10}/M^{-1}

(Adapted from Takamatsu, J., Refetoff, S., Charbonneau, M., et al.: Two new inherited defects of the thyroxine-binding globulin (TBG) molecule presenting as partial TBG deficiency. J. Clin. Invest. 79:833-840, 1987.)

have been postulated to have a defect in hepatic TBG synthesis, but the molecular mechanism remains obscure.

THYROXINE-BINDING GLOBULIN EXCESS

Subjects with increased levels of TBG have increased total serum T_4 concentrations with normal TSH levels. Serum T_3 concentrations are modestly increased. In these subjects, as in those with low TBG concentrations, TBG production rates and serum levels are correlated, suggesting that the mechanism for the high TBG concentrations is increased production, presumably by the liver. TBG levels are increased fourfold to fivefold in affected individuals. Early reports suggested a dominant mode of inheritance, but subsequent studies are compatible with an X-linked mode of inheritance.

FAMILIAL DYSALBUMINEMIC HYPERTHYROXINEMIA

Several groups of investigators have reported euthyroid subjects with increased serum T_4 concentrations but normal free T_4, total serum T_3, and TSH levels (Ruiz et al., 1982). There is increased binding of T_4 to albumin, and the albumin in these patients has an affinity for T_4 binding intermediate between TBG and TBPA. T_3 is less avidly bound, accounting for the preferential increase in serum T_4 concentration. Patients with the disorder are euthyroid with normal thyroid hormone production rates. The abnormal albumin seems to be transmitted as an autosomal dominant trait.

Diagnosis in these patients is confirmed by protein electrophoresis of serum containing labeled T_4. The fraction of T_4 label associated with TBG, TBPA, or albumin is measured, and the albumin-bound T_4 can be calculated and related to normal values. Measurements of TBG and TBPA concentrations also are useful. Antithyroid therapy is not necessary in these patients, but it is important to make the diagnosis to avoid a misdiagnosis of hyperthyroidism.

Finally, although the emphasis of neonatal thyroidology is on early detection and appropriate therapy of the hypothyroid state, hyperthyroid states do occur and are associated with significant morbidity.

NEONATAL THYROTOXICOSIS

Neonatal Graves disease is rare, probably due to the low incidence of thyrotoxicosis in pregnancy (one to two cases per 1000 pregnancies) and the fact that the neonatal disease occurs only in about one of 70 cases of thyrotoxic pregnancy (Burrow, 1974). In most cases, the disease is due to transplacental passage of thyroid-stimulating antibody (TSA) from a mother with active or inactive Graves disease or Hashimoto thyroiditis. Thus, prediction of neonatal Graves disease from the maternal clinical status is not always possible. However, it is possible to predict the occurrence of Graves disease in newborns on the basis of maternal TSA titers. In a report by Zakarija and co-workers (1986), all women with TSA titers exceeding 500 per cent of control values (measured by stimulation of cAMP in human thyroid slices) delivered thyrotoxic infants, whereas those with lower titers delivered euthyroid infants. In some infants, both TSH-receptor–stimulating and TSH-receptor–blocking antibodies are acquired from the mother, and the blocking antibodies have been reported to block the effect of the stimulating antibodies for 4 to 6 weeks so that a previously unrecognized infant develops late-onset neonatal Graves disease (McKenzie et al., 1978).

Graves disease in the newborn is manifested by irritability, flushing, tachycardia, hypertension, poor weight gain, thyroid enlargement, and exophthalmos. Thrombocytopenia, hepatosplenomegaly, jaundice, and hypoprothrombinemia also have been observed. Arrhythmias, cardiac failure, and death may occur if the thyrotoxicity is severe and the treatment is inadequate. Mortality approaches 25 per cent in disease severe enough to be diagnosed. In some infants the onset of symptoms and signs may be delayed as long as 8 to 9 days. This is due to the postnatal depletion of transplacentally acquired blocking doses of maternal antithyroid drugs and to the abrupt increase in conversion of T_4 to active T_3 shortly after birth in the newborn. The diagnosis is confirmed by measuring high levels of T_4, free T_4, and T_3 in postnatal blood. Cord blood values may be normal or near normal while levels at 2 to 5 days may be markedly increased; the serum TSH is low. Neonatal Graves disease resolves spontaneously as maternal TSA in the newborn is degraded. The usual clinical course of neonatal Graves disease extends 3 to 12 weeks.

The treatment of hyperthyroidism in the newborn includes sedatives and digitalis as necessary. Iodide or antithyroid drugs are administered to decrease thyroid hormone secretion. These drugs have additive effects with regard to inhibition of hormone synthesis; in addition, iodide rapidly inhibits hormone release. Lugol solution (5 per cent iodine and 10 per cent potassium iodide; 126 mg of iodine per milliliter) is given in doses of one drop (about 8 mg) three times daily. Methimazole, carbimazole, or propylthiouracil are administered in doses of 0.5 to 1 mg, 0.5 to 1 mg, or 5 to 10 mg, respectively, per kilogram daily in divided doses at 8-hour intervals. A therapeutic response should be observed within 24 to 36 hours. If a satisfactory response is not observed, the dose of antithyroid drug and iodide can be increased by 50 per cent. Corticosteroids in anti-inflammatory doses and propranolol (1 to 2 mg/kg/day) also may be helpful. Radiographic contrast agents (ipodate, 200 mg/kg/d) also may be useful in treatment either alone or in conjunction with antithyroid drug treatment.

■ REFERENCES

Bernal, J., and Pekonen, F.: Ontogenesis of nuclear 3,5,3′ triiodothyronine receptors in human fetal brain. Endocrinology 114:667–679, 1984.

Brown, A. L., Fernhoff P M, Milner J, et al: Racial differences in the incidence of congenital hypothyroidism. J Pediatr 99:934–937, 1981.

Burrow, G. N.: The Thyroid Gland in Pregnancy. Philadelphia, W. B. Saunders Company, 1974, pp. 83–100.

Chowdry, P., Scanlon, J. W., Auerbach, R., et al.: Results of a controlled double-blind study of thyroid replacement in very low birth weight premature infants with hypothyroxinemia. Pediatrics 73:301–304, 1984.

Dammacco, F., Dammacco, A., Cavallo, T., et al.: Serum thyroglobulin and thyroid ultrasound studies in infants with congenital hypothyroidism. J. Pediatr. 106:451–453, 1985.

Delange, F., Bourdoux, P., and Ermans, A. M.: Transient disorders of thyroid function and regulation in preterm infants, In Delange, F., Fisher, D. A., and Malvaux, P. (Eds.): Pediatric Thyroidology. Basel, Karger, 1985, pp. 369–393.

Drexhage, H. A., and Bottazzo, G. F.: The thyroid and autoimmunity. In Delange, F., Fisher, D. A., and Malvaux, P. (Eds.): Pediatric Thyroidology. Basel, Karger, 1985, pp. 90–105.

Dussault, J. H., Letarte, J., Guyda, H., et al.: Lack of influence of thyroid antibodies on thyroid function in the newborn infant and on a mass screening program for congenital hypothyroidism. J. Pediatr. 96:385–387, 1980.

Fisher, D. A.: Thyroid hormone and thyroglobulin synthesis and secretion. In Delange, F., Fisher, D. A., and Malvaux, P. (Eds.): Pediatric Thyroidology. Basel, Karger, 1985, pp. 44–56.

Fisher, D. A., and Klein, A. H.: Thyroid development and disorders of thyroid function in the newborn. N. Engl. J. Med. 304:702–708, 1981.

Fort, P., Lifschitz, F., Bellisario, R., et al.: Abnormalities of thyroid function in infants with Down syndrome. J. Pediatr. 104:545–549, 1984.

Frasier, S. D., Penny, R., and Synder, R.: Primary congenital hypothyroidism in Spanish-surnamed infants in Southern California. J. Pediatr. 101:315–317, 1982.

Gonzales, L. A., and Ballard, P. L.: Identification and characterization of nuclear 3,5,3′-triiodothyronine binding sites in fetal human lung. J. Clin. Endocrinol. Metab. 53:21–28, 1981.

Hadeed, A. J., Asay, L. D., Klein, A. H., et al.: Significance of transient hypothyroxinemia in premature infants with and without respiratory distress syndrome. Pediatr. Res. 68:494–497, 1981.

Harada, A., and Hershman, J. M.: Extraction of human chorionic thyrotropin (hCT) from term placentas: Failure to recover thyrotropic activity. J. Clin. Endocrinol. Metab. 47:681–685, 1978.

Hollander, C. S., Bernstein, G., and Oppenheimer, J. H.: Anomalies in thyroid hormone transport proteins, In Delange, F., Fisher, D. A., and Malvaux, P. (Eds.): Pediatric Thyroidology. Basel, Karger, 1985, pp. 394–406.

Jacobsen, B. B., and Brandt, N. J.: Congenital hypothyroidism in Denmark. Arch. Dis. Child. 56Z:134–136, 1981.

Kruse, K., Suss, A., Busse, M., et al.: Monomeric serum calcitonin and bone turnover during anticonvulsant treatment and in congenital hypothyroidism. J. Pediatr. 111:57–63, 1987.

LaFranchi, S. H., Hanna, C. E., Krainz, P. L., et al.: Screening for congenital hypothyroidism with specimen collection at two time periods: Results of the Northwest Regional Screening Program. Pediatrics 76:734–740, 1985.

Lever, E. G., Medeiros-Neto, G. A., and DeGroot, L. J.: Inherited disorders of thyroid metabolism. Endocr. Rev. 4:213–247, 1983.

McCrossin, R. B., Sheffield, L. J., and Robertson, E. F.: Persisting abnormality in the pituitary-thyroid axis in congenital hypothyroidism. In Nagetaki, S., and Stockgit, J. H. R. (Eds.): Thyroid Research VIII. Canberra, Australian Academy of Science, 1980, pp. 37–40.

McKenzie, J. M., and Zakarija, M.: Pathogenesis of neonatal Graves' disease. J. Endocrinol. Invest. 2:183–187, 1978.

Marchant, B., Brownlie, B. E. W., Hant, D. M., et al.: The placental transfer of propylthiouracil, methimazole and carbimazole. J. Clin. Endocrinol. Metab. 45:1187–1193, 1977.

Matsurra, N., Yamamoto, Y., Nohara, Y., et al.: Familial neonatal transient hypothyroidism due to maternal TSH-binding inhibitor immunoglobulins. N. Engl. J. Med. 303:733–741, 1980.

Miyai, K., Amino, N., Nishi, K., et al.: Transient infantile hyperthyrotropinemia. Arch. Dis. Child. 54:965–967, 1979.

Padbury, J. F., Polk, D. H., Newnham, J. P., et al.: Neonatal adaptation: Greater sympathoadrenal response in preterm than full-term fetal sheep at birth. Am. J. Physiol.: Endocrinol. Metab. 11:E443–E447, 1985.

Polk, D. H., Callegari, C. C., Newnham, J. P., et al.: Effect of fetal thyroidectomy on newborn thermogenesis in lambs. Pediatr. Res. 21:453–457, 1988a.

Polk, D. H., Wu, S. Y., Wright, C., et al.: Ontogeny of thyroid hormone effect on tissue 5′ monodeiodinase activity in fetal sheep. Am. J. Physiol.: Endocrinol. Metab. 17:E337–341. 1988b.

Refetoff, S., and Larsen, P. R.: Transport, cellular uptake and metabolism of thyroid hormone. In DeGroot, L. J., et al.: (Eds.): Endocrinology. Philadelphia, W. B. Saunders Company, 1989, pp. 541–561.

Roti, E., Gnudi, A., Braverman, L. E., et al.: Human cord blood concentrations of thyrotropin, thyroglobulin and iodothyronines after maternal administration of thyrotropin-releasing hormone. J. Clin. Endocrinol. Metab 53:813–817, 1981.

Roti, E.: Regulation of thyroid-stimulating hormone (TSH) secretion in the fetus and neonate. J. Endocrinol. Invest. *11*:145–150, 1988.

Ruiz, M., Rajatanavin, R., Young, R. A., et al.: Familial dysalbuminemic hyperthyroxinemia. N. Engl. J. Med. *306*:635–639, 1982.

Stanbury, J. B., and Dumont, J. E.: Familial goiter and related disorders. *In* Stanbury, J. B., et al. (Eds.): The Metabolic Basis of Inherited Disease. New York, McGraw Hill, 1983, pp. 231–269.

Takamatsu, J., Refetoff, S., Charbonneau, M., et al.: Two new inherited defects of the thyroxine-binding globulin (TBG) molecule presenting as partial TBG deficiency. J. Clin. Invest. *79*:833–840, 1987.

Theodoropoulos, T., Bravermam, L. E., and Vagenakis, A. G.: Iodide-induced hypothyroidism: A potential hazard during perinatal life. Science *205*:502–503, 1979.

Zakarija, M., and McKenzie, J. M.: Pregnancy-associated changes in the thyroid stimulating antibody of Graves' disease and the relationship to neonatal hyperthyroidism. J. Clin. Endocrinol. Metab. *57*:1036–1039, 1983.

Zakarija, M., McKenzie, J. M., and Hoffman, W. H.: Prediction and therapy of intrauterine and late onset neonatal hyperthyroidism. J. Clin. Endocrinol. Metab. *62*:368–374, 1986.

DISORDERS OF CARBOHYDRATE METABOLISM

Daniel H. Polk

■ DISORDERS OF CARBOHYDRATE METABOLISM

While abnormalities of carbohydrate metabolism represent a wide spectrum of pathophysiologic states (inborn errors of metabolism, abnormal endocrine responses, nonspecific hypermetabolic states), they are included in this section on perinatal endocrine function because of the critical integration that must occur among a variety of organs in order to achieve glucose homeostasis. This section outlines the major endocrine pathways that regulate glucose levels and the pathophysiologic states that affect neonatal glucose metabolism. Because of the impact maternal diabetes mellitus plays in altering neonatal glucose homeostasis, a discussion of infants born to mothers whose pregnancies are complicated by diabetes is also included.

PATTERNS OF PERINATAL GLUCAGON, INSULIN, AND SOMATOSTATIN SECRETION

The pancreas appears during the 4th week of gestation in the human fetus. Development of the islets of Langerhans is classically divided into primary and secondary transition phases. During primary transition, the various secretory products of the alpha cell (glucagon), beta cell (insulin), and D cell (somatostatin) are immunohistochemically demonstrable. Through the influence of as yet uncharacterized pancreatic mesenchymal differentiation factor(s), further differentiation of these cell lines occurs. The phase of secondary transition involves the organization of these various cell types into mature islets.

While the pancreatic insulin concentration is higher in the fetus than adult and blood levels are comparable, the regulation of insulin secretion between the two varies markedly. Acute changes in fetal plasma glucose are not associated with significant changes in the pattern of plasma insulin levels (Menon and Sperling, 1988). This lack of insulin response is most likely due to defects in the c-AMP generating system of the β-cell; phosphodiesterase inhibitors seem to augment an insulin response. Insulin receptors are abundant in many fetal tissues, representing the largely anabolic role of insulin in the fetus. The chronic effect of hyperglycemia on fetal insulin secretion is well known. Hypertrophy and hyperplasia of pancreatic islets and increased pancreatic insulin content are classically described in infants born to mothers whose own glucose

metabolism is impaired as a result of diabetes mellitus. These infants also have a more mature pattern of insulin secretion in utero (Oakley et al., 1972). It is likely this maturational effect is due to a variety of influences including amino acids, catecholamines, and poorly understood influences of the fetal hypothalamic-pituitary axis (Grasso et al., 1973; Sperling et al., 1980a; Van Assche et al., 1970). Thus, while insulin is readily demonstrable in the developing fetus, control of secretion and patterns of receptor ontogeny suggest the largely trophic function of this hormone in the fetus. The relative contribution of insulin receptors and related insulin-like growth factor receptors in fetal growth remains to be demonstrated.

Pancreatic glucagon is detectable in the fetal pancreas between the 6th and 8th week of gestation in the human (Schaeffer et al., 1973). The human placenta is impermeable to glucagon, and fetal plasma glucagon levels rise steadily from about the 15th week of gestation until term (Adam et al., 1972; Sperling et al., 1977). The fetal glucagon response, like that of insulin, is also relatively insensitive to acute changes in fetal glucose concentrations (when compared to responses in the adult). Hyperglycemia does not suppress glucagon levels in fetal sheep, and chronic but not acute hypoglycemia modulates fetal glucagon levels in the rat (Fiser et al., 1974; Girard et al., 1974). Amino acids (particularly alanine and arginine) are potent secretagogues for fetal pancreatic glucagon, as are acetylcholine and epinephrine (Sperling et al., 1980a). Fetal glucagon responses are also impaired. Physiologic doses of glucagon do not result in fetal hepatic glucose production, probably because of a paucity of fetal hepatic glucagon receptors. Incomplete glucagon receptor linking to c-AMP in the fetus has also been proposed (Menon and Sperling, 1988).

The role of somatostatin in the maintenance of fetal glucose homeostasis is not well documented. In adults, somatostatin infusion suppresses both insulin and glucagon secretion. This is accompanied by an initial decrease in plasma glucose concentrations (due to the initial glucagon deficiency) which then normalize. These observations have been extended to the newborn lamb (Menon and Sperling, 1988). The role for fetal somatostatin remains to be described.

■ FETAL GLUCOSE METABOLISM

In the basal nonstressed state, placental transport of glucose from mother to fetus meets all of the fetal glucose requirements. This observation is supported by several investigators. Using glucose tracer techniques, Kalhan and co-workers (1979) have shown that no net glucose production can be demonstrated in the human fetus at term. Hay and associates (1983) have used the Fick principle and glucose isotope dilution techniques to show that umbilical vein glucose uptake equals fetal glucose utilization. Finally, in fetal sheep, no gluconeogenesis is demonstrable under basal, nonstressed conditions (Sperling et al., 1980b). In all species studied, fetal glucose concentrations are related to, but lower than, maternal glucose concentrations. The rate of glucose utilization in the human fetus is uncertain; values of 6 to 10 mg/kg/minute have been described in studies of fetal sheep.

Glucose may not be the sole energy source for the fetus. Basal measurements of placental substrates and fetal oxygen consumption suggest that as much as 50 per cent of the substrates used for fetal respiration are derived from lactate and amino acids (Battaglia and Meschia, 1978). This proportion may change in response to maternal starvation as well as during periods of fetal stress. In vivo measurements of oxygen consumption in various organs suggest that the majority of glucose is used to support fetal brain metabolism. The relative dependence of the fetus on maternal sources of glucose may be altered during fetal stress. Catecholamines, particularly epinephrine, are released in large quantities following a variety of physiologic states including fetal hypotension and hypoxia. Fetal epinephrine infusion at physiologic concentrations results in significant increases in fetal glucose and fatty acid levels due to stimulation of hepatic and adipocyte beta-adrenergic receptors. Of interest is the observation that the substrate-mobilizing threshold for this catecholamine effect is much lower than the level of epinephrine required for fetal insulin or glucagon stimulation (Padbury et al., 1987).

GLUCOSE HOMEOSTASIS AT PARTURITION

At birth, a variety of events occur that permit the newborn to assume its own glucose homeostasis. In general, changes in circulatory insulin and glucagon levels as well as changes in their related receptors are accompanied by increases in enzyme activities essential for glycogenolysis and gluconeogenesis. Both serum glucagon and catecholamines increase threefold to fivefold in response to umbilical cord-cutting (Padbury et al., 1981; Sperling et al., 1980a). Circulating insulin levels usually fall in the immediate newborn period and remain low for several days. The high epinephrine, high glucagon, and low insulin state may be related: epinephrine both stimulates pancreatic glucagon release and inhibits the release of insulin. The dependence of normal neonatal glucose homeostasis on adrenal epinephrine release has been demonstrated in adrenalectomized newborn sheep (Padbury et al., 1987). Thus, the depressed serum insulin and elevated glucagon and epinephrine levels (along with elevated serum growth hormone levels) at birth favor glycogenolysis, lipolysis, and gluconeogenesis. This is supported by observations in newborns. After a transient decrease immediately after birth, serum glucose levels rise, hepatic glycogen stores deplete, and plasma fatty acid concentrations reflecting lipolysis increase. Gluconeogen-

esis (predominantly from alanine), which is difficult to demonstrate in the fetus, becomes evident in the newborn.

Changes in various hormonal receptors also modulate these processes. Hepatic glucagon receptors increase in number and become functionally linked with c-AMP responses (Ganguli et al., 1983). The functional significance of the decrease in insulin receptors that occurs during this time is unknown, but it parallels the decrease in postnatal serum insulin levels.

Neonatal glucose homeostasis also requires appropriate enzyme maturation and response in the newborn. The neonatal liver, in contrast to that of the fetus, is characterized by an increase in glycogen phosphorylase activity and a decrease in glycogen synthetase activity, consistent with the rapid depletion of hepatic glycogen seen during the newborn period. Phosphoenolpyruvate carboxykinase activity, which is the rate-limiting enzyme required for gluconeogenesis, also increases during the immediate postnatal period. This is likely a response to the changes in glucagon and insulin that occur during the immediate postnatal period (Girard, 1986; Granner et al., 1983). Gluconeogenesis provides about 10 per cent of the glucose metabolized in the newborn during the hours following birth (Frazier et al., 1981). Thus, hormonal, receptor, and enzyme activities in the fetus provide for anabolism and substrate accretion, while those in the newborn period predominantly provide for the maintenance of glucose homeostasis in response to the abrupt interruption of maternal glucose supply. As can be inferred, many pathophysiologic states may impact this balance leading to hypo- or hyperglycemia in the newborn.

■ HYPOGLYCEMIA

DEFINITION AND DIAGNOSIS

In adults, brain metabolism accounts for nearly 80 per cent of the total glucose consumption. This value may be higher in newborns in whom the brain represents a proportionally larger tissue mass. Thus, glucose utilization is highest in the preterm infant when compared with term-infant and adult values. The rate of glucose utilization in preterm infants is approximately 6 to 8 mg/kg/minute, while adult values range from 2 to 4 mg/kg/minute (Bier et al., 1977). That the brain is the primary site for glucose utilization and uses glucose as a primary energy source leads to the predominance of neurologic symptoms that accompany hypoglycemia (Table 110–1). Of interest is the observation of relative glucose intolerance and hyperglycemia in infants sustaining major hypoxic encephalopathy; other agents (such as catechols and steroid hormones) may further mediate this response.

Blood glucose values in term and preterm infants after birth are shown in Figure 110–1. There is no consensus agreement defining a blood glucose level diagnostic of

TABLE 110–1. Symptoms in Neonatal Hypoglycemia

Jitteriness
Lethargy
Feeding intolerance
Apnea
Cyanosis
Seizures

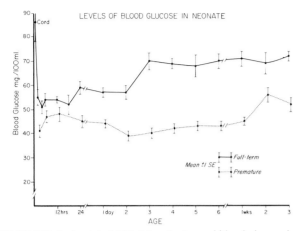

FIGURE 110–1. *A total of 206 determinations of blood glucose levels was obtained in 179 full-sized infants (>2.5 kg), and a total of 442 determinations was made in 104 low-birth-weight infants (<2.5 kg) throughout the neonatal period. (From Cornblath, M. and Reisner, S.: N. Engl. J. Med. 273:378, 1965. Reprinted, by permission of the New England Journal of Medicine.)*

hypoglycemia. Earlier data defining hypoglycemia as blood glucose levels of 30 mg/dl in term infants and 20 mg/dl in preterm infants relied on measurements in fasted infants and are probably not valid. Other concerns about the long-term effects of asymptomatic neonatal hypoglycemia, first raised by Pildes and co-workers (1974), have led to efforts to aggressively diagnose and treat this entity. There are limited data correlating the length of the hypoglycemic period with outcome or the relative risk of symptomatic versus asymptomatic hypoglycemia (Lucas et al., 1988). Because of these concerns and uncertainties, it seems prudent to aggressively screen infants at risk for hypoglycemia and treat those with values <40 mg/dl (Pagliaria et al., 1973). In most nurseries, this consists of heel-stick whole blood determinations of glucose using a commercially available indicator (Dextrostix or Chemstrip). Although useful, these methods have limitations. Various agents including fluoride, uric acid, bilirubin, acetaminophen, and isopropyl alcohol have been shown to interfere with these determinations. Additionally, low glucose values as reported by the reagent strips tend to underestimate the degree of hypoglycemia present. Values close to those representing hypoglycemia (<40 mg/dl) or hyperglycemia (>125 mg/dl) should be confirmed by actual laboratory chemical analysis. Initial therapies, especially in asymptomatic infants, should not be postponed in borderline cases, but continuation of therapy should be based on reliable laboratory glucose values. Because the onset and duration of hypoglycemia is variable in infants at risk, repeated routine screening of these infants should continue until the risk period for developing hypoglycemia has passed. Certain pathophysiologic states (infants of diabetic pregnancies or infants who are small for gestational age) may require screening over several days (Koh et al., 1988).

CONDITIONS ASSOCIATED WITH NEONATAL HYPOGLYCEMIA

In general, hypoglycemia develops in newborns as a result of one or more of three basic mechanisms: (1) limited glycogen stores, (2) hyperinsulinism, or (3) dimin-

ished glucose production. Each of these categories is associated with several different disease states (Table 110–2). In addition, various other conditions are associated with hypoglycemia through unknown mechanisms.

LIMITED GLYCOGEN STORES

Preterm Infants. The majority of hepatic glycogen accumulation occurs in the 3rd trimester of pregnancy. Prematurity is associated with decreased hepatic stores of glycogen and thus may predispose infants to hypoglycemia. As many as 15 per cent of preterm infants develop hypoglycemia in the first hours of birth. As preterm infants may further develop a variety of other conditions associated with a risk of hypoglycemia (e.g., sepsis, feeding intolerance, and hypothermia), there may be additive effects on the duration and course of their hypoglycemia. The relatively increased proportion of brain tissue in preterm infants may also contribute to increased glucose requirements. Because hypoglycemia is so prevalent in preterm infants, routine blood glucose screening while the infant is sick or until feedings are well established is critical. The onset of hypoglycemia after the immediate newborn period in an otherwise stable preterm infant should prompt an evaluation for other associated conditions (i.e., sepsis).

Perinatal Distress. Infants who are stressed in utero or intrapartum are at risk for hypoglycemia. Hypoxia and acidosis lead to increased catecholamine activity which promotes hepatic glycogenolysis. Hypoxia also accelerates glucose utilization due to the effects of anaerobic metabolism. Roughly 18 times more glucose is required to produce comparable amounts of ATP during anaerobic metabolism. There is evidence that neurologic outcome in stressed fetuses requiring resuscitation at birth is improved by early glucose administration (Dawes et al., 1963).

Disorders of Glycogen Metabolism. Three disorders of glycogen metabolism may present with hypoglycemia in the newborn period. Glucose-6-phosphatase deficiency,

TABLE 110–2. Conditions Associated with Neonatal Hypoglycemia

Limited Glycogen Supply
Prematurity
Perinatal stress
Starvation
Glycogen storage disease
Hyperinsulinism
Infant of a diabetic mother
Beckwith-Wiedemann syndrome
Maternal drug therapy
Islet cell adenoma or nesidioblastosis
Erythroblastosis fetalis
Diminished Glucose Production
Small-for-gestation-age infants
Inborn errors of metabolism
Others
Hypothermia
Sepsis
Hypothalamic or hypopituitary disorders
Adrenal insufficiency
Polycythemia

amylo-1,6-glucosidase deficiency, and phosphorylase deficiency limit either glycogen metabolism or glucose release resulting in excess glycogen stores, hepatomegaly, and hypoglycemia. Diagnosis of these disorders ultimately rests on laboratory analysis of biopsy material in children with characteristic phenotypes (cherubic face, truncal obesity, and hepatomegaly). These disorders are inherited primarily in an autosomal recessive manner.

HYPERINSULINISM

Infant of a Diabetic Mother. A variety of disorders leading to neonatal hypoglycemia are the result of fetal or neonatal hyperinsulinism. The prototype for this condition is the infant of a diabetic mother. These children are at risk for neonatal hypoglycemia due to the persistence of fetal hyperinsulinism in the face of an interrupted supply of maternal glucose. Other maternal metabolic substrates (amino acids and lipids) may also play a role in maintaining the fetal hyperinsulinemic state. The fetal hyperinsulinemic state is induced by these abnormal quantities and types of metabolic fuels transplacentally acquired resulting in fetal pancreatic β-cell hypertrophy. Hypoglycemia in affected infants frequently occurs 4 to 6 hours after birth, although the coexistence of other complications may impact this timing. These infants also manifest augmented pancreatic β-cell sensitivity to glucose, which persists for several days after birth, and thus continue to be at risk for hypoglycemia during this time (Molsted-Petersen and Jorgensen, 1972) (see also Chapter 9).

The persistent fetal hyperinsulinemia leads to effects on all insulin-sensitive tissues, giving rise to the myriad of clinical signs and symptoms seen in these infants (Table 110–3). In addition to the disorders of carbohydrate metabolism, these infants are at significant risk for other types of perinatal morbidity. The observed increased incidence of respiratory distress in these infants is the result of many factors; the influences of glucose and insulin on surfactant and pulmonary function have been extensively studied. This work is outlined in Chapters 5 and 53. Of particular note is the observation that affected infants may exhibit all of the manifestations of respiratory distress syndrome despite advanced gestational age or documented amniotic fluid lecithin-to-sphingomyelin ratios of more than 2:1.

The effects of chronic stimulation of insulin and insulin-like growth factor receptors in many fetal tissues including placenta, liver, heart, and adipose tissues may lead to large-for-gestational-age infants with their attendant difficulties during labor and delivery. The increased incidence of intrapartum fetal distress and third trimester fetal demise

TABLE 110–3. Associated Conditions in Infants of Diabetic Mothers

Congenital malformations
Macrosomia
Fetal distress
Sudden fetal demise
Hypoglycemia
Hypocalcemia
Hyperviscosity
Hyperbilirubinemia
Respiratory distress
Feeding difficulties

may result from placental dysfunction due to abnormal substrate accretion and decreased diffusion capacity. Perinatal stress may have an additive effect on the degree of hypoglycemia via effects of catecholamines, glucocorticoids, and glycogen depletion. Plethora and hyperviscosity due to increased red blood cell mass may further compromise these infants who are at risk of developing venous thromboses. Erythropoietin levels are elevated in the infants of diabetic mothers, but the relative contributions of placental insufficiency, perinatal stress, and insulin to increased red blood cell mass are not well characterized. Hyperbilirubinemia may be present as a result of the increased red cell mass or secondary to placental or hepatic dysfunction. These infants may also manifest hypocalcemia—again, reflecting reduced placental function; hypoxia and perinatal stress probably also contribute to neonatal hypocalcemia in affected infants. A subgroup of infants born to diabetic mothers have marked hypertrophy of the cardiac septum and present with congestive heart failure. The increased incidence of other structural heart lesions may complicate the differential diagnosis of these infants; specific diagnosis is usually confirmed by cardiac ultrasound.

The observed increase in congenital malformations in infants of diabetic mothers led to the hypothesis that alterations in maternal glucose metabolism in the first weeks of pregnancy may cause defects in organogenesis. The work by Miller and co-workers (1981) correlated excess maternal glucose levels during the first trimester with an increased incidence of congenital malformations in their infants. Insulin does not seem to be teratogenic, but hyperglycemia, hyperketonemia, and hyperosmolality have all been shown to disrupt organogenesis in animal models. Increased attention to maternal glucose homeostasis later in pregnancy has dramatically improved perinatal mortality; the same may be true for early attention ameliorating associated congenital malformations (Reece et al., 1988) (see discussion in Chapter 9). Of interest are the observations that transient hypoglycemia may also disrupt organogenesis as well as affect later fetal growth indices; both extremes of maternal hyperglycemia and hypoglycemia are therefore to be avoided (Buchanan et al., 1986).

In certain instances, the phenotype and clinical symptomatology of hyperinsulinemic infants are so striking as to suggest the diagnosis of maternal diabetes mellitus. This diagnosis is supported by the finding of increased maternal levels of circulating glycosylated hemoglobin (Hb A_1c). While glucose homeostasis frequently returns toward normal in the days following delivery in women with gestational diabetes mellitus, Hb A_1c levels remain elevated for weeks after delivery. Because of the impact of this condition on subsequent pregnancies, this diagnosis should be actively pursued in pregnancies complicated by inadequate prenatal care and large-for-gestational-age infants.

Mothers with severe long-standing diabetes associated with vasculopathy or retinopathy (White class F) may give birth to infants who are small for gestational age and prone to all the perinatal complications described. This condition is more fully described in Chapters 9 and 32.

Other Causes of Hyperinsulinism. In rare instances, primary abnormalities of pancreatic β-cell development result in sustained neonatal hyperinsulinism and hypoglycemia. Nesidioblastosis is characterized by a proliferation of pancreatic β cells. In addition, discrete islet-cell adenomas may mimic most of the features of nesidioblastosis. Because these abnormalities may be present during fetal development, affected infants may initially be indistinguishable from infants of diabetic mothers, but the persistence of prolonged hypoglycemia usually suggests the diagnosis. Inappropriately elevated blood insulin–to–glucose ratios (plasma insulin >10 μU/ml when plasma glucose is <40 mg/dl) or increased calculated glucose requirements (typically >15 mg/kg/minute) frequently are present, although these findings are not specific for primary pancreatic β-cell disorders. Medical management (steroids, diazoxide, or somatostatin) may ameliorate these conditions, but surgery may offer a definitive means of both diagnosis and treatment.

Beckwith-Wiedemann Syndrome. Infants with the syndrome of exopthalmos, macroglossia, and gigantism often have associated omphaloceles, macrosomia, and neonatal hypoglycemia. This condition is associated with pancreatic β-cell hypertrophy and hyperinsulinism; the metabolic defect is unknown. While most cases of Beckwith-Wiedemann syndrome are sporadic, there is some evidence that it may be inherited as an autosomal dominant trait (Engstrom et al., 1988). Early recognition and treatment of the attendant hypoglycemia is likely to improve the intellectual outcome of these infants.

Erythroblastosis Fetalis. Infants with erythroblastosis fetalis complicating Rh incompatibility may also manifest hypoglycemia secondary to hyperinsulinism. Pancreatic β-cell hyperplasia is demonstrable, but the underlying biochemical defect is unknown. Although unrelated, infants undergoing exchange transfusion for any cause are at risk for hypoglycemia afterward because of the transient stimulation of endogenous insulin by the added dextrose in citrated stored blood products. The insulin response then leads to rebound hypoglycemia as the infused glucose is metabolized (Schiff et al., 1971). Heparinized blood contains no added glucose, but may lead to hypoglycemia owing to limited substrate availability during a double-volume exchange procedure.

Maternal Drug Effects on Neonatal Glucose Metabolism. Maternal chlorpropamide and benzothiazides increase fetal insulin secretion and predispose the newborn to hypoglycemia. The teratogenicity of chlorpropamide precludes most fetal exposure. Propranolol may also induce neonatal hypoglycemia via inhibition of catecholamine-induced glycogenolysis. Beta-sympathomimetics, commonly used in the prophylaxis of preterm labor, have been occasionally associated with neonatal hypoglycemia (Ogata, 1981). This may be due to both direct effects on fetal insulin secretion as well as effects mediated via abnormal maternal glucose concentrations. Obviously, inappropriate intrapartum maternal glucose administration may also lead to transient fetal hyperinsulinism and attendant neonatal hypoglycemia. This is particularly important as a consequence of inappropriate fluid management in the treatment of epidural anesthesia-associated hypotension.

DIMINISHED GLUCOSE PRODUCTION

Small for Gestational Age. Infants born small for gestational age not only have decreased glycogen stores but impaired gluconeogenesis. Elevated levels of gluconeogenic precursors (particularly alanine) have been reported in the blood of these infants. Defects in phosphoenolpyruvate carboxykinase activity (the rate-limiting enzyme for gluconeogenesis) have been suggested (Bussey et al., 1985). While insulin and glucagon secretion are similar in appropriate and small-for-gestational-age infants, the plasma amino acid response to glucagon may be altered in hypoglycemic small-for-gestational-age infants. Commonly, several days are required for these infants to maintain normal glucose homeostasis; thus, they remain at risk for hypoglycemia for an extended time after birth.

Inborn Errors of Metabolism. Rarely, aminoacidopathies (particularly those amino acids involved in gluconeogenesis) may be associated with neonatal hypoglycemia. The diagnosis rests on the demonstration of abnormal concentrations of amino acids in blood or urine samples.

OTHER CAUSES ASSOCIATED WITH NEONATAL HYPOGLYCEMIA

Hypothermia has been associated with hypoglycemia in part through the augmented effects of circulating catecholamines. The infants most likely at risk for hypothermia are those who are least able to support their own glucose requirements; thus, preterm stressed infants requiring resuscitation are at major risk for hypoglycemia. Infants exhibiting temperature instability should have their glucose status evaluated as well. Cortisol and growth hormone deficiencies are associated with hypoglycemia secondary to effects on hepatic glycogenolysis and gluconeogenesis. Polycythemia may lead to hypoglycemia as a direct result of increased glucose consumption by the red cell mass as well as secondary to effects on the intestinal absorption of substrates. Postprandial hypoglycemia has been noted in infants who are leucine-sensitive. This may be mediated by leucine effects on insulin secretion. Appropriate alteration of feeding schedules usually obviates these effects.

■ DIAGNOSIS AND TREATMENT OF NEONATAL HYPOGLYCEMIA

All infants at risk for developing neonatal hypoglycemia should be monitored, as anticipation and prevention are much more effective in the improvement of neonatal outcome than treatment. Blood glucose values <40 mg/dl should be verified and treated. Anticipation requires that screening continue for several days in infants of diabetic mothers and those born small for gestational age. Preterm infants should also be routinely monitored until feedings are well established.

The treatment of hypoglycemia depends on several factors. Infants who are asymptomatic with borderline glucose levels and capable of enteral feeds may receive either formula or 5 per cent dextrose in water as an initial therapy. Hypoglycemia may progress or persist in these infants, and they should continue to be closely monitored. Infants with symptomatic hypoglycemia should be treated with intravenous glucose solutions. The author favors an initial bolus of 100 mg/kg of 10 per cent dextrose in water solution (1 ml/kg). This is followed by a continuous infusion of 6 mg/kg/minute of 10 per cent dextrose in water. This method is associated with a much lower incidence of rebound hyper- or hypoglycemia than previous approaches based on 20 or 50 per cent dextrose solutions (Lilien et al., 1980). The rate of infusion can be titrated to provide for normal blood glucose levels. The use of a peripheral vein for infusion is preferable to an umbilical vessel, particularly for prolonged infusions. Infusions of glucose into an umbilical artery have been associated with hyperinsulinism via direct pancreatic stimulation via the infused glucose.

In circumstances of extremely high glucose utilization associated with hyperinsulinism, corticosteroids, glucagon, diazoxide, and somatostatin have all been suggested as additional adjunctive therapy. Although successful, their use should be restricted to isolated cases, or in collaboration with endocrine consultants.

HYPERGLYCEMIA

Hyperglycemia, defined as a blood glucose >125 mg/dl, is most commonly encountered in the very low birth weight (<1500 g) infant receiving intravenous glucose infusions. The glucose infusion rate may inadvertently exceed 6 to 8 mg/kg/minute as the fluids are advanced if the concentration of glucose is not adjusted accordingly. The osmotic diuresis and resultant dehydration can be quite marked in these cases; the resultant hyperosmolar state has been associated with intraventricular hemorrhage.

Sepsis and stress have also been associated with hyperglycemia in any infant. This is probably due to multiple influences of catecholamines, cortisol, and acid-base status on the mobilization of glycogen, gluconeogenesis, and insulin responses. Endotoxins have been proposed to have direct effects on insulin actions in septic infants.

A transient state of neonatal diabetes mellitus has also been described. In about a third of the cases there is a positive family history of diabetes mellitus. Some of these infants are thought to have a deficiency in pancreatic β-cell adenylcyclase activity, which improves with time (Haymond et al., 1989). The defect in the remaining infants is unknown. Many of these infants are small for gestational age and present with polyuria, glucosuria, and hyperglycemia. They may progress to severe dehydration, acidosis, and ketonemia. These infants require prompt attention to maintain their fluid and electrolyte balance and insulin therapy. The syndrome is usually self-limiting, and normal glucose homeostasis after the neonatal period is common. Rarely, hyperglycemia may be noted in infants receiving methylxanthines (theophylline). It is speculated that the increased levels of c-AMP associated with this therapy activate hepatic glucose output.

Finally, several pitfalls in the diagnosis of neonatal hyperglycemia have been described. Glucose values of blood samples obtained from umbilical catheters concurrently used for glucose infusion are unreliable unless strict attention is paid to inadvertent glucose contamination. In cases of concern, heel-stick blood may provide a more reasonable value.

Tests using Benedict solution (alkaline solution of cupric-citrate ions) for carbohydrate determination in urine are not glucose-specific and react with any reducing sugar (notably galactose). Thus, glycosuria can be inadvertently diagnosed and galactosemia missed unless specific glucose or galactose determinations are made. In the same manner, urine dipstick methods employing glucose oxidase are specific for glucose as a substrate; galactose does not react with this agent.

REFERENCES

Adam, P. A. J., King, K. C., Schwartz, R., et al.: Human placental barrier to ^{125}I-glucagon early in gestation. J. Clin. Endocrinol. Metab. 34:772–775, 1972.

Battaglia, F. C., and Meschia, G.: Principal substrates of fetal metabolism. Physiol. Rev. 58:499–531, 1978.

Bier, D. M., Leake, R. D., Haymond, M. W., et al.: Measurement of "true" glucose production rates in infancy and childhood with 6,6-dideuteroglucose. Diabetes 26:1016–1023, 1977.

Buchanan, T., Schweiner, J. K., and Freinkel, N.: Embryotoxic effects of brief maternal insulin-hypoglycemia during organogenesis in the rat. J. Clin. Invest. 78:643–649, 1986.

Bussey, M. E., Finley, S., and Ogata, E. S.: Hypoglycemia in the newborn growth-retarded rat. Delayed phosphoenol pyruvate carboxylase induction despite increased glycogen availability. Pediatr. Res. 19:363–367, 1985.

Dawes, G. S., Jacobsen, H. N., Moh, J. C., et al.: The treatment of asphyxiated mature foetal lambs and rhesus monkeys with intravenous glucose and sodium carbonate. J. Physiol. 169:167–184, 1963.

Engstrom, W., Lindham, S., and Schofield, P.: Wiedmann-Beckwith syndrome. Eur. J. Pediatr. 147:450–457, 1988.

Fiser, R. H., Erenberg, A., Sperling, M. A., et al.: Insulin-glucagon substrate interrelations in the fetal sheep. Pediatr. Res. 8:951–953, 1974.

Frazier, T. E., Karl, I. E., Hillman, L. S., et al.: Direct measurement of gluconeogenesis from (2,3,[13]C2) alanine in the human newborn. Am. J. Physiol. 240:E615–621, 1981.

Ganguli, S., Sinha, M. K., Sterman, B., et al.: Ontogeny of hepatic insulin and glucagon receptors and adenylate cyclase in the rabbit. Am. J. Physiol. 244:E624–631, 1983.

Girard, J.: Gluconeogenesis in late fetal and early neonatal life. Biol. Neonate 50:237–258, 1986.

Girard, J. R., Kervan, A., Soufflet, E., et al.: Factors affecting the secretion of insulin and glucagon by the rat fetus. Diabetes 23:310–314, 1974.

Granner, D., Andreone, T., Sabitie, K., et al.: Inhibition of transcription of the phosphoenol pyruvate carboxykinase gene by insulin. Nature 305:549–551, 1983.

Grasso, S., Messina, A., DiStefano, G., et al.: Insulin secretion in the premature infant: Response to glucose and amino acids. Diabetes 22:349–353, 1973.

Hay, W. W., Jr., Sparks, J. W., Wilkening, R. B., et al.: Fetal glucose uptake and utilization as functions of maternal glucose concentration. Am. J. Physiol. 245:E347–350, 1983.

Haymond, M. H., Pagliara, A. S., and Bier, D. M.: Endocrine and metabolic aspects of fuel homeostasis in the fetus and neonate. In DeGroot, L. J., Besser, G. M., Cahill, G. F., et al. (Eds.): Endocrinology. Philadelphia, W. B. Saunders Company, 1989, pp. 2215–2241.

Kalhan, S. C., D'Angelo, L. J., Savin, S. M., et al.: Glucose production in pregnant women at term gestation. J. Clin. Invest. 63:388–394, 1979.

Koh, T. H. H. G., Aynsley-Green, A., Tarbit, M., et al.: Neonatal hypoglycaemia: The controversy regarding definition. Arch. Dis. Child. 63:1386, 1988.

Lilien, L. D., Pildes, R., Srinivasan, G., et al.: Treatment of neonatal hypoglycemia with minibolus and intravenous glucose infusion. J. Pediatr. 97:295–298, 1980.

Lucas, A., Morley, R., and Cole, J. J.: Adverse neurodevelopmental outcome of moderate neonatal hyperglycaemia. Br. Med. J. 297:304, 1988.

Menon, R. K., and Sperling, M. A.: Carbohydrate metabolism. Semin. Perinatol. 12:157–162, 1988.

Miller, E., Hare, J. W., Cloherty, J. P., et al.: Elevated maternal hemoglobin A_{1c} in early pregnancy and major congenital anomalies in infants of diabetic mothers. N. Engl. J. Med. *304*:1331–1334, 1981.

Molsted-Peterson, L., and Jorgensen, K. R.: Aspects of carbohydrate metabolism in newborn infants of diabetic mothers. III. Plasma insulin during intravenous glucose tolerance test. Acta Endocrinol. *71*:115–126, 1972.

Oakley, N. W., Beard, R. W., and Turner, R. C.: Effect of sustained maternal hyperglycemia on the fetus in normal and diabetic pregnancies. Br. Med. J. *1*:466–473, 1972.

Ogata, E. S.: Isoxysuprine infusion in the rat: Maternal fetal and neonatal glucose homeostasis. J. Perinat. Med. *9*:293–301, 1981.

Oppenheimer, E. H., and Esterly, J. R.: Thrombosis in the newborn: Comparison between infants of diabetic and non-diabetic mothers. J. Pediatr. *67*:549, 1965.

Padbury, J., Roberman, B., Oddie, T. H., et al.: Fetal catecholamine release in response to labor and delivery. Obstet. Gynecol. *60*:607–611, 1981.

Padbury, J., Agata, Y., Ludlow, J., et al.: Effect of fetal adrenalectomy on catecholamine release and physiologic adaptation at birth of sheep. J. Clin. Invest. *80*:1096–1103, 1987.

Pagliaria, A., Karle, I. E., Haywood, M. W., et al.: Hypoglycemia in infancy and childhood, parts I and II. J. Pediatr. *82*:365–370, 558–575, 1973.

Pildes, R. S., Cornblath, M., Warren, I., et al.: A prospective controlled study of neonatal hypoglycemia. Pediatrics *54*:5–14, 1974.

Reece, E. A., Gabrielli, S., and Abdalla, M.: The prevention of diabetes-associated birth defects. Semin. Perinatol. *12*:292–301, 1988.

Schaeffer, L. D., Wilder, M. L., and Williams, R. H.: Secretion and content of insulin and glucagon in human fetal pancreas slices in vitro. Proc. Soc. Exp. Biol. Med. *143*:314–318, 1973.

Schiff, D., Aranda, J. V., Colle, E., et al.: Metabolic effects of exchange transfusions II. Delayed hypoglycemia following exchange transfusion with citrated blood. J. Pediatr. *79*:589–593, 1971.

Sperling, M. A., Christiansen, R. A., Artal, R., et al.: The nature and significance of amniotic fluid (AF) glucagon. Pediatr. Res. *11*:412 (Abstract), 1977.

Sperling, M. A., Christiansen, R., Ganguli, S., et al.: Adrenergic modulation of pancreatic hormone secretion in utero: Studies in fetal sheep. Pediatr. Res. *14*:203–208, 1980a.

Sperling, M. A.: Carbohydrate metabolism: Glucagon, insulin and somatostatin. *In* Tulchinsky, D., and Ryan, K., (Eds.): Maternal-Fetal Endocrinology. Philadelphia, W. B. Saunders Company, 1980b, pp. 333–353.

Van Assche, F. A., Gepts, W., and DeGasparo, M.: The endocrine pancreas in anencephalics: A histological, histochemical and biological study. Biol. Neonate *14*:374–377, 1970.

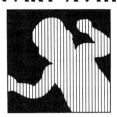

PART XVIII

DERMATOLOGIC CONDITIONS

CONGENITAL AND HEREDITARY DISORDERS OF THE SKIN

=111=

Nancy B. Esterly and Lawrence M. Solomon

Numerous heritable disorders can cause diverse aberrations of pigmentation, texture, elasticity, and structural integrity of the integument of the newborn. Some of these entities are confined to the skin, but others produce anomalies of several organ systems. Although, fortunately, most of these disorders are relatively uncommon, we have included the more frequently encountered, particularly those that have a prominent cutaneous component.

■ ICHTHYOSES

The ichthyoses are a group of heritable and acquired skin disorders in which the presence of visible scaling serves as a hallmark. Several of the heritable forms are evident in the neonatal period.

HARLEQUIN BABY

This severe type of congenital ichthyosis may represent the extreme form of lamellar ichthyosis (nonbullous ichthyosiform erythroderma) or may be a distinct entity. It is inherited as an autosomal recessive trait.

Etiology. The cause of harlequin baby is unknown. Although abnormalities of keratinization and epidermal lipid metabolism have been reported, few affected infants have been studied, and no single defect has been identified consistently.

Clinical Findings. The appearance and consistency of the skin of these infants has inspired innumerable metaphors. It has been likened to a baked apple, tree bark, a loosely built wall, elephant or rhinoceros skin, a coat of mail, and Moroccan leather. The skin is hard, discolored, cracked, and rigid, flattening the nose, ears, and digits. Moist granular fissures develop over areas of movement, particularly the thorax, joints, groin, axillae, and neck. The inelastic skin results in flexion of all joints and lends a waxy appearance to the hands and feet. Chemosis of the conjunctivae obscures the globes, the lips are gaping, and the nails and hair are hypoplastic or absent (Fig. 111–1). The viscera are usually normal.

Diagnosis. The diagnosis is made by the striking clinical picture. The histologic findings are relatively nonspecific, although certain features are supportive of the diagnosis.

Prognosis and Treatment. Treatment consists of a humid, temperature-controlled environment and lubrication; nevertheless, these infants almost invariably succumb to the disease because of inability to feed and ventilate adequately. Until recently, survival beyond 6 weeks was extremely unusual. Genetic counseling for the families of these infants is mandatory.

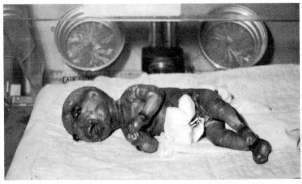

FIGURE 111–1. *Harlequin fetus. (Courtesy of Dr. Marvin Cornblath.)*

New Approaches. Several affected infants have been treated with oral retinoids and survived the neonatal period. They appear to have nonbullous ichthyosiform erythroderma (Lawlor, 1988; Roberts, 1989; Rogers, 1989).

COLLODION BABY

This rare congenital disorder resembles harlequin baby but is milder in degree. Collodion babies occur uncommonly, although not as rarely as the harlequin baby.

Clinical Findings. The infant is born tightly encased in a shiny membrane resembling parchment or oiled silk, which is perforated by scalp and lanugo hair. To some observers, the infant looks as if he had been varnished or lacquered. The tautness of the membrane holds the face immobile and distorts the features. The resultant ectropion, eclabium, and flattened, crumpled ears cause these infants to resemble one another within the first few days of life (Fig. 111–2). Motion of the limbs is restricted. Within a day or two, the membrane begins to fissure and peel, especially about the thorax and joints. In some instances, the skin beneath the membrane has a beefy-red color, and it may continue to scale or form a new membrane. No abnormality of the internal organs has been associated with these infants.

Etiology. The collodion baby probably represents a phenotype for several genotypes. Most of these infants undergo a gradual transition to lamellar ichthyosis or nonbullous ichthyosiform erythroderma, but collodion membranes have also been observed in patients with

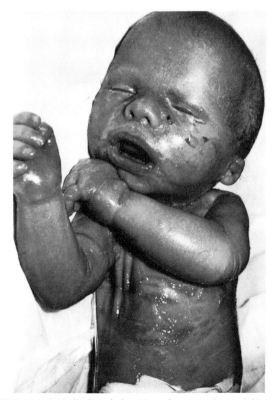

FIGURE 111–2. Collodion baby. Note the ectropion, eclabium, and areas of rupture in the membrane over the anterior thorax.

other forms of ichthyosis. Occasionally, an affected infant is observed to have normal skin subsequent to shedding of the membrane.

Prognosis and Treatment. The mortality rate for infants with collodion membrane is relatively low as compared with that of the harlequin baby (Williams, 1983). These infants have an increased incidence of premature birth. Complications include marked temperature instability, defective barrier function, increased insensible water loss predisposing to hypernatremic dehydration, and pneumonia secondary to aspiration of squamous material in the amniotic fluid. Cutaneous infections from gram-positive organisms and *Candida albicans* are a common problem; however, overzealous administration of antibiotics may lead to gram-negative infections and subsequent septicemia. A prolonged period of observation may be required to determine the outcome and prognosis. As soon as a secure diagnosis has been made, genetic counseling should be provided.

Treatment consists of careful monitoring of fluid and electrolytes, a humid environment, and lubrication with a bland emollient until the membrane has been desquamated.

MAJOR TYPES OF ICHTHYOSIS

Several distinct types of ichthyosis have been delineated on the basis of their clinical and histologic features and their patterns of genetic transmission (Williams, 1983 and 1986). Many of these disorders are apparent at birth. The more common conditions can be outlined briefly as follows.

ICHTHYOSIS VULGARIS

This is the most common form of ichthyosis and is inherited as an autosomal dominant trait. Onset is usually after the first 3 months of life. Scaling is most prominent on the extensor surfaces of the limbs. The flexural areas are spared, but the palms and soles are affected.

X-LINKED ICHTHYOSIS

This variant affects males only and may be present at birth. The scales are large and dark and prominent on the neck and limbs. The palms and soles are spared, but variable sparing of the flexural areas occurs. A deep corneal dystrophy may be detected by slit-lamp examination but usually is not apparent until late childhood or adolescence. Cryptorchidism may be present in up to 25 per cent of the affected males. Patients with this disorder have been shown to lack the enzyme steroid sulfatase (Williams, 1986); absence of enzyme activity has been demonstrated in leukocytes, hair bulbs, stratum corneum, and cultured fibroblasts and keratinocytes.

LAMELLAR ICHTHYOSIS AND NONBULLOUS CONGENITAL ICHTHYOSIFORM ERYTHRODERMA

Lamellar ichthyosis and nonbullous congenital ichthyosiform erythroderma (CIE) may be subtypes of a single entity or may represent distinct entities. Both conditions are present at birth and are characterized by erythroderma and a variable degree of generalized scaling. In lamellar ichthyosis the scales are large, dark, and platelike (Fig. 111–3) and accompanied by palmar-plantar keratoderma and ectropion. In CIE the scales are finer and whiter but also cover the entire integument, including the flexures, palms, and soles. Both disorders are inherited as an autosomal recessive trait. Recently an autosomal dominant form of lamellar ichthyosis has also been described.

EPIDERMOLYTIC HYPERKERATOSIS

Also affected at birth, patients with epidermolytic hyperkeratosis (bullous congenital ichthyosiform erythroderma) have a generalized erythroderma and small, thick, yellow, shotty scales. Scaling is accentuated in the flexural areas, and the palms and soles may be involved. The eruption of bullae, most frequently on the lower legs, is characteristic of the disease in infancy and childhood. Transmission is by an autosomal dominant gene.

ICHTHYOSIS LINEARIS CIRCUMFLEXA

This rare dermatosis is present at birth and transmitted as an autosomal recessive disorder. It is characterized by migratory, polycyclic lesions with a peripheral double-edged scale and hyperkeratosis of the flexural areas.

ERYTHROKERATODERMIA VARIABILIS

This type of ichthyosis is also very rare; it is inherited in an autosomal dominant fashion and can be detected in infancy. Affected individuals have transient migratory areas of discrete macular erythema as well as fixed hyperkeratotic plaques.

Prognosis and Treatment. It is important to distinguish

the various forms of ichthyosis so that the physician can offer a prognosis and appropriate genetic counseling to the family. The prognosis is related to the severity of the condition and the type of ichthyosis. Frequently, the clinical picture and pedigree data provide sufficient information on which to base a diagnosis; however, at times a period of observation beyond the first 4 weeks of life is required to assess the situation accurately. A skin biopsy may help solve a diagnostic dilemma, as all types of ichthyosis have a fairly characteristic histologic pattern and/or electron microscopic findings (Schachner and Hansen, 1988).

Therapy is restricted to topical preparations. Hydration of the stratum corneum is important and can be accomplished by bathing with a water-dispersible bath oil. Lubrication with a bland adherent emollient, such as petrolatum, Aquaphor, or Eucerin, should be provided immediately following the bath and whenever necessary throughout the day. Urea-containing emollients (10 to 25 per cent) are also effective preparations. Other available modalities, such as vitamin A acid, and preparations containing propylene glycol or keratolytics such as the alpha-hydroxy acids are not required in early infancy and should be reserved for older patients. Irritating soaps and detergents should be avoided. Extremes in temperature and excessively dry indoor heating also impose undue hardship on these individuals.

Studies using orally administered aromatic derivatives of retinoic acid have shown promising results in the management of several types of ichthyosis. However, these drugs have significant side effects and the risk-benefit ratio must be considered before recommending their use.

SYNDROMES WITH ICHTHYOSIS AS A FEATURE

Several syndromes, identifiable in infants, have ichthyosis as a major feature (Schachner and Hansen, 1988). Brief descriptions of several follow:

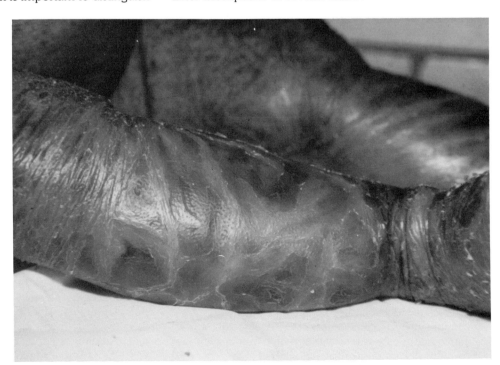

FIGURE 111–3. Large dark scales of lamellar ichthyosis on the leg of an affected infant.

Netherton Syndrome. Ichthyosis (lamellar or linearis circumflexa), hair shaft defects, and atopic diathesis.

Sjögren-Larsson Syndrome. Lamellar ichthyosis, spastic diplegia, and mental retardation.

Rud Syndrome. Ichthyosis, epilepsy, mental retardation, and sexual infantilism.

Chondrodysplasia Punctata. Patterned scaling, stippled epiphyses, cataracts, and bony anomalies.

Keratitis, Ichthyosis, Deafness (KID) Syndrome. Atypical ichthyosiform erythroderma, vascularizing keratitis, sensorineural deafness, and nail and hair abnormalities.

CHILD Syndrome. Congenital hemidysplasia, unilateral ichthyosiform erythroderma, and limb defects.

Chanarin-Dorfman Syndrome. Generalized ichthyosis, myopathy, vacuolated leukocytes, neurosensory deafness, and cataracts.

■ ALBINISM

The term "oculocutaneous albinism" refers to a group of congenital disorders of pigmentation that is clinically manifest by hypomelanosis of the skin, hair, and eyes, with associated photophobia and nystagmus. All races are affected; estimates of gene frequency vary depending on the population under consideration. As with many genetic disorders, the incidence of affected individuals is increased in certain racial isolates in which there is a high percentage of consanguineous marriages (Witkop et al., 1989).

Etiology. All forms of oculocutaneous albinism but one are inherited in an autosomal recessive fashion. The presence of genetic heterogeneity has been well documented in this condition. The characteristic pigmentary changes are probably due to a spectrum of biochemical defects that interfere with melanin synthesis.

Diagnosis. Some types of oculocutaneous albinism can be distinguished on the basis of subtle clinical differences and by a hair bulb tyrosine test (King and Olds, 1985). Oculocutaneous albinism should be distinguished from simple ocular albinism, which has sex-linked, autosomal dominant and autosomal recessive forms.

Clinical Findings. Affected infants, whatever their race, have a marked decrease in skin pigment and brown, red, yellow, or white hair. The irides are brown, hazel, bluish-gray, or pink in reflected light. Photophobia and nystagmus of variable degree are present, depending on the type of albinism. Visual acuity is almost always impaired. Patients with tyrosine-negative oculocutaneous albinism have the most severe form of visual impairment. Associated abnormalities may include hemorrhagic diathesis (Hermansky-Pudlak syndrome), small stature, and defective mentation. Deafness can occur in association with oculocutaneous albinism as well as with a number of other pigmentary disorders (Konigsmark, 1972).

Prognosis and Treatment. In patients with some forms of albinism, e.g., the tyrosinase-positive and yellow, platinum, brown, and rufous forms, some pigment may accumulate with increasing age. Concomitant with the development of pigment in the irides, visual acuity may improve significantly. There is no treatment for albinism, but regular use of sunscreen preparations is mandatory to protect against excessive exposure to sunlight. Such patients are predisposed to sun-induced carcinogenesis and should be examined yearly by a dermatologist.

Piebaldism

Although there are few reported families with piebaldism, or partial albinism, the disease is believed to be more common than the literature would indicate. Piebaldism is a heritable disorder transmitted by an autosomal dominant gene. Ultrastructural studies show an absence of melanocytes in the depigmented areas of skin and normal melanocytes in the uninvolved skin (Jimbow et al., 1975). A genetic defect in melanoblast differentiation has been proposed to account for these findings.

Clinical Findings. Partial albinism is present at birth but may be relatively inconspicuous if the infant is very fair-skinned. The amelanotic areas predominate on the ventral skin, with relative sparing of the dorsal surface. A favored site of involvement is the central forehead, where a triangular or diamond-shaped defect extends to the scalp to produce a white forelock. Similar depigmented patches may be found on the eyebrows, chin, trunk, midarm, and midleg. Within these areas, smaller normally pigmented or hyperpigmented patches may be evident (Fig. 111–4).

Diagnosis. The disorder is readily differentiated from albinism, in which the absence of pigment is uniform. Vitiligo may have a similar appearance, but it is not congenital and usually does not remain fixed. Waardenburg syndrome may also cause confusion. Occasional families may have associated defects such as sensorineural deafness and mental retardation (Telfer et al., 1971).

Prognosis and Treatment. The defects remain constant throughout life and are not amenable to treatment, although adequate cosmetic results may be achieved with the use of hair dyes and cosmetics (e.g., Dermablend, Covermark).

■ APLASIA CUTIS CONGENITA

The congenital absence of skin is a rare developmental anomaly that occurs most often on the scalp but that also may involve the skin of the trunk and extremities.

Etiology. Although most instances of aplasia cutis congenita are sporadic, there are several well-documented pedigrees demonstrating autosomal dominant and autosomal recessive transmission of the defect (Sybert, 1985). Association with other developmental abnormalities, such as cutaneous organoid nevi, cleft lip and palate, syndactyly, clubbing of hands and feet, congenital heart disease, vascular lesions, and malformations of the brain, also have

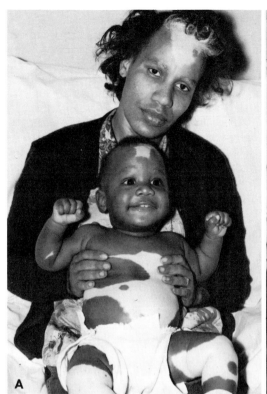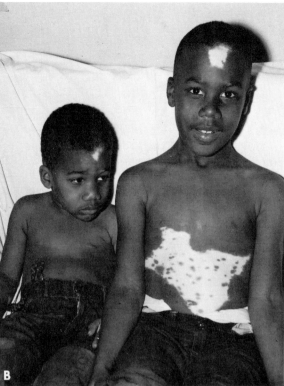

FIGURE 111–4. A, Mother and child with partial albinism. Both have patches on the forehead, although of different sizes and shapes. The areas of nonpigmentation on the infant's trunk and extremities are unusually extensive. B, Siblings with different degrees of partial albinism. (From Jahn, H. M., and McIntire, M. S.: Am. J. Dis. Child. 88:481, 1954. © American Medical Association.)

been recorded (Frieden, 1986; Sybert, 1985). In addition, scalp defects are frequently found in infants with malformation syndromes such as trisomy 13, Johanson-Blizzard syndrome, amniotic band disruption complex, and the ectodermal dysplasias.

The cause of aplasia cutis congenita is unknown. Basically, it is a physical finding signifying disruption of the skin in utero and probably attributable to numerous causes. The findings of a twin fetus papyraceous and/or a placental infarct have suggested vascular thrombosis as a cause in infants with lesions on the trunk and limbs (Levin et al., 1980).

Clinical Findings. The defects are usually along the midline of the scalp in the parietal or occipital areas and may be solitary or multiple, measuring up to several centimeters in diameter (Fig. 111–5). Multiple defects, particularly those on the trunk and extremities, may be strikingly symmetric in distribution (Levin et al., 1980). The lesion is sharply marginated, often oval or round, and can be ulcerated, bullous, cicatricial, or covered with a tough membrane. The depth of the base can vary from the level of the dermis to that of the arachnoid, with defects in the calvarium and dura.

Histologic examination of tissue from the defect demonstrates an absent epidermis and a diminished number of appendageal structures and dermal elastic fibers or, in deeper lesions, the absence of all layers of the integument. No evidence of inflammation or pathogenic organisms is usually detectable.

Prognosis and Treatment. Healing of the lesions is

usually uneventful, resulting in an atrophic or hypertrophic scar, which is always hairless. The repair process takes weeks to months, during which time little treatment is required. Secondary infections will respond to compresses and an antibiotic ointment; if there is an associated bony defect, the patient must be observed for the possibility of a complicating meningitis. Those lesions that fail to heal or produce cosmetically unacceptable scars can be excised with primary closure (Kosnik and Sayers, 1975). Punch-graft hair transplant or scalp reduction for larger lesions may be attempted as an alternative procedure.

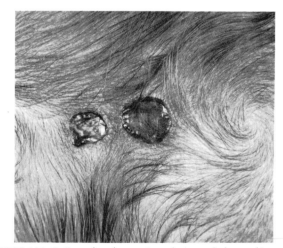

FIGURE 111–5. Two sharply marginated areas of absent skin on the scalp of a normal newborn male infant whose mother's labor and delivery were normal. The defects extended to the subcutaneous tissue and healed in 3 weeks with the formation of thin, white atrophic scars.

■ INCONTINENTIA PIGMENTI

Also known as the Bloch-Sulzberger syndrome, incontinentia pigmenti is now widely recognized as a multisystem disease affecting structures of both ectodermal and mesodermal origin.

Etiology. This heritable disorder is restricted almost exclusively to females, although a few affected males have been reported. The abnormal gene is believed to be transmitted on the X chromosome, with a dominant effect in females and a lethal effect in males. Several well-documented pedigrees demonstrating mother-daughter transmission have been recorded; an increased incidence of spontaneous abortions has been noted in these kindreds.

Clinical Findings. The most striking feature of this disorder is the bizarre skin eruption that, in most patients, can be divided into three stages that persist for variable periods (O'Brien and Feingold, 1985). The bullous phase, which generally lasts for the first several months, is characterized by widespread inflammatory vesicular lesions in a linear distribution on the scalp, trunk, and extremities (Fig. 111–6A). The infant is otherwise well, although a peripheral eosinophilia as high as 50 per cent may be associated. The vesicular phase is superseded by the verrucous phase, in which warty lesions appear in roughly the same distribution as the blisters but are most pronounced on the hands and feet. The third stage, most familiar to pediatricians, consists of macular gray or brown pigmentation in whorls, stripes, and feathered patterns that are independent of the sites of previous lesions (Fig.

111–6B). The pigmentary lesions usually fade in later years and may disappear by adulthood. In an occasional infant, the typical pigmentary changes are present at birth, and the first two stages are never evident (Lerer et al., 1973). Fourth-stage lesions seen in some affected women consist of hypopigmented, atrophic, anhidrotic streaks, usually localized to the legs (Moss and Ince, 1987).

It is important to recognize the particular anomalies that accompany the skin changes in about 80 per cent of affected individuals. Central nervous system aberrations include seizures, microcephaly, retardation, and spastic paralysis. Patchy alopecia, defective dentition, ocular abnormalities, and less commonly, bony defects have all been documented repeatedly in affected children (Carney, 1976).

Diagnosis. Differential diagnosis sometimes poses a serious problem during the neonatal period. Although the linear blisters are often so characteristic that they permit instant recognition of the disorder, at times certain procedures must be performed to exclude other bullous abnormalities (Solomon and Esterly, 1973). Skin biopsy during the bullous phase, although not pathognomonic, will show intraepidermal vesicles filled with eosinophils. Alterations in the epidermal melanocytes and dermal deposits of melanin are apparent in the later phases of the disease (Schachner and Hansen, 1988).

Prognosis and Treatment. Treatment of the skin lesions is not necessary. Occasionally, vesicular lesions become extremely inflamed or secondarily infected. In the latter instance, cool tap water compresses and antibiotic therapy may be required. If other anomalies are present,

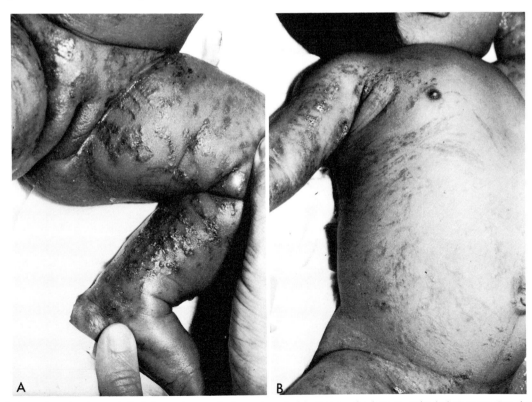

FIGURE 111–6. Incontinentia pigmenti: A, Inflammatory vesicular and crusted lesions on the legs. B, Whorled pigmentation developing on the trunk of a 1-month-old infant who still has inflammatory lesions on the limbs.

on-going care should be provided by the appropriate specialists.

■ CUTIS LAXA

Cutis laxa is a rare, genetically determined disorder in which the skin hangs in pendulous folds, producing a lugubrious facies and a grotesque, prematurely aged appearance (Fig. 111–7). Both autosomal dominant and autosomal recessive forms have been described (Beighton, 1972). Males and females are affected equally. An X-linked form has also been delineated (Byers et al., 1980). It should be noted that cutis laxa can be found in many disorders (e.g., combined immunodeficiency disease and the Prader-Willi and Langer-Giedion syndromes).

Clinical Features. The facies of a patient with cutis laxa is characteristic, with hooked nose, everted nostrils, a long upper lip, and sagging cheeks. The infant may have a strikingly hoarse cry due to redundant laryngeal tissue. Individuals with the autosomal dominant form of cutis laxa suffer few ill effects, apart from their altered appearance, and enjoy good health and a normal life span. Pulmonary and cardiovascular manifestations are absent or minimal. In contrast, patients with the recessive form of the disorder are often seriously compromised and may die in childhood of pulmonary or cardiovascular complications. Systemic manifestations include diverticula of the gastrointestinal and urogenital tracts, rectal prolapse, multiple hernias, pulmonary emphysema, and cardiac disease (Mehregan et al., 1978). A few infants have been reported who manifested additional defects, such as skeletal anomalies, dislocation of the hips, and intrauterine growth retardation (Sakati et al., 1983).

Diagnosis. Although the basic defect is unknown, all the manifestations are attributable to abnormalities of the elastic tissue. Elastic fibers are diminished in the papillary and upper dermis, whereas those in the lower dermis undergo fragmentation and granular degeneration (Mehregan et al., 1978). Similar changes occur in the elastic tissue of affected viscera.

Treatment. Plastic surgery can improve the physical

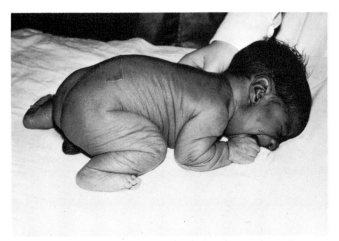

FIGURE 111–7. *Newborn infant with dwarfism and cutis laxa.*

appearance of these patients. The internal manifestations are not amenable to therapy.

■ EHLERS-DANLOS SYNDROME

In contrast to patients with cutis laxa, those with Ehlers-Danlos syndrome have skin that is hyperextensible rather than loose-fitting and that, when stretched, snaps back into place readily. Fragility of the skin is also characteristic, leading to easy bruising and bleeding; minor trauma may produce gaping wounds, which heal with cigarette-paper–like scars that are often detectable over the forehead, knees, elbows, and anterior lower legs. Other cutaneous findings include redundant skin on the palms and soles, molluscoid pseudotumors over pressure points, and small, lipid-containing cysts that may calcify and are identifiable radiologically as subcutaneous. Hypermobility of the joints with skeletal deformity and ocular manifestations such as epicanthal folds, blue sclerae, microcornea, retinal detachment, and subluxation of the lens are frequently present. Although diverticula and hernias can occur, they are by no means as common as in cutis laxa (McKusick, 1972).

Etiology. Genetic heterogeneity has been well established for Ehlers-Danlos syndrome; 10 forms have been delineated on the basis of differences in clinical, genetic, and biochemical findings (Schachner and Hansen, 1988). It has been postulated that all forms of the Ehlers-Danlos syndrome are due to a defect in the biogenesis of collagen of the skin and other affected organs. Types I, II, and III are autosomal dominant with unknown biochemical defects. Type IV Ehlers-Danlos syndrome is characterized by a type III collagen deficiency, type V by lysyl oxidase deficiency, type VII by procollagen peptidase deficiency or defective conversion of procollagen to collagen, type VI by lysyl hydroxylase deficiency, type IX by reduced activity of lysyl oxidase, and type X by fibronectin deficiency. These specific defects can be identified by culture of dermal fibroblasts from a skin biopsy.

Treatment. There is no effective treatment for the various forms of Ehlers-Danlos syndrome. These patients tolerate surgical procedures poorly because of difficulty in healing and frequent dehiscence of surgical wounds. Repair of cutaneous wounds may require the services of a plastic surgeon and progressive joint disease, ongoing orthopedic care.

■ EPIDERMOLYSIS BULLOSA

Epidermolysis bullosa (EB) is a group of diseases that are all characterized by vesiculobullous lesions that arise in response to minimal trauma or shearing force to the skin, and are most easily classified based on the level of cleavage within the skin, available genetic information, and the clinical features. Four main groups are delineated: simplex, junctional, dominant dystrophic, and recessive dystrophic epidermolysis bullosa. Many patients have been described with variants of these major forms, and more than 20 subtypes have been delineated (Fine, 1986; Haber, 1985). Involvement of other organ systems occurs in patients with certain of these disorders (Briggaman, 1983; Workshop Proceedings, 1988).

EPIDERMOLYSIS BULLOSA SIMPLEX

Epidermolysis bullosa simplex has both localized and generalized forms, and as many as nine separate subtypes have been described. The three most common subtypes are described as follows.

GENERALIZED EPIDERMOLYSIS BULLOSA SIMPLEX, KOEBNER VARIANT

This form of EB, inherited as an autosomal dominant trait, is present at birth or early in infancy. Bullae arise most frequently over pressure points, such as the elbows and knees as well as on the legs, feet, and hands. Mucous membrane involvement occurs primarily during infancy. The extensive erosions that sometimes result from the trauma of birth may be mistaken for aplasia cutis. Nails may be lost but almost always regrow. The blister cleavage plane is through the basal layer of the epidermis and, for this reason, the disease does not cause scarring. The prognosis is relatively good, and the propensity to blister may decrease with age.

GENERALIZED EPIDERMOLYSIS BULLOSA, DOWLING-MEARA VARIANT

This variant of EB simplex causes generalized, often extensive, blistering in the neonatal period and early years of life. Herpetiform grouping of the blisters is characteristic. Additional findings include nail dystrophy, palmoplantar keratoderma as a late feature, and improvement with age.

LOCALIZED EPIDERMOLYSIS BULLOSA, WEBER-COCKAYNE VARIANT

The blisters in this disease are usually limited to the hands and feet, although they occasionally occur elsewhere on the body. This type of epidermolysis bullosa, which is inherited in an autosomal dominant fashion, usually does not occur during the neonatal period. Cleavage is at the basilar level; therefore, healing proceeds without the formation of scars.

JUNCTIONAL EPIDERMOLYSIS BULLOSA

Junctional EB has at least six variants. Several are relatively localized and benign. The most severe form is described below.

JUNCTIONAL EPIDERMOLYSIS BULLOSA, HERLITZ TYPE

Although patients with junctional EB, Herlitz type (letalis), exhibit varying degrees of severity, in general this diagnosis implies an ominous prognosis, and many of these patients die in infancy. The disorder is transmitted as an autosomal recessive trait. Bullae and moist erosions occur on the scalp, in the perioral area, and over pressure points elsewhere on the body (Fig. 111–8A). Some of these erosions become the sites of vegetating granulomas. The hands and feet are relatively spared, and digital fusion, inevitable in the recessive dystrophic type of epidermolysis bullosa, does not occur. Nails are affected and may be lost permanently. Mucous membrane erosions are inconspicuous and rarely cause distress of any significance; however, defective dentition is the rule. These patients grow poorly, appear malnourished, and have chronic recalcitrant anemia. The cleavage plane in the skin lesions occurs between the plasma membrane of the basal cell and the basement membrane. The hemidesmosomes responsible for attachment of the basal cells to the basement membrane are reduced in number and abnormally structured. Since the separation does not involve the dermis, uncomplicated blisters heal without scarring.

RECESSIVE DYSTROPHIC EPIDERMOLYSIS BULLOSA

Recessive dystrophic EB is inherited as an autosomal recessive trait and, as might be expected, consanguineous marriages are frequent in affected kindreds. There are two forms, the most severe of which is described below.

RECESSIVE DYSTROPHIC EPIDERMOLYSIS BULLOSA, HALLOPEAU-SIEMENS VARIANT

Infants with recessive dystrophic EB, Hallopeau-Siemens variant, often have extensive denuded lesions at birth and during the neonatal period. Bullae may be hemorrhagic and occur on all surfaces, including the hands and feet; loss of the nails is usual. Over subsequent years the mobility of the fingers and toes becomes severely restricted, as fusion of digits, bone resorption and the inevitable mittenlike deformity of the hands and feet ensue. Mucous membrane involvement may be severe, resulting in esophageal strictures and serious impairment of nutrition due to the restriction of oral intake. These bullae are subepidermal and always eventuate in scarring. On electron microscopy, there are diminished or absent anchoring fibrils associated with marked degeneration of collagen in the papillary portion of the dermis. Also evident is excess abnormal collagenase in fibroblast cultures.

DOMINANT DYSTROPHIC EPIDERMOLYSIS BULLOSA

There are several localized forms of dominant dystrophic epidermolysis bullosa as well as two generalized variants. The localized forms may cause blistering only in very specific areas and may become less pronounced with increasing age.

The two generalized forms of dominant dystrophic epidermolysis bullosa (Cockayne-Touraine and Pasini variants) tend to be less severe than recessive dystrophic epidermolysis bullosa. Of the two, the Pasini variant is more troublesome. The bullae are subepidermal and heal with scarring, but the process may be relatively limited, involving mainly hands, feet (Fig. 111–8B), and skin over bony protuberances or may be generalized, particularly in the Pasini variant. Nails may be lost. Milia are common and may appear in profusion in the soft, wrinkled scars; pigmentary changes are also usual. Mucous membrane lesions, if present, are mild, and general health may be unimpaired. The appearance of albopapuloid lesions on the trunk during adolescence is a unique feature of the Pasini variant.

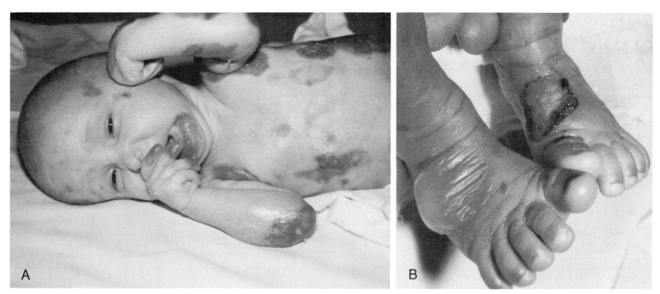

FIGURE 111–8. A, *Large bullae on the feet of an infant with a scarring form of epidemolysis bullosa.* B, *Multiple moist erosions characteristic of junctional epidermolysis bullosa. Note involvement of fingers and perioral skin.*

Diagnosis. The diagnosis of infants with this group of diseases is not always easy. Bullous impetigo is probably the most commonly confused entity. A positive culture may indicate either secondary infection of epidermolysis bullosa or impetigo. Absence of organisms is suggestive of epidermolysis bullosa. The distribution of the lesions may be a diagnostic aid. Those of impetigo more often begin in the diaper region and spread peripherally; in epidermolysis bullosa, the earliest lesions occur on extremities and those points that make closest contact with the crib sheets, such as the heels, wrists, knees, and sacrum. The fluid within the bullae is more likely to be clear or hemorrhagic in epidermolysis bullosa, but turbid contents do not positively gainsay this diagnosis. A careful family history for blistering diseases should, of course, be obtained. A biopsy of an induced blister for light and electron microscopy as well as immunofluorescence mapping and monoclonal antibody studies may help confirm the diagnosis (Fine, 1986 and 1988). It is important to appreciate that, once the diagnosis of epidermolysis bullosa has been made, further classification may be fraught with error due to the many phenotypic variations that are now being recognized. Classification is particularly difficult during the neonatal period when many of these conditions share identical clinical features.

Treatment. There is no specific therapy for this group of disorders. Systemic corticosteroids have been ineffective except in the prevention of severe stricture formation in the esophagus from lesions of recessive dystrophic disease. Oral administration of vitamin E is also ineffective in most cases. The infant should be protected from trauma as much as possible. For the newborn, attention to environmental (isolette) temperature is critical as overheating may result in extensive blistering. The infant should be placed on a soft material (sheepskin or linen), and clothing with metal closures should be avoided. If mucous membranes are involved, soft nipples, bulb syringes, and devices used for feeding infants with cleft palates should be employed. Bathing may have to be restricted to avoid excessive handling. Compresses with normal saline or 0.25 to 0.5

per cent silver nitrate for eroded areas may be helpful in some instances. Hot water should never be used, since warm temperatures increase the tendency to blister. Blisters should be decompressed by several punctures in the surface, but the blister tops should not be removed. Petrolatum or nonsensitizing topical antibiotic ointments, such as Polysporin and Bactroban, should be applied to oozing or crusted areas to prevent adherence of the skin to clothing and sheets. Denuded areas can be covered with one of the hydrocolloid dressings or vaseline gauze. Dressings can be secured with a soft gauze wrap. Adhesive tape should never be applied as large areas of epidermis may be torn off with its removal. Cribs, high chairs, and infant seats should be well padded, and only soft toys offered for play.

Every attempt should be made to ensure adequate nutrition, but growth may be impaired despite these efforts. Anemia should be anticipated in patients with severe disease, and high doses of supplemental iron may be indicated from early infancy (Workshop Proceedings, 1988).

New Approaches. Studies are in progress with several potentially beneficial drugs, including phenytoin and oral retinoids. Successful skin-grafting has been accomplished in selected patients using autologous epidermal cell culture-derived grafts. A national EB Registry has been created in order to facilitate data collection. The support group Dystrophic Epidermolysis Bullosa Research Association (D.E.B.R.A.), D.E.B.R.A. of America, Inc., 141 Fifth Avenue, Suite 7-S, New York, N.Y. 10010, provides helpful information and can direct families of affected children to the appropriate regional center.

■ NEONATAL LUPUS ERYTHEMATOSUS

Infants born to mothers with acute, subacute, and clinically latent systemic lupus erythematosus or other connective tissue disorders can manifest transient cutaneous lesions, hematologic abnormalities, congenital heart block, and serologic evidence of lupus erythematosus during the first few months of life (Lee and Weston, 1984; Provost et al., 1987).

Etiology. Neonatal lupus erythematosus is almost invariably associated with the presence of Ro (SS-A) and La (SS-B) autoantibodies in mother and infant. With the exception of congenital heart block, the manifestations of neonatal lupus resolve with disappearance of maternal antibody, suggesting an important role for these antibodies in pathogenesis. An association with HLA-DR$_3$ in the mother but not the infant has also been documented (Lee and Weston, 1984). Ro-positive, HLA-DR$_2$ mothers, in contrast, produce unaffected infants (Provost et al., 1987).

Clinical Findings. Characteristic cutaneous lesions resembling those of subacute lupus may be present with or without congenital heart block and evidence of systemic disease (Hardy et al., 1979). The lesions are usually localized to the scalp, face, and shoulders, although they can be more widespread and are erythematous, scaly, and sharply demarcated, often with mild atrophy (Fig. 111–9). Annular and polycyclic lesions are common, but follicular plugging, telangiectasia, and scarring are absent. The eruption has a predilection for sun-exposed areas, and a history of intense sun exposure preceding the eruption can often be obtained. Skin lesions develop from birth to 3 months of age and generally begin to resolve at

about 6 months concurrent with the disappearance of maternal antibodies. Additional but uncommon manifestations include hematologic aberrations, particularly thrombocytopenia, pneumonitis, and hepatosplenomegaly. Congenital heart block is the most frequent extracutaneous finding.

Diagnosis. These lesions can be mistaken for several cutaneous disorders including seborrheic dermatitis, dermatophytosis, atopic dermatitis, and psoriasis. A skin biopsy may demonstrate the histopathologic features of lupus, and direct immunofluorescent study of a snap-frozen skin biopsy specimen may demonstrate deposition of immunoglobulin, most often IgG and complement, at the dermal-epidermal junction. More reliable, however, is the detection of Ro (SS-A) and/or La (SS-B) antibody in serum from the infant and mother.

Prognosis and Treatment. During the spring and summer months, affected infants should be protected from undue exposure to sunlight by application of one of the many commercially available sunscreen preparations. The activity of the skin lesions may be controlled by local treatment with a corticosteroid cream. The skin lesions are self-limiting; however, long-term prognostic studies are not available, so a predictable outcome cannot be assured. Two infants with neonatal lupus reported many years ago have been observed to develop systemic lupus erythematosus in early adulthood.

It is also important to recognize that asymptomatic mothers are at risk for connective tissue disorders later in life and that offspring of subsequent pregnancies may be affected with neonatal lupus (Gawkrodger and Beveridge, 1984; McCune et al., 1987).

■ ECTODERMAL DYSPLASIAS

The term "ectodermal dysplasia" connotes abnormalities of the skin and its appendages, the sweat glands, sebaceous glands, and hair follicles, but it also has been applied to disease entities in which abnormalities of nails, hair, and teeth are a prominent feature. This variation in approach has caused some confusion in the literature, and for this reason, we believe it is most helpful to define or qualify the type of ectodermal defect, if possible, when describing a particular entity (Solomon and Keuer, 1980). A recent monograph describes more than 100 such syndromes classified by the particular structures affected (hair, teeth, nails, and sweat glands) (Freire-Maia and Pinheiro, 1984). Because these conditions are rare and because these families share similar problems, much can be gained from the support and educational materials available through the National Foundation for Ectodermal Dysplasias, 219 E. Main St., Mascouteh, IL, 62258.

Although a number of entities might thus be included under this heading, we will confine our discussion to three of the more common conditions: hidrotic ectodermal dysplasia, hypohidrotic ectodermal dysplasia, and the EEC syndrome.

HIDROTIC ECTODERMAL DYSPLASIA

Sweating response is normal in this form of ectodermal dysplasia. Hypoplasia, absence or dystrophy of the nails,

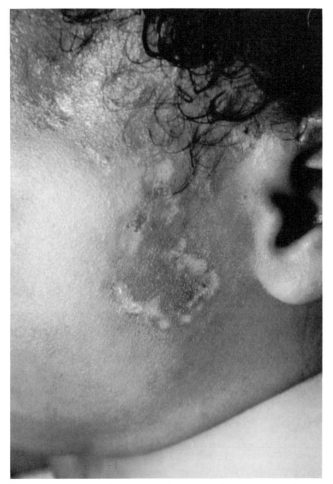

FIGURE 111–9. *Newborn with cutaneous lesions of neonatal lupus erythematosus.*

sparse hair, and hyperkeratosis of the palms and soles are characteristic. The teeth are usually normal but may be small and subject to decay. The disorder is inherited as an autosomal dominant trait.

HYPOHIDROTIC ECTODERMAL DYSPLASIA

The hypohidrotic (anhidrotic) form of ectodermal dysplasia is probably of greater interest to the neonatologist and pediatrician, as it may cause considerable difficulty during the first year of life. The most serious disturbance is the absence or diminution of sweating, due to rudimentary or absent eccrine sweat glands, which results in marked heat intolerance and episodes of hyperpyrexia during infancy (Richards and Kaplan, 1969). If the possibility of this disorder is not considered, such infants may undergo numerous hospitalizations and tests until the true nature of the problem is appreciated.

Clinical Features. Patients with hypohidrotic ectodermal dysplasia have several identifiable features that permit correct diagnosis later in life but may be difficult to appreciate in the newborn. Severe peeling or scaling skin appears to be a common finding in affected newborns. This skin change, which is often misconstrued as an indication of postmaturity, may provide a valuable clue to the diagnosis (Executive and Scientific Advisory Boards of the NFED, 1989). Thereafter, the skin may appear relatively pale and dry, with a prominent venous pattern over most of the body, but hyperpigmented and wrinkled in the periorbital area (Fig. 111–10).

The facial characteristics of frontal bossing, depression of the central face, saddle nose, thick protruding lips, and prominent chin are not readily apparent in the newborn. Likewise, the sparse, unruly, light-colored hair and scanty brows and lashes are also difficult to appreciate in the first few months. The changes in dentition cannot, of course, be detected until late infancy. Hypodontia with conical, poorly formed teeth is the rule; these changes can be identified on radiographs of the jaws prior to eruption of the teeth. Atrophic rhinitis, diminished lacrimation, hoarseness, and hypoplastic or absent mucous glands in nasotracheobronchial passages are also frequent findings in

these patients (Reed et al., 1970). If the diagnosis is in doubt, a skin biopsy may demonstrate absent or hypoplastic eccrine sweat glands. Techniques used to elicit sweating, such as pilocarpine iontophoresis or examination of the sweat pores on the palm with O-phthalaldehyde, can also be utilized to demonstrate the defect (Esterly et al., 1973). Atopic dermatitis occurs frequently in these children (Reed et al., 1970), as well as a decrease in T-cell function (Davis and Solomon, 1976).

In most families, the disorder is transmitted as an X-linked recessive trait, with the fully expressed disease appearing only in males. Carrier females may be detected by minor clinical stigmata and by decreased sweat pore counts and abnormal dermatoglyphic findings (Crump and Danks, 1971; Esterly et al., 1973). However, females with the complete syndrome have been carefully documented, and in these families, an autosomal recessive gene appears to be operating (Gorlin et al., 1970).

Once the diagnosis is made, it is important to educate parents so that these children are protected from overexertion and undue exposure to heat. Defective lacrimation can be palliated by the use of artificial tears. The nasal mucosa should be treated with saline irrigations for removal of adherent crusts, followed by application of petrolatum. Regular dental evaluations should be started early in life and dentures fitted for maintenance of good nutrition and improvement in the appearance of the child before starting school. Some of these children also require a wig and reconstructive procedures later in life to improve facial configuration.

EEC SYNDROME

The EEC syndrome consists of ectodermal dysplasia, ectrodactyly, and cleft lip and palate. This syndrome affects both ectodermal and mesodermal tissues and is inherited as an autosomal dominant trait. The cutaneous and appendageal anomalies include diffuse hypopigmentation affecting both skin and hair, scanty scalp hair and eyebrows, dystrophic nails and small teeth with enamel hypoplasia. Sweating appears to be intact, and sweat glands are present on skin biopsy. The clefting of the lip is usually complete and bilateral, and the palate has a median cleft. Dry granulomatous lesions in the corners of the mouth consistently yield *Candida albicans* on culture. Anomalies of the hands and feet include lobster claw deformity, syndactyly, and clinodactyly. Other findings include scarred lacrimal ducts, blepharitis and conjunctivitis, xerostomia, conductive hearing loss, and retardation. Although incomplete forms of this syndrome have been documented, the fully developed EEC syndrome should not be confused with other types of ectodermal dysplasia (Pries et al., 1974).

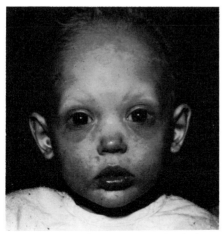

FIGURE 111–10. *Female with fully expressed anhidrotic ectodermal dysplasia. Note the sparse, wispy hair, hyperpigmentation around the eyes, depressed nasal bridge, and protruding lips and ears.*

■ REFERENCES

Beighton, P.: The dominant and recessive forms of cutis laxa. J. Med. Genet. 9:216, 1972.

Byers, P. H., Siegel, R. C., Holbrook, K. A., et al.: X-linked cutis laxa. N. Engl. J. Med. 303:61, 1980.

Briggaman, R. A.: Hereditary epidermolysis bullosa with special emphasis on newly recognized syndromes and complications. Dermatol. Clin. 1:263, 1983.

Carney, R. G., Jr.: Incontinentia pigmenti. A world statistical analysis. Arch. Dermatol. *112*:535, 1976.

Clarke, A., Sarfarazi, M., Thomas, N. S., et al.: X-linked hypohidrotic ectodermal dysplasia: DNA probe linkage analysis and gene localization. Hum. Genet. *75*:378, 1987.

Cooper, T. W., and Bauer, E. A.: Epidermolysis bullosa: A review. Pediatr. Dermatol. *1*:181, 1984.

Crump, J. A., and Danks, D. M.: Hypohidrotic ectodermal dysplasia. J. Pediatr. *78*:466, 1971.

Davis, J. R., and Solomon, L. M.: Cellular immunodeficiency in anhidrotic ectodermal dysplasia. Acta Dermatol. Venereol. *56*:115, 1976.

Esterly, N. B., Pashayan, H. M., and West, C. E.: Concurrent hypohidrotic ectodermal dysplasia and X-linked ichthyosis. Am. J. Dis. Child. *126*:539, 1973.

Executive and Scientific Advisory Boards of the National Foundation for Ectodermal Dysplasia: Scaling skin in the newborn: A clue to the early diagnosis of X-linked hypohidrotic ectodermal dysplasia (Christ-Siemens-Touraine syndrome). J. Pediatr. *114*:600, 1989.

Fine, J.-D.: Epidermolysis bullosa. Clinical aspects, pathology, and recent advances in research. Internat. J. Dermatol. *25*:143, 1986.

Fine, J.-D.: Changing clinical and laboratory concepts in inherited epidermolysis bullosa. Arch. Dermatol. *124*:523, 1988.

Franco, H. L., Weston, W. L., Peebles, C., et al.: Autoantibodies directed against sicca syndrome antigens in the neonatal lupus syndrome. J. Am. Acad. Dermatol. *4*:67, 1981.

Freire-Maia, N., and Pinheiro, M.: Ectodermal Dysplasias: A Clinical and Genetic Study. New York, Alan R. Liss, 1984.

Frieden, I. J.: Aplasia cutis congenita: A clinical review and proposal for classification. J. Am. Acad. Dermatol. *14*:646, 1986.

Gawkrodger, D. J., and Beveridge, G. W.: Neonatal lupus erythematosus in four successive siblings born to a mother with discoid lupus erythematosus. Br. J. Dermatol. *111*:683, 1984.

Gorlin, R. J., Old, T., and Anderson, V. E.: Hypohidrotic ectodermal dysplasia in females. A critical analysis and argument for genetic heterogeneity. Z. Kinderheilkd. *108*:1, 1970.

Haber, R. M., Hanna, W., Ramsay, C. A., et al.: Hereditary epidermolysis bullosa. J. Am. Acad. Dermatol. *13*:252, 1985.

Hardy, J. D., Solomon, S., Barwell, G. S., et al.: Congenital complete heart block in the newborn associated with maternal systemic lupus erythematosus and other connective tissue disorders. Arch. Dis. Child. *54*:7, 1979.

Jimbow, K., Fitzpatrick, T. B., Szabo, G., et al.: Congenital circumscribed hypomelanosis: A characterization based on electron microscopic study of tuberous sclerosis, nevus depigmentosus and piebaldism. J. Invest. Dermatol. *64*:50, 1975.

King, R. A., and Olds, D. P.: Hairbulb tyrosinase activity in oculocutaneous albinism: Suggestions for pathway control and block location. Am. J. Med. Genet. *20*:49, 1985.

Konigsmark, B.: Hereditary childhood hearing loss and integumentary system disease. J. Pediatr. *80*:909, 1972.

Kosnik, E. J., and Sayers, M. P.: Congenital scalp defects: Aplasia cutis congenita. J. Neurosurg. *42*:32, 1975.

Lawlor, F.: Harlequin fetus progression to nonbullous ichthyosiform erythroderma. Pediatrics *82*:870, 1988.

Lee, L. A., and Weston, W. L.: New findings in neonatal lupus syndrome. Am. J. Dis. Child. *138*:233, 1984.

Lerer, R. J., Ehrenhranz, R. A., and Campbell, A. G. M.: Pigmented lesions of incontinentia pigmenti in a neonate. J. Pediatr. *83*:503, 1973.

Levin, D. L., Nolan, K. S., and Esterly, N. B.: Congenital absence of skin. J. Am. Acad. Dermatol. *2*:203, 1980.

McCune, A. B., Weston, W. L., and Lee, A. A.: Maternal and fetal outcome in neonatal lupus erythematosus. Ann. Int. Med. *106*:518, 1987.

McKusick, V. A.: Heritable Disorders of Connective Tissue. St. Louis, C. V. Mosby, 1972.

Mehregan, A. H., Lee, S. C., and Nabai, H.: Cutis laxa (generalized elastolysis). A report of four cases with autopsy findings. J. Cutan. Pathol. *5*:116, 1978.

Moss, C., and Ince, P.: Anhidrotic and achromians lesions in incontinentia pigmenti. Br. J. Dermatol. *116*:839, 1987.

O'Brien, J. E., and Feingold, M.: Incontinentia pigmenti. A longitudinal study. Am. J. Dis. Child. *139*:712, 1985.

Pinnell, S. R., Krane, S. M., Kenzora, J., et al.: A new heritable disorder of connective tissue with hydroxylysine-deficient collagen. N. Engl. J. Med. *286*:1013, 1972.

Pries, C., Mittleman, D., Miller, M., et al.: The EEC syndrome. Am. J. Dis. Child. *127*:840, 1974.

Provost, T. T., Watson, R., Gaither, K. K., et al.: The neonatal lupus erythematosus syndrome. J. Rheumatol. *14*(Suppl. 13):199, 1987.

Reed, W. B., Lopez, D. A., and Landing, B.: Clinical spectrum of anhidrotic ectodermal dysplasia. Arch. Dermatol. *102*:134, 1970.

Richards, W., and Kaplan, M.: Anhidrotic ectodermal dysplasia: An unusual cause of hyperpyrexia in the newborn. Am. J. Dis. Child. *117*:597, 1969.

Roberts, L. J.: Long-term survival of a harlequin fetus. J. Am. Acad. Dermatol. *21*:335, 1989.

Rogers, M., and Scarf, C.: Harlequin baby treated with etretinate. Pediatr. Dermatol. *6*:216, 1989.

Rosenfeld, S., and Smith, M. E.: Ocular findings in incontinentia pigmenti. Ophthalmology *92*:543, 1985.

Sakati, N. O., Nyhan, W. L., Shear, C. S., et al.: Syndrome of cutis laxa, ligamentous laxity, and delayed development. Pediatrics *72*:850, 1983.

Schachner, L. A., and Hansen, R. C. (Eds.): Pediatric Dermatology. New York, Churchill Livingstone, 1988.

Solomon, L. M., and Esterly, N. B.: Neonatal Dermatology. Philadelphia, W. B. Saunders Company, 1973.

Solomon, L. M., and Keuer, E. J.: The ectodermal dysplasias. Arch. Dermatol. *116*:1295, 1980.

Sybert, V. P.: Aplasia cutis congenita: A report of 12 new families and a review of the literature. Pediatr. Dermatol. *3*:1, 1985.

Telfer, M. A., Sugar, A., Jaeger, E. A., et al.: Dominant piebald trait (white forehead and leukoderma) with neurological impairment. Am. J. Hum. Genet. *23*:383, 1971.

Williams, M. L.: The ichthyoses—pathogenesis and prenatal diagnosis: A review of recent advances. Pediatr. Dermatol. *1*:1, 1983.

Williams, M. L.: A new look at the ichthyoses: Disorders of lipid metabolism. Pediatr. Dermatol. *3*:476, 1986.

Witkop, C. J., Jr., Quevedo, W. C., Jr., Fitzpatrick, T. B., and King, R. A.: In Scriver, C. R., Beaudet, A. L., Sly, W. S., and Volle, D. (Eds.): The Metabolic Basis of Inherited Disease. 6th ed. New York, McGraw-Hill, 1989, p. 2905.

Workshop Proceedings: Pathogenesis, clinical features and management of the nondermatologic complications of epidermolysis bullosa. Arch. Dermatol. *124*:705, 1988.

INFECTIONS OF **112** THE SKIN

Nancy B. Esterly and Lawrence M. Solomon

The newborn skin may be the site of a variety of lesions of infectious origin. Some types represent localized disease, whereas others are a reflection of generalized disease. Although certain systemic infections such as disseminated herpes simplex (see Chapter 36), varicella-zoster (see Chapter 36), and *Pseudomonas* sepsis produce characteristic skin lesions, these lesions have been described elsewhere in this text as a feature of the total clinical picture. Other systemic infections, such as cytomegalic inclusion disease, toxoplasmosis, and rubella, cause less distinctive skin lesions that are not specific for the particular disease entity; these, also, are described in other chapters. In this chapter, we confine our discussion to those infections that are primarily cutaneous in nature.

▪ BULLOUS IMPETIGO

Impetigo is one of the most common infections that plague the infant and neonatologist (Hebert and Esterly, 1986). The disease may occur sporadically in an individual infant, or it may involve a number of infants simultaneously or sequentially in an epidemic form. Although usually not life-threatening, the possibility of bacteremic spread to visceral organs should not be overlooked. Constant surveillance of nursing techniques in the nursery is essential to preventing the initiation of epidemics. The appearance of a single case demands immediate investigation and possible revision of these techniques.

The number of cases originating in a given nursery is related to the physical facilities and adequacy of care in handling the infants. Overcrowding, insufficient nursery personnel, carelessness in the simple matters of washing and gowning on the part of both nurses and physicians, and other infractions of elementary rules of hygiene may lead to an increased incidence of impetigo. This is particularly true now that hexachlorophene bathing has been abandoned as standard nursery procedure because of the potential neurotoxicity of the compound if it is absorbed. If modern nursery procedures are fastidiously observed, however, the recommendations for skin care proposed by the American Academy of Pediatrics Committee on the Fetus and Newborn (Guidelines for Perinatal Care, 1983) should be adequate to prevent the occurrence of impetigo (Table 112–1). Furthermore, it appears that enforced aseptic techniques actually may be more effective in preventing superficial skin infection than is the routine use of hexachlorophene bathing (Gehlbach et al., 1975).

Etiology. Bullous impetigo is caused by coagulase-positive hemolytic *Staphylococcus aureus*. Most often, the organism can be classified as one of the group 2 phage types (Albert et al., 1970), although occasional infections can be attributed to organisms in other phage groups (Curran and Al-Salihi, 1980).

Clinical Findings. In contrast to the lesions of some of the congenital blistering diseases, those of bullous impetigo usually appear during the latter part of the 1st week or as late as the 2nd week of life. The diaper region is most frequently involved, but bullae may arise anywhere on the body surface. The blisters may vary considerably in size and may spread to contiguous areas, often forming arcs or circles, but they usually do not exhibit the characteristic grouping in grapelike clusters seen in the cutaneous eruptions of herpes simplex infection. Staphylococcal bullae are flaccid, filled with straw-colored or turbid fluid, and rupture easily, leaving a red, moist, denuded base, which then becomes covered by a thin varnish-like crust (Fig. 112–1). These lesions are very superficial, re-epithelialize rapidly, and do not result in scars.

Diagnosis. The diagnosis is suggested by the demonstration of gram-positive cocci on smears of the blister fluid and is confirmed by identification of the organism on culture of material from the blister.

Treatment. Treatment should be instituted promptly, and strict isolation maintained until the lesions have resolved. Compresses with sterile water, normal saline, or Burow solution applied every few hours causes maceration, rupture, and drying of blisters. Extremely limited infections may be treated with a topical antibiotic ointment. More extensive lesions require a systemically administered antibiotic that will effectively eradicate a penicillinase-producing strain of *Staphylococcus*. Ultimately, the sensi-

TABLE 112–1. Recommendations for Skin Care in the Newborn Nursery

1. Cleaning of the newborn's skin should be deferred until body temperature has stabilized
2. Sterile cotton pledgets soaked with warm water (with or without a mild soap) may be used to remove blood and meconium
3. Careful drying and removal of blood minimize risk of infection; the vernix need not be removed
4. Iodophors and chlorhexidine should not be used for bathing or localized skin care during nursery stay to prevent infection
5. The cord may be treated with triple dye or a topical antimicrobial (bacitracin); alcohol is not adequate for the prevention of cord colonization and infection
6. Agents applied to newborn skin should be dispensed in single-use containers

(From Guidelines for Perinatal Care. AAP Committee on the Fetus and Newborn. ACOG Committee on Obstetrics; Maternal and Fetal Medicine, 2nd ed., 1988.)

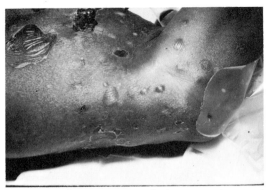

FIGURE 112–1. *Bullous impetigo. Multiple intact and ruptured bullae on the abdomen, hip, and thigh of a newborn infant. No underlying erythema is present.*

tivities of the organism cultured should determine the choice of antibiotics.

■ STAPHYLOCOCCAL SCALDED SKIN SYNDROME

Formerly called Ritter disease when it occurred in the newborn infant, the exfoliative form of this disorder is now included with nonstreptococcal scarlatiniform eruption and bullous impetigo under the rubric of staphylococcal scalded skin syndrome (Elias et al., 1977; Melish and Glasgow, 1971). Although a somewhat similar cutaneous reaction pattern may result from drug hypersensitivity in the older child or adult, scalded skin syndrome in the infant is virtually always caused by *Staphylococcus*. As might be expected because of their common origin, all three forms of the scalded skin syndrome may be seen simultaneously in a nursery epidemic of staphylococcal disease.

Etiology. Although initial reports suggested that all patients with scalded skin syndrome were infected with group 2 phage type staphylococci (Albert et al., 1970; Anthony et al., 1972; Melish and Glasgow, 1971), later evidence suggests that strains in other phage groups are also capable of causing this clinical picture (Curran and Al-Salihi, 1980). These organisms produce an erythrogenic exotoxin called *exfoliatin*, which causes the intraepidermal separation responsible for the clinical manifestations of blistering and exfoliation of large sheets of skin. The toxin has been isolated, purified, and partially characterized and has been studied extensively in the murine model (Elias et al., 1974; Melish and Glasgow, 1970).

Clinical Findings. The onset of scalded skin syndrome is often abrupt, and the disease may progress with astonishing rapidity. Affected infants have an intense, generalized erythema that most often starts on the face and spreads to the contiguous skin. Facial edema may be striking. Oozing from the conjunctival area and crusting around the nose and mouth give the infant a characteristic "sad mask" appearance. The reddened skin is exquisitely sensitive to touch, and the formation of flaccid bullae may precede widespread exfoliation in which the skin peels in large sheets, leaving a moist, red, denuded surface (Fig. 112–2). The denudation, which can be induced by light

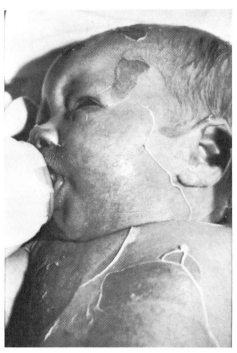

FIGURE 112–2. *Staphylococcal scalded skin syndrome (Ritter disease). Intense erythema and peeling of large areas of epidermis.*

stroking with the examining finger, is called the Nikolsky sign, and it can always be elicited in the exfoliative form of the disease. Separation usually occurs first on the face and in the flexural areas and may be incomplete, leaving a rolled edge of epidermis at the junction of the unpeeled and desquamated areas. The skin over the hands and feet may be shed in a glovelike fashion. Infants with scalded skin syndrome may be toxic or appear relatively well, but fluctuations in body temperature, poor feeding, and irritability due to skin tenderness are usual manifestations of the infection (Sheagren, 1984). With rapid, widespread denudation, fluid balance may become a serious problem. Conjunctivitis, omphalitis, or other localized inflammatory lesions may be prominent, depending on the portal of entry of the organism.

Approximately 2 to 3 days after onset, the denuded areas become dry, and a flaky desquamation ensues. Resolution occurs in another 3 to 5 days, leaving no residual lesions. Since the intraepidermal cleavage plane is at the level of the granular layer, scarring occurs only in instances of secondary complications.

The infant with the less severe form of this disease, the scarlatiniform eruption, also exhibits a generalized type of erythema, but Nikolsky sign is absent. The skin has a sandpaper-like texture similar to that of the skin of the patient with streptococcal scarlet fever; however, the palatal enanthem, strawberry tongue, and perioral pallor are lacking. Instead, perioral erythema with subsequent fissuring and crusting result in the rather characteristic facial appearance. A dry, flaky desquamative phase also occurs at the end of the 1st week in this form of the disease.

Diagnosis. The only helpful laboratory procedures are bacterial cultures. Blood cultures should be obtained, since sepsis, although uncommon, may supervene. In the exfoliative form, fluid from intact bullae is sterile; however, exudate from denuded or crusted areas may yield the organism. Purulent drainage from any area, such as the conjunctival sac, is also a good source of *Staphylococcus,* as are nasopharyngeal and throat cultures. Phage typing is of interest and should be obtained if possible. Gram stains of material obtained for culture may be used to confirm the clinical diagnosis if clumps of gram-positive cocci can be demonstrated. Polymorphonuclear leukocytes may be sparse or absent on smear. The presence of a peripheral leukocytosis is not a reliable indication of infection.

The differential diagnosis includes severe seborrheic dermatitis, epidermolytic hyperkeratosis (bullous congenital ichthyosiform erythroderma), epidermolysis bullosa, erythema multiforme, and diffuse cutaneous mastocytosis. Further studies, including a skin biopsy, may be required in confusing situations, but the clinical picture of scalded skin syndrome is usually sufficiently characteristic to suggest the diagnosis. Although extremely uncommon, it should be appreciated that boric acid poisoning in the young infant causes a clinical picture indistinguishable from that of scalded skin syndrome. Appropriate toxicology studies must be performed for confirmation of this diagnosis (Rubenstein and Mesher, 1970).

Treatment. Because most of the staphylococcal strains that cause this syndrome are penicillinase-producing organisms, systemic administration of a penicillinase-resistant penicillin is the therapy of choice (Rudolph et al., 1974). Fluid and electrolyte replacement and measures for maintenance of normal body temperature may be required. Crusted and denuded areas may be treated with compresses of Burow or normal saline solution. Application of a bland emollient may accelerate the return of the skin to normal during the flaky desquamative phase.

■ OTHER STAPHYLOCOCCAL SKIN LESIONS

Staphylococci may also cause superficial pustulosis, folliculitis, or localized cutaneous abscesses. Superficial lesions, if limited, may respond to compresses and topical antibiotic therapy. Deeper lesions require systemic antibiotic therapy and, occasionally, surgical intervention. Procedures such as fetal monitoring may induce scalp dermatitis, abscess formation, and associated osteomyelitis (Wagner, 1984). *Staphylococcus epidermidis* also has been implicated in this type of lesion (Overturf and Balfour, 1975).

■ CANDIDIASIS

Candidal infections during the neonatal period are most often manifest as mucosal lesions (thrush) or as localized or generalized dermatitis. Rarely, umbilical cord granulomas or a widespread systemic mycosis may occur.

THRUSH

Etiology. The relatively high incidence of localized mucosal or cutaneous lesions can be attributed to the acquisition of *Candida albicans* as normal flora in the oral cavity and gastrointestinal tract by a significant number of infants. One longitudinal study of infants from birth through 1 year of age demonstrated a maximal isolation peak in infants 4 weeks of age, when 82 per cent of infants were found to have *Candida* in the mouth (Russell and Lay, 1973). *Candida albicans* is not a saprophyte of normal skin. In infants, the yeast is deposited on the surface of the integument via the saliva and feces. The original source of the yeast, in most instances, is the mother, who may be a vaginal or intestinal carrier of the organism or who may have had overt disease during her pregnancy (Hebert and Esterly, 1986).

Clinical Findings. The peak incidence of thrush occurs during the beginning of the 2nd week of life. The lesions are readily recognized as plaques of white, friable, pseudomembranous material on an erythematous base distributed over the tongue, palate, buccal mucosa, and gingivae.

Diagnosis. Both yeast and mycelial fungal elements can be demonstrated on a potassium hydroxide preparation of surface material removed from a typical lesion. The diagnosis may be confirmed by identification of the organism on culture.

Treatment. Oral lesions usually respond promptly to a course of nystatin suspension, 100,000 to 200,000 units, administered by mouth four times daily for 10 to 14 days. In refractory cases, an increased dosage of nystatin or alternative approaches may have to be instituted (Hebert and Esterly, 1986).

LOCALIZED CUTANEOUS CANDIDIASIS

Clinical Findings. Localized candidal infections of skin are also common in infants. Intertriginous areas, particularly the diaper area (Fig. 112–3A), are most commonly affected, but even facial eruptions can occur, presumably by the infant's acquiring the organism while passing through the vagina. Multiple tiny vesicopustules erode and merge, forming bright, erythematous, scaly plaques, often with a scalloped edge bordered by a fringe of epithelium. Scattered satellite vesicopustules develop beyond the margins of the plaque and are one of the hallmarks of cutaneous candidiasis. Eruptions in the diaper area usually result from contamination of the perineal skin with feces containing *C. albicans;* therefore, it is usual to have involvement of perirectal skin. The moisture and maceration of the diaper and flexural areas encourage proliferation of the yeast; pruritus and burning associated with the dermatitis may cause extreme discomfort.

Occasionally, a widespread cutaneous dermatitis occurs either as a result of spread from an untreated localized plaque or by contamination of the entire integument during the process of birth (Fig. 112–3B). Superficial vesicopustules rupture, leaving a denuded surface with a ring of detached epidermis. The lesions spread peripherally, forming confluent plaques of dermatitis with generalized scaling. Mucous membrane involvement may be associated. Extensive cutaneous lesions may occur in normal newborns; in infants with an underlying dermatologic disease, such as acrodermatitis enteropathica or ichthyosis; in patients with immunodeficiency disease; and

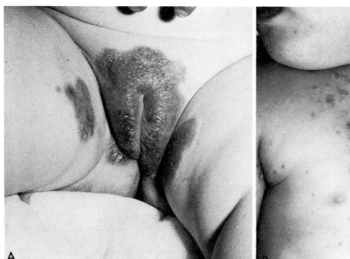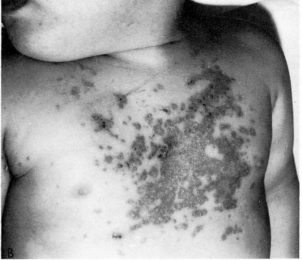

FIGURE 112–3. A, *Sharply demarcated erythematous scaly candidal rash in the groin.* B, *Candidal eruption on the central chest of an infant.*

in those with chronic mucocutaneous candidiasis and endocrinopathies.

Diagnosis. When it involves the perineal skin, cutaneous candidiasis may be confused with superficial staphylococcal infection or with a primary irritant diaper dermatitis. More extensive disease may resemble other types of infection, including congenital syphilis as well as seborrheic dermatitis. Potassium hydroxide preparations of scrapings from involved skin disclose budding yeasts and mycelia, which is confirmatory evidence of yeast infection, but cultures should be obtained if there is any doubt as to the causative agent.

Treatment. Localized cutaneous candidiasis should be treated with a specific candidicidal agent, such as nystatin or one of the imidazoles (e.g., miconazole, clotrimazole, or ketoconazole) in a cream, ointment, lotion, or powder. Generally, ointments are the most soothing and best tolerated. Normal infants respond rapidly to application of anticandidal topical agents; patients with underlying disease may be refractory to therapy.

CONGENITAL CUTANEOUS CANDIDIASIS

Intrauterine infection with *C. albicans* may result in lesions of the placenta and fetal membranes and characteristic granulomas of the umbilical cord (Hebert and Esterly, 1986; Schirar et al., 1974). The cord lesions are multiple yellow-white papules, usually measuring 1 to 3 mm in diameter. A mixed inflammatory cell infiltrate and fungal elements are demonstrable on histologic sections of the cord lesions prepared with the appropriate stains. Although most of these infants have been born prior to term, premature or prolonged rupture of the membranes is extremely rare. Some affected infants have been delivered by cesarean section.

Etiology. Ascending infection from the mother's vagina or cervix is believed to be the route of invasion. The amniotic fluid is often turbid in appearance and is found positive for *C. albicans* when it is smeared and cultured. There is no correlation between severity of involvement

of the fetal adnexa and extent of involvement of the newborn infant's skin.

Clinical Findings. The eruption of congenital cutaneous candidiasis may be sparse or widespread and consists of papules and vesicopustules on an erythematous base. The face is relatively spared as are the oral mucous membranes, and there is no predilection for the diaper area. Palmar and plantar pustules are a hallmark of this infection (Fig. 112–4). Nail dystrophy occurs occasionally secondary to paronychial involvement. Desquamation is usually a late feature but may also be prominent early in the course of the disease (Fig. 112–5).

Rarely, disseminated infection has occurred in the lungs and gastrointestinal tract, presumably as the result of aspiration or swallowing of infected amniotic fluid. Infants at risk for visceral infection are those weighing less than 1500 g at birth and those with early-onset severe respiratory distress (Johnson et al., 1981). Function of the immune system was normal in those infants studied.

Diagnosis. The differential diagnosis includes several of the vesiculopustular eruptions of the newborn including staphylococcal pustulosis, erythema toxicum, and transient neonatal pustular melanosis. Generally, the organism is readily demonstrated on potassium hydroxide preparations and cultures of scrapings from involved skin.

Prognosis and Treatment. The eruption may resolve spontaneously or may become more widespread if left untreated. However, infants without visceral involvement respond rapidly to topical anticandidal agents. Visceral involvement portends a poor prognosis and requires intravenous therapy with an appropriate antifungal agent.

■ STREPTOCOCCAL INFECTIONS

Cutaneous streptococcal infections occur in the newborn but are less common than staphylococcal infections. *Group A streptococci* may cause disease of epidemic proportions (Dillon, 1966; Peter and Hazard, 1975) following the introduction of the organism into the nursery by maternal carriers or nursery personnel. The umbilicus

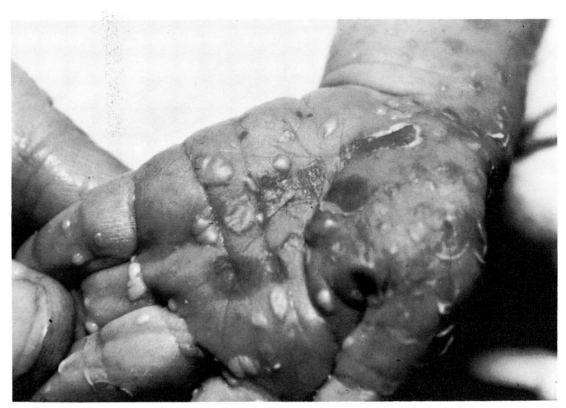

FIGURE 112–4. *Congenital cutaneous candidiasis—pustular stage—in a 6-day-old infant. A maculopapular rash was present at birth. (Courtesy of P. J. Kozinn, N. Rudolf, A. A. Tariq, M. R. Reale, and P. K. Goldberg.)*

is a frequent site of infection, which becomes manifest by seropurulent drainage from the umbilical stump and erythema and pustules on the contiguous abdominal skin. Conjunctivitis, paronychia, vaginitis, and an erysipelas-like eruption have also been described (Dillon, 1966; Geil et al., 1970; Isenberg et al., 1984). Because sepsis and meningitis may result, infected infants should be treated promptly and strict isolation should be instituted. As with staphylococcal infection, serious efforts should be made to identify the source of the organism. Several nursery outbreaks have been difficult to terminate because colonized infants may show little evidence of disease (Lehtonen et al., 1984). Isolation and treatment of infected infants; disinfection of the umbilical stump, the most likely reservoir of the organism; and penicillin prophylaxis for carriers and exposed infants have been the most effective measures. The infections respond readily to penicillin, which should be administered over a 10-day course.

Group B streptococci are now one of the most frequently encountered pathogens in the newborn nursery. Early-onset disease (during the 1st week of life), probably acquired in utero or during delivery, most commonly becomes manifest as septicemia with respiratory distress and shock. Late-onset disease (after the 1st week of life) is acquired postpartum and more often takes the form of meningitis. Patients with early-onset disease may harbor the organism on the skin; however, the presence of this agent on the skin is short lived as compared with other sites (Baker, 1977).

Skin infections caused by group B streptococcus are uncommon but have been documented (Belgaumkar, 1975; Hebert and Esterly, 1986; Howard and McCrackin,

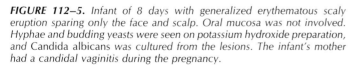

FIGURE 112–5. *Infant of 8 days with generalized erythematous scaly eruption sparing only the face and scalp. Oral mucosa was not involved. Hyphae and budding yeasts were seen on potassium hydroxide preparation, and Candida albicans was cultured from the lesions. The infant's mother had a candidal vaginitis during the pregnancy.*

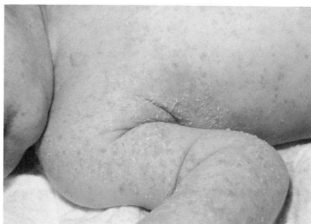

1974). Vesiculopustular lesions, cellulitis, and small abscesses have all been noted. A 10-day course of procaine penicillin is considered the treatment of choice.

■ REFERENCES

Albert, S., Baldwin, R., Czekajewski, S., et al.: Bullous impetigo due to group II *Staphylococcus aureus*. Am. J. Dis. Child. *120*:10, 1970.

Anthony, B. F., Giuliano, D. M., and Oh, W.: Nursery outbreak of staphylococcal scalded skin syndrome. Am. J. Dis. Child. *124*:41, 1972.

Baker, C. J.: Summary of workshop on infections due to group B streptococcus. J. Infect. Dis. *136*:137, 1977.

Belgaumkar, T. K.: Impetigo neonatorum congenita due to group B beta-hemolytic streptococcus infection. J. Pediatr. *86*:982, 1975.

Curran, J. P., and Al-Salihi, F. L.: Neonatal staphylococcal scalded skin syndrome: Massive outbreak due to an unusual phage type. Pediatrics *66*:285, 1980.

Dillon, H. C., Jr.: Group A Type 12 streptococcal infection in a newborn nursery. Am. J. Dis. Child. *112*:177, 1966.

Elias, P. M., Fritsch, P., and Epstein, E. H., Jr.: Staphylococcal scalded skin syndrome. Clinical features, pathogenesis, and recent microbiological and biochemical developments. Arch. Dermatol. *113*:207, 1977.

Elias, P. M., Mittermayer, H., Tappeiner, G., et al.: Staphylococcal toxic epidermal necrolysis (TEN): The expanded mouse model. J. Invest. Dermatol. *63*:467, 1974.

Gehlbach, S. H., Gutman, L. T., Wilfert, C. M., et al.: Recurrence of skin disease in a nursery: Ineffectuality of hexachlorophene bathing. Pediatrics *55*:422, 1975.

Geil, C. C., Castle, W. K., and Mortimer, E. A., Jr.: Group A streptococcal infections in newborn nurseries. Pediatrics *46*:489, 1970.

Guidelines for Perinatal Care. AAP Committee on the Fetus and Newborn. ACOG Committee on Obstetrics: Maternal and Fetal Medicine, 2nd ed. 1988.

Hebert, A. A., and Esterly, N. B.: Bacterial and candidal cutaneous infections in the neonate. Dermatol. Clin. *4*:3, 1986.

Howard, J. B., and McCrackin, G. H., Jr.: The spectrum of group B streptococcal infections in infancy. Am. J. Dis. Child. *128*:815, 1974.

Isenberg, H. D., Tucci, V., Lipsitz, P., et al.: Clinical laboratory and epidemiological investigations of a *Streptococcus pyogenes* cluster epidemic in a newborn nursery. J. Clin. Microbiol. *19*:366, 1984.

Johnson, D. E., Thompson, T. R., and Ferrieri, P.: Congenital candidiasis. Am. J. Dis. Child. *135*:273, 1981.

Kam, L. A., and Giacoia, G. P.: Congenital cutaneous candidiasis. Am. J. Dis. Child. *129*:1215, 1975.

Lehtonen, O. P., Ruuskanen, O., Karo, P., et al.: Group-A streptococcal infection in the newborn. Lancet *2*:1473, 1984.

Melish, M. E., and Glasgow, L. A.: Staphylococcal scalded skin syndrome—development of an experimental model. N. Engl. J. Med. *282*:1114, 1970.

Melish, M. E., and Glasgow, L. A.: Staphylococcal scalded skin syndrome: The expanded clinical syndrome. J. Pediatr. *78*:958, 1971.

Overturf, B. D., and Balfour, G.: Osteomyelitis and sepsis: Severe complications of fetal monitoring. Pediatrics *55*:244, 1975.

Peter, G., and Hazard, J.: Neonatal group A streptococcal disease. J. Pediatr. *87*:454, 1975.

Rubenstein, A. D., and Mesher, D. M.: Epidemic boric acid poisoning simulating staphylococcal toxic epidermal necrolysis of the newborn infant: Ritter's disease. J. Pediatr. *77*:884, 1970.

Rudolph, N., Tariq, A. A., Reale, M. R., et al.: Congenital cutaneous candidiasis. Arch. Dermatol. *113*:1101, 1977.

Rudolph, R. I., Schwartz, W., and Leyden, J. J.: Treatment of staphylococcal toxic epidermal necrolysis. Arch. Dermatol. *110*:559, 1974.

Russell, C., and Lay, K. M.: Natural history of *Candida* species and yeasts in the oral cavities of infants. Arch. Oral Biol. *18*:957, 1973.

Schirar, A., Rendu, C., Vielh, J. P., and Gautray, J. P.: Congenital mycosis *(Candida albicans)*. Biol. Neonate *24*:273, 1974.

Sheagren, J. N.: *Staphylococcus aureus*: The persistent pathogen (Parts I and II). N. Engl. J. Med. *310*:1368, 1437, 1984.

Wagner, M. M., Rycheck, R. R., Yee, R. B., et al.: Septic dermatitis of the neonatal scalp and maternal endomyometritis with intrapartum internal fetal monitoring. Pediatrics *74*:81, 1984.

COMMON BENIGN SKIN DISORDERS 113

Lawrence M. Solomon and Nancy B. Esterly

In this chapter, we discuss a number of mysterious cutaneous disorders that cause concern to the physician or parents. Most of these disorders are self-limited, some are serious, and the pathogenesis of only one of them (miliaria) is understood. They share one common characteristic: All may be diagnosed with certainty, and, for this reason, a clear concept of the clinical process and the requisites for establishing a diagnosis are essential for pediatricians.

■ SEBORRHEIC ECZEMA

Perhaps a word about terminology is appropriate because of the commonly expressed bewilderment about what the terms eczema, dermatitis, and seborrhea mean. Some authors consider the term eczema to be synonymous with dermatitis. For the purposes of discussion, we would like to consider the term dermatitis to represent a family of diseases, whereas eczema may be considered a genus and atopic eczema a species of cutaneous disorder. The qualifying adjective seborrheic describes a type of inflammatory skin disease that has a particular appearance and evolution (Solomon and Rostenberg, 1978), although it may simply reflect a form of childhood atopic eczema rather than a distinct disorder.

The primary lesion of seborrheic eczema is a greasy, yellow, flaky scale on an erythematous base. The scales coalesce to form plaques that may, in flexural areas such as the ear folds, erode and leave weeping fissures that may become infected. Other areas that may become involved are the neck folds, arm and leg folds, and the diaper area.

Etiology. The cause of seborrheic eczema is unknown, but it is one of the group of eczemas that appear to be endogenous in origin, as opposed to the exogenous eczemas caused by, for example, primary irritants, infections, or topical allergens. There has been considerable speculation as to the relationship of seborrheic eczema to atopic eczema, a disease that occurs in the older infant (Podmore et al., 1986). Certainly, the cutaneous lesions and distribution of both conditions are often similar. Furthermore, occasional cases of seborrheic eczema that are diagnosed with assurance when first seen in the 1-month-old infant may, on prolonged observation, evolve into typical atopic eczema. It is almost impossible, on strictly morphologic grounds, to say that any one child with seborrheic eczema will not develop atopic eczema. Some observers consider the greasy, scaling eruption of seborrhea as an early stage of atopic eczema.

Clinical Findings. Seborrheic eczema is a common disorder having two peaks of occurrence in early infancy. It appears during the 1st week or two of life as cradle cap, or milk crust, and then again from the end of the 1st month to the 3rd month, this time as a more widespread process involving the scalp, ears, forehead, and flexural areas, including the perineum (Fig. 113–1).

Most infants with seborrheic eczema seem perfectly well except for the dermatitis.* The eruption may last 3 to 6 weeks or longer and then heal and never reappear, or it may, as mentioned previously, evolve into atopic dermatitis. In the rare infant, seborrheic eczema may become a generalized process with full-blown exfoliative erythroderma (Leiner disease).

Treatment. For cradle cap, frequent shampooing is the secret for effective management of the condition. A zinc pyrithione or salicylic acid/sulfur–containing shampoo should control the problem and may be used daily or two or three times a week, depending on the severity of the scaling. When the scaling persists, 1 per cent salicylic acid or 3 per cent sulfur in an ointment vehicle may be applied to the scalp following the shampoo.

For seborrheic eczema in flexures or the diaper area, bathe the infant with tepid water containing a small amount of water-dispersible oil (advise the mother to expect a slippery infant). Any mild or superfatted soap will do. Dress the infant in cotton clothing, avoiding wool, nylon, or abrasive synthetic fabrics. Absorbent, disposable diapers are acceptable but should be changed frequently. The perineum may be protected with simple zinc oxide paste.† The soiled paste can be removed with mineral oil at each diaper change, then fresh paste can be applied. One per cent hydrocortisone cream may be used twice per day for brief periods, periodically (8 to 14 days), to accelerate resolution. It is frequently wise to culture the perineal area, where pustules or ulceration may herald supervening infection with Candida or pathogenic bacteria. Appropriate treatment should be instituted if pathogenic organisms are identified. The infant's room should be humidified in winter and air-conditioned in summer, because infants with widespread dermatitis may have difficulty tolerating extremes of heat, dryness, or humidity. Superabsorbent diapers are acceptable provided they are not used as an excuse to avoid changing the soiled diaper.

---

*The presence of purpura and systemic manifestations, such as listlessness, poor feeding, failure to thrive, recurrent fever, mouth lesions, or hepatosplenomegaly, should alert the physician to the possibility of a serious underlying illness, such as Wiskott-Aldrich syndrome or histiocytosis (Solomon and Esterly, 1973a; Fitzpatrick, 1981).

†Zinc oxide 30 per cent, talc 30 per cent, and petrolatum 40 per cent.

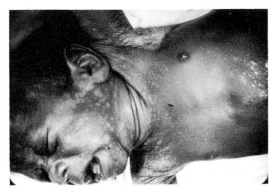

FIGURE 113–1. *Infant with seborrheic eczema on the face and neck and in the axillae. Note the scaling and hypopigmentation. Temporary hypopigmentation is common in black infants with this disorder.*

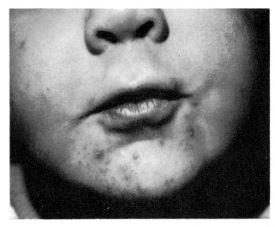

FIGURE 113–2. *Papules, pustules, and comedones (acne) on the chin and cheeks of an infant male.*

■ HARLEQUIN COLOR CHANGE

This condition should not be confused with an entirely different disorder called harlequin fetus. Harlequin color change, first described by Neligan and Strang in 1952, is characterized by reddening of one-half of the body and simultaneous blanching of the other half. A sharp line of demarcation runs from the center of the forehead, down the face and trunk, very nearly in the midline. Occasionally, the line of demarcation may be incomplete, sparing the face and genitalia. Harlequin color change occurs most frequently in low-birth-weight infants, but may be seen in about 10 per cent of term infants on the 3rd and 4th days of life and occasionally earlier or later. Apparently the color change is accentuated by gravitational force, because turning the body from one side to the other induces blanching of the upper half and reddening of the lower half. The total duration of these episodes may range from a few minutes to several hours. Harlequin color change occurs most often during the first 4 days of life (Mortensen and Stougard-Andresen, 1959), but some infants may still experience such episodes up to 3 weeks of age. There is no accompanying change in respiratory rate, pupillary reflexes, muscle tone, or response to external stimuli. Harlequin color change probably represents a state of vascular instability related to temporary inadequacy of the autonomic nervous system. It has no pathologic significance, requires no treatment, and can be expected to disappear no later than the 3rd week of life.

■ ACNE NEONATORUM

Clinical Findings. Acne neonatorum is usually a self-limited process but has most interesting physiologic, genetic, and pathologic implications. The lesions can be found at birth or may not be noticed until several weeks postnatally. They appear in crops on the cheeks, nose, chin, and, occasionally, the forehead. Open comedones (blackheads), closed comedones (granular, pale papules), and inflammatory papules and pustules are characteristic (Fig. 113–2). Cystic lesions very rarely occur. Affected infants are almost always boys. In infantile acne, which occurs after 3 months of age, there is only a small preponderance of males over females.

Etiology. The cause of acne neonatorum has not been elucidated, but certain elements that may contribute to

the process have been studied. In most instances, the infant does not suffer from an endocrine disturbance because the urinary excretion of 17-ketosteroids is normal (Tromovitch et al., 1963). There is, however, a strong genetic component to the process, as a familial tendency for acne is frequently present (Hellier, 1954). The fact that infants with acne tend to develop severe acne later in life (Hellier, 1954) suggests that the acnegenic process in the infant is related to a genetically determined end-organ (pilosebaceous unit) hyperresponsiveness to androgens that have crossed the placental barrier (Forest et al., 1973). Androgens produced by the male infant are probably also contributory factors. It is also interesting to note that infants with the feminizing testis syndrome, who are unable to respond to testosterone, never develop infantile (or adolescent) acne.

Treatment. In most instances, given the self-limited nature of the process, no special treatment of neonatal acne is required. In severe cases, a mild, sulfur-containing lotion or water-based benzoyl peroxide will suffice. Creams, ointments, and topical steroids should be avoided. Caution is necessary in using irritating scrubs or topical agents such as retinoic acid or concentrated benzoyl peroxides on infants with very fair skin, because the inflammatory reaction may be stimulated to a severe degree. Similarly, irritants used on black skin may cause unwanted hyperpigmentation or hypopigmentation at treatment sites.

■ MILIA AND SEBACEOUS GLAND HYPERPLASIA

Clinical Findings. Milia (single lesions are called milium) are found in about 40 per cent of full-term infants (Gordon, 1959). They are 1- to 2-mm keratin-filled pearly lesions that occur on the face of the newborn. The sites of predilection are the cheeks, forehead, ears, chin, and periorbital areas (Fig. 113–3). Large milia (larger than 2 mm) are found in infants with the oral-facial-digital syndrome (Solomon et al., 1970). Rarely, milia may occur in unusual sites, such as on the arms, legs, or the foreskin.

Histologically, a milium represents a defect in formation of the pilosebaceous apparatus. An invagination of epidermal tissue forms a keratin-producing pocket that even-

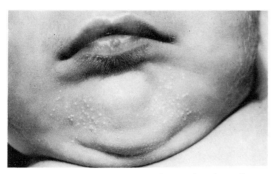

FIGURE 113–3. Numerous grouped milia on the chin of a newborn infant.

tually may lose its canalicular attachment to the surface and, thereby, become a cyst lined by several layers of keratin-producing cells. The expressed contents of milial cysts resemble tiny white pearls and consist mostly of keratin.

The most frequent confusion in the diagnosis of the condition stems from the resemblance of milia to the lesions of sebaceous gland hyperplasia, which occur in much the same areas. The papules of sebaceous gland hyperplasia are smaller (pinpoint), more yellow, and contain expressible sebaceous material. Milia usually exfoliate spontaneously within a few weeks. Even the large milia of the oral-facial-digital syndrome exfoliate in 3 to 4 months, but these lesions may leave pitted scars. Sebaceous hyperplasia also resolves spontaneously within the first few weeks of life.

■ EPSTEIN PEARLS

Clinical Findings. These tiny cystic lesions occur in about 85 per cent of newborn infants and are usually found on the palate, particularly along the mid-palatine raphe and at the junction of the hard and soft palate. The lesions are usually grouped, firm, and movable, and are an opaque white color. They are probably derived from entrapped epithelial remnants that become keratin-filled cysts. Epstein pearls are self-limited but may take several months to resolve (Solomon and Esterly, 1973a).

■ ERYTHEMA TOXICUM NEONATORUM

Clinical Findings. Erythema toxicum is an inflammatory cutaneous disease of unknown origin that affects about half of all full-term newborns (Berg and Solomon, 1987). It occurs more frequently among term-weight infants and less frequently among preterm infants (Carr et al., 1966; Taylor and Bondurant, 1957). In the majority of infants, the lesions develop between 24 and 48 hours of life but may occur as late as 2 weeks postpartum. No predilection of the disorder for race, sex, season, or geographic location has been noted.

The basic lesion in erythema toxicum is a small (1 to 3 mm) papule that becomes a sterile vesicopustule, usually white and firm and surrounded by a prominent halo of erythema and edema. An entire lesion may measure 1 to 3 cm across (Fig. 113–4). The number of lesions present may vary from a few to dozens. The areas most frequently involved are the chest and back, but the arms, legs, buttocks, and face may not be spared. Individual lesions

may persist only a few hours, but the eruption usually lasts 3 to 6 days and disappears spontaneously.

Etiology. On examination of histologic sections prepared from a lesion of erythema toxicum, one finds eosinophil-filled intraepidermal vesicles and an intradermal inflammatory component, which is also heavily infiltrated with eosinophils but contains other polymorphonuclear leukocytes and a few lymphocytes. These cells, usually accompanied by edema, tend to localize around the superficial portion of the pilosebaceous organ. The eosinophilic infiltrate has suggested to some authors that erythema toxicum is a disease of hypersensitivity, but studies attempting to incriminate chemical or microbiologic substances, acquired either transplacentally or vaginally from the mother, drugs, topical irritants, sebum, or milk, have failed to provide support for this hypothesis. At present, all that can be said with certainty is that erythema toxicum is a benign inflammatory disease of unknown cause.

Diagnosis. The differential diagnosis of erythema toxicum may occasionally raise some troublesome doubts. Entities that may be considered as possible alternatives to the diagnosis include transient neonatal pustular melanosis, miliaria rubra, pyoderma, and candidiasis. Miliaria rubra usually affects the flexures, face, arms, and legs, and it rarely disappears as rapidly as does erythema toxicum. The pustules of pustular melanosis lack an erythematous base and contain no eosinophils. Pyoderma and cutaneous candidiasis may be identified by gram stain and KOH preparation and culture of the pustular contents. Furthermore, polymorphonuclear leukocytes predominate in the pustule of pyoderma. A useful diagnostic procedure to follow when the diagnosis is in doubt consists of using a preparation of a Wright- or Giemsa-stained smear of intralesional contents. The presence of large numbers of eosinophils may be considered strong evidence to support a diagnosis of erythema toxicum if the infant is otherwise well.

Treatment and Prognosis. Erythema toxicum requires

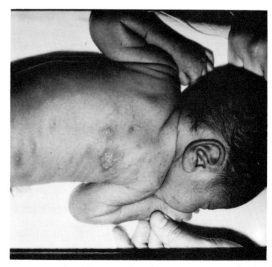

FIGURE 113–4. Florid lesions of erythema toxicum on the back of a newborn infant. The pustules are large and surrounded by an erythematous halo. Smears of the pustular contents showed only eosinophils.

no treatment, because it resolves spontaneously within a brief period. Not infrequently, however, parents may worry about the eruption, and reassurance should be provided. Recurrence is rare. There is no evidence of systemic manifestations accompanying the process, other than peripheral blood eosinophilia of varying degrees.

■ MILIARIA

Etiology. Miliaria is a cutaneous eruption caused by a functional disturbance in sweat secretion. In the days before air-conditioned nurseries were commonplace, miliaria was a frequent occurrence; however, with the advent of environmental humidity and temperature control, it has decreased sharply in frequency. Lately, with the use of phototherapy for hyperbilirubinuria, we are once more observing an increase in this minor cutaneous nuisance.

Clinical Findings. Miliaria takes two principal clinical forms, depending on the site of obstruction in the sweat duct. The less serious form, miliaria crystallina, consists of small, very superficial, clear, thin-walled, noninflammatory vesicles, resulting from retention of sweat localized in the epidermis just below the stratum corneum. Miliaria rubra consists of small, erythematous, grouped papules and results from rupture of the intraepidermal portion of the sweat duct. The lesion is found at the level of the basal layer of the epidermis and may be surrounded by many inflammatory cells. The papules may become pustular if there is a prominent inflammatory component. Miliaria is usually accentuated in the intertriginous areas, but the face, scalp, and shoulders also are commonly involved.

Diagnosis. During the first few days of life, the differential diagnosis of miliaria includes erythema toxicum, candidal infection, and pyoderma. Culture, gram stain, and KOH preparation of vesicular contents should resolve the question regarding the presence of yeast or bacteria. The vesicopustules of erythema toxicum are usually full of eosinophils.

Treatment. Treatment of miliaria should be conservative. The infant should be lightly clothed and placed in a cooler, less humid environment. No topical preparations are necessary because the eruption resolves spontaneously.

■ SCLEREMA NEONATORUM

Clinical Findings. Sclerema neonatorum is a rare but serious cutaneous change occurring in the 1st, or less commonly, the 2nd week of life in debilitated or preterm newborns. It results in widespread stone-hard, nonpitting induration of the skin. The infant is immobilized and feels cold to the touch. The face is fixed in a mask-like expression (Fig. 113–5); the joints are stiff. The skin change is a manifestation of a systemic process that may include sepsis, pneumonia, gastroenteritis, and, occasionally, multiple congenital anomalies. Body temperature and blood pressure are unstable, feeding is poor, and apneic spells are common. Complications such as central nervous system depression, cyanosis, respiratory distress, and convulsions frequently supervene. Changes in blood urea

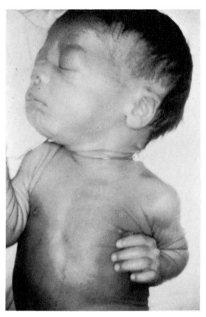

FIGURE 113–5. *Sclerema neonatorum. Note the masklike expression on the face, "pseudotrismus" of the partially immobilized mouth, and thickening of the skin over the face, arms, and hands. (From the Collection of the American Academy of Pediatrics. Reproduced with permission of the officers of the Academy.)*

nitrogen and potassium and a decrease in blood carbon dioxide (Levin and Milunsky, 1965) may reflect severe constitutional stress.

Etiology. The mechanism responsible for sclerema is unknown, but biochemical and crystalline changes in the subcutaneous fat of affected infants have suggested a shift in its composition toward an increase in triglycerides (Horsefield and Yardley, 1965) and in the ratio of saturated to unsaturated fats. Specifically, palmitin and stearin were found to be increased, with abnormal excess formation of large crystalline structures of these substances in the subcutaneous fat (Kellum et al., 1968).

The histologic changes in sclerema are not highly specific; surprisingly little inflammation is evident. On examination of sections from biopsies, one usually sees edema and thickening of the interlobular septa of the panniculus.

Treatment. The treatment of sclerema neonatorum is essentially that of management of a very sick infant. Maintenance of normal body temperature, control of infection, adequate nutrition, and balance of fluid and electrolytes are required. Corticosteroid therapy has been advocated for this disorder, but controlled studies have not shown steroids to be effective in altering the mortality rate (Levin et al., 1961), which approaches 50 per cent.

■ SUBCUTANEOUS FAT NECROSIS

The lesions of subcutaneous fat necrosis are similar to those of sclerema neonatorum, and the pathogenesis leading to the two diseases may be identical. However, the subcutaneous fat necrosis is highly localized, whereas sclerema neonatorum is diffuse; sclerema is a very serious illness, whereas subcutaneous fat necrosis is usually a benign self-limited process (Fretzin and Arias, 1987).

Clinical Findings. Subcutaneous fat necrosis commonly develops within the first 2 weeks of life, most frequently between the 5th and 10th days, but may be found as early as the 2nd or as late as the 24th day. The lesions are sharply circumscribed, often tender nodules or plaques, which are hard and have a dusky reddish-purple hue. They are found in areas in which a fat pad is present: buttocks, back, arms, and thighs (Fig. 113–6). The affected area may have an uneven surface and a sharp margin delineating it from surrounding normal skin. The lesions may become the site of dystrophic calcification, and rarely, hypercalcemia may accompany the process. When cutaneous calcification is present, radiographic examination of the skin may provide supportive evidence for the diagnosis. Extensive calcification may lead to extrusion and drainage of a liquefied material from the discharging lesion. The drainage site (usually sterile) often heals with scarring.

Although most infants appear to suffer few systemic complications of subcutaneous fat necrosis, a few vomit, fail to thrive, become irritable, develop fever, and refuse to feed. Rarely, visceral calcification may supervene (Sharlin and Koblenzer, 1970).

Etiology. Numerous causes have been ascribed to subcutaneous fat necrosis. Most prominent among these are obstetric trauma, intrauterine asphyxia (Chen et al., 1981), and hypothermia. Obstetric trauma is commonly observed without the consequences of fat necrosis, and the maintenance of normal body temperature is a common problem in healthy preterm infants, so one must take a reserved attitude toward these suppositions. It is probable that if these factors contribute to fat necrosis, they do so only in infants susceptible to the disease.

Treatment. The management of subcutaneous fat ne-

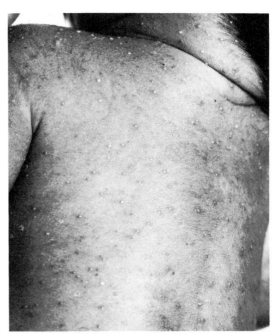

FIGURE 113–7. Numerous superficial pustules on the neck and back of a 1-day-old infant. A few pustules have ruptured, leaving a collarette of scale.

crosis depends on the severity of the process, the presence of draining ulcerations, and systemic complications. In all cases, warm or hot packs applied to the lesions should be avoided. In most infants, the process is self-limited and resolution occurs over a period of weeks to months without much residual atrophy or scarring. Where fluctuant areas are present, careful needle aspiration may reduce scarring. In infants with hypercalcemia (Norwood-Galloway et al., 1987) or visceral calcification, restriction of oral calcium intake, a decrease in vitamin D intake, and the administration of corticosteroids systemically may aid in resolving the process.

■ TRANSIENT NEONATAL PUSTULAR MELANOSIS

Clinical Findings. This benign disorder occurs relatively frequently in the newborn and is present at birth (Ramamurthy et al., 1976). It appears to be more common in black infants. Characteristic lesions consist of small, superficial pustules that rupture easily, leaving a collarette of fine scale and hyperpigmented macules that are often discernible at the sites of unroofed pustules (Fig. 113–7). The macules visible at birth may represent end-stage lesions of pustules that have ruptured in utero (Fig. 113–8). The lesions may be profuse or sparse and can involve all body surfaces, including the palms, soles, and scalp. Areas of predilection are the forehead, anterior neck and submental area, lower back, and shins.

Etiology. The cause of the eruption is unknown. Affected infants are otherwise well. Gram stains and bacterial cultures obtained from intact pustules uniformly fail to disclose the presence of organisms. Wright-stained smears of pustular fluid contain cellular debris, polymorphonuclear leukocytes, and few or no eosinophils. The differential diagnosis includes erythema toxicum, candidiasis,

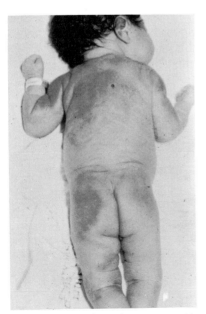

FIGURE 113–6. Rear view of newborn showing several large discolored areas of subcutaneous fat necrosis. They were irregular in size and shape, felt firm, and were not hot or tender.

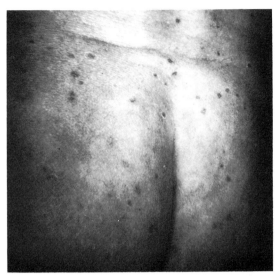

FIGURE 113–8. *Transient neonatal pustular melanosis. Hyperpigmented macules on the lower back and buttocks, some of which are encircled by scale. (From Ramamurthy, R. S., Reveri, M., Esterly, N. B., et al.: Transient neonatal pustular melanosis. J. Pediatr. 88:831, 1976.)*

and staphylococcal pyoderma, which can usually be distinguished with the aforementioned studies. The pustules last about 48 hours; the macules may persist for up to 3 months. The disorder is transient and self-limited and requires no therapy.

■ REFERENCES

Berg, F. J., Solomon, L. M.: Erythema neonatorum toxicum. Arch. Dis. Child. *62*:327, 1987.

Carr, J. A., Hodgeman, J. E., Freedman, R. J., and Levan, N. E.: Relationship between toxic erythema and infant maturity. Am. J. Dis. Child. *112*:129, 1966.

Chen, T. H., Shewmake, S. W., Hansen, D. D., and Lacey, H. L.: Subcutaneous fat necrosis of the newborn. Arch. Dermatol. *117*:36, 1981.

Fitzpatrick, R., Rapaport, M. S., and Silva, D. G.: Histiocytosis X. Arch. Dermatol. *117*:253, 1981.

Forest, M. G., Cathiard, A. M., and Bertrand, G. H.: Evidence of testicular activity in early infancy. G. Clin. Endocrinol. Metab. *37*:148, 1973.

Fretzin, D. F., and Arias, A. M.: Sclerema neonatorum and subcutaneous fat necrosis of the newborn. Pediatr. Dermatol. *4*:112, 1987.

Gordon, J.: Miliary sebaceous cysts and blisters in the healthy newborn. Acta Obstet. Gynaecol. Scand. *38*:352, 1959.

Hellier, F. F.: Acneiform eruptions in infancy. Br. J. Dermatol. *66*:25, 1954.

Horsefield, G. J., and Yardley, H. J.: Sclerema neonatorum. J. Invest. Dermatol. *44*:326, 1965.

Kellum, R. E., Ray, T. L., and Brown, G. R.: Sclerema neonatorum. Report of case analysis of subcutaneous and epidermal-dermal lipids by chromatographic methods. Arch. Dermatol. *97*:372, 1968.

Levin, S. E., Bakst, C. M., and Isserow, L.: Sclerema neonatorum treated with corticosteroids. Br. Med. J. *2*:1533, 1961.

Levin, S. E., and Milunsky, A.: Urea and electrolyte levels in the serum in sclerema neonatorum. J. Pediatr. *67*:812, 1965.

Mortensen, O., and Stougard-Andresen, P.: Harlequin color change in the newborn. Acta Obstet. Gynaecol. Scand. *38*:352, 1959.

Neligan, G. W., and Strang, L. B.: A "harlequin" colour change in the newborn. Lancet *2*:1005, 1952.

Norwood-Galloway, A., Lebwohl, M., Phelps, R. G., et al.: Subcutaneous fat necrosis of the newborn and hypercalcemia. J. Am. Acad. Dermatol. *16*:435, 1987.

Podmore, P., Burrows, D., Eedy, D. J., and Stanford, C. F.: Seborrhoeic eczema—a disease entity or a clinical variant of atopic eczema? Br. J. Dermatol. *115*:341, 1986.

Ramamurthy, R. S., Reveri, M., Esterly, N. B., et al.: Transient neonatal pustular melanosis. J. Pediatr. *88*:831, 1976.

Sharlin, D. N., and Koblenzer, P.: Necrosis of subcutaneous fat with hypercalcemia. A puzzling and multifaceted disease. Clin. Pediatr. *9*:290, 1970.

Solomon, L. M., and Esterly, N. B.: Eczema in Neonatal Dermatology. Philadelphia, W. B. Saunders Co., 1973a, p. 125.

Solomon, L. M., and Esterly, N. B.: Transient Cutaneous Lesions in Neonatal Dermatology. Philadelphia, W. B. Saunders Co., 1973b, p. 43.

Solomon, L. M., Fretzin, D., and Pruzansky, S.: Pilosebaceous dysplasia in the oral-facial-digital syndrome. Arch. Dermatol. *102*:596, 1970.

Solomon, L. M., and Rostenberg, A., Jr.: Atopic dermatitis and infantile eczema. In Samter, M., Talmadge, D. W., Rose, B., et al. (Eds.): Immunological Diseases. 3rd ed. Boston, Little, Brown, and Co., 1978, p. 953.

Taylor, W. B., and Bondurant, C. P.: Erythema neonatorum allergicum. Arch. Dermatol. *76*:591, 1957.

Tromovitch, T. A., Abrams, A. A., and Jacobs, P. H.: Acne in infancy. Am. J. Dis. Child. *106*:230, 1963.

NEVI AND CUTANEOUS TUMORS

114

Lawrence M. Solomon and Nancy B. Esterly

There is no universally accepted or even satisfying definition of the word nevus. By common usage, it has come to mean a cutaneous malformation represented by a localized collection of cells in a variably advanced state of differentiation. The distinction between hamartoma and nevus is not clear. In a nevus, the aggregation of cells in the skin may originate from any tissue normally found in the skin and may attempt to become functional (i.e., produce pigment or keratin) or may form imperfect versions of their destined structures (i.e., abortive hair follicles, blood vessels, sebaceous glands).

In 1969, Pinkus and Mehregan suggested that nevi are derived from pluripotential epithelial germ buds in the basal layer of the epidermis that undergo aberrant development. It is possible that a disturbance in tissue growth factors may play a significant role in their genesis.

The clinical forms of cutaneous nevi are extremely numerous, and a discussion of each would be beyond the scope of this chapter. For this reason, we have summarized the spectrum of nevi to be found in Table 114–1. We will discuss the most common and important nevi in this chapter.

■ HEMANGIOMAS AND OTHER VASCULAR MALFORMATIONS

In two recent treatises on the subject (Esterly, 1987; Mulliken and Young, 1988) a more definitive classification of vascular lesions has been proposed: Hemangiomas include raised lesions of the capillary (strawberry) type, capillary-cavernous, and pure cavernous lesions (Fig. 114–1A; Table 114–2). The term malformation is reserved for lesions present at birth, such as nevus flammeus, port-wine stain, deep venous malformations, and others to be discussed later. Their origin may be capillary, venous, lymphatic, or arteriovenous.

Etiology. The cause of a neovascular formation or a vascular malformation is not known. However, it is reasonable to speculate that angiogenic factors play a role both in promotion of neovascularization and vascular organization in the dermal structures (Folkman, 1986).

Clinical Findings. Localized vascular malformations and hemangiomas occur extremely frequently in the pediatric population. The incidence of all vascular nevi is probably about 6 to 25 per cent. We believe that for the numbers to be more accurately considered they should be separated into capillary hemangiomas, raised above the surface (about 5 to 10 per cent), and nevus flammeus, flat lesions (about 30 per cent) (Harris et al., 1975). Hemangiomas may be superficial (about 65 per cent), subcutaneous (15 per cent), or mixed (20 per cent) (Alper and Holmes, 1983). The clinical appearance of the lesion may not correspond exactly to a histopathologic classification (Wade et al., 1978). Capillary hemangiomas consist of dilated vessels, which are often associated with endo-

TABLE 114–1. Spectrum of Nevi

Epidermal
Keratinocytic (Epidermal) Nevi
Nevus unius lateris
Systematized verrucous nevi
Small verrucous nevi
Ichthyosis hystrix
Unilateral congenital ichthyosiform erythroderma
Epidermal nevus syndrome
Benign congenital acanthosis nigricans
Porokeratosis of Mibelli
Inflammatory linear verrucous epidermal nevus (Ilven)

Appendageal (Organoid) Nevi

Sebaceous nevi ⎤
Hair follicle nevi ⎬ comedo nevi
Apocrine duct nevi ⎦
  (nevus syringocystadenoma papilliferus)

Melanocytic Nevi

Dermal
Melanocytic Nevi
Vascular Nevi
Connective Tissue Nevi
Collagen
Elastic tissue
Digital fibroma
Juvenile fibromatosis
Osteoma cutis
                    Nervous Tissue Nevi
Nasal glioma
Meningioma

Subcutaneous Tissue
Lipoma
Nevus lipomatosis cutaneus superficialis
Michelin tire baby
Encephalocraniocutaneous lipomatosis

Mixed
Benign teratomas (dermoids)

(From Solomon, L. M., and Esterly, N. B.: Neonatal Dermatology. Philadelphia, W. B. Saunders Co., 1973.)

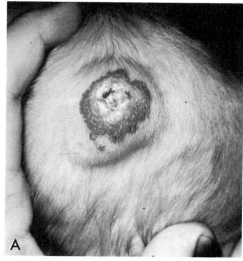

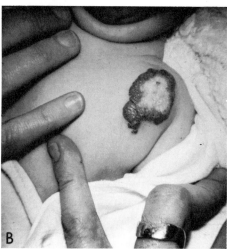

FIGURE 114–1. A, *Mixed capillary and cavernous hemangioma with small central ulceration on the scalp of an infant. B, Involuting strawberry hemangioma with central gray fibrotic area.*

TABLE 114–2. Characteristics of Vascular Birthmarks

	HEMANGIOMA	MALFORMATION
Clinical		
	Usually nothing seen at birth, 30 per cent present as red macule	All present at birth; may not be evident
	Rapid postnatal proliferation and slow involution	Commensurate growth; may expand as a result of trauma, sepsis, hormonal modulation
	Female:male 3:1	Female:male 1:1
Cellular		
	Plump endothelium, increased turnover	Flat endothelium, slow turnover
	Increased mast cells	Normal mast cell count
	Multilaminated basement membrane	Normal thin basement membrane
	Capillary tubule formation in vitro	Poor endothelial growth in vitro
Hematologic		
	Primary platelet trapping: thrombocytopenia (Kasabach-Merritt syndrome)	Primary stasis (venous); localized consumptive coagulopathy
Radiologic		
	Angiographic findings: well-circumscribed, intense lobular-parenchymal staining with equatorial vessels	Angiographic findings: diffuse, no parenchyma
		Low-flow: phleboliths, ectatic channels
		High-flow: enlarged, tortuous arteries with arteriovenous shunting
Skeletal		
	Infrequent "mass effect" on adjacent bone; hypertrophy rare	Low-flow: distortion, hypertrophy, or hypoplasia
		High-flow: destruction, distortion, or hypertrophy

(From Mulliken, J. B., and Young, A. E.: Vascular Birthmarks, Hemangiomas and Malformations. Philadelphia, W. B. Saunders, 1988, p 35.)

thelial proliferation. They develop fibrotic changes as they resolve. Cavernous hemangiomas have, in the lower dermis, large irregular spaces filled with blood, lined by a single layer of endothelial cells and by a fibrous wall of varying thickness. Both pathologic changes may be found in different portions of many hemangiomas. It is important to note that a biopsy and pathologic study of a localized area or section of the lesion may not always distinguish the differences between congenital and acquired vascular nevi, or between nevi and other reactive vascular phenomena. A useful clinical consideration is whether the lesions are strictly cutaneous or are associated with other abnormalities. Finally, the rate of endothelial mitosis may be the most important distinguishing feature among hemangiomas (Mulliken and Glowacki, 1982).

TELANGIECTATIC NEVI (MALFORMATIONS)

These lesions are among the most frequent abnormalities of the skin of the newborn infant. They are designated nevus flammeus as a group but may be subdivided into salmon patch, nuchal nevus, and port-wine stain (Tan, 1972). The typical lesion is flat and bright to dark red and has a sharp border. Those found at the base of the skull tend to remain throughout life. A paler variety of nevus flammeus may be found over the eyelids, between the eyes, and on the mid-forehead (salmon patch). Hemangiomas in these sites tend to be less apparent as the skin becomes less translucent, and they usually fade completely. However, in moments of anger or during intense exercise or flushing, the lesion may become visible. Telangiectatic nevi on other sites, such as the cheeks, usually do not fade but instead acquire a purplish hue, which gave rise to the term port-wine stain. Port-wine stains occur much less frequently than nuchal nevi. They may be associated with ocular complications when they are located in the area of the ophthalmic portion of the trigeminal nerve. In 1980, Barsky and co-workers found glaucoma to occur in 10 per cent of such patients. Nevus flammeus may, in fact, be found almost anywhere on the body or on any mucosal surface.

Macular telangiectatic nevi occur in the following conditions with varying frequency: trisomy 13, Rubinstein-Taybi syndrome, Beckwith-Wiedemann syndrome, and the epidermal nevus syndrome.

Treatment for uncomplicated telangiectatic nevi is primarily cosmetic. The nevi grow only proportionately with the individual and are not invasive. Many are estrogen sensitive; therefore, the adolescent should be aware that contraceptives may have an adverse effect on telangiectasias. Make-up may hide the lesions. The pulsed dye laser treatment of these lesions on visible areas in infants and children shows promise of improving their appearance.

STURGE-WEBER SYNDROME

A nevus flammeus affecting that area of skin innervated by the ophthalmic portion of the trigeminal nerve may be a sign of Sturge-Weber syndrome (Paller, 1987). This syndrome represents a congenital malformation (not hereditary) of the vessels of the skin, meninges, and frequently, the orbit. The malformation is most often unilateral, but bilateral involvement is not rare (about 1 in 10 cases).

Clinical Features. The clinical features are port-wine nevus, leptomeningeal angioma, cortical calcifications, seizures, hemiparesis, and mental retardation. Ocular complications include glaucoma, buphthalmos, choroidal angiomas, and optic atrophy. The nevus flammeus may also involve the mouth, tongue, and buccal mucosa. Nevus flammeus is also frequently present elsewhere on the body (Paller, 1987).

Careful neurologic and ophthalmologic examination should be performed during infancy as a basis for future evaluations (Gordon et al., 1981). Computed tomography (CT) or magnetic resonance imaging (MRI) studies of the skull may detect epicortical vascular anomalies at a very early age, i.e., before 2 years. Periodic assessment of the intelligence and behavior and radiographic examination of the skull not only may confirm the diagnosis but, more importantly, may also indicate the degree of severity of the process. In some patients, only minimal central nervous system involvement will occur, whereas in others the disorder may cause profound retardation and the frequent occurrence of seizures. Longitudinal observation of the patient is required before an appropriate prognosis can be made.

Prognosis. The radiographic finding of double-contoured (tram-line) calcifications in the cerebral cortex is not seen during infancy but develops during childhood. Unilateral depression of cortical activity and episodes of spike discharges are the most characteristic electroencephalographic changes seen in this disorder.

Treatment. Treatment measures for Sturge-Weber syndrome include anticonvulsant drugs, management of glaucoma, and a masking screen (Covermark) for the skin lesions. Argon, copper flash laser (in the postadolescent period) or pulsed dye laser treatment of the cutaneous lesions may be feasible if the lesion is not too large. In severely affected infants, neurosurgical procedures aimed at removal of abnormal meningeal and cortical tissue have been palliative. Plastic repair of gingival overgrowth due to either hemangioma or anticonvulsant therapy also may be indicated.

CAPILLARY (STRAWBERRY) AND CAVERNOUS HEMANGIOMAS

These hemangiomas may be single or multiple and most often begin after birth. The lesions are raised and may be felt as a mass in the skin or deeper tissues. The borders can be either well or poorly defined. Superficial lesions are bright red, lobulated, and somewhat compressible. Deeper lesions may have a bluish hue or may be flesh toned if the overlying skin is not significantly involved. About one-fourth of the lesions are present at birth as an area of blanched skin with a few superficial dilated vessels. Approximately 1 per cent of newborn infants are affected (Hidano and Nakajima, 1972), with a somewhat higher incidence in preterm infants (Amir et al., 1986; Harris et al., 1975).

Clinical Findings. Most of these lesions increase in size during the first 3 to 6 months of life. A subsequent stationary interval is followed by involution, which may take a variable period of time. The vast majority of hemangiomas resolve by 7 to 9 years of age without treatment (Margileth, 1971). Involution of an individual strawberry hemangioma is heralded by the appearance of gray fibrotic plaques on the surface, a change in color to a darker hue, and softening of the mass (Fig. 114–1B). As healing progresses, the skin may return to its normal color or may be streaked by a few telangiectatic vessels. The texture of the healing skin is flabby at first but improves with time. Those patients we have followed whose hemangiomas have been allowed to involute spontaneously have achieved a more successful cosmetic result than those subjected to surgical or radiologic intervention.

Diagnosis. Most cases of hemangioma are diagnosed clinically. However, the extent of involvement may not be readily discerned without technical aid. CT scan, Doppler ultrasound (Oates et al., 1985), Tc-99m, tagged red cell visualization (Gordon et al., 1981), and angiography (Burrows et al., 1983) are some techniques that are proving helpful in this regard.

Complications. The following complications may occur in cavernous and capillary hemangiomas:

1. Local problems include necrosis, ulceration, hemorrhage, and infection.
2. Impingement on particular vital structures may result in obstruction of vision, interference with respiration, hearing impairment, and interference with nutrition.
3. Systemic problems may result in hemangiomas residing in internal organs, congestive heart failure, thrombocytopenia, and disseminated intravascular coagulation.
4. Complications following treatment with radiation, surgery, or injection of sclerosing agents include scarring, ulceration, damage to internal organs, and local impairment of growth.
5. Psychological and social problems may result from facial or other visible deformities.

Treatment. For uncomplicated hemangiomas (cavernous and capillary hemangiomas), the treatment of choice is patient observation. The lesion should be measured regularly and its growth recorded and followed. In our experience, parents inevitably show signs of anxiety and a need for constant reassurance. Demonstration of before-and-after photographs of involuted lesions in other children often alleviates parental concern. Local compression of accessible lesions has been advocated (Mangus, 1973) and is helpful.

1. Treatment of local complications: Massive hemorrhage is rare, but when it occurs it becomes a management

problem. Minor episodes of bleeding respond to compression. Necrotic, ulcerated, and infected areas should be cultured and treated with appropriate antibiotics, either topically or systemically. The ulcers will heal, but scarring may result.

2. When large hemangiomas interfere with vital functions or sight, surgical intervention or the use of systemically administered corticosteroids (prednisone, 2 to 4 mg/kg in a single daily morning dose or in an alternate-day regimen) for 6 to 12 weeks may halt expansion and initiate involution of the lesion (Fig. 114–2) (Brown et al., 1972; Fost and Esterly, 1968).

3. Hemangiomatous involvement of the subglottic area or internal organs, such as the liver, gastrointestinal tract,

and bladder, resulting in high-output congestive heart failure and Kasabach-Merritt syndrome (see later) are life-threatening conditions that require active intervention (Berman and Lim, 1978; Esterly, 1987). Prednisone in large doses has been helpful in some infants, but unfortunately not all patients respond. Interferon-α is being studied as a form of treatment in these seriously affected infants.

4. A major complication of therapy is scarring. Regrowth of a hemangioma after surgery is not uncommon. All one can do in such instances is to wait for involution and follow with plastic repair and cosmetic screens such as Covermark or Dermablend.

5. A small number of hemangiomas simply do not

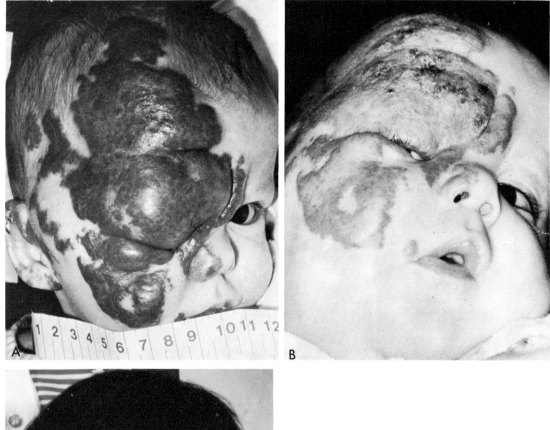

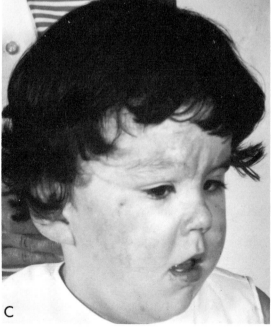

FIGURE 114–2. A, A flat hemangioma was noted at birth and by 3 weeks of age had expanded, as shown in the figure. After 11 weeks of prednisone (20 mg per day), the lesion had regressed, as shown in B. C, Nearly complete regression is evident by age 4 years. She is a normally intelligent child whose only residual problem is strabismus.

resolve in spite of all the physician may do. For this reason, a prognosis of resolution may be premature. The subsequent psychological and social problems of these individuals require constant support from the physician and social agencies. We have found that if patients or parents are willing to express their feelings openly, they seem to cope with the issue somewhat better. On rare occasions, psychiatric help should be sought.

KLIPPEL-TRENAUNAY-WEBER SYNDROME

Clinical Findings. Klippel-Trenaunay-Weber syndrome consists of a nonhereditary vascular nevus involving an entire limb or large area associated with hypertrophy of skin, subcutaneous tissue, muscle, and bones. The cutaneous lesion, which is usually visible at birth, affects boys more often than girls (Mullins et al., 1962). Associated deformities include venous varicosities, capillary or cavernous hemangiomas, and rarely, arteriovenous fistulas (the "Weber" component of the syndrome).

Treatment. Treatment is not very effective, and surgical repair (Glovitzki et al., 1983) and occasionally amputation may have to be considered, owing to severe deformity and functional loss of a limb.

DIFFUSE NEONATAL HEMANGIOMATOSIS (DISSEMINATED HEMANGIOMATOSIS, VISCERAL HEMANGIOMATOSIS, MILIARY HEMANGIOMATOSIS)

Clinical Findings. Disseminated hemangiomatosis may be present without visceral involvement, in which case it is preceded by the descriptive adjective benign. Unfortunately, one can never be certain of the strictly cutaneous nature of the lesions, and careful clinical evaluation of the entire patient must be made.

Numerous cutaneous lesions may be present at birth or may develop within the first few weeks of life. The most commonly involved organ systems are the central nervous system, liver, gastrointestinal tract, and lungs, although any organ may be involved. Affected infants may develop high-output congestive failure, pulmonary obstruction, neurologic deficit, or gastrointestinal hemorrhage leading to early death (Holden and Alexander, 1970). In 1978, Berman and Lim reviewed the literature and found that untreated patients had a mortality rate of 81 per cent, whereas treated patients had a mortality rate of 29 per cent. The difference may be due to benign versus visceral types, but in our experience, treatment with systemic steroids is definitely effective in halting the appearance of new lesions and healing old lesions.

The cutaneous lesions are small, button-shaped or dome-shaped, red or dark blue protrusions. The presence of a profusion of hemangiomas in the skin should alert the physician to search for internal involvement. Work-up should include a careful total physical examination and CT examination of the skull. Some physicians rely only on the physical examination, awaiting clinical findings before ordering CT scans and other studies.

Treatment. For visceral involvement, 2 to 4 mg prednisone/kg/day is the treatment of choice. The prognosis is

improving with carefully individualized therapy (Esterly et al., 1984; Golitz et al., 1986). Recombinant interferon-α_{2a} may be effective (White et al., 1989).

KASABACH-MERRITT SYNDROME

Clinical Findings. During the first few months of life, a rapidly expanding cavernous hemangioma may be complicated by the development of thrombocytopenia. A few infants have developed this complication with lesions as small as 5 and 6 cm in diameter. Thrombocytopenia can be followed by bleeding and anemia. Bleeding is believed to be caused by a trapping of platelets in the hemangioma and a depletion of circulating clotting factors (Rodriguez-Erdmann et al., 1971). Hypofibrinogenemia and decreased factors II, V, VII, and VIII may be found. Fibrin split products are elevated, an indication of the consumption coagulopathy. Red blood cell and platelet survivals are also shortened.

Treatment. The prognosis of Kasabach-Merritt syndrome is serious, and the results of various forms of treatment are difficult to evaluate. Administration of systemic corticosteroids, compression of the lesion, and surgical extirpation have been followed by improvement in the hematologic status (Esterly, 1983). A severe consumption coagulopathy may require heparin for control. Aspirin and other antiplatelet drugs have also been advocated. Radiation to the hemangioma has been effective in some cases, but the hazards of such therapy must be carefully weighed. A surgical approach has also been advocated and may be appropriate in individual cases.

CUTIS MARMORATA TELANGIECTATICA CONGENITA (CONGENITAL GENERALIZED PHLEBECTASIA)

Clinical Findings. Cutis marmorata telangiectatica congenita may describe several clinically similar diseases. The process is certainly a malformation that has two major characteristics: It can lead to thrombosis-infarction of the skin, and it seems to improve with age in most, if not all patients (Cohen and Zalar, 1988; Powell and Su, 1984). In its most common form, a lower limb and part of the trunk demonstrate vascular reticulation in a bluish-red network (Fig. 114–3) (Way et al., 1974). Thrombosed nodular lesions lead to superficial ulcerations that then undergo healing and leave a scarred defect with a netlike distribution. Overall, the prognosis is fairly good. Most children recover from the disorder with minimal cutaneous dysfunction; a few suffer some associated anomalies, but these represent more diffuse involvement and are rarely seen in the localized form.

Improvement in appearance is usual but is not always pleasing to the observer. If hypertrophy of a limb results, this condition is difficult to distinguish from Klippel-Trenaunay-Weber syndrome.

CIRSOID ANEURYSM (ARTERIOVENOUS FISTULAR MALFORMATION)

Clinical Findings. This rare lesion may be found anywhere on the body but is usually located on the scalp.

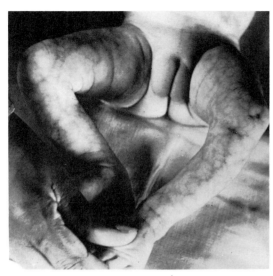

FIGURE 114–3. *Cutis marmorata telangiectatica congenita. Note the striking network of dilated vessels most distinct over the extremities. (Humphries, J. M.: J. Pediatr. 40:486, 1952.)*

The lesion may be several centimeters in size, is elevated and warm, and often pulsates. A murmur may be auscultated in the area of involvement. Angiography may identify one or more central feeding vessels. These vessels should be tied or the lesion should be surgically extirpated at some time during early childhood. A fistulous aneurysm may complicate a cavernous hemangioma (Mulliken and Young, 1988).

BLUE RUBBER BLEB NEVUS SYNDROME

Clinical Findings. This interesting and extremely rare syndrome (Fretzin and Potter, 1965; Munkvad, 1983) consists of multiple hemangiomas of skin, mucous membrane, bowel, and less frequently, spleen, liver, and central nervous system. Numerous lesions may be present at birth. They range in size from 1 mm to several centimeters and have three peculiar characteristics: They look like blue nodules and resemble the blueberry muffin lesions seen in other disorders, such as cytomegalovirus infection. They are tender on palpation, and they are surmounted by droplets of sweat.

Treatment. Since spontaneous gastrointestinal or central nervous system bleeding are two major complications of this disorder, a complete evaluation of the affected child is mandatory. Treatment is restricted to resection of involved areas of bowel. Blue rubber bleb hemangiomas do not resolve spontaneously.

RARE VASCULAR NEVI

Other rare vascular tumors that may occur in the newborn include linear verrucous hemangioma, benign juvenile hemangioendothelioma, hemangiopericytoma, multiple glomus tumors, Gorham syndrome, and Bannayan syndrome (Esterly, 1987).

LOCALIZED MALFORMATION OF THE LYMPHATIC VESSELS

Localized nevoid tumors of lymphatic vessel origin (lymphangiomas) are less common than hemangiomas in infants. A mixed tumor consisting of lymphatic and blood vessels may also occur; however, at times it is difficult to distinguish the tissue of origin of a vascular tumor, especially if bleeding into a lymphatic bleb has occurred. Four morphologic forms of lymphangioma have been distinguished. The histologic features of all are basically similar: They consist of dilated lymph channels forming cystic structures of varying size that are lined by a simple endothelium, characteristic of a lymphatic vessel.

LYMPHANGIOMA CIRCUMSCRIPTUM

Lymphangioma circumscriptum is the most common variant of lymphangioma encountered in the infant (Peachy et al., 1970). It is usually located on the upper portion of the limbs, in the axillary or inguinal folds, and on the oral mucosa. The lesion consists of a grapelike cluster of very thin-walled translucent vesicles filled with a clear or somewhat bloody fluid. The surrounding skin may have a red to wine color and may be somewhat verrucous. Although most of the lesions appear to be very superficial, most often there is an associated anomaly of the deeper vessels (Mulliken and Young, 1988) consisting of deep thick-walled cisterns that may pulsate and transmit pressure changes to the connecting channels (Browze et al., 1986). Biopsy or incision of a group of vesicles may result in chronic drainage that may be repaired only by excision of the entire lesion and application of full-thickness grafts. This form of lymphangioma may recur even after extensive surgery. The most serious frequent complication is recurring infectious cellulitis.

SIMPLE LYMPHANGIOMA

The simple lymphangioma is extremely rare and occurs as a skin-colored nodule on the head, thorax, or oral mucosa. Chronic drainage and recurrence following surgical excision may complicate management.

DIFFUSE LYMPHANGIOMA

The diffuse lymphangioma is a large, ill-defined, soft tissue mass involving skin, subcutaneous tissue, and muscle on the trunk, extremities, face, lips, or tongue. Marked enlargement of the affected area may result from invasion by the cystic lymphatics complicated by stasis and infection. Surgical intervention is often extremely difficult to perform in these cases but may be the only alternative if oral lesions interfere with feeding.

CYSTIC HYGROMA (CAVERNOUS LYMPHANGIOMA)

More localized but in many ways similar to diffuse lymphangioma, the hygroma is a large, multiloculated, translucent lesion that may involve any part of the body but most frequently affects the face, trunk, and shoulder-girdle area. It expands rapidly. Surgery may be curative (Saijo et al., 1975), and an attempt at excision should be made before the lesion reaches unmanageable proportions.

LYMPHEDEMA

Lymphedema is swelling as a result of lymphatic stasis. A widespread defect (or aplasia) of lymphatic channels may result in the characteristic brawny edema. Females are affected more frequently than males. The lower limbs are the most common sites, but other sites may also be involved, and rarely, chylothorax or ascites may be present. When the legs are involved and an autosomal dominant form of transmission can be demonstrated, the eponym Milroy disease may be applied. Patients with diffuse lymphatic malformations require extensive radiologic contrast studies for adequate evaluation and lifetime vascular supportive treatment to the affected areas. It should be stressed that the underlying defect in many of the lymphedemas is unclear and that arteriovenous dysfunction may also be involved in the pathogenesis of the swelling. Lymphedema of the hands, feet, and legs also occurs in the Turner (XO) syndrome.

PIGMENTED NEVI

Noninflammatory pigmented localized lesions occur in about 1 to 4 per cent of newborns. Localized pigmented lesions can be caused by hyperactivity of the pigment-forming cells (melanocytes) in the epidermis, by collections of cells of melanocytic origin in the basal areas of the epidermis and high in the dermis (melanocytic nevus cells), or by collections of spindle-shaped melanocytic cells deep in the dermis (dermal melanocytes). The location of the melanocytic cells in the skin, the degree of melanin production, and the numbers of cells present are the variables that determine the size, shape, surface, and color of the nevus. Not all known types of melanocytic lesions occur in this age group. Some of them are described in the following sections.

CAFE-AU-LAIT SPOTS

Cafe-au-lait spots are flat lesions of light brown color in whites and of darker brown color in blacks. They vary in size from a few millimeters in their largest diameter to much larger lesions that cover a significant portion of the surface anatomy (Fig. 114–4). The surface is usually uniform in color, but minor variations may occur. Small single lesions (under 2 cm) are found in 19 per cent of normal children under 5 years of age (Whitehouse, 1966). Much larger lesions or the presence of six or more cafe-

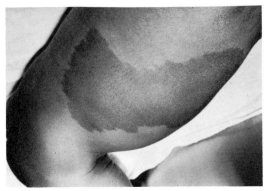

FIGURE 114–4. Large cafe-au-lait spot on the trunk of a newborn infant.

au-lait spots connotes an existing underlying pathologic condition, usually neurofibromatosis or the Albright syndrome (McCune-Albright syndrome).

NEUROFIBROMATOSIS

Etiology. Neurofibromatosis (NF) has been demonstrated to consist of a number of disorders, most of which are transmitted as an autosomal dominant trait. The gene for NF-1 has been localized to chromosome 17 and the gene for NF-2 to chromosome 22 (National Institutes for Health Consensus Conference, 1988).

The cause of neurofibromatosis at the biochemical level has yet to be identified, but isolated elements of the disorder are coming to the fore. The disorder is probably multicellular in origin, and there may exist a defect in ganglioside metabolism in tumors more likely to undergo malignant degeneration (Tsuchida et al., 1984).

Clinical Findings and Diagnosis. Riccardi (1981) has devised a classification system that includes a number of definable subtypes. Of special interest to the pediatrician are types that may be identifiable in the newborn period. These include the classic or von Recklinghausen variety (NF-1), bilateral acoustic neurofibromatosis (NF-2), the segmental form (NF-5), and the form that strictly involves only cafe-au-lait spots (NF-6). The other forms are mixtures more difficult to differentiate on clinical grounds. The incidence of neurofibromatosis is approximately 1 in 3000 live births. NF-1 accounts for the vast majority of neurofibromatosis patients.

The cutaneous manifestations in the newborn infant of Types 1, 2, and 6 are limited to the presence of a few cafe-au-lait spots, which become more numerous as the child grows older. The presence of more than six cafe-au-lait spots (≥ 0.5 cm in diameter) in a child under 5 years of age is highly suggestive of neurofibromatosis. Axillary freckling is also a very common feature of NF-1 in the older child. Lisch nodules, hyperpigmented excrescences of the iris seen by binocular ophthalmoscopy, are found in 94 per cent of patients with NF-1 over age 6 years (Lewis and Riccardi, 1981). The protuberant cutaneous tumors, consisting of perineural elements, usually appear in late childhood and adolescence, although they may be seen earlier. Neurofibromatosis is a complex disease with multiorgan involvement, and patients with this condition should be carefully observed for other manifestations of the disease (Riccardi, 1981; Riccardi and Eichner, 1986). The physician faced with the need to discriminate between the cafe-au-lait spots of neurofibromatosis and those of other conditions is often in a quandary. Overall assessment of the patient is more likely to be of help than any laboratory test, including examination of the melanocytic melanosome.

Macromelanosomes are found in a wide variety of conditions other than neurofibromatosis; therefore, one must not consider their presence as diagnostic (Eady et al., 1975). Cafe-au-lait spots may also be found in the Bloom syndrome, the Russell-Silver syndrome, the epidermal nevus syndrome, and the LEOPARD syndrome, among other disorders. Perhaps it is also wise to remember that up to 2 per cent of black infants may have 1 to 3 cafe-au-lait spots that are of no significance (Alper et al., 1979).

Prognosis. The prognosis is variable, depending on the severity of involvement and the type of neurofibromatosis. Central nervous system involvement occurs in about one-third of patients with NF-1 (Riccardi, 1982) and may include difficulties in speech or seizures. Mental retardation is a less common phenomenon (2 to 5 per cent), whereas many other neurologic problems are strictly dependent on the site of tumor growth and impingement on neighboring structures. The bones may have localized or diffuse involvement. Kyphoscoliosis is a frequent affliction after the onset of puberty in these patients. There is an increased incidence of malignancies, including sarcomas of varying origins. Pheochromocytoma occurs in 1 per cent of patients. Arterial anomalies occur in 10 per cent of 46 affected children below the age of 12 years (Fienman, 1970).

Treatment. Surgical removal of neurofibromas is often difficult to achieve because of their unencapsulated nature; however, surgery often palliates the presence of annoying or symptomatic lesions. Genetic counseling is imperative, particularly now that the identification of linked markers make prenatal diagnosis a possibility. Work-up should include a complete history and complete physical examination and further studies predicated on the clinical findings (National Institutes of Health Consensus Conference, 1988; Riccardi and Eichner, 1986). Patients may benefit from membership in one of the neurofibromatosis support groups.

ALBRIGHT SYNDROME (McCUNE-ALBRIGHT SYNDROME)

Albright syndrome consists of polyostotic fibrous dysplasia, endocrine dysfunction (D'Armiento et al., 1983), sexual precocity (in females), and large cafe-au-lait spots. The cafe-au-lait lesions in this syndrome may be unilateral, have irregular borders, are elongated and very large, and usually contain melanocytes with normal-appearing melanosomes. Bony involvement is often centered on the long bones and jaw but may also occur elsewhere. The first sign of bony involvement is often a pathologic fracture; therefore, in the presence of the typical large ragged cafe-au-lait spot, a CT scan of the skeleton may be indicated.

MELANOCYTIC NEVI

Melanocytic nevi, by definition, include several lesions, all of which have a common feature: the presence of cells of melanocytic origin derived from the neural crest, situated in the dermis, placed either high at the junction between the epidermis and dermis or deeper in the dermis. Paradoxically, the lesions found just under or adjacent to the dermis are flat and are called junctional nevi. The deeper lesions tend to be bulkier, are raised above the skin surface, and are called intradermal nevi. Mixtures of the two are known as compound nevi. The lesions are further divided into three categories of size: Small (< 2 cm), large (2 to 20 cm), and giant (> 20 cm or 120 cm² surface area) (Zitelli et al., 1984). If the lesions are made

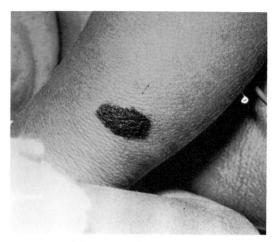

FIGURE 114–5. Dark brown irregular congenital nevus on the limb of an infant.

up of cells that have an elongated, almost fibrocytic character, they are called blue nevi or dermal melanocytosis. There are many variants of these lesions, but the basic features can be found in this categorization no matter what the lesion is called. A lentigo has no nevus cells. It consists of a localized hyperactivity or increase in the number of normal melanocytes found in the basal layer.

Clinical Findings. Flat, dark brown to black, sharply demarcated melanocytic nevi are found in about 2 per cent of newborn infants (Alper et al., 1979). They vary in size and grow proportionally with the infant. Most frequently, one may find one or two lesions in normal infants (Fig. 114–5), but more numerous melanocytic nevi are found in a number of syndromes (such as the epidermal nevus syndrome) or accompanying a giant nevus. The presence of these lesions in profusion, either at birth or within the 1st month of life, usually signifies a more widespread disorder. Flat nevi have a characteristic histologic appearance. They consist of nests of cuboidal cells clustered at the base of the epidermis, at the junction with the dermis. The presence of these lesions on the skin of the newborn should be charted.

GIANT NEVI

Giant nevi are, from the perspective of the neonatologist, the most important of the congenital pigmented nevi. This is true because of their potential for malignant degeneration (Reed et al., 1965). These nevi vary in size from lesions of several centimeters to massive deformities covering half the body (Fig. 114–6). Extremely large lesions involving the back, thorax, and abdomen are called "bathing-trunk nevi." The lesion is invariably noticed at birth, is raised and fleshy, has a brown to black color, and has a leathery surface. The pigment may appear to spill over at the borders, staining the surrounding skin with a junctional halo. Coarse hair grows in the area in many children but may not be apparent until later in childhood. Histologically, the lesion consists of a plethora of melanocytic nevus cells. These cells may be pigment laden or clear and cuboidal or spindle shaped and invade the entire cutis, subcutaneous tissue, and even muscle, fascia, and periosteum. The meninges may also be involved, resulting

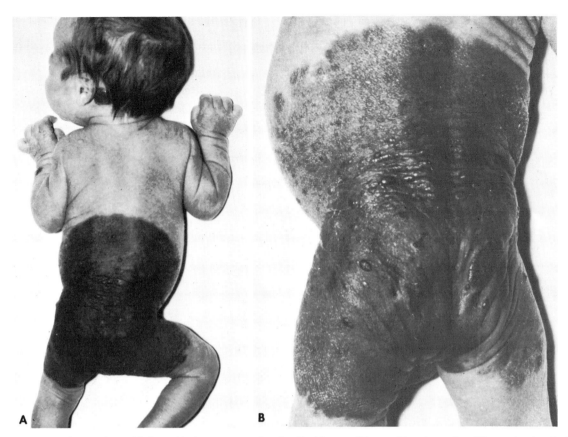

FIGURE 114–6. A, Newborn infant with large black nevus covering the "bathing trunk" area. The closer view (B) permits visualization of the nodular surface typical of giant nevi.

in central nervous system disorders and leptomeningeal melanocytosis (Hoffman and Freeman, 1967; Reed et al., 1965).

BLUE NEVUS

Blue nevi are so called because of their deep Prussian blue color and are, on occasion, found at birth (Lund and Kraus, 1962) on the scalp, face, arms, or buttocks. These are oval, dome-shaped tumors that protrude above the skin surface in contrast to the flat bluish nevi described in the succeeding paragraphs. Two histologic types of blue nevi have been described: In one, the melanocytic component is similar to that found in mongolian spot, and in the second, the melanocytes take the form of cuboidal cells with a pale vacuolated cytoplasm.

MONGOLIAN SPOTS, NEVI OF OTA AND ITO

More than 90 per cent of black and Oriental infants, but less than 5 per cent of white children (Pratt, 1953), are born with mongolian spots, deep brown to slate-gray or blue-black, large macules of varying size located most commonly in the lumbosacral area. Although the buttock area is the most frequent site, multiple lesions involving the lower limbs, back, flanks, and shoulders are not uncommon. Mongolian spots represent collections of spindle-shaped melanocytes located deep in the dermis. Most mongolian spots gradually fade during the 1st year of life.

Nevus of Ota is a blue or grey discoloration involving

the orbital and zygomatic area. The sclera and fundus on the affected side also may appear to be stained. When the lesion is located in the deltotrapezius area, it is called nevus of Ito. Treatment of nevus of Ota is only of concern after the child starts school and should include an adequate cosmetic cover (such as Covermark or Dermablend) for the affected area. When the eye itself is involved, periodic examination by an ophthalmologist is warranted.

Diagnosis. The differential diagnosis of nevi may include urticaria pigmentosa, postinflammatory hyperpigmentation, and juvenile lentigines. Freckles are not seen at birth or during the first few months of life. The lentiginous spots found in the LEOPARD syndrome appear after the first year of life, and those in the Peutz-Jeghers syndrome appear at about puberty. In generalized hereditary lentiginosis, an autosomal dominant disease that is associated with mental retardation and nystagmus, the numerous lentigines are present at birth.

Treatment. The treatment of melanocytic nevi depends, in part, on their location and the age at which they appear. The most frequent concern of parents and pediatricians is the lesion's potential for malignant transformation (Arons and Hurwitz, 1983). The risk for small lesions (1 to 2 cm) is probably small, but the risk is greater for congenital lesions than for lesions that appear after birth (Rhodes and Melski, 1982; Rhodes et al., 1982; Solomon, 1980). For this reason, there is an increasing tendency to remove congenital melanocytic nevi by surgical excision (Alper, 1985; Elder, 1985; Illig et al., 1985). The pediatrician should advise the parents on what stage of growth the infant can best tolerate the procedure physically and psychologically.

About 10 to 15 per cent of patients with giant pigmented hairy nevi of the bathing-trunk type develop malignant melanoma. For this reason, it is desirable to remove these lesions surgically. The postoperative course in patients undergoing extensive procedures may be difficult, but the risk for malignant transformation in giant nevi warrants a drastic surgical approach.

DYSPLASTIC NEVUS SYNDROME

Familial or sporadic malignant melanoma may occur in some patients with acquired nevi of the dysplastic type. These nevi usually develop gradually during adolescence (Elder et al., 1980). In the presence of, or with a history of, dysplastic nevi or malignant melanoma in the family, it is absolutely necessary to advise total avoidance of sunburn in infants and children (Greene et al., 1984; Sober, 1987).

WHITE MACULES

Localized areas of hypopigmentation on the skin of the newborn infant may be prognostically significant. A distinction must first be made between complete depigmentation (vitiligo or piebaldism) and hypopigmentation. The depigmented lesion is pure white when fully developed, and may be seen in ordinary daylight, even in fair-skinned infants. The hypopigmented lesion is lighter in color than the surrounding skin and, in fair-skinned children, may require exposure of the skin to a Wood light to be made apparent. Simple hypopigmented macules may be seen as an innocent unchanging localized defect in melanocyte function (achromic nevus), in congenital giant halo nevi containing a junction nevus surrounded by an area of postinflammatory hypopigmentation, as a pale vascular anomaly called nevus anemicus, or as evidence of an incipient hemangioma.

Small oval areas of hypopigmentation, often in the shape of a European-mountain-ash leaflet (Fig. 114–7), are found at birth on the thorax and limbs of approximately 90 per cent of infants with tuberous sclerosis,

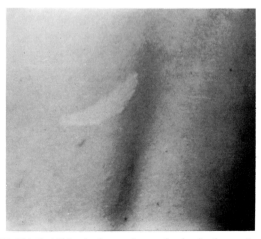

FIGURE 114–7. *White leaf macule on the back of a patient with tuberous sclerosis.*

especially if the skin is carefully examined under a Wood light. The number of white spots may be variable, but their presence should alert the pediatrician to the need for a careful genetic history and thorough examination of the infant and all members of the family for further evidence of tuberous sclerosis. When a question exists about the nature of a hypopigmented macule, a biopsy specimen taken from it and prepared for electron microscopic examination may help resolve the issue. In vitiligo and partial albinism, few or no melanocytes may be found. Melanocytes are present in the white macule of tuberous sclerosis, but the melanosomes are poorly pigmented.

Tuberous sclerosis is an autosomal dominant disease characterized by the development of multiple fibroangiomas, which ultimately may affect the skin (digital fibromas, adenoma sebaceum); the central nervous system (intercerebral tubers), leading to intracerebral calcification and seizure disorders; and the eye (retinal glial tumors). Moderate to severe mental retardation and seizures may be associated with the condition. The prognosis depends on the number of organs involved and the extent of fibroangiomatous involvement of individual organs. Serious complications of tuberous sclerosis include hamartomas of the lung and kidney and rhabdomyomas of the heart.

■ EPIDERMAL NEVI

Nomenclature and Clinical Findings. Epidermal (epithelial, verrucous) nevi represent congenital growth disturbances in cells involved in keratin production and hypertrophy of the epidermis. The resulting lesions may be present at birth and continue to spread during the 1st or 2nd decade of life. Infrequently, they appear after the neonatal period. A spectrum of epidermal lesions may be seen on different anatomic areas of the same patient. The lesions may be deeply or slightly pigmented, be well or poorly demarcated, and have either a unilateral or bilateral distribution. Affected skin varies from warty to scaly. Given the morphologic variability of epidermal nevi, it is not surprising to find a host of Latin names describing them. Until evidence is accumulated to distinguish these lesions on other than strictly morphologic grounds, we prefer to consider epidermal nevi as a group. A brief description of some of the common morphologic variants follows:

1. Nevus unius lateris: A linear, highly verrucous lesion that streaks across a variable portion of the anatomy (Fig. 114–8). The lesion may be strictly unilateral on one surface and cross the midline on another surface of the body. If the limbs are affected, nail deformity is frequent. When the scalp, face, or neck is involved, the adnexal tissues, such as the sebaceous glands, may be involved by becoming enlarged. If a large part of the body is affected, the process may be referred to as systematized epithelial nevus. When the sebaceous gland element on the scalp is very prominent, some authors prefer the term linear nevus sebaceous.

2. Verrucous nevus: A more localized form that consists of a short (6 to 10 cm) warty streak across the thorax, arm, or abdomen. Occasionally (in the neck or axilla), the warty element is so localized as to result in a narrow string of small, soft tumors. Smaller (2 to 3 cm) epidermal nevi

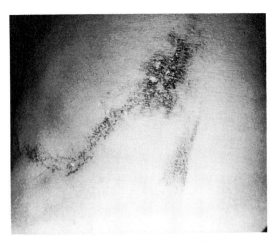

FIGURE 114–8. *Linear hyperkeratotic epidermal nevus on the back and lateral thorax.*

on the scalp or face may be mistaken for a melanocytic nevus.

3. Ichthyosis hystrix: A scaly eruption often involving both sides of the body but in some areas stopping abruptly at the midline. The patterns formed result in an appearance of marbling, feathery streaks, sheets, or whorls of discolored thickened skin. The linear character of these lesions suggests that they result from a hereditary disorder with partial expression in some cells but not others and that they are a form of mosaicism.

EPIDERMAL NEVUS SYNDROME

Clinical Findings. The epidermal nevus syndrome (Rogers et al., 1989; Solomon, 1985; Solomon and Esterly, 1975), consists of widespread epidermal nevi (any of the aforementioned types); bony abnormalities, including kyphoscoliosis, hemihypertrophy, discordance in limb length, and vertebral anomalies; central nervous system disorders, including seizures, mental retardation, and hemiplegia; and vascular disorders, primarily hemangiomas of skin and of the central nervous system. We have seen one patient with Wilms tumor with epidermal nevus but without hemihypertrophy. Other malignancies also occur in this syndrome with a greater than expected frequency, both in the affected skin and in other organ systems such as the brain, salivary glands, and kidney.

Prognosis. Epidermal nevi that evolve in any area except the scalp and face are unpredictable. Continued spread may persist until well after puberty. We have seen none resolve spontaneously. Affected infants should have a thorough physical examination and appropriate radiologic and electroencephalographic studies if defects in bony structure or neurologic function are detected.

Treatment. The optimal treatment of epidermal nevi of small dimension is simple excision down to the subcutaneous tissue. Lesions recur if underlying dermis is not removed. Since malignant degeneration (usually basal cell epitheliomas) may occur at a later date (Swint and Klaus, 1970), it is preferable to excise smaller lesions, but large lesions are difficult to treat surgically and it may be impractical to attempt surgery in all but exposed areas.

One of us (LMS) has treated such severely affected adults with 13-*cis*-retinoic acid with very modest success.

■ JUVENILE XANTHOGRANULOMA

Clinical Findings. Xanthogranulomas are benign tumors of fat-laden histiocytic cells and Touton giant cells associated with a chronic inflammatory process. About one-fifth of infants with juvenile xanthogranuloma have visible lesions at birth, and in two-thirds they are present by 6 months of age (Nomland, 1959). In the majority of affected infants, the lesions are confined to the skin of the upper half of the body (Fig. 114–9). Usually, they are firm, red-yellow papules or nodules (Esterly et al., 1972).

Prognosis. Most of the lesions resolve spontaneously within 6 to 12 months of onset, but occasionally they leave residual pigmentary or atrophic changes. The vast majority of infants are otherwise healthy and have no abnormalities of serum lipids; however, an increased incidence of familial cafe-au-lait spots and neurofibromatosis has been documented in infants with juvenile xanthogranuloma (Crocker, 1979).

Ocular involvement is the only complication of concern. Cellular infiltrates may invade the iris, ciliary body, episclera, or entire orbit. The ocular tumors may occur as an isolated finding or may coincide with or follow the onset of skin lesions. They may be present as unilateral glaucoma, hyphema, uveitis, heterochromia iridis, or proptosis (Gaynes and Cohen, 1967; Zimmerman, 1965).

Treatment. Treatment of ocular lesions by radiation therapy or systemically administered corticosteroids may be necessary for prevention of serious sequelae (Gaynes and Cohen, 1967; Smith and Ingram, 1968). Very rarely, lesions have developed in the lung, testis, or pericardium. The cutaneous lesions do not require treatment.

■ MASTOCYTOSIS (URTICARIA PIGMENTOSA)

Etiology. Mastocytosis is a disease of undetermined origin. Although pedigrees of affected individuals have

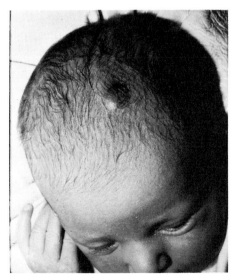

FIGURE 114–9. *Solitary juvenile xanthogranuloma on the scalp, a typical site for these lesions.*

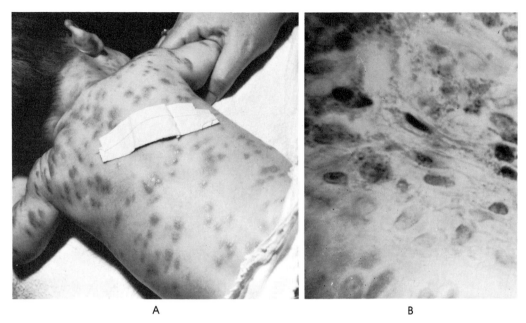

A   B

FIGURE 114–10. A, *Deeply pigmented nodules and macules on the back of an infant with urticaria pigmentosa. A group of vesicles is visible just below the bandage that covers the biopsy site. B, Microscopic section from biopsy of patient stained with Giemsa. The mast cells can be identified as spindle-shaped cells containing granules that are located in the upper dermis.*

been carefully studied (Selmanowitz et al., 1970), the question of genetic transmission remains unresolved (Cainelli et al., 1983; Fowler et al., 1986).

Clinical Findings. Mast cells may infiltrate the skin and result in a variety of lesions of differing prognostic significance. Infants may have solitary lesions, a generalized maculopapular eruption (Fig. 114–10), or rarely, diffuse thickening of the skin (Sagher and Evan-Paz, 1967; Solomon and Esterly, 1973).

The solitary tumor may be discovered at birth or may develop shortly thereafter. The lesion is often oval, pink, yellow, or light brown, and it measures under 6 cm in length. It is raised, has a pebbly surface, and feels rubbery and may appear anywhere on the body surface. If rubbed or traumatized, mastocytomas develop a wheal (Darier sign), and in the newborn infant, may blister or become hemorrhagic. A blister may be the sole presenting sign of a localized mast cell infiltrate.

All forms of the disease are due to an infiltrate of mast cells in the dermis that may be demonstrated by Giemsa stain. Symptoms are due to release of histamine from the mast cells. Itching is usual, and with widespread lesions and occasionally with solitary lesions, massive histamine release may result in episodes of flushing, irritability, tachycardia, respiratory distress, and hypotension. Coagulopathy may occur rarely. In the systemic form of the disease, the liver, spleen, lymph nodes, bone marrow, and gastrointestinal tract may show evidence of mast cell invasion (Sagher and Evan-Paz, 1967).

Prognosis. Solitary cutaneous lesions usually have no systemic component and may be treated conservatively without recourse to extensive studies and with every expectation that the lesion will resolve spontaneously within a few years. The maculopapular form also has a relatively good prognosis in childhood. Systemic involvement carries a poor prognosis.

Treatment. In patients with any form of mastocytosis, the following should be avoided: trauma to the lesions, hot baths, excessive rubbing, alcohol-containing elixirs, aspirin, codeine, polymyxin B, and procaine (all histamine releasers). Hydroxyzine and cyproheptadine hydrochloride in regular doses may offer some relief when symptoms become bothersome. Cimetidine and oral disodium cromoglycate are useful in the management of patients with severe manifestations.

■ REFERENCES

Alper, J.: Congenital nevi—the controversy rages on. Arch. Dermatol. *121*:734, 1985.

Alper, J., and Holmes, L. B.: The incidence of birthmarks in a cohort of 4,641 newborns. Pediatr. Dermatol. *1*:58, 1983.

Alper, J., Holmes, L. B., and Mihm, M. C.: Birthmarks with serious medical significance: Nevocellular nevi, sebaceous nevi, and multiple cafe-au-lait spots. J. Pediatr. *95*:696, 1979.

Amir, T., Krikler, R., Metzker, A., et al.: Strawberry hemangioma in preterm infants. Pediatr. Dermatol. *3*:331, 1986.

Arons, M. S., and Hurwitz, S.: Congenital nevocellular nevus: A review of the treatment controversy and a report of 46 cases. Plast. Reconstr. Surg. *72*:355, 1983.

Barsky, S. H., Rosen, S., Geer, D. E., et al.: The nature and evolution of port wine stains: A computer assisted study. J. Invest. Dermatol. *74*:154, 1980.

Berman, B., and Lim, H. W. P.: Concurrent cutaneous and hepatic hemangiomata in infancy. Report of a case and a review of the literature. J. Cutan. Surg. Oncol. *4*:869, 1978.

Brown, S. H., Jr., Neerhout, R. C., and Fonkalsrud, E. W.: Prednisone therapy in the management of large hemangiomas in infants and children. Surgery *71*:168, 1972.

Browze, N. L., Whimster, I., Stewart, G., et al.: The surgical management of lymphangioma circumscriptum. Br. J. Surg. *73*:535, 1986.

Burman, D., Mansell, P. W. Q., and Warin, R. P.: Miliary hemangiomata in the newborn. Arch. Dis. Child. *42*:193, 1967.

Burrows, D. E., Mulliken, J. B., Fellows, K. E., et al.: Childhood hemangiomas and vascular malformations: Angiographic differentiation. Am. J. Roentgenol. *141*:483, 1983.

Cainelli, T., Marchesi, L., Pasquali, F., et al.: Monozygotic twins discordant for cutaneous mastocytosis. Arch. Dermatol. *119*:1021, 1983.

Cates, C. P., William, E. D., Ward-Booth, R. P., et al.: Doppler ultrasound: A valuable diagnostic aid in a patient with facial hemangioma. Oral Surg. *59*:458, 1985.

Cohen, P. R., and Zalar, G. L.: Cutis marmorata telangiectatica congenita: Clinico-pathologic characteristics and differential diagnosis. Cutis *42*:418, 1988.

Crocker, A. L.: The histiocytosis syndromes. *In* Fitzpatrick, T. B., Eisen, A. A., Wolff, K., et al. (Eds.): Dermatology in General Medicine. 2nd ed. New York, McGraw-Hill, 1979, p. 1171.

D'Armiento, M., Reda, E., Camagna, A., et al.: McCune-Albright syndrome: Evidence for autonomous multiendocrine hyperfunction. J. Pediatr. *102*:585, 1983.

Eady, P. A. J., Sparrow, G. P., and Grice, K.: Naevoid pigmentation with giant melanosomes. Two cases. Proc. R. Soc. Med. *68*:759, 1975.

Elder, D. E.: The blind men and the elephant—Different views of small congenital nevi. Arch. Dermatol. *121*:1263, 1985.

Elder, D. E., Goldman, L. I., Goldman, S. C., et al.: Dysplastic nevus syndrome. Cancer *46*:1787, 1980.

Esterly, N. B.: Cutaneous hemangiomas, vascular stains and associated syndromes. Curr. Prob. Pediatr. *17*:1, 1987.

Esterly, N. B.: Kasabach-Merritt syndrome in infants. J. Am. Acad. Dermatol. *8*:504, 1983.

Esterly, N. B., Margileth, A. M., Kahn, G., et al.: The management of disseminated eruptive hemangiomata in infants. Special Symposium, Pediatr. Dermatol. *1*:312, 1984.

Esterly, N. B., Sahihi, T., and Medenica, M.: Juvenile xanthogranuloma: An atypical case with study of ultrastructure. Arch. Dermatol. *105*:99, 1972.

Fienman, N. L., and Yakovac, W. C.: Neurofibromatosis in childhood. J. Pediatr. *76*:339, 1970.

Folkman, J.: How is blood vessel growth regulated in normal and neoplastic tissue? Cancer Res. *46*:467, 1986.

Fost, N. C., and Esterly, N. B.: Successful treatment of juvenile hemangiomas with prednisone. J. Pediatr. *72*:351, 1968.

Fowler, J. F., Porsley, W., and Cotter, P. G.: Familial urticaria pigmentosa. Arch. Dermatol. *122*:80, 1986.

Fretzin, D. F., and Potter, B.: Blue rubber bleb nevus. Arch. Intern. Med. *116*:924, 1965.

Gaynes, P. M., and Cohen, G. S.: Juvenile xanthogranuloma of the orbit. Am. J. Ophthalmol. *63*:755, 1967.

Glovitzki, P., Hallier, C. H., Telander, R. L., et al.: Surgical implications of Klippel-Trenaunay syndrome. Ann. Surg. *192*:353, 1983.

Golitz, L. E., Ruchkoff, J., and O'Meara, P.: Diffuse neonatal hemangiomatosis. Pediatr. Dermatol. *3*:145, 1986.

Gordon, L., Vujic, I., and Spicer, K. M.: Visualization of cutaneous hemangiomas with Tc-99m tagged red cells. Clin. Nucl. Med. *4*:468, 1981.

Greeley, P. W., Middleton, A. G., and Curtain, J. W.: Incidence of malignancy in giant pigmented nevi. Plast. Reconstr. Surg. *36*:26, 1965.

Greene, M. H., Clark, W. H., Jr., Tucker, J. H., et al.: Managing the dysplastic naevus syndrome. Lancet *1*:166, 1984.

Harris, L. E., Stayura, L. A., Ramirez-Talavera, P. F., and Annegers, J. F.: Congenital and acquired abnormalities observed in liveborn and stillborn neonates. Mayo Clin. Proc. *50*:85, 1975.

Hidano, A., and Nakajima, S.: Earliest features of the strawberry mark in the newborn. Br. J. Dermatol. *87*:138, 1972.

Hoffman, H. J., and Freeman, A.: Primary leptomeningeal melanoma in association with giant hairy nevi. Report of two cases. J. Neurosurg. *26*:62, 1967.

Holden, K. R., and Alexander, R.: Diffuse neonatal hemangiomatosis. Pediatrics *46*:411, 1970.

Illig, W., Weidner, F., Hundeiker, M., et al.: Congenital nevi ≤ 10 cm precursors to melanoma: 52 cases, a review, and a new conception. Arch. Dermatol. *121*:1274, 1985.

Lewis, R. A., and Riccardi, V. M.: Von Recklinghausen neurofibromatosis: Incidence of iris hamartomata. Ophthalmology *88*:348, 1981.

Lund, H. A., and Kraus, J. M.: Melanotic tumors of the skin. Fascicle 3, Atlas of Tumor Pathology. Washington, D.C., Armed Forces Institute of Pathology, 1962.

Mangus, D. J.: Continuous compression therapy of hemangiomas: Evaluation in two cases. Plast. Reconstr. Surg. *49*:490, 1973.

Margileth, A. M.: Developmental vascular abnormalities. Med. Clin. North Am. *18*:773, 1971.

Mulliken, J. B., and Glowacki, J.: Hemangiomas and vascular malformations in infants and children: A classification based on endothelial characteristics. Plast. Reconstr. Surg. *69*:421, 1982.

Mulliken, J. B., and Young, A. E.: Vascular Birthmarks, Hemangiomas, and Malformations. Philadephia, W. B. Saunders Company, 1988.

Mullins, J. F., Naylor, D., and Pedetski, J.: The Klippel-Trenaunay-Weber syndrome (nevus vasculosus osteohypertrophicus). Arch. Dermatol. *86*:202, 1962.

Munkvad, M.: Blue rubber bleb nevus. Dermatologica *163*:307, 1983.

National Institutes of Health Consensus Development Conference: Neurofibromatosis. Arch. Neurol. *45*:575, 1988.

Nomland, R.: Nevoxanthoendothelioma, a benign xanthomatous disease of infants and children. J. Invest. Dermatol. *22*:207, 1959.

Oates, C. P., Williams, E. D., Ward-Booth, R. P., et al.: Doppler ultrasound: A valuable diagnostic aid in a patient with a facial hemangioma. Oral Surg. *59*:958, 1985.

Paller, A. S.: The Sturge-Weber syndrome. Pediatr. Dermatol. *4*:300, 1987.

Peachy, R. D. G., Lim, C. C., and Whimster, J. W.: Lymphangioma of skin. A review of 65 cases. Br. J. Dermatol. *83*:419, 1970.

Pinkus, H., and Mehregan, A. H.: A Guide to Dermatohistopathology. New York, Appleton-Century-Crofts, Inc., 1969, pp. 352–354.

Powell, S. T., and Su, W. P. D.: Cutis marmorata telangiectasia congenita: Report of nine cases and review of the literature. Cutis *34*:305, 1984.

Pratt, A. G.: Birthmarks in infancy. Arch. Dermatol. *67*:302, 1953.

Reed, W. B., Becker, S. W., Sr., Becker, S. W., Jr., and Nickel, W. R.: Giant pigmented nevi, melanoma and leptomeningeal melanocytosis. Arch. Dermatol. *91*:100, 1965.

Rhodes, A. R., and Melski, J. W.: Small congenital nevocellular nevi and the risk of cutaneous melanoma. J. Pediatr. *100*:219, 1982.

Rhodes, A. R., Sober, A. J., Day, C. L., et al.: The malignant potential of small congenital nevocellular nevi: An estimate of association based on a histologic study of 234 primary cutaneous melanomas. J. Am. Acad. Dermatol. *6*:620, 1982.

Riccardi, V. M.: Von Recklinghausen neurofibromatosis. N. Engl. J. Med. *305*:1617, 1981.

Riccardi, V. M., and Eichner, J. E.: Neurofibromatosis, Phenotype, Natural History and Pathogenesis. Baltimore, Johns Hopkins University Press, 1986.

Riccardi, V. M.: Early manifestations of neurofibromatosis: Diagnosis and management. Compr. Ther. *8*:35, 1982.

Rogers, M., McCrossin I., and Commens, C.: Epidermal nevi and the epidermal nevus syndrome: A review of 131 cases. J. Am. Acad. Dermatol. *20*:476, 1989.

Rodriguez-Erdmann, F., Button, L., Murray, J. E., and Moloney, M.: Kasabach-Merritt syndrome: Coagulo-analytical observations. Am. J. Med. Sci. *261*:9, 1971.

Sagher, F., and Evan-Paz, Z.: Mastocytosis and the Mast Cell. Chicago, Year Book Medical Publishers, 1967.

Saijo, M., Munroe, I. R., and Mancer, K.: Lymphangioma: Long-term follow-up study. Plast. Reconstr. Surg. *56*:642, 1975.

Sanchez, N. P., Rhodes, A. R., Mandell, F., and Mihm, M. C.: Encephalocraniocutaneous lipomatosis: A new syndrome. Br. J. Dermatol. *104*:89, 1981.

Selmanowitz, V. J., Orentreich, N., Tiangco, C. C., and Demis, D. J.: Uniovular twins discordant for cutaneous mastocytosis. Arch. Dermatol. *102*:34, 1970.

Smith, J. L. S., and Ingram, R. M.: Juvenile oculodermal xanthogranuloma. Br. J. Ophthalmol. *52*:696, 1968.

Sober, A. J.: Solar exposure in the etiology of cutaneous melanoma. Photodermatology *4*:23, 1987.

Solomon, L. M.: The management of congenital melanocytic nevi. Arch. Dermatol. *116*:1017, 1980.

Solomon, L. M.: Epidermal nevi: A study of 300 cases. *In* Fabrizi, G., and Serri, F. (Eds.): Dermatologia Pediatrica. Transactions of a symposium on pediatric dermatology. Rome, Italy, CILAG S.p.A., 1985.

Solomon, L. M., and Esterly, N. B.: Neonatal Dermatology. Philadelphia, W. B. Saunders Company, 1973.

Solomon, L. M., and Esterly, N. B.: Epidermal and other congenital organoid nevi. Curr. Probl. Pediatr. *6*:1, 1975.

Solomon, L. M., Fretzin, D. F., and De Wald, R. L.: The epidermal nevus syndrome. Arch. Dermatol. *97*:273, 1968.

Swint, R. B., and Klaus, S. W.: Malignant degeneration of an epithelial nevus. Arch. Dermatol. *101*:56, 1970.

Tan, K. L.: Nevus flammeus of the nape, glabella, and eyelids. Clin. Pediatr. *11*:112, 1972.

Tsuchida, T., Oksuka, H., Riimura, M., et al.: Biochemical study of gangliosides in neurofibroma and neurofibrosarcomas of Recklinghausen's disease. J. Dermatol. (Tokyo) *11*:129, 1984.

Wade, T. R., Kamino, H., and Ackerman, A. B.: A histologic atlas of vascular lesions. J. Dermatol. Surg. Oncol. *4*:845, 1978.

Way, B. H., Hermana, J., Gilbert, E. F., et al.: Cutis marmorata telangiectatica congenita. J. Cutan. Pathol. *1*:10, 1974.

White, C. W., Sondheimer, H. M., Crouch, E. C., et al.: Treatment of pulmonary hemangioma tests with recombinant interferon alfa-2a. N. Engl. J. Med. *320*:1197, 1989.

Whitehouse, D.: Diagnostic value of the cafe-au-lait spot in children. Arch. Dis. Child. *41*:316, 1966.

Zimmerman, L. C.: Ocular lesions of juvenile xanthogranuloma. Am. J. Ophthalmol. *60*:1011, 1965.

Zitelli, G. A., Grant, M. G., Abell, E., et al.: Histologic patterns of congenital nevocytic nevi and implications for treatment. J. Am. Acad. Dermatol. *11*:402, 1984.

PART XIX

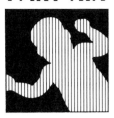

DISORDERS OF THE EYE

DISORDERS OF 115 THE EYE*

Creig S. Hoyt, William Good, and Robert Petersen

During the past decade ophthalmologists have been asked by pediatricians and neonatologists with increasing regularity to examine newborns, especially low-birth-weight, premature, and at-risk infants. The primary reason has been the return of and, indeed, a new epidemic of retinopathy of prematurity. As ophthalmologists have become more adept at examining premature infants, it has become clear that these children are also at risk for a number of other ocular disorders, including strabismus, amblyopia, and high refractive errors.

Nevertheless, the primary factor of this increased interest in detailed ophthalmologic examination of the young infant is the growing awareness of "critical" or "sensitive" periods in normal development with a convergence of interest among clinician and research neurobiologists in the problems of visual development. Experimentally induced disorders of the visual system caused by visual deprivation or unusual kinds of experience early in life have relevance to the clinical problem of amblyopia that is estimated to affect 3 per cent of full-term infants in the United States. For example, the experimental evidence that irreversible morphologic changes can take place in both the visual cortex and the lateral geniculate body of monocular-deprived infant animals implies the necessity for early therapeutic intervention in infants with monocular congenital cataracts, corneal opacities, or other disorders of the visual media.

Although examination of the eyeball itself and recognition of such common disorders as retinal hemorrhages in the newborn are not especially difficult for either ophthalmologists or pediatricians with an interest in ophthalmic disorders, some fundamental phenomenologic questions—such as "Does this child see?" or "Will this baby grow out of this muscle imbalance?"—are challenging issues for even the experienced examiner of preverbal, noncooperative young infants. As in other aspects of developmental biology, the definition of normal behavior and function for a given age is the essential prerequisite for the diagnosis of abnormalities in the infant visual

system. In recent years our understanding of what is "normal" visual function in young infants has undergone radical revision, and our knowledge is still expanding about this critical period of development.

■ DEVELOPMENT OF THE EYE

The formation of the eye begins at about the 22nd day of fetal life in the human. During the next 6 to 8 weeks, development is nearly complete.

The eye begins as a neuroectodermal evagination of the forebrain with a contribution from the mesoderm. The surface ectoderm is the precursor of the lens whose fibers develop from its nucleus in concentric layers. A vascular system, known as the hyaloid system, is a transitory group of vessels that surrounds the lens, both anteriorly and posteriorly, and nourishes it during development. The system normally atrophies by 35 weeks' gestation.

The iris continues undergoing development through the first 6 months of postnatal life. At term birth, the surface has both crypts and hillocks, which progress through the first 6 months of life. The color of the iris in white infants is usually gray or blue and may become darker as the melanocytes produce pigments. The vessels may change in caliber and course over the first 6 months. The eyes of dark-skinned babies tend to be gray or blue at birth but become darker brown during the first months after birth.

The eyelids are fused usually until 25 weeks, but they may rarely remain fused until 30 weeks.

MATURATION OF VISION

A pupillary light reaction is present at approximately 30 weeks' gestation but becomes better developed during the first month after birth (Table 115–1). True blinking in response to an object approaching the eyes is not often developed until 2 to 5 months after term birth.

It is estimated that the visual acuity of full-term infants is approximately 20/400. This is because the macula of the retina is not mature. Furthermore, the optic nerve is

---

*This chapter includes portions from 5th ed. by Dr. Lawrence W. Hirst.

TABLE 115–1. Maturation of Vision and the Eye

DESCRIPTION	AGE
Pupillary light reaction present	30-week gestation
Pupillary light reaction well developed	1 month
Lid closure in response to bright light	30-week gestation
Blink response to visual threat	2–5 months
Visual fixation present	Birth
Fixation well developed	2 months
Conjugate horizontal gaze well developed	Birth
Conjugate vertical gaze well developed	2 months
Vestibular eye rotations well developed	34-week gestation
Optokinetic nystagmus well developed	Birth
Visual following well developed	3 months
Accommodation well developed	4 months
Visual evoked potential acuity at adult level	6 months
Grating acuity preferential looking at adult level	2 years
Snellen letter acuity at adult level	2 years
End of critical period for monocular visual deprivation	10 years
Ocular alignment stable	1 month
Fusional convergence well developed	6 months
Stereopsis well developed	6 months
Stereoacuity (Titmus) at adult level	7 years
Eyeball 70 per cent of adult diameter	Birth
Eyeball 95 per cent of adult diameter	3 years
Cornea 80 per cent of adult diameter	Birth
Cornea 95 per cent of adult diameter	1 year
Differentiation of fovea completed	4 months
Myelination of optic nerve completed	7 months–2 years
Iris stromal pigmentation well developed	6 months

(From Isenberg, S. J.: The Eye in Infancy. Chicago, Year Book Medical Publishers, 1989.)

not completely myelinated until approximately 1 year of age. The eye continues to develop synapses in the visual cortex during the first 10 years after birth. Visual acuity, however, is normally 20/20 by 2 years of age.

Tears are not normally present with crying until 1 to 3 months of age in a full-term infant (Spierer et al., 1989).

■ EXAMINATION OF THE EYE

Examination of the eye should begin with examination of the lids to ascertain their movement and any possible irregularities. The eyes of a healthy, normal newborn are rarely aligned. During the first few weeks of life, they frequently shift between orthotropia and esotropia or exotropia. The exact frequency with which these deviations occur as well as the anatomic and physiologic correlates of these transient neonatal heterotropias has yet to be defined. Nevertheless, it is clear that most full-term infants establish normal ocular alignment within the first 8 weeks of life. Any apparent misalignment of the visual axes after this period of time should be considered pathologic.

Examination of the pupils involves their response to light, which begins only after 29 weeks' gestation and remains incomplete until 1 month of age.

The anterior segment of the eye can be inspected with a flashlight, with or without magnification, or with a portable slit lamp. The cornea should be examined for clarity and the presence of any opacities. The lens and vitreous humor are similarly examined for opacities. If the cornea is enlarged, it could be the earliest sign of glaucoma and requires urgent consultation with an ophthalmologist.

The posterior segment is best examined after the pupils

have been maximally dilated. For term infants, a sympathomimetic agent, such as phenylephrine (1 per cent) is usually sufficient. For preterm infants (or those at term), the parasympatholytic agent cyclopentolate in a concentration of 1 per cent or less works well. The fundus is best examined with the indirect ophthalmoscope and lens. The optic nerve is somewhat paler in the newborn than in the adult regardless of race. It is important to examine the periphery of the eye because the earliest signs of retinopathy of prematurity (ROP) develop in the temporal periphery. Any alterations in pigmentation of the retina or loss of the red reflex suggests more serious disease and should mandate a consultation with an ophthalmologist. See discussion of ROP later in this chapter.

■ DISORDERS OF MOTILITY

STRABISMUS

Strabismus (meaning "to squint or look obliquely") may be evident in any field of gaze and can be intermittent or constant. It is present in 2 per cent of the general population but is more frequent in a number of genetically determined central nervous system (CNS) disorders as well as in infants affected by ROP.

By far the most common form of strabismus in early infancy is congenital or infantile esotropia (eyes are convergent). The term "congenital" is probably inappropriate, since this ocular motor disorder does not become apparent in most children until a few weeks postpartum (Fig. 115–1). Congenital esotropia is a characteristic disorder in which there is a large angle of deviation that is usually grossly apparent without even an attempt to evaluate the child's fixation or quantitatively evaluate the size of the disorder with a cover test. In addition, the child has a tendency to cross-fixate using the right eye in left gaze and the left eye in right gaze. This results in a pseudoabduction deficit in each eye, which can be readily mistaken for a bilateral VI nerve palsy. However, it should be pointed out that VI nerve palsies in the neonatal period, even in the severely traumatized newborn, are extremely unusual.

Congenital esotropia is a persistent disorder that does not spontaneously resolve. It requires surgical correction for realignment and, because of a high associated risk of amblyopia, patching may also be necessary. Moreover, at least one-third to one-half of all patients successfully operated upon with congenital esotropia require a spectacle correction postoperatively in order to maintain good ocular alignment. Prompt referral of these patients to an ophthalmologist within the first few months of life is appropriate. However, there are no data at the present time to suggest that surgical correction in the 1st year of life carries any better long-term visual outcome than in the 2nd year of life. Most authorities feel these children should be carefully evaluated on several occasions before surgical intervention is recommended.

An alternate to surgery is the use of botulinum toxin injection, which has been advocated by Magoon (1987). The toxin is used to paralyze the overactive muscle. This procedure may be helpful if surgery is contraindicated for any reason, or if it fails to provide optimal correction.

The child who presents with a smaller angle of esotropia

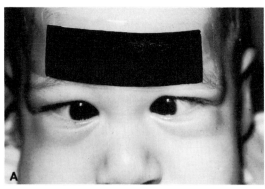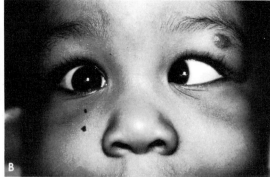

FIGURE 115–1. *Strabismus. A, Congenital esotropia with alternating fixation. B, Congenital esotropia with constant in-turning of the left eye. There is also a hemangioma of the left upper eyelid. At surgery, the medial rectus muscles in cases of congenital esotropia are often somewhat tight, presumably not because of a defect in the muscle, but rather from physiologic contracture. (From the collection of Dr. Arnall Patz.)*

or, more frequently, an apparent esotropia only intermittently is more difficult to evaluate. Many young infants who are believed to be cross-eyed by their parents or grandparents in fact have no ocular motor disorder whatsoever. They suffer from nothing more than the pseudostrabismus that is associated with the prominent epicanthal folds of infancy (Fig. 115–2). Characteristically, the apparent esotropia is noted particularly in lateral gaze where the adducting eye becomes occluded by the epicanthal fold. Nevertheless, the differential between pseudostrabismus and the early onset of accommodative esotropia is sometimes a difficult clinical dilemma. It is now clear that full accommodative amplitudes are present in the 3-month-old infant, and the onset of accommodative esotropia may occur in the first few months of life. Even if the pediatrician feels that a child's apparent esotropia is likely to be a pseudostrabismus, it is probably prudent to refer the patient for complete ophthalmologic examination, including a psychoplegic refraction, to make certain that the child is not a high hyperope. If any additional risk factors exist, including a family history of strabismus, the presence of Prader-Willi syndrome (Hered et al., 1988), albinism, or premature birth, then a higher suspicion for strabismus should be maintained (Hoyt et al., 1982).

NYSTAGMUS

A less common but far more serious ocular motor disorder is congenital nystagmus. "Congenital" nystagmus is usually not apparent until approximately 8 to 12 weeks of life in the full-term infant. Although a distinct clinical entity referred to as "congenital motor nystagmus" has been characterized and pedigrees of this disorder have been described (Gelbart and Hoyt, 1988), congenital nystagmus should always be considered a sign of bilateral visual loss until proved otherwise. Recent studies have documented that in excess of 80 per cent of infants who present with congenital nystagmus have another disorder involving the visual pathways as the underlying etiology. In some cases, such as a child with bilateral cataracts, corneal opacities, or glaucoma, the cause is readily apparent. In other cases the underlying sensory defect may require additional testing, including electroretinography, in order to detect disorders of the retina or the optic nerve. Subtle forms of tyrosinase-positive ocular albinism present a particularly difficult clinical problem in evaluation, particularly in the blond, fair-skinned young infant.

Although congenital nystagmus is usually considered to be a horizontally directed nystagmus symmetric in both eyes and commonly with a latent component, it may show unusual features, particularly in the first few months of life, that superficially mimic nystagmus associated with specific neurologic disorders. For example, upbeat nystagmus, see-saw nystagmus, and even monocular nystagmus may be associated with visual loss in early infancy rather than being a specific sign of neurologic dysfunction. Indeed, nystagmus of any type with an onset in the first 6 months of life should be considered a sign of a visual disorder rather than evidence for neurologic disease. Careful ophthalmologic examination of all children under the age of 6 months of age with nystagmus is essential in order to establish the etiologic cause.

TRANSIENT MOTILITY DISORDERS

Several transient disorders of the ocular motor system in infancy have been described. Opsoclonus, or flutter-like movements, in newborns may be self-limiting and imply no serious ocular or systemic abnormality and should not be mistaken for congenital nystagmus as the movement in this disorder is much more rapid and usually smaller in amplitude. This transient ocular motor defect usually resolves spontaneously within the first few weeks of life. More perplexing are those infants who present with transient downward deviation of the eyes (a more infrequent form with transient upward deviation has also been reported). Transient downward deviation of the eyes may superficially mimic the so-called setting-sun sign associated with hydrocephalus. This disorder, however, may be distinguished from its more serious kin by the fact that

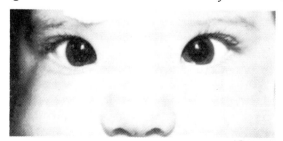

FIGURE 115–2. *Child with pseudoesotropia. Note wide bridge of nose and prominent epicanthal folds simulating esotropia. Flashbulb reflection is centered in each pupil, showing that the eyes are indeed straight. (From Patz, A.: The management of some common pediatric eye problems. Md. Med. J. 8:600, 1959.)*

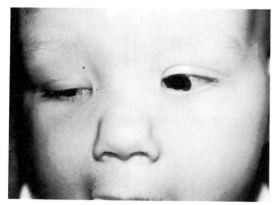

FIGURE 115–3. Unilateral congenital ptosis. (From the collection of Dr. Arnall Patz.)

transient downward deviation is not a true upgaze palsy, and therefore, vesticular ocular responses will demonstrate that the upgaze in these children is entirely intact. Transient downward deviation of the eyes may persist for months with only a gradual improvement. Neurologic and neuroradiographic investigation of these infants has failed to show any underlying neurologic disorder to account for this curious ocular motor disturbance.

CONGENITAL PTOSIS

Congenital ptosis is the inability to raise one or both of the upper eyelids and may occur as a solitary defect or in association with the inability to rotate the eye upward. The condition is associated with the incomplete development of the superior rectus muscle and the elevator of the lid, the levator palpebrae superioris.

Congenital ptosis should be distinguished from facial nerve palsy in which the problem is principally the inability to close the lid tightly, rather than the inability to open it (Figs. 115–3 and 115–4). Both conditions need to be distinguished from myasthenia gravis, which is rarely associated with ptosis in the newborn. Congenital ptosis as an isolated defect is usually transmitted as a dominant trait. Treatment consists of a plastic surgical procedure on the upper eyelid.

Acquired ptosis can occur with any systemic neuromuscular disorder characterized by muscle weakness. Infant botulism is one such condition associated with *Clostridium botulinum* infection. It usually resolves by 1 to 2 years of age.

MÖBIUS SYNDROME

Möbius syndrome is a supranuclear horizontal gaze palsy that is often associated with a facial myopathy. The only horizontal movement is convergence. The condition is associated with flattening of the nasolabial folds and hemiatrophy of the tongue, which may lead to poor feeding.

■ AMBLYOPIA AND REFRACTIVE ERRORS

Amblyopia may be defined as a reduction in visual acuity in the absence of obvious ocular structural abnormality to account for it. An important concept in the definition of amblyopia is that it is a consequence of the interference of normal visual experience during a critical developing sensory period and, in appropriate cases, is reversible with appropriate therapeutic measures.

Attempts to reverse amblyopia once the sensitive period has passed will be doomed to failure. It is imperative therefore that each form of amblyopia and its sensitive period be clearly defined. Although there are at least four or five distinct forms of amblyopia, three forms constitute the majority of cases seen. These may be defined as strabismic, anisometropic, and form deprivation amblyopia. Strabismic amblyopia is the visual loss associated with patients with strabismus who choose to fixate with one eye and allow the other eye to be constantly deviated. Anisometropic amblyopia arises as the result of unequal refractive errors in both eyes. In its most severe form, this is usually associated with high degrees of myopia or hyperopia. Form deprivation amblyopia occurs as the result of complete obstruction of the visual axis. For example, complete ptosis of the eyelid, corneal opacification, or a congenital cataract will result in form deprivation amblyopia. The sensitive period for each of these forms of amblyopia is distinctly different. For example, in the case of congenital monocular cataracts, successful visual rehabilitation requires identification within the first few weeks of life, immediate referral to an opthalmologist, surgical correction, and aphakic rehabilitation, all completed within the first 3 to 4 months of life. In contrast, strabismic amblyopia may be treatable well up until 6 to 7 years of age and anisometropic amblyopia may be treatable into the early teens. Each form of amblyopia therefore requires a different degree of suspicion in early infancy, and from a public health point of view, form deprivation amblyopia is the one of most concern to the neonatologist and the pediatrician. Careful examination of the infant to be certain that ptosis does not occlude the pupil and a careful search for a good, clear red-light reflex

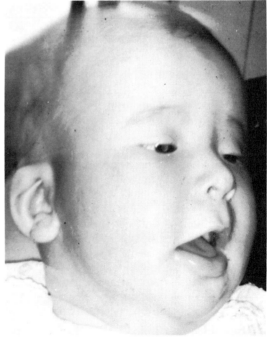

FIGURE 115–4. Bilateral congenital ptosis of the upper lids.

to be certain that the visual axis is clear in each eye are imperative if these severe forms of amblyopia are to be treated successfully within the first few weeks of life.

The practical problems of measuring the refraction of infants even in the hands of a well-trained pediatric ophthalmologist are considerable. Nevertheless, cycloplegic refraction utilizing retinoscopy allows an ophthalmologist to detect severe refractive errors even within the first few months of life. This is particularly important in the case of severely premature infants in whom a high incidence of severe degrees of myopia has been detected early. It is not practical nor advisable for all healthy newborns to be referred for a refractive examination. However, in the case of the premature infant, early cycloplegic refraction should be undertaken in order to detect treatable refractive errors, even in patients who have not suffered from retinopathy of prematurity.

■ RETINOPATHY OF PREMATURITY

Retinopathy of prematurity (ROP), originally called retrolental fibroplasia by Terry in 1942, primarily affects premature infants weighing less than 1500 g at birth with a prevalence rate inversely proportional to birth weight. In infants <1000 g, some signs of retinopathy may be found in 40 to 70 per cent of the survivors (Table 115–2). ROP is a vasoproliferative retinal disorder that since its recognition in the 1950s has produced blindness in tens of thousands of premature infants. It is estimated that retinopathy of prematurity is responsible for producing some degree of visual loss in approximately 1300 children and severe visual loss in 500 children each year in the United States (Phelps, 1981).

Epidemiology. In 1951 Campbell published an uncontrolled clinical study that first suggested intensive oxygen therapy is an important etiologic factor. Subsequently, it became evident that infants at risk were rarely born after 33 weeks' gestational age and that some of them, particularly the most immature, could develop the changes of retinopathy of prematurity even in room air. There does not appear to be a given level of oxygen at which retinopathy has not occurred that is still compatible with postnatal life. It is, however, clear that the greater the duration of elevated oxygen tensions in the blood, the greater the risk of injury to the developing vascular structure of the retina (Kinsey et al., 1977). Attempts to restrict oxygen in very immature infants have led to an increase in mortality from their pulmonary immaturity and subsequent cyanosis (Avery and Oppenheimer, 1960). At least one infant whose congenital heart disease prevented arterial oxygen tensions to reach even normal levels was reported to have retrolental fibroplasia (Kalina et al., 1980).

Data collected during the recent multicenter, randomized prospective trial of cryotherapy in the treatment of acute retinopathy of prematurity clearly demonstrate variable frequencies of this disorder from one area of the country to another as well as from one hospital to another. It is unclear what economic, sociologic, or environmental factors may account for this dramatic difference in the incidence of retinopathy of prematurity.

Pathogenesis. The classic theory of pathogenesis of retinopathy of prematurity was proposed by Patz and colleagues (1953) and Ashton (1953). The proposal involves the following sequence of events: (1) vasoconstriction of the immature retinal vessels triggered by significantly elevated arterial Po_2 levels from supplemental oxygen administration; (2) vascular closure and subsequent permanent vascular occlusion if vasoconstriction is sustained; (3) upon return of the arterial Po_2 to levels from inspired ambient air, there is marked endothelial proliferation from residual vascular complexes adjacent to the vessels closed during the period of hyperoxia; (4) subsequent extension of these vasoproliferative elements within the retina and in some cases into the vitreous produces hemorrhages, promotes fibrous and glial tissue ingrowth with subsequent vitreoretinal traction, and ultimately, retinal detachment. This theory of pathogenesis has been tested in experimental animal models involving newborn kittens and dogs.

An alternative theory proposed by Kretzer and Hittner (1988) notes the importance of spindle cells in the vitreal neovascularization process. A complete understanding of the pathogenesis of this disorder awaits our isolation of factor S, which promotes neovascularization in the retina.

Diagnosis. The single most essential aspect of ophthalmic care in the newborn nursery is effective screening for retinopathy of prematurity and, when appropriate, treatment of the acute disorder with cryotherapy. Various recommendations regarding the timing of ocular examinations of infants have been proposed.

The American Academy of Pediatrics has recommended screening all infants of under 36 weeks' gestation or less than 2000 g who have received oxygen therapy. All infants under 1000 g at birth, even if they have not received oxygen therapy, should have an eye examination with indirect ophthalmoscopy between 4 and 8 weeks postnatally with a follow-up every 2 to 3 weeks if there is active disease. This recommendation has imposed an enormous burden on the ophthalmologists associated with neonatal intensive care units and probably is overly stringent. The question of whom to screen has been addressed by Brown and co-workers (1987), who found that cicatricial retinopathy of prematurity was found in 1.9 per cent of infants under 2 kg birth weight. They found no patients over 1.6 kg who had cicatricial disease unless exposed to oxygen in excess of room air for over 50 days. By changing the criteria for screening to less than 1.6 kg or to oxygen exposure over 50 days in larger infants, the

TABLE 115–2. Relation of Birth Weight to the Development of Retinopathy of Prematurity

BIRTH-WEIGHT GROUP (g)	n	SURVIVORS (per cent)	EXAM (per cent)	ROP (per cent)
501–750	343	40	89	81
751–1000	380	70	90	53
1001–1250	478	89	75	29
1251–1500	554	94	64	14

Note: 17 per cent of the infants with ROP had ≥ Stage 3.
(Results of 7-center study. Bandstra, E. S., Bauer, C. R., Onstad, L., et al.: Retinopathy of prematurity: Prevalance and clinical correlates in very-low-birth-weight (VLBW) infants. Pediatr. Res. (abstract) 27:239A, 1990.)

burden could be significantly reduced without endangering the vision of any infant. Although it is important to recognize the disease in its earliest stages, examination before 4 weeks' postnatal age is not essential since most infants are first detected between 7 and 9 weeks of age, and only 4.3 per cent after 15 weeks (Fig. 115–5).

Screening of premature infants for retinopathy of prematurity requires a dilated examination of the retina utilizing an indirect ophthalmoscope. Most authorities recommend a combination of Cyclomydril and phenylephrine in order to obtain pupillary dilatation.

Classification. In 1987, an international classification of retinopathy of prematurity was established replacing the earlier classification of Reese. This classification allows the examiner to specify two parameters of the disease: (1) its location and (2) the extent of developing vasculature involved.

Three zones of retinal involvement are recognized; each zone is centered on the optic disc rather than the macula. Zone 1 involves the posterior pole or inner zone, consisting of a circle whose radius subtends the angle of 30 degrees and extends from the disc to twice the distance from the disc to the center of the macula. Zone 2 is a middle area that extends from the edge of Zone 1 peripherally to a position tangential to the nasal ora serrata and around to an area near the temporal anatomic equator. Zone 3 is the outermost area that is the residual crescent of retina anterior to Zone 2. This area is primarily seen in the temporal retina, although it extends to the superior and inferior quadrants as well. This is the zone that is vascularized last in the eyes of premature infants, and it is the most frequently involved with retinopathy of prematurity.

The extent of involvement of the retinal vasculature may be indicated by the number of hours of the clock in which acute changes are noted. This is important in the staging of the disease and in determining whether or not it is appropriate to recommend therapy.

In staging the acute changes of retinopathy of prematurity the new classification identifies 5 distinct stages (Fig. 115–6): (1) a demarcation line, the initial feature of retinopathy of prematurity, is a thin but definite structure that separates the avascular retina anteriorly from the vascular retina posteriorly. (2) Stage 2, the ridge, the demarcation line Stage 1 now grows, exhibits height and width, and occupies a volume. It extends up onto the plane of the retina. (3) Stage 3, the ridge with extraretinal

fibrovascular proliferation. At the next level of severity, extraretinal fibrovascular proliferation tissue is seen in addition to the ridge. This is the most important stage to identify, as the new data from cryotherapy studies suggest that this is the appropriate stage in which to consider therapy. (4) Stage 4, retinal detachment. At this level of severity there is unequivocal detachment of the retina. The retinal detachment may be associated with exudative traction or fluid changes. (5) Total retinal detachment, Stage 5, is always a funnel-shaped total retinal detachment. In addition to these changes the term "plus disease" is used to identify those cases in which an inflammatory-like component of the disorder is noted. In these patients poor pupillary dilatation, often secondary to iris vascular engorgement, and synechiae are noted. The vitreous may be extremely hazy, and detailed examination of the retina difficult. Most studies indicate that patients with plus disease have a much more severe outcome than those who do not show these changes.

Prevention. An effective means for totally preventing retinopathy of prematurity remains to be found. Efforts aimed at monitoring oxygen tension in the newborn are discussed in Chapter 52. Respiratory monitoring guidelines are listed in Table 115–3. Although the careful control of oxygen therapy obviously has some effect on the prevalence rate of retinopathy of prematurity, this factor alone does not account for the disease. Recent trials of vitamin E, selenium, and steroids in the nursery have not proven to be efficacious in the prevention of retinopathy of prematurity.

Treatment. A randomized trial sponsored by the Cryotherapy for ROP Cooperative Group (1988) for the investigation of cryotherapy in the treatment of acute retinopathy of prematurity found that those patients who reach Stage 3 should undergo careful cryotherapy treatment. Preliminary data suggest that the incidence of retinal detachment is reduced by 50 per cent with this therapy. Although long-term functional results of this trial are still awaited, the preliminary anatomic results justify the judicious use of cryotherapy in the treatment of acute retinopathy of prematurity that reaches the threshold criteria established by the study. Additional studies are under way to investigate whether therapy should be initiated earlier than Stage 3 in selected patients. Moreover, some authorities in this country feel that the endolaser technology may provide more effective means of treating the disease and eventually replace cryotherapy.

Although the data from the cryotherapy study are encouraging, 25 per cent of the treated patients went on to experience some significant retinal detachment. The use of vitrectomy techniques to approach the cicatricial phase of retinopathy of prematurity has produced mixed results. Successful anatomic reattachment of the retina may be accomplished in some of these severely damaged eyes, but functional results from these patients have been disappointing. At the present time the use of vitrectomy, lensectomy, and buckling therapy techniques has proved to be disappointing. Some patients without complete funnel retinal detachment may be benefited by surgery.

Prognosis. A significant number of infants with ROP

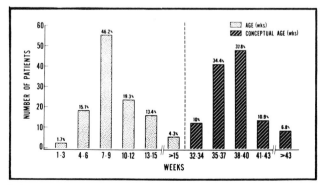

FIGURE 115–5. Time of diagnosis of retinopathy of prematurity (postnatal age-light shading; postconceptual age-dark shading). (From Flynn, J. T.: J. Pediatr. Ophthalmol. Strabismus 24:215, 1987.)

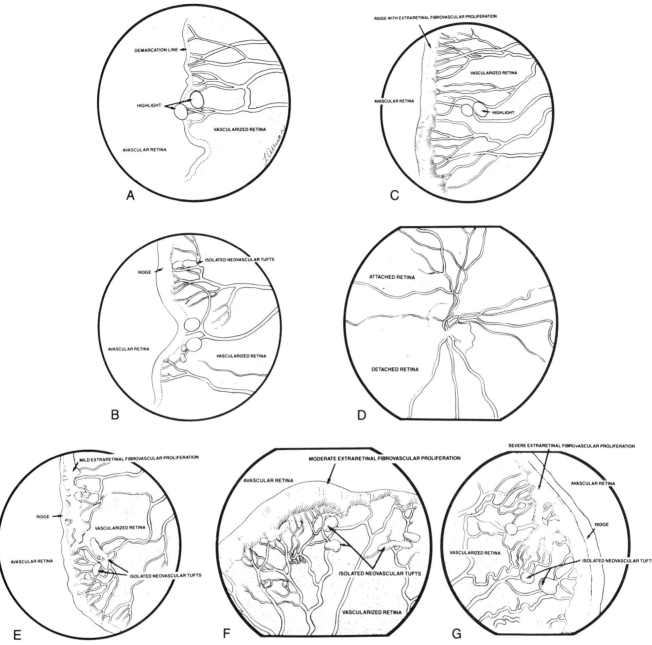

FIGURE 115–6. *Line drawings of stages 1–4 retinal lesions in retinopathy of prematurity. A, Stage 1. B, Stage 2. C, Stage 3. D, Stage 4. E, Mild stage 3. F, Moderate stage 3. G, Severe stage 3. (Reproduced with permission from Patz, A.: An international classification of retinopathy of prematurity. Pediatrics 74:127, 1984.)*

will have regression of their disease without therapy. However, the question of the long-term ophthalmologic morbidity of premature infants with and without retinopathy of prematurity was studied by Cats and Tan (1989) in 42 infants age 6 to 10 years, who had had regression of their retinopathy of prematurity, compared with 42 infants of like birth weight (1075 g versus 1160 g), who did not have any retinopathy detected in the newborn period. They found that 55 per cent of the preterm infants with regressed retinopathy of prematurity in follow-up had strabismus, amblyopia, or significant refraction anomalies. They were surprised to note that 36 per cent of the matched controls also had similar vision problems, con-

firming the general impression that all preterm infants are at risk for later visual problems. Therefore, it is imperative that all small preterm infants, particularly those with any degree of ROP, be followed carefully by an ophthalmologist familiar with the complications of ROP (Cats and Tan, 1989).

■ CONGENITAL CATARACTS

True congenital cataracts, defined as an opacity in the lens that limits vision, are rare at birth. Although the vast majority are sporadic, cataracts may occur as an isolated genetically determined abnormality that may be either

TABLE 115–3. Guidelines for Use of Blood Gas Monitoring

CLINICAL SITUATION	PREFERRED TECHNOLOGY	SUPPLEMENTAL MONITORING	RATIONALE
Acutely ill premature infant	Pulse oximetry: $StcO_2$ 87–92 optimal	ABG via arterial line $PtcO_2$ if $StcO_2$ >95 per cent	Major concern is hypoxemia. Pulse oximetry minimizes invasiveness and cost, but risks hyperoxia; supplemental monitoring is therefore essential.
Chronically ill premature infants with bronchopulmonary dysplasia	Pulse oximetry: $StcO_2$ 87–92 optimal, 85–95 acceptable	Periodic arterial blood gases (ABGs) by arterial puncture to correlate. Complete blood gases (CBGs) if only CO_2 is of concern	Major concern is hypoxemia. Hyperoxia less worrisome if ROP risk low, but chronic excessive oxygen must be avoided. $PtcO_2$ shown to be less accurate in older infants.
Premature infant with normal lung function on room air (e.g., apnea)	Pulse oximetry: $StcO_2 \geq 87$	ABG or CBG to correlate and to check CO_2	Hyperoxia risk negligible. Pulse oximetry to monitor for hypoxemia. Periodic blood gases to evaluate CO_2.
Acutely ill term infants with pneumonia/aspiration	Transcutaneous: $PtcO_2$ 60–80, or pulse oximetry $StcO_2$ 87–92	Pre- and postductal $PtcO_2$ if concerned about pulmonary hypertension. ABGs by arterial line to correlate and monitor CO_2. $PtcCO_2$ may be helpful if hyperventilating.	Higher PaO_2 goals used in treating pulmonary hypertension make $PtcO_2$ preferable. Dual pre- and postductal monitoring informative of shunt.

(From Richardson, D. K., and Stark, A. R.: Blood gas monitoring. *In* Cloherty, J. R., and Stark, A. R. (Eds.): Manual of Neonatal Care. 3rd ed. Boston, Little, Brown & Co. (in press).)

dominant or recessive. More commonly, cataracts are associated with chromosomal disorders, particularly trisomies 13, 18, and 21, and occasionally the Turner syndrome. Congenital infections, especially rubella, are notorious for their association with cataracts, and in the case of rubella, also glaucoma.

Metabolic disorders may be associated with cataracts, particularly galactosemia, which are, in turn, associated with galactose-1-phosphate uridyl transferase deficiency. Occasionally, cataracts are found in association with ectodermal dysplasia and congenital ichthyosis. When sporadic congenital cataracts are found, the chance of their appearance in subsequent siblings is about 1 in 40 (Fig. 115–7).

Natural History. Cataracts associated with galactosemia may be prevented with early diagnosis and a strict elimination diet. In a follow-up study, Burke and co-workers (1989) reported that cataracts had been prevented in 13 of 17 children with transferase-deficient galactosemia.

Treatment. With monocular congenital cataracts, surgical removal should be undertaken as soon as diagnosis is made to prevent loss of vision in the affected eye (Robb and Rodier, 1987). In the instance of bilateral cataracts, early removal in the most affected eye is also encouraged. Young infants manage to tolerate contact lenses as early as 3 or 4 weeks of age, or as soon as the cataract is removed.

Prognosis. In a review of a 32-year experience with 97 children in British Columbia who were visually impaired as the result of a primary diagnosis of bilateral cataracts, 90 were diagnosed as having congenital cataracts, and seven were acquired. Prenatal infection was the leading cause (35 cases), and 22 were hereditary, 9 were metabolic or traumatic, and 30 were of unknown cause. Since the wide use of rubella vaccine, prenatal infection is an uncommon cause of cataracts. A full neurodevelop-

mental assessment in childhood is warranted in any child with congenital cataracts. In retrospect, this Canadian experience shows the peak time of diagnosis to be between 2 and 3 months, most frequently on the basis of parental suspicion (Pike et al., 1989). (See also the discussion of amblyopia in this chapter.)

■ INFECTIOUS DISEASES

CONJUNCTIVITIS

Although the incidence of acute conjunctivitis in the newborn has been drastically reduced in the past several decades, the potentially devastating visual consequences of acute conjunctival infections in the first few days of life cannot be minimized. The etiologic cause of conjunctivitis in the newborn may be bacterial, viral, or a chemical response to the prophylactic use of 1 per cent silver nitrate. Knowing the time of onset of the conjunctivitis is occasionally helpful in establishing the appropriate diagnosis (Table 115–4). Silver nitrate conjunctivitis typically occurs within the first 24 hours after birth. Gonococcal conjunctivitis, in contrast, usually is not apparent until the 2nd or 3rd day of life. Cases that have been delayed beyond this period of time have, however, been reported,

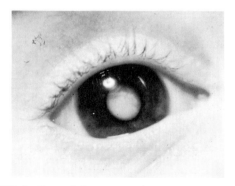

FIGURE 115–7. *Congenital cataract. The opaque lens stands out sharply. (From the collection of Dr. Arnall Patz.)*

TABLE 115–4. Differential Diagnostic Features of Conjunctivitis

AGENT	ONSET	RESOLVES	COMMENT
AgNO₃	Several hours after instillation	24–36 hours	AgNO₃ effective against gonococcus but not *Chlamydia*
Bacterial gonococcus	2–4 days after birth	In days with treatment	Marked purulent discharge and edema
Chlamydia	5–12 days after birth	Days to a few weeks	Mild mucopurulent discharge, basophilic intracytoplasmic inclusions in scrapings; may be associated with pneumonia (later onset)
Other bacteria	Any time	In days with treatment	Mild "sticky lids" to acute purulent inflammation, one or both eyes
Viral	Any time, initially in one eye	4 days to 2 weeks	May be associated with corneal changes
Herpes simplex	Any time, unilateral	About 1 week or may be recurrent	Often associated with skin lesions, steroids contraindicated
Allergic	In association with other symptoms most common in spring	As allergies resolved—about 1 week	Itching followed by mild redness and tearing; "ropy" secretions; cobblestone papillas in vernal type

(From Avery, M. E., and First, L. R.: Pediatric Medicine. Baltimore, Williams & Wilkins, 1989.)

particularly if the patient has received silver nitrate prophylaxis. Other forms of bacterial conjunctivitis usually become apparent after 3 or more days of life. Chlamydial conjunctivitis occurs 5 to 21 days after birth. As will be readily apparent in studying these figures, there is enough overlap in the time of onset of conjunctivitis with different etiologic causes to mandate that all newborns with conjunctivitis be carefully evaluated with conjunctival cultures and that specific therapy be prescribed when indicated. Because of the rapid penetration of gonococcal infection in the eye often leading to perforation of the globe within 24 hours, all forms of conjunctivitis must be considered bacterial until proved otherwise, and gonococcal prophylaxis needs to be initiated even while specific cultures, scrapings, and bacterial and microscopic examinations of the exudate are examined.

Considerable controversy surrounds the routine use of silver nitrate drops as prophylaxis to prevent gonococcal infection. The emergence of chlamydial infection as a major cause of neonatal ophthalmic infection, an infection resistant to silver nitrate, has prompted neonatologists, pediatricians, and ophthalmologists to review the policy of routine use of silver nitrate in the nursery. Acceptable alternative prophylactic agents include erythromycin, 0.1 to 0.5 per cent ointment or drops, and tetracycline, 1 per cent ointment or drops, given as a single topical application to the eyes immediately post partum. Nevertheless, recent reports have clearly indicated that, even with appropriate use of these prophylactic agents, serious ophthalmic infections may still occur.

GONOCOCCAL CONJUNCTIVITIS

The most severe form of bacterial conjunctivitis in the neonatal period is secondary to *N. gonorrheae* (Fig. 115–8). This is a hyperacute purulent conjunctivitis characterized by bilateral involvement, marked edema of the lids with chemosis, and copious discharge of pus. Perforation of the globe may occur within the first 24 hours, and the eye may be affected by an infection that involves all layers of the external and internal portions of the eye. Conjunctival smears and scrapings show gram-negative intracellular diplococci, clearly distinguishing this infection from chlamydial or staphylococcal diseases. Most authorities recommend the use of intravenous aqueous penicillin, 50,000 to 100,000 U/kg/day in two to four doses for one

week. Second- and third-generation cephalosporin antibiotics may be appropriate in cases of penicillinase-producing gonococcal infections. Pseudogonococcal infection may occur with *Branhamella catarrhalis*. Any common bacterial pathogen may also cause conjunctivitis in the newborn period (Table 115–5).

STAPHYLOCOCCAL CONJUNCTIVITIS

Staphylococcal conjunctivitis, which is usually nosocomially acquired, may occur within the 1st postnatal week and is usually manifested by profuse mucoid discharge and conjunctival hyperemia and chemosis. Treatment consists of lid hygiene and 0.5 per cent erythromycin ophthalmic ointment or bacitracin eye ointment applied six times per day for 2 weeks. Despite the usually innocuous course of this conjunctivitis, corneal infection after mild corneal epithelial trauma may lead to rapid corneal perforation. The scalded skin syndrome has been reported following staphylococcal conjunctivitis.

CHLAMYDIAL CONJUNCTIVITIS

An obligate intracellular organism is now the most common infectious cause in the newborn. *Chlamydia* is resistant to silver nitrate. Although the disease is characterized by a purulent discharge, this is usually not as

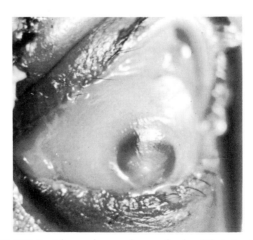

FIGURE 115–8. Advanced case of gonorrheal ophthalmia. Note the intense panophthalmitis with reddening and thickening of both the bulbar and the tarsal conjunctivae and ulceration of the cornea and sclera. (From the collection of Dr. Arnall Patz.)

TABLE 115–5. Frequency of Bacterial and Chlamydial Isolation in Cases of Infectious Ophthalmia Neonatorum*

PATHOGEN	REPORTED INCIDENCE (per cent)
Chlamydia trachomatis	10–43
Staphylococcus aureus	5–27
Neisseria gonorrhoeae	4–14
Streptococcus sp. viridans group	1–29
Hemophilus species	5–14
Streptococcus pneumoniae	5–6
Escherichia coli	2–5
Branhamella catarrhalis	1–5
Mycoplasma hominis	3
Streptococcus sp. group D	3
Corynebacterium sp	2
Pseudomonas aeruginosa	1

*Includes pathogens isolated from cases of ophthalmia neonatorum in the absence of other organisms and that have been reported in more than one series or identified in more than one patient in single large series.

(From Holland, G. N.: Infectious diseases. *In* Isenberg, S. J. (Ed.): The Eye in Infancy. Chicago, Year Book Medical Publishers, 1989.)

marked as in gonococcal infections. Premature infants appear to be particularly susceptible to this disorder. Conjunctival scrapings show a basophilic granular intracytoplasmic inclusion in epithelial cells in more than 90 per cent of the cases. Ocular sequelae are unusual. A mild conjunctival scarring may occur. Because of the risk of associated pneumonitis, treatment of affected infants usually includes both topical and systemic therapy. Intravenous erythromycin, 50 mg/kg/day in four divided doses for at least 2 weeks, and topical 1 per cent tetracycline or 0.5 per cent erythromycin ointment, four times a day for 2 weeks, is recommended.

HERPES SIMPLEX KERATOCONJUNCTIVITIS

The incidence of herpes simplex in neonatal conjunctivitis is low but is increasing with the increased incidence of genital herpes infection. The herpes simplex virus type 2 responsible for this conjunctivitis may result in unilateral or bilateral conjunctivitis (nonfollicular in the newborn), which may be associated with lid vesicles and corneal epithelial dendritic figures. The occurrence of either of these conditions should establish the clinical diagnosis, which may be supported by demonstration of cytopathic effects on cell cultures inoculated by a cottontip swab drawn across the conjunctival surface and transported immediately in viral transport media to the laboratory. Scrapings taken from the conjunctival surface may reveal giant cells with intracytoplasmic inclusions. Sequential serology may reveal a rising neutralizing antibody titer. Treatment should consist of administration of 3 per cent vidarabine ointment, five times per day for 10 days, or 1 per cent idoxuridine ointment, five times per day for 10 days, or 1 per cent trifluorothymidine drops every 2 hours, seven doses per day for 10 days. The association of recurrent corneal herpetic disease following a primary follicular conjunctivitis with herpes simplex virus type 2 infection is unclear.

PERIORBITAL AND ORBITAL CELLULITIS

Orbital cellulitis is an infection presenting with reduced ocular motility, proptosis, and chemosis of the conjunctiva;

pain should initiate a radiologic search for sinus infection. Intravenous antibiotics should be administered and are usually sufficient. If an abscess is suspected, drainage should be performed as a matter of urgency.

Periorbital cellulitis is more frequent and denotes infection around the eye, including the lid and adjacent tissues. It is almost always unilateral and can occur at any age. When it is present in the first month of life, *Hemophilus* species (often *H. influenzae* type B) is most common, but beta-hemolytic *Streptococcus* or *Staphylococcus aureus* and a wide variety of other organisms may be etiologic.

In a series of 30 cases in infants under 1 month of age reported from Harbor-UCLA, 10 per cent were secondary to local skin lesions, 63 per cent were preceded by upper respiratory infections, 7 per cent had a ruptured dacryocele, and 3 per cent had dacryocystitis. Seventeen per cent were of unknown cause. Eight of the 30 infants had bacteremia (Molarte and Isenberg, 1989).

Except in very mild cases, intravenous antibiotics are appropriate in order to avoid orbital spread of infection. Treatment should continue until resolution is complete, which is usually a few days in periorbital infection or 7 to 10 days in orbital infection. If the cellulitis responds promptly, no further studies are indicated. If the response is poor, CT scans may demonstrate spread to other areas.

UVEITIS

Uveitis, or chorioretinitis, is a chronic prenatal or perinatal intraocular inflammation with a group of organisms considered under the acronym TORCH. The most common of these is congenital toxoplasmosis, which may produce systemic disease in addition to the chorioretinitis, which is present in about 80 per cent of diagnosed cases. Most affected infants are asymptomatic at birth, but identified several months or years later (Sever et al., 1988). In addition to toxoplasmosis, the TORCH complex includes rubella, cytomegalic inclusion disease, and herpes simplex virus infections as well as congenital syphilis (the fetus is at risk of infection with *Treponema pallidum* between the 5th and the 9th months of pregnancy).

Although rarely seen in recent years, a resurgence in congenital syphilis may be noted soon because 41,300 new cases of syphilis in adults were reported by the CDC in 1989.

Diagnosis. Chorioretinitis may be seen at birth but often is not evident until approximately 10 days of age, by which time the red reflexes from the retina are likely to be diminished. Many of these infections have major systemic problems, including hepatosplenomegaly and bone lesions, and often microphthalmos is a complication of the eye infection. Occasionally, glaucoma may coexist with infection of the uveal tract. It occurs in about 10 per cent of those infants with congenital rubella syndrome.

The laboratory work-up of an infant suspected of having one of the TORCH infections would be IgM ELISA for toxoplasmosis, a urine culture for cytomegalic virus, and pharyngeal and conjunctival cultures for herpes simplex. A genital culture from the mother is also appropriate if herpes is suspected. The infant should have a CSF examination because of the possible coexistence of encephalomyelitis and a skull film for the presence of intracranial calcifications.

Treatment. The treatment of uveitis is with cycloplegics to lessen the incidence of synechiae and topical steroid therapy to suppress inflammation.

Pyrimethamine and sulfonamides are the most commonly used chemotherapeutic agents for infants over 1 week of age with toxoplasmosis. Although treatment may halt the progression of lesions, recurrences may appear even into adulthood.

■ TUMORS

Tumors of the eyelids are rarely noted at birth. Facial hemangiomas (port wine stains), such as those found in the distribution of the fifth cranial nerve on one side (as in Sturge-Weber syndrome), may involve the lid or conjunctiva on the same side. Glaucoma often occurs in the affected eye. If glaucoma is present, goniotomy is the initial procedure of choice.

Angiomatous tumors may be small "strawberry" marks (capillary hemangiomas) or large "cauliflower-like" masses that typically progress over the first months of life and then become static, fluctuate, and eventually regress between 3 and 7 years of age. When they involve the upper eyelid, they can cause amblyopia. If they interfere with vision, local or systemic glucocorticoid therapy may be considered and is associated with a prompt regression in about a third of the tumors. Dexamethasone (2 mg/kg/day) for 2 to 3 weeks will reduce the size of the hemangiomas and can then be slowly tapered. If there is no change after 3 weeks, other forms of therapy are indicated.

Interferon alfa-2a has been effective in reducing the size of tumors in pulmonary hemangiomatosis and is being evaluated for possible beneficial effect in facial hemangiomas (White et al., 1989).

Neurofibromas, dermoid cysts, and rhabdomyosarcomas should be considered when an abnormal mass appears in the orbit or lids in infancy.

■ OTHER NEONATAL DISORDERS OF THE EYE

INFANTILE GLAUCOMA

Glaucoma occurring in the newborn is a potentially blinding disease and requires emergency treatment. It is considered to be of a multifactorial inheritance pattern, although there are certain congenital anomalies (e.g., Sturge-Weber syndrome, aniridia, and mesodermal dysgenesis) that have a definite inheritance pattern, which is usually autosomal dominant. Corneal diameter measurements are also imperative (Fig. 115–9). Unfortunately, two of the principal parameters in adult glaucoma either cannot be obtained or are not reliable in congenital infantile glaucoma. First, the cup-to-disc ratio in the eye may be greater than 1:3 in normal children, and the disc is frequently not grossly excavated until advanced glaucoma is present. Second, visual field testing cannot be performed in young infants. A generally accepted upper level of intraocular pressure, as measured by applanation tonometry, is 17 mm Hg in newborns.

Treatment of this condition is primarily surgical. Goniotomy is the principal mode of operative therapy and is aimed at increasing the facility of outflow of aqueous humor through the angle structures, since obstruction of this flow is thought to be the primary cause of the glaucoma. Whether this blockage is due to an abnormal membrane across the angle of the eye or to developmental anomalies, such as abnormal insertions of ciliary muscles, remains unclear.

Children with this form of glaucoma require careful and frequent follow-up examinations performed after the administration of general anesthesia. Of those children tested after the age of 5 years, approximately 40 per cent obtain better than 20/40 vision if pressure is satisfactorily controlled. Early surgical therapy would appear to control the pressure in 85 per cent of the children in whom the diagnosis is made and in whom treatment is initiated before the age of 1 year.

EVERSION OF THE EYELIDS

The eyelids of the newborn may be everted at birth secondary to microphthalmos, buphthalmos, lid defects, or other abnormalities of the eyes. Primary eversion, without a discoverable contributing cause, has been reported only a few times. The tarsal conjunctivae, facing outward, are chemotic and hyperemic (Fig. 115–10). There is no history of obstetric difficulties or other ocular abnormalities. The lids return to normal in a few weeks, following the application of an ophthalmic ointment and moist, sterile gauze dressings.

NASOLACRIMAL DUCT OBSTRUCTION

The infant with a mucopurulent discharge must be carefully distinguished from the infant who demonstrates only excessive tearing with no apparent involvement of infection of the eye. The child with excessive tearing most likely represents a patient with nasolacrimal duct obstruction, although the possibility of glaucoma must always be ruled out. Congenital obstruction of the nasolacrimal duct is an extremely common disorder with a high spontaneous resolution rate. It is said to occur in 1 to 6 per cent of newborns and is most common in firstborn children. Obstruction is commonly unilateral or asymmetric. As a consequence of obstruction, secondary infection may occur with a dacryocystitis resulting (Fig. 115–11). This presents as a tender swelling of the skin overlying the lacrimal sac and adjacent eyelids. Pressure on the lacrimal sac causes a reflux of pus from the punctum in these cases. Acute or chronic conjunctivitis and keratitis may therefore be associated in these cases. Congenital obstruction of the nasolacrimal drainage system usually resolves spontaneously within the 1st year of life. Conservative management is indicated if dacryocystitis is not noted. Parental massage of the lacrimal sacs several times a day and the use of a topical antibiotic for conjunctival irritation, if noted, is usually effective. When the obstruction fails to resolve by 9 to 12 months of age, referral to an ophthalmologist for consideration of nasolacrimal duct probing should be undertaken.

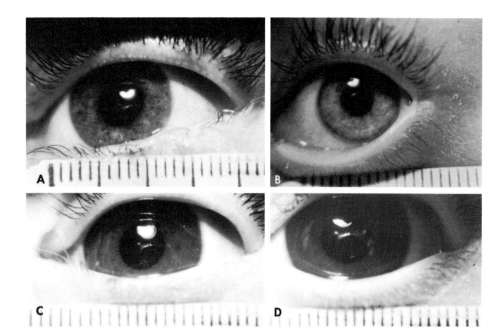

FIGURE 115–9. A, Normal eyeball with cornea of normal size. It measures 10 mm in diameter. B, Small eyeball with microcornea, measuring 6.5 mm across. This photograph is included for comparison and contrast. C, Early glaucoma, without hazing of cornea or tearing of Descemet membrane. The cornea is 13.5 mm wide. D, Early glaucoma; cornea is 14.0 mm in diameter. (From the collection of Dr. Arnall Patz.)

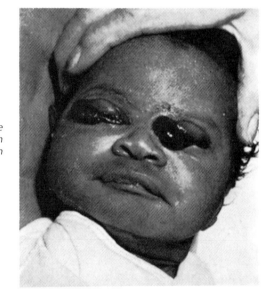

FIGURE 115–10. At 10 days of life, note the marked edema of both conjunctivae of the upper lids while the eversion of the lids has practically returned to normal. (From Stillerman, M. L., Emanuel, B., and Padorr, M. P.: Eversion of the eyelids in the newborn without an apparent cause. J. Pediatr. 69:656, 1966.)

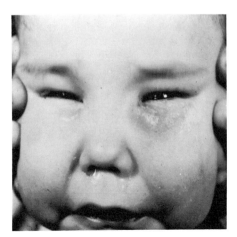

FIGURE 115–11. Acute dacryocystitis. Note the swollen, reddened lower lid and the cystic swelling in the angle between the eye and the bridge of the nose. (From the collection of Dr. Arnall Patz.)

TABLE 115–6. Colobomas Associated with Multisystem Disease

NAME	INHERITANCE	OTHER FINDINGS
Lenz syndrome	X-linked recessive	Microphthalmos, dysmorphic ears, short stature, mental retardation.
Aicardi syndrome	X-linked dominant (only in females)	Optic disc colobomas, microphthalmos, vertebral anomalies, absent corpus callosum.
Warburg syndrome	Autosomal recessive	Many ocular and CNS abnormalities, profound mental retardation, poor prognosis for life.
Meckel syndrome	Autosomal recessive	Retinal dysplasia, microcephaly, polycystic kidney, liver and pancreatic disease.
CHARGE association	Mostly sporadic	Coloboma, *heart defect*, atresia choanae, *retarded growth*, genital hypoplasia, ear anomalies, deafness.
Trisomy 13, Patau syndrome		Severe CNS abnormalities.
Cat-eye syndrome (extra fragments chromosomes 22 and 13 or 14)		Imperforate anus and renal malformations.
Trisomy 18 (Edwards syndrome)		Hypertelorism, microphthalmos, corneal opacities, glaucoma, rocker-bottom feet, low-set ears.
Triploidy (69 chromosomes)		Marked craniofacial abnormalities, syndactyly, heart defects, renal dysplasia.
Rubinstein-Taybi syndrome		Cataracts, broad thumb and big toe, beaked nose, hypoplasia of the maxilla.
Goldenhar syndrome (sporadic)		Epibulbar dermoid, accessory auricular appendages, aural fistula, microphthalmos.

(Modified from Pagon, R.: Ocular coloboma. Surv. Ophthalmol. 25:223–236, 1981.)

COLOBOMA

A notch or gap in the iris, called a coloboma, is a congenital defect that results from arrest of normal embryonic fissure closure at 4 to 6 weeks' gestation. Most colobomas are inferior in location and rarely disturb vision. They are usually sporadic, but some are transmitted as an autosomal dominant trait. They may be associated with multisystem disorders (Table 115–6) (Singh and Gupta, 1986).

■ REFERENCES

Ashton, N., Ward, B., Serpell, G., et al.: Role of oxygen in the genesis of retrolental fibroplasia. Brit. J. Ophthalmol. 37:513–520, 1953.

Avery, M. E., and First, L. R.: Pediatric Medicine. Baltimore, Williams & Wilkins, 1989.

Avery, M. E., and Oppenheimer, E. H.: Recent increase in mortality from hyaline membrane disease. J. Pediatr. 57:553, 1960.

Baker, J. D., and Parks, N. M.: Early onset accommodative esotropia. Am. J. Ophthalmol. 90:11–15, 1980.

Bandstra, E. S., Bauer, C. R., Onstad, L., et al.: Retinopathy of prematurity: Prevalence and clinical correlates in very-low-birth-weight (VLBW) infants. Pediatr. Res. (abstract) 27:239A, 1990.

Beller, R., Hoyt, C. S., Marg, E., et al.: Good visual function after neonatal surgery for congenital monocular cataracts. Am. J. Ophthalmol. 91:559–567, 1981.

Brown, D. R., Biglan, A. W., and Stretavsky, M. A. M.: Screening criteria for the detection of retinopathy of prematurity in patients in a neonatal intensive care unit. J. Pediatr. Ophthal. Strabis. 24:212, 1987.

Burke, J. P., O'Keefe, M., Bowell, R., et al.: Ophthalmic findings in classical galactosemia—a screened population. J. Pediatr. Ophthal. Strabis. 26:165, 1989.

Campbell, K.: Intensive oxygen therapy as a possible cause of retrolental fibroplasia: A clinical approach. Med. J. Aust. 2:48–50, 1951.

Cats, B. P., and Tan, K. E. W. P.: Prematures with and without regressed retinopathy of prematurity: Comparison of long-term (6–10 years) ophthalmological morbidity. J. Pediatr. Ophthal. Strabis. 26:271, 1989.

Clarke, W. N., Bastianelli, F., and Noel, L. P.: Lacrimal hypersecretion in children. J. Pediatr. Ophthalmol. Strabis. 24:204, 1987.

Cryotherapy for Retinopathy of Prematurity Cooperative Group: Multicenter trial of cryotherapy for retinopathy of prematurity. Arch. Ophthalmol. 106:471, 1988.

Dear, P. R. F.: Monitoring oxygen in the newborn: Saturation or partial pressure. Arch. Dis. Child. 62:879, 1987.

Eisenberg, S. J., and Apt, L.: Bacterial flora of the conjunctiva at birth. J. Pediatr. Ophthalmol. 23:284–288, 1986.

Gelbart, S. S., and Hoyt, C. S.: Congenital nystagmus: A clinical perspective in infancy. Graefes's Arch. Clin. Exp. Ophthalmol. 226:178–180, 1988.

Gibson, D. L., Sheps, S. B., Uh, S. H.: Retinopathy of prematurity–induced blindness: Birth weight–specific survival the new epidemic. Pediatrics 86:405, 1990.

Gund, T. R.: Risk factor in retrolental fibroplasia. Pediatrics 6:1096–1098, 1980.

Hammerschlag, M. R.: Neonatal ocular prophylaxis. Pediatr. Inf. Dis. 7:81, 1988.

Hammerschlag, M. R., Cummings, C., Roblin, P. M., et al.: Efficacy of neonatal ocular prophylaxis for the prevention of chlamydial and gonococcal conjunctivitis. N. Engl. J. Med. 320:769, 1989.

Hered, R. W., Rogers, S., Zang, U. F., et al.: Ophthalmologic features of Prader-Willi syndrome. J. Pediatr. Ophthal. Strabis. 25:145, 1988.

Holland, G. N.: Infectious Diseases. In Isenberg, S. J. (Ed.): The Eye in Infancy. Chicago, Year Book Medical Publishers, 1989.

Hoyt, C. S., Mousel, D. K., and Weber, A. A.: Transient supranuclear disturbances of gaze in healthy neonates. Am. J. Ophthalmol. 89:708–713, 1980.

Hoyt, C. S., Nickel, B. L., and Billson, F. A.: Ophthalmologic examination of the infant. Developmental aspects. Surv. Ophthalmol. 26:177–189, 1982.

International Classification of Retinopathy of Prematurity. Arch. Ophthal. 105:906, 1987.

Isenberg, S. J.: The Eye in Infancy. Chicago, Year Book Medical Publishers, 1989.

Kalina, R. E.: Treatment of retrolental fibroplasia. Surv. Ophthalmol. 24:229–236, 1980.

Kinsey, V. E., Arnold, H. J., Kalina, R. E., et al.: PaO$_2$ levels and retrolental fibroplasia: A report of the cooperative study. Pediatrics 60:655, 1977.

Kretzer, F. L., and Hittner, H. M.: Retinopathy of prematurity. Arch. Dis. Child 63:1151, 1988.

Magoon, E. H., and Scott, A. B.: Botulinum toxic chemodenervation in infants and children: an alternative to incisional strabismus surgery. J. Pediatr. 110:719, 1987.

Maskin, S. L., and Yee, R. W.: Use of impression cytology in neonatal chlamydial conjunctivitis. Arch. Ophthalmol. 105:1626–1639, 1987.

Molarte, A. B., and Isenberg, S. J.: Periorbital cellulitis in infancy. J. Pediatr. Ophthal. Strabis. 26:232, 1989.

Molgaard, I. L., Nielsen, P. B., and Kaern, J.: A study of the incidence of neonatal conjunctivitis and its bacterial causes, including chlamydia. Acta Ophthalmol. 62:461–471, 1984.

Multicenter trial of cryotherapy for retinopathy of prematurity. Three month outcome. Arch. Ophthal. 108:195, 1990.

Neumann, E., Friedman, Z., and Abel-Peleg, B.: Prevention of strabismic amblyopia of early onset with special reference to the optimal age for screening. J. Pediatr. Ophthal. Strabis. 24:106, 1987.

Palmer, E. A.: Multicenter trial of cryotherapy for retinopathy of prematurity. Pediatrics 77:428, 1986.

Patz, A., Eastham, A., Higginbotham, D. H., et al.: Oxygen studies in retrolental fibroplasia in experimental animals. Am. J. Ophthalmol. 36:1511, 1953.

Petersen, R. A., and Robb, R. M.: The natural course of congenital obstruction of the nasolacrimal duct. J. Pediatr. Ophthalmol. Strabis. 15:246, 1978.

Phelps, D. L.: Retinopathy of prematurity: An estimate of visual loss in the United States, 1979. Pediatrics 67:924–926, 1981.

Pike, M. G., Jan, J. E., and Wong, P. K. H.: Neurological and developmental findings in children with cataracts. Am. J. Dis. Child. 143:706, 1989.

Raisner, S. H., and Perlman, N.: Transient lateral rectus paresis in the newborn infant. J. Pediatr. 78:461–464, 1971.

Rathy, I.: Development of a simultaneous fixation from the divergent anatomic eye position of the neonate. J. Pediatr. Ophthalmol. 6:92–95, 1969.

Reese, A. B., King, M. T., Owens, A.: Classification of retrolental fibroplasia. Am. J. Ophthalmol. 36:1333, 1953.

Robb, R. M., and Rodier, D. W.: The variable clinical characteristics and course of early infantile esotropia. J. Pediatr. Ophthal. Strabis. 24:276, 1987.

Sever, J. L., Ellenberg, J. H., Ley, A. C., et al.: Toxoplasmosis: Maternal and pediatric findings in 23,000 pregnancies. Pediatrics 82:181, 1988.

Silverman, W. A.: A New Affliction in Premature Infants in Retrolental Fibroplasia: A Modern Parable. New York, Grune & Stratten, 1983.

Singh, Y. P., and Gupta, S. L.: Congenital ocular abnormalities of the newborn. J. Pediatr. Ophthalmol. Strabis. 17:162, 1986.

Spierer, A., Isenberg, S. J., and Inkelis, S. H.: Characteristics of the iris in 100 neonates. J. Pediatr. Ophthal. Strabis. 26:28, 1989.

Stenson, S., and Newman, R.: Conjunctivitis in the newborn. Observations on incidence, cause, and prophylaxis. Ann. Ophthalmol. 13:329–334, 1981.

Tasman, W.: The natural history of active retinopathy of prematurity. Ophthalmology 91:1499–1503, 1984.

Terry, T. L.: Extreme prematurity and fibroplastic overgrowth of persistent vascular sheath behind each crystalline lens. I. Preliminary report. Am. J. Ophthalmol. 25:203, 1942.

White, C. W., Sondheimer, H. M., Crouch, E. C., et al.: Treatment of pulmonary hemangiomatosis with recombinant interferon alfa-2a. N. Engl. J. Med. 320:1197, 1989.

PART XX

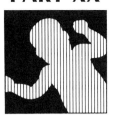

OTHER NEOPLASMS AND MISCELLANEOUS CONDITIONS

CONGENITAL MALIGNANT DISORDERS 116

Katherine K. Matthay*

Neonatal malignancies differ in incidence, clinical behavior, and heritable features from the cancers seen in older children. Exposure to potential carcinogens or teratogens during the prenatal period may be related etiologically. Special consideration must also be given to treatment problems peculiar to the newborn age group, including differences in drug metabolism and pharmacokinetics from older children and the possible intolerance of rapidly growing and developing normal tissues to the inhibitory effects of antineoplastic chemotherapy and radiation. Late effects on reproductive capacity, intellectual development, and induction of secondary malignancy are also of heightened concern in treating the newborn. The epidemiology of neonatal malignancy is reviewed here, followed by disease-specific discussions of the most commonly encountered malignancies in the newborn. Other malignancies specific to individual organ systems are discussed in appropriate sections of this book.

■ EPIDEMIOLOGY

INCIDENCE AND MORTALITY

A study of death certificates by Fraumeni and Miller during the 5-year period ranging from 1960 to 1964 revealed that the death rate from malignant diseases in infants younger than 28 days of age was 6.25 per 1 million live births (Table 116–1). Over one-half of cancer deaths in the neonatal period occurred in the first week of life, and over one-third occurred on the first day (Fraumeni and Miller, 1969).

Basing their report on the Third National Cancer Survey (1969–1971), Bader and Miller (1979) found the incidence of malignant neoplasms in the United States to be 183.4 per 1 million live births in infants younger than 1

year and 36.5 per 1 million live births in newborns younger than 29 days. The cancer incidence in those younger than 1 year was almost three and one-half times greater than mortality determined from death certificates from 1960 to 1969. When mortality of infants younger than age 1 year is used as an indicator of frequency, leukemia appears to be the most common cancer, followed by neuroblastoma, central nervous system tumors, and renal tumors. When ranked by incidence, neuroblastoma is most common, followed by leukemia, renal tumors, sarcomas, retinoblastomas, and central nervous system tumors. Because retinoblastoma is so often cured, the incidence is 159 times greater than the mortality.

Among newborns, the incidence of neuroblastoma is more than ten times greater than the mortality for this tumor, whereas the incidence of leukemia is less than two times greater than its mortality. Thus, a study of mortality differs markedly from one of incidence, since certain malignancies are rapidly fatal, others lead to death beyond the neonatal period, and a large number are curable or undergo spontaneous regression. Data from the Third National Cancer Study indicate that approximately 653 cancers are diagnosed annually in infants in the United States and that 130 of these cancers are found in newborns. A summary of incidence, mortality, and types of malignancies seen in the newborn and infant is shown in Table 116–2. A summary of four recently reported surveys from Los Angeles (Isaacs, 1985), Toronto (Campbell et al., 1987a), Memphis (Crom et al., 1989), and San Francisco (1990) is shown in Table 116–3. The relative frequencies of most types of malignancy are unchanged from those reported earlier (see Table 116–2), except for retinoblastoma, which is seen to occur more frequently than shown in Table 116–2, perhaps because of referral patterns at University of California—San Francisco and Hospital for Sick Children, Toronto.

*Revised from the chapter originally written by Allan P. Schwartz.

TABLE 116–1. Mortality From Malignant Neoplasms in United States Children Younger Than 5 Years As Compared with Those Younger Than 28 Days of Age, 1960–1964

| NEOPLASM | NO. DEATHS IN CHILDREN AGED YOUNGER THAN 5 YEARS | NO. DEATHS IN CHILDREN AGED YOUNGER THAN 28 DAYS | | |
		No.	Rate Per 10^6 Live Births	Per Cent*
Leukemia	4592	44	2.11	1.0
Neuroblastoma	1049	27	1.30	2.6
Brain tumor	1035	7	0.34	0.7
Wilms tumor	696	9	0.43	1.3
Liver cancer, primary	196	10	0.48	5.1
Teratoma	111	9	0.43	8.1
Sarcoma, type specified	1940	12	0.58	1.2
Other		12	0.58	
TOTAL	9619	130	6.25	1.4

*Percentage of neonatal deaths among type-specific cancers in patients younger than 5 years of age (e.g., for leukemia = [44 × 100]/4592 = 1.0).

(From Fraumeni, J. F., and Miller, R. W.: Cancer deaths in the newborn. Am. J. Dis. Child. *117*:186, 1969.)

■ PATHOGENESIS

TRANSPLACENTAL TUMOR PASSAGE

Few cases of malignant melanomas of the mother with spread to the fetus have been reported and reviewed (Anderson et al., 1989; Campbell et al., 1987b). The infant reported by Cavell (1963) recovered from the metastatic disease. Factors found to suggest an unfavorable fetal/infant outcome are maternal age younger than 30 years, primiparity, leg primary lesion, onset of disease more than 3 years prior to pregnancy, metastatic status prior to pregnancy, birth at more than 36 weeks' gestation, and male sex. Kasdon (1949) recorded two instances of Hodgkin's disease occurring in infants of mothers with the disorder. Maternal virilizing tumors have resulted in fetal virilization due to transplacental passage of androgens secreted by the neoplasm, but the tumors have not spread to the fetus (Haymond and Weldon, 1973). Multiple myeloma has been reported in a small number of pregnant women (Lergier et al., 1974). In two instances no abnormal myeloma protein was found in the infants, but a transient abnormal protein believed to be passively transferred from the mother was demonstrated in two others. None of the infants had evidence of disease.

Leukemia has not been found in newborns of women with this malignancy, although two children of affected mothers developed the disease at 5 and 9 months of age. In these instances, both mothers and children had acute lymphoblastic leukemia (Bernard et al., 1964; Cramblett et al., 1958). Although leukemia in mice can be transmitted to their offspring by viruses in breast milk, there is no evidence that leukemia is passed to the human infant in this manner.

The development of choriocarcinoma in an infant as a complication of placental choriocarcinoma is rare. In at least four instances, both mother and infant have been affected. This represents tumor transmission from the fetus to the mother because the trophoblast, the site of origin,

is composed of fetal rather than maternal tissue. In all the recorded cases, summarized by Witzleben and Bruninga (1968), there was either a recognized placental choriocarcinoma or absence of a primary site in the infants with disseminated malignancy. These authors stressed the characteristic presentation of hematemesis or hemoptysis, anemia, hepatomegaly, and pulmonary metastasis in the infant. The diagnosis is established by the demonstration of an elevated urinary or plasma gonadotropin.

ENVIRONMENTAL FACTORS

The review by Fraumeni and Miller (1969) showed no significant annual variation or aggregation of cases of neonatal cancers in the United States. A number of authors have reported that abdominal radiation to the mother during pregnancy increases the risk of the child in utero subsequently developing leukemia (Bithell and Stewart, 1975; Diamond et al., 1973), whereas others do not substantiate the existence of a relationship between prenatal x-ray exposure and childhood cancer (Totter and MacPherson, 1981). Children exposed prenatally to the atomic bombs in Hiroshima and Nagasaki have no significant excess of mortality from leukemia or other cancers. An epidemiologic study of 234 cases of childhood leukemia/lymphoma (McKinney et al., 1987) failed to reveal any significant association with prenatal x-ray exposure, maternal drug ingestion and smoking, or parental medical conditions or occupations.

In 1977, Herbst and co-workers reported that large doses of diethylstilbestrol (DES) given to pregnant women were related to the development of adenocarcinoma of the vagina in their daughters of that pregnancy from 14 to 22 years later. A relationship between exposure in utero to DES and its close synthetic analogues during the first half of pregnancy and the later development of clear cell adenocarcinoma of both vagina and cervix is now well established. According to the 1977 calculations of Herbst and colleagues, the risk of developing such tumors is 0.14 to 1.4 per 1000 DES-exposed females up until the age of 24 years. Melnick and co-workers (1987) reported the risk up to age 34 is 1 case per 1000. The tumors are rare in females younger than 14 years of age, but the frequency rises rapidly to a peak at age 17 to 22 years, after which there is a precipitous drop. In addition to neoplastic changes, several nonmalignant epithelial and structural alterations of the lower genital tract have been noted (Robboy et al., 1979), as have deformities of the endometrial cavity. Other authors have reported an increased risk of unfavorable outcome of pregnancy in daughters exposed to in utero DES. Detailed studies of males exposed in utero to DES showed increased frequencies of testicular hypoplasia, cryptorchidism, epididymal cysts, microphallus, increased abnormal sperm forms, and lowered sperm counts. An estimated 30 per cent of the males studied are probably infertile (Bibbo et al., 1977; Gill et al., 1979), and a few have been found to have seminomas (Conley et al., 1983).

A number of other agents known to cross the placenta may possibly be carcinogenic to the offspring. In utero exposure to phenytoin or possibly other antiepileptic drugs is associated with a syndrome in the newborn that includes hypoplasia of the midface, tapering of the fingers and

TABLE 116–2. Incidence and Mortality of Malignant Tumors in United States Newborns and Infants

TUMOR TYPE	INCIDENCE				MORTALITY				RATIO (A/B)
	<29 Days		12 Mos.		<29 Days		12 Mos.		
	No.	Rate	No.	Rate* (A)	No.	Rate	No.	Rate* (B)	
Leukemia	5	4.7	34	31.8	101	2.6	807	20.8	1.5
Neuroblastoma	21	19.7	67	62.7	70	1.8	302	7.8	8.0
Central nervous system	1	0.9	15	14.0	12	0.3	257	6.6	2.1
Kidney	5	4.7	21	19.7	21	0.5	141	3.6	5.4
Reticuloendotheliosis	0	0	3	2.8	7	0.2	131	3.4	—
Sarcoma	4	3.7	19	17.8	29	0.7	129	3.3	5.4
Liver	0	0	8	7.5	15	0.4	99	2.6	2.9
Lymphoma	1	0.9	2	1.9	2	<0.1	60	1.5	1.3
Teratoma	0	0	3	2.8	11	0.3	28	0.7	4.0
Carcinoma	1	0.9	6	5.6	6	0.2	18	0.5	11.2
Germ cell, excluding teratoma	0	0	0	0	0	0	6	0.2	
Retinoblastoma	0	0	17	15.9	1	<0.1	4	0.1	159.0
Other	1	0.9	1	0.9	20	0.5	62	1.6	
TOTAL	39	36.4	196	183.4	295	7.6	2044	52.7	3.5

*Per one million live births per year.

(From Bader, J. I., and Miller, R. W.: U.S. cancer incidence and mortality in the first year of life. Am. J. Dis. Child. *133*:157, 1979. Copyright 1979, American Medical Association.)

toes, and hypoplasia or aplasia of the nails. At least five children with this syndrome have been reported to have neuroblastoma (Ehrenbard and Chaganti, 1981; Jiminez et al., 1981), and one has been found to have an extrarenal Wilms tumor (Taylor et al., 1980). One young adult with a history of exposure in utero to phenytoin has developed a malignant mesenchymoma (Blattner et al., 1977).

The fetal alcohol syndrome, a disorder occurring in the children of mothers who consume excessive amounts of alcohol, is characterized by developmental delay, growth deficiency, and multiple minor anomalies. One child with this syndrome has been reported with neuroblastoma (Kinney et al., 1980), a second with hepatoblastoma, and a third with adrenocortical carcinoma, but there is no evidence of increased incidence.

The association of neoplasms with other environmental agents has been inconclusive. Jick and associates (1981) noted an increase in pregnancies ending in spontaneous abortion and in congenital anomalies in live infants born to women presumed to have used vaginal spermicides near the time of conception. Two of the children were found to have neoplasms shortly after birth. A case-control study of neuroblastoma suggested increased risk associated with use in pregnancy of neurally active drugs, diuretics, and hair dyes and with alcohol consumption and

sex hormone exposure (Kramer et al., 1987), and paternal exposure to electromagnetic fields has been suggested as a risk factor (Spitz and Johnson, 1985).

Agents implicated in childhood neoplasia following in utero exposure also often have teratogenic effects (Table 116–4). In the case of DES, the same organ appears to be at risk for both the oncogenic and teratogenic effects of the drug. It is of interest that phenytoin exposure in the adult has been associated with the development of lymphomas, whereas phenytoin exposure in utero has been associated with neuroblastomas. Thus, an agent may have various teratogenic or oncogenic effects, depending on the susceptibility of the target organ at the time of exposure, prenatally or well into adulthood. The same toxic agent has been shown in animals to be teratogenic to the fetus in the second quarter of pregnancy and carcinogenic in the latter half of pregnancy (Napalkov, 1973). Experimental evidence in animals suggests that maternal chemical carcinogen exposure may result in an increased incidence of tumors not only in the offspring but also in later generations of untreated descendants (Tomatis, 1979).

HOST FACTORS

Certain host factors seem to predispose a person to the development of neoplastic disease. There is an increased

TABLE 116–3. Diagnoses in 221 Cases of Neonatal Malignancy

CENTER (DATES)	NEUROBLASTOMA	LEUKEMIA	RETINOBLASTOMA	SARCOMA	WILMS	CENTRAL NERVOUS SYSTEM	OTHER*
CHLA, Los Angeles[a] (1955–82)	14	11	2	8	3	2	6
HSC, Toronto[b] (1922–82)	48	8	17	12	4	9	4
SJCRH, Memphis[c] (1962–88)	19	6	3	0	2	0	4
UCSF, San Francisco[d] (1942–87)	11	4	9	2	5	1	7
TOTAL (No.)	92	29	31	22	14	12	21
TOTAL (%)	42%	13%	14%	10%	6%	5%	10%

*Includes 8 malignant germ cell tumors or teratomas, 3 hepatoblastomas, 2 melanomas, 1 blue nevus, 3 carcinomas, 2 histiocytoses, 1 schwannoma, and 1 unspecified.

CHLA, Children's Hospital of Los Angeles; HSC, Hospital for Sick Children; SJCRH, St. Jude's Children's Research Hospital; UCSF, University of California-San Francisco.

(From [a]Isaacs, 1985; [b]Campbell, 1987a; [c]Crom et al., 1989; [d]Matthay, unpublished. Courtesy of the Cancer Patient Data Program, Cancer Research Institute, and the Cancer Registry of UCSF, 1990.)

TABLE 116–4. Drugs Associated with Teratogenic and Carcinogenic Disorders Following in Utero Exposure

DRUG	TERATOGENIC EFFECTS	CARCINOGENIC EFFECTS
Diethylstilbestrol	Structural alterations on genital tract	Vaginal and cervical adenocarcinoma
Phenytoin	Fetal hydantoin syndrome	Neuroblastoma* Wilms tumor*
Alcohol	Fetal alcohol syndrome	Neuroblastoma* Hepatoblastoma* Adrenocortical carcinoma*
Vaginal spermicides	Limb reduction deformities* Chromosomal abnormalities* Hypospadias*	Medulloblastoma* Nesidioblastosis*
Phenobarbital	Microcephaly*	Brain tumors*

*Present data are only suggestive of an etiologic association.

incidence of leukemia in persons with Down syndrome, Fanconi aplastic anemia, and Bloom syndrome and of leukemia and lymphoreticular malignancies in persons born with immunodeficiency disorders such as ataxia-telangiectasia, Wiskott-Aldrich syndrome, and severe combined immunodeficiency. Of interest are the observations that phenytoin depresses immune function (Sorrell et al., 1971) and that immune deficiency occurs in children with the fetal alcohol syndrome (Johnson et al., 1981). Miller (1963) found Down syndrome to be more common than usual among siblings of children with leukemia. Both Down syndrome and leukemia occur more frequently among children of older mothers. Others have reported cytogenic variants of prezygotic origin in 4 of 25 non-mongoloid children with acute leukemia and suggested that the aneuploid cell might be more susceptible to malignant change.

Although the risk of developing leukemia is increased slightly in a dizygotic twin or other sibling of a child who has the disease, the chance of developing leukemia is greatest in a monozygotic twin. If one monozygotic twin has leukemia, the co-twin has approximately a 25 per cent chance of developing leukemia, usually within weeks or months of the diagnosis of the sibling.

A small number of well-defined hereditary disorders such as neurofibromatosis, tuberous sclerosis, and basal cell carcinoma syndrome are associated with an increased incidence of certain neoplasms. The neoplastic diseases, however, seldom present during infancy. Kindreds have been reported in which multiple members developed the types of malignant diseases that usually occur in sporadic fashion. Although the number of such families is small, it is hard to escape the conclusion that, at least in some instances, heredity plays an important role in the development of malignancy.

CONGENITAL DEFECTS

An unexpectedly large number of childhood tumors occur in association with certain congenital defects. Children with Wilms tumor have an increased incidence of congenital aniridia. Aniridia is a rare anomaly, found in only 1 of 75,000 persons. It is about 1000 times more likely to occur in children with Wilms tumor (1 in 75). The association with a deletion in chromosome 11 has

been described in at least 20 patients (Yunis and Ramsay, 1980). The majority of these patients also have genitourinary abnormalities and mental retardation. From the clinical perspective, if an infant has aniridia, chromosome analysis should be undertaken. If a deletion of chromosome 11 is found, the child should be monitored for Wilms tumor with serial ultrasonographic studies of the kidneys. Approximately half of these patients will develop Wilms tumor.

Other problems associated with Wilms tumor include anomalies of the genitourinary tract. Congenital hemihypertrophy occurs excessively with Wilms tumor, adrenocortical neoplasia, and hepatoblastoma, and it is also associated with hamartomas and with the visceral cytomegaly syndrome described by Beckwith (Sotelo-Avila et al., 1980). Hamartomas occur commonly in children with Wilms tumor and adrenocortical neoplasia. One child has been reported with hepatoblastoma and Wilms tumor; another, with congenital hemihypertrophy, had an adrenocortical adenoma and years later developed a Wilms tumor. Of interest is the fact that Beckwith visceral cytomegaly syndrome affects the kidney, adrenal cortex, and liver, the three organs that develop the malignancies associated with hemihypertrophy. These relationships among hemihypertrophy, visceral cytomegaly syndrome, hamartomas, and malignancy have been reviewed by Miller (1963). The associations of congenital anomalies with childhood neoplasias again emphasize the close relationship between oncogenesis and teratogenesis.

■ CONGENITAL LEUKEMIA

Leukemia rarely occurs during the first month of life. Only 3 per cent of all children with acute lymphoblastic leukemia are younger than 1 year of age; of 115 infants entered on Children's Cancer Study Group protocols, only 2 had congenital leukemia (Reaman et al., 1985). Most of the neonatal cases reported have acute nonlymphoblastic leukemia, in contrast to the predominance of acute lymphoblastic leukemia found in later childhood. In the Children's Cancer Study Group, 18 per cent of all children treated for acute nonlymphoblastic leukemia were infants (< 1 year). No child born to a mother with leukemia has been found to have the disease during the neonatal period. Instances of familial neonatal leukemia are extremely rare. Campbell and co-workers (1962) described male and female siblings who died at 10 and 8 weeks of age, respectively, of myelogenous leukemia and a third female in the family who died at 4 weeks of age with a clinical course similar to that of her siblings, although a definite diagnosis was not made.

Congenital leukemia is occasionally associated with a number of congenital anomalies (Miller et al., 1969) and with chromosomal disorders such as Down syndrome, trisomies D and E, and a number of nonspecific chromosomal abnormalities. Subtle cytogenetic abnormalities may occur more commonly than was previously believed in affected infants and their parents when studied with newer cytogenetic techniques.

CLINICAL MANIFESTATIONS

The clinical signs of leukemia may be evident at birth, with hepatosplenomegaly, petechiae, and ecchymoses.

Leukemic cell infiltration into the skin (leukemia cutis) results in nodular fibroma-like masses. These tumors are freely movable over the subcutaneous tissue and result in a blue or gray discoloration of the overlying skin (Fig. 116–1). Such cutaneous lesions are commonly found when the disease appears at birth and have been noted in stillborn premature infants with leukemia. They may be the first clinical signs of the disease. At birth, many of the infants have respiratory distress due to either leukemia infiltration in the lungs or atelectasis. Severe respiratory difficulty may develop soon after birth from pulmonary hemorrhage secondary to thrombocytopenia.

In those infants who develop signs of the disease within the first month but in whom no detectable signs of leukemia were noted at birth, the symptoms are often ill defined, with low-grade fever, diarrhea, hepatomegaly, and failure to gain weight. Hemorrhagic manifestations are often the first signs of the disease, and leukemia cutis is less common.

Hemoglobin levels are often normal at first, but they soon fall to low levels. Total white blood cell counts may be within normal limits or diminished, but leukocytosis is usually present. White blood cell counts of 150,000 to 250,000/mm^3 or more are not unusual, and counts as high as 1.3 million/mm^3 have been recorded. Leukocyte counts often rise progressively before death. There is usually a predominance of blast cells and immature granulocytes. Auer rods may be present in the blast cells (Fig. 116–2). These intracellular inclusions are composed of lysosomes and are considered to be pathognomonic of acute myelogenous leukemia.

DIFFERENTIAL DIAGNOSIS

A number of newborns reported in the earlier literature who were originally believed to have leukemia were later found to have other diseases. The predominance of myelogenous leukemia in this age group has contributed to the difficulty in differentiating the disorder from leukemoid reactions. Confusion with infections such as congenital syphilis, cytomegalovirus infection, toxoplasmosis, and bacterial septicemia may occur because of the leukocytosis, organomegaly, and thrombocytopenia that may accompany these diseases. The low platelet counts and leukemoid reactions reported in infants with congenital amegakaryocytic thrombocytopenia may also lead to an incorrect diagnosis of leukemia, but the absence of radii commonly seen in these children is a major clue to the correct diagnosis.

Severe erythroblastosis fetalis can mimic leukemia. Such infants usually have hepatosplenomegaly, large numbers of nucleated erythroblasts in the peripheral blood, and, occasionally, thrombocytopenia. Small infiltrates of extramedullary erythropoiesis may appear in the skin and superficially resemble leukemia cutis.

Infants with neonatal neuroblastoma often have hepatomegaly and may also have discolored tumor nodules in the subcutaneous tissue (see Figs. 116–4 and 116–7). Their blood cell counts are usually normal without circulating blasts, and specimens of bone marrow, if involved, reveal small clusters of neuroblastoma cells (see Fig. 116–5). Although these cells may resemble leukemia blast cells, their tendency to occur in clumps in an otherwise normal bone marrow distinguishes them from leukemic cells, which usually completely replace the normal bone marrow. In cases of complete bone marrow replacement, increased excretion of catecholamine metabolites and the presence of an abdominal mass or other primary lesion are clues to the diagnosis of neuroblastoma.

Congenital human immunodeficiency virus infection may also rarely be confused with leukemia. Clonal B-cell expansions in such patients may cause lymphadenopathy. One newborn has been reported by Voelkerding and co-workers (1988) who presented with thrombocytopenia

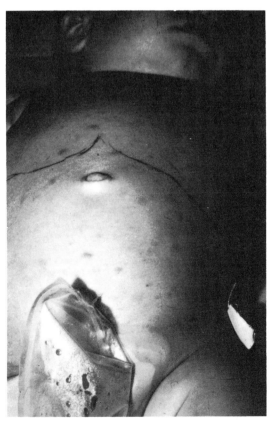

FIGURE 116–1. Leukemia cutis in a newborn infant.

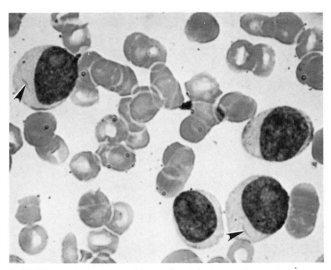

FIGURE 116–2. Malignant blast cells with Auer rods (arrows) present in cytoplasm diagnostic of acute myelogenous leukemia.

and had lymphocyte clusters in the bone marrow that were of B-cell lineage, clonal as defined by immunoglobulin gene arrangement and positive for the common acute lymphocytic leukemia antigen. However, the patient was well and without evidence of lymphoproliferative disease a year later.

A marked but transient leukemoid reaction may occur in the newborn following in utero exposure to betamethasone (Anday and Harris, 1982). Lack of the usual clinical and laboratory findings of leukemia and a history of maternal drug exposure usually exclude the diagnosis of leukemia.

PATHOLOGY

Biopsy or autopsy shows heavy infiltration of many immature leukocytes into extrahematopoietic tissues. The bone marrow is hypercellular, with a marked predominance of the immature cells of the series affected, either myeloid or lymphoid. Cirrhosis of the liver has been noted at autopsy in several infants.

CELLULAR MORPHOLOGY, IMMUNOPHENOTYPE, AND CHROMOSOMES

Both acute lymphoblastic and acute nonlymphoblastic leukemia may be found in newborns. These diseases are differentiated on the basis of typical morphologic characteristics, such as the presence of granules or Auer rods and nuclear and cytoplasmic morphology and by cytochemical stains. Periodic acid–Schiff stain will show large aggregates of glycogen in the blast cells in acute lymphoblastic leukemia, whereas the pattern in acute nonlymphoblastic leukemia will be finely granular and diffuse. Most acute lymphoblastic leukemia cells will stain positively for terminal deoxynucleotidyl transferase, a DNA polymerase that catalyzes the polymerization of deoxynucleotides in thymocytes. This enzyme is present in 90 per cent of acute lymphoblastic leukemia, but less than 5 per cent of acute nonlymphoblastic leukemia. Activity can be measured by enzyme-linked immunosorbent assay, immunofluorescence, immunoperoxidase stain, and enzyme assay (Diamond and Matthay, 1988). Both types of leukemia are now subclassified according to an international French-American-British classification (FAB) based on cell morphology and histochemistry and are divided into subtypes based on morphologic characteristics (Bennett et al., 1976; Table 116–5). The most common subtype by far in infantile and neonatal acute nonlympho-

blastic leukemia is the monocytic variety (Odom and Gordon, 1984; van Wering and Kamps, 1986).

Immunophenotype determined using a panel of monoclonal antibodies against differentiation antigens and detected by fluorescence is helpful both in differentiating the lymphoid and nonlymphoid leukemias and in further subtyping (Crist et al., 1986; Katz et al., 1988; Pui et al., 1987). Most of the neonatal and infant acute lymphoblastic leukemia cells exhibit an early pre-B-cell phenotype, including Ia positivity, negativity for CD10 (common acute lymphoblastic leukemia antigen), unlike most childhood acute lymphoblastic leukemia, and positivity for CD19 and CD24 (early B-cell markers). The frequent rearrangements of the immunoglobulin heavy-chain gene, and occasionally the light-chain gene but almost never the T-cell receptor gene, may also be helpful in subclassification and understanding the biology of neonatal acute lymphoblastic leukemia (Felix et al., 1987; Ludwig et al., 1989). The acute nonlymphoblastic leukemia surface antigen expression is shown in Table 116–5.

Chromosomal abnormalities in the leukemic cells have gained increasing importance in subclassification and prognosis of both acute lymphoblastic and acute nonlymphoblastic leukemia. A number of chromosomal translocations and deletions have been found to carry an unfavorable prognosis, such as the t(4;11), which is commonly present in infants with leukemia (Nagasaka et al., 1983). The most common chromosome involved in translocations in infantile acute lymphoblastic leukemia and acute nonlymphoblastic leukemia is the 11q23, found in at least 50 per cent of infant leukemia and in a predominance of neonatal cases (Kaneko et al., 1988).

TREATMENT AND PROGNOSIS

The course of the disease has usually been one of rapid deterioration and death from hemorrhage or infection. Although the length of survival has been significantly prolonged in children with leukemia, success has been very limited in treating the newborn. The infant with leukemia frequently presents with hyperleukocytosis (blast cell count in excess of 100,000/mm³). This syndrome may result in sludging of blast cells in capillaries with resultant intracranial hemorrhage, respiratory distress, or problems from tumor lysis with hyperkalemia, hyperphosphatemia, hypocalcemia, hyperuricemia, and renal failure. These metabolic problems must be corrected prior to initiation

TABLE 116–5. Classification of Acute Nonlymphoblastic Leukemias

FAB	COMMON NAME	HISTOCHEMISTRY	ANTIGEN EXPRESSION
M1	Acute myeloblastic leukemia, undifferentiated	MPO+	Ia, MY7, MY9
M2	Acute myeloblastic leukemia, with differentiation	MPO+	Ia, MY7, MY9
M3	Acute promyelocytic leukemia	MPO+	MY7, MY9
M4	Acute myelomonocytic leukemia	MPO+, NSE+	Ia, MY4, MY7, MY8, MY9
M5	Acute monocytic leukemia	NSE+	Ia, MY4, MY8, MY9
M6	Acute erythroleukemia	MPO+, PAS+	MY7, MY9
M7	Acute megakaryoblastic leukemia	PPO+	Platelet glycoproteins Ib, IIb/IIIa, or factor VIII related antigen

MPO = myeloperoxidase; NSE = nonspecific esterase; PAS = periodic acid–Schiff; PPO = platelet peroxidase by electron microscopy; FAB = French-American-British morphologic classification.
(Bennett, J. M., Catovsky, D., Daniel, M. T., et al.: Proposals for the classification of the acute leukaemias: French-American-British [FAB] Co-Operative Group. Br. J. Hematol. *33*:451, 1976.)

of chemotherapy. In the infant, exchange transfusion is the easiest way to accomplish this and simultaneously lower the white blood cell count, which will further decrease tumor lysis problems once chemotherapy is begun. Disseminated intravascular coagulation is another common complication seen in hyperleukocytosis and infantile leukemia, where monocytic subtypes are common. The monoblasts release procoagulants and cause consumptive coagulopathy, which may initially be exacerbated owing to further blast cell lysis with chemotherapy and require heparinization. Central nervous system involvement is very common in infants with acute lymphoblastic leukemia and those with monocytic leukemia. Evaluation of cerebrospinal fluid and intrathecal prophylactic chemotherapy should be a routine part of treatment.

The current improved success of remission induction with treatment of acute nonlymphoblastic leukemia in infants under 1 year is similar to that in older children, using intensive combination chemotherapy regimens (Lampkin et al., 1984). The experience with newborns is limited, but between 1984 and 1989, 5 of 12 newborns with acute nonlymphoblastic leukemia sustained complete remissions with chemotherapy; all were in the myelomonocytic or monocytic category (Kaneko et al., 1988; Odom and Gordon, 1984). However, in acute lymphoblastic leukemia, the treatment outcome is significantly poorer in infants younger than 1 year at diagnosis (23 per cent disease-free survival compared with 70 per cent for older children) and may be even lower in newborns. Fewer than 15 per cent of newborns with acute lymphoblastic leukemia have remissions lasting more than a few months.

Although exchange transfusions may cause clinical improvement by rapidly decreasing an extremely high white blood cell count, the response is usually transient. The same chemotherapeutic agents used for older children with acute lymphoblastic leukemia may be used in infants, with the precaution that dosages may need to be altered to prevent undue toxicity. Furthermore, dosages should be calculated on the basis of body weight, rather than by the surface area calculation used in an older child. Infants have been shown to experience excessive neurotoxicity with vincristine, with hypotonia, a poor cry, inability to feed, and flaccid paralysis (Reaman et al., 1985). Radiation therapy, used for central nervous system leukemia, may also result in more marked neurotoxicity than in older children. The relatively lower renal function and biliary excretion in newborns may also result in unexpected toxicity of certain drugs. Accordingly, many of the drugs commonly used in the treatment of infantile leukemias will require dosage modifications, including vincristine, anthracyclines, cyclophosphamide, epipodophyllotoxins (etoposide, teniposide), prednisone, cytarabine, 6-mercaptopurine, and methotrexate (Reaman, 1989). Spontaneous remissions, which occur in Down syndrome infants with leukemia, are rarely experienced by the normal child. Sansone (1989) reported an infant with myelomonocytic leukemia who relapsed after initial chemotherapy and then had a spontaneous remission persisting for more than 3 years at the time of the report.

■ LEUKEMIA WITH DOWN SYNDROME

An increased incidence of acute leukemia in children with Down syndrome (10- to 30-fold increased risk) is now well recognized (Fong and Brodeur, 1987). A review of the world literature by Rosner and Lee (1972) revealed 227 children with both disorders; 31 per cent had acute myeloblastic leukemia, and 69 per cent had acute lymphoblastic leukemia. Among 47 such infants with leukemia, 58 per cent had myeloblastic leukemia and 42 per cent had lymphoblastic leukemia. Eighteen additional Down syndrome infants who had a transient disorder initially indistinguishable from acute myelogenous leukemia experienced complete clinical and hematologic recovery. In those with "transient leukemia" who died of other causes, no evidence of leukemia could be found at postmortem examination. It has been suggested by Ross and associates (1963) that the transient leukemoid reaction is due to a defect in the regulation of granulocyte multiplication and maturation, possibly related to the chromosomal abnormality. The same transient myeloproliferative disorder may be seen in trisomy 21 mosaicism (Seibel et al., 1984). The increased incidence of neonatal polycythemia in Down syndrome patients observed by Weinberger and Oleinick (1970) has led these investigators to propose that the abnormality in the regulation of hematopoiesis is not limited to granulocyte production. Miller and Cosgriff (1983) found a hematologic abnormality in 28 of 81 newborns with Down syndrome (35 per cent). The most common problem was polycythemia (21), the second most common, thrombocytopenia (7), with transient leukocytosis (2), third. However, a number of infants with transient leukemia have had recurrence of their disease leading to death, indicating that the disorders of marrow dysfunction and neonatal leukemia may not be separate entities but may be intimately related.

Attempts to differentiate the transient myeloproliferative disorder from a true leukemia have been made clinically, morphologically, through cell culture, and by chromosomal analysis. The self-limited transient myeloproliferative disorder is usually not associated with anemia, neutropenia, or thrombocytopenia, despite the presence of blast cells in the peripheral blood; the percentage of blast cells is greater in the blood than in the bone marrow; and the blast cells demonstrate trisomy 21 with no other cytogenetic abnormalities. Suda and co-workers (1987) showed that bone marrow blast cells cultured from such a patient resulted in colony formation with differentiation into normal basophils, neutrophils, eosinophils, macrophages, and erythrocytes. This differs from true acute nonlymphoblastic leukemia, in which in vitro colony formation is abnormal with lack of maturation. Hayashi and colleagues (1988) studied the chromosomes of 13 patients with Down syndrome and acute leukemia compared with 15 patients with Down syndrome and transient myeloproliferative disorder. Clonal chromosomal abnormalities were found in the cells of all patients with leukemia but not in the cells of those with the transient myeloproliferative disorder. However, Lazarus and co-workers (1981) reported one infant with transient myeloproliferative disorder whose cells demonstrated chromosomal abnormalities including −22,t(Xp;8q),t(21q;22q), which disappeared as the syndrome resolved spontaneously.

The high incidence of spontaneous remission of leukemia in infants with Down syndrome makes it difficult to interpret their response to antileukemic therapy. It may be most prudent to withhold the use of chemotherapeutic agents in this unusual group of newborns unless the clinical course is one of rapid deterioration.

NEUROBLASTOMA

Neuroblastoma is the most common malignant tumor in infancy. The neoplasm originates from neural crest cells that normally give rise to the adrenal medulla and sympathetic ganglia. In infancy, the first clinical manifestations in more than half the cases are usually due to the presence of metastatic disease rather than to the primary tumor. Yet despite the occurrence of widespread disease, the prognosis in the newborn is remarkably good.

CLINICAL MANIFESTATIONS

Neuroblastoma may present as a tumor mass anywhere that sympathetic neural tissue normally occurs. Over half of affected children have the primary tumor within the abdomen, arising in the adrenal medulla or a sympathetic ganglion. The tumor may arise in the posterior mediastinum, and because of bronchial obstruction the symptoms may be either increasing dyspnea or pulmonary infection. The neoplasm may also arise in the neck or pelvis. Involvement of the stellate ganglion may result in Horner syndrome, which includes sinking in of the eyeball, ptosis of the upper eyelid, slight elevation of the lower lid, constriction of the pupil, narrowing of the palpebral fissure, and anhidrosis (Fig. 116–3). The neoplasm arising from a paravertebral sympathetic ganglion has an unusual tendency to grow into the intervertebral foramina, causing spinal cord compression and resultant paralysis. Careful periodic neurologic evaluation should be performed on the child with a neuroblastoma arising from this location, since the onset of cord compression may necessitate emergency neurosurgical intervention. The late diagnosis of this complication has resulted in permanent paraplegia.

Metastatic lesions, especially of the skin and liver, are common presenting findings during the neonatal period. Often the primary site cannot be discovered. Hawthorne and co-workers (1970) found that the skin nodules may first become erythematous for 2 or 3 minutes after palpation and then blanch, presumably owing to vasoconstriction from release of catecholamines from the tumor cells. This may be a diagnostic sign of subcutaneous neuroblastoma.

The liver often bears the brunt of metastatic dissemi-

nation, becoming studded with innumerable foci of tumor growth. The infant will present with a distended abdomen and respiratory distress (Fig. 116–4) from the rapidly growing hepatic neoplasm. Rarely, stippled calcifications occur in the liver metastases. The liver may be large enough at the time of birth to cause dystocia. The massive liver involvement common in newborns with disseminated neuroblastoma causing respiratory distress and coagulopathy is responsible for the higher mortality seen in newborns compared with older infants (Nickerson et al., 1985).

Neuroblastomas arising from sympathetic ganglia lower in the abdomen give rise to the clinical pictures consistent with their locations. Thus, presacral neuroblastomas may simulate presacral teratomas and be distinguished from them only by biopsy.

UNUSUAL PRESENTATIONS

Several children with neuroblastoma have been reported whose sole presenting symptom was persistent, intractable diarrhea. The children were believed to have had either cystic fibrosis or celiac syndrome before roentgenographic discoveries of calcified masses were made. Their symptoms dramatically abated following surgical removal of the tumors. It is thought that such symptoms are due to excessive excretion by the tumor of a vasoactive intestinal peptide (Swift et al., 1975).

The association of acute myoclonic encephalopathy and neuroblastoma has been described by numerous authors. This usually consists of rapid multidirectional eye

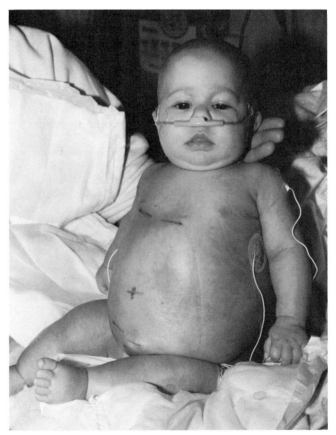

FIGURE 116–4. Stage 4S neuroblastoma causing abdominal distention and respiratory distress due to hepatic infiltration.

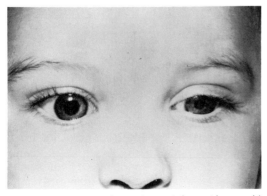

FIGURE 116–3. Horner syndrome in an infant with neuroblastoma arising from the left cervical sympathetic ganglion.

movements (opsoclonus), myoclonus, and truncal ataxia in the absence of increased intracranial pressure. Removal of the tumor may not result in improvement in neurologic signs and symptoms. In general, the prognosis for survival of children with opsomyoclonus is excellent, although long-term neurologic deficits are common.

A report from the Netherlands suggests that there may be signs and symptoms in mothers whose fetuses have neuroblastoma. Voûte and co-workers (1970) reported six women who had sweating, pallor, headaches, palpitations, hypertension, and tingling in the feet and hands during the eighth and ninth months of pregnancy. All the women were delivered of children who were diagnosed as having neuroblastoma shortly after birth or during the first few months of life. Because the mothers' symptoms disappeared postpartum, the authors proposed that they were caused by fetal catecholamines entering the maternal circulation.

Occasionally, a newborn with congenital neuroblastoma may be thought to have erythroblastosis. Severe jaundice with hepatosplenomegaly and an increase of nucleated red blood cells have been noted. Anders and co-workers (1973) described two newborns with congenital neuroblastoma that had metastasized to the liver and placenta who were thought to have hydrops fetalis. In one, the diagnosis was established by histologic examination of the placenta.

DIAGNOSIS

Neuroblastoma of the newborn most commonly manifests by enlargement of the liver alone (65 per cent), followed by subcutaneous metastases (32 per cent). These figures differ strikingly from those for older infants and children (Table 116–6). Metastases to lungs, bones, skull, and orbit are rare in the newborn, although clumps of tumor cells are often found if one carefully examines bone marrow aspiration specimens (Fig. 116–5). Otherwise, a localized primary tumor may be palpable or cause symptoms from spinal cord compression or Horner syndrome. Metastatic evaluation should include computed tomography or magnetic resonance imaging of the primary lesion, magnetic resonance imaging of the spine for paraspinal and posterior mediastinal lesions, bone scan, bone marrow aspirate and biopsy, and an ^{123}I or ^{131}I metaiodobenzyl-

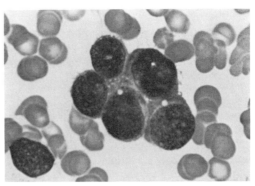

FIGURE 116–5. *Clump of neuroblastoma cells found in bone marrow aspiration.*

guanidine (MIBG) scan. MIBG is a norepinephrine analogue specifically taken up by neuroblastoma both in bone and soft tissue and provides a sensitive modality for disease localization (Feine et al., 1987; Geatti et al., 1985). Immunocytologic staining of bone marrow with antineuroblastoma monoclonal antibodies can increase sensitivity of detection of bone marrow disease (Moss et al., 1985).

BIOCHEMICAL FEATURES

In 1957, Mason and colleagues reported an increased excretion of pressor amines in the urine of an infant with neuroblastoma. Subsequent studies in children with neuroblastoma have shown elevated levels of norepinephrine as well as its biochemical precursors and their metabolites in the urine, including dopa, dopamine, normetanephrine, homovanillic acid (HVA), and vanillylmandelic acid (VMA). As many as 95 per cent of patients have an elevated urinary excretion of VMA or HVA or both. Currently, accurate VMA and HVA determinations can be made on random urine samples when normalized for creatinine concentration. In occasional cases, however, there is no elevation of catecholamines necessitating a 24-hour urine collection. It is therefore important to measure urinary catecholamines in a child prior to surgical removal of a neuroblastoma or initiation of therapy to determine whether it is a catecholamine-producing tumor. This unique property of the neoplasm can be used not only as a diagnostic aid but also as a means of assessing the response to therapy or detecting the recurrence of tumor.

Urinary excretion of cystathionine is detectable in most patients with neuroblastoma but is also found in a number of other childhood neoplasms. Plasma carcinoembryonic antigen levels are also elevated in many cases, but this finding also is nonspecific. Serum lactic acid dehydrogenase levels increase with advanced disease, fall with remission, and rise with recurrence. The degree of initial elevation may have prognostic significance in patients with advanced disease (Quinn et al., 1980).

NEWBORN SCREENING

Urinary catecholamine screening for neuroblastoma has been proposed by Woods and co-workers (1987) since the incidence of 8.7 per 1 million children per year is comparable to or higher than that of other congenital diseases for which screening is already in place, such as hypothyroidism, galactosemia, and phenylketonuria.

TABLE 116–6. Incidence of Metastases in the Newborn with Neuroblastoma

SITE	NUMBER	PERCENTAGE	PER CENT
Liver	20	64.6	24.3
Subcutaneous	10	32.3	2.6
Marrow	3	9.7	
Lung	2	6.5	13.2
Spleen	2	6.5	2.0
Kidney	2	6.5	2.0
Pancreas	2	6.5	
Brain	2	6.5	15.8
Bone	1	3.2	47.4
Nodes	1	3.2	32.2
Pleura	1	3.2	
Myocardium	1	3.2	
Periadrenal	1	3.2	

(From Schneider, K. M., Becker, J. M., and Krasna, I. H.: Neonatal neuroblastoma. Pediatrics 36:359, 1965.)

Rapid quantitative screening methods have been developed that have a high degree of sensitivity and specificity. Using such methods, researchers in Japan have demonstrated a dramatic improvement in the survival of infants detected on screening for neuroblastoma compared with those who were diagnosed clinically (Sawada et al., 1984). The prevalence of neuroblastoma was identical during both periods, suggesting that these results were not due to detection of patients with occult disease who would have had spontaneous regression. Studies are under way in North America with mass urinary screening at 3 weeks and 6 months to further determine the usefulness of this test (Lemieux et al., 1989).

PATHOLOGY

The most primitive histologic subgroup of this tumor, the neuroblastoma, is very cellular and is composed of small round cells with scant cytoplasm. The ganglioneuroma, its more benign counterpart, is composed of large, mature ganglion cells with abundant cytoplasm, whereas the ganglioneuroblastoma is intermediate in the degree of cellular differentiation. However, the histologic appearance of an individual tumor may show various degrees of cellular maturation. Past attempts at correlation of prognosis with histologic grading have been contradictory. However, Shimada and co-workers (1984) have developed a system of histologic grading based on the amount of stroma, the degree of differentiation, and the nuclear morphology (mitosis and karyorrhexis). Using this classification, one can separate patients who have a favorable prognosis from those who do not, although the classification is most helpful in patients with stage 1, 2, 3, and 4S, since most of the patients with stage 4 disease in this initial report had unfavorable histopathology. A study of patients with stage 3 and 4 disease from the Children's Cancer Study Group (Chatten et al., 1988) confirms the value of the Shimada classification for both these stages of disease with a highly significant difference in survival of patients with favorable versus unfavorable histopathology.

PROGNOSIS

The outcome for patients with neuroblastoma has long been known to depend on the age at diagnosis and the stage of disease (Fig. 116–6). However, these two variables alone do not define a homogeneous group with respect to outcome. Additional characteristics that have been correlated with prognosis include serum ferritin, serum neuron-specific enolase, N-*myc* oncogene amplification, cellular DNA content, and histopathology.

Although different staging systems have been used for neuroblastoma, the system now internationally accepted, which was modified from the system of Evans and the Children's Cancer Study Group, is shown in Table 116–7. Patients with stage 1 neuroblastoma have a 96 to 100 per cent survival with surgery alone, as shown in cooperative studies reported by Evans and co-workers (1984). Similarly, for stage 2 neuroblastoma, surgery alone is sufficient to provide a 90 per cent disease-free survival. Initial cooperative studies showed no benefit from the addition of chemotherapy to surgery with local irradiation for patients with stage 2 disease; our subsequent review

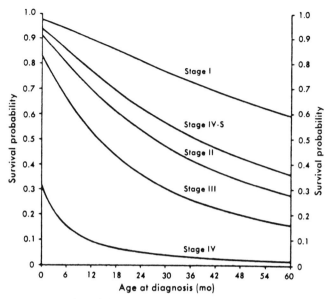

FIGURE 116–6. *Probability of survival in neuroblastoma according to age and stage of disease. (From Breslow, N., and McCann, B.: Statistical estimation of prognosis for children with neuroblastoma. Cancer Res. 31:2098–2103, 1971. Reprinted by permission.)*

of 156 children with stage 2 neuroblastoma showed no significant benefit from the addition of radiation therapy to surgery alone, even in patients with microscopic or gross residual disease (Matthay et al., 1989). Infants with stage 3 and 4 disease have a poorer survival, even with aggressive chemotherapy, although the outcome, with better than 50 per cent surviving overall, is far better than the 10 to 20 per cent reported for older children.

Stage 4S comprises a unique group of patients with disseminated disease but a good prognosis, occurring almost exclusively in infants younger than 1 year old. This special group of children have remote spread of tumor involving the liver, skin, and/or bone marrow without

TABLE 116–7. International Staging System for Neuroblastoma

STAGE	DESCRIPTION
Stage 1	Localized tumor confined to the area of origin; complete gross excision, with or without microscopic residual disease; identifiable ipsilateral and contralateral lymph nodes negative microscopically.
Stage 2A	Unilateral tumor with incomplete gross excision; identifiable ipsilateral and contralateral lymph nodes negative microscopically.
Stage 2B	Unilateral tumor with complete or incomplete gross excision, with positive ipsilateral regional lymph nodes; identifiable contralateral lymph nodes negative microscopically.
Stage 3	Tumor infiltrating across the midline with or without regional lymph node involvement; or, unilateral tumor with contralateral regional lymph node involvement; or, midline tumor with bilateral regional lymph node involvement.
Stage 4	Dissemination of tumor to distant lymph nodes, bone, bone marrow, and liver and/or other organs (except as defined in stage 4S).
Stage 4S	Localized primary tumor as defined for stage 1 or 2 with dissemination limited to liver, skin, and bone marrow.

(From Brodeur, G. M., Seeger, R. C., Barrett, A., et al.: International criteria for diagnosis, staging, and response to treatment in patient with neuroblastoma. J. Clin. Oncol. 6:1874, 1988.)

roentgenographic evidence of skeletal metastases. The primary tumor may be unidentifiable or else no more extensive than defined by stage 1 or stage 2. Eighteen of 20 infants younger than the age of 1 year with stage 4S disease reported by D'Angio and associates (1971) were cured of their disease. The 2-year survival rate of all of those with stage 4S disease was 84 per cent as compared with 5 per cent survival of all children with stage 4 disease, or the 50 per cent survival of infants younger than 1 year with stage 4 disease. Haas and colleagues (1988) reviewed 212 infants with stage 4S neuroblastoma and found that only 13 per cent died of disease progression while 12 per cent died of therapy-related causes. Recently, biologic differences have been demonstrated between stages 4S and 4 neuroblastoma, with lack of elevation of serum ferritin levels in stage 4S compared with stage 4. E-rosette inhibitory factor was present frequently in the serum of patients with stage 4 disease but was seldom present in the serum of patients with stage 4S disease, and there is usually lack of N-*myc* oncogene amplification in stage 4S tumors compared with stage 4 tumors.

Levels of two serum markers, ferritin and neuron-specific enolase, have been shown to be elevated in the serum of patients with advanced neuroblastoma. Analysis of these markers at diagnosis has been shown to be helpful in distinguishing those patients with stage 3 and 4 disease who may have a more favorable survival and therefore require less intensive treatment. Hann and co-workers (1981) initially showed that ferritin levels were elevated in 15 of 17 children with stage 4 disease, but in none of 13 children with stage 4S disease. Subsequently, they demonstrated that ferritin was a prognostic factor independent of age and stage for children with stage 3 and 4 neuroblastoma: progression-free survival at 24 months of follow-up for patients with stage 3 tumor with normal ferritin levels was 76 per cent versus 23 per cent with elevated ferritin levels, while for stage 4 disease survival was 27 per cent versus 3 per cent, respectively (Hann et al., 1985). Zeltzer and co-workers (1986) demonstrated similar findings for neuron-specific enolase, a cytoplasmic protein found in normal neural tissue and present in elevated quantities in the serum of patients with neuroblastoma. In patients with stage 3 and 4 neuroblastoma, only 5 per cent survived who had neuron-specific enolase levels greater than 100 ng/ml, while 63 per cent survived with neuron-specific enolase levels less than 100 ng/ml.

Amplification of the N-*myc* oncogene in primary neuroblastoma has also been shown to correlate with advanced stage disease and with rapid tumor progression regardless of stage (Brodeur et al., 1984; Seeger et al., 1985). Estimated progression-free survival was 68, 30, and 0 per cent, respectively, for patients whose tumors had 1, 3 to 10, or more than 10 copies of the N-*myc* oncogene. Patients with stage 1 or 4S disease have N-*myc* amplification only very rarely; when present, it has been associated with rapid disease progression in these usually favorable stages (Cohn et al., 1987). Approximately 10 per cent of patients with stage 2 disease have amplification; all of such patients to date have developed rapid disease progression and death within 2 years of diagnosis. Thus, N-*myc* amplification is a significant prognostic factor that is independent of stage. It will be most helpful in detecting the newborns with high-risk disease.

Total cellular DNA content may also predict response to therapy in infants with neuroblastoma (Look et al., 1984). Infants with hyperdiploid tumors had a significantly better response to therapy than did those with diploid tumors. Furthermore, hyperdiploidy correlated with stage 4S. Subsequently, others confirmed the poor prognosis of patients with diploid (euploid) tumors and correlated tumor DNA with histologic grading and clinical stage (Gansler et al., 1986; Hayashi et al., 1989). Tumor karyotype may also influence outcome in neuroblastoma: abnormalities of the short arm of chromosome 1 are more common in patients with metastatic disease but are rare in patients with stage 1, 2, and 4S disease (Christiansen and Lampert, 1988; Fong et al., 1989).

A number of children have experienced spontaneous tumor regression despite the presence of metastases, most commonly in infants with stage 4S disease. In other instances, malignant neuroblastomas have apparently undergone maturation into benign ganglioneuromas. The case (Haas et al., 1988) shown in Figure 116–7 is an example of spontaneous maturation and regression.

The diagnosis of neuroblastoma was made before the age of 6 months in 21 of 29 case reports collected by Everson and Cole (1966) in which spontaneous regression occurred. The remainder were diagnosed in patients between 6 and 24 months of age. This relationship of spontaneous regression to age has also been noted by Evans and co-workers (1971), who found that the majority of those with tumor regression were younger than 6 months of age and were usually those with stage 2 or stage 4S disease. Some patients with spontaneous regression of stage 4 disease have been reported (Sitarz et al., 1975). Patients with stage 1 disease, however, could not be evaluated because the tumor was usually completely resected.

The mechanism of the spontaneous regression is uncertain, although in our case and at least two others in the literature, pathologic differentiation and maturation to ganglioneuroma have been documented. The incidence of spontaneous regression of neuroblastoma may be more common than is clinically evident. Beckwith and Perrin (1963) detected the presence of microscopic clusters of neuroblastoma cells, termed *neuroblastoma in situ,* in the adrenal glands of a significant number of infants younger than the age of 3 months with no clinical evidence of tumor on whom postmortem examinations were performed. These investigators estimated the incidence of neuroblastoma in situ to be about 40 times greater than the number of cases of clinically diagnosed disease. Basing their theory on these findings, they proposed that the great majority of these tumors either degenerated or underwent differentiation to normal tissue. Turkel and Itabashi (1974), however, believe that such neuroblastic nodules represent normal changes in the developing adrenal gland and noted their presence in 100 per cent of 169 fetal adrenal glands they examined. Whether or not neuroblastoma in situ is a true neoplasm, it completely disappears after 3 months of life under normal circumstances.

TREATMENT

The unpredictable course of neuroblastoma, with its occasional spontaneous maturation or regression, not only

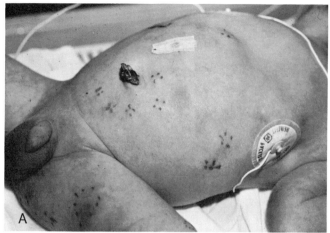
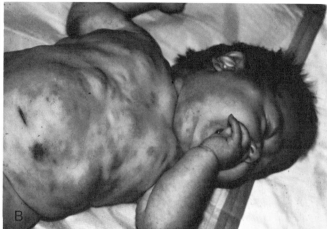
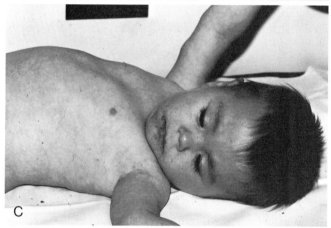

FIGURE 116–7. A newborn with Stage 4S neuroblastoma who developed progression followed by spontaneous maturation and regression. (A) birth, (B) 3 months, (C) 10 months.

makes the tumor unusual but also causes difficulty in evaluating therapy. The type and intensity of treatment can now be based on the ability to define infants with relatively good, intermediate, and poor prognoses based on stage, pathology, ferritin level, neuron-specific enolase level, and N-*myc* amplification. Patients who have localized disease (stage 1 or 2) without amplification of N-*myc* will have a 90 to 100 per cent survival with surgery alone, even if the tumor is not completely resected. Such patients should have surgical resection or partial resection, but they will probably not derive any additional benefit from postoperative radiation or chemotherapy. An exception to this rule would be in the case of spinal cord compression, where prompt decompression either with osteoplastic laminotomy, limited chemotherapy, or local radiation therapy may be used to preserve function. The combination of extensive laminectomy with postoperative irradiation should be avoided, since later spinal deformity is almost inevitable in the infant. If a recurrence should develop after local therapy in stage 2 neuroblastoma, such patients are almost always salvageable with further treatment (Matthay et al., 1989).

Patients with stage 4S disease have a highly favorable prognosis and may require minimal therapy. Since many patients undergo spontaneous regression without chemotherapy, and the disease-free survival overall is 85 to 90 per cent, therapy should be directed toward supportive care with minimal chemotherapy and surgery. The main cause of death is massive hepatic involvement resulting in respiratory insufficiency or compromise of renal or gas-

trointestinal function. In a review of 212 cases in the literature, 21 patients died of local disease progression, 20 died of therapy-related causes, while only 7 died of progression to a stage 4 tumor. The hepatic tumor will often regress with low-dose radiation therapy at a dose of 450 cGy given in three fractions through across-table, opposed ports angled to avoid the kidneys, spine, and ovaries. Concomitant low-dose cyclophosphamide will often hasten tumor regression. No benefit has been shown to result from resection of the primary tumor, despite anecdotal case reports. Nutritional and blood product support may also be necessary until the lesions begin to resolve. Only in the rare 3 per cent of cases in which progression to a stage 4 lesion occurs will intensive antineoplastic treatment be required.

Infants with the less favorable stages, 3 and 4, are usually treated with combination chemotherapy and local surgery and radiation therapy as necessary to eradicate residual disease. It is possible that the use of the newer prognostic factors, pathology, N-*myc*, ferritin levels, and neuron-specific enolase levels, may obviate the need for intensive therapy for patients with favorable stages. Active drugs that are currently most commonly employed in treatment programs for advanced neuroblastoma include cisplatin, etoposide, doxorubicin, cyclophosphamide, vincristine, and ifosfamide. A few infants with a very unfavorable prognosis include patients with stage 2, 3, and 4 disease with amplification of the N-*myc* oncogene; it is possible that for such patients, as in older children with neuroblastoma, standard chemotherapy regimens will be insufficient for cure. In these high-risk patients, myeloablative therapy followed by bone marrow infusion is being tested (Philip et al., 1987; Seeger et al., 1988).

■ MELANOTIC NEUROECTODERMAL TUMORS

Melanotic neuroectodermal tumors of infancy are uncommon neoplasms derived from cells of the neural crest. These melanin-containing tumors usually are diagnosed between 1 and 8 months of age and most commonly appear overlying the maxilla. With few exceptions, the tumor behaves in a benign manner (Cutler et al., 1981).

■ WILMS TUMOR

Wilms tumor, or nephroblastoma, the most common intra-abdominal tumor of childhood, occurs in 1 in 8000 children. In some children with aniridia, for instance, the risk is much higher. In contrast to neuroblastoma, this neoplasm, with optimal treatment, is associated with an increasing rate of cure that has been one of the dramatic success stories in the field of cancer therapy. The National Wilms Tumor Study, established in 1969, has helped in the rapid accumulation of information regarding the prognosis and treatment of this tumor, which results in death if untreated.

CLINICAL MANIFESTATIONS

The majority of children with Wilms tumor have either an abdominal mass or an increase in abdominal size noted as the first clinical evidence of disease. This is often first discovered by a parent and brought to the attention of the physician. The tumor lies deep in the flank, is attached to the kidney or is part of it, and is usually firm and smooth. It seldom extends beyond the midline, even though it may grow downward beyond the iliac crest. In 5 to 10 per cent of all cases, tumors involve both kidneys. Gross hematuria is a rare presenting symptom, but microscopic hematuria is found in approximately one-fourth of cases. However, hematuria in Wilms tumor is not a poor prognostic sign, as it is in adults with hypernephroma. Hypertension, occasionally noted in older infants and children, has not been observed in the newborn. The tumor may sometimes present with abdominal pain and be discovered at laparotomy, and occasionally acute hemorrhage into the tumor may result in a rapidly enlarging mass, usually associated with anemia and fever.

Wilms tumor is seldom diagnosed at birth or during the neonatal period, although several renal tumors have been so large as to have caused dystocia during delivery. Of the 77 children with Wilms tumor treated at the M.D. Anderson Hospital and Tumor Institute over a period of 18 years, only one case of Wilms tumor was diagnosed during the first month of life (Sullivan et al., 1973). Characteristics associated with an earlier presentation include bilaterality or associated aniridia or hypospadias (Pastore et al., 1988).

Rare cases of Wilms tumor associated with polycythemia have been reported. This finding is secondary to an increased production of erythropoietin by the neoplasm. The demonstration of elevated plasma erythropoietin levels in nonpolycythemic children with Wilms tumor studied preoperatively led to the suggestion that this test may be useful in the diagnosis and evaluation of response to therapy.

DIFFERENTIAL DIAGNOSIS

The other intra-abdominal tumor that may be easily confused with Wilms tumor is neuroblastoma. Although Wilms tumor distorts the kidney while neuroblastoma displaces it, preoperative distinction may be difficult when neuroblastoma arises within kidney substance. Less common intrarenal neoplasms that may be seen are rhabdoid tumor, mesoblastic nephroma, renal cell carcinoma, rhabdomyosarcoma, hemangiopericytoma, and lymphoma. Benign processes that may simulate Wilms tumor include multicystic kidneys, hematomas, and renal carbuncles.

HEREDITARY ASSOCIATIONS AND CONGENITAL ANOMALIES

The association among Wilms tumor, hemihypertrophy, congenital aniridia, hamartomas, and genitourinary defects has been discussed earlier in this chapter. The finding of hemihypertrophy should alert the physician to observe the child for the possible development of Wilms tumor, adrenal cortical tumor, or hepatoma. Some of these patients may have incomplete forms of the Beckwith-Wiedemann syndrome (Sotelo-Avila et al., 1980). It is interesting that abnormalities of chromosome 11 are seen in tumor cells from Wilms tumor, rhabdomyosarcoma, and hepatoblastoma, all tumors associated with Beckwith-Wiedemann syndrome (Cowell and Pritchard, 1987). A number of cases of pseudohermaphroditism, nephron disorders (diffuse mesangial sclerosis), and Wilms tumor have also been reported (Gallo and Chemes, 1987). Occasionally, certain members of a family may have the congenital anomaly and others may have the neoplasm. Meadows and coworkers (1974) reported one family in which a mother had congenital hemihypertrophy, three of the children had Wilms tumor, and a fourth had a urinary tract anomaly.

Aniridia is usually inherited in an autosomal dominant pattern with high penetrance and little variability of phenotypic expression. The child with aniridia who has Wilms tumor does not have this usual inheritance pattern but has sporadic congenital aniridia. Pilling (1975) reported 26 children with aniridia, 20 of whom had the sporadic type. Seven of the 20 developed Wilms tumor. It appears that the risk of developing Wilms tumor is higher if the sporadic aniridia is accompanied by a major genitourinary tract anomaly, severe mental retardation, or both. The Wilms tumor–aniridia syndrome, a combination of mental retardation, microcephaly, bilateral aniridia, anomalies of the pinna, Wilms tumor, and ambiguous genitalia, is associated with a small deletion of chromosome 11 (11p13–14.1). In some tumor tissues, the same section of DNA deleted from one chromosome may be duplicated on another. The behavior is compatible with a recessive oncogene. Although usually sporadic, this syndrome may occasionally be familial (Yunis and Ramsay, 1980). Rarely, affected persons may demonstrate all the findings except the Wilms tumor (Riccardi et al., 1978). There are two reports of aniridia in monozygous twins in which only one member of each pair developed Wilms tumor (Maurer et al., 1979; Miller, 1979). Bloom syndrome, a rare autosomal recessive disease previously associated with a high risk of cancer, has been reported to predispose to Wilms tumor (Cairney et al., 1987). Reports of tumors occurring in siblings, identical twins, parent–child pairs, and cousins with no malformations indicate that hereditary factors at times may play a major role in the development of this neoplasm. However, heritability of the unilateral sporadic form of Wilms tumor was examined by Li and associates (1988) in 96 long-term survivors. No Wilms tumor developed in 179 offspring of these patients, confirming the low likelihood of heritability in the sporadic form.

PROGNOSTIC FACTORS

Three factors seem to influence the response to therapy and ultimate prognosis of the child with Wilms tumor: the histologic pattern, the age of the patient at the time of diagnosis, and the extent of disease (Breslow et al., 1978). Tumors with better differentiation, showing glomeruloid and tubular formation, indicate a better chance for survival than do those with anaplastic and sarcomatous patterns. Patients younger than 2 years of age at diagnosis have fewer relapses, especially to distant sites, than do older children. Age, however, seems to be of little prognostic significance regarding mortality. Specimens weighing over 250 g and positive regional lymph nodes, however, are often important predictors of both relapse and mortality.

The most common staging system now in use is that devised by the National Wilms Tumor Study, which is being used for the fourth study (Table 116–8). The clinical staging is an important factor in predicting survival; those with more extensive spread have a poorer prognosis. Therefore, adequate evaluation of the extent of tumor involvement is essential and should include computed tomography of the abdomen and chest to fully evaluate both kidneys, the inferior vena cava for tumor thrombus, and the liver and lungs, which are the most commonly involved areas of hematogenous spread (Fig. 116–8). Other commonly involved sites of metastatic spread are the retroperitoneum, peritoneum, mediastinum, and pleurae. If the histology shows a clear cell sarcoma, bone metastases may occur, so a bone scan should be included in the evaluation; rhabdoid tumors, which frequently metastasize to brain, mandate computed tomography or magnetic resonance imaging of the brain.

TABLE 116–8. Clinicopathologic Staging of Wilms Tumor

Stage I:	Tumor limited to the kidney and completely resected.
Stage II:	Tumor extending beyond the kidney but completely resected. The tumor may have been biopsied, or there may have been local spillage.
Stage III:	Residual nonhematogenous tumor confined to the abdomen, including any of the following: lymph node involvement in the abdomen, diffuse peritoneal spillage or tumor growth that has penetrated the peritoneal surface, peritoneal implants, gross or microscopic extension beyond surgical margins, or unresectable because of infiltration into vital structures.
Stage IV:	Hematogenous metastases. Deposits beyond stage III (i.e., lung, liver, bone, and brain).
Stage V:	Bilateral renal involvement at diagnosis.

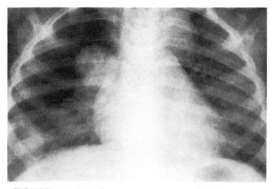

FIGURE 116–8. *Pulmonary metastases of Wilms tumor.*

TREATMENT AND PROGNOSIS

Prior to 1950, the two major modalities of therapy for Wilms tumor, surgical removal and radiation therapy, resulted in cure rates approaching 50 per cent. The advantage of treatment with the chemotherapeutic agent dactinomycin was demonstrated in 1966 by Farber, who reported an 89 per cent survival rate in children who had no evidence of metastatic disease at the time of diagnosis and who were followed for at least 2 years, and a 53 per cent survival rate in those presenting with evidence of metastatic disease. The drug therapy appeared to prevent clinical hematogenous metastases following surgical removal and radiation to the tumor bed by presumably destroying nondetectable, microscopic tumor foci, especially in the lungs. Vincristine also has striking activity against Wilms tumor and appears to be at least as effective as dactinomycin. Other single agents shown to have activity against this tumor include doxorubicin, cyclophosphamide, ifosfamide, and bleomycin.

Infants younger than 12 months of age have experienced undue toxicity to the liver, hematopoietic system, and lungs from the prescribed doses of dactinomycin, vincristine, and doxorubicin. On the earlier National Wilms Tumor Studies, 47 per cent of infants had severe hematologic toxicity and there were toxic deaths in 6 per cent. Dosages were subsequently reduced to 50 per cent of the usual per kilogram dose given to older children, with a decrease in hematologic toxicity to 13 per cent and elimination of toxic deaths. It is interesting that the dosage reduction did not compromise therapeutic effect as judged by the 2-year relapse-free survival figures (Morgan et al., 1988).

Results of the first two National Wilms Tumor Studies show that treatment with vincristine and dactinomycin is superior to treatment with either drug alone. Postoperative radiation therapy adds little benefit to those with totally excised tumors, and 6 months of therapy with two drugs appears to be as effective as 15 months of therapy in such patients. Patients with more advanced disease fared better following treatment with three drugs (dactinomycin, vincristine, doxorubicin) than with two (dactinomycin, vincristine). Patients with unfavorable histology had a significantly poorer prognosis than did those with favorable histology, as did those with positive nodes (D'Angio et al., 1981). Current treatment results from the third National Wilms Tumor Study (D'Angio et al., 1989) in children with Wilms tumor according to stage and histology are shown in Table 116–9. Thus, Wilms tumor, a neoplasm that is fatal if untreated, presently has a cure rate overall approaching 90 per cent. The use of newer therapeutic agents may continue to improve these remarkably successful results. It has been suggested that infants with small, totally resected tumors may not need any more treatment than surgery.

■ OTHER RENAL NEOPLASMS

A number of neonatal renal tumors have been confused with the typical Wilms tumor in the past. Now that these neoplasms have been recognized as separate entities, they are more commonly diagnosed during the neonatal period than is the classic nephroblastoma, which very rarely occurs during the first month of life.

RHABDOID TUMOR OF KIDNEY

Rhabdoid tumor of the kidney is an uncommon renal tumor of children that is one of the most lethal neoplasms of early neonatal life, with a mortality rate exceeding 80 per cent. It has a predilection for males, with a male-to-female ratio of 1.5:1, and for infants, with median age at diagnosis of 11 months. Overall, rhabdoid tumors comprised 1.8 per cent of all malignant childhood renal tumors entered on the National Wilms Tumor Study. Rhabdoid tumors frequently present simultaneously with embryonal primary tumors of the central nervous system, such as medulloblastoma (Bonnin et al., 1984). Originally believed to represent a "rhabdomyosarcomatoid" pattern of Wilms tumor, it subsequently was shown to lack any evidence of myoblastic differentiation or any morphologic or clinical linkage to Wilms tumor. Review of 111 cases by Weeks and co-workers and the National Wilms Tumor Study (1989) showed several findings suggesting that rhabdoid tumors may arise from cells involved in formation of the renal medulla but that they have no histogenic relationship to Wilms tumor. The prognosis is poor, particularly for infants with evidence of dissemination. The only patients who survived were those with completely resected disease and negative lymph nodes (50 per cent), whereas all those with metastases died.

MESOBLASTIC NEPHROMA

The congenital mesoblastic nephroma, or fetal mesenchymal hamartoma, was clearly distinguished from Wilms

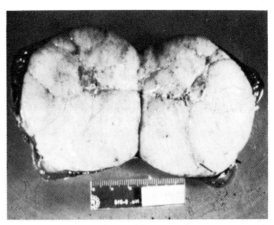

FIGURE 116–9. *Congenital mesoblastic nephroma compressing and nearly totally replacing the kidney.*

tumor in 1967 by Bolande and co-workers, who emphasized its benign nature. The involved kidney is usually greatly enlarged and distorted by the tumor, but, contrary to the findings with Wilms tumor, there is usually no lobulation, necrosis, hemorrhage, or discrete capsule between neoplasm and compressed kidney (Fig. 116–9). Polyhydramnios and premature labor occur with increased frequency in women whose infants have mesoblastic nephroma. The tumor may be diagnosed prenatally with ultrasonography, which helps to differentiate it from Wilms tumor because of its typical sonographic appearance of concentric echogenic and echo-poor ring pattern (Chan et al., 1987). The histologic picture is of a preponderance of interlacing bundles of spindle-shaped cells within which dysplastic tubules and glomeruli are irregularly scattered. Extrarenal infiltration is common, especially into the perihilar connective tissues. Since that initial description, a cellular or atypical variant of congenital mesoblastic nephroma with focal hemorrhage, necrosis, hypercellularity, and a high mitotic index was described. The atypical variants usually present at a later age (mean 5.3 months) than the classic type (mean 16 days) (Pettinato et al., 1989). Despite pathologic variation, efforts to predict clinical behavior on this basis have failed. In the 16 cases of congenital mesoblastic nephroma reported by Pettinato and associates, all of the patients survived with surgery alone, despite frequent extension into psoas and perirenal fat and despite atypical histology in 10 tumors.

The vast majority of all patients have been cured by nephrectomy alone, even in the presence of localized extrarenal extension. There is good evidence that more patients with mesoblastic nephroma have died as a result of aggressive chemotherapy and irradiation than from the tumor itself. Radical nephrectomy alone is the treatment of choice; however, in very rare instances the tumor has been unusually aggressive.

PERSISTENT RENAL BLASTEMA AND NEPHROBLASTOMATOSIS

Accumulations of immature renal tissue are not normally found beyond 36 weeks' gestation, the time at which nephrogenesis normally ceases. Nodular renal blastema is characterized by microscopic nests of primitive cells in the subcapsular renal cortex resembling the blas-

TABLE 116–9. Treatment Results of the Third National Wilms Tumor Study According to Stage and Histology

| STAGE | HISTOLOGY | NO. | % RELAPSE-FREE | | % ALIVE |
			2 Yr	4 Yr	4 Yr
I	Favorable	607	91.6	90.4	96.5
II	Favorable	278	90.4	88.1	92.3
III	Favorable	275	79.8	79.0	87.0
IV	Favorable	120	76.0	74.9	82.5
I–III	Unfavorable	130	69.7	64.8	68.4
IV	Unfavorable	29	55.6	55.6	55.3
All patients		1439	85.0	83.3	89.1

(Data from D'Angio, G. J., Breslow, N., Beckwith, B., et al.: Treatment of Wilms' tumor: Results of the Third National Wilms' Tumor Study. Cancer 64:349, 1989.)

ternal cells of Wilms tumor but lacking mitoses. Although benign, these nodules are believed to have the potential for neoplastic transformation. They are found in one of every 200 to 400 postmortem examinations of infants younger than 4 months of age, but they are discovered in the kidneys of children older than 4 months of age only in cases of Wilms tumor. When nodular renal blastema becomes massive and confluent and replaces the cortex, it is referred to as "nephroblastomatosis" (Bove and McAdams, 1976). Kumar and associates (1978) reported the nodular renal blastema–nephroblastomatosis complex in 8 of 118 patients (6.8 per cent) with Wilms tumor. Five of these eight patients had bilateral tumors. Children with this disorder may also have the congenital anomalies associated with Wilms tumor (Fig. 116–10). The fact that nodular renal blastema is rarely found in older children suggests that the majority of these lesions regress, a situation analogous to the course of neuroblastoma in situ. It is believed that those that persist give rise to Wilms tumor, whereas a small number progress to diffuse nephroblastomatosis. Complete progression of nodular renal blastema to nephroblastomatosis to Wilms tumor has been documented (Kulkarni et al., 1980). Children with massive bilateral involvement will often respond to therapy used for Wilms tumor. Although persistent renal blastema is not a true malignancy, it probably has been confused with Wilms tumor in the past, and it appears in many instances to be a precursor of this malignancy.

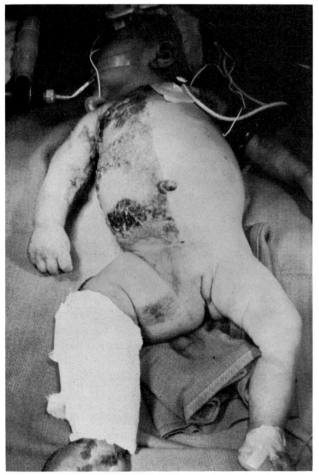

FIGURE 116–10. Congenital epidermal nevus in association with hemihypertrophy and nephroblastomatosis.

CYSTIC PARTIALLY DIFFERENTIATED NEPHROBLASTOMA

A renal neoplasm in infants is known by a variety of names: polycystic nephroblastoma, benign multilocular cystic nephroma, well-differentiated polycystic Wilms tumor, and cystic partially differentiated nephroblastoma. It is a cystic encapsulated tumor occurring before 2 years of age. The cysts are lined by epithelium and show a mixture of partially differentiated and undifferentiated metanephrogenic blastema that differentiates this lesion from multilocular cysts of the kidney. The tumor appears to have a benign course, and nephrectomy is the treatment of choice (Joshi et al., 1977). These neoplasms probably represent a differentiated form of nephroblastoma.

■ RETINOBLASTOMA

Retinoblastoma is a malignant ocular tumor that arises in embryonic retinal cells. The incidence of retinoblastoma in the United States is approximately 1:18,000 live births. Bilateral involvement is observed in 20 to 35 per cent of retinoblastomas; in as many as one-fourth of these patients, the tumor is initially detected in only one eye.

GENETICS

The gene for retinoblastoma, located on chromosome 13q14, has now been cloned and belongs to a class of tumor suppressor genes whose function is to control cellular growth. When the gene is inactivated, either by a mutation or deletion, the block to cellular proliferation is removed, leading to tumor formation. Mutations at the retinoblastoma locus can be inherited in an autosomal dominant pattern or arise spontaneously. The Knudson "two hit" hypothesis postulates that the first gene change can occur in a germ cell (inherited cases) or in a retinoblast (in sporadic cases); only when the second gene change develops in a somatic target cell (retinoblast) already carrying a first hit will that cell be transformed. All patients with bilateral retinoblastoma have a new germinal mutation or an inherited one. Approximately 80 per cent of unilateral retinoblastomas occur as a result of a somatic nonheritable mutation (Cowell and Pritchard, 1987). The germinal trait responsible for retinoblastoma is a dominant one with 80 to 96 per cent penetrance. There are also a small number of patients (5 per cent of retinoblastoma) born with a constitutional deletion of chromosome 13, 13q−, who have the associated anomalies of microencephaly, macrognathia, malformed ears and thumbs, hypertelorism, microphthalmia, ptosis, protruding upper incisors, short stature, cleft palate, developmental delay, and psychomotor retardation (Knudson et al., 1976). Children with the bilateral and hereditary form are diagnosed at an earlier age, since the chromosomal abnormality is present at birth, providing a greater susceptibility to tumorigenesis. It is now possible, using DNA restriction-fragment length polymorphisms, to predict susceptibility to retinoblastoma (Cavenee et al., 1986; Wiggs et al., 1988).

CLINICAL MANIFESTATIONS

Retinoblastoma commonly presents either with leukocoria or "cat's eye" on ocular examination or because of strabismus due to loss of vision in the affected eye. Multifocal retinal involvement is common, occurring in 84 per cent of patients. Intraocular spread may fill the vitreous body by extension or seeding, while exophytic tumors arise from the outer retinal layer and cause retinal detachment. Extraocular spread is seen in less than 15 per cent of patients, usually occurring by direct invasion of the optic nerve and eventually leading to subarachnoid involvement and intracranial spread. In such cases the cerebrospinal fluid may contain tumor cells. Rarely, tumors may spread by invasion of the orbit or by hematogenous dissemination to bones and bone marrow.

The diagnosis is made by ophthalmoscopic examination under anesthesia. Computed tomography or magnetic resonance imaging of the eye is useful to determine tumor extent and optic nerve involvement. A lumbar puncture for cerebrospinal fluid cytology should be obtained if there is optic nerve invasion; bone scan and bone marrow biopsy will detect hematogenous spread. Tumors are then staged according to the Reese-Ellsworth classification based on the number and size of the lesions and whether they extend anterior to the ora serrata. In addition, any extraocular extension must be specified.

TREATMENT

Since extraocular spread and death from dissemination are rare, the main goal of treatment is local control and preservation of vision. Surgical enucleation is employed only when there is no chance for useful vision, if glaucoma is present, or if conservative measures fail to control tumor. External beam radiation therapy, administered by experienced clinicians using careful positioning and general anesthesia, is the standard treatment for cure of retinoblastoma. Doses range from 3500 to 5000 cGy given in three fractions per week. Occasionally, radioactive plaques are used for local recurrences. If local extension has occurred, the field must be enlarged to include the orbit or a craniospinal field for meningeal or brain involvement (Donaldson and Smith, 1989). Small tumors confined to the retina, occurring either before or after radiation therapy, can often be controlled with cryotherapy and photocoagulation. Chemotherapy, including agents such as vincristine, doxorubicin, cyclophosphamide, cisplatin, and etoposide, has achieved responses and may be indicated in patients with disseminated disease. Thus far, no advantage has been demonstrated for the use of chemotherapy as adjuvant treatment given in addition to radiation therapy or enucleation.

The prognosis for children with unilateral retinoblastoma is excellent, with cure rates of 85 to 90 per cent using conservative local treatment. However, patients with bilateral disease have a much lower long-term survival, not because of the retinoblastoma but because of a high predisposition to second malignancy, which may occur from 5 years up to the rest of the patient's life. Local extension also confers a poor prognosis, with survival less than 40 per cent with optic nerve invasion and less than 10 per cent with orbital extension or distant dissemination.

■ HEPATIC MALIGNANCIES

Primary malignant tumors of the liver are uncommon in infants and children. The most common malignant neoplasm involving the liver in infancy is metastatic neuroblastoma. The two major histologic types of hepatomas are hepatoblastoma and hepatocellular carcinoma. Hepatoblastomas usually occur in infants and are rarely seen after 3 years of age. In the 129 cases reported by Exelby and co-workers (1975), almost half of the patients were 18 months of age or younger, 11 were younger than 6 weeks of age, and 3 were newborns. Hepatocellular carcinomas, however, appear to have a bimodal age distribution, occurring either in very young children younger than 4 years of age or in patients between the ages of 12 and 15 years. Both types of tumors occur more commonly in males.

The most common presenting symptoms of hepatic tumors are an upper abdominal mass and an enlarging abdomen. Anorexia, weight loss, and pain also frequently occur. Laboratory studies of liver function are rarely helpful in establishing a diagnosis and are usually normal. Alpha-fetoprotein, an alpha$_1$-globulin that occurs normally in the fetus and disappears in the first few weeks of life, is often present in the serum of the child with hepatic malignancy. A number of children with hepatoblastoma have elevated levels of the amino acid cystathionine in their urine. If present, cystathioninuria may allow one to differentiate among hepatoblastoma and a number of benign and malignant disorders, but elevated levels of cystathionine also occur in about 50 per cent of patients with neuroblastoma.

Hepatic calcification is demonstrated in 20 per cent of cases on the plain abdominal roentgenogram. Radioisotopic liver scanning usually demonstrates the presence of a neoplasm by an area of decreased uptake of labeled isotope and is useful in following regeneration of the liver after hepatic lobectomy and in diagnosing tumor recurrence. Angiography is useful in determining whether both lobes of the liver are involved. If one lobe is free of malignancy and there is no evidence of distant metastatic disease, a lobectomy of the involved portion of the liver should be performed despite the high operative mortality. At the present time, surgery appears to be the only means for cure. In the aforementioned large series, there was no evidence that radiation therapy or chemotherapy controlled disease that could not be totally resected. When incomplete excision was performed, no patient survived, but 60 per cent of those with hepatoblastoma and 33 per cent with hepatocellular carcinoma were cured if the tumor could be completely excised. The subgroup with pure "fetal" histology and complete resection have 100 per cent survival (Weinberg and Finegold, 1983). However, a number of cases have been reported since in which initially inoperable tumors could be removed and the patient cured by a second surgical procedure following reduction in tumor size by the use of chemotherapy and radiation therapy (Weinblatt et al., 1982). Chemotherapy after total gross tumor resection may increase survival rates (Evans et al., 1982). Three patients with unresectable disease, including one with pulmonary metastases, were rendered disease free with cisplatin and doxorubicin and remained in remission off treatment (Quinn et al., 1985).

In addition to hepatomas, a variety of very rare liver tumors have been reported in infants. Angiosarcomas are believed to be the malignant form of infantile hemangioendotheliomas. One interesting case occurred in a 20-month-old child following in utero exposure to arsenic (Falk et al., 1981), a toxin implicated in hepatic angiosarcomas in adults. Seventeen cases of hepatic teratomas have been reported in children, the majority occurring in females younger than 3 years of age. About one-half of hepatic teratomas are malignant.

SACROCOCCYGEAL TERATOMAS

Teratomas are neoplasms that contain derivatives of more than one of the three primary germ layers of the embryo. Although these tumors are often benign, one or more of the germ layer derivatives may develop malignant characteristics. Teratomas arise in a wide variety of locations of the body but usually occur along the axial midline during early childhood. After puberty, teratomas most frequently occur in the gonads, particularly the ovary.

The sacrococcygeal region is the most common site of teratomas in the first year of life, and the sacrococcygeal teratoma is the most common solid tumor in the newborn, although it is rarely malignant. Females are affected two to four times more frequently than males. The earliest detection of a teratoma may occur prenatally or at birth. Polyhydramnios, nonimmune fetal hydrops, and dystocia have all been described in association with germ cell tumors. Congenital anomalies are often present in association with sacrococcygeal teratomas, including genitourinary, hind gut, and lower vertebral malformations. Most tumors present as a mass protruding between the coccyx and rectum and may be quite large (Fig. 116–11). About 10 per cent are found by rectal examination. Nearly all arise at the tip or inner surface of the coccyx and can be diagnosed early in life by the pediatrician who makes the rectal examination a routine part of the physical examination.

Sacrococcygeal teratomas may be confused with meningomyeloceles, rectal abscesses, pelvic neuroblastomas, pilonidal cysts, and a variety of very rare neoplasms that may occur in that region. The majority of benign teratomas in this area produce no functional difficulties, even when marked intrapelvic extension is present. Thus, bowel or bladder dysfunction, painful defecation, and vascular or lymphatic obstruction suggest that the lesion is malignant.

Treatment of sacrococcygeal tumors is primarily surgical. They should be excised as soon as possible because small, undifferentiated foci may proliferate and become aggressive. They are attached to the coccyx, and therefore

removal of the entire coccyx is a necessary part of the surgical procedure. Failure to remove the coccyx results in a 30 to 40 per cent risk of local recurrence.

Sixty to 70 per cent of sacrococcygeal teratomas in newborns are unequivocally benign, as determined by the presence of mature tissues. Embryonic or immature somatic tissues are present in 10 to 15 per cent of cases, and the remaining tumors contain malignant elements as defined by the presence of an endodermal sinus tumor or highly undifferentiated neoplasm resembling neuroblastoma (Dehner, 1983). Local recurrence or metastasis of teratoma is very rare but may occur when immature elements are present. In an early series reported by Gonzalez-Crussi and associates (1978), there were two of four recurrences in immature teratomas. However, there were no recurrences in eight infants with immature neuroepithelial or renal elements in a later series of 68 sacrococcygeal teratomas reported by Valdiserri and Yunis (1981). However, nine patients with endodermal sinus tumor in the same series all had metastases and all died. Alpha-fetoprotein is usually markedly elevated in the serum of patients with endodermal sinus tumor and provides a useful marker of disease status. This must be interpreted with careful reference to normal values in infants, whose serum levels are normally high but decline with age in a predictable fashion (Blair et al., 1987). In the series of 398 cases reported by Altman and associates (1974), 60 per cent of the patients with malignant tumors died within 10 months of surgery, 21 per cent were alive with residual disease, 11 per cent were alive without apparent disease, and 9 per cent were lost to follow-up. These findings contrast markedly to the mortality rate reported for children with benign lesions, which was approximately 5 per cent.

A topographic classification for sacrococcygeal tumors appears valuable in predicting potential for metastatic behavior and survival (Fig. 116–12). An internal location predisposes the tumor to metastatic behavior, possibly because the delay in diagnosis is associated with a greater risk of malignant transformation. Therapy for children with malignant sacrococcygeal teratoma is far from optimal. Even those who have localized tumor that is grossly completely excised usually have recurrence. The tumor may respond to combination chemotherapy and radiation therapy in similar regimens to those used for germ cell tumors in general, and occasional cures, even in those patients with metastatic and unresectable disease, have been reported. The addition of regimens containing cisplatin, etoposide, and bleomycin to the therapy for disseminated germ cell tumors has improved the disease-free survival to as much as 50 per cent (Flamant et al., 1984; Logothetis et al., 1985). Unfortunately, some children have died of the complications of the intensive therapy (Raney et al., 1981).

SARCOMAS

Soft tissue sarcomas are rarely seen in newborns, accounting for only 2 per cent of all childhood sarcomas in a study of 357 patients in Germany (Koscielniak et al., 1989) and in the Intergroup Rhabdomyosarcoma Study (Ragab et al., 1986). Fibrosarcomas account for one-fifth of these tumors in infants, a 10-fold excess compared with

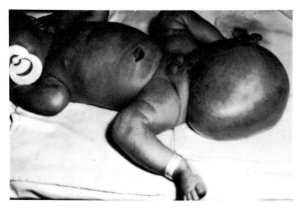

FIGURE 116–11. Large sacrococcygeal teratoma in a newborn girl.

TYPE I

Predominantly external
with minimal presacral
component

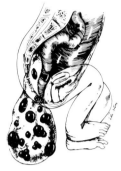

Frequency 46.6%
Metastatic rate 0%
Mortality rate 11%

TYPE II

Presenting externally
but significant intrapelvic
extension

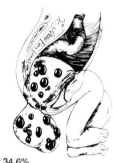

Frequency 34.6%
Metastatic rate 6%
Mortality rate 18%

TYPE III

Predominant mass
pelvic with extension
into abdomen

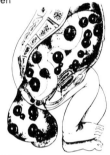

Frequency 8.8%
Metastatic rate 20%
Mortality rate 28%

TYPE IV

Entirely presacral with
no external presentation

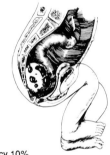

Frequency 10%
Metastatic rate 8%
Mortality rate 21%

FIGURE 116–12. Location of sacrococcygeal teratoma in 398 patients. (From Altman, R. P., et al.: Sacrococcygeal teratoma: American Academy of Pediatrics Surgical Section Survey–1973. J. Pediatr. Surg. 9:389, 1974. Reprinted by permission.)

those in older children. The other subtypes seen are rhabdomyosarcoma (67 per cent) and undifferentiated sarcoma (5 per cent). The most common sites affected are the genitourinary tract and the extremities. However, any site may be affected, and rare cases of chest wall tumors (Shamberger et al., 1989) or pericardial tumors (Lazarus et al., 1989) have been reported. A case of Kaposi sarcoma has been reported in a 6-day-old infant with congenital human immunodeficiency virus infection (Gutierrez-Ortega et al., 1989). The prognosis in infantile sarcomas is at least as good as that for older children, who have a 5-year overall survival of approximately 50 per cent. The outlook is particularly favorable for infantile fibrosarcomas; five such patients survived in the series reported by Koscielniak and co-workers (1989). The majority of sarcomas are unresectable at diagnosis and therefore require combination chemotherapy and, occasionally, radiation. As in treatment of other infantile malignancies, it is necessary to decrease the doses by 50 per cent to prevent excessive toxicity. The value of adjuvant therapy for fibrosarcomas is uncertain, since all those completely resected did well without further treatment. Radiation therapy for residual disease is problematic in the newborn, because of the possible deleterious effects on growth.

■ MELANOMA

Congenital malignant melanoma may be acquired transplacentally from the mother or may arise de novo. Those in the latter group may be associated with a congenital melanocytic nevus. Transplacentally acquired melanoma from an affected mother is usually evident at birth. The placenta may have a mottled brown-black discoloration. Malignant cells are evident on microscopic examination of the intervillous space and have been reported in cord blood. The tumor may involve any part of the body, may be manifest as an external mass or organ enlargement, or may involve the neural axis. Those with congenital de novo melanoma usually (seven of eight cases) develop metastases during the first year of life (Prose et al., 1987). Prior to 1965, the outcome was uniformly poor for newborns with malignant melanoma, whether it was maternal in origin or de novo (Campbell et al., 1987b). However, in four of the seven cases in the literature since then the patients had a prolonged (5- to 18-year) survival even with metastases, suggesting that such lesions may have a more favorable prognosis in infancy than later childhood. Local excision is the currently accepted therapy, with chemotherapy if dissemination is present.

■ CENTRAL NERVOUS SYSTEM TUMORS

Central nervous system malignancies are a mixed group in newborns, which altogether comprise less than 5 per cent of newborn cancers. The usual presentation is with enlarging head circumference. Supratentorial locations are more common than infratentorial, unlike the pattern in older children (Campbell et al., 1987a). Many types of brain tumors have been reported in newborns, including astrocytoma, peripheral neuroectodermal tumor, teratoma, medulloblastoma, ependymoma, choroid plexus papilloma, craniopharyngioma, myxofibrosarcoma, and vascular tumors (Dehner, 1983). The most common in a series of 103 neonatal brain tumors was teratoma (53 per cent), usually occurring in the region of the pineal gland. Treatment for residual disease with radiation is again especially problematic in the newborn, whose brain development is likely to be more susceptible to radiation damage than that of an older child. For such patients in cases in which tumors are likely to be responsive to cytotoxic drugs, chemotherapy as a primary modality may be preferable to radiation for local control in unresectable cases.

■ HISTIOCYTOSES

The histiocytoses represent a spectrum of rare, poorly understood disorders of histiocytes ranging from benign to clearly malignant. These diseases have recently been classified by an international group, The Histiocyte Society, on the basis of pathology (1987). The cytologically benign end of the spectrum (class I disease) comprises the childhood histiocytic syndromes, formerly called histiocytosis X (encompassing eosinophilic granuloma, Letterer-Siwe disease, and Hand-Schüller-Christian disease), now known as Langerhans cell histiocytosis. It is postulated that an immunologic stimulus to a normal antigen-processing cell, the Langerhans cell, results in uncontrolled proliferation. Langerhans cells with cleaved nuclei and Birbeck granules are seen by electron microscopy; cell surface antigens include S-100 and CD-1, and multinucleated giant cells are sometimes seen. The class II histiocytoses include the familial erythrophagocytic lymphohistiocytosis and the infection-associated hemophagocytic syndrome. They are believed to be a secondary histiocytic reaction to an unknown antigenic stimulation or infectious agent, with erythrophagocytosis possibly reflecting foreign antigens adsorbed on erythrocytes or activation of macrophages by excess lymphokine production because of abnormal immunoregulation. The lesions are characterized by morphologically normal, reactive macrophages without Birbeck granules and with prominent erythrophagocytosis, and the process involves the entire reticuloendothelial system. The infiltrates are mixed lymphohistiocytic, unlike class I disease, in which either mixed histiocytic-eosinophilic or pure histiocytic infiltrates are seen. The class III histiocytoses are the truly malignant disorders of mononuclear phagocytes, including acute monocytic leukemia, malignant histiocytosis, and histiocytic lymphoma. These represent a local or disseminated clonal proliferation of neoplastic macrophages or their precursors.

LANGERHANS CELL HISTIOCYTOSIS

Although traditionally Langerhans cell histiocytosis has been regarded as malignant, the high incidence of spontaneous remission, the histologic features, and the lack of clonality argue against this view. Studies have suggested that the disease has an immunologic basis. Most patients with Langerhans cell histiocytosis have a deficiency of circulating suppressor lymphocytes and an increased peripheral blood helper-suppressor cell ratio, suggesting immune dysregulation as the cause of the abnormal macrophage behavior. In some patients there is histologic evidence of an abnormal thymus.

Langerhans cell histiocytosis will occasionally be seen in the newborn, generally in the disseminated (Letterer-Siwe) form or as an isolated spontaneously resolving cutaneous involvement, which has been called congenital self-healing reticulohistiocytosis or Hashimoto-Pritzker disease. The infant with Langerhans cell histiocytosis will often present with extensive hepatosplenomegaly, lymphadenopathy, and skin infiltration. Fever and jaundice are often present. Lytic bone lesions will eventually be seen, although they may not always be present at diagnosis in the infants. These lesions most typically involve the skull, ribs, pelvis, and scapula but may also be seen in the long bones and spine. Exophthalmos may result from a tumor mass in the orbit, and otitis media with drainage is often associated with destruction of the mastoid and petrous portion of the temporal bone. Pulmonary involvement may cause interstitial infiltrates and respiratory compromise. The disseminated form with multiple organ dysfunction has a poor prognosis, with less than 40 per cent survival (Raney and D'Angio, 1989). In contrast, many infants have now been described who present with isolated skin lesions of Langerhans cell histiocytosis that resolve over months to years without dissemination or any specific therapy (Kanitakis and colleagues, 1988). These infants present soon after birth with red-violaceous or brown, firm nodules scattered over the scalp and face, where they are more numerous, and also over the trunk and proximal part of the limbs. No systemic manifestations are present, and health is good. Sometimes the cutaneous form may present as an erythematous, scaly maculopapular rash on the scalp and intertriginous areas, which may include vesicular and crusted lesions. It is often confused with seborrhea, but the reddish-brown or purpuric papules are typical of histiocytosis. Histochemical and cell surface phenotype of the cutaneous self-healing and systemic disease appear to be indistinguishable.

Although Langerhans cell histiocytosis appears to respond to radiation and to many chemotherapeutic agents, including vincristine, vinblastine, prednisone, 6-mercaptopurine, chlorambucil, methotrexate, and cyclophosphamide, investigators have been unable to show any definitive improvement in cure rates using these modalities. The rarity of the disease combined with the high rate of self-healing has made prospective studies problematic. Langerhans cell histiocytosis will respond locally to low-dose radiation therapy, 600 to 1000 cGy, which can be used for troublesome bone lesions that threaten well-being. For life-threatening disseminated histiocytosis with organ dysfunction, single-agent or combination chemotherapy has produced responses. In general, the minimal therapy that will control the disease is advised. For isolated skin lesions, topical corticosteroid preparations and expectant care only are recommended.

FAMILIAL ERYTHROPHAGOCYTIC LYMPHOHISTIOCYTOSIS

Like infants with Letterer-Siwe disease, infants with familial erythrophagocytic lymphocytosis also become ill within the first few months of life, with fever, anorexia, and wasting. However, this disease is differentiated by the presence of hemophagocytosis and a positive family history. This rare and fatal disease has an autosomal recessive pattern of inheritance, although a genetic marker is as yet unidentified. The proliferating histiocytes in familial erythrophagocytic lymphohistiocytosis have a phenotype similar to that of normal reactive sinusoidal histiocytes and lack the typical S-100 protein, CD-1, and Birbeck granules found in Langerhans cell histiocytosis (Wieczorek et al., 1986).

Patients present with fever, wasting, hepatosplenomegaly, and progressive pancytopenia. Central nervous symptoms with seizures, disorientation, and coma with elevated cerebrospinal fluid protein levels and pleocytosis are common. Biopsy specimens of lesions found in the liver, spleen, lymph nodes, lungs, or bone marrow show marked erythrophagocytosis and a lymphohistiocytic infiltrate. The disease usually has a fulminant downhill course, with death in virtually all patients regardless of treatment. Etoposide and other antineoplastic drugs have induced temporary remission but have not changed the outcome. Plasmapheresis has also been tested with only temporary clinical improvement and correction of depressed cellular immune responses; bone marrow transplantation has also been used successfully in one patient (Ladisch and Jaffe, 1989).

MALIGNANT HISTIOCYTOSIS

Malignant histiocytosis has been reported occasionally in newborns (Ishii et al., 1987). It is characterized clinically by a similar symptomatology to familial erythrophagocytic lymphohistiocytosis, with fever, hepatosplenomegaly, lymphadenopathy, and pancytopenia. However, the family history is negative and pathologic examination shows malignant cells with large nuclei and prominent nucleoli that have histochemical features of histiocytes (stain positively with α-naphthyl butyrate esterase). Erythrophagocytosis may be present but less prominent than in familial erythrophagocytic lymphohistiocytosis. The disease is more responsive to chemotherapy regimens containing cyclophosphamide, prednisone, doxorubicin, vincristine, etoposide, and cytarabine. Such regimens have been reported to produce 3-year disease-free survival in 40 to 50 per cent of patients.

■ REFERENCES

Allan, R. A., Wadsworth, L. D., Kalousek, D. K., and Massing, B. G.: Congenital erythroleukemia: A case report with morphological, immunophenotypic, and cytogenetic findings. Am. J. Hematol. 31:114, 1989.

Allen, J. E.: Teratomas in infants and children. In Holland, J. F., and Frei, E., III (Eds.): Cancer Medicine. Philadelphia, Lea & Febiger, 1973.

Alpert, M. E., and Seeler, R. A.: Alpha fetoprotein in embryonal hepatoblastoma. J. Pediatr. 77:1058, 1970.

Altman, R. P., Randolph, J. G., and Lilly, J. R.: Sacrococcygeal teratomas: American Academy of Pediatrics Surgical Section Survey—1973. J. Pediatr. Surg. 9:989, 1974.

Anday, E. K., and Harris, M. C.: Leukemoid reaction associated with antenatal dexamethasone administration. J. Pediatr. 101:614, 1982.

Anders, D., Kindermann, G., and Pfeifer, U.: Metastasizing fetal neuroblastoma with involvement of the placenta simulating fetal erythroblastosis. J. Pediatr. 82:50, 1973.

Anderson, J. F., Kent, S., and Machin, G. A.: Maternal malignant melanoma with placental metastasis: A case report with literature review. Pediatr. Pathol. 9:35, 1989.

Bader, J. L., and Miller, R. W.: U.S. cancer incidence and mortality in the first year of life. Am. J. Dis. Child. 133:157, 1979.

Barnes, A. B., Colton, T., Gundersen, J., et al.: Fertility and outcome of pregnancy in women exposed in utero to diethylstilbestrol. N. Engl. J. Med. 302:609, 1980.

Beckwith, J. B.: Mesenchymal renal neoplasms of infancy revisited. J. Pediatr. Surg. 9:803, 1974.

Beckwith, J. B., and Perrin, E. V.: In situ neuroblastoma: A contribution to the natural history of neural crest tumors. Am. J. Pathol. 43:1089, 1963.

Bell, R. J. M.: Fetal virilisation due to maternal Krukenberg tumour. Lancet 1:1162, 1977.

Bennett, J. M., Catovsky, D., Daniel, M. T., et al.: Proposals for the classification of the acute leukaemias: French-American-British (FAB) Co-Operative Group. Br. J. Hematol. 33:451, 1976.

Bernard, J., Jacquillat, C., Chavalet, F., et al.: Leucemie aigue d'une enfant de 5 mois née d'une mere atteinte de leucemie aigue au moment de l'accouchement. Nouv. Rev. Fr. Hematol. 4:140, 1964.

Bibbo, M., Gill, W. B., Azizi, F., et al.: Follow-up study of male and female offspring of DES-exposed mothers. Obstet. Gynecol. 49:1, 1977.

Bithell, J. F., and Stewart, A. M.: Prenatal irradiation and childhood malignancy: A review of British data from the Oxford survey. Br. J. Cancer 31:271, 1975.

Blair, J. I., Carachi, R., Gupta, R., et al.: Plasma α-fetoprotein reference ranges in infancy: Effect of prematurity. Arch. Dis. Child. 62:362, 1987.

Blattner, W. A., Henson, D. E., Young, R. C., and Fraumeni, J. F., Jr.: Malignant mesenchymoma and birth defects, prenatal exposure to phenytoin. J.A.M.A. 238:334, 1977.

Bolande, R. P., Brough, A. J., and Izant, R. J.: Congenital mesoblastic nephroma of infancy: A report of eight cases and the relationship to Wilms' tumor. Pediatrics 40:272, 1967.

Bonnin, J. M., Rubinstein, L. J., Palmer, N. F., and Beckwith, J. B.: The association of embryonal tumors originating in the kidney and in the brain: A report of seven cases. Cancer 54:2137, 1984.

Bove, K. E., and McAdams, A. J.: The nephroblastomatosis complex and its relationship to Wilms' tumor: A clinicopathologic treatise. Perspect. Pediatr. Pathol. 3:185, 1976.

Breslow, N. E., Palmer, N. F., Hill, L. R., et al.: Wilms' tumor: Prognostic factors for patients without metastases at diagnosis. Cancer 41:1577, 1978.

Broadbent, V., and Pritchard, J.: Histiocytosis X—current controversies. Arch. Dis. Child. 60:605, 1985.

Brodeur, G. M., Seeger, R. C., Barrett, A., et al.: International criteria for diagnosis, staging, and response to treatment in patient with neuroblastoma. J. Clin. Oncol. 6:1874, 1988.

Brodeur, G. M., Seeger, R. C., Schwab, M., et al.: Amplification of N-myc in untreated human neuroblastoma correlates with advanced disease stage. Science 224:1121, 1984.

Cairney, A. E. L., Andrews, M., Greenberg, M., et al.: Wilms tumor in three patients with Bloom syndrome. J. Pediatr. 111:414, 1987.

Campbell, A. N., Chan, H. S. L., O'Brien, A., et al.: Malignant tumours in the neonate. Arch. Dis. Child. 62:19, 1987a.

Campbell, W. A., Macafee, A. L., and Wade, W. B.: Familial neonatal leukaemia. Arch. Dis. Child. 37:93, 1962.

Campbell, W. A., Storlazzi, E., Vintzileos, A. M., et al.: Fetal malignant melanoma: Ultrasound presentation and review of the literature. Obstet. Gynecol. 70:434, 1987b.

Cavell, B.: Transplacental metastasis of malignant melanoma. Acta Paediatr. Suppl. 146:37, 1963.

Cavenee, W. K., Murphree, A. L., Shull, M. M., et al.: Prediction of familial predisposition to retinoblastoma. N. Engl. J. Med. 314:1201, 1986.

Chan, H. S. L., Cheng, M-Y., Mancer, K., et al.: Congenital mesoblastic nephroma: A clinicoradiologic study of 17 cases representing the pathologic spectrum of the disease. J. Pediatr. 111:64, 1987.

Chatten, J., Shimada, H., Sather, H. N., et al.: Prognostic value of histopathology in advanced neuroblastoma: A report from The Children's Cancer Study Group. Hum. Pathol. 19:1187, 1988.

Christiansen, H., and Lampert, F.: Tumour karyotype discriminates between good and bad prognostic outcome in neuroblastoma. Br. J. Cancer 57:121, 1988.

Cohn, S. L., Herst, C. V., Maurer, H. S., and Rosen, S. T.: N-myc amplification in an infant with Stage IVS neuroblastoma. J. Clin. Oncol. 5:1441, 1987.

Coldman, A. J., Fryer, C. J. H., Elwood, J. M., and Sonley, M. J.: Neuroblastoma: Influence of age at diagnosis, stage, tumor site, and sex on prognosis. Cancer 46:1896, 1980.

Conley, G. R., Sant, G. R., Ucci, A. A., and Mitcheson, H. D.: Seminoma and epididymal cysts in a young man with known diethylstilbestrol exposure in utero. J.A.M.A. 249:1325, 1983.

Cowell, J., and Pritchard, J.: The molecular genetics of retinoblastoma and Wilms' tumor. Science 7:153, 1987.

Cramblett, H. G., Friedman, J. L., and Najjar, S.: Leukemia in an infant born of a mother with leukemia. N. Engl. J. Med. 259:727, 1958.

Crist, W., Pullen, J., Boyett, J., et al.: Clinical and biologic features predict a poor prognosis in acute lymphoid leukemias in infants: A Pediatric Oncology Group Study. Blood 67:135, 1986.

Crom, D. B., Williams, J. A., Green, A. A., et al.: Malignancy in the neonate. Med. Pediatr. Oncol. 17:101, 1989.

Cutler, L. S., Chaudry, A. P., and Topazian, R.: Melanotic neuroectodermal tumor of infancy: An ultrastructural study, literature review, and reevaluation. Cancer 48:257, 1981.

D'Angio, G. J., Breslow, N., Beckwith, B., et al.: Treatment of Wilms' tumor: Results of the Third National Wilms' Tumor Study. Cancer 64:349, 1989.

D'Angio, G. J., Evans, A., Breslow, N., et al.: The treatment of Wilms' tumor: Results of the second National Wilms' Tumor Study. Cancer 47:2302, 1981.

D'Angio, G. J., Evans, A. E., and Koop, C. E.: Special pattern of widespread neuroblastoma with a favorable prognosis. Lancet 1:1046, 1971.

Dehner, L. P.: Neoplasms of the fetus and neonate. In Naeye, R. L., Kissane, J. M., and Kaufman, N. (Eds.): Perinatal Diseases. International Academy of Pathology Monograph No. 22. Baltimore, Williams & Wilkins Company, 1981, p. 286.

Dehner, L. P.: Gonadal and extragonadal germ cell neoplasia of childhood. Hum. Pathol. 14:493, 1983.

Diamond, C. A., and Matthay, K. K.: Childhood acute lymphoblastic leukemia. Pediatr. Ann. 17:156, 1988.

Diamond, E. L., Schmerler, H., and Lilienfeld, A. M.: The relationship of intrauterine radiation to subsequent mortality and development of leukemia in children: A prospective study. Am. J. Epidemiol. 97:283, 1973.

Donaldson, S., and Smith, L. M.: Retinoblastoma: Biology, presentation, and current management. Oncology 3:45, 1989.

Dryja, T. P., Cavenee, W., White, R., et al.: Homozygosity of chromosome 13 in retinoblastoma. N. Engl. J. Med. 310:550, 1984.

Ehrenbard, L. T., and Chaganti, R. S. K.: Cancer in the fetal hydantoin syndrome. Lancet 2:97, 1981.

Esseltine, D. W., De Leeuw, N. K. M., and Berry, G. R.: Malignant histiocytosis. Cancer 52:1904, 1983.

Evans, A. E., d'Angio, G. J., and Randolph, J. R.: A proposed staging for children with neuroblastoma: A report for The Children's Cancer Study Group. Cancer 27:374, 1971.

Evans, A. E., Brand, W., and deLorimier, A.: Results in children with local and regional neuroblastoma managed with and without vincristine, cyclophosphamide, and imidazolecarboxamide. Am. J. Clin. Oncol. 6:3, 1984.

Evans, A. E., Land, V. J., Newton, W. A., et al.: Combination chemotherapy (vincristine, adriamycin, cyclophosphamide, and 5-fluorouracil) in the treatment of children with malignant hepatoma. Cancer 50:821, 1982.

Everson, T. C., and Cole, W. H.: Spontaneous Regression of Cancer: A Study and Abstract of Reports in the World Medical Literature and of Personal Communications Concerning Spontaneous Regression of Malignant Disease. Philadelphia, W. B. Saunders Company, 1966, pp. 88–163.

Exelby, P. R., Filler, R. M., and Grosfeld, J. L.: Liver tumors in children in particular reference to hepatoblastoma and hepatocellular carcinoma: American Academy of Pediatrics Surgical Section Survey—1974. J. Pediatr. Surg. 10:325, 1975.

Falk, H., Herbert, J. T., Edmonds, L., et al.: Review of four cases of childhood hepatic angiosarcoma: Elevated environmental arsenic exposure in one case. Cancer 47:382, 1981.

Farber, S.: Chemotherapy in the treatment of leukemia and Wilms' tumor. J.A.M.A. 108:826, 1966.

Feine, U., Muller-Schauenburg, W., Treuner, J., and Klingebiel, T.: Metaiodobenzylguanidine (MIBG) labeled with $^{123}I/^{131}I$ in neuroblastoma diagnosis and follow-up treatment with a review of the diagnostic results of the International Workshop of Pediatric Oncology held in Rome, September 1986. Med. Pediatr. Oncol. 15:181, 1987.

Felix, C. A., Reaman, G. H., Korsmeyer, S. J., et al.: Immunoglobulin and T cell regulator gene configuration in acute lymphoblastic leukemia of infancy. Blood 70:536, 1987.

Finklestein, J. Z.: Neuroblastoma: The challenge and frustration. Hematol. Oncol. Clin. North Am. 1:675, 1987.

Flamant, F., Schwartz, L., Delons, E., et al.: Nonseminomatous malignant germ cell tumors in children: Multidrug therapy in Stages III and IV. Cancer 54:1687, 1984.

Fong, C., and Brodeur, G. M.: Down syndrome and leukemia: Epidemiology, genetics, cytogenetics and mechanisms of leukemogenesis. Cancer Genet. Cytogenet. 28:55, 1987.

Fong, C., Dracopoli, N. C., White, P. S., et al.: Loss of heterozygosity for the short arm of chromosome 1 in human neuroblastomas: Correlation with N-myc amplification. Proc. Natl. Acad. Sci. USA 86:3753, 1989.

Fraumeni, J. F., and Miller, R. W.: Cancer deaths in the newborn. Am. J. Dis. Child. 117:186, 1969.

Gallo, G. E., and Chemes, H. E.: The association of Wilms' tumor, male pseudohermaphroditism and diffuse glomerular disease (Drash syndrome): Report of eight cases with clinical and morphologic findings and review of the literature. Pediatr. Pathol. 7:175, 1987.

Gansler, T., Chatten, J., Varello, M., et al.: Flow cytometric DNA analysis of neuroblastoma. Cancer 58:2453, 1986.

Geatti, O., Shapiro, B., Sisson, J. C., et al.: Iodine-131 metaiodobenzylguanidine scintigraphy for the location of neuroblastoma: Preliminary experience in ten cases. J. Nucl. Med. 26:736, 1985.

Gill, W. B., Schumacher, G. F. B., Bibbo, M., et al.: Association of diethylstilbestrol exposure in utero with cryptorchidism, testicular hypoplasia, and semen abnormalities. J. Urol. 122:36, 1979.

Gonzalez-Crussi, F., Winkler, R. F., and Mirkin, D. L.: Sacrococcygeal teratomas in infants and children. Arch. Pathol. Lab. Med. 102:420, 1978.

Greenberger, J. S., Crocker, A. C., Vawter, G., et al.: Results of treatment of 127 patients with systemic histiocytosis (Letterer-Siwe syndrome, Schüller-Christian syndrome, and multifocal esoinophilic granuloma). Medicine 60:311, 1981.

Gutierrez-Ortega, P., Hierro-Orozco, S., Sanchez-Cisneros, R., and Montano, L. F.: Kaposi's sarcoma in a 6-day-old infant with human immunodeficiency virus (letter). Arch. Dermatol. 125:432, 1989.

Haas, D., Ablin, A. R., Miller, C., Zoger, S., and Matthay, K. K.: Complete pathologic maturation and regression of Stage IVS neuroblastoma without treatment. Cancer 62:818, 1988.

Haicken, B. N., and Miller, D. R.: Simultaneous occurrence of congenital aniridia, hamartoma, and Wilms' tumor. J. Pediatr. 78:497, 1971.

Hann, H. L., Evans, A. E., Cohen, I. J., and Leitmeyer, J. E.: Biological differences between neuroblastoma stages IV-S and IV: Measurement of serum ferritin and E-rosette inhibition in 30 children. N. Engl. J. Med. 305:425, 1981.

Hann, H. L., Evans, A. E., Siegel, S. E., et al.: Prognostic importance of serum ferritin in patients with Stages III and IV neuroblastoma: The Children's Cancer Study Group experience. Cancer Res. 45:2843, 1985.

Hawthorne, H. C., Nelson, J. S., Witzleben, C. L., and Giangiacomo, J.: Blanching subcutaneous nodules in neonatal neuroblastoma. J. Pediatr. 77:297, 1970.

Hayashi, Y., Eguchi, M., Sugita, K., et al.: Cytogenetic findings and clinical features in acute leukemia and transient myeloproliferative disorder in Down syndrome. Blood 72:15, 1988.

Hayashi, Y., Kanda, N., Inaba, T., et al.: Cytogenetic findings and prognosis in neuroblastoma with emphasis on marker chromosome 1. Cancer 63:126, 1989.

Haymond, M. W., and Weldon, V. V.: Female pseudohermaphroditism secondary to a maternal virilizing tumor: Case report and review of the literature. J. Pediatr. 82:682, 1973.

Herbst, A. L., Cole, P., Colton, T., et al.: Age-incidence and risk of diethylstilbestrol-related adenocarcinoma of the vagina and cervix. Am. J. Obstet. Gynecol. 128:43, 1977.

Isaacs, H., Jr.: Perinatal (congenital and neonatal) neoplasms: A report of 110 cases. Pediatr. Pathol. 3:165, 1985.

Ishii, E., Hara, T., Okamura, J., et al.: Malignant histiocytosis in infants: Surface marker analysis of malignant cells in two cases. Med. Pediatr. Oncol. 15:102, 1987.

Jablon, S., and Kato, H.: Childhood cancer in relation to prenatal exposure to atomic-bomb radiation. Lancet 2:1000, 1970.

Jick, H., Walker, A. M., Rothman, K. J., et al.: Vaginal spermicides and congenital disorders. J.A.M.A. 245:1329, 1981.

Jiminez, J. F., Brown, R. E., Seibert, R. W., Seibert, J. J., and Char, F.: Melanotic neuroectodermal tumor of infancy and fetal hydantoin syndrome. Am. J. Pediatr. Hematol. Oncol. 3:9, 1981.

Johnson, S., Knight, R., Marmer, D. J., and Steele, R. W.: Immune deficiency in fetal alcohol syndrome. Pediatr. Res. 15:908, 1981.

Joshi, V. V., Banenee, A. K., Yadav, K., and Pathak, I. C.: Cystic partially differentiated nephroblastoma. Cancer 40:789, 1977.

Kaneko, Y., Shikano, T., Maseki, N., et al.: Clinical characteristics of infant acute leukemia with or without 11q23 translocations. Leukemia 2:672, 1988.

Kanitakis, J., Zambruno, G., Schmitt, D., et al.: Congenital self-healing histiocytosis (Hashimoto-Pritzker). Cancer 61:508, 1988.

Kasdon, S. C.: Pregnancy and Hodgkin's disease. Am. J. Obstet. Gynecol. 57:282, 1949.

Katz, F., Malcolm, S., Gibbons, B., et al.: Cellular and molecular studies on infant null acute lymphoblastic leukemia. Blood 71:1438, 1988.

Kinney, H., Faix, R., and Brazy, J.: The fetal alcohol syndrome and neuroblastoma. Pediatrics 66:130, 1980.

Knudson, A. F., Meadows, A. T., Nichols, W. W., and Hill, R.: Chromosomal deletion in retinoblastoma. N. Engl. J. Med. 295:1120, 1976.

Kojima S., Mimaya, J., Tonouchi, T., et al.: Identification of myeloid origin in undifferentiated congenital leukemia by in vitro marrow culture study. Am. J. Pediatr. Hematol. Oncol. 11:337, 1989.

Koscielniak, E., Harms, D., Schmidt, D., et al.: Soft tissue sarcomas in infants younger than 1 year of age: A report of the German Soft Tissue Sarcoma Study Group (CSW-81). Med. Pediatr. Oncol. 17:105, 1989.

Kramer, S., Ward, E., Meadows, A. T., and Malone, K. E.: Medical and drug risk factors associated with neuroblastoma: A case-control study. J.N.C.I. 78:797, 1987.

Kretschmar, C. S., Frantz, C. N., Rosen, E. M., et al.: Improved prognosis for infants with Stage IV neuroblastoma. J. Clin. Oncol. 2:799, 1984.

Kulkarni, R., Bailie, M. P., Bernstein, J., and Newton, B.: Progression of nephroblastomatosis to Wilms' tumor. J. Pediatr. 96:178, 1980.

Kumar, A. P. M., Pratt, C. B., Coburn, T. P., and Johnson, W. W.: Treatment strategy for nodular renal blastema and nephroblastomatosis associated with Wilms' tumor. J. Pediatr. Surg. 13:281, 1978.

Ladisch, S., and Jaffe, E. S.: The histiocytoses. In Pizzo, P. A., and Poplack, D. G. (Eds.): Pediatric Oncology. Philadelphia, J. B. Lippincott, 1989, pp. 491–504.

Lampkin, B., Buckley, J., Nesbit, M., Hammond, D., and Children's Cancer Study Group (CCSG), Los Angeles: Clinical and laboratory findings and responses to therapy in infants less than one year of age with acute non-lymphoblastic leukemia (ANLL). Proc. Am. Soc. Clin. Oncol. 3:201, 1984.

Lazarus, K. H., D'Orsogna, D. E., Bloom, K. R., and Rouse, R. G.: Primary pericardial sarcoma in a neonate. Am. J. Pediatr. Hematol. Oncol. 11:343, 1989.

Lazarus, K. H., Heerema, N. A., Palmer, C. G., and Baehner, R. L.: The myeloproliferative reaction in a child with Down syndrome: Cytological and chromosomal evidence for a transient leukemia. Am. J. Hematol. 11:417, 1981.

Lemieux, B., Auray-Blais, C., Giguere, R., and Scriver, C. R.: Neuroblastoma screening: The Canadian experience. Med. Pediatr. Oncol. 17:279, 1989.

Lergier, J. E., Jiminez, E., Maldonado, N., and Veray, F.: Normal pregnancy in multiple myeloma treated with cyclophosphamide. Cancer 34:1018, 1974.

Li, F. P., Williams, W. R., Gimbrere, K., et al.: Heritable fraction of unilateral Wilms tumor. Pediatrics 81:147, 1988.

Logothetis, C. J., Samules, M. L., Selig, D. E., et al.: Chemotherapy of extragonadal germ cell tumors. J. Clin. Oncol. 3:316, 1985.

Look, A. T., Hayes, F. A., Nitschke, R., et al.: Cellular DNA content as a predictor of response to chemotherapy in infants with unresectable neuroblastoma. N. Engl. J. Med. 311:231, 1984.

Ludwig, W-D., Bartram, C. R., Harbott, J., et al.: Phenotypic and genotypic heterogeneity in infant acute leukemia: I. Acute lymphoblastic leukemia. Leukemia 3:431, 1989.

MacMahon, B., and Levy, M. A.: Prenatal origin of childhood leukemia: Evidence from twins. N. Engl. J. Med. 270:1082, 1964.

Martin, E. S., and Griffith, J. F.: Myoclonic encephalopathy and neuroblastoma. Am. J. Dis. Child. 122:257, 1971.

Mason, G. A., Hart-Mercer, J., Miller, E. J., et al.: Adrenaline-secreting neuroblastoma in an infant. Lancet ii:322, 1957.

Matthay, K. K., Sather, H. N., Seeger, R. C., et al.: Excellent outcome of Stage II neuroblastoma is independent of residual disease and radiation therapy. J. Clin. Oncol. 7:236, 1989.

Maurer, H. S., Pendergrass, T. W., Borges, W., and Honig, G. R.: The role of genetic factor in the etiology of Wilms' tumor: Two pairs of monozygous twins with congenital abnormalities (aniridia; hemihypertrophy) and discordance for Wilms' tumor. Cancer 43:205, 1979.

McKinney, P. A., Cartwright, R. A., Saiu, J. M. T., et al.: The interregional epidemiological study of childhood cancer (IRESCC): A case control study of aetiological factors in leukaemia and lymphoma. Arch. Dis. Child. 62:279, 1987.

Meadows, A. T., Lichtenfeld, J. L., and Koop, C. E.: Wilms' tumor in three children of a woman with congenital hemihypertrophy. N. Engl. J. Med. 291:23, 1974.

Melnick, S., Cole, P., Andersen, D., and Herbst, A.: Rates and risks of diethylstilbestrol-related clear-cell carcinoma of the vagina and cervix: An update. N. Engl. J. Med. 316:514, 1987.

Miller, D. R., Newstead, G. J., and Young, L. W.: Perinatal leukemia with a possible variant of Ellis–van Creveld syndrome. J. Pediatr. 74:300, 1969.

Miller, M., and Cosgriff, J. M.: Hematological abnormalities in newborn infants with Down syndrome. Am. J. Med. Genet. 16:173, 1983.

Miller, R. W.: Down syndrome (mongolism), other congenital malformations and cancers among the sibs of leukemic children. N. Engl. J. Med. 268:393, 1963.

Miller, R. W.: Persons at exceptionally high risk of leukemia. Cancer Res. 27:2420, 1967.

Miller, R. W.: Relation between cancer and congenital defects: An epidemiologic evaluation. J.N.C.I. 40:1079, 1968.

Miller, R. W.: Discordance for Wilms' tumor in MZ twins with aniridia. Childhood Cancer Etiol. Newsletter No. 56, 1979.

Moe, P. G., and Nellhaus, G.: Infantile polymyoclonia-opsoclonus syndrome and neural crest tumors. Neurology 20:756, 1970.

Morgan, E., Baum, E., Breslow, N., et al.: Chemotherapy-related toxicity in infants treated according to the Second National Wilms' Tumor Study. J. Clin. Oncol. 6:51, 1988.

Moss, T. J., Seeger, R. C., Kindler-Rohrbora, A., et al.: Immunohistologic detection and phenotyping of neuroblastoma cells in bone marrow using cytoplasmic neuron-specific enolase and cell surface antigens. In Evans, A. E., D'Angio, G. J., and Seeger, R. C. (Eds.): Advances in Neuroblastoma Research. New York, Alan R. Liss, 1985, pp. 367–378.

Murphree, A. L., and Benedict, W. F.: Retinoblastoma: Clues to human oncogenesis. Science 223:1028, 1984.

Nagasaka, M., Maeda, S., Maeda, H., et al.: Four cases of t(4;11) acute leukemia and its myelomonocytic nature in infants. Blood 61:1174, 1983.

Napalkov, N.: In Tomatis, L., Mohr, U., and Davis, W. (Eds.): Transplacental Carcinogenesis. International Agency for Research on Cancer Scientific Publication No. 4, 1973.

Nesbit, M. D., Jr., O'Leary, M., Dehner, L. P., and Ramsay, N. K. C.: The immune system and the histiocytosis syndromes. Am. J. Pediatr. Hematol. Oncol. 3:141, 1981.

Nickerson, H. J., Nesbit, M. E., Grosfeld, J. L., et al.: Comparison of Stage IV and IV-S neuroblastoma in the first year of life. Med. Pediatr. Oncol. 13:261, 1985.

Odom, L. F., and Gordon, E. M.: Acute monoblastic leukemia in infancy and early childhood: Successful treatment with an epipodophyllotoxin. Blood 64:875, 1984.

Padilla, R. S., McConnell, T. S., Gribble, J. T., and Smoot, C.: Malignant melanoma arising in a giant congenital melanocytic nevus. Cancer 62:2589, 1988.

Parkin, D. M., Stiller, C. A., Draper, G. J., and Bieber, C. A.: The international incidence of childhood cancer. Int. J. Cancer 42:511, 1988.

Pastore, G., Carli, M., Lemerle, J., et al.: Epidemiological features of Wilms' tumor: Results of studies by the International Society of Paediatric Oncology (SIOP). Med. Pediatr. Oncol. 16:7, 1988.

Pettinato, G., Manivel, J. C., Wick, M. R., and Dehner, L. P.: Classical and cellular (atypical) congenital mesoblastic nephroma: A clinicopathologic, ultrastructural, immunohistochemical, and flow cytometric study. Hum. Pathol. 20:682, 1989.

Philip, T., Bernard, J. L., Zucker, J. M., et al.: High-dose chemoradiotherapy with bone marrow transplantation as consolidation treatment in neuroblastoma: An unselected group of Stage IV patients over 1 year of age. J. Clin. Oncol. 5:266, 1987.

Pierce, M. I.: Leukemia in the newborn infant. J. Pediatr. 54:691, 1959.

Pilling, G. P.: Wilms' tumor in seven children with congenital aniridia. J. Pediatr. Surg. 10:87, 1975.

Prose, N. S., Laude, T. A., Heilman, E. R., and Coren, C.: Congenital malignant melanoma. Pediatrics 79:967, 1987.

Pui, C-H., Raimondi, S. C., Murphy, S. B., et al.: An analysis of leukemic cell chromosomal features in infants. Blood 69:1289, 1987.

Quinn, J. J., Altman, A. J., and Frantz, C. N.: Serum lactic dehydrogenase, an indicator of tumor activity in neuroblastoma. J. Pediatr. 97:89, 1980.

Quinn, J. J., Altman, A. J., Robinson, H. T., et al.: Adriamycin and cisplatin for hepatoblastoma. Cancer 56:1926, 1985.

Ragab, A. H., Heyn, R., Tefft, M., et al.: Infants younger than one year of age with rhabdomyosarcoma. Cancer 58:2606, 1986.

Raney, R. B., Jr., Chatten, J., Littman, P., et al.: Treatment strategies for infants with malignant sacrococcygeal teratoma. J. Pediatr. Surg. 16:573, 1981.

Raney, R. B., Jr., and D'Angio, G. J.: Langerhans' cell histiocytosis (histiocytosis X): Experience at the Children's Hospital of Philadelphia, 1970–1984. Med. Pediatr. Oncol. 17:20, 1989.

Reaman, G.: Special considerations for the infant with cancer. In Pizzo, P. A., and Poplack, D. G. (Eds.): Pediatric Oncology. Philadelphia, J. B. Lippincott, 1989, pp. 263–274.

Reaman, G., Zeltzer, P., Bleyer, W. A., et al.: Acute lymphoblastic leukemia in infants less than one year of age: A cumulative experience of the Children's Cancer Study Group. J. Clin. Oncol. 3:1513, 1985.

Reinberg, Y., Anderson, G. F., Franciosi, R., et al.: Wilms tumor and the VATER association. J. Urol. 140:787, 1988.

Riccardi, V. M., Sujansky, E., Smith, A. C., and Francke, U.: Chromosomal imbalance in the aniridia–Wilms' tumor association: 11p interstitial deletion. Pediatrics 61:604, 1978.

Robboy, S. J., Kauffman, R. H., Prat, J., et al.: Pathologic findings in women enrolled in the National Cooperative Diethylstilbestrol Adenosis (DESAD) Project. Obstet. Gynecol. 53:309, 1979.

Rosner, F., and Lee, S. L.: Down syndrome and acute leukemia: Myeloblastic or lymphoblastic? Report of forty-three cases and review of the literature. Am. J. Med. 53:203, 1972.

Ross, J. D., Moloney, W. C., and Desforges, J. F.: Ineffective regulation of granulopoiesis masquerading as congenital leukemia in a mongoloid child. J. Pediatr. 63:1, 1963.

Sansone, R., Haupt, R., Stigini, P., et al.: Congenital leukemia: Persistent spontaneous regression in a patient with an acquired abnormal karyotype. Acta Haematol. 81:48, 1989.

Sawada, T., Kidowaki, T., Sakamoto, I., et al.: Neuroblastoma: Mass screening for early detection and its prognosis. Cancer 53:2731, 1984.

Schneider, K. M., Becker, J. M., and Krasna, I. H.: Neonatal neuroblastoma. Pediatrics 36:359, 1965.

Schneiderman, H., Wu, A. Y-Y., Campbell, W. A., et al.: Congenital melanoma with multiple prenatal metastases. Cancer 60:1371, 1987.

Schoeck, V. W., Peterson, R. D. A., and Good, R. A.: Familial occurrence of Letterer-Siwe disease. Pediatrics 32:1055, 1963.

Schwartz, A. D., Dadash-Zadeh, M., Lee, H., and Swaney, J. J.: Spontaneous regression of disseminated neuroblastoma. J. Pediatr. 85:760, 1974.

Seeger, R. C., Brodeur, G. M., Sather, H., et al.: Association of multiple copies of the N-myc oncogene with rapid progression of neuroblastomas. N. Engl. J. Med. 313:1111, 1985.

Seeger, R. C., Moss, T. J., Feig, S. A., et al.: Bone marrow transplantation for poor prognosis neuroblastoma. In Gale, R. P., and Champlin, R. (Eds.): Bone Marrow Transplantation: Current Controversies. Prog. Clin. Biol. Res. 271:203, 1988.

Seibel, N. L., Sommer, A., and Miser, J.: Transient neonatal leukemoid reactions in mosaic trisomy 21. J. Pediatr. 104:251, 1984.

Shamberger, R. C., Holcombe, E. G., Weinstein, H. J., et al.: Chest wall tumors in infancy and childhood. Cancer 63:774, 1989.

Shimada, H., Chatten, J., Newton, W. A., Jr., Marsden, H. B., and Misugi, K.: Histopathologic prognostic factors in neuroblastic tumors: Definition of subtypes of ganglioneuroblastoma and an age-linked classification of neuroblastomas. J.N.C.I. 73:405, 1984.

Sitarz, A. L., Santulli, T. V., Wigger, H. J., and Berdon, W. E.: Complete maturation of neuroblastoma with bone metastases in documented stages. J. Pediatr. Surg. 10:533, 1975.

Solis, V., Pritchard, J., and Cowell, J. K.: Cytogenetic changes in Wilms' tumors. Cancer Genet. Cytogenet. 34:223, 1988.

Sorrell, T. C., Forbes, I. J., Burness, F. R., and Rischbieth, R. H. C.: Depression of immunological function in patients treated with phenytoin sodium (sodium diphenylhydantoin). Lancet 2:1233, 1971.

Sotelo-Avila, C., Gonzalez-Crussi, F., and Fowler, J. W.: Complete and incomplete forms of Beckwith-Wiedemann syndrome: Their oncogenic potential. J. Pediatr. 96:47, 1980.

Spear, G. S., Hyde, T. P., Gruppo, R. A., and Slusser, R.: Pseudohermaphroditism, glomerulonephritis with the nephrotic syndrome and Wilms' tumor in infancy. J. Pediatr. 79:677, 1971.

Spitz, M., and Johnson, C. C.: Neuroblastoma and paternal occupation: A case-control analysis. Am. J. Epidemiol. 121:924, 1985.

Stark, B., Hershko, C., Rosen, N., et al.: Familial hemophagocytic lymphohistiocytosis (FHLH) in Israel: I. Description of 11 patients of Iranian-Iraqi origin and review of the literature. Cancer 54:2109, 1984.

Stark, B., Vogel, R., Cohen, I. J., et al.: Biologic and cytogenetic characteristics of leukemia in infants. Cancer 63:117, 1989.

Stark, C. R., and Mantel, N.: Effects of maternal age and birth order on the risk of mongolism and leukemia. J.N.C.I. 37:687, 1966.

Suda, J., Eguchi, M., Akiyama, Y., et al.: Differentiation of blast cells from a Down syndrome patient with transient myeloproliferative disorder. Blood 69:508, 1987.

Sullivan, M. P., Hussey, D. H., and Ayala, A. G.: Wilms' tumor. In Sutow, W., Vietti, T., and Fernbach, D. (Eds.): Clinical Pediatric Oncology. St. Louis, C. V. Mosby Company, 1973, p. 359.

Swift, P. G. F., Bloom, S. R., and Harris, F.: Watery diarrhea and ganglioneuroma with secretion of vasoactive intestinal peptide. Arch. Dis. Child. 50:896, 1975.

Takaku, A., Kodama, N., Ohara, H., and Hori, S.: Brain tumor in newborn babies. Child's Brain 4:365, 1978.

Taylor, W. F., Myers, M., and Taylor, W. R.: Extrarenal Wilms' tumour in an infant exposed to intrauterine phenytoin. Lancet ii:481, 1980.

Tomatis, L.: Prenatal exposure to chemical carcinogens and its effect on subsequent generations. NCI Monogr. 51:159, 1979.

Totter, J. R., and MacPherson, H. G.: Do childhood cancers result from prenatal x-rays? Health Physics 40:511, 1981.

Touran, T., Applebaum, H., Frost, D. B., et al.: Congenital metastatic cervical teratoma: Diagnostic and management considerations. J. Pediatr. Surg. 24:21, 1989.

Turkel, S. B., and Itabashi, H. H.: The natural history of neuroblastic cells in the fetal adrenal gland. Am. J. Pathol. 76:225, 1974.

Valdiserri, R. O., and Yunis, E. J.: Sacrococcygeal teratomas: A review of 68 cases. Cancer 48:217, 1981.

van Wering, E. R., and Kamps, W. A.: Acute leukemia in infants: A unique pattern of acute nonlymphocytic leukemia. Am. J. Pediatr. Hematol. Oncol. 8:220, 1986.

Voelkerding, K. V., Sandhaus, L. M., Belov, L., et al.: Clonal B-cell proliferation in an infant with congenital HIV infection and immune thrombocytopenia. Am. J. Clin. Pathol. 90:470, 1988.

Voûte, P. A., Jr., Wadman, S. K., and van Putten, W. J.: Congenital neuroblastoma: Symptoms in the mother during pregnancy. Clin. Pediatr. 9:206, 1970.

Weeks, D. A., Beckwith, J. B., Mierau, G. W., and Luckey, D. W.: Rhabdoid tumor of kidney. Am. J. Surg. Pathol. 13:439, 1989.

Weinberg, A. G., and Finegold, M. J.: Primary hepatic tumors of childhood. Hum. Pathol. 14:512, 1983.

Weinberger, M. M., and Oleinick, A.: Congenital marrow dysfunction in Down syndrome. J. Pediatr. 77:273, 1970.

Weinblatt, M. E., Siegel, S. E., Siegel, M. M., et al.: Preoperative chemotherapy for unresectable primary hepatic malignancies in children. Cancer 50:1061, 1982.

Wieczorek, R., Greco, M. A., McCarthy, K., et al.: Immunophenotypic, immunohistochemical, and ultrastructural demonstration of the relation to sinus histiocytes. Hum. Pathol. 17:55, 1986.

Wiggs, J., Nordenskjold, M., Yandell, D., et al.: Prediction of the risk of hereditary retinoblastoma, using DNA polymorphisms within the retinoblastoma gene. N. Engl. J. Med. 318:151, 1988.

Witzleben, C. L., and Bruninga, G.: Infantile choriocarcinoma: A characteristic syndrome. J. Pediatr. 73:374, 1968.

Woods, W. G., and Tuchman, M.: Neuroblastoma: The case for screening infants in North America. Pediatrics 79:869, 1987.

Yunis, J. J., and Ramsay, N. K. C.: Familial occurrence of the aniridia–Wilms' tumor syndrome with deletion 11p13–14.1. J. Pediatr. 96:1027, 1980.

Zeltzer, P. M., Marangos, P. J., Evans, A. E., and Schneider, S. L.: Serum neuron-specific enolase in children with neuroblastoma. Cancer 57:1230, 1986.

APPENDIX 1
DRUGS

Pharmacopeia for the Newborn Period

ABBREVIATIONS:

IM—intramuscularly	PR—by rectum
IT—intratracheal	SC—subcutaneously
IV—intravenously	Top—topical
PO—by mouth	

DRUG	ROUTE AND DOSE	ADVERSE EFFECTS, CAUTIONS
Acetazolamide	PO: 5 mg/kg/dose q 6–8 h; increase as needed to 25 mg/kg/dose (*temporarily effective*)	Hyperchloremic metabolic acidosis, hypokalemia, drowsiness, paresthesias
ACTH	IM, IV, SC: 3–5 units/kg/day in 4 divided doses, usual maximum of 30 units/day	Hypertension, immunosuppression, electrolyte imbalance, cataracts, growth retardation, GI ulcers or dysfunction
Acyclovir	IV: 5–10 mg/kg/dose q 8 h, infuse over 1 h	Transient renal dysfunction; lengthen dose interval with renal failure
Albumin, 5 per cent	IV: 1.0 gm/kg slowly	Hypovolemia, heart failure; monitor blood pressure
Albuterol	Aerosol: 0.1–0.5 mg/kg/dose q 2–6 h PO: 0.1–0.3 mg/kg/dose q 6–8 h	Tachycardia, arrhythmias, tremor, irritability
Amikacin	IV, IM: 7.5 mg/kg/dose q 8–12 h; q 12 h for <1200 gm for 4 weeks	Nephrotoxicity; ototoxicity; blood level monitoring recommended (desirable levels: peak = 10–25 μg/ml; trough = 3–5 μg/ml)
Aminophylline	See Theophylline	
Amphotericin B	IV: 0.25–1.0 mg/kg/dose/day; on day 1, diluted and infused over 4–6 h (*do not use filters with pore size <1.0 micron*); total dosage 30–35 mg/kg over 6 wk	Nephrotoxicity; fever; flushing; anemia; hypotension; hyposthenuria; hypokalemia; protect bottle and tubing from light with foil
Ampicillin	IM, IV: newborns <7 days = 25–50 mg/kg/dose q 8–12 h; >7 days old = 25–50 mg/kg/dose q 6–8 h Double dose for meningitis Maintain q 12 h for 4 weeks for <1200 gm	
Amrinone	Initial: 0.75 mg/kg over 2–3 min; maintenance 5–10 mg/kg/min	Fluid balance; electrolytes; renal function
Ascorbic acid	See Vitamin C	
Atropine	IV, IM, IT, SC: 0.01–0.03 mg/kg, repeat q 2 h prn	Hyperthermia, tachycardia, urinary retention
Bacitracin	Top: as ointment (500 units/gm), q 4–8 h	
Bethanecol	PO: 0.1–0.2 mg/kg/dose q 6–8 h or 3 mg/m²/dose q 8 h 20 min before feeding	Diarrhea, jitteriness, tremors, sleeplessness, bronchoconstriction, increased tracheobronchial secretions
Caffeine	PO, IV: loading dose = 10 mg/kg; maintenance dose = 2.5 mg/kg/dose q 24 h (*doses are for the nonsalt form of drug—caffeine base*). Therapeutic plasma concentration = 5–20 μg/ml free base	Restlessness, emesis, tachycardia
Calcium chloride 10% (27 mg elemental Ca++/ml)	IV: 0.35–0.70 ml (9–19 mg Ca++)/kg/dose for acute hypocalcemia	Bradycardia if injected too quickly; necrosis from extravascular leakage
Calcium glubionate 6.47% (23 mg elemental Ca++/ml)	PO: treatment = 500 mg/kg/day q 3–4 h; supplement = 150 mg/kg/day q 3–4 h	High osmotic load of syrup may cause diarrhea
Calcium gluconate 10 per cent (9.3 mg elemental Ca++/ml)	IV: 1–2 ml (9–19 mg Ca++)/kg/dose for acute hypocalcemia PO: 3–9 ml/kg/day in 2–4 divided doses (30–80 mg/Ca++/kg/day) for chronic use	Bradycardia if injected too quickly; necrosis from extravascular leakage; gastric necrosis and calcification if it is too concentrated; diarrhea may potentiate digitalis effect
Calcium lactate 13% (130 mg elemental Ca++/gm powder)	PO: 0.5 gm/kg/day in divided doses	See Calcium gluconate; GI irritation
Captopril	PO: 0.01–0.05 mg/kg/dose q 6–24 h; increase dose q d to control blood pressure	High initial doses may cause hypotension and renal insufficiency
Carbenicillin	IV: newborns <7 days = 100 mg/kg/dose q 12 h; >7 days = 100 mg/kg/dose q 6–8 h	Sodium content is 4.7 mEq/gm, monitor electrolytes

Table continued on following page

Pharmacopeia for the Newborn Period *Continued*

ABBREVIATIONS:	IM—intramuscularly	PR—by rectum
	IT—intratracheal	SC—subcutaneously
	IV—intravenously	Top—topical
	PO—by mouth	

DRUG	ROUTE AND DOSE	ADVERSE EFFECTS, CAUTIONS
Cefotaxime	IV: 25–50 mg/kg/dose <7 days = q 12 h; >7 days = q 8 h	
Ceftazidime	IV, IM: 30–50 mg/kg/dose q 12 h up to 1 month	
Ceftriaxone	IV, IM: 50 mg/kg/dose; preterm q days till 4 wk; term < 7 days qd; term >7 days = 75 mg/kg/dose qd	
Cefuroxime	25 mg/kg/dose; <7 days q 12 h; >7 days q 8 h	
Cephalothin	20 mg/kg/dose; preterm <7 days q 12 h (till 4 wk for <1200 gm) >7 days q 8 h; term <7 days q 8 h; >7 days q 6 h	
Chloral hydrate	PO, PR: Sedative = 10–30 mg/kg/day div. q 6–8 h; hypnotic = 50 mg/kg as single dose	Gastric irritation; caution with hepatic, renal, cardiac, or pulmonary disease. Provides *no* analgesia
Chloramphenicol	IV, PO: loading dose = 20 mg/kg; maintenance = 5 mg/kg/dose q 6 h; maintenance doses vary 2.5–12.5 mg/kg/dose q 6 h; 25 mg/kg q 24 h for 4 wk for <1200 gm	Hematologic and blood level monitoring mandatory (usual therapeutic level 10–25 μg/ml). Cardiac toxicity, "gray baby" syndrome, dose-related bone marrow suppression, idiosyncratic aplastic anemia
Chlorothiazide	PO: 10–20 mg/kg/dose q 12–24 h	Hypokalemia; hyponatremia decreases calcium excretion; hyperglycemia
Chlorpromazine	PO, IM, IV: 0.2–0.5 mg/kg/dose prn withdrawal symptoms	Extrapyramidal symptoms; potentiates hypnotics and narcotics; hypotension
Cimetidine	PO, IV: 2.5–5 mg/kg/dose q 6 h according to gastric pH	H2 antagonist that has rarely been tried in newborns. Decreases drug clearance by hepatic cytochrome P450
Clindamycin	PO, IV: 5 mg/kg/dose preterm <1 wk = q 12 h, term <1 wk = q 8 h, term >1 wk = q 6 h, maintain q 12 h till 4 wk for <1200 gm	Pseudomembranous colitis is rare in newborns. Limited experience in newborns. Hepatic metabolism
Cortisone	PO: 0.5–2 mg/kg/day, divided q 6 h	Treatment of more than 7–10 days requires gradual dosage reduction to avoid adrenal insufficiency. Immunosuppression, hyperglycemia, growth delay, leukocytosis, gastric irritation
Desoxycorticosterone acetate (DOCA)	IM: 1 mg q 12 h the first day, then 0.5–1 mg/day	
Dexamethasone	IM, IV: bronchopulmonary dysplasia—0.25 mg/kg/dose q 8–12 h for 3–7 days	See Cortisone
Diazepam	PO, IV, IM: sedative = 0.02–0.3 mg/kg/dose q 6–8 h; seizure = 0.3–0.75 mg/kg/dose slow IV push	Diluted injection may precipitate; IM absorption is poor; respiratory depression, hypotension
Dicloxacillin	4–8 mg/kg/dose (PO) q 6 h	
Digoxin	IV: Acute digitalization*	Risk of arrhythmias is increased during digitalization. IV formulation is twice as concentrated as oral. Conduction defects, emesis, ventricular arrhythmias

IV: Acute digitalization*

	Loading dose (TDD)**
Prematures	10–20 μg/kg
<1.5 kg	20 μg/kg
1.5–2.5 kg	30 μg/kg
Term newborns	35 μg/kg
Infants (1–12 mo)	

Maintenance dose: 1/8 TDD q 12 h
Begin 12 h after last digitalization dose

DRUG	ROUTE AND DOSE	ADVERSE EFFECTS, CAUTIONS
Diphenhydramine	PO: 5 mg/kg/day q 6 h	Somnolence
Diphenylhydantoin	See Phenytoin	
Diphtheria antitoxin	IM, IV: 20,000–50,000 units/day for 2–3 successive days	Hypersensitivity reaction
Dobutamine	IV: 2–15 μg/kg/min	Tachycardia, hypotension
Dopamine	IV: 2–20 μg/kg/min	Extravasation may lead to necrosis. (Phentolamine is an antidote.) High dose may constrict renal arteries
Edrophonium	Tensilon test for myasthenia gravis SC, IM: 0.5 mg/kg; IV: preliminary test dose = 0.04 mg slow push, test dose = 0.16 mg/kg (1 min later)	Cardiac arrhythmia, diarrhea, tracheal secretions may require atropine antagonism

*PO dose increased 20 per cent.
**TDD (loading dose): 1/2, 1/4, 1/4 dose q 8 h.

Pharmacopeia for the Newborn Period *Continued*

ABBREVIATIONS:	IM—intramuscularly	PR—by rectum
	IT—intratracheal	SC—subcutaneously
	IV—intravenously	Top—topical
	PO—by mouth	

DRUG	ROUTE AND DOSE	ADVERSE EFFECTS, CAUTIONS
Epinephrine	Resuscitation: IV, ET–1:10,000: 0.1 ml/kg q 10–15 min Hypotension: 0.01–0.1 μg/kg/min	Tachycardia, arrhythmia
Erythromycin	PO, IV: 10 mg/kg/dose, <7 days = q 12 h, >7 days = q 8 h Eye prophylaxis at birth: ophthalmic 0.5 per cent—in each eye	IV administration is painful. May affect theophylline serum levels.
Ethacrynic acid	IV: 0.5–1.0 mg/kg/dose q 12–24 h	Ototoxicity with aminoglycosides: hypokalemia and hyponatremia
Fentanyl	IV, SC: 1 μg/kg/dose, q 4–6 h prn	50–100 times the potency of morphine. Muscle rigidity ("stiff man" syndrome) may occur.
Fibrinogen	IV: 50 mg/kg: repeated prn as determined by clotting time	
Flucytosine	PO: 20–40 mg/kg q 6 h	Monitor levels. Effective antifungal concentration: 35–70 μg/ml. Bone marrow dysfunction: >100 μg/ml. Renal dysfunction decreases clearance
Fludrocortisone	PO: 0.025–0.2 mg/day	Mineralocorticoid replacement
Folic acid	PO: 50 μg/day for preterm newborns after feeding is established	
Furosemide	IM, IV: 0.5–2 mg/kg/dose q 12–24 h PO: 1–4 mg/kg/dose q 12–24 h Bioavailability reduced by cor pulmonale	Hypokalemia, hyponatremia, hypochloremia. Half-life prolonged in premature newborns
Gentamicin	IV, IM: 2.5 mg/kg q 8–24 h, adjust for gestation and age, maintain q 12 h, or more for 4 wk for <1200 gm	Blood level monitoring indicated for efficacy; toxicity is rare in newborn (desirable levels: trough <2 μg/ml; peak 5–10 μg/ml)
Gentian violet	Top (skin): as 1–2 per cent aqueous solution, bid. Top (oral): as 1 per cent aqueous solution, bid	
Glucagon	IM, IV: 30–100 μg/kg; may be repeated after 6–12 h; infant of diabetic mother may require 300 μg/kg	Maximum dose 1 mg; higher doses possibly toxic
Heparin	IV: Initial dose—50 units/kg; maintenance dose—100 units/kg q 4 h or 20–25 units/kg/h continuous infusion. Titrate dose to 1½–2 times baseline whole-blood clotting time or activated partial thromboplastin time	Intractable bleeding (reversible with protamine); heparin half-life: prematures < term < adults
Hydralazine	PO, IM, IV: 0.15 mg/kg every 6 h; increase as needed in 0.1 mg/kg increments up to 4 mg/kg/day	
Hydrochlorothiazide	PO: 2.0–2.5 mg/kg every 12 h	Hypercalcemia, hypokalemia, hyperglycemia
Hydrocortisone	PO, IM, IV: adrenal crisis, 3–10 mg/kg/day; PO: physiologic replacement, 1 mg/kg/day or 15–25 mg/m²/day	See Cortisone
Immunoglobulin intravenous, human	IV: 400–750 mg/kg/dose infused over 2–6 h	Studies in newborns are preliminary. Necrotizing enterocolitis, volume overload
Indomethacin	PO, IV: 0.1–0.2 mg/kg/dose q 12–24 h	Transient renal dysfunction, decreased platelet aggregation
Insulin (Regular)	IV: hyperglycemia infusion dose, 0.01–0.1 units/kg/h; SC: intermittent dose, 0.1–0.2 units/kg q 6–12 h	
Iron	PO: 6 mg/kg/day elemental iron	
Isoniazid	PO: 10 mg/kg/day, single dose	Newborns do not require pyridoxine supplement. Follow liver function tests
Isoproterenol	IV: 0.05–0.5 μg/kg/min	Arrhythmias, systemic vasodilation, tachycardia, hypotension, hypoglycemia
Kanamycin	IM, IV: 7.5–10 mg/kg/dose; <7 days = q 12 h; >7 days = q 8 h	Nephrotoxicity, ototoxicity. Monitoring of blood levels useful (optimal serum peak concentrations 15–25 μg/ml)
Kayexalate	See Sodium polystyrene sulfonate	
Lidocaine	IV: 1 mg/kg infused over 5–10 min; may be repeated q 10 min 5 times, prn; infusion dose 10–50 μg/kg/min or 1 mg/kg/h	Monitoring of blood levels useful (therapeutic range 1–6 mg/ml plasma)
Lorazepam	IV: 0.05–0.1 mg/kg infused over 2–5 min	Limited data in newborns, preparations may contain benzyl alcohol. Dilute

Table continued on following page

Pharmacopeia for the Newborn Period *Continued*

ABBREVIATIONS:	IM—intramuscularly	PR—by rectum
	IT—intratracheal	SC—subcutaneously
	IV—intravenously	Top—topical
	PO—by mouth	

DRUG	ROUTE AND DOSE	ADVERSE EFFECTS, CAUTIONS
Magnesium sulfate	IM, IV: 25–50 mg/kg q 4–6 h for 3–4 doses prn; 50 per cent solution IM; 1 per cent solution IV	Hypotension, central nervous system depression; monitor serum concentration; calcium gluconate should be available as an antidote
Medium-chain triglyceride (MCT)	PO: 1–8 ml/24 h divided in feedings (7.7 cal/ml)	
Meperidine	IV, IM, PO: 0.5–1.5 mg/kg/dose q 4 h prn	Respiratory depression reversible with naloxone; underdosage increases pain perception
Methyldopa	IV, PO: 2–3 mg/kg q 6–8 h; increased as needed at 2-day intervals; maximum dosage 12–15 mg/kg	Sedation, fever, false-positive Coombs' test, hemolysis; sudden withdrawal of methyldopa may cause rebound hypertension
Metoclopramide	PO, IV: 0.03–0.2 mg/kg/dose q 6–8 h or prior to each feeding	Dystonic reactions, irritability, diarrhea, decreases glomerular filtration rate in adults
Methylene blue	IV: 0.1–0.2 mg/kg of 1 per cent solution for methemoglobinemia, infused slowly	
Methylprednisolone	IV, IM: 10–30 mg/kg/dose, q 6 h	Hydrocortisone preferred for physiologic replacement
Mezlocillin	75 mg/kg/dose <7 days q 12 h; >7 days q 8 h; maintain q 12 h for 4 wk for <1200 gm	Urinary retention
Midazolam	IV, IM: 0.07–0.20 mg/kg/dose q 2–4 h prn for sedation	Limited experience in newborns. Respiratory depression, apnea
Morphine sulfate	IV, IM, SC: 0.1–0.2 mg/kg/dose q 2–6 h prn	Respiratory depression reversible with naloxone
Mycostatin	PO: 100,000–200,000 units q 6 h Topical: as 2 per cent ointment (in liquid petrolatum 95 per cent polyethylene 5 per cent) 3–4 times daily	
Nafcillin	IV, IM: 25 mg/kg/dose, newborns 0–7 days = q 12 h, infants >7 days = q 6–8 h; double dosage for meningitis; maintain q 12 h for 4 wk for <1200 gm	Agranulocytosis; granulocytopenia; hepatic dysfunction; may require dosage adjustment
Naloxone	IV, IM, SC: 0.1 mg/kg/dose; may be repeated as necessary; delivery room, minimum = 0.5 mg for term newborn	Onset of action may be delayed 15 + min after IM or SC administration. Narcotic effects may outlast naloxone antagonism
Neomycin	PO: 10–25 mg/kg/dose q 6 h Topical: 0.5 per cent ointment, 3–4 times daily	Renal toxicity and ototoxicity if absorbed
Neostigmine	IM: Test for myasthenia gravis—0.1 mg/kg PO: Treatment for myasthenia gravis = 2 mg/kg/day q 3–6 h	Cardiac arrhythmia (atropine should be kept available)
Nitroprusside	IV: begin in dose of 0.5 μg/kg/min and vary as needed to control blood pressure	Profound hypotension possible; requires arterial line to monitor blood pressure; thiocyanate toxicity with long-term use or renal insufficiency
Oxacillin	IV, IM: 25 mg/kg/dose Preterm <1200 gm q 12 h for 4 wk; 1200–2000 gm q 12 h for 7 days; 1200–2000 gm q 8 h for 7 days; Term 25–40 mg/kg/dose <7 days, q h; >7 days, q 6 h	Sterile abscess formation, nephrotoxicity; monitor liver enzymes and complete blood count
Pancreatin	PO: 0.3–0.5 mg with each feeding PR and into colostomy: 0.3–0.5 gm in sufficient liquid (for meconium ileus)	
Pancuronium	IV: 0.03–0.1 mg/kg/dose q 1–4 h prn	Ensure adequate oxygenation and ventilation. Tachycardia, bradycardia, hypotension, hypertension. Potentiated by acidosis, hypothermia, neuromuscular disease
Paraldehyde	PR: 0.3 ml/kg q 4–6 h IM: 0.15 ml/kg q 4–6 h IV: loading dose = 200 mg/kg, infusion 20 mg/kg/h (10% solution)	Reserve for refractory status epilepticus. Local irritation, pulmonary edema, hemorrhage. Hepatic dysfunction decreases clearance. Avoid IM if possible. Do not give by arterial catheter. Avoid plastic containers
Penicillin G	IV, IM: sepsis 25,000–50,000 units/kg/dose, meningitis 75,000–100,000 units/kg/dose, q 8–12 h; <7 days, q 6–8 h; >7 days; *Use higher doses for group B streptococcus infections* Maintain q 12 h for 4 wk for <1200 gm	Use for susceptible organisms such as streptococci; syphilis
Pentobarbital	PO, IM, IV: 2–6 mg/kg prn	Blood level monitoring helpful (sedative level 0.5–3 μg/ml). Higher doses may depress respirations. Monitor blood pressure

Pharmacopeia for the Newborn Period

ABBREVIATIONS:	IM—intramuscularly	PR—by rectum
	IT—intratracheal	SC—subcutaneously
	IV—intravenously	Top—topical
	PO—by mouth	

DRUG	ROUTE AND DOSE	ADVERSE EFFECTS, CAUTIONS
Phenobarbital	IV, IM, PO: anticonvulsant loading dose—15–20 mg/kg, may repeat 10 mg/kg/dose twice for status epilepticus; maintenance dose: 3–5 mg/kg/day q 12–24 h, begin 12–24 h after load dose: Sedation: 2–3 mg/kg q 8–12 h prn	Blood level monitoring helpful (therapeutic range 15–40 µg/ml). Half-life 40–200 h in infants, prolonged by asphyxia
Phentolamine	SC: dilute to 0.5 mg/ml, inject 0.2 ml at 5 sites around dopamine infiltration	
Phenytoin	IV: loading dose, 15–20 mg/kg, infused <0.5 mg/kg/min PO, IV: maintenance, 4–8 mg/kg/dose q 24 h. Higher doses q 8 h >7 days. Flush IV with saline before/after dose	Therapeutic blood level monitoring indicated (desirable level 10–20 µg/ml). Infant clearance may be high
Phosphate	PO: supplement formula phosphorus intake to 75 mg/kg/day; diluted solution contains 3.3 mg phosphorus/ml	Large amounts may cause catharsis; increase gradually to full supplementation
Piperacillin	IM, IV: 50–100 mg/kg/dose—preterm <7 days q 12 h, preterm >7 days q 8 h, term <7 days q 8 h, term >7 days q 6 h	
Pitressin	See Vasopressin	
Plasma	IV: 5–10 ml/kg; repeated prn	Volume overload, viral infection risk
Prednisone	PO: 0.5–3 mg/kg/dose, q 6 h	See Cortisone
Procainamide	IV: 1.5–2.5 mg/kg infused over 10–30 min; may be repeated in 30 min if needed PO: 40–60 mg/kg/day q 4–6 h	Asystole, myocardial depression, anorexia, vomiting, nausea. Blood level monitoring helpful (therapeutic range: procainamide, 3–10 µg/ml; N-acetyl procainamide, 5–30 µg/ml)
Propranolol	IV: 0.01–0.2 mg/kg infused over 10 min; may be repeated in 10 min PO: 0.05–2 mg/kg q 6 h	Relatively contraindicated in low-output congestive heart failure and patients with bronchospasm
Propylthiouracil	PO: 2–4 mg/kg q 8 h. Increase to maximum of 10 mg/kg/dose. Onset of action may be delayed days to weeks	
Prostaglandin E₁	IV: 0.05–0.1 µg/kg/min. Often, dose may be reduced by ½ after initial response. Intra-arterial infusion offers no advantage	Apnea, seizures, fever, disseminated intravascular coagulation, diarrhea, cutaneous vasodilatation, decreased platelet aggregation, cortical bone proliferation during prolonged infusion
Protamine sulfate	IV: 1.0 mg for each 100 units heparin in previous 4 h	Excessive doses induce coagulopathy
Pyridoxine	See Vitamin B₆	
Quinidine gluconate	PO, IM: 2–10 mg/kg/dose q 2–6 h until desired effect or toxicity occurs. IV dosing not recommended	Check electrocardiogram before each dose; discontinue if QRS interval increases 50 per cent or more. Maintain level of 2–6 µg/ml. Nausea, vomiting, diarrhea, fever, A-V block
Ranitidine	PO, IV: 1–2 mg/kg q 8–12 h	H2 antagonist minimally studied in newborns. Minimal inhibition of hepatic P450 enzymes.
Ribavirin	Nebulized in hood from solution 20 mg/ml 12–18 h/day for 3–7 days	May precipitate in endotracheal tube; avoid exposure of pregnant staff; possible teratogenic effects
Silver nitrate (1 per cent solution)	Prophylaxis: 1 drop each eye	Chemical conjunctivitis
Sodium bicarbonate (0.5 mEq/ml)	IV: 1–2 mEq/kg/dose infused slowly only if infant ventilated adequately	Intravascular hemolysis may be associated with rapid infusion
Sodium polystyrene sulfonate (Kayexalate)	PO, PR: 1 gm/kg; approximately q 6 h	Usually administered as a solution with 20 per cent sorbitol to prevent intestinal obstruction; 20 per cent sorbitol solution may injure intestinal mucosa of very-low-birth-weight newborns; may decrease serum calcium or magnesium
Spironolactone	PO: 1–3 mg/kg/day q 8–24 h	Contraindicated with hyperkalemia; onset of action delayed; drowsiness; nausea; vomiting; diarrhea; androgenic effects in females; gynecomastia in males
Streptomycin	IM: 20–30 mg/kg/day q 12 h	Nephotoxicity, ototoxicity. Use in newborns as part of triple therapy for tuberculosis
Sulfisoxazole	PO, IV: 25 mg/kg q 6 h	In prematures or in presence of jaundice, may lead to kernicterus

Table continued on following page

Pharmacopeia for the Newborn Period

ABBREVIATIONS:	IM—intramuscularly	PR—by rectum
	IT—intratracheal	SC—subcutaneously
	IV—intravenously	Top—topical
	PO—by mouth	

DRUG	ROUTE AND DOSE	ADVERSE EFFECTS, CAUTIONS
Tetanus antitoxin	IM, IV: 10,000–20,000 units/day for 2 successive days	Optimal dosage not established for newborns
Tetanus immune globulin	IM: 3000–6000 units	Optimal dosage not established for newborns
Tetracyclines	PO: 50 mg/kg/day q 6–8 h IV, IM: 50 mg/kg/day q 8–12 h	Rarely used; may stain teeth permanently
Theophylline	PO, IV: loading dose: 5–6 mg/kg; maintenance dose: 1–2.5 mg/kg/dose q 6–12 h; aminophylline (PO) dose = theophylline (IV) dose x 1.25	Blood level monitoring indicated (therapeutic range: apnea, 7–12 µg/ml; bronchospasm, 10–20 µg/ml). Tachycardia at 15–20 µg/ml, seizures >40 µg/ml. Avoid rectal dosing owing to variable absorption. Clearance decreased by asphyxia and prematurity
Thiamine	See Vitamin B₁	
Thyroxine (Synthroid)	PO: starting dose 10 µg/kg/day (round off to nearest 12.5, 25.0, or 37.5 µg to coincide with pill size). Increase by 12.5–25 µg/24 h every 2 weeks	Adjust dosage on 3–6 wk schedule by clinical response and T4. Optimal T4 range 8–11 µg/dl
Ticarcillin	IM, IV: 75 mg/kg/dose <7 days q 12 h, >7 days q 8 h; maintain q 12 h for 4 wk for <1200 gm	Contains 5.2 mEq Na⁺/gm; may inhibit platelet function
Tobramycin	See Gentamicin dosing guidelines	
Tolazoline	Loading dose: 0.5–1 mg/kg IV over 10 min; maintenance dose 0.2–2 mg/kg/h, IV	Hypotension; gastrointestinal and pulmonary bleeding; renal dysfunction. Accumulates with oliguria; no antidote
Vancomycin	PO: 10 mg/kg, q 6 h IV: Post/Conceptional Age—< 27 wk—27 mg/kg q 36 h, 27–30 wk—24 mg/kg q 24 h, 31–36 wk—18 mg/kg/dose q 12–18 h, 37+ wk—22.5 mg/kg/dose q 12 h. Infuse dose over 60 min or more Cerebrospinal fluid: 4–5 mg q 48–72 h (cerebrospinal fluid trough <20 µg/ml)	Nephrotoxicity; ototoxicity. (Therapeutic levels: peak = <25–40 µg/ml; trough = 5–10 µg/ml). Rapid infusion may cause cutaneous vasodilatation and shock
Vasopressin (20 units/ml)	SC: 1–3 ml/day, divided into 3 equal doses	
Vasopressin in oil (5 units/ml)	IM: 0.2 ml/dose q 1–3 days	
Vecuronium	IV: 0.08–0.1 mg/kg/dose, repeat prn	Neuromuscular blockade potentiated by calcium channel blockers such as verapamil
Verapamil	IV: 0.1–0.2 mg/kg infused over 2 min; if response is inadequate, repeat in 30 min	Monitor ECG during infusion. Bradycardia, A-V block, asystole. Contraindicated in patients with 2nd or 3rd degree A-V block and during treatment with beta blockers
Vitamin A	PO: preventive, 600–1500 units/day	
Vitamin B₁	PO: preventive, 0.5–1.0 mg q day; PO: therapeutic, 5–10 mg q 6–8 h	
Vitamin B₆	PO: preventive, 100 µg/l of ingested formula; therapeutic for deficiency = 2–5 mg/day q 6 h; test dose for dependency = 50–100 mg IV	
Vitamin C	PO: preventive, 25–50 mg/day (term infants); 100 mg/day (premature infants); PO, IM: therapeutic = 100 mg q 4 h	
Vitamin D	PO: preventive, 400–1000 IU/day (premature infants), 40–100 IU/day (term infants)	
Vitamin E	PO: prevention of hemolysis—25 IU/day (1 IU = 1 mg)	Some preparations are hyperosmolar
Vitamin K₁	IM: preventive, 0.5–1.0 mg, single dose; therapeutic, 2.5–5.0 mg/kg/dose q 6–12 h according to prothombin time	With thombocytopenia, slow intravenous infusion at same dose. Anaphylaxis observed with rapid injection intravenously

References
1. Bhatt, D.R., Furman, G.I., Wirtschaften, D.D., and Reber, D.J.: Neonatal Drug Formulary, 1987–1988. Coving, CA, California Perinatal Association, 1988.
2. Gilman, A.G., Goodman, L.S., Rall, T.W., and Murad, F.: Goodman and Gilman's The Pharmacological Basis of Therapeutics, 7th ed. New York, Macmillan Publishing Company, 1985.
3. Roberts, R.J.: Drug Therapy in Infants. Philadelphia, W.B. Saunders Company, 1984.
4. Young, T.E., and Mangum, O.B.: Neofax. 3rd ed. Columbus, OH, Ross Laboratories, 1990.

Concentration of Various Drugs in Maternal Blood and Breast Milk Under Normal pH Conditions

DRUG ADMINISTERED (THERAPEUTIC DOSAGE)	DRUG LEVELS (units/100 ml)		ADMINISTERED DRUG APPEARING IN MILK (%/day)
	Plasma or Serum (pH 7.4)	Milk (pH 7.0)	
Aspirin	1–5 mg	1–3 mg	0.5
Bishydroxycoumarin	11–16.5 mg	0.2 mg	0.5
Chloral hydrate	0–3 mg	0–1.5 mg	0.6
Chloramphenicol	2.5–5 mg	1.5–2.5 mg	1.3
Chlorpromazine	0.1 mg	0.03 mg	0.07
Colistin sulfate	0.3–0.5 mg	0.05–0.09 mg	0.07
Cycloserine	1.5–2 mg	1–1.5 mg	0.6
Diphenylhydantoin	0.3–4.5 mg	0.6–1.8 mg	1.4
Erythomycin	0.1–0.2 mg	0.3–0.5 mg	0.1
Ethanol	50–80 mg	50–80 mg	0.25
Ethyl biscoumacetate	2.7–14.5 mg	0–0.17 mg	0.1
Folic acid	3 μg	0.07 μg	0.1
Imipramine hydrochloride	0.2–1.3 mg	0.1 mg	0.1
Iodine-131	0.002 μc	0.13 μc	2–5
Isoniazid	0.6–1.2 mg	0.6–1.2 mg	0.75
Kanamycin sulfate	0.5–3.5 mg	0.2 mg	0.05
Lincomycin	0.3–1.5 mg	0.05–0.2 mg	0.025
Lithium carbonate	0.2–1.1 mg	0.07–0.4 mg	0.12
Meperidine hydrochloride	0.07–0.1 mg	trace (<0.1 mg)	<0.1
Methotrexate	3 μg	0.3 μg	0.01
Nalidixic acid	3–5 mg	0.4 mg	0.05
Novobiocin	1.2–5.2 mg	0.3–0.5 mg	0.15
Penicillin	6–120 μg	1.2–3.6 μg	0.03
Phenobarbital	0.6–1.8 mg	0.1–0.5 mg	1.5
Phenylbutazone	2–5 mg	0.2–0.6 mg	0.4
Pyrilamine maleate	—	0.2 mg	0.6
Pyrimethamine	0.7–1.5 mg	0.3 mg	0.3
Quinine sulfate	0.7 mg	0.1 mg	0.05
Rifampin	0.5 mg	0.1–0.3 mg	0.05
Streptomycin sulfate	2–3 mg	1–3 mg	0.5
Sulfapyridine	3–13 mg	3–13 mg	0.12
Tetracycline hydrochloride	80–320 μg	50–260 μg	0.03
Thiouracil	3–4 mg	9–12 mg	5

(Modified from Vorherr, H.: The Breast: Morphology, Physiology, and Lactation. New York, Academic Press, Inc., 1974.)

■ TRANSFER OF DRUGS AND OTHER CHEMICALS INTO HUMAN MILK*

Since the first publication of this statement, much new information has been published conerning the transfer of drugs and chemicals into human milk. This information, in addition to other research published before 1983, makes a revision of the previous statement necessary. In this revision, lists of the pharmacologic or chemical agents transferred into human milk and their possible effects on the infant or on lactation, if known, are provided (Tables 1 to 7). The fact that a pharmacologic or chemical agent does not appear in the tables is not meant to imply that it is not transferred into human milk or that it does not have an effect on the infant but indicates that there are no reports in the literature. These tables should assist the physician in counseling a nursing mother regarding breast-feeding when the mother has a condition for which a drug is medically indicated.

The following questions should be considered when prescribing drug therapy for lactating women. (1) Is the drug therapy really necessary? Consultation between the pediatrician and the mother's physician can be most useful. (2) Use the safest drug—for example, acetaminophen rather than aspirin for oral analgesia. (3) If there is a possibility that a drug may present a risk to the infant (eg, phenytoin, phenobarbital), consideration should be given to measurement of blood concentrations in the nursing infant. (4) Drug exposure to the nursing infant may be minimized by having the mother take the medication just after completing a breast-feeding and/or just before the infant has his or her lengthy sleep periods.

Data have been obtained from a search of the medical literature. Because methodologies used to quantitate drugs in milk continue to improve, this current information will require continuous updating. Brand names are listed in Table 8 in accordance with the current *AMA Drug Evaluation*, the *USAN*, and *USP Dictionary of Drug Names*. The reference list is not inclusive of all articles published.

Physicians who encounter adverse effects in infants fed drug-contaminated human milk are urged to document these effects in a communication to the AAP Committee on Drugs and the US Food and Drug Administration. Such communication should include the generic and

*This paper is from the American Academy of Pediatrics Committee on Drugs: The transfer of drugs and other chemicals into human breast milk. Pediatrics 84:924, 1989. Copyright © 1989 by the American Academy of Pediatrics.

The recommendations in this statement do not indicate an exclusive course of treatment to be followed. Variations, taking into account individual circumstances, may be appropriate.

brand names of the drug, the maternal dose and mode of administration, the concentrations of the drug in milk and maternal and infant blood in relation to time of ingestion, the age of the infant, and the method used for laboratory identification. Such reports may significantly increase the pediatric community's fund of knowledge regarding drug transfer into human milk and the potential or actual risk to the infant.

■ ACKNOWLEDGMENT

We thank Linda Harnden for her work in reference identification, document retrieval, and manuscript preparation.

Drugs cited in the following seven tables are listed in alphabetical order by generic name.

Committee on Drugs, 1988–1989
- Robert J. Roberts, MD, PhD, Chairman
- Jeffrey L. Blumer, MD
- Richard L. Gorman, MD
- George H. Lambert, MD

- Barry H. Rumack, MD
- Wayne Snodgrass, MD

Liaison Representatives
- Donald R. Bennett, MD, PhD, American Medical Association
- Jose F. Cordero, MD, MPH, Centers for Disease Control
- John C. Petricciani, MD, Pharmaceutical Manufacturers' Association
- Sam A. Licata, MD, National Health and Welfare, Health Protection Branch, Canada
- Mary Lund Mortensen, MD, Centers for Disease Control
- Martin L. Pernoll, MD, American College of Obstetricians and Gynecologists
- Gloria Troendle, MD, Food and Drug Administration
- Sumner J. Yaffe, MD, National Institute of Child Health and Human Development

AAP Section Liaison
- Cheston M. Berlin, MD, Section on Clinical Pharmacology

Consultants
- Ralph E. Kauffman, MD
- Anthony R. Temple, MD

TABLE 1. Drugs That Are Contraindicated During Breast-Feeding*

DRUG	REPORTED SIGN OR SYMPTOM IN INFANT OR EFFECT ON LACTATION
Bromocriptine	Suppresses lactation
Cyclophosphamide	Possible immune suppression; unknown effect on growth or association with carcinogenesis; neutropenia
Cyclosporine	Possible immune suppression; unknown effect on growth or association with carcinogenesis
Doxorubicin†	Possible immune suppression; unknown effect on growth or association with carcinogenesis
Ergotamine	Vomiting, diarrhea, convulsions (doses used in migraine medications)
Lithium	⅓ to ½ therapeutic blood concentration in infants
Methotrexate	Possible immune suppression; unknown effect on growth or association with carcinogenesis; neutropenia
Phenindione	Anticoagulant; increased prothrombin and partial thromboplastin times in 1 infant (not used in USA)

*The Committee on Drugs believes strongly that nursing mothers should not ingest any illicit drugs, or use cigarettes or alcohol. Not only are they hazardous to the nursing infant but they are detrimental to the physical and emotional health of the mother.
†Drug is concentrated in human milk.

TABLE 2. Radiopharmaceuticals That Require Temporary Cessation of Breast-Feeding*

DRUG	RECOMMENDED ALTERATION IN BREAST-FEEDING PATTERN
Gallium-67 (^{67}Ga)	Radioactivity in milk present for 2 wk
Indium-111 (^{111}In)	Small amount present at 20 h
Iodine-125 (^{125}I)	Risk of thyroid cancer; radioactivity in milk present for 12 d
Iodine-131 (^{131}I)	Radioactivity in milk present for 2–14 d depending on study
Radioactive sodium	Radioactivity in milk present for 96 h
Technetium-99m (^{99m}Tc), ^{99m}Tc macroaggregates, ^{99m}TcO$_4$	Radioactivity in milk present for 15 h to 3 d

*Consult nuclear medicine physician before performing diagnostic study so that a radionuclide with the shortest excretion time in breast milk can be used. Before study, the mother should pump her breast and store enough milk in freezer for feeding the infant; after study, the mother should pump her breast to maintain milk production but discard all milk pumped for the required time that radioactivity is present in milk.

TABLE 3. Drugs Whose Effect on Nursing Infants Is Unknown but May Be of Concern

DRUG	EFFECT
Psychotropic drugs	Special concern when given to nursing mothers for long periods of time
Antianxiety	
Diazepam	None
Lorazepam	None
Prazepam*	None
Quazepam	None
Antidepressant	
Amitriptyline	None
Amoxapine	None
Desipramine	None
Dothiepin	None
Doxepin	None
Imipramine	None
Trazodone	None
Antipsychotic	
Chlorpromazine	Galactorrhea in adult; drowsiness and lethargy in infant
Chlorprothixene	None
Haloperidol	None
Mesoridazine	None
Chloramphenicol	Possible idiosyncratic bone marrow suppression
Metoclopramide*K	None described; potent central nervous system drug
Metronidazole	In vitro mutagen; may discontinue breast-feeding 12–24 h to allow excretion of dose when single-dose therapy given to mother
Tinidazole	See Metronidazole

*Drug is concentrated in human milk.

TABLE 4. Drugs That Have Caused Significant Effects on Some Nursing Infants and Should Be Given to Nursing Mothers With Caution*

DRUG	EFFECT
Aspirin (salicylates)	Metabolic acidosis (dose related); may affect platelet function; rash
Clemastine	Drowsiness, irritability, refusal to feed, high-pitched cry, neck stiffness (1 case)
Phenobarbital	Sedation; infantile spasms after weaning from milk containing phenobarbital, methemoglobinemia (1 case)
Primidone	Sedation, feeding problems
Salicylazosulfapyridine (sulfasalazine)	Bloody diarrhea in 1 infant

*Measure blood concentration in the infant when possible.

TABLE 5. Maternal Medication Usually Compatible With Breast-Feeding*

DRUG	REPORTED SIGN OR SYMPTOM IN INFANT OR EFFECT ON LACTATION
Anesthetics, sedatives	
Alcohol	Drowsiness, diaphoresis, deep sleep, weakness, decrease in linear growth, abnormal weight gain; maternal ingestion of 1 g/kg daily decreases milk ejection reflex
Barbiturate	See Table 4
Bromide	Rash, weakness, absence of cry with maternal intake of 5.4 g/d
Chloral hydrate	Sleepiness
Chloroform	None
Halothane	None
Lidocaine	None
Magnesium sulfate	None
Methyprylon	Drowsiness
Secobarbital	None
Thiopental	None
Anticoagulants	
Bishydroxycoumarin	None
Warfarin	None
Antiepileptics	
Carbamazepine	None
Ethosuximide	None; drug appears in infant serum
Phenobarbital	See Table 4
Phenytoin	Methemoglobinemia (1 case)
Primidone	See Table 4
Thiopental	None
Valproic acid	None

Table continued on following page

TABLE 5. Maternal Medication Usually Compatible With Breast-Feeding* *Continued*

DRUG	REPORTED SIGN OR SYMPTOM IN INFANT OR EFFECT ON LACTATION
Antihistamines, decongestants, and bronchodilators	
Dexbrompheniramine maleate with *d*-isoephedrine	Crying, poor sleep patterns, irritability
Dyphylline†	None
Iodides	May affect thryoid activity; see Miscellaneous, iodine
Pseudoephedrine†	None
Terbutaline	None
Theophylline	Irritability
Triprolidine	None
Antihypertensive and cardiovascular drugs	
Acebutolol	None
Atenolol	None
Captopril	None
Digoxin	None
Diltiazem	None
Disopyramide	None
Hydralazine	None
Labetalol	None
Lidocaine	None
Methyldopa	None
Metoprolol†	None
Mexiletine	None
Minoxidil	None
Nadolol†	None
Oxprenolol	None
Procainamide	None
Propranolol	None
Quinidine	None
Timolol	None
Verapamil	None
Anti-infective drugs (all antibiotics transfer into breast milk in limited amounts)	
Acyclovir†	None
Amoxicillin	None
Aztreonam	None
Cefadroxil	None
Cefazolin	None
Cefotaxime	None
Cefoxitin	None
Ceftazidine	None
Ceftriaxone	None
Chloroquine	None
Clindamycin	None
Cycloserine	None
Dapsone	None; sulfonamide detected in infant's urine
Erythromycin†	None
Ethambutol	None
Hydroxychloroquine†	None
Isoniazid	None; acetyl metabolite also secreted; ? hepatoxicity
Kanamycin	None
Moxalactam	None
Nalidixic acid	Hemolysis in infant with glucose-6-phosphate deficiency (G-6-PD)
Nitrofurantoin	Hemolysis in infant with G-6-PD
Pyrimethamine	None
Quinine	None
Rifampin	None
Salicylazosulfapyridine (sulfasalazine)	See Table 4
Streptomycin	None
Sulbactam	None
Sulfapyridine	Caution in infant with jaundice or G-6-PD, and in ill, stressed, or premature infant. Appears in infant's urine
Sulfisoxazole	Caution in infant with jaundice or G-6-PD, and in ill, stressed or premature infant. Appears in infant's urine
Tetracycline	None; negligible absorption by infant
Ticarcillin	None
Trimethoprim/sulfamethoxazole	None

TABLE 5. Maternal Medication Usually Compatible With Breast-Feeding* *Continued*

DRUG	REPORTED SIGN OR SYMPTOM IN INFANT OR EFFECT ON LACTATION
Antithyroid drugs	
Carbimazole	Goiter
Methimazole (active metabolite of carbimazole)	None
Propylthiouracil	None
Thiouracil	None mentioned; drug not used in USA
Cathartics	
Cascara	None
Danthron	Increased bowel activity
Senna	None
Diagnostic agents	
Iodine	Goiter; see Miscellaneous, iodine
Iopanoic acid	None
Metrizamide	None
Diuretic agents	
Bendroflumethiazide	Suppresses lactation
Chlorothiazide, hydrochlorothiazide	None
Chlorthalidone	Excreted slowly
Spironolactone	None
Hormones	
^{3}H-norethynodrel	None
19-norsteroids	None
Clogestone	None
Contraceptive pill with estrogen/progesterone	Rare breast enlargement; decrease in milk production and protein content (not confirmed in several studies)
Estradiol	Withdrawal, vaginal bleeding
Medroxyprogesterone	None
Prednisolone	None
Prednisone	None
Progesterone	None
Muscle relaxants	
Baclofen	None
Methocarbamol	None
Narcotics, nonnarcotic analgesics, anti-inflammatory agents	
Acetaminophen	None
Butorphanol	None
Codeine	None
Dipyrone	None
Flufenamic acid	None
Gold salts	None
Hydroxychloroquine	None
Ibuprofen	None
Indomethacin	Seizure (1 case)
Mefenamic acid	None
Methadone	None if mother receiving ≤20 mg/24 h
Morphine	None
Nefopam	None
Phenylbutazone	None
Piroxicam	None
Prednisolone, prednisone	None
Propoxyphene	None
Salicylates	See Table 4
Suprofen	None
Tolmetin	None
Stimulants	
Caffeine	Irritability, poor sleep pattern, excreted slowly; no effect with usual amount of caffeine beverages
Vitamins	
B$_1$ (thiamine)	None
B$_6$ (pyridoxine)	None
B$_{12}$	None
D	None; follow infant's serum calcium if mother received pharmacologic doses
Folic acid	None
K$_1$	None
Riboflavin	None
Miscellaneous	
Acetazolamide	None
Atropine, scopolamine	None
Cimetidine†	None
Cisapride	None
Cisplatin	Not found in milk

Table continued on following page

TABLE 5. Maternal Medication Usually Compatible With Breast-Feeding* Continued

DRUG	REPORTED SIGN OR SYMPTOM IN INFANT OR EFFECT ON LACTATION
Domperidone	None
Iodine (povidone-iodine; vaginal douche)	Elevated iodine levels in breast milk, odor of iodine on infant's skin
Metoclopramide	See Table 4
Noscapine	None
Pyridostigmine	None
Tolbutamide	? Jaundice

*Drugs listed have been reported in the literature as having the effects listed or no effect. The word "none" means that no observable change was seen in the nursing infant while the mother was ingesting the compound. It is emphasized that most of the literature citations concern single case reports of small series of infants.

†Drug is concentrated in human milk.

TABLE 6. Food and Environmental Agents and Their Effect on Breast-Feeding

AGENT	REPORTED SIGN OR SYMPTOM IN INFANT OR EFFECT ON LACTATION
Aflatoxin	None
Aspartame	Caution if mother or infant has phenylketonuria
Bromide (photographic laboratory)	Potential absorption and bromide transfer into milk; see Table 6, Anesthetics, sedatives
Cadmium	None reported
Chlordane	None reported
Chocolate (theobromine)	Irritability or increased bowel activity if excess amounts (16 oz/d) consumed by mother
DDT, benzenehexachlorides, dieldrin, aldrin, hepatachlorepoxide	None
Fava beans	Hemolysis in patient with glucose-6-phosphate deficiency (G-6-PD)
Fluorides	None
Hexachlorobenzene	Skin rash, diarrhea, vomiting, dark urine, neurotoxicity, death
Hexachlorophene	None; possible contamination of milk from nipple washing
Lead	Possible neurotoxicity
Methyl mercury, mercury	May affect neurodevelopment
Monosodium glutamate (MSG)	None
Polychlorinated biphenyls and polybrominated biphenyls	Lack of endurance, hypotonia, sullen expressionless facies
Tetrachlorethylene-cleaning fluid (perchloroethylene)	Obstructive jaundice, dark urine
Vegetarian diet	Signs of B_{12} deficiency

TABLE 7. Trade Names of Generic Drugs*

GENERIC	TRADE	GENERIC	TRADE
acebutolol	Sectral	ceftriaxone	Rocephin
acetaminophen	Tylenol, Tylenol Extra Strength, Tempra, Phenaphen	chloramphenicol	Chloromycetin
		chloroquine	Aralen
acetazolamide	Diamox	chlorothiazide	Diuril, Chlotride
amitriptyline	Elavil, Endep	chlorpromazine	Thorazine
amoxapine	Asendin	chlorthalidone	Hygroton, Combipres
amoxicillin	Amoxyl	cimetidine	Tagamet
amphetamine (dexamphetamine)	Dexedrine	cisapride	Benzamide
		cisplatin	Platinol
aspartame	Nutrasweet	clemastine	Tavegil, Tavist
atenolol	Tenormin	clindamycin	Cleocin
aztreonam	Azactam	cyclophosphamide	Cytoxan
baclofen	Lioresal	cycloserine	Seromycin
bendroflumethiazide	Naturetin	danthron	Dorbane, Modane
bromocriptine	Parlodel	dapsone	
butorphanol	Stadol	desipramine	Norpramin, Pertofrane
captopril	Capoten	dexbrompheniramine maleate with d-isoephedrine	Drixoral, Disophrol, Chronotab
carbamazepine	Tegretol		
carbimazole	Neo-mercazole	diazepam	Valium
cefadroxil	Duricef	dicumarol	
cefazolin	Ancef, Kefzol	digoxin	Lanoxin, SK-Digoxin
cefotaxime	Claforan	diltiazem	Cardizem
ceftazidime	Fortaz		

TABLE 7. Trade Names of Generic Drugs* *Continued*

GENERIC	TRADE	GENERIC	TRADE
dipyrone	Novaldin	nitrofurantoin	Furadantin, Nitrofor, Macrodantin
disopyramide	Norpace	³H-norethynodrel	Enovid
domperidone		noscapine	Tusscapine
dothiepin	Prothiaden	oxprenolol	
doxepin	Adapin, Sinequan	phenindione	Hedulin, Eridione
doxorubicin	Adriamycin	phenylbutazone	Azolid, Butazolidin
dyphylline	Dilor	phenytoin	Dilantin
ergotamine tartrate with caffeine	Cafergot	piroxicam	Feldene
		prazepam	Centrax
estradiol	Estrace	prednisolone	Delta-Cortef, Sterane
ethambutol	Myambutol	prednisone	Deltasone, Meticorten, SK-Prednisone
ethosuximide	Zarontin		
flufenamic acid	Arlef	primidone	Mysoline
gold sodium thiomalate	Myochrysine	procainamide	Pronestyl
haloperidol	Haldol	propoxyphen	Darvon, SK65, Donlene
hydralazine	Apresoline	propranolol	Inderal
hydrochlorothiazide	Hydrodiuril	propylthiouracil	Propacil
hydroxychloroquine	Plaquenil	pseudoephedrine	Actifed
ibuprofen	Motrin	pyrimethamine	Daraprim
imipramine	Tofranil, SK-Pramine, Imavate	pyridostigmine	Mestinon
indomethacin	Indocin	quazepam	Dormalin
iopanoic acid	Telepaque	quinine	Quine
isoniazid	INH	rifampin	Rifamycin, Rifadin, Rimactane
kanamycin	Kantrex		
labetalol	Normodyne, Trandate	salicylazosulfapyridine	Azulfidine
lidocaine	Xylocaine	secobarbital	Seconal, Seco-8
lorazepam	Ativan	senna	Senokot
medroxyprogesterone	Provera	spironolactone	Aldactone
mefenamic acid	Ponstel	sulbactam	Unasyn
mesoridazine	Lidanar	sulfisoxazole	Gantrisin
methadone	Westadone	suprofen	Suprol
methimazole	Tapazole	terbutaline	Bricanyl, Brethine
methocarbamol	Robaxin	tetracycline	Achromycin, SK-Tetracycline
methotrexate (amethopterin)	Folex	theophylline	Theo-Dur, Elixophyllin, Slo-Phyllin, Bronkodyl
methyprylon	Noludar		
metoclopramide	Reglan	thiopental	Pentothal
metoprolol	Lopressor	thiouracil	Thiouracil
metrizamide	Amipaque	ticarcillin	Timentin
metronidazole	Flagyl	timolol	Blocadren, Timoptic
mexiletine	Mexitil	tolbutamide	Orinase, SK-Tolbutamide
minoxidil	Loniten	tolmetin	Tolectin
monosodium glutamate	MSG, Accent, Adolph's Meat Tenderizer	trazodone	Desyrel
		trimethoprim with sulfamethoxazole	Bactrim, Septra, Septra DS
moxalactam	Moxam	triprolidine	Actifed
nadolol	Corgard	valproic acid	Depakene
nalidixic acid	NegGram	verapamil	Calan
nefopam	Acupan	warfarin	Coumadin, Panwarfin

*For convenience, one or more examples of the trade name are given.

APPENDIX 2
FORMULAS

20-Calorie Formulas

	MATURE TERM HUMAN MILK†[1]	SIMILAC® AND SIMILAC® WITH IRON 20	ENFAMIL® AND ENFAMIL® WITH IRON 20	SMA® AND SMA® WITH IRON 20	SIMILAC® SPECIAL CARE® 20	ENFAMIL® PREMATURE FORMULA® 20	"PREEMIE" SMA® 20	SIMILAC® PM 60/40 20
ENERGY, Cal	680§	676	670	676	676	670	676	676
PROTEIN, g	10.5	15	15	15	18.3	20	20	15.8
% of total Calories	6	9	9	8.9	11	12	11.9	9
Source	Mature Term Human Milk	Cow's Milk	Reduced Minerals, Whey & Nonfat Milk	Nonfat Milk & Demineralized Whey	Cow's Milk & Whey	Whey Protein Concentrate & Nonfat Milk	Nonfat Milk & Demineralized Whey	Whey & Caseinate
Amino Acids, mg								
Histidine	230	310	290	360	360	390	510	330
Isoleucine	580	730	910	830	970	1160	1370	970
Leucine	1050	1410	1560	1480	1800	1940	2470	1730
Lysine	680	1070	1040	1170	1450	1510	2080	1350
Tryptophan	210	190	230	240	210	310	350	230
Phenylalanine	430	730	590	620	600	760	1080	570
Threonine	520	640	790	800	1070	1100	1410	970
Valine	650	810	930	890	990	1220	1470	950
Methionine	200	420	290	370	450	450	470	430
Cystine	185[2]	130	180	280	290	220	370	240
FAT, g	39	36.3	38	36	36.7	34	35	37.6
% of total Calories	52	48	50	48.2	47	44	46.7	50
Source	Mature Term Human Milk	Soy & Coconut Oils	Coconut & Soy Oils	Oleo, Coconut, Oleic & Soy Oils	Medium-Chain Triglycerides, Soy & Coconut Oils	Medium-Chain Triglycerides, Soy & Coconut Oils	Coconut, Oleic, Oleo & Soy Oils & Medium-Chain Triglycerides	Soy & Coconut Oils
Fatty Acids								
Polyunsaturated, g	4.8§	13	11	4.9	7	8	5.2	14
Saturated, g	17.4§	16	18#	15	21	9#	16.3	16
Monounsaturated, g	14.9§	6	6	14	4	4	11.8	6
Linoleic acid, mg	3971§	8790	7400	3300	4730	6700	3300	8790
E:PUFA Ratio*	0.5§	1.1	1.3	1.3	2.5	2.6	3.0	1.0
CARBOHYDRATE, g	72	72.3	69	72	71.7	74	70	69
% of total Calories	42	43	41	42.9	42	44	41.5	41
Source	Lactose	Lactose	Lactose	Lactose	Lactose & POLYCOSE® Glucose Polymers	Corn Syrup Solids, Lactose	Lactose & Glucose Polymers	Lactose

MINERALS		mEq		mEq		mEq		mEq		mEq		mEq		mEq		mEq
Calcium, mg	280	14.0	510	25.4	460	23	420	20.9	1220	60.8	790	40	750	37.4	380	19.0
Phosphorus, mg	140		390		310		280		610		400		380		190	
Magnesium, mg	35		41		52		45		81		68		70		41	
Iron, mg	0.3		12(1.5)††		12.7(1.1)‡		12.0(1.5)‡‡		2.5		1.7		3		1.5	
Zinc, mg	1.2		5.1		5.2		5		10.1		6.8		8		5.1	
Manganese, µg	6		34		105		150		80		88		200		34	
Copper, µg	252		610		630		470		1690		1080		700		610	
Iodine, µg	110		100		68		60		40		54		83		41	
Sodium, mg	180	7.8	190	8.3	181	8	150	6.5	290	12.6	260	11	320	13.9	160	7.0
Potassium, mg	525	13.4	730	18.7	720	18	560	14.3	870	22.3	750	19	750	19.2	580	14.8
Chloride, mg	420	11.9	450	12.7	420	12	375	10.6	550	15.5	570	16	530	14.9	400	11.3

20-Calorie Formulas *Continued*

	MATURE TERM HUMAN MILK†[1]	SIMILAC® AND SIMILAC® WITH IRON 20	ENFAMIL® AND ENFAMIL® WITH IRON 20	SMA® AND SMA® WITH IRON 20	SIMILAC® SPECIAL CARE® 20	ENFAMIL® PREMATURE FORMULA® 20	"PREEMIE" SMA® 20	SIMILAC® PM 60/40 20
VITAMINS								
Vitamin A, IU	2230	2030	2100	2000	4600	8100	3200	2030
Vitamin D, IU	20	410	420	400	1010	2200	510	410
Vitamin E, IU	2.3 (mg)	20	21	9.5	27	31	15	20
Vitamin K, μg	2.1	54	58	55	81	88	70	54
Thiamine (vitamin B$_1$), μg	210	680	520	670	1690	1690	800	680
Riboflavin (vitamin B$_2$), μg	350	1010	1050	1000	4190	2300	1300	1010
Vitamin B$_6$, μg	205	410	420	420	1690	1690	500	410
Vitamin B$_{12}$, μg	0.5	1.7	1.5	1.3	3.7	2.0	2	1.7
Niacin, μg	1500	7100	8400	5000	33,800	27,000	6300	7100
Folic acid (folacin), μg	50	100	105	50	250	230	100	100
Pantothenic acid, μg	1800	3040	3100	2100	12,840	8100	3600	3040
Biotin, μg	4	30	15.4	15	250	13.5	18	30
Vitamin C (ascorbic acid), mg	40	60	54	55	250	230	70	60
Choline, mg	92	108	105	100	68	51	127	81
Inositol, mg	149[3]	32	31	32	37	32	30	162
OTHER NUTRIENTS								
Cholesterol, mg	150	11	~7	33	21	~7	NA	22
Taurine, mg	40	45	40	40	45	40	48	45
Water, g	880	900	900	904	900	900	904	910
OSMOTIC CHARACTERISTICS								
Renal solute load,** mosm	75.1	99.7	98	91.4	123.6	126	128	96.3
Osmolality, mosm/kg water	290	300	300	300	250	240	268	280
Osmolarity, mosm/liter	255	270	270	271	230	220	242	250

Nutrients per liter: Values calculated and rounded from nutrient values per 100 Calories   Courtesy of Ross Laboratories, 1989.

*E:PUFA ratio $= \dfrac{\text{d-alpha tocopherol (mg)}}{\text{polyunsaturated fatty acids (g)}}$

**Estimated renal solute load = [Protein (g) × 4] + [Na (mEq) + K (mEq) + Cl (mEq)].

†Composition of human milk varies with stage of lactation, within feedings, diurnally and among mothers.

††Similac® Low-Iron Infant Formula.

‡Enfamil® Low-Iron Infant Formula.

‡‡SMA® Lo-Iron Infant Formula.

§Values recalculated from reference.

\\\Similac® Special Care® 24-Low-Iron Premature Infant Formula.

‖Values listed are for Similac Natural Care® only; designed for use as a human milk fortifier.

¶Values listed are for 1:1 dilution with water. However, standard dilution is one part formula base to one part prescribed carbohydrate and water solution. If carbohydrate is not added to this product, a 1:1 dilution with water provides approximately 12 Cal/fl oz (40.6 Cal/100 ml).

#Medium-chain fatty acids are not included in total saturated fatty acids.

NOTE: Values listed are subject to change. Refer to product label or packaging for most current information.

NA = not available.

References

1. Committee on Nutrition, American Academy of Pediatrics: Pediatric Nutrition Handbook, ed 2. Elk Grove Village, Illinois, American Academy of Pediatrics, 1985, pp 363–368.
2. Composition of Foods: Dairy and Egg Products, Raw, Processed, Prepared, Agriculture Handbook No. 8-1. US Dept. of Agriculture, Agricultural Research Service, rev 1976, Item No. 01–107.
3. Ogasa K, Kuboyama M, Kiyosawa I, et al: The content of free and bound inositol in human and cow's milk. J. Nutr. Sci. Vitaminol. *21*:129–135, 1975.

Enriched Calorie Formulas

	SIMILAC® AND SIMILAC® WITH IRON 24	ENFAMIL® AND ENFAMIL® WITH IRON 24	SMA® AND SMA® WITH IRON 24	SIMILAC® 27	SMA® AND SMA® WITH IRON 27	SIMILAC® SPECIAL CARE® 24 AND WITH IRON 24	ENFAMIL® PREMATURE FORMULA® 24	"PREEMIE" SMA® 24
ENERGY, Cal	812	810	811	913	913	812	810	810
PROTEIN, g	22	17.8	18	24.7	20.3	22	24	20
% of total Calories	11	9	8.9	11	8.9	11	12	9.6
Source	Cow's Milk	Reduced Minerals, Whey & Nonfat Milk	Nonfat Milk & Demineralized Whey	Cow's Milk	Nonfat Milk & Demineralized Whey	Cow's Milk & Whey	Whey Protein Concentrate & Nonfat Milk	Nonfat Milk & Demineralized Whey
Amino Acids, mg								
Histidine	450	350	430	510	490	430	470	510
Isoleucine	1070	1080	1000	1210	1120	1160	1390	1370
Leucine	2060	1850	1780	2320	2000	2170	2300	2470
Lysine	1570	1240	1400	1760	1580	1740	1810	2080
Tryptophan	280	270	290	320	320	250	380	350
Phenylalanine	1070	700	740	1210	840	720	920	1080
Threonine	940	940	960	1060	1080	1280	1320	1410
Valine	1190	1100	1070	1340	1200	1190	1460	1470
Methionine	610	350	440	680	500	540	540	470
Cystine	190	210	340	210	380	350	260	370
FAT, g	42.8	45	43.2	48.1	48.6	44.1	41	44
% of total Calories	47	50	48.2	47	48.2	47	44	48.5
Source	Soy & Coconut Oils	Coconut & Soy Oils	Oleo. Coconut, Oleic & Soy Oils	Soy & Coconut Oils	Oleo, Coconut, Oleic & Soy Oils	Medium-Chain Triglycerides, Soy & Coconut Oils	Medium-Chain Triglycerides, Soy & Coconut Oils	Coconut, Oleic, Oleo & Soy Oils & Medium-Chain Triglycerides
Fatty Acids								
Polyunsaturated, g	15	13	6	17	7	8	9	6.4
Saturated, g	19	21#	18	21	20	25	11#	20.3
Monounsaturated, g	7	7	17	8	19	5	5	14.7
Linoleic acid, mg	10,560	8900	3960	11,870	4455	5680	8100	4000
E:PUFA Ratio*	1.1	1.3	1.3	1.1	1.3	2.5	2.6	1.6
CARBOHYDRATE, g	85.3	83	86.4	95.9	97.2	86.1	89	86
% of total Calories	42	41	42.9	42	42.9	42	44	41.9
Source	Lactose	Lactose	*Lactose	Lactose	Lactose	Lactose & POLYCOSE® Glucose Polymers	Corn Syrup Solids, Lactose	Lactose & Glucose Polymers

MINERALS		mEq		mEq		mEq		mEq		mEq		mEq		mEq		mEq
Calcium, mg	730	36.4	560	28	504	25.1	820	41.0	567	28.2	1460	72.8	950	47	750	37.4
Phosphorus, mg	570		380		336		640		378		730		480		400	
Magnesium, mg	57		63		54		64		61		100		81		70	
Iron, mg	15(1.8)††		15.2(1.3)‡		14.4(1.8)#		2.0		16.2(2.0)#		15(3.0)\\\		2		3	
Zinc, mg	6.1		6.3		6		6.9		6.8		12.2		8.1		8	
Manganese, μg	41		126		180		46		203		100		106		200	
Copper, μg	730		730		564		820		635		2030		1300		700	
Iodine, μg	120		81		72		140		81		50		64		83	
Sodium, mg	280	12.2	220	10	180	7.8	310	13.5	203	8.8	350	15.2	320	14	320	13.9
Potassium, mg	1070	27.4	870	22	672	17.2	1210	31.0	756	19.3	1050	26.9	900	23	750	19.2
Chloride, mg	660	18.6	500	14	450	12.7	740	21.0	506	14.3	660	18.6	690	20	530	14.9

Enriched Calorie Formulas *Continued*

	SIMILAC® AND SIMILAC® WITH IRON 24	ENFAMIL® AND ENFAMIL® WITH IRON 24	SMA® AND SMA® WITH IRON 24	SIMILAC® 27	SMA® AND SMA® WITH IRON 27	SIMILAC® SPECIAL CARE® 24 AND WITH IRON 24	ENFAMIL® PREMATURE FORMULA® 24	"PREEMIE" SMA® 24
VITAMINS								
Vitamin A, IU	2440	2500	2400	2740	2700	5520	9700	2400
Vitamin D, IU	490	510	480	550	540	1220	2600	480
Vitamin E, IU	24	25	11.4	27	13	32	37	15
Vitamin K, μg	65	70	66	73	74	100	106	70
Thiamine (vitamin B_1), μg	810	650	804	910	905	2030	2000	800
Riboflavin (vitamin B_2), μg	1220	1300	1200	1370	1350	5030	2900	1300
Vitamin B_6, μg	490	490	504	550	567	2030	2000	500
Vitamin B_{12}, μg	2.0	1.9	1.6	2.3	1.8	4.5	2.4	2.0
Niacin, μg	8530	10,100	6000	9590	6750	40,600	33,000	6300
Folic acid (folacin), μg	120	126	60	140	68	300	290	100
Pantothenic acid, μg	3650	3800	2520	4110	2835	15,430	9700	3600
Biotin, μg	36	18.6	18	40	20	300	16.3	18
Vitamin C (ascorbic acid), mg	70	66	66	80	74	300	290	70
Choline, mg	130	126	120	146	135	81	61	127
Inositol, mg	38	38	38	43	43	45	38	32
OTHER NUTRIENTS								
Cholesterol, mg	15	~9	40	16	45	25	~9	NA
Taurine, mg	54	49	48	61	54	54	49	48
Water, g	885	880	885	870	872	890	880	880
OSMOTIC CHARACTERISTICS								
Renal solute load,** mosm	146.2	117	109.5	164.4	123.4	148.7	153	128.0
Osmolality, mosm/kg water	380	360	364	430	416	300	300	280
Osmolarity, mosm/liter	340	320	322	370	362	270	260	246

Nutrients per liter: Values calculated and rounded from nutrient values per 100 Calories

Courtesy of Ross Laboratories, 1989.

*E:PUFA ratio = $\dfrac{\text{d-alpha tocopherol (mg)}}{\text{polyunsaturated fatty acids (g)}}$

**Estimated renal solute load = [Protein (g) × 4] + [Na (mEq) + K (mEq) + Cl (mEq)].

†Composition of human milk varies with stage of lactation, within feedings, diurnally, and among mothers.

††Similac® Low-Iron Infant Formula.

‡Enfamil® Low-Iron Infant Formula.

‡‡SMA® Lo-Iron Infant Formula.

§Values recalculated from reference.

\\\Similac® Special Care® 24-Low-Iron Premature Infant Formula.

║Values listed are for Similac Natural Care® only; designed for use as a human milk fortifier.

¶Values listed are for 1:1 dilution with water. However, standard dilution is one part formula base to one part prescribed carbohydrate and water solution. If carbohydrate is not added to this product, a 1:1 dilution with water provides approximately 12 Cal/fl oz (40.6 Cal/100 ml).

#Medium-chain fatty acids are not included in total saturated fatty acids.

NOTE: Values listed are subject to change. Refer to product label or packaging for most current information.

NA = not available.

References

1. Committee on Nutrition, American Academy of Pediatrics: Pediatric Nutrition Handbook, ed 2. Elk Grove Village, Illinois, American Academy of Pediatrics, 1985, pp 363–368.
2. Composition of Foods: Dairy and Egg Products, Raw, Processed, Prepared, Agriculture Handbook No. 8-1. US Dept. of Agriculture, Agricultural Research Service, rev 1976, Item No. 01–107.
3. Ogasa K, Kuboyama M, Kiyosawa I, et al: The content of free and bound inositol in human and cow's milk. J. Nutr. Sci. Vitaminol. *21*:129–135, 1975.

Special Formulas

	SIMILAC® 13		ISOMIL® 20		ISOMIL® SF 20		PROSOBEE® 20		NURSOY® 20		ALIMENTUM®		NUTRAMIGEN® 20		PREGESTIMIL® 20		RCF® ¶		ADVANCE®		PEDIASURE®	
ENERGY, Cal	440		676		676		670		676		676		670		670		405		540		1000	
PROTEIN, g	11.9		18		18		20		21		18.6		19		19		20		20		30	
% of total Calories	11		11		11		12		12.3		11		11		11		20		15		12	
Source	Cow's Milk		Soy Protein Isolate		Soy Protein Isolate		Soy Protein Isolate		Soy Protein Isolate		Casein Hydrolysate, Cystine, Tyrosine & Tryptophan		Casein Hydrolysate, Cystine, Tryosine & Tryptophan		Casein Hydrolysate, Cystine, Tyrosine & Tryptophan		Soy Protein Isolate		Cow's Milk & Soy Protein Isolate		Low-Lactose Whey Protein & Sodium Caseinate	
Amino Acids, mg																						
Histidine	250		420		420		460		560		480		570		570		475		490		720	
Isoleucine	580		780		780		920		1090		1000		1140		1140		870		920		1440	
Leucine	1120		1440		1440		1520		1820		1640		1940		1940		1580		1730		2880	
Lysine	850		1035		1035		1200		1220		1600		1630		1630		1210		1350		2280	
Tryptophan	150		190		190		240		310		260		300		270		210		230		390	
Phenylalanine	580		900		900		980		1100		820		910		910		990		890		1440	
Threonine	510		680		680		640		850		870		930		930		710		810		1440	
Valine	650		750		750		920		1060		1320		1420		1420		875		1030		1710	
Methionine	330		400		400		360		530		500		590		590		435		430		840	
Cystine	100		200		200		180		290		300		300		280		200		160		270	
FAT, g	23.2		36.9		36.9		36		36		37.5		26		38		36		27		50	
% of total Calories	47		49		49		48		47.4		48		35		48		80		45		44	
Source	Soy & Coconut Oils		Soy & Coconut Oils		Soy & Coconut Oils		Coconut & Soy Oils		Oleo, Coconut, Oleic & Soy Oils		Medium Chain Triglycerides, Safflower & Soy Oils		Corn Oil		Medium-Chain Triglycerides, Corn & High-Oleic Safflower Oils		Soy & Coconut Oils		Soy & Corn Oils		High-Oleic Safflower & Soy Oils & Medium-Chain Triglycerides	
Fatty Acids																						
Polyunsaturated, g	8		14		14		11		4.7		12.8		16		6		13		15		13	
Saturated, g	10		16		16		17#		14.9		18.2		4#		2#		15		5		13	
Monounsaturated, g	4		6		6		6		14.2		2.6		7		8		6		6		21	
Linoleic acid, mg	5720		8790		8790		6700		3300		10,816		13,400		5000		8790		12,420		11,400	
E:PUFA Ratio*	1.1		1.0		1.0		1.4		1.3		1.1		0.9		2.7		1.0		0.9		1.2	
CARBOHYDRATE, g	46.2		68.3		68.3		68		69.0		68.9		91		69		0.04		55.1		110	
% of total Calories	42		40		40		40		40.3		41		54		41		0		40		44	
Source	Lactose		Corn Syrup & Sucrose		POLYCOSE® Glucose Polymers		Corn Syrup Solids		Sucrose		Sucrose & Modified Tapioca Starch		Corn Syrup Solids & Modified Cornstarch		Corn Syrup Solids, Modified Cornstarch & Dextrose		Selected by Physician		Corn Syrup & Lactose		Corn Syrup Solids & Sucrose	
MINERALS		mEq		mEq		mEq		mEq		mEq		mEq		mEq		mEq		mEq		mEq		mEq
Calcium, mg	400	20.0	710	35.4	710	35.4	630	31	600	29.9	710	35.4	630	31	630	31	700	34.9	510	25.4	970	48.4
Phosphorus, mg	310		510		510		500		420		510		420		420		500		390		800	
Magnesium, mg	31		51		51		74		67		51		74		74		50		41		200	
Iron, mg	1.0		12		12		12.7		11.5		12		12.7		12.7		1.5		10		14	
Zinc, mg	3.3		5.1		5.1		5.3		5		5.1		5.3		6.3		5		4.9		12	
Manganese, μg	22		200		200		169		200		200		210		210		200		32		2500	
Copper, μg	400		510		510		630		470		510		630		630		500		590		1000	
Iodine, μg	66		100		100		69		60		100		48		48		100		97		97	
Sodium, mg	150	6.5	300	13.0	300	13.0	240	10	200	8.7	300	13.0	320	14	320	14	300	13.0	190	8.3	380	16.5
Potassium, mg	580	14.8	730	18.7	730	18.7	820	21	700	17.9	800	20.5	740	19	740	19	730	18.7	790	20.2	1310	33.5
Chloride, mg	360	10.2	420	11.9	420	11.9	560	16	375	10.6	540	15.3	580	16	580	16	420	11.9	480	13.6	1010	28.5

Special Formulas *Continued*

	SIMILAC® 13	ISOMIL® 20	ISOMIL® SF 20	PROSOBEE® 20	NURSOY® 20	ALIMENTUM®	NUTRAMIGEN® 20	PREGESTIMIL® 20	RCF® ¶	ADVANCE®	PEDIASURE®
VITAMINS											
Vitamin A, IU	1320	2030	2030	2100	2000	2030	2100	2500	2030	1620	2570
Vitamin D, IU	260	410	410	420	400	410	420	510	410	320	510
Vitamin E, IU	13	20	20	21	9.5	20	21	25	20	16	23
Vitamin K, μg	35	100	100	106	100	100	106	127	100	43	34
Thiamine (vitamin B_1), μg	440	410	410	520	670	410	520	520	410	650	2700
Riboflavin (vitamin B_2), μg	660	610	610	630	1000	610	630	630	610	920	2100
Vitamin B_6, μg	260	410	410	420	420	410	420	420	410	410	2600
Vitamin B_{12}, μg	1.1	3.0	3.0	2.1	2	3	2.1	2.1	3.0	1.6	6
Niacin	4620	9130	9130	8500	5000	9130	8500	8500	9030	7020	17,000
Folic acid (folacin), μg	66	100	100	106	50	100	106	106	100	100	370
Pantothenic acid, μg	1980	5070	5070	3200	3000	5070	3200	3200	5020	3020	10,000
Biotin, μg	19	30	30	53	35	30	53	53	30	24	320
Vitamin C (ascorbic acid), μg	40	60	60	55	55	60	55	79	55	50	100
Choline, mg	70	54	54	53	85	54	90	90	53	86	300
Inositol, mg	21	34	34	32	27	34	32	32	32	25	80
OTHER NUTRIENTS											
Cholesterol, mg	8	0	0	0	10	<10	~7	~7	0	7	21
Taurine, mg	30	45	45	40	40	45	40	40	45	36	72
Water, g	940	900	900	900	898	900	900	910	948	920	844
OSMOTIC CHARACTERISTICS											
Renal solute load,**mosm	79.1	115.6	115.6	127	122.2	123.2	125	125	123.6	122.1	198.5
Osmolality, mosm/ kg water	200	240	150	200	296	370	320	320	74	200	300
Osmolarity, mosm/liter	190	220	140	170	266	330	290	290	70	180	254

Nutrients per liter: Values calculated and rounded from nutrient values per 100 Calories

684

$$*E{:}PUFA\ ratio = \frac{d\text{-alpha tocopherol (mg)}}{\text{polyunsaturated fatty acids (g)}}$$

**Estimated renal solute load = [Protein (g) × 4] + K (mEq) + [Na (mEq) + Cl (mEq)].

†Composition of human milk varies with stage of lactation, within feedings, diurnally and among mothers.

††Similac® Low-Iron Infant Formula.

†Enfamil® Low-Iron Infant Formula.

‡‡SMA® Low-Iron Infant Formula.

§Values recalculated from reference.

\\\Similac® Special Care® 24 Low-Iron Premature Infant Formula.

‖Values listed are for Similac Natural Care® only; designed for use as a human milk fortifier.

¶Values listed are for 1:1 dilution with water. However, standard dilution is one part formula base to one part prescribed carbohydrate and water solution. If carbohydrate is not added to this product, a 1:1 dilution with water provides approximately 12 Cal/fl oz (40.6 Cal/100 ml).

#Medium-chain fatty acids are not included in total saturated fatty acids.

NOTE: Values listed are subject to change. Refer to product label or packaging for most current information.

NA = not available.

Courtesy of Ross Laboratories, 1989.

References

1. Committee on Nutrition, American Academy of Pediatrics: Pediatric Nutrition Handbook, ed 2. Elk Grove Village, Ill, American Academy of Pediatrics, 1985, pp 363–368.
2. Composition of Foods: Dairy and Egg Products, Raw, Processed, Prepared, Agriculture Handbook No. 8-1. US Dept. of Agriculture, Agriculture Research Service, rev 1976, Item No. 01-107.
3. Ogasa K, Kuboyama M, Kiyosawa I, et al: The content of free and bound inositol in human and cow's milk. J. Nutr. Sci. Vitaminol. *21*:129–135, 1975.

Estimated Daily Requirements of Premature Infants:*†
Growth and Non-Growth

	BODY WEIGHT INTERVALS (gm)								
	750–1000	1000–1250	1250–1500	1500–1750	1750–2000	2000–2250	2250–2500	2500–2750	2750–3000
Energy									
Growth (kcal)	21	46	68	79	93	104	114	111	108
Nongrowth									
(kcal)	71	94	117	133	156	180	204	215	239
Total (kal/kg)	105	124	127	130	133	133	134	124	121
Protein									
Growth (g)	1.78	3.45	4.44	4.79	4.85	4.90	4.68	4.27	3.77
Nongrowth (g)	0.87	1.12	1.37	1.62	1.87	2.12	2.37	2.62	2.87
Total (g/kg)‡	3.02	4.06	4.22	3.94	3.58	3.30	2.96	2.62	2.30
Sodium									
Growth (mEq)	0.95	1.68	2.10	2.21	2.21	2.21	2.10	1.89	1.57
Nongrowth (mEq)	0.18	0.23	0.28	0.34	0.39	0.44	0.49	0.55	0.60
Total (mEq/kg)	1.29	1.69	1.73	1.56	1.38	1.24	1.09	0.92	0.75
Potassium									
Growth (mEq)	0.31	0.73	1.05	1.15	1.26	1.36	1.36	1.36	1.15
Nongrowth (mEq)	0.20	0.26	0.32	0.38	0.43	0.49	0.55	0.61	0.66
Total (mEq/kg)	0.58	0.88	0.99	0.94	0.90	0.87	0.80	0.75	0.63
Calcium									
Growth (mg)	148	317	442	530	592	632	660	627	592
Nongrowth (mg)	—	—	—	—	—	—	—	—	—
Total (mg/kg)	169	282	321	326	316	300	278	239	206
Phosphorus									
Growth (mg)	49	110	148	172	188	197	202	194	177
Nongrowth (mg)	12	27	37	43	47	49	50	49	44
Total (mg/kg)	70	121	135	132	125	116	106	93	77
Magnesium									
Growth (mg)	9.0	18.5	25.5	30.0	33.5	35.5	37.0	35.5	32.5
Nongrowth (mg)	—	—	—	—	—	—	—	—	—
Total (mg/kg)	10.3	16.4	18.6	18.5	17.8	16.7	15.6	13.5	11.3

*Assuming extent of intestinal absorption as follows: energy: 75 per cent absorption for infants weighing 750 to 1500 gm, 80 per cent for those weighing 1500–2500 gm, and 85 per cent for those weighing more than 2500 gm; protein: 75 per cent absorption at 750–1250 gm, 77 per cent at 1250–1500 gm, 80 per cent at 1500–2250 gm, 83 per cent at 2250–2500 gm, and 85 per cent above 2500 gm; sodium and potassium, 95 per cent absorption throughout; calcium, 40 per cent, phosphorus, 80 per cent, and magnesium, 20 per cent throughout.

†See also chapter on nutrition.

‡Based on arithmetic mean weight for the weight interval. (Data of O'Donnell, A. M., Ziegler, E. E., and Fomon, S. J., reproduced with permission of Dr. Fomon.)

APPENDIX 3
ILLUSTRATIVE FORMS AND NORMAL VALUES

ESTIMATION OF GESTATIONAL AGE BY MATURITY RATING
Symbols: X - 1st Exam   O - 2nd Exam

NEUROMUSCULAR MATURITY

	0	1	2	3	4	5
Posture						
Square Window (Wrist)	90°	60°	45°	30°	0°	
Arm Recoil	180°		100°-180°	90°-100°	< 90°	
Popliteal Angle	180°	160°	130°	110°	90°	< 90°
Scarf Sign						
Heel to Ear						

Gestation by Dates _____ wks

Birth Date _____ Hour _____ am / pm

APGAR _____ 1 min _____ 5 min

MATURITY RATING

Score	Wks
5	26
10	28
15	30
20	32
25	34
30	36
35	38
40	40
45	42
50	44

PHYSICAL MATURITY

	0	1	2	3	4	5
SKIN	gelatinous red, transparent	smooth pink, visible veins	superficial peeling &/or rash, few veins	cracking pale area, rare veins	parchment, deep cracking, no vessels	leathery, cracked, wrinkled
LANUGO	none	abundant	thinning	bald areas	mostly bald	
PLANTAR CREASES	no crease	faint red marks	anterior transverse crease only	creases ant. 2/3	creases cover entire sole	
BREAST	barely percept.	flat areola, no bud	stippled areola, 1–2 mm bud	raised areola, 3–4 mm bud	full areola, 5–10 mm bud	
EAR	pinna flat, stays folded	sl. curved pinna, soft with slow recoil	well-curv. pinna, soft but ready recoil	formed & firm with instant recoil	thick cartilage, ear stiff	
GENITALS Male	scrotum empty, no rugae		testes descending, few rugae	testes down, good rugae	testes pendulous, deep rugae	
GENITALS Female	prominent clitoris & labia minora		majora & minora equally prominent	majora large, minora small	clitoris & minora completely covered	

SCORING SECTION

	1st Exam=X	2nd Exam=O
Estimating Gest Age by Maturity Rating	_____ Weeks	_____ Weeks
Time of Exam	Date _____ Hour _____ am/pm	Date _____ Hour _____ am/pm
Age at Exam	_____ Hours	_____ Hours
Signature of Examiner	_____ M.D.	_____ M.D.

(Scoring system: From Ballard J., et al.: A simplified assessmesnt of gestational age. Pediatr. Res. 11:37, 1977. Figures adapted from Sweet, A. Y.: Classification of the low birth weight infant. In Klaus, M. H., Fanaroff A. A. (Eds.): Care of the High-Risk Infant. 2nd ed. Philadelphia, W. B. Saunders Co., 1979, p. 79.)

Physical criteria alone are preferable to neurologic or combined criteria for assessment of gestational age in low birth weight infants. (Constantine, N. A., Kraemer, H. C., Kendall-Tackett, K. A., et al.: Use of physical and neurologic observations in assessment of gestational age in low birth weight infants. J. Pediatr.110:921, 1987.)

Correlations Between Gestation Length and Embryonic and Fetal Bodily Dimensions

WEEK OF GESTATION	CROWN-RUMP LENGTH (cm)	WEIGHT (gm)	BIPARIETAL DIAMETER (cm)
6	0.5		
7	0.8	0.07	
8	1.5	0.22	
9	2.5	0.88	
10	3.5	3.5	
11	4.6	6.0	
12	5.7	11.0	
13	6.8	19.0	
14	8.1	33.0	
15	9.4	55.0	
16	10.7	80.0	
17	12.1	120.0	3.7
18	13.6	170.0	4.0
19	15.3	253.0	4.4
20	16.4	316.0	4.8
21	17.5	385.0	5.2
22	18.6	460.0	5.5
23	19.7	542.0	5.75
24	20.8	630.0	5.95
25	21.8	723.0	6.1
26	22.8	823.0	6.2
27	23.8	930.0	6.35
28	24.7	1045.0	6.5
29	25.6	1174.0	6.65
30	26.5	1323.0	6.85
31	27.4	1492.0	7.1
32	28.3	1680.0	7.3
33	29.3	1876.0	7.6
34	30.2	2074.0	7.8
35	31.1	2274.0	8.1
36	32.1	2478.0	8.35
37	33.1	2690.0	8.6
38	34.1	2914.0	8.9
39	35.1	3150.0	9.2
40	36.2	3405.0	9.55
41		3600.0	9.8
42		3650.0	9.85
		3750.0	10.0
		3900.0	10.2
		4000.0	10.3
		4200.0	10.6

(Data based on the study of Bartolucci, L.: Am. J. Obstet. Gynecol. *122*:439, 1975. Courtesy of Iffy, L., et al.: Pediatrics *56*:173, 1975.)

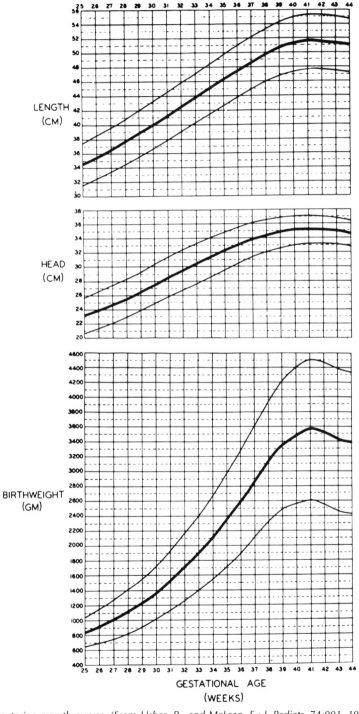

Intrauterine growth curves. (From Usher, R., and McLean, F.: J. Pediatr. 74:901, 1969.)

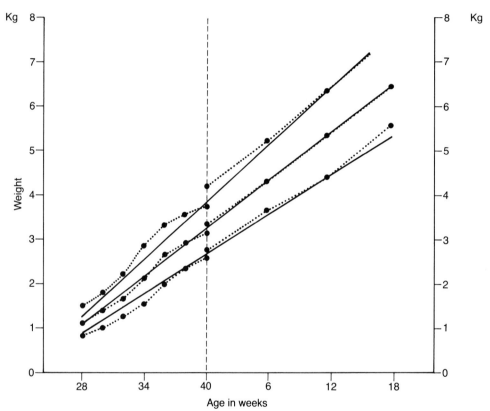

Fetal growth curves (10th, 50th, 90th percentiles) of Lubchenco et al. and early growth curves of Tanner as superimposed on The Bristol Perinatal Growth Chart of Dunn.

Distribution of Measurements for White Newborn Male Infants (Controls) by Percentiles According to Gestational Ages

PERCENTILE*	GESTATIONAL AGE, wk					
	37	38	39	40	41	42–43
	Crown-Heel Lengths, cm					
95	52.0	53.0	54.0	54.5	55.0	55.3
90	51.5	52.5	53.5	54.0	54.5	54.8
75	50.5	51.5	52.5	53.0	53.5	54.0
50	50.0	50.7	51.5	52.0	52.5	53.0
25	49.0	49.7	50.5	51.0	51.5	52.0
10	48.0	48.7	49.5	50.0	50.5	51.0
5	47.5	48.2	49.0	49.5	50.0	50.5
	Occipitofrontal Circumference, cm					
95	35.5	36.0	36.4	36.8	37.2	37.4
90	35.2	35.6	35.9	36.3	36.7	37.2
75	34.6	34.9	35.3	35.7	36.0	36.2
50	34.0	34.3	34.6	34.9	35.2	35.5
25	33.4	33.7	34.0	34.3	34.7	35.0
10	32.8	33.2	33.5	33.8	34.2	34.5
5	32.4	32.7	33.1	33.4	33.8	34.2
	Birth Weights, First-born Infants, kg					
95	3.63	3.82	3.97	4.10	4.23	4.34
90	3.50	3.70	3.86	4.00	4.13	4.24
75	3.30	3.48	3.65	3.78	3.92	4.03
50	3.10	3.27	3.43	3.57	3.70	3.82
25	2.85	3.00	3.13	3.26	3.38	3.49
10	2.70	2.84	2.96	3.08	3.18	3.28
5	2.62	2.76	2.88	3.00	3.10	3.20
	Birth Weights, Infants of Multiparas, kg					
95	3.66	4.00	4.20	4.39	4.50	4.60
90	3.47	3.70	3.90	4.08	4.24	4.37
75	3.30	3.50	3.70	3.87	4.03	4.15
50	3.10	3.27	3.44	3.61	3.75	3.85
25	2.85	3.02	3.18	3.34	3.50	3.62
10	2.71	2.86	3.02	3.19	3.34	3.45
5	2.63	2.78	2.94	3.08	3.31	3.32

(From Miller, H. C.: Intrauterine growth retardation: an unmet challenge. Am. J. Dis. Child. *135*:946, 1981.)

Distribution of Measurements for White Newborn Female Infants (Controls) by Percentiles According to Gestational Ages

PERCENTILE	GESTATIONAL AGE, wk					
	37	38	39	40	41	42–43
	Crown-Heel Lengths, cm					
95	51.5	52.5	53.5	54.0	54.5	54.5
90	51.0	52.0	53.0	53.5	54.0	54.0
75	50.0	51.0	52.0	52.5	52.8	53.1
50	49.0	50.0	50.7	51.3	51.7	52.0
25	48.0	48.9	49.5	50.0	50.5	51.0
10	47.5	48.5	49.0	49.5	50.0	50.5
5	47.0	47.9	48.6	49.1	49.5	50.0
	Occipitofrontal Circumferences, cm					
95	35.0	35.5	35.9	36.2	36.5	36.8
90	34.5	35.0	35.4	35.7	36.1	36.3
75	33.9	34.3	34.7	35.1	35.5	35.8
50	33.2	33.6	34.1	34.5	34.8	35.2
25	32.5	32.9	33.4	33.8	34.2	34.5
10	32.0	32.4	32.8	33.2	33.6	33.9
5	31.8	32.2	32.6	32.9	33.3	33.6
	Birth Weights, First-born Infants, kg					
95	3.44	3.72	3.90	4.03	4.12	4.20
90	3.30	3.60	3.80	3.92	4.02	4.10
75	3.17	3.38	3.57	3.70	3.82	3.94
50	3.00	3.15	3.30	3.43	3.56	3.66
25	2.79	2.93	3.07	3.18	3.29	3.37
10	2.55	2.72	2.85	2.97	3.09	3.17
5	2.46	2.61	2.76	2.89	3.01	3.10
	Birth Weights, Infants of Multiparas, kg					
95	3.60	3.86	4.02	4.14	4.23	4.31
90	3.50	3.67	3.84	3.95	4.07	4.15
75	3.26	3.48	3.64	3.75	3.85	3.95
50	3.00	3.20	3.34	3.50	3.62	3.72
25	2.80	2.95	3.08	3.23	3.35	3.45
10	2.67	2.80	2.93	3.05	3.16	3.26
5	2.52	2.67	2.80	2.92	3.04	3.15

(From Miller, H. C.: Intrauterine growth retardation: an unmet challenge. Am. J. Dis. Child. *135*:946, 1981.)

Distribution of Measurements for Black Male Newborn Infants (Controls) by Percentiles According to Gestational Ages

PERCENTILE	GESTATIONAL AGE, wk					
	37	38	39	40	41	42–43
	Crown-Heel Lengths, cm					
95	51.5	52.5	53.5	54.5	54.5	54.5
90	51.0	52.0	52.7	53.5	54.0	54.0
75	50.5	51.5	52.0	52.5	53.0	53.0
50	49.5	50.0	50.5	51.0	51.5	52.0
25	48.5	49.0	49.5	50.0	50.5	51.0
10	47.5	48.0	48.5	49.0	49.5	50.0
5	47.0	47.5	48.0	48.5	49.0	49.5
	Occipitofrontal Circumferences, cm					
95	35.3	35.8	36.2	36.7	37.0	37.0
90	35.0	35.5	35.9	36.3	36.7	36.8
75	34.6	34.9	35.3	35.6	36.0	36.3
50	33.6	34.0	34.4	34.7	35.1	35.5
25	33.1	33.4	33.8	34.1	34.5	34.9
10	32.4	32.8	33.1	33.4	33.8	34.1
5	32.1	32.5	32.8	33.1	33.4	33.7
	Birth Weights, kg					
95	3.44	3.71	3.97	4.13	4.29	4.40
90	3.38	3.62	3.84	3.97	4.10	4.15
75	3.30	3.46	3.62	3.72	3.82	3.92
50	3.08	3.18	3.30	3.40	3.50	3.60
25	2.83	2.93	3.03	3.13	3.22	3.32
10	2.63	2.73	2.82	2.90	2.99	3.08
5	2.54	2.68	2.72	2.82	2.95	3.00

(From Miller, H. C.: Intrauterine growth retardation: an unmet challenge. Am. J. Dis. Child. *135*:947, 1981.)

Distribution of Measurements for Black Newborn Female Infants (Controls) by Percentiles According to Gestational Ages

PERCENTILE	GESTATIONAL AGE, wk					
	37	38	39	40	41	42–43
	Crown-Heel Lengths, cm					
95	51.0	51.7	52.5	53.3	54.0	54.0
90	50.3	51.0	51.8	52.5	53.5	53.0
75	49.5	50.5	51.0	51.5	52.0	52.5
50	49.0	49.5	50.0	50.5	51.0	51.5
25	48.0	48.5	49.0	49.5	50.0	50.5
10	47.0	47.5	48.0	48.5	49.0	49.5
5	46.5	47.0	47.5	48.0	48.5	49.0
	Occipitofrontal Circumferences, cm					
95	35.0	35.1	35.6	35.9	36.2	36.5
90	34.3	34.8	35.3	35.6	35.8	36.0
75	34.1	34.3	34.6	34.8	35.1	35.3
50	33.4	33.6	33.9	34.1	34.4	34.7
25	32.7	33.0	33.2	33.5	33.7	34.0
10	32.1	32.3	32.6	32.8	33.1	33.3
5	31.7	32.0	32.2	32.5	32.8	33.0
	Birth Weights, kg					
95	3.44	3.65	3.83	3.97	4.00	4.15
90	3.32	3.53	3.73	3.88	3.98	4.05
75	3.14	3.32	3.48	3.60	3.73	3.85
50	2.93	3.07	3.22	3.34	3.46	3.58
25	2.70	2.83	2.95	3.08	3.03	3.32
10	2.53	2.65	2.77	2.89	3.01	3.10
5	2.43	2.54	2.65	2.77	2.89	3.01

(From Miller, H. C.: Intrauterine growth retardation: an unmet challenge. Am. J. Dis. Child. *135*:947, 1981.)

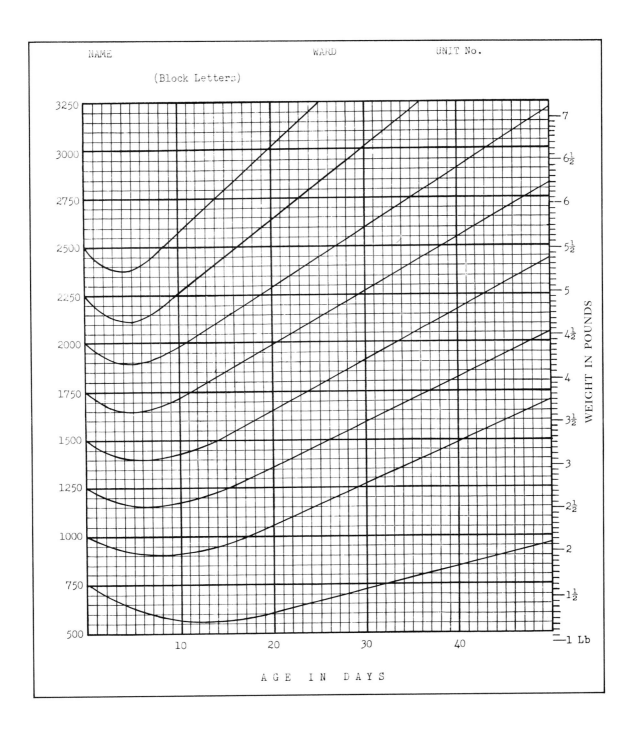

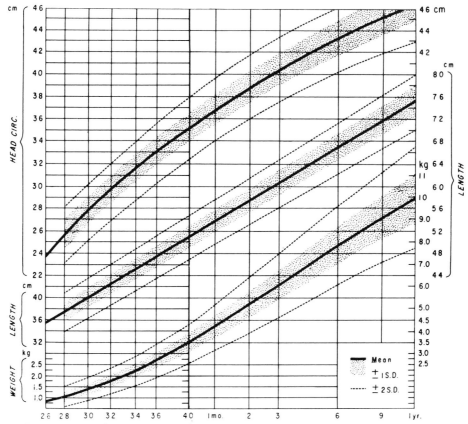

Extrauterine growth curves. (From Babson, S. G., and Benda, G. I.: Pediatrics 89:814, 1976.)

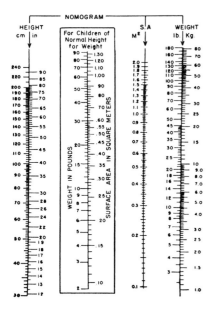

The West nomogram for the estimation of body surface area. The surface area is indicated where a straight line connecting height and weight intersects the surface area column. If the patient is roughly of average size, the surface area can also be estimated from the weight alone (enclosed area). (From Shirkey, H. C.: Drug therapy. In Vaughan, V. C. III, McKay, R. J. [Eds.]: Nelson Textbook of Pediatrics, 10th ed. Philadelphia, W. B. Saunders, 1975.)

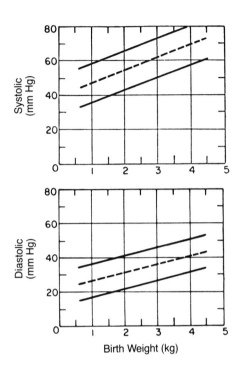

Linear regressions (broken lines) and 95 per cent confidence limits (solid lines) of systolic (top) and diastolic (bottom) aortic blood pressures on birth weight in 61 healthy newborn infants during the first 12 hours after birth. For systolic pressure, y = 7.13x + 40.45; r = 0.79. For diastolic pressure, y = 4.81x + 22.18; r = 0.71. For both, n = 413 and P < 0.001. (From Versmold, H. T., et al.: Pediatrics 67:607, 1981. Reproduced by permission of Pediatrics © 1981.)

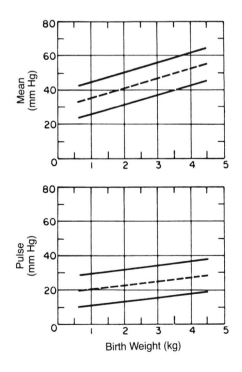

Linear regressions (broken lines) and 95 per cent confidence limits (solid lines) of mean pressures (top) and pulse pressures (systolic-diastolic pressure amplitudes) (bottom) on birth weight in 61 healthy newborn infants during the first 12 hours after birth. For mean pressure, y = 5.16x + 29.80; n = 443; r = 0.80. For pulse pressure, y = 2.31x + 18.27; n = 413; r = 0.45. For both, P < 0.001. (From Versmold, H. T., et al.: Pediatrics 67:607, 1981. Reproduced with permission of Pediatrics © 1981.)

Average Blood Pressure, Heart Rate, Hemoglobin, and Weight During First Week of Life

			DAY						
			1	2	3	4	5	6	7
Systolic pressure	Awake	Mean	67.9	71.9	74.3	77.5	74.2	76.8	76.2
		(2 SD)	(30.8)	(33.6)	(31.4)	(37.0)	(29.2)	(31.0)	(29.6)
	Asleep	Mean	65.0	72.0	77.0	71.0	74.8	76.9	73.7
		(2 SD)	(27.2)	(33.0)	(31.4)	(41.2)	(27.2)	(33.8)	(27.0)
Diastolic pressure	Awake	Mean	43.5	48.3	49.3	52.5	49.0	51.8	47.6
		(2 SD)	(28.8)	(30.2)	(31.6)	(31.8)	(28.6)	(30.0)	(27.2)
	Asleep	Mean	41.4	48.9	52.7	50.7	49.3	53.0	46.7
		(2 SD)	(24.6)	(31.0)	(32.0)	(28.2)	(26.8)	(33.0)	(25.4)
Mean arterial pressure	Awake	Mean	57.7	59.6	63.7	65.0	61.9	63.5	63.5
		(2 SD)	(31.8)	(29.6)	(30.2)	(35.4)	(31.6)	(30.8)	(28.4)
	Asleep	Mean	55.8	60.9	64.8	62.6	61.7	64.4	61.0
		(2 SD)	(27.2)	(31.0)	(34.2)	(30.0)	(28.2)	(33.6)	(28.4)
Heart rate	Awake	Mean	169.2	164.6	167.2	173.2	169.2	172.9	170.9
		(2 SD)	(63.2)	(78.4)	(64.4)	(66.8)	(50.2)	(57.2)	(60.8)
	Asleep	Mean	177.5	173.1	169.1	176.4	166.3	173.1	168.9
		(2 SD)	(67.8)	(77.2)	(61.0)	(69.6)	(56.0)	(54.2)	(74.2)
PVC (per cent)		Mean	61.0		53.7				50.8
		(2 SD)	(18.2)		(21.2)				(16.8)
Hemoglobin (gm/dl)		Mean	20.2		17.9				17.0
		(2 SD)	(6.0)		(7.0)				(5.2)
Wt (gm)		Mean	1221.8		1171.1				1155.2
		(2 SD)	(342.8)		(314.0)				(382.8)

Right upper arm morning blood pressure, heart rate, packed volume of cells (PVC), hemoglobin (Hb), and weight in the first week of life for infants under 34 weeks' gestation and under 1500 grams birth weight.
(From Tan, K. L.: J. Pediatr. *112*:266, 1988.)

Colloid Osmotic Pressure (Torr) in Infants' Blood

Term, vaginal delivery	19.5 ± 2.1 (SD)
Term, C-section	16.1 ± 2.0
Term, vaginal (sick) (sepsis, asphyxia, heart failure, abdominal surgery)	19.5 ± 3.1
Pre-term (700–1980 gm) (hyaline membrane disease, asphyxia, necrotizing entero- colitis, etc.)	12.5 ± 2.5

(Data from Sola, A., and Gregory, G. A.: Critical Care Med. 9:568, 1981.)

Normal Blood Chemistry Values, Term Infants

DETERMINATION	SAMPLE SOURCE	CORD	1–12 H	12–24 H	24–48 H	48–72 H
Sodium, mEq/l*	Capillary	147 (126–166)	143 (124–156)	145 (132–159)	148 (134–160)	149 (139–162)
Potassium, mEq/l		7.8 (5.6–12)	6.4 (5.3–7.3)	6.3 (5.3–8.9)	6.0 (5.2–7.3)	5.9 (5.0–7.7)
Chloride, mEq/l		103 (98–110)	100.7 (90–111)	103 (87–114)	102 (92–114)	103 (93–112)
Calcium, mg/100 ml		9.3 (8.2–11.1)	8.4 (7.3–9.2)	7.8 (6.9–9.4)	8.0 (6.1–9.9)	7.9 (5.9–9.7)
Phosphorus, mg/100 ml		5.6 (3.7–8.1)	6.1 (3.5–8.6)	5.7 (2.9–8.1)	5.9 (3.0–8.7)	5.8 (2.8–7.6)
Blood urea nitrogen, mg/100 ml		29 (21–40)	27 (8–34)	33 (9–63)	32 (13–77)	31 (15–68)
Total protein, gm/100 ml		6.1 (4.8–7.3)	6.6 (5.6–8.5)	6.6 (5.8–8.2)	6.9 (5.9–8.2)	7.2 (6.0–8.5)
Blood sugar, mg/100 ml		73 (45–96)	63 (40–97)	63 (42–104)	56 (30–91)	59 (40–90)
Lactic acid, mg/100 ml		19.5 (11–30)	14.6 (11–24)	14.0 (10–23)	14.3 (9–22)	13.5 (7–21)
Lactate, mm/L†		2.0–3.0	2.0			

*(Acharya and Payne: Arch. Dis. Child. *40*:430, 1968.)
†(Daniel, Adamsons, and James: Pediatrics *37*:942, 1966.)

Serum Electrolyte Values in Preterm Infants

CONSTITUENT	AGE 1 WEEK Mean	SD	Range	AGE 3 WEEKS Mean	SD	Range	AGE 5 WEEKS Mean	SD	Range	AGE 7 WEEKS Mean	SD	Range
Na (mEq/L)	139.6	±3.2	133–146	136.3	±2.9	129–142	136.8	±2.5	133–148	137.2	±1.8	133–142
K (mEq/L)	5.6	±0.5	4.6–6.7	5.8	±0.6	4.5–7.1	5.5	±0.6	4.5–6.6	5.7	±0.5	4.6–7.1
Cl (mEq/L)	108.2	±3.7	100–117	108.3	±3.9	102–116	107.0	±3.5	100–115	107.0	±3.3	101–115
CO_2 (mM/L)	20.3	±2.8	13.8–27.1	18.4	±3.5	12.4–26.2	20.4	±3.4	12.5–26.1	20.6	±3.1	13.7–26.9
Ca (mg/dl)	9.2	±1.1	6.1–11.6	9.6	±0.5	8.1–11.0	9.4	±0.5	8.6–10.5	9.5	±0.7	8.6–10.8
P (mg/dl)	7.6	±1.1	5.4–10.9	7.5	±0.7	6.2–8.7	7.0	±0.6	5.6–7.9	6.8	±0.8	4.2–8.2
BUN (mg/dl)	9.3	±5.2	3.1–25.5	13.3	±7.8	2.1–31.4	13.3	±7.1	2.0–26.5	13.4	±6.7	2.5–30.5

(From Klaus, M. H., and Fanaroff, A. A.: Care of the High Risk Neonate. 3rd ed. Philadelphia, W. B. Saunders, 1986. Adapted from Thomas, J., and Reichelderfer, T.: Clin. Chem. *14*:272, 1968.)

THYROID FUNCTION IN FULL-TERM AND PRETERM INFANTS

Serum T$_4$ Concentration in Premature and Term Infants

	ESTIMATED GESTATIONAL AGE (wk)				
	30–31	32–33	34–35	36–37	Term
Cord					
Mean	6.5*	7.5	6.7†	7.5	8.2
SD	1.0	2.1	1.2	2.8	1.8
n	3	8	18	17	37
12–72 hr					
Mean	11.5‡	12.3‡	12.4‡	15.5†	19.0
SD	2.1	3.2	3.1	2.6	2.1
n	12	18	17	15	6
3–10 days					
Mean	7.7‡	8.5‡	10.0‡	12.7†	15.9
SD	1.8	1.9	2.4	2.5	3.0
n	7	8	9	9	29
11–20 days					
Mean	7.5†	8.3‡	10.5	11.2	12.2
SD	1.8	1.6	1.8	2.9	2.0
n	5	11	9	9	8
21–45 days					
Mean	7.8‡	8.0‡	9.3†	11.4	12.1
SD	1.5	1.7	1.3	4.2	1.5
n	11	17	13	5	5
46–90 days	(30 to 73 weeks)				
Mean		9.6			10.2
SD		1.7			1.9
n		16			17

(From Cuestas, R. A.: J. Pediatr. 92:963, 1982.)
*p < 0.05.
†p < 0.005 } for the comparison of premature vs. term infants (t test)
‡p < 0.001

Serum Free T$_4$ Index in Premature and Term Infants

	ESTIMATED GESTATIONAL AGE (wk)				
	30–31	32–33	34–35	36–37	Term
Cord					
Mean			5.6	5.6	5.9
SD			1.3	2.0	1.1
n			12	10	14
12–72 hr					
Mean	13.1*	12.9*	15.5†	17.1	19.7
SD	2.4	2.7	3.0	3.5	3.5
n	12	14	14	14	6
3–10 days					
Mean	8.3*	9.0*	12.0‡	15.1	16.2
SD	1.9	1.8	2.3	0.7	3.2
n	6	9	5	4	11
11–20 day					
Mean	8.0§	9.1‡	11.8	11.3	12.1
SD	1.6	1.9	2.7	1.9	2.0
n	5	8	8	4	8
21–45 days					
Mean	8.4§	9.0‡	10.9		11.1
SD	1.4	1.6	2.8		1.4
n	11	17	5		5
46–90 days	30 to 35 weeks				
Mean		9.4			9.7
SD		1.4			1.5
n		13			10

(From Cuestas, R. A.: J. Pediatr. 92:963, 1982.)
*p 0.001
†p 0.025 } for the comparison of premature vs. term infants (t test)
‡p 0.01
§p 0.005

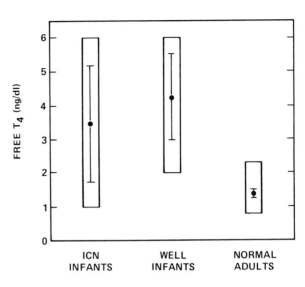

Free thyroxine (T₄) levels in sick infants, healthy term infants, and normal adults. The center • represents the mean ± SD. (From Wilson, D. M., et al.: J. Pediatr. 101:113, 1982.)

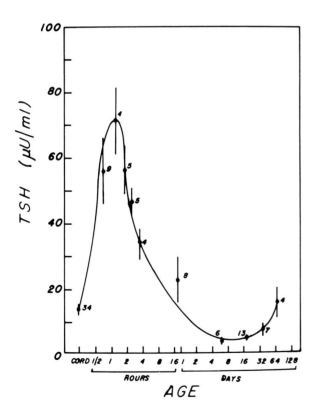

Thyroid-stimulating hormone levels in healthy preterm infants. Mean, standard error of the mean, and sample size are shown. (From Cuestas, R. A.: J. Pediatr. 92:963, 1982.)

Normal Values for Cerebrospinal Fluid

	TERM BABIES
Color	Clear or xanthochromic
White cell count	6–8 (range 0–34)
Protein	45 mg per 100 ml (range 30–102)

(Data from Samson: Ergebn. d. inn. Med. u. Kinderh. *41*:553, 1931; Otilia: Acta Paed. 35: Suppl. 8, 1948; Bauer, et al.: J. Pediat. 66:1017, 1965; Wolf and Hoepffuer: World Neurol. *2*:871, 1961; and Widell: Acta Paed. 47: Suppl. *115*, 1958).

CSF Values in VLBW Infants on Basis of Birth Weight

	GROUP 1 (≤1000 gm) (n = 38*)		GROUP 2 (1001–1500 gm) (n = 33*)		
	Mean ± SD	Range	Mean ± SD	Range	*p*
Birth weight (gm)	763 ± 115	550–980	1278 ± 152	1020–1500	
Gestational age (wk)	26 ± 1.3	24–28	29 ± 1.4	27–33	
Leukocytes/mm³	4 ± 3	0–14	6 ± 9	0–44	NS
Erythrocytes/mm³	1027 ± 3270	0–19,050	786 ± 1879	0–9750	
PMNs (%)	6 ± 15	0–66	9 ± 17	0–60	NS
MN leukocytes (%)	86 ± 30	34–100	85 ± 28	13–100	
Glucose (mg/dl)	61 ± 34	29–217	59 ± 21	31–109	NS
Protein (mg/dl)	150 ± 56	95–370	132 ± 43	45–227	NS

NS, Not significant ($p > 0.05$); MN, mononuclear.
*Number of CSF specimens.
(From Rodriguez, A. F., Kaplan, S. L., and Mason, E. O.: Cerebrospinal fluid values and the very LBW infant. J. Pediatr. *116*:971, 1990.)

CSF Values in VLBW Infants, by Chronologic Age: Group 1 (Birth Weight ≤ 1000 gm)

	POSTNATAL AGE (DAYS)					
	0–7 (6 Infants; n = 6*)		8–28 (12 Infants; n = 17)		29–84 (10 Infants; n = 15)	
	Mean ± SD	*Range*	*Mean ± SD*	*Range*	*Mean ± SD*	*Range*
Birth weight (gm)	822 ± 116	630–980	752 ± 112	550–970	750 ± 120	550–907
Gestational age at birth (wk)	26 ± 1.2	24–27	26 ± 1.5	24–28	26 ± 1.0	24–27
Leukocytes/mm³	3 ± 3	1–8	4 ± 4	0–14	4 ± 3	0–11
Erythrocytes/mm³	335 ± 709	0–1780	1465 ± 4062	0–19,050	808 ± 1843	0–6850
PMNs (%)	11 ± 20	0–50	8 ± 17	0–66	2 ± 9	0–36
Glucose (mg/dl)	70 ± 17	41–89	68 ± 48	33–217	49 ± 22	29–90
Protein (mg/dl)	162 ± 37	115–222	159 ± 77	95–370	137 ± 61	76–260

*Number of CSF specimens.
(From Rodriguez, A. F., Kaplan, S. L., and Mason, E. O.: Cerebrospinal fluid values and the very LBW infant. J. Pediatr. *116*:971, 1990.)

CSF Values in VLBW Infants, by Chronologic Age: Group 2 (Birth Weight ≥ 1001 to 1500 gm)

	POSTNATAL AGE (DAYS)					
	0–7 (8 Infants; n = 8*)		8–28 (11 Infants; n = 14)		29–84 (6 Infants; n = 11)	
	Mean ± SD	*Range*	*Mean ± SD*	*Range*	*Mean ± SD*	*Range*
Birth weight (gm)	1428 ± 107	1180–1500	1245 ± 162	1020–1480	1211 ± 86	1080–1300
Gestational age at birth (wk)	31 ± 1.5	28–33	29 ± 1.2	27–31	29 ± 0.7	27–29
Leukocytes/mm³	4 ± 4	1–10	7 ± 11	0–44	8 ± 8	0–23
Erythrocytes/mm³	407 ± 853	0–2450	1101 ± 2643	0–9750	661 ± 1198	0–3800
PMNs (%)	4 ± 10	0–28	10 ± 19	0–60	11 ± 19	0–48
Glucose (mg/dl)	74 ± 19†	50–96	59 ± 23	39–109	47 ± 13	31–76
Protein (mg/dl)	136 ± 35	85–176	137 ± 46	54–227	122 ± 47	45–187

*Number of CSF specimens.
†$p = 0.004$. Infants up to 7 days of age had significantly higher value compared with those older than 29 days.
(From Rodriguez, A. F., Kaplan, S. L., and Mason, E. O.: Cerebrospinal fluid values and the very LBW infant. J. Pediatr. *116*:971, 1990.)

CSF Analysis From Previous Studies in Premature Infants with Birth Weight ≤ 2500 gm

AUTHOR	NO. OF INFANTS	POSTNATAL AGE	MEAN CSF CELLS/mm³ (RANGE)	MEAN PROTEIN (mg/dl) (RANGE)
Samson	NR	Up to 1 mo	4	55
Otila	46	Up to 1 mo	10	101
Wolf and Hoepffner	22	1–3 days	2 (0–13)	105 (50–180)
Gyllenswärd and Malmström	36	1–40 days	7 (1–37)	115 (55–292)
Sarff et al.	30	1–6 days	9 (0–29)	115 (65–150)

NR, Not recorded.
(From Rodriguez, A. F., Kaplan, S. L., and Mason, E. O.: Cerebrospinal fluid values and the very LBW infant. J. Pediatr. *116*:971, 1990.)

TERM NEWBORN

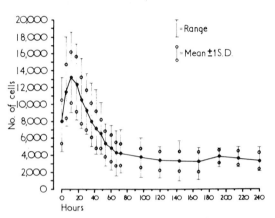

Means, ranges, and means ± 1 SD of neutrophils of 15 full-term healthy babies during the first 10 days of life.

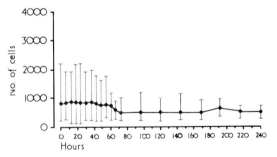

Means and ranges of the eosinophils of full-term babies during the first 10 days of life.

PREMATURES

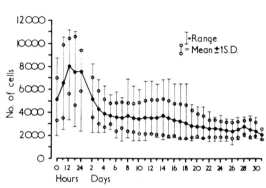

Means, ranges, and means ± 1 SD of neutrophils of 14 healthy babies during the first month of life (13 premature + 1 small for dates).

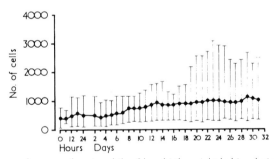

Means and ranges of eosinophils of low-birth-weight babies during the first month of life.

(Data of Xanthou, M.: Arch. Dis. Child. 45:242, 1970.)

TERM NEWBORN

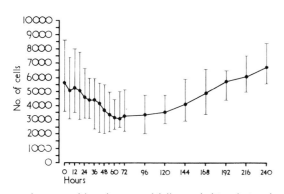

Means and ranges of lymphocytes of full-term babies during the first 10 days of life.

PREMATURES

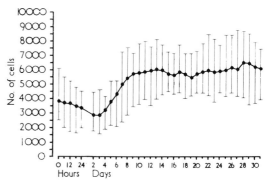

Means and ranges of lymphocytes of low birth weight babies during the first month of life.

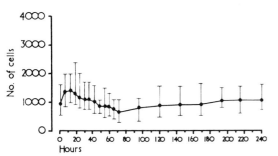

Means and ranges of the monocytes of healthy full-term babies during the first 10 days of life.

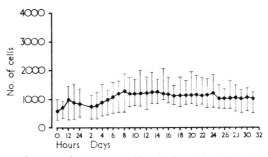

Means and ranges of monocytes of low birth weight babies during the first month of life.

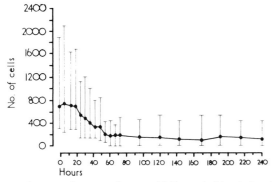

Means and ranges of metamyelocytes of full-term babies during the first 10 days of life.

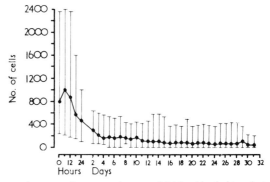

Means and ranges of metamyelocytes of 14 healthy babies during the first month of life.

(Data of Xanthou, M.: Arch. Dis. Child. 45:242, 1970.)

Nucleated RBCs in Normal Infants and Infants of Diabetic Mothers

Variables	CONTROL INFANTS n = 102	INFANTS OF DIABETIC MOTHERS	
		No Perinatal Asphyxia n = 54	Perinatal Asphyxia n = 25
Gestational age (weeks)	39.5 ± 1.5	38.0 ± 1.0*	37.9 ± 1.2*
Birth weight (kg)	3.3 ± 0.3	3.5 ± 0.6*	3.6 ± 0.6*
Leukocyte count†	27.3 ± 9.2	17.1 ± 5.1*	16.8 ± 6.1*
NRBCs (absolute count)	0.4 ± 1.3	1.4 ± 3.1*	1.8 ± 2.3*
NRBCs/100 leukocytes	1.7 ± 6.2	8.3 ± 17.8*	13.0 ± 18.9*

*Significantly different from control infant values (p at least <0.05).
†Data are expressed as × 10⁹/liter.
(Adapted from Green, D. W., and Mimouni, F.: J. Pediatr. *116*:129, 1990.)

Blood Gases: Representative Values in Normal Infants at Term

	Umbilical Vein	30 min	1–4 hr	12–24 hr	24–48 hr	96 hr	Reference
			Arterial Blood				
pH	7.33		7.30	7.30	7.39	7.39	
P_{CO_2}, mm Hg	43		39	33	34	36	Reardon et al. (1960)
HCO_3, mEq/liter	21.6		18.8	19.5	20	21.4	Oliver et al. (1961)
P_{O_2}, mm Hg	28±8		62±13.8	68	63–87		Nelson et al. (1962, 1963)
O_2 saturation			95%	94%	94%	96%	
Crying vital capacity, ml (for 3 kg infant)		77 range (56–110)			92 (69–128)	100	Sutherland and Ratcliff (1961)
Functional residual capacity ml/kg		22 ± 8	25 ± 8	21 ± 1	28 ± 7	39 ± 9	Klaus et al. (1962)
Lung compliance, ml/cm H_2O/kg		1.5 ± 0.05		2.0 ± 0.4		1.7	Cook et al. (1957)
Lung compliance/FRC, ml/cm H_2O/ml			0.04 ± 0.10	0.053 ± 0.009		0.065	Chu et al. (1964) Cook et al. (1957)
Right to left shunt, percentage cardiac output			22% (range 11–29%)	24% (17–32%)			Prod'hom et al. (1964)

		Comment	Reference
Respiratory frequency	34/min. (range 20–60)	1–2 days 1–11 days	Cook et al. (1955) Cross (1949)
Resistances, cm H_2O/liter/sec	29, 26 18 ± 6/3	Total lung resistance Airway resistance	Cook et al. (1949), Swyer et al. (1960), Polgar (1962)
Flow rates, ml/sec	48–37 161–106	Max. insp., max. exp. rest crying	Swyer et al. (1957), Long and Hull (1961)
Ventilation, ml/kg/min	200		Cook et al. (1955), Nelson et al. (1962)
Dead space, ml	4.4–9.2	Term infants	Nelson et al. (1962), Cook et al. (1955), Strang (1961)
Alveolar ventilation, ml/kg/min	120–145	First 3 days of life	Nelson et al. (1962)
O_2 consumption, ml/kg/min	6.2	At neutral temperature	Oliver and Karlberg (1963)
CO_2 production, ml/kg/min	5.1	At neutral temperature	Oliver and Karlberg (1963)
Alveolar-arterial O_2 differences, mm Hg	28 ± 10, room air 311 ± 70, 100% O_2	Age 7 hr to 42 days Age 6 to 58 hr, 3 infants	Nelson et al. (1963)
Arterial-alveolar CO_2 differences, mm Hg	1.8 ± 3.8	Age 3 to 74 hr	Nelson et al. (1962)

(From Avery, M. E., and Normand, C.: Anesthesiology 26:510, 1965.)

Body Composition of the Reference Fetus

Gestational Age (wk)	Body Weight (gm)	Water (gm)	Protein (gm)	Lipid (gm)	Other (gm)	Water (gm)	Protein (gm)	Ca (mg)	P (mg)	Mg (mg)	Na (mEq)	K (mEq)	Cl (mEq)
		per 100 gm body weight				per 100 gm fat-free weight							
24	690	88.6	8.8	0.1	2.5	88.6	8.8	621	387	17.8	9.9	4.0	7.0
25	770	87.8	9.0	0.7	2.5	88.4	9.1	615	385	17.6	9.8	4.0	7.0
26	880	86.8	9.2	1.5	2.5	88.1	9.4	611	384	17.5	9.7	4.1	7.0
27	1010	85.7	9.4	2.4	2.5	87.8	9.7	609	383	17.4	9.5	4.1	6.9
28	1160	84.6	9.6	3.3	2.4	87.5	10.0	610	385	17.4	9.4	4.2	6.9
29	1318	83.6	9.9	4.1	2.4	87.2	10.3	613	387	17.4	9.3	4.2	6.8
30	1480	82.6	10.1	4.9	2.4	86.8	10.6	619	392	17.4	9.2	4.3	6.8
31	1650	81.7	10.3	5.6	2.4	86.5	10.9	628	398	17.6	9.1	4.3	6.7
32	1830	80.7	10.6	6.3	2.4	86.1	11.3	640	406	17.8	9.1	4.3	6.6
33	2020	79.8	10.8	6.9	2.5	85.8	11.6	656	416	18.0	9.0	4.4	6.5
34	2230	79.0	11.0	7.5	2.5	85.4	11.9	675	428	18.3	8.9	4.4	6.4
35	2450	78.1	11.2	8.1	2.6	85.0	12.2	699	443	18.6	8.9	4.5	6.3
36	2690	77.3	11.4	8.7	2.6	84.6	12.5	726	460	19.0	8.8	4.5	6.1
37	2940	76.4	11.6	9.3	2.7	84.3	12.8	758	479	19.5	8.8	4.5	6.0
38	3160	75.6	11.8	9.9	2.7	83.9	13.1	795	501	20.0	8.8	4.5	5.9
39	3330	74.8	11.9	10.5	2.8	83.6	13.3	836	525	20.5	8.7	4.6	5.8
40	3450	74.0	12.0	11.2	2.8	83.3	13.5	882	551	21.1	8.7	4.6	5.7

Data of Ziegler, E. E., et al., University of Iowa, Iowa City, 1975.

Plasma Immunoglobulin Concentrations in Premature Infants (25 to 28 weeks' gestation)

Age (months)	n	IgG* (mg/dl)	IgM* (mg/dl)	IgA* (mg/dl)
0.25	18	251 (114–552)†	7.6 (1.3–43.3)	1.2 (0.07–20.8)
0.5	14	202 (91–446)	14.1 (3.5–56.1)	3.1 (0.09–10.7)
1.0	10	158 (57–437)	12.7 (3.0–53.3)	4.5 (0.65–30.9)
1.5	14	134 (59–307)	16.2 (4.4–59.2)	4.3 (0.9–20.9)
2.0	12	89 (58–136)	16 (5.3–48.9)	4.1 (1.5–11.1)
3	13	60 (23–156)	13.8 (5.3–36.1)	3 (0.6–15.6)
4	10	82 (32–210)	22.2 (11.2–43.9)	6.8 (1–47.8)
6	11	159 (56–455)	41.3 (8.3–205)	9.7 (3–31.2)
8–10	6	273 (94–794)	41.8 (31.1–56.1)	9.5 (0.9–98.6)

From Ballow, M., et al.: Pediatr. Res 20:899, 1986.
*Geometric mean.
†The normal ranges in parentheses were determined by taking the antilog of (mean logarithm ± 2 SD of the logarithms).

Plasma Immunoglobulin Concentrations in Premature Infants (29 to 32 weeks' gestation)

Age (months)	n	IgG* (mg/dl)	IgM* (mg/dl)	IgA* (mg/dl)
0.25	42	368 (186–728)†	9.1 (2.1–39.4)	0.6 (0.04–1)
0.5	35	275 (119–637)	13.9 (4.7–41)	0.9 (0.01–7.5)
1	26	209 (97–452)	14.4 (6.3–33)	1.9 (0.3–12)
1.5	22	156 (69–352)	15.4 (5.5–43.2)	2.2 (0.7–6.5)
2	11	123 (64–237)	15.2 (4.9–46.7)	3 (1.1–8.3)
3	14	104 (41–268)	16.3 (7.1–37.2)	3.6 (0.8–15.4)
4	21	128 (39–425)	26.5 (7.7–91.2)	9.8 (2.5–39.3)
6	21	179 (51–634)	29.3 (10.5–81.5)	12.3 (2.7–57.1)
8–10	16	280 (140–561)	34.7 (17–70.8)	20.9 (8.3–53)

From Ballow, M., et al.: Pediatr. Res 20:899, 1986.
*Geometric mean.
†The normal ranges in parentheses were determined by taking the antilog of (mean logarithm ± 2 SD of the logarithms).

Temperature Equivalents

Celsius	Fahrenheit	Celsius	Fahrenheit
34.0	93.2	38.6	101.4
34.2	93.6	38.8	101.8
34.4	93.9	39.0	102.2
34.6	94.3	39.2	102.5
34.8	94.6	39.4	102.9
35.0	95.0	39.6	103.2
35.2	95.4	39.8	103.6
35.4	95.7	40.0	104.0
35.6	96.1	40.2	104.3
35.8	96.4	40.4	104.7
36.0	96.8	40.6	105.1
36.2	97.1	40.8	105.4
36.4	97.5	41.0	105.8
36.6	97.8	41.2	106.1
36.8	98.2	41.4	106.5
37.0	98.6	41.6	106.8
37.2	98.9	41.8	107.2
37.4	99.3	42.0	107.6
37.6	99.6	42.2	108.0
37.8	100.0	42.4	108.3
38.0	100.4	42.6	108.7
38.2	100.7	42.8	109.0
38.4	101.1	43.0	109.4

To convert Celsius to Fahrenheit:

$$9/5 \times \text{Temperature} + 32$$

Example: To convert 40° Celsius to Fahrenheit

$$9/5 \times 40 = 72 + 32 = 104° \text{ Fahrenheit}$$

To convert Fahrenheit to Celsius:

$$(\text{Temperature} - 32) \times 5/9$$

Example: To convert 98.6° Fahrenheit to Celsius

$$98.6 - 32 = 66.6 \times 5/9 = 37° \text{ Celsius}$$

Conversion of Pounds and Ounces to Grams

Ounces	1 lb	2 lb	3 lb	4 lb	5 lb	6 lb	7 lb	8 lb
				Grams				
0	454	907	1361	1814	2268	2722	3175	3629
1	482	936	1389	1843	2296	2750	3204	3657
2	510	964	1418	1871	2325	2778	3232	3686
3	539	992	1446	1899	2353	2807	3260	3714
4	567	1021	1474	1928	2381	2835	3289	3742
5	595	1049	1503	1956	2410	2863	3317	3771
6	624	1077	1531	1985	2438	2892	3345	3799
7	652	1106	1559	2013	2466	2920	3374	3827
8	680	1134	1588	2041	2495	2948	3402	3856
9	709	1162	1616	2070	2523	2977	3430	3884
10	737	1191	1644	2098	2552	3005	3459	3912
11	765	1219	1673	2126	2580	3033	3487	3941
12	794	1247	1701	2155	2608	3062	3515	3969
13	822	1276	1729	2183	2637	3090	3544	3997
14	851	1304	1758	2211	2665	3119	3572	4026
15	879	1332	1786	2240	2693	3147	3600	4054

Conversion of Inches to Centimeters

Inches	cm	Inches	cm	Inches	cm
10	25.40	15	38.10	20	50.80
10½	26.67	15½	39.37	20½	52.07
11	27.94	16	40.64	21	53.34
11½	29.21	16½	41.91	21½	54.61
12	30.48	17	43.18	22	55.88
12½	31.75	17½	44.45	22½	57.15
13	33.02	18	45.72	23	58.42
13½	34.29	18½	46.99	23½	56.69
14	35.56	19	48.26	24	60.96
14½	36.83	19½	49.53		

APPENDIX 4
COMMUNITY AND AGENCY RESOURCES

■ CHILDREN'S SERVICES

The Maternal-Child Health Division of most states' Department of Health and Human Services (DHHS) provides financial assistance for follow-up of certain infants whose families meet state-established financial criteria. These services are variously named, e.g., Crippled Children's Services (CCS), California Children's Services (CCS). Services vary from state to state, but usually include diagnostic and treatment services, laboratory tests, appliances, equipment, and others if a family's insurance will not pay for needed services. Some CCS programs also provide or will contract for services such as physical or occupational therapy. Inquiries can be made by calling the state or local Maternal-Child Health Division of the Department of Health and Human Services.

■ EASTER SEALS SOCIETY

Each community served by the Easter Seals Society defines what services are needed for that community. Physical and occupational therapy programs are common. The cost of services is based on ability to pay, and no one is denied services because of financial limitations. The national office address is: National Easter Seals Society, 2023 West Ogden Avenue, Chicago, IL 60612.

■ HOME CARE AGENCIES

Many communities have local home care agencies that offer services, such as oxygen and stoma care, for infants with special needs. Some are privately operated, while others contract with local county health or social service departments. Fees vary with location and services. When an infant with special medical home care needs is to be discharged, the local health department is the best place to begin to locate such an agency.

■ INFANT PROGRAMS

Most areas have specialized infant programs that provide services to infants and their families until age 3 years.

(From Headlee, J.: Community and Agency Resources. *In* Ballard, R. A.: Pediatric Care of the ICN Graduate. Philadelphia, W. B. Saunders, 1988.)

These programs may be state, locally, or privately funded and provide a range of services. Infant programs are a good resource for conferring with infant specialists from various disciplines.

■ MARCH OF DIMES BIRTH DEFECTS FOUNDATION

There are 650 March of Dimes chapters nationally, with the goal of achieving healthy babies, born free of handicapping or fatal problems caused by birth defects or prematurity. Their focus is on preventing birth defects, and the Foundation funds scientific research, medical services, and professional and public health education. Some chapters provide specialized services, such as special day care programs for children with cerebral palsy or other handicapping conditions.

■ SUPPORT GROUPS FOR PARENTS OF CHILDREN WITH DOWN AND OTHER SYNDROMES

Numerous support groups exist for parents of children with Down and other genetic syndromes or congenital anomalies. Information for the respective groups can be obtained by writing or calling:

- American Cleft Palate Association, 331 Salk Hall, University of Pittsburgh, Pittsburgh, PA 15261
- Down Syndrome Congress, 1640 W. Roosevelt Road, Chicago, IL 60808
- National Down Syndrome Society, 70 West 40th Street, New York, NY 10018
- Little People of America, PO Box 633, San Bruno, CA 94066
- Osteogenesis Imperfecta Foundation, Box 838, Manchester, NH 03105
- Turner Syndrome Support Group, PO Box 9082, Morristown, NJ 07960

The support organization for trisomy 18/13 (SOFT), established in Utah in 1980, is a national organization for families who have a child with the more serious autosomal trisomies:

- Support Organization for Trisomy 18/13, c/o Debbie Stutz, 3646 West Valley West Drive, West Jordan, UT 84084 or 478 Terrace Lane, Tooele, UT 84074

■ **PARENTS OF PREMATURES AND HIGH-RISK INFANTS (PPHRI)**

This is a nationwide clearinghouse for parents of premature infants. Listings are maintained for local parent support groups, reading materials, clothing, and breast-feeding information related to premature and high-risk infants. This information is published in *The Resource Directory*, which can be obtained by calling PPHRI (212-869-2818).

■ **PUBLIC HEALTH NURSES**

Every county has a public health department. For premature and high-risk infants, a home visit by a public health nurse before discharge is encouraged to assess the parents' readiness for the homecoming and the home situation. Public health nursing home visits are free of charge, and some health departments also provide home care services for at-risk infants. Usually the public health nurse will visit once a week until the family and nurse mutually agree the visits are no longer necessary. The teaching done by the nurses should be coordinated with the pediatrician or family physician; therefore, an ongoing dialogue between the nurse and the physician is encouraged. Finally, local health departments also provide immunization and well-child clinics at no or very low cost.

■ **REGIONAL CENTERS**

Most state health departments also provide regional centers, which offer services to children up to 3 years of age. These state-funded programs usually serve children who are developmentally delayed or have cerebral palsy, epilepsy, autism, or other long-term handicapping disabilities. The centers usually provide comprehensive assessment, referral to local programs most appropriate to a child's needs, and case management services.

■ **SCHOOL DISTRICTS**

Every school district is required to provide special educational services to children with severe learning disabilities or significant handicap at 3 years of age. A parent can request an Individualized Education Plan (IEP) conference, which will assess the child's learning needs and if a special classroom environment is required. These IEP conferences are free; however, long waiting periods may occur. The local school district administrative office can provide specific guidelines for scheduling an IEP conference.

■ **WOMEN, INFANTS, AND CHILDREN (WIC) PROGRAM**

This is a federal supplemental food program, funded through the United States Department of Agriculture and administered by local health departments. WIC offers nutrition education and supplemental food to financially eligible pregnant women and children up to 5 years of age who are assessed as being at risk.

■ **PARENTERAL NUTRITION**

The Lifeline Foundation provides education concerning parenteral or enteral nutrition and publishes a free newsletter for patients on home nutrition programs. For information write to:

● The Lifeline Foundation, 2 Osprey Road, Sharon, MA 02067

■ **EYE DISORDERS**

● PACK (Parents and Cataract Kids), P.O. Box 73, Southeastern, PA 19399, 215-352-0719
● National Association for Parents of the Visually Impaired, P.O. Box 18-806, Austin, TX 78718
● Eye Research Institute, 20 Staniford St., Boston, MA 02114, 617-742-3140

■ **SKIN DISORDERS**

● NFED (National Foundation for Ectodermal Dysplasias), 108 North First, Suite 311, Mascoutah, IL 62258, 618-566-2020
● National Arthritis and Musculoskeletal and Skin Diseases Information Clearinghouse, Box AMS, Bethesda, MD 20892, 301-468-3235

■ **GENETIC COUNSELING**

● The National Birth Defects Center, 30 Warren St., Brighton, MA 02135, 617-787-5958
● March of Dimes Birth Defects Foundation, 1275 Mamaroneck Ave., White Plains, NY 10605, 914-428-7100

■ **GENERAL**

● NORD (National Organization for Rare Disorders, Inc.), P.O. Box 8923, New Fairfield, CT 06812, 203-746-6518
● Exceptional Parent Magazine, 605 Commonwealth Ave., Boston, MA 02215
● The Alliance of Genetic Support Groups, National Center for Education in Maternal and Child Health,* 38th and R Street, N.W., Washington, DC 20057, 202-625-8400 or 202-625-8410

---

*The center updated its 170-page *Guide to Selected National Genetic Voluntary Organizations* in 1988. The directory lists over 150 national voluntary organizations that provide services for individuals with genetic disorders. For a free copy, request publication number G50 at the address above.

THE CHILDRENS HOSPITAL
INFANT FOLLOW-UP PROGRAM
EVERY-VISIT DATA CODING FORM

CONTACT INFORMATION

Complete for ALL Patients

1. Last Name _____

2. First Name _____ (1–2)

3. DOB _____ / _____ / _____

4. Insurance _____ (3–4)

DEMOGRAPHIC DATA

Complete for ALL NEW IFUP Patients Only

4. Reason/s for IFUP Visit (indicate all)
   <1250 gm birth weight ___ Neuro ___ BPD

   Research Project, Specify _____ (5–8)
   Other, Specify _____
5. Maternal *Race* _____ (9)
   1 = Caucasian
   2 = Black
   3 = Hispanic
   4 = Other, Specify _____ (10)
6. Last Grade *Mother* Completed
   in School   _____ (11)
   1 = Less than 9th Grade
   2 = 9th Through 12th Grade
   3 = High School Graduate
   4 = Completed Some College
   5 = College Graduate
7. *Eyes* Examined Before NICU Discharge?
   (0 = No Exam, 1 = Normal,
   2 = Abnormal, 3 = Suspect,
   4 = Unknown)   _____ (12)
8. *Audiology* Exam Before NICU Discharge?
   (0 = No Exam, 1 = Normal,
   2 = Abnormal, 3 = Suspect,
   4 = Unknown)   _____ (13)

■ VISIT DATA

Complete for ALL Patients

9. *Date of this visit*   _____ / _____ /
                                           (14)
10. *Height* (cm)   _____ _____ . _____ (15)
11. *Weight* (gm)   _____ _____ . _____ (16)
12. *Head Circumference* (cm) ___ ___ . ___ (17)

13. *# Hospitalizations* Since NICU
    Discharge   _____ (18)
14. *Exam Outcomes*
    (1 = Normal, 2 = Abnormal, 3 = Suspect,
    4 = Not Assessed)
    A. Developmental Assessment _____ (19)
    B. Pediatric Assessment   _____ (20)
    C. Neurological Assessment   _____ (21)
    D. Behavior/Temperament   _____ (22)
    E. Maternal-Infant Interaction _____ (23)
    F. Major Social Problems   _____ (24)
    G. Language   _____ (25)
    H. Gross Motor   _____ (26)
    I. Fine Motor   _____ (27)
15. Have *Eyes* (ROP) Been Examined?
    (Check **One**)
    After NICU Discharge   _____ (28)
    Followed Regularly   _____ (29)
    Needs Eye Exam   _____ (30)
    Not Necessary   _____ (31)
16. Has *Hearing* Been Tested? (Check **One**)
    After NICU Discharge   _____ (32)
    Followed Regularly   _____ (33)
    Needs Hearing Exam   _____ (34)
    Not Necessary   _____ (35)
17. What Were the Results of the *Psychological
    Exam* Today?
    (1 = Normal, 2 = Abnormal, 3 = Suspect,
    4 = No Exam)   _____ (36)
18. What Were the Results of the *Physical Ther-
    apy Exam* Today?
    (1 = Normal, 2 = Abnormal, 3 = Suspect,
    4 = No Exam)   _____ (37)
19. List **Current** Major *Diagnoses*

    A. _____ (38)

    B. _____ (39)

    C. _____ (40)

■ RECONTACT INFORMATION

Complete for ALL Patients

20. *When* Does This Child Need Another IFUP
    Clinic Visit?   _____ (41)
    6 Months corrected age   _____ (42)
    12 Months corrected age   _____ (43)
    24 Months corrected age   _____ (44)
    Do Not Reschedule   _____ (45)
    Other Time Period   _____ (46)
    If *Other,* Specify in _____ Months

Index

Note: Page numbers in *italics* refer to illustrations; page numbers followed by "t" refer to tables.